VOLUME I

RINCIPLES AND PRACTICE OF
SURGICAL
PATHOLOGY

SECOND EDITION

Edited by

Steven G. Silverberg, M.D.

*Professor
Department of Pathology
The George Washington University School of
Medicine and Health Sciences
Director
Division of Anatomic Pathology
The George Washington University Medical Center
Washington, D.C.*

CHURCHILL LIVINGSTONE
New York   Edinburgh   London   Melbourne

Library of Congress Cataloging in Publication Data

Principles and practice of surgical pathology/edited by Steven G. Silverberg. —2nd ed.
    p.   cm.
    Includes bibliographical references.
    ISBN 0-443-08692-3 (set)
    1. Pathology, Surgical.   I. Silverberg, Steven G., date.
    [DNLM: 1. Pathology, Surgical.   WO 142 P957]
RD57.P73   1990
617'.07—dc20
DNLM/DLC
for Library of Congress   89-22048
                                             CIP

Distributed in the United Kingdom by Churchill Livingstone, Robert Stevenson House, 1–3 Baxter's Place, Leith Walk, Edinburgh EH1 3AF, and by associated companies, branches, and representatives throughout the world.

The Publishers have made every effort to trace the copyright holders for borrowed material. If they have inadvertently overlooked any, they will be pleased to make the necessary arrangements at the first opportunity.

Acquisitions Editor: *Robert A. Hurley*
Copy Editor: *Marian Ryan*
Production Designer: *Marci Jordan*
Production Supervisor: *Sharon Tuder*

Printed in the United States of America

First published in 1990

To Kiyoe

Contributors

Jorge Albores-Saavedra, M.D.
Professor, Department of Pathology, University of Miami School of Medicine, Miami, Florida

Ronald W. Alexander, M.D.
Department of Pathology, Monroe Regional Medical Center, Ocala, Florida

Vernon W. Armbrustmacher, M.D.
Colonel, USAF, MC, Deputy Director, Armed Forces Institute of Pathology, Washington, D.C.

Alberto G. Ayala, M.D.
Professor, Department of Pathology, University of Texas Medical School at Houston; Department of Pathology, M. D. Anderson Hospital and Tumor Institute, Houston, Texas

Leona W. Ayers, M.D.
Associate Professor, Department of Pathology, Ohio State University College of Medicine; Director, Department of Microbiology, Ohio State University Hospital, Columbus, Ohio

Leon Barnes, M.D.
Associate Professor, Department of Pathology, University of Pittsburgh School of Medicine; Chief, Division of Head and Neck Pathology, Presbyterian-University Hospital; Chief, Division of Head and Neck Pathology, Eye and Ear Hospital, Pittsburgh, Pennsylvania

John G. Batsakis, M.D.
Professor, Department of Pathology, University of Texas Medical School at Houston; Chairman, Department of Pathology, M. D. Anderson Hospital and Tumor Institute, Houston, Texas

Paul A. Bloustein, M.D.
Director, Division of Anatomic Pathology, The Jewish Hospital, Cincinnati, Ohio

Fred T. Bosman, M.D., Ph.D.
Professor and Chairman, Department of Pathology, University of Limburg Faculty School of Medicine, Maastricht, The Netherlands

Barrett D. Brantley, M.D.
Clinical Fellow, Department of Pathology, Vanderbilt University School of Medicine, Nashville, Tennessee

Peter G. Bullough, M.D.
Professor, Department of Pathology, Cornell University Medical College; Director, Department of Laboratory Medicine, The Hospital for Special Surgery, New York, New York

Ian Carr, M.D., Ph.D.
Professor, Department of Pathology, University of Manitoba Faculty of Medicine; Director, Electromicroscopy Unit, Department of Pathology, St. Boniface General Hospital, Winnipeg, Manitoba, Canada

David Chad, M.D.
Associate Professor, Department of Neurology, University of Massachusetts Medical School; Department of Neurology, University of Massachusetts Medical Center, Worcester, Massachusetts

Bernard Czernobilsky, M.D.
Professor, Department of Pathology, Medical School of the Hebrew University and Hadassah, Jerusalem; Chief, Department of Pathology, Kaplan Hospital, Rehovot, Israel

Umberto DeGirolami, M.D.
Professor, Departments of Pathology and Neurology, University of Massachusetts Medical School; Neuropathologist, Department of Pathology, University of Massachusetts Medical Center, Worcester, Massachusetts; Neuropathologist, Department of Pathology, New England Deaconess Hospital, Boston, Massachusetts

Ronald A. DeLellis, M.D.
Professor, Department of Pathology, Tufts University School of Medicine; Senior Attending Pathologist, Department of Pathology, New England Medical Center Hospital, Boston, Massachusetts

Ralph C. Eagle, Jr., M.D.
Professor, Department of Ophthalmology, Jefferson Medical College of Thomas Jefferson University; Director, Department of Pathology, Wills Eye Hospital, Philadelphia, Pennsylvania

Horatio T. Enterline, M.D.
Emeritus Professor, Department of Pathology and Laboratory Medicine, University of Pennsylvania School of Medicine, Philadelphia, Pennsylvania

Robert A. Erlandson, Ph.D.
Associate Professor, Department of Pathology, Cornell University Medical College; Attending Electron Microscopist, Department of Pathology, Memorial Sloan-Kettering Institute for Cancer Research, New York, New York

Daniel Faverly, M.D.
Assistant, Department of Pathology, Jules Bordet Institute, Free University of Brussels, Brussels, Belgium

Robert E. Fechner, M.D.
Professor, Department of Pathology, University of Virginia School of Medicine; Director, Division of Surgical Pathology, University of Virginia Health Sciences Center, Charlottesville, Virginia

CONTRIBUTORS

Cecilia M. Fenoglio-Preiser, M.D.
Professor and Vice Chairman, Department of Pathology, University of New Mexico School of Medicine, Albuquerque, New Mexico

Victor J. Ferrans, M.D., Ph.D.
Chief, Ultrastructure Section, Pathology Branch, National Heart, Lung and Blood Institute, National Institutes of Health, Bethesda, Maryland

Gerald Fine, M.D.
Consultant Pathologist, Department of Pathology, Grace Hospital; Consultant Pathologist, Department of Pathology, Holy Cross Hospital; Former Chief, Division of Anatomic Pathology, Henry Ford Hospital, Detroit, Michigan; Consultant Pathologist, Department of Pathology, St. Joseph's Hospital, Mt. Clemens, Michigan

Mary Ann S. Frable, M.D.
Professor, Department of Otolaryngology, Virginia Commonwealth University Medical College of Virginia School of Medicine, Richmond, Virginia

William J. Frable, M.D.
Director, Departments of Surgical Pathology and Cytopathology, Virginia Commonwealth University Medical College of Virginia School of Medicine, Richmond, Virginia

Yao Shi Fu, M.D.
Professor, Department of Pathology, University of California, Los Angeles, UCLA School of Medicine, Los Angeles, California

Loren E. Golitz, M.D.
Professor, Departments of Dermatology and Pathology, University of Colorado Health Sciences Center School of Medicine; Chief, Department of Dermatology, Denver General Hospital, Denver, Colorado

Claude Gompel, M.D.
Professor Emeritus and Honorary Chairman, Department of Pathology, Jules Bordet Institute, Free University of Brussels, Brussels, Belgium

Victor E. Gould, M.D.
Ortho S.A. Sprague Professor, Department of Pathology, Rush Medical College of Rush University; Senior Attending Pathologist, Department of Pathology, Rush-Presbyterian-St. Luke's Medical Center, Chicago, Illinois

Robert O. Greer, Jr., D.D.S., Sc.D.
Professor, Department of Pathology, University of Colorado Health Sciences Center School of Medicine; Professor and Chairman, Division of Oral Pathology and Oncology, University of Colorado School of Dentistry, Denver, Colorado

John M. Hardman, M.D.
Professor and Chairman, Department of Pathology, University of Hawaii, John A. Burns School of Medicine, Honolulu, Hawaii

William H. Hartmann, M.D.
Pathologist-in-Residence, University of California, Irvine, California College of Medicine, Irvine, California; Medical Director, Department of Pathology, Long Beach Memorial Medical Center, Long Beach, California

Bruce C. Horten, M.D.
Associate Professor, Department of Pathology, Cornell University Medical College; Attending Pathologist, Department of Pathology, Lenox Hill Hospital, New York, New York

Eva Horvath, Ph.D.
Associate Professor, Department of Pathology, University of Toronto Faculty of Medicine; Research Associate, Department of Pathology, St. Michael's Hospital, Toronto, Ontario, Canada

Harry L. Ioachim, M.D.
Clinical Professor, Department of Pathology, Columbia University College of Physicians and Surgeons; Director, Department of Pathology, Lenox Hill Hospital, New York, New York

Kamal G. Ishak, M.D., Ph.D.
Clinical Professor, Department of Pathology, Uniformed Services University School of the Health Sciences F. Edward Hébert School of Medicine, Bethesda, Maryland; Chairman, Department of Hepatic Pathology, Armed Forces Institute of Pathology, Washington, D.C.

Saul Kay, M.D.
Professor Emeritus, Department of Pathology, Virginia Commonwealth University Medical College of Virginia School of Medicine, Richmond, Virginia

Urmila Khettry, M.D.
Assistant Professor, Department of Pathology, Harvard Medical School; Department of Pathology, New England Deaconess Hospital; Department of Pathology, New England Baptist Hospital, Boston, Massachusetts

Elmer W. Koneman, M.D.
Associate Professor, Department of Pathology, University of Illinois College of Medicine; Director, Department of Clinical Pathology, University of Illinois Hospital, Chicago, Illinois

Kalman Kovacs, M.D., Ph.D., D.Sc., F.R.C.P.C., F.C.A.Path.
Professor, Department of Pathology, University of Toronto Faculty of Medicine; Department of Pathology, St. Michael's Hospital, Toronto, Ontario, Canada

Frederick T. Kraus, M.D.
Professor (Visiting Staff), Department of Pathology, Washington University School of Medicine; Chairman, Department of Pathology and Laboratory Medicine, St. John's Mercy Medical Center, Saint Louis, Missouri

Ernest E. Lack, M.D.
Professor, Department of Pathology, Georgetown University School of Medicine; Director, Division of Surgical Pathology, Department of Pathology, Georgetown University Hospital, Washington, D.C.

Frederick D. Lee, M.D.
Consultant Pathologist, Department of Pathology, Glasgow Royal Infirmary, Glasgow, Scotland

CONTRIBUTORS

Merle A. Legg, M.D.
Associate Professor, Department of Pathology, Harvard Medical School; Consultant, Department of Anatomic Pathology, New England Deaconess Hospital, Boston, Massachusetts

Beatriz Lifschitz-Mercer, M.D.
Senior Pathologist, Department of Pathology, Kaplan Hospital, Rehovot, Israel

Trevor A. Macpherson, M.B., Ch.B., M.R.C.O.G.
Associate Professor, Department of Pathology, University of Pittsburgh School of Medicine; Chief, Department of Pathology, Magee Women's Hospital, Pittsburgh, Pennsylvania

John Maksem, M.D.
Assistant Professor, Department of Pathology, Case Western Reserve University School of Medicine; Attending Pathologist, Department of Pathology, St. Vincent's Charity Hospital, Cleveland, Ohio

Scott A. Martin, M.D.
Clinical Associate Professor, Department of Anatomic Pathology, Saint Louis University School of Medicine; Director, Department of Anatomic Pathology, St. John's Mercy Medical Center, Saint Louis, Missouri

Hugh A. McAllister, Jr., M.D.
Clinical Professor, Department of Pathology, Baylor College of Medicine; Clinical Professor, Department of Pathology, University of Texas Medical School at Houston; Chief, Department of Pathology, Texas Heart Institute; Chief, Department of Pathology, St. Luke's Episcopal Hospital, Houston, Texas

W.T. Elliott McCaughey, M.D.
Professor, Department of Pathology, University of Ottawa School of Medicine; Consultant, Canadian Reference Centre for Cancer Pathology; Chief, Department of Laboratory Medicine, Ottawa Civic Hospital, Ottawa, Ontario, Canada

Thomas A. Merrick, M.D.
Laboratory Director, Department of Pathology, Denver Presbyterian Hospital, Denver, Colorado

Nabila E. Metwalli, M.B., B.Ch., Ph.D.
Lecturer, Department of Pathology, University of Alexandria School of Medicine, Alexandria, Egypt

Roberta R. Miller, M.D., F.R.C.P.C.
Clinical Associate Professor, Department of Pathology, University of British Columbia Faculty of Medicine; Consultant Pathologist, Department of Pathology, Vancouver General Hospital, Vancouver, British Columbia, Canada

A. Scott Mills, M.D.
Associate Professor, Department of Pathology, Virginia Commonwealth University Medical College of Virginia School of Medicine, Richmond, Virginia

Joseph Montedonico, J.D., Esq.
Senior Trial Attorney, Montedonico & Mason, Chartered, Specialists in Defense of Medical Malpractice, Washington, D.C.

Azorides R. Morales, M.D.
Professor and Chairman, Department of Pathology, University of Miami School of Medicine; Director, Pathology Laboratories, University of Miami-Jackson Memorial Hospital Medical Center, Miami, Florida

Pamela J. Murari, M.D.
Acting Chairman, Department of Hematopathology, Armed Forces Institute of Pathology, Washington, D.C.

Mehrdad Nadji, M.D.
Professor, Department of Pathology, University of Miami School of Medicine; Director, Division of Anatomic Pathology, University of Miami-Jackson Memorial Hospital Medical Center, Miami, Florida

Lucien E. Nochomovitz, M.D.
Associate Professor, Department of Pathology, The George Washington University School of Medicine and Health Sciences, Washington, D.C.

Jan M. Orenstein, M.D.
Professor, Department of Pathology, The George Washington University School of Medicine and Health Sciences; Director, Diagnostic Electron Microscopy Laboratory, The George Washington University Medical Center, Washington, D.C.

Robert R. Pascal, M.D.
Professor and Vice Chairman, Department of Pathology and Laboratory Medicine, Emory University School of Medicine; Director, Division of Anatomic Pathology, Emory University Hospital, Atlanta, Georgia

Karl H. Perzin, M.D.
Professor, Division of Clinical Surgical Pathology, Department of Pathology, Columbia University College of Physicians and Surgeons, New York, New York

Norman M. Pettigrew, M.D.
Associate Professor, Department of Pathology, University of Manitoba Faculty of Medicine; Department of Pathology, University of Manitoba Health Sciences Centre, Winnipeg, Manitoba, Canada

Eduardo Quant, M.D.
Department of Pathology, Humana Hospital Bennett, Plantation, Florida

Usha B. Raju, M.D.
Department of Pathology, Henry Ford Hospital, Detroit, Michigan

James W. Reagan, M.D.
Late Professor, Departments of Pathology and Reproductive Biology, Institute of Pathology, Case Western Reserve University School of Medicine, Cleveland, Ohio

Richard J. Reed, M.D.
Professor, Department of Pathology, Tulane University School of Medicine; Senior Surgical Pathologist, Department of Pathology, Tulane Medical Center, New Orleans, Louisiana

Nicholas Romas, M.D.
Professor, Department of Urology, Columbia University College of Physicians and Surgeons; Chief, Department of Urology, St. Luke's-Roosevelt Hospital Center; Attending Urologist, Department of Urology, Columbia-Presbyterian Medical Center, New York, New York

Sanford I. Roth, M.D.
Professor, Department of Pathology, Northwestern University Medical School; Attending Pathologist, Department of Pathology, Northwestern Memorial Hospital, Chicago, Illinois

Frank R. Rudy, M.D.
Clinical Assistant Professor, Department of Pathology, Pennsylvania State University College of Medicine, Hershey, Pennsylvania; Associate Pathologist, Department of Pathology, Polyclinic Medical Center, Harrisburg, Pennsylvania

Mario J. Saldana, M.D.
Professor, Department of Pathology, University of Miami School of Medicine; Attending Pathologist, Department of Pathology, University of Miami-Jackson Memorial Hospital Medical Center, Miami, Florida

Diane Cereghino Salyer, M.D.
Director, Division of Anatomic Pathology, Samuel Merritt Hospital, Oakland, California

William Ray Salyer, M.D.
Director, Division of Anatomic Pathology, Alta Bates Hospital-Herrick Hospital Health Center, Berkeley, California

Scott H. Saul, M.D.
Associate Professor, Department of Pathology and Laboratory Medicine, University of Pennsylvania School of Medicine; Staff Pathologist, Section of Surgical Pathology, Hospital of the University of Pennsylvania, Philadelphia, Pennsylvania

James J. Sciubba, D.M.D., Ph.D.
Professor, Department of Oral Biology and Pathology, State University of New York at Stony Brook Health Sciences Center School of Medicine, Stony Brook, New York; Chairman, Department of Dentistry, Long Island Jewish Medical Center, New Hyde Park, New York

Maria Shevchuk, M.D.
Associate Professor, New York Medical College, Valhalla, New York; Associate Attending Pathologist, Lenox Hill Hospital, New York, New York

Robert H. Shikes, M.D.
Professor and Vice Chairman, Department of Pathology, University of Colorado Health Sciences Center School of Medicine, Denver, Colorado

Steven G. Silverberg, M.D.
Professor, Department of Pathology, The George Washington University School of Medicine and Health Sciences; Director, Division of Anatomic Pathology, The George Washington University Medical Center, Washington, D.C.

Thomas W. Smith, M.D.
Associate Professor, Departments of Pathology and Neurology, University of Massachusetts Medical School; Neuropathologist, Department of Pathology, University of Massachusetts Medical Center; Neuropathologist, Department of Pathology, St. Vincent Hospital, Worcester, Massachusetts

Harlan J. Spjut, M.D.
Professor, Department of Pathology, Baylor College of Medicine; Senior Attending Pathologist, Department of Pathology, The Methodist Hospital, Houston, Texas

Francis H. Strauss II, M.D.
Professor, Department of Pathology, University of Chicago Pritzker School of Medicine, Chicago, Illinois

F. Wayne Stromeyer, M.D.
Clinical Associate Professor, Department of Pathology, Louisiana State University School of Medicine in New Orleans, New Orleans, Louisiana; Vice Chief, Department of Pathology, Our Lady of the Lake Regional Medical Center, Baton Rouge, Louisiana

Nora C.J. Sun, M.D.
Associate Professor, Department of Pathology, University of California, Los Angeles, UCLA School of Medicine, Los Angeles, California; Head, Division of Hematopathology, Harbor-UCLA Medical Center, Torrance, California

Aron E. Szulman, M.B., F.R.C.Path.
Professor, Department of Pathology, University of Pittsburgh School of Medicine; Department of Pathology, Magee Women's Hospital, Pittsburgh, Pennsylvania

Myron Tannenbaum, M.D.
Professor, Departments of Pathology and Urology, Mount Sinai School of Medicine of the City University of New York; Attending Pathologist, Department of Pathology, The Mount Sinai Hospital, New York, New York; Chief, Departments of Pathology and Cytology, Bronx Veterans Administration Hospital, Bronx, New York

John Jones Thompson, M.D.
Director of Laboratories, Kaiser-Permanente Laboratory, Clackamas, Oregon

William M. Thurlbeck, M.B., F.R.C.P.C., F.R.C.Path.
Professor, Department of Pathology, University of British Columbia Faculty of Medicine; Consultant Pathologist, Department of Pathology, Children's Hospital, Vancouver, British Columbia, Canada

Peter G. Toner, M.D.
Musgrave Professor, Department of Pathology, Royal Victoria Hospital, Belfast, Northern Ireland

Virginia M. Walley, M.D.
Assistant Professor, Department of Pathology, University of Ottawa School of Medicine; Chief, Division of Anatomic Pathology, Department of Laboratory Medicine, Ottawa Civic Hospital, Ottawa, Ontario, Canada

CONTRIBUTORS

Nancy E. Warner, M.D.
Hastings Professor, Department of Pathology, University of Southern California School of Medicine; Surgical Pathologist, Department of Pathology, Norris Cancer Hospital, Los Angeles, California

James E. Wheeler, M.D.
Professor, Department of Pathology and Laboratory Medicine, University of Pennsylvania School of Medicine, Philadelphia, Pennsylvania

James M. Woodruff, M.D.
Associate Professor, Department of Pathology, Cornell University Medical College; Attending Pathologist, Memorial Sloan-Kettering Institute for Cancer Research, New York, New York

Hong-Yi Yang, M.D.
Professor, Department of Pathology, University of Hawaii John A. Burns School of Medicine, Honolulu, Hawaii

Preface to the Second Edition

This is an exciting and challenging time to be a surgical pathologist. The clinical indications for the performance of various biopsy and operative procedures are changing rapidly, and the types of specimens generated and sent to the surgical pathologist are changing accordingly. Many practices are becoming more and more oriented to smaller and smaller specimens, including the results of fine needle aspiration procedures. Paradoxically, as the specimens diminish in volume, the demands for clinically important or basic science-oriented (or both) uses to which tissues may be subjected continue to increase. Thus, pathologists often find themselves functioning as triage officers for specimens, a role in which they must choose the disposition of tissue that will be most beneficial to the patient, will allow the progress of medical science to continue, and will be consistent with the current—and in all likelihood, progressively more stringent—climate of cost containment.

Both this new triage role and the classic diagnostic role of the surgical pathologist demand that practicing pathologists—more than ever before—be aware of the clinical and epidemiologic implications of their cases and, furthermore, that they be familiar with the new research techniques rapidly finding application in diagnostic surgical pathology. The use of electron microscopy and immunohistochemistry is by now widely accepted, although specimens are still sometimes sent by small laboratories to referral centers for undergoing these techniques. Other analyses, such as flow cytometry, gene rearrangement studies, and in situ hybridization, are routinely utilized far less often, but will probably quickly become more extensively applied to at least some specific diagnostic and prognostic situations. In all of these, intelligent light microscopic differential diagnosis still remains the key. In this edition, the chapter authors and I attempt to provide the reader with up-to-date information in all of these areas; as in the first edition, the expertise of the authors guarantees the most current treatment of the numerous topics covered.

The organization of the book is essentially the same as in the first edition. Two new chapters (Chapter 4, Surgical Pathology of Immunodeficiency Disorders, and Chapter 6, Immunohistochemical Techniques) have been added, and two chapters from the first edition have been deleted, with material formerly found in them now integrated into other chapters. All other chapters have been extensively revised, mostly by the original authors, in a few instances by entirely new authors, and in many cases by a combination of original authors and newly associated colleagues. This retention of our original expertise, combined with the introduction of new points of view, is a source of great personal satisfaction for me. I must mention with sadness, however, the untimely loss of two of our first edition authors—Jim Reagan, who was able to contribute to the current edition before his death, and Arkadi Rywlin, who was not. Both of these fine gentlemen are deeply missed by their many friends and colleagues. Other giants in our field who were close to me have also passed away while the current work was in progress, including Frank Foote (one of my mentors at Memorial Sloan-Kettering) and Joe Eggleston (a classmate at Johns Hopkins and long-time friend). Although not contributors to this book, both of these superb surgical pathologists certainly influenced my career up to and including its preparation, and I remain in their debt.

The production and publication of this book has passed from John Wiley & Sons to Churchill Livingstone Inc., but fortunately for me Bob Hurley has moved there as well, so I can again thank him for his assistance. Sidney Landau at Wiley, and Nancy Terry and Marian Ryan at Churchill Livingstone have also been important and valued colleagues. Order has been created from chaos by Betty Hallinger, who constructed the index. Dorothy Molero has typed, pleaded, harangued, consoled, and cried as appropriate. Colleagues, including residents and fellows, at The George Washington University have been subjected to my frequent disappearances and inappropriate mood swings during the preparation of this work, and some—especially Eric Wargotz, Tucker Burks, Barry Brown, and Andra Frost—have provided valuable editorial assistance and advice. My parents, Bertram and Esther Silverberg, have continued to be a source of support. Finally, as with the first edition, the greatest sacrifice has been made by my long-suffering wife, Kiyoe, to whom I again offer my deepest gratitude.

Steven G. Silverberg, M.D.

Preface to the First Edition

Why another textbook of surgical pathology? The raison d'être of this project is two-fold: first, to provide a thorough and authoritative survey of the field; second, to present information in a practical format that is useful to the pathologist in training or practice.

To accomplish the first goal, the authors chosen represent an international array of experts, most of whom have written recent monographs or major review articles on the subjects that they have covered here. The subject assigned to each author or team of authors is narrow enough to be covered in depth. Toward the second goal, most chapters include introductory sections on specimen handling, clinical correlations, and normal gross and microscopic anatomy. The chapters are in part specimen-oriented rather than disease-oriented: thus, for example, lesions likely to be encountered as medical biopsy specimens of lung, liver, and kidney are discussed in separate chapters from those encountered primarily in surgical resection specimens of the same organs. Organ site chapters, with the exception of Chapters 24 and 26, are arranged so that Volume 2 contains all topographic sites from SNOMED code 56000 (SNOP code 56) on, and Volume 1 contains sites with lower code numbers. Finally, common problems, particularly of differential diagnosis, are emphasized over rare ones.

Several chapters at the beginning of the first volume are provided as introductory material for the student of surgical pathology. These include discussions of some problems (e.g., infections and metastatic tumors) that are not unique to any one organ or organ system and are thus applicable to many of the specific site chapters. I recommend that these chapters be read once in their entirety rather than merely referred to when a specific problem arises in the laboratory.

The main credit for this work must go to the individual authors, many of whom must have regretted ever having agreed to work with such an unreasonable and arbitrary editor as myself. It is a tribute to the development of the field of surgical pathology that there are so many pathologists expert in so many fields. Only a few years ago, the majority of authors of a work of this sort would have been clinicians who doubled as pathologists in their own limited fields but had no broad background in general pathology.

My thanks also go to a few people who provided special assistance with respect to the conceptual development and physical production of the entire work. Drs. Richard J. Reed, William J. Frable, Robert W. McDivitt, Andrew G. Huvos, and Richard J. Kempson served as editorial consultants and provided valuable suggestions in the planning phase. John de Carville, Robert Hurley, Scott Klein, and Charles Kyreakou at John Wiley & Sons provided constant encouragement, advice, and hard work from beginning to end. LaVonne King functioned diligently and uncomplainingly as my editorial assistant, and Luann Bergquist typed some of my chapters and pertinent correspondence. Howard Mitchell provided his usual excellent artistic and photographic assistance. Many of my colleagues and especially residents at the University of Colorado offered invaluable criticism during the process of writing and editing and certainly always showed patience and understanding when I was unavailable for other tasks because of an editing deadline.

Finally, two special words of thanks. The inspiration to undertake a task of this magnitude developed over many years largely as a result of my association with many talented surgical pathologists, first as a trainee, later as a colleague, and most recently as a mentor and consultant. I could hardly hope to list all those colleagues whose ability, enthusiasm, and dedication have promoted my own development over the years; but I should certainly single out Drs. Fred Stewart, Frank Foote, Saul Kay, and my good friend and partner in yet another opus, Claude Gompel. The late Drs. Abou Pollack, William Barriss McAllister, Jr., Harry Greene, and Averill Liebow also deserve the thanks that I never conveyed adequately when they were still with me. Ultimately, however, the main burden of an undertaking such as this falls on the loved ones who make personal sacrifices to free time from other activities for the many hours of work involved. For this and all other support, I offer my deepest gratitude to my wife, Kiyoe.

Steven G. Silverberg, M.D.

Contents

Volume II

1

General Philosophy and Principles of Surgical Pathology

Steven G. Silverberg

What is surgical pathology? Probably the best definition is that surgical pathology is the discipline that deals with the anatomic pathology of tissues removed from living patients. Many surgical pathologists expand this definition to include smears, aspirates, and body fluids as well, so cytopathology is usually considered within the domain of surgical pathology.

By this definition, surgical pathology differs from autopsy pathology in (1) the nature of the specimens seen most frequently and (2) the usual immediacy of the decisions to be made and their relation to the subsequent management of an individual patient. The latter distinction is perhaps more immediately apparent. The tissue diagnosis made by the surgical pathologist often precedes the treatment of the patient and, in fact, in such instances usually influences or even determines what such treatment will be. On the other hand, the role of the autopsy pathologist, or morbid anatomist, invariably begins after treatment has ended and includes an assessment of the appropriateness and adequacy of the therapeutic regimens employed.

The first difference listed above between surgical and autopsy pathology is also an important one to remember, however. As an example, diagnostic material from the heart forms a fairly small (but currently increasing) portion of the workload of the surgical pathologist, whereas it is a major (if not the major) consideration in the practice of autopsy pathology. By contrast, the skin and the female genital tract are usually not studied extensively at autopsy, yet together they comprise more than one half

the specimens seen in most practices of surgical pathology. Thus, it is apparent that the reading and continuing education that must be undertaken to keep up to date in the two fields is quite different, almost justifying their characterization as entirely separate disciplines. On the other hand, the basic skills essential to the practice of surgical pathology are the same as those learned in the performance of autopsies, and there are few practicing surgical pathologists who do not continue their involvement with autopsy pathology as well.

PRACTICE OF SURGICAL PATHOLOGY

Whether working in an academic medical center or a small community hospital, the surgical pathologist always functions as a teacher and often as a researcher, but the main role is still essentially the practice of medicine. It is sometimes easy for the pathologist—particularly the pathologist who does not regularly see living patients—to forget this and, when this happens, the result may be disastrous for both the pathologist and the patient. The role of the surgical pathologist should be that of a consultant to the clinician for the ultimate benefit of the patient, and this role must be remembered even when the pathologist is in the laboratory, far from direct contact with either the clinician or the patient.

Furthermore, despite the traditional name of the field, *surgical* pathology, the practitioner in this field soon

1

learns that service to, and contact with, general and specialty surgeons comprises only a small part of the total practice. The workload of the modern surgical pathologist also includes specimens from dermatologists, gynecologists, gastroenterologists, pediatricians, nephrologists, and physicians in many other specialties, so the surgical pathologist must have some familiarity with each of these fields and the clinical problems encountered therein. This need again points out that the formative and continuing education of the surgical pathologist must consist of training not only in morphologic interpretation but also in the clinical practice of medicine. The most effective surgical pathologists are often those who have had some advanced clinical training after their undergraduate medical education, and thus are best able to place the specimens they receive into the proper clinical context.

Consultative Role of the Surgical Pathologist

Recalling the relationship between the surgical pathologist and the clinician and patient, the general principles of the approach to a specimen are greatly simplified. Surgical pathologists should deal with each specimen as if they were the clinician—or better yet, the patient—awaiting the surgical pathology report. Questions such as whether to photograph a gross specimen, how many sections to submit of a particular lesion, how carefully to search for lymph nodes in a radical procedure, whether to order recuts or special stains, whether to write or dictate a microscopic description, and so forth, all become answerable in terms of the single basic question, "Were I either the clinician or the patient in this case, what information would I need about this specimen, and how can that information best be supplied?"

Given this approach, the answers to different but similar questions about the same specimen may initially appear to be at odds, but this apparent contradiction is easily resolved when the ultimate benefit to the patient is considered. For example, the question of whether to perform radiography on a breast resection specimen is usually answered in the affirmative, since the information obtained from this procedure will assist the surgical pathologist in guaranteeing that the clinically suspicious lesion has been removed and that no other grossly inapparent but clinically important lesions are present in the same specimen.[1] On the other hand, the question of whether to perform laborious fat-clearing procedures for the axillary contents received as part of a mastectomy specimen is usually resolved negatively, since the information that may be obtained from this procedure (detection of additional small lymph nodes and perhaps even

additional micrometastases) does not appear to influence significantly either the prognosis or the treatment.[2]

Thus, the approach to any specimen received in the surgical pathology laboratory obviously depends on the specific clinical problem to be resolved by the interpretation of that specimen. Therefore, it is essential that each specimen be accompanied by an adequate description of what it represents, as well as an appropriate clinical history. The surgical pathologist should design the request form so the clinician filling out the form is sure to appreciate the need for supplying this information. If adequate clinical information is not received with a particular specimen, the surgical pathologist is completely justified in not processing that specimen until the appropriate information is obtained. The telephone should also be an important part of the surgical pathologist's equipment. Submitting physicians should be called promptly if there is any question about any specimen submitted.

Similarly, the responsibility of the surgical pathologist does not end when a diagnosis has been made and recorded on the surgical pathology report. If the diagnosis differs significantly from what was clinically suspected, or if it requires any immediate response by the clinician, the clinician should be contacted promptly rather than waiting for the report by the usual route of distribution. Similarly, if the diagnosis made is an uncommon one, the significance of which is not likely to be understood by the clinician, the surgical pathologist should be sure that the meaning of the term is explained and a pertinent reference provided, either verbally or in the body of the surgical pathology report, and preferably both.

The importance of communication between the clinician and the pathologist is often underestimated by both parties. This is particularly true of surgical pathologists, who perhaps become too familiar with the "What do you think of this slide without any history?" type of quiz they often receive during residency. It is essential to remember, however, that the practice of surgical pathology is not an intellectual game, but rather a serious facet of the practice of medicine, often with life or death implications. Thus, when dealing with any living patient, all the available clinical information should be presented to the surgical pathologist responsible for the case. This is obviously of less importance in some cases than in others, but it is easier to invoke it as a general rule to which occasional exceptions will be made than to face a constant struggle in obtaining clinical information when it is urgently needed.

These comments pertaining to communication between the clinician and the surgical pathologist are indicative of the role of the surgical pathologist as a clinical consultant. The clinician would certainly not think of calling in a gynecologist as a consultant to evaluate a possible pelvic mass without providing both adequate clinical data and the reason for the consultation, and similarly the clinician should not obtain a consultation from the surgical pathologist without the same courtesy. To continue the same analogy, just as the clinician would not demand that the gynecologic consultant perform a specific diagnostic or therapeutic procedure, the surgical pathologist should not be required to perform a particular stain or other procedure on the tissues submitted. The other side of the coin is that it then becomes the role of the surgical pathologist to decide what special stains or other studies to perform based on an interpretation of all the clinical and pathologic data available in a given case, and it is the surgical pathologist's responsibility to be sure that all this information has indeed been supplied.

Interpathologist Consultation in Surgical Pathology

The question of consultations in surgical pathology is one that is frequently puzzling for the novice. It is always difficult to find the proper middle ground between the hesitancy to ever ask for a consultation and the temptation to seek consultation on virtually every case that is not entirely routine. We who practice surgical pathology are fortunate that it is far easier to transport slides to an expert consultant than to transport the patient; therefore, there is never really an excuse for not obtaining a consultation in situations in which it is indicated, and thus we are safer in erring on the side of overutilization rather than underutilization of this service.

Internal consultation should always be used in questionable cases. Thus, if three members of a group at a particular institution practice surgical pathology, all three should review such a case, and the final report should express the consensus diagnosis. If such a consensus is unobtainable, or if doubt remains, outside consultation is then sought. A good general rule to follow is that one outside consultant should be used for each case. Nothing is more disturbing to the practicing pathologist than to send slides from a case to three different eminent consultants and get three different answers. The consultant should be chosen for expertise in a particular field of surgical pathology or because the referring pathologist has previous favorable experience with that consultant—not because the consultant is located at a famous institution, although the person chosen may lack the credentials of an expert consultant in the particular case to be referred.

Having chosen the consultant, it is essential to provide that individual with the same courtesies that we expect our clinicians to provide to us. Thus, the name, age, and sex of the patient, the hospital and/or surgical pathology number, and the pertinent clinical history should be submitted, as well as a copy of the surgical pathology report in which the gross pathologic features of the case are described. The slides submitted should be adequate in both quantity and quality, since the function of a consultant is not to overcome someone else's inadequate histotechnique. Specially stained slides, if pertinent, should also be submitted, or at least unstained slides on which the consultant may perform the stains that he deems necessary. Referring pathologists should always include their own diagnoses, or the differential if a final diagnosis has not been reached. If there are questions about the clinical management of the case, these should be asked directly in the referring letter. Unless there is some compelling reason for wanting these slides returned (such as the lesion being seen on only one slide or the block being unavailable), the consultant should be permitted to retain the submitted slides. When the report of the consultant is received by the referring pathologist, it should always be made available to the clinician, even (or especially) if it is at variance with the referring pathologist's original diagnosis.

The surgical pathologist should always be willing to send a case for consultation if so requested by the clinician, but certainly the surgical pathologist is free to state that a consultation is not really necessary if such is the case. If the clinician requests a specific consultant, and the pathologist believes that that individual is inappropriate for the case in question, the clinician should be so informed. If the clinician still insists on that consultant, the pathologist should probably acquiesce but is certainly entitled to send the case to another consultant as well. This is one of the few acceptable reasons for violating the "one consultant per case" rule mentioned earlier.

The consultant pathologist is entitled to adequate clinical information and histologic material and in most instances should be able to retain the slides for clinical records (especially if the patient is being treated in his institution). If these slides or the clinical data submitted are in any way inadequate, consultant pathologists should feel free to make the same demands of the referring pathologist that they would make of their clinicians or of their laboratory, and they should not make a diagnosis on the basis of inadequate clinical or pathologic data. This may require requesting the paraffin blocks or fixed tissues for processing in the consultant's laboratory, but the fear of insulting the referring pathologist by asking for this material should not outweigh the responsibility to the patient of rendering a diagnosis only on optimal preparations.

The same responsibility applies to the surgical pathologist in the laboratory. Histotechnologists who seem incapable of producing interpretable slides should be educated, and if they prove ineducable should be fired. This may sound cruel, but in the long run it is less cruel than the alternative of patients having breasts, extremities, and other parts removed for nonexisting cancers that are misdiagnosed because of inadequate histotechnique.

Intraoperative Consultation in Surgical Pathology

This question of "false positive" diagnoses is particularly relevant with respect to frozen section examinations. Older reports of frozen section results[3–5] in breast lesions, for example, have generally indicated that the frequency of false positive diagnoses (something being called cancer that in reality is benign) should be zero, that false negative diagnoses comprise about 1 percent of cases, and that diagnosis must be deferred to permanent sections in 1 to 2 percent of the cases. Several points should be emphasized with reference to these figures. Firstly, those who publish results of frozen section examination (or, for that matter, of anything) are invariably those who have a great deal of experience with the technique, and the surgical pathologist who performs 100 frozen section examinations per year is likely to have considerably poorer results than one who performs 1,000 examinations per year. Secondly, the frequency of false positive diagnoses is inversely related to that of deferred diagnoses, so the attempt to "force" a diagnosis in a difficult situation is likely to lead to the feared result of a false positive interpretation. Thus, there should be no shame in equivocating in such a situation, and in certain situations (e.g., intralobular and intraductal mammary lesions, questionable lymphomas), discretion is usually the better part of valor. Thirdly, most false negative interpretations are probably due to sampling error and are thus unavoidable. By taking one or two sections from a 10 cm specimen, despite our competence in gross pathology, we will invariably encounter situations in which the definitive diagnosis is not made until many more sections are examined the following day.

Finally, my colleagues and I[6–8] as well as others[9,10] have commented on recent changes in both the indications for frozen section examination and the specimens most frequently encountered. In almost one half of our cases, the examination is performed not primarily for a diagnosis, but rather to comment on the adequacy of the specimen for subsequent diagnosis, to select tissue for special studies (e.g., hormone receptors, lymphoid cell markers, flow cytometry) or to demonstrate gross pathology and thus ensure better communications. Thus, the proportion of cases with a deferred diagnosis has increased considerably since the early reports. Similarly, the proportion of breast cases (still the most frequent organ site involved) with occult or "minimal" cancer has also increased markedly, contributing as well to an elevated proportion of both deferred and false negative diagnoses.

In actuality, "frozen section" examination is a poor term, since many intraoperative consultations (the preferred term) do not result in frozen section examinations actually being performed. It is the responsibility of the surgical pathologist as the consultant in this situation to decide exactly what needs to be done, and if the gross appearance of the specimen is characteristic, or the diagnosis can be made by the imprint or smear technique alone, the performance of a frozen section examination may be unnecessary. Similarly, freezing of tissues may not only be unnecessary but may actually be contraindicated in certain situations. For example, if the specimen submitted is so small that frozen section examination would be likely to exhaust the tissue completely, and if the frozen section diagnosis is likely to be either difficult to make or unnecessary for the immediate management of the patient, then certainly this procedure should not be performed.

The role of the frozen section examination in providing instant gratification for the surgeon should be commented on further at this point. Since most departments of pathology charge the patient an additional fee for these examinations, it should be understood by both the clinician and the pathologist that they should be performed only when they will provide information that will be of immediate or ultimate value in patient management. Thus, a breast biopsy specimen should certainly be frozen if immediate mastectomy is contemplated (a rare event today in our hospital), but the tissue should probably not be frozen if the surgeon plans to delay the mastectomy by several days even if the results of the biopsy are positive for carcinoma. However, intraoperative consultation still may be indicated to obtain fresh tumor tissue for estrogen and progesterone receptor assays and/or for flow cytometric analysis. As another example, in a case of suspected malignant lymphoma, intraoperative consultation may be requested to determine whether diagnostic tissue has indeed been removed before the incision is closed but should not be requested to provide a definitive diagnosis unless the physician plans to institute therapy immediately (e.g., in a case of spinal cord compression or superior vena cava syndrome).

Special mention should be made of the surgical practice of requesting frozen section examination to determine the adequacy of margins in a resection for cancer. This is done most frequently in the head and neck area, where the tissues are often difficult to freeze and section because of the high content of fat. In addition, it is apparent that in a large resection specimen, only a limited number of frozen section examinations can be performed perpendicular to the tumor and its resection margins while the patient is still waiting under anesthesia. Thus, a report of a positive margin is of great value, but a negative report does not by any means guarantee that tumor will not be found when permanent sections of the adjacent tissues are examined. Thus, I usually remind our surgeons at The George Washington University Medical Center that frozen section examinations in this situation are analogous to the old bumper sticker in that, if you need this, "you are too darn close."

Margins on tumor resections, incidentally, are one of those situations in which cytologic preparations do not add significantly to the information obtained by performing a classic frozen section examination. Unless massive amounts of tumor are present at a resection margin (usually enough to be visible grossly), the results of the imprint will probably still be negative for tumor cells. On the other hand, we have found these preparations of considerable assistance as a complement to frozen section examination in many situations, and in some cases, they even supplant the frozen section examination itself. For example, false negative results on a lymph node containing a small volume of metastatic cancer are more likely to be obtained from a frozen section examination than from an imprint preparation of that lymph node. The main reason is that multiple cut surfaces of the node can be processed on one slide using the imprint technique, as opposed to the multiple frozen sections that would be necessary to examine the node as thoroughly without the use of imprints. Also, since freezing artifact is not a factor in the imprint preparation, a few cancer cells are more easily distinguished from the surrounding population of lymphocytes and histiocytes than they are in the artifactually distorted frozen section. Imprints or smears also are often of more value than the classic frozen section in the case of a tumor that is largely necrotic, in which a few malignant cells can be lost in the sea of necrosis on the frozen section but are usually easily visible on the cytologic preparation.

There are relatively few other situations in which the imprint is of more value than the frozen section examination, but there are many in which it is of equal (or at least complementary) value. When only a small tissue sample is provided and the possibility exists that a frozen section examination would exhaust the specimen and leave none available for permanent sections, a positive imprint can preclude the necessity of performing the frozen section examination, and thus preserve the tissue in its entirety. Since imprints are also quicker to perform, time is saved in the operating room, where it is obviously an essential consideration. Toward this end, I have used imprints extensively in the intraoperative evaluation of cases of hyperparathyroidism, and have found that they are at least as accurate as the frozen section examination in distinguishing parathyroid tissue from thyroid, lymph node, thymus, or adipose tissue.[11] In other non-neoplastic situations as well, the cytologic technique has been helpful; for example, I have been able to identify ganglion cells in smears from sympathetic ganglia that were submitted for intraoperative evaluation. A more complete summary of the technique and our experience with it is available elsewhere.[12]

Before leaving the topic of intraoperative cytology entirely, it is worthy of mention that this technique can prepare the surgical pathologist for the interpretation of fine needle aspiration specimens. The fine needle aspiration, long a popular clinical technique in Europe, has finally found its way across the Atlantic, and more and more surgical pathologists in the United States are being asked to interpret this material today. Although fuller discussions of fine needle aspiration and its interpretation are found in textbooks of cytopathology, and, therefore, the subject is not covered in detail in this text, one may certainly note that this, like any other new procedure, should not be entered into lightly by the surgical pathologist who is unfamiliar with this material and its interpretation. An excellent way for surgical pathologists to prepare for reading specimens of this sort is to perform touch preparations or smears on all tumors received fresh in the operating room, and for that matter even to perform needle aspirations of these tissues themselves before beginning to accept in vivo specimens from their clinicians. As in the case of frozen section examinations, discretion is often the better part of valor, and the results of an aspiration should never be reported as positive without absolute certainty that tumor is indeed present. As in other cytologic techniques, the emphasis should be on reporting in terms of the anticipated histopathologic diagnosis, rather than using a "negative–suspicious–positive" or a numerical grading system.

The Surgical Pathology Report

The subject of special stains and their uses and abuses is obviously a very important one in surgical pathology. The question of which (if any) special stains to perform in a particular case is best resolved by a consideration of the clinical significance of the report in that case. Since special stains are performed most frequently in the search for and interpretation of either infectious or neoplastic disease, their use in these two situations is covered in more detail in Chapters 3 and 7, respectively. Similarly, questions of how many sections to submit from a particular gross specimen, how these sections should be taken and labeled, whether multiple or serial sections are required, and similar considerations are best decided with reference to an individual case. Thus, such questions are dealt with in the individual chapters of this text relating to specific organs and organ systems. In general terms, however, perhaps the most important single consideration is that of consistency in the practice of surgical pathology within a given laboratory. Thus, if one surgical pathologist in the laboratory does not use the letter "I" as a designation for tissue sections because of its possible confusion with the Roman numeral "I," none of the pathologists submitting tissue in that laboratory should use that designation. If one pathologist uses a particular designation for resection margins, then all colleagues should use the same designation. Only in this manner can submitting clinicians be guaranteed that the terms of a surgical pathology report that they receive on a Monday will mean the same as the terms of the report they receive on Tuesday. Similarly, when all the surgical pathologists in that laboratory have gone elsewhere, their successor or successors will be able to review old slides and old reports and be aware of exactly what they signify.

This brings us to the topic of the correct way to prepare a surgical pathology report, but the best statement that can be made is that there is no single best way to prepare a surgical pathology report. The most important thing to remember is that the report should be prepared with the best interests of the clinician and the patient in mind. Thus, the most important features are clarity, brevity, and careful attention to those details that may influence the management of the patient. In general terms, those portions of the clinical history that are relevant to the specimen should always be included in the final report, as should the exact source of the specimen and the condition in which it is received (e.g., in formalin, fresh, unfixed and poorly preserved, intact, or previously opened). All necessary measurements should be performed before the specimen is dissected, and these measurements (including weight) should be recorded. The description of the gross pathology encountered should proceed from the general to the specific; for example, the presence of a tumor must be noted before its characteristics are described in detail. In general terms, the portion of a specimen (or multiple specimens) described first should be that in which the clinician is most interested, although there may be exceptions to this rule, as in the situation in which peripheral specimens are received first for frozen section examination and thus are described first in the gross description. If anything has been done to the specimen before its gross examination and sectioning, this should be mentioned in the surgical pathology report. Thus, if a frozen section examination has been performed, the final report should mention this fact, should contain the exact (i.e., word-for-word) frozen section report rendered to the clinician and should indicate who performed the frozen section examination and rendered the report (in many instances, the pathologist who performed the frozen section examination may not be the same pathologist who cuts, examines, and eventually

signs out the case). Similarly, if portions of tissue have been removed for electron microscopic examination, hormone receptor analysis, virologic or other cultures, or any study other than histologic examination, this should also be noted in the final report.

If the gross specimen is a complex one, a photograph may add immeasurably to the dictated or written gross description. Photographs should be taken before the specimen is extensively dissected and may be repeated if necessary during and after the process of dissection as well. Important gross details should be adequately labeled in the photograph, and a Polaroid or other instant photographic technique may be extremely valuable for this purpose. Finally, the gross dictation should always include the eventual disposition of the specimen, since this is the only way that future reviewers of the case will have of knowing what each slide represents. This rule should be followed whether the specimen is a single, small piece of tissue that is submitted in toto or a radical resection for cancer, in which 100 or more sections may be submitted, with the relationship of the label for each section to its exact source duly recorded in a "slide key" accompanying the gross description.

In addition to the possible benefit mentioned earlier for future reviewers, the advantage of a careful recording of the disposition of the gross specimen may be more immediate. Thus, in the unfortunate event that a specimen is lost or confused with another specimen, the gross dictation and slide key may resolve the possible serious confusion resulting in this situation. Similarly, if the gross description indicates that four pieces of tissue were submitted from a particular biopsy, and only three appear on the slide produced by the histotechnologist, the pathologist knows instantly that the block should be inspected and sections of deeper levels ordered.

The same rules of reason that pertain to gross descriptions and dictations apply equally to both the microscopic description and the final diagnosis. In both sections of the report, the clinically most significant lesions should precede the incidental findings, even if the portion of the specimen containing the latter was processed grossly before the former. As a general rule, what is visible with the scanning lens of the microscope should be described before what is visible with the high-power objective. For example, the pushing versus infiltrating character of the margin of a tumor should always be described before its degree of nuclear pleomorphism or mitotic activity. The microscopic description should be just that, rather than a diagnosis or prognostic commentary. Thus, a phrase such as "a tumor that appears to be of low-grade malignancy" should never appear in the microscopic description but should be reserved for a comment appended to the final diagnosis. Information included in the microscopic description should be as specific as possible, so "vascular invasion" should be replaced by an exact characterization of the type of vessel (e.g., artery, vein, capillary, lymphatic) invaded, and "chronic inflammation" should yield to an enumeration of the specific cells (lymphocytes, histiocytes, plasma cells) comprising the infiltrate.

Similarly, the final diagnosis should be as specific as possible, should list diagnoses in their order of clinical importance, and should be inclusive of all the specimens received (not forgetting, for example, the unremarkable appendix received with the hysterectomy specimen for cervical cancer). Terminology will vary with the individual laboratory, but again some attempt should be made at standardization. For example, tumors may be subdivided as well, moderately, or poorly differentiated or as grade I, II, or III, but not as both on different days or by different pathologists. The diagnosis should also be clinically relevant; so for a squamous cell carcinoma of the cervix, possibly neither of the above grading systems would be used, but perhaps an indication as to whether the tumor is keratinizing, large cell nonkeratinizing, or small cell. If terminology used is likely to be confusing to the clinician, it should be clearly defined in an appended comment, perhaps with a suitable bibliographic reference. Better yet, the clinician should also be contacted in person or by telephone to be sure that he fully understands the information the pathologist is seeking to convey.

Although the essentials of a microscopic description have been detailed above, it should be noted that there has been a great deal of debate in recent years over the necessity for any microscopic description at all in a surgical pathology report. In our laboratory, my colleagues and I have adopted the middle ground between those who demand a microscopic description on every specimen and those who consider it totally unnecessary. Normal appendices, cervical biopsy specimens showing only chronic cervicitis, unremarkable hernia sacs, and the like are described grossly and given a diagnosis, with the microscopic features omitted, while the time saved by this maneuver is put to good use in ensuring that the microscopic descriptions for diagnostic biopsy specimens, tumor resections, and other "nonroutine" specimens are complete to the point of containing all the pertinent normal observations.

NEW ADJUNCTS TO THE PRACTICE OF SURGICAL PATHOLOGY

The history of the field of surgical pathology contains innumerable techniques that were initially developed as basic research tools and subsequently became adapted to the diagnostic armamentarium. Many of the techniques we now think of as routine (e.g., cryostat procedures for frozen section preparation, electron microscopy, immunohistochemistry, and fine needle aspiration cytology) were at one time a novelty—to our antecedents, or even to us. This section briefly discusses a few of the new adjuncts already in place in some surgical pathology laboratories and some that may become commonplace while this volume is still in use.

Flow Cytometry

Flow cytometry was developed during the early 1970s, but because of the great expense and special environmental accommodations necessary to maintain the equipment, it did not become popular for clinical applications until the early to mid-1980s.[13,14] The basic equipment is a machine that can create a single-file stream of cells from a cell suspension and can then measure specific quantitative determinants of these individual cells or even of portions of cells. The first—and still the most widespread—clinical application of flow cytometry has been in the immunophenotyping of lymphoid and myeloid cells, initially in leukemias and lymphomas and subsequently in the spectrum of disease associated with the human immunodeficiency virus (HIV).

Another important application of flow cytometry in surgical pathology concerns DNA analysis. Flow cytometry is capable of determining whether cells in a solid tumor are diploid or aneuploid, as well as calculating the percentage of cells in the different phases of the cell cycle. It is generally expected that aneuploid tumors in general—and especially tumors with increased fraction of cells in S-phase—are more likely to be malignant or, if already known to be malignant, are likely to have a poorer prognosis. Unfortunately, there are still many exceptions to both rules, and the specific measurements that are clinically significant vary from one tumor type to another, and often from one laboratory to another. Much of the literature thus far has concentrated on tumors of the urinary bladder, breast, and colon but, with the recent development of a technique to analyze cells from paraffin-embedded tissue,[14] many other tumors are being studied as well. In some of these situations, flow cytometry will probably be no more than an expensive way of confirming evidence already supplied by routine light microscopy, but in tumors in which routine microscopy is not highly predictive, flow cytometry will probably prove to be of greatest value. It is also possible that flow cytometry may provide the key to the subsequent behavior of certain premalignant lesions[15] and in some instances may help resolve the question of whether two synchronous or metachronous tumors at different sites represent separate primaries or a single primary and its metastases.[16]

Genotyping

At a less developed stage than flow cytometry is the study of gene rearrangements and their applications to human disease.[17] Analysis of the genotype of lymphoid cells has already proved a valuable tool in the diagnosis and accurate characterization of cases of leukemia and lymphoma.[18] By analyzing the entire pattern of gene rearrangements in a particular lymphocytic population, the presence of malignancy (i.e., monoclonality) and the cell of origin of the neoplasm can be determined in most cases. However, there is not a perfect correlation between clonality and neoplasia; therefore, the results of these studies must be correlated with other clinical and laboratory data in their interpretation. I have nonetheless seen cases in which the DNA probe analysis has proved to be the deciding factor in the interpretation of a difficult case.

Another application of DNA analysis is in the study of oncogene activation.[19] Activated oncogenes have been detected in both experimentally induced and clinical human neoplasms. Since oncogenes can be detected even when only very few neoplastic cells are present, they may be of use in the diagnosis of minimal residual or metastatic disease. In addition, there are early suggestions that they may also provide an indication of the natural history and prognosis of some human malignant tumors. These studies are still in a very early phase.

In Situ Hybridization

The technique of in situ hybridization represents a direct application of DNA probe technology to tissue pathology. Using various methodologies, biologic stains for specific DNA sequences can be performed.[20,21] Currently, these techniques are applied predominantly in the field of infectious disease pathology, in which they have been used to detect both viral (herpes simplex virus, CMV, human papillomavirus, hepatitis B virus, and HIV) and nonviral (e.g., *Chlamydia, Mycoplasma, Mycobacterium*) agents. These studies can be performed on both cytologic and tissue preparations and are capable of detecting these agents with more sensitivity and specificity than several other available techniques. This methodology is rapidly evolving as an alternative to standard immunohistochemical techniques.

Morphometry

The term *morphometry* can be used to describe any quantitative determination on microscopically examined tissues and thus can vary from such pseudoquantitative activities as measuring depth or counting mitotic figures to highly sophisticated measurements requiring complicated and expensive equipment.[22,23] The latter techniques include digital imaging analysis,[23] which consists of a highly computerized cell counting and measuring system with properties of spatial resolution and photometry. It has thus far been used primarily in quantitative cytopathology. These techniques have been found to provide valuable prognostic information in neoplasms for which behavior is difficult to predict by standard light microscopy alone but, because they are expensive and labor-intensive, they have failed to gain wide acceptance in many diagnostic laboratories. Many of the classic morphometric techniques are gradually being integrated with flow cytometry.

Computerization

In addition to the use of computers in several of the specialized techniques described above, I refer here to computerization of the surgical pathology laboratory itself. I continue to list this as a new technique because, although computerization of clinical laboratories has progressed rapidly, the development of functional software programs for surgical pathology laboratories is still in its infancy. In our laboratory, experience with computers in surgical pathology has thus far been less impressive than that of the other techniques summarized above, but the literature suggests that various computerized systems can be of great use in such aspects of data management as file searches, standardized format reporting, ensuring follow-up of selected cases, reporting results to distant terminals, and documentation of quality assurance programs.[24–27]

Telepathology

The term *telepathology* was coined by Weinstein[28] to describe programs involving the transfer by video of images of pathologic specimens from one site to another. Variations of this technique have been in use for a number of years for in-house transmission of both gross and microscopic images,[29] but it has been demonstrated more recently that the technology is now also capable of transmitting high-quality images from one hospital to another, and even from one city to another.[28] We believe that the potential of these techniques for providing rapid consultation to geographically isolated pathologists is enormous, although—as in most of the technologies discussed in this section—the cost-benefit ratio remains to be established.

QUALITY ASSURANCE

Quality assurance has become an important facet of surgical pathology in the modern era of accountability. The relation of quality assurance to malpractice liability is discussed in Chapter 2, but a few words are in order on general principles. We do not believe that quality assurance is meaningful if quality is absent, and much of what has already been discussed above—communication with the clinician, the role of internal and external consultation, correlation of intraoperative with final diagnoses, preparation of the surgical pathology report, the use of new techniques, and so forth—provides the framework of quality. The essence of quality assurance, then, is the documentation that these activities are actually taking place.[25-27] Complete and up-to-date procedure manuals (containing procedures that are really being followed), written recording of consultations and communications, and careful review of reports in general and diagnoses in particular form the essence of a quality assurance program. Ways of achieving these goals are too numerous to detail here, but attention to the items discussed in this chapter and in Chapter 2, as well as material available from local and national pathology societies, should provide a framework on which to build.

TRAINING IN SURGICAL PATHOLOGY

It is difficult to be very specific about training in surgical pathology without first defining the ultimate goal of the individual to be trained. For example, the resident who desires to become an academic surgical pathologist should spend a minimum of three years of training in anatomic pathology, with at least two of those years devoted to surgical pathology and cytology. Ideally, at least one more year is advisable, as is training in more than one institution (both because of the variety of specimens seen in different institutions and the exposure to several different philosophies). A prolonged period of exposure to specialized techniques (electron microscopy, immunoperoxidase, needle aspiration cytology) and/or fields of study (dermatopathology, hematopathology, gynecologic pathology) is also advisable. The neophyte academic surgical pathologist is also well advised to undertake and complete some research project or projects during train-

ing and to experience the difficulties and triumphs resulting from the presentation and publication of the results thereof.

On the other hand, the training program in surgical pathology for the resident who spends a total of two years in anatomic and two years in clinical pathology before taking the board examinations and entering clinical practice must, by virtue of the length of time on surgical pathology rotations, be considerably different. At our own institution, in which training is received in several different hospital laboratories, many of our residents follow the latter path. Although the nature of the surgical pathology workload differs both quantitatively and qualitatively from one laboratory to the next within our training program, the directors of these laboratories believe that the principles to be developed by the trainee are similar in each laboratory. Thus, we have formulated the following list of fundamentals that we expect our residents to master during training:

1. Cognizance of their own role in the clinical situation in relation to both the clinician and the patient. Residents are responsible for the surgical specimen from the time it is obtained from the patient until the final report is received by the clinician. They should ensure that the specimen is received in time and in proper condition for processing, that the slides are prepared to their satisfaction, and that the diagnosis is received and understood as early as possible by the clinician.
2. Ability to perform in a reasonable time a technically adequate frozen section examination and to deliver an appropriate interpretation. Residents should be able to communicate in this situation with the surgeon in order to obtain and to deliver pertinent information. Residents should also be aware of the limitations of frozen section technique and know when a diagnosis must be deferred and be able to apply special techniques such as imprints, which complement or supplant the frozen section examination.
3. Ability to identify, describe, and submit appropriate sections from specimens commonly encountered in surgical pathology practice. Trainees should establish which cases need to be processed first in a day's workload. They should be able to dictate the gross descriptions of the great majority of cases in final form at the cutting table; to identify the specimens received, how they are processed, and what each section submitted represents, in clear enough fashion that this information is immediately evident to anyone subsequently reading the report; and to recognize the importance of maintaining the specimen for subsequent diagnostic workup and for teaching.
4. Cooperation with investigators studying human tissues, to the extent that patient care is not compromised.
5. Ability to determine whether slides received are ade-

quate in number and quality and to take appropriate remedial steps if they are not. Residents should be aware of uses and abuses of special stains, recuts, and similar techniques; should be able to assign priorities for the earlier and more extensive investigation of more important cases; and should be able to write a clinically relevant, concise but complete, organized and intelligible microscopic description on every case for which such a description is required.

6. Ability to diagnose correctly the great majority of commonly encountered lesions, awareness of the existence of other lesions, and knowledge of when and how to seek consultation. Trainees should develop a systematic approach to slide examination, to ensure that lesions, even if not always correctly interpreted, will at least not be overlooked. They should also be able to relate the histologic findings to the clinical and gross features of the case.

7. Cognizance of new and specialized techniques in such fields as histochemistry, electron microscopy, immunopathology, and specimen radiography and their applications to diagnostic surgical pathology; knowledge of when it is appropriate to submit tissues for these and other studies, and in what form the tissue must be submitted for the studies to be successful.

8. Understanding the clinical manifestations and natural history of lesions encountered. This demands independent reading, beginning with standard textbooks and progressing to familiarity with and critical reading of current clinical and pathologic literature.

9. Familiarity with the technical aspects of histopathology as related to surgical pathology. This includes techniques of sectioning, embedding, and staining, comparative values of different fixatives, operation and servicing of microtomes and cryostats, and similar problems.

Although this list of goals might easily be modified in different institutions training residents in surgical pathology, we believe that some goals should be established by each institution for its own training program. Both trainees and those who are responsible for their training should be aware of these goals and should monitor the program carefully to be sure that they are being met.

A word should also be said about training in surgical pathology for nonpathologists. Although it is our strong conviction that surgical pathology should be practiced by pathologists, we also believe that, just as the pathologist with advanced clinical experience is often a better pathologist, the general surgeon, gynecologist, dermatologist, or other clinical specialist who has been exposed to a rotation in surgical pathology during his or her training is often the better for this experience as well. These rotations by clinical trainees through the surgical pathology service will often be limited to one or a few months, and

the goals of the training in this situation should be (1) to instill an appreciation of the role of the surgical pathologist as a consultant in the appropriate clinical field; (2) to develop a recognition of the importance of adequate communication (including the provision by the clinician of appropriate clinical histories and specimen descriptions) in the performance of this consultative role of the surgical pathologist; (3) to develop a respect for the specimen as the primary vehicle for this communication, together with an appropriate appreciation of proper techniques of fixation and submission of specimens; (4) to develop a realization of what the surgical pathologist cannot do, so as to expect fewer miracles from him in subsequent clinical practice; (5) to develop some concept of basic principles of gross pathology, so inflammatory, neoplastic, traumatic, and other processes can be distinguished in the operating room or the clinic; and (6) to develop the same sort of familiarity with microscopic interpretation, and with the clinical and pathologic significance of the main entities encountered in the individual field of clinical practice, so a surgical pathology report may be interpreted and slides reviewed with the surgical pathologist with more confidence in the future.

RESEARCH IN SURGICAL PATHOLOGY

According to the *Random House Dictionary of the English Language,* research is defined as ''diligent and systematic inquiry or investigation into a subject in order to discover or revise facts, theories, applications, etc.'' We have emphasized that most surgical pathologists do indeed perform research as defined in this manner.[30] We have classified the types of research performed by the surgical pathologist and directly related to surgical pathology as (1) observational; (2) manipulative with human tissues; (3) experimental with nonhuman models; and (4) technical, instructional, and delivery. A few comments will now be offered on each of these categories of research in surgical pathology.

The first of these, designated observational research, is probably the most common, and certainly the most common outside the university or academic setting. The role of the surgical pathologist in this form of research is the observation of the results of an experiment of nature. The subject chosen depends on the material available in one's own institution, although collaborative relationships with other pathologists and/or other institutions may add to the volume of material observed. The results of this form of research may range from the report of a single case to a major clinical–pathologic–epidemiologic review.

Although this type of project—particularly the case report—has often been denigrated, it is worth noting that many new and important entities in the surgical pathology literature were originally described in the form of a single case report, and many new and important observations on previously described entities have been made in the same format. This does not mean that every case report is equally valuable, and certainly many have added nothing but verbiage and paper to the world's resources. (The same statement, of course, can equally be made of many other research projects, including many that have been well funded by tax dollars.)

In the second category of research in surgical pathology are those studies that involve some degree of manipulation with human tissues. The importance of the role of the surgical pathologist in making such tissues available for study has been commented on briefly earlier and should be emphasized again at this time. It is equally important for the surgical pathologist to remember, however, that his primary role is that of a diagnostician, and he must be careful not to give away so much tissue for research that the amount retained is inadequate for the provision of the diagnostic and prognostic information for which it was originally sent.

In this type of research, the surgical pathologist may serve merely as the collector of tissues for others, or may be the primary researcher himself. Human tissues obtained from living patients may be used for organ or cell culture, transplantation into animals, study by DNA spectrophotometry or flow microfluorimetry, immunohistochemistry, transmission or scanning electron microscopy, genotyping, or other studies.[31] If any of these techniques is found to be of diagnostic importance for the patient, this sort of research may not only provide interesting biologic data but also may add new tools to the diagnostic armamentarium of the surgical pathologist.

In the category of experimental research with nonhuman models, I refer to those studies that are carried out in vitro or in animals but are related directly to human disease. Again, the surgical pathologist may personally perform this research or may function as a consultant to, or collaborator with, a basic scientist. The morphologic skills of surgical pathologists are often invaluable to the basic scientist who is working in this sort of system and cannot by themselves transpose these histologic observations to the appropriate human disease.

Finally, research in the technical, instructional, and delivery aspects of surgical pathology is a rapidly expanding field. This includes such projects as developing and perfecting new techniques that can be applied to the diagnosis of human disease, developing new models for training in surgical pathology, and developing new techniques for providing better service in surgical pathology to clinicians and referring pathologists alike. Many of the currently accepted standard techniques in the field arose

from someone's pioneering research of this sort in the past.

One of the most attractive aspects of the field of pathology in general, and surgical pathology in particular, is the fact that this wide diversity of research models enables interesting and satisfying research to be performed outside the traditional academic setting. Thus, many surgical pathologists in community hospital practice situations perform significant research, and no doubt this trend will be magnified in the future. The image of research in surgical pathology as being somehow unable to compete for academic stature with more basic experimental research is fortunately being supplanted by an appreciation of the fact that both good and bad research are performed in both fields, and that the quality and significance of research in surgical pathology are often equal to those of more "fundamental" studies.

Funding has often been a problem for research in surgical pathology in the past, but my colleagues and I firmly believe that good research in surgical pathology should be as fundable by the grant mechanism as good research in any other field. The emphasis in this statement, however, should be placed on the word "good," and surgical pathologists must be sure that the scientific reasoning and methodology applied to their research can stand up to criticism by full-time scientists as well as by other surgical pathologists. Time and physical facilities are also important to the performance of research in surgical pathology, and those who are responsible for providing these must be made aware of the importance of research to both the practice and teaching of surgical pathology.

REFERENCES

1. Schwartz GF, Feig SA, Patchefsky AS: Clinicopathologic correlations and significance of clinically occult mammary lesions. Cancer 41:1147, 1978
2. Morrow M, Evans J, Rosen PP, Kinne DW: Does clearing of axillary lymph nodes contribute to accurate staging of breast cancer? Cancer 53:1329, 1984
3. Ackerman LV, Ramirez GA: The indications for and limitations of frozen section diagnosis. Br J Surg 46:336, 1959
4. Holaday WJ, Assor D: Ten thousand consecutive frozen sections. Am J Clin Pathol 61:769, 1974
5. Nakazawa H, Rosen P, Lane N, Lattes R: The frozen section experience in 3000 cases. Am J Clin Pathol 49:41, 1968
6. Silverberg SG: The role of the pathologist in oncology. p. 174. In McKenna RJ, Murphy GP (eds): Fundamentals of Surgical Oncology. Macmillan, New York, 1986
7. Esteban JM, Zaloudek C, Silverberg SG: Intraoperative diagnosis of breast lesions. Am J Clin Pathol 88:681, 1987
8. Oneson RH, Minke JA, Silverberg SG: Intraoperative path-

ologic consultation: An audit of 1,000 recent consecutive cases. Am J Surg Pathol 13:237, 1989

9. Agnantis NJ, Apostolikas N, Christodoulou I, et al: The reliability of frozen section diagnosis in various breast lesions: A study based on 3452 biopsies. Recent Results Cancer Res 90:205, 1984

10. Fessia L, Ghiringhello B, Arisio R, et al: Accuracy of frozen section diagnosis of breast cancer detection. A review of 4436 biopsies and comparison with cytodiagnosis. Pathol Res Pract 179:61, 1984

11. Sasano H, Geelhoed GW, Silverberg SG: Intraoperative cytologic evaluation of lipid in the diagnosis of parathyroid adenoma. Am J Surg Pathol 12:282, 1988

12. Bloustein PA, Silverberg SG: Rapid cytologic examination of surgical specimens. Pathol Annu 12(pt 2):251, 1977

13. Lovett EJ, Schnitzer B, Keren DF, et al: Application of flow cytometry to diagnostic pathology. Lab Invest 50:115, 1984

14. Coon JS, Landay AL, Weinstein RS: Biology of disease. Advances in flow cytometry for diagnostic pathology. Lab Invest 57:453, 1987

15. Banner BF, Chacho MS, Roseman DL, Coon JS: Multiparameter flow cytometric analysis of colon polyps. Am J Clin Pathol 87:313, 1987

16. Symonds DA, Johnson DP, Wheeless CR Jr: Feulgen cytometry in simultaneous endometrial and ovarian carcinoma. Cancer 61:2511, 1988

17. Fenoglio-Preiser CM, Willman CL: Molecular biology and the pathologist: General principles and applications. Arch Pathol Lab Med 111:601, 1987

18. Cossman J, Uppenkamp M, Sundeen J, et al: Molecular genetics and the diagnosis of lymphoma. Arch Pathol Lab Med 112:117, 1988

19. Garrett CT: Oncogenes: A critical review. Clin Chim Acta 156:1, 1986

20. Grody WS, Cheng L, Lewin KJ: In-situ viral DNA hybridization in diagnostic surgical pathology. Hum Pathol 18:535, 1987

21. Nagai N, Nuovo G, Friedman D, Crum CP: Detection of papillomavirus nucleic acids in genital precancers with the in situ hybridization technique. Int J Gynecol Pathol 6:366, 1987

22. Baak JPA, Oort JO: A Manual of Morphometry in Diagnostic Pathology. Springer-Verlag, Berlin, 1983

23. Hall TL, Fu YS: Applications of quantitative microscopy in tumor pathology. Lab Invest 53:5, 1985

24. Rosenheim SH, Volz JH: Use of an automated microfilm system in the surgical pathology laboratory. Am J Clin Pathol 79:467, 1983

25. Cechner RL: A multifunction network of computers in a large pathology department. Integration of word processing, database management and general purpose computing using network principles. Am J Clin Pathol 79:472, 1983

26. Rickert RR: Peer review and quality control in anatomic pathology: Approach of the I and A Commission. Pathologist 32:483, 1978

27. Murphy MSN, Derman H: Quality assurance in surgical pathology: Personal and peer assessment. Am J Clin Pathol 75:462, 1981

28. Weinstein RS: Prospects for telepathology. Hum Pathol 17:434, 1986

29. Hutter RVP, Kim DU, Carter HW, Rickert RR: Video intercom: Operating room consultation and frozen section with screen display of gross and microscopic findings. Pathologist 33:599, 1979

30. Silverberg SG: The surgical pathologist as researcher. Am J Clin Pathol 75:453, 1981

31. Trump BF, Harris CC: Human tissues in biomedical research. Hum Pathol 10:245, 1979

2

Medicolegal Principles and Problems

Joseph Montedonico

Much has been written about the medical malpractice crisis during the past 10 years. Blame has been assigned to physicians, consumers, lawyers, and insurance companies with equal frequency. While the causes of the sharp increase in malpractice cases in recent years are complex and still open to debate, the effects are more clearly definable. The physician today needs not only to be a competent professional but to have a basic understanding of medicolegal principles in order to effectively decrease the risk of a lawsuit.

The purpose of this chapter is to introduce surgical pathologists to the basic legal rules that apply to their practice and to illustrate areas in which surgical pathologists may be particularly vulnerable to lawsuit. While each state has particular laws, regulations, and precedent governing these issues, the following general discussion is meant to provide practitioners with a framework to be remembered and applied to day-to-day problems confronting them in their practice.

MEDICAL MALPRACTICE: AN OVERVIEW

The patient who sues a surgical pathologist for medical malpractice has to prove each of the following elements in order to get the case to the jury. The plaintiff has to clear the hurdles of proving (1) that the pathologist failed to meet the applicable standard of care, (2) that such failure caused an injury, and (3) the nature and extent of the injury. In showing a violation of a standard of care, the plaintiff must first establish what is the applicable standard. This is done through expert witness testimony.

In cases for which there are established national standards (such as specialty boards) the practitioner may be held to a national standard of care; therefore, the plaintiff may bring in an expert witness from any type of institution in the country in order to establish the standard and to testify that the surgical pathologist deviated from the range of acceptable practice.

As one might imagine, proving violation of a standard of care is not an exact science. First of all, *standard of care* is a broad term and, while written guidelines, by the College of American Pathologists and Joint Commission on Accreditation of Hospitals, primarily, may specifically govern the conduct in question, it is more likely that the issue will be a judgment call based on the particular conditions at the time of occurrence. As a result, there will be significant latitude for the testimony of various physician experts, both for and against the conduct. Adding to the uncertainty is the fact that an increasing number of physicians are testifying against their colleagues; many of those "hired gun" experts spend most of their time reviewing and giving testimony in malpractice cases, resulting in the relative ease with which parties on either side may obtain standard of care expert testimony. With conflicting testimony among appropriate standard of care experts in a given case, the jury will decide what is the appropriate standard on the basis of the testimony that is most convincing to the jury.

Having set forth expert testimony that a standard of care in the field of surgical pathology has been breached, the plaintiff's burden is then to prove that an injury resulted from that breach. If, for example, a pathologist misreads a specimen and reports a benign condition, but the patient is correctly diagnosed with cancer 3 months later and medical testimony shows that no physical injury, in fact, resulted during the 3 month delay (no change in prognosis), the plaintiff does not prevail. Despite what may be a fairly clear case of negligence, the plaintiff suffered no injury as a result, and there can be no recovery. Most often, expert testimony will be required to prove that the injury was caused by the negligent conduct. More than one negligent act may be found to have caused an injury.

DAMAGES

The plaintiff has the burden of proving that, as a result of the alleged violation of a standard of care, some physical damage resulted. An award of damages in a medical malpractice case is intended to make the injured party "whole again." Once physical injury is established, the patient can then recover related damages, including pain and suffering, loss of income, and past and future medical expenses. In addition, a spouse or child of a deceased may be able to recover on behalf of an injured or deceased patient for the loss of the patient's affections or services.

LEGAL CONSIDERATIONS OF SURGICAL PATHOLOGY

Statute of Limitations

Each state has its own rules for limiting the time in which a patient may bring a lawsuit. This is based on the public policy rationale that the right to bring a lawsuit should expire after a few years if not filed in a timely fashion, thus giving some finality to events. Most U.S. statutes of limitation for negligence are 2 to 3 years. It is important to know when the period of time begins. In most jurisdictions, it commences on the date of the alleged negligent act; however, most jurisdictions defer the commencement of the statutory period until the patient actually discovers, or should have discovered, the negligent act. For example, in a case in which a sponge is left in during surgery, with the patient remaining asymptomatic for several years but later developing abdominal pain caused by the retained sponge, the period of time for filing the lawsuit begins at the time the sponge is discovered and not on the date of surgery. The statute of limitations does not begin for a minor until he/she reaches the age of adulthood—in most states, 18 years of age. Other events that might alter the running of the time within which lawsuits must be filed are a patient's incompetency or a physician's fraud or concealment of record evidence. Another condition that extends the regular 2 or 3 year period is a finding that negligence occurred as a result of a

"continuous course of treatment" over a number of years. In this situation, the statute does not commence until the course of treatment is completed; the effect may be to include care within the statutory period that occurred many years earlier than the 2 or 3 year period. In certain cases, such as when a pathologist reasonably expects that his work will be relied on by other practitioners in determining the mode of treatment, it is appropriate to impute to that pathologist constructive participation in that treatment as long as it continues; the pathologist may be included in the suit although it may be more than the 2 or 3 years since the evaluation had passed.

Liability of the Surgical Pathologist

The surgical pathologist faces certain unique problems with regard to liability. The primary distinction between the pathologist and other physicians that affects the risk of suit is lack of patient contact. Since there is no opportunity to develop a relationship of trust and support with the patient, the pathologist becomes a more likely target for a lawsuit than do other physicians, especially once the patient has been advised by counsel that there is a valid cause of action.

Standard of Care

Surgical pathologists must familiarize themselves with the standard of care against which they will be measured in the event of a claim. Written guidelines such as those set forth by the College of American Pathologists and other professional associations must be introduced by the plaintiff as evidence of the rules. It is difficult to defend a case governing pathology practice in which physicians have clearly violated guidelines set by their own professional group. The Joint Commission on Accreditation of Hospitals (JCAH) sets requirements for pathology services in the hospital; violation of JCAH requirements will also evidence negligence. In addition, violation of a hospital's own internal written policies and procedures will be considered evidence of negligence. Surgical pathologists should familiarize themselves with any written guidelines pertaining to their profession.

MEDICAL STAFF RELATIONSHIPS

Early appellate court decisions held that the hospital could not be liable for medical negligence because it merely provided the facility for the physicians and nurses and therefore did not actually deliver health care services. The hospital was regarded as having no control over those who rendered patient care. During the 1960s, the modern concept of the hospital emerged—that is, that the hospital is responsible for the health care rendered within its walls and has a duty to provide the care and skill of hospitals generally considered reasonable, as evidenced by federal and state health statutes and regulations, the patient admissions contract, licensing regulations, and so forth.

Theories supporting hospital and institutional liability for medical staff negligence have centered on *vicarious liability* and *corporate liability*. Under vicarious liability, the negligent act or omission by a hospital employee is imputed to the employer (hospital). Employees are responsible as well for their own negligent acts, nevertheless, and the plaintiff can sue either the hospital or the employee, or both, for the injury. The key to imposing vicarious liability on the hospital lies in the relationship of the parties; it usually applies to a "master-servant" relationship, derived from English common law (i.e., employer–employee or some other relationship wherein the negligent acts are under the direction and control of the party to whom they are imputed, as in the principal–agent relationship).

While some pathologists may be employees of the hospital in which they practice, it is often the case that a pathology group will contract with an institution for its services; the pathologist receives a percentage of the service fee or some fee arrangement other than a direct salary from the hospital. In most cases, that pathologist will be considered an independent contractor, not under the direct control of the institution; institutions will not be vicariously liable for the negligent act of the pathologist.

The modern trend, however, has been to find the hospital or institution responsible for the acts of independent contractors under a theory of *ostensible* or *apparent agency*. Under this theory, the hospital does not avoid liability when the patient's logical assumption is that the pathology services are provided by the hospital and under its auspices. Courts have recently been finding it too harsh a rule to require patients to inquire about the backgrounds of the various physicians providing services in an institution; therefore they have been ruling that the institution will share each physician's liability to the patient.

Finally, the theory of *corporate liability* has been applied to hospitals in the area of medical staff competency, so that hospitals may be liable for the negligence of non-staff physicians when there is evidence that the hospital's internal mechanism for checking credentials was inadequate in identifying certain incompetent practitioners and suspending their privileges.

In many situations, then, pathologists' acts may impose concurrent liability on the institution in which they practice. Pathologists may also be held liable for the negligent acts of other staff, including residents, medical students, nurses, and laboratory technologists. The negligence of those persons will be imputed to pathologists to the extent that they act under that physician's direction and control.

Although residents, technicians, and other staff members are usually employees of the institution, and not of the pathologist, some courts have considered them to function as "borrowed servants" who, for the time they are involved in a procedure, are under the direct control and supervision of the pathologist. In such cases, the pathologist may be held liable for their acts of negligence.

EXAMPLES OF SURGICAL PATHOLOGY MALPRACTICE

The claims unique to surgical pathology fall into categories of misdiagnosis, mixed or lost specimens, and communications failures.

Misdiagnosis

Generally, pathologists can be found liable if they misdiagnose a condition that could have been correctly diagnosed if ordinary and customary practices had been followed. In some instances, a deviation from the ordinary and customary practices can be easily proven and the pathologist found liable.

An example occurred in a case in which a hospital pathologist misdiagnosed a biopsy and advised the surgeon that the patient had cancer of the cervix. Following this advice, the surgeon performed a hysterectomy. The diagnosis was later proved incorrect and this pathologist was held liable for negligence.

In another malpractice case, a state laboratory pathologist was found negligent in diagnosing as benign a malignant melanoma in a specimen of an excised mole. This erroneous diagnosis and the ensuing delay in treatment caused the patient, who subsequently died, to fall from a category of persons who statistically would have been expected to survive to a category in which there was almost no chance of survival.

In another case, a hospital was held liable for $2.5 million after its pathologist mistakenly diagnosed an esophageal biopsy as showing poorly differentiated adenocarcinoma. The patient then underwent an operation for removal of part of the esophagus and stomach, leaving him with long-term complications.

It is important to note, however, that pathologists will not always be liable for misdiagnosis. The determining factor is always whether they followed the applicable standard of care when making their misdiagnosis.

For example, in a suit alleging that a pathologist was negligent in failing to diagnose as malignant a tissue sample taken from a mass in a boy's throat, the court found no evidence that the pathologist was negligent. The court stated that the evidence did not show that a pathologist who met the requisite degree of competence would have reasonably been expected to have read the slides of tissue as showing a malignant tumor.

In an action by a patient against a pathologist who erroneously diagnosed tissue removed from the patient's breast as malignant, when in fact it was benign, the court was persuaded by expert witness testimony in making its decision that the pathologist was not negligent. The expert witness, a well known pathologist, testified that it was not unreasonable for a pathologist to have diagnosed the tissue as malignant. For liability to result, the court explained, "a pathologist must have failed to exercise that degree of skill ordinarily employed, under similar circumstances, by members of the profession in good standing in the community". The court noted that the expert medical testimony indicated that the pathologist had followed customary procedure in preparing the frozen section of tissue for microscopic examination and it was not unreasonable for this pathologist to have diagnosed the frozen tissue section as malignant.

Lost Specimen

It is much more difficult for the pathologist to defend a case in which the specimen has been lost. The results of this type of accident are often so shocking to both the jury and the judge that pathologists are almost always held liable. In these instances, a physician becomes hard-pressed to explain how this specimen was lost, even though "customary procedures were followed."

A startling case occurred when a patient's orbital contents were removed and sent to a university medical center's pathology department for expert analysis of the type of tumor present. While the resident was washing the specimen prior to examining it, the eye fell down the sink drain and could not be recovered. The patient therefore could not know whether the malignant tumor was of a type likely to spread and cause his death. The patient won his suit for physical injury, and the jury verdict reflected a sizable award for related mental anguish.

Mixed Specimens

Pathologists are often held liable in cases in which the specimens have been mixed rather than lost. The same trial problem exists as with lost specimens, that is that juries are shocked by such an accident and its potential dire consequences despite the fact that it may not be negligent to lose or mix a statistically minute number of samples per year. As a case in point, a patient had cysts in both of her breasts. A surgeon removed the cysts and sent them to the pathology laboratory in one container. The pathologist dissected both without making inquiries as to which specimen came from which breast. Only one cyst was malignant but, because it could not be determined after dissection which breast was involved, both breasts had to be removed. Both the pathologist and the surgeon were found negligent.

Communications Failures

Another area of liability exposure particular to the pathologist is that of communications failures. Consider the case in which a pathologist is referred a breast biopsy from a 35-year-old patient with a strong family history of breast cancer and a suspicious mammogram. In reporting his findings, the pathologist notes on the report the absence of microcalcifications. The pathologist then goes on to state in the report, "recommend rebiopsy as soon as possible." The surgeon following this patient does not perform another biopsy. Nine months later, the patient is diagnosed with metastatic breast cancer and her prognosis is poor. An expert for the plaintiff states that had a biopsy been performed nine months earlier, she would have had a greater than 50 percent chance of full recovery and cure. The lawsuit against the hospital includes as named defendants both the surgeon and the pathologist. The allegations against the pathologist state that the pathologist, having recommended rebiopsy, knew or should have known that one was not in fact carried out in a timely manner. The pathologist had a duty to follow up on his recommendation and to attempt to override the surgeon's decision. Ultimately, a settlement is reached that includes contribution from both the surgeon's and pathologist's insurance companies.

This case illustrates the fact that the pathologist who takes on the role of recommending treatment may in fact be extending the scope of potential liability as a result. A pathologist who makes a practice of recommending follow-up treatment should be aware that this may lead to personal responsibility for that recommendation. Whether the pathologist's duty to a patient is evolving to one in which such recommendations need to be made depends again on the national practice among pathologists, which in turn defines the standard of care.

SAFEGUARDS

It is important to remember that, although pathologists do not treat patients in the conventional sense, they still are considered to have an ongoing relationship with the patients imputed to them. Out of that special relationship arises legal duties from which liability may rise. Pathologists should, moreover, also always expect that their work will be relied on by the treating doctors.

Many of the safeguards pathologists should employ to avoid liability are common sense methods that aid in efficiency as well as liability protection. Pathologists should always require the treating (referring) doctor to submit an adequate tissue specimen and descriptive background before rendering a definitive diagnosis. If this has not been done, pathologists should avoid making an unequivocal diagnosis and should request the additional specimen or information if possible.

Good documentation is a must. It is wise to use extensive written documentation. Telephone conversations with clinicians and consultants should be documented. Documented consultations should be suggested in difficult cases. It is also important to make sure the treating doctor understands the submitted report and to keep in communication with the treating doctor. Diagnoses should be formulated with the utmost care, and over-diagnosis should be avoided (since patients can also receive damages due to mental anguish). In difficult cases, it is best to state that one is unsure and to suggest a conservative course of action. In these situations, outside consultations should be obtained and documented. If a respected consultant has agreed with the referral diagnosis, this will constitute conformity with the standards of care on the part of the referring pathologist, even if this diagnosis is subsequently proved to have been incorrect. To my knowledge, there are no cases in which the consultant was held negligent in this situation.

RETENTION AND MAINTENANCE OF RECORDS

Pathology reports should be completed promptly and filed in the medical record. Only written requests for specimen examinations should be accepted.

Procedures in the laboratory should be written and must outline the ordering of tests; the methods used for preparation and collection of specimens; any special procedures; and methods for identification, storage, and preservation of specimens. Laboratory reports should include the date, time of reporting, the name of the laboratory, and the condition of any unsatisfactory specimen. A system should be established that ensures the ability to identify the individual responsible for performing and/or completing the procedure. All diagnoses should be indexed for retrieval, and all records should be kept for a minimum of 2 years; however, 10 years is a safer period of retention. Even typographical errors can be critical; in one case, the mistyped gross description of a specimen as an ovary and cyst rather than as an ovarian cyst was the eventual key element.

All tissue sections should be readily available for reference and consultation. Slides, paraffin blocks, bone marrow aspirates, and needle biopsy specimens should be retained as long as needed for patient care and in accordance with the federal and state requirements. Gross tissue specimens should be kept for at least 7 days after all microscopic sections have been examined.

PATIENT ACCESS TO RECORDS

An interesting issue arises as to the patient's right to review and/or obtain records and pathology specimens. It is clear from case law as well as written medical standards that hospital patients have the right to review their records and diagnostic reports. This includes the right to obtain copies of these materials, although it is generally understood that the patient should be required to pay for the copies if he/she can afford to do so. According to the JCAH,

> The patient has the right to obtain from the practitioner responsible for coordinating his care, *complete and current information concerning his diagnosis, treatment and any known prognosis.* This information should be communicated in terms the patient can reasonably be expected to understand. When it is not medically advisable to give such information to the patient, information should be made available to a legally authorized individual.

While patients have a right to obtain certain information, case law supports the fact that the original medical record is owned by the hospital or doctor, and therefore the patient is not entitled to acquire or keep it. Since professional standards require record retention for continuity of patient care and other administrative purposes, it is not feasible or appropriate to dispense original medical documents. There is a dearth of case law regarding the ownership rights to medical materials other than hospital records, such as radiographs, specimens, slides, and paraffin blocks. The best analogy to case law suggests that patients would have a right to review and inspect these materials and to speak to a physician with regard to them and would also have a right to obtain copies or duplicates if such specimen lends itself to copying or duplication. This again would be at the patient's expense. A good case can be made that the original materials themselves remain in the ownership and possession of the institution according to their normal protocol for retention and/or destruction of such materials.

A helpful way to clarify the respective ownership rights to these materials is to include a statement in the hospital admissions contract to the effect that any gross tissue or other specimens are the property of the hospital and not the patient.

CONCLUSION

Health care professionals today are facing increased exposure for liability suits based on a complex set of factors, the most significant of which may be the recent advances in medical technology, which have raised patient's expectations as to medical results, coupled with the depersonalization that results from increased specialization in health care. Pathologists are particularly vulnerable to lawsuits, since they have no personal relationship with the patient to offset a disappointing or less than optimal result. The pathologist must therefore be particularly sensitive to those factors that may either discourage a lawsuit or minimize liability if one should arise. Good medical record documentation is a critical first step, in that record documentation is admissable in court as evidence of the care rendered. There is a legal presumption, in fact, that what is not recorded in the record was not done. The pathology reports and documentation should be documented thoroughly and contemporaneously with the event.

In order to prevail in a malpractice case, the patient/plaintiff must demonstrate that the pathologist deviated from the applicable standard of care, that an injury resulted and that the injury was caused by the negligent act. Conformity with the existing professional standards for pathology services will protect the practitioner from allegations of negligence. These standards are set forth in JCAH guidelines, state regulations, professional society guidelines, and actual national pathology practice. Along with maintaining good documentation and careful communication with referring and treating physicians, practitioners need to become familiar with any written regulations within their own institutions. Following all these recommendations will certainly not guarantee prevention of a successful malpractice suit, but it should reduce the risk considerably.

3

Surgical Pathology of Infectious Diseases

Leona W. Ayers
Elmer W. Koneman
Thomas A. Merrick

The inflammatory, necrotic, hyperplastic, and neoplastic lesions in human tissues produced by microorganisms can be so varied as to challenge even the most experienced surgical pathologist. Infectious diseases are produced by a wide variety of microbes ranging from those that are common to those that are rarely encountered in clinical practice. Body tissues are limited in the types of responses to these various agents. Because of the differing conditions of human hosts, the expected responses may vary considerably. The challenge for the tissue consultant in infectious diseases is to be able to define the process, to suggest a differential diagnosis of probable infectious agents, and to pursue appropriately the identity of the infectious agent. To meet this challenge successfully, the surgical pathologist should acquire a knowledge of the elements in the specific diagnosis of infectious diseases.

Many primary pathogens (virulent organisms) produce a disease in a remarkably consistent "natural history" sequence, with predictable progression of the morphologic lesions and the presentation of microbes with distinct morphologic features. With these diseases, the challenge may be to recognize the specific disease process during the "unfolding" period, before the completion of morphologic lesions. An early, noncaseating granuloma, for example, requires a broader differential diagnosis than does the well developed granuloma with central caseous necrosis. With other primary pathogens, the morphologic alterations produced may be nonspecific, but the pattern of tissue reaction may suggest a group of

diseases that can be explored by nontissue techniques such as serologic studies, culture, and electron microscopy. Atypical lymphoid hyperplasias, for example, may suggest a serologic investigation for antibodies to the antigens of *Toxoplasma gondii*, Epstein-Barr virus (EBV), and cytomegalovirus (CMV). Certain lymphomas have a clear association with viruses such as EBV (Burkitt's) and HTLV I and can be investigated by the direct demonstration of viral antigens or genomes or by serologic response to the virus.

The rapidity and the specificity with which tissue reactions evolve are a function of the virulence of the organism and the integrity of the host defense systems. The recognition of a given infectious disease may be complicated by alterations in the visual tissue presentation due to (1) extensive invasion and in vivo multiplication of the microbe; (2) the action of enzymes and toxins produced by the microbe locally or from distant sites; (3) the immediate inflammatory reaction of the host to tissue injury; (4) the humoral or cell-mediated immune response; and (5) the vigor and composition of the host elements of repair. Partial or inadequate therapy may also modify the presentation of the morphologic lesion.

Tissue diagnosis of infectious disease in immunosuppressed hosts is a relatively new consideration for the surgical pathologist (see Ch. 4). Factors favoring infection exist in many patients due to both the effects of debilitating intrinsic disease and vigorous medical and surgical management.

Some of the important factors associated with in-

19

creased incidence of infection are (1) granulocytopenia with invasion of the tissues by bacteria normally associated with body surfaces or abnormally colonized onto body surfaces; (2) cellular immune dysfunction with diminished ability to contain microbes such as *Salmonella* sp., *Listeria monocytogenes, Mycobacterium tuberculosis,* and the atypical mycobacteria, *Nocardia asteroides,* herpesvirus, CMV, *Pneumocystic carinii, T. gondii,* and many species of fungi; (3) humoral immune dysfunction with the loss of opsonins and the invasion of encapsulated organisms such as *Streptococcus pneumoniae* and *Hemophilus influenzae;* and (4) damage to physical barriers such as mucosal surfaces by cytotoxic chemotherapy and surgical and diagnostic procedures allowing direct invasion or introduction of environmental organisms.

Several modes of treatment other than direct immunosuppressive therapy are associated with increased risk of infection. Antibiotic therapy can facilitate superinfections with opportunistic organisms not normally considered human pathogens; transfusion of whole blood and products such as leukocytes and plasma can transmit CMV, *T. gondii,* and viral hepatitis to hosts made susceptible by diseases and their treatment. Treatment with steroids, aspirin, and total parenteral nutrition have a variety of depressive effects on phagocytosis, intracellular bacterial killing, blood clotting, and lymphocyte function.

The patient with depressed cell-mediated immunity (e.g., acquired immunodeficiency syndrome [AIDS][1] [see Ch. 4]) is most likely to present with a diagnostic problem requiring the special skills of the surgical pathologist. The usual techniques for the diagnosis of infectious disease, such as culture and serologic studies, may not provide the needed timely diagnosis in these patients because of rapid disease progression. The surgical pathologist and cytopathologist provide valuable information through the microscopic examination of material obtained by biopsy, bronchoalveolar lavage, translaryngeal aspiration, and bronchial brushing.[2] A knowledge of the clinical setting is critical in the management of these specimens. The interpretation of altered or atypical tissue responses and organism morphologic characteristics in bacterial, viral, fungal, and parasitic infections may provide the immediate basis for patient management. The identification of a tissue process alone may be invaluable in that the range and type of additional special studies are defined.

A final challenge for the surgical pathologist is to recognize tissue responses as clearly inflammatory or reactive rather than neoplastic. This differentiation is usually not difficult; however, there are certain morphologic reactions in which even experienced surgical pathologists must use caution in the interpretation of stained tissue sections. For example, granulomatous prostatitis can simulate carcinoma of the prostate gland. The mononuclear cell response to an arthropod bite can suggest ma-

lignant lymphoma cutis.[3] *Histoplasma capsulatum* or other mycotic agents can cause pseuodoepitheliomatous hyperplasia of the skin or mucous membranes simulating squamous cell carcinoma, and *Leishmania donovanii* or other intracellular organisms can produce cellular proliferations resembling malignant histiocytosis.[4]

To establish the infectious etiology of a given lesion, a number of procedural steps must be followed. The following sections in this chapter discuss in some detail the various steps in the processing, management, and interpretation of surgical tissue specimens used to arrive at a diagnosis of an infectious disease.

GROSS APPEARANCE OF TISSUE SPECIMENS

Visual examination of a tissue specimen along with gentle palpation should be sufficient to detect obvious pathologic processes. The discovery of a collection of pus within a well demarcated abscess generally indicates an infectious process and is one of the prime indications for the surgical pathologist to obtain a culture; however, it must be remembered that purulent microabscesses frequently complicate malignant neoplasms. Infectious processes, whether in the form of abscesses, granulomas, focal areas of necrosis or fibrosis, or healed calcific nodules, tend to be well demarcated from the adjacent tissue. In contrast, malignant neoplasms tend to invade tissues and become fixed to surrounding structures. Necrosis may be common to both benign infectious and malignant processes, although the presence of caseous necrosis, in which the tissue assumes the appearance and consistency of cottage cheese, is more consistent with infection. Since there are no rigid gross criteria to define an infectious process, microscopic examination of stained tissue sections is virtually always necessary.

CULTURE OF TISSUE SPECIMENS

Direct recovery of the causative microorganism from the affected tissue is necessary to make a definitive diagnosis of an infectious disease. Unfortunately, prosectors often fail to obtain cultures of surgical specimens because they are not alerted to the possibility of infection. Later regret over this oversight can be avoided in a number of ways. In some institutions, the physician obtaining the biopsy specimen or performing the surgical procedure takes the primary responsibility of submitting tissues for culture. Although this relieves the prosector of this duty, the practice has the disadvantage that the tissue selected for culture may be less appropriate than tissue selected by the surgical pathologist on the basis of careful, complete gross examination. Even if it is known that the surgeon has submitted tissue for culture, the surgical pathologist should obtain additional cultures when infection is suspected.

It is the current practice of many surgical pathologists to save for future culture a small portion of fresh tissue from lesions that appear grossly infected until microscopic examination discloses the true nature of the process. A small piece of tissue can be removed with a sterile surgical blade, placed in a small sterile container with a tight lid, and stored in the refrigerator at 4°C for 48 hours. The only exceptions are tissues suspected of harboring temperature-labile viruses such as CMV, which should be processed immediately. Specimens sent to referral laboratories can be transported on ice (melting ice bath at 4°C).

If a long storage period is required, or if the tissue is to be referred to a distant laboratory, initial freezing at −60°C or below is necessary. The specimen must be kept frozen until ready for processing, since repeated freezing and thawing is detrimental to the recovery of many species of organisms. Standard frost-free refrigerator/freezers are not recommended for frozen storage of tissues because fluctuations in temperature due to the frost-free process may cause microbe death and tissue dehydration. Viruses are poorly preserved at −20°C or lower, particularly if the temperature varies, and have better survival with limited storage and transportation at 4°C (ice).

On occasion, gross specimens will be delivered to the laboratory already immersed in fixative. If the specimen is relatively large and the time of contact with the fixative is relatively short (an hour or two), recovery of microorganisms from the central portion of the specimen may be possible.

Gross morphology or tissue reactions in frozen sections may suggest the presence of infectious agents and invoke special requirements for specimen sampling, transportation, smear preparation, and/or culture inoculation. For example, when an abscess is encountered in the dissection of a tissue specimen, the liquid material should be aspirated by needle into a syringe. Air bubbles should always be removed after aspiration, and the syringe should be tightly capped to maintain relative anaerobiosis. Subsequent smears and appropriate anaerobic, as well as routine, cultures can be made from this specimen. After the abscess has been evacuated, a portion of the cavity wall should be sampled for histologic examination and culture because the microorganisms at the interface with viable tissue may be different from those populating the necrotic center. In an amoebic abscess or a tuberculous cavity, the viable organisms are far more likely to be visualized and cultured from the cavity wall

than from the central necrotic debris. In actinomycosis or a mixed pyogenic abscess, by contrast, the organisms are found within the liquid debris and may not be found within the cavity wall. Taking both specimens in advance reduces the likelihood of failing to demonstrate the causative agent.

In general, portions of tissue can be minced into small fragments and ground with a mortar and pestle or in a tissue grinder. If a mortar and pestle are used, a small amount of sterile saline free of preservatives can be added to produce a tissue eluate that can conveniently be transferred to appropriate culture media. The addition of a small amount of sterile sand aids in macerating the tissue during grinding. However, if the tissue appears burned, charred, or necrotic, suggesting an infection with one of the members of the zygomycetes (*Mucor* sp., *Rhizopus* sp.) subclass of fungi, vigorous grinding should be avoided. Rather, the tissue to be cultured should be delicately teased or lightly minced so as not to destroy the nonseptate hyphae and thus ensure the recovery of viable fungal elements.

The junction between the areas of necrosis and recognizable viable tissue is the optimal site for sampling, both in selecting material for culture and for tissue sections. Extremely small biopsy specimens should be submitted for sectioning only. A second biopsy specimen should be obtained for culture if the tissue reaction suggests the presence of an infectious agent that can only be identified by culture.

The methods of obtaining tissue or organ biopsy specimens for culture from autopsies may also be applied to large surgical specimens. The technique described in detail by deJongh and associates[5] is summarized below:

1. All cultures should be obtained immediately, before organs are manipulated.
2. A small entry surface area on the organ to be cultured is sterilized by applying a red-hot, thin steel spatula blade. A 1 cm^3 block of tissue for culture is removed with sterile forceps and scissors from beneath the seared area. A separate set of sterile instruments is used for each culture biopsy specimen.
3. Each tissue block for culture is ground in a tissue grinder or with mortar and pestle and the supernatant eluate is used to inoculate appropriate bacteriologic culture media.

Medical laboratories vary greatly in the range and depth of available microbiology services. In small laboratories, the surgical pathologist may participate directly in culture processing. In large laboratories, the microbiology service may be directed by another pathologist or a microbiologist. Under the latter circumstance, the surgical pathologist should become aware of available services so the laboratory can be used to full advantage. Reference laboratories are also available to complement the individual laboratory service. The pathologist should keep on hand a directory of available services at local and regional medical centers, state health laboratories, and the Centers for Disease Control (CDC) in Atlanta, Georgia, so appropriate consultations may be obtained.

In initiating cultures or in recommending cultures in consultation, the pathologist should be aware of the culture isolation requirements of the pathogen or group of pathogens sought. A number of specimen manipulations are necessary to isolate ordinary microbes, and individual special cultures are needed to isolate many of the primary pathogens encountered within tissues. The pathologist must be aware of the level of isolation provided

by routine cultures and must recognize those instances in which special specimen management must be requested. For example, special techniques are needed for the recovery of *Campylobacter pylori*,[6] as described in Table 3-1, which provides a guide for the culture evaluation of tissue specimens.

DIRECT TECHNIQUES FOR IMMEDIATE PRESUMPTIVE DIAGNOSIS

The surgical pathologist should be aware of the importance of direct microscopic examinations of tissue specimens to make immediate presumptive diagnoses in select cases. Perhaps the most urgent clinical indication for direct smear examination is suspected infectious disease in the immunosuppressed patient. Pneumonia caused by *Pneumocystis carinii* is the most common infection in patients with AIDS and prompt identification of the organism is of considerable importance. Touch preparations or direct smears may be prepared from different specimen types, including induced sputum,[7] bronchoalveolar lavage fluid,[2] transbronchial biopsies, brushes and washings, and open lung biopsies.[8] Rapid staining techniques such as the Giemsa, Wright's or Diff-Quick stains, are required to visualize the cytoplasm and nuclei of the trophozoites; however, they do not stain the cyst wall. Gomori methenamine silver and toluidine blue O stains can be used to identify the cyst wall, and rapid methods for performing these stains were recently described.[9–11]

Effective therapy exists for fungal infections in immunosuppressed patients, and direct examination of specimens can provide a tentative and sometimes definitive diagnosis. Modified Gram stains, such as the Brown and Brenn and Brown-Hopps procedures, may be used to identify the Gram-positive filaments of the agents of actinomycosis and nocardiosis (bacteria) as well as certain yeasts (notably *Candida* sp.) and the fungi causing eumycotic mycetoma. Fungal hyphae and yeasts can be identified in direct saline mounts with a light or phase contrast microscope or by using potassium hydroxide digestion, lactophenol cotton blue, or calcofluor white stains.[12] Calcofluor white, a textile whitener, and Ulitex 28 are colorless dyes that fluoresce brightly when reacting with the cellulose and chitin in cell walls of yeast cells, hyphae, algae, and amoebic cysts.[13–17] An acid-fast or auramine-rhodamine stain can be used to identify mycobacteria.

Newer methods for the rapid diagnosis of infectious agents rely on the use of either monoclonal antibodies or nucleic acid probes. Nonradioactive DNA probe technology can be used for in situ hybridization in cytologic preparations and tissue sections. These techniques will

TABLE 3-1. Culture Guide for Surgical Pathology Specimens

Type of Culture	Culture Media
Routine Isolations: bacterial aerobes, facultative anaerobes, aerotolerant anaerobes	5% sheep blood agar; chocolate blood agar; macConkey agar (MAC) or eosin methylene blue agar (EMB)
Incubation: 37°C, atmospheric air or air + 6% CO_2, 2–7 days	Colistin naladixic acid agar (CNA)
Anaerobic Isolations: fastidious and O_2-sensitive anaerobic bacteria, including the actinomycetes	Blood agar with vitamin K, kanamycin, and vancomycin
Incubation: 37°C, 80% N_2, 10% CO_2, and 10% H_2, 4–7 days	Chopped-meat glucose broth or supplemented thioglycollate broth (vitamin K + hemin or equivalent)
Special—Gastric biopsy[6] Isolations: *Campylobacter pylori*	Chocolate blood agar and BHIA with 5% horse blood and antibiotics or comparable media
Incubation: 37°C and "campy" gas mixture, 4–7 days	
Fungal Isolations: pathogenic dimorphic fungi, yeasts, and "opportunists"	Inhibitory mold agar, SABHI agar or equivalent Brain–heart infusion agar with cycloheximide and chloramphenicol (C & C)
Incubation: 30°C, atmospheric air, 30 days	
Mycobacteria Isolations: rapid-, intermediate-, and slow-growing mycobacteria	Lowenstein-Jensen medium and/or Middlebrook $7H_{11}$ agar
Incubation: 37°C in 10% CO_2, 3–6 weeks	
Virus Isolations: common endemic and epidemic viruses	Primary cell line Diploid cell line Heteroploid cell line
Incubation: 37°C, atmospheric air, 4 days to 3 weeks	

permit the detection of a variety of viral agents, such as CMV, herpes simplex virus (HSV), hepatitis B virus (HBV), human papillomavirus (HPV), and human immunodeficiency virus (HIV),[18] as well as bacteria (*Legionella* sp., *Mycobacteria* sp., and *Chlamydia* sp.).

IMMUNOHISTOCHEMISTRY AS AN AID TO PRESUMPTIVE DIAGNOSIS[19]

Some microorganisms fortunately are directly visualized by routine tissue microscopy and can be identified by their morphologic characteristics. Special histochemical stains may be used to ease the field-by-field search and to confirm the identity of the organism. Recognition, however, becomes more difficult when organisms are not directly visible and can only be suspected by the surgical pathologist, so special techniques such as histochemical or immunochemical staining or electron microscopy may be used. In these cases, analysis of the tissue reaction is followed by special procedures designed to visualize the suspected organism.

Microbial antigens can be detected directly in smears/imprints, cryostat sections, and paraffin-embedded sections by monoclonal antibodies tagged for visualization.

The choice of visualization method will depend on the availability of commercially or in-house prepared reagents. Immunoperoxidase techniques are broadly applicable in diagnostic tissue work and may represent the method of choice. This stain and the DNA probe technique provide two choices for the precise localization of microbes in tissues.

To make the most efficient use of special staining techniques, the pathologist should have an organized approach to their application. The commonly used stains, their probable modes of action, the specific organisms stained, and the staining reactions are summarized in Table 3-2. The histology laboratory should maintain control smears or tissues with known organisms, and these smears should be processed each time a special stain is performed. Good control sections can frequently be obtained from autopsy material, from the Armed Forces Institute of Pathology (AFIP),[6] in Washington, D.C., and from the CDC, in Atlanta, Georgia.

DNA PROBES

Microorganisms can be directly identified in fluids, smears, or formalin-fixed, paraffin-embedded tissue sections by labeled DNA probes. The DNA probe is a frag-

TABLE 3-2. Stains Commonly Used to Demonstrate Microorganisms in Tissues and Smears

Type	Microorganisms	Action and Reactions

Inclusion body stains
  Giemsa
  Hematoxylin and eosin (H&E)
  Lendrum's phloxine tartrazine
	Adenovirus
	CMV
	Herpes simplex (HSV)
	Measles virus
	Molluscum contagiosum
	Poliovirus
	Poxvirus (Guarnieri bodies)
	Rabies (Negri bodies)
	Respiratory syncytial virus (RSV)
	Varicella-zoster (HVS)
		Most viral inclusions can be recognized in routine H&E stains, where they appear as discrete intranuclear or cytoplasmic eosinophilic, amphophilic or basophilic bodies. Small round eosinophilic intranuclear inclusions that are surrounded by a clear halo in turn marginated by nuclear chromatin are designated Cowdry type A inclusions. Small eosinophilic bodies approximating the size of nucleoli are designated Cowdry type B inclusions. Other viral inclusions may occupy most of the nucleus, producing a ground-glass (HSV) or a deep basophilic "smudge" (adenovirus) appearance. Many stains have been developed to demonstrate the variety of viral inclusion bodies; however, no one stain demonstrates all inclusions. Phloxinophilic inclusions (red) may be nicely displayed in tissue sections, but immunofluorescent staining and tissue electron microscopy are the desirable specific tools for smear and tissue identification of virus-infected cells. Inclusion bodies may also be caused by *Chlamydia* (which can be stained by Giemsa) and may be seen in noninfectious processes such as lead poisoning.

Silver impregnation stains
  Warthin-Starry
  Warthin-Faulkner
  Dieterle
  Steiner-Steiner
	Spirochetes
	Klebsiella rhinoscleromatis (rhinoscleroma)
	Legionella pneumophilia
	Legionella-like bacilli
	Campylobacter pylori
		Selected microorganisms that are difficult to visualize by simple routine techniques can be impregnated with silver nitrate. Following impregnation the silver nitrate is developed to form a visible metallic deposit. Underdevelopment of this process may fail to demonstrate the organism or can result in a field-to-field variation in organism staining. Nuclei and certain pigments with a high affinity for silver may also interfere with the staining of adjacent organisms. Overdevelopment of the staining procedure will lead to background precipitates and will cause the organisms to appear thickened and overstained. Correct processing should reveal delicate black organisms against a pale yellow to brown background. A good spirochete control tissue is required to evaluate each staining effort.

(continued)

TABLE 3-2. *Continued*

Type	Microorganisms	Action and Reactions
Acid-fast stains Ziehl-Neelsen Kinyon Wade-Fite Auramine-Rhodamine	Ascospores of *Saccharomyces* sp. *Mycobacterium* sp. *Nocardia* sp.	Microorganisms having prominent cell wall lipids may retain basic aniline dyes such as carbolfuchsin, new fuchsin, and auramine O by resisting the elution of these dyes with dilute solutions of mineral acids in alcohol. This phenomenon of dye retention following an acid wash is called acid fastness. The degree of dye retention varies with some organisms such as lepra bacilli, which require protection from lipid solvents by the use of solvent-oil mixtures during tissue deparaffinization. Other organisms (*Nocardia* sp.) require the use of weaker solutions of mineral acids and stain "partially acid fast." Organisms appear red, violet, or dark blue or emit a bright yellow fluorescence, depending on the staining method used. The background varies with the counterstain used but should be sufficiently pale to permit good visualization of the acid-fast organisms.
Carbohydrate stains Gomori's methenamine-silver nitrate (GMS) (Grocott's modification) Periodic acid-Schiff (PAS) PAS with diastase Gridley fungus Hotchkiss-McManus	Fungi, including yeasts and mycelial forms Actinomycetes, including *Nocardia* sp. *Pneumocystis carinii* cysts Amoeba (glycogen) CMV (glycogen in cytoplasmic inclusions) Macrophages with mycobacteria and Whipple's disease agent Fungi, yeasts, and mycelia *Actinomyces* sp.	Microorganisms rich in a variety of polysaccharides, neutral mucopolysaccharides, mucoproteins, and glycoproteins can be oxidized by chromic or periodic acids to release aldehyde groups which in turn react with ammoniacal-silver complexes or Schiff reagent. The silver complex, when reduced to a metallic silver, renders the organism gray to black, and the Schiff reagent produces a magenta-to-purple coloration of the organism. Pretreatment of the tissue with diastase removes the polysaccharide glycogen and improves the differential staining of fungi in the PAS method, particularly in tissues rich in glycogen. The silver method is preferred as a routine fungal stain because dead or damaged organisms may still be stained. Also, the initial chromic acid treatment removes the low-level background reactive substances to leave only those structures with large quantities of reactive groups such as the fungi. Where tissue cellular detail is needed, the silver preparation may be counterstained by the routine H&E method.
Toluidine Blue O stain (TBO)	Cysts of *Pneumocystis carinii* Fungal hyphae and pseudo-hyphae Yeasts	Microorganisms with large amounts of carbohydrates in the cell wall can be subjected to a sulfation reaction which prepares the wall to be stained by TBO, a stain related to methylene blue and azure A. The sulfation step uses strong acids which, in addition to preparing the cell wall, digest away most of the cellular background. The stain is most applicable to cell sediments or imprints for rapid examination for the cysts of *Pneumocystis carinii* (5–20 min). Fungi, with the exception of *Histoplasma capsulatum*, are regularly preserved and also stain with TBO.
Mayer's mucicarmine	*Cryptococcus neoformans* (capsule)	The aluminum in the mucicarmine stain is believed to act as a mordant in chelating complexes of the acid groups of mucin to which the carmine is then attached in a dyelike form. The mucopolysaccharide capsules of cryptococci are stained a deep rose to red, while there is little staining of the connective tissue mucin. Tissue nuclear detail is enhanced by iron hematoxylin and a yellow background provides good contrast for the rose-colored capsules. This stain has limited utility but may be helpful in the identification of *Cryptococcus neoformans* in tissue sections, where the organism often has atypical morphologic characteristics.
Fluorescent stains Auramine-rhodamine Acridine orange	Fungi Mycobacteria Plasmodia *Campylobacter pylori*	Fluorescent dyes are used for the selective staining of microbes or the selective staining of cell constituents. The dyes can be excited by an ultraviolet light source, and each dye fluoresces with its own color according to a particular chemical interaction. Auramine O, for example, is retained by acid-fast bacteria and fluoresces a bright yellow. Acridine orange fluoresces red with RNA and green with DNA. Plasmodial cells show a bright red fluorescence, while fungi show a red-green fluorescence. These dyes have been used in rapid staining techniques and for facilitating the search for small numbers of organisms.
Fluorochrome-conjugated immunoglobulins	Bacteria including *Legionella pneumophilia* Fungi Helminths Protozoa Viral antigens Viral inclusions	Antigen-specific, high-titered antibodies are conjugated with fluorescent dyes such as fluorescein-isothiocyanate or rhodamine B to allow specific immunologic identification of microorganisms in smears and tissues. The method preferred is a procedure where a high-titered antibody is directly conjugated to the fluorescent dye. This reagent is then directly reacted with the tissue antigen (direct immunofluorescence). This method gives the highest intensity of fluorescence. A second method is to react the high-titered antibody with the antigen and then react this

(continued)

TABLE 3-2. *Continued*

Type	Microorganisms	Action and Reactions
		complex with a fluorescein anti-gamma globulin complex (indirect immunofluorescence). Commercial reagents are available for a variety of direct immunofluorescent tests for the identification of microorganisms. A bright yellow-to-apple-green fluorescence indicates a positive reaction.
Fluorescent Whiteners Calcofluor white Uvitex 28	Acanthamoeba cysts Algae Fungal hyphae and pseudo-hyphae Yeasts	Microorganisms rich in cell wall cellulose and chitin will fluoresce brightly when stained by these colorless dyes and exposed to long-wave ultraviolet light. Yeast cells, pseudohyphae, hyphae, algae, and amoebic cysts display a specific bright apple green or blue-white fluorescence in response to the filter system used in the fluorescent microscope. The stain can be performed as a wet preparation. This type of stain is particularly useful for rapid testing, screening for low numbers of organisms, or clarifying ambiguous reactions presented by less specific stains.
Giemsa stain Wolbach's modification	*Babesia* sp. *Bartonella* sp. *Campylobacter pylori* *Chlamydia trachomatis* inclusions Giardia (trophozoites) Gram-negative bacilli *Leishmania* sp. *Plasmodium* sp. *Pneumocystis carinii* (trophozoites) *Rickettsia* sp. *Trypanosoma* sp. *Toxoplasma* sp.	Microorganisms stain according to their affinity for basic or acidic dye components of methylene blue-eosinate, azure B-eosinate, azure A-eosinate, and methylene blue chloride. Tissues stain better at a beginning acid pH and produce a variety of colors within the so-called Romanowsky color range. The Giemsa stain along with others of the Romanowsky group are valued for the variety of microorganisms that can be stained, ranging from blue to red-purple to violet, against a pink background.
Gram stains Brown and Brenn Brown-Hopps Gram-Weigert MacCallum-Goodpasture Taylor's	Bacteria including *Actinomyces* sp. and *Nocardia* sp. Fungi, especially yeasts	A crystal violet–iodine complex is formed within some bacterial and yeast cells, which resists elution by alcohol or acetone. The exact mechanism of this resistance to elution is unknown but is probably related to permeability characteristics of the cell and to the stability of the dye complex. Dead or damaged cells will not retain the dye complex and are only stained by counterstain. Those organisms retaining the dye are defined as Gram-positive and appear blue-black. The Gram-negative organisms are stained red to brown, depending on the counterstain. Methods such as Brown and Brenn give excellent definition of Gram-positive cells but poorer definition of those that are Gram-negative. Other methods give better definition of Gram-negative cells but may not stain the Gram-positive organisms as distinctly. Each user must determine the performance characteristics of the routine method chosen and understand the limitations of that method. Some bacteria will not be visualized in Gram stains and a Giemsa or silver impregnation method may be required.

DNA probes
Biotinylated
Radioisotopic
	Viruses
	  Adenovirus
	  CMV
	  EBV
	  HBV
	  HIV
	  Papillomavirus
	Selected bacteria
		Microorganisms can be directly identified in fluids, smears, and formalin-fixed, paraffin-embedded tissue sections by labeled DNA probes. The DNA probe is a fragment of nucleic acid that can identify and bind itself to nucleic acid complementary sequences. Since all microorganisms have unique sequences of DNA, in situ hybridization permits specific identification of the organism. Visualization of the tag component controls the sensitivity of the stain. This is an important technique for those viruses that can cause serious disease, and can be associated with significant treatment alternatives, but are difficult to isolate consistently in culture.

ment of nucleic acid that can identify and bind itself to nucleic acid complementary sequences.[20] Since all microorganisms have unique sequences of DNA, in situ hybridization theoretically allows for the specific identification of virtually all organisms.

Using biotin-labeled probes and a direct colorimetric detection with avidin-alkaline phosphatase complexes, Unger et al.[21] were able to identify cytomegalovirus and adenovirus genetic information in tissue sections. DNA probes were also used by Hilborne et al.[22] to identify CMV in bronchoalveolar lavage smears and in embedded tissue by Loning et al.[23] The detection of HSV in brain tissue with a DNA probe was reported by Forghani et al.[24] Thus, the technique is evolving as a practical alternative to standard immunochemistry methods.

Ross et al.[25] see DNA probes as a means for distinguishing submicroscopic features with the light microscope and as a means of potentially revealing the cell lineage of neoplastic processes, for those who do not have access to expensive equipment or the resources to perform sophisticated techniques. Probes also are an important technique in detecting those viruses that can cause serious disease and that can be associated with significant treatment alternatives, but that are difficult to isolate consistently in culture.

SPECIFIC TISSUE REACTIONS IN INFECTIOUS DISEASE

The purpose of this section is to present the several morphologic types of host reactions that may be seen in stained tissue sections and to discuss some of the microorganisms that must be considered in making a differential diagnosis for each reaction type. It must be remembered that the tissue reaction produced by a given microbe may vary depending on the virulence of the microbe, the length of time the infective agent has been present, and the immunologic competence of the host. The types of tissue reactions that may be observed are limited and rarely pure, and the same species of microorganism may produce different morphologic patterns in varying organs and hosts. Nevertheless, the following classification of morphologic types of tissue reactions will serve as a helpful guideline in suggesting specific microorganisms or groups of microorganisms that should be considered when a given reaction is observed:

1. Acute inflammation (exudative)
   Purulent
   Hemorrhagic
   Serous
   Fibrinous
   Ulcerative
2. Chronic inflammation (proliferative)
   Nonspecific
   Granulomatous
3. Acellular (inert) inflammation
4. Hyperplasia (reactive)

Before discussing the nature of these inflammatory and reactive lesions, the following definitions are necessary.

Acute inflammation is a nonimmunologic acute vascular reaction characterized by vascular congestion and exudation of fluids, protein, and cells from the vascular channels. In effect, exudation is that component of an acute inflammatory response that originates from cellular and molecular constituents within the circulation. By definition, exudative inflammation is always acute and occurs only in tissues that have a microcirculation.

Chronic inflammation is characterized by the later delivery of mononuclear cells and lymphocytes to the inflammatory site. These mononuclear cells, together with capillary buds and fibroblasts, accumulate and proliferate in situ to produce one of the proliferative inflammatory reaction patterns listed above. Humoral and cell-mediated immunity are important in the production of these patterns. Among morphologists, there is an inconsistency in terminology in reference to the mononuclear inflammatory cells that contribute to the proliferative reactions. This chapter identifies and names the lymphocytes, plasma cells, and monocytes according to their classic morphologic characteristics. The term macrophage is used to describe the large eosinophilic cells representing the tissue phase of the mononuclear phagocyte complex. These cells begin as monocytes in the bone marrow and are known by different names in different organs: Kupffer cells in the liver, alveolar macrophages in the lung, reticulum cells in the lymph nodes and spleen, microglial cells in the central nervous system, and histiocytes in the skin. The whole system of cells is known as the macrophage system or the reticuloendothelial system. Reticulum cells (fixed macrophages) are cytologically identical with histiocytes (free macrophages). The term epithelioid cell will refer to those macrophages that have abundant eosinophilic cytoplasm, giving them the appearance of epithelial cells, and that demonstrate characteristic clusters in tissue. A discussion of the derivation and physiology of these cells is beyond the scope of this chapter; however, Lasser[26] has provided an up-to-date review, including a discussion of the various chemical mediators that orchestrate the activation and interaction of cells comprising the inflammatory and reparative responses, as well as various enzyme markers that can be identified to assess the adequacy of the immune reaction.

Acellular or inert inflammation is characterized by the virtual absence of nucleated inflammatory cells within the lesion. Varying degrees of edema, congestion, hem-

TABLE 3-3. Tissue Reactions Associated with Microorganisms

Class	Microorganisms	Tissue Reactions
Bacteria Extracellular	*Staphylococcus aureus*, streptococci, *Hemophilus* sp., pathogenic *Neisseria* sp., enteric bacilli, *Pseudomonas* sp., *Nocardia asteroides*, other actinomycetes, *Legionella pneumophilia*	Acute inflammation Purulent
	Exotoxins of *Bacillus anthracis*, clostridia, hemolytic streptococci, *Corynebacterium diphtheriae*	Acute inflammation Hemorrhagic Necrotic Purulent
Facultative intracellular parasites	*Mycobacterium tuberculosis* and atypical mycobacteria, *Brucella* sp., *Francisella tularensis*, *Yersinia pestis*, *Salmonella typhi*, *Listeria monocytogenes*	Granulomatous inflammation Chronic nonspecific inflammation Acute inflammation Purulent Hemorrhagic Necrotic
Spirochetes Extracellular parasites	*Borellia* sp., *Leptospira* sp., *Treponema pallidum*, other treponemes	Hemorrhage, necrosis Chronic nonspecific inflammation (plasma cells)
Spirilla	*Spirillum minor*, *Campylobacter fetus*	Acute inflammation Purulent Hemorrhagic
Mycoplasma Extracellular parasites	*Mycoplasma pneumoniae*	Acute inflammation Purulent
Chlamydia Intracellular parasites	*Chlamydia trachomatis*, *Chlamydia psittaci*	Acute inflammation Purulent Chronic nonspecific inflammation Granulomatous inflammation (necrobiotic)
Rickettsiae Intracellular parasites	*Rickettsia rickettsii* (Rocky Mountain spotted fever), *Rickettsia prowazekii* (epidemic typhus), *Coxiella burnettii* (Q fever), *Rickettsia mooseri* (murine typhus)	Chronic nonspecific inflammation Hemorrhage, necrosis Vascular proliferation
Viruses Intracellular parasites	*Herpes simplex*, cytomegalovirus, varicella-zoster virus, adenovirus, papillomavirus, rabies virus	Chronic nonspecific inflammation Hyperplasia Viral inclusions Necrosis
	Influenza virus, Epstein-Barr virus, hepatitis virus, measles virus, yellow fever virus, coxsackievirus, echovirus	Chronic nonspecific inflammation Lymphocytosis Necrosis, hemorrhage
Fungi Extracellular parasites	*Candida albicans*, *Candida* sp., *Torulopsis glabrata*, *Blastomyces dermatitidis*, *Sporothrix schenckii*	Acute inflammation Purulent
Facultative intracellular parasites	*Histoplasma capsulatum*, *Coccidioides immitis*, *Blastomyces dermatitidis*, *Paracoccidioides brasiliensis*, *Cryptococcus neoformans*	Granulomatous inflammation
Opportunists	*Candida* sp., *Aspergillus fumigatus*, *Cryptococcus neoformans*, *Mucor* sp., *Rhizopus* sp., *Absidia* sp.	Acellular reaction Necrosis Hemorrhage Edema
Parasites Extracellular	*Entamoeba histolytica*, *Balantidium coli*, *Giardia lamblia*, *Enterobius vermicularis*, *Trichuris trichiura*, *Taenia* sp., *Ascaris lumbricoides*, *Schistosoma* sp., *Necator americanus*, *Strongyloides stercoralis*, *Trichinella spiralis*	Acute inflammation Ulcerative Chronic nonspecific inflammation (eosinophils) Granulomatous inflammation
Intracellular	*Plasmodium* sp., *Babesia* sp., *Toxoplasma gondii*, *Leishmania* sp., (amastigotes)	Hemolysis, necrosis Chronic nonspecific inflammation (macrophages)

orrhage, and fibrin deposition may be present, and necrosis may be a significant component of this type of reaction pattern.

Hyperplasia of various cell types may be seen in all the above inflammatory reactions. In some instances, particularly when microorganisms cannot be demonstrated in the tissue sections, or during a stage in the inflammatory process when the cellular infiltrate has subsided and fibrosis has not yet occurred, cellular hyperplasia may serve as the only clue that an infectious process is present. These reactions include the proliferation of reticuloendothelial cells or parenchymal cells of the organ involved, including glandular elements or mucosal or cutaneous epithelium (the latter is a process called pseudoepitheliomatous hyperplasia).

Hyperplasia may also be the primary response to individual cell parasitization by selected agents. Viral agents of the papilloma group, for example, directly stimulate epithelial cell hyperplasia. Discrete lesions, such as verrucae, must be recognized and differentiated from noninfectious hyperplasias and from neoplasms.

Table 3-3, which lists the classes and genera of microorganisms found in the various types of infectious tissue reactions listed above, will serve as a guide to the detailed discussion and illustrations of these reactions that follow. Table 3-3 is only a guide to the reactions as they commonly occur and does not exclude the possibility that reactions other than those listed may be found on occasion in a given lesion.

Acute Inflammation

Purulent Inflammation

Purulent inflammation is characterized by the accumulation of polymorphonuclear leukocytes and is most commonly associated with acute or continuing tissue injury by extracellular microorganisms. Staphylococci, streptococci (including *S. pneumoniae*), various species of Gram-negative bacilli, and pathogenic strains of *Neisseria* are among the organisms most commonly producing purulent or suppurative inflammation. When this type of acute exudative inflammation is observed, a direct Gram stain and culture should be performed to identify a causative organism and to separate the infectious from the noninfectious causes of such a purulent lesion.

The location of the purulent inflammation may be helpful in developing a differential diagnosis. Purulent lesions of the skin (Fig. 3-1) immediately implicate skin bacteria such as staphylococci or streptococci, which have immediate access to the skin as a portal of entry. The presence of intraepithelial microabscesses, particularly in the presence of marked pseudoepitheliomatous hyperplasia, should alert the microscopist to the possibility of cutane-

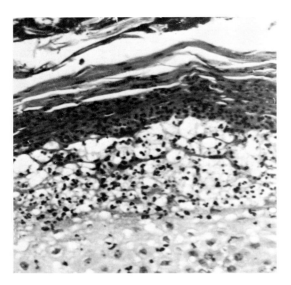

Fig. 3-1. Acute inflammation, skin. Note the neutrophils infiltrating the subcorneal layer of the epidermis.

ous blastomycosis, and special stains to identify the broad-based budding yeast form should be performed. The differentiation between infectious pyodermas and noninfectious pyodermas and noninfectious pustular dermatoses is not made through routine histologic examination alone but requires supporting clinical information, Gram's stains, and/or culture. Purulent lesions in other parts of the body may suggest entirely different microbes based on known microbe-host associations. Purulent reactions associated with mucosal surfaces will often be associated with the microorganisms commonly found at those surfaces.

The purulent reaction may be differentiated not only by anatomic location but, on occasion, also by the presence of certain characteristic associated structures. The presence of structures known as granules (Fig. 3-2) suggests a distinct group of diseases: botryomycosis, actinomycosis, and mycetoma. Special histochemical stains are needed to clarify the probable infectious agents. Gram stain is the best method to characterize the granules formed by the actinomycetes. The branching Gram-positive filaments and the presence of prominent "clubs" at the periphery of the granule (Fig. 3-3) suggest that the structure is an actinomycotic granule. However, it must be remembered that radiating eosinophilic deposits (clubs or rays) may surround fungi, helminth ova, and bacterial colonies (the asteroid body of sporotrichosis) (Fig. 3-4). This reaction, called the Splendore-Hoeppli phenomenon, was traditionally considered to result from the condensation of products of antigen-antibody complexes with degenerating inflammatory cells. However, Bhagavan et al.[27] question whether immune complexes are involved; rather, in analyzing "pseudoactinomycotic"

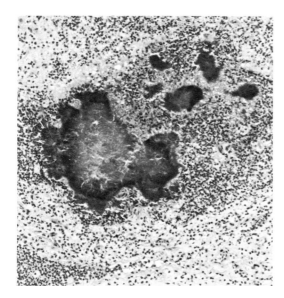

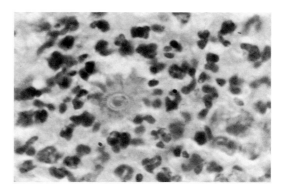

Fig. 3-4. Asteroid body, skin microabscess. A central yeast cell 5 to 10 μm in diameter is surrounded by the homogeneous eosinophilic-staining "rays" of the Splendore-Hoeppli phenomenon. *Sporotrichum schenckii* was cultured from the tissue.

Fig. 3-2. Actinomycosis. Microabscess containing multiple basophilic lobulated granules with homogeneous centers and eosinophilic peripheral clubbed projections, bordered by macrophages and fibroconnective tissue.

granules they encountered in female genital tract lesions, they found only neutral glycoproteins, lipid moieties, and calcium, possibly derived from lysosomes released by degranulating or disintegrating leukocytes.

The dense aggregates of Gram-positive cocci or less common Gram-negative bacilli seen in botryomycotic granules can also be demonstrated by Gram stain. Eumy-

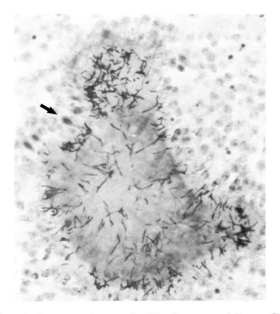

Fig. 3-3. Actinomycotic granule. The Brown and Brenn Gram stain shows branching, Gram-positive filaments within the granule radiating to the peripheral clubs (arrow).

cotic granules are best recognized by the natural brown pigment of the dermataceous fungi that produce them or by silver stains, which outline the hyphal elements within the granules. *Nocardia* sp. may be associated with similar clinical syndromes but do not produce the typical granule with clubs or rays. Rather, clumps of branching filaments form "grains," which are much smaller than granules. Individual or branching filaments are usually dispersed throughout the purulent exudate and appear Gram-positive. If the filaments are partially acid-fast, *Nocardia* sp. are clearly suggested.[28] Successful culture of *Nocardia* requires an adequate sample of the exudate, whereas actinomycetes are more often recovered from a crushed granule inoculated directly into anaerobic culture media.

The proliferative tissue changes associated with the ongoing acute inflammatory process may obscure the active centers of infection. Chronic nonspecific inflammation, fibrosis, and epithelial hyperplasia eventually accompany persistent purulent reactions and should be appreciated as an index to the chronicity of the disease process. The microscopist's eye, however, should quickly move to acute tissue changes where the infectious agent is most likely to be found. An intraepithelial microabscess (Figs. 3-5 and 3-6), for example, is a likely location to seek the infectious agent. The size of suspected microbial forms can be estimated in tissue sections by comparing the structures observed with the surrounding inflammatory cells. An individual lobe of a neutrophil measures about 2 μm, the nucleus of a small lymphocyte about 5 to 6 μm, an erythrocyte about 7 μm, and the nucleus of a reticuloendothelial cell about 10 μm. Budding yeast cells seen within a purulent exudate that measure 10 μm or more in diameter are highly suspicious of *Blastomyces dermatitidis*. This diagnosis can be virtually confirmed in tissue sections if the characteristic yeast

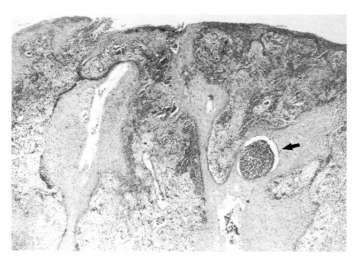

Fig. 3-5. Blastomycosis, skin. Note the marked pseudoepitheliomatous hyperplasia and the presence of an intraepidermal abscess (arrow). The dermis shows chronic nonspecific inflammation in this section but may contain microabscesses and Langhans giant cells.

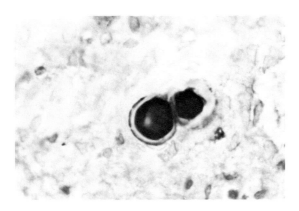

Fig. 3-7. *Blastomyces dermatitidis*, GMS stain. Note the spherical yeast cell with a thick refractile cell wall and single bud arising from a broad base. Individual yeast cells range from 8 to 15 μm in diameter.

cell with a thick doubly refractile wall and a broad-based single bud can be identified (Fig. 3-7). Yeast forms can be best demonstrated by Gomori's methenamine-silver nitrate (GGMS) or Gridley's fungal stains. The yeast forms of most other fungal organisms are smaller (2 to 7 μm) than those of *B. dermatitidis*. Exceptions are the blastoconidia (chlamydospores) of *Candida albicans* (7 to 10 μm), in which pseudohyphae are usually present. Immature *Coccidioides immitis* spherules (10 to 20 μm) generally are not found within a purulent reaction, although focal accumulations of polymorphonuclear leukocytes may be seen in areas immediately adjacent to where endospores are released from mature spherules into the sur-

rounding tissue. According to Vanek and associates,[29] the tissue response to *B. dermatitidis* is classically characterized by the combination of suppuration and epithelioid cell granulomatous reactions. Giant cells and chronic nonspecific inflammation are seen in older lesions.

Hemorrhagic Inflammation

Hemorrhagic inflammation refers to the tissue reaction in which there is marked vascular congestion with extravasation of fluid and erythrocytes into the tissues. This reaction most commonly results from direct injury to small blood vessels with disruption of the vessel walls and diapedesis or leakage of red cells and fluid. The direct vascular damage may be associated with bacteria that produce potent toxins such as histotoxic *Clostridium* sp., *Bacillus anthracis,* and *Yersinia pestis*. These toxins can also destroy phagocytes, explaining why polymorphonuclear leukocytes are conspicuously absent in this reaction. *Escherichia coli* serotype 0157:H7 has been associated with several outbreaks and sporadic cases of hemorrhagic diarrhea, particularly in newborns and young children.[30] A lymph node biopsy specimen showing hemorrhage and necrosis with edema and a remarkable absence of a cellular response (Fig. 3-8) should lead immediately to a careful search for the type of agents associated with this reaction pattern. In addition to Gram stain of tissue, other histochemical stains such as Giemsa, and possibly silver impregnation, should also be used in the evaluation of this type of reaction, because Gram stains of tissue will not always adequately visualize Gram-negative bacteria.

Direct vascular damage may also be associated with organisms that invade vessel walls. For example, certain fungi, notably the zygomycetes (*Mucor* sp. and *Rhizopus* sp.) and certain species of *Aspergillus*, notoriously in-

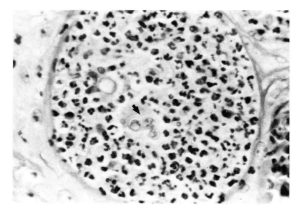

Fig. 3-6. Intraepidermal abscess, cutaneous blastomycosis. Note the dense accumulation of neutrophils surrounding the large yeast-like budding cells (arrow). These forms suggest *Blastomyces dermatitidis*.

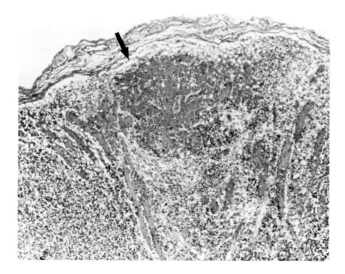

Fig. 3-8. Bubonic plaque, inguinal lymph node. Prominent vascular congestion, edema and an area of subcapsular hemorrhage and necrosis (arrow). Brown and Brenn Gram stain revealed large, plump Gram-negative bacilli consistent with *Yersinia pestis* within the areas of hemorrhage and necrosis.

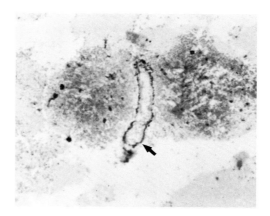

Fig. 3-9. Acute falciparum malaria: ring hemorrhage, brain. Perivascular hemorrhages are associated with small vessels congested by parasitized erythrocytes. Note the heavy deposition of malarial pigments along the endothelial lining of the arteriole (arrow).

vade blood vessels with resulting hemorrhagic necrosis and infarction. Intracellular microbes, such as viruses and rickettsiae, may have a clinical presentation in which hemorrhage (e.g., dermal, mucosal, scleral) is a prominent feature, with or without hypotension and shock. The hemorrhagic fevers, caused by viruses transmitted by arthropods, may only manifest hemorrhage and focal tissue necrosis with varying amounts of edema. A specific diagnosis may be suggested by exposure within a known endemic area and the absence of other causes of hemorrhage. Support for either viral or rickettsial agents comes from careful tissue examination, special stains for rickettsiae, serologic testing, and viral culture.

Falciparum malaria is an infectious disease in which hemorrhage may be caused by a mechanism that differs from that described earlier. The infected erythrocytes stick to capillary endothelium and block the capillary lumina. Stasis with dilatation and weakening of the vessel walls occurs as a result of hypoxia. Erythrocytes leak into the surrounding tissue, causing perivascular hemorrhage (so-called "ring hemorrhages") and ischemic necrosis (Fig. 3-9). Malarial pigment, if present, will be seen ringing the capillaries. Other organs, including the liver and spleen, will show congestion and reticuloendothelial hyperplasia with phagocytic cells containing malarial pigment, parasites, and parasitized erythrocytes.[31]

Serous Inflammation

Serous exudation is characterized by the outpouring of a low specific gravity fluid derived from plasma or from the secretion of serous mesothelial cells, depending on the site of reaction. The effect is the collection of clear, straw-colored fluid in body cavities and spaces such as the pericardial sac, the pleural spaces, the abdominal cavity, and joint spaces. These effusions are more commonly caused by neoplastic, metabolic, or immunologic diseases. Among infectious agents, viruses are a common cause; although less common, tuberculous pleuritis or peritonitis must be considered.

Fibrinous Inflammation

Fibrinous inflammation results from the outpouring of larger molecular weight proteins, specifically fibrinogen, into the inflammatory exudate. The subsequent conversion of the fibrinogen into fibrin or fibrinoid degradation products may result in the formation of a shaggy (fibrinous) exudate covering serous membranes. Fibrinous pericarditis, often caused by viral agents or seen in poststreptococcal rheumatic fever, and fibrinous pleuritis or pericarditis associated with pneumococcal lobar pneumonia are classic examples.

Ulcerative Inflammation

Superficial or deep ulceration of mucosal surfaces is a common manifestation of several infectious diseases, secondary to a variety of mechanisms. In particular, the cutaneous lesions of *Leishmania tropica* are ulcerative, and certain fungi (*Sporothrix schenckii, Blastomyces dermatitidis,* and *Paracoccidioides brasiliensis*) produce papulopustular and ulcerative lesions of the skin. In fact, one should think of fungal infections with any nonhealing ulcer or draining sinus of the skin or mucous membranes,

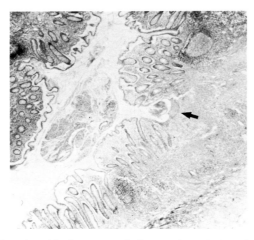

Fig. 3-10. Amebiasis, mucosal ulcer, colon. A sharply defined mucosal ulcer with a crater containing necrotic tissue (arrow) is shown.

and appropriate direct examinations and special stains of exudates and tissue sections should be performed.

Mycobacterium marinum can also cause ulcerative lesions of the skin; therefore, acid-fast stains may also be in order in undiagnosed cases.

Entamoeba histolytica, the agent of acute amoebic dysentery, may cause ulcers of the large intestine by direct invasion and focal destruction of the mucosa by motile trophozoites, which are capable of releasing proteolytic enzymes. A classic lesion is the "buttonhole" ulcer in acute amoebic dysentery (Fig. 3-10). The inflammatory reaction seen in amoebic dysentery may closely simulate the changes seen in other inflammatory bowel diseases such as ulcerative colitis.[32,33] Special stains such as trichrome, iron hematoxylin, or periodic acid-Schiff (PAS) may be useful in demonstrating the presence of amoebic trophozoites and in differentiating them from host mono-

nuclear phagocytes (Fig. 3-11). Although amoebic trophozoites may be present within an exudate, commonly the reaction is necrotic and fibrinoid in nature, not cellular.

Mucosal ulcerations of the intestine may also be seen in shigellosis, tuberculous enteritis, and typhoid fever, the latter resulting from hyperplasia of the mononuclear elements in Peyer's patches. Nonspecific ulcerations of the intestinal mucosa and pseudomembranous colitis may be caused by cytotoxin-producing *Clostridium difficile* and have been associated with the use of certain broad-spectrum antibiotics.[34]

Chronic Nonspecific Inflammation

Chronic nonspecific inflammation (Fig. 3-12) is characterized by the accumulation of lymphocytes, plasma cells, macrophages, and possibly a few neutrophils and eosinophils. These cells are accompanied by the proliferation of the components of repair, capillary buds and fibroblasts, with the production of granulation tissue and fibrosis. The type and extent of the proliferative components are characteristic for the tissue and will reflect the chronicity of the inflammatory lesion. Cultures or special tissue stains usually fail to reveal microorganisms within this advanced stage of inflammatory tissue. Depending on the class of infecting agent, the composition of the host tissue, and the chronicity of the process, one or more of the cellular components of chronic nonspecific

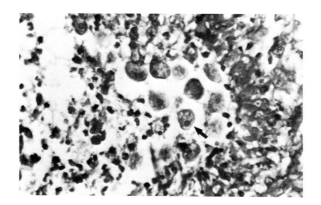

Fig. 3-11. Amebiasis, colon ulcer shown in Figure 3-10. Invasive trophozoites (arrow) with finely granular cytoplasm, small round nuclei, and central karyosomes consistent with *Entamoeba histolytica.* Note the mild acute inflammation associated with the tissue invasion.

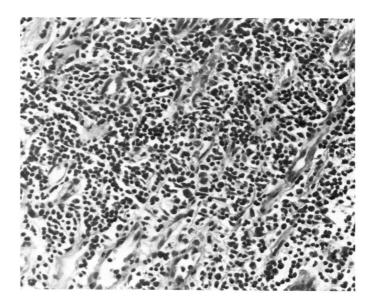

Fig. 3-12. Chronic nonspecific inflammation. The characteristic tissue infiltration with lymphocytes, plasma cells, and a few monocytes (macrophages) is shown. Note the prominence of newly formed blood vessels (granulation tissue).

inflammation may occur prominently and can present a histologic pattern that suggests classes of etiologic agents.

Lymphocytes

The presence of lymphocytes is an important but clearly nonspecific finding. Their predominance suggests the possibility of viral infection and indicates the need for evaluation of both the pattern of distribution within the tissues and the presence of specific morphologic changes. For example, the accumulation of lymphocytes within the supporting tissue of organs and around blood vessels in association with individual parenchymal cell degeneration or necrosis is strong evidence for a viral etiology.

Within the central nervous system, the distinct perivascular cuffing of lymphocytes (Fig. 3-13) may be distant from the specific virus-induced changes within neuronal cells and the reactive changes of microglial proliferation with gliosis, demyelination of white matter, and hypertrophy of astrocytes within the substance of the brain. Virus-infected neurons may show early degenerative changes or may be necrotic and surrounded by collections of astrocytes, microglia, and macrophages, a phenomenon called neuronophagia. This focal collection of neurons and reactive cells, called a glial nodule or node (Fig. 3-14), is found in a variety of viral, as well as some nonviral, encephalitides. This morphologic arrangement, then, is a nonspecific finding unless characteristic viral inclusions can be identified, as in the nodule illustrated.

Rabies, for example, can be suspected on the basis of the clinical history, plus perivascular lymphocyte cuffing and glial nodules (Babes nodes). For presumptive diagno-

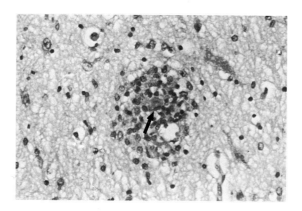

Fig. 3-14. Glial nodule, brain. Note the perineuronal cuffing with reactive glial cells, cerebral macrophages, and astrocytes. The large inclusion within the neuron (arrow) suggests cytomegalovirus.

sis, the typical eosinophilic, round or oval virus inclusions called Negri bodies must be identified. They are usually found within large neurons such as the Purkinje cells of the cerebellum (Fig. 3-15). The specific diagnosis of rabies is made by demonstrating fluorescent antibody staining of the viral inclusions.

Rubeola (measles) is another viral disease that may be immediately suspected on the basis of characteristic morphologic features in tissue sections or stained smears. Large multinucleated giant cells, the Warthin-Finkeldey giant cells of reticuloendothelial cell origin, with or without intranuclear and intracytoplasmic inclusions, are present in lymphoid tissues such as adenoids, spleen, Peyer's patches, and the vermiform appendix (Fig. 3-16). Giant multinucleated cells, infected with the measles virus, may also be seen at other sites such as skin, mucosa, and pulmonary alveolar lining cells.

An infiltrate with a preponderance of lymphocytes may also be seen with infectious agents that are more commonly associated with other reaction patterns. For exam-

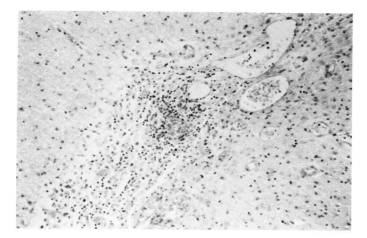

Fig. 3-13. Lymphocytic perivascular cuffing, Virchow-Robin space, brain. A cellular infiltrate composed largely of mature lymphocytes and a few plasma cells around blood vessels, as seen here, is suggestive of viral encephalitis.

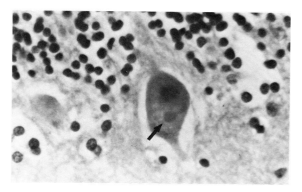

Fig. 3-15. Negri body, Purkinje cell, cerebellum. The large neuron contains a distinct round intracytoplasmic Negri body (arrow), a viral inclusion characteristic of rabies.

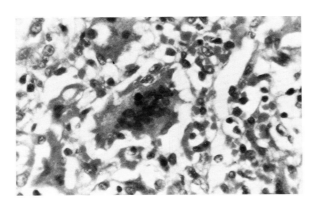

Fig. 3-16. Warthin-Finkeldey cell, lymphoid tissue. This multinucleated giant cell of reticuloendothelial cell origin is often found in hyperplastic lymphoid tissue during the prodromal stage of measles (rubeola).

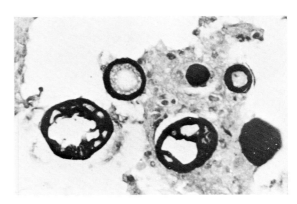

Fig. 3-18. Coccidioidomycosis, GMS stain. Note the characteristic thick-walled spherules (sporangia), which vary from 15 to 80 μm in diameter. Some contain endospores (sporangiospores).

ple, nonproliferating or resting forms of microorganisms may be associated with little more than a mild lymphocytic infiltrate. This nonspecific lymphocytic accumulation when seen alone is of no assistance in suspecting an etiology. Some agents, however, can be directly visualized in the routine tissue section. *Coccidioides immitis* spherules, for example, in the nonproliferating or resting form (Figs. 3-17 and 3-18) are sufficiently large and stain well enough to be visualized in routine tissue sections. The tissue reaction in active coccidioidomycosis is most commonly granulomatous[35]; however, when the mature spherules rupture, the released endospores (sporangiospores) may lead to an acute purulent exudate.

Eosinophils

When eosinophils are the predominant cell type in an inflammatory reaction, the presence of tissue parasites should be suspected. For example, in trichinosis the diag-

nostic larval forms may be identified within striated muscle fibers surrounded by eosinophils. The absence of eosinophils, however, does not exclude a parasitic infection, and the surgical pathologist should not abandon the search for parasitic forms purely on the basis of the absence of this typical inflammatory response. In hyperinfestation syndromes and in overwhelming lethal parasitic infections, eosinophils may be reduced or absent.

In fatal cases of trichinosis, there may be a conspicuous absence of eosinophils both in the peripheral circulation and in association with the migrating larvae of *Trichinella spiralis*.[36] The muscle tissue may show extensive muscle fiber atrophy and focal lymphocyte accumulations around degenerating muscle fibers. The diagnosis is made by a strong suspicion leading to a careful tissue survey to demonstrate larvae inside degenerating muscle fibers (Fig. 3-19). Detection of the larvae may be en-

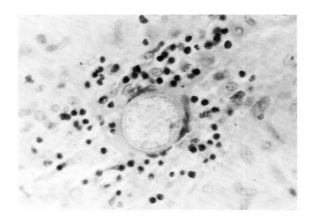

Fig. 3-17. Spherule of *Coccidioides immitis*. Note the smooth, round outline, immature endospores, and mild infiltration of mononuclear cells into the adjacent tissue.

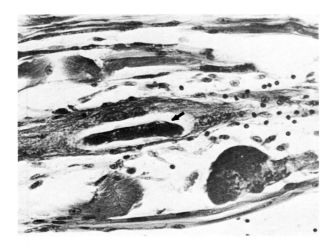

Fig. 3-19. *Trichinella spiralis*, skeletal muscle. The uncoiled larva (arrow) is found within a swollen, degenerating muscle fiber surrounded by a sparse mononuclear cell infiltrate.

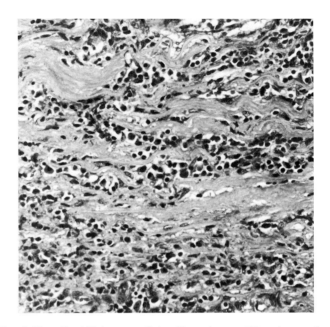

Fig. 3-20. Syphilitic vasculitis. Vascular proliferation and a mononuclear cellular infiltrate composed chiefly of plasma cells are characteristic. Spirochetes are usually difficult to demonstrate.

hanced by the use of a trichrome stain, which will accentuate the muscle fiber changes.

Plasma Cells

Plasma cells are prominent in many chronic nonspecific inflammations where a viable infectious agent persists in the tissue and stimulates a humoral immune response. In syphilis and related spirochetal diseases, plasma cells and lymphocytes appear early in the lesion, with plasma cells usually predominating (Fig. 3-20). In addition to the predominance of plasma cells, the presence of vascular proliferation and endothelial cell swelling or hyperplasia should suggest the possibility of syphilis, leading to serologic evaluation. In active spirochetal lesions (primary or secondary) the loosely coiled spirochetes may be demonstrated in tissue sections by Dieterle or Warthin-Starry silver impregnation techniques. *Treponema pallidum* may also be visualized by immunohistochemical staining in active human infections.[37]

Macrophages

Mononuclear phagocytes (macrophages) are generally regarded as the first line of defense against facultative and obligate intracellular parasites such as *Mycobacterium tuberculosis* and *M. leprae*,[8] *Salmonella* sp., *Listeria monocytogenes*, *Francisella tularensis*, *Brucella* sp., *T. gondii*, *Pneumocystis carinii*, and *H. capsulatum*.

In typhoid fever the causative bacterium, *Salmonella typhi*, invades the intestinal mucosa and produces hyperplasia of lymphoid elements in the small bowel and mesenteric lymph nodes. Early in typhoid fever, macrophages actively proliferate within Peyer's patches and contain intracellular phagocytized Gram-negative bacilli and erythrocytes. Focal collections of these macrophages accompanied by a variable number of lymphocytes and plasma cells form the so-called "typhoid" nodules, which may be found within a variety of organs as well as in the gastrointestinal (GI) tract, which is the primary target organ (Fig. 3-21).

During the fastigium of typhoid fever, local endotoxemia and systemic toxemia are present, and necrosis of the mononuclear infiltrate becomes an increasingly prominent feature.[38] Hemorrhages and microthrombi may also be present, and Zenker's degeneration of active skeletal muscles may be so severe as to produce extraordinary elevation in the serum creatine phosphokinase (CPK) levels.

The alveolar exudate in selected pneumonias may show a predominance of macrophages. The sequence of the development of this mononuclear cellular infiltrate differs with different classes of infectious agents, although the tissue morphologic features may appear to be similar.

In viral pneumonias, one may see a diffuse interstitial pneumonitis with hyaline membrane formation and characteristic intranuclear inclusion bodies within alveolar lining cells.[39] Macrophages also may predominate during certain stages of the pneumonic process.

In the pneumonia of Legionnaires' disease, on the other hand, the process begins as an acute fibrinopurulent alveolitis indistinguishable from other acute pneumo-

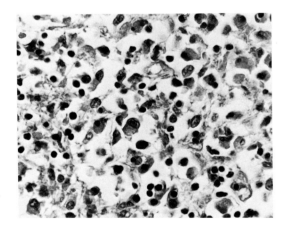

Fig. 3-21. Typhoid cells, typhoid fever. Macrophages containing Gram-negative bacilli, *Salmonella typhi*, are the predominant inflammatory cells accompanied by a variable number of plasma cells and lymphocytes. Note the abscence of neutrophils in this bacterial infection.

nias.[40] At this acute stage, there are mixtures of neutrophils and macrophages. As the pneumonia progresses, however, lysis of the inflammatory exudate occurs. The exudate may come to consist largely of intra-alveolar macrophages with amorphous debris and only rare neutrophils.[41] The bacterial agent, *L. pneumophilia,* is usually clustered within these intra-alveolar macrophages and can be visualized by the Dieterle silver impregnation stain or Wohlbach's modification of the Giemsa stain.[42] Specific identification can be made by direct immunofluorescent techniques on smears or tissue.

Focal collections of large eosinophilic macrophages within hyperplastic lymph nodes may implicate specific disease processes. In the acute acquired lymphadenitis due to *T. gondii,* there is prominent follicular hyperplasia associated with increased immunoblasts within the medullary cords and focal or diffuse infiltration with monocytoid B-lymphocytes.[43] Located within the perifollicular zones and sometimes within the follicles are small, tight clusters of "epithelioid" macrophages. The recognition of this pattern of macrophage accumulation within this type of lymphoid hyperplasia, along with the demonstration of a rising or high serologic titer, gives specificity to the diagnosis by the surgical pathologist of toxoplasmic lymphadenitis.[44]

It is important to note, however, that collections of large eosinophilic macrophages may also be seen with other lymphoid hyperplasias. In the lymphadenopathy associated with EBV disease (infectious mononucleosis), collections of eosinophilic macrophages, immunoblasts, and plasma cells may be seen within distended sinuses of

Fig. 3-22. Hyperplastic lymph node. Note the sinusoidal hyperplasia with obliteration of normal architecture and the clusters of large, pale-staining histiocyte-like cells mixed with large lymphoid cells (immunoblasts).

hyperplastic lymph nodes.[45] Similar changes are also seen in antigenically stimulated lymph nodes, whether due to viral infections, to vaccinations, or hypersensitivity to drugs such as diphenylhydantoin[46] (Fig. 3-22). The focal accumulation of macrophages within lymph nodes is nonspecific; however, if this is observed together with lymphoid hyperplasia in the context of the appropriate patient history, toxoplasmosis can be strongly suspected by the surgical pathologist.

Fibrosis

If the microbial agent is not removed by the inflammatory process and remains for extended periods of time within the tissue, the chronic process progresses to fibrosis and mineralization (calcification). Chitinous parasitic ova such as those in schistosomiasis survive in tissue despite acute purulent, eosinophilic, and granulomatous inflammatory reactions. The continuous antigenic challenge by these ova eventually triggers modulating effects that suppress the host response and reduce the tissue stimulation.[47] Eventually, mineralized ova are seen in bland areas of mature fibrous tissue with only a few remaining lymphocytes (Fig. 3-23).

The finding of squamous metaplasia or neoplasia in the adjacent epithelial surface is an important observation in the evaluation of tissues in these chronic parasitic infections. Squamous carcinoma of the urinary bladder has been associated with *Schistosoma haematobium* infestation, and urinary schistosomiasis is thought to be a cocarcinogen or promoter of urothelial cancer.[48]

Other tissue parasites, such as *Trichinella spiralis,* may encyst within the tissue by stimulating the host to lay down a hyaline layer around the parasite cyst. The parasite is then protected to some extent from the host defenses and may survive for long periods. This hyaline layer, however, can be penetrated by macrophages, and the encysted larvae can be completely destroyed and removed. The residual site of the encysted larvae persists as an oval area of dense fibrosis with mineralization (Fig. 3-24), often seen as an incidental finding in biopsy specimens of striated muscle.

Granulomatous Inflammation

Granulomatous inflammation is a chronic inflammatory tissue response characterized by discrete, nodular collections of large, eosinophilic macrophages. When the process of delayed hypersensitivity with cell-mediated immunity is prominent, the macrophages take on an epithelial appearance and are called epithelioid cells. These epithelioid cells, together with characteristic mul-

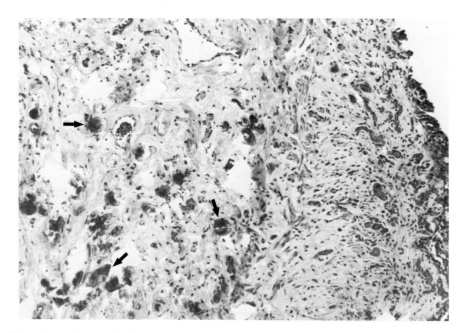

Fig. 3-23. Chronic schistosomiasis, urinary bladder. Mineralized ova of *Schistosoma haematobium* (arrows) are seen within a dense fibrotic tissue reaction. Note the marked reactive hyperplasia of adjacent mucosa.

tinucleated giant cells, peripheral lymphocytes, and fibrous tissue, form the typical lesion (Fig. 3-25).

This pattern of reaction is associated with microorganisms that can elicit cellular immunity and that are able to survive phagocytosis by neutrophils and live intracellularly within macrophages. The discrete lesions formed are called infectious granulomas. This pattern may also be associated with poorly digestible foreign material, in which case the discrete lesions are called foreign body granulomas.

Granulomatous inflammation is classically associated with the agent *M. tuberculosis.* van den Oord and associates[49] have characterized the cellular composition of the granulomas seen in tuberculosis and sarcoidal lymphadenitis. OKM1 and OK1a epithelioid histiocytes and multinucleated giant cells are seen centrally, with a few

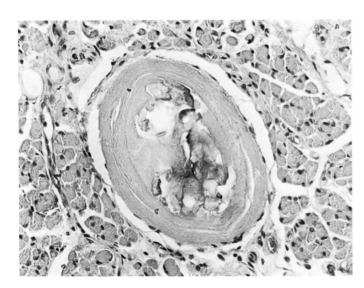

Fig. 3-24. Healed *Trichinella spiralis* cyst, muscle of tongue. The encysted larva is completely calcified within the distinct fibrous capsule.

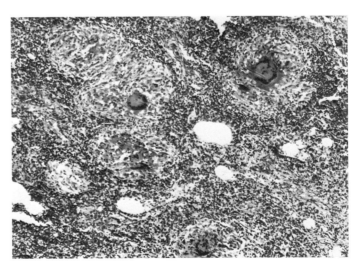

Fig. 3-25. Granulomatous inflammation. Note the centrally placed Langhans multinucleated giant cells within focal accumulations of epithelioid macrophages surrounded by a lymphocytic infiltrate.

OKT4⁺ admixed. B-lymphocytes are absent. Many OKT8⁺ suppressor/cytotoxic T-lymphocytes were demonstrated between the perigranulomatous cuff and the central aggregation of histiocytes. These investigators believe that the multinucleated giant cells seen in these granulomas have more to do with antigen processing than phagocytosis and digestion of organisms and foreign material. Cell-mediated immunity to tuberculoprotein is prominent, and the granulomas are discrete lesions, often referred to as tubercles (Fig. 3-25). Central caseous necrosis is a prominent feature and is useful in separating some infectious granulomas from noncaseating granulomas such as those seen in sarcoidosis.

The tubercle in tuberculosis, however, may be difficult to differentiate from the granulomas seen in histoplasmosis, tuberculoid leprosy, coccidioidomycosis, blastomycosis, and syphilis (gumma). Most granulomas seen in surgical pathologic material are found in cases of sarcoid, mycobacteriosis, mycoses, and rheumatoid arthritis. The granulomas seen in sarcoid and in mycobacterial infections have a predominance of epithelioid histiocytes with minimal necrosis; extensive necrosis is more likely to be seen in the lesions associated with rheumatoid arthritis.[50] Acid-fast and silver stains for organism visualization are very important in the differential evaluation of this type of reaction pattern. Isolation of the organism in culture is required for definitive diagnosis.

Many of the primary granulomatous infections do not progress in the immunologically competent host. When the organism reaches the host tissue, a nonspecific inflammatory response is noted initially. Exudation and active phagocytosis of the organisms, first by neutrophils and then by macrophages, is part of the early process;

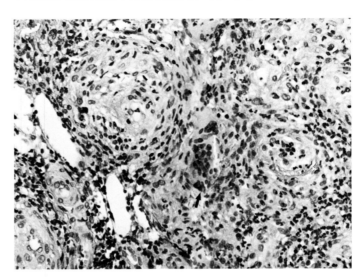

Fig. 3-27. Atypical granulomatous inflammation, skin. This inflammatory reaction is characterized by diffuse infiltration with monocytes (macrophages), lymphocytes, and scattered multinucleated giant cells (arrow). The reaction shown was caused by an infection with *Mycobacterium chelonei.*

however, engulfment does not kill the organisms. Multiplication continues intracellularly at the site of original inoculation, or the organism may be transported within the macrophages into the regional lymphatics and subsequently to regional or distant lymph nodes. With the development of specific cell-mediated immune mechanisms, multiplication and spread of the organism is stopped by enhanced intracellular killing by activated macrophages, epithelioid cells, and cytotoxic lymphocytes. The tubercles and granulomas formed are termed productive and usually represent successful containment of the organism. The lesion may progress to caseous necrosis, but this inflammatory process generally subsides as the organisms are eliminated, and the lesion heals by peripheral fibrosis and eventual mineralization (dystrophic calcification) of the caseous center (Fig. 3-26).

If the cellular immunity is less pronounced, the epithelioid and lymphocytic reaction is less sharply defined, and the reaction may be increasingly difficult to distinguish from chronic nonspecific inflammation. A less well defined infiltration in which macrophages, multinucleated giant cells, and lymphocytes can still be identified should also be classified as granulomatous and should be evaluated for similar pathogens (Fig. 3-27). Atypical mycobacteria and borderline lesions of leprosy, for example, have a less distinct granulomatous pattern. The atypical mycobacteria can further confuse the microscopist by producing mixed inflammatory infiltrates with different areas showing acute purulent inflammation, chronic nonspecific inflammation, and chronic granulomatous inflammation. The granulomas formed by *M. avium-intracellulare*

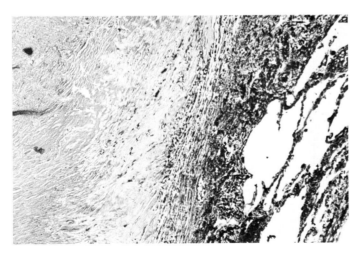

Fig. 3-26. Tuberculoma, lung. The outer layer of a large fibrocaseous mass is shown. Note the caseous necrosis (left), the thick, acellular fibrous capsule, and the dense infiltration of mononuclear cells in the tissue adjacent to the capsule.

SURGICAL PATHOLOGY OF INFECTIOUS DISEASES

(MAI) are more likely to show necrotic areas filled with inflammatory cells and nuclear debris rather than acellular areas of caseation. The palisading ring of histiocytes and the presence of Langhans giant cells, so characteristic of *M. tuberculosis* granulomas, are usually inconspicuous in MAI lesions. In AIDS there tends to be a poor granulomatous response with the production of massive numbers of intracellular organisms resembling the lesions of lepromatous leprosy.[51]

The morphologic development of the granulomatous lesions in cat-scratch fever[52] lymphogranuloma venereum, tularemia, listeriosis, brucellosis, melioidosis, and mesenteric lymphadenitis due to *Yersinia pseudotuberculosis*[53] differs from that of the typical "tubercle." The morphologic progression of these lesions, also associated with cell-mediated immunity, can be divided into early, intermediate, and late lesions. As the inflammation progresses through the early, intermediate, and late stages, a shift toward a preponderance of cytotoxic OKT8+ cells occurs, resulting in necrosis. Necrosis may also result from the formation of immune complexes from the production of antibodies by the surrounding plasma cells. The appearance of the individual lesion will vary somewhat depending on the particular agent, but each shares certain common characteristics.

In lymphoid tissue, the follicles become prominent with large, active germinal centers, and there is a proliferation of immunoblasts and macrophages. Focal tissue necrosis with deposition of fibrin and infiltration of neutrophils represents the earliest lesion (Fig. 3-28). Infiltra-

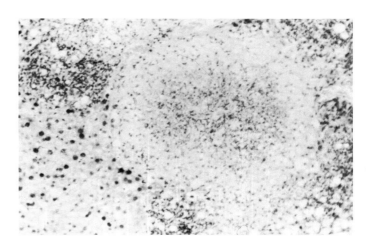

Fig. 3-29. Listeriosis, liver. An intermediate stage of a stellate abscess or necrobiotic granuloma with a central collection of neutrophils and cellular debris surrounded by a well developed zone of epithelioid cells.

tion of neutrophils may progress to the formation of microabscesses; a peripheral accumulation of macrophages may also be appreciated at this early stage. In acute melioidosis, lethal neonatal listeriosis, and acute mesenteric lymphadenitis, numerous microorganisms can be demonstrated within the necrotic foci by Gram stains of tissue, and culture of this tissue should provide excellent isolation of the organism. In other infections associated with these lesions, negative cultures and appropriate serologic tests demonstrating a rising antibody titer are important diagnostic tools at this stage of disease.

The intermediate lesions have been variously termed granulomatous abscess formation, necrobiotic granuloma, and stellate abscess.[54] The lesion is characterized by a well demarcated "abscess" containing central debris with fragmented neutrophil nuclei and a distinct rim of palisading "epithelioid" macrophages and occasional multinucleated giant cells (Fig. 3-29). This reaction is distinguished from the caseating granuloma, in which there is complete destruction of central cellular structures producing granular, amorphous debris without neutrophilic infiltration. The outer zone of the lesion is composed of lymphocytes, plasma cells, and some fibroblasts.

The fully mature or late lesion has the appearance of a caseating granuloma (Fig. 3-30), and in many instances is histologically indistinguishable from the granuloma of tuberculosis. The continued presence of the distinct zone of central necrosis (which becomes increasingly acellular), palisading of epithelioid macrophages, and the peripheral zone of lymphocytes, plasma cells, and active fibrosis, is helpful in the recognition of this morphologic entity (Fig. 3-31). Organisms at times may be demonstrated in mature caseous granulomas with the GGMS and acid-fast stains; however, organisms usually are not

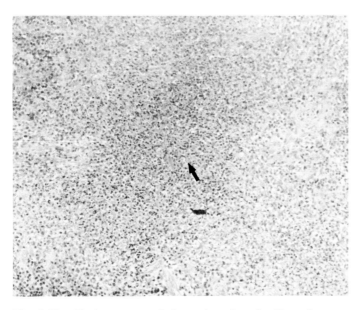

Fig. 3-28. Early cat-scratch fever, lymph node. Note the non-specific lymphoid hyperplasia with a beginning area of necrosis (arrow) lightly infiltrated by neutrophils and bordered by a subtle accumulation of large mononuclear cells.

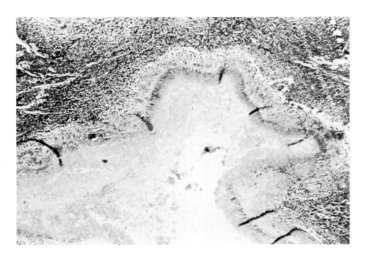

Fig. 3-30. Lymphogranuloma venereum, lymph node. A mature stellate abscess or necrotic granuloma with central necrosis and a distinct rim of palisading epithelioid cells.

present within the mature necrobiotic granulomas. An accurate history and serologic testing may be most helpful in the differential evaluation of this mature lesion.

Cavities may be formed within deep tissues and draining sinus tracts from superficial lymph nodes or subcutaneous tissue may develop after the rupture of caseating granulomata onto adjacent surfaces. The inflammatory debris from the infected walls of the cavity collects within the cavity and is discharged to the surface. Cavitation is a significant development in granulomatous disease caused by primary pathogens such as *M. tuberculosis*.

The open cavity poses a number of opportunities for complications in the evolution of the disease. Treatment is less efficient because the wall of the cavity that remains open is usually rigid from fibrosis, and the organisms remain viable within the avascular cavity. Colonization of the cavity by saprophytes may complicate management by confusing the results of cultures taken from tracts leading into the cavity or by the development of a significant secondary infection. Surgical removal or biopsy may become necessary for diagnosis or treatment.

A well recognized complication of open cavities, natural as well as postinflammatory, is the colonization of the cavity by aspergillus spores, which subsequently develop into a large fungal colony known as a fungal ball or aspergilloma (Fig. 3-32). The fungal growth may cause no symptoms or may erode the residual intracavitary blood vessels causing hemorrhage. Uncontrolled bleeding is a common indication for the surgical removal of these saprophytic growths.

Histiocytic inflammation is characterized by the extensive proliferation of large foamy or vacuolated macrophages (histiocytes). The masses of macrophages may be accompanied by a variable number of plasma cells and lymphocytes; Langhans-type giant cells and necrosis are usually absent. Accumulation of macrophages within tissue often begins around blood vessels and around dermal appendages in skin lesions. Because of the mononuclear cell population and the nodular appearance of the infiltrate, the term histiocytic granuloma is frequently used.

Most organisms associated with this pattern of reaction can produce tuberculoid granulomas in immunocompe-

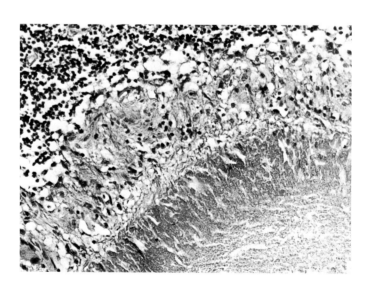

Fig. 3-31. Rim of the stellate abscess shown in Figure 3-30. Note the distinct zone of necrosis with no residual neutrophils and the palisading of epithelioid monocytes with a peripheral accumulation of lymphocytes.

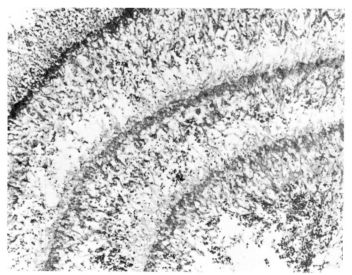

Fig. 3-32. Aspergilloma, old tuberculous cavity, lung. Cross section of a fungus ball found within a fibrotic lung cavity. Note the laminated growth pattern of the *Aspergillus* fungal colony, composed of branching hyphal elements.

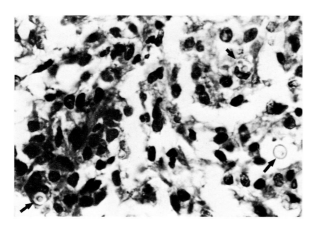

Fig. 3-33. Cryptococcal granuloma, brain. Histiocytes (monocytes or macrophages) predominate within the infiltrate, accompanied by a few lymphocytes and plasma cells. Note the presence of encapsulated, budding yeast cells, 4 to 7 μm (arrows), consistent with *Cryptococcus neoformans*.

tent hosts. The encapsulated yeast cells of *Cryptococcus neoformans,* for example, may be associated with a typical tuberculoid granuloma, with a histiocytic granuloma (Fig. 3-33), or with an inert reaction, depending on the level of integrity of the host immune system. A similar variety of responses is seen in leprosy, in which the host capable of demonstrating cell-mediated immunity to the lepromin skin test antigen produces tuberculoid granulomas and demonstrates few organisms within lesions, whereas in hosts who have skin anergy, infiltrates composed primarily of macrophages filled with microorganisms (lepra cells) are usually observed (Fig. 3-34).[55]

Macrophage proliferations and skin test anergy to the specific antigen have also been associated with mycobacteria other than *M. leprae* (Fig. 3-35). In early cases of

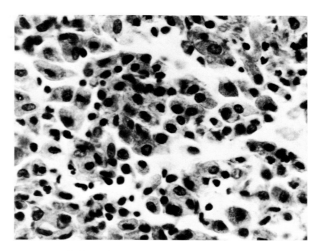

Fig. 3-35. Histiocytic granuloma, lung. This lesion demonstrates sheets of foamy histiocytes or macrophages admixed with a few other inflammatory cells and a little fibroblastic activity at the periphery. Acid-fast staining reveals numerous acid-fast bacteria within the phagocytes. *Mycobacterium intracellulare* was cultured from this lesion.

anergic cutaneous leishmaniasis, tuberculoid granulomas may be produced initially, later progressing to massive histiocytic proliferation (Fig. 3-36). Histoplasmosis caused by the fungus *H. capsulatum* produces primarily a tuberculoid reaction indistinguishable histologically from tuberculosis. A histiocytic form also occurs, particularly in the immunocompromised host, with a histologic pattern very similar to that seen in anergic leishmaniasis (Fig. 3-37).

Intracellular containment of microbes without intracellular killing, then, appears to represent the host response

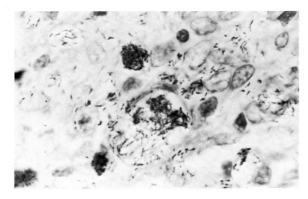

Fig. 3-34. Lepra cells, acid-fast stain. Note the large intracellular masses of *Mycobacterium leprae* within vacuolated histiocytes or macrophages called lepra cells. This photomicrograph was taken from a skin biopsy specimen of lepromatous leprosy. Similar mycobacteria-packed macrophages are also seen in *M. avium-intracellulare* infections in patients with AIDS.

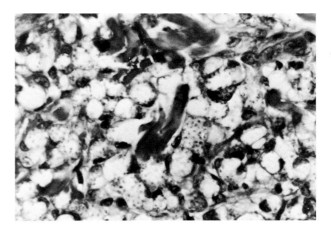

Fig. 3-36. Anergic leishmaniasis, skin. Large histiocytes containing leishmanial forms crowd the field, separated only by scattered bundle of collagen, lymphocytes, plasma cells, and blood vessels. The intracellular organisms must be distinguished from organisms found in similar reaction patterns by the demonstration of a nucleus and a kinetoplast.

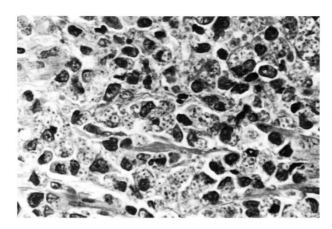

Fig. 3-37. Histoplasmosis, lung. Note the similarity of the large histiocytes containing the small (1 to 3 μm in diameter) spores of *Histioplasma capsulatum* to those containing leishmanial forms in Figure 3-36.

to a wide variety of agents including bacteria, protozoans, and fungi in the absence of cell-mediated immunity.

Morphologic discrimination among the histiocytic reactions requires the evaluation of two types of manifestations. In the first, massive accumulations of foamy or vacuolated macrophages occur with no visible microorganisms in reactions associated with chronic nonspecific inflammation, atypical mycobacterioses, lepromatous leprosy with lepra cells, and rhinoscleroma with very similar appearing Mikulicz cells. Special stains are required both to visualize and to identify the intracellular organisms, if present. An acid-fast stain separates the atypical mycobacterioses and leprosy from the others, and a silver impregnation stain has the greatest reliability in visualizing the remaining intracellular organisms.

In the second type of manifestation, accumulations of macrophages are filled with visible organisms in histoplasmosis anergic leishmaniasis, and, occasionally, cryptococcosis. The size and shape of the individual organisms can be estimated in a Giemsa preparation; however, to differentiate among this group, a silver stain may be utilized to demonstrate the kinetoplasts of the leishmania, a mucicarmine stain to demonstrate the capsule of the cryptococcus, and a GGMS or Gridley's fungal (GF) stain to characterize the histoplasma cells.

Acellular Inflammation

The acellular (or inert) reaction is characterized by an exudate composed chiefly of edema, hemorrhage, and fibrin deposition. The occurrence of this pattern of reaction is associated with a number of predictable clinical settings, and the surgical pathologist must be alert to the variety of infectious agents that may be identified. Be-

cause there is a lack of tissue-reactive centers to attract the attention of the surgical pathologist, a careful, consistent microscopic study of stained tissue sections is necessary. Special stains may be used to aid in the low-power search for characteristic organisms.

Bacterial agents are most commonly associated with exudative lesions; however, when the tissue is naturally avascular or gangrenous, bacteria may proliferate to form microcolonies. These organisms can produce absorbable toxins or may directly seed the bloodstream. Careful tissue examination may be of value in a number of clinical settings. The eschar of burns may be examined to determine the level of bacterial colonization; gangrenous tissue may be examined for the presence of the large Grampositive bacilli of *Clostridium* sp.; and a number of naturally avascular tissues may be removed for evaluation of infectious processes. In infective endocarditis, for example, either on the natural valve or on a mechanical or xenograft valve replacement, chronic progressive infection may require tissue removal for cure. Bacterial or fungal colonies may be buried deep within the acellular vegetation (Fig. 3-38). The bacteria can be characterized by the Gram stain reaction (Fig. 3-39), and fungi can be characterized by the GGMS stain (Fig. 3-40). Care should be taken to ensure that appropriate culture evaluations have been made.

Fungal infections associated with acellular reactions have become increasingly important in immunosuppressed hosts. Because leukopenic patients are unable to produce a significant response to infection, frequent and protracted courses of antibiotic are used, with subsequent overgrowth of resistant microbial forms such as yeast and fungi.

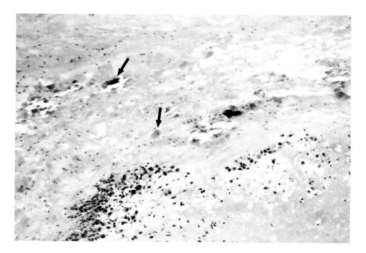

Fig. 3-38. Infective endocarditis, cardiac valve xenograft. Bacterial colonies (arrows) are shown embedded within the acellular deposits of the valve surface. Chronic bacteremia resulting from infection with an antibiotic-resistant *Corynebacterium* sp. required removal of the valve.

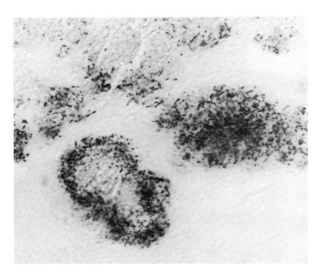

Fig. 3-39. Bacterial colonies, Gram stain of Figure 3-38. Discrete colonies of pleomorphic Gram-positive bacilli present within the acellular debris are morphologically consistent with *Corynebacterium* sp.

Disseminated candidiasis may follow colonization and infection of the gastrointestinal tract, with metastatic lesions appearing throughout parenchymal organs.[56] Pseudohyphae may be prominent in the areas of invasion, requiring differentiation from filamentous fungi (Fig. 3-41).

Vascular invasion by fungi may result in thrombosis and infarction of tissue with an acellular response.[57] The wall of the blood vessel and the thrombus may be extensively infiltrated by fungal hyphae (Fig. 3-42). In the evaluation of tissue with an acellular reaction, the fungal

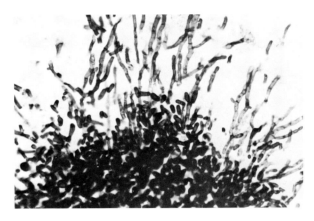

Fig. 3-41. Candidiasis, GGMS stain. Note the presence of both round and oval yeast forms, as well as filamentous pseudohyphae. Distribution of these elements may vary, but in deep lesions pseudohyphae are commonly seen radiating from a focus of yeast cells as shown. *Candida albicans* is the species most commonly isolated in humans.

thrombus may be distant from the apparently involved tissue. Blood vessels that appear expanded by thrombus should be carefully examined for hyphal elements. When hyphae are located, general separation into genera such as *Aspergillus* (Fig. 3-43) and *Mucor* (Fig. 3-44) can be made on the basis of hyphal morphologic characteristics using special stains. Culture remains, however, the only mechanism to confirm the identity of the fungal species.

Cryptococcus neoformans may proliferate extensively throughout body tissues in the immunosuppressed patient, producing no cellular reaction or necrosis. *C. neoformans* may fail to induce an inflammatory reaction because the capsule prevents exposure of protein anti-

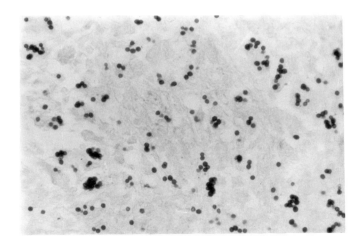

Fig. 3-40. *Histoplasma capsulatum,* GMS stain. Note the small yeast cells which appear larger than in Figure 3-37 because of the staining of the entire spore by GMS.

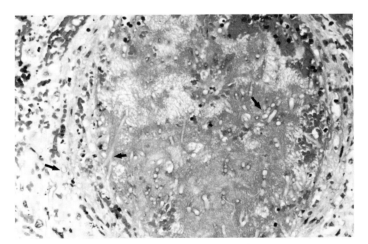

Fig. 3-42. Vascular thrombosis, invasive aspergillosis. Note the blood vessel distended by thrombus. Fungal hyphae, in longitudinal and cross sections, can be seen (arrows) in the vessel wall and scattered within the thrombus.

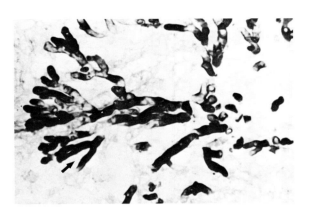

Fig. 3-43. Aspergillosis, GGMS stain. Note the characteristic septate hyphae that dichotomously branch at 45-degree angles (arrow). These hyphal filaments stain heavily with GGMS but poorly in Gram stains.

gen; in fact, intense inflammation may be seen in infections with nonencapsulated strains.[58] Grossly, mucinous nodules may be present. Microscopically, the tissue elements may appear to be pushed apart, separated by clear spaces, which result from the production of abundant capsular material by the organism. Because there is no cellular response, the tissue morphology (Fig. 3-45) can simulate mucin-secreting carcinoma. The GGMS stain, however, stains the cells nicely and illustrates the characteristic irregularity in the size of the yeast-cell bodies and the abundant capsular material (Fig. 3-46). A mucicarmine stain demonstrates directly the capsular material

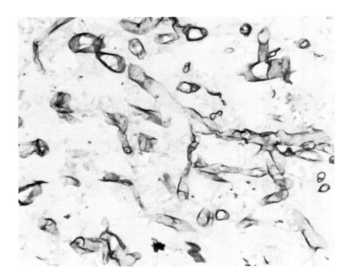

Fig. 3-44. Zygomycosis, GGMS stain. Note the characteristic broad, aseptate hyphae that appear wrinkled and folded. This fungus stains lightly with GGMS stain and can be easily overlooked in tissue sections if only the thin-walled hyphae cut in a transverse diameter are present. *Mucor, Rhizopus,* and *Absidia* are the genera most commonly isolated.

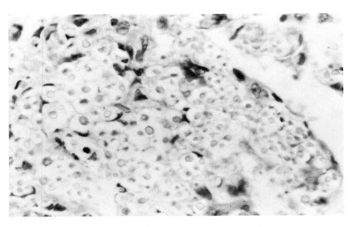

Fig. 3-45. Cryptococcosis. Gelatinous mass showing massive proliferation of the characteristic encapsulated 4 to 7 μm yeast cells of *Cryptococcus neoformans*. Note that the yeast cells are irregular in size and thin-walled, and many have a single bud with a narrow base. The yeast cells are widely separated from one another by the abundant capsular material.

and is particularly useful in atypical cases. The Fontana-Masson stain may be used to stain the cell walls of *C. neoformans* regardless of the presence or absence of capsular material. The stain detects the melanin produced by virtually all strains of *C. neoformans*.[59]

A variety of protozoan agents have taken on new importance. *Pneumocystis carinii,* in the immunosuppressed host, produces a spectrum of histopathologic changes including interstitial pneumonitis, fibrosis, and rarely granulomas. Typically, the pneumonia is characterized by a foamy or honeycombed intra-alveolar exu-

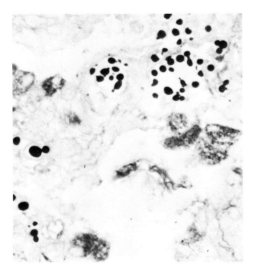

Fig. 3-46. *Cryptococcus neoformans,* GGMS stain. GGMS stain is useful for locating fungal forms in low numbers within tissue. Note the distinct visualization of the irregular-sized, encapsulated, budding yeast cells in this photomicrograph.

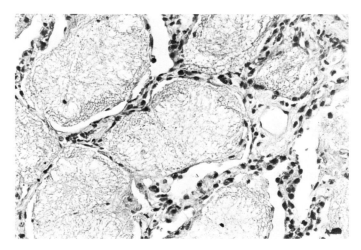

Fig. 3-47. Pneumocystosis, lung. The characteristic foamy or meshlike, acellular, eosinophilic intra-alveolar exudate is shown. Note the relative absence of inflammatory cells within the alveolar septa in this severely immunosuppressed patient.

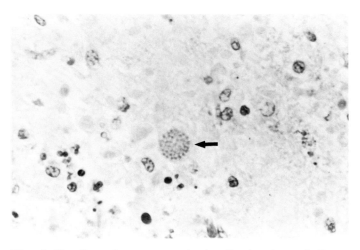

Fig. 3-49. *Toxoplasma* cyst, brain. Bradyzoites of *Toxoplasma gondii* are packed tightly within the cyst (arrow) and multiply slowly during this chronic asymptomatic phase in the immune host.

date with minimal inflammatory response (Fig. 3-47). Lung biopsy material with these morphologic features should be studied by stains such as GGMS and Giemsa, to demonstrate the characteristic organisms[60] (Fig. 3-48). Care must be taken to differentiate pneumocystis cysts from the yeast cells of *Histoplasma capsulatum,* which will also stain with the GGMS. A demonstration of the pneumocystis trophozoites in a Giemsa stained preparation may be helpful in making this differentiation.

Toxoplasmosis, caused by the protozoan *T. gondii,* has long been recognized as a worldwide subclinical infection. The common tissue presentation is the toxoplasmal cyst, usually found in brain, skeletal muscle, or eye, where the reaction is usually inert (Fig. 3-49). The disease is not active at this stage, but the organisms may still be viable within the cyst. Immunosuppressed patients, presumably previously infected, can develop fatal infections. Sheibani et al.[43] describe aggregates of "monocytoid" cells in cases of toxoplasma lymphadenitis. These cells are pale staining and generally larger than the typical small mature-appearing lymphocytes seen in other inflammatory reactions. These investigators conclude

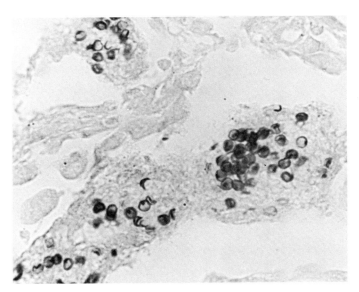

Fig. 3-48. *Pneumocystis carinii* cysts, GGMS stain, tissue in Figure 3-47. The cyst wall is clearly stained by GGMS and reveals forms 3 to 7 μm in diameter with round-to-oval or folded, cuplike shapes. The trophozoites which adhere to the alveolar walls are not stained by GMS and can be best demonstrated by the Giemsa stain.

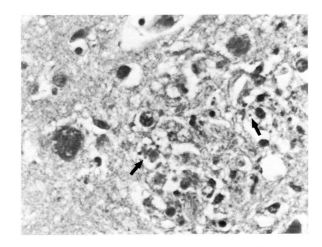

Fig. 3-50. *Toxoplasma* encephalitis. Note the focal necrosis with numerous tachyzoites (arrows) and cysts of *Toxoplasma gondii.* Except for a few scattered monocytoid lymphocytes, no inflammatory response is seen.

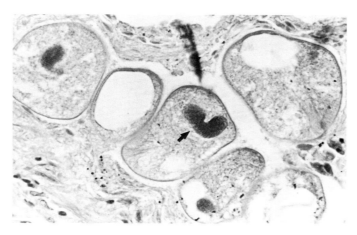

Fig. 3-51. Balantidiasis, colon. Superficial mucosal invasion by trophozoites of *Balantidium coli* in an immunosuppressed host. Note the characteristic large (40 to 80 μm in broadest diameter) trophozoites with foamy cytoplasm, a macronucleus (arrow), and a thin cell membrane covered by cilia.

that these monocytoid cells are probably not derived from monocyte/histiocyte cell lines based on the absence of peanut agglutinin activity as determined by a biotinylated DNA probe. These monocytoid cells are most likely lymphocytes. In toxoplasmic encephalitis (Fig. 3-50), large areas of necrosis containing free tachyzoites or tachyzoites within mononuclear cells are seen. Direct immunofluorescent techniques will aid in the diagnosis.[61] Vasculitis with thrombosis and infarction may occur or,

more commonly, areas of acellular necrosis or organ infiltration may be observed. A collection of tachyzoites within myofibers must be differentiated from the amastigotes of Chagas' disease. Because the yeast forms of histoplasmosis may be of a similar size, this differential diagnosis should also be considered.

Intestinal parasites may provide unexpected complications in the immunosuppressed host and may go undiagnosed because of the absence of the usual peripheral blood eosinophilia. Colon ulceration and even perforation and peritonitis may occasionally occur from nonpathogenic protozoans such as *Balantidium coli* (Fig. 3-51). Vague general symptoms of abdominal pain and progressive hypoxia can occur with progressive infestation due to autoinfection in strongyloidiasis (Fig. 3-52).[35] In all such parasitic hyperinfestations, few clues other than direct visualization of the organisms may be available to explain the clinical findings.

Viral infections within the general population are quite common and usually are associated with little mortality. In the immunosuppressed host, susceptibility to reactivation of latent viral infections and to acquiring latent viral infection from organ transplants and blood transfusions poses a significant problem. Tissue culture isolation techniques for viruses and direct specific immunofluorescent specimen testing are well developed. However, the surgical pathologist frequently examines tissues infected with viruses and should be able to recognize the clues to this class of infectious agents.

Individual cell necrosis and viral inclusions are impor-

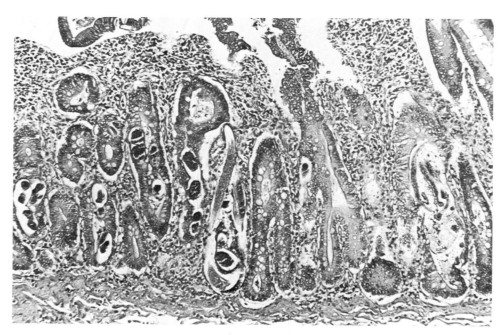

Fig. 3-52. Strongyloidiasis, jejunum. Note the large number of characteristic eggs and adult nematodes of *Strongyloides stercoralis* in hyperinfective strongyloidiasis.

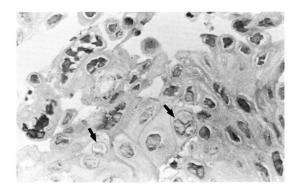

Fig. 3-53. Herpes virus inclusions, epithelium. Homogeneous, intranuclear viral inclusions (arrows) consistent with Herpes simplex infection are shown within degenerating epithelial cells.

tant clues to the presence of viral infection. For example, HSV produces characteristic inclusions in cells (Fig. 3-53), and the inclusions together with the pattern of necrosis indicate the presumptive diagnosis.[62] Early viral inclusions may not be obvious, although nuclear enlargement and cytoplasmic vacuolization may suggest a viral etiology. Well developed viral inclusions, such as those seen with CMV (Fig. 3-54), leave little doubt as to the diagnosis.[63]

Inclusion bodies are divided into two groups on the basis of their location within the cell. The inclusion bodies of the pox group of diseases (e.g., variola, vaccinia) are found in the cytoplasm of the infected cell. Those associated with other virus diseases are intranuclear and are of two kinds. The Cowdry type A inclusion body is a relatively large body that disrupts the structure of the nucleus and is found in cells infected with viruses such as herpes and varicella. These appear as prominent nonnucleolar eosinophilic bodies surrounded by a distinct zone of pallor ("halo") caused by margination and

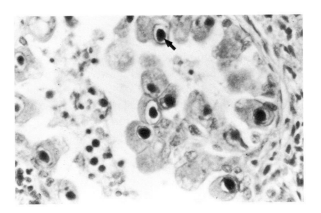

Fig. 3-54. CMV infection, kidney. Note the enlarged renal epithelial cells with prominent intranuclear inclusions (arrow) separated from the compressed nuclear chromatin by a distinct halo.

clumping of nuclear chromatin. The Cowdry type B inclusion body is much smaller and occurs in an otherwise normal-appearing nucleus. It is found in such viral diseases as poliomyelitis.

The adenoviruses characteristically produce Cowdry type A inclusions and also large purple intranuclear inclusion bodies that appear to fill the nucleus and blue its margin ("smudge cells"). These latter inclusions should be distinguished from the large basophilic intranuclear inclusion bodies seen in cells infected with CMV. Marked cellular enlargement and numerous small intracytoplasmic inclusion bodies help distinguish CMV infection from adenovirus infection.

Hyperplasia

Some groups of viruses cause a hyperplastic response within the cells and must be differentiated from other causes of hyperplasia on the basis of tissue morphology and the presence of viral inclusions. Viral infections of squamous epithelial cells produce a variety of common hyperplastic lesions. Verrucae (or "warts") are the most common. The wart virus (papilloma group) replicates within the nucleus of the epithelial cell. In verruca vulgaris, intranuclear basophilic viral inclusions may be seen within the cells of the granular layer or the upper stratum malpighii. Little inflammation occurs within the adjacent dermis.

There is remarkable acanthosis and papillomatosis of the epithelium in response to this infection. Condylomata acuminata, the venereal member of this "wart" group, are occasionally removed because of concern about malignant transformation.[64] Occasionally, the hyperplastic (acanthotic) lesions of condylomata lata (secondary syphilis) may be confused grossly with condylomata acuminata. The syphilitic lesion is easily differentiated by the prominent dermal perivascular infiltrate of plasma cells and the proliferation of vascular tissues. Spirochetes are also easily demonstrated by the impregnation stain.

Molluscum contagiosum (Fig. 3-55) represents one of the most striking forms of epithelial cell hyperplasia with the presence of viral inclusions. The large eosinophilic molluscum inclusion bodies (poxvirus group) form in the lower epidermis, predominantly within the cytoplasm of epithelial cells. They later mature into basophilic molluscum bodies, which displace the cell nucleus in the upper epidermis. This lesion differs from Milker's nodules (paravaccinia virus, which also has large eosinophilic viral inclusions) by the absence of an inflammatory infiltrate within the adjacent dermis.

Rarely, epithelial hyperplasia due to individual cell parasitization by viruses or local infections such as cuta-

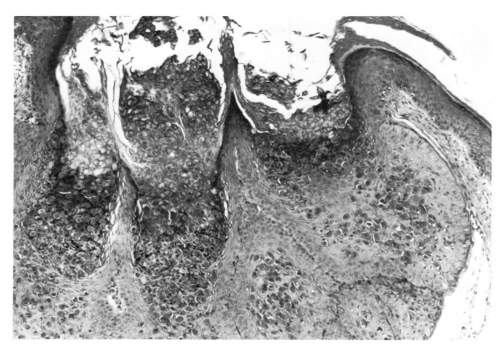

Fig. 3-55. Molluscum contagiosum, skin. Warty epithelial cell hyperplasia with numerous intracytoplasmic eosinophilic inclusion bodies is seen. Note the transition of the large inclusions to molluscum bodies at the surface of the lesion. The infectious agent belongs to the poxvirus group.

neous blastomycosis will produce a pseudocarcinomatous hyperplasia. The differential diagnosis of pseudocarcinoma from actual malignancy is obviously critical. Malignant tumors have rarely been noted to arise in these infectious hyperplasias.

NEOPLASIA

Viruses have long been sought as etiologic agents of neoplasia or as co-agents in the initiation of neoplasms. The number of neoplasms associated with viruses is increasing, so that today selected diagnoses infer infection with specific viruses. The following associations are recognized: Burkitt's lymphoma/EBV; central nervous system lymphoma/retrovirus; T-cell lymphoma/retrovirus; Kaposi's sarcoma/CMV, and squamous cell carcinoma/papilloma virus.

Both the tissue evaluation for malignancy and for the presence of the suspect virus may become standard practice in the future.

CONCLUSIONS

With the advent of medical progress, we had come to expect that diseases caused by infectious agents would decline, and that their place in diagnostic considerations would diminish. Unfortunately, the success in the eradication of highly pathogenic organisms by immunization, sanitation, and antibiotic therapy has been offset by an increase in the incidence of infections caused by other organisms.

Organisms once thought to be nonpathogenic, such as *Serratia marcescens, Mucor* sp., and *Aspergillus* sp., are now regularly involved in the production of serious and fatal disease in immunosuppressed patients. New infectious agents have been discovered for old diseases. Slow viruses ("viroids") are now associated with Creutzfeldt-Jakob disease, Broad Street pneumonia now has the agent *L. pneumophilia,* and defective viruses have been implicated in a variety of diseases such as subacute sclerosing panencephalitis, multiple sclerosis, and progressive multifocal leukoencephalopathy. The recent discovery of the association of peptic ulcer disease and gastritis with *C. pylori* is yet another example of how new infectious disease syndromes continue to evolve. Finally, the increased mobility of world populations through travel and emigration have brought exposure to infectious diseases once thought to be exotic.

Surgical pathologists can expect, then, that a portion of their practice will relate to infectious diseases and that the more compromised the patients and the more cosmopolitan the patient population, the greater this portion will become.

There are two potential serious pitfalls for the surgical

pathologist to avoid in rendering an infectious disease diagnosis. The first is the failure to maintain strict criteria in the morphologic identification of visible microorganisms in tissues. In each instance of presumptive identification, there should be a mental check to ensure that (1) tissue reaction is compatible with the identification; (2) the size and morphologic characteristics are consistent with the suspected etiologic agent; (3) the staining characteristics in both the routine and special stains are consistent with the agent; and (4) specific identification methods are used, if available. This mental checklist should prevent the misinterpretation as infectious agents of a variety of other structures that may be observed in tissue sections. Calcospherites, for example, have a superficial resemblance to yeast cells (Fig. 3-56). These structures, however, stain basophilic in routine sections, are smaller than most yeasts, and have a laminated structure rather than a true cell body. Calcospherites stain positive in GGMS and PAS stains, which can be misleading if one does not also perform a calcium stain, which will also be positive.

Second is the failure to recognize a rarely encountered organism, either by dismissing the observation as being artifact, or by naming a similar but more common agent instead. Rare or new discoveries are made by keeping an open, inquisitive attitude toward observations that do not immediately fit into a recognized pattern. The recognition of human protothecosis (Fig. 3-57), for example, requires a general appreciation of the morphologic features of the rarely pathogenic algae. Once the morphologic characteristics have been appreciated, recognition and identification of rare organisms are ensured. When unfamiliar tissue reactions are encountered, the pathologist has a variety of reference sources available to aid with definitive identification. If the pathologist does not appreciate

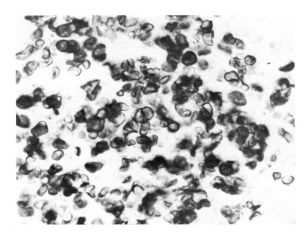

Fig. 3-57. Protothecosis, GGMS stain. The single, oval-to-round, folded, nonbudding alga cells of *Prototheca* sp. are shown. The cells vary from 2 to 18 μm in diameter and are accompanied by little tissue reaction.

the unusual morphologic features, identification or clarification of the process will not occur.

REFERENCES

1. Rotterdam H: Tissue diagnosis of selected AIDS-related opportunistic infections. Am J Surg Pathol 11(suppl 1):3, 1987
2. Martin WJ, Smith TF, Sanderson DR, et al: Role of bronchoalveolar lavage in the assessment of opportunistic pulmonary infections: Utility and complications. Mayo Clin Proc 62:549, 1987
3. Fisher ER, Park EJ, Wechsler HL: Histologic identification of malignant lymphoma cutis. Am J Clin Pathol 65:149, 1976
4. Matzner Y, Behar A, Elliot B, et al: Systemic leishmaniasis mimicking malignant histiocytosis. Cancer 43:398, 1979
5. deJongh DS, Loftis JW, Green SG, et al: Postmortem bacteriology: A practical guide for routine use. Am J Clin Pathol 49:424, 1968
6. Goodwin CS, Blincow E, Warren JR, et al: Evaluation of cultural techniques for isolating *Campylobacter pyloridis* from endoscopic biopsies of gastric mucosa. J Clin Pathol 38:1127, 1985
7. Bigby TD, Margolskee D, Curtis JL, et al: The usefulness of induced sputum in the diagnosis of *Pneumocystis carinii* pneumonia in patients with the acquired immunodeficiency syndrome. Am Rev Respir Dis 133:515, 1986
8. Cockerill FR, Wilson WR, Carpenter HA, et al: Open lung biopsy in immunocompromised patients: Arch Intern Med 145:1398, 1985
9. Gosey LL, Howard RM, Witebsky FG, et al: Advantages of a modified toluidine blue O stain and bronchoalveolar lavage for the diagnosis of *Pneumocystis carinii* pneumonia. J Clin Microbiol 22:803, 1985

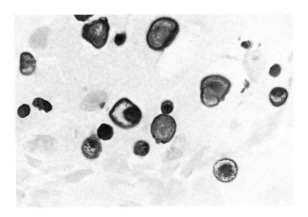

Fig. 3-56. Calcospherites, GGMS stain. Note the superficial resemblance of the calcospherites (arrows) to yeast cells. These structures stain intensely PAS-positive and stain strongly for calcium.

10. Regan MC, Ayers LW: A five minute toluidine blue-O stain for *Pneumocystis carinii*. Am J Clin Pathol 88:533, 1987

11. Shimono LH, Hartman B: A simple and reliable rapid methenamine silver stain for *Pneumocystis carinii* and fungi. Arch Pathol Lab Med 110:855, 1986

12. Elder BL, Roberts GD: Rapid methods for the diagnosis of fungal infections. Lab Med 17:591, 1986

13. Monheit JG, Brown G, Kott MM: Calcofluor white detection of fungi in cytopathology. Am J Clin Pathol 85:222, 1986

14. Hegeage GJ, Harrington BJ: Use of calcofluor white in clinical mycology. Lab Med 15:109, 1984

15. Hollander I, Keilig W, Bauer J, Rothmund E: A reliable fluorescent stain for fungi in tissue sections and clinical specimens. Mycopathologia 88:131, 1984

16. Koch HH, Pimsler M: Evaluation of Uvitex 2B: A nonspecific fluorescent stain for detecting and identifying fungi and algae in tissue. Lab Med 18:603, 1987

17. Wilhelmus KR, Osato MS, Font RL, et al: Rapid diagnosis of Acanthamoeba keratitis using calcofluor white. Arch Ophthalmol 104:1309, 1986

18. Grody WW, Cheng L, Lewin KJ: In-situ viral DNA hybridization in diagnostic surgical pathology. Hum Pathol 18:535, 1987

19. DeLellis RA (ed): Diagnostic Immunohistochemistry. Masson Publishing USA, Paris 1981

20. Brigati DJ, Myerson D, Leary JJ, et al: Detection of viral genomes in cultured cells and paraffin-embedded tissue sections using biotin-labeled hybridization probes. Virology 126:32, 1983

21. Unger ER, Budgeon LR, Myerson D, et al: Viral diagnosis by in-situ hybridization. Am J Surg Pathol 10:1, 1982

22. Hilborne LH, Nieberg RK, Cheng L, et al: Direct in-situ DNA hybridization for rapid detection of cytomegalovirus in bronchoalveolar lavage. Lab Invest 54:26A, 1986

23. Loning T, Milde K, Foss HD: In-situ hybridization for detection of cytomegalovirus infection. Application of biotinylated CMV-DNA probes on paraffin embedded specimens. Virchows Arch [A] 490:777, 1986

24. Forghani B, Dupius KW, Schmidt NJ: Rapid detection of herpes simplex virus DNA in human brain tissue by in-situ hybridization. J Clin Microbiol 22:656, 1985

25. Ross D: Surgical pathology and DNA probes. Arch Pathol Lab Med 111:20, 1987

26. Lasser A: The mononuclear phagocytic system. A review. Hum Pathol 14:108, 1983

27. Bhagavan BS, Ruffier J, Shinn B: Pseudoactinomycotic radiate granules in the lower female genital tract: Relationship to the Splendore-Hoeppli phenomenon. Hum Pathol 13:898, 1982

28. Robboy SJ, Vickery AL: Tinctorial and morphologic properties distinguishing actinomycosis and nocardiosis. N Engl J Med 282:593, 1970

29. Vanek J, Schwarz J, Hakin S: North American blastomycosis: A study of ten cases. Am J Clin Pathol 54:383, 1970

30. Riley LW, Remis RS, Helgerson SD, et al: Outbreaks of hemorrhagic colitis associated with a rare *Escherichia coli* serotype. N Engl J Med 308:681, 1983

31. Connor DH, Neafie RC, Hochmeyer WT: Malaria. p. 273.

In Binford CH, Connor DH (eds): Pathology of Tropical and Extraordinary Diseases. Atlas of Pathology. Vol. 1 Armed Forces Institute of Pathology, Washington, DC, 1976

32. Tucker PC, Webster PD, Kilpatrick ZM: Amebic colitis mistaken for inflammatory bowel disease. Arch Intern Med 135:681, 1975

33. Pittman FE, Hennigar GR: Sigmoidoscopic and colonic mucosal biopsy findings in amebic colitis. Arch Pathol Lab Med 97:155, 1974

34. Gerding DN, Olson MM, Peterson LR, et al: *Clostridium difficile*-associated diarrhea and colitis in adults. Arch Intern Med 146:95, 1986

35. Dippische LM, Donowho EM: Pulmonary coccidioidomycosis. Am J Clin Pathol 58:489, 1972

36. Jacobson ES, Jacobson HG: Trichinosis in an immunosuppressed human host. Am J Clin Pathol 68:791, 1977

37. Beckett JH, Bighee JW: Immunoperoxidase location of *Treponema pallidum*. Arch Pathol Lab Med 103:135, 1979

38. Hornick RB, Greisman S: On the pathogenesis of typhoid fever. Arch Intern Med 138:357, 1978

39. Landry ML, Fond CLY, Neddermann K: Disseminated adenovirus infection in an immunocompromised host. Am J Med 83:555, 1987

40. Carrington CB: Pathology of Legionnaires' disease. Ann Intern Med 90:496, 1979

41. Winn WC, Myerowitz RL: The pathology of the legionella pneumonias. Hum Pathol 12:401, 1981

42. Frenkel JK, Baker LH, Chanko AM: Autopsy diagnosis of Legionnaires' disease in immunosuppressed patients. Ann Intern Med 90:559, 1979

43. Sheibani K, Fritz RM, Winberg CD, et al: "Monocytoid" cells in reactive follicular hyperplasia with and without multifocal histiocytic reactions: An immunohistochemical study of 21 cases including suspected cases of toxoplasmic lymphadenitis. Am J Clin Pathol 81:453, 1984

44. Dorfman RF, Remington JS: Value of lymph-node biopsy in the diagnosis of acute acquired toxoplasmosis. N Engl J Med 289:878, 1973

45. Childs CC, Parham DM, Berard CW: Infectious mononucleosis. The spectrum of morphologic changes simulating lymphoma in lymph nodes and tonsils. Am J Surg Pathol 11:122, 1987

46. Dorfman RF, Warnke R: Lymphadenopathy simulating the malignant lymphomas. Hum Pathol 5:519, 1974

47. Boros DL, Pelley RP, Warren KS: Spontaneous modulation of granulomatous hypersensitivity in *Schistosoma mansoni*. J Immunol 114:1437, 1975

48. Smith JH, Christie JD: The pathobiology of *Schistosoma haematobium* infection in humans. Hum Pathol 17:333, 1986

49. van der Oord JJ, de Wolf-Peeters C, Facchetti F, et al: Cellular composition of hypersensitivity-type granulomas: Immunohistochemical analysis of tuberculosis and sarcoidal lymphadenitis. Hum Pathol 15:559, 1984

50. Woodard BH, Rosenberg SI, Farnham R, Adams DO: Incidence and nature of primary granulomatous inflammation in surgically removed material. Am J Surg Pathol 6:119, 1982

51. Farhi DC, Mason UG, Horsburgh CR: Pathologic findings in disseminated *Mycobacterium avium-intracellulare* infection. Am J Clin Pathol 85:67, 1986

52. Osborne BM, Butler JJ, MacKay B: Ultrastructural observations in cat scratch disease. Am J Clin Pathol 87:739, 1987

53. El-Marogli NRH, Man NS: The histopathology of enteric infection with *Yersinia pseudotuberculosis*. Am J Clin Pathol 71:631, 1979

54. van den Oord JJ, de Wolf-Peeters C, Desmet VJ: Cellular composition of suppurative granulomas: An immunohistochemical study of suppurative granulomatous lymphadenitis. Hum Pathol 16:1009, 1985

55. VanVoorhis WC, Kaplan G, Sarno EN, et al: The cutaneous infiltrates of leprosy. Cellular characteristics and the predominant T-cell phenotypes. N Engl J Med 307:1593, 1982

56. Myerowitz RL, Pazin GJ, Allen CM: Disseminated candidiasis. Am J Clin Pathol 68:29, 1977

57. Meyer RP, Rosen PP, Armstrong D: Phycomycosis complicating leukemia and lymphoma. Ann Intern Med 77:871, 1972

58. Kaplan MH, Rosen PP, Armstrong D: Cryptococcosis in a cancer hospital. Cancer 39:2265, 1977

59. Ro JY, Lee SS, Ayala AG: Advantage of Fontana-Masson stain in capsule-deficient cryptococcal infection. Arch Pathol Lab Med 111:53, 1987

60. Marchevsky A, Rosen MJ, Chrystal G, Kleinerman J: Pulmonary complications of the acquired immunodeficiency syndrome. A clinico-pathologic study of 70 cases. Hum Pathol 16:659, 1985

61. Sun T, Greenspan J, Tenenbaum M, et al: Diagnosis of cerebral toxoplasmosis using fluorescein-labeled antitoxoplasma monoclonal antibodies. Am J Surg Pathol 10:312, 1986

62. Nakamura Y, Yamamoto S, Tanaka S, et al: *Herpes simplex* viral infection in human neonates: An immunohistochemical and electron microscopic study. Hum Pathol 16:1091, 1985

63. Morgello S, Cho ES, Nielsen S, et al: Cytomegalovirus encephalitis in patients with acquired immunodeficiency syndrome. Hum Pathol 18:289, 1987

64. Ferenczy A, Mitao M, Nagai N, et al: Latent papillomavirus and recurring genital warts. N Engl J Med 313:784, 1985

4

Surgical Pathology of Immunodeficiency Disorders

Harry L. Ioachim

The immune system is a complex combination of specialized cells, tissues, and organs that protects organisms against infections and neoplasms. Deficiencies in the system occur occasionally, resulting in its deregulation and subsequent failure to control aggressive environmental agents. Owing to the complexity of the system, a great variety of deficiencies can occur. Some are primary or congenital, others secondary or acquired. They are expressed by specific pathologic alterations involving various components of the immune system. In addition, as a result of the components' failure to respond to infectious and carcinogenic agents, a broad spectrum of lesions involving different organs is present. Infections and neoplasms are not only more frequent in immunodeficient persons, but their clinicopathologic manifestations differ from those of the same diseases in normal immunocompetent persons.[1] Of the numerous viruses, bacteria, fungi, and protozoa that are pathogenic for humans, some are particularly apt to induce lesions in the immunodeficient host. These are the opportunistic infections that, in the general population, produce rare and generally mild symptoms, whereas in those with compromised immunity they cause severe and often fatal diseases. Opportunistic infections in immunodeficient hosts are likely to (1) present in uncommon locations, (2) show unusual pathology, (3) be more aggressive, (4) disseminate, (5) recur, and (6) be resistant to treatment. Immunodeficient hosts also have a markedly increased incidence of malignant tumors. Like the infections, the types of tumors that predominate in immunocompromised hosts are not those that occur more commonly in the normal population. And again, malignant tumors in these persons, regardless of the type of immunodeficiency, show a tendency toward unusual locations, high grade histology, generalization, relapse, and short survival.[1] This chapter describes the pathologic changes associated with the various types of immunodeficiency, as well as the pathology of their infectious and neoplastic complications.

The classification of immunodeficiency disorders presents difficulties because individual cases show a great variety of immunologic findings. Two major categories are recognized: primary and secondary. In primary immunodeficiencies, various components of the immune system fail to develop. Most primary immunodeficiencies are congenital; therefore, the majority of patients are children. In secondary immunodeficiencies, the immune system is basically intact; however, as a result of disease processes or medical intervention, the host immune defenses are temporarily or permanently impaired.

PRIMARY IMMUNODEFICIENCIES

Primary immunodeficiencies constitute a large group of great diversity, indicating that they are the result of multiple causes. They can be simply classified into immunodeficiencies of T-cell type, in which the deficiency is basically affecting cellular immunity, and immunodeficiencies of B-cell type, in which humoral immunity is mostly affected. In fact, in most immunodeficiencies, both arms of the immune system are affected due to their

54

PRINCIPLES AND PRACTICE OF SURGICAL PATHOLOGY

intimate relationships, and therefore more complex classifications with multiple specific subtypes have been proposed.[2] Immunodeficiencies involving the B-cell system, expressed as antibody immunodeficiencies, are more common, representing about 50 percent of all primary immunodeficiencies. T-cell immunodeficiencies form 40 percent of primary immunodeficiencies; however, three fourths have associated B-cell deficiencies and are therefore far more severe, such as the combined immunodeficiency. Phagocytic immunodeficiencies represent 6 percent of the total and comprise impairments of both polymorphonuclear leukocytes and of mononuclear phagocytes. Disorders of the complement system make up the remaining 4 percent of primary immunodeficiencies.[2] Almost all primary immunodeficiencies are congenital, and many of these are hereditary. They are more common in males, and most are diagnosed in infants and children under 15 years of age.[3]

B-Cell (Antibody) Immunodeficiencies

B-cell (antibody) immunodeficiencies form a spectrum of disorders with decreased formation of immunoglobulins (Ig) ranging from the absence of all classes to selective deficiency of a single Ig class. Patients in the first category become symptomatic earlier and are susceptible to more frequent and more severe diseases than those in the second category.[4]

X-Linked Agammaglobulinemia

Also known as Bruton's type of immunodeficiency, X-linked agammaglobulinemia is the result of a failure in the development of B-cell precursors, probably the gut-associated lymphoid tissue, which in mammals is the equivalent of the bursa of Fabricius. The disease affects boys only and has a recessive mode of inheritance.[5] Clinically, it is manifested by numerous severe recurrent pyogenic infections, including cutaneous abscesses, draining ears, and sinusitis, which may progress to severe bronchopneumonia, purulent meningitis, and sepsis.[5]

The infections usually begin after 6 months of age, when the infant is no longer protected by the waning, passively transferred maternal antibodies.[4,5] Patients with this syndrome lack plasma cells, which are entirely absent from the peripheral blood and bone marrow.[5] Serum Ig of all classes are low or absent, and the affected persons are unable to make antibodies in response to an antigenic challenge. The lymph nodes are usually very small, and on section the nodal parenchyma appears diminished.[5,6] Lymphoid follicles are rare, and germinal centers are totally absent.[5,7] The reticulum is dense, the sinuses barely visible, and the capsule thickened by fibro-

sis. There are no plasma cells, only small lymphocytes and few scattered pyroninophilic cells (some large with prominent nucleoli) in the paracortex. Occasional clusters of epithelioid cells may be also present.[7] Meanwhile, the thymus appears unaltered, and T-cells are present in usual numbers in the peripheral blood.[8] The cellular immunity appears to be unaffected, as T-cells maintain their functions both in vivo, as expressed by cutaneous reactions to antigens, and in vitro by cell transformation in response to lectins.[5] Children with X-linked gammaglobulinemia may not survive the acute early infections. Those who survive or are treated with globulin replacement may develop chronic lung disease.[4] Late development of acute lymphoblastic leukemia has been also described.[7]

Dysgammaglobulinemias

Dysgammaglobulinemias are deficiencies of the B-cell system in which the synthesis of one class of Ig is selectively inhibited while the others are present in normal amounts. IgA deficiency is the most common, occurring in about 1 of 700 persons.[9] Autoimmune diseases, including lupus erythematosus, thyroiditis, and rheumatoid arthritis, are frequently associated with IgA immunodeficiency. Persons with this disorder may also suffer from allergies and recurrent infections as well as from malignant tumors, particularly gastrointestinal (GI) carcinomas and lymphomas.[9,10] IgM deficiency is rare and few cases, mostly in boys, have been described. The lymph nodes and spleen have hypoplastic follicles that lack germinal centers, and serum IgM is less than 20 mg/dl or entirely absent.[8] Recurrent and often fatal infections and lymphomas have been reported to occur in these patients.

T-Cell (Cellular) Immunodeficiencies

Pure T-cell immunodeficiency is rare, as it is usually associated with some B-cell abnormality expressed by an impairment of antibody formation.

Congenital Thymic Aplasia

Also known as the DiGeorge syndrome, congenital thymic aplasia is the result of a defect in the development of the third and fourth pharyngeal pouches during embryogenesis.[5] This maldevelopment causes thymic hypoplasia or aplasia, hypoparathyroidism, congenital heart disease, and a variety of malformations of the face.[11] The thymus, when not entirely absent, is small and devoid of corticomedullary architecture and of Hassall's corpus-

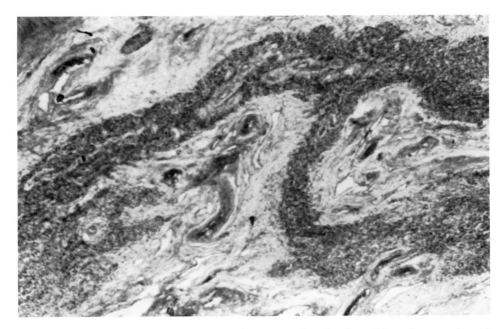

Fig. 4-1. Congenital thymic hypoplasia and dysplasia. Narrow bands of small lymphocytes devoid of corti-comedullary architecture and Hassall's corpuscles within a mass of fibrovascular tissues. (×25)

cles[12] (Fig. 4-1). The lymph nodes have follicles with germinal centers, but the paracortical areas are largely depleted of lymphocytes.[6] Symptoms occur during the neonatal period, and children die early of heart failure. Those who survive develop recurrent severe chronic infections with fungi and protozoa. Survival is too short for the development of tumors; however, a case of glioma associated with the DiGeorge syndrome has been reported.[9]

Combined Immunodeficiencies

The full development of B-cells is dependent on the thymus and therefore the two immune systems, cellular and humoral, are strongly interrelated, which explains why most primary immunodeficiencies are of combined types affecting both B- and T-cell immunity.

Severe Combined Immunodeficiency Disease

Also known as Swiss-type agammaglobulinemia, this most severe and probably most frequent hereditary immunodeficiency disease involves cellular and humoral immunity. Clinically, it becomes apparent soon after birth with recurrent septic episodes, including bacterial pneumonitides related to the B-cell defect as well as esophageal candidiasis, *Pneumocystis* pneumonitis, cytomegalovirus (CMV) enteritis, and viral leukoencephalitides related to the T-cell defect. Short-limbed dwarfism

is sometimes associated with this syndrome. Overwhelmed by repeated complications caused by infections with a variety of agents to which no immune response is mounted, infants with severe combined immunodeficiency usually do not survive beyond 2 years of age.[9] Pathognomonic are the lesions of the thymus, which may be entirely absent or markedly diminished. Histologically, the thymic architecture is unrecognizable, with almost total lymphocyte depletion and absence of Hassall's corpuscles. Other lymphatic tissues, particularly the lymph nodes, are also composed mainly of reticulum cells and severely depleted of lymphocytes. The intestinal mucosa shows atrophy of lymphatic tissues, explaining the frequent GI infections.[5] Although an infrequent disease associated with a very short life span, severe combined immunodeficiency is able to provide a favorable environment for the development of malignant tumors, which have been reported to occur in a disproportionately high incidence among these children. The Immunodeficiency Cancer Registry recorded 42 such cases by 1987, representing 8 percent of the total 522 neoplasms in patients with primary immunodeficiencies.[13] Thirty-one of 42 tumors were non-Hodgkin's lymphomas, in sharp contrast with the virtual absence of lymphomas in immunologically normal children of this age.[13] As in all neoplasms associated with immunodeficiencies, tumors in children with severe combined immunodeficiency were of high histologic grade, unusually invasive, and most often already generalized at diagnosis. They were consistently of B-cell phenotype and usually associated with Epstein-Barr virus (EBV) infection.[13]

Ataxia-Telangiectasia Syndrome

Ataxia-telangiectasia syndrome consists of the characteristic triad of progressive cerebellar ataxia, mucocutaneous telangiectasia, and recurrent sinopulmonary infections. The disease is inherited in an autosomal-recessive manner and has its clinical onset at about 2 years of age.[4] The ataxia begins as early as 9 months and as late as 6 years and progresses slowly but relentlessly to include posture, gait, and speech.[4] The cerebellum shows loss of the Purkinje and granular cell layers, while the spinal cord presents with degenerative and demyelinating lesions.[14] Telangiectases are usually present by 2 years of age, first on the bulbar conjunctiva (Fig. 4-2) and later on the bridge of the nose, skin of the ears, malar eminences, and antecubital fossae.[4,5] Severe respiratory infections with a variety of bacteria and viruses affect 85 percent of patients, leading to bronchiectasis, fibrosis, and early death.[15] Atrophy of ovaries and testes is common, and secondary sexual characteristics rarely develop in those patients who survive beyond puberty.[9,15] At this time, most of those affected also develop mental retardation. The thymus at autopsy shows the features of dysplasia previously described, with effacement of architecture, lymphocyte depletion, and absence of Hassall's corpuscles. The lymph nodes show lymphoid follicles without peripheral mantles and T-cell depletion of the paracortical areas. Later, the lymph nodes become entirely burnt

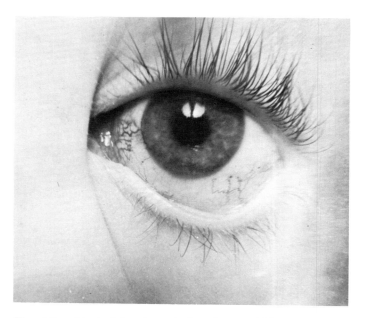

Fig. 4-2. Ataxia-telangiectasia in a 3-year-old boy. Markedly dilated capillaries are visible in the bulbar conjunctiva.

out and atrophic.[7,15,16] Ig abnormalities are also present, with IgA deficiency in up to 72 percent of cases, low or absent IgE, and generally high IgM.[10] The pathogenesis of ataxia-telangiectasia is complex and poorly understood, probably related to a defect in tissue differentiation occurring at a very early stage. A high frequency of chromosomal breakages is seen in 80 percent of cases. Malignant tumors are often associated with ataxia-telangiectasia, as with other immunodeficiency diseases. A review of 263 cases showed that tumor incidence was increased in white patients 61 times and in black patients 184 times over that recorded in the age-matched general population.[17] Of these tumors, as in all immunodeficiencies, lymphomas were the most common, with their frequency increased 252 times in whites and 750 times in blacks over those in normal controls. The lymphomas in these patients generally showed the unfavorable histologic and clinical features previously described.[13] Although hematologic neoplasms were the most common, tumors of other organs, including glioma, medulloblastoma, gastric carcinoma, hepatoma, and ovarian dysgerminoma, were also recorded.[13,16,18,19]

Wiskott-Aldrich Syndrome

Wiskott-Aldrich syndrome is well defined and consists of thrombocytopenia, eczema, and severe recurrent and frequently fatal infections. It is genetically transmitted and X-linked. Female carriers appear healthy and cannot be detected.[5] The syndrome can be diagnosed by demonstration of thrombocytopenia in a male infant with a positive family history, usually after a bleeding episode occurring in the first 6 months of life. Eczema, often atopic and secondarily infected, is usually present by 1 year of age. Later, lymphadenopathy, splenomegaly, and hepatomegaly develop, followed by otitis, pneumonia, and other bacterial and viral infections. Patients with Wiskott-Aldrich syndrome have defective T-cell function, poor antibody response to polysaccharide antigens, and a characteristic pattern of serum Ig with low levels of IgM and high levels of IgA and IgE.[9] Pathologic changes involve primarily the thymus, which is hypoplastic, and the lymph nodes, which show diminished follicles and depletion of T-cells from the paracortical zones.[20,21] The pathogenesis of Wiskott-Aldrich syndrome is related to defects of differentiation of various components of the immune system and is therefore not well understood. Children with this immunodeficiency syndrome are also susceptible to the development of neoplasia. The risk of malignancy in a series of 301 cases of Wiskott-Aldrich syndrome was 126 times greater than in the age-matched general population.[22] This risk of cancer appears to be the highest of all primary immunodeficiencies, estimated to be more than 10 percent of all patients.[10] Again, lymphomas, most often extranodal and showing a predilection for the brain, are the predominant tumors.[13] They are of high histologic grade and are of B-cell phenotype.[23] Persistent benign lymphadenopathies have often preceded the lymphomas by several years.[24]

X-Linked Lymphoproliferative Syndrome

X-linked lymphoproliferative (XLP) syndrome, first described in 1975, consists of severe, usually fatal, lymphoproliferative disease.[25] Since the original case report, in which six brothers in the Duncan kindred died of infectious mononucleosis and of lymphomas, 105 males in 26 kindreds with XLP syndrome have been described.[26] Because of a special form of immunodeficiency, males with XLP syndrome are unable to control B-cells infected by EBV, which proliferate without restriction, eventually giving rise to lymphomas.[26] The inborn immunodeficiency that makes this possible is transmitted by females and affects males exclusively. Its characteristic feature is a selective depletion of T-cells in the thymus, liver, and spleen.

Common Variable Immunodeficiency

Common variable immunodeficiency is a heterogeneous group of immunodeficiencies characterized by adult onset, in which the clinical manifestations occur after years of apparently normal immunologic function.

The patients have a high incidence of immune disorders, particularly autoimmune diseases, among members of their families.[10] Clinically, there may be bronchopulmonary infections, noncaseating granulomas of the lung, bronchiectasis, or GI involvement with a sprue-like syndrome, diarrhea, and characteristic nodular hyperplasia of the lymphoid tissue in the intestinal mucosa.[10,27] Patients have various Ig deficiencies related to intrinsic B-cell defects. One of the most common types is IgA and IgG hypogammaglobulinemias accompanied by normal or increased IgM.[7] The lymph nodes contain few plasma cells and sometimes hyperplastic follicles containing numerous IgM-expressing lymphocytes.[7] Lymphocyte depletion may be seen at a later stage (Fig. 4-3). The incidence of neoplasms among patients with common variable immunodeficiency is increased by four times.[17] Lymphomas are the most common; however, other tumors, particularly of the GI tract, are also frequent. Gastric carcinoma in one studied series was 47 times more frequent in patients with this type of immunodeficiency than in comparable normal persons.[28]

SECONDARY IMMUNODEFICIENCIES

The normal immune system can be compromised as a result of infections or exposure to physical and chemical agents. Some infectious agents, particularly viral, are

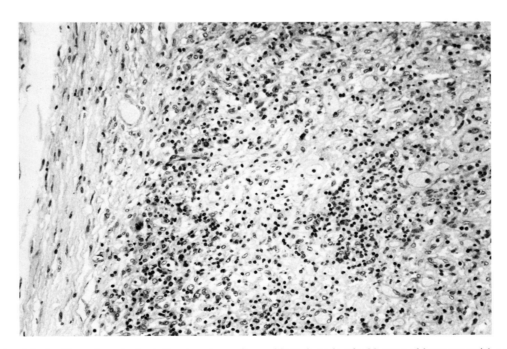

Fig. 4-3. Marked lymphocyte depletion in retroperitoneal lymph node of a 22-year-old woman with common variable immune deficiency. (×200)

lymphotropic and thus able to infect and destroy particular types of lymphoid cells, producing temporary or permanent immunodeficiencies. The best known example is the recently discovered human immunodeficiency virus (HIV), that selectively destroys T-helper lymphocytes, giving rise to the acquired immune deficiency syndrome (AIDS). Autoimmune diseases, some of them also caused by viruses, represent states of immune deregulation usually characterized by excessive activity of B-cells with production of autoantibodies that are destructive to the host's own cells and tissues.

Medically Induced Immunosuppression

Among physical agents, ionizing radiation is particularly destructive for cycling cells; therefore, lymphoid cells are at greatest risk. Whole body exposure to x-rays, whether accidental or medically applied for the treatment of neoplasia, induces immunodeficiencies of various intensities and durations. A number of chemical compounds and hormones are also used in the treatment of tumors and in the suppression of rejection reactions to transplants. The cytotoxic drugs may interfere with DNA, RNA, or protein synthesis and thus block the metabolism and growth of many cell types, particularly hemopoietic and lymphopoietic. Among hormones, the corticosteroids, which are the most commonly used, have multiple target cells and mechanisms of action. The immature T-cell is particularly affected, as well as the ability of macrophages to take up and process antigens. As a result of injuries to various components of the immune system by any of these agents, different conditions of immunodeficiency may be created. With partial or total suppression of its immunity, the organism is immunocompromised and thus vulnerable to a host of opportunistic infections and neoplasms.

The opportunistic infections are the most common complications of immunosuppression.[29] Infectious agents may come from exogenous sources or from the reactivation of previously dormant infections. Infections with staphylococci and Gram-negative bacilli are most frequent during the first phase of leukocytopenia that follows the cytotoxic and immunosuppressive treatments. In transplant recipients, the graft-versus-host reaction (which is often severe) and the inadequate reconstitution of the affected immune system further increase the susceptibility to opportunistic infectious agents. When antibiotic therapy is added, Gram-negative bacteria such as *Pseudomonas* may develop resistance and become predominant. If the graft-versus-host reaction progresses and the transplant rejection occurs, further infections with viruses, fungi, or protozoa may develop. Most common, life-threatening opportunistic infections affecting patients with such acquired immunodeficiencies are viral

infections with CMV; fungal infections with *Candida, Aspergillus, Cryptococcus*, and *Nocardia;* and protozoal infections with *Pneumocystis* and *Toxoplasma*. Combined infections with more than one agent are not uncommon. Interstitial pneumonitis may occur in up to 50 percent of organ transplant recipients within the first 5 months after transplantation. About 50 percent of pneumonitides in these patients are caused by CMV and 10 percent by *Pneumocystis carinii* (PC).[29] Infections with CMV are particularly severe in the absence of any effective therapy. Up to 50 percent of cases may be fatal; even in successful transplants, active CMV infection may persist for a long time.[29] Toxoplasmic encephalitis is another grave complication of medically induced immunosuppression. Infection with *Toxoplasma* is widespread, with up to 30 percent of military recruits in the United States having antibodies to it, but it remains occult in the general population. The infection may be reactivated by prolonged antineoplastic or immunodepressant treatments, particularly with corticosteroids. Onset in such cases is subtle and the symptoms uncharacteristic; the most common location is the brain, in which toxoplasmic encephalitis or abscesses may develop.[30]

Persons with acquired immunodeficiencies, like those with congenital immunodeficiencies, not only are highly vulnerable to opportunistic infections but are also at high risk for the development of malignant neoplasms.[1] Case reports in the medical literature and in the Renal Transplant Registry during the past 20 years show a significant increase in the risk of cancer among the recipients of renal transplants. The incidence of tumors in large series of renal transplant recipients varies from 2 to 7 percent, 100 times greater than in the age-matched general population.[31,32] The risk of cancer increases with the length of survival after the transplant, reaching 11 percent after 5 years in one reported series.[33] Of all the tumors observed in transplant recipients, non-Hodgkin's lymphomas are by far the most common. Various surveys show increases in the incidence of lymphomas from 35- to 49-fold over that observed in age-matched controls.[34,35] Hodgkin's disease is the more common type of lymphoma in the general population, while in immunosuppressed recipients of renal and cardiac transplants non-Hodgkin's lymphomas are far more frequent.[36] The location of these tumors is also different. In contrast to the general population (in which lymphomas usually originate in lymph nodes), extranodal lymphomas constitute 78 percent of lymphomas in the recipients of transplanted organs.[32] Of these, the GI tract and the central nervous system (CNS) are the common locations. While primary lymphomas of the brain represent only 0.04 to 1.5 percent of all lymphomas in the population at large, in patients with organ transplants the incidence may be as high as 73 percent.[37] Almost all lymphomas occurring in immunosuppressed persons are of high histologic grade. In different reports, they were predominantly classified as large cell noncleaved, immunoblastic, or undifferentiated, to some extent explaining their highly malignant behavior.[1] The immunophenotype has been invariably of B-cell type. The age of immunosuppressed patients with lymphoma (39 years on average) is generally younger than those in the general population with lymphoma and the time interval from transplantation to tumor appearance is remarkably short (1 to 153 months, with an average of 23 months).[36,38]

Lymphomas are not the only tumors showing an increased incidence in transplant recipients. Carcinomas of the skin and lip, melanomas, and particularly Kaposi's sarcoma are also more commonly seen. The latter, formerly an infrequent tumor with distribution characteristically limited to Africa and the Mediterranean area, occurred 150 to 200 times more often in patients who underwent kidney transplantation.[39] As in the case of lymphomas, the intervals for tumor development were short, averaging 16 months from the time of transplantation, and the tumor aggressiveness was high, with a tendency toward generalization and a mortality rate about 10 times greater than in the epidemic forms.[39,40]

The treatment of various types of cancer by ionizing radiation, cytotoxic drugs, or combinations of both modalities has become increasingly efficient. As a result, the disease-free survival of patients has markedly increased. The success in the treatment of neoplasia, however, has been accompanied by an increasing occurrence of new cancers in surviving patients. Although more difficult to assess than the incidence of tumors following organ transplantation, it has been documented that patients with various autoimmune diseases of long duration, as well as patients treated with x-rays, corticosteroid hormones, and cytotoxic drugs, are at increased risk of the development of cancer.[41,42] The clinicopathologic features of such neoplasms are entirely similar to those occurring in persons with other forms of immunodeficiency, as previously described.

An interesting new feature in the course of such tumors is the observation of their potential reversibility. Recent reports describe regression and sometimes complete disappearance of tumor masses in the case of lymphomas and Kaposi's sarcomas upon withdrawal of the immunosuppressive treatment that had been applied during the course of organ transplantation.[43]

Acquired Immune Deficiency Syndrome

Severe opportunistic infections and neoplasias in homosexual men, which are considered a characteristic aspect of AIDS, were first reported in 1981.[44] In the following years, AIDS has made rapid and dramatic progress, growing into a worldwide epidemic that is still expanding. On July 1, 1988, the World Health Organization was reporting 250,000 cases in 138 countries.[45] In the United States there were over 90,000 cases, including 600 in children. The gravity of its complications and the mortality rate of more than 50 percent have raised great general concern and have stimulated extensive research on AIDS. In a relatively short time, much has been learned about the etiology, pathogenesis, and clinical manifestations of this new disease. In an unprecedented fashion, the immune system is the target of a specific viral infection, while its subsequent deficiency becomes the cause of the devastating complicating diseases.[46]

An infection with HIV, a newly discovered retrovirus, is acquired by direct contamination with infected body fluids. Homosexual men, IV drug abusers, and recipients of contaminated blood transfusions have been the populations at greatest risk of infection. In many persons, the initial HIV infection remains asymptomatic and is accompanied only by the appearance of circulating anti-HIV antibodies. Currently, over 100,000 persons in the United States and 1 million worldwide are believed to show seroconversion, indicating their infection with HIV.[45] At variable intervals after the initial infection, some may experience general symptoms such as fever, fatigue, weight loss, or diarrhea, others a characteristic swelling of lymph nodes. The latter finding, known as persistent generalized lymphadenopathy (PGL), involves two or more lymph nodes that are markedly enlarged, palpable, indolent, and persistent for long periods of time.[47] Such nodes are frequently biopsied in order to rule out suspected neoplastic involvement. Histologically, in the early, acute stage of the HIV infection, the lymph nodes show markedly enlarged lymphoid follicles with hyperplastic germinal centers[48] (Fig. 4-4). These are often coalescent with serpentine or hourglass shapes, showing extensive cytolysis, phagocytosis of nuclear debris by tingible-body macrophages, and cellular regeneration with frequent cells in mitosis (Fig. 4-5). There are multiple focal hemorrhages and aggregates of characteristic large cells with clear cytoplasm designated monocytoid cells and identified as activated B-lymphocytes (Fig. 4-6). Polymorphonuclear leukocytes are usually associated with the monocytoid cells, and on occasion scattered multinucleated giant cells of the type commonly seen in measles infection[48] (Fig. 4-7).

Immunohistochemical studies using monoclonal antibodies have documented in lymph node tissues a diminished number of helper, and relatively increased number of suppressor, T-lymphocytes, reflecting the reversed ratios of lymphocyte subsets in the peripheral blood.[49]

The etiologic agent of PGL can be also detected in the involved lymph nodes. The presence of viral antigen was demonstrated with the aid of monoclonal antibodies in the form of deposits on the processes of dendritic cells

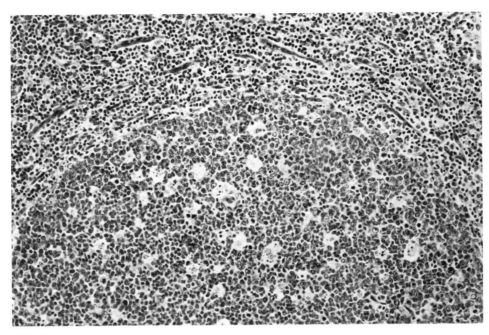

Fig. 4-4. HIV lymphadenopathy, acute phase, axillary lymph node. Enlarged lymphoid follicle with hyperplastic germinal center containing numerous tingible-body macrophages. (×200)

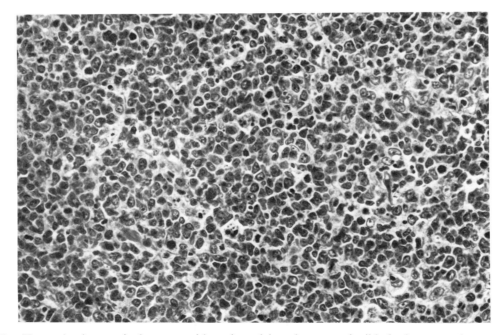

Fig. 4-5. Hyperplastic germinal center with activated lymphocytes, tingible-body macrophages and frequent mitoses; same node shown in Fig. 4-4. (×400)

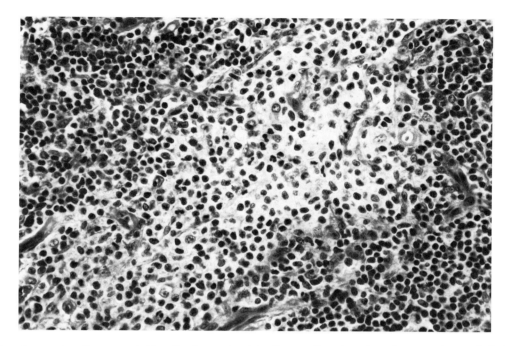

Fig. 4-6. Aggregate of monocytoid cells. In contrast to the small mature lymphocytes (upper left, lower right), these cells have sharp borders, abundant clear cytoplasm, and central nuclei; same node shown in Fig. 4-4. (×400)

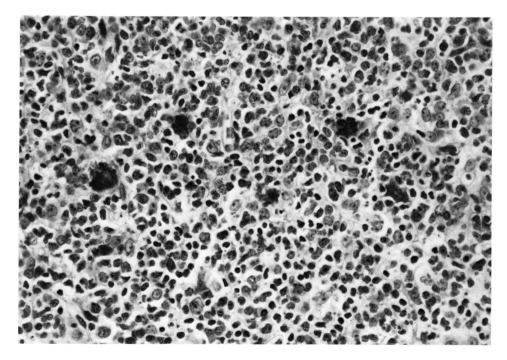

Fig. 4-7. Multinucleated giant cells with darkly stained, grape-like clusters of nuclei (Warthin-Finkeldey type); same node shown in Fig. 4-4. (×400)

and viral particles consistent with the morphology of HIV were visualized in the same location.[50,51] As the lymph node lesions progress, the morphologic appearance changes from that of an acute, hyperreactive process to that of an atrophic, burnt-out organ. The follicles are involuted and the germinal centers replaced by fibrosis (Fig. 4-8). An unusually extensive proliferation of blood vessels, accumulations of plasma cells, and focal areas of hyalinization are seen[48] (Fig. 4-9). Clinical follow-up of patients with PGL shows that a majority progress to AIDS over variable periods of time and that those with the involuted, burnt-out histologic pattern are more likely to make this transition and therefore to have a poorer prognosis.[48,52–54] Lymphocytic interstitial pneumonitis (LIP), more common in children than in adults, is also a manifestation of HIV infection, as demonstrated by the presence of HIV particles, HIV-RNA, and HIV antibodies in the affected pulmonary tissues.[55] The thymus shows severe dysplastic changes in children and adults with the HIV infection. The hematopoietic bone marrow is also frequently affected by the HIV infection, resulting in anemia, leukopenia, thrombocytopenia, or pancytopenia. Bone marrow biopsies often performed in these cases show marked hypoplasia and dysplasia with characteristic alterations, particularly of megakaryocytes.[56]

In the HIV infection, the virus manifests, in addition to its critical lymphotropism, a tendency to severely affect the CNS. Histopathologic studies show that up to 74 percent of patients with AIDS have neurologic lesions at autopsy.[57,58] About 30 percent of the neurologic diseases associated with AIDS are focal processes produced by opportunistic infections and tumors, such as cerebral toxoplasmosis, cryptococcal meningitis, progressive multifocal leukoencephalopathy, and lymphoma. The most common neurologic syndrome in patients with AIDS, however, is a particular form of subacute encephalitis that leads to cerebral atrophy and progressive dementia and is the direct result of the HIV infection. The brain biopsy in such cases shows areas of demyelination affecting both the white and gray matter, deposition of iron and calcium in vessel walls, and perivascular collections of cells that include lymphocytes, macrophages, and multinucleated giant cells similar to those seen in the HIV lymphadenopathies[58] (Fig. 4-10).

Once the profound immune deregulation of AIDS is established, a host of pathogenic microorganisms are able to induce severe infections. Their tendency is to be highly aggressive, to become generalized, and to resist treatment. They comprise viral, bacterial, fungal, and protozoal diseases, some of them rarely encountered in the population at large. The most common viral infection in AIDS patients is that with CMV. It may be systemic or localized to a variety of organs, manifested most commonly as GI ulcers, interstitial pneumonia, glomerulonephritis, chorioretinitis, and encephalitis. In the GI tract of patients with AIDS, CMV infection is common, and characteristic viral inclusions can be easily seen in routine paraffin sections.[56] They appear as (1) nuclear amphophilic inclusions surrounded by a clear halo with a

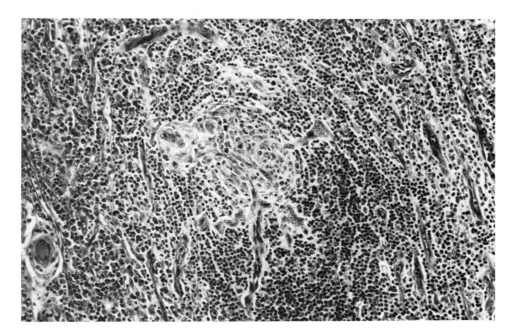

Fig. 4-8. HIV lymphadenopathy, chronic phase, cervical lymph node. Atrophic, burnt-out follicle with central, penetrating arteriole, perivascular hyalinization, and perifollicular vascular proliferation. (×200)

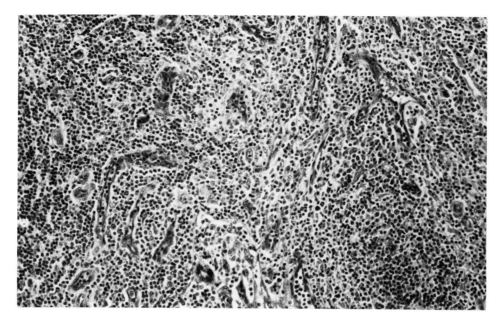

Fig. 4-9. Effacement of follicular architecture and extensive proliferation of blood vessels; same case depicted in Fig. 4-8. (×200)

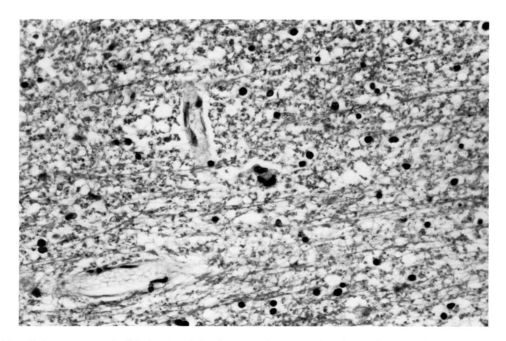

Fig. 4-10. Subacute encephalitis in HIV infection showing extensive demyelination of cortical white matter and multinucleated giant cell (center) near blood vessel (upper left). (×400)

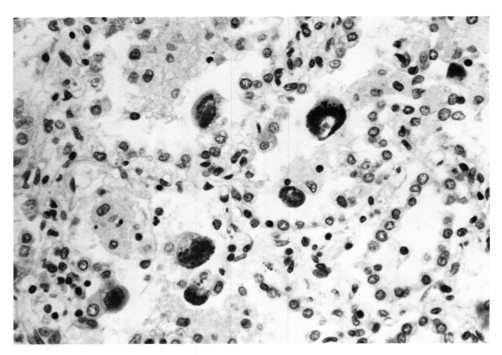

Fig. 4-11. CMV pneumonitis. Intracytoplasmic granular staining with anti-CMV monoclonal antibody and peroxidase-antiperoxidase stain of infected alveolar cells. (×400)

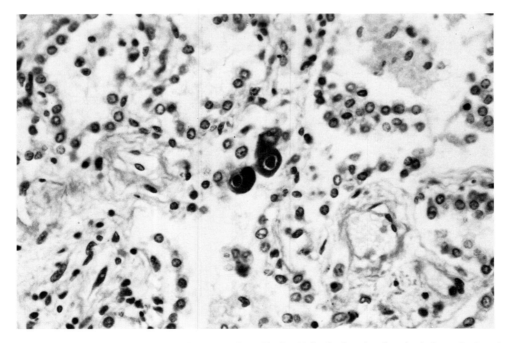

Fig. 4-12. CMV pneumonitis. Intranuclear "owl-eye" CMV inclusion bodies in infected alveolar cells stained with peroxidase-antiperoxidase stain after hybridization with CMV probe. (×400)

typical "owl-eye" appearance, (2) cytoplasmic granular acidophilic inclusions, or (3) cells markedly enlarged without clearly defined inclusions (Figs. 4-11 and 4-12). In the lung, there is a diffuse dissemination of CMV-infected cells, diffuse interstitial pneumonitis, and frequent foci of tissue necrosis. Hemorrhage, necrosis, and cells with inclusion bodies may also be seen in the adrenals, the retina, and the brain. In fact, no organs are spared from the CMV infection, which in AIDS patients often coexists with infections by other agents, such as PC. Herpes simplex virus (HSV) may be the cause of characteristic cutaneous and mucosal vesicles and ulcers. In immunocompromised hosts, the ulcers tend to be large, confluent, long-lasting, and secondarily infected by bacteria or fungi. Herpetic encephalitis may occur as a fulminant disease, with necrotizing lesions more often located in the temporal and frontal regions of the brain. Progressive multifocal leukoencephalopathy—a subacute, progressive, demyelinating disease of the CNS, previously known as a viral complication of patients with leukemia and Hodgkin's disease—also occurs in those with AIDS. The lesions as seen in a brain biopsy consist of multiple asymmetric foci of demyelination surrounded by inflammatory cells, including some bizarre, hyperchromatic astrocytes often resembling neoplastic cells.[59] Another lesion indicative of immunodeficiency described in AIDS patients is oral hairy leukoplakia. It consists of white, corrugated, hair-like excrescences on the lateral and ventral borders of the tongue. The microscopic picture is that of a flat condyloma, as commonly seen in the anogenital area; the cause similarly appears to be a member of the papillomavirus family.[60]

Among bacterial pathogens, mycobacteria are most commonly the etiologic agents of infections in persons with AIDS. By contrast, to the general population, in which *M. tuberculosis* and *M. leprae* are frequent causes of disease, in AIDS the organisms of the *Mycobacterium avium-intracellulare* (MAI) complex are usually seen. They cause a severe disseminated infection, recognized as one of the most common opportunistic infections favored by the immunodeficiency of the host and included in the definition of the syndrome.[61] In countries in which tuberculosis is endemic, persons afflicted with AIDS may show reactivation of earlier infections with *M. tuberculosis* that, like most complications of AIDS, will be more aggressive, more often in extrapulmonary locations, and more prone to generalization.

Fungal diseases are frequently seen in AIDS patients. Candidiasis, cryptococcosis, and aspergillosis are the most common, while histoplasmosis and coccidioidomycosis occur predominantly in persons with AIDS who have lived in areas in which these fungal infections are endemic.[62,63] Again, as with other infections in AIDS patients, even less pathogenic fungi such as *Candida,* which is part of the normal flora, invade the blood vessels and disseminate to deep-seated organs, causing infarcts, abscesses, and miliary lesions that are frequently fatal (Fig. 4-13).

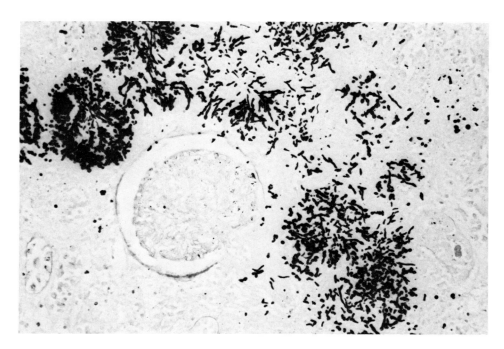

Fig. 4-13. Mycelial colonies in renal cortex surrounding glomerulus in 24-year-old homosexual man with disseminated candidiasis. (GMS stain, ×200)

The most common opportunistic infection of AIDS, as well as the one responsible for most of its fatalities, is pulmonary involvement by PC. Its incidence in AIDS patients is 65 percent, and as high as 84 percent in hemophilia-associated AIDS.[64] Each episode of PC pneumonia carries a mortality of approximately 30 percent, and more than 25 percent of cases experience recurrences. The infectious agent is a protozoan with worldwide distribution that is an animal parasite but very rarely a human pathogen. Infections with PC are asymptomatic, and occult infections may result from which reactivation occurs during the course of acquired immunodeficiency. The clinical disease usually develops insidiously during the course of days or weeks, with low fever, dry cough, and tachypnea. The radiographic patterns are fairly typical, with bilateral reticulonodular infiltrates. The hilar lymph nodes and the pleura are generally not involved. The lungs in PC pneumonia are heavy, consolidated, and noncrepitant. Microscopically, the characteristic feature is an alveolar thick, foamy, eosinophilic, and generally acellular exudate that stains strongly with periodic acid-Schiff (PAS) stain (Figs. 4-14 and 4-15). Within the exudate, parasite cysts aggregated in small clusters are present. They are round or collapsed in semilunar forms, 3.5 to 7 μm in diameter, and selectively stained with methenamine silver stain (Fig. 4-16). Cellular infiltrates, granulomas, and fibrosis are uncommon. Association

with pulmonary CMV, HSV, or Kaposi's sarcoma (Fig. 4-14) is relatively frequent, reflecting the severe cellular immunodeficiency of the host. For a definitive diagnosis, the identification of PC cysts by silver staining is required, and the specimens routinely submitted may be obtained by bronchial brushings, bronchoalveolar lavage, transbronchial biopsy, or open lung biopsy.[56]

Toxoplasma gondii is another ubiquitous protozoan that causes inapparent infections in the general population and life-threatening diseases in the immunodeficient host. In patients immunosuppressed for the treatment of leukemias and lymphomas, particularly in those with AIDS, *Toxoplasma* infection may result in acute dissemination with involvement of the CNS.[58,65] In the brain, *Toxoplasma* causes foci of coagulative or hemorrhagic necrosis with pseudocysts or free tachyzoites and intense inflammation[66] (Fig. 4-17). The lesions can be diffuse or circumscribed in the form of abscesses that are commonly localized in the gray matter of the basal ganglia or of the cerebral and cerebellar cortices. The image of toxoplasmic abscesses on contrast-enhanced computed tomography (CT) scans is characteristic, in the form of single or multiple ring-enhancing cystic structures in the gray matter.[65] The lung, the myocardium, and the retina may be also affected, showing free tachyzoites or cysts and inflammatory infiltrates with lymphocytes and sometimes eosinophils. As with other pathogens in AIDS, se-

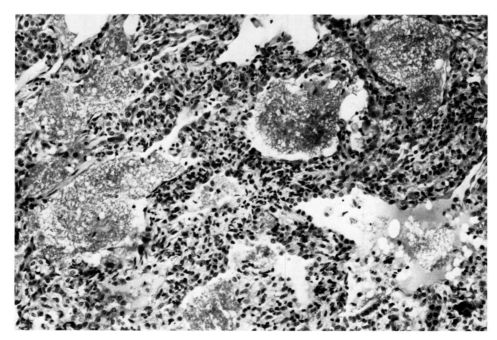

Fig. 4-14. *Pneumocystis* pneumonia and Kaposi's sarcoma in lung of AIDS patient. Alveoli are filled with foamy, acellular exudate and interalveolar septa are thickened by the infiltrates of Kaposi's sarcoma cells. ($\times$200)

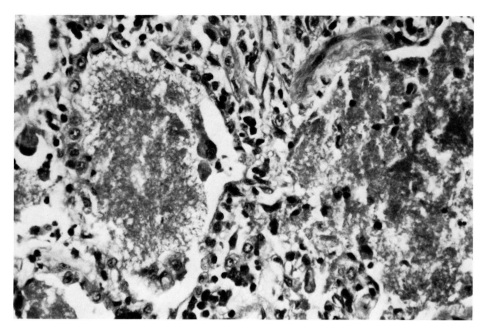

Fig. 4-15. *Pneumocystis* pneumonia in 34-year-old homosexual man. Alveoli are filled with thick, foamy, PAS-positive acellular exudate. Foreign body giant cells at the borders of alveolar exudates. (×400)

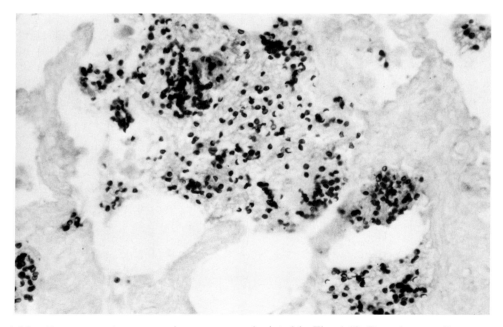

Fig. 4-16. *Pneumocystis* pneumonia, same case depicted in Fig. 4-18. Round or semilunar parasite cysts, singly and in clusters, stained with methenamine silver, within alveolar exudates. (×400)

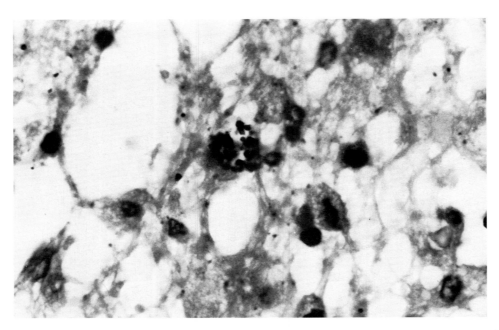

Fig. 4-17. Cerebral toxoplasmosis in AIDS patient. Cluster of free tachyzoites (center) in area of severe edema and necrosis of cerebral cortex. (×1,000)

rologic diagnoses may not be reliable, and biopsies of the affected organs are necessary for definitive diagnoses.[56]

Two GI protozoan parasites, *Cryptosporidium* and *Isospora,* may cause severe acute disease in AIDS patients, manifested mainly by chronic diarrhea, electrolyte imbalance, and weight loss. In cryptosporidiosis, biopsies of the small intestine, cecum, or colon reveal the small, oval organisms concentrated along the apical poles of the intestinal epithelial cells (Fig. 4-18).[67] In isosporiasis, saline wet mounts or smears stained with Kinyoun acid-fast stain are most effective in showing the characteristic large, oval, bright-red cysts.

As in all other categories of immunodeficiency, persons with AIDS are at high risk for the development of neoplasia. Kaposi's sarcoma, non-Hodgkin's lymphoma, and squamous cell carcinoma of the oral cavity and the anus occur far more frequently in homosexual men and in IV drug abusers, the two population groups at highest risk of HIV infection and AIDS, than in the general population.[44,68–72] It appears that the immunodeficiency resulting from HIV infection provides the background for a second infection, not only with a host of opportunistic microorganisms producing severe systemic diseases but also with oncogenic viruses capable of inducing specific types of neoplasia.[1,46]

Kaposi's sarcoma, outside the homosexual population, is a rare tumor, with an incidence of only 0.02 to 0.06 cases per 100,000 in America and Western Europe, although endemic areas are known to exist in equatorial

Africa. It is associated with an ethnic background, particularly Jewish and Italian, and manifests itself predominantly as skin lesions with a slow and indolent course.[73] In AIDS patients, Kaposi's sarcoma has emerged as the second most common manifestation of the disease and the most common type of neoplasia. Its incidence is highest in homosexual men with AIDS, in whom its frequency has been estimated to be as high as 40 percent.[68,69,73] Kaposi's sarcoma involves the skin, mucosal surfaces, lymph nodes, and internal organs. The skin lesions are the most common and noticeable. Sizes range from 1 to 2 mm to 2 to 3 cm. They can be single or multiple, widely spread over one area or the entire body. Often they are symmetric and bilateral in a linear pattern following the skin creases.[68] The lesions are of three types: patches, papules, and nodules, probably representing stages of progression. In AIDS patients, Kaposi's sarcoma also involves mucosal surfaces (particularly GI), other viscera, and lymph nodes. Early lesions in the mouth appear as macules or papules on the mucosa of the hard palate. Red-purple patches and plaques may also develop on the gums, tonsils, pharynx, esophagus, stomach, colon, rectum, and anus. The lungs may be also involved (Fig. 4-19), producing symptomatic pulmonary disease with dyspnea, hemoptysis, and pleural effusions. Histologically, all types of Kaposi's sarcoma—whether in their classic sporadic form or in the AIDS epidemic form—are similar, regardless of location. They consist of exuberant proliferations of neoplastic spindle-shaped

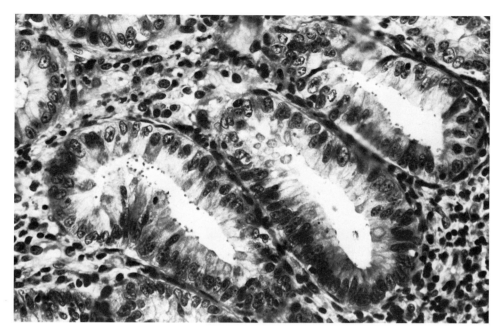

Fig. 4-18. Cryptosporidiosis of colon in 26-year-old homosexual man. Biopsy of descending colon showing three crypts with sporozoites of cryptosporidiosis attached to the apical poles of lining epithelial cells. Plasma cells and lymphocytes in lamina propria. (×400)

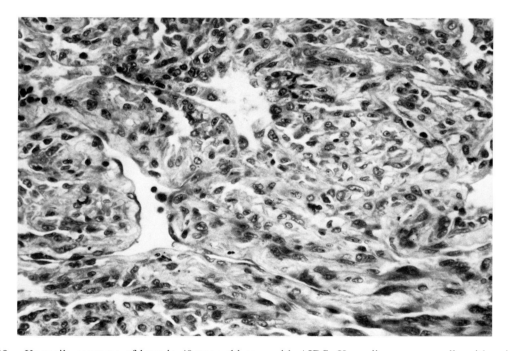

Fig. 4-19. Kaposi's sarcoma of lung in 49-year-old man with AIDS. Kaposi's sarcoma cells with spindle-shaped nuclei expand the interalveolar septa, compressing and obliterating the alveoli. (×400)

cells arranged in bundles or whorls with formation of capillary-like slits and clefts that contain a variable amount of red blood cells. Nuclear pleomorphism is moderate, but mitoses are present. The neoplastic cells of Kaposi's sarcoma originate in endothelial cells of lymphatic or blood vessels, as indicated by their selective immune staining with antibody to factor VIII-related antigen. Deposition of hemosiderin and inflammatory infiltrates of plasma cells and lymphocytes is usually associated with the neoplastic cells. In the lung, large tumor nodules, frequently perivascular, distend the interalveolar septa and compress the alveolar spaces. Opportunistic infections such as PC pneumonia may be associated with pulmonary Kaposi's sarcoma[56] (Fig. 4-14). Lymph nodes may be largely replaced by Kaposi's sarcoma. Their involvement, however, does not represent metastases, as they may be affected in the absence of other localizations. The foci of Kaposi's sarcoma in lymph nodes are not always located in the marginal sinuses like metastatic tumors but seem to arise de novo in multiple foci. Although Kaposi's sarcoma is sensitive to radiotherapy and chemotherapy, the prognosis remains poor, with a mortality of about 40 percent, due to the background of immunodeficiency.[73]

Lymphomas occur frequently in patients with AIDS and exhibit a number of distinctive features. In contrast to the general population, in which Hodgkin's disease is prevalent in young adults, in the population at risk for AIDS non-Hodgkin's lymphoma is by far the most com-

mon form of lymphoma.[74] In AIDS patients, lymphomas are also more likely to be situated in extranodal locations, while in the adult population at large, lymphomas more commonly originate in the lymph nodes.[70,71,74] The GI tract and the brain (Fig. 4-20) are the predominant sites for non-Hodgkin's lymphoma in AIDS. Primary lymphomas arising in some unusual sites, such as the eyes, salivary glands, and anus (Fig. 4-21), have been reported. All lymphomas associated with AIDS tend to be highly aggressive, to invade extensively, and to disseminate to multiple sites, including organs not commonly involved, such as the myocardium, the kidneys, and the testes. Histologically, non-Hodgkin's lymphomas in most cases of high-grade types are characterized as diffuse, undifferentiated, Burkitt's or large cell noncleaved[70,71] (Fig. 4-22). Chromosomal studies in some cases showed a predominance of t (8:14) translocation usually seen in the Burkitt's lymphomas.[75] The phenotype has been invariably of B-cell type.[71,74] Nonneoplastic lymphadenopathies associated with the HIV infection, particularly in their atrophic, involuted phase, frequently precede the lymphomas of AIDS. The potential of lymph nodes reactive to the HIV infection to develop lymphoma justifies the biopsy of enlarged lymph nodes in patients at risk for AIDS. Reflecting the high-grade histologic types and the defective immune response, the course of lymphomas in AIDS patients has been highly malignant despite initial response to a variety of chemotherapy regimens.

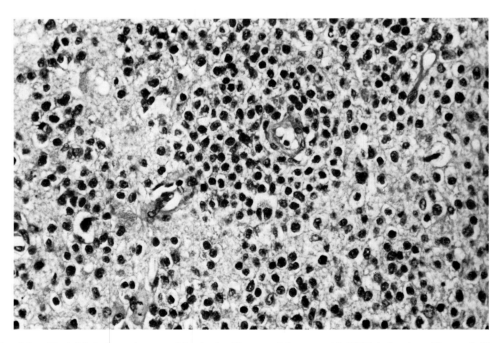

Fig. 4-20. Non-Hodgkin's lymphoma of brain in 50-year-old man with HIV infection. Dense infiltrate of lymphoma cells surrounds a blood vessel (center) and replaces cerebral tissue in temporal lobe. (×400)

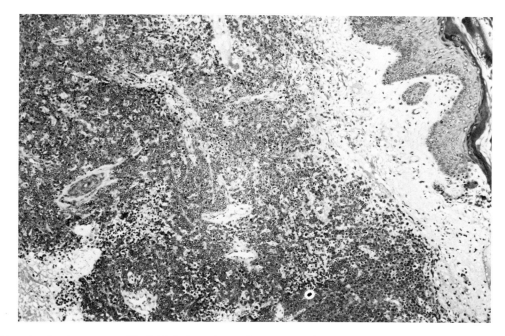

Fig. 4-21. Anal primary non-Hodgkin's lymphoma in 33-year-old homosexual man. Sheets of lymphoma cells invade and replace the wall of anal canal without penetrating into the covering squamous epithelium (upper right) and its underlying stroma. (×200)

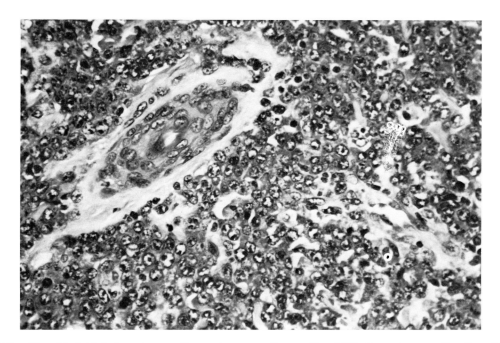

Fig. 4-22. Non-Hodgkin's lymphoma of anus (same section as Fig. 4-23). Lymphoma cells of undifferentiated Burkitt's cell type with scarce cytoplasm, round nuclei, conspicuous nucleoli and numerous mitoses. Evenly scattered macrophages with engulfed nuclear debris produce a "starry-sky" pattern. (×400)

Homosexual men at risk for AIDS frequently have anal traumatic, infectious, and neoplastic lesions. Among the latter are anal condylomas, dysplasias, and squamous cell carcinomas. Condylomas are characterized, as in other locations, by the presence of koilocytotic atypia involving the upper third of the epithelium. Squamous cell dysplasia and carcinoma in situ in this location usually take the form of Bowen's disease, which appears microscopically as band-like hyperplasia accompanied by cell disorientation and lack of cellular maturation. There is marked cytoplasmic basophilia and nuclear pleomorphism, including giant nuclei and atypical mitoses. The subjacent stroma, which is not invaded by tumor, is infiltrated by lymphocytes and plasma cells. Invasive squamous cell carcinoma of the anorectum has also been reported in the population of homosexual men at risk for AIDS.[76] Neoplastic lesions of the anus in these patients are frequently associated with the koilocytotic changes of condyloma, thus indicating their etiologic relationship with the papillomaviruses.

The diagnosis of lesions and diseases in patients with immunodeficiencies raises special problems for pathologists. The background of immunodeficiency provides a far greater variety of microorganisms with the opportunity of becoming pathogenic. As a result, pathology in patients with immunodeficiencies is more diverse, more peculiar, and more unfavorable than in the immunocompetent patients of the general population.

ACKNOWLEDGMENT

The assistance of Dr. Renate Dische of Mount Sinai Hospital, New York, who provided Figures 4-1 and 4-2, is gratefully acknowledged.

REFERENCES

1. Ioachim HL: Neoplasms associated with immune deficiencies. Pathol Annu 2:147, 1987
2. Stiehm RE: Immunodeficiency disorders—General considerations. p. 183. In Stiehm RE, Fulginiti VA (eds): Immunologic Disorders in Infants and Children. WB Saunders, Philadelphia, 1980
3. Medical Research Council Working Party: Hypogammaglobulinemia in the United Kingdom. Lancet 1:163, 1969
4. Ammann AJ, Fudenberg HH: Immunodeficiency diseases. p. 333. In Fudenberg HH, et al (eds): Basic and Clinical Immunology. Appleton & Lange, East Norwalk, CT, 1976
5. Hitzig WH: Congenital immunodeficiency diseases: Pathophysiology, clinical appearance and treatment. Pathobiol Annu 5:163, 1976

6. Cottier H, Buerki K, Hess MW, et al: Pathological considerations of immunologic deficiency diseases in man. In Bergsma D, Good RA (eds): Immunologic Deficiency Diseases in Man. Birth Defects 4(1):152, 1968
7. Paradinas F: Primary and secondary immune disorders. p. 159. In Stansfeld AG (ed): Lymph Node Biopsy Interpretation. Churchill Livingstone, New York, 1985
8. Ochs HD, Wedgwood RJ: Disorders of the B-cell system. p. 239. In Stiehm RE, Fulginiti VA (eds): Immunologic Disorders in Infants and Children. WB Saunders, Philadelphia, 1980
9. Amman AJ, Hong R: Disorders of the T-cell system. p. 291. In Stiehm RE, Fulginiti VA (eds): Immunologic Disorders in Infants and Children. WB Saunders, Philadelphia, 1980
10. Waldman TA, Strober W, Blaese RM: Immunodeficiency disease and malignancy. Ann Intern Med 77:605, 1972
11. Conley ME, Beckwith JB, Maneer JFK, et al: The spectrum of Di George's syndrome. J Pediatr 94:883, 1979
12. Borzy MS, Schulte-Wissermann H, Gilbert E, et al: Thymic morphology in immunodeficiency diseases: Results of thymic biopsies. Clin Immunol Immunopathol 12:31, 1979
13. Filipovich AH: Symposium on immunodeficiency and cancer. Am J Pediatr Hematol 9:178, 1987
14. Boder E, Sedgwick R: Ataxia-telangiectasia: A review of 101 cases. Cerebellum posture and cerebral palsy. Little Club Clin Devel Med Natl Spastic Soc (Lond) 8:110, 1963
15. Peterson RDA, Kelly WD, Good RA: Ataxia-telangiectasia. Its association with a defective thymus, immunological-deficiency disease and malignancy. Lancet 1:1189, 1964
16. Truman JT, Richardson EP, Dvorak HF: Young man with telangiectases, glioma and peripheral lymphadenopathy. N Engl J Med 292:1231, 1975
17. Morrell D, Cromartie E, Swift M: Mortality and cancer incidence in 263 patients with ataxia-telangiectasia. J Natl Cancer Inst 77:89, 1986
18. Kersey JH, Spector BD, Good RA: Primary immunodeficiency diseases and cancer: The immunodeficiency-cancer registry. Int J Cancer 12:333, 1973
19. Shuster J, Hart Z, Stimson CW, et al: Ataxia-telangiectasia with cerebellar tumor. Pediatrics 37:776, 1966
20. Cooper MD, Chase HP, Lowman JT, et al: Wiskott-Aldrich syndrome: Immunologic deficiency disease involving the afferent limb of immunity. Am J Med 44:499, 1968
21. Snover DC, Frizzera G, Spector BD, et al: Wiskott-Aldrich syndrome: Histopathologic findings in the lymph nodes and spleens of 15 patients. Hum Pathol 12:821, 1981
22. Perry GS, Spector BD, Schumann LM, et al: The Wiskott-Aldrich syndrome in the United States and Canada (1892–1979). J Pediatr 92:72, 1980
23. Frizzera G, Rosai J, Dehner LP, et al: Lymphoreticular disorders in primary immunodeficiencies: New findings based on an up-to-date histologic classification of 35 cases. Cancer 46:692, 1980
24. Gatti RA, Good RA: Occurrence of malignancy in immunodeficiency disease. Cancer 28:89, 1971
25. Purtilo DT, Cassel C, Yang JPS, et al: X-linked recessive progressive combined variable immunodeficiency (Duncan's disease). Lancet 1:935, 1975
26. Purtilo DT, Sakamoto L, Saemundsen A, et al: Documen-

tation of Epstein-Barr virus infection in immunodeficient patients with life-threatening lymphoproliferative diseases by clinical, virological and immunopathological studies. Cancer Res 41:4226, 1981

27. Rosen FS, Cooper MD, Wedgwood RJP: The primary immunodeficiencies. N Engl J Med 311:300, 1984

28. Kinley LJ, Webster AD, Bird AG, et al: Prospective study of cancer in patients with hypogammaglobulinemia. Lancet 1:263, 1985

29. Wells JV, Ries CA: Hematologic Diseases. p. 390. In Fudenberg HH, et al (eds): Basic and Clinical Immunology. Appleton & Lange, East Norwalk, CT, 1976

30. Frenkel JK, Nelson BM, Arias-Stella J: Immunosuppression and toxoplasmic encephalitis. Hum Pathol 6:97, 1975

31. Penn I: Development of cancer as a complication of clinical transplantation. Transplant Proc 9:1121, 1977

32. Penn I: Tumor incidence in human allograft recipients. Transplant Proc 9:1047, 1979

33. Sheil ACR: Cancer in renal allograft recipients in Australia and New Zealand. Transplant Proc 9:1133, 1977

34. Hoover R, Fraumeni JF Jr: Risk of cancer in renal-transplant recipients. Lancet 2:55, 1973

35. Kinlen L: Cancer Surv 1:565, 1982

36. Penn I: Lymphomas complicating organ transplantation. Transplant Proc 15:2790, 1983

37. Schneck SA, Penn I: De-novo brain tumours in renal-transplant recipients. Lancet 1:983, 1971

38. Matas AJ, Hertel BF, Rosai J, et al: Post-transplant malignant lymphoma. Distinctive morphologic features related to its pathogenesis. Am J Med 61:716, 1976

39. Harwood AR: Kaposi's sarcoma in renal transplant patients. p. 41. In Friedman-Kien AE, Laubenstein LJ (eds): AIDS: The Epidemic of Kaposi's Sarcoma and Opportunistic Infections. Masson, New York, 1984

40. Stribling J, Weitzner S, Smith GV: Kaposi's sarcoma in renal allograft recipients. Cancer 42:442, 1978

41. Coleman CN, Williams CJ, Flint A, et al: Hematologic neoplasia in patients treated for Hodgkin's disease. N Engl J Med 297:1249, 1977

42. Krikorian JG, Burke JS, Rosenberg SA, et al: Occurrence of non-Hodgkin's lymphoma after therapy for Hodgkin's disease. N Engl J Med 300:452, 1979

43. Starzl TE, Porter KA, Iwatsuki S, et al: Reversibility of lymphomas and lymphoproliferative lesions developing under cyclosporin-steroid therapy. Lancet 1:583,1984

44. Centers for Disease Control: Kaposi's sarcoma and pneumocystis pneumonia among homosexual men—New York City and California. MMWR 30:305, 1981

45. Monn JM, Chin J: AIDS: A global perspective. NEJM 319:302, 1988

46. Ioachim HL: Acquired immune deficiency disease after three years: The unsolved riddle (editorial). Lab Invest 51:1, 1984

47. Ioachim HL, Lerner VC, Tapper ML: Lymphadenopathies in homosexual men: Relationships with the acquired immune deficiency syndrome. JAMA 250:1306, 1983

48. Ioachim HL, Lerner CW, Tapper ML: The lymphoid lesions associated with the acquired immunodeficiency syndrome. Am J Surg Pathol 7:543, 1983

49. Biberfeld P, Porwit-Ksiazek A, Bottiger B, et al: Immunohistopathology of lymph nodes in HTLV-III infected homosexuals with persistent adenopathy or AIDS. Cancer Res 45(suppl):4665s, 1985

50. Tenner-Racz K, Racz P, Bofill M, et al: HTLV-III/LAV viral antigens in lymph nodes of homosexual men with persistent generalized lymphadenopathy and AIDS. Am J Pathol 123:9, 1986

51. Le Tourneau A, Audouin J, Diebold J, et al: LAV-like viral particles in lymph node germinal centers in patients with the persistent lymphadenopathy syndrome and the acquired immunodeficiency syndrome-related complex. Hum Pathol 17:1047, 1986

52. Guarda LA, Butler JJ, Mansell P, et al: Lymphadenopathy in homosexual men. Morbid anatomy with clinical and immunologic correlations. Am J Clin Pathol 79:559, 1983

53. Byrnes RK, Chan WC, Spira TJ, et al: Value of lymph node biopsy in unexplained lymphadenopathy in homosexual men. JAMA 250:1313, 1983

54. Ioachim HL, Roy M, Cronin W: Histologic patterns of lymphadenopathies in AIDS: Correlations with progress of disease. p. 188. Abstracts. Third International Conference on AIDS, Washington DC, 1987

55. Morris JC, Rosen MJ, Marchevsky A, et al: Lymphocytic interstitial pneumonia in patients at risk for the acquired immune deficiency syndrome. Chest 91:63, 1987

56. Pehta J, Cooper MC, Ioachim HL: Abnormal hematopoiesis in acquired immune deficiency syndrome (AIDS) and AIDS-related complex (ARC). American Association of Clinical Pathology, National Conference, October 1986, Orlando, FL (abst)

57. Anders KH, Guerra WF, Tomiyasu U, et al: The neuropathology of AIDS. UCLA experience and reviews. Am J Pathol 124:537, 1986

58. Petito CK, Cho E-S, Lemann W, et al: Neuropathology of acquired immunodeficiency syndrome (AIDS): An autopsy review. J Neuropathol Exp Neurol 45:635, 1986

59. Moskowitz LB, Hensley GT, Chan JC, et al: Brain biopsies in patients with acquired immune deficiency syndrome. Arch Pathol Lab Med 108:368, 1984

60. Greenspan D, Conant M, Silverman S Jr, et al: Oral "hairy" leucoplakia in male homosexuals: Evidence of association with both papillomavirus and a herpes-group virus. Lancet 2:813, 1984

61. Masur H: Mycobacterium avium-intracellulare: Another scourge for individuals with the acquired immunodeficiency syndrome. JAMA 248:3013, 1982

62. Wheat LJ, Slama TG, Zeckel ML: Histoplasmosis in the acquired immune deficiency syndrome. Am J Med 78:203, 1985

63. Bronnimann DA, Adam RD, Galgiani JN, et al: Coccidioidomycosis in the acquired immunodeficiency syndrome. Ann Intern Med 106:372, 1987

64. Centers for Disease Control: Changing patterns of acquired immunodeficiency syndrome in hemophilia patients—United States MMWR 34:241, 1985

65. Snider WD, Simpson DM, Nielsen S, et al: Neurological complications of acquired immune deficiency syndrome: Analysis of 50 patients. Ann Neurol 14:403, 1983

66. McLeod R, Berry PF, Marshall WH, et al: Toxoplasmosis presenting as brain abscesses. Am J Med 67:711, 1979

67. Soave R, Danner RL, Honig CL, et al: Cryptosporidiosis in homosexual men. Ann Intern Med 100:504, 1984

68. Friedman-Kien AE, Laubenstein LJ, Rubinstein P, et al: Disseminated Kaposi's sarcoma in homosexual men. Ann Intern Med 96:693, 1982

69. Centers for Disease Control: Diffuse, undifferentiated non-Hodgkin's lymphoma among homosexual males—United States. MMWR 31:277, 1982

70. Ziegler JL, et al: Non-Hodgkin's lymphoma in 90 homosexual men: Relationship to generalized lymphadenopathy and acquired immunodeficiency syndrome (AIDS). N Engl J Med 311:565, 1984

71. Ioachim HL, Cooper MC, Hellman GC: Lymphomas in men at high risk for acquired immune deficiency syndrome (AIDS): A study of 21 cases. Cancer 56:2831, 1985

72. Cooper HS, Patchefsky AJ, Marks G: Cloacogenic carcinoma of the anorectum in homosexual men: An observation of four cases. Dis Colon Rect 22:557, 1979

73. Safai B, Johnson KE, Myskowski Pl, et al: The natural history of Kaposi's sarcoma in the acquired immunodeficiency syndrome. Ann Intern Med 103:744, 1985

74. Ioachim HL, Cooper MC: Lymphomas of AIDS. Lancet 1:96, 1986

75. Kalter SP, Riggs SA, Cabanillas F, et al: Aggressive non-Hodgkin's lymphomas in immunocompromised homosexual males. Blood 66:655, 1985

76. Lauwers G, Weinstein MA, Sohn N, Ioachim HL: Condyloma, Bowen's disease, and squamous cell carcinoma in homosexual men. Mod Pathol 2:51A, 1989

5

The Surgical Pathology of Iatrogenic Lesions

Robert E. Fechner

The clinical application of hundreds of new therapeutic and diagnostic agents in the past few decades has added iatrogenic problems as a new dimension to the practice of medicine. The surgical pathologist sees iatrogenic changes in many different situations ranging from hyperplastic endometrium from women taking estrogen to life-threatening radiation-induced malignancies.

The pathologist is also involved in the problem of adverse drug reactions. Caranasos et al.[1] noted that nearly 3 percent of patients admitted to a medical service were hospitalized for complications of drug therapy. Iatrogenic illness was considered to contribute to the death of 2 percent of patients in a university hospital.[2]

In most cases of suspected adverse drug reaction, the diagnosis is made on clinical grounds, but sometimes a biopsy is done in an effort to distinguish a drug-induced reaction from some other cause. Since the morphologic alterations in such a case are often closely similar or even identical to those of other diseases, the differential diagnosis of drug-induced changes in the liver, kidney, skin, and lung is discussed in the chapters dealing with these organs.

REACTION TO DIAGNOSTIC PROCEDURES

Trauma of Biopsy

Distortion of tissue due to the physical trauma at the moment of biopsy can alter the architectural pattern and/or the cytologic detail. When a small piece of benign glandular mucosa is twisted or compressed, the evenly spaced distribution of normal glands is lost, and the irregular pattern may be worrisome. The problem is compounded if cytologic atypia is present, as in atrophic gastritis. Perhaps the most common mechanical distortion of glandular epithelium is seen in endometrial curettings where telescoping of the epithelium may be mistaken for adenomatous hyperplasia. The loss of stroma between glands also gives a false impression of hyperplastic crowding (Fig. 5-1).

Mechanical compression and disruption of nuclei are especially common in small biopsy specimens along the edge of the tissue where cup forceps have severed the fragment from the parent organ. Lymphocytes and neutrophils are susceptible to this alteration, as well as epithelium. The cells of oat cell carcinoma of the lung are particularly prone to this type of damage. Nonetheless, even when much of the biopsy specimen is distorted, it is usually possible to identify a few intact cells and to make a cytologic diagnosis.

Thermal artifacts are found in a variety of cauterized specimens, but they are most frequent in tissue from the urinary bladder or prostate obtained via the urethroscope. The changes are most severe at the edges but can reach the central portion of thin prostatic fragments since the heat affects the entire surface. It is sometimes possible to reach unaffected tissue by deeper sectioning beyond the surface thermal changes. The line of demarcation between the damaged area and normal tissue is quite abrupt. In one illustration of a high-power field of perineural invasion by prostatic carcinoma, one half the circumference of the nerve was uninterpretable due to thermal damage, whereas the other half had completely intact cells with good nuclear detail that allowed a firm diagno-

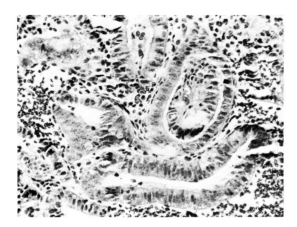

Fig. 5-1. Mechanical distortion of normal proliferative endometrium due to curettage. Note telescoping of epithelium within glandular lumens and loss of stroma between glands. There is no cytologic atypia, nor is this the pattern of true architectural abnormality of hyperplasia.

sis of carcinoma.[3] Tissue removed by laser will have a thin rim of thermal change identical to thermal changes from electrocautery.

A signet ring configuration of lymphocytes and stromal cells in transurethral resections may be mistaken for carcinoma. This artifact is probably thermal.[4]

Tissue removed by surgical resection after a recent biopsy can have many alterations in the normal parenchyma and stroma at the biopsy site. The site is usually readily identified by the necrosis and hemorrhage along the edges of the incised tissue or needle track. In addition, there may be changes several millimeters away due to disruption of the blood supply beyond the area of direct trauma. Completely necrotic parenchyma is easily recognized, but epithelium that is still viable can have

enlarged nuclei, and when these cells are set in a degenerating collapsing stroma, the normal architecture may be severely altered (Fig. 5-2). Reactive fibroblasts and endothelial cells further complicate the picture. The latter form small solid buds or cords of cells lacking a lumen or having an irregularly shaped lumen. The individual cells often have large vesicular nuclei with huge nucleoli and frequent mitoses. By cytologic criteria, the reactive cells raise the possibility of malignancy. Small aggregates of atypical cells in foci of hemorrhage or necrosis must not be diagnosed as epithelial unless there is unequivocal evidence of specialized functions such as keratin formation or mucin secretion. Even when recognized as epithelial, cells in these foci must be interpreted with extreme caution, since regenerative and degenerative changes of normal epithelium are often prominent.

Necrosis of fat after an incisional or needle biopsy may be confusing, especially in the breast. The nuclei of degenerating fat cells or reactive histiocytes range from hyperchromatic to vesicular but usually are small and lack the large nucleoli seen in reactive fibroblasts and endothelial cells. Occasionally, they are arranged in small nests or in a circular configuration that mimics adenocarcinoma.

Necrosis of parenchymal elements after a biopsy is often accompanied by vigorous repair. Re-epithelialization of the endometrium or endocervix after curettage is characterized by cells of variable size having nuclei that are dense and angulated and lack polarity (Fig. 5-3). These changes are most marked on the surface but may be seen in the underlying glands as well. The surface location of most of the atypical cells is the most helpful feature distinguishing them from adenocarcinoma. If the glands are involved, their even distribution with intervening stroma helps separate them from neoplastic glands, which are crowded, lack a regular pattern of distribution, and have little or no normal stroma between the glands.

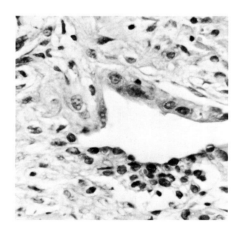

Fig. 5-2. Breast duct has cells with irregularly enlarged nuclei. Tissue obtained by incisional biopsy 3 days after a needle biopsy through this area. Degeneration of stroma is also evident. The same duct was normal 1 mm away.

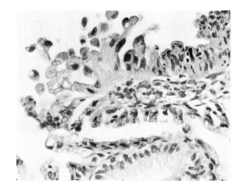

Fig. 5-3. Endocervical epithelium 12 days after endometrial curettage. Surface is lined by elongated cells with pleomorphic dense nuclei intermixed with neutrophils. Normal endocervical gland is at bottom.

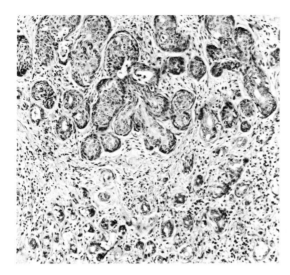

Fig. 5-4. Tissue from resection of palate showing squamous metaplasia in minor salivary gland tissue 8 days after incisional biopsy specimen detected squamous carcinoma. Degeneration of acini with loss of lobular pattern is seen in lower half of field, while squamous epithelium fills acini and ducts in upper half of field. The epithelium is cytologically bland.

Surgical specimens of mucosa from the oral cavity obtained after a biopsy may contain reactive changes in the minor salivary glands. The trauma of the original biopsy produces degeneration of the salivary gland lobules, which then undergo squamous metaplasia (Fig. 5-4). The squamous cells distend acini and ducts forming complex branching arrangements that simulate either squamous or mucoepidermoid carcinoma. The cytologic blandness of the squamous cells coupled with the surrounding remnants of degenerated acini permit recognition of these changes as reactive rather than malignant. The appearance is identical to that described in the spontaneously occurring entity of necrotizing sialometaplasia of the palate.[5] Squamous metaplasia of acini has also been described in the major salivary glands after biopsy.[6]

Hambrick[7] described the fate of colonoscopic polypectomy sites. Initially, there is acute inflammation in the submucosa, and over a period of two weeks granulation tissue covers the defect as the inflammation subsides. By the end of 3 weeks, the site is completely resurfaced by normal colonic mucosa. There is no mention of atypical epithelial changes.

Granulomas with a central necrobiotic zone surrounded by palisading histiocytes occur in the prostate, kidney, cervix, salpinx, and ovaries of patients who have had previous surgical procedures.[8-12] Electrocautery has been used in many of the operations, but the pathogenesis of these granulomas is unknown. The granulomas have been found from 1 week to 3 years after surgery.

Implantation of Normal Epithelium

Symptomatic intradural extramedullary squamous-lined cysts measuring up to 2 cm in size have occurred at the site of lumbar punctures carried out 1 to 23 years previously. It appears that the pathogenesis is the use of needles with improperly fitting stylets that carry skin into the spinal canal.[13] Squamous epithelium has also been implanted in the meniscus of a joint.[14]

Radiographic Media

Barium sulfate is seen on the enteric mucosa as chalky white strands. Microscopically it consists of fine, fairly uniform golden granules. They are not doubly refractile. Barium elicits little inflammatory reaction when it reaches an extraluminal location through a perforated diverticulum or fistula. It lies free or is found in histiocytes. Rarely, there are foreign body giant cells but without well formed granulomas. When barium is found in areas of severe inflammatory and fibrous reaction, the response is due to concomitant fecal contamination rather than to barium per se. In one case, there was sufficient reaction to cause ureteral obstruction.[15] Occasionally, barium is forced into the rectal mucosa at the time of barium enema and produces a polypoid mass.[16] In another report, barium entered the peritoneal cavity through a perforated duodenal ulcer and was still visible on radiographs 4 years later.[17]

The medium used for lymphangiography is an organic iodine compound in a lipid vehicle. It accumulates mainly in the peripheral and deeper sinuses of the lymph node but is occasionally seen within germinal centers as well. Since the vehicle is dissolved with organic solvents, the droplets are empty spaces in tissue sections. Within 24 hours, the medium provokes a neutrophilic reaction that reaches a peak after about 4 days. Eosinophils are frequently prominent, and small numbers of plasma cells are common. By the end of 1 week, the neutrophils and eosinophils have nearly disappeared, and a histiocytic response is evident. Mononuclear and multinucleated histiocytes are seen along the edge of the droplets and frequently appear to be "stretched" over the oil (Fig. 5-5). During the next several months, the material is gradually resorbed, and the histiocytic response diminishes. Small droplets may persist for at least as long as 30 months, but the node retains a normal architecture without fibrosis.[18]

Lymph nodes are often removed during staging laparotomies for lymphoma shortly after a lymphangiogram has been performed, and the question is frequently raised about the certainty of the diagnosis of lymphoma in these nodes. If the nodes are involved with either Hodgkin's or

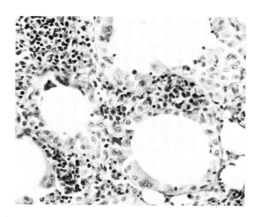

Fig. 5-5. Lymph node from retroperitoneum 7 days after lymphangiography. The dye was in the empty spaces, which are rimmed by histiocytes.

non-Hodgkin's lymphoma, the tumor is nearly always clearly identifiable because it obliterates the sinuses, and the nests of lymphoma are not significantly penetrated or distorted by dye. Even if there is only focal involvement of the nodes by lymphoma, the tumor remains recognizable despite the accumulation of lymphangiographic material around the neoplasm.[19]

The media used in hysterosalpingograms are also oil-based iodine-containing compounds. The dye may be retained, and in one patient was visualized in a salpinx 25 years after the salpingogram.[20] In another patient, foreign body granulomas of the peritoneum were found that were attributed to extravasated medium.[21] The condition referred to as xanthomatous or lipoid salpingitis is characterized by a submucosal accumulation of foam cells, and, occasionally, a history of a salpingogram will be obtained.

REACTION TO PHYSICAL AND CHEMICAL AGENTS
Starch, Cotton Lint, Cellulose, Gelfoam

Rubber surgical gloves were introduced by Halsted to protect the hands of his scrub nurse from irritating disinfectants used in the operating room and later were found to protect the patient from infection as well.[22] Talcum powder was used to facilitate the donning of the gloves. By the 1940s, it was clear that the powder caused intestinal adhesions, fecal fistulas, delayed wound healing, and occasionally led to death. Since the 1950s, cornstarch mixed with 2 percent magnesium oxide (Bio-sorb) has become the most widely used agent, but rice starch is also available, and both can produce a granulomatous reaction.[23] Most symptomatic cases are due to peritoni-

tis. Starch may be introduced into the abdomen by vaginal examination[24] and paracentesis,[25] as well as at laparotomy. Granulomatous reactions have also occurred in the pleura, middle ear, oral cavity, and brain.[26]

Symptoms of starch peritonitis usually begin in the second or third week after an otherwise uneventful recovery from surgery. There are often low-grade fever and signs of peritonitis, which gradually resolve after several days. If an exploratory laparotomy is done, the peritoneum is found to be focally or diffusely studded with granulomas ranging from 1 mm to more than 1 cm in size. Omental necrosis or matting of the fat into discrete masses may be found.

The histologic response to the starch ranges from scattered histiocytes, lymphocytes, and neutrophils to well formed granulomas containing foreign body giant cells. The larger granulomas may have central necrosis.[25] The starch particles are seen on hematoxylin and eosin sections as faintly eosinophilic particles averaging 3 to 10 μm in size. They stain deeply with periodic acid-Schiff (PAS) reagent, and under polarized light have a Maltese-cross birefringence (Fig. 5-6). Peritoneal or pleural fluid contains the granules, and the diagnosis can be made by examination with polarized light.[27]

In one patient, who underwent exploratory laparotomy because of starch peritonitis and then underwent surgery 18 months later, starch granules were found in calcified foreign body granulomas.[28]

Lint from cotton gauze sponges also produces a granulomatous or fibrous reaction.[29] Initially, the fragments of lint are up to 50 μm in width and are several times longer. They are ragged, irregularly shaped particles that are pale pink or violaceous in hematoxylin and eosin (H&E) sections and are shown to better advantage with polarized light. Over a period of time, they disintegrate and exist as tiny particles requiring polarized light to be seen. At this stage, the distinction from starch granules is based on the formation of Maltese crosses in the latter, whereas the cotton lint lacks this property (Fig. 5-6).

In fibrous adhesions from patients who have had previous surgery, foreign material is almost invariably identified, whether it be glove powder or cotton lint.[29] Absorbable hemostatics and the vehicles of antimicrobial agents are other potential irritants that may enhance adhesion formation.[30]

Cellulose fibers are the major component of disposable surgical gowns and drapes. The fibers have produced symptomatic granulomatous peritonitis, as well as other complications.[31] They are 5 to 15 μm in width and up to several hundred microns in length with twists at many levels that result in obliquely transverse folds. On cross section, they are donut-shaped with a central empty space surrounded by the fiber wall. The material is faintly pink in H&E sections, PAS positive, doubly refractile,

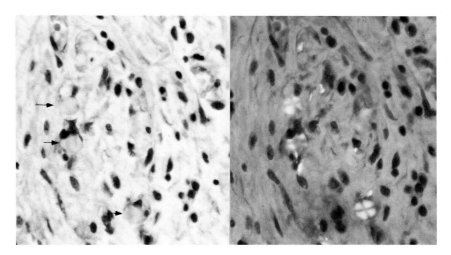

Fig. 5-6. Spherical particles of Bio-sorb (arrows) in subserosal fibrous tissue. Specimen was obtained at time of closure of colostomy 5 weeks after previous surgery (left). Identical field under polarized light shows Maltese-cross configuration of Bio-sorb. The small irregular shreds of doubly refractile material probably represent cotton lint from gauze sponges or packs (right).

and is found inside multinucleated giant cells or embedded in fibrous tissue.

Gelfoam is an absorbable material that is used for hemostasis and to embolize highly vascular tumors. Microscopically it is basophilic and has a spiculated configuration (Fig. 5-7). It may produce a severe foreign body reaction in the brain.[32]

Myospherulosis

In 1977 Kyriakos[33] reported that tissue removed from paranasal sinuses or the middle ear had small sacs containing spherules about the size of erythrocytes (Fig. 5-8). The name myospherulosis was chosen because of the identification of the findings with previously described cases from Africa, which occurred in muscle. All of the patients of Kyriakos had had previous operations which included packing with gauze impregnated with antibiotic ointment. Rosai[34] and Travis et al.[35] proved that the spherules are erythrocytes that become enveloped in a sac. Wheeler et al.[36] demonstrated that erythrocytes undergo the same change in vitro when incubated with human fat. This accounts for myospherulosis in soft tissues at injection sites.[37] Myospherulosis has also been demonstrated in the brain.[38]

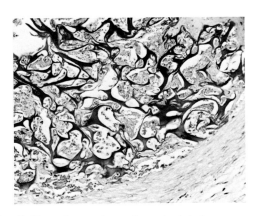

Fig. 5-7. Gelfoam has an irregular spiculated appearance. The material is in an artery injected before resection of a hemangioma in this region.

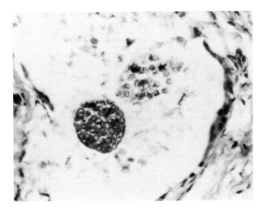

Fig. 5-8. Myospherulosis consists of an aggregate of altered red cells surrounded by a membrane. A fibrous and histiocytic inflammatory change is seen at the periphery. Patient had previous surgery for sinusitis that included packing with petroleum-impregnated gauze. (Courtesy of Thomas M. Wheeler, M.D.)

80

Steroid Injection

A granulomatous reaction resembling rheumatoid nodules develops in the nasal mucosa after injection with steroids. The central amorphous area is apparently the injected substance itself.[39] A similar reaction occurs in keloids injected with steroids.[40] Rupture of tendons sometimes follows steroid injection, but histologic findings are not specific.[41]

Oleogranuloma

Oleogranulomas (lipid granuloma, oleoma, paraffinoma) are reactive masses that occur as a reaction to a variety of oils that have been injected, topically applied, or used as a lubricant during dilatation of the cervix. The histiocytic response may not produce a clinically detectable mass until years later, at which time rapid enlargement is possible.[42] Lesions have been reported in the rectum, parametrium, and pleural space.[43,44]

Silicone

Silicone injections of the breast are no longer used, but many women still carry this substance and have symptoms that sometimes lead to biopsy. The reaction is fibrous and histiocytic. Many of the histiocytes have an irregular configuration, and the silicone produces a fine to coarse cytoplasmic vacuolization. Such cells may be mistaken for malignant lipoblasts (Fig. 5-9). Regional lymph nodes can have large histiocytes that contain silicone.

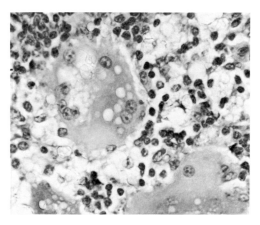

Fig. 5-10. Axillary lymph node from patient with silicone-gel prosthesis of the breast. The translucent strands and globules of the gel are found within giant cells, as well as in extracellular locations. (Courtesy of Richard J. Hausner, M.D.)

Silicone-gel-filled prostheses leak even when the envelope is intact.[45] Vacuolated histiocytes containing the weakly refractile gel are in the fibrous capsule at the edge of the prosthesis. Identical material is in giant cells in the axillary nodes (Fig. 5-10). Cases of carcinoma have been reported in patients with prostheses, but there is no evidence thus far that there is an increased incidence of cancer unless the patient had been irradiated.[46]

Symptomatic splenomegaly due to macrophages filled with silicone has been reported in a patient undergoing hemodialysis. The silicone was presumably from the roller pumps.[47] It may also be found in the liver and kidney.

Silicone lymphadenopathy is seen in nodes draining joints that have silicone prostheses. The adenopathy can occur in the absence of synovitis or malfunction of the prosthesis.[48-50]

Intrauterine Devices

Intrauterine devices (IUD) produce epithelial erosion and acute inflammation at the point of contact with the endometrium. Squamous metaplasia and foreign body granulomas are encountered rarely.[51] Secretory development is delayed by 3 days or more in about 30 percent of women wearing these devices.[52]

Serious complications include perforation of the uterus and extrauterine infection consisting usually of tubo-ovarian abscess. Inexplicably, the abscesses are nearly always unilateral, unlike "ordinary" pelvic inflammatory disease, which is almost always bilateral.[53] A disproportionate number of abscesses are secondary to actinomyces with its characteristic inflammatory response of a purulent exudate mixed with foamy histiocytes. Actino-

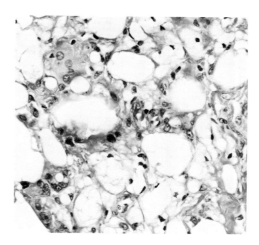

Fig. 5-9. Biopsy specimen of an irregular breast mass from a woman who had had silicone injections 12 years previously. Irregular empty spaces, as well as vacuolated cytoplasm, contained silicone, which is removed by tissue processing. The histiocytes have irregular nuclei, but the vacuolated and convoluted appearance of nuclei in malignant lipoblasts is not seen.

myces may also be seen in cervicovaginal smears, and their presence should be reported in an effort to forestall more serious internal infection.[54] Actinomycosis of the urinary bladder, not associated with genital disease, has also been reported in a device user.[55] Pseudo-sulfur granules, which are probably fragments of the device, must be distinguished from actinomyces organisms.[56]

Cryotherapy

The degree of damage to tissue by intense cold depends on the temperature and duration applied. In the uterine cervix, the epithelium becomes contracted and degenerates almost instantly. The sharp line of demarcation is only a few cells wide. Blood vessels regenerate a new endothelial lining after about 2 weeks. After a few months the only marker of previous cryosurgery is the hyalinized but patent blood vessels.[57] Bizarre cells are exfoliated for about 6 weeks until re-epithelialization is complete.[58]

Orthopedic Hardware

A variety of materials are used in prosthetic devices. The identification of the materials used and tissue reactions are discussed in detail in Chapter 14. The carcinogenic effect of the various materials has been of concern, since the substances used in prostheses produce sarcomas in rodents. The relevance of these studies to humans remains to be determined. Thus far there have been only three cases of sarcoma developing at the site of a hip prosthesis. One patient was a 77-year-old woman who developed pain 2 years after arthroplasty, who had malignant fibrous histiocytoma.[59] Another patient had an osteosarcoma 5 years after surgery,[60] and one other patient had a malignant fibrous histiocytoma 4 years after insertion of a prosthesis.[61] Between 1956 and 1980, five sarcomas were reported in sites where metal plates had been inserted for traumatic fracture.[62,63] Even if there is a cause-and-effect relation in some of these cases, they attest to the rarity of neoplasms associated with the 300,000 to 400,000 total joint replacements inserted each year worldwide.[64]

Teflon Paste and Proplast

A paste containing the polymer polytetraflorethane (Teflon) is used to correct vocal cord paralysis. Microscopically, it consists of shiny yellow particles in a myriad of shapes and sizes ranging from 6 to 100 μm (Fig. 5-11). The injected bolus becomes surrounded by a fi-

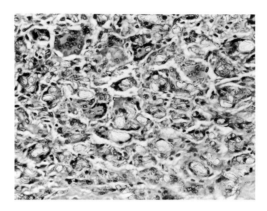

Fig. 5-11. Teflon paste within vocal cord. Irregular particles provoke a fibrous and histiocytic reaction.

brous rim with some penetration between the particles. There is also a histiocytic response of mononuclear and multinucleated histiocytes. In several patients, the material has entered the anterior neck through the cricothyroid cartilage and has mimicked a thyroid tumor.[65] Whether the Teflon migrated or was initially deposited there because of misplacement of the needle is unclear. The overlying epithelium of the vocal cord has not shown atypical changes nor have there been any other recognizable adverse reactions despite the presence of small particles within the lymphatics or blood vessels.

Proplast is a polymer of Teflon and carbon used mainly in cosmetic surgery for filling soft tissue defects. Its porosity permits ingrowth of capillaries and connective tissue, which helps anchor the material in place. Occasionally, the material may shift so the desired cosmetic effect is lost, and the implant is removed. The soft tissue around the prosthesis contains foreign body giant cells, some of which have small punctate particles of the carbon component.[66]

Suture Materials

The thoughtful pathologist always removes suture material before submitting a block of tissue for embedding. Nevertheless, small fragments of suture may be buried in the middle of the block or may be in a stage of disintegration and not grossly detectable. On occasion, a surgeon asks whether suture is present in an excised focus of inflammation, and if so, he may wish to know the type of material.

Sutures are divided into two groups, absorbable and nonabsorbable. Absorbable sutures include catgut (derived from sheep or beef intestines), collagen, polyglycolic acid, and polyglactin 910, which is a copolymer of glycolic and lactic acids in a ratio of 9:1. The nonabsorbable sutures are nylon, cotton, polyester (Dacron), polypropylene, steel, and silk. Silk is generally placed in this category although it disintegrates and eventually disappears after a period of many months to years.[67]

All sutures provoke a tissue response. Catgut is destroyed by the proteolytic enzymes of neutrophils and, therefore, requires inflammation to be absorbed. The absorbable synthetic polymers are hydrolyzed by water and do not require enzymatic degradation, but nonetheless they evoke a histiocytic and fibrous reaction.[68] The response to silk and cotton includes neutrophils, lymphocytes, or macrophages and eventually ends with a fibrous reaction accompanied only by macrophages. All the other materials excite a histiocytic response with minimal fibrosis.[69]

On microscopic examination some sutures are always specifically identifiable (e.g., catgut), whereas others can only be placed in a general category (e.g., multifilamentous synthetic agents). Silk, Dacron, and cotton are always multifilamentous. Nylon and steel are produced in either a mono- or multifilamentous form. Polypropylene is manufactured only as a monofilament. Catgut, whether plain or chromic, is a homogeneous faintly eosinophilic or amphophilic substance (Fig. 5-12). The multiple filaments of silk are of similar size but are round, square, or triangular when seen in cross section (Fig. 5-13). Each of the filaments in the multifilament synthetic sutures are round and of identical size (Fig. 5-14). Randomly scattered tiny black specks are seen both in Dacron and nylon. Polyglactin and polypropylene tend to have a glossy, transparent appearance.[69] Some sutures are covered on the surface with Teflon to decrease the abrasive effect, and minute fragments may be flaked off into the adjacent tissue.

On occasion, the inflammatory reaction to suture after resection of a portion of the gastrointestinal (GI) tract

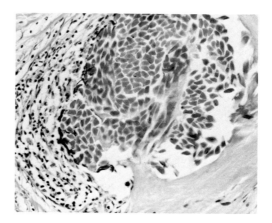

Fig. 5-13. Silk suture is always multifilamentous with irregularly shaped, dark filaments.

produces a mass sufficiently large to be seen as a filling defect on barium examination. A few patients have undergone re-exploration because the defect was believed to be a recurrence of neoplasm at the suture line or a new primary in another organ into which suture had migrated.[70,71]

Vascular Prosthesis

Three patients with sarcoma arising in the region of a Dacron or Teflon-Dacron graft have been reported. The strongest case for a cause-and-effect relationship is presented by Weinberg and Maini despite the fact that the tumor arose only 14 months after the insertion of the graft.[72]

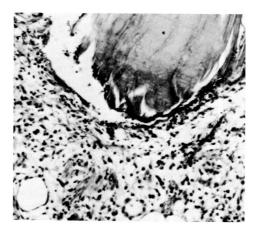

Fig. 5-12. Catgut suture is fairly homogeneous material with inflammatory response including many neutrophils.

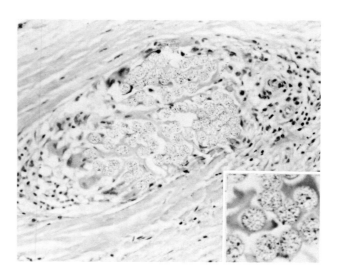

Fig. 5-14. Cross section of Dacron, which had been in place for 2 years and has foreign body giant cells between the individual filaments.

Monsel's Solution

Monsel's solution (20 percent ferric subsulfate) is commonly used by dermatologists as a styptic or hemostatic after superficial skin biopsies. The compound may be in spindle cells with large vesicular nuclei[73] and may seep as deeply as skeletal muscle.[74] If the diagnosis on the biopsy specimen is melanoma and the area is subsequently excised, the interpretation of the depth of invasion is hampered by the distorted cells and pigment.

UNTOWARD RESULTS OF SURGICAL PROCEDURES

Implantation of Normal Tissue

Normal colonic mucosa deep in the wall of the bowel was found when a colostomy was closed after 8 years. Presumably it was implanted at the original procedure.[75] Six of 19 patients with localized colitis cystica profunda of the rectum had a history of previous rectal surgery.[76] It is possible that the procedure implanted mucosa or altered the muscularis mucosae to permit downward extension of glands.

Thyroid tissue has been described in the lateral neck after prior surgery. The adjacent suture material suggests mechanical implantation.[77] Omentum has been implanted in the endometrium following operative perforation of the uterus.[78]

The fallopian tube is sometimes caught in the incision at the time of vaginal hysterectomy and can produce a vaginal mass on subsequent examination. The biopsy specimen shows tubal architecture with its normal complement of cells; degenerative and regenerative cytologic alterations can be seen in the form of cells with enlarged or dense nuclei. Stratification of the cells can be prominent.

Postintubation Granulation Tissue

Endotracheal intubation sometimes provokes the formation of bulky granulation tissue on the vocal cords requiring excision. Donnelly[79] showed that all patients intubated for 3 or more hours had denuded epithelium over the vocal processes. The endotracheal tube presumably compresses the mucosa against unyielding cartilage and thus produces ischemic necrosis. This explains the higher frequency in patients undergoing operations in a prone position, in which the cuff would be even more forcibly lodged against the posterior commissure.[80] Histologically, plump endothelial cells and fibroblasts are seen. Active epithelial regeneration occurs at the base of the protruding mass, but awareness of the clinical history should preclude any difficulty in interpretation. These lesions are not true pyogenic granulomas.[81]

Alterations at the Site of Anastomoses

Numerous alterations, including roughly 50 adenocarcinomas, have been reported in the colon in the immediate area of ureterosigmoidostomies. Some are adenomatous polyps with prominent submucosal cysts resembling colitis cystica profunda. The carcinomas are weighted by undifferentiated and mucin-producing tumors. The neoplasms are related closely to the length of time that the patients have had the ureterosigmoidostomy (an average of about 20 years). One patient developed cancer at age 17.[82] This argues strongly in favor of a causal relationship for the urinary stream producing premalignant changes and ultimately a malignant neoplasm.[83,84] Carcinoma can occur even after early external diversion.[85]

Gastric polyps around gastroenterostomy stomas have included small discrete masses as well as completely circumferential proliferations, which on occasion have prolapsed into the lumen. Microscopically, dilated glands protrude through the muscularis and the term *gastritis cystica polyposa* has been proposed.[86]

Even in the absence of a gross polyp, sections from the gastric mucosa at the anastomotic site may have abnormalities, including dilated glands and a decrease in chief and parietal cells. If there is an erosion or ulcer, the adjacent epithelium can have regenerating, immature cells with a high nuclear-cytoplasmic ratio that line irregular glands of variable sizes.[87,88] There is an increased incidence of gastric cancer in patients with gastroenterostomies,[89] and the tumors may arise in the polyps.[90]

Postoperative Abdominal Cysts

Peritoneal cysts may develop several months to five years after surgery, particularly in patients who have had a postoperative course with signs of peritonitis or wound infection.[91] The cysts may be free floating, may be embedded in the retroperitoneum, or may be attached to any of the abdominal viscera. They are unilocular or multilocular and contain clear, yellow, or green-brown fluid. The cysts are lined by low cuboidal or flattened mesothelium-like cells, squamous epithelium, or no cells at all. The wall is fibrous with variable vascularity and inflammation. The pathogenesis is not clear but possibly relates to walled-off areas of inflammation. The rapid growth that sometimes occurs may be due to osmotic forces secondary to hemorrhage.

The formation of lymphocysts is a complication of pelvic or renal surgery. The cyst contains a clear slightly yellow fluid and is devoid of lining cells. Symptoms are related to a mass compressing the ureter, bladder, colon, or vessels resulting in edema of the lower extremities. The origin from lymphatic channels is documented by numerous reports in which lymphangiography medium has filled the mass.[92] Meticulous attention to ligation of lymphatic trunks at the time of the original surgery minimizes cyst formation.[93]

Mesenteric cysts, usually lined by luteal cells, can follow surgery of the ovary. Presumably minute portions of ovary are dislodged and implant on the peritoneum, where they survive and enlarge.[94]

Reactions Resembling Neoplasms

Proppe et al.[95] described a highly cellular spindle cell proliferation with numerous mitotic figures that occurred in the vagina after a variety of surgical procedures. The largest mass was 4 cm in diameter. A similar proliferation has occurred in the prostatic urethra and urinary bladder following transurethral resections and in the endocervix.[96] The lesions appear 2 weeks to 3 months after surgery.

A highly cellular fibrohistiocytic proliferation with nu-

clear atypia resembling liposarcoma has occurred in sites in which sclerosing agents were used for the repair of hernia. Silica has been identified in these foci. Although this material is no longer used, the interval between injection and lesion has ranged up to 40 years; therefore, this lesion may still be seen.[97] Broad aggregates of histiocytes with eosinophilic granular cytoplasm may accumulate at the site of surgical trauma and resemble granular cell tumor. The granular cytoplasm is lipofuscin, which is usually acid-fast.[98]

Unilocular or multilocular cysts that raise the possibility of malignant neoplasm have been found in women who have undergone previous surgery.[99] Entrapped, markedly atypical mesothelial cells with mitotic activity mimic adenocarcinoma (Fig. 5-15).

Malignant Neoplasms

A few malignant tumors have arisen in the site of previous surgery. One of the 200 malignant fibrous histiocytomas reported by Weiss and Enzinger[100] arose 8 years later, at the excision site for a lipoma. Two additional cases, one at an amputation site and the other in a hernioplasty scar, were recently reported.[101] Whether these are coincidental is arguable.

REACTIONS TO CYTOTOXIC DRUGS AND IMMUNOSUPPRESSION

Chemotherapy for cancer and some nonmalignant conditions involves potent agents that may have morphologic as well as physiologic effects on a variety of normal tissues. The toxicity of the various agents is diverse. Much of the morbidity consists of GI symptoms, bone marrow suppression, cutaneous alterations, and hepatic or renal impairment. The surgical pathologist is uncommonly involved in these problems with some notable exceptions. For example, perforation of the small intestine in patients with widespread lymphoma was a rare event prior to chemotherapy but now occurs due to drug-induced massive necrosis of tumor within the bowel wall.[102] There are also changes in the behavior of some tumors, such as unusual sites of metastases,[103–105] or a more widespread distribution.[106–108] Whether this reflects immune suppression that facilitates spread of the tumor or is due to an increased duration of survival is uncertain. Cavitation of pulmonary metastases can occur due to chemotherapy and can be confused with inflammatory lesions.[109] Hepar lobatum results from chemotherapeutic effect on breast cancer metastatic to the liver.[110]

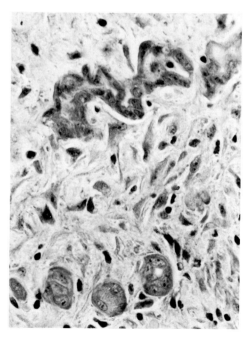

Fig. 5-15. Entrapped mesothelial cells mimic adenocarcinoma. This is from the wall of a postoperative peritoneal inclusion cyst. (Courtesy of Philip B. Clement, M.D.)

Changes in Normal Epithelium

The alkylating agents are especially likely to produce abnormalities in the epithelium of virtually every organ.[111,112] Cytologic specimens from cervicovaginal smears, urine, or sputum may contain altered cells, raising the possibility of metastases or a new neoplasm. The hallmark of drug-induced cytopathy is a gigantically enlarged cell with the volume of both the nucleus and cytoplasm increased (Fig. 5-16). The nucleus may have an even distribution of chromatin and a rather bland appearance, or it may be hyperchromatic with large nucleoli. There is usually a broad range of sizes. One can trace a continuum of cells from minimally enlarged, but recognizably non-neoplastic, cells to the gigantic cells, but the cells are more or less qualitatively similar regardless of size. This provides a clue that the abnormal cells are not neoplastic.

Histologic Maturation After Chemotherapy

Cytotoxic drug therapy may alter the histologic pattern of residual neoplasms. Testicular mixed germ cell tumors can have only benign-appearing elements in metastases after chemotherapy.[113] Many ovarian immature teratomas and a few adenocarcinomas have shown maturation after drug therapy.[114] A plausible explanation is based on the premise that neoplasms have heterogeneous subpopulations that react differently to the same therapeutic agent, with the less well differentiated component being more susceptible. This phenomenon has been reported frequently since the advent of chemotherapy, but it should be kept in mind that an identical maturation of metastatic germ cell tumors was reported prior to the chemotherapy era.[115]

Resected germ cell tumors that contain predominantly benign mature elements must be examined carefully, because they may also have small foci of malignancy. The malignancy can be present even when previously elevated serum markers have returned to normal.[113] Cytologic atypia, as opposed to obviously invasive malignancy, does not seem to be an adverse prognostic factor in males.[116]

Residual rhabdomyosarcoma of childhood sometimes has a high proportion of rhabdomyoblasts and strap cells after chemotherapy. It occurs only when similar cells are focally present in the original tumor.[117,118] Other types of soft tissue sarcomas also have a lower histologic grade after chemotherapy (with or without concomitant radiation therapy).[119] This again suggests that high-grade populations of cells are more susceptible to therapy than low-grade clones.

An autopsy study of patients with choriocarcinoma disclosed that a few patients had residua consisting only of atypical cytotrophoblasts.[120] Similar trophoblast can be seen in surgically resected choriocarcinomas after chemotherapy. These cells resemble intermediate trophoblast and may reflect an insensitivity of this stage of trophoblastic differentiation to chemotherapy.

Persistent Non-neoplastic Tumor Mass

A tumor mass can persist after chemotherapy, radiotherapy, or a combination of the two. It can be interpreted as a therapeutic failure and result in additional, unnecessary therapy. After an adequate course of therapy, persistent tumor masses that are resected often consist only of inflamed fibrous tissue with necrotic areas lacking any neoplasm. It has been reported in lymph nodes from patients with Hodgkin's disease,[121] histiocytic lymphoma,[122] and testicular embryonal carcinoma.[123,124] This phenomenon has also occurred in the spleen.[122]

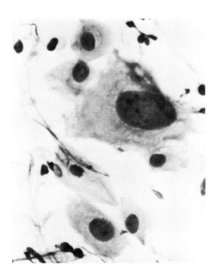

Fig. 5-16. Cells in sputum of a patient receiving busulfan for leukemia. He had pneumonia but no pulmonary neoplasm. The wide variation in size of qualitatively similar cells is the characteristic spectrum for this cytopathy.

Thymic Hyperplasia

The thymus may become hyperplastic after chemotherapy and mimic a mediastinal neoplasm. The cause is unknown.[125,126]

Non-neoplastic Lymphadenopathy

Enlarged lymph nodes following therapy for malignant neoplasm always raise the possibility of metastatic disease. In one instance, a man developed rapidly enlarging axillary nodes 1 month after completion of chemotherapy for lymphoma. The node consisted only of a narrow rim of lymphoid tissue surrounding normal mature fat.[127] Fatty replacement is commonly seen in nodes removed during axillary dissections for carcinoma of the breast, but rapid growth is not a feature of such nodes.[128]

Geis et al.[129] reported five renal transplant recipients in whom gigantic systemic lymphadenopathy developed shortly after transplantation. It rapidly resolved with no evidence of residual disease from 6 to 15 months later. These patients had received antithymocyte globulin and presumably had a transient reaction to this agent. The biopsies were indistinguishable from diffuse histiocytic lymphoma. In another report, a similar reaction developed in the soft tissue at the site of antilymphocytic globulin injection.[130]

Drug-Associated Neoplasms

Ironically, some drugs used in the treatment of cancer are carcinogenic in themselves. Alkylating agents such as cyclophosphamide, melphalan, and chlorambucil have been associated with acute myelogenous leukemia and carcinoma of the urinary bladder. These tumors have followed successful chemotherapy for Hodgkin's disease, non-Hodgkin's lymphoma, multiple myeloma, ovarian carcinoma, and polycythemia vera. Leukemia has also been reported after alkylating agents were used in the treatment of rheumatoid arthritis or multiple sclerosis.[131] Leukemia developed 30 to 90 months after the onset of therapy in 0.3 percent of nearly 6,000 women treated for ovarian cancer.[132]

Carcinoma of the urinary bladder has occurred 1 to 10 years after chemotherapy. Most patients were being treated with cyclophosphamide for lymphoma. Dysplastic lesions, some interpreted as carcinoma in situ, were present in addition to invasive carcinoma. Some of the carcinomas were of unusual types, such as mucus-secreting carcinoma,[133] spindle cell carcinoma,[134] and a disproportionate number of squamous cancers.[135] A leiomyosarcoma of the bladder occurred in a 17-year-old boy treated at age 4 with cyclophosphamide.[136] A fibrosarcoma-like tumor has also been seen.[137] A second group of patients at increased risk for neoplasms are recipients of kidney and heart transplants who are on prolonged immunosuppressive therapy with azathioprine and prednisone. One hazard is to receive a donor organ containing carcinoma and then develop metastases from the trans-planted neoplasm.[138] More importantly, there is a risk of developing a primary neoplasm estimated to be 80 times greater than in the general population.[139] Neoplasms have been reported in more than 2,000 renal transplant recipients, occurring at a much younger age than in persons with similar tumors in the general population.[140] Diffuse large cell lymphoma, Kaposi's sarcoma, and squamous carcinoma of the cervix, lip, tongue, and anogenital region have been the main offenders. The squamous carcinomas, including the cutaneous tumors, are capable of widespread metastases. Some lymphomas have been extranodal, including the renal pelvis of a transplanted kidney,[141] colon,[142] stomach,[143] and brain. Epstein-Barr virus (EBV) may play a role in these lymphomas.[144] One sarcoma, malignant fibrous histiocytoma of bone, has been reported in a renal transplant patient.[145]

Radiation Recall by Drugs

The ability of a cytotoxic drug to cause signs or symptoms localized to a previously irradiated area constitutes the radiation recall phenomenon. The changes produced by the drug are clinically and pathologically indistinguishable from radiation damage occurring in the absence of drug therapy. In most instances, the administration of the drug has produced erythema or necrosis in previously irradiated skin. In addition, recall has been seen in the small intestine,[146] esophagus,[147] and lung.[148]

IONIZING RADIATION

The surgical pathologist receives irradiated tissue in four main clinical situations: (1) planned surgical resections in patients treated with preoperative radiation; (2) biopsy specimens from patients treated by radiation with the intent to cure but who have possible postirradiation persistent tumor; (3) nonneoplastic tissue resected because of late radiation damage; and (4) resection or biopsy specimens of postirradiation neoplasms.

High-energy radiation capable of producing ionization within living cells is generated either in the form of x-rays from a vacuum tube external to the body or in the form of β- and γ-rays emitted from the nuclei of radioactive atoms that are placed into the organ containing the neoplasm. The physiologic and morphologic changes are identical regardless of the source.

Radiation in therapeutic doses injures every living tissue to some degree. The beneficial result in cancer therapy is based on the difference in the sensitivity and regenerative capacity of normal versus malignant cells. Indeed, it is the deleterious effect of radiation on nonneoplastic tissue that limits the radiation dose.

The clinical effect of radiation on normal tissue can be divided into early and late phases. The temporal cutoff is arbitrary, but "early" is usually defined as any alteration occurring up to eight weeks after initiation of therapy, and "late" is any time thereafter. Late changes may follow continuously on early changes, or there may be a symptom-free interval of weeks to many years before late changes declare themselves clinically.

The histologic alterations during the early phase include epithelial damage and connective tissue changes. Exquisitely sensitive cells such as those in the crypts of the small intestine show nuclear swelling and clumping of chromatin within minutes after receiving 50 to 100 rads. Cytoplasmic changes are manifest optically by increases in volume and altered shape. These correlate ultrastructurally with swelling of mitochondria, dilatation of the endoplasmic reticulum, the formation of vesicles, an accumulation of lipid, and an increase in lysosome-like bodies. In addition, there may be disintegration of the Golgi apparatus, mitochondria, cytoplasmic filaments, and centrioles.

Stromal changes are probably triggered by damage to the endothelium of capillaries. The endothelial cytoplasm becomes swollen and vacuolated, and there is nuclear enlargement. These damaged cells result in an alteration of the histohematic barrier manifest by edema and a fibrinous exudate. A patchy fibrous reaction ensues, and the combination of collagen and persisting fibrin produces eosinophilic hyalinized areas. Ultrastructurally, the hyalinized areas are a mixture of collagen bundles and cytoplasmic fragments that are cemented together by an amorphous finely granular protein substance. Large fibroblasts are often conspicuous, with proportionately enlarged nuclei that are either vesicular or hyperchromatic. Sometimes fibroblasts stand out due to basophilia secondary to abundant rough endoplasmic reticulum. Occasionally, there are angulated tapering cytoplasmic projections, which have been called swallow-tail fibroblasts or radiation fibroblasts (Fig. 5-17). Fibroblasts with this appearance are not found exclusively in irradiated tissue, however. Areas of intense inflammation due to any cause may have bizarre fibroblasts, especially when infection is present. There is nothing pathognomonic for radiation damage.[149]

Endothelial damage is also seen in arterioles and muscular arteries but apparently does not acutely affect their function because of the large lumen. Within several weeks, however, intimal and medial fibrosis or hyalinization may drastically alter the configuration of the muscular arteries, and rarely there is an intimal accumulation of foam cells, which compromises the lumen (Figs. 5-18 to 5-20). The changes along the course of a vessel may be spotty so in any one tissue section relatively few sites of vascular damage are seen even though extensive connec-

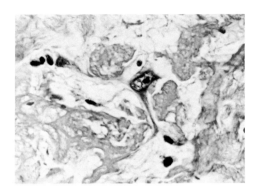

Fig. 5-17. Greatly enlarged fibroblasts with long cytoplasmic processes are typical, but not pathognomonic, of radiation damage. The stroma shows the splotchy, amorphous, hyalinized stroma characteristic of radiation effect.

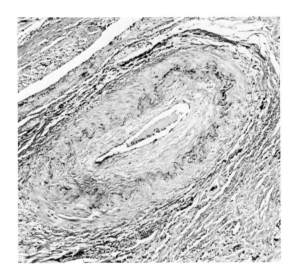

Fig. 5-18. Artery from soft tissue of neck 1 year after patient received 6,000 rads. The internal elastica is discontinuous, there is intimal fibrous thickening, and the adventitia is fibrotic.

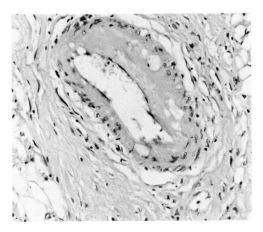

Fig. 5-19. Small artery with vacuolated and hyalinized media. This can be either an early or late radiation change.

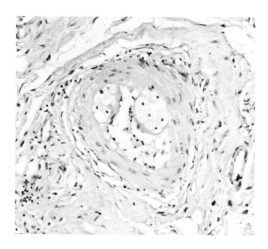

Fig. 5-20. Intimal foam cells are covered with endothelium. The change can be found at the completion of radiotherapy (as in this case) or can be seen many years later.

tive tissue changes are evident. Arteries are affected far more often than veins, except for the unique sensitivity of hepatic veins.

Traditionally, late radiation damage has been attributed to progressive arterial sclerosis accompanied by stromal fibrosis. Epithelial changes such as ulceration of the rectum or skin are considered secondary to vascular insufficiency rather than a persisting direct effect on the epithelial cells per se. The compromised vasculature presumably makes an irradiated tissue permanently susceptible to devastating damage if it becomes infected or is traumatized.[150]

Effect on Neoplasms

The effect of radiation on the gross and microscopic appearance of a tumor is unpredictable. For example, if two laryngeal squamous cancers with the same histologic pattern and clinical stage of the disease are given preoperative radiation, one tumor may be completely absent in the resected specimen, whereas the other persists and is identical to the original biopsy. More often, the tumor is altered, with the most frequent change being necrosis. Intact tumor cells, however, can undergo nuclear and cytoplasmic enlargement similar to that seen in normal epithelium. Sometimes, the cells assume gigantic size with grotesquely shaped, densely hyperchromatic nuclei. The tumor pattern or degree of differentiation may be altered. Squamous carcinoma frequently has more keratin in the postirradiated tumor, which may or may not be associated with intact tumor cells.[151] This phenomenon probably reflects the sensitivity of poorly differentiated

(immature) cells to radiation, whereas postmitotic cells are capable of maturing and carrying out specialized functions before dying.

Generally, residual adenocarcinoma is histologically unchanged. This has been especially well documented for endometrial and prostatic carcinoma.[152,153] Occasionally, however, the malignant cells have grotesque cytologic features with gigantic nuclei and a degree of pleomorphism far greater than the original tumor (Fig. 5-21).

Squamous metaplasia has been described in adenocarcinomas of the breast and endometrium and in oat cell carcinoma of the lung after irradiation.[154] However, squamous metaplasia can be seen in nonirradiated tumors of these types, and one must raise the question of sampling deficiencies in the small amounts of tissue available before irradiation. In an extensive study of irradiated uteri, Silverberg and DeGiorgi[152] found that squamous elements were first seen after irradiation in five cases, but in three others the squamous elements were noted in sections of the initial biopsy specimen and not in sections of the uterus after hysterectomy. They concluded that this was more likely a result of sampling variation than a direct effect of irradiation.

Transitional cell carcinomas of the urinary bladder tend to have more nuclear pleomorphism after irradiation, whereas carcinoma in situ is not altered. Squamous differentiation in the carcinoma has been described, but raises the same questions as described above.[155]

Residual carcinoma in a specimen resected as part of a combined radiotherapeutic and surgical approach is not unexpected because of the short interval between completion of radiotherapy and surgery. The prognostic sig-

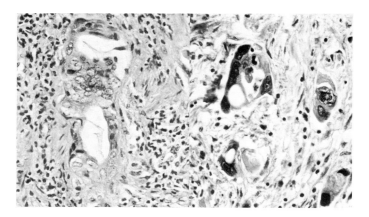

Fig. 5-21. Well differentiated adenocarcinoma of prostate before irradiation (left). Immediately after the conclusion of 5,500 rads, the tumor in the resected specimen showed bizarre nuclei and minimal formation of lumens (right). The postirradiation section came from the immediate area of the original biopsy, and none of the residual tumor resembled the preradiation pattern.

nificance of residual tumor is frequently raised, but there are few data to answer this question. Residual carcinoma of the endometrium does not seem to adversely affect the prognosis if the tumor is in a favorable stage, namely, confined to the endometrium.[152] For laryngeal carcinoma, patients without residual tumor have a better survival, but this again probably correlates with a more favorable initial clinical stage.[156]

A far more perplexing problem arises when intact tumor cells are found in tissue from a patient irradiated for cure and for whom surgery was not planned. What is the reproductive capacity of these cells? Intact tumor cells with normal staining characteristics must be sufficiently metabolically active to maintain their appearance. Nonetheless, this intactness does not assure their capability for completing the next cell division or the one after that. Suit and Gallager[157] showed that irradiated tumor samples histologically identical to the original tumor failed to grow when transplanted into other animals, whereas nonirradiated samples of the tumor grew when transplanted. Viability as measured by histologically intact cells is not to be equated with further growth potential. This has been demonstrated in uteri removed after irradiation[152] and in serial biopsies of patients with prostatic carcinoma who have been radiated.[153] Thus, the pathologist should limit his interpretation of tumor cells to the observation that "morphologically intact tumor cells are present," because an accurate prediction of future growth cannot be made. As a rule of thumb, however, one might assume that the presence of intact tumor cells more than 6 months after completion of radiotherapy is evidence of a radioresistant tumor capable of further cell division, particularly when this is accompanied by clinical evidence of persistent tumor.

The problem of persistent tumor after irradiation for cure comes up most often in squamous cancers of the head and neck. Some carcinomas of the larynx undergo regression accompanied by mucosal healing, but edema continues to be present at the site of the tumor. The difficulty in finding carcinoma in biopsy specimens from the edematous area is frustrating. Goldman et al.[158] found that tumor in postradiation resected specimens often consisted only of scattered microscopic foci less than 0.5 mm in diameter. Furthermore, when the mucosa is intact, the tumor will not be reached, unless there is a deep biopsy. Even in the absence of tumor in a biopsy, progressive edema 3 to 6 months after radiation therapy may be an indication for surgical resection. Tumor will be found in almost all these resection specimens.[159,160]

Paradoxically, cutaneous metastases may be sharply confined to the field of previous irradiation. This may be due to increased vasculature secondary to the radiation.[161] The effects on normal tissues that are commonly irradiated will now be considered.

Skin and Mucous Membranes

The early phase of radiation dermatitis is occasionally seen when skin is excised en bloc after preoperative radiotherapy. The epidermis and dermis are edematous, and the capillaries are dilated and lined by swollen endothelial cells. The cells of the pilosebaceous apparatus and sweat glands may be enlarged or focally necrotic.

In the late phase, the epidermis is atrophic in some areas and acanthotic in others. Hyperkeratosis is common. Atypical nuclei and individual cell keratinization are similar to those seen in solar keratosis. The dermal collagen bundles are swollen and often hyalinized, with variable staining. Fibrocytes associated with "new" collagen are irregularly distributed. The capillaries are usually ectatic and appear to be held rigidly open by the dense stroma about them. The pilosebaceous apparatus is usually absent altogether, but sweat glands may persist. Inflammation is negligible unless the skin is ulcerated.[162] Mucous membranes show the same changes as the skin except for damage to the minor salivary glands in place of the skin appendages.

Salivary Glands

The acute effect of radiation on salivary glands is manifest clinically by mucositis, and microscopically there is distention of the ducts and acini with secretions. By the end of a course of radiation therapy, however, the lobular architecture is destroyed because of a loss of acini and a chronic inflammatory infiltrate. Ducts and acini may contain cells with enlarged nuclei (two to three times normal size), which may be either vesicular or hyperchromatic (Fig. 5-22). Fibrous tissue is increased particularly within the lobules, but the broad bands of fibrosis seen in cases of obstruction are not attained.[163] It was also found that intralobular fat persisted in irradiated glands, whereas it

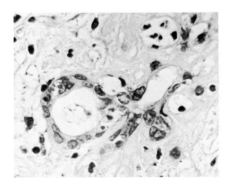

Fig. 5-22. Salivary gland at completion of 5,800 rads of therapy for carcinoma of the oral cavity. Most acini are destroyed, and the remaining cells have pleomorphic nuclei.

was absent in glands with obstructive disease. The epithelium of both ducts and acini may be partly replaced by squamous epithelium, and, occasionally, it irregularly distends the ducts and acini to a point where they may be confused with squamous carcinoma.[164] This may be particularly problematic if an enlarged, hard submandibular gland is removed because it is thought to be a lymph node with metastases.

Intestine

Either the small or large intestine may require surgical intervention for late radiation damage, which may appear within a few months after completion of therapy or may not be seen until more than 10 years later. Radiation enterocolitis manifests symptoms of obstruction due to a narrowed segment that ranges from 0.5 to 5 cm in length but is usually 1.5 to 2 cm long. Lesser degrees of edema and fibrosis extend away for 3 to 4 cm. The mucosa is usually ulcerated, but there may be partial re-epithelialization. Vascular damage is spotty but is invariably

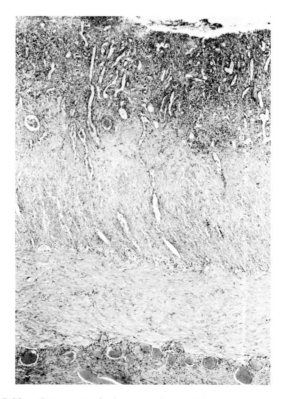

Fig. 5-23. Segment of obstructed small intestine removed 4 years after radiotherapy for carcinoma of cervix. The stenotic segment has ulcerated mucosa, greatly thickened and fibrotic submucosa, focal necrosis and fibrosis of the circular muscle layer, a normal longitudinal muscle layer, and serosal fibrosis with ectatic vessels.

present both within the bowel wall and the adjacent mesentery. The circular muscular layer is particularly susceptible to destruction and fibrous replacement, whereas the outer longitudinal layer is almost always spared (Fig. 5-23). Since radiation damage is a progressive, continuing process, there is also edema and inflammation.[165]

Colonic glands may be located in the muscularis as a late change. The epithelium of the glands is normal or atrophic, and its appearance is identical to that seen in colitis cystica profunda.[166]

Modest doses (2,000 to 2,500 rads) of preoperative radiation produce marked atypia in non-neoplastic colonic mucosa. The changes are not permanent, since biopsy specimens from colostomy sites after 2 months do not show the change even though the line of resection had atypia at the time of the operation.[167] Similar cytologic changes plus villous atrophy occur in the small intestinal mucosa. Doses as low as 1,000 rads produce severe but transient alterations.

Liver

Radiation damage to the liver is unique because the major site of vascular injury is to veins, namely, the small radicles of the hepatic venous system. Sclerosis of the portal vein is rare, and arterial lesions have not been reported.[168] The central veins and small sublobular hepatic veins undergo an intimal thickening that is unrelated to overt thrombosis.

Kidney

Radiation damage to the glomeruli, tubules, and vessels of the kidney is not accompanied by much inflammation, and, therefore, the term radiation nephropathy is preferable to the more widely used term radiation nephritis. Luxton and Kunkler[169] followed 54 patients up to 12 years and grouped them into five major clinical groups: (1) acute radiation nephropathy; (2) chronic radiation nephropathy; (3) asymptomatic proteinuria; (4) benign hypertension; (5) malignant hypertension. From a morphologic viewpoint, Mostofi[170] divided radiation changes into four categories that serve to emphasize the different changes that are seen in the clinical groups. These categories are (1) mild sclerosing nephrosis; (2) severe sclerosing nephrosis with mild to severe nephrosclerosis; (3) mild to severe sclerosing nephrosis with hypertensive necrotizing vasculitis; and (4) nephroglomerulosis. Sclerosing nephrosis consists of small or collapsed tubules intermixed with interstitial fibrosis (Fig. 5-24). Nephroglomerulosis is predominantly a glomerular affliction, and in contrast to most cases in the other groups, it

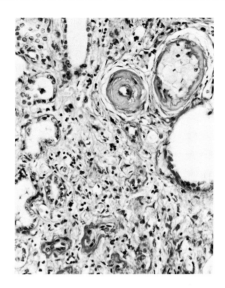

Fig. 5-24. Sclerosing nephrosis secondary to radiation consists of atrophic tubules separated by fibrous tissue. A markedly hyalinized arteriole is present, as well as an artery with intimal foam cells. The patient had been irradiated 10 years previously for testicular carcinoma.

begins within 3 to 12 months after irradiation. The dominant change is in the glomeruli, almost all of which have decreased lobulation and thickening of the capillary walls simulating membranous glomerulonephritis. By electron microscopy disruption of hypertrophic endothelial and epithelial cells from the basement membrane is seen.[171] In a few instances, the affected zone has been sharply demarcated, and the remainder of the kidney was normal, presumably because only a portion of the kidney was lying in the field of radiation. This possibility must be kept in mind because of the potential for sampling error at the time of needle biopsy.

Urinary Bladder

Transitional epithelium is readily damaged by radiation, and almost all patients will exfoliate abnormal cells whether the therapy is directed to a primary cancer of the bladder or an adjacent organ. The cells are enlarged and the cytoplasm is often vacuolated.[172] Nuclei are enlarged more or less in proportion to the cytoplasmic increase and tend to be multiple. These alterations disappear within two months after completion of therapy in virtually every patient.[173] Abnormal cells noted beyond that time can be evaluated using standard criteria. The presence of malignant-appearing cells in transitional epithelium from a patient who has been irradiated for primary bladder carcinoma probably reflects radioresistant invasive carcinoma or carcinoma in situ. The latter is a likely

source for the later development of invasive carcinoma.[173,174]

The rich vasculature of the bladder and its abundant submucosal connective tissue renders this organ susceptible to late complications of radiation. Approximately 1 to 3 percent of long-term survivors will develop chronic devastating damage to the bladder in the form of deep ulceration, fibrotic contraction, or fistula formation in the absence of tumor.

Prostate

Biopsies of men whose prostatic carcinoma has been radiated often show squamous metaplasia with marked cytologic atypia in the nonneoplastic glands, larger prostatic ducts, and prostatic urethra. In other glands, necrotic epithelium exposes corpora amylacea to the stroma, eliciting a giant cell reaction. The seminal vesicles become atrophic and fibrotic.[175]

Uterus

Intracavitary radiation for endometrial carcinoma produces changes in the cervix, endometrium, and myometrium. The squamous lining of the exocervix is often obliterated, and only a fibrinous exudate lies on the surface. The endocervical epithelium may be pleomorphic, with either hyperchromatic or vacuolated nuclei that frequently lie in the middle or luminal end of the cell. Mucin is diminished. The distinction from adenocarcinoma involving the endocervix is readily made because, despite their cytologic changes, the glands are normally spaced.

Nuclear and cytoplasmic alterations are especially common in the endometrium treated with intracavitary radium. Markedly abnormal cells are found not only in the endometrium but in foci of adenomyosis. The latter might be diagnosed incorrectly as invasive adenocarcinoma. Misinterpretation can be avoided by knowing that residual endometrial adenocarcinoma characteristically shows little change when compared with preoperative biopsy material,[152] whereas the nonneoplastic endometrium is severely altered. The epithelium forms an irregular layer one to four cells thick with some cells protruding above the surface and attached to the epithelial lining only by a thin strand of cytoplasm (see Fig. 5-25). Most cells are greatly enlarged and have a polygonal, round, or extremely attenuated shape rather than the normal cuboidal or low columnar configuration. The cytoplasm ranges from a powdery ground-glass appearance through a finely or coarsely eosinophilic granularity. Vacuolization is present in some cells as either tiny droplets or large vacuoles. Nuclei are occasionally normal, but most are en-

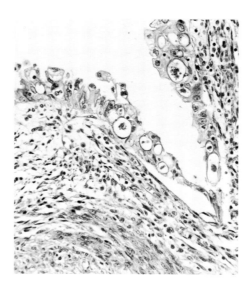

Fig. 5-25. Focus of adenomyosis after intracavitary radium therapy for endometrial carcinoma. The epithelium is stratified, and a few cells are attached only by a strand of cytoplasm. Many cells are vacuolated, and there is nuclear pleomorphism. The endometrial stroma beneath the epithelium is edematous and inflamed, but the stromal cells are not atypical. Normal myometrium is at the bottom of the field.

larged and may be round, angulated, or have an irregular contour due to numerous folds and convolutions. Small nucleoli are frequent. The endometrial stromal cells do not undergo these cytologic changes although there is invariably inflammation and edema. Thus, the presence of bizarre endometrial cells adjacent to endometrial stromal cells is virtual proof that the epithelial cells are non-neoplastic. In rare cases, myometrial cells are enlarged and vacuolated after intracavitary radiation.[176]

Thyroid

Numerous changes are found in the thyroid, including colloid nodules with foci of hyperplasia identical to those seen in nonirradiated thyroid. Small foci of hyperplasia are also scattered throughout the parenchyma with the columnar cells forming small tufts. Occasionally, a nodule is composed of small fingers of thyroid tissue forming tiny lumens. Large, dense nuclei may be found either in hyperplastic nodules or within individual follicles. Oxyphilic cells are frequent and are often associated with a lymphocytic infiltrate.[177]

Many nodules have been classified as adenomas, since they have a trabecular pattern. When nuclear abnormalities are superimposed, the possibility of carcinoma is raised. In the absence of invasion, such nodules are probably best considered atypical adenomas.[178]

Breast

Patients treated for breast cancer with primary radiation therapy may subsequently develop clinical or mammographic abnormalities that are biopsied. In some instances, fat necrosis has mimicked a primary tumor on physical examination. It may be located near the biopsy site and may result in fixation of the skin.[179] The most characteristic radiation affect is the presence of atypical epithelial cells in the terminal duct/lobular unit, accompanied by atrophy and lobular fibrosis. Occasionally, epithelial atypia is seen in larger ducts.[180]

RADIATION-ASSOCIATED TUMORS

Tumors associated with radiation have occurred in patients receiving high-dose therapy for malignancy, low-dose therapy for benign conditions, multiple diagnostic exposure, and internal radiation due to deposition of isotopes used in diagnostic procedures (thorium dioxide) and therapeutic procedures (^{131}I).[181]

There may not be a threshold below which radiation has no effect, a concept summarized in the following manner by Rubin and Casarett:[182] (1) There is a finite probability that the smallest amount of radiation can cause a significant change in a cell such as gene mutation; (2) there is a finite probability that such a cell alteration may be an event in a complex multievent mechanism of carcinogenesis; (3) the probability that such a single event will complete the carcinogenic mechanism in an individual of a population depends on the size of the exposed population and on the number of individuals in it that are so predisposed; (4) it is therefore reasonable to assume that there is no threshold dose in a population in which there is not at least one individual who requires merely this one cell change to complete a carcinogenic event.

The following principles must be kept in mind when assigning radiation as the probable cause of a neoplasm. The new tumor must have been in the field of radiation. The organ in which it arises must have been previously documented as being normal. There should be a symptom-free period after radiation, which is conventionally considered to be at least five years. In point of fact, however, strong arguments can be made for radiation-induced tumors arising within two or three years after irradiation.

Most tumors attributed to radiation are malignant although a few benign osseous and neurogenic neoplasms appear to have been radiation-induced.[183,184] Generally speaking, the gross and microscopic appearances of radiation-induced tumors are not distinctive, and their behavior parallels the course of disease that would be expected for the same histologic type of tumor arising in a nonirradiated organ. The few exceptions to these statements will be noted in the subsequent sections. Radiation damage to normal structures may or may not be found in the region of the tumor, and the presence of radiation damage in the surrounding nonneoplastic tissue is not a requisite for the diagnosis of a radiation-induced tumor.

Skin

Postirradiation basal or squamous cell carcinomas of the skin are most common on the face and usually become manifest 20 or more years after irradiation for benign conditions.[185] The latency period varies from 3 to 64 years, however.[186] The role of radiation is securely established by the occurrence of cancers in unusual locations such as the antecubital fossa or forearm after irradiation of these areas for dermatitis.[187] Multiple lesions are the rule, both synchronously and metachronously. Their number far exceeds the multiple lesions that are also characteristic of cutaneous cancers in nonirradiated patients. The squamous carcinomas are more aggressive than those arising in actinic keratosis. Nonetheless, skin damaged by radiation need not inevitably develop cancer even when the injury is severe enough to produce necrosis.[186]

Atypical fibroxanthomas have arisen in skin that had been irradiated.[188] Most appeared more than 15 years after irradiation, but a few were seen in less than 5 years.

Salivary Gland

Low-dose radiation to the head in childhood increases the incidence of mixed tumors. In one study, 2 of 971 persons who received radiation had mixed tumors, whereas the expected number was 0.04 cases.[189] Other tumors include Warthin's tumor, mucoepidermoid tumor, or unclassified carcinoma.[190–192] A few patients receiving high-dose radiation therapy for carcinoma have later developed malignant tumors of the parotid gland.

Intestine

About 35 colorectal carcinomas have been reported in patients who had previous irradiation, usually of the uterine cervix. Castro et al.[193] analyzed 24 patients with colorectal carcinoma who were long-term survivors (5 to 28 years) of uterine cancer treated with radiotherapy. They found that in 13 cases the segment of bowel bearing the tumor had vascular and stromal changes consistent with

radiation injury. Moreover, 13 patients had colloid carcinoma, which otherwise constitutes only about 10 percent of colon cancers. Qizilbash[194] described a treacherous combination wherein a papillary adenocarcinoma surrounded the margin of an ulcerated radiation-induced stricture. Colloid carcinoma has occurred in a child in the field of irradiation for Wilms' tumor.[195]

Angiosarcoma of the small intestine developed in a woman 8 years after postoperative irradiation for ovarian carcinoma.[196] I have seen one case of small intestinal angiosarcoma 12 years after radiation for squamous cancer of the cervix.

Uterus

Several hundred cases of endometrial malignancy have been reported after irradiation of the uterus for endometrial bleeding from benign disease. It is uncertain how many of these are radiation induced, since many of the cases received radiation for abnormal endometrial bleeding and may have been predisposed to adenocarcinoma. Furthermore, many of the postirradiation lesions were diagnosed as adenocarcinoma in situ, and the almost universal lack of illustrations leaves the exact nature of the lesions in question. It is possible that some of the cases may have been postirradiation cytopathy of normal endometrium.

The frequency of bona fide endometrial malignancy in patients receiving radiation for squamous cancer of the cervix was studied by Fehr and Prem,[197] who found 12 examples in 2,294 patients, which was more than double the expected number. The proportion of mixed müllerian sarcomas was striking. Looking at it from another direction, Norris and Taylor[198] found that 15 percent of 477 patients with uterine sarcomas had a history of irradiation. The tumors included mixed müllerian sarcomas, endometrial stromal sarcomas, and unclassified sarcoma. Leiomyosarcoma did not seem to be related. The behavior of postirradiation mixed müllerian sarcomas has been reported as more aggressive than spontaneous tumors in one study,[199] but not in another study.[200] Postirradiation endometrial adenocarcinoma has a dismal outlook.[201]

Bone

Approximately 200 sarcomas have been reported at the site of a benign bone lesion that was irradiated. About three fourths of these patients received what would now be considered unacceptably high doses. Moreover, most of the irradiated lesions (such as giant cell tumors) would currently be treated with newer surgical techniques. Postirradiation tumors have included osteosarcomas, fibrosarcomas, chondrosarcomas, and malignant fibrous histiocytomas.[202] The latent period has varied from slightly less than 3 years to 30 years, with an average of 6 years for tumors occurring in weight-bearing bones and 14 years in nonweight-bearing bones.[203]

A new complication appears to be emerging from the successful treatment of Ewing's sarcoma by local irradiation to the primary coupled with systemic chemotherapy. Four of 10 patients who had lived 5 or more years after the initial diagnosis of Ewing's sarcoma developed an osteosarcoma at the site of the original tumor.[204]

Postirradiation sarcoma in previously normal bone is a rare event. A review of about 6,000 patients treated for malignant disease disclosed 2 osteosarcomas arising in bone that had been normal at the time of treatment 5 and 11 years previously.[205] This is 0.03 percent of all patients treated or 0.1 percent of the 5-year survivors. In another study, Tountas et al.[206] found 10 postradiation sarcomas, representing 0.035 percent of 5 year survivors. In children, genetic factors seem to play a role.[207]

Benign osseous tumors in the field of high-dose radiotherapy have all been osteochondromas. They occur when the radiation is given in childhood.[183,208]

Soft Tissue

Most sarcomas in irradiated soft tissues are on the chest or shoulder 4 to 16 years after radiation for breast carcinoma.[209,210] Most have metastasized. The lesions have had the conventional histologic patterns of malignant fibrous histiocytoma,[211] fibrosarcoma, chondrosarcoma, or a mixture of the latter two. One fibrosarcoma had large, bizarre cells resembling so-called radiation fibroblasts interspersed among more typical foci of fibrosarcoma, a pattern that is occasionally seen even in the absence of prior radiation.[212] Postradiation sarcomas of the head and neck are rare. Malignant schwannomas have occurred in radiated soft tissues and have pursued a highly aggressive course. About one half have been in patients with von Recklinghausen's disease.[213] Angiosarcoma is a rare postirradiation sarcoma.[214,215]

Breast

Cancer of the breast has been reported in women in their 20s who received radiation to the chest during the first two decades of life, either for metastatic tumor[216] or benign conditions.[217] Adult women receiving radiation for mastitis or other benign breast disease have shown a twofold increase in frequency of breast cancer,[218] as have women undergoing repeated, prolonged fluoroscopic examination of the chest during therapy for tuberculosis.[219] Cancers in irradiated women tend to have less desmopla-

sia than cancers in controls.[220] Carcinoma of the male breast has been reported at age 46 after irradiation at puberty for gynecomastia[221] and at age 35 after low-dose irradiation in infancy.[222] The possible tumorigenic effect of repeated mammograms remains to be determined.[223]

Central Nervous System

The most frequent radiation-induced tumor in the CNS is the so-called pituitary sarcoma, which is actually a fibrosarcoma with abundant collagen formation in some foci. Remnants of the irradiated adenoma are often scattered within the sarcoma. The latent period between irradiation and symptoms referable to the sarcoma ranges from 2.5 to 21 years, with an average of 7 years. The tumors do not metastasize and death occurs from local growth.[224]

Donahue et al.[225] described two patients with neurofibromas of the spinal cord 11 and 13 years after radiation to the mediastinum in childhood.

Meningiomas have been found in a few patients receiving either high-dose or low-dose irradiation. Watts[226] reported meningiomas 15 and 25 years after therapeutic irradiation for glioma. Three meningiomas occurred in a group of more than 5,000 patients receiving radiation to the scalp in childhood for tinea capitis, whereas none was present in the control group.[227] Radiation has been incriminated as a cause of malignant gliomas.[228] A spinal cord glioma arose in a region irradiated for Hodgkin's disease.[229]

Thyroid and Parathyroid

In 1950 Duffy and Fitzgerald[230] suggested an association between thyroid carcinoma in childhood and a prior history of irradiation to the thymus in infancy. The practice of using radiation to treat benign conditions such as acne or tonsillitis largely ceased by 1960, but there is a continuing occurrence of thyroid cancer in these patients. As many as 7 percent of the persons who received radiation to the head or neck have been found to have thyroid carcinoma.[231] In one report, 40 percent of the adults operated on for thyroid cancer between 1968 and 1972 had a history of irradiation.[232]

Virtually all the cancers have been classified as papillary, follicular, or mixed.[233] In one patient, medullary carcinoma was found in a gland also containing papillary cancer.[234] There is one report of a case of anaplastic carcinoma in a 32-year-old man who was irradiated at age 7.[235]

The thyroid gland removed from a patient with a history of irradiation almost always contains multiple nodules. As often as not, the clinically palpable nodule is either an adenoma or colloid nodule, and the carcinoma is present elsewhere. The cancers may be small, and in one series nearly one half the malignancies were not found at the time of frozen section examination. Extensive sampling was required to disclose foci of carcinoma, which were 2 to 3 mm in size.[178] Frozen section interpretation is also complicated when nonneoplastic follicles with nuclear atypia are trapped within inflammatory fibrous areas. Multifocal bilateral cancers are common.[236]

Nearly a dozen cases of thyroid cancer have been reported in patients receiving relatively high doses of ^{131}I for Graves' disease.[237] Nuclear pleomorphism, oncocytic change, and multiple small adenomas are also seen.[238]

Patients treated with radiation for medulloblastoma receive an estimated 200 to 3,000 rads to the thyroid and several carcinomas have been reported.[239] Doses in excess of this are probably not associated with a markedly increased risk of cancer, perhaps because more of the injured thyroid cells are rendered incapable of division.[240] Nonetheless, several cases of papillary cancer have occurred after high-dose radiation for Hodgkin's disease.[241,242]

The possibility that low-dose irradiation may produce adenomas or hyperplasia in parathyroid glands has been raised. Several investigators have obtained a history of low-dose irradiation in 14 to 30 percent of patients with hyperparathyroidism.[243] The irradiated glands do not have special histologic features, except for a possible increase in the proportion of oncocytes.[244] The latter has not been the subject of an adequately controlled study. The association of thyroid carcinoma and hyperparathyroidism (excluding medullary carcinoma and patients with syndromes of multiple endocrine adenomas) may in part be explained by irradiation. Nonetheless, in one series of 40 patients with coexistent parathyroid adenoma and thyroid carcinoma, only one had a history of prior irradiation.[244]

Mesothelium

Ten pleural or peritoneal mesotheliomas have occurred 7 to 31 years after medium- to high-dose radiation. An especially convincing argument for radiation as a causative agent can be made in a woman in whom mesothelioma developed at age 28, who had a lung lesion radiated when she was 4 years old.[245]

Thorium Dioxide

Thorotrast is the trade name for a radioactive suspension of thorium dioxide used between 1930 and 1950 as a contrast medium. More than 50,000 persons received the

agent,[246] including at least 4,300 Americans.[247] More than 90 percent of the Thorotrast remains in the reticuloendothelial system for life, as brown, shiny, granules. In the liver, it is found in Kupffer cells or in histiocytes. At the site of arterial injection, a progressive fibrous reaction around extravasated dye can continue for years, and sarcomas have been reported.[248,249] More than 200 neoplasms have been reported overall.[250] More than one half of the tumors are hepatic: approximately one third angiosarcomas, one third cholangiocarcinomas and one third hepatocellular carcinomas.[251] Rarely all three types occur simultaneously.[252] The occurrence of tumors as long as 36 years after exposure indicates a lifelong risk.[253] Several osteosarcomas have been reported.[254] A detailed bibliography of Thorotrast-associated neoplasms has been published.[246]

Thermal Therapy

Numerous studies on the use of hyperthermia have shown that it enhances radiation therapy and/or chemotherapy.[255] Hyperthermia alone damages small vessels and presumably contributes to cytotoxic effects.[256] Alterations in experimental and human tumors are not specific. There may be an increased quantity of necrosis or increased frequency of absent tumor in the resected specimen when compared with resected specimens from patients treated with either radiation or chemotherapy alone.[257–259]

REFERENCES

1. Caranasos GJ, Stewart RB, Cluff LE: Drug-induced illness leading to hospitalization. JAMA 228:713, 1974
2. Steel K, Gertman PM, Crescenzi C, et al: Iatrogenic illness on a general medical service at a university hospital. N Engl J Med 304:638, 1981
3. Tannenbaum M: Differential diagnosis in uropathology. II. Urologic artifact and/or pathologist's dilemma. Urology 4:485, 1974.
4. Alguacil-Garcia A: Artifactual changes mimicking signet ring cell carcinoma in transurethral prostatectomy specimens. Am J Surg Pathol 10:795, 1986
5. Fechner RE: Necrotizing sialometaplasia. A source of confusion with carcinoma of the palate. Am J Clin Pathol 67:315, 1977
6. Batsakis JG: Sialometaplasia (letter). Arch Otolaryngol 102:191, 1976
7. Hambrick E: The fate of colonoscopic polypectomy sites. Dis Colon Rect 19:400, 1976
8. Evans SC, Goldman RL, Klein HZ, et al: Necrobiotic granulomas of the uterine cervix. Probable post-operative reaction. Am J Surg Pathol 8:841, 1984

9. Herbold DR, Frable WJ, Kraus FT: Isolated noninfectious granulomas of the ovary. Int J Gynecol Pathol 2:380, 1984

10. Balogh K: Palisading granuloma in the kidney after open biopsy. (Letter.) Am J Surg Pathol 10:441, 1986

11. Spagnolo DV, Waring PM: Bladder granulomata after bladder surgery. Am J Clin Pathol 86:430, 1986

12. Epstein JI, Hutchins GM: Granulomatous prostatitis: Distinction among allergic, nonspecific, and posttransurethral resection lesions. Hum Pathol 15:818, 1984

13. Batnitzky S, Keucher TR, Mealey J Jr, et al: Iatrogenic intraspinal epidermoid tumors. JAMA 237:148, 1977

14. Strauchen JA, Strefling AM: Epidermal inclusion cyst of the meniscus. J Bone J Surg 64A:290, 1982

15. Elliot JS, Rosenberg ML: Ureteral occlusion by barium granulomata. J Urol 71:692, 1954

16. Lewis JW Jr, Kerstein MD, Koss N: Barium granuloma of the rectum: An uncommon complication of barium enema. Ann Surg 181:418, 1975

17. Hayden RS: Perforation of duodenal ulcer during fluoroscopy. Disposition of barium sulfate in the abdominal cavity. Radiology 57:214, 1951

18. Ravel R: Histopathology of lymph nodes after lymphangiography. Am J Clin Pathol 46:335, 1966

19. Dorfman RF, Warnke R: Lymphadenopathy simulating the malignant lymphomas. Hum Pathol 5:519, 1974

20. Fox RM, Malter IJ: Prolonged oviduct retention of iodized contrast medium. Obstet Gynecol 40:221, 1972

21. Kantor HI, Kamholz JH, Smith AL: Foreign-body granulomas following the use of Salpix. Report of a case simulating intraabdominal tuberculosis. Obstet Gynecol 7:171, 1956

22. Coder DM, Olander GA: Granulomatous peritonitis caused by starch glove powder. Arch Surg 105:83, 1972

23. Taft DA, Lasersohn JT, Hill JD: Glove starch granulomatous peritonitis. Am J Surg 120:231, 1970

24. Paine CG, Smith P: Starch granulomata. J Clin Pathol 10:51, 1957

25. Davies JD, Neely J: The histopathology of peritoneal starch granulomas. J Pathol 107:265, 1972

26. Aarons J, Fitzgerald N: The persisting hazards of surgical glove powder. Surg Gynecol Obstet 138:385, 1974

27. Sobel HJ, Schiffman RJ, Schwarz R, et al: Granulomas and peritonitis due to starch glove powder. Arch Pathol Lab Med 91:558, 1971

28. Holmes EC, Eggleston JC: Starch granulomatous peritonitis. Surgery 71:85, 1972

29. Sturdy JH, Baird RM, Gerein AN: Surgical sponges. A cause of granuloma and adhesion formation. Ann Surg 165:128, 1967

30. Saxén L, Myllärniemi H: Foreign material and postoperative adhesions. N Engl J Med 279:200, 1968

31. Dragan MJ: Wood fibers from disposable surgical gowns and drapes. JAMA 241:2297, 1979

32. Knowlson GTG: Gel-foam granuloma in the brain. J Neurol Neurosurg Psychiatry 37:971, 1974

33. Kyriakos M: Myospherulosis of the paranasal sinuses, nose and middle ear. A possible iatrogenic disease. Am J Clin Pathol 67:118, 1977

34. Rosai J: The nature of myospherulosis of the upper respiratory tract. Am J Clin Pathol 69:475, 1978

35. Travis WD, Li C-Y, Weiland LH: Immunostaining for hemoglobin in two cases of myospherulosis. Arch Pathol Lab Med 110:763, 1986

36. Wheeler TM, Sessions RB, McGavran MH: "Myospherulosis": A preventable iatrogenic nasal and paranasal entity. Arch Otolaryngol 106:272, 1980

37. White JT: Myospherulosis. South Med J 72:485, 1979

38. Mills SE, Lininger JR: Intracranial myospherulosis. Hum Pathol 13:596, 1982

39. Wolff M: Granulomas in nasal mucous membranes following local steroid injections. Am J Clin Pathol 62:775, 1974

40. Santa Cruz DJ, Ulbright TM: Mucin-like changes in keloids. Am J Clin Path 75:18, 1981

41. Ford LT, DeBender J: Tendon rupture after local steroid injection. South Med J 72:827, 1979

42. Hutton L: Oleothorax: Expanding pleural lesion. AJR 142:1107, 1984

43. Hoare AM, Alexander-Williams J: Oleogranuloma of the rectum produced by Lasonil ointment. Br Med J 2:997, 1977

44. Ghosh A: Lipogranuloma of the uterine parametrium. Br J Obstet Gynecol 83:409, 1976

45. Hausner RJ, Schoen FJ, Mendez-Fernandez MA, et al: Migration of silicone gel to axillary lymph nodes after prosthetic mammoplasty. Arch Pathol Lab Med 105:371, 1981

46. Frantz P, Herbst CA Jr: Augmentation mammoplasty, irradiation, and breast cancer. A case report. Cancer 36:1147, 1975

47. Bommer J, Ritz E, Waldherr R: Silicone-induced splenomegaly. Treatment of pancytopenia by splenectomy in a patient on hemodialysis. New Eng J Med 305:1077, 1981

48. Christie AJ, Weinberger KA, Dietrich M: Silicone lymphadenopathy and synovitis. Complications of silicone elastomer finger joint prostheses. JAMA 237:1463, 1977

49. Christie AJ, Weinberger KA, Dietrich M: Recurrence of silicone lymphadenopathy. JAMA 245:1314, 1981

50. Travis WD, Balogh K, Abraham JL: Silicone granulomas: Report of three cases and review of the literature. Hum Pathol 16:19, 1985

51. Ober WB: Effects of oral and intrauterine administration of contraceptives on the uterus. Hum Pathol 8:513, 1977

52. Czernobilsky B, Rotenstreich L, Mass N, et al: Effect of intrauterine device on histology of endometrium. Obstet Gynecol 45:64, 1975

53. McCormick JF, Scorgie RDF: Unilateral tubo-ovarian actinomycosis in the presence of an intrauterine device. Am J Clin Pathol 68:622, 1977

54. Bhagavan BS, Gupta PK: Genital actinomycosis and intrauterine contraceptive devices. Cytopathologic diagnosis and clinical significance. Hum Pathol 9:567, 1978

55. King DT, Lam M: Actinomycosis of the urinary bladder. Association with an intrauterine contraceptive device. JAMA 240:1512, 1978

56. O'Brien PK, Roth-Moyo LA, Davis BA: Pseudo-sulfur granules associated with intrauterine contraceptive devices. Am J Clin Pathol 75:822, 1981

57. Ostergard DR, Townsend DE, Hirose FM: Treatment of chronic cervicitis by cryotherapy. Am J Obstet Gynecol 102:426, 1968

58. Crisp WE, Smith MS, Asadourian LA, et al: Cryosurgical treatment of premalignant disease of the uterine cervix. Am J Obstet Gynecol 107:737, 1970

59. Bago-Granell J, Aguirre-Canyadell M, Nardi J, et al: Malignant fibrous histiocytoma of bone at the site of a total hip arthroplasty. J Bone Joint Surg 66B:38, 1984

60. Penman HG, Ring PA: Osteosarcoma in association with total hip replacement. J Bone Joint Surg 66B:632, 1984

61. Swann M: Malignant soft-tissue tumour at the site of a total hip replacement. J Bone Joint Surg 66B:629, 1984

62. Fechner RE: Bone and joints. p. 79. In Riddell RH (ed): Pathology of Drug-Induced and Toxic Diseases. Churchill Livingstone, New York, 1982

63. Lee YS, Rho RWH, Nather A: Malignant fibrous histiocytoma at site of metal implant. Cancer 54:2286, 1984

64. Goldring SR, Schiller AL, Roelke M, et al: The synovial-like membrane at the bone-cement interface in loose total hip replacements and its proposed role in bone lysis. J Bone Joint Surg 65A:575, 1983

65. Stephens CB, Arnold GE, Stone JW: Larynx injected with polytef paste. Arch Otolaryngol 102:432, 1976

66. Freeman BS: Proplast, a porous implant for contour restoration. Br J Plast Surg 29:158, 1976

67. Peacock EE Jr, Van Winkle W JR: Wound Repair. 2nd Ed. WB Saunders, Philadelphia, 1976

68. Postelthwait RW: Tissue reaction to surgical sutures. p. 263. In Dunphy JE, Van Winkle W Jr (ed): Repair and Regeneration. The Scientific Basis for Surgical Practice. McGraw-Hill, New York, 1968

69. Salthouse TN, Matlaga BS, Wykoff MH: Comparative tissue response to six suture materials in rabbit cornea, sclera, and ocular muscle. Am J Opththal 84:224, 1977

70. Shauffer IA, Sequeira J: Suture granuloma simulating recurrent carcinoma. AJR 128:856, 1977

71. Belleza NA, Lowman RM: Suture granuloma of the stomach following total colectomy. Radiology 127:84, 1978

72. Weinberg DS, Maini BS: Primary sarcoma of the aorta associated with a vascular prosthesis: A case report. Cancer 46:398, 1980

73. Amazon K, Robinson MJ, Rywlin AM: Ferrugination caused by Monsel's solution. Clinical observations and experimentations. Am J Dermatopathol 2:197, 1980

74. Olmstead PM, Lund HZ, Leonard DD: Monsel's solution. A histologic nuisance. J Am Acad Dermatol 3:492, 1980

75. Rosen Y, Vaillant JG, Yerkmakov V: Submucosal mucous cysts at a colostomy site: Relationship to colitis cystica profunda and report of a case. Dis Colon Rect 19:453, 1976

76. Wayte DM, Helwig EB: Colitis cystica profunda. Am J Clin Pathol 48:159, 1967

77. Rosai J: Ackerman's Surgical Pathology. 7th Ed. CV Mosby, St. Louis, 1989

78. Armin A-R, Moradi A, Winters G: Posttraumatic intrauterine omental implantation mimicking lipomatous lesion 16 years later. Int J Gynecol Pathol 6:89, 1987

79. Donnelly WH: Histopathology of endotracheal intubation. An autopsy study of 99 cases. Arch Pathol Lab Med 88:511, 1969

80. Barton RT: Observation on the pathogenesis of laryngeal granuloma due to endotracheal anesthesia. N Engl J Med 248:1097, 1953

81. Fechner RE, Cooper PH, Mills SE: Pyogenic granuloma of larynx and trachea. A causal and pathologic misnomer for granulation tissue. Arch Otolaryngol 107:30, 1981

82. Recht KA, Belis JA, Kandzari J, et al: Ureterosigmoidostomy followed by carcinoma of the colon. Cancer 44:1538, 1979

83. Harford FJ, Fazio VW, Epstein LM, et al: Rectosigmoid carcinoma occurring after ureterosigmoidostomy. Dis Colon Rectum 27:321, 1984

84. Iannoni C, Marcheggiano A, Pallone F, et al: Abnormal patterns of colorectal mucin secretion after urinary diversion of different types: Histochemical and lectin binding studies. Hum Pathol 17:834, 1986

85. Schipper H, Deckter A: Carcinoma of the colon arising at uretero-implant sites despite early external diversion. Pathogenetic and clinical implications. Cancer 47:2062, 1981

86. Littler ER, Gleibermann E: Gastritis cystica polyposa. (Gastric mucosal prolapse at gastroenterostomy site, with cystic and infiltrative epithelial hyperplasia.) Cancer 29:205, 1972

87. Koga S, Watanabe H, Enjoji M: Stomal polypoid hypertrophic gastritis. A polypoid gastric lesion at gastroenterostomy site. Cancer 43:647, 1979

88. Stemmermann GN, Nayashi T: Hyperplastic polyps of the gastric mucosa adjacent to gastroenterostomy stomas. Am J Clin Pathol 71:341, 1979

89. Morgenstern L, Yamakawa T, Seltzer D: Carcinoma of the gastric stump. Am J Surg 125:29, 1973

90. Bogomoletz WV, Potet F, Barge J, et al: Pathological features and mucin histochemistry of primary gastric stump carcinoma associated with gastritis cystica polyposa. A study of six cases. Am J Surg Pathol 9:401, 1985

91. Monafo W, Goldfarb W: Postoperative peritoneal cyst. Surgery 53:470, 1963

92. Steinberg AO, Madayag MA, Bosniak MA, et al: Demonstration of 2 unusually large pelvic lymphocysts by lymphangiography. J Urol 109:477, 1973

93. Basinger GT, Gittes RF: Lymphocyst: Ultrasound diagnosis and urologic management. J Urol 114:740, 1975

94. Payan HM, Gilbert EF: Mesenteric cyst-ovarian implant syndrome. Arch Pathol Lab Med 111:282, 1987

95. Proppe KH, Scully RE, Rosai J: Postoperative spindle cell nodules of genitourinary tract resembling sarcomas. A report of eight cases. Am J Surg Pathol 8:101, 1984

96. Kay S, Schneider V: Reactive spindle cell nodule of the endocervix simulating uterine sarcoma. Int J Gynecol Pathol 4:255, 1985

97. Weiss SW, Enzinger FM, Johnson FB: Silica reaction simulating fibrous histiocytoma. Cancer 42:2738, 1978

98. Sobel HJ, Avrin E, Marquet E, et al: Reactive granular cells in sites of trauma. A cytochemical and ultrastructural study. Am J Clin Pathol 61:223, 1974

99. McFadden DE, Clement PB: Peritoneal inclusion cysts

with mural mesothelial proliferation. A clinicopathologic analysis of six cases. Am J Surg Pathol 10:844, 1986

100. Weiss SW, Enzinger FM: Malignant fibrous histiocytoma: An analysis of 200 cases. Cancer 41:2250, 1978

101. Inoshita T, Youngberg GA: Malignant fibrous histiocytoma arising in previous surgical sites. Report of two cases. Cancer 53:176, 1984

102. Sherlock P, Oropeza R: Jejunal perforations in lymphoma after chemotherapy. Arch Intern Med 110:102, 1962

103. Hartmann WH, Sherlock P: Gastroduodenal metastases from carcinoma of the breast. An adrenal steroid-induced phenomenon. Cancer 14:426, 1961

104. Mayer RJ, Berkowitz RS, Griffiths CT: Central nervous system involvement by ovarian carcinoma. A complication of prolonged survival with metastatic disease. Cancer 41:776, 1978

105. Gercovich FG, Luna MA, Gottlieb JA: Increased incidence of cerebral metastases in sarcoma patients with prolonged survival from chemotherapy. Report of cases of leiomyosarcoma and chondrosarcoma. Cancer 36:1843, 1975

106. Telles NC, Rabson AS, Pomeroy TC: Ewing's sarcoma: An autopsy study. Cancer 41:2321, 1978

107. Lockwood WB, Broghamer WL Jr: The changing prevalence of secondary cardiac neoplasms as related to cancer therapy. Cancer 45:2659, 1980

108. Espana P, Chang P, Wiernik PH: Increased incidence of brain metastases in sarcoma patients. Cancer 45:337, 1980

109. Thalinger AR, Rosenthal SN, Borg S, et al: Cavitation of pulmonary metastases as a response to chemotherapy. Cancer 46:1329, 1980

110. Qizilbash A, Kontozoglou T, Sianos J, et al: Hepar lobatum associated with chemotherapy and metastatic breast cancer. Arch Pathol Lab Med 111:58, 1987

111. Koss LG, Melamed MR, Mayer K: The effect of busulfan on human epithelia. Am J Clin Pathol 44:385, 1965

112. Nelson BM, Andrews GA: Breast cancer and cytologic dysplasia in many organs after busulfan (Myleran). Am J Clin Pathol 42:37, 1964

113. Tiffany P, Morse MJ, Bosl G, et al: Sequential excision of residual thoracic and retroperitoneal masses after chemotherapy for stage III germ cell tumors. Cancer 57:978, 1986

114. Hong SJ, Lurain JR, Tsukada Y, et al: Cystadenocarcinoma of the ovary in a four-year old: Benign transformation during therapy. Cancer 45:2227, 1980

115. Willis GW, Hajdu SI: Histologically benign teratoid metastasis of testicular embryonal carcinoma: Report of five cases. Am J Clin Pathol 59:338, 1973

116. Davey DB, Ulbright TM, Loehrer PJ, et al: The significance of atypia within teratomatous metastases after chemotherapy for malignant germ cell tumors. Cancer 59:533, 1987

117. Molenaar WM, Oosterhuis JW, Kamps WA: Cytological "differentiation" in childhood rhabdomyosarcomas following polychemotherapy. Hum Pathol 15:973, 1984

118. Molenaar WM, Oosterhuis JW, Oosterhuis AM, et al: Mesenchymal and muscle-specific intermediate filaments (vi-

mentin and desmin) in relation to differentiation in childhood rhabdomyosarcomas. Hum Pathol 16:838, 1985

119. Wilson RE, Antman KH, Brodsky G, et al: Tumor-cell heterogeneity in soft tissue sarcomas as defined by chemoradiotherapy. Cancer 53:1420, 1984

120. Mazur MT, Lurain JR, Brewer JI: Fatal gestational choriocarcinoma. Clinicopathologic study of patients treated at a trophoblastic disease center. Cancer 50:1833, 1982

121. Durkin W, Durant J: Benign mass lesions after therapy for Hodgkin's disease. Arch Intern Med 139:333, 1979

122. Stewart FM, Williamson BR, Innes DJ, et al: Residual tumor masses following treatment for advanced histiocytic lymphoma. Diagnostic and therapeutic implications. Cancer 55:620, 1985

123. Einhorn LH, Donohue J: Cis-diamminedichloroplatinum, vinblastine and bleomycin combination chemotherapy in disseminated testicular cancer. Ann Intern Med 87:293, 1977

124. Lamm DL, Wepsic HT, Feldman P, et al: Importance of alpha-fetoprotein in patients with seminoma. Urology 10:233, 1977

125. Shin M, Hoo K: Diffuse thymic hyperplasia following chemotherapy for nodular sclerosing Hodgkin's disease. Cancer 51:30, 1983

126. Carmosino L, DiBenedetto A, Feffer S: Thymic hyperplasia following successful chemotherapy. A report of two cases and review of the literature. Cancer 56:1526, 1985

127. Smith T: Fatty replacement of lymph nodes mimicking lymphoma relapse. Cancer 58:2686, 1986

128. Werbin N: Fatty changes and metastases in axillary lymph nodes. J Surg Oncol 25:145, 1984

129. Geis WP, Iwatsuki S, Molnar Z, et al: Pseudolymphoma in renal allograft recipients. Arch Surg 113:461, 1978

130. Deodhar SD, Kuklinca AG, Vidt DG, et al: Development of reticulum-cell sarcoma at the site of antilymphocyte globulin injection in a patient with renal transplant. N Engl J Med 280:1104, 1969

131. Tchernia G, Mielot F, Subtil E, et al: Acute myeloblastic leukemia after immunodepressive therapy for primary nonmalignant disease. Blood Cells 2:67, 1967

132. Reimer RR, Hoover R, Fraumeni JR Jr, et al: Acute leukemia after alkylating-agent therapy of ovarian cancer. N Engl J Med 297:177, 1977

133. Dale GA, Smith RB: Transitional cell carcinoma of the bladder associated with cyclophosphamide. J Urol 112:603, 1974

134. Casko SB, Keuhnelian JG, Gutowski III, et al: Spindle cell cancer of bladder during cyclophosphamide therapy for Wegener's granulomatosis. Am J Surg Pathol 4:191, 1980

135. Wall RL, Clausen KP: Carcinoma of the urinary bladder in patients receiving cyclophosphamide. N Engl J Med 293:271, 1975

136. Seo IS, Clark SA, McGovern FD, et al: Leiomyosarcoma of the urinary bladder thirteen years after cyclophosphamide therapy for Hodgkin's disease. Cancer 55:1597, 1985

137. Carney CN, Stevens PS, Fried FA, et al: Fibroblastic tu-

mor of the urinary bladder after cyclophosphamide therapy. Arch Pathol Lab Med 106:247, 1982

138. Peters MS, Stuard DI: Metastatic malignant melanoma transplanted via a renal homograft. A case report. Cancer 41:2426, 1978

139. Penn I, Starzl TE: Malignant tumors arising de novo in immunosuppressed organ transplant recipients. Transplantation 14:407, 1972

140. Penn I: Cancers of the anogenital region in renal transplant recipients. Analysis of 65 cases. Cancer 58:611, 1986

141. Maeda K, Hawkins ET, Oh HK, et al: Malignant lymphoma in transplanted renal pelvis. Arch Pathol Lab Med 110:626, 1986

142. Cosson DN, Ross BH, Ansell ID: A large bowel lymphoma complicating renal transplantation. Br J Radiol 54:418, 1981

143. Jamieson NV, Thiru S, Calne RY, et al: Gastric lymphomas arising in two patients with renal allografts. Transplantation 31:224, 1981

144. Leech SH, Kumar P: Epstein-Barr virus-induced B-cell lymphoma after renal transplantation. N Engl J Med 307:896, 1982

145. Barenfange J, Mazur JM, Mody N, et al: Malignant fibrous histiocytoma of bone in a renal-transplant patient. J Bone Joint Surg 62A:297, 1980

146. Stein RS: Radiation-recall enteritis after actinomycin-D and adriamycin therapy. South Med J 71:960, 1978

147. Greco FA, Brereton HD, Kent H, et al: Adriamycin and enhanced radiation reaction in normal esophagus and skin. Ann Intern Med 85:294, 1976

148. Cassady JR, Richter M, Piro AJ, et al: Radiation-adriamycin interactions: Preliminary observations. Cancer 36:946, 1975

149. Fajardo LF, Berthrong M: Radiation injury in surgical pathology. Part I. Am J Surg Pathol 2:159, 1978

150. White DC: The histopathologic basis for functional decrements in late radiation injury in diverse organs. Cancer 37:1126, 1976

151. Skolnik EM, Soboroff BJ, Tardy ME Jr, et al: Preoperative radiation of larynx. Analysis of serial sections. Ann Otol Rhinol Laryngol 79:1049, 1970

152. Silverberg SG, DiGiorgi LS: Histopathologic analysis of preoperative radiation therapy in endometrial carcinoma. Am J Obstet Gynecol 119:698, 1974

153. Cox JD, Stoffel TJ: The significance of needle biopsy after irradiation for Stage C adenocarcinoma of the prostate. Cancer 40:156, 1977

154. Gray SR, Hahn IS, Cornog JL Jr: Short-term effect of radiation on human neoplasms. Arch Pathol Lab Med 97:74, 1974

155. Neumann MP, Limas C: Transitional cell carcinomas of the urinary bladder. Effects of preoperative irradiation on morphology. Cancer 58:2758, 1986

156. Weymuller ER Jr: Prognostic importance of the tumor-free laryngectomy specimen. Arch Otol 104:505, 1978

157. Suit HD, Gallager HS: Intact tumor cells in irradiated tissue. Arch Pathol 78:648, 1964

158. Goldman JL, Cheren RV, Zak FG, et al: Histopathology of larynges and radical neck specimens in a combined radiation and surgery program for advanced carcinoma of the larynx and laryngopharynx. Ann Otol Rhinol Laryngol 75:313, 1966

159. Flood LM, Brightwell AP: Clinical assessment of the irradiated larynx. Salvage laryngectomy in the absence of histological confirmation of residual or recurrent carcinoma. J Laryngol Otol 98:493, 1984

160. Calcaterra TC, Stern F, Ward PH: Dilemma of delayed radiation injury of the larynx. Ann Otol Rhinol Laryngol 81:501, 1972

161. Diehl LF, Hurwitz MA, Johnson SA, et al: Skin metastases confined to a field of previous irradiation. Report of two cases and review of the literature. Cancer 53:1864, 1984

162. Tessmer CF: Radiation effects in skin. p. 146. In Berdjis CC (ed): Pathology of Irradiation. Williams & Wilkins, Baltimore, 1971

163. Harwood TR, Staley CJ, Yokoo H: Histopathology of irradiated and obstructed submandibular salivary glands. Arch Pathol Lab Med 96:189, 1973

164. Kashima HK, Kirkham WR, Andrews JR: Postirradiation sialadenitis. A study of the clinical features, histopathologic changes and serum enzyme variations following irradiation of human salivary glands. AJR 94:271, 1965

165. Perkins DE, Spjut HJ: Intestinal stenosis following radiation therapy. AJR 88:953, 1962

166. Gardiner GW, McAuliffe N, Murray D: Colitis cystica profunda occurring in a radiation-induced colonic stricture. Hum Pathol 15:295, 1984

167. Weisbrot IM, Liber AF, Gordon BS: The effects of therapeutic radiation on colonic mucosa. Cancer 36:931, 1975

168. Lewin K, Millis RR: Human radiation hepatitis. A morphologic study with emphasis on the late changes. Arch Pathol Lab Med 96:21, 1973

169. Luxton RW, Kunkler PB: Radiation nephritis. Acta Radiol Ther Phys Biol 2:169, 1964

170. Mostofi FK: Radiation effects on the kidney. p. 338. In Mostofi FK, Smith DE (eds): The Kidney. Williams & Wilkins, Baltimore, 1966

171. Kapur S, Chandra R, Antonovych T: Acute radiation nephritis. Light and electron microscopic observations. Arch Pathol Lab Med 101:469, 1977

172. Loveless KJ: The effects of radiation upon the cytology of benign and malignant bladder epithelia. Acta Cytol (Baltimore) 17:355, 1973

173. Eposti PL, Edsmyr F, Moberger G, et al: Cytologic diagnosis in bladder carcinoma treated by supervoltage irradiation. Scand J Urol Nephrol 3:201, 1969

174. Tweeddale DN: Urinary Cytology. Little, Brown, Boston, 1977

175. Bostwick DG, Egbert BM, Fajardo LF: Radiation injury of the normal and neoplastic prostate. Am J Surg Pathol 6:541, 1982

176. Mazur MT, Kraus FT: Histogenesis of morphologic variations in tumors of the uterine wall. Am J Surg Pathol 4:59, 1980

177. Spitalnik PF, Straus FH: Patterns of human thyroid paren-

chymal reaction following low-dose childhood irradiation. Cancer 41:1098, 1978

178. Komorowski RA, Hanson GA: Morphologic changes in the thyroid following low-dose childhood radiation. Arch Pathol Lab Med 101:36, 1977

179. Clarke D, Curtis JL, Martinez A, et al: Fat necrosis of the breast simulating recurrent carcinoma after primary radiotherapy in the management of early stage breast carcinoma. Cancer 52:442, 1983

180. Schnitt SJ, Connolly JL, Harris JE, et al: Radiation-induced changes in the breast. Hum Pathol 15:545, 1984

181. Hutchison GB: Late neoplastic changes following medical irradiation. Cancer 37:1102, 1976

182. Rubin P, Casarett GW: Clinical Radiation Pathology. WB Saunders, Philadelphia, 1968

183. Katzman H, Waugh T, Berdon W: Skeletal changes following irradiation of childhood tumors. J Bone Joint Surg 51A:825, 1969

184. Schore-Freedman E, Abrahams C, Recant W, et al: Neurilemomas and salivary gland tumors of the head and neck following childhood irradiation. Cancer 51:2159, 1983

185. van Vloten WA, Hermans J, van Daal WAJ: Radiation-induced skin cancer and radiodermatitis of the head and neck. Cancer 59:411, 1987

186. Martin H, Strong E, Spiro RH: Radiation-induced skin cancer of the head and neck. Cancer 25:61, 1970

187. Lazar P, Cullen SI: Basal cell epithelioma and chronic radiodermatitis. Arch Dermatol 88:172, 1963

188. Hudson AW, Winkelmann RK: Atypical fibroxanthoma of the skin: A reappraisal of 19 cases in which the original diagnosis was spindle-cell squamous carcinoma. Cancer 29:413, 1972

189. Harzen RW, Pifer JW, Toyooka ET, et al: Neoplasms following irradiation of the head. Cancer Res 26:305, 1966

190. Walker MJ, Chaudhuri PK, Wood DC, et al: Radiation-induced parotid cancer. Arch Surg 116:329, 1981

191. Smith DG, Levitt SH: Radiation carcinogenesis: An unusual familial occurrence of neoplasia following irradiation in childhood for benign disease. Cancer 34:2069, 1974

192. Little JW, Rickles NH: Malignant papillary cystadenoma lymphomatosum. Report of a case, with a review of the literature. Cancer 18:851, 1965

193. Castro EB, Rosen PP, Quan SHQ: Carcinoma of large intestine in patients irradiated for carcinoma of cervix and uterus. Cancer 31:45, 1973

194. Qizilbash AH: Radiation-induced carcinoma of the rectum. A late complication of pelvic irradiation. Arch Pathol Lab Med 98:118, 1974

195. Sabio H, Teja K, Elkon D, et al: Adenocarcinoma of the colon following treatment of Wilms' tumor. J Pediatr 95:424, 1979

196. Chen KTK, Hoffman KD, Hendricks EJ: Angiosarcoma following therapeutic irradiation. Cancer 44:2044, 1979

197. Fehr PE, Prem KA: Malignancy of the uterine corpus following irradiation-therapy for squamous cell carcinoma of the cervix. Am J Obstet Gynecol 119:685, 1974

198. Norris HJ, Taylor HB: Postirradiation sarcomas of the uterus. Obstet Gynecol 26:689, 1965

199. Meredith RF, Eisert DR, Kaka Z, et al: An excess of uterine sarcomas after pelvic irradiation. Cancer 58:2003, 1986

200. Varella-Duran J, Nochomovitz LE, Prem KA, et al: Postirradiation mixed mullerian tumors of the uterus. A comparative clinicopathologic study. Cancer 45:1625, 1980

201. Kwon TH, Prempree T, Tang C-K, et al: Adenocarcinoma of the uterine corpus following irradiation for cervical cancer. Gynecol Oncol 11:102, 1981

202. Huvos AG, Woodard HQ, Heilweil M: Postradiation malignant fibrous histiocytoma of bone. A clinicopathologic study of 20 patients. Am J Surg Pathol 10:9, 1986

203. Weatherby RP, Dahlin DC, Ivins JC: Postradiation sarcoma of bone. Review of 78 Mayo Clinic cases. Mayo Clin Proc 56:294, 1981

204. Chan RC, Sutow WW, Lindberg RD, et al: Management and results of localized Ewing's sarcoma. Cancer 43:1001, 1979

205. Phillips TL, Sheline GE: Bone sarcomas following radiation therapy. Radiology 81:992, 1963

206. Tountas AA, Fornasier VL, Harwood AR, et al: Postirradiation sarcoma of bone. A perspective. Cancer 43:182, 1979

207. Meadows AT, Strong LC, Li FP, et al: Bone sarcoma as a second malignant neoplasm in children: Influence of radiation and genetic predisposition. Cancer 46:2603, 1980

208. Rutherford H, Dodd GD: Complications of radiation therapy: Growing bone. Semin Roentgenol 9:15, 1974

209. Oberman HA, Oneal RM: Fibrosarcoma of the chest wall following resection and irradiation of carcinoma of the breast. Am J Clin Pathol 53:407, 1970

210. Travis EL, Kreuther A, Young T, et al: Unusual postirradiation sarcoma of chest wall. Cancer 38:2269, 1976

211. Langham MR Jr, Mills AS, DeMay RM, et al: Malignant fibrous histiocytoma of the breast. A case report and review of the literature. Cancer 54:558, 1984

212. Senyszyn JJ, Johnston AD, Jacox HW, et al: Radiation induced sarcoma after treatment of breast cancer. Cancer 26:394, 1970

213. Sordillo PP, Helson L, Hadju SI, et al: Malignant schwannoma-Clinical characteristics, survival, and response to therapy. Cancer 47:2503, 1981

214. Goette DK, Detlefs RL: Postirradiation angiosarcoma. J Am Acad Dermatol 12:922, 1985

215. Ulbright TM, Clark SA, Einhorn LH: Angiosarcoma associated with germ cell tumors. Hum Pathol 16:268, 1985

216. Ivins JC, Taylor WF, Wold LE: Elective whole-lung irradiation in osteosarcoma treatment: Appearance of bilateral breast cancer in two long-term survivors. Skel Radiol 16:133, 1987

217. Iknayan HF: Carcinoma associated with irradiation of the immature breast. Radiology 114:431, 1975

218. Baral E, Larsson LE, Mattsson B: Breast cancer following irradiation of the breast. Cancer 40:2905, 1977

219. Mackenzie I: Breast cancer following multiple fluoroscopies. Br J Cancer 19:1, 1965

220. Dvoretsky PM, Woodard E, Bonfiglio TA, et al: The pa-

thology of breast cancer in women irradiated for acute postpartum mastitis. Cancer 46:2257, 1980

221. Lowell DM, Martineau RG, Luria SB: Carcinoma of the male breast following radiation. Report of case occurring 35 years after radiation therapy of unilateral prepubertal gynecomastia. Cancer 22:581, 1968

222. Curtin CT, McHeffy B, Kolarsick AJ: Thyroid and breast cancer following radiation. Cancer 40:2911, 1977

223. Bailer JC III: Screening for early breast cancer: Pros and cons. Cancer 39:2783, 1977

224. Powell HC, Marshall LF, Ignelzi AR: Post-irradiation pituitary sarcoma. Acta Neuropathol (Berl) 39:165, 1977

225. Donahue WE, Jaffe FA, Newcastle NB: Radiation-induced neurofibromata. Cancer 20:589, 1967

226. Watts C: Meningioma following irradiation. Cancer 38:1939, 1976

227. Modan B, Baidatz D, Mart H, et al: Radiation-induced head and neck tumours. Lancet 1:277, 1974

228. Marus G, Levin CV, Rutherford GS: Malignant glioma following radiotherapy for unrelated primary tumors. Cancer 58:886, 1986

229. Clifton MD, Amromin GD, Perry MC, et al: Spinal cord glioma following irradiation for Hodgkin's disease. Cancer 45:2051, 1980

230. Duffy BJ Jr, Fitzgerald PJ: Thyroid cancer in children: A report of 28 cases. J Clin Endocrinol 10:1296, 1950

231. Refetoff S, Harrison J, Karanfilski BT, et al: Continuing occurrence of thyroid carcinoma after irradiation to the neck in infancy and childhood. N Engl J Med 292:171, 1975

232. DeGroot L, Paloyan E: Thyroid carcinoma and radiation. A Chicago endemic. JAMA 225:487, 1973

233. Greenspan FS: Radiation exposure and thyroid cancer. JAMA 237:2089, 1977

234. Cerletty JM, Guansing AR, Engbring NH, et al: Radiation-related thyroid carcinoma. Arch Surg 113:1072, 1978

235. Komorowski RA, Hanson GA, Garancis JC: Anaplastic thyroid carcinoma following low-dose irradiation. Am J Clin Pathol 70:303, 1978

236. Schneider AB, Pinsky S, Bekerman C, et al: Characteristics of 108 thyroid cancers detected by screening in a population with a history of head and neck irradiation. Cancer 46:1218, 1980

237. McDougall IR, Kennedy JS, Thomson JA: Thyroid carcinoma following iodine-131 therapy. Report of a case and review of literature. J Clin Endocrinol 33:287, 1971

238. Sheline GE, Lindsay S, McCormack KR, et al: Thyroid nodules occurring late after treatment of thyrotoxicosis with radioiodine. J Clin Endocrinol 22:8, 1962

239. Roggli VL, Estrada R, Fechner RE: Thyroid neoplasia following irradiation for medulloblastoma. Report of two cases. Cancer 43:2232, 1979

240. Maxon HR, Thomas SR, Saenger EL, et al: Ionizing irradiation and the induction of clinically significant disease in the human thyroid gland. Am J Med 63:967, 1977

241. McDougall IR, Coleman CN, Burke JS, et al: Thyroid carcinoma after high-dose external radiotherapy for Hodgkin's disease: Report of three cases. Cancer 45:2056, 1980

242. McHenry C, Jarosz H, Calandra D, et al: Thyroid neoplasia following radiation therapy for Hodgkin's lymphoma. Arch Surg 122:684, 1987

243. Russ JE, Scanlon EF, Sener SF: Parathyroid adenomas following irradiation. Cancer 43:1078, 1979

244. LiVolsi VA, LoGerfo P, Feind CR: Coexistent parathyroid adenomas and thyroid carcinoma. Can radiation be blamed? Arch Surg 113:285, 1978

245. Austin MB, Fechner RE, Roggli VL: Pleural malignant mesothelioma following Wilms' tumor. Am J Clin Pathol 86:227, 1986

246. Grampa G: Radiation injury with particular reference to Thorotrast. Pathol Annu 6:147, 1971

247. Telles NC: Follow-up of thorium dioxide patients in the United States. Ann NY Acad Sci 145:674, 1967

248. Kamiho A, Okabe K, Hirose T: Thorium dioxide granuloma of the neck with resultant fatal hemorrhage. Arch Otol 105:45, 1979

249. Hasson J, Hartman KS, Milikow E, et al: Thorotrast-induced extraskeletal osteosarcoma of the cervical region. Report of a case. Cancer 36:1827, 1975

250. Levy DW, Rindsberg S, Friedman AC, et al: Thoratrast-induced hepatosplenic neoplasia: CT identification. AJR: 146:997, 1986

251. Smoron GL, Battifora HA: Thorotrast-induced hepatoma. Cancer 30:1252, 1972

252. Kojiro M, Kawano Y, Kawasaki H, et al: Thoratrast-induced hepatic angiosarcoma, and combined hepatocellular and cholangiocarcinoma in a single patient. Cancer 49:2161, 1982

253. Underwood JCE, Huck P: Thorotrast associated hepatic angiosarcoma with 36 years latency. Cancer 42:2610, 1978

254. Sindelar WF, Costa J, Ketcham AS: Osteosarcoma associated with Thorotrast administration. Report of two cases and literature review. Cancer 42:2604, 1978

255. Stewart JR, Gibbs FA Jr: Hyperthermia in the therapy of cancer. Perspectives on its promise and its problems. Cancer 54:2823, 1984

256. Badylak SF, Babbs CF, Skojal TM, et al: Hyperthermia-induced vascular injury in normal and neoplastic tissue. Cancer 56:991, 1985

257. Sugimachi K, Kai H, Matsufuji H, et al: Histopathological evaluation of hyperthermo-chemo-radiotherapy for carcinoma of the esophagus. J Surg Oncol 32:82, 1986

258. Sugaar S, LeVeen HH: A histopathologic study on the effects of radiofrequency thermotherapy on malignant tumors of the lung. Cancer 43:767, 1979

259. Skibba JL, Quebbeman EJ: Tumoricidal effects and patient survival after hyperthermic liver perfusion. Arch Surg 121:1266, 1986

6

Immunohistochemical Techniques

Mehrdad Nadji
Azorides R. Morales

Immunohistochemical techniques are a group of immunolabeling procedures that are capable of demonstrating various substances (antigens) in cells and tissues. These techniques are based on the ability of specific antibodies to localize and bind to corresponding antigens. Depending on the nature of the immunohistochemical method and the type of label used, the antibody-antigen reaction is then visualized by light, fluorescent, or electron microscopy.

This chapter first examines the technical aspects of the immunohistochemical methods, including a brief discussion on the principles of the various procedures; some technical notes related to the specimen, fixation, staining procedure, reagents, and controls; as well as potential technical pitfalls and means to avoid them. Second, the application of this technique to diagnostic surgical pathology is reviewed and selection of markers, interpretation of results, and potential analytical pitfalls discussed as they relate to different immunohistochemical markers. Details concerning each marker and their use in specific diagnostic situations are discussed in Chapter 7 and in other chapters devoted to pathologic lesions of specific organs. Although the principles of various immunohistochemical methods are presented here briefly, this chapter addresses primarily immunoperoxidase techniques. This is because most immunohistochemical techniques used in diagnostic surgical pathology today are the immunoperoxidase procedures.[1-4]

HISTORY

Labeled antibodies that permit visualization of specific substances in tissue sections have been in use for nearly half a century. Fluorescein isothiocyanate and other fluorescent compounds were the first substances to be bound to antibodies.[5] Colloidal metals such as ferritin and mercury were next to be conjugated with antibodies.[6,7] It was only after the introduction of enzyme-labeled antibodies that immunohistochemical techniques were accepted as simple, versatile, and practical tools in diagnostic histopathology.[8,9] Today, great advances have been made in the development and refinement of various immunohistologic methods. The introduction of monoclonal antibodies into the realm of immunohistochemistry has ensured the availability of an unlimited source of highly specific reagents for histologic demonstration of various cell and tissue antigens.[4,10] Numerous commercial sources offer good quality antibodies, conjugates, and immunohistochemical staining kits. Diagnostic immunohistochemistry has become an important part of a pathology laboratory, and one can safely predict that it will continue to remain valuable for many years to come.

METHODOLOGY

Different Immunohistologic Techniques

Antigen-antibody binding is not visible under the light or electron microscope, unless the antibody is tagged with a label that permits its visualization. Common labels in immunohistochemistry either absorb or emit light and thus produce a color.

Fluorescein compounds, when excited by ultraviolet (UV) light, emit light within the visible wavelengths. The color of the emitted light depends on the nature of the compound. Fluorescein isothiocyanate, for example, emits green light, whereas rhodamine produces red fluorescence. Efforts are under way to introduce other fluorescein substances that emit light of other colors. As a group, immunofluorescence methods require the use of fresh or unfixed fresh frozen tissue. The reaction results are visualized on a dark background. The requirement for a fluorescent microscope and fresh tissue, together with the lack of morphologic detail, have severely limited the use of immunofluorescence methods in diagnostic pathology; nevertheless, they remain the procedure of choice for evaluation of immunologic disorders of kidney and skin.

Various metals, such as iron (ferritin), gold, and mercury, have been used as labels for immunohistochemical methods.[6,7,11] All produce sufficient electron opacity for visualization by light and electron microscopy. The poor penetration of metal conjugates and their nonspecific deposition in the background is the major drawback of immunometal methods. Immunogold methods are the most popular of these techniques and are used predominantly for ultrastructural localization of various substances such as hormones. The immunogold-silver staining technique is one of the most sensitive immunohistochemical procedures.[11]

Enzymes are the most widely used labels in immunohistochemistry. Peroxidase, alkaline phosphatase, and glucose oxidase are the commonly used enzymes, with peroxidase being the label of choice in more than 90 percent of immunohistochemical procedures currently employed in diagnostic histopathology.[12,13] Enzyme-antibody complexes retain both their immunologic and enzymatic properties and are therefore able to bind to specific antigens in tissues and to change the color of a suitable chromogen.

In immunohistochemistry, the labels are either directly bound to the primary, secondary, or tertiary antibodies, or they are indirectly introduced into the reaction by the use of other substances such as haptens, biotin, or protein A. Currently available immunohistochemical techniques are a large, heterogeneous group of procedures that differ from one another by the type of label, the number of antibodies, and the type of nonimmunologic substances used. In the following summary, the major categories of immunohistochemical methods are discussed briefly. We use the general term *label* in the description of these methods to imply that any one of the above described immunohistochemical labels may be used, although certain labels are used more commonly in certain procedures, such as enzymes in label-antilabel methods.

Labeled Antibody Methods

In labeled antibody procedures, the label is conjugated with the primary (direct) or secondary (indirect) anti-body.[14,15] The direct labeled antibody methods are the least sensitive of all immunohistochemical techniques. Although relatively simple to perform, they usually manifest nonspecific background staining. Furthermore, a panel of different conjugated antibodies is required to detect various respective antigens.

In indirect labeled antibody methods, the primary antibody is unconjugated and is followed in the staining sequence by a labeled antibody directed against the primary antibody. The indirect techniques are more sensitive than direct methods. They are also more versatile, since a single labeled secondary antibody can be used against a number of different primary antibodies from the same species of animal.

Unlabeled Antibody Procedures

Unlabeled antibody techniques were devised to increase the sensitivity and to circumvent some of the problems inherent to the conjugation of antibodies with label.[14-16] Frequently, the conjugation process is not complete, and the unlabeled antibody reduces the sensitivity of the procedure by competing with labeled antibody and by adding to the undesirable background staining.

Hybrid Antibody Method

In the hybrid antibody technique the antibody against the antigen under study and an antilabel antibody developed in the same animal species are enzymatically split and then reconstituted in such a manner that each antibody contains one valency against the antigen and one against the label, usually an enzyme.[17] In the second step of the staining procedure, free enzyme is added. This method is not widely accepted because of the difficulty in preparing the hybrid antibody. The presence of nonhybrid antibodies that are competing for the antigenic sites also reduces the sensitivity of this technique.

The Immunoglobulin-Label Bridge Method

Application of the primary antibody in this method is followed by a second antibody and an antilabel antibody, usually an antienzyme. The second antibody reacts as a bridge between the first antibody and the antienzyme that is raised in the same animal as the first antibody. In the final stage, free enzyme is added.[18,19] Although very sensitive, this technique is one of the most time-consuming immunoenzymatic methods.

Label-Antilabel Method

The label-antilabel technique is a modification of the label bridge method. The label is usually an enzyme, but haptens have also been used.[20,21] The prototype of these procedures is the peroxidase-antiperoxidase (PAP) method introduced by Sternberger's group.[20] In this technique, the last two steps of the enzyme bridge methods are combined by reacting free enzyme and antienzyme antibody to form a soluble complex. The enzyme-antienzyme technique is one of the most sensitive immunoenzymatic procedures presently used.

Other Immunohistochemical Methods

Labeled Antigen Method

Mason and Sammons developed the labeled antigen technique, in which the specific primary antibody is followed by antigen conjugated with the label, horseradish peroxidase (HRP).[22] The primary antibody acts bivalently to link the labeled antigen to antigen in the tissue. The major advantage of this procedure is that contaminating antibodies cannot cause nonspecific reactions, since they do not have affinity for the labeled antigen. This technique is also less time-consuming.

Protein A-Label Method

Protein A, a cell wall protein from *Staphylococcus aureus*, binds specifically to the Fc portion of immunoglobulin G (IgG); its coupling with other substances, such as enzymes and metals, does not affect this biologic property.[23] In the two-stage method, the primary antibody is followed by the protein A conjugated with a label, whereas in the three-stage technique, protein A acts as a bridge between the primary antibody and the label-antilabel complex.[16]

Hapten-Labeled Antibody Method

In the indirect method, a hapten-labeled primary antibody is followed by an enzyme-labeled antibody with specificity against the hapten.[16] The three-stage technique depends on the addition of an excess of antihapten to bridge between hapten-labeled primary antibody and the haptenated enzyme-antienzyme complex.[21]

Biotin-Avidin Procedure

In the biotin-avidin technique, the intense affinity of avidin (an egg white protein) for biotin (a low molecular weight vitamin) is used to introduce the label into the immunologic reaction.[24] In the direct method, the primary antibody conjugated with biotin (biotinylated) is followed by labeled avidin. In the indirect method, the primary antibody is followed by a biotinylated secondary antibody and then by labeled avidin. Endogenous biotin in various tissues may cause nonspecific background staining that should be circumvented by appropriate blocking techniques.

Avidin-Biotin Conjugate Method

In the avidin-biotin conjugated (ABC) procedure, a preformed complex of avidin-biotin-label is added to either a biotinylated primary antibody (direct) or biotinylated secondary antibody (indirect).[25] The latticework formed by ABC complexes contains several molecules of the label, hence ABC methods have one of the highest sensitivities of all immunohistochemical techniques.

Combination Methods

In an attempt to increase the sensitivity of immunohistochemical procedures, a variety of combination techniques have been described. In some of these techniques, the steps of a given procedure, such as PAP, are repeated two times or more,[26] whereas in others a combination of two different techniques, such as PAP and ABC, is recommended.[27] These combination techniques are generally more time-consuming. In addition, they may cause increased nonspecific background staining.

Simultaneous Staining for Two or More Antigens

More than 20 different immunohistochemical methods for concurrent localization of two or more antigens in the same tissue section have been described.[2] They result in the production of two or more colors, each of which signals the presence of a different antigen. Although most of these techniques are relatively simple to perform, in our experience there is no practical value in demonstrating two or more antigens in the same histologic section. Furthermore, in most cases, the color reaction of one chromogen overshadows the other, and the recognition of double or triple staining in one cell or area becomes difficult, if not impossible.

Technical Considerations

From the moment of biopsy to that of histologic examination of the stained sections, numerous factors may influence immunohistochemical results and lead to diagnostic problems or errors in interpretation.[28–30] This section examines a number of these factors and suggests guidelines to circumvent potential technical problems. Because most immunohistochemical techniques currently used in diagnostic histopathology are immunoperoxidase methods, this discussion is limited to that group of procedures.

Specimen

Immunoperoxidase procedures are applicable to both cytologic and histologic material; the latter may be a frozen section or a fixed and embedded block.

Cytologic Specimens

Cell smears, imprints, filter and cytocentrifuge preparations, cell suspensions, and cell blocks are all used for immunoperoxidase staining.[31] Cell block preparations are processed and handled in the same manner as are histologic samples. Cell suspensions are seldom used for routine immunocytochemistry, although the technique can be very useful in demonstrating cell surface antigens. Conventional filter preparations produce an undesirable background staining, probably because of nonspecific absorption of reagents by the filter. Unless alternative filters suitable for immunocytochemistry become available, they are not recommended for routine immunostaining.

Cell surface membrane antigens can be demonstrated readily in smears, imprints, and cytocentrifuge preparations with a sensitivity equal to, or greater than, that of histologic sections. By contrast, intracytoplasmic and intranuclear antigens may be more difficult to demonstrate in cytologic material. This is probably because despite the increased permeability of cytoplasmic membranes produced by various methods of fixation, they remain structurally intact and do not allow for easy penetration of immunologic reagents into the cells. False negative immunoperoxidase results for intracellular antigens are therefore more common in cytologic samples than in histologic specimens.[32]

Frozen Sections

Cell and tissue antigens are best preserved in either fresh or fresh frozen specimens. There is ample evidence that routine fixation and processing reduce the amount of immunohistochemically detectable antigens.[1–4] For example, some monoclonal antibodies react only on frozen sections. Many cell surface antigens are present in small amounts in fresh tissue and may be completely lost during routine processing and embedding. Cryostat sections are therefore preferable for demonstration of many cytoplasmic membrane antigens, including those found on the surfaces of hematopoietic cells.[33,34] Freezing a portion of each biopsy specimen in its fresh state ensures the availability of an optimal sample should the need for localization of such antigens arise.

Cell and tissue antigens are best preserved when the specimen is immediately and rapidly frozen. This can be accomplished by rapid immersion of a block of tissue, no larger than $1.0 \times 1.0 \times 0.3$ cm, in liquid nitrogen (snap freezing). Slow freezing of the specimens by placing them in a freezer will result in considerable antigen loss and poor morphologic detail. Thawing and refreezing the specimens also has a negative impact on histologic detail and preservation of tissue antigens.

Paraffin-Embedded Specimens

Ideal morphologic detail is obtained in sections of routinely processed paraffin-embedded tissue. The applicability of immunohistochemical procedures to paraffin-embedded tissue is responsible for their popularity and widespread use in diagnostic pathology. Every pathology file is now a potential source for numerous retrospective studies.

There is no conclusive evidence as to the degree of deleterious effect that different types of commercially available paraffin may have on various antigens. There is ample evidence, however, that infiltration of specimens by melted paraffin warmer than 60°C will result in denaturation of many antigens. When fixed and processed tissue is embedded in paraffin, immunohistochemically detectable tissue antigens remain intact in the block for many years and will not decrease during prolonged storage.

Plastic-Embedded Tissue

Thin sections from tissues embedded in different plastics, such as araldite, epoxy resin (Spurr), and methacrylate, demonstrate excellent morphologic detail. For immunohistochemistry, it is necessary to remove the resin with sodium ethoxide and to digest the tissue with trypsin to re-expose the antigens.[35] Unfortunately, even with these additional steps, immunohistochemical reactions in plastic-embedded tissue have yielded unpredictable, usually negative, results. Therefore, plastic sections are not recommended for routine immunohistochemistry in diagnostic pathology. A number of pre- and postembedding methods have been described for immunoelectron microscopy; however, a discussion of those procedures is beyond the scope of this review.

Fixative

It is safe to say that currently there are no ideal fixatives for immunohistochemistry. All fixatives, in one way or another, adversely affect the immunohistochemically detectable cell and tissue antigens. Among the factors that influence the choice of fixative are its availability, price, safety, and suitability for one or more antigens. In fact, cell and tissue substances differ in their susceptibility to various fixatives. An optimal fixative for intermediate filaments, for example, may cause deterioration of plasma proteins. In prospective studies, therefore, the choice of fixative depends on the type of antigens that are to be detected immunohistochemically. This section briefly examines the advantages and limitations of some of the more commonly used fixatives.

Formalin

Although 10 percent neutral formalin is the most widely available and economical fixative, it is not the best for immunohistochemistry.[36,37] The deteriorating effect of formalin is more evident with certain substances such as plasma proteins, including light and heavy chain immunoglobins, α-fetoprotein, and factor VIII-related antigen. Many other cytoplasmic antigens, however, withstand formalin fixation and can be demonstrated adequately either directly or by the use of proteolytic enzymes.

Alcohol-Containing Fixatives

Alcoholic fixatives, such as ethanol, methanol, Carnoy's, and methacarn, have the advantage of penetrating tissue rapidly. They are the fixatives of choice for a number of cell markers, including all intermediate filaments and other substances, such as synaptophysin.[38,39] However, the tissue fixed in alcoholic solutions shrinks and hardens quickly and may exhibit poor morphology.

Picric Acid-Containing Fixatives

Bouin's and Zamboni's are the two most commonly used fixatives in this group.[1,28,40] With the exception of intermediate filaments and immunoglobulins, most other cytoplasmic antigens can be demonstrated successfully in Bouin's fixed tissue. Bouin's fixation is particularly advantageous in preserving viral antigens, peptide hor-

mones, and some normal tissue substances such as prostatic acid phosphatase and prostatic-specific antigen. Zamboni's solution (picric acid, paraformaldehyde) is also suitable for electron microscopy.[40]

Mercuric Fixatives

B5 and other mercuric chloride-containing fixatives, such as Zenker's and Susa's, are better than formalin in preserving histologic detail, particularly nuclear morphology. These fixatives are also the best for immunohistochemical demonstration of immunoglobulins as well as some B- and T-cell surface markers, such as the LN, MB, and MT series, in paraffin-embedded tissues.[41–43] Mercuric fixatives, however, are not recommended for the majority of other cellular antigens. These fixatives produce undesirable background staining and may result in erroneous interpretation of immunohistochemical reactions.

Fixation Process

To achieve the highest quality immunohistochemical results, the tissue should be fixed promptly, thoroughly, and adequately, for no less or no more than necessary. Delay in fixation, inadequate fixation, and overfixation are all equally detrimental to good immunohistochemistry and may cause analytic errors.[1,30] Adequate penetration of the fixative can be achieved only by trimming the histologic specimen properly before fixation. Optimal fixation time for a $1.0 \times 1.0 \times 0.3$ cm block of tissue in formalin is between 12 and 18 hours. For fixatives containing alcohol, picric acid, and mercuric chloride, the optimal fixation time is 2 to 5 hours, and the tissue block should be no larger than $0.5 \times 0.5 \times 0.2$ cm.[2] Prolonged fixation results in a progressive loss in immunohistochemically detectable antigens. This is particularly true of overfixation in formalin, which then often necessitates protease digestion to unmask susceptible proteins.[44]

Rapid fixation of tissue can be achieved by using a conventional microwave oven.[45] Fixation time in formalin, for example, can be reduced to a few seconds, preserving both morphology and stainable tissue antigens.[45] Rapid microwave fixation will also obviate the need for protease digestion.

Specimen Preparation, Processing, and Embedding

Optimal specimen preparation and controlled processing and embedding are all prerequisites for good immunohistochemical staining. This section describes guidelines for proper handling of the specimen prior to the immuno-histochemical procedure. These recommendations are for cytologic samples as well as frozen sections and paraffin-embedded tissues.

Cytologic Samples

Cytoplasmic membranes in cell smears, imprints, and cytocentrifuge preparations are relatively intact; consequently, the immunologic reagents do not penetrate the cells as readily as they do in histologic sections.[31] This may result in lower sensitivity of the technique in demonstrating intracellular antigens and an increase in false negative results.[32] Pretreatment of slides with a 0.10 to 0.20 percent solution of Triton X-100 for 5 to 10 minutes will increase the permeability of the membranes, thus enhancing the sensitivity of the technique in smears, imprints, and cytocentrifuged specimens.[46] Overnight incubation of the slides with the primary antibody also helps to increase the sensitivity for demonstration of cytoplasmic antigens.

Cytocentrifugation of cellular specimens with a high content of protein may produce a precipitated film of protein over cellular material, which decreases the penetration of reagents into the cells. To prevent this, gentle washing of the cells before cytocentrifugation with a solution of phosphate-buffered saline is recommended. In order to reduce the detachment of cells from the slides during the immunoperoxidase procedure we coat them with poly-D-lysine before preparing smears and other cytologic specimens.

A large number of fixatives and fixation procedures for cytologic material have been reported in the literature. Some of the more commonly used fixatives include 95 percent ethanol, buffered formalin, cold (4°C) acetone, and buffered formol-acetone. One to 3 minutes of exposure to any of these solutions will be adequate for fixation of most cytologic specimens. Again, there is no universal optimal fixative for various cellular antigens. Some antigens, such as intermediate filaments, are best preserved in alcohol-based fixatives. For most other antigens, we have used buffered formol-acetone solution with good results.[31]

Cell preparations can either be fixed immediately or they can be first air-dried and fixed later. The latter option is particularly suitable for demonstrating cytoplasmic membrane antigens. Air-dried slides can also be wrapped in aluminum foil and stored indefinitely at −20°C. Frozen smears, however, should be brought back to room temperature before fixation and immunostaining.

On many occasions, the consideration for immunoperoxidase study on cytologic material comes about after examination of fixed and stained preparations. In such circumstances the coverglass is removed and the slide

carried through the immunocytochemical steps.[31] Destaining of the preparation is not necessary.

Histologic Sections

Whether of cryostat or paraffin origin, histologic sections of good quality are essential for optimal immunohistochemical reactions. Because necrotic tissue and blood in sections may lead to undesired background staining, tissue blocks should be selected from areas with little or no necrosis or hemorrhage.[1,28] In our experience, 4 to 5 μm thick sections of frozen or paraffin-embedded tissues provide the best preparations for immunostaining. Thicker sections, folded sections, and sections with tears or nicks from the microtome are undesirable for immunohistochemistry.[28,30] Histologic sections such as these are easily washed off during the procedure. To prevent this problem, we recommend one of the two following procedures:

1. *Subbed slides:* Dissolve 0.5 g of gelatin powder in 100 ml distilled water at low heat. Add 1.0 ml 5 percent potassium dichromate and cool to room temperature. Coat alcohol-cleaned slides by dipping them in the gelatin solution. Drain and dry well before using. Subbed slides can be stored for later use.
2. *Glue-coated slides:* Dissolve 4 to 5 drops Elmer's Glue-All in 50 ml distilled water at 56°C for 1 to 2 hours. Mix the solution well, then dip precleaned slides in it. Dry slides overnight at 37°C. Glue-coated slides can be used for frozen sections as well.

Preparation of Frozen Sections

Fresh tissue should be frozen immediately and rapidly. Snap-freezing of a 1.0 × 1.0 × 0.3 cm block of fresh tissue can be accomplished by immersing it in liquid nitrogen. A mixture of isopentane and liquid nitrogen will result in a more uniform freezing of tissue, and hence the best preservation of histomorphology.[2] A supporting embedding compound such as OCT (Ames) will facilitate preparation of good quality frozen sections. Because there is evidence that OCT-embedded frozen tissues gradually lose their cellular antigens, prolonged storage of OCT-embedded histologic material in the frozen state is not recommended. Snap-frozen fresh tissue, without supporting media, however, can be stored at −70°C for long periods of time without appreciable antigen loss.

In order to maximize the adherance of frozen sections to the slides, subbed or glue-coated slides should be used. Fifteen second irradiation in a microwave oven at 320 W will also produce excellent adherence of frozen sections to glass slides without loss of antigens.[47]

A number of different fixatives have been recommended for frozen sections. Cell surface antigens are best preserved in sections fixed briefly in cold acetone (5 minutes at 4°C).[3] Good results are also obtained in frozen sections fixed for a few minutes in ethanol, formalin, and picric acid paraformaldehyde. Sections can be either fixed immediately or air-dried first and fixed later. If fixation is apt to mask or denature the antigen under study, it can be delayed until after the primary antibody has been applied. Immunohistochemistry of unfixed frozen tissue will result in poor morphological results, diffusion of the antigens, and increased background staining.[2]

Paraffin-Embedded Tissues

Processing and embedding appear to have little effect on immunostaining of fixed tissue, provided processing and embedding temperatures do not exceed 60°C. Routinely fixed, paraffin-embedded specimens combine good morphology with localization of various cell and tissue markers. Some cell surface antigens, however, may be completely lost during routine processing and embedding. In recent years, several alternative tissue processing and paraffin-embedding techniques have been described that result in an improved preservation of cell surface antigens for immunostaining.[48,49] For example, a procedure in which the tissue is freeze-dried and then embedded directly in paraffin is likely to produce staining results with an intensity equal to, or greater than, that observed in frozen sections.[49]

Decalcification

Different decalcifying solutions, such as EDTA, formic acid, and nitric acid, do not significantly alter the antigenicity of various cell and tissue substances.[50] However, tissues should not be left in decalcifying solutions any longer than necessary. If antigen loss is anticipated during decalcification, the specimen should be fixed first and then placed in decalcifying solution.

Protease Digestion

Trypsin and other proteolytic enzymes have been advocated to enhance immunohistochemical reactions by unmasking antigens and increasing the contrast between the specific reaction and nonspecific background staining.[51] In addition to trypsin, pepsin, pronase, ficin, proteases type VII, VIII, and XIV, collagenase and DNase have all been used in immunohistochemistry.[52,53] The following facts should be known before proteolytic digestion of histologic sections is attempted:

1. Enzymatic predigestion is not for all antigens; it may enhance detection of a few markers but no enhancement or false negative staining may occur with a number of others.[54]
2. There is no universal optimal proteolytic enzyme. The choice of enzyme depends on the type of antigen (e.g., intermediate filaments), its location (cytoplasm, nucleus), and the type of fixative and embedding medium being used. Trypsin, for example, is a good enzyme to enhance the immunohistochemistry of keratins in formalin-fixed, paraffin-embedded tissues. It may, however, have an adverse effect on the demonstration of keratins in ethanol-fixed tissues.[44]
3. The length of the enzymatic digestion period should be adjusted to the extent of tissue exposure to the fixative. Tissue that has been fixed in formalin for several weeks requires a longer digestion period than that of similar tissue fixed for 1 or 2 days.[44]
4. It is easy to overdigest tissue, thus affecting morphology adversely and even causing detachment of the sections from the glass slide. The quality of enzyme predigestion, therefore, should be carefully controlled to achieve optimal sensitivity for demonstration of those antigens that benefit from the use of proteolytic enzymes.
5. Enzyme digestion is not recommended for cytologic samples except for cell block preparations. Cell blocks are treated in the same manner as are histologic specimens.

Melanin Bleaching

The peroxidase label is usually visualized using diaminobenzidine as chromogen, with the formation of orange-brown granules. Pigments of similar color, such as melanin, when present in excessive amounts may interfere with correct interpretation of immunoperoxidase results. Of all the methods described for the removal of melanin, treatment of the sections with potassium permanganate and oxalic acid before beginning the immunoperoxidase procedure appears to be the least damaging to stainable antigens and tissue morphology.[55]

Staining Procedure

Although immunoperoxidase staining is simple enough for any qualified technician to perform, every step of the procedure may harbor a potential pitfall. The following are recommendations for the improvement of staining results and prevention of technical mishaps during the procedure.

Attachment of Sections to Slides

Use of subbed or glue-coated slides decreases the possibility of specimen detachment. For freshly cut paraffin sections, overnight incubation in a 37°C oven minimizes the loss of tissues during the procedure.

Clearing and Rehydration

These steps are for removal of the paraffin by a clearing agent such as xylene and rehydration of tissue by their immersion in decreasing grades of ethanol. Short cuts in these steps will result in poor morphologic resolution of the final product.

Inhibition of Endogenous Peroxidase Activity

The activity of endogenous peroxidase can be inhibited by several means. The technique most commonly used is immersion of the slides in a freshly prepared 1 : 4 solution of 3 percent hydrogen peroxidase in absolute methanol.[56] If it is not inhibited, the peroxidase and peroxidase-like activity of various cells may interfere with interpretation of stains, particularly in frozen sections. Some workers, however, choose not to block endogenous peroxidase and to use its activity as an internal control for evaluation of the chromogen reaction.

Reduction of Nonspecific Background Staining

Nonspecific background staining of some tissues such as collagen, smooth and skeletal muscle, and certain mitochondrion-rich cells, such as hepatocytes and oncocytes, is a common nuisance of immunoperoxidase techniques.[1,28,30,56] These nonspecific background stains are more common when conventional polyclonal antisera are used, although some monoclonal antibodies, particularly those of mouse ascites origin, may produce similar results. Preincubation of histologic sections with a high concentration of a protein solution, such as nonimmune serum or albumin, may reduce undesirable background staining, although ordinarily it cannot be avoided completely.[56] Use of the primary antibody, in its highest possible dilution, may also help reduce this unwanted reaction.

Incubation with the Primary Antibody

The optimal incubation time for most primary antibodies is 20 to 30 minutes at room temperature (20 to 22°C). Overnight (18 hour) incubation of sections at 4°C will increase the sensitivity of the procedure with some monoclonal antibodies, particularly those against cell membrane antigens. To accomplish this, adequate amounts of the primary antibody are applied, the section is covered with a coverglass, and the slide is stored horizontally in a regular refrigerator. It is also possible to decrease the incubation time to 5 to 10 minutes by increasing the temperature to 37°C. Immunostaining in higher temperatures, however, is unpredictable and may cause false negative results.

The optimal concentration of a primary antibody should be determined by applying serial dilutions of that antibody to several sections of a known positive tissue.[1] The slide with the best specific reaction and the least background staining reflects the optimal dilution for that antibody. Prediluted antibodies, such as those in commercial staining kits, are usually titrated for a tissue with an average amount of antigen and may not be suitable for tissues containing either more or less than that amount. Etching a circle around the tissue section with a diamond pen will prevent diffusion of reagent over the entire slide, thus saving precious antibody.

Linking Antibodies and Peroxidase Conjugates

Once the optimal dilutions are determined for a batch of linking antibody and peroxidase-containing complex, such as PAP and avidin-biotin-peroxidase, they remain constant for their use with all primary antibodies. The optimal incubation time for linking antibodies and peroxidase conjugates is 30 to 60 minutes at room temperature.

Color Development

Common chromogens for peroxidase are diaminobenzidine (DAB) and aminoethylcarbazole (AEC). DAB and AEC solutions should be made fresh immediately before their use. Failure to add hydrogen peroxide to either of these solutions is a common oversight, particularly for beginners; it results in total lack of staining of all slides, including positive controls.

Counterstaining

Hematoxylin and eosin (H&E) is the most popular nuclear counterstain for immunoperoxidase-stained tissues. It should not be used, however, when antigen localization is expected to be in the nucleus. The choice of the type of hematoxylin (Harris's or Mayer's) depends on the type of chromogen used. Since AEC is soluble in organic solvents, it should be used with Mayer's hematoxylin, which is not alcohol-based.[2] To obtain maximum contrast in black and white photography of immunoperoxidase-stained slides, it is advisable to use only light nuclear counterstaining. The color of DAB granules can also be darkened by rapid dipping of the slides in a 0.5 percent solution of osmium tetroxide.

Other Technical Notes

All washes and dilutions are made with phosphate-buffered saline (PBS) with a pH of 7.2 to 7.6. Although slight variation in pH is not critical to the outcome of an immunoperoxidase procedure, periodic checks of the pH of stock PBS solution are recommended. All incubations should take place in a humidity chamber to reduce the possibility of reagent evaporation. At no time between incubations and washes should the sections be left to dry.

They should be immersed in PBS if delay in staining is inevitable. Dried sections will show poor morphologic resolution as well as false negative or false positive reactions.

Automated Immunohistochemistry

Automation is only an expected development for a new analytic procedure, such as immunohistochemistry, composed, as it is, of well defined steps and standardized variables such as volume, time, and temperature. The limiting factor for automated immunohistochemistry has always been the requirement for reagent volume control. Recent innovations have solved this important problem by using either capillary action or pipettes to deliver immunologic reagents to the glass slides.[57,58] The entire process is controlled by a computer. The advantages of automated immunohistochemistry are better standardization of the staining procedure, improved reproducibility of the results, and reduction in technician time.[57]

Reagents

The crucial element in any reliable immunoperoxidase system is a good quality monospecific antibody.[1–4] The use of conventional polyclonal antisera in immunohistochemistry is gradually decreasing in favor of utilization of monoclonal antibodies.[4] Monoclonal antibodies are relatively easy to produce, and specific, with little batch-to-batch variation. By contrast, because their reactivity is usually against an epitope rather than the whole antigen, they may result in lesser sensitivity of antigen detection in histologic sections. In addition, since different types of antigens may share common epitopes, monoclonal antibodies may recognize and bind to a number of unrelated antigens. This specific pattern of cross-reactivity of monoclonal antibodies is best demonstrated by the apparent reactivity of certain monoclonal antibodies reactive against lymphocyte antigens with cells of other lineage, such as epithelial cells. It should be remembered therefore, that monoclonal antibodies are generally epitope-specific and their use does not guarantee antigen specificity. In immunohistochemistry, there is usually a tradeoff between the better defined specificity of monoclonal antibodies and the higher affinity of polyclonal antisera.

The stability and shelf life of most immunologic reagents used in immunohistochemistry are ordinarily indicated by the supplier. Many such reagents are normally stored at 4°C, and they will ultimately lose their reactivity. Most frequently used reagents may be frozen in small portions and used after thawing. Frozen reagents have an indefinite shelf life, but repeated thawing and freezing diminishes their reactivity.[28,30]

Chromogens are another important group of reagents in immunohistochemistry. Diaminobenzidine is the most widely used chromogen for the immunoperoxidase technique. It produces orange-brown granules at the reaction site that are not soluble in organic solvents. The intensity of the reaction remains unchanged for years in storage if DAB is used as the chromogen. Because of the suspected carcinogenicity of DAB, other chromogens for peroxidase have been introduced.[30,59,60] One of the most popular of these alternative chromogens is AEC. It produces a cherry-red color that, unlike DAB, is soluble in alcohol and clearing reagents. Therefore, it requires special aqueous mounting media to coverslip the slides, and that reduces the morphologic resolution of histologic sections. In addition, AEC-stained slides gradually lose their intensity in storage. Since AEC is also a suspected carcinogen, there is no valid reason for its use as an alternative to DAB.[30,59] Other chromogens for peroxidase are less popular because of technical difficulties that complicate their use.[60] Furthermore, many have the same disadvantages as AEC. All chromogens for peroxidase should be disposed of according to the supplier's instructions.

Because of the increasing popularity of immunohistochemical techniques, there are now many commercial sources for antibodies, conjugates, and staining kits. Most of these reagents and kits have proved reliable, but it is ultimately the responsibility of the user to ensure their diagnostic specificity and to control their quality.

Controls

As with other immunologic techniques, the results of immunohistochemical reactions are not valid unless proper controls and standards are used and evaluated in each procedure. For standard immunoperoxidase procedures, two important control slides should be included.

1. Positive control. A positive control is a histologic section that is known to contain the antigen under study. For a negative reaction to be considered truly negative, the known positive slide must be positive. The use of positive controls of intermediate intensity is preferable, because they become negative if the sensitivity of the reaction is reduced,[30] whereas a strongly positive control may still be positive and thus cause a false negative interpretation of the case under study.
2. Antibody control. Antibody control (sometimes erroneously referred to as negative control) should also be included in every immunoperoxidase procedure. Its negativity validates positive results. Replacement of the primary antibody on an adjacent slide by the same antibody preabsorbed with the antigen under study is the most reliable antibody control. In most instances, however, a less desirable but more practical antibody control is used

by replacing the primary antibody with either nonimmune serum or another antibody with irrelevant specificity.

3. Other controls. Controls for linking antibodies, PAP complex, and avidin-biotin reagents are not ordinarily included in routine immunoperoxidase staining. Similarly, sections of tissues known to be negative for the antigen under study are not required to be included in every procedure provided that the specificity of the antibodies is predetermined. Panels of known negative and positive tissues, however, are an integral part of evaluation of the specificity of every newly acquired antibody. In addition, different cellular components of immunohistochemically stained tissue serve as reliable built-in positive and negative controls (e.g., endothelium and smooth muscle of normal blood vessels associated with a neoplasm that is being investigated).

Several rapid and simple methods for antibody testing have been introduced that use multiple tissue samples embedded in a single paraffin block.[61,62] These multitissue approaches simplify the screening of newly developed monoclonal antibodies to a considerable degree. These methods also consume smaller amounts of antibodies and other reagents compared to conventional methods using several different tissue sections.

With the exception of cell blocks, for all other cytologic samples both the known positive and the antibody controls should consist of cytologic specimens.[31] One can ensure the availability of known positive cytologic slides by organizing a file of imprints from normal and neoplastic tissues known to contain various antigens. For antibody controls, however, duplicate slides of the case under study may not be available. In that situation, two separate circles can be etched with a diamond pen on the same cytologic slide. The primary antibody is added to one circle, while the other is covered with control antibody.[31]

DIAGNOSTIC APPLICATION

Relative Value of Different Immunohistochemical Markers

Immunohistochemical markers can be divided into two groups: specific markers and nonspecific markers. Specific markers are those whose expression is limited to one cell line; their localization in a cell population signals a specific line of differentiation. Prostatic-specific antigen and thyroglobulin, expressed respectively by prostatic glandular epithelium and follicular cells of the thyroid, are examples of specific markers. By contrast, most of the currently used cell and tissue markers are nonspecific and are expressed by more than one type of cell. Nevertheless, these markers are still valuable in diagnostic immunohistochemistry, as they allow for general categorization of a cellular population (e.g., epithelial, lymphoid).

The diagnostic value of different immunohistochemical markers depends upon a number of factors, two of the most important of which are the specificity of the marker and its stability during fixation and processing. Although there are no general rules to predict the extent of damage various antigens incur during routine fixation and processing, it appears that some cell products, such as immunoglobulins and factor VIII-related antigen, suffer most, whereas other substances, such as peptide hormones, are less susceptible.[1,30] Therefore, although factor VIII-related antigen is a highly specific marker for endothelial cells, its lack of durability during different stages of tissue handling decreases its potential diagnostic value.

On the basis of their specificity and durability, we arbitrarily divide cell and tissue markers into three groups:

1. Very useful markers. Antigens in this category are not only cell-specific, but they are expressed by their respective cells with a high frequency, and their detection in different tissues is not affected by variations in specimen handling, fixation, and processing. These markers are therefore diagnostically important both when they are present and when they are absent. Prostatic-specific antigen qualifies for inclusion in this category. Using currently available antibodies, this marker is found exclusively in normal and neoplastic prostatic epithelium. Most (more than 97 percent, in our experience) prostatic carcinomas express this antigen. It is also a fairly durable antigen, as it is not easily destroyed or masked by improper handling of tissue. Unfortunately, not many markers provide such a high degree of diagnostic specificity and sensitivity.

2. Useful markers. This category comprises the majority of currently detectable immunohistochemical markers. Some of these antigens are very specific for a cell type but are either not expressed with a high frequency or are easily damaged by slight variations in the treatment of the tissue. Myoglobin, for instance, is a specific marker for rhabdomyoblasts but several studies have shown that it is not expressed by all proven rhabdomyosarcomas. Similarly, although leukocyte common antigen is a specific marker for lymphoreticular cells, it is not demonstrable in all malignant lymphomas. The reason for this is that lymphomas occasionally do not express this antigen. In addition, with currently available antibodies one may sometimes observe false negative results in formalin-fixed, paraffin-embedded tissue, even when enhancement steps, such as overnight incubation, and amplification procedures are undertaken. These markers are therefore diagnostically useful when present, but of limited value when not detectable.

Another subgroup of useful markers are those which

are not specific to a single cell line but whose demonstration in a group of cells helps to classify the cells in a general category. Most intermediate filaments (with the exception of vimentin) fall into this group of antigens. In general, the diagnostic value of this group of antigens is greatest when used as part of a panel of markers.

3. Markers of borderline or no diagnostic value. The markers in this category, whether present or absent, provide little important diagnostic information. Vimentin and α_1-antichymotrypsin are typical examples. They are expressed by such a wide range of different cells and tissues that their immunohistochemical detection is of extremely limited diagnostic value, even when they are used with a panel of other markers. In other words, what is diagnostically important in the evaluation of a spindle cell tumor is the presence or absence of useful markers, such as keratins, S-100 protein, and desmin, and not the presence or absence of vimentin.

Antibody Panels

The use of antibody panels in diagnostic immunohistochemistry will increase the diagnostic specificity and sensitivity. It also saves time and reduces the expense because it usually obviates further study of a case for additional markers. The number of antibodies used in a panel is entirely dependent on the differential diagnoses entertained. Generally, one or two antibodies are used as the main diagnostic reagents while an additional one or more antibodies play a confirmatory role. It is important to remember that the intelligent use of panels in immunohistochemistry is the use of two or more antibodies in a specific differential diagnosis based on a reasonable histologic and clinical judgement; it is not the indiscriminate use of a number of irrelevant antibodies without consideration of histomorphology or clinical history (the buckshot approach). Antibody panels are used most commonly in the following diagnostic situations[1,63]:

1. Undifferentiated malignant neoplasms composed of large, small, or spindle cells
2. Lymphoproliferative processes including reactive and neoplastic lymphoid proliferations of B- and T-cell types
3. Soft tissue sarcomas
4. Neuroendocrine tumors, the panels for which may include general neuroendocrine markers like neurofilaments and chromogranin, or specific endocrine products such as hormones
5. Nervous system neoplasms, including those arising from both the central and peripheral nervous systems
6. Gonadal and extragonadal germ cell tumors and gestational trophoblastic diseases
7. Viral, bacterial, fungal, and protozoal diseases
8. Specific differential diagnoses (bladder versus prostate neoplasms, hepatocellular carcinoma versus metastatic carcinomas, adenocarcinoma versus mesothelioma, intraepidermal skin tumors)
9. All other instances when one needs to differentiate specific disease entities

How to Choose Markers

The selection of appropriate immunohistologic markers, to aid in the histologic diagnosis of a specific disease process of uncertain nature, depends on a number of factors, including clinical findings, the histologic appearance of the lesion, the differential diagnosis, and the availability of markers for those disease entities included in the differential diagnosis. Since diagnostic immunohistochemistry is used most commonly in the diagnosis and classification of neoplasms, we review briefly the influence of each of these factors in selecting appropriate markers for the diagnosis of tumors only.

Clinical History

Information regarding the patient's age, sex, past and present clinical history, the site of biopsy, and any history of previous tumors or treatments is important for the histologic evaluation of a neoplasm and the selection of appropriate immunohistochemical markers. For example, the choice of antibodies for the histologic diagnosis of a small cell malignant tumor varies depending on whether the patient is a child or an adult. Similarly, in a patient with metastatic poorly differentiated carcinoma in bone, it is important to know that the patient has had previous surgery for a thyroid carcinoma, because with this knowledge one would include thyroglobulin in the panel.

Histomorphology of the Tumor

The histologic appearance of a tumor is the basis for selection of related markers. Here the experience of the observer plays an important role. Immunohistochemistry may only compound the problem if the original histologic interpretation is totally erroneous. For instance, the results of immunohistochemical stains for subtyping of a "carcinoma" in bone may be confusing and even misleading if the correct histologic diagnosis is an epithelioid hemangioendothelioma.

Differential Diagnosis

A reasonable differential diagnosis is based on the histomorphology of the tumor, clinical information, and the probability of occurrence of certain neoplasms in that age group and in that anatomic location. Thus, the differential diagnosis can be broad or limited. The differential diagnosis of a large cell undifferentiated neoplasm, for example, is rather wide and may include carcinoma, sarcoma, melanoma, lymphoma, and even germinoma (seminoma). This differential diagnosis obviously requires a large number of markers in the panel, whereas the differential diagnosis of an adenocarcinoma involving both the urinary bladder and the prostate is a narrow one requiring only a limited number of markers.[63]

Availability of Markers

With presently available antibodies against various cellular antigens, it is not possible to classify all primary and metastatic neoplasms. In fact, the most prevalent human carcinomas do not have specific markers. This limits severely the choice of markers in a number of diagnostic situations, including classification of common adenocarcinomas. For example, with currently available immunohistochemical markers, it is not possible to separate adenocarcinomas of breast, lung, pancreas, gastrointestinal (GI) tract, and biliary system from one another.[1] In these situations, based on the degree of clinical and histologic suspicion and the results of staining for few nonspecific markers, one can place the tumor in a general category, such as carcinoembryonic antigen-positive adenocarcinoma, and suggest the most likely sites of origin.[1]

Evaluation of the Results

From the moment of examination of the H&E-stained sections to the time of interpretation of immunohistochemical reactions, the skill and experience of the pathologist is the most important determining factor in the diagnostic value of the technique. The observer should not only be familiar with the characteristics of a true positive reaction, but also the possibility of variability in results and potential sources of technical and analytical errors.

True Positive Reaction

When DAB is used as a chromogen, a true positive immunoperoxidase reaction not only stains cells brown but has several characteristics as well, familiarity with which will help the observer avoid false positive interpretations. The most important quality of a true positive reaction is its heterogeneity in distribution within single cells, among a group of cells, or throughout a neoplasm. In individual cells, the crisp brown granules of DAB may occupy all of the cytoplasm, the perinuclear area alone, or simply one of the poles of a cell.[1,30] Diffuse, pale brown, or a single-tone yellow staining of neoplastic cells

is, in all likelihood, nonspecific.[1,30] The only exception to this rule is the specific but diffuse and homogeneous pattern of staining for neuronal enolase.

The site of positive reaction within a cell is another clue to the specificity of the staining. Most immunohistochemical markers are localized either intracytoplasmically and/or on cytoplasmic membranes. Both cytoplasmic and nuclear staining of variable proportions are seen with some viral antigens, neuronal enolase, estrogen and progesterone receptor proteins, and S-100 protein. In fact, in the absence of nuclear staining, one should question the validity of a positive reaction for S-100 protein. Distinctive patterns of the localization of antigens in certain normal and neoplastic cells will also help verify a true positive reaction. For example, familiarity with the characteristic perinuclear staining and its accentuation in the Golgi area of immunoglobulins in large cell lymphomas aids in separating it from nonspecific homogeneous staining of the entire cytoplasm which occurs in degenerative and necrotic cells.

Negative Reaction

True negative reactions are difficult to verify in immunohistochemistry, even when appropriate controls are used. When faced with a negative immunohistochemical reaction, there are two possible questions to ask: Do the cells elaborate the antigen under study but we are unable to demonstrate it? Or, do the cells not express the antigen?[32]

When cells express an antigen and we are unable to demonstrate it by immunohistochemistry, we are dealing with a false negative result. A false negative reaction may be because of a technical problem related to the specimen, fixation, processing, the procedure, or the reagents used, or it could be due to the sensitivity of the method, being lower than the threshold necessary to detect trace amounts of the antigen. Technical problems leading to false negative results can be identified and corrected if appropriate positive controls, both built-in and external, are used and evaluated in each procedure.[32] True negative reactions, however, are more difficult to prove, even when positive controls are positive, and consequently, negative results in immunohistochemistry are not usually as meaningful as positive reactions.

Potential Sources of Problems

The potential pitfalls of immunoperoxidase procedures can be divided into technical problems and errors in interpretation of results.[1,28] The two, however, are closely related because any technical mishap will eventually appear under the microscope and may thus lead to an error in interpretation.

Technical Problems

Every step of the immunoperoxidase technique, from the moment of biopsy to microscopic examination of the stained section, may harbor a problem. Many of these have been discussed above. The following discussion summarizes the most common technical problems associated with the immunoperoxidase technique.[1,28,30,64,65]

Specimen

Whether it is snap-frozen or fixed, the specimen should be as fresh as possible. A delay in freezing or fixation may cause false negative results. Delay in fixation may also cause drying of the surfaces of the tissue and produce a nonspecific positive reaction at the periphery of the section.

Fixation

Inadequate fixation of the histologic material for any reason, particularly large size of the block, the presence of a fibrous capsule, or an insufficient period of time for fixation, may lead to artefactual positive or negative staining of unfixed areas. Overfixation causes an exponential loss of antigen and leads to false negative results.

Staining Procedure

Failure to block the activity of endogenous peroxidase or undesirable nonspecific background staining may lead to false positive interpretations. Unintentional omission of any of the immunologic reagents, improperly prepared buffers, and failure to add hydrogen peroxide to the DAB solution all lead to false negative reactions. Any short cuts in the procedure, such as shortening of the incubation time, may reduce the sensitivity of the technique and lead to negative results.

Reagents

Low affinity primary antibodies, or antibodies that are outdated or excessively diluted, may lead to false negative results. Some polyclonal antisera, and occasionally monoclonal antibodies derived from ascitic fluid, may cause unacceptable background staining. The specificity of each newly acquired antibody should be determined before it is used for diagnostic purposes. Attention to built-in and external controls will help to identify most technical sources of problems.

Problems in Interpretation

In evaluation of the results of immunohistochemical techniques, the observer should not only be familiar with the characteristics of a true positive reaction but also with many potential causes of misinterpretation. Com-

mon causes of false positive interpretations are reviewed briefly here.[1,30]

Crushed cells, degenerated and necrotic cells, and histiocytes and macrophages all absorb reagents nonspecifically, and may therefore lead to erroneous interpretation. This phenomenon is responsible for false positive readings of Ig stains in malignant lymphomas because those tumors commonly contain degenerated and necrotic cells. Similarly, cells in mitosis, tumor giant cells, and neoplastic cells with active phagocytosis and cannibalism stain nonspecifically for a variety of antigens, particularly for circulating substances. Nonspecific staining is also seen in intermediate and superficial cells of keratinizing and nonkeratinizing squamous epithelia.[66]

The free edges of histologic sections at times exhibit nonspecific positive reactions.[67] Also, cells which float in fluids, such as body cavity effusions or the contents of vesicles or pustules, may show nonspecific membrane staining for antigens present in that fluid. Undissolved granules of DAB or other chromogens produce spots of nonspecific positive reaction in histologic sections. Passive diffusion of an antigen from tissues containing large amounts of that substance to adjacent negative cells is another source of false positive results.[67]

It is not unusual to observe complete lack of staining for different antigens in tissues known to contain them in a condensed or consolidated form. For example, the keratin layer of skin, Russell bodies in plasma cells,[68] and colloid in thyroid follicles may not stain for keratin, immunoglobulins, or thyroglobulin, respectively.[30] The inability of reagents to penetrate these solidified structures is the explanation for this phenomenon. This view is supported by the presence of a rim of positivity in their more penetrable peripheries and by enhancement of staining after protease digestion. Another cause of false negative staining in tissues known to contain the substance under study is the prozone effect. This occurs when the tissue contains unusually large concentrations of antigen to the extent that the antigen-antibody reaction does not take place unless the antibody is substantially diluted (Nadji M, Morales AR, unpublished observations). A plasmacytoma, for example, may not stain for the expected immunoglobulin with usual concentrations of the antibody, whereas a lower concentration of the same antibody will produce satisfactory results.

Diagnostic Sensitivity and Specificity

The sensitivity of an immunohistochemical method is the smallest amount of an antigen that it can detect.[69] This is usually represented by the lowest staining intensity that will distinguish the antigen from the background. Although current immunohistochemical techniques are sensitive enough to provide useful information about a variety of diagnostic problems, even the most sensitive methods have limits below which the reaction cannot be detected. Therefore, negative immunohistochemical results for a given antigen in certain tissues must be accepted cautiously.[69]

Although closely related, diagnostic sensitivity and technical sensitivity for detection of an antigen are not the same. No matter how sensitive a technique might be, one cannot achieve the highest diagnostic sensitivity if the target antigen is not uniformly expressed by all the cells or tissues that are expected to contain it. Therefore, in addition to the technical sensitivity, the diagnostic sensitivity is also dependent on the pattern of distribution and the frequency of expression of an antigen.

The specificity of a diagnosis derived from the immunohistochemical staining for an antigen depends not only on the technical specificity but also on the specificity of that antigen for the suspected diagnosis. Therefore, regardless of how specific the method and the antibody might be, one cannot achieve acceptable diagnostic specificity if the antigen is not specific for that diagnosis.

Technical specificity may also be discussed in terms of specificity of the method as well as of the antibody.[69,70] Testing for the nonspecificity of the method is relatively simple; it is accomplished by omitting each reagent, one at a time, to pinpoint the source of the nonspecific staining.[69]

As discussed before, both conventional and monoclonal antibodies may recognize and bind specifically to epitopes (sites) rather than whole antigen molecules. Thus, an antibody that is site-specific may be antigen-nonspecific, if the antigenic site is common to several unrelated molecules. Preabsorption of such antibodies by their respective antigens, therefore, will not serve as appropriate tests of specificity.[69] Although there are various methods to evaluate the specificity of an antibody, it must be recognized that in routine diagnostic pathology these additional tests are both cumbersome and impractical. In such instances, one normally relies on other information such as clinical history, histomorphology, histochemistry, and electron microscopy to validate the specificity of the results.

REFERENCES

1. Nadji M, Morales AR: Immunoperoxidase Techniques. A Practical Approach to Tumor Diagnosis. American Society of Clinical Pathologists Press, Chicago, 1986
2. Taylor CR: Immunomicroscopy: A Diagnostic Tool for the Surgical Pathologists. WB Saunders, Philadelphia, 1986
3. Tubbs R, Petras RE, Gephardt GN: Atlas of Immunohistology. American Society of Clinical Pathologists Press, Chicago, 1986
4. Wick MR, Siegal GP (eds): Monoclonal Antibodies in Diagnostic Immunohistochemistry. Marcel Dekker, New York, 1988
5. Coons AH, Creech HJ, Jones RN: Immunological properties of an antibody containing a fluorescent group. Proc Soc Exp Biol Med 47:200, 1941
6. Singer SJ: Preparation of an electron-dense antibody conjugate. Nature (Lond) 183:1523, 1959
7. Zhdanoff VM, Azdova NB, Kulberg AY: The use of antibody labeled with an organic mercury compound in electron microscopy. J Histochem Cytochem 13:684, 1965
8. Avrameas S, Uriel J: Methode de marquage d'antigènes et d'anticorps avec des enzymes et son application en immunodiffusion. CR Acad Sci 262:2543, 1966
9. Nakane PK, Pierce GB Jr: Enzyme-labeled antibodies: Preparation and application for the localization of antigens. J Histochem Cytochem 14:929, 1966
10. Kohler G, Milstein C: Continuous culture of fused cells secreting antibody of predefined origin. Nature (Lond) 256:495, 1975
11. Holgate CS, Jackson P, Cowen PN, Bird CC: Immunogold-silver staining: New method of immunostaining with enhanced sensitivity. J Histochem Cytochem 31:938, 1983
12. Mason DY, Sammons R: Alkaline phosphatase and peroxidase for double immunoenzymatic labeling of cellular constituents. J Clin Pathol 31:454, 1978
13. Suffin SC, Muck KB, Young JC: Improvement of the glucose oxidase immunoenzyme technique. Use of tetrazolium whose formazan is stable without heavy metal chelation. Am J Clin Pathol 71:492, 1979
14. Taylor CR: Immunoperoxidase techniques. Practical and theoretical aspects. Arch Pathol Lab Med 102:113, 1978
15. Heyderman E: Immunoperoxidase techniques in histopathology: Application, methods and controls. J Clin Pathol 32:971, 1979
16. Falini B, Taylor CR: New developments in immunoperoxidase techniques and their application. Arch Pathol Lab Med 107:105, 1983
17. Hammerling U, Aoki T, Wood HA, et al: New visual markers of antibody for electron microscopy. Nature (Lond) 223:1158, 1969
18. Sternberger LA: Some new developments in immunocytochemistry. Microskopie 25:346, 1969
19. Mason TE, Phifer RF, Spicer SS, et al: An immunoglobulin-enzyme bridge method for localizing tissue antigens. J Histochem Cytochem 17:563, 1969
20. Sternberger LA, Hardy PH Jr, Cuculis JJ, Mayer HG: The unlabeled antibody-enzyme method of immunohistochemistry. Preparation and properties of soluble antigen-antibody complex (horseradish peroxidase-antihorseradish peroxidase) and its use in identification of spirochetes. J Histochem Cytochem 18:315, 1970
21. Jasani B, Thomas DW, Williams ED: Use of monoclonal antihapten antibodies for immunolocalization of tissue antigens. J Clin Pathol 34:1000, 1981
22. Mason DY, Sammons RE: The labeled antigen method of immunoenzymatic staining. J Histochem Cytochem 27:832, 1979

23. Goding JW: Use of staphylococcal protein A as an immunological reagent. J Immunol Methods 20:241, 1978

24. Warnke R, Levy R: Detection of T and B cell antigens with hybridoma monoclonal antibodies: A biotin-horseradish peroxidase method. J Histochem Cytochem 28:771, 1980

25. Hsu SM, Raine L, Fanger H: Use of avidin-biotin peroxidase complex (ABC) in immunoperoxidase techniques: A comparison between ABC and unlabeled antibody (PAP) procedures. J Histochem Cytochem 29:577, 1981

26. Lansdorp PM, Van der Kwast TH, DeBoer M, Zeijlemaker WP: Stepwise amplified immunoperoxidase staining. I Cellular morphology in relation to membrane markers. J Histochem Cytochem 32:172, 1984

27. Kamiya H, Imamura M: Sensitive immunohistochemical demonstration of human lymphocyte cell surface antigens in tissue sections by using a combined PAP-avidin-biotin and repeated PAP method. Clin Immunol Jpn 14(suppl. 5):191, 1982

28. Nadji M, Morales AR: Immunoperoxidase. Part I. The technique and its pitfalls. Lab Med 14:767, 1983

29. Lewis RE Jr, Johnson WW, Cruse JM: Pitfalls and caveats in the methodology for immunoperoxidase staining in surgical pathologic diagnosis. Surv Synth Pathol Res 1:134, 1983

30. Nadji M: Immunoperoxidase techniques. Facts and artifacts. Am J Dermatopathol 8:32, 1986

31. Nadji M: The potential value of immunoperoxidase techniques in diagnostic cytology. Acta Cytol (Praha) 24:442, 1980

32. Nadji M: The negative immunocytochemical result: What does it mean? Diagn Cytopathol 2:81, 1986

33. Warnke RA, Rouse RV: Limitations encountered in the application of tissue section immunodiagnosis to the study of lymphomas and related disorders. Hum Pathol 16:326, 1985

34. Magidson JG, Cheng L, Hannah JB, Lewin KJ: Immunoperoxidase study of lymphomas. Comparison of a one-step frozen section technique with indirect methods on paraffin sections. Am J Clin Pathol 84:166, 1985

35. Pedraza MA, Mason D, Doslu FA, et al: Immunoperoxidase methods with plastic-embedded materials. Lab Med 15:113, 1984

36. Miller HRP: Fixation and tissue preservation for antibody studies: A review. Histochem J 4:305, 1972

37. Puchtler H, Meloan SN: On the chemistry of formaldehyde fixation and its effect on immunohistochemical reactions. Histochemistry 82:201, 1985

38. Gown AM, Vogel AM: Monoclonal antibodies to human intermediate filament proteins. II. Distribution of filament proteins in normal human tissues. Am J Pathol 114:309, 1984

39. Gould VE, Cheifec G, Rosen ST, et al: Fixation methods alter the immunohistochemical demonstrability of synaptophysin. Lab Invest 58:35A, 1988

40. Somogyi P, Takagi H: A note on the use of picric acid-paraformaldehyde-glutaraldehyde fixative for correlated light and electron microscopic immunocytochemistry. Neuroscience 7:1779, 1982

41. Bosman FT, Lindeman J, Kuiper G, et al: The influence of fixation on immunoperoxidase staining of plasma cells in paraffin sections of intestinal biopsy specimens. Histochemistry 53:57, 1977

42. Leathem A, Atkins N: Fixation and immunohistochemistry of lymphoid tissue. J Clin Pathol 33:1010, 1980

43. Okon E, Felder B, Epstein A, et al: Monoclonal antibodies reactive with B-lymphocytes and histiocytes in paraffin sections. Cancer 56:95, 1985

44. Battifora H, Kopinski M: The influence of protease digestion and duration of fixation on the immunostaining of keratins. A comparison of formalin and ethanol fixation. J Histochem Cytochem 34:1095, 1986

45. Login GR, Schmitt SJ, Dvorak AM: Rapid microwave fixation of human tissues for light microscopic immunoperoxidase identification of diagnostically useful antigens. Lab Invest 57:585, 1987

46. Li CY, Lazcano-Villareal O, Pierre RU, Yam LT: Immunocytochemical identification of cells in serous effusions. Technical considerations. Am J Clin Pathol 88:696, 1987

47. Leong AS-Y, Milios J: Rapid immunoperoxidase staining of lymphocyte antigens using microwave irradiation. J Pathol 148:183, 1986

48. Sato Y, Mukai K, Watanabe S, Goto M, Shimosato Y: The AMeX method. A simplified technique of tissue processing and paraffin embedding with improved preservation of antigens for immunostaining. Am J Pathol 125:431, 1986

49. Stein H, Gatter K, Asbahr H, Mason DY: Use of freeze-dried, paraffin-embedded sections for immunohistologic staining with monoclonal antibodies. Lab Invest 52:676, 1985

50. Mukai K, Yoshimura S, Anzai M: Effects of decalcification on immunoperoxidase staining. Am J Surg Pathol 10:413, 1986

51. Curran RC, Gregory J: The unmasking of antigens in paraffin sections of tissue by trypsin. Experientia 33:1400, 1977

52. Taschini PA, MacDonald DM: Protease digestion step in immunohistochemical procedures: Ficin as a substitute for trypsin. Lab Med 18:532, 1987

53. Mauro A, Bertolotto I, Germano I, et al: Collagenase in immunohistochemical demonstration of laminin, fibronectin and factor VIII/RAg in nervous tissue after fixation. Histochemistry 80:157, 1984

54. Ordonez NG, Manning JT, Brooks TE: Effect of trypsinization on the immunostaining of formalin-fixed, paraffin-embedded tissues. Am J Surg Pathol 12:121, 1988

55. Alexander RA, Hiscott PS, Hart RL, Grierson I: Effect of melanin bleaching on immunoperoxidase, with reference to ocular tissues and lesions. Med Lab Sci 43:121, 1986

56. Burns J: Immunohistochemical methods and their application in the routine laboratory. p. 337. In Anthony PP, Woolf N (eds): Recent Advances in Histopathology. Churchill Livingstone, London, 1978

57. Brigati DJ, Budgeon LR, Unger ER, et al: Immunocytochemistry is automated. The development of a robotic workstation based upon the capillary action principle. J Histotechnol 11:165, 1988

58. Stark E, Faltimat D, Von der Fecht R: An automated device for immunocytochemistry. J Immunol Methods 107:89, 1988

59. Bioassay of 3-amino-9-ethylcarbazole hydrochloride for possible carcinogenicity. p. 1. In Carcinogenesis. Technical Report Series No. 93. National Cancer Institute, Bethesda, MD, 1978

60. Sheibani K, Tubbs RR: Enzyme immunohistochemistry: Technical aspects. Semin Diagn Pathol 1:235, 1984

61. Battifora H: The multitumor (sausage) tissue block: Novel method for immunohistochemical antibody testing. Lab Invest 55:244, 1986

62. Wan W-H, Fortuna MB, Furmanski P: A rapid and efficient method for testing immunohistochemical reactivity of monoclonal antibodies against multiple tissue samples simultaneously. J Immunol Methods 103:121, 1987

63. Nadji M, Morales AR: Immunoperoxidase. Part II. Practical applications. Lab Med 15:33, 1984

64. Angel E, Nagle RG: Magic markers: Practical problems in the use of immunoperoxidase histochemistry. Pathologist November, p 13, 1985

65. Erlandson RA: Diagnostic immunohistochemistry of human tumors. An interim evaluation. Am J Surg Pathol 8:615, 1984

66. Coruh G, Mason DY: Serum proteins in human squamous epithelium. Br J Dermatol 102:497, 1980

67. Reid WA, Branch T, Thompson WD, Kay J: The effect of diffusion on the immunolocalization of antigen. Histopathology 11:1277, 1987

68. Hsu S-M, Hsu P-L, McMillan PN, Fanger H: Russel bodies. A light and electron microscopic immunoperoxidase study. Am J Clin Pathol 77:26, 1982

69. Petrusz P: Essential requirements for the validity of immunocytochemical staining procedures. J Histochem Cytochem 31:177, 1983

70. Van der Sluis PJ, Boer GJ: The relevance of various tests for the study of specificity in immunocytochemical staining: A review. Cell Biochem Function 4:1, 1986

7

Differential Diagnosis of Metastatic Tumors

Fred T. Bosman
Jan M. Orenstein
Steven G. Silverberg

The differential diagnosis of metastatic tumors is a problem that has long perplexed surgical pathologists. Although as morphologists we have always endeavored to be as specific as possible in characterizing a neoplasm, whether primary or metastatic, until recently the correct identification of the primary site of a metastasis has been of only minor clinical importance. Within the past few years, however, the development of chemotherapeutic regimens that are fairly specific for certain primary sites has made it imperative that the surgical pathologist provide this information if at all possible. Fortunately, some of our diagnostic techniques have also improved simultaneously, so although many mysteries still remain after thorough investigation, we are indeed often able to provide more information commensurate with clinical expectations.

This chapter is divided into several sections, which are presented in the usual order in which the surgical pathologist deals with these problems. The first section is concerned with a discussion of some of the most common clinicopathologic problems in this area, with general recommendations for preliminary resolution of these problems by the interpretation of clinical and routine histopathologic data. The second section concerns the application of histochemical methods, including the so-called special stains, while the third reviews the use of the newer but still relatively inexpensive immunohistochemical methods. Finally, the fourth section presents what at the present time is the final technique applied for differential diagnosis—ultrastructural analysis.

THE CLINICOPATHOLOGIC PROBLEM

The exact proportion of malignant tumors presenting as distant metastases with an occult primary source is difficult to determine, with figures as divergent as 1.5 percent[1] and 6.5 percent[2] available in the recent literature. For the surgical pathologist, however, these cases must be added to those in which a primary site is known or clinically suspected but histologic material from the primary tumor is not available for review. In these latter cases as well, the surgical pathologist must be able to state whether the appearance of the metastatic disease is consistent with the known or suspected primary site.

Sites

The most common site of a metastatic cancer with an unknown primary source is a lymph node, particularly a cervical lymph node, and occasionally bone.[1-5] The most common histologic type of tumor seen in the cervical lymph nodes is squamous cell carcinoma,[1] and in this situation the primary site, if it is discovered, usually is in the head and neck region.[5-7] Lindberg[6] illustrated the specific nodal groups most likely to be involved by tumors originating in different sites in this region. Thus, it is particularly helpful to know the exact site of the lymph node submitted. It is also worth remembering that approximately 40 percent of metastases to cervical lymph nodes will be from subclavicular primary sites such as lung, gastrointestinal (GI) tract, pancreas, prostate, and breast.[7]

Another important point worth noting about cervical lymph node metastases is that they can often show a lymphoepithelioma pattern, in which individual tumor cells are intimately admixed with lymphocytes, often giving the false impression of a primary malignant lymphoma.[8] Reed-Sternberg-like cells have been reported in these cases, particularly when the primary site was in the nasopharynx. It has been shown[9] that patients with this primary malignancy are likely to have antibodies to Epstein-Barr virus (EBV)-associated antigens in their sera, and this information can be applied to immunoperoxidase stains or in situ hybridization (see Ch. 1) of the lymph nodes as well.

After the cervical lymph nodes, metastases from unknown primary sites are next most frequently seen in axillary,[10] inguinal,[11] and supraclavicular[12] lymph nodes. Each of these again has its own characteristic pattern for the most likely primary tumor sites. For example, metastatic carcinoma in axillary nodes in women is far and away most likely to be from the breast. Indeed, unless the histologic characteristics of the tumor are totally inconsistent with a primary breast tumor, ipsilateral mastectomy will usually be performed in these cases even if an obvious primary lesion is not detectable. It should be remembered, however, that carcinomas arising in the axillary tail of the breast can occasionally be mistaken for axillary lymph node metastases, especially when they contain a marked lymphocytic infiltrate, as in the case of medullary carcinoma (Fig. 7-1). In this instance, what is originally thought to be a metastasis may really be the primary tumor, and, of course, no other primary lesion will be found even after careful study of the mastectomy specimen. This situation (primary tumor in an unusual site initially thought to be metastatic) has been commented on in other sites as well.[13] If the possibility of a mammary primary tumor can be eliminated, the other common sources of axillary lymph node metastases are lung carcinomas and malignant melanomas.

In the case of inguinal lymph node metastases, the most common occult primary sites in women are the cervix, endometrium, and ovary. Vulvar carcinoma, although common, usually has a clinically evident primary tumor. In men, the most frequent sites are prostate, anus, and rectum.[7] Supraclavicular lymph nodes are unique in that they can attract metastases from almost anywhere in the body, ranging from head and neck to mammary, pulmonary, GI, and genitourinary primary sites.

After lymph nodes, there is no clear-cut second most common site of metastasis from an unknown primary source. In most series, however, the second most fre-

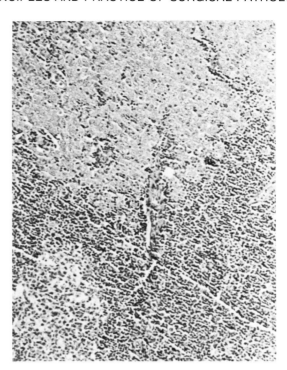

Fig. 7-1. Metastatic medullary carcinoma of breast in axillary lymph node. Sharp demarcation of tumor (above) from lymphoid tissue (below) suggests metastatic carcinoma rather than primary lymphoma. Germinal centers (below) and subcapsular sinus (not illustrated) indicate that this is a node rather than a lymphoid infiltrate in a primary carcinoma of the axillary tail of the breast.

quent anatomic location (and occasionally the most frequent) is bone.[1,14] Metastases to long bones and the vertebral column are about equally frequent, and are followed by those to ribs and the skull. The radiologist may be of help in establishing the primary site, since certain metastatic tumors, such as those from the prostate, kidney, thyroid, and neuroblastoma, are said to have distinctive radiologic features.[14] By contrast, the fact that these lesions often must be decalcified before sectioning may make histologic interpretation more difficult. It is always worthwhile to try to dissect out some uncalcified tissues for submission for histologic examination before decalcification of the major portion of the specimen.

After bone, the most frequent sites of metastases from occult primary lesions are (roughly in descending order) the lungs, liver, central nervous system, pleura, intestine, and skin.[1,2] Actually more frequent than several of these, but not listable as a single metastatic site, are those occult primary tumors manifesting as generalized or abdominopelvic peritoneal carcinomatosis. Fairly few rules are applicable to determining the primary source of metastases in these various sites, with the exception that common tumors (such as breast in women and lung in men) should obviously be thought of first. However, unusual metastatic patterns may often be demonstrated.

It can also not be overemphasized that malignant melanoma is the great clinical and pathologic mimic in this situation and should always be considered in the differential diagnosis of any metastatic tumor without a known primary source. Indeed, for unusual sites of metastatic disease (e.g., heart, gallbladder, prostate), melanoma is frequently the most common primary tumor found.

It should also be remembered that in most cases manifesting with metastases from an occult source, the primary site will never be found.[2,7,15] This is often true even after investigation at autopsy.[2] Thus, the question of how extensively to investigate these cases before treatment is instituted is still debatable and may eventually depend on a cost-benefit analysis.[2-15] In most series, metastatic squamous or undifferentiated carcinomas in cervical lymph nodes are associated with fairly good survival rates after radiation therapy,[1] and only 10 to 15 percent of other metastases from unknown primary sites turn out to be of treatable type by currently available chemotherapeutic regimens.[2-4] Routine light microscopy is often not helpful in predicting the favorable responses,[4] and the relative roles of immunohistochemistry[2] and electron microscopy[3,4,13] are still being evaluated.

Adenocarcinoma

Within the clinical spectrum of metastatic tumors from unknown primary sites, by far the most common histologic features are those of carcinoma, and if the cervical lymph node metastases are excluded, the overwhelmingly most common type is adenocarcinoma.[2-4] One of the main problems for the surgical pathologist in sites in which metastatic adenocarcinomas are frequently seen is the distinction of a metastasis from a primary tumor at that site.[13,16] The lung and liver are excellent examples of this problem. Needle biopsies, aspirations, or even resections often raise the question of metastatic carcinoma versus primary pulmonary or hepatic carcinoma. In the lung, a bronchiolo-alveolar histologic pattern or an admixture of squamous elements favors a primary lesion, whereas nodular circumscription of the tumor favors metastatic disease. In the liver, the appearance of primary hepatocellular carcinoma is often distinctive, particularly if bile or hyaline globules can be demonstrated. Immunologic markers such as α-fetoprotein (AFP) may be demonstrable either in the serum or by immunoperoxidase study in the tumor. If these methods fail, ultrastructural examination may show characteristic hepatic morphologic features, with intercellular bile canaliculi and intracellular voluminous smooth endoplasmic reticulum. In the case of primary bile duct adenocarcinomas of the liver, however, distinction from a metastatic carcinoma is often impossible, particularly if the metastasis is of a ductal type (e.g., pancreas, common bile duct). Radiologic studies may be helpful, but often exploratory surgery will be necessary to make this distinction.

In other organs, the diagnostic problem may be that of distinguishing a metastatic adenocarcinoma from a histologically similar primary tumor that is not adenocarcinoma. Common problems here include mesotheliomas of the pleura, peritoneum, and pericardium and papillary ependymomas and choroid plexus papillomas of the central nervous system (CNS). Another potential, but far less common, problem of similar type involves the so-called adamantinoma of bone, most frequently seen in the tibia. The distinction in the case of both mesothelioma and the central nervous system tumors is best made on the basis of histochemical and/or ultrastructural findings, which are discussed later in this chapter and in the appropriate organ-site chapters of this book.

A problem distinctive to the female genital tract concerns the differential diagnosis of endometrioid carcinoma of the ovary from a metastasis from a primary carcinoma of the endometrium. If the endometrium can be proven benign, the ovarian tumor can clearly be accepted as a primary endometrioid carcinoma. Similarly, if origin can be shown in a focus of endometriosis in the ovary, the tumor can also safely be considered primary. However, in many instances neither of these situations will pertain, and the primary or secondary nature of the ovarian tumor is then not clear. It is our impression that, although endometrial carcinoma does metastasize to the ovary, this situation is far less common than that of separate primary tumors in ovary and endometrium. A recent addition to the techniques used to make this distinction is flow cytometry; different ploidy levels in the two tumors strongly favor separate primaries.[17] This subject is discussed in more detail in Chapters 41 and 42.

A similar situation exists with other metastatic tumors to the ovary, which may be mistaken for primary lesions and vice versa. Particularly difficult is the distinction between a primary ovarian mucinous carcinoma and a metastasis from the colon or rectum. Since the primary mucinous ovarian carcinomas are usually of colorectal type, we know of no foolproof way at the present time of making this distinction. Bilaterality suggests metastatic disease, but certainly does not rule out the possibility of bilateral primary ovarian tumors or a single ovarian primary lesion with metastasis to the contralateral ovary. On the other hand, if the tumor being considered is a carcinoid, bilaterality is virtually a guarantee of origin outside the ovary, while unilateral tumor is almost always primary and benign. Again, the reader is referred to Chapter 42 for a more complete discussion of these problems (see also discussion of tumor alkaline phosphatase below).

Another problem posed by the ovary, as well as other paired organs such as breast, lung, and kidney, is that of whether bilateral disease represents multiple primary foci or a single primary focus with contralateral metastasis. Again, this question is often impossible to answer with complete certainty, but both clinical and pathologic features of the individual case may help. For example, bilateral paired organ tumors without evidence of other dissemination suggest that both lesions are primary, whereas widespread disseminated disease suggests metastasis, or at least makes the problem a purely academic one. The presence of preneoplastic or preinvasive neoplastic changes associated with the tumor (e.g., in situ lobular or intraductal carcinoma associated with an infiltrating carcinoma of the breast) suggests strongly that the associated invasive tumor is primary at that site. Circumscription of most tumors suggests metastatic disease, whereas an infiltrating margin usually suggests a primary origin at that site. Strong histologic dissimilarity between the two tumors being considered suggests separate primary sources, while histologic identity suggests (but certainly does not prove) the possibility that one may be a metastasis from the other. Flow cytometry (identical versus different ploidy levels) may help here as well, as may studies of gene rearrangements. Finally, in some organs, primary and metastatic lesions occupy somewhat different locations. For example, primary breast tumors occur within mammary tissue, whereas metastases to the breast may often be found in the subcutaneous fat. Similarly, although endobronchial metastases certainly exist, they are relatively uncommon, and thus this location might suggest a primary rather than a metastatic lung tumor.

Other Tumors

Although thus far we have considered the question of primary versus metastatic disease only in relation to adenocarcinomas, this differential diagnosis often must be considered in other types of malignant tumors as well. With respect to squamous cell carcinomas, the problem most frequently arises when a tumor is found in the lung of a patient who has previously been treated for squamous cell carcinoma of the head and neck region, esophagus, cervix, or other primary site. Again in this instance, the clinical history will often be of primary importance. For example, late metastases from esophageal carcinomas are almost unknown, so a patient fortunate enough to survive 5 or more years after treatment for this disease who then develops a squamous cell carcinoma in the lung

can safely be assumed to have a new primary tumor. The precise location of the tumor is also helpful, in that primary squamous cell carcinoma of the lung usually arises centrally from a major bronchus, whereas metastatic cancers to the lung tend to be more peripheral. As mentioned earlier, the circumscribed versus infiltrating character of the tumor margins also helps in the differential diagnosis. Finally, an admixture of other histologic types, such as oat cell or adenocarcinoma, also suggests a primary lung tumor. If doubt still persists after all these criteria are applied, and if disseminated disease is not present elsewhere, the patient is probably best treated for a new primary pulmonary carcinoma.

A fairly recent observation is that the same situation exists in the mediastinum and retroperitoneum of men when malignant germ cell tumors are found.[4] As discussed in more detail in Chapter 24, the differential diagnosis between germ cell tumors and thymoma, lymphoma, and metastatic carcinoma in these sites may be a difficult one, and even when a malignant germ cell tumor is diagnosed with confidence, a primary lesion in the testis must be ruled out with care. In women, this is less of a problem, since primary mediastinal and retroperitoneal germ cell tumors are vanishingly rare.

The differentiation between germ cell tumors and lymphoma, thymoma and metastatic carcinoma can be greatly facilitated by immunohistochemical methods. Carcinomas and most thymomas express cytokeratins, and lymphomas express common leucocyte antigen, as well as more cell-type-specific antigens, whereas germ cell tumors often express AFP or human chorionic gonadotropin (hCG). This is discussed in more detail in the section on immunohistochemistry and in Chapters 37 and 42.

The question of primary versus metastatic disease often arises when malignant melanoma is diagnosed as well, whether it be in the skin or in the much less common mucosal, meningeal, or ocular locations. The presence of either junctional activity (in skin or mucous membranes) or benign precursor cells (e.g., nevus cells) strongly suggests the primary origin of a melanoma at the site in question. The absence of these features on the initial sections—particularly if no history of a prior or concurrent primary melanoma elsewhere is available—mandates multiple sectioning of the tissue block in question. In all considerations of this problem, it should be remembered that melanomas frequently metastasize widely from occult primary sites, or as a delayed phenomenon many years after the primary source has been apparently successfully treated.

Since the suggestion of a primary site for a metastatic tumor depends in large measure on the histologic type of the tumor, the distinction between, for example, squamous and adenocarcinoma is an important but often difficult problem. The well-differentiated squamous carcinoma showing keratin pearls and intercellular bridges does not pose this problem, nor does the well-differentiated adenocarcinoma containing glands or ducts with lumina and obvious mucin production. On the other hand, the metastatic tumor composed of solid nests or sheets of anaplastic cells without the above-mentioned attributes is often difficult to classify. Special stains may be of value, but in our experience if the tumor is so undifferentiated that mucin, for example, is not detected or at least suspected with the routine hematoxylin and eosin stain, it usually is not present in sufficient quantity to be detectable with a more specific stain.

Even in these poorly differentiated tumors, however, certain morphologic features may be of value. For example, a spindled appearance of some of the cells is more suggestive of squamous than adenocarcinoma, while extremely large solitary nucleoli are more frequently seen in adenocarcinomas. Electron microscopy can also be extremely helpful in these cases. It has been shown, for example, that so-called undifferentiated or poorly differentiated carcinomas of the cervix[18] and lung[19] can usually be identified as being of either squamous or glandular origin when examined with the electron microscope. More specific details of this differentiation will be discussed later.

The differentiation between adenocarcinoma and squamous cell carcinoma can also be facilitated through the study of the expression of cell type-specific cytokeratins. Adenocarcinomas, for example, express cytokeratin 18, which is absent in squamous cell carcinomas, which express cytokeratin 10. This approach is discussed in more detail in the section on immunohistochemistry.

In many instances, metastatic or primary malignant tumors can be characterized by their pattern of growth, and a differential diagnosis can be formulated therefrom. Often the differential diagnosis includes not only different types of carcinoma, as discussed earlier, but noncarcinomatous neoplasms as well. For example, when the pattern of growth is that of a spindle cell tumor, the diagnostic possibilities include carcinoma, sarcoma, and melanoma. In the case of a primary tumor, the site involved may be the most important diagnostic criterion. For example, although both malignant melanoma and various types of sarcoma have been reported in the larynx, a spindle cell tumor in that organ, particularly if it grows as a polypoid mass elevating the mucosa, is most likely to be a metaplastic squamous cell carcinoma ("pseudosarcoma"), and a careful search should be made for foci of in situ or invasive squamous cancer. In metastatic sites, of course, this sort of criterion is more difficult to apply, so a spindle cell tumor metastatic to the lung with no known primary site, for example, could equally be carcinoma, sarcoma, or melanoma. Although reticulin and tri-

chrome stains are said to be of value in distinguishing spindle cell carcinomas from spindle cell sarcomas, we have rarely found this to be the case, and we prefer to rely on immunohistochemistry in combination with electron microscopy, if suitable tissue is available for study. Expression of cytokeratin practically rules out the possibility of sarcoma or melanoma, although in some sarcomas (*e.g.*, epithelioid sarcoma and synovial sarcoma) cytokeratin expression has been reported. Melanomas almost without exception express S-100 protein, but this marker is by no means specific for melanoma. Various melanoma-specific monoclonal antibodies have been reported, but none of these appears to be entirely specific.

Lack of cohesiveness of the spindled tumor cells, a tendency for them to aggregate in nests, and, of course, the presence of stainable melanin also suggest that the spindle cell tumor in question is a malignant melanoma. Since sarcomas usually manifest as bulky primary tumors rather than as precocious metastases from occult primary sites, in practical terms they are far less likely than either carcinoma or melanoma to be the source of unexplained metastatic disease.

Another type of tumor cell morphologic pattern that is seen frequently, particularly in lymph nodes, is that of tumors composed of large round to polygonal cells (Table 7-1). This differential diagnosis is most common in adults, and the three most likely possibilities are carcinoma, lymphoma, and melanoma. As mentioned earlier in the discussion of spindle cell tumors, the presence of poor tumor cell cohesiveness, nesting, and/or stainable melanin is suggestive of melanoma, as is the presence of scattered multinucleate giant cells and of numerous intranuclear inclusions of cytoplasm. In a lymph node, tumor cells in the subcapsular sinus and/or sharply defined from normal lymphoid structures of the node suggest a metastatic carcinoma or melanoma. A diffuse infiltrate replacing and blending in with the surrounding lymphoid tissues (if any remain) is more suggestive of malignant lymphoma. Markedly convoluted or cleaved nuclei are likely to be seen in lymphoma cells as well. The presence of any glandular or squamous differentiation establishes the di-

TABLE 7-1. Large Round to Polygonal Cell Tumors

Carcinoma

Lymphoma

Melanoma

Plasmacytoma

Eosinophilic granuloma

Histiocytoma

Germinoma

TABLE 7-2. Small Round Cell Tumors

Lymphoma

Oat cell/carcinoid

Neuroblastoma

Ewing's sarcoma

Embryonal rhabdomyosarcoma

Plasmacytoma

Lobular carcinoma (breast)

TABLE 7-3. Giant Cell Tumors

Carcinoma
  Lung
  Pancreas
  Thyroid

Giant cell tumor of bone

Soft tissue sarcomas

Choriocarcinoma

Glioblastoma

agnosis of carcinoma. These three diagnostic possibilities, as well as the others listed in Table 7-1, are often better distinguished by histochemical or ultrastructural studies as discussed later. Here again, immunohistochemistry may be helpful. In this differential diagnosis leukocyte common antigen (LCA), which will be expressed by all lymphoid cells, will assist in the identification of lymphoma, while the markers mentioned above may identify carcinoma or melanoma.

The problem of small round cell tumors (Table 7-2) is one that is encountered in the pediatric age group. Any tissue may be involved, but here bone is a particularly puzzling site, since both Ewing's sarcoma and malignant lymphoma may be both primary tumors or metastatic lesions in bone. All the tumors listed in Table 7-2 can also be encountered in adults, with lymphomas, plasmacytomas, oat cell and lobular carcinomas, and carcinoid tumors being encountered more frequently in adults. The nuclei of plasmacytomas should be distinctive, as may those of some malignant lymphomas. Rosettes in neuroblastomas and brightly eosinophilic cytoplasm with or without cross-striations in embryonal rhabdomyosarcomas are, of course, also distinctive. Lobular carcinoma of the breast metastasizes in a "sinus catarrh"-like pattern in axillary lymph nodes (see Ch. 11), and may show a characteristic single-file linear arrangement of tumor cells in other sites, such as the skin. In these small round cell tumors as well, special stains and immunohistochemical and ultrastructural studies may provide the definitive answer.

Immunohistochemical analysis here may include antibodies to cytokeratins, which will identify carcinomas; LCA, which will identify lymphoma; neurofilaments, which occur in neuroblastomas and occasionally also in carcinoids; neuron-specific enolase, which occurs in neuroblastomas, oat cell carcinomas and carcinoids; desmin, which characterizes myogenic differentiation; and finally immunoglobulins, which characterize plasmacytomas.

At the other end of the size spectrum, giant cell tumors (Table 7-3) may also pose diagnostic problems. For the most part, however, the tumors listed in Table 7-3 will

manifest clinically obvious primary sites rather than distant metastases from an occult primary site. Giant cell carcinomas of the lung and pancreas, however, may represent an exception to this rule. Giant cell glioblastomas rarely metastasize but may be difficult to distinguish in their primary situation in the brain from metastatic giant cell carcinomas or sarcomas. Giant cell carcinomas, whether originating in lung, pancreas, thyroid, or other organs, frequently show a sarcomatoid histologic pattern and may be identified as epithelial neoplasms only on immunohistochemical or ultrastructural examination, and even then often with difficulty. For this differential diagnosis, an immunohistochemical workup will include antibodies to cytokeratin, hCG and GFAP.

A much more frequent diagnostic problem in the clinical situation of a metastasis from an occult primary site is that of tumors characterized by numerous clear cells (Table 7-4). Histochemical and ultrastructural studies have shown that the clear appearance of these cells by light microscopy may represent three different subcellular characteristics: (1) large amounts of intracytoplasmic glycogen; (2) organelle-poor cytoplasm with little or no glycogen; and (3) fixation or other artifact.[20] Obviously, the determination of which of these three mechanisms is responsible for the clear cell morphologic features will influence the final diagnosis. Far and away the most com-

TABLE 7-4. Clear Cell Tumors

Carcinoma
  Kidney
  Liver
  Adrenal
  Salivary gland
  Sweat gland
  Lung
  Thyroid
  Female genital tract

Clear cell sarcoma of tendon sheath

Leiomyoblastoma

Germinoma

mon of the clear cell tumors—as well as the most likely to metastasize from an occult primary source—is primary carcinoma of the kidney, or hypernephroma. The cells of this tumor contain both glycogen and lipid and have a characteristic ultrastructural appearance. Clear cell sarcomas of tendon sheath may contain melanin (in which case some surgical pathologists prefer to diagnose them as clear cell melanomas). Leiomyoblastomas infrequently metastasize, and if they do, they should have an obvious primary tumor, usually in the gastrointestinal tract or the uterus. They should also show evidence of smooth muscle origin at the histochemical or ultrastructural level. Germinomas (seminoma in men, dysgerminoma in women) are a classic example of cells that appear clear because of a paucity of organelles. They contain little or no stainable glycogen (or, for that matter, anything else) and frequently show nucleoli with Chinese character-like nucleonemata. Immunohistochemical studies for the differentiation between these tumor types will include antibodies to cytokeratins, cytokeratin subtypes (which may assist in characterizing the organ site of the primary carcinoma), desmin (for leiomyoblastoma), and placental alkaline phosphatase (for germinoma).

Although clear cell carcinomas are characteristically adenocarcinomas, squamous carcinomas may also show this appearance, either focally or diffusely. This has recently been pointed out in cases of so-called clear cell carcinomas of the lung, and it has been suggested that this is indeed not a distinct entity.[21]

As in the case of clear cell tumors, an eosinophilic granular cell tumor may owe its light microscopic appearance to an increase in any one of several different organelles, including (1) mitochondria; (2) smooth endoplasmic reticulum; (3) dense lysosomelike bodies; (4) secretory granules; and (5) others.[22] Examples of each of these mechanisms can be found in the list of tumors in Table 7-5. For example, true oncocytomas of salivary gland and other organs (which are rarely malignant) show marked mitochondrial hyperplasia demonstrable by phosphotungstic acid hematoxylin (PTAH) stain and by electron microscopy. Steroid-hormone-secreting tumors, such as hepatic and adrenal cortical carcinomas and ovarian or testicular hilar or Leydig cell tumors and luteomas, characteristically demonstrate hyperplastic smooth endoplasmic reticulum.

Secretory granules are present in paragangliomas and pheochromocytomas, lysosomelike bodies in granular cell myoblastomas, and rhomboid crystals in alveolar soft part sarcomas. Other tumors in this group may show a combination of these features. In any event, probably the single most common tumor listed in Table 7-5 that manifects initially with metastatic disease is malignant melanoma. Metastatic renal carcinomas are more frequently of the clear cell type, as described earlier, and the other

TABLE 7-5. Eosinophilic Granular Cell Tumors

Carcinoma
Kidney
Liver
Adrenal cortex
Apocrine (breast, sweat gland)
Hürthle cell (thyroid)
Glassy cell (cervix)
Sarcoma
Epithelioid
Alveolar soft parts
Melanoma
Paraganglioma/pheochromocytoma
Oncocytomas
Granular cell myoblastoma
Gemistocytic astrocytoma
Hilar/Leydig cell tumors
Luteomas
Decidua

entities listed either rarely manifest initially with metastatic disease or are benign (luteoma, decidual polyp) or are so low-grade malignant (oncocytomas, granular cell myoblastoma, gemistocytic astrocytoma, hilar/Leydig cell tumors) that they rarely metastasize at all. The immunohistochemical distinction of melanoma from carcinoma has been discussed above.

HISTOCHEMISTRY

General Histochemical Methods

Histochemistry permits identification and histotopographic localization of substances in tissue sections. Its advantage over biochemical analysis of tissue homogenates is that the chemical composition of histologic structures can be studied in parallel with morphologic evaluation. Therefore, histochemical methods can provide parameters that are very valuable for the differential diagnosis of primary or metastatic tumors. Histochemical methods, however, have some inherent limitations. Special tissue processing may be required for optimal results, and, therefore, many techniques cannot be applied to routinely fixed and embedded specimens. Furthermore, many histochemical methods are not specific for one chemically defined substance but stain groups of more or less related molecules. Many of these components occur in more than one type of cell or tissue, and, therefore, very few histochemical methods are specific for a single cell type or tissue component.

Histochemistry includes special histologic staining methods, enzyme histochemical methods, and immunohistochemical methods, which will be discussed in a separate section. Special stains often are not, but can be, quite specific, even though the chemical basis of many methods is still unclear. Enzyme-histochemical methods generally are specific with regard to the interaction of a given enzyme with a given substrate. Most enzymes, however, are not cell or organ specific, and when organ-specific isoenzymes have been found, methods for their histologic detection have rarely been developed. Often the differences will be quantitative rather than qualitative. For this reason, semiquantitative assessment of patterns of staining of different enzymes in tumors usually gives more information than the reaction of a single enzyme. Consequently, thus far enzyme histochemistry has been of limited significance in the differential diagnosis of tumors. Nonetheless, in selected cases enzyme histochemistry can provide valuable information about the nature and origin of neoplastic tissue.

Many excellent texts exhaustively describe the existing staining methods and enzyme histochemical techniques.[23–26] Therefore, only a few general remarks will be made.

Tissue processing frequently affects the chemical composition of cells or intercellular structures. Fortunately, most of the special staining reactions can be successfully performed on routinely processed (i.e., formalin-fixed and paraffin-embedded) tissues. For some staining techniques special fixatives are recommended. In some cases, postfixation of a rehydrated section will be sufficient, but in others special tissue processing is essential. Lipid histochemical studies, for example, are practically impossible on paraffin sections because of the removal of most of the lipids by the organic solvents that are used in the embedding cycle. Formaldehyde-induced fluores-

cence of catecholamines[27] can be performed on immersion-fixed tissues, but optimal results are obtained by freeze-drying of fresh frozen tissue and special paraffin embedding, because of the high solubility of these substances.

With very few exceptions, routinely processed tissues are not suitable for enzyme histochemical studies. For almost all enzyme histochemical methods, cryostat sectioning of unfixed frozen tissue is the best processing method. The sections can subsequently be fixed according to the requirements for the enzyme of interest. Therefore, whenever differential diagnostic problems are anticipated and unfixed tissue is available, a representative sample should be snap frozen (preferably in isopentane quenched in liquid nitrogen) and stored at −70°C.

Selected special staining methods and enzyme histochemical methods are listed in Tables 7-6 and 7-7, respectively. These methods are detailed in references 23–26.

Applications

A significant number of substances can be stained by means of a histochemical reaction. In many instances, positive staining indicates the presence of a category of substances rather than one chemically defined molecule (e.g., diastase-resistant PAS-positivity indicates the presence of a macromolecule with free hexose groups but is not specific for any single type of carbohydrate molecule). Therefore, at best, both staining techniques and enzyme histochemical reactions can give an indication of tissue type (e.g., epithelium versus connective tissue) or differentiation (e.g., squamous versus adenocarcinoma) rather than pointing toward an organ of origin.

TABLE 7-6. Histochemical Staining Methods in Tumor Diagnosis

	Method	Substance	Diagnostic Application
Fibrillary proteins	Congo red; thioflavine	Amyloid	Medullary thyroid carcinoma
	van Gieson	Collagen	Carcinoma, sarcoma, lymphoma
Carbohydrates	PAS, diastase degradable	Glycogen	Rhabdomyosarcoma, Ewing's sarcoma, renal adenocarcinoma
	PAS, diastase resistant	Neutral mucosubstances	Carcinomas, lymphomas of B-cell type, hepatoma
	Alcian blue	Acid mucosubstances	Carcinomas, mesothelioma
Lipids	Oil red O	All lipid material	Liposarcoma, adrenal carcinoma, ovarian stromal cell tumors
	Perchloric acid-naphthoquinone	Cholesterol and derivatives	Adrenal carcinoma, ovarian stromal cell tumors
Nucleic acids	Methyl green-pyronine (MGP)	RNA and DNA	Lymphomas of B-cell type
Pigments	Schmorl	Melanin	Melanoma
	Fouchet	Bile	Hepatoma
Neuroendocrine granules	Grimelius	Argyrophil granules	Neuroendocrine-type carcinoid tumors
	Masson-Fontana	Argentaffin granules	Neuroendocrine-type carcinoid tumors
	Formaldehyde-induced fluorescence	Catecholamines	Neuroendocrine-type carcinoid tumors

TABLE 7-7. Enzyme Histochemical Methods in Tumor Diagnosis

Enzyme		Diagnostic Application
Phosphatases	Alkaline	Adenocarcinoma of lung, endometrium, kidney
	Acid	Prostatic carcinoma
		Carcinoid-type tumors
		Monocytic leukemia
		Histiocytic sarcoma
		Convoluted lymphoma
	Acid, tartrate resistant	Hairy cell leukemia
	Adenosine triphosphatase (ATPase)	Rhabdomyosarcoma
Oxidases	Dihydroxyphenylalanine (DOPA) oxidase	Melanoma
Dehydrogenases	Nicotinamide adenine dinucleotide tetrazolium reductase (NADH-TR)	Rhabdomyosarcoma
Sulphatases	Arylsulphatase	Digestive tract adenocarcinoma
Esterases	α-Naphthyl(nonspecific) esterase	Carcinoid-type tumors
		Monocytic leukemia
		Histiocytic sarcoma
Peptidases	Aminopeptidase	Adenocarcinoma of stomach, bile duct, urinary bladder, kidney

Endocrine Tumors

Steroids in endocrine neoplasms, regardless of the tissue of origin, can be stained with general lipid staining methods such as oil red 0. In addition, cholesterol and related substances can be stained by the perchloric acid-naphthoquinone reaction.[28] This reaction should be performed on fresh frozen sections and does not distinguish between different types of cholesterol esters.

Neoplasms derived from cells of the diffuse neuroendocrine system[29] can be diagnosed and, to a certain extent, can also be differentiated according to the cell type of origin with different staining techniques.[30-32] In general, whenever a carcinoid-type tumor consisting of solid nests or cords of monomorphic cells is encountered, the silver impregnation techniques serve as a method of screening. Argentaffin methods[33] stain cells that can reduce ammoniacal silver solutions, resulting in a brown silver precipitate. Argyrophil cells have to be treated with a reducing substance before they can react with the silver solution.[34] Absence of silver reactivity, however, does not preclude neuroendocrine origin. Although in the normal situation the neuroendocrine cells can be differentiated into different types according to their staining properties, these characteristics often are not valid for neoplastic cells because these may show abnormal patterns of reaction. For example, normal β-cells in pancreatic islets are not argyrophilic, but neoplastic β-cells often are.[35] In general, carcinoid-type tumors in organs derived from the foregut tend to be argyrophilic, whereas mid- and hindgut carcinoids are argentaffin or areactive.[32] In addition to the aforementioned silver staining methods, the aldehyde fuchsin, lead hematoxylin, and diazonium methods are useful for the visualization of neuroen-

docrine cells. Formaldehyde-induced fluorescence[27] is an elegant method for the demonstration of biologic amine content. Originally described for the demonstration of norepinephrine in the adrenal medulla, this method allows detection of many different related amines, which are converted into a fluorophore with a specific fluorescence emission spectrum through formaldehyde condensation.[36] Enzyme histochemistry of neuroendocrine tumors is not very specific. Nonspecific esterases and acid phosphatases occur frequently[37] but are also found in many other neoplasms.

Parafollicular or C cells of the thyroid also belong to the diffuse neuroendocrine system. The cells in parafollicular or medullary carcinoma of the thyroid frequently are argyrophilic. A rather characteristic feature of these tumors is the presence of amyloid. Unfortunately, this typical feature is often lost in metastases. The amyloid stains with Congo red or thioflavine. The dimethylaminobenzaldehyde method for tryptophane allows differentiation between the so-called APUD-amyloid in neuroendocrine tumors and immunoamyloid, because the former does not contain tryptophane.[38]

Melanocytes stain with many of the above-mentioned methods and are therefore regarded as belonging to the diffuse neuroendocrine system.[29] As a result, in addition to the Schmorl method for melanin, argyrophil and argentaffin methods are also helpful for the diagnosis of melanoma, but only if melanin is present. Consequently, the diagnosis of amelanotic melanoma can be very difficult. Fortunately, the enzyme DOPA-oxidase is quite specific for melanocytes and can often be demonstrated even in the absence of melanin. The reaction, which has to be applied to cryostat sections of unfixed tissue, can be of great help in the diagnosis of melanoma.

Lymphomas

Histochemical methods are useful for the characterization of neoplastic cells in leukemia and lymphoma. In addition, several of these methods can be helpful in distinguishing lymphoma from nonlymphoid neoplasms.

Special stains of interest are the methyl green-pyronine (MGP) method and the periodic acid-Schiff (PAS) method. Pyronine in the MGP method stains the cytoplasm of immunoglobulin-synthesizing plasmacytoid and mature plasma cells. However, pyronine binds to RNA, and, therefore, all cells actively engaged in protein synthesis will be stained. Nevertheless, pyroninophilic cytoplasm of poorly differentiated diffusely growing cells in a tumor mass suggests plasmacytoid differentiation and therefore is supportive evidence for a lymphoma of B-cell type. PAS staining provides comparable information. Stored immunoglobulins in lymphoma cells can be found as globular or diffuse cytoplasmic PAS-positive diastase-resistant staining.[39] This pattern of staining, therefore, also supports the diagnosis of lymphoma of B-cell type. Carcinoma cells, however, can also be PAS-positive.

Several enzyme histochemical methods are helpful in the diagnosis of lymphoma and for further subtyping of lymphomas. Enzyme histochemical evaluation of lymphomas can be done on cryostat sections, but better results are obtained on imprint cytologic preparations of fresh specimens. The α-naphthyl (nonspecific) esterase method[40] shows diffuse cytoplasmic staining in monocytic and histiocytic cells but staining of one or more spotlike granules in the cytoplasm of T lymphocytes.[41] Diffuse cytoplasmic staining of this enzyme therefore will be found in monocytic leukemia, in true histiocytic lymphoma or sarcoma, and in histiocytosis X or malignant histiocytosis.

Acid phosphatase shows a pattern of staining similar to that of nonspecific esterase. Of particular interest is its focal granular staining pattern in so-called convoluted lymphoma,[42] which can be of help in the differential diagnosis of mediastinal masses. Tartrate-resistant acid phosphatase is virtually diagnostic of hairy cell leukemia.[43]

Carcinomas

In the differential diagnosis of metastatic carcinoma, histochemistry can contribute first to the differential diagnosis between carcinoma and other neoplasms, especially sarcoma, and second to the determination of the type of differentiation within a carcinoma and, if possible, the origin of the neoplasm. Unfortunately, with regard to the latter, the results are usually rather poor.

In distinguishing between anaplastic carcinoma and sarcoma or lymphoma, the arrangement of the tumor cells can be of help. With few exceptions, carcinoma cells tend to grow in solid nests and cords surrounded by connective tissue stroma, whereas sarcomas and lymphomas tend to grow diffusely. Reticulin and van Gieson stains will reveal the pattern of reticulin and collagen fibers and thereby accentuate the growth pattern of the neoplastic cells.

As mentioned earlier, MGP staining can be useful in the differentiation of undifferentiated large cell carcinoma from immunoblastic sarcoma of B-cell type, with the restriction that all cells actively engaged in protein synthesis will be pyroninophilic. For the differentiation of carcinoma from lesions derived from histiocytes, such as histiocytic sarcoma or histiocytosis X, enzyme histochemical staining for α-naphthyl (nonspecific) esterase and acid phosphatase can be helpful. These enzymes occurs diffusely in the cytoplasm of cells of monocytic and histiocytic origin.

The production of mucopolysaccharides in an anaplastic carcinoma is an argument in favor of adenocarcinoma. In general, diastase-resistant PAS staining indicates the presence of neutral mucosubstances, but—as in lymphomas—also of glycoproteins, whereas alcian blue staining indicates the presence of acid mucosubstances. More extensive histochemical differentiation of mucosubstances can be obtained by applying blocking procedures and enzyme digestion before staining. These methods, however, are of little help in the classification of neoplasms. An exception is the hyaluronidase-labile alcian blue staining of hyaluronic acid in mesothelioma. Although not entirely specific (chondroitin sulfate in cartilage is also degradable by hyaluronidase), this reaction can be useful for the diagnosis of mesothelioma.[44]

In very few cases, general histochemical methods will determine the final classification of carcinoma. Whenever hepatocellular carcinoma is suspected, the presence of diastase-resistant, PAS-positive hyaline intracytoplasmic globules is useful supportive evidence for this diagnosis.[45] In addition, in these tumors bile pigments can be stained with standard histochemical methods.

In some cases, enzyme histochemistry can help in establishing the origin of a metastatic carcinoma. Unfortunately, no enzymes have so far been found that are completely specific for a single cell or tissue type. This implies that in addition to qualitative differences in enzyme content, quantitative differences have to be taken into account. Furthermore, the absence or presence of a given enzyme will usually be compatible with several different tissues of origin, and, therefore, staining for multiple enzymes will result in more specific information.

Acid phosphatase can be found in a wide variety of tumors. Extremely high activity of this enzyme in an adenocarcinoma, however, is almost diagnostic of prostatic origin.[37] The presence of alkaline phosphatase in adenocarcinoma strongly favors pulmonary, endometrial, ovarian, or renal origin and virtually excludes the intestinal tract as the primary site.[37] Determination of the activity of this enzyme in an ovarian neoplasm can therefore be helpful in distinguishing between a primary carcinoma of the ovary or metastatic endometrial carcinoma on the one hand and metastasis of breast or intestinal adenocarcinoma on the other.[46] Conversely, arylsulfatase activity in an adenocarcinoma strongly favors intestinal origin.[47] Aminopeptidase is mostly found in adenocarcinoma of the stomach, bile ducts, urinary bladder, or kidney.[37] Many other enzymes have been studied,[48–50] but the lack of specificity and the enormous variability limit the diagnostic significance of these methods.

Mesenchymal Tumors

Special stains and histochemical methods have few useful applications in this area. Primary and metastatic localizations of soft tissue sarcomas not infrequently cause differential diagnostic problems, but in most cases, histochemical methods will be of little help. The same holds true for metastatic localizations of undifferentiated round cell neoplasms of bone (Ewing's sarcoma and malignant lymphomas). Nonetheless, in some differential diagnostic problems special stains can provide useful information and therefore deserve brief discussion.

In a localization of undifferentiated pleomorphic sarcoma a differentiation will have to be made between malignant schwannoma, rhabdomyosarcoma, liposarcoma, and malignant fibrous histiocytoma. The presence of α-naphthyl esterase activity suggests histiocytic origin. Demonstration of intracytoplasmic lipid droplets with an oil red 0 stain will support the diagnosis of liposarcoma. One should however realize that reactive phagocytic cells, especially in tumors with necrosis, also contain lipid material. The rare cross-striated contractile elements in a rhabdomyosarcoma can be stained with the phosphotungstic acid hematoxylin (PTAH) method. In addition, quite often PAS-positive diastase-degradable glycogen deposits can be found in the tumor cells. Enzyme histochemical techniques applied to fresh cryostat sections of tumor tissue can provide evidence of muscular origin in undifferentiated sarcomas. Although not entirely specific for muscular tissue, the presence of NADH-TR and ATPase strongly supports a diagnosis of rhabdomyosarcoma.[51]

It should be stressed that among soft tissue tumors PAS staining is by no means unique for rhabdomyosarcoma. In alveolar soft part sarcoma the tumor cells usually show granular diastase-resistant PAS staining, while in synoviosarcoma the mucosubstances in the slit-like spaces in the tumor are also PAS-positive. For the differential diagnosis of these tumors, therefore, the PAS reaction is of little value. However, this method can be

essential for the diagnosis of Ewing's sarcoma. In undifferentiated round cell neoplasms of bone, Ewing's sarcoma will have to be differentiated from malignant lymphoma and metastatic neuroblastoma. Of these, only Ewing's sarcoma always contains numerous PAS-stainable glycogen granules.[52] In addition, both malignant lymphoma and neuroblastoma contain a fibrillar stroma, stainable with routine reticulin methods, which is not found in Ewing's sarcoma.

IMMUNOHISTOCHEMISTRY

Diagnostic pathology of neoplastic disease has benefitted tremendously from the development of immunohistochemical techniques and the availability of a wide range of specific (polyclonal and monoclonal) antibodies against diagnostically useful antigens. In oncologic research, considerable emphasis has been placed on the development of tumor-specific or tumor-type-specific monoclonal antibodies. Tumor-specific antigens have not been detected, and even purportedly tumor-type- or cell-type-specific monoclonal antibodies frequently have limited specificity. Nonetheless, the hybridoma methodology for the development of monoclonal antibodies[53] has resulted in a multitude of diagnostically useful reagents.

Methodologic Considerations

The immunohistochemical methods and the principles of their application in surgical pathology are extensively reviewed in Chapter 6. It is of importance, however, to re-emphasize some essential considerations here because the reliability of diagnostic immunohistochemistry rests entirely on the quality of the applied immunohistochemical techniques and on the validity of the applied working hypotheses. In using immunoreactivity patterns for various antigens as a diagnostic tool, some general rules have to be strenuously applied. These can be summarized in the following questions.

1. Were the applied techniques valid?
   In assessing the validity of the applied techniques proper attention should be paid to tissue processing procedures and antibody specificity. Proper tissue processing is of paramount importance for reliable immunohistochemistry. In principle, for each antigen an appropriate tissue processing protocol has to be developed. Fortunately, however, for many antigens routine processing (including formalin fixation and paraffin embedding), if necessary in combination with enzyme pretreatment, is compatible with reliable im-

munohistochemistry.[54] For each newly acquired antibody (especially for monoclonal antibodies this is rather important) the compatibility with the local tissue processing conditions has to be ascertained.

Antibody specificity is another crucial element in reliable immunohistochemistry. In most diagnostic histology laboratories, facilities for extensive immunochemical specificity testing are not available, making appropriate tissue controls absolutely essential, as outlined below.

2. Were the controls adequate?

With all immunostaining procedures positive and negative controls should be utilized with material that has been processed similarly to the case material. Negative controls should include checks for nonspecific binding of the detection system (e.g., conjugates, PAP, ABC complex) as well as the primary antibody (nonimmune serum or absorbed antiserum).[55] Omission of controls may lead to serious misinterpretation of case material.

3. Is the distribution of the antigen known in sufficient detail?

This aspect is of particular importance when monoclonal antibodies (MA) are used. The specificity of many MAs is largely defined on the basis of tissue reactivity tests, and therefore these can almost never be too exhaustive. This is demonstrated by the Leu-7 MA, which was originally claimed to react only with natural killer cells, but was subsequently found to react also with endocrine cells.[56] Also illustrating the importance of extensive testing is the CAM 5.2 monoclonal anticytokeratin antibody, which recently appeared to react as well with an epitope occurring in smooth muscle cells.[57] Similarly, some antigens were originally claimed to be specific for one organ or cell type but subsequently proved to be more widely distributed. Examples are neuron-specific enolase, which has been demonstrated in a variety of nonneural and nonneuroendocrine tissues,[58] and prostatic acid phosphatase, which occurs not only in the prostate but also in some normal and neoplastic endocrine cells.[59]

4. Are markers of differentiation of normal cells also valid as markers of differentiation of neoplastic cells?

Marker-based classification relies on the assumption that neoplastic cells usually and perhaps always differentiate along the same lines as their normal counterparts and that markers of differentiation of normal cells will retain their differentiational specificity in neoplastic cells. Unfortunately, tumors tend to break rules. Many case reports illustrate the potential for aberrant differentiational behavior of neoplastic cells and call for cautious interpretation of marker patterns in the classification of tumors. Within this context, histogenetic concepts of tumor development have proved rather limited. The number of neoplasms of which the histogenesis has been conclusively established is restricted. Most histogenetic concepts have been inferred from circumstantial evidence.

Events such as the occurrence of endocrine cells in a considerable number of adenocarcinomas of various organs,[59,60] of vimentin immunoreactivity in certain carcinoma cells,[61] of keratin immunoreactivity in some smooth muscle tumors[57] and of chorionic gonadotropin in a variety of carcinomas[62] are illustrations of the important basic notion that patterns of differentiation dominate the morphology and immunophenotype of neoplasms, rather than the ontogenetic derivation of the tissue in which the neoplasm developed.

Applications

Diagnostic immunohistochemistry of malignant neoplasms calls for a systematic approach. It is absolutely essential to perform detailed morphologic studies before immunohistochemistry is applied. The morphologic analysis should lead to an exact identification of the diagnostic problem, preferentially phrased as a question to which marker immunohistochemistry might provide an answer. The markers should be carefully chosen to allow an answer to the question, and the potential results of the marker studies should actually be anticipated in the decision as to which markers to choose. In reading the immunostained slides, the methodologic considerations should be taken into account before a final conclusion can be drawn.

One of the most difficult problems in surgical pathology is that of an undifferentiated metastatic tumor with an unknown primary. Careful and stepwise application of marker immunohistochemistry according to the following questions can be of tremendous help in this situation. The first question is whether or not the tumor expresses markers of carcinoma. If so, the tumor can either be a carcinoma or a biphasic neoplasm (e.g., epithelioid sarcoma, mesothelioma or synovial sarcoma). If the lesion is a carcinoma, subsequently it must be decided which type of carcinoma it is and where the primary tumor might be located. If it is a biphasic neoplasm, further classification will have to be performed. If the tumor does not express markers of carcinoma the second question will be whether the lesion might be a lymphoma, a melanoma or a sarcoma. If it is a lymphoma, further morphologic and immunophenotypic classification will be performed. If it is a sarcoma, the tumor will also have to be further classified. Markers for these different groups are listed in Table 7-8. Obviously, this approach is rather general. For specific situations more detailed or better tailored approaches might be envisaged.

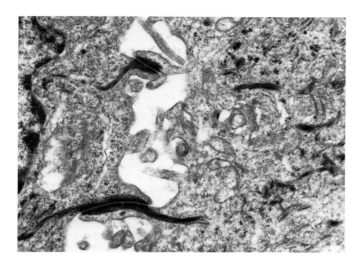

Fig. 7-2. Electron micrograph of a squamous cell carcinoma of the lung showing typical desmosomes with keratin tails (intercellular bridges) and bundles of tonofilaments. Villous processes between desmosomes can be mistaken for microvilli. ×25,000.

adenocarcinomas, will prevent confusing poorly differentiated adenocarcinomas and squamous cell carcinomas. It will also prevent overdiagnosing adenosquamous carcinomas. Neuroendocrine cell tumors are characterized by varying concentrations of dense core, neuroendocrine-type, neurosecretory granules within processes or in the subplasmalemma (Fig. 7-3). Combinations of the three

paths of differentiation are commonly encountered at the TEM level, especially in certain locations, such as lung.[132,145]

Adenocarcinomas, whether clearly identified by light microscopy or only at the electron microscopic level, often present initially or subsequently as metastases. The electron microscopist is regularly asked whether there are ultrastructural features that suggest the primary site.[146] Not only does determining the source of a metastasis help in honing the therapy, but also in minimizing the time and extent of the diagnostic workup. The distinction between primary and metastasis is always to be considered in any lung lesion, while the lesion is clearly a metastasis in the brain, bones, and lymph nodes—the most common sites for metastases. In our experience, most adenocarcinomas of the *lung,* primary or metastatic, consist of cells resembling the nonciliated Clara cell, which is characterized by a bulging apical cytoplasm containing large, dense, often laminated granules, sometimes resembling surfactant granules, with varying amounts of apical glycogen, and relatively little mucin.[147,148] (Fig. 7-4) *Breast* cancers typically have so-called intracytoplasmic microvillus-lined lumina surrounded by tonofilaments and dense secretory vacuoles

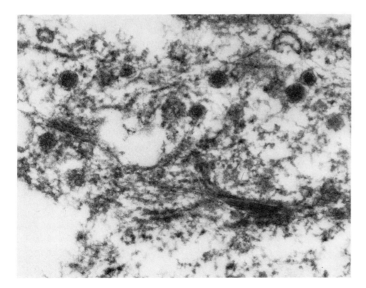

Fig. 7-3. Electron micrograph of a bronchial biopsy from a small cell carcinoma of the lung. Even though the tissue was fixed in formalin and embedded in paraffin and displays extremely poor general preservation, dense core granules measuring roughly 120 nm are still discernible. The structure in the lower right may represent a junction. ×51,000.

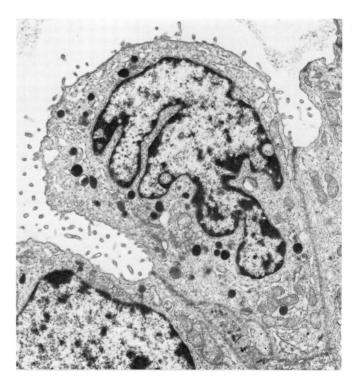

Fig. 7-4. Electron micrograph of a recurrent adenocarcinoma of the lung with a bronchioloalveolar growth pattern. Typical of Clara cells, there are relatively large dense bodies surrounding an irregular nucleus. The apical portion of the cell bulges into the lumen above the lateral junctions. ×7,000.

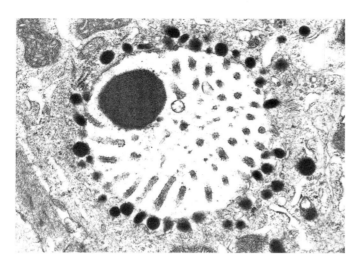

Fig. 7-5. Electron micrograph of a chest wall recurrence of an adenocarcinoma of the breast. The intracytoplasmic lumen is surrounded by small, dense secretory vacuoles and intermediate filaments. The lumen contains secretions while the microvilli lack core rootlets. ×24,000.

which can be confused with dense core granules[149–151] (Fig. 7-5). The microvilli in each of these two common tumors are often described as nonspecific, irregular, pleomorphic, and lacking features characteristic of the alimentary tract, especially the *colorectum*. The latter include long core rootlets that extend deep into the apical cytoplasm and a prominent glycocalyx and abundant glycocalyceal bodies.[152] Although these features are espe-

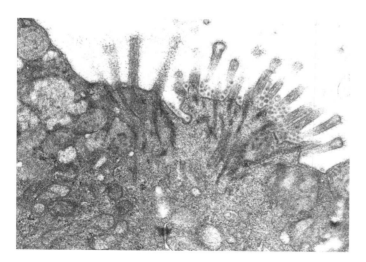

Fig. 7-6. Electron micrograph of a moderately differentiated mucinous adenocarcinoma of the right upper lobe of the lung (single lesion, 9 negative lymph nodes, no other primaries at 24 months). The ''rigid'' microvilli have prominent core rootlets, glycocalyx, and glycocalyceal bodies. Typical flocculent mucinous vacuoles are present (lower field). ×32,000.

cially common and prominent in tumors of the colorectal region, they can be seen in tumors from all portions of the alimentary tract, as well as in some mucinous tumors of the ovary and even the lung (Fig. 7-6), where they resemble adenocarcinomas of the nasopharynx.[153] If the cells in a metastatic adenocarcinoma are dominated by glycogen and lipid, a *renal* primary should be considered.[154] Both features are nonspecific, even together, but their presence in relatively large amounts, in the proper setting, is highly suggestive. Lipid is a common sign of degeneration, and thus especially observed in association with necrosis in any tumor. Further subdivision of squamous cell carcinomas is presently not possible on the basis of TEM. Therefore, the location of the metastasis takes on special importance.

Anterior Mediastinal Tumors

Tumors of the anterior mediastinum can usually be distinguished by TEM.[155] Thymomas characteristically have well formed desmosomes and bundles of tonofilaments. Neuroendocrine tumors have characteristic dense core granules. Adenocarcinomas have glandular lumina, and when no primary can be found, one should consider an extragonadal germ cell tumor, a lesion that responds well to therapy.[156] Identification of circulating or intratumoral AFP and/or hCG will confirm this diagnosis. Lymphomas lack junctions and this diagnosis can be supported by the absence of other findings. Germinoma is suggested by characteristic Chinese character-appearing nucleoli, although they are not unique to this lesion.

Soft Tissue Tumors

TEM plays a major role in the distinction of soft tissue sarcomas from one another and from other spindle cell tumors (squamous, renal-cell, and other metaplastic carcinomas and malignant melanoma). Since soft tissue tumors rarely present as metastatic lesions, they are not discussed in detail here, and the reader is referred to Chapter 10.

Diagnostic Features

Relatively few ultrastructural features are pathognomonic for a particular lesion. Electron microscopists have searched for such features as they have for clear histogenetic patterns.[157,158] It has become appreciated that tumor cells are capable of differentiating along multiple pathways or combinations of pathways, regardless of their presumed cell of origin.[157] Tumors can vary in appearance due to time and therapy, and the phenotype of a lesion does not necessarily reflect a particular embryonal layer. Tumor cells share the same genetic information and, in parallel with the neoplastic state, distinctions recede and unusual combinations and patterns appear.

Within the proper context, the presence of premelanosomes and melanosomes is diagnostic of melanoma, but they can also be seen in other tumors derived from the neural crest, such as melanocytic schwannoma (Fig. 7-7) and soft tissue tumor of tendon sheath or clear cell sarcoma of soft parts (soft tissue melanoma).[159] When dealing with melanosomes in which the typical transversely oriented striations may be obscured by the pigment, one must always ascertain that the melanosomes are in the tumor cells and not in macrophages, especially in a lymph node.

Although in their normal cellular counterparts, the size, appearance, and even shape of secretory granules/vacuoles can tell something about their contents and thus the cell type, this does not necessarily hold true for tumors. The crystalline appearance of insulin granules may be maintained, as well as the large halos with central or eccentric dense cores in epinephrine- and norepinephrine-containing pheochromocytomas, respectively. The Weibel-Palade body characteristic of endothelial cells[160] is an elongated body with longitudinally oriented striated or tubular contents. Unfortunately, these structures tend to be retained only in the more differentiated endothelial cell tumors. Characteristic crystalline inclusions are seen in certain rare tumors, such as alveolar soft parts sarcomas, juxtaglomerular or renin-secreting tumors, hilus cell tumors of the ovary, and interstitial or Leydig cell tumors of the testis. Birbeck or Langerhans bodies or granules are characteristic of variants of histiocytosis X, such as eosinophilic granuloma.[161] Lamellar surfactant granules or myelinoid bodies are diagnostic for alveolar type II pneumocytes of the lung. Ribosome-lamellar complexes are especially common in hairy cell leukemia.

At times the appearance of organelles can be helpful. Mitochondria of steroid-secreting cells and their tumorous counterparts (e.g., adrenocortical tumors) have tubulovesicular cristae. Plasma cells have stacks of rough endoplasmic reticulum that fill the cytoplasm to varying degrees, depending on the level of differentiation. The nucleus and nucleolus, which provide such critical information at the light microscopic level, are relatively uninformative at the ultrastructural level, although plasma cell neoplasms may maintain their cartwheel or clockface pattern. The nuclear morphology is more helpful in mycosis fungoides/Sézary syndrome, where the nuclei are highly contorted and have a cerebriform appearance. However, complicated nuclei are not unique to this syndrome and must be considered in context.

REFERENCES

1. Snee MP, Vyrnmuthu N: Metastatic carcinoma from unknown primary site: The experience of a large oncology centre. Br J Radiol 58:1091, 1985
2. Kirsten F, Chi CH, Leary JA, et al: Metastatic adeno- or undifferentiated carcinoma from an unknown primary site—Natural history and guidelines for identification treatable subsets. Q J Med 62:143, 1987
3. Hamilton CS, Langlands AO: ACUPS (adenocarcinoma of unknown primary site): A clinical and cost benefit analysis. Int J Radiat Oncol Biol Phys 13:1497, 1987
4. Hainsworth JD, Wright EP, Gray GF Jr, Greco FA: Poorly differentiated carcinoma of unknown primary site: Correlation of light microscopic findings with response to Cisplatin-based combination chemotherapy. J Clin Oncol 5:1275, 1987
5. MacComb WS: Diagnosis and treatment of metastatic cervical cancerous nodes from an unknown primary site. Am J Surg 124:441, 1972
6. Lindberg R: Distribution of cervical lymph node metastases from squamous cell carcinoma of the upper respiratory and digestive tracts. Cancer 29:1446, 1972
7. Krementz ET, Cerise EJ: Metastatic lesions of undetermined source. Hosp Med 6:91, 1970
8. Giffler RF, Gillespie JJ, Ayala AG, et al: Lymphoepithelioma in cervical lymph nodes of children and young adults. Am J Surg Pathol 1:293, 1977
9. Pearson GR, Weiland LH, Neel HB III, et al: Application of Epstein-Barr virus (EBV) serology to the diagnosis of North American nasopharyngeal carcinoma. Cancer 51:260, 1983
10. Copeland EM, McBride CM: Axillary metastases from unknown primary sites. Ann Surg 178:25, 1973

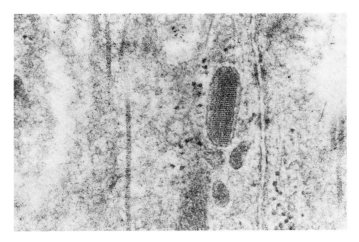

Fig. 7-7. Electron micrograph of malignant melanocytic nerve sheath tumor (malignant melanocytic Schwannoma) apparently arising from the myenteric plexus of the stomach of a 24-year-old woman. Transversely striated premelanosomes are located in a long process joined to a second process by several small nonspecific junctions. ×60,000.

11. Zaren HA, Copeland EM: Inguinal node metastases. Cancer 41:919, 1978

12. Agliozzo CM, Reingold IM: Scalene lymph nodes in necropsies of malignant tumors: Analysis of one hundred sixty-six cases. Cancer 20:2148, 1967

13. Hammar S, Bockus D, Remington F: Metastatic tumors of unknown origin: An ultrastructural analysis of 265 cases. Ultrastruct Pathol 11:209, 1987

14. Copeland MM: Metastases to bone from primary tumors in other sites. Proc Natl Cancer Conf 6:743, 1970

15. Stewart JF, et al: Unknown primary adenocarcinoma: Incidence of overinvestigation and natural history. Br Med J 1:1530, 1979

16. Viadana E, Au K-L: Patterns of metastases in adenocarcinomas of man. An autopsy study of 4,728 cases. J Med 6:1, 1975

17. Symonds DA, Johnson DP, Wheeless CR Jr: Feulgen cytometry in simultaneous endometrial and ovarian carcinoma. Cancer 61:2511, 1988

18. Auersperg N, Erber H, Worth A: Histologic variation among poorly differentiated invasive carcinomas of the human uterine cervix. J Natl Cancer Inst 51:1461, 1973

19. Churg A: The fine structure of large cell undifferentiated carcinoma of the lung: Evidence for its relation to squamous cell carcinomas and adenocarcinomas. Hum Pathol 9:143, 1978

20. Batsakis JG, Regezi JA: Selected controversial lesions of salivary tissues. Otolaryngol Clin North Am 10:309, 1977

21. Katzenstein A-LA, Prioleau PG, Askin FB. The histologic spectrum and significance of clear-cell change in lung carcinoma. Cancer 45:943, 1980

22. Askew JB Jr, Fechner RE, Bentinck DC, et al: Epithelial and myoepithelial oncocytes: Ultrastructural study of a salivary gland oncocytoma. Arch Otolaryngol 93:46, 1971

23. Steward PJ, Polak JM (eds): Histochemistry: The Widening Horizon of its Applications in Biomedical Sciences. John Wiley & Sons, London, 1981

24. Filipe MI, Lake BD: Histochemistry in Pathology. Churchill Livingstone, Edinburgh, 1983

25. Spicer SS (ed): Histochemistry in Pathologic Diagnosis. Marcel Dekker, New York, 1987

26. Lojda Z, Gossrau R, Schiebler TH: Enzymhistochemische Methoden. Springer-Verlag, Berlin, 1976

27. Falck B, Hillarp NA, Thieme G, et al: Fluorescence of catecholamines and related compounds condensed with formaldehyde. J Histochem Cytochem 10:348, 1962

28. Adams CWM: A Perchloric acid-naphthoquinone method for the histochemical localization of cholesterol. Nature (Lond) 192:331, 1961

29. Pearse AGE: The diffuse neuroendocrine system and the APUD concept: Related peptides in brain, intestine, pituitary, placenta and apocrine cutaneous glands. Med Biol 55:115, 1977

30. Jones RA, Dawson IMP: Morphology and staining patterns of endocrine cell tumours in the gut, pancreas and bronchus and their possible significance. Histopathology 1:137, 1977

31. Dawson IMP: The endocrine cells of the gastrointestinal tract and the neoplasms which arise from them. p. 222. In Morson BC (ed): Pathology of the Gastrointestinal Tract. Current Topics in Pathology Vol. 63. Springer-Verlag, New York, 1976

32. Grimelius L, Wilander E: Silver impregnation and other nonimmunocytochemical methods. p. 95. In Polak JM, Bloom SR (eds): Endocrine Tumours. Churchill Livingstone, Edinburgh, 1985

33. Singh I: A modification of the Masson-Hamperl method for staining of argentaffin cells. Anat Anz 115:81, 1964

34. Grimelius L: A silver nitrate stain for α_2-cells in human pancreatic islets. Acta Soc Med Uppsal 73:243, 1968

35. Nieuwenhuijzen Kruseman AC, Knijnenburg G, Brutel de la Rivière G, et al: Morphology and immunohistochemically defined endocrine function of pancreatic islet cell tumors. Histopathology 2:389, 1978

36. Ewen SB, Rost FDW: The histochemical demonstration of catecholamines and tryptamines by acid and aldehyde-induced methods. Microspectrofluorimetric characterization of the fluorophores in models. Histochem J 4:59, 1972

37. Willighagen RGJ: Histochemistry in pathologic diagnosis. Beitr Pathol 141:280, 1970

38. Westermark P, Grimelius L, Polak JM, et al: Amyloid in peptide hormone-producing tumors. Lab Invest 37:212, 1977

39. Stein H, Lennert K, Parwaresch MR: Malignant lymphomas of B-cell type. Lancet 2:855, 1972

40. Leder LD: Der Blutmonocyt. Springer-Verlag, Berlin, 1967

41. Grossi CE, Webb SR, Zicca A, et al: Morphological and histochemical analysis of 2 human T-cell subpopulations bearing receptors for IgM or IgG. J Exp Med 147:1405, 1978

42. Stein H, Petersen N, Gaedicke G, et al: Lymphoblastic lymphoma of convoluted or acid phosphatase type—A tumor of T precursor cells. Int J Cancer 17:292, 1976

43. Katayama I, Yang JPS: Reassessment of a cytochemical test for differential diagnosis of leukemic reticuloendotheliosis. Am J Clin Pathol 68:268, 1977

44. Wagner JC, Munday DE, Harington JS: Histochemical demonstration of hyaluronic acid in pleural mesotheliomas. J Pathol 84:73, 1962

45. Norken SA, Campagna-Pinto D: Cytoplasmic hyaline inclusions in hepatomas. Arch Pathol 86:25, 1968

46. Willighagen RGJ, Thiery M: Enzyme histochemistry of ovarian tumors. Am J Obstet Gynecol 100:393, 1968

47. Koudstaal J: The histochemical demonstration of arylsulphatase in human tumors. Eur J Cancer 11:809, 1975

48. Wachstein M: Histochemistry of enzymes in tumours. In Handbuch der Histochemie. Vol. VII. Gustav Fischer, Stuttgart, 1962

49. Koudstaal J, Makkink B, Overdiep SH: Enzyme histochemical patterns in human tumours. I. Hydrolytic enzymes in carcinoma of the colon and the breast. Eur J Cancer 2:105, 1975

50. Koudstaal J, Makkink B, Overdiep SH: Enzymehistochemical patterns in human tumours. II. Oxidoreductases in carcinoma of the colon and the breast. Eur J Cancer 2:111, 1975

51. Sarnat HB, de Millo DE, Siddiqui SY: Diagnostic value of histochemistry in embryonal rhabdomyosarcoma. Am J Surg Pathol 3:177, 1979

52. Schajowicz F: Ewing sarcoma and reticulum cell sarcoma of bone. With special reference to the histochemical demonstration of glycogen as an aid to differential diagnosis. J Bone Joint Surg 41A:349, 1959

53. Köhler G, Milstein C: Continuous cultures of fused cells secreting antibodies of predefined specificity. Nature (Lond) 256:495, 1975

54. Curran RC, Gregory J: Demonstration of immunoglobulin in cryostat and paraffin sections of human tonsil by immunofluorescence and immunoperoxidase techniques. Effects of processing on immunocytochemical performance of tissues and on the use of proteolytic enzymes to unmask antigens in sections. J Histochem Cytochem 31:974, 1978

55. Lee AK, DeLellis R: Immunohistochemical techniques and their applications to tissue diagnosis. p. 31. In Spicer SS (ed): Histochemistry in Pathological Diagnosis. Marcel Dekker, New York, 1987

56. Bunn PA Jr, Linnoila I, Minna JD, et al: Small cell lung cancer, endocrine cells of the fetal bronchus and other neuroendocrine cells express the leu-7 antigenic determinant present on natural killer cells. Blood 65:764, 1985

57. Norton AJ, Thomas JA, Isaacson PG: Cytokeratin-specific monoclonal antibodies are reactive with tumors of smooth muscle cells. An immunocytochemical and biochemical study using antibodies to intermediate filament cytoskeletal proteins. Histopathology 11:487, 1987

58. Schmechel DE: Gamma subunits of the glycolytic enzyme enolase: Non-specific or neuron-specific. Lab Invest 52:239, 1985

59. Choe BK, Pontes EJ, Rose NR, et al: Expression of human prostatic acid phosphatase in a pancreatic islet cell carcinoma. Invest Dermatol 15:312, 1978

60. Bosman FT: Neuroendocrine cells in non-neuroendocrine tumors. p. 519. In Falkmer S, Hakanson R, Sundler F (eds): Evolution and Tumor Pathology of the Diffuse Neuroendocrine System. Elsevier, Amsterdam, 1983

61. Roholl PJM, Ramaekers FCS, Bosman FT: Markers of carcinomas and sarcomas. Diagnostic implications. p. 227. In den Otter W, Ruitenberg EJ (eds): Tumor Immunology—Mechanisms, Diagnosis, Therapy. Elsevier, Amsterdam, 1987

62. Fukuyama M, Hayashi Y, Koike M, et al: Human chorionic gonadotrophin in lung and lung tumors. Immunohistochemical study on unbalanced distribution of subunits. Lab Invest 55:433, 1987

63. Wang E, Fishman D, Lieu RKH, Sun T-T (eds): Intermediate filaments. Ann NY Acad Sci Vol. 455, 1985

64. Gabbiani G, Kapanci Y, Barazzone P, et al: Immunochemical identification of intermediate sized filaments in human neoplastic cells: A diagnostic aid for the surgical pathologist. Am J Pathol 104:206, 1981

65. Osborn M, Weber K: Tumor diagnosis by intermediate filament typing: A novel tool for surgical pathology. Lab Invest 48:372, 1983

66. To A, Coleman DV, Dearnley DP, et al: Use of antisera to epithelial membrane antigen for the cytodiagnosis of malignancy in serous effusions. J Clin Pathol 34:1326, 1981

67. Miettinen M: Chordoma. Antibodies to epithelial antigen and carcinoembryonic antigen in differential diagnosis. Arch Pathol Lab Med 10:891, 1984

68. Moll R, Cowin P, Kapprell H-P, et al: Desmosomal proteins: New markers for identification and classification of tumors. Lab Invest 54:4, 1986

69. Miettinen M, Lehto V-P, Virtanen I: Keratin in the epithelial-like cells of classical biphasic synovial sarcoma. Virchows Arch [B] 40:157, 1982

70. Mullink H, Henzen-Logmans SC, Alons-van Kordelaar JJM, et al: Simultaneous immunoenzyme staining of vimentin and cytokeratins with monoclonal antibodies as an aid in the differential diagnosis of malignant mesothelioma from pulmonary adenocarcinoma. Virchows Arch [B] 52:55, 1986

71. Churg A: Immunohistochemical staining for vimentin and keratin in malignant mesothelioma. Am J Surg Pathol 9:360, 1985

72. Blewitt RW, Aparicio SRG, Bird CC: Epithelioid sarcoma: A tumor of myofibroblasts. Histopathology 7:573, 1983

73. Herman CJ, Moesker O, Kant A, et al: Is renal cell ("Grawitz") tumor a carcinosarcoma? Evidence from analysis of intermediate filament types. Virchows Arch [Cell Pathol] 44:73, 1983

74. Miettinen M, Franssila K, Passivuo R, et al: I. Expression of intermediate filaments in thyroid gland and thyroid tumors. Lab Invest 50:262, 1984

75. Caselitz J, Osborn M, Seifert G, et al: Intermediate sized filaments (prekeratin, vimentin, desmin) in the normal parotid gland and parotid gland tumours. Virchows Arch [A] 393:273, 1981

76. Altmansberger M, Osborn M, Schafer H, et al: Distinction of nephroblastomas from other childhood tumours using antibodies to intermediate filaments. Virchows Arch [Cell Pathol] 45:113, 1985

77. Marshall RJ, Herbert A, Braye SG, et al: Use of antibodies to carcinoembryonic antigen and human milk fat globule to distinguish carcinoma, mesothelioma, and reactive mesothelium. J Clin Pathol 37:1215, 1984

78. Gosh AK, Gatter KC, Dunnill MS, et al: Immunohistochemical staining of reactive mesothelium, mesothelioma and lung carcinoma with a panel of monoclonal antibodies. J Clin Pathol 40:19, 1987

79. Miettinen M, Foidart J-M, Ekblom P: Immunohistochemical demonstration of laminin, the major glycoprotein of basement membranes, as an aid in the diagnosis of soft tissue tumors. Am J Clin Pathol 79:306, 1983

80. Quinlan RA, Schiller DL, Hartfeld M, et al: Patterns of expression and organization in cytokeratin intermediate filaments. Ann NY Acad Sci 455:282, 1985

81. Moll R, Franke WW, Schiller DL, et al: The catalog of human cytokeratins: Patterns of expression in normal epithelia, tumors and cultured cells. Cell 31:11, 1982

82. Debus E, Weber K, Osborn M: Monoclonal cytokeratin

antibodies that distinguish simple from stratified squamous epithelia: Characterization on human tissues. EMBO J 1:1641, 1982

83. Ramaekers FCS, Huijsmans A, Moesker O, et al: Monoclonal antibody to keratin filaments specific for glandular epithelia and their tumors: Use in surgical pathology. Lab Invest 49:353, 1983

84. Debus E, Moll R, Franke WW, et al: Immunohistochemical distinction of human carcinomas by cytokeratin typing with monoclonal antibodies. Am J Pathol 114:121, 1984

85. van Muijen GNP, Ruiter DJ, Franke WW, et al: Cell type heterogeneity of cytokeratin expression in complex epithelia and carcinoma as demonstrated by monoclonal antibodies specific for cytokeratins 4 and 13. Exp Cell Res 162:97, 1986

86. Jöbsis AC, De Vries GP, Anholt RRH, et al: Demonstration of the prostatic origin of metastasis: An immunohistochemical method for formalin-fixed embedded tissue. Cancer 41:1788, 1978

87. Kimura N, Sasano N: Prostate specific acid phosphatase in carcinoid tumours. Virchows Arch [A] 410:247, 1986

88. McCarthy KS Jr., Miller LS, Cox EB, et al: Estrogen receptor analyses. Correlation of biochemical and immunohistochemical methods using monoclonal antireceptor antibodies. Arch Pathol Lab Med 109:716, 1985

89. Burt A, Goudie RB: Diagnosis of primary thyroid carcinoma by immunohistological demonstration of thyroglobulin. Histopathology 3:279, 1979

90. Goldenberg DM, Neville AM, Carter AM, et al: CEA (Carcinoembryonic antigen): Its role as a marker in the management of cancer. J Cancer Res Clin Oncol 101:239, 1981

91. Muraro R, Wunderlich D, Thor A, et al: Definition by monoclonal antibodies of a repertoire of epitopes of carcinoembryonic antigen differentially expressed in human colon carcinomas versus normal adult tissues. Cancer Res 45:5769, 1985

92. Kuhlmann WD: Alpha-fetoprotein: Cellular origin of a biological marker in rat liver under various experimental conditions. Virchows Arch [A] 393:9, 1981

93. Beilby JOW, Horne CHW, Milne GD, et al: Alpha-fetoprotein, alpha-1-antitrypsin, and transferrin in gonadal yolk-sac tumours. J Clin Pathol 32:455, 1979

94. Bast RC, Feeney M, Lazarus H, et al: Reactivity of a monoclonal antibody with human ovarian carcinoma. J Clin Invest 68:1331, 1981

95. Kawabat SE, Bast RC, Bhan AK, et al: Tissue distribution of a coelomic-epithelium-related antigen recognized by the monoclonal antibody OC 125. Int J Gynecol Pathol 2:275, 1983

96. Moon TD: A highly restricted antigen for renal cell carcinoma defined by a monoclonal antibody. Hybridoma 4:163, 1985

97. Oosterwijk E, Ruiter DJ, Wakka JC, et al: Immunohistochemical analysis of monoclonal antibodies to renal antigens: Applications in the diagnosis of renal cancers. Am J Pathol 123:301, 1986

98. De Ley L, Broers R, Ramaekers FCS, et al: Monoclonal antibodies in clinical and experimental pathology of lung cancer. p. 191. In Ruiter DJ, Fleuren GJ, Warnaar SO (eds): Applications of Monoclonal Antibodies in Tumor Pathology. Martinus Nijhof, Dordrecht, 1987

99. Marangos PJ: Clinical utility of neuron-specific enolase as a neuroendocrine tumor marker. p. 181. In Polak JM, Bloom SR, (eds): Endocrine Tumours. Churchill Livingstone, Edinburgh, 1985

100. Bishop AE, Polak JM, Facer P, et al: Neuron specific enolase: A common marker for the endocrine cells and innervation of the gut and the pancreas. Gastroenterology 83:902, 1982

101. Tapia RJ, Polak JM, Barbosa AJA, et al: Neuron specific enolase is produced by neuroendocrine tumours. Lancet 2:808, 1981

102. Gu J, Polak JM, van Noorden S, et al: Immunostaining of neuron-specific enolase as a diagnostic tool for Merkel cell tumours. Cancer 52:1039, 1983

103. Fischer-Colbrie R, Fischenschlager I: Immunological characterization of secretory proteins of chromaffin granules: Chromogranins A, chromogranin B and enkephalin-containing peptides. J Neurochem 44:1854, 1985

104. Fischer-Colbrie R, Hagn C, Kilpatrick L, et al: Chromogranin C: A third component of the acidic proteins in chromaffin granules. J Neurochem 47:318, 1986

105. O'Connor DT, Burtin D, Deftos LJ: Immunoreactive human chromogranin A in diverse polypeptide hormone producing human tumors and normal endocrine tissues. J Clin Endocrinol Metab 57:1084, 1984

106. Wiedenmann B, Franke WW, Kuhn C, et al: Synaptophysin: A marker protein for neuroendocrine cells and neoplasms. Proc Natl Acad Sci USA 83:3500, 1987

107. Ramaekers FCS, Puts JJG, Moesker O, et al: Antibodies to intermediate filament proteins in the immunohistochemical identification of human tumours. An overview. Histochem J 15:691, 1983

108. Warnke RA, Gatter KC, Falini B, et al: Diagnosis of human lymphoma with monoclonal antileucocyte antibodies. N Engl J Med 309:1275, 1983

109. Nakajima T, Watanabe S, Sato Y, et al: Immunohistochemical demonstration of S-100 protein in malignant melanoma and pigmented nevus, and its diagnostic application. Cancer 50:912, 1981

110. Nakajima T, Watanabe S, Sato Y, et al: An immunoperoxidase study of S-100 protein distribution in normal and neoplastic tissues. Am J Surg Pathol 6:715, 1982

111. Kahn HJ, Marks A, Thorn H, et al: Role of antibody to S-100 protein in diagnostic pathology. Am J Clin Pathol 79:341, 1983

112. Van Duinen SG, Ruiter DJ, Hageman PH, et al: Immunohistochemical and histochemical tools in the diagnosis of amelanotic melanoma. Cancer 53:1566, 1984

113. Ruiter DJ, Dingjan M, Steijlen PM, et al: Monoclonal antibodies selected to discriminate between malignant melanomas and nevocellular nevi. J Invest Dermatol 66:145, 1986

114. Atkinson B, Ernst CS, Ghrist BFD, et al: Identification of

melanoma-associated antigens using fixed tissue screening for antibodies. Cancer Res 44:2577, 1984

115. Martinez-Hernandez A, Amenta P: The basement membrane in pathology. Lab Invest 48:656, 1983

116. Bosman FT, Havenith M, Cleutjens J: Basement membranes in cancer. Ultrastruct Pathol 8:291, 1985

117. Birembaut P, Caron Y, Adnet JJ, et al: Usefulness of basement membrane markers in tumoral pathology. J Pathol 145:283, 1985

118. Roholl PJM, Kleyne J, Pijpers HW, et al: Comparative immunohistochemical investigation of markers for malignant histiocytes. Hum Pathol 16:763, 1985

119. Roholl PJM, De Jong ASH, Ramaekers FCS: Application of markers in soft tissue tumors. Histopathology 9:1019, 1985

120. Roholl PJM, Kleyne J, van Basten CDH, et al: A study to analyze the origin of tumor cells in malignant fibrous histiocytomas. Cancer 56:2809, 1985

121. Roholl PJM, Kleyne J, van Unnik JAM: Characterization of tumor cells in malignant fibrous histiocytoma and other soft tissue tumours in comparison with malignant histiocytes. II. Immunohistochemical studies in cryostat sections. Am J Pathol 121:269, 1985

122. Sehested M, Hou-Jensen K: Factor VIII related antigen as an endothelial cell marker in benign and malignant diseases. Virchows Arch [Pathol Anat] 391:217, 1981

123. Ordonez NG, Batsakis JG: Comparison of Ulex Europaeus I lectin and factor VIII related antigen in vascular lesions. Arch Pathol Lab Med 108:129, 1984

124. De Jong ASH, van Vark M, Albus-Lutter ChE, et al: Myosin and myoglobin as tumor markers in the diagnosis of rhabdomyosarcomas: A comparative study. Am J Surg Pathol 8:521, 1984

125. De Jong ASH, van Kessel-van Vark M, Albus-Lutter ChE, et al: Skeletal muscle actin as tumor marker in the diagnosis of rhabdomyosarcoma in childhood. Am J Surg Pathol 9:467, 1985

126. De Jong ASH, van Kessel-van Vark M, Albus-Lutter ChE, et al: Creatine kinase subunits M and B as markers in the diagnosis of poorly differentiated rhabdomyosarcomas in children. Hum Pathol 16:924, 1985

127. Mogollon R, Penneys N, Albores-Saavedra J, et al: Malignant Schwannoma presenting as a skin mass. Confirmation by the demonstration of myelin basic protein within tumor cells. Cancer 53:1190, 1984

128. Russo J, Sommers SC (eds): Tumor Diagnosis by Electron Microscopy. Vol. 1. Field, Rich, and Associates, New York, 1986

129. Mackay B (ed): Clinics in Laboratory Medicine; Diagnostic Electron Microscopy of Tumors. Vol. 7. WB Saunders, Philadelphia, 1987

130. Mason D, Pedraza MA, Doslu FA, et al: Ultrastructural and immunological methods in diagnostic pathology in a community hospital. Ultrastruct Pathol 2:373, 1981

131. Wang N-S, Minassian H: The formaldehyde-fixed and paraffin-embedded tissues for diagnostic transmission electron microscopy. A retrospective study. Hum Pathol 18:715, 1987

132. Neal MH, Kosinski R, Cohen P, et al: Atypical endocrine tumors of the lung: A histologic, ultrastructural, and clinical study of 19 cases. Hum Pathol 17:1264, 1986

133. Wills EJ, Carr S, Philips J: Electron microscopy in the diagnosis of percutaneous fine needle aspiration specimens. Ultrastruct Pathol 11:361, 1987

134. Mackay B, Fanning T, Brunner JM, et al: Diagnostic electron microscopy using fine needle aspiration biopsies. Ultrastruct Pathol 11:659, 1987

135. Herrera GA, Wilkerson JA: Ultrastructural studies of malignant cells in fluids. Diagn Cytopathol 1:272, 1985

136. Triche TJ, Askin FB: Neuroblastoma and the differential diagnosis of small-, round-, blue-cell tumors. Hum Pathol 14:569, 1983

137. Mierau GW, Berry PJ, Orsini EN: Small round cell neoplasms: Can electron microscopy and immunohistochemical studies accurately classify them? Ultrastruct Pathol 9:99, 1985

138. Mierau GW, Favara BE: Rhabdomyosarcoma in children: Ultrastructural study of 31 cases. Cancer 46:2035, 1980

139. Mahoney JP, Alexander RW: Ewing's sarcoma. A light- and electron-microscopic study of 21 cases. Am J Surg Pathol 2:283, 1978

140. Llombart-Bosch A, Blache R, Peydro-Olaya A: Ultrastructural study of 28 cases of Ewing's sarcoma: Typical and atypical forms. Cancer 41:1362, 1978

141. Cavazzana AO, Miser JS, Jefferson J, et al: Experimental evidence for a neural origin of Ewing's sarcoma of bone. Am J Pathol 127:507, 1987

142. Warhol MJ, Corson JM: An ultrastructural comparison of mesotheliomas with adenocarcinomas of the lung and breast. Hum Pathol 16:50, 1985

143. Dardick I, Jabi M, Elliot M, et al: Diffuse epithelial mesothelioma: A review of the ultrastructural spectrum. Ultrastruct Pathol 11:503, 1987

144. Auerbach O, Frasca JM, Parks VR, et al: A comparison of World Health Organization (WHO) classification of lung tumors by light and electron microscopy. Cancer 50:2079, 1982

145. McDowell EM, Trump BF: Pulmonary small cell carcinoma showing tripartite differentiation in individual cells. Hum Pathol 12:286, 1981

146. Dvorak AM, Monahan RA: Metastatic adenocarcinoma of unknown primary site. Diagnostic electron microscopy to determine the site of tumor origin. Arch Pathol Lab Med 106:21, 1982

147. Kimura Y: A histochemical and ultrastructural study of adenocarcinoma of the lung. Am J Surg Pathol 2:253, 1978

148. Ogata T, Endo K: Clara cell granules of peripheral lung cancers. Cancer 54:1635, 1984

149. Sobrinho-Simoes M, Johannessen JV, Gould VE: The diagnostic significance of intracytoplasmic lumina in metastatic neoplasms. Ultrastruct Pathol 2:327, 1981

150. Clayton F, Sibley RK, Ordonez NG, et al: Argyrophilic breast carcinomas. Evidence of lactational differentiation. Am J Surg Pathol 6:323, 1982

151. Nesland JM, Memoli VA, Holm R, et al: Breast carcino-

mas with neuroendocrine differentiation. Ultrastruct Pathol 8:225, 1985

152. Hickey WF, Seiler MW: Ultrastructural markers of colonic adenocarcinoma. Cancer 47:140, 1981

153. Batsakis JG, Mackay B, Ordonez NG: Enteric-type adenocarcinoma of the nasal cavity. Cancer 54:855, 1984

154. Mackay B, Ordonez NG, Khoursand J, et al: The ultrastructure and immunohistochemistry of renal cell carcinoma. Ultrastruct Pathol 11:483, 1987

155. Carlson G, Sibley RK: Anterior mediastinal neoplasms: An ultrastructural review. p. 253. In Russo J, Sommers SC (eds): Tumor Diagnosis by Electron Microscopy. Vol. 1. Field, Rich, and Associates, New York, 1986

156. Richardson RL, Schoumacher RA, Fer MF, et al: The unrecognized extragonadal germ cell cancer syndrome. Ann Intern Med 94:181, 1981

157. Gould VE: Histogenesis and differentiation: A re-evaluation of these concepts as criteria for the classification of tumors. Hum Pathol 17:212, 1986

158. Sidhu GS: The endodermal origin of digestive and respiratory tract APUD cells. Histopathologic evidence and a review of the literature. Am J Pathol 96:5, 1979

159. Burns DK, Silva FG, Forde KA, et al: Primary melanocytic Schwannoma of the stomach: Evidence of dual melanocytic and Schwannian differentiation in an extra-axial site in a patient without neurofibromatosis. Cancer 52:1432, 1983

160. Carstens PHB: The Weibel-Palade body in the diagnosis of endothelial tumors. Ultrastruct Pathol 2:315, 1981

161. Favara BE, McCarthy RC, Mierau GW: Histiocytosis X. Hum Pathol 14:663, 1983

8

Inflammatory Diseases of the Skin

Loren E. Golitz

HANDLING AND PROCESSING OF SKIN BIOPSY SPECIMENS

It is important in the diagnosis of the inflammatory dermatoses to select the proper site for biopsy. In many diseases, such as lichen planus and psoriasis, biopsy of an older lesion may provide the most histologic information. Care should be taken, however, to avoid lesions that show excoriation and secondary infection. In the bullous dermatoses, it is preferable to biopsy an early vesicle since secondary changes in an older lesion may obscure the characteristic findings. In most cases of dermatitis, the inclusion of normal skin in the biopsy specimen is not necessary and may result in the oversight of important changes if the specimen is sectioned through the area of normal skin.

Three types of skin biopsies are most often used in the diagnosis of the inflammatory dermatoses. The excisional biopsy obtains a generous amount of tissue and is the most desirable form of skin biopsy from the pathologist's point of view. A good excisional biopsy is elliptical and includes subcutaneous fat. This form of biopsy may be necessary for the interpretation of inflammatory changes in the subcutaneous fat such as erythema nodosum. The disadvantages of the excisional biopsy are the time required to perform the procedure and the necessity for sutures. A second form of skin biopsy is the punch biopsy. Most punch biopsy specimens are 4 mm in diameter; however, they vary from 2 to 8 mm in diameter. The punch biopsy obtains a round plug of skin, which frequently includes the superficial portion of the subcutaneous fat. In general, the punch biopsy is adequate for most inflammatory dermatoses with the exception of those that involve the fat and deep fascia. The punch biopsy is

quick and easy to perform and does not require sterile technique or sutures; however, the resulting round scar is less desirable than the linear scar of an excisional biopsy. A third type of biopsy, the shave biopsy, may be preferable for those disorders that involve predominantly the epidermis and superficial dermis. The shave biopsy usually obtains a larger piece of epidermis than the 4 mm punch biopsy and is ideal for diseases such as psoriasis and lichen planus that do not involve the fat. The shave biopsy is performed quickly without the use of sterile technique or sutures. A fourth type of biopsy, the curette biopsy, is used for a variety of tumors by some clinicians but is generally unacceptable for the inflammatory dermatoses since it may provide an inadequate specimen or excessively traumatize the tissue. In all forms of skin biopsies, but particularly with the punch biopsy, care should be taken not to compress the tissue with the forceps since this tends to distort the histologic changes.

The ideal fixative for skin biopsy specimens is 10 percent phosphate-buffered neutral formalin. A minimum of 8 hours should be allowed for fixation, although 24 hours is ideal. Large specimens should be sectioned to 4 mm or less in thickness to allow adequate fixation. In cold climates where tissue is sent through the mail, a fixative solution containing alcohol may be desirable to prevent the formation of ice crystals in the tissue.

When processing biopsy specimens of the inflammatory dermatoses, the epidermal surface should be inspected grossly, and the tissue should be bisected through the area of greatest alteration. For disorders with focal changes such as scabies, this may mean the difference between an accurate diagnosis and a nonspecific one. Most punch biopsy and shave biopsy specimens should be bisected and embedded with the cut surfaces down. Two mm punch biopsy specimens are small and should be embedded intact. While excisional biopsy specimens of tumors are usually bisected through the narrow axis, more information may be obtained in the inflammatory dermatoses if they are bisected longitudinally. Hair shafts that protrude from the surface of the skin should be trimmed before embedding to avoid dulling the microtome blade and scratching the surface of the sections. Excessive fat should be trimmed from the specimen if the inflammatory process does not involve the subcutaneous fat.

HISTOLOGY OF NORMAL SKIN

The outer layer of the epidermis is known as the stratum corneum, keratin layer, or horny layer. This layer often shows a loose basketweave pattern, but on the palms and soles it is thick and compact. Skin from acral portions of the body may show a clear zone or stratum lucidum immediately beneath the keratin layer. Deep to the stratum lucidum is the granular cell layer, which is formed by partially flattened cells that contain deeply basophilic keratohyaline granules. The thickness of the granular cell layer varies from 1 to 10 cells and is usually proportional to the thickness of the stratum corneum. Beneath the granular cell layer is the stratum malpighii, also known as the squamous cell layer or prickle cell layer. The cells in this layer are polygonal and contain round to oval nuclei. The malpighian cells are attached to each other by modifications of their cell membranes known as prickles or desmosomes. The deepest layer of the epidermis is the basal cell layer. The basal cell layer contains two types of cells, epidermal basal cells and melanocytes. The basal cells are columnar and are attached to the underlying basement membrane by hemidesmosomes. Basal cells divide and daughter cells become the cells of the stratum malpighii. Almost all mitotic activity occurs in the basal cell layer; however, mitoses occur rarely one or two layers above the basal cell layer. About 28 to 30 days are required for a cell to move from the basal cell layer to the outer portion of the keratin layer where it is shed off. Approximately every tenth cell in the basal cell layer is a melanocyte, which produces a granular pigment known as melanin. Melanocytes have elongated dendritic processes that extend into the malpighian layer. Melanin pigment moves through the dendrites and is eventually found in the cytoplasm of the malpighian cells where it functions to screen the nucleus of these cells from ultraviolet radiation. A second type of dendritic cell, the Langerhans' cell, occurs within the malpighian layer. This cell, which is not obvious in routinely stained sections, constitutes 3 to 8 percent of

the epidermal cells and functions as a macrophage by processing and presenting antigens to inflammatory cells such as T lymphocytes.[1]

The epidermis and dermis interface in an undulating pattern. The projections of epidermis are known as rete ridges. The intervening projections of dermal connective tissue are known as dermal papillae. The dermis is divided into papillary dermis and reticular dermis. The papillary dermis occurs between the rete ridges and extends for a short distance beneath the tips of the rete ridges. The papillary dermis stains pale pink with the hematoxylin and eosin stain and contains delicate collagen fibers, some of which are oriented perpendicularly or obliquely to the surface of the epidermis. Beneath the papillary dermis, the reticular dermis contains thick, deeply eosinophilic collagen fibers that are oriented parallel to the surface of the skin. Deep to the reticular dermis is the subcutaneous fat, which is divided into distinct lobules by thin septa of connective tissue. Fascia is immediately deep to the subcutaneous fat.

A superficial vascular plexus of arterioles, venules, and capillaries is present in the superficial dermis. A deep vascular plexus of arteries and veins occurs in the deep dermis and superficial subcutaneous fat and is connected to the superficial plexus by connecting vessels. The dermal vessels are often accompanied by nerves.

A distinctive feature of skin is the presence of a variety of adnexal structures. Eccrine sweat glands are widely distributed and function to control body temperature through the evaporation of sweat. They are composed of an intraepidermal duct, which empties directly onto the skin surface; a dermal duct; and a glandular portion, which is located in the deep dermis. The coiled glandular portion is surrounded by a narrow zone of subcutaneous fat. The apocrine sweat glands are most numerous in the axillae and the groin. The glandular portion of the apocrine sweat glands is larger and has larger lumina than the eccrine glands. The apocrine duct empties into the upper portion of a hair follicle or directly onto the skin surface. The third major adnexal structure of the skin is the pilosebaceous apparatus, which is composed of a hair follicle, a sebaceous gland, an arrector muscle, and in some parts of the body an apocrine gland. Sebaceous glands are numerous on the face but are also present on all parts of the body except the palms and soles. The multilobular glands have a single peripheral row of germinative cells that divide and produce the sebaceous cells that make up the bulk of the lobules. Sebaceous cells have a small centrally placed nucleus and foamy cytoplasm. Sebaceous glands are holocrine glands; that is, the sebaceous cells degenerate and become the secretory material that is discharged into the follicular lumen. The deepest portion of the hair follicle is the hair bulb, which surrounds a dermal hair papilla containing blood vessels and nerves.

Just above the hair papilla is the matrix, a rapidly dividing area that produces the hair shaft. The hair follicle is surrounded by an inner root sheath and an outer root sheath. The arrector muscle extends from the deep portion of the hair follicle or hair bulb to the undersurface of the epidermis. Contractions of these smooth muscles produce the clinical appearance of goosebumps. Smooth muscle also occurs in the areola of the nipples and the tunica dartos of the external genitalia. Striated muscle in the skin is generally limited to the facial and platysma muscles.

CLINICOPATHOLOGIC CORRELATION

In no other area of anatomic pathology is the correlation of clinical information more important in arriving at the correct diagnosis than in the inflammatory dermatoses. Many cases that appear to be nonspecific dermatitis histologically can be accurately diagnosed when clinical information is used. For example, lichen striatus histologically shows a subacute or chronic dermatitis. However, a linear pruritic rash extending down the entire length of an arm or leg in a young individual, when combined with these histologic features, is typical of lichen striatus. The subepidermal bullae in dermatitis herpetiformis at times are nonspecific. However, a clinical history of grouped, pruritic vesicles on the elbows and interscapular area is characteristic of dermatitis herpetiformis and should stimulate a search for neutrophils within dermal papillae at the margins of the subepidermal bullae. When histologic changes do not support the clinical information, additional levels through the tissue or additional biopsies may be indicated. At times, the clinical differential diagnosis may be incorrect, and the pathologist should not hesitate to discuss impressions with the clinician before issuing the pathology report.

GENERAL RULES FOR EXAMINING THE SLIDE

The histologic diagnosis of an inflammatory dermatosis is best made by examining the pattern of inflammation and categorizing it with a specific group of diseases. In most cases, the inflammatory pattern is best evaluated by looking at the slide at low magnification. To prevent confusion, high magnification should be used only when something specific is being observed in greater detail. A few general rules are helpful in evaluating biopsy specimens of the inflammatory skin diseases: (1) Look at all slides as unknowns, (2) evaluate the slide grossly against a contrasting background and note the inflammatory pattern, (3) look at all sections on each slide, and (4) look at each slide in a systematic manner, starting with the stratum corneum and progressing to the subcutaneous fat.

INFLAMMATORY REACTION PATTERNS

Epidermal Reaction Patterns

Spongiotic Dermatitis

Spongiotic dermatitis is characterized by intercellular edema that produces separation of the cells of the malpighian layer, often resulting in the formation of microabscesses or bullae. The prickles or desmosomes between epidermal cells appear prominent and stretched in the presence of spongiosis. The epidermis is often mildly acanthotic, whereas the dermis shows vascular dilatation and a patchy perivascular infiltrate of mononuclear cells. Skin diseases that commonly produce spongiotic dermatitis include allergic contact dermatitis, nummular eczema, pityriasis rosea, id reactions, dyshidrotic eczema, incontinentia pigmenti, and a variety of other eczematous processes.

Allergic Contact Dermatitis

The prototype of spongiotic dermatitis is allergic contact dermatitis caused by skin contact with allergens such as poison ivy, nickel in jewelry, or topical medications. Typically, the skin is erythematous and edematous with small vesicles and crusting. The distribution of the rash in contact dermatitis is often characteristic with nickel dermatitis occurring on the earlobes, neck, fingers, and wrists in areas of contact with jewelry. Poison ivy occurs on exposed portions of the body and often shows linear vesicles where the broken leaf or stem of the plant has brushed against the skin. Allergic contact dermatitis of the hands and feet typically involves the dorsal aspects with sparing of the keratotic palms and soles. It should be kept in mind that any allergen can be transferred to the eyes or genitalia after contact with the hands. Of equal importance is the fact that the allergen may be something to which the patient has been exposed for years. Once contact allergy to a chemical develops, the potential to react to that chemical persists for many years.

The epidermis shows hyperkeratosis and parakeratosis with mild to moderate acanthosis and spongiosis. The prickles between epidermal cells are easily visible and intraepidermal spongiotic microabscesses occur (Fig. 8-1). The surface of the epidermis may be covered with crust and cellular debris. The small vessels of the papillary dermis are dilated, and a perivascular infiltrate of

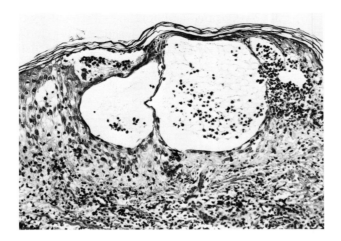

Fig. 8-1. Spongiotic dermatitis (acute dermatitis). Intraepidermal spongiotic vesicles contain acute and chronic inflammatory cells. A patchy infiltrate of mononuclear cells surrounds small vessels in the upper dermis.

lymphocytes and histiocytes is present. Occasionally, eosinophils may be present but often they are absent. Spongiosis and exocytosis of lymphocytes into the epidermis are present within 6 hours after exposure to an allergen in experimental contact dermatitis.[2]

Nummular Eczema

Nummular eczema shows coin-shaped patches of dermatitis involving predominantly the extremities in a symmetrical pattern. The legs and the dorsal aspects of the hands are commonly affected. The coin-shaped areas, which appear swollen and elevated above the surface of the surrounding skin, are often studded with tiny vesi-

cles, which can be seen clinically. Crusting and secondary infection are common. Often the surrounding skin appears dry and scaly.

The epidermis shows hyperkeratosis and crusting. A characteristic change is the presence of spotty parakeratosis manifested by small mounds of parakeratotic scale occurring in an interrupted pattern across the surface of the epidermis. Moderate acanthosis and spongiosis occur, often with the formation of spongiotic microabscesses (Fig. 8-2). The dermal changes are nonspecific, showing only a patchy perivascular infiltrate of lymphocytes and histiocytes in the upper dermis. Diseases associated with spotty parakeratosis include nummular eczema, pityriasis rosea, chronic guttate parapsoriasis, seborrheic dermatitis, id reactions, guttate psoriasis and pityriasis rubra pilaris.

Pityriasis Rosea

Pityriasis rosea typically involves the trunk and proximal extremities of young healthy adults in the second or third decade of life. An initial lesion known as a herald patch often precedes the main rash by one to several days. Multiple scaly papules and plaques with an oval appearance tend to show a symmetric dermatome pattern. When the patient's back is observed from a distance the rash may have a characteristic "Christmas tree" distribution. Individual oval plaques have a peripheral collarette of fine scale. The rash of pityriasis rosea generally lasts 4 to 6 weeks and rarely recurs. Although a viral etiology has been suggested, the exact cause remains unknown.

The stratum corneum shows mild hyperkeratosis and spotty parakeratosis (Fig. 8-3). The epidermis is mildly

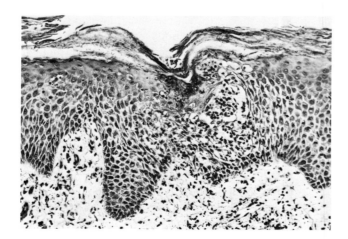

Fig. 8-2. Nummular eczema. There is both acanthosis and spongiosis with exocytosis of lymphocytes into the epidermis. Spongiosis causes the prickles between epidermal cells to appear prominent and small spongiotic microabscesses are present.

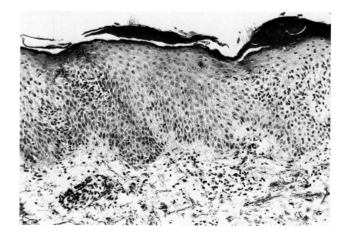

Fig. 8-3. Pityriasis rosea. Small mounds of parakeratosis (spotty parakeratosis) are associated with mild acanthosis, spongiosis and exocytosis of inflammatory cells. A superficial perivascular infiltrate of lymphocytes is often associated with extravasation of red blood cells.

INFLAMMATORY DISEASES OF THE SKIN

acanthotic with elongation of rete ridges. Spongiosis is usually focal and may occur deep to the areas of parakeratosis. Small spongiotic vesicles occur in half of the cases.[3] A patchy infiltrate of lymphocytes surrounds dilated dermal vessels, which often show extravasation of red blood cells (RBC).

Autosensitization Dermatitis

An id reaction is thought to represent an allergic eczematous reaction to an acute dermatitis on another part of the body, although the specific antigens have not been identified.[4] Often the primary process is stasis dermatitis[5] or acute vesicular tinea pedis. When the primary eruption is treated, the id reaction clears spontaneously. Common manifestations of an id reaction are facial eczema and a vesicular eruption of the hands and forearms. When the primary dermatitis involves the hands and feet, the id reaction may extend proximally up the extremities. Erythema, edema, vesicles, and crusting are common.

The epidermis is often crusted and shows spotty parakeratosis. There is variable acanthosis associated with spongiotic vesicles and exocytosis of lymphocytes. Edema of the papillary dermis is prominent and may resemble early subepidermal bulla formation. A perivascular infiltrate within the superficial dermis consists of lymphocytes and histiocytes with occasional eosinophils.

Dyshidrotic Eczema

Dyshidrotic eczema or dyshidrosis is a common form of eczema that is characterized by tiny deep-seated vesicles along the margins of the fingers and toes and on the palms and soles.[6] The rash is characterized by a waxing and waning course that often shows exacerbations during times of emotional stress. The vesicular lesions progress through pustular, erosive, and scaly stages and finally resolve within a period of 1 to 3 weeks, only to recur at a later time.

There is focal hyperkeratosis with parakeratosis. Spongiosis is often prominent with the formation of small and large intraepidermal vesicles. Erosions and crusting may be present. A perivascular infiltrate within the superficial dermis consists of lymphocytes, histiocytes, and occasional neutrophils and eosinophils.

Dermatophyte Infection

Dermatophyte infections, particularly of the feet and intertriginous areas, may show vesicles and pustules with or without accompanying scale. Small pustules are also occasionally seen with monilia infections.

Hyperkeratosis and parakeratosis are often associated with subcorneal pustules or intraepidermal spongiotic vesicles.[7] Neutrophils are numerous within the vesicles,

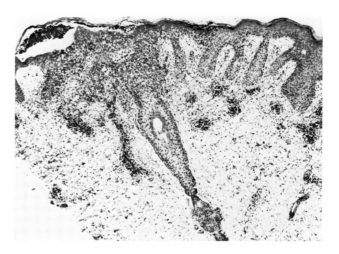

Fig. 8-4. Pustular tinea infection. A subcorneal pustule contains neutrophils. The adjacent epidermis shows acanthosis, spongiosis and exocytosis of inflammatory cells. PAS stain demonstrated hyphae within the pustule and the stratum corneum.

often producing frank pustules (Fig. 8-4). The perivascular infiltrate within the superficial dermis includes lymphocytes, histiocytes, and some neutrophils. Periodic acid-Schiff (PAS) stain demonstrates fungal hyphae within the stratum corneum and the pustules.

Incontinentia Pigmenti

Incontinentia pigmenti is a sex-linked dominant disorder that affects predominantly females.[8] Males are involved so severely that they usually die in utero. The skin eruption, which has three stages, begins between birth and 2 weeks of age with erythema and linear vesiculation that involves mainly the extremities. The second stage, from 2 to 6 weeks of age, is characterized by verrucous nodules predominantly on the extremities that may heal with atrophy and hypopigmentation. Atypical cases may present with verrucous lesions at birth. The third stage, which begins between 12 and 26 weeks of age, shows splashes of macular pigmentation on the trunk and less often the extremities. The brown pigmentation is often arranged in a whorled pattern resembling marble cake. By early adulthood, most of the pigmentary changes have resolved. Incontinentia pigmenti may be associated with severe mental retardation and with other congenital abnormalities of the skeletal system, central nervous system (CNS), eyes, and teeth.[9]

Hyperkeratosis and parakeratosis are absent or mild. There is mild acanthosis associated with prominent spongiosis of the epidermis and exocytosis of large numbers of eosinophils into the spongiotic vesicles (Fig. 8-5). A smaller number of mononuclear cells may also be present

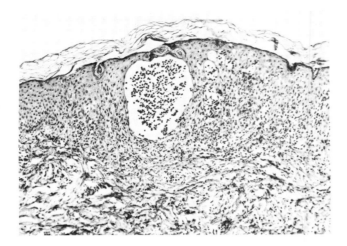

Fig. 8-5. Incontinentia pigmenti. An intraepidermal spongiotic vesicle contains numerous eosinophils. Spongiosis and exocytosis of eosinophils are present in the adjacent epidermis.

within the epidermis. Dyskeratotic keratinocytes are often scattered within the epidermis. The superficial dermis shows mild papillary edema and a perivascular infiltrate of lymphocytes, histiocytes, and numerous eosinophils.

Differential Diagnosis of Spongiotic Dermatitis

It is often not possible to distinguish between allergic contact dermatitis, dyshidrotic eczema, id reactions, and nummular eczema on the basis of the histologic changes. With clinical correlation, however, the distinction can usually be made. Small mounds of parakeratosis (spotty parakeratosis) are seen predominantly in pityriasis rosea, nummular eczema, chronic guttate parapsoriasis, seborrheic dermatitis, and id reactions. Eosinophilic spongiosis is a reaction pattern characterized by eosinophils within a spongiotic epidermis.[10] While this reaction is characteristic of incontinentia pigmenti, it may also be seen in bullous pemphigoid, in early stages of pemphigus vulgaris,[11] and in allergic contact dermatitis, acute arthropod bite reactions, and herpes gestationis.

Psoriasiform Dermatitis

Psoriasiform dermatitis is characterized by prominent parakeratosis and by acanthosis with uniform elongation and clubbing of rete ridges. Neutrophils can often be seen extravasating from dilated vessels of the papillary dermis.[12] Exocytosis of neutrophils into the epidermis is associated with parakeratosis and Munro's microabscesses. Although a large number of inflammatory dermatoses may show a psoriasiform reaction pattern, psoriasiform changes are most characteristics of psoriasis,

Reiter's syndrome, seborrheic dermatitis, pityriasis rubra pilaris, and chronic neurodermatitis.[13]

Psoriasis

Psoriasis is a chronic papulosquamous disease that typically involves the scalp, groin, and extensor aspects of the extremities.[14] Occasionally patients with psoriasis develop generalized erythroderma.[15] The typical lesion is a beefy-red plaque of the elbows or knees that is covered by a thick silvery scale. Kinetic studies of skin in patients with psoriasis show a rapid turnover rate of psoriatic epidermis.[16,17] Psoriasis may occur in areas of trauma such as scratches (Koebner phenomenon). Discrete pitting of the fingernails and toenails is common. Psoriatic arthritis characteristically affects the distal interphalangeal joints, but larger joints may also be involved. The rheumatoid factor test is negative. Variants of psoriasis include a pustular eruption localized to the palms and soles (pustular psoriasis of Barber)[18] and an acute widespread pustular eruption associated with marked constitutional symptoms (pustular psoriasis of von Zumbusch).[19]

A biopsy specimen of a plaque of psoriasis shows marked hyperkeratosis, parakeratosis, and a thin or absent granular cell layer. There is uniform acanthosis with elongation, clubbing, and fusion of rete ridges. Dermal papillae appear edematous and contain dilated vessels. The malpighian layer is thinned over the dermal papillae, and exocytosis of neutrophils frequently occurs in this area. In about 75 percent of the biopsy specimens, Munro's microabscesses containing pyknotic neutrophils are present in the stratum corneum.[20] A patchy perivascular infiltrate of lymphocytes, histiocytes and a variable number of neutrophils is localized to the superficial dermis. The classic changes just described are only present in a relatively small percentage of biopsy specimens.[21] In pustular psoriasis, numerous neutrophils are present in the superficial malpighian layers and the stratum corneum. There are subcorneal pustules containing neutrophils and Munro's microabscesses may be numerous. Neutrophils within the superficial malpighian layer often produce a spongelike appearance due to intracellular edema and the presence of residual plasma membranes of keratinocytes. These multilocular pustules seen in pustular psoriasis have been referred to as spongioform pustules of Kogoj (Fig. 8-6).

Reiter's Syndrome

Reiter's syndrome is characterized by the triad of arthritis, urethritis, and conjunctivitis. Some cases may be associated with diarrhea rather than with urethritis. Approximately 80 percent of affected patients have mucocutaneous lesions including an acral eruption that resem-

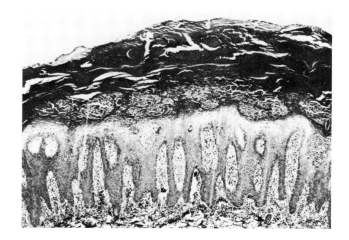

Fig. 8-6. Pustular psoriasis. There is marked hyperkeratosis, parakeratosis and regular acanthosis of the epidermis with clubbing and fusion of rete ridges. Immediately superficial to the stratum malpighii are numerous spongioform pustules of Kogoj.

bles pustular psoriasis of the palms and soles.[22] The eruption of the palms and soles has been called keratoderma blenorrhagica. Additional characteristic features include nail dystrophy, geographic tongue, and an erythematous, pustular eruption of the corona of the glans penis known as balanitis circinata. Arthritis is frequently the most prominent component of the syndrome. Reiter's syndrome, pustular psoriasis, and psoriatic arthritis are associated with an increased incidence of HLA-B27 antigen.[14]

The histologic changes in Reiter's syndrome are indistinguishable from pustular psoriasis (Fig. 8-7). Spongioform pustules are common. Biopsy specimens of geo-

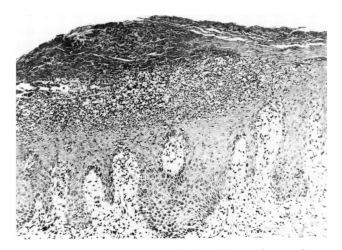

Fig. 8-7. Reiter's syndrome. The hyperkeratosis, parakeratosis and spongioform pustules within the superficial epidermis are indistinguishable from pustular psoriasis.

graphic tongue and balanitis circinata also show spongiotic pustules.[23-25]

Seborrheic Dermatitis

Seborrheic dermatitis produces an erythematous scaly eruption of the scalp and less often of the eyebrows, nasolabial folds, presternal area, and groin. Dandruff and itching are the main symptoms. Severe seborrheic dermatitis is occasionally associated with Parkinson's disease.

The histologic changes resemble psoriasis but are less well developed.[26] The epidermis shows hyperkeratosis and parakeratosis, which may be spotty in nature. Mild to moderate acanthosis is produced by rete ridge elongation; however, clubbing and fusion are less marked than in psoriasis. Small vessels in the papillary dermis are dilated, and there may be exocytosis of neutrophils and lymphocytes into the epidermis. Lymphocytes and histiocytes surround small vessels in the superficial dermis.

Pityriasis Rubra Pilaris

Pityriasis rubra pilaris (PRP) often begins as a scaly eruption of the face and scalp resembling seborrheic dermatitis.[27] Patients develop pink, finely scaly plaques of the trunk and extremities that coalesce leaving intervening islands of normal skin. Other characteristic features include a prominent keratoderma of the palms and soles and the presence of spiny papules at the openings of hair follicles, which are most prominent on the dorsal aspects of the fingers and in the scalp. Like psoriasis, the epidermal turnover rate is increased.[28] A familial form of PRP has its onset in childhood, whereas the more common acquired type usually begins in middle age. The familial form persists for years, whereas the acquired form improves or clears in 75 percent of patients.[29]

There is hyperkeratosis; however, parakeratosis may be mild or absent. Keratin plugs within hair follicles may project above the surface of the adjacent stratum corneum. The epidermis at the margins of involved hair follicles shows spotty parakeratosis and mild to moderate acanthosis with rete ridge elongation. The acanthosis is less marked than in psoriasis, and the granular layer is present. The neutrophils and microabscesses of psoriasis are usually absent. There is a mild perivascular infiltrate of lymphocytes and histiocytes in the superficial dermis.

Chronic Neurodermatitis

Chronic neurodermatitis or lichen simplex chronicus shows sharply demarcated plaques of scaly, lichenified, hyperpigmented skin with excoriations. A common site of involvement in men is the lateral leg above the ankle, while in women the posterior neck and lateral aspects of the arms are more commonly affected.

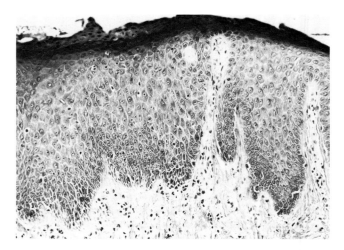

Fig. 8-8. Neurodermatitis. There is hyperkeratosis, parakeratosis and irregular acanthosis without significant spongiosis. There is focal exocytosis of lymphocytes into the epidermis.

There is hyperkeratosis with variable parakeratosis. Moderate to marked acanthosis is present, but spongiosis is usually absent or minimal (Fig. 8-8). The acanthosis is often of a psoriasiform type with elongation and clubbing of rete ridges. Neutrophilic microabscesses generally do not occur,[30] and the perivascular infiltrate in the superficial dermis is predominantly mononuclear. There is focal exocytosis of lymphocytes into the epidermis. A characteristic feature is thickening of collagen fibers in the papillary dermis. These reactive fibers are oriented perpendicular to the skin surface.

Differential Diagnosis of Psoriasiform Dermatitis

While the histologic changes in psoriasis and Reiter's syndrome are indistinguishable, the clinical features usually allow the proper diagnosis to be made. Spotty parakeratosis in the presence of psoriasiform epidermal changes suggests the diagnosis of seborrheic dermatitis or guttate psoriasis. The histologic diagnosis of pityriasis rubra pilaris can be made 40 to 50 percent of the time based predominantly on follicular plugging and spotty parakeratosis at the shoulders of hair follicles. Thickened collagen fibers in the papillary dermis favor the diagnosis of neurodermatitis. Other disorders such as nummular eczema, dyshidrotic eczema, and atopic dermatitis may also produce psoriasiform changes.

Lichenoid Dermatitis

Disorders classified as lichenoid dermatitis have epidermal basal cell damage as a primary event and may be associated with other features of lichen planus such as a bandlike infiltrate of inflammatory cells that interacts with the epidermis.[31,32] Because of damage to basal zone melanocytes, pigmentary incontinence is common.

Lichen Planus

Lichen planus is characterized by pruritic flat-topped papules that may coalesce to form small plaques. The margins of the papules are often angulated, giving them a polygonal shape. The papules of lichen planus are violaceous and often have a surface with a lacy, white pattern known as Wickham's striae.[33] Koebner's phenomenon, the reproduction of the rash by minor trauma such as scratching, occurs in lichen planus as it does in psoriasis. Lichen planus most often involves the volar aspects of the wrists, the trunk, and the mucous membranes of the mouth and genitalia. Approximately two thirds of the patients with clinically typical lichen planus experience spontaneous involution with a duration of approximately 8 to 15 months.[34-36] Atypical forms of lichen planus may be chronic.

A number of variants of lichen planus have been described: (1) annular lichen planus, which appears to be somewhat more common in blacks; (2) hypertrophic lichen planus,[37] which occurs as persistent, lichenified plaques of the pretibial areas; (3) atrophic lichen planus; (4) bullous lichen planus, which is most often seen in individuals with acute eruptive lichen planus; (5) follicular lichen planus (lichen planopilaris), which produces scarring alopecia of the scalp and a spiny follicular eruption of the trunk and extremities due to keratin plugging of hair follicles; (6) mucosal lichen planus,[38] which produces a lacy white pattern or a white speckled pattern on the buccal mucosa with or without painful oral erosions; (7) ulcerative lichen planus,[39] which involves the soles of the feet and may be associated with typical lichen planus elsewhere; and (8) ungual lichen planus, which affects approximately 10 percent of patients and produces longitudinal ridging, pterygium formation, or even complete nail destruction.

The histologic changes of lichen planus are often diagnostic. There is hyperkeratosis; however, parakeratosis is uncommon, occurring in less than 15 percent of cases. When parakeratosis is present, it is usually mild. Hypergranulosis is present, and occasionally the granular layer may be up to one half the thickness of the malpighian layer. The acanthosis is platelike, and the lower margin of the epidermis shows an irregular sawtooth pattern. A key feature, liquefaction degeneration of the basal zone, is present in almost every case.[40] The dermal infiltrate is composed of lymphocytes and histiocytes and has a band-like distribution immediately beneath the basal zone (Fig. 8-9). Plasma cells, neutrophils, and eosinophils are usually absent. Extensive liquefaction degener-

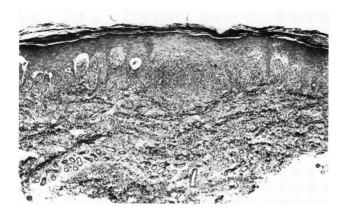

Fig. 8-9. Lichen planus. There is hyperkeratosis, plate-like acanthosis and a band-like infiltrate of mononuclear cells. Liquefaction degeneration of the basal zone has produced small clefts (Max Joseph spaces) at the dermal-epidermal junction.

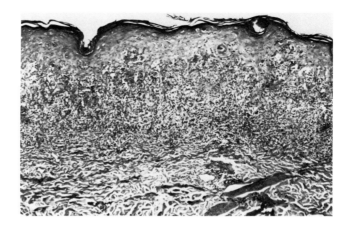

Fig. 8-10. Lichenoid drug eruption (gold). Plate-like acanthosis, liquefaction degeneration of the basal zone, and a band-like infiltrate of chronic inflammatory cells may be indistinguishable from lichen planus. The presence of parakeratosis and eosinophils are helpful distinguishing features.

ation may produce small clefts beneath the basal cell layer known as Max Joseph spaces. Colloid bodies, which measure 5 to 20 μm in diameter, are present in approximately 40 percent of cases of lichen planus as round eosinophilic bodies in the lower epidermis or papillary dermis. Melanin pigment is present within macrophages in the superficial dermis or free in the papillary dermis. Dilated dermal blood vessels, pigmentary incontinence, and the thickened granular layer account for the violaceous color of lichen planus papules. Immunofluorescence studies of skin show globular deposits of immunoglobulin below the dermal epidermal junction in 95 percent of cases of lichen planus.[33]

Lichenoid Drug Eruption

Lichenoid drug eruptions are associated with gold therapy for rheumatoid arthritis.[33,41] Thiazide diuretics, chloroquine, quinidine, streptomycin, and arsenicals may also produce a lichenoid dermatitis. The lichenoid dermatitis caused by drugs produces a widespread violaceous papulosquamous eruption that may closely mimic lichen planus.

There is hyperkeratosis with variable parakeratosis. The parakeratosis is often extensive and is a key feature in distinguishing lichenoid drug eruptions from lichen planus. There may be hypergranulosis; however, in the presence of extensive parakeratosis, the granular layer is usually thinned. Plate-like acanthosis of the epidermis is associated with liquefaction degeneration of the basal zone (Fig. 8-10), melanin pigment incontinence, the presence of colloid bodies, and a bandlike dermal infiltrate. In addition to lymphocytes and histiocytes, the dermal infiltrate in lichenoid drug eruptions may contain a variable

number of eosinophils and occasional plasma cells. The mixture of cell types is helpful in distinguishing lichenoid drug eruptions from lichen planus.

Lupus Erythematosus

Discoid lupus erythematosus is a chronic scarring cutaneous eruption of sun-exposed areas.[42,43] Plaques of discoid lupus erythematosus typically show central hypopigmentation with a peripheral margin of hyperpigmentation. There is erythema, atrophy, telangiectasia, and keratin plugging of hair follicles. Discoid lupus erythematosus often produces scarring alopecia. Most patients with discoid lupus erythematosus do not have evidence of systemic disease, although approximately 10 to 15 percent of patients with systemic lupus erythematosus may have discoid skin lesions. The skin lesions in systemic lupus erythematosus are characterized by erythematous papules and plaques on sun-exposed skin.[44] Scarring is usually not a feature of the cutaneous lesions of systemic lupus erythematosus, which often appear more urticarial.

A typical skin biopsy specimen of discoid lupus erythematosus shows hyperkeratosis with absent or minimal parakeratosis. Keratin plugging is often present within dilated hair follicles, which show atrophy of follicular epithelium (Fig. 8-11). The epidermis is usually atrophic but acanthosis occasionally occurs. There is prominent liquefaction degeneration of the basal zone with melanin pigment incontinence.[45] Colloid bodies are usually present within the epidermis or the papillary dermis. A dermal infiltrate of lymphocytes and histiocytes interacts with the basement membrane zone of the epidermis. The

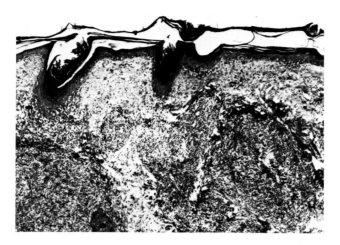

Fig. 8-11. Lupus erythematosus. There is hyperkeratosis with keratin plugging of hair follicles. Liquefaction degeneration is present at the basement membrane zone.

dermal infiltrate shows a patchy perivascular pattern in the superficial dermis and surrounds hair follicles in the deep and superficial dermis (Fig. 8-12). The basement membrane zone often appears pink and thickened, a feature that is demonstrated even better with PAS stain. The cutaneous lesions of systemic lupus erythematosus may show little or no hyperkeratosis and follicular plugging, but epidermal atrophy is typically present. There is liquefaction degeneration of the basal zone associated with pigmentary incontinence and colloid body formation; however, the perivascular and perifollicular dermal infiltrate is usually less marked than in discoid lupus erythematosus. Prominent vascular dilation and edema of the papillary dermis are often features of systemic lupus erythematosus.

Lichen Nitidus

Lichen nitidus is an uncommon cutaneous disorder that affects children and young adults.[46] It is characterized by pinhead-sized, white, shiny papules that tend to be grouped on the extremities, genitals, abdomen, and breasts. Oral lesions do not occur.

Individual papules of lichen nitidus are often slightly elevated and show hyperkeratosis and parakeratosis. The epidermis over the center of the papule is atrophic and shows liquefaction degeneration of the basal zone (Fig. 8-13). At the margins of the papules, elongated rete ridges extend downward around the dermal infiltrate, producing a claw-like pattern. The dermal infiltrate is composed predominantly of lymphocytes and histiocytes with occasional multinucleate giant cells and epithelioid cells. The papules are usually small, occupying a space approximately the size of two to four contiguous dermal papillae. Dermal-epidermal separation over the center of the papule may occur. Immunofluorescence microscopy of skin lesions reveals deposits of subepidermal immunoglobulins similar to those of lichen planus in 80 percent of cases of lichen nitidus.[33]

Secondary Syphilis

Although secondary syphilis may mimic a great number of cutaneous disorders, it is most often papulosquamous in character with a predilection for the palms and soles. Widespread cutaneous lesions of secondary syphilis resemble pityriasis rosea, although pruritus is usually minimal or absent. Mucous membrane lesions are common. The primary chancre is still present in approximately one third of persons at the time the cutaneous rash occurs.

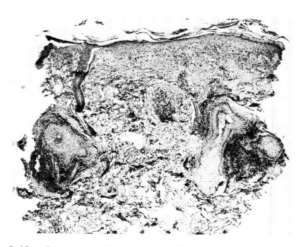

Fig. 8-12. Lupus erythematosus. The distribution of the dermal infiltrate is perivascular and periadnexal.

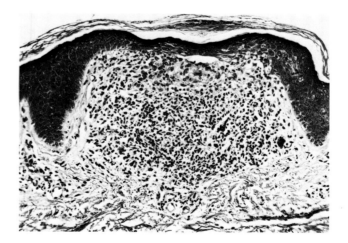

Fig. 8-13. Lichen nitidus. A focal collection of lymphocytes, histiocytes and multinucleate cells is present between elongated rete ridges. The epidermis shows hyperkeratosis, parakeratosis, atrophy and liquefaction degeneration.

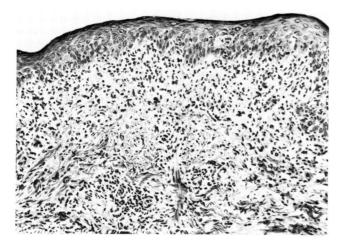

Fig. 8-14. Secondary syphilis. Mild acanthosis and a band-like infiltrate of mononuclear cells interact with the epidermis. A variable number of plasma cells are present.

There is variable hyperkeratosis with parakeratosis and irregular acanthosis of the epidermis. An infiltrate of inflammatory cells often obscures the dermoepidermal junction[47] (Fig. 8-14). Liquefaction degeneration of the basal zone is common. Deep to the band-like infiltrate, the inflammatory cells surround blood vessels that show swollen endothelial cells. Plasma cells are usually present, but in early cases of secondary syphilis they may be absent. The Warthin-Starry stain may demonstrate *Treponema pallidum* within the epidermis or in perivascular areas of the dermis. Although other patterns of inflammation occur with secondary syphilis,[47] the lichenoid pattern is most common.

Lichenoid Keratosis

Clinically, a lichenoid keratosis (lichenoid actinic keratosis, solitary lichen planuslike keratosis) may resemble an actinic keratosis or seborrheic keratosis.[48] The characteristic lesion is a flat topped, slightly scaly, tan to pink keratosis, which can often be clinically distinguished from other types of keratoses. The clinical history of a solitary keratotic lesion is very helpful in distinguishing a lichenoid keratosis from true lichen planus. Lichenoid keratoses appear to be caused by inflammation of pre-existing actinic keratoses or other forms of keratoses.

Originally described as solitary lichen planus,[49] lichenoid keratoses may exactly mimic the changes in lichen planus. In many cases, however, there is focal parakeratosis and proliferation of rete ridges with atypical keratinocytes. The atypical keratinocytes involve predominantly the deeper layers of the epidermis and are associated with loss of normal polarity of epidermal cells and individual cell dyskeratosis. Solar elastosis of dermal

connective tissue is present in 70 percent of cases.[48] The liquefaction degeneration of the basal zone and the band-like infiltrate of chronic inflammatory cells closely resemble lichen planus; however, eosinophils or plasma cells are more likely to be present in a lichenoid keratosis.

Differential Diagnosis of Lichenoid Dermatitis

The pigmented purpuric dermatoses (*progressive pigmentary purpura, Schamberg's disease, lichen aureus*) may have a prominent lichenoid inflammatory infiltrate associated with extravasation of RBC.[50] Cases of *graft versus host disease* often show epidermal atrophy with liquefaction degeneration, colloid bodies, and a lichenoid inflammatory infiltrate.[51] The helpful differential feature is the sparse nature of the infiltrate in graft vs. host disease due to severe immunosuppression. *Poikiloderma atrophicans vasculare*[52] and *dermatomyositis*[53] (Fig. 8-15) may cause diagnostic confusion with systemic lupus erythematosus. They generally show a sparse lichenoid infiltrate with prominent liquefaction degeneration, pigment incontinence, and vascular dilatation. In cases of poikiloderma that are precursors of myocosis fungoides, atypical mononuclear cells may be present. *Halo nevus*[54] should be included in the differential diagnosis of lichenoid dermatitis since the dense bandlike infiltrate may destroy and obscure the nevus cells.

The differential diagnosis of lupus erythematosus includes *lichen sclerosis et atrophicus* (LS and A).[55] More than 80 percent of cases of LS and A occur in women. The disorder is characterized by pruritic, white atrophic papules that coalesce into plaques. Individual papules are polygonal and flat topped and may show keratin plugging of hair follicles. The genitalia, neck, and trunk are sites of

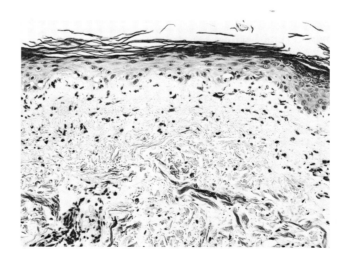

Fig. 8-15. Dermatomyositis. There is liquefaction degeneration of the basal zone associated with melanin pigment incontinence and moderate edema of the papillary dermis.

156

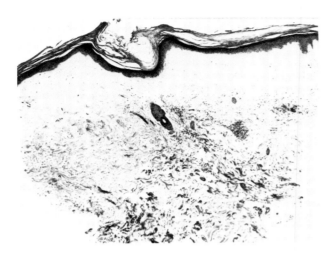

Fig. 8-16. Lichen sclerosis et atrophicus. There is hyperkeratosis, follicular plugging, and epidermal atrophy. A band of pale-staining edematous connective tissue is present within the superficial dermis.

predilection. When LS and A involves the female genitalia, it is called *kraurosis vulvae*. Involvement of the glans penis is known as *balanitis xerotica obliterans*. Histologically, LS and A shows prominent hyperkeratosis, resulting in a stratum corneum that may be thicker than the atrophic malpighian layer (Fig. 8-16). Follicular plugging is a common finding. Liquefaction degeneration of the basal zone is associated with incontinence of melanin pigment and in some cases with subepidermal bulla formation. There is pronounced edema of the superficial third of the dermis, producing a pale pink amorphous zone. Dilated blood vessels and a few inflammatory cells may be present in the edematous area. Deep to the area of edema is a bandlike infiltrate of mononuclear cells.

Intraepidermal Bullous Dermatoses

Intraepidermal blisters may be produced by a variety of mechanisms: (1) epidermal necrolysis in the staphylococcal scalded skin syndrome; (2) acantholysis in pemphigus, benign chronic familial pemphigus, keratosis follicularis, and transient acantholytic dermatosis; and (3) spongiosis in allergic contact dermatitis, discussed earlier. Viral blisters may show necrolysis, acantholysis and spongiosis. When biopsying a bullous disease, a newly formed blister should always be selected.

Impetigo

While most cases of impetigo were previously produced by β-hemolytic streptococci,[56] *Staphylococcus aureus* has now become the most common causative agent. The superficial pustules (which occur most often on the

face and hands) rapidly break, leaving erosions with honey-colored crusts. The disorder affects predominantly children and young adults. Streptococcal impetigo may be associated with glomerulonephritis if caused by a group A streptococcus with an M antigen.[57] Staphylococcal impetigo is more likely to cause frank bullae.

The roof of the blister is formed by delicate stratum corneum. The bulla contains numerous neutrophils and within the first few hours after onset is more properly termed a pustule (Fig. 8-17). A few acantholytic epidermal cells may be seen in the blister cavity. The malpighian layer shows moderate spongiosis and exocytosis of lymphocytes and neutrophils. A patchy perivascular infiltrate of lymphocytes, histiocytes, and neutrophils is present in the superficial dermis. Older lesions may show only erosions covered by crust and cellular debris.

Staphylococcal Scalded Skin Syndrome

This acute febrile disease is seen predominantly in infants and children.[58] It is produced by coagulase-positive staphylococci, which are often of phage group 2, type 71. The organisms are present in the nasopharynx or throat and produce a toxin that produces painful erythema, followed by desquamation of large sheets of epidermis.[59] When treated with appropriate antibiotics, the prognosis in infants and children is good. Staphylococcal scalded skin syndrome occurs rarely in adults[60,61] in which case the prognosis for survival is guarded since the patients may be immunosuppressed or have a serious underlying disease.

The stratum corneum, stratum granulosum, and superficial portion of the malpighian layer show extensive necrosis and are often separated from the remainder of the

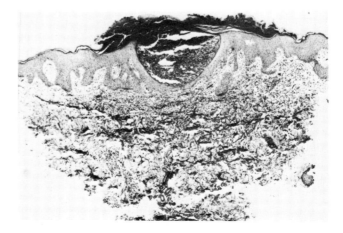

Fig. 8-17. Impetigo. A subcorneal pustule contains numerous neutrophils. The epidermis is covered by a layer of crust.

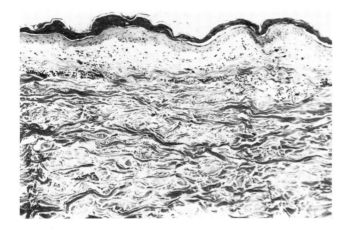

Fig. 8-18. Staphylococcal scalded skin syndrome. The superficial portion of the epidermis is necrotic and amorphous. A sparse perivascular infiltrate of lymphocytes is present in the superficial dermis.

epidermis (Fig. 8-18). The roof of the blister appears eosinophilic and necrotic. In areas in which necrosis is less severe, there may be necrosis of individual keratinocytes. The malpighian layer at the floor of the blister is relatively uninvolved, and the dermis shows only a scant inflammatory infiltrate. The use of exfoliative cytology or frozen sections makes possible rapid distinction from Stevens-Johnson syndrome, which shows full-thickness epidermal necrosis.[62]

Pemphigus Erythematosus and Pemphigus Foliaceus

Pemphigus erythematosus produces a crusted erythematous rash predominantly on the face and scalp.[63] The eruption is often confused clinically with seborrheic dermatitis or lupus erythematosus. In pemphigus foliaceus, the individual lesions are similar[64]; however, more extensive areas of the scalp, face, and trunk may be involved, at times producing a resemblance to exfoliative dermatitis. It is likely that pemphigus erythematosus represents a limited form or initial stage of pemphigus foliaceus. Oral lesions are uncommon in both pemphigus erythematosus and pemphigus foliaceus, and the prognosis is much better than in pemphigus vulgaris.

The histologic changes in pemphigus erythematosus and pemphigus foliaceus are identical. Acantholysis of epidermal cells produces a superficial blister, which usually occurs just beneath the granular cell layer.[65] The roof of the blister may be lost in processing. Acantholytic cells are few in number. Often, small collections of pyknotic, dyskeratotic cells are seen in the granular layer, particularly at the openings of hair follicles or sweat ducts. The small vessels of the superficial dermal plexus are surrounded by variable numbers of lymphocytes, histiocytes, and eosinophils. The pattern seen on immunofluorescence microscopy is similar to that seen in pemphigus vulgaris. The intercellular fluorescence in pemphigus erythematosus and foliaceus, however, may be limited to the superficial portion of the epidermis. Some cases of pemphigus erythematosus also have shown a granular pattern of immunofluorescence at the basement membrane zone, suggesting a relationship between this disorder and lupus erythematosus.[66]

Pemphigus Vulgaris

In approximately one third of cases, pemphigus vulgaris begins as painful oral blisters that rapidly ulcerate. The oral lesions show little tendency to heal and are associated with difficulty eating and drinking, resulting in weight loss and dehydration. The cutaneous rash may be limited to a few lesions or may involve large areas of skin. Since the blister roofs are thin, the blisters appear flaccid and break easily leaving areas of erosions and crusts. Rubbing the skin gently at the margin of a blister often causes it to extend (Nikolsky sign). Before the advent of systemic corticosteroids and other immunosuppressive agents, pemphigus vulgaris was considered to be uniformly fatal. Patients with pemphigus have an increased incidence of thymoma and myasthenia gravis.[67]

Early changes in a nonbullous area may show spongiosis and exocytosis of eosinophils[11] known as eosinophilic spongiosis (Fig. 8-19). Intact blisters demonstrate, acantholysis of epidermal cells producing a blister cavity that forms immediately above the basal cell layer.[68] The roof of the blister usually appears viable; however, older lesions may show necrosis and crusting. The blister cav-

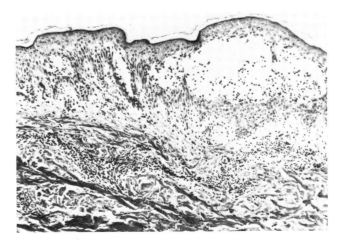

Fig. 8-19. Pemphigus vulgaris with eosinophilic spongiosis. An intraepidermal blister containing numerous eosinophils shows both spongiosis and acantholysis. The adjacent epidermis shows prominent spongiosis and exocytosis of eosinophils.

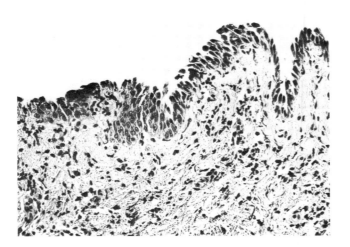

Fig. 8-20. Pemphigus vulgaris. The floor of an intraepidermal blister shows villi lined by one or two layers of epithelial cells.

ity contains individual acantholytic cells and clumps of acantholytic cells. Inflammatory cells within the blister cavity include lymphocytes and a variable number of eosinophils and neutrophils. Dermal papillae lined by a single row of basal cells, known as villi, project into the base of the blister cavity (Fig. 8-20). The single row of basal cells often becomes separated from each other laterally producing the appearance of a "row of tombstones." The dermal inflammatory infiltrate is usually mild and consists of lymphocytes, histiocytes, and a few eosinophils. Direct immunofluorescence microscopy shows an intercellular immunofluorescence pattern.[69] The autoantibodies are usually of the IgG class and complement is often present. Circulating autoantibodies can also be identified by the indirect immunofluorescence technique; however, their serum levels do not necessarily parallel the course of the disease.[69]

Benign Familial Chronic Pemphigus

Benign familial chronic pemphigus or *Hailey-Hailey disease* is a chronic bullous eruption that involves predominantly flexural areas such as the neck, axillae, and groin.[70] The disorder is inherited as an autosomal dominant trait and usually begins during the second decade of life. The blisters rapidly break, forming superficial crusted erosions, which become secondarily infected. The disease, which is chronic and recurrent, is aggravated by friction from tight clothing and is often worse in the summer due to heat and maceration.

The acantholysis in Hailey-Hailey disease is marked and may involve almost the entire thickness of the epidermis. The acantholysis of large sheets of epidermal cells often produces a "dilapidated brick wall" appearance. The acantholysis typically occurs above the basal cell layer, and, as in pemphigus vulgaris, there may be

dermal papillae lined by a single layer of basal cells (villi), which extend into the base of the blister cavity. The outer root sheath of hair follicles may be involved with the acantholytic process (Fig. 8-21). Dyskeratosis of individual keratinocytes similar to that seen in Darier's disease may be present but is usually mild. The roof of the blister is viable, and few inflammatory cells are present in the blister cavity unless secondary infection is present. A mild perivascular infiltrate of lymphocytes and histiocytes is present in the superficial dermis. The results of immunofluorescence microscopy in benign familial chronic pemphigus are negative.

Keratosis Follicularis

Keratosis follicularis or *Darier's disease* is an autosomal dominant disorder that usually has its onset about the time of puberty. It is characterized by keratotic greasy papules and papulovesicles of the face, neck, chest, upper back, axillae, and inguinal areas.[71] In severe cases, the entire body surface may be affected. Involvement of the oral mucosa[72] and nails also occurs. The disease is chronic and progressive.

There is hyperkeratosis associated with parakeratosis and variable acanthosis of the epidermis. Small clefts containing acantholytic cells occur above the basal cell layer (Fig. 8-22). Two types of dyskeratotic cells are characteristic of Darier's disease. Corps ronds are large dyskeratotic cells with a central basophilic nucleus surrounded by a clear halo, and a cytoplasm that appears densely pink and homogeneous. Grains are densely basophilic with an elongated rectangular or fusiform shape, and resemble a parakeratotic cell of the stratum cor-

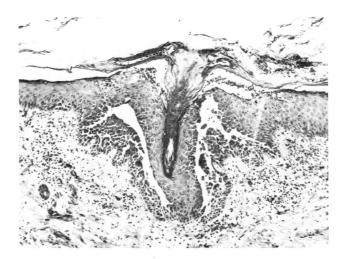

Fig. 8-21. Benign familial chronic pemphigus. Prominent acantholysis extends along the outer root sheath of a hair follicle.

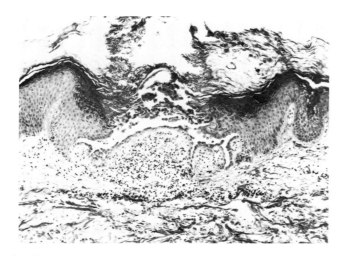

Fig. 8-22. Keratosis follicularis. A suprabasal acantholytic cleft is associated with hyperkeratosis, parakeratosis and dyskeratotic cells.

neum. Upward projections of dermal papillae lined by a single layer of basaloid cells are prominent in keratosis follicularis. In hypertrophic areas of Darier's disease, the epidermis may proliferate producing pseudoepitheliomatous hyperplasia. The vesicles in Darier's disease usually remain small. Histologic changes essentially identical to Darier's disease may occur in a solitary lesion known as a *warty dyskeratoma*.[73] A warty dyskeratoma resembles an enlarged hair follicle with acanthotic epithelium in which acantholytic and dyskeratotic changes of keratosis follicularis occur[74] (Fig. 8-23). The results of immunofluorescence microscopy are negative in Darier's disease and warty dyskeratoma.

Transient Acantholytic Dermatosis

Transient acantholytic dermatosis or *Grover's disease* typically occurs on the trunk of middle-aged or elderly men as discrete papulovesicular lesions that may itch intensely.[75,76] The patient's general health is good, and no evidence of pemphigus, Hailey-Hailey disease, or Darier's disease is present. While original reports suggested that all cases resolved within weeks to months, it is now apparent that some cases may persist for several years.[77]

The characteristic change in transient acantholytic dermatosis is a tiny suprabasal cleft containing acantholytic cells and occasionally dyskeratotic cells (Fig. 8-24). Three histologic patterns have been described, with the histologic changes resembling either pemphigus vulgaris, benign familial chronic pemphigus, or keratosis follicularis.[77] The changes in Grover's disease differ from these three disorders by showing multiple tiny discrete foci of epidermal involvement. More than one pattern may be present in an individual patient, and focal areas of spongiosis are occasionally noted. The results of immunofluorescence microscopy are generally negative.

Varicella, Herpes Zoster, and Herpes Simplex

Varicella or chickenpox is characterized by a widespread vesicular eruption that usually occurs in children or young adults. The vesicles and bullae are located predominantly on the trunk and face, although there may be spread to the extremities. Lesions are in all stages of development and resolution. Re-exposure to the varicella virus or reactivation of latent varicella virus in individuals previously infected results in herpes zoster. In most

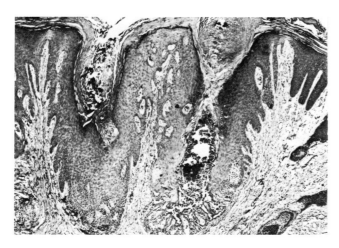

Fig. 8-23. Warty dyskeratoma. Suprabasalar acantholysis and dyskeratotic cells are present within the epithelium of a hair follicle.

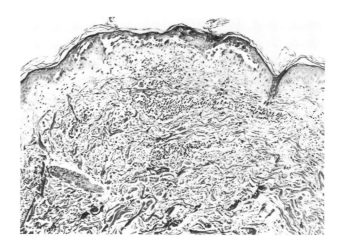

Fig. 8-24. Transient acantholytic dermatosis. Tiny suprabasalar acantholytic clefts occur in an interrupted pattern within the epidermis.

cases, the virus appears to extend from cranial nerve ganglia or spinal nerve ganglia to the peripheral nerves of the skin. Usually, only one or two peripheral nerves are involved, producing a linear rash extending from the spinal cord in a dermatome distribution or involving one or more of the three branches of the trigeminal nerve. The characteristic lesions are grouped vesicles on an erythematous base, which rapidly become pustular. The pustules heal over a 1 to 2 week period, often leaving varioliform scars. Recurrent herpes simplex infection most often involves the lips or genitalia. After the initial infection, which may be extensive or completely asymptomatic, recurrent lesions are typically localized to small groups of vesicles and pustules on an edematous swollen base. Periodic recurrence of the lesions often is associated with fatigue, sunburn, windburn, or upper respiratory infection. Sexual contact may stimulate recurrence of genital lesions. Like herpes zoster, the virus is believed to reside in cranial nerve ganglia or dorsal root ganglia of the spinal cord with subsequent extension to the cutaneous nerves and skin.

The histologic changes in varicella, herpes zoster, and herpes simplex are essentially identical with the exception that the associated dermal inflammatory infiltrate tends to be less marked in varicella and most severe in recurrent herpes simplex.[78] An intraepidermal blister shows severe necrosis of epidermal cells with areas of spongiosis and acantholysis (Fig. 8-25). The necrosis of epidermal cells may be secondary to ballooning degeneration, which produces a marked increase in homogeneous eosinophilic cytoplasm. The ballooned epidermal cells lose their intercellular bridges and become acantholytic. Reticular degeneration results from marked intracellular edema with rupture of cell walls producing a reticulated multilocular blister. Large multinucleate viral giant cells are common in all three disorders. Eosinophilic intranuclear viral inclusions are often seen in the ballooned cells and in the multinucleate cells. The inclu-

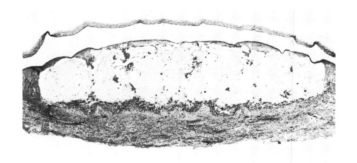

Fig. 8-25. Herpes zoster. An intraepidermal blister shows severe necrosis of epidermal cells associated with acantholysis. Multinucleate viral giant cells are often present within the vesicle.

sions are approximately 5 μm in diameter. An intense infiltrate of lymphocytes, histiocytes, and neutrophils associated with prominent vascular dilation is most marked in herpes simplex but is also seen in herpes zoster and varicella. The intense infiltrate at the base of the blister may resemble vasculitis.

Differential Diagnosis of Intraepidermal Bullous Dermatoses

Suprabasilar acantholysis often occurs in actinic keratoses and should not be confused with acantholytic diseases such as pemphigus or Darier's disease.[79] An important distinguishing feature is the presence of atypia of the cells of the deeper epidermis in actinic keratosis and the presence of associated actinic changes in the underlying connective tissue. It should be kept in mind that any cutaneous eruption with numerous neutrophils can produce acantholysis possibly due to the effects of lysosomal enzymes on the cohesion of epidermal cells. Pemphigus vulgaris, benign familial chronic pemphigus, and keratosis follicularis may be difficult to distinguish histologically. Of the three disorders, benign familial chronic pemphigus shows the most striking acantholysis with involvement of the full thickness of epithelium, whereas keratosis follicularis shows the most prominent dyskeratosis. In addition, keratosis follicularis shows hyperkeratosis, parakeratosis, and papillomatosis, which are often lacking in the other two disorders. In pemphigus vulgaris, the acantholysis is often limited to the suprabasal layer and areas of eosinophilic spongiosis may be seen. Spongiotic bullae, discussed earlier in this chapter (see Fig. 8-1), are among the most common causes of intraepidermal blisters.

Subepidermal Bullous Dermatoses

When selecting a biopsy site in a patient with a bullous disease, a small relatively new lesion should be selected, and skin adjacent to the blister should be included in the biopsy specimen. Older lesions that have become necrotic, pustular, and crusted tend to show less characteristic changes. A biopsy for immunofluorescence microscopy should be from perilesional skin and should not include the blister.

Bullous Pemphigoid

Bullous pemphigoid has also been referred to as bullous disease of the aged because of its propensity to affect older individuals. Pemphigoid is a chronic, relatively benign disease that produces large tense blisters on normal-appearing or erythematous skin.[68] Large urticarial plaques are common. A clinical variant of pemphigoid has small grouped vesicles resembling dermatitis herpetiformis.[80] The blisters tend to involve the axillae and groin and may become quite large. Blister fluid may be clear or hemorrhagic and, unlike pemphigus vulgaris, ruptured blisters show a tendency to heal. Oral lesions are present in one third of cases,[69] but the mouth is rarely the initial site of involvement. The duration of bullous pemphigoid is from a few months to several years, and it is uncommon for patients to die of the disease unless it is extensive. Patients with pemphigoid appear to have a higher incidence of rheumatoid arthritis; however, the previously reported association with internal malignancy was apparently related to the elderly population affected by pemphigoid and cancer.[67]

A subepidermal blister shows a roof that is formed by the entire epidermis. Unlike erythema multiforme, the roof of the blister in bullous pemphigoid remains viable with minimal necrosis of epidermal cells. (Fig. 8-26). The blister cavity contains serum and a variable number of inflammatory cells, which characteristically include a large percentage of eosinophils. The extent of dermal inflammation depends on whether the blister occurred clinically on erythematous or normal-appearing skin.[81] A marked infiltrate of lymphocytes, eosinophils, and neutrophils is often present in blisters that occur in erythematous skin. Eosinophilic spongiosis is a common finding in perilesional skin, particularly if an urticarial plaque is biopsied. Blisters located on normal-appearing skin typically show a sparse perivascular infiltrate of lymphocytes and eosinophils. Immunofluorescence microscopy of skin from patients with bullous pemphigoid shows deposition of predominantly IgG, IgM, and complement in a linear pattern at the basement membrane zone.[69] Autoantibodies can also be demonstrated in the patients' serum by indirect immunofluorescence techniques.

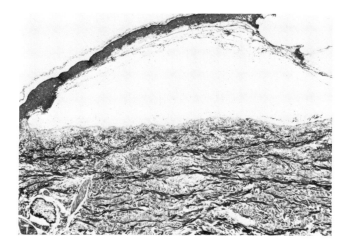

Fig. 8-26. Bullous pemphigoid. A subepidermal bulla has a roof of viable epidermis. A variable number of eosinophils are present within the blister cavity.

Erythema Multiforme

As the name implies, erythema multiforme may show a variety of clinical lesions, including persistent erythematous plaques, migratory erythemas, polycyclic lesions, vesicles and bullae, target lesions, and extensive mucous membrane involvement. Erythema multiforme is most common between 10 and 30 years of age and frequently follows prodromal symptoms of an upper respiratory infection. The classic cutaneous lesion of erythema multiforme is the target lesion, which has a dusky bluish center and an erythematous margin. The hands and feet are sites of predilection. Severe erythema multiforme with mucous membrane involvement has been called *Stevens-Johnson syndrome*. Occasionally, severe Stevens-Johnson syndrome may show sloughing of large areas of the skin resembling staphylococcal scalded skin syndrome. Erythema multiforme has multiple causes including infections with mycoplasma,[82] *Histoplasma capsulatum*, and herpes simplex or reactions to drugs such as penicillin and sulfonamides. The most common cause of erythema multiforme is recurrent herpes simplex, which usually precedes the erythema multiforme by 1 to 4 days. The erythema multiforme may recur with each episode of herpes simplex.[83]

So-called epidermal and dermal types of erythema multiforme[84] probably do not occur but represent different stages in the development of lesions. Target lesions may show different zones of involvement with predominantly epidermal or dermal changes.[85] Early or nonbullous lesions may show a relatively normal-appearing epidermis; however, dyskeratotic epidermal cells are usually present. Spongiosis with exocytosis of lymphocytes and liquefaction degeneration of the basal zone are often early changes. The spongiosis may cause epidermal cells to appear stretched perpendicular to the skin surface.[86] In early lesions or in the erythematous margin of a target lesion, there is prominent edema of the papillary dermis (Fig. 8-27). A perivascular infiltrate of lymphocytes and histiocytes is present in the upper dermis. Bullous lesions or the dusky centers of target lesions show subepidermal bullae with prominent necrosis of the blister roof (Fig. 8-28). Individual dyskeratotic cells may be seen in the blister roof. The blister cavity contains predominantly lymphocytes, although a mixture of inflammatory cells may be present. While extravasation of RBC is common, true vasculitis is not seen. A variable infiltrate of lymphocytes and histiocytes surrounds small vessels in the upper dermis. Lateral to the blister cavity, the changes may resemble those described for early or nonbullous lesions. Immunofluorescence microscopy of skin biopsy specimens shows granular deposits of immunoglobulins and complement within small vessels of the papillary dermis.[87]

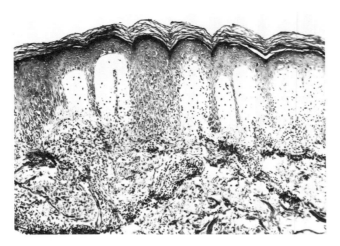

Fig. 8-27. Erythema multiforme. Biopsy of a nonbullous lesion shows marked edema of the papillary dermis associated with exocytosis of lymphocytes and individual dyskeratotic epidermal cells.

Dermatitis Herpetiformis

Dermatitis herpetiformis is characterized clinically by grouped papulovesicles that are extremely pruritic.[88] Vesicles are located symmetrically on the elbows, buttocks, and interscapular areas. Excoriations are common, and intact vesicles may be difficult to find. The eruption clinically resembles scabies. Dermatitis herpetiformis has a chronic course with exacerbations and remissions. Men are affected twice as often as women. Although the oral mucosa is not involved, over half the patients have a syndrome characterized by gluten sensi-

tivity, malabsorption, and villous atrophy of the jejunal mucosa. The villous atrophy and steatorrhea are corrected by a gluten-free diet, and if the diet can be maintained for a prolonged period of time, the cutaneous rash may also improve.[89] Sulfapyridine or sulfone drugs are effective in controlling the rash of dermatitis herpetiformis. Improvement is so dramatic that treatment with these drugs has been used as a diagnostic test. The drugs have no effect on the small bowel symptoms.

The subepidermal blisters of older lesions may be difficult to distinguish from bullous pemphigoid. Characteristic changes, however, are seen in new lesions. A subepidermal vesicle shows a viable roof of epidermis. Early vesicles may appear multilocular. The diagnostic changes occur just lateral to the blister where there are accumulations of neutrophils within dermal papillae (Fig. 8-29). The connective tissue of the dermal papillae may show basophilic necrosis and early separation of the epidermis and dermis producing a crescent-moon-shaped space. Fragmented nuclei are often seen in the dermal papillae. While eosinophils may be present, it is the neutrophil that is the most characteristic cell in the dermal papillae and the blister cavity. Within the superficial dermis, a patchy infiltrate of neutrophils, lymphocytes, and eosinophils is often noted. Immunofluorescence microscopy of a skin specimen shows deposition of IgA in a granular pattern at the basement membrane zone and/or in the papillary dermis.[90] Circulating IgA autoantibodies have recently been demonstrated.[91] It has been suggested that the autoantibodies in dermatitis herpetiformis are antigluten antibodies, which may precipitate in the skin as immune complexes.[90]

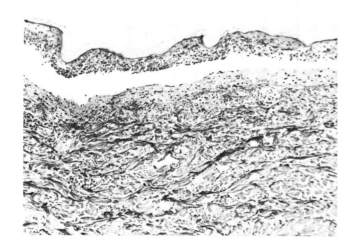

Fig. 8-28. Erythema multiforme. Biopsy of a target lesion from a patient with drug-induced Stevens-Johnson syndrome shows a subepidermal bulla with marked necrosis of the roof. Individual dyskeratotic keratinocytes can be seen in the bulla roof.

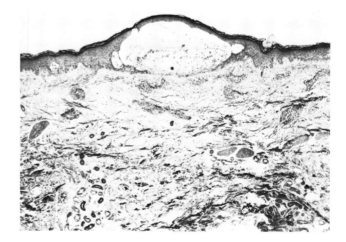

Fig. 8-29. Dermatitis herpetiformis. Adjacent to a subepidermal blister, small collections of neutrophils are present within an edematous dermal papilla. Necrosis of the connective tissue of the dermal papilla has resulted in separation from the epidermis.

Linear IgA Dermatosis

Many cases of the disorder were earlier called chronic bullous disease of childhood.[92] Linear IgA dermatosis occurs mainly in preschool children but may also affect adults. It clinically resembles dermatitis herpetiformis but more often has annular erythematous patches and grouped bullae which may be sausage-shaped. Gluten sensitivity is absent and the therapeutic response to sulfones is not as good as in dermatitis herpetiformis.

Neutrophils are present along the dermal-epidermal junction, with the formation of microabscesses at the tips of dermal papillae. The resulting blisters are subepidermal and contain neutrophils. The changes may be indistinguishable from those of dermatitis herpetiformis. However, immunofluorescence microscopy shows a linear pattern of IgA along the basement membrane zone in contrast to the granular IgA pattern seen with dermatitis herpetiformis.

Porphyria Cutanea Tarda

Porphyria cutanea tarda is characterized by blisters and erosions of sun-exposed skin with secondary scarring, hyperpigmentation, and the formation of milia.[93] Facial hypertrichosis is common. The skin of the chest may develop a sclerotic appearance resembling scleroderma. The photosensitivity appears to be secondary to activation of porphyrin compounds by 4,000 Å ultraviolet light (Soret band). Patients with porphyria cutanea tarda have decreased activity of hepatic uroporphyrinogen decarboxylase.[94]

Since the eruption is common on the dorsa of the hands, the stratum corneum is often thickened in a manner characteristic of acral skin. The subepidermal blister shows a viable epidermal roof and a blister cavity that is often devoid of inflammatory cells.[95] Inflammation is also sparse or absent in the superficial dermis. Dermal papillae protrude into the base of the blister cavity producing fingerlike projections (Fig. 8-30). This finding, called "festooning," may also be seen in bullous pemphigoid, cicatricial pemphigoid, and epidermolysis bullosa. A characteristic finding in porphyria cutanea tarda is the presence of pink, hyalinized material around the small vessels of the dermal papillae. The material is PAS-positive and diastase-resistant and is formed by reduplications of the basement membrane of small vessels and the periodic extravasation of immunoglobulins, complement, fibrin and other serum proteins. Immunofluorescence microscopy shows immunoglobulins and complement surrounding the small vessels of the papillary dermis[93]; however, these changes appear to be secondary to vessel wall damage.

Epidermolysis Bullosa Dystrophica

Epidermolysis bullosa represents a group of genetically determined diseases that have been referred to as the mechanobullous diseases because of the production of cutaneous blisters and erosions by minor mechanical trauma.[95] The two severe dystrophic forms of the disease are inherited as either autosomal-dominant or autosomal-recessive traits. The onset of both diseases is shortly after birth, with erosions occurring on the hands, feet, knees, and diaper area after minor trauma. Similar blisters occur in the mouth and pharnyx, and many infants die within the first year of life of secondary infection or inability to sustain nutrition. In individuals who survive, there may be severe scarring with fusion of fingers producing club-like hands. Scarring of the esophagus may produce esophageal stenosis.[96] Growth retardation, iron deficiency anemia, and recurrent infections are common. Squamous cell carcinomas may develop in cutaneous scars.[97]

The light microscopic changes in the dominant and recessive forms of epidermolysis bullosa dystrophica are essentially identical. The subepidermal blister shows a roof of intact and viable epidermis. There is minimal inflammation, either in the blister cavity or in the underlying dermis. Festooning may be prominent with elongated rete ridges projecting into the base of the blister cavity. Electron microscopy of the recessive form of epidermolysis bullosa shows the separation to occur just beneath the basal lamina associated with an absence of anchoring fibrils.[98] Another form of the disease, *epidermolysis bullosa letalis,* which occurs at birth and has identical light microscopic changes, shows separation between the plasma membrane of the basal cells and the basal lamina

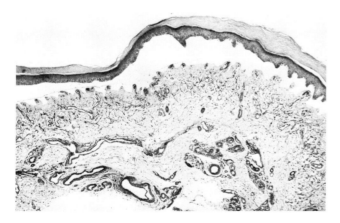

Fig. 8-30. Porphyria cutanea tarda. A biopsy of acral skin shows a subepidermal blister with festooning of dermal papillae into the floor of the blister. This PAS stain demonstrates a hyaline material around the small vessels of the dermal papillae.

by electron microscopy. The results of immunofluorescence microscopy are negative in all forms of the disease.

Epidermolysis Bullosa Simplex

This form of epidermolysis bullosa is inherited as an autosomal dominant trait and often does not appear until early childhood. However, blisters may be present at birth. The mechanically induced blistering is milder than with the dystrophic forms and is typically limited to the feet and hands. The blisters heal without scarring. Biopsies of fresh lesions or of experimentally induced lesions shows cytolysis and vacuolization of the basal cells with the subsequent bulla located above the basement membrane.[99]

Differential Diagnosis of Subepidermal Bullous Dermatoses

Cicatricial pemphigoid or benign mucous membrane pemphigoid may represent a variant of bullous pemphigoid with predominant involvement of the mucous membranes and secondary scarring.[100] The histologic changes are essentially identical to bullous pemphigoid, although dermal fibrosis may be more prominent. Herpes gestationis, a bullous eruption that occurs most often during the last trimester of pregnancy, produces a subepidermal blister that is usually indistinguishable from bullous pemphigoid. Immunofluorescence microscopy of skin biopsies in herpes gestationis shows deposition of the third component of complement and, less often, IgG at the dermoepidermal junction.[101] The important distinguishing features of the bullous diseases are the prominence of eosinophils in the blister cavity in bullous pemphigoid, the necrosis of the blister roof with individual dyskeratotic cells in erythema multiforme, the presence of neutrophils in necrotic dermal papillae in dermatitis herpetiformis, and the presence of PAS-positive diastase-resistant material around small vessels in the papillary dermis in porphyria cutanea tarda. In addition, the characteristic immunofluorescence microscopy changes are of great value in distinguishing the various subepidermal bullous diseases.

Dermal Reaction Patterns

Perivascular Dermatitis

Perivascular dermatitis is differentiated from spongiotic, psoriasiform, and lichenoid dermatitis by a relative absence of epidermal changes. The histologic patterns are often referred to as superficial perivascular dermatitis or superficial and deep perivascular dermatitis.[102] Clinically, they are often manifested as red annular lesions or red plaques, which have been referred to in general terms as reactive erythemas or gyrate erythemas.

Most of these disorders appear to have an allergic basis but clinically and histologically have many overlapping features.

Urticaria is characterized by annular to polycyclic erythematous lesions that typically come and go over periods of hours.[103] Arthropod bite reactions are often referred to as papular urticaria since they show a papular area of erythema and edema with a central puncta at the site of the bite. Drug eruptions and viral exanthems typically produce widespread erythematous macular eruptions that may have an annular configuration.

When gyrate erythemas appear to be rather fixed and change slowly over days to weeks, they have been referred to as erythema annulare centrifugum[104] or erythema perstans. These disorders have a distinct annular erythematous border, which may be palpable. Erythema chronicum migrans is a specific form of reactive erythema that is usually solitary and spreads centrifugally from a central tick bite.[105] The lesions of erythema chronicum migrans, which enlarge up to 30 cm in diameter, are more common in Europe but do occur in the United States.[106] Cases in the United States are usually associated with Lyme disease (described in Lyme, Connecticut), which includes arthritic, neurologic, and cardiac manifestations. The tick Ixodes dammini has been shown to transmit a spirochete, Borrelia burgdorferi, which causes the cutaneous and systemic symptoms.[107] Erythema gyratum repens consists of multiple waves of gyrate erythema, which produce a pattern resembling the grain of wood. The eruption is almost always associated with internal malignancy.[108] Polymorphous light eruption occurs as erythematous plaques, particularly on the face and arms after sunlight exposure.[109] The eruption, which is more common in the summer, usually occurs within hours after sunlight exposure.[110] A familial form of polymorphous light eruption is common in American Indians.

Superficial perivascular dermatitis is characterized histologically by a perivascular infiltrate of inflammatory cells localized to the superficial dermal plexus. Urticaria (Fig. 8-31), arthropod bite reactions, drug eruptions, and viral exanthems are examples of this type of reaction. In urticaria, the infiltrate is sparse with a mixture of cell types including lymphocytes, histiocytes, eosinophils, and occasionally neutrophils. The pattern of superficial perivascular dermatitis with eosinophils should always suggest the possibility of an arthropod bite reaction or drug eruption. The infiltrate is predominantly lymphocytic in viral exanthems. Viral exanthems, drug eruptions, and arthropod bite reactions may also show spongiosis.

The other clinical disorders described above are more often associated with both superficial and deep perivascular dermatitis with an almost pure infiltrate of lymphocytes (Fig. 8-32). The infiltrate may be very dense and obscure the vascular lumina and endothelial cells. The

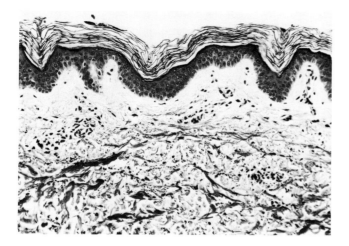

Fig. 8-31. Urticaria. The epidermis is unremarkable. Edema of the papillary dermis is associated with a sparse perivascular infiltrate of lymphocytes, histiocytes and eosinophils.

presence of a dense perivascular infiltrate in the superficial and deep dermis in a biopsy specimen of facial skin with numerous pilosebaceous structures and solar elastosis should suggest the possibility of polymorphous light eruption. Cases of erythema annulare centrifugum that clinically show a peripheral collarette of scale may histologically demonstrate spotty parakeratosis and spongiosis, similar to pityriasis rosea.

Differential Diagnosis of Perivascular Dermatitis

Before a diagnosis of perivascular dermatitis is made, an attempt should be made to rule out other more specific causes of this reaction pattern. *Tinea versicolor* is a common superficial fungus infection in which the short hy-

phae and spores are refractile and can often be seen on routinely stained sections (Fig. 8-33). *Dermatophyte infections* such as tinea corporis also produce a superficial perivascular dermatitis but often show small foci of parakeratosis. The hyphae of dermatophytes usually cannot be seen with hematoxylin and eosin (H & E)-stained sections but require the use of PAS or silver methenamine stains. *Progressive pigmented purpura of Schamberg* shows a superficial perivascular dermatitis with focal hemorrhage and small amounts of hemosiderin pigment. Macular forms of *urticaria pigmentosa* show a superficial perivascular infiltrate of mononuclear cells, which on closer examination have a centrally placed nucleus and granular gray to purple cytoplasm.[111] A Giemsa stain is helpful in demonstrating the characteristic mast cell granules. *Lymphoma cutis* and *leukemia cutis* often produce a superficial and deep perivascular infiltrate. In chronic lymphocytic leukemia or in well differentiated lymphocytic lymphoma, the lymphocytes do not appear atypical, and it may be extremely difficult to make the correct diagnosis without additional clinical information. *Jessner's lymphocytic infiltrate* is often listed in the differential diagnosis of superficial and deep perivascular dermatitis. It is possible that Jessner's lymphocytic infiltrate, which produces erythematous plaques or annular infiltrated lesions of the upper trunk or face, represents a variant of *polymorphous light eruption* (Fig. 8-34) or discoid lupus erythematosus.[112] Occasionally, biopsy specimens of the lesions of lupus erythematosus show little or no epidermal change.

Vasculitis

Vasculitis, which is characterized by the inflammation of small or large blood vessels, may have a broad spec-

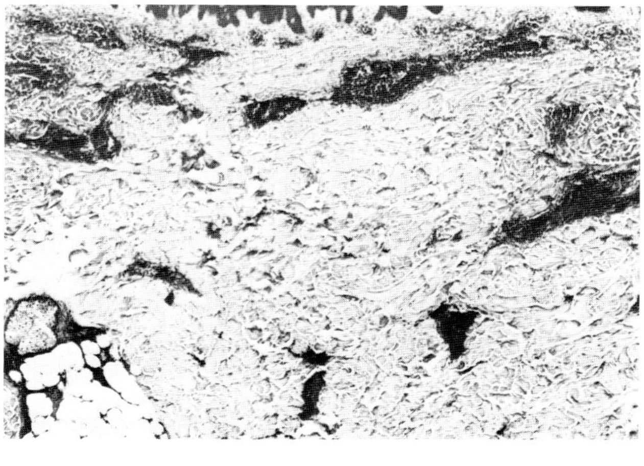

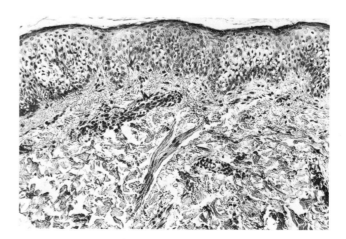

Fig. 8-32. Erythema annulare centrifugum. The epidermis is unremarkable. Dense perivascular cuffing of lymphocytes is present within both the superficial and deep dermis.

Fig. 8-33. Tinea versicolor. There is mild hyperkeratosis, acanthosis, and spongiosis of the epidermis. PAS stain revealed spores and short plump hyphae.

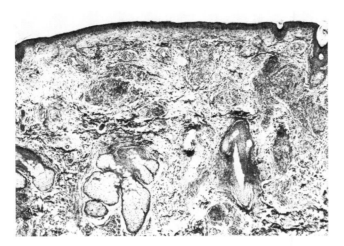

Fig. 8-34. Polymorphous light eruption. The epidermis is unremarkable. Dense patchy infiltrate of lymphocytes is oriented around blood vessels of the superficial and deep dermis.

trum of clinical manifestations involving the skin and/or internal organs. In addition to primary destruction of vessel walls, secondary changes such as hemorrhage, thrombosis, and necrosis of tissue supplied by the vessels occur. Vasculitis may be subclassified based on the type of inflammation: (1) neutrophilic, (2) lymphocytic, or (3) granulomatous. Types of vasculitis that involve predominantly neutrophilic inflammation of vessels include leukocytoclastic vasculitis, erythema elevatum diutinum, infectious vasculitis, and periarteritis nodosa. Lymphocytic vasculitis appears to be a feature of some cases of pityriasis lichenoides et varioliformis acuta (Mucha-Habermann disease). Granulomatous vasculitis is seen in allergic granulomatosis, Wegener's granulomatosis, and giant cell arteritis.

Leukocytoclastic Vasculitis

Leukocytoclastic vasculitis or allergic vasculitis is characterized by two major clinical syndromes. *Henoch-Schönlein purpura* is a disorder of children in which prodromal symptoms are followed by abdominal pain, joint pain, and palpable purpura of the skin, mainly of the lower extremities. *Leukocytoclastic vasculitis of adults* has a more varied clinical picture. It may involve only the skin, only visceral organs, or both. The numerous causes include bacterial, viral, and mycoplasma infections; drug eruptions; and collagen vascular diseases.[113] The characteristic skin lesion in both children and adults is palpable purpura, which has a predilection for the legs. Urticarial vasculitis shows relatively fixed urticarial lesions with fine purpura. Serum complement levels are typically depressed.

The epidermis in leukocytoclastic vasculitis varies from normal to necrotic depending on the severity of the vascular changes. The characteristic vascular changes involve the small postcapillary venules of the superficial vascular plexus. Vessel walls are necrotic, neutrophils are present within and around vessel walls, and the walls appear to be thickened by deposits of eosinophilic fibrin (Fig. 8-35). Leukocytoclasis or nuclear dust results from the fragmentation of the nuclei of neutrophils. Often, there is hemorrhage and thrombosis of the small vessels. At times, there may be evidence of perivascular fibrosis. In severe cases, the adjacent connective tissue and epidermis may be completely necrotic. Leukocytoclastic vasculitis is an immune-complex disease that results when antigen and immunoglobulin combine with complement producing complexes within vascular lumina. Direct immunofluorescence of skin samples in leukocytoclastic vasculitis shows granular deposits of IgM or IgG and complement within small vessels of the superficial dermis.[109] In Henoch-Schönlein purpura, the immunoglobulin deposited in the vessel walls is predominantly IgA.

Erythema Elevatum Diutinum

Erythema elevatum diutinum is a rare disease that appears to represent a chronic form of leukocytoclastic vasculitis. Red to brown plaques and nodules involve the dorsa of the hands and feet, as well as the elbows and knees.[114] The disease tends to persist for a number of years.[115]

The epidermis shows variable acanthosis (Fig. 8-36). Neutrophils and nuclear dust are present around and within the walls of small dermal vessels. A few lympho-

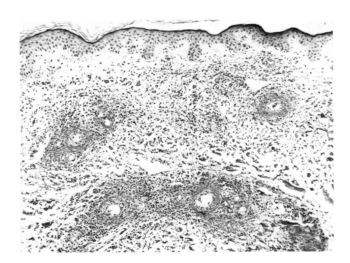

Fig. 8-35. Leukocytoclastic vasculitis. Small blood vessels of the superficial dermis show necrosis of their walls, which are infiltrated by neutrophils. The vessel walls contain fibrin and the surrounding dermis shows leukocytoclasis (nuclear dust).

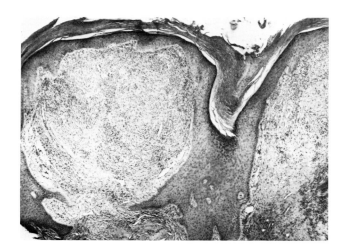
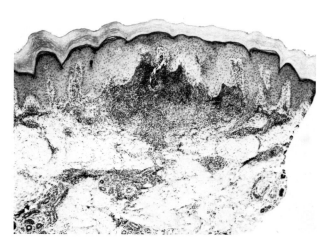

Fig. 8-36. Erythema elevatum diutinum. There is hyperkeratosis, acanthosis, and papillomatosis of the epidermis associated with a dense perivascular dermal infiltrate of neutrophils. The dermal connective tissue appears fibrotic.

Fig. 8-37. Gonococcemia. Biopsy of acral skin shows intense neutrophilic infiltration and hemorrhage in the superficial dermis.

cytes, eosinophils, and plasma cells may also be present. Endothelial cells appear swollen, and there are deposits of fibrin within vessel walls. Focal extravasation of RBC may be noted. Fibrosis of dermal connective tissue is more marked than in classic leukocytoclastic vasculitis, and in the late stages of erythema elevatum diutinum the fibrosis may replace the inflammatory infiltrate.

Infectious Vasculitis

Gonococcal and meningococcal infections may produce an acute febrile illness with cutaneous lesions characterized by acral pustules on an erythematous base. Tiny purpura may be present around the edges of the pustules.

The epidermis is often necrotic and infiltrated by neutrophils. Small vessels of the superficial dermis and middermis are surrounded and infiltrated by massive collections of neutrophils associated with nuclear dust, hemorrhage, and vessel wall necrosis (Fig. 8-37). Hemorrhagic subepidermal bullae may occur.[116] Organisms are usually not demonstrable by special stains but can be demonstrated by immunofluorescence microscopy.

Pseudomonas or staphylococcal septicemia occurs most often in terminally ill or immunosuppressed individuals. Necrotic ulcers known as ecthyma gangrenosum are characteristic of pseudomonas sepsis.

The epidermis and superficial dermis may be necrotic and pale staining. Inflammatory cells are characteristically sparse or absent. Vessel walls appear thickened and necrotic and have a hazy blue appearance with hematoxylin and eosin stain[117] (Fig. 8-38). There may be extensive hemorrhage. Closer examination of the vessel walls

with a tissue Gram stain (Brown and Brenn) shows that the bluish color noted on hematoxylin and eosin stain is caused by the presence of massive numbers of organisms.

Periarteritis Nodosa

Periarteritis nodosa is a form of leukocytoclastic vasculitis that involves small- and medium-sized muscular arteries. The disorder, which is more common in men, affects the kidneys, heart, GI tract, liver, lungs, and CNS. Approximately 10 percent of cases of systemic pe-

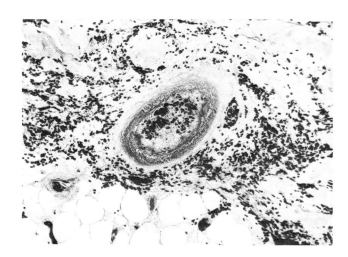

Fig. 8-38. Pseudomonas vasculitis. Blood vessel in the deep dermis shows a hazy thickening of its wall due to infiltration by organisms. The surrounding dermis shows marked hemorrhage but only a sparse inflammatory infiltrate.

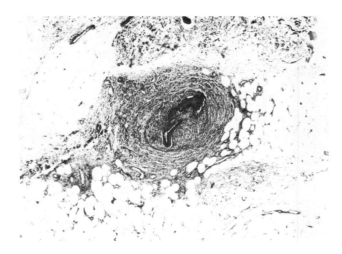

Fig. 8-39. Periarteritis nodosa. Muscular artery within the subcutaneous fat is infiltrated by neutrophils and lymphocytes with partial occlusion of its lumen. There is prominent perivascular fibrosis.

riarteritis nodosa involve the skin, although a purely cutaneous form of the disease also occurs.[118] Immune complexes of hepatitis B surface antigen may play a role in the pathogenesis of some cases of periarteritis nodosa.[119]

The epidermis varies from normal to ulcerated. At the junction of the deep dermis and subcutaneous fat, small- and medium-sized arteries show increased thickness of their walls, which are infiltrated with neutrophils (Fig. 8-39). The vessel walls are partially necrotic, and there is thrombosis, hemorrhage, and nuclear dust. The media of the vessels may be replaced by granulation tissue or fibrosis, and the lumina may be partly or completely obliterated. The vascular inflammation is often segmental, with intervening segments of normal-appearing vessel wall

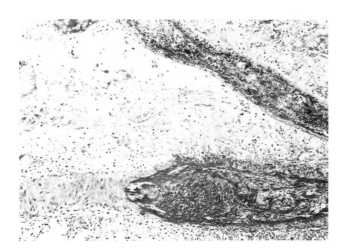

Fig. 8-40. Periarteritis nodosa. Blood vessels in the deep dermis are sectioned longitudinally and show the segmental nature of the involvement.

(Fig. 8-40). The surrounding connective tissue shows a mixed inflammatory infiltrate, which often includes many eosinophils.

Pityriasis Lichenoides et Varioliformis Acuta

Pityriasis lichenoides et varioliformis acuta (PLEVA) or Mucha-Habermann disease often begins in children and young adults. Papulovesicular lesions become hemorrhagic and necrotic and heal over a period of approximately two weeks leaving small scars. New lesions continue to develop for years.

The epidermis varies from normal to necrotic (Fig. 8-41). When inflammation is intense, a wedge-shaped area of necrosis of epidermis and superficial dermal connective tissue is present. A dense infiltrate of lymphocytes often completely obscures blood vessels of the superficial dermis and middermis.[120] Lymphocytes and extravasated RBC extend into the overlying epidermis. The basement membrane zone may be involved in a pattern suggestive of lichen planus.

Allergic Granulomatosis

Allergic granulomatosis of Churg and Strauss is characterized by asthma, pulmonary infiltrates, blood and tissue eosinophilia, and a cutaneous rash composed of papules, nodules, purpuric lesions, and ulcers.[121,122] Cardiac involvement, renal failure, and central nervous system disease are common causes of death.

The walls of small- and medium-sized muscular arteries are infiltrated by neutrophils and show fibrinoid necrosis. Granulomas containing a central area of necrotic

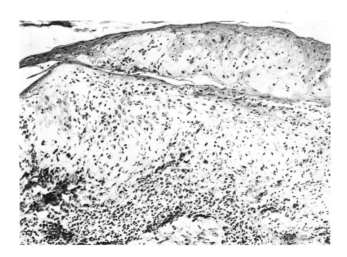

Fig. 8-41. Pityriasis lichenoides et varioliformis acuta. Focally necrotic epidermis is covered with crust and cellular debris. Dense infiltrates of lymphocytes obscure dermal blood vessels and are associated with exocytosis of lymphocytes and red blood cells.

collagen and cellular debris are present in the dermis and subcutaneous fat. The necrotic areas are surrounded by epithelioid cells, multinucleate giant cells, and mononuclear inflammatory cells. Eosinophils are often numerous.[123] A small necrotic vessel may be seen in the center of the granulomatous inflammation.

Wegener's Granulomatosis

Necrotizing lesions of the upper and lower respiratory tract, widespread necrotizing vasculitis, and necrotizing glomerulitis with death from renal failure are the main features of Wegener's granulomatosis. The disease may begin as ulcerative lesions of the nose and oral cavity. Cutaneous papulonecrotic lesions and ulcers are present in 25 to 50 percent of cases.[124,125]

Depending on the degree of dermal inflammation, the epidermis may be normal or necrotic. Neutrophils are present within the walls of small arteries and veins. Surrounding connective tissue contains granulomas with extensive tissue necrosis and a mixed infiltrate of eosinophils, plasma cells, and lymphocytes. Multinucleate giant cells are common. A variable amount of hemorrhage is often present.

Giant Cell Arteritis

Pain and erythema over the temporal arteries of elderly individuals are the classic symptoms of giant cell arteritis.[126] Inflammation of the vessels may result in extensive areas of scalp necrosis.[127] Involvement of the retinal arteries can produce blindness. Vessels of the heart and brain may also be involved.

The arteries show destruction of internal elastic lamina with partial or complete occlusion of the lumina. Macrophages and multinucleate giant cells are present within the vessel walls and appear to surround altered elastic tissue. Different segments of the vessel walls appear to be involved unevenly in the inflammatory process. The Verhoeff-van Gieson elastic stain is helpful in defining the presence of altered elastic tissue.

Differential Diagnosis of Vasculitis

Three disorders not discussed in the previous sections should be considered in the differential diagnosis of neutrophilic vasculitis. *Granuloma faciale* consists clinically of solitary or multiple infiltrated facial nodules with a red-brown color and prominent follicular openings.[128] Ectatic vessels in the superficial dermis are surrounded by a ''sea of neutrophils'' with a lesser number of eosinophils and mononuclear cells. The infiltrate is separated from the epidermis and appendages by grenz zones of uninvolved collagen. Although nuclear dust is common, true vessel wall inflammation and necrosis are generally absent.

Acute febrile neutrophilic dermatosis (Sweet's syndrome), which affects mainly women, is characterized by multiple tender red plaques of the face and/or extremities associated with fever and leukocytosis.[129,130] A dense dermal infiltrate of neutrophils may be angiocentric but is often diffuse. A few eosinophils and mononuclear cells are present. Although there may be considerable nuclear dust, true vasculitis is absent. *Livedo vasculitis (atrophic blanch, segmental hyalinizing vasculitis)* produces recurrent painful ulcerations of the ankles and lower legs that heal with white atrophic scars and patchy hyperpigmentation.[131] The course is chronic, with exacerbations during the winter or summer. Small vessels of the superficial dermis show marked thickening of their walls by a dense pink hyalin material that is PAS-positive and diastase-resistant. There is often endothelial proliferation and thrombosis, but the inflammatory infiltrate is sparse and predominantly mononuclear.

Granulomatous Dermatitis

Granulomatous dermatitis can be subclassified into necrobiotic, sarcoidal, and infectious types. The three major forms of necrobiotic granulomas are granuloma annulare, necrobiosis lipoidica, and rheumatoid nodules. Sarcoidal granulomas may be produced by sarcoidosis, tuberculoid leprosy, and reactions to silica, beryllium, and zirconium. Certain foreign body granulomas may be confused with sarcoidosis. Infectious granulomas produce a characteristic epithelial and granulomatous reaction pattern. This pattern is seen mainly in deep fungal infections, in atypical acid-fast bacterial infections and in noninfectious disorders such as iododerma and bromoderma.

Granuloma Annulare

Granuloma annulare (GA) is characterized by flesh-colored asymptomatic papules that often occur in a ring-like or circinate pattern on the dorsal aspects of the hands or feet. Generalized,[132] perforating,[133] and subcutaneous forms,[134] of granuloma annulare also occur. The disorder affects mainly children and young adults, and most cases clear spontaneously within approximately 2 years.

The epidermis in granuloma annulare is usually normal. Discrete stellate areas of necrobiosis within the superficial dermis are surrounded by lymphocytes, histiocytes, and epithelioid cells in a palisaded pattern (Fig. 8-42). The necrobiotic collagen varies from granular to wispy and stains somewhat basophilic with the hematoxylin and eosin stain. Remnants of collagen fibers can be recognized in the necrobiotic areas. Multinucleate giant cells are often present but are usually few in number. A dense lymphocytic cuffing of small vessels in the su-

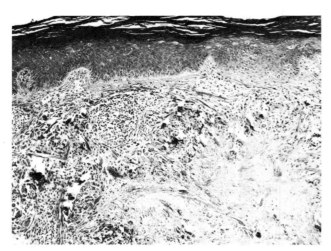

Fig. 8-42. Granuloma annulare. Stellate area of necrobiotic collagen within the upper dermis is surrounded by histiocytes and lymphocytes.

perficial dermis is a common feature. If a biopsy is obtained from a younger lesion, the dermis may show only a single-file arrangement of lymphocytes and histiocytes between collagen bundles in association with small indistinct areas of necrobiotic collagen (Fig. 8-43). IgM and complement have been found in small dermal vessels in about one-third of the cases.[135]

Necrobiosis Lipoidica

Necrobiosis lipoidica may begin as erythematous nodules on the lower extremities resembling erythema nodosum. With time the skin becomes atrophic and yellow, producing confluent plaques with hyperpigmented margins. Telangiectatic vessels can be seen beneath the skin

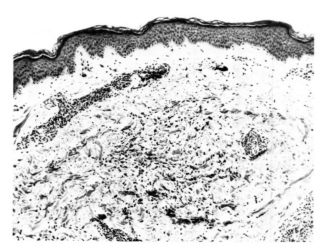

Fig. 8-43. Granuloma annulare. Single-file arrangement of mononuclear cells between collagen bundles is associated with indistinct areas of necrobiosis.

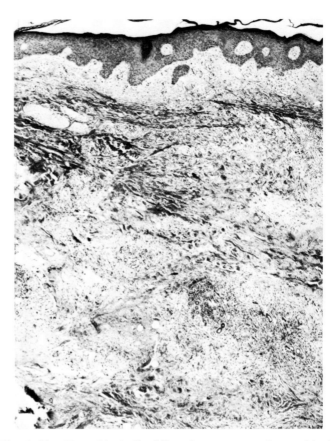

Fig. 8-44. Necrobiosis lipoidica. Large areas of necrobiosis within the deep dermis and subcutaneous fat are oriented parallel to the surface epithelium.

surface. In approximately 15 percent of cases, areas other than the legs are involved such as the arms, trunk, and face.[136] Diabetes mellitus is present or will eventually develop in 60 to 80 percent of patients with necrobiosis lipoidica.[136]

The necrobiosis in necrobiosis lipoidica is located in the deep dermis and subcutaneous fat (Fig. 8-44). Large elliptical areas of necrobiosis are oriented parallel to the surface of the skin. The necrobiotic connective tissue varies from a wispy bluish appearance to necrotic to eosinophilic and hyalinized in various cases. Granulomatous inflammation with multinucleate giant cells and vascular changes characterized by dense perivascular infiltrates of mononuclear cells are more prominent than in granuloma annulare (Fig. 8-45). Plasma cells are often present.

Rheumatoid Nodule

Rheumatoid nodules occur in adults with seropositive rheumatoid arthritis and active joint disease. They are rare in children with Still's disease. Rheumatoid nodules

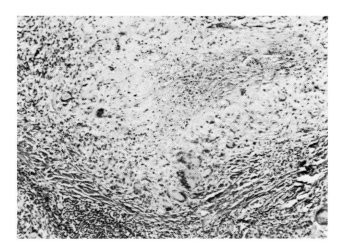

Fig. 8-45. Necrobiosis lipoidica. Area of necrobiotic connective tissue is surrounded by a palisaded infiltrate of epithelioid cells and multinucleate giant cells.

are nontender and occur over extensor aspects of joints. Similar nodules have been found in the lung, meninges, and heart valves. Rheumatoid nodules may occur in lupus erythematosus.[137] The lesions of subcutaneous granuloma annulare (pseudorheumatoid nodules) in children[138] show histologic features which may be confused with rheumatoid nodules.

The necrobiotic connective tissue in rheumatoid nodules is deeper than in granuloma annulare or necrobiosis lipoidica, and the epidermis is often not present in the biopsy specimen. The areas of necrobiosis are large and sharply circumscribed (Fig. 8-46). Palisading of epithelioid cells around the necrobiotic area is usually well developed. The necrobiosis tends to be complete, with few

collagen fibers remaining. Occasionally, small amounts of calcium may be present within the necrobiotic tissue.

Sarcoidosis

Sarcoidosis is a systemic granulomatous disease of unknown etiology that affects predominantly lymph nodes, lung, eyes, and skin. Cutaneous lesions most often occur as papules and nodules on the face and head. Translucent raised brown papules around the eyes or on the nose are characteristic. Scarring alopecia is an unusual complication.[139]

The epidermis is normal or is effaced by the underlying granulomas. Distinct granulomas composed predominantly of epithelioid cells are surrounded by a narrow rim of lymphocytes (Fig. 8-47). Caseation necrosis is usually absent, but small foci of caseation necrosis occasionally occur. Multinucleate giant cells are common and may contain asteroid bodies.[140] Round, laminated, calcified Schaumann bodies occasionally are present within the giant cells. The granulomatous infiltrate may fill the dermis and extend into the subcutaneous fat.

Tuberculoid Leprosy

Tuberculoid leprosy is a variant of leprosy in which host cell-mediated immunity is generally intact and the number of organisms are few.[141] Clinical lesions are characterized by annular plaques with central clearing and variable hypopigmentation. The margins of the plaques are scaly, and there is cutaneous anesthesia in the center of the plaque. Peripheral nerves that run through the plaque may be palpably enlarged. Patients with pure tuberculoid leprosy often have only one or a few lesions.

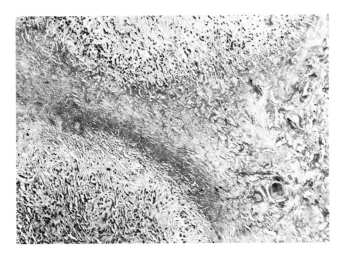

Fig. 8-46. Rheumatoid nodule. Zone of relatively complete necrobiosis is surrounded by histiocytes and epithelioid cells in a palisaded pattern. Multinucleate giant cell is present.

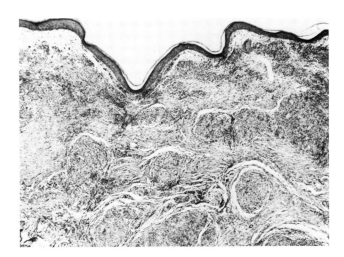

Fig. 8-47. Sarcoidosis. Numerous distinct granulomas are present throughout the dermis. Lymphocytes are sparse, and caseation necrosis is absent.

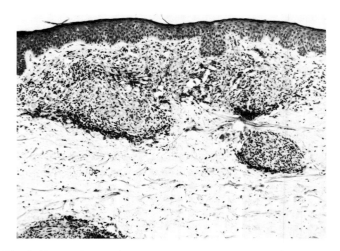

Fig. 8-48. Tuberculoid leprosy. Granulomas surrounded by a narrow rim of lymphocytes are present in the superficial dermis. Exocytosis of lymphocytes into the epidermis is present.

The prognosis for cure with appropriate drug therapy is excellent.

The epidermis is normal or shows mild hyperkeratosis and parakeratosis. Well circumscribed sarcoidal granulomas are present throughout the dermis (Fig. 8-48). The granulomas are surrounded by a sparse infiltrate of lymphocytes. A small number of lymphocytes may extend from the dermis into the epidermis. Cutaneous nerves in the deep dermis are almost completely obliterated by the granulomatous process. Fite's acid-fast stain may demonstrate a rare organism, but often it is negative.

Silica, Beryllium, and Zirconium Granulomas

Silica granulomas result from the contamination of wounds with particles of glass or soil that contain silicon dioxide or from the contamination of surgical wounds with talcum powder, which contains magnesium silicate. Typically, the inflammatory response does not occur until months or years after the exposure.[142] Zirconium contained in deodorant preparations[143] or poison ivy medications[144] is a rare cause of a papular eruption. Systemic berylliosis resulting from the inhalation of beryllium particles may produce a papular skin rash. Localized beryllium granulomas due to contamination of lacerations with beryllium from fluorescent light tubes are now quite rare.

Silica granulomas may be indistinguishable from sarcoidosis, although typically the granulomatous inflammation is more diffuse, with histiocytes, epithelioid cells, and multinucleate giant cells. Often, crystalline particles of silica can be observed in the dermis. Polarized light examination enhances the identification of the particles, which are doubly refractile. The granulomas produced by zirconium are indistinguishable from those of sarcoido-

sis, but the small zirconium particles are not detectable by polarized light examination. The cutaneous granulomas of systemic berylliosis are also indistinguishable from sarcoidosis.[145] Beryllium granuloma secondary to inoculation of beryllium into the skin often shows extensive areas of caseation necrosis surrounded by a tuberculoid granulomatous infiltrate. The epidermis may be acanthotic or ulcerated.

Foreign Body Granulomas

The most common cause of granulomatous inflammation on the face is a foreign body reaction to keratin secondary to a ruptured epidermoid cyst or acne lesion. The diagnosis of sarcoidosis should not be made when a single biopsy specimen from the face shows granulomatous inflammation.

Within the dermis are collections of epithelioid cells, histiocytes, lymphocytes, and foreign body giant cells (Fig. 8-49). The multiple nuclei of foreign body giant cells tend to be clustered in one portion of the cytoplasm. Foreign material may be present within the cytoplasm of

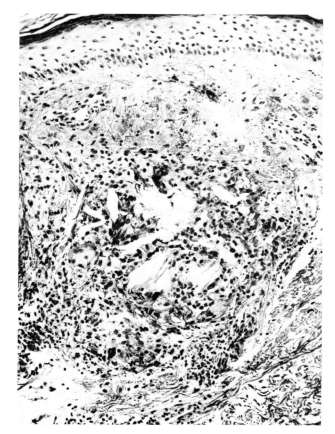

Fig. 8-49. Foreign body granuloma secondary to keratin. Fibrillar collections of keratin are surrounded by lymphocytes, histiocytes, and foreign body giant cells.

multinucleate giant cells or within the granulomatous infiltrate. The keratin fibers are often fibrillar in appearance. Epithelium from the wall of the ruptured cyst and occasionally microabscesses containing acute inflammatory cells may be present. Although the keratin of the stratum corneum is doubly refractile, the small amounts of keratin in a foreign body reaction may be difficult to demonstrate with polarized light.

Infectious Granulomas

Infectious granulomas of the skin produced by deep fungal infections typically produce verrucous nodules or plaques that may have small pustules studding their surfaces. An excellent review of this subject has been published by Conant et al.[146] Systemic ingestion of halogens such as iodide[147] and bromide produce cutaneous lesions that are clinically and histologically similar to deep fungal granulomas (Fig. 8-50).

The epidermis shows hyperkeratosis, parakeratosis, and papillomatosis. Marked irregular acanthosis produces pseudoepitheliomatous hyperplasia (Fig. 8-51). Microabscesses containing neutrophils and mononuclear inflammatory cells are present within the acanthotic epithelium and within the dermis. The dermis contains scattered epithelioid cells, multinucleate giant cells, histiocytes, and lymphocytes. Distinct granulomas are occasionally seen; however, caseation necrosis is uncommon in deep fungal infections. The organisms that produce deep fungal infections are often visible on H & E-stained sections but are easier to identify with the silver methenamine stain and with the PAS reaction following predigestion with diastase to remove glycogen particles.

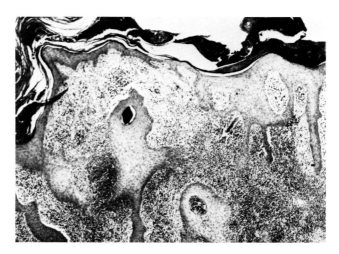

Fig. 8-51. Sporotrichosis. There is hyperkeratosis, acanthosis, and pseudoepitheliomatous hyperplasia of the epidermis. Intraepithelial microabscesses contain neutrophils. Organisms are difficult to identify in the granulomatous infiltrate with special stains.

Differential Diagnosis of Granulomatous Dermatitis

Tuberculosis verrucosa cutis may show epitheliomatous and granulomatous changes similar to the deep fungal infections. In cutaneous tuberculosis, however, the granulomatous inflammation tends to be less polymorphous than in the deep fungal infections. In tuberculosis verrucosa cutis, caseation necrosis may be slight to moderate, and organisms usually cannot be identified with acid-fast stains.[148] Foreign body granulomas may show a mixed inflammatory infiltrate similar to that of deep fungal infections and halogen eruptions. However, the presence of foreign material and/or the presence of distinctive foreign body giant cells should help to distinguish foreign body reactions from deep fungal infections. *Swimming pool granuloma* due to infection with *Mycobacterium marinum*[149] also produces chronic verrucous cutaneous plaques that show epithelial hyperplasia, neutrophilic microabscesses within the epidermis, and a mixed inflammatory infiltrate in the dermis (Fig. 8-52). Epithelioid cells and giant cells are often present; however, distinct tubercle formation is uncommon and caseation necrosis is slight or absent. *M. marinum* is difficult to identify in tissue with the Ziehl-Neelsen stain but is easily cultured on Lowenstein-Jensen media at 32°C.

Folliculitis

Bacterial Folliculitis

Most cases of folliculitis are the result of infection with *Staphylococcus aureus*. Folliculitis can be divided into superficial and deep forms. Superficial folliculitis is char-

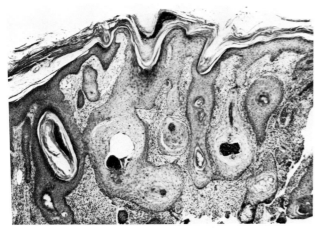

Fig. 8-50. Iododerma. Hyperkeratosis, papillomatosis and irregular acanthosis are associated with intraepidermal neutrophilic microabscesses and a granulomatous dermal infiltrate.

174

PRINCIPLES AND PRACTICE OF SURGICAL PATHOLOGY

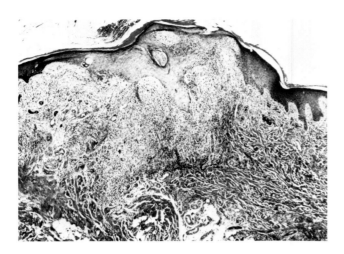

Fig. 8-52. Swimming pool granuloma. Irregular acanthosis of the epidermis is associated with a dermal infiltrate of lymphocytes, histiocytes, epithelioid cells, and multinucleate giant cells.

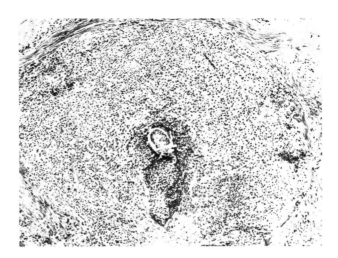

Fig. 8-53. Deep folliculitis. Intradermal hair shaft surrounded by a neutrophilic microabscess and a lymphohistiocytic infiltrate.

acterized by small pustules situated at the openings of hair follicles and frequently pierced by a hair shaft. This form of folliculitis is known as impetigo Bockhart. More often, staphylococcal folliculitis also involves a deeper portion of the follicle and adjacent dermis. A red tender nodule centered around a hair follicle is referred to as a *furuncle*. Recurrent furunculosis tends to involve the buttocks and thighs and may be associated with diabetes mellitus. A larger furuncle, which involves several hair follicles producing a boggy purulent mass, is known as a *carbuncle*.

Superficial folliculitis produces a subcorneal pustule located at the mouth of the hair follicle. This pustule is often pierced by a hair shaft, but this is difficult to demonstrate histologically. An inflammatory infiltrate of neutrophils, lymphocytes, and histiocytes surrounds the upper portion of the follicle and may infiltrate follicular epithelium. In deep folliculitis, a dense perifollicular infiltrate of neutrophils, lymphocytes, and histiocytes extends into the follicular epithelium. The follicular epithelium may rupture with extrusion of the hair shaft and keratin into the surrounding dermis and the formation of neutrophilic microabscesses and a foreign body granulomatous reaction (Fig. 8-53). In carbuncles, a massive dermal infiltrate of acute and chronic inflammatory cells, including plasma cells and foreign body giant cells, is centered around several hair follicles, which show destruction of follicular epithelium.

Fungal Folliculitis

Dermatophyte infections may involve the hair follicles of the scalp or head. The manifestations vary from a dry scaly eruption with breakage of hair shafts to a severe inflammatory process with boggy infiltrated plaques (*kerion*) and subsequent scarring alopecia. Distinct erythematous perifollicular papules and nodules occurring on the extremities or scalp secondary to a dermatophyte infection of hair follicles are known as *Majocchi's granulomas*.

The epidermis shows hyperkeratosis, parakeratosis, and variable acanthosis. Fungal hyphae and/or arthrospores are seen on or within the hair shaft (Fig. 8-54). Occasionally, hyphae are also seen in the adjacent stratum corneum with special stains. The location of arthrospores on the surface of the hair shaft (ectothrix) or within the hair shaft (endothrix) and the size of the arthrospores (small or large) are important clues for species identification. Follicular epithelium is often acanthotic

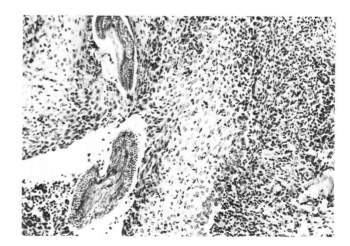

Fig. 8-54. Fungal folliculitis. Small spores can be seen within the hair shaft of an inflamed follicle.

and is infiltrated by inflammatory cells. Focal rupture of follicular epithelium is associated with neutrophilic abscesses and foreign body granulomatous inflammation in the adjacent dermis.[150] Special stains such as silver methenamine or the PAS reaction are helpful in further delineating the extent of the fungal infection.

Folliculitis Decalvans

Folliculitis decalvans occurs predominantly on the scalp of black men and is characterized by perifollicular papules, pustules, and abscesses that produce boggy masses and destruction of hair follicles. Draining sinuses, inflammatory nodules, and cutaneous atrophy are common features.

Numerous hair follicles within the dermis show inflammation of follicular epithelium with lymphocytes, histiocytes, and neutrophils. There is rupture of follicular epithelium, and hair shafts are present in the dermal connective tissue. Lymphocytes, plasma cells, epithelioid cells, and foreign body giant cells surround the displaced hair shafts. Microabscesses containing neutrophils and sinus tracts with walls composed of acanthotic epithelium are often present. There is considerable fibrosis of dermal connective tissue with the formation of hypertrophic scars or keloids.

Differential Diagnosis of Folliculitis

Pityrosporum ovale is a common yeast that occupies hair follicles of the head and upper trunk. Pityrosporum folliculitis shows follicular hyperkeratosis, inflammation of follicular epithelium, dermal abscesses and PAS-positive budding yeast in the follicular lumen and in the dermis.[151] It is important to recognize *pityrosporum ovale* and not to confuse it with dermatophyte infections. *Folliculitis keloidalis* (acne keloidalis) characteristically produces inflammatory papules at the nape of the neck in black men. *Pseudofolliculitis barbae* results from ingrown hairs and subsequent inflammation in the beard areas of black males. The histologic changes in folliculitis keloidalis and pseudofolliculitis barbae may be identical to folliculitis decalvans.

Cutaneous Deposits

Systemic Amyloidosis

Primary Systemic Amyloidosis. The cutaneous lesions of primary systemic amyloidosis are characterized by coalescing papules and nodules with a smooth surface and a translucent appearance.[152] Lesions are commonly located around the eyes and in the perianal area. Petechiae and purpura may follow minor cutaneous trauma. The distribution of amyloid in primary systemic amyloidosis and in

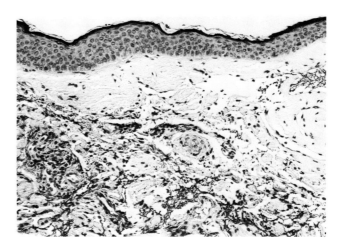

Fig. 8-55. Primary systemic amyloidosis. Amorphous masses of amyloid are present within the superficial dermis.

myeloma-associated amyloidosis is identical and includes the skin, tongue, heart, gastrointestinal tract, nerves, and carpal ligaments. The skin is involved in approximately 25 percent of cases, while the tongue is infiltrated and enlarged in 40 percent.[153]

Eosinophilic masses of amorphous material are deposited within the dermis and subcutaneous fat (Fig. 8-55). The dermal papillae appear enlarged and rounded due to fissured masses of amyloid which may press against the basement membrane zone. A few fibroblasts may be present within the amyloid. Melanin pigment is often present in macrophages in the papillary dermis. Deposits of amyloid surround dermal vessels and encase eccrine sweat glands. There is often extravasation of red blood cells from the affected vessels. In the subcutaneous fat, amyloid infiltrates the walls of blood vessels (Fig. 8-56)

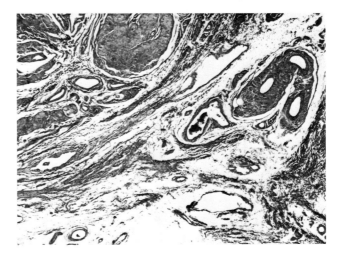

Fig. 8-56. Primary systemic amyloidosis. Blood vessels in the deep dermis are encased by dense deposits of amyloid.

and surrounds individual fat cells producing characteristic amyloid rings. A number of recent articles have described the structure and origin of the amyloid fibrils.[154,155]

Secondary Systemic Amyloidosis. Skin lesions are rare in secondary systemic amyloidosis. Amyloid deposits are typically found in the kidneys, liver, spleen, and adrenals.[156,157] Patients may develop hepatomegaly, proteinuria, and uremia. Secondary systemic amyloidosis is associated with a chronic inflammatory process such as tuberculosis, leprosy, rheumatoid arthritis, osteomyelitis, stasis ulcers, hidradenitis suppurativa, or epidermolysis bullosa.

Skin biopsy specimens usually do not show deposits of amyloid in secondary systemic amyloidosis.

Localized Amyloidosis

Lichen amyloidosus usually involves the pretibial areas, where it produces a scaly, papular, confluent rash that may be intensely pruritic.[158] The eruption persists for many years and is refractory to treatment.

The epidermis shows a variable amount of hyperkaratosis and acanthosis. Small globules of amyloid are limited to the papillary dermis (Fig. 8-57). The amyloid may be separated from the epidermis by a narrow grenz zone of collagen or appear to be in direct contact with the epidermal basement membrane. Small amounts of melanin are present in dermal macrophages. Occasionally, the amyloid deposits in several adjacent dermal papillae coalesce to form larger aggregates. The amyloid is often fissured and contains a few fibroblasts and capillaries.

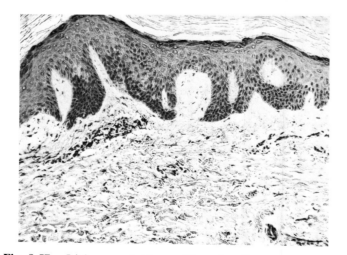

Fig. 8-57. Lichen amyloidosus. There is mild hyperkeratosis and acanthosis of the epidermis. Dermal papilla is enlarged and club-shaped due to small deposits of amyloid.

In *macular amyloidosis*, the interscapular or pretibial areas are involved with pruritic, symmetric, brownish, reticulated macules. This type of localized amyloidosis appears to represent an early stage of lichen amyloidosus.[159] Rubbing or scratching the lesions of macular amyloidosis may produce the hyperkeratotic papules of lichen amyloidosus. In contrast to systemic forms of amyloidosis, the amyloid in the lichenoid and macular forms of cutaneous amyloidosis results from filamentous degeneration of epidermal cells which are discharged into the papillary dermis.[160]

The epidermis is normal. The small amounts of amyloid that are deposited at the tips of dermal papillae resemble colloid bodies. The histologic changes are subtle and easily overlooked. The presence of melanin pigment in dermal macrophages is a helpful sign and should stimulate a careful search for amyloid deposits.

In *nodular (tumefactive) amyloidosis* one or several nodules occur mainly on the legs, but they have also been reported on the trunk and genitalia. There is no evidence of systemic amyloidosis or myeloma.

Large masses of amyloid are present within the dermis and subcutaneous fat.[158,161] The changes are usually indistinguishable from primary systemic amyloidosis and myeloma-associated amyloidosis.

A variety of cutaneous tumors such as basal cell carcinoma, Bowen's disease, and seborrheic keratosis may contain deposits of amyloid.[158] Clinically, the lesions are not distinguishable from tumors that do not contain amyloid.

Small amounts of amyloid are typically present in the stroma of the tumors. Amyloid deposits are not present in blood vessels in the surrounding dermis.

Special Stains and Procedures for Amyloidosis

In addition to the characteristic distribution and the pale pink fissured appearance of amyloid, several special stains and procedures may be helpful in distinguishing amyloid from other material. With polarized light examination, collagen is birefringent, whereas amyloid is not. With the Giemsa stain, collagen is pink and amyloid is blue. The Verhoeff–van Gieson stain stains collagen red and amyloid yellow. With the PAS reaction, collagen is pale pink, whereas amyloid is red. Amyloid stains metachromatically (red) with crystal violet or methyl violet stains. With the alkaline Congo red stain, amyloid is orange. A very helpful diagnostic feature is the apple green color (dichromatic) of amyloid with the alkaline Congo red stain and polarized light. Amyloid is brightly fluorescent with the thioflavin T stain utilizing fluorescence microscopy. Waldenström's macroglobulinemia may produce cutaneous deposits that mimic amyloid. However, by immunofluorescence microscopy the material can be shown to be predominantly IgM.

Colloid Milium

Colloid milium is a sunlight-induced disease that produces translucent papules on the dorsa of the hands and face of adults. A rare juvenile form is not related to sunlight exposure.[162]

The epidermis is often elevated and effaced by large masses of homogeneous fissured material in the dermal papillae. The colloid is separated from the epidermis by a thin grenz zone of connective tissue. The eosinophilic fissured aggregates may contain small vessels and a variable number of fibroblasts. Amyloid and colloid can be differentiated by electron microscopy. The straight, nonbranching fibrils of amyloidosis are 70 to 100 Å in diameter. Colloid fibers are of a similar width but show branching and anastomosing. Colloid is most likely produced by fibroblasts.[163] The staining properties of colloid are similar to amyloid.[164]

Hyalinoses

Lipoid proteinosis (hyalinosis cutis et mucosae) is an autosomal recessive disorder that usually begins in infancy. Translucent waxy papules are present along the eyelid margins and around the mouth. The tongue, mucous membranes, and vocal cords are infiltrated, and the infants have a characteristic hoarse cry. Similar deposits affect the gastrointestinal tract, vagina, testis, eye, brain, and kidney.[165]

The epidermis is often hyperkeratotic and papilloma-tous. A pink hyalin material surrounds blood vessels, sweat glands, and hair follicles (Fig. 8-58). Rarely, diffuse dermal involvement is noted. Because of the periadnexal distribution of the hyalin material, it is often oriented perpendicular to the epidermis. The deposits produce a positive PAS reaction and are diastase resistant. The material is metachromatic with the toluidine blue stain. Fat stains on frozen sections show small droplets of fat within the hyalin material.

Erythropoietic protoporphyria is inherited as an autosomal-dominant trait. It manifests in childhood as burning and itching of the skin after ultraviolet light exposure. Sun-exposed skin becomes papular, lichenified, and indurated. The dorsa of the hands and face are typical sites of involvement. Massive deposits of protoporphyrin in the liver may result in fatal cirrhosis.[166]

The epidermis shows hyperkeratosis and papillomatosis. Large deposits of a pink hyalin material are present around blood vessels in the superficial dermis (Fig. 8-59). There is little tendency for the hyalin to surround adnexal structures as in lipoid proteinosis.[167] Unlike porphyria cutanea tarda, subepidermal bullae are rare in erythropoietic protoporphyria. The hyalin material stains red with the PAS reaction and is diastase resistant. *Porphyria cutanea tarda, variegate porphyria,* and *coproporphyria* show much smaller amounts of hyalin material around small vessels in the papillary dermis. Immunofluorescence of the hyalin material in the porphyrias is positive for immunoglobulin and complement but is felt to be a secondary phenomenon related to damage and reduplication of the basement membrane of small dermal vessels associated with the leakage of serum proteins.[168]

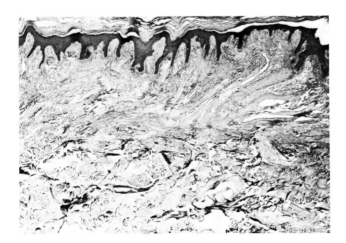

Fig. 8-58. Lipoid proteinosis. Deposits of hyaline material surround dermal vessels and are oriented perpendicular to the epidermis.

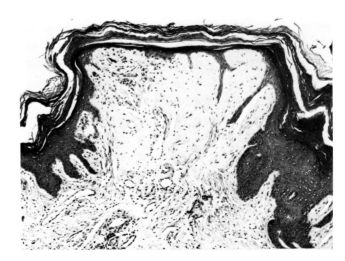

Fig. 8-59. Erythropoietic protoporphyria. Collections of hyaline material encase small vessels of the papillary dermis. Epidermis appears hyperkeratotic and papillomatous.

Mucinoses

Pretibial Myxedema

Pretibial myxedema occurs in patients with hyperthyroidism (Graves' disease), especially in those individuals with exophthalmos and increased serum levels of long-acting thyroid stimulator (LATS).[169] Yellow, waxy, indurated nodules and plaques of the pretibial area often occur after successful treatment of the hyperthyroidism. The surface of the skin lesion may appear dimpled or scaly. The presence of a thick, stringy, dermal mucin may be obvious at the time of the biopsy.

The epidermis may show hyperkeratosis and acanthosis but is often normal. The rete ridge pattern tends to be effaced by large amounts of dermal mucin. A narrow, subepidermal grenz zone of relatively normal connective tissue separates the epidermis from massive amounts of mucin within the dermis. Collagen fibers and fibroblasts are few in number, and the dermis appears to be replaced by a pale blue wispy material or by empty spaces where mucin has been removed during processing (Fig. 8-60). The fibroblasts have a delicate fusiform or stellate shape. The mucin, which is hyaluronic acid, stains blue with the alcian blue stain at pH 2.5 but does not stain at pH 0.4. The mucin is metachromatic with the toluidine blue stain at pH 3.0 and stains positively for mucin with the colloidal iron and mucicarmine stains.

Generalized Myxedema

Patients with hypothyroidism or generalized myxedema have a dull appearance with puffy facies and pale, dry, often scaly skin. They have dry brittle hair and loss of lateral eyebrows. Their palms are yellow due to deposition of carotene in the keratin layer.

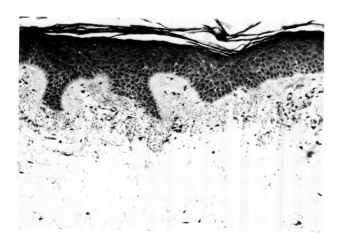

Fig. 8-60. Pretibial myxedema. The epidermis is unremarkable. Except for a narrow zone immediately deep to the epidermis, the entire dermis appears pale staining and contains fusiform and stellate fibroblasts.

Routinely stained sections appear relatively normal except for mild hyperkeratosis. Careful examination shows slightly increased spaces between dermal collagen fibers. Occasionally, a bluish wispy material is seen in these spaces, but the mucin is often removed during processing. The presence of dermal hyaluronic acid can usually be demonstrated with the special stains described for pretibial myxedema.[170]

Papular Mucinosis

Clinical variants of papular mucinosis are known as scleromyxedema and lichen myxedematosus. *Scleromyxedema* shows leonine facies and diffuse thickening of the skin.[171] In contrast to scleroderma, the skin is freely movable. In *papular mucinosis,* discrete papules are present, whereas in lichen myxedematosus the papular eruption may have a lichenified appearance. In all forms of papular mucinosis, an abnormal IgG with a slow electrophoretic migration is present in the serum.[172] The abnormal immunoglobulin, which is thought to be produced in the bone marrow by plasma cells, almost always has λ-type light chains.[173]

The epidermis may be normal or show hyperkeratosis and acanthosis. Focal collections of mucin are present within the superficial dermis and are often separated by intervening areas of relatively normal connective tissues. In contrast to the other mucinoses, the number of fibroblasts is significantly increased in the areas of mucin deposition. The mucin is hyaluronic acid and stains similarly to that described for pretibial myxedema. At autopsy, the mucin content of the internal organs is not found to be increased.

Scleredema of Buschke

Scleredema of Buschke, also known as *scleredema adultorum,* is characterized by diffuse nonpitting induration of the skin of the face, neck, and upper trunk and often follows an infectious episode such as influenza. In most patients, the eruption resolves over a period of months. Diabetes mellitus is a commonly associated disease.[174,175]

The dermis appears normal on superficial examination. The overall thickness of the dermis is often greatly increased, and spaces are present between collagen fibers similar to those seen in generalized myxedema. The spaces contain hyaluronic acid, which is demonstrated with special stains as described for pretibial myxedema. Often the amount of mucin is so small that the special stains fail to demonstrate any abnormality. The secretory portions of eccrine sweat glands are located in the mid-dermis, and it appears that new collagen is laid down beneath the glands, replacing a portion of the subcutaneous fat.

Digital Mucous Cyst

A solitary translucent, slightly fluctuant cyst on the distal finger proximal to the fingernail or directly over the distal interphalangeal joint is characteristic of a digital mucous cyst. The cysts may be slightly tender and, if punctured, drain a thick mucinuous material. Injection of the interphalangeal joint with methylene blue dye demonstrates a communication between the cysts and the joint space.[176]

The epidermis is effaced by a large area of pale-staining mucin within the superficial dermis and middermis. Fusiform and stellate fibroblasts are present within the mucin, which may appear bluish and stringy. Older lesions tend to develop cleftlike spaces between the mucin and the surrounding connective tissue producing a large, sharply circumscribed cyst.[177] Occasionally, the cystic space is lined by macrophages or granulation tissue. In lesions that have drained to the surface periodically, the cyst may have the appearance of being partly intraepidermal.

Mucous Cyst of Oral Mucosa

A solitary translucent cyst of the lower lips is characteristic of a mucous cyst (mucocele).[178] Minor trauma, such as biting the lip, causes rupture of a salivary duct, resulting in the extravasation of sialomucin into the surrounding connective tissue. The translucent papules often resolve spontaneously.

Ill defined areas of mucin are present within the connective tissue. The mucin has a bluish amorphous to stringy appearance. In older lesions, a cystic space is lined by a wall of granulation tissue and inflammatory cells. Much mucin may be removed during processing. Mucin is phagocytized by macrophages, giving them a foamy appearance. Often a salivary duct can be seen entering the cyst. The sialomucin stains positively with the PAS reaction and is diastase-resistant. The alcian blue stain is positive at pH 2.5 but negative at pH 4.0. The material is not metachromatic with the toluidine blue stain. It is resistant to digestion with hyaluronidase but is removed with sialidase.

Cutaneous Focal Mucinosis

Cutaneous focal mucinosis or cutaneous myxoma occurs as a solitary asymptomatic nodule on the head, trunk, or extremities.[179] There is no association with systemic disease and surgical excision is curative.

The epidermis is effaced by a nonencapsulated collection of mucin within the upper dermis and middermis. The mucinous area is pale staining and contains fusiform and stellate fibroblasts. Mucin that has not been removed during processing has a pale blue, wispy or stringy appearance. The histologic appearance is similar to that of a digital mucous cyst except that there is less tendency to form a sharply circumscribed cystic space with retraction of the mucin from the surrounding connective tissue. The mucin is hyaluronic acid and stains with special stains as described for pretibial myxedema.

Follicular Mucinosis

Follicular mucinosis or *alopecia mucinosa* occurs mainly on the face, neck, and upper trunk and is characterized by grouped follicular papules or red, raised, boggy plaques.[180] Alopecia is not obvious if the eruption occurs on glabrous skin. About 20 percent of cases of follicular mucinosis are associated with an underlying lymphoma, most often mycosis fungoides. Follicular mucinosis that is not associated with mycosis fungoides usually resolves in two months to two years.[181]

The epithelium of hair follicles appears greatly thickened and infiltrated by a pale-staining, bluish, wispy material (Fig. 8-61). Large cystic spaces often develop within the follicular epithelium. Fusiform cells are seen in the follicular epithelium. The mucin is hyaluronic acid and stains in a manner similar to that described for pretibial myxedema. In cases of follicular mucinosis associated with lymphoma, atypical cells are present within the surrounding dermis. In mycosis fungoides, Pautrier's microabscesses are often present within the epidermis associated with a bandlike dermal infiltrate of atypical mononuclear cells and a variable number of eosinophils.

Calcinosis Cutis

Dystrophic Calcification

In dystrophic calcification, the serum calcium and phosphorus levels are normal, and the calcification oc-

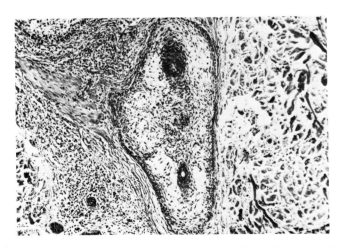

Fig. 8-61. Follicular mucinosis. The epithelium of a hair follicle shows pale-staining areas of mucin deposition associated with fusiform cells.

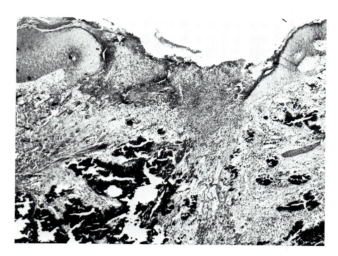

Fig. 8-62. Dystrophic calcification. Dark-staining deposits of calcium are being eliminated from the skin through an ulcerated epidermis.

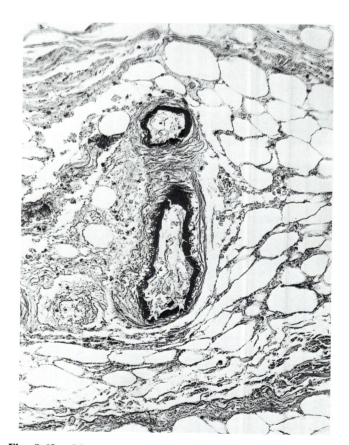

Fig. 8-63. Metastatic calcification. Blood vessels within the subcutaneous fat show large amounts of calcium within their media.

curs secondary to previous tissue damage. Scleroderma, dermatomyositis,[182] granulomatous inflammation, and subcutaneous fat necrosis are often associated with dystrophic calcification.

Irregular deposits of a granular basophilic material are present in the dermis or subcutaneous fat (Fig. 8-62). Granulomatous inflammation may be present around some calcium particles.

Metastatic Calcification

The serum calcium and/or phosphorus levels are elevated and their product is usually over 80. Metastatic calcification may be associated with primary hyperparathyroidism, hypervitaminosis D, the milk alkali syndrome, osteomyelitis, metastatic carcinoma to bone, and renal failure with secondary hyperpparathyroidism.[183] Massive calcium deposits within blood vessels of the extremities may be visible on radiographs. In renal failure with secondary hyperparathyroidism, the deposits of calcium within the media of vessels may be associated with extensive areas of skin necrosis.[184] In patients with metastatic calcification, the vessels of the kidneys, lungs, and spleen are involved more often than the skin.

Calcium deposits are present within the media of dermal and subcutaneous blood vessels (Fig. 8-63). Focal collections of calcium may be present in the surrounding connective tissue. In cases associated with skin necrosis, the connective tissue is necrotic and amorphous.

Subepidermal Calcified Nodule

A solitary, hard, painless nodule on the face or extremities of a child is characteristic of a subepidermal calcified nodule. It has been suggested that this lesion represents dystrophic calcification in a pre-existing nevus or adnexal tumor. An elevated concentration of calcium in sweat has been reported.[185]

Focal collections of calcification within the upper dermis occur in nests resembling the pattern of a nevus. Occasionally, residual nuclei are visible within the calcified material. A foreign body granulomatous reaction may occur.

Scrotal Calcinosis

Solitary or multiple firm nodules of the scrotum are usually noted during the first or second decade of life. Clinically, the lesions resemble epidermoid cysts, which also occur on the scrotum.

Although originally considered idiopathic,[186] scrotal calcinosis appears to represent dystrophic calcification occurring in ruptured or in inflamed epidermoid cysts.[187]

INFLAMMATORY DISEASES OF THE SKIN

Several patients have now been observed showing both epidermoid cysts and scrotal calcification with transitions occurring between the two disorders.

Special Stains for Calcium

The von Kossa stain is often used to identify calcium; however, it is nonspecific since it stains carbonate and phosphate salts of calcium and other minerals. Uric acid may therefore stain with the von Kossa stain. Carbonate and phosphate salts stain black with the von Kossa stain. A more specific stain for calcium is the alizarin red stain, which stains calcium red or orange-red.

Gout

Gouty tophi occur on the fingers, toes, elbows, and ears. Large tophi may discharge a chalky white material. Tophi are radiolucent but may show secondary calcification.[188]

The epidermis may be normal or may show hyperkeratosis and acanthosis. Occasionally, the epidermis is ulcerated, and uric acid is discharged to the surface. Formalin fixation removes uric acid from the tissues and produces an amorphous pale-staining appearance in the areas of uric acid deposition (Fig. 8-64). Often, however, residual uric acid is present as gray-black, needle-shaped crystals that are present in circumscribed masses. The masses of uric acid are usually surrounded by a foreign-body granulomatous reaction. Uric acid crystals are brightly birefringent with polarized light. The von Kossa stain for carbonate and phosphate salts may be positive.

Xanthomas

Cutaneous xanthomas associated with hyperlipidemia may be due to an inherited defect of lipid metabolism.[189] More often, the lipid abnormality is secondary to another systemic disease such as diabetes mellitus, pancreatitis, nephrotic syndrome, hypothyroidism, or liver disease. Only about one third of the patients with *xanthelasma* have elevated serum lipids. *Eruptive xanthomas,* characterized by erythematous yellow papules that appear suddenly over the trunk and extremities, are consistently associated with hypertriglyceridemia.[190] *Plane xanthomas* are often seen with biliary cirrhosis. Diffuse normolipemic plane xanthomas may be a cutaneous sign of multiple myeloma.[191]

It is usually not possible to distinguish between the various types of xanthomas based on the histologic changes. The epidermis shows effacement of the rete ridge pattern by the dermal infiltrate, which contains many histiocytes with foamy cytoplasm (foam cells, xanthoma cells). The cytoplasm of the histiocytes is pale staining, increased in amount, and vacuolated due to the presence of numerous lipid droplets. Sudan black B, oil red O, scarlet red stains of frozen sections demonstrate that the cytoplasmic droplets are lipid. Xanthomas may contain a variable number of fibroblasts, lymphocytes, and multinucleate giant cells. An objective diagnosis of xanthelasma can often be made if the epidermis shows the delicate features of eyelid skin and striated muscle is present deep to the infiltrate of foamy histiocytes. Two features that should suggest the possibility of the eruptive form of xanthomas are the presence of a significant lymphocytic infiltrate and extracellular lipid (Fig. 8-65). The

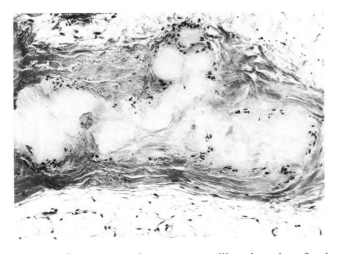

Fig. 8-64. Gout. Amorphous to crystalline deposits of uric acid are surrounded by epithelioid cells.

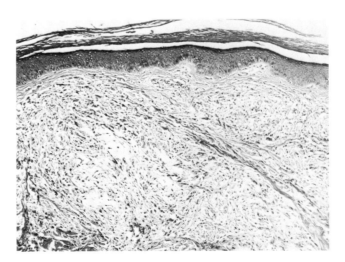

Fig. 8-65. Eruptive xanthoma. Small collections of extracellular lipid are associated with an infiltrate of lymphocytes and foamy histiocytes.

differential diagnosis of xanthomas includes lepromatous leprosy, solitary or eruptive histiocytomas,[192,193] juvenile xanthogranuloma, and histiocytosis X.

Subcutaneous Reaction Patterns

Panniculitis

Erythema Nodosum

Erythema nodosum is characterized by painful, tender nodules mainly on the anterior aspects of the lower legs.[194] Females are involved three times as often as males, and the 15- to 25-year-old age group is most commonly affected. The tender cutaneous nodules are often associated with prodromal symptoms of fever, arthralgia, or leg pain. The nodules rarely ulcerate and heal without scarring. Beta-hemolytic streptococcal infection and sarcoidosis are the most common causes of erythema nodosum in the United States, although in approximately 50 percent of cases there is no demonstrable cause. Deep fungal infections such as coccidioidomycosis and histoplasmosis are also causes of erythema nodosum. Drugs appear to be much less common causative agents than infection.

The epidermis and upper portions of the dermis are usually normal. Biopsy specimens of early lesions show lymphocytes and neutrophils in the interlobular septa of the subcutaneous fat. The walls of small veins may be thickened and surrounded by inflammatory cells, but true vasculitis is usually absent. In more mature lesions of erythema nodosum, the septa between fat lobules become greatly thickened with fibrous connective tissue. Lymphocytes, epithelioid cells, and multinucleate giant cells occur within the thickened septa. Lymphocytes and histiocytes predominate, and neutrophils are usually absent. The inflammatory process typically extends only for a short distance into the fat lobules. In late lesions, fibrosis of fat septa may occur with trapping of giant cells; however, there is no significant atrophy of fat lobules.

Subacute Nodular Migratory Panniculitis

Subacute nodular migratory panniculitis occurs mainly in women as nodules and plaques on the lower legs. Lesions persist for several years, and nodules may enlarge to form plaques.[195] The eruption is said to be unilateral more often than erythema nodosum.

The histologic changes in subacute nodular migratory panniculitis are essentially indistinguishable from erythema nodosum, and it is likely that the former is a chronic variant of erythema nodosum.[196]

Weber-Christian Disease

Weber-Christian disease or relapsing febrile nodular nonsuppurative panniculitis produces recurrent crops of nodules and plaques that may involve the trunk as well as the extremities. The nodules are tender and resemble abscesses. Individual lesions heal, leaving depressed scars.[197] Patients are ill with fever, malaise, and arthralgias. Inflammation of visceral fat may produce symptoms of an acute abdomen. Anemia, leukopenia, and focal liver necrosis have been reported.

Early lesions show infiltration of entire fat lobules predominantly with neutrophils, producing changes that resemble an acute infection (Fig. 8-66). Later, macrophages predominate and ingest fat from damaged lipocytes, producing abundant foamy cytoplasm.[198] Interlobular septa are generally intact. In late stages, the fat lobules may be replaced by fibrous tissue. Blood vessels within the subcutaneous fat show thickening of their walls and are surrounded by patchy infiltrates of lymphocytes. A few multincleate giant cells may be present.

Erthema Induratum

Erythema induratum is a rare form of panniculitis that produces inflammatory nodules on the calves. The nodules tend to break down and drain puruient material. Erythema induratum is considered a form of cutaneous tuberculosis in which *Mycobacterium tuberculosis* or its products disseminate during transient bacteremia to areas of vascular stasis.[199] Evidence of previous pulmonary tuberculosis may be present, but most patients do not have clinically active disease. Delayed skin test reactions to mycobacterial antigens are positive. The term *nodular*

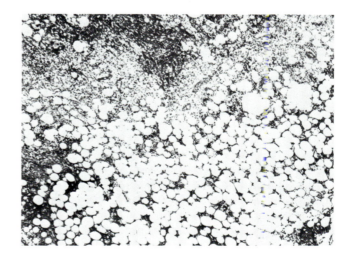

Fig. 8-66. Weber-Christian disease. Panlobular infiltrate of inflammatory cells surrounds individual lipocytes.

vasculitis has been suggested for those cases in which there is no evidence of tuberculosis.[200]

The epidermis and upper dermis are often normal. A granulomatous infiltrate containing lymphocytes, histiocytes, epithelioid cells, and giant cells extends into fat lobules and replaces subcutaneous fat. Distinct tubercles may be present. There are focal areas of caseation necrosis and vascular changes characterized by vessel wall thickening, fibrinoid necrosis, and vascular inflammation. Some veins and venules may be surrounded by granulomatous inflammation.

Subcutaneous Fat Necrosis of the Newborn

Otherwise healthy infants of either sex may be affected during the neonatal period by subcutaneous fat necrosis.[201] Deep-seated nodules and plaques involve the back, cheeks, arms, thighs, and buttocks.[202] Some lesions are movable and have sharply defined margins. Several cases of subcutaneous fat necrosis have been associated with hypercalcemia.[203]

The epidermis and upper dermis are normal. Basophilic areas of fat necrosis are associated with the presence of needlelike crystals within fat cells. When clusters of fat cells are involved, the crystals have a radial arrangement. The fat is infiltrated by lymphocytes, histiocytes, epithelioid cells, and multinucleate giant cells. Interlobular septa are often thickened, and deposits of calcium occur within the fat lobules. In frozen sections, the crystals within fat cells are seen to be doubly refractile by polarized light examination. The von Kossa stain may be helpful in demonstrating the presence of calcium deposits.

Sclerema Neonatorum

This uncommon disorder affects premature or debilitated infants within the first few days of life. The skin is smooth, cool, tense, hard, and purplish. Firm induration of the skin begins on the thighs and legs but may involve the entire body except for the palms, soles, and scrotum.[204] Body movement and respiration may be hindered, and infants frequently develop pneumonia. In the past, up to 75 percent of infants with this disorder died; however, preventing a reduction in body temperature by using heated incubators for premature infants may prevent sclerema neonatorum.

The histologic changes in the fat in sclerema neonatorum are similar to subcutaneous fat necrosis of the newborn except that fat necrosis is minimal or absent. Clusters of fat cells are filled with needle-like clefts, which on frozen section are shown to be occupied by doubly refractile crystals. The crystals do not stain with fat stains. Interconnecting bands of fibrous tissue and focal collections of mononuclear inflammatory cells are seen in the fat. Calcium deposits are usually absent in sclerema neonatorum.

Pancreatic Fat Necrosis

Pancreatitis or pancreatic carcinoma may result in elevated levels of serum lipase with the resulting breakdown of fat in the skin, joints, and viscera. Tender nodules and plaques on the lower extremities tend to break down and drain an oily material. Polyarthritis, pleural effusions, and abdominal pain may result from widespread inflammation of fat.[205]

The subcutaneous fat shows focal areas of fat necrosis associated with the presence of ghost-like fat cells with thickened walls and no nuclei.[206] The basophilic areas of fat necrosis often contain calcium granules. The areas of fat necrosis may contain extravasated RBC, as well as a polymorphic infiltrate of neutrophils, lymphocytes, histiocytes, and foreign body giant cells.

Lupus Panniculitis

Unlike the other forms of panniculitis, lupus panniculitis (lupus profundus) shows a predilection for the face, upper arms, and buttocks.[207] Most cases are associated with systemic lupus erythematosus, although cases associated with discoid lupus erythematosus also occur. Cutaneous lesions may be preceded by trauma. The skin overlying the inflammatory nodules and plaques may be normal or show scaly atrophic lesions characteristic of discoid lupus erythematosus. Nodules that resolve leave clinically depressed areas in the skin secondary to atrophy of subcutaneous fat.

The epidermis may be normal or may show changes of discoid lupus erythematosus, which include hyperkeratosis, follicular plugging, and atrophy of the epidermis. Liquefaction degeneration of the basal zone is associated with melanin pigment incontinence and the presence of colloid bodies within the epidermis or superficial dermis. A patchy infiltrate of lymphocytes surrounds small dermal blood vessels and pilosebaceous structures. Two patterns of inflammation are seen in the subcutaneous fat. Early lesions may show only a dense patchy infiltrate of lymphocytes surrounding blood vessels in the deep dermis and upper subcutaneous fat. More advanced lesions show necrosis of fat lobules with replacement by eosinophilic hyalinized connective tissue (Fig. 8-67). The hyalinized connective tissue may run in thick bands that tend to be oriented parallel to the surface of the skin. Inflamed vessels are seen within the subcutaneous fat, and a variable number of plasma cells are present. Immunofluorescence microscopy often shows the deposition of immunoglobulins and complement in a granular pattern along the basement membrane zone.

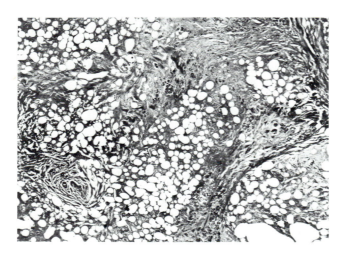

Fig. 8-67. Lupus erythematosus panniculitis. Panlobular infiltrate of inflammatory cells is associated with hyalinization of connective tissue and replacement of fat lobules.

Scleroderma

Localized scleroderma or *morphea* characteristically produces indurated erythematous to hyperpigmented plaques on the trunk.[208] Plaques are often surrounded by an erythematous, purple border. In systemic scleroderma, the indurated skin is not well circumscribed as in morphea and more often involves the face and acral portions of the extremities.[209] The skin over the fingers appears shiny and smooth, and there may be ulcerations of the fingertips. Cutaneous telangiectasia and calcium deposits occur. Sclerosis of the esophagus causes difficulty in swallowing, and there may be involvement of the GI tract, lungs, and kidneys with malabsorption, dyspnea, and uremia.

The most characteristic changes in the subcutaneous fat occur in morphea. Dense patches of lymphocytes occur around small vessels and eccrine sweat glands at the dermal-subcutaneous junction. In later lesions of morphea and in systemic scleroderma, the inflammatory infiltrate is mild, and the upper subcutaneous fat is replaced by dense fibrous connective tissue, which surrounds and entraps eccrine sweat glands.[210] The normal layer of fat around sweat glands is absent. The connective tissue deep to the sweat glands may stain pale pink with the H & E stain, suggesting new collagen. Hair follicles are often destroyed, and the overall thickness of the dermis appears increased. The dermal collagen appears compact and homogeneous with few spaces between collagen fibers. Electron microscopic examination of the deep dermis reveals active fibroblasts and an increased percentage of young collagen fibrils.[211] The young collagen fibrils show less of a tendency to be oriented parallel to the surface of the skin than the more mature collagen of the reticular dermis.

Factitial Panniculitis

Factitial panniculitis may result from mechanical trauma, thermal injuries, or injection of foreign material into the subcutaneous fat.[212] Although any part of the body may be involved, bizarre cases of inflammation of the fat of breasts and genitalia should raise suspicion of factitial panniculitis. Foreign material such as milk, paraffin oil, drugs, and paint have been injected.

Inflammation within fat lobules may show a mixture of abscesses containing neutrophils associated with areas of granulomatous inflammation. The presence of foreign material in the subcutaneous fat is diagnostic but may be difficult to document. Polarized light examination should be used in all cases of undiagnosed panniculitis.[212] Collections of calcium may be seen in the subcutaneous fat with the von Kossa stain. Paraffin oil injected into the skin shows numerous clear vacuoles with the appearance of Swiss cheese. A mixed inflammatory infiltrate may surround individual vacuoles. The oil is dissolved from the vacuoles during processing. Sclerosis of connective tissue associated with the oil vacuoles produces a reaction pattern referred to as *sclerosing lipogranuloma*[213] (Fig. 8-68). Drugs such as pentazocine are particularly likely to produce sclerosis of subcutaneous fat.

Differential Diagnosis of Panniculitis

There is considerable overlap in the histologic changes seen in panniculitis, and a specific diagnosis cannot be made in many cases. It is helpful to subclassify panniculitis into septal panniculitis and lobular panniculitis. Septal panniculitis is exemplified by erythema nodosum, by far the most common cause of panniculitis, and subacute

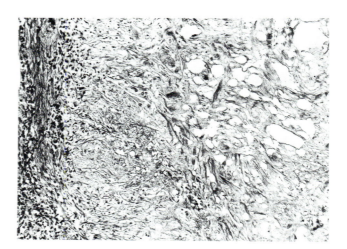

Fig. 8-68. Sclerosing lipogranuloma. Empty vacuoles from which an oily material has been dissolved during processing are associated with hyalinization of connective tissue and a granulomatous infiltrate.

INFLAMMATORY DISEASES OF THE SKIN

nodular migratory panniculitis, which may be a variant of erythema nodosum. The other forms of panniculitis discussed in the previous sections are lobular. Lobular panniculitis often results in replacement of fat cells with clinical atrophy. Many cases initially diagnosed as Weber-Christian disease have been found to be factitial panniculitis,[214] so a careful search for foreign material and polarized light examination should be a part of the evaluation of every case of panniculitis. In some cases, a descriptive diagnosis such as lobular panniculitis with granulomatous inflammation may be the most specific diagnosis that can be made. *Superficial migratory thrombophlebitis* may mimic panniculitis but shows an inflammatory infiltrate within the wall of a large vein at the border of the dermis and subcutaneous fat.[200] The lumen of the vessel is often filled with thrombus.

Fasciitis

Fasciitis with eosinophilia (Shulman syndrome) is characterized by the sudden onset of edema and induration of the skin of the hands, arms, and legs with sparing of the face and fingers.[215] The skin changes are often

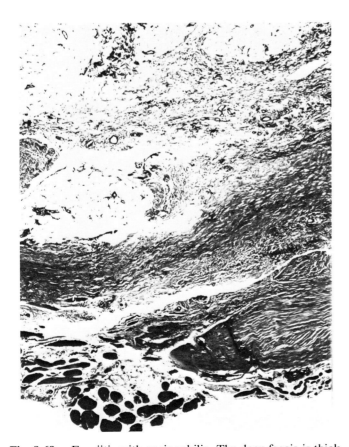

Fig. 8-69. Fasciitis with eosinophilia. The deep fascia is thickened and contains a sparse infiltrate of mononuclear cells.

preceded by some form of strenuous physical exercise. The involved skin often has a cobblestoned or dimpled appearance and cannot be mobilized. The skin may show pigmentary changes and loss of hair. Associated clinical findings include an increased number of circulating eosinophils, an elevated erythrocyte sedimentation rate, and hypergammaglobulinemia.

Skin biopsies in fasciitis with eosinophilia should be deep enough to include the full thickness of the subcutaneous fat and deep fascia. A patchy infiltrate of lymphocytes, histiocytes, and plasma cells may be present at the junction of the deep dermis and subcutaneous fat. In 15 to 20 percent of cases, there is fibrosis of the deep dermis beneath the level of eccrine sweat glands similar to that seen in scleroderma. The most typical histologic changes are a marked thickening of the deep fascia and infiltration of the fascia with lymphocytes, histiocytes, and a variable number of plasma cells[215] (Fig. 8-69). In less than half the cases, a few eosinophils are present in the fascia. The thickened fascia tends to replace the overlying subcutaneous fat.

Differential Diagnosis of Fasciitis

Fasciitis with eosinophilia is generally considered a variant of scleroderma. At least 50 percent of deep biopsy specimens of scleroderma also show thickening of the subcutaneous fascia.[216]

GLOSSARY OF TERMS

Only the most commonly used pathologic terms in dermatopathology will be defined.

- *Acantholysis:* Loss of cohesion of cells of the malpighian layer. The rupture of desmosomes connecting epidermal cells results in intraepidermal vesicles.
- *Acanthosis:* Increased thickness of the malpighian layer.
- *Adnexal structures:* The pilosebaceous units, eccrine sweat glands, and apocrine sweat glands. Also known collectively as adnexa or appendages.
- *Apoptosis:* A distinctive mode of cell death that typically affects individual epithelial cells and does not evoke an inflammatory response. The colloid bodies of lichen planus and lupus erythematosus are apoptotic bodies.[217]
- *Basement membrane zone:* A narrow zone present immediately deep to the epidermal basal cells, which is visible by light microscopy using the periodic acid-Schiff reaction. The basement membrane zone is not identical to the basal lamina, which is visible by electron microscopy.

- *Bulla:* A cavity or blister within or beneath the epidermis. A bulla smaller than 5 mm in diameter is called a vesicle.
- *Colloid bodies:* Deeply eosinophilic, round to oval bodies within the epidermis or the superficial dermis. Most, if not all, colloid bodies appear to result from the degeneration of epidermal cells. Synonyms include hyaline bodies, eosinophilic bodies, and Civatte bodies.
- *Crust:* Tissue fluid that has coagulated on the skin surface. Most often seen in acute inflammatory diseases.
- *Dyskeratosis:* Abnormal keratinization of squamous cells. May occur as individual cell dyskeratosis or dyskeratosis of groups of cells. Seen in inflammatory diseases and in benign or malignant tumors.
- *Exocytosis:* The migration of inflammatory cells into the epidermis.
- *Festooning:* The projection of prominent dermal papillae into the base of a subepidermal bulla cavity.
- *Follicular plugging:* The occlusion and dilatation of the openings of hair follicles by increased amounts of keratin.
- *Grenz zone:* A marginal zone of uninvolved connective tissue that often separates the epidermis or the adnexa from an inflammatory or infiltrative process.
- *Hyperkeratosis:* Thickening of the stratum corneum.
- *Liquefaction degeneration:* Degeneration of the basal cells and the basement membrane zone with the formation of clear vacuoles. Also called hydropic degeneration.
- *Microabscesses:* Small abscesses within the epidermis that are not visible grossly. Munro's microabscesses of psoriasis contain pyknotic neutrophils and most often occur in the keratin layer. Spongiotic microabscess characteristic of acute dermatitis occurs within the malpighian layer due to intercellular edema. Pautrier's microabscesses of mycosis fungoides are sharply circumscribed spaces within the malpighian layer containing atypical mononuclear cells.
- *Necrobiosis:* An alteration of dermal collagen characterized by basophilia and incomplete necrosis so the fibrillar nature of the connective tissue may still be appreciated. Necrobiosis differs from caseation necrosis, which produces more complete tissue death and in which the necrotic tissue appears amorphous. A third form of cell death, apoptosis, usually affects individual epithelial cells and results in the formation of colloid bodies.
- *Papillomatosis:* Irregular undulation of the outer surface of the epidermis produced by outward projection of epidermis and associated connective tissue.
- *Parakeratosis:* Retention of nuclei within the stratum corneum.
- *Pigmentary incontinence:* A displacement of melanin pigment from the basal cell layer into dermal macrophages or into the connective tissue of the superficial dermis. It follows liquefaction degeneration or other alteration of the basement membrane zone.
- *Pseudoepitheliomatous hyperplasia:* Marked reactive proliferation of epidermis mimicking carcinoma.
- *Pustule:* An intraepidermal or subepidermal cavity containing neutrophils. May result from secondary changes in a pre-existing bulla.
- *Pyknosis:* Shrinkage of nuclei.
- *Spongiosis:* Edema occurring between epidermal cells that may progress to spongiotic microabscesses and bullae.
- *Villi:* Elongated dermal papillae that project into the floor of a bulla cavity and are covered by a single layer of basal cells.

REFERENCES

1. Katz SI: The role of Langerhans' cells in immunity. Arch Dermatol 116:1361, 1980
2. Fisher JP, Cooke RA: Experimental toxic and allergic contact dermatitis. II. A histopathologic study. J Allergy 29:411, 1958
3. Bunch LW, Tilley JC: Pityriasis rosea. Arch Dermatol 84:79, 1961
4. Walzer RA: Autoimmunity and cutaneous disease. Med Clin North Am 49:769, 1965
5. Whitfield A: Lumelian lectures on some points in the aetiology of skin diseases. Lancet 2:122, 1921
6. Young E: Dyshidrotic (endogenous) eczema. Dermatologica 129:306, 1964
7. Graham JH: Superficial fungal infections. p. 137. In Graham JH, Johnson WC, Helwig EB (eds): Dermal Pathology. Harper & Row, Hagerstown, MD, 1972
8. Wiklund DA, Weston WL: Incontinentia pigmenti: A four-generation study. Arch Dermatol 116:701, 1980
9. Carney RG Jr: Incontinentia pigmenti: A world statistical analysis. Arch Dermatol 112:535, 1976
10. Knight AG, Black MM, Delaney TJ: Eosinophilic spongiosis: A clinical, histological, and immunofluorescent correlation. Clin Exp Dermatol 1:141, 1976
11. Emmerson RW, Wilson-Jones E: Eosinophilic spongiosis in pemphigus. Arch Dermatol 97:252, 1968
12. Pinkus H: Psoriasiform tissue reactions. Aust J Dermatol 8:31, 1965
13. Pinkus H, Mehregan AH: A Guide to Dermatohistopathology. Appleton & Lange, E. Norwalk, CT, 1976, p. 125
14. Crám DL: Psoriasis: Current advances in etiology and treatment. J Am Acad Dermatol 4:1, 1981
15. Abrahams J, McCarthy JT, Sander SL: 101 cases of exfoliative dermatitis. Arch Dermatol 87:96, 1963
16. Weinstein GD, Van Scott EJ: Autoradiographic analysis of turnover times of normal and psoriatic epidermis. J Invest Dermatol 45:257, 1965
17. Weinstein GD, Frost P: Abnormal cell proliferation in psoriasis. J Invest Dermatol 50:254, 1968

18. Barber HW: Acrodermatitis continua vel perstans (dermatitis repens) and psoriasis pustulosa. Br J Dermatol 42:500, 1930
19. Baker H, Ryan TJ: Generalized pustular psoriasis: A clinical and epidemiological study of 104 cases. Br J Dermatol 80:771, 1968
20. Gordon M, Johnson WC: Histopathology and histochemistry of psoriasis. I. The active lesion and clinically normal skin. Arch Dermatol 95:402, 1967
21. Cox AJ, Watson W: Histologic variations in lesions of psoriasis. Arch Dermatol 106:503, 1972
22. Engleman EP, Weber HM: Reiter's syndrome. Clin Orthop 57:19, 1968
23. Weinberger HJ, Ropes MW, Kulka JP, et al: Reiter's syndrome—Clinical and pathological observations: A long-term study of 16 cases. Medicine (Baltimore) 41:35, 1962
24. Kulka JP: The lesions of Reiter's syndrome. Arthritis Rheum 5:195, 1962
25. Pindborg GR, Gorlin RJ, Asboe-Hansen G: Reiter's syndrome. Oral Surg 16:551, 1963
26. Pinkus H, Mehregan AH: The primary histologic lesion of seborrheic dermatitis and psoriasis. J Invest Dermatol 46:109, 1966
27. Gross DA, Landau JW, Newcomer VD: Pityriasis rubra pilaris: Report of a case and analysis of the literature. Arch Dermatol 99:710, 1969
28. Porter D, Shuster S: Epidermal renewal and amino acids in psoriasis and pityriasis rubra pilaris. Arch Dermatol 98:339, 1968
29. Davidson CL Jr, Winkelmann RK, Kierland RR: Pityriasis rubra pilaris: A followup study of 57 patients. Arch Dermatol 100:175, 1969
30. Shaffer B, Beerman H: Lichen simplex chronicus and its variants. Arch Dermatol Syph 64:340, 1951
31. Pinkus H: Lichenoid tissue reactions: A speculative review of the clinical spectrum of epidermal basal cell damage with special reference to erythema dyschromicum perstans. Arch Dermatol 107:840, 1973
32. Pinkus H, Mehregan AH: A Guide to Dermatohistopathology. Appleton & Lange, East Norwalk, CT, 1976, p. 141
33. Fellner MJ: Lichen planus. Int J Dermatol 19:71, 1980
34. Altman J, Perry HO: The variations and course of lichen planus. Arch Dermatol 84:47, 1961
35. Samman PD: Lichen planus: An analysis of 200 cases. Trans St Johns Hosp Dermatol Soc 46:36, 1961
36. Tompkins JK: Lichen planus: A statistical study of 41 cases. Arch Dermatol 71:515, 1955
37. Haber H, Sarkany I: Hypertrophic lichen planus and lichen simplex. Trans St Johns Hosp Dermatol Soc 41:61, 1958
38. Shklar G: Erosive and bullous oral lesions of lichen planus. Arch Dermatol 97:411, 1968
39. Cram DL, Kierland RR, Winkelmann RK: Ulcerative lichen planus of the feet. Arch Dermatol 93:692, 1966
40. Black MM: What is going on in lichen planus? Clin Exp Dermatol 2:303, 1977
41. Pennys NS, Ackerman AB, Gottlieb NL: Gold dermatitis. Arch Dermatol 109:372, 1974
42. Baer RL, Harber LC: Photobiology of lupus erythematosus. Arch Dermatol 92:124, 1965
43. Prystowsky SD, Herndon JH Jr, Gillian JN: Chronic cutaneous lupus erythematosus: A clinical and laboratory investigation of 80 patients. Medicine (Baltimore) 55:183, 1976
44. Tuffanelli DL, Dubois EL: Cutaneous manifestations of systemic lupus erythematosus. Arch Dermatol 90:377, 1964
45. Tuffanelli DL, Kay D, Fukuyama K: Dermal-epidermal junction in lupus erythematosus. Arch Dermatol 99:652, 1969
46. Weiss RM, Cohen AD: Lichen nitidus of the palms and soles. Arch Dermatol 104:538, 1971
47. Jeerapaet P, Ackerman AB: Histologic patterns of secondary syphilis. Arch Dermatol 107:373, 1973
48. Goette DK: Benign lichenoid keratosis. Arch Dermatol 116:780, 1980
49. Lumpkin LR, Helwig EB: Solitary lichen planus. Arch Dermatol 93:54, 1966
50. Abramovits W, Landau JW, Lowe NJ: A report of two patients with lichen aureus. Arch Dermatol 116:1183, 1980
51. Krüger GRF, Berard CW, DeLellis RA, et al: Graft-versus-host disease: Morphologic variation and differential diagnosis in 8 cases of HL-A matched bone marrow transplantation. Am J Pathol 63:179, 1971
52. Wolf DJ, Selmanowitz VJ: Poikiloderma vasculare atrophicans. Cancer 25:682, 1970
53. Janis JF, Winkelmann RK: Histopathology of the skin in dermatomyositis. Arch Dermatol 97:640, 1968
54. Wayte DM, Helwig EB: Halo nevi. Cancer 22:69, 1968
55. Bergfeld WF, Lesowitz SA: Lichen sclerosus et atrophicus. Arch Dermatol 101:247, 1970
56. Dajani AS, Ferrieri P, Wanamaker L: Endemic superficial pyoderma in children. Arch Dermatol 108:517, 1973
57. Kaplan EL, Anthony BF, Chapman SS, et al: Epidemic acute glomerlonephritis associated with type 49 streptococcal pyoderma. Am J Med 48:9, 1970
58. Lowney ED, Baublis JV, Kreye GM, et al: The scalded skin syndrome in small children. Arch Dermatol 95:359, 1967
59. Melish ME, Glasgow LA: The staphylococcal scalded-skin syndrome. N Engl J Med 282:1114, 1970
60. Levine J, Nooden CW: Staphylococcal scalded-skin syndrome in an adult. N Engl J Med 287:1339, 1972
61. Rothenberg R, Renna FS, Drew TM, et al: Staphylococcal scalded skin syndrome in an adult. Arch Dermatol 108:408, 1973
62. Elias PM, Fritsch P, Epstein EH Jr: Staphylococcal scalded skin syndrome. Clinical features, pathogenesis, and recent microbiological and biochemical developments. Arch Dermatol 113:207, 1977
63. Bean SF, Lynch FW: Senear-Usher syndrome (pemphigus erythematosus). Arch Dermatol 101:642, 1970
64. Perry HO: Pemphigus foliaceus. Arch Dermatol 83:52, 1961
65. Furtado TA: Histopathology of pemphigus foliaceus. Arch Dermatol 80:66, 1959
66. Chorzelski T, Jablonska S, Blaszczyk M: Immunopatho-

logical investigation in Senear-Usher syndrome (coexistence of pemphigus and lupus erythematosus). Br J Dermatol 80:211, 1968

67. Callen JP: Internal disorders associated with bullous disease of the skin. J Am Acad Dermatol 3:107, 1980

68. Lever WF: Pemphigus and Pemphigoid. Charles C Thomas, Springfield, IL, 1965

69. Lever WF: Pemphigus and pemphigoid. A review of the advances made since 1964. J Am Acad Dermatol 1:2, 1979

70. Palmer DD, Perry HO: Benign familial chronic pemphigus. Arch Dermatol 86:493, 1962

71. Gottlieb SK, Lutzner MA: Darier's disease. Arch Dermatol 107:225, 1973

72. Weathers DR, Olansky S, Sharpe LO: Darier's disease with mucous membrane involvement. Arch Dermatol 100:50, 1969

73. Szymanski FJ: Warty dyskeratoma. Arch Dermatol 75:567, 1957

74. Tanay A, Mehregan AH: Warty dyskeratoma. Dermatologica 138:155, 1969

75. Grover RW: Transient acantholytic dermatosis. Arch Dermatol 101:426, 1970

76. Grover RW: Transient acantholytic dermatosis. Arch Dermatol 104:26, 1971

77. Chalet M, Grover R, Ackerman AB: Transient acantholytic dermatosis. Arch Dermatol 113:431, 1977

78. McSorley HE, Shapiro L, Brownstein MH, et al: Herpes simplex and varicella-zoster: Comparative histopathology of 77 cases. Int J Dermatol 13:69, 1974

79. Pinkus H, Mehregan AH: A Guide to Dermatohistopathology. Appleton & Lange, East Norwalk, CT, 1976, p. 502

80. Gruber GG, Owen LG, Callen JP: Vesicular pemphigoid. J Am Acad Dermatol 3:619, 1980

81. Eng AM, Moncada B: Bullous pemphigoid and dermatitis herpetiformis: Histopathologic differentiation of bullous pemphigoid and dermatitis herpetiformis. Arch Dermatol 110:51, 1978

82. Cannell H, Churcher GM, Milton-Thompson GJ: Stevens-Johnson syndrome associated with Mycoplasma pneumoniae infection. Br J Dermatol 81:196, 1969

83. Howland WW, Golitz LE, Huff JC, Weston WL: Erythema multiforme: Clinical, histopathologic and immunologic study. J Am Acad Dermatol 10:438, 1984

84. Orfanos CE, Schaumburg-Lever G, Lever WF: Dermal and epidermal types of erythema multiforme. Arch Dermatol 109:682, 1974

85. Ackerman AB, Pennys NS, Clark WH: Erythema multiforme exudativum: Distinctive pathological process. Br J Dermatol 84:554, 1971

86. Pinkus H, Mehregan AH: A Guide to Dermatohistopathology. Appleton & Lange, East Norwalk, CT, 1976, p. 160

87. Kazmierowski JA, Wuepper KD: Erythema multiforme: Immune complex vasculitis of the superficial cutaneous microvasculature. J Invest Dermatol 71:366, 1978

88. Alexander JOD: Dermatitis Herpetiformis. WB Saunders, London, 1975

89. Fry L, Seah PP, Riches DJ, et al: Clearance of skin lesions in dermatitis herpetiformis after gluten withdrawal. Lancet 1:288, 1973

90. Katz SI, Strober W: The pathogenesis of dermatitis herpetiformis. J Invest Dermatol 70:63, 1978

91. Yaoita H, Katz SI: Circulating IgA anti-basement membrane zone antibodies in dermatitis herpetiformis. J Invest Dermatol 69:558, 1977

92. Chorzelski TP, Jablonska S: IgA linear dermatosis of childhood (chronic bullous disease of childhood). Br J Dermatol 101:535, 1979

93. Epstein JH, Tuffanelli DL, Epstein WL: Cutaneous changes in the porphyrias. Arch Dermatol 107:689, 1973

94. Elder GH, Lee GB, Tovery JA: Decreased activity of hepatic uroporphyrinogen decarboxylase in sporadic porphyria cutanea tarda. N Engl J Med 299:274, 1978

95. Bauer EA, Briggaman RA: The mechanobullous diseases (epidermolysis bullosa). p. 334. In Fitzpatrick TB, Eisen AZ, Freedberg IM, et al. (eds): Dermatology in General Medicine. McGraw-Hill, New York, 1979

96. Schuman BM, Arciniegas E: The management of esophageal complications of epidermolysis bullosa. Am J Dig Dis 17:875, 1972

97. Reed WB, College J Jr, Frances MJO, et al: Epidermolysis bullosa dystrophica with epidermal neoplasms. Arch Dermatol 110:894, 1974

98. Bruggaman RA, Wheeler CE: Epidermolysis bullosa dystrophica—recessive: A possible role of anchoring fibrils in the pathogenesis. J Invest Dermatol 65:203, 1975

99. Haneke E, Anton-Lamprecht I: Ultrastructure of blister formation in epidermolysis bullosa hereditaria: V. Epidermolysis bullosa simplex localisata type Weber-Cockayne. J Invest Dermatol 78:219, 1982

100. Bean SF: Cicatricial pemphigoid. Arch Dermatol 110:552, 1974

101. Harrington CI, Bleehen SS: Herpes gestationis: Immunopathologic and ultrastructural studies. Br J Dermatol 100:389, 1979

102. Ackerman AB: Histologic Diagnosis of Inflammatory Skin Diseases. Lea & Febiger, Philadelphia, 1978

103. Monroe EW, Jones HE: Urticaria. Arch Dermatol 113:80, 1977

104. Shelley WB: Erythema annulare centrifrigum due to Candida albicans. Br J Dermatol 77:383, 1965

105. Scrimenti RJ: Erythema chronicum migrans. Arch Dermatol 102:104, 1970

106. Mast WE, Burrows WM: Erythema chronicum migrans in the United States. JAMA 236:859, 1976

107. Hardin JA, Steere AC, Malawista SE: Immune complexes and the evolution of Lyme arthritis. N Engl J Med 301:1358, 1979

108. Thompson J, Stankler L: Erythema gyratum repens: Reports of two further cases associated with carcinoma. Br J Dermatol 82:406, 1970

109. Epstein JH: Polymorphous light eruption. J Am Acad Dermatol 3:329, 1980

110. Jansén CT: The natural history of polymorphous light eruptions. Arch Dermatol 115:165, 1979

111. Fine J: Mastocytosis. Int J Dermatol 19:117, 1980

112. Gottlieb B, Winkelmann RK: Lymphocytic infiltration of the skin. Arch Dermatol 86:626, 1962

113. Sams WM Jr: Necrotizing vasculitis. J Am Acad Dermatol 3:1, 1980
114. Haber H: Erythema elevatum diutinum. Br J Dermatol 67:121, 1955
115. Laymon CW: Erythema elevatum diutinum: A type of allergic vasculitis. Arch Dermatol 85:62, 1962
116. Ackerman AB: Hemorrhagic bullae in gonococcemia. New Engl J Med 282:793, 1970
117. Morgaretten W, Nakai H, Landing BH: Significance of selective vasculitis and the ''bone marrow'' syndrome in pseudomonas septicemia. N Engl J Med 265:773, 1961
118. Diaz-Perez JL, Winkelmann RK: Cutaneous periarteritis nodosa. Arch Dermatol 110:407, 1974
119. Michalak T: Immune complexes hepatitis B surface antigen in the pathogenesis of periarteritis nodosa. Am J Pathol 90:619, 1978
120. Szymanski FJ: Pityriasis lichenoides et varioliformis acuta. Arch Dermatol 79:7, 1959
121. Churg J, Strauss L: Allergic granulomatosis, allergic angiitis, and periarteritis nodosa. Am J Pathol 27:277, 1951
122. Sokolov RA, Rachmaninoff N, Kaine HD: Allergic granulomatosis. Am J Med 32:131, 1962
123. Strauss L, Churg J, Zak FG: Cutaneous lesions of allergic granulomatosis. J Invest Dermatol 17:349, 1951
124. Fauci AS, Wolff SM: Wegener's granulomatosis: Studies in eighteen patients and a review of the literature. Medicine (Baltimore) 52:535, 1973
125. Reed WB, Jensen AK, Konwaler BE, et al: The cutaneous manifestations in Wegener's granulomatosis. Acta Dermatoven 43:250, 1963
126. Hamilton CR Jr, Shelley WM, Tumulty PA: Giant cell arteritis: Including temporal arteritis and polymyalgica rheumatica. Medicine 50:1, 1971
127. Barefoot SW, Lund HZ: Temporal (giant-cell) arteritis associated with ulcerations of the scalp. Arch Dermatol 93:79,1966
128. Pedace FJ, Perry HO: Granuloma faciale: A clinical and histopathologic review. Arch Dermatol 94:387, 1966
129. Sweet RD: An acute febrile dermatosis. Br J Dermatol 76:349, 1964
130. Goldman GC, Moschella SL: Acute febrile neutrophilic dermatosis (Sweet's syndrome). Arch Dermatol 103:654, 1971
131. Bard IW, Winkelman RK: Livedo vasculitis. Arch Dermatol 96:489, 1967
132. Dicken CH, Carrington SG, Winkelmann RK: Generalized granuloma annulare. Arch Dermatol 99:556, 1969
133. Owens DW, Freeman RG: Perforating granuloma annulare. Arch Dermatol 103:64, 1971
134. Rubin M, Lynch FW: Subcutaneous granuloma annulare. Arch Dermatol 93:416, 1966
135. Dahl MV, Ullman S, Goltz RW: Vasculitis in granuloma annulare: Histopathology and direct immunofluorescence. Arch Dermatol 113:463, 1977
136. Muller SA, Winkelmann RK: Necrobiosis lipoidica diabeticorum. Arch Dermatol 93:272, 1966
137. Duboid EL, Friou GJ, Chandor S: Rheumatoid nodules and rheumatoid granulomas in systemic lupus erythematosus. JAMA 220:515, 1972
138. Draheim JH, Johnson LC, Helwig EB: A clinicopathologic analysis of ''rheumatoid'' nodules occurring in 54 children. Am J Pathol 35:678, 1959
139. Golitz LE, Shapiro L, Hurwitz E, et al: Cicatricial alopecia of sarcoidosis. Arch Dermatol 107:758, 1973
140. Azar HA, Lunardelli C: Collagen nature of asteroid bodies of giant cells in sarcoidosis. Am J Pathol 57:81, 1969
141. Ridley DS, Jopling WH: Classification of leprosy according to immunity: A five-group system. Int J Leprosy 34:255, 1966
142. Shelley WB, Hurley HJ: The pathogenesis of silica granulomas in man: A non-allergic colloidal phenomenon. J Invest Dermatol 34:107, 1960
143. Shelley WB, Hurley HJ: The allergic origin of zirconium deodorant granulomas. Br J Dermatol 70:75, 1958
144. Baler GR: Granulomas from topical zirconium in poison ivy dermatitis. Arch Dermatol 91:145, 1965
145. Stoeckle JD, Hardy HL, Weber AL: Chronic beryllium disease. Am J Med 46:545, 1967
146. Conant NF, Smith DT, Baker RD, et al: Manual of Clinical Mycology, 3rd Ed. WB Saunders, Philadelphia, 1971
147. Rosenberg FR, Einbinder J, Walzer RA, et al: Vegetating iododerma. Arch Dermatol 105:900, 1972
148. Montgomery H: Histopathology of the various types of cutaneous tuberculosis. Arch Dermatol Syph 35:698, 1937
149. Jolly HW Jr, Seabury JH: Infections with *Mycobacterium marinum*. Arch Dermatol 106:32, 1972
150. Graham JH, Johnson WC, Burgoon CF Jr, et al: Tinea capitis: A histopathological and histochemical study. Arch Dermatol 89:528, 1964
151. Potter BS, Burgoon CF Jr, Johnson WC: Pityrosporum folliculitis. Arch Dermatol 107:388, 1973
152. Brownstein MH, Helwig EB: The cutaneous amyloidoses. II. Systemic forms. Arch Dermatol 102:20, 1970
153. Rukawina JG, Block WD, Jackson CE, et al: Primary systemic amyloidosis. Medicine 35:239, 1956
154. Glenner GG: Amyloid deposits and amyloidosis. N Engl J Med 302:1282; 302:1333, 1980
155. Hashimoto K, Kobayashi H: Histogenesis of amyloid in the skin. Am J Dermatopathol 2:165, 1980
156. Brownstein MH, Helwig EB: Systemic amyloidosis complicating dermatoses. Arch Dermatol 102:1, 1970
157. Brownstein MH, Helwig EB: Secondary systemic amyloidosis: Analysis of underlying disorders. South Med J 64:491, 1971
158. Brownstein MH, Helwig EB: The cutaneous amyloidoses. I. Localized forms. Arch Dermatol 102:8, 1970
159. Brownstein MH, Hashimoto K: Macular amyloidosis. Arch Dermatol 106:50, 1972
160. Kumakiri M, Hashimoto K: Histogenesis of primary localized cutaneous amyloidosis: Sequential change of epidermal keratinocytes to amyloid via filamentous degeneration. J Invest Dermatol 73:150, 1979
161. Ratz JL, Bailin PL: Cutaneous amyloidosis. J Am Acad Dermatol 4:21, 1981
162. Edner H, Gebhart W: Colloid milium: Light and electron microscopic investigations. Clin Exp Dermatol 2:217, 1977
163. Hashimoto K, Katzman RL, Kang AH, et al: Electron

microscopical and biochemical analysis of colloid milium. Arch Dermatol 111:49, 1975

164. Graham JH, Marques AS: Colloid milium: A histochemical study. J Invest Dermatol 49:497, 1967

165. Caplan RM: Visceral involvement in lipoid proteinosis. Arch Dermatol 95:149, 1967

166. Wells MM, Golitz LE, Bender BJ: Erythropoietic protoporphyria with hepatic cirrhosis. Arch Dermatol 116:429, 1980

167. van der Walt JJ, Heyl T: Lipoid proteinosis and erythropoietic protoporphyria. Arch Dermatol 104:501, 1971

168. Haber LC, Bickers DR: The porphyrias: Basic science aspects, clinical diagnoses and management. p. 9. In FD Malkinson, RW Pearson (eds): Year Book of Dermatology. Year Book Medical Publishers, Chicago, 1975

169. Lynch PJ, Maize JC, Sisson JC: Pretibial myxedema and nonthyrotoxic thyroid disease. Arch Dermatol 107:107, 1973

170. Gabrilove JL, Ludwig AW: The histogenesis of myxedema. J Clin Endocrinol 17:925, 1957

171. Feldman P, Shapiro L, Pick AI, et al: Scleromyxedema. Arch Dermatol 99:51, 1969

172. McCarthy JT, Osserman E, Lombardo PC, et al: An abnormal serum globulin in lichen myxedematosus. Arch Dermatol 89:446, 1964

173. Harris RB, Perry HO, Kyle RA, et al: Treatment of scleromyxedema with Melphalan. Arch Dermatol 115:295, 1979

174. Cohn BA, Wheeler CE Jr, Briggaman RA: Scleredema adultorum of Buschke and diabetes mellitus. Arch Dermatol 101:27, 1970

175. Fleischmajer R, Faludi G, Krol S: Scleredema and diabetes mellitus. Arch Dermatol 101:21, 1970

176. Newmeyer WL, Kilgore ES Jr, Graham WP III: Mucous cysts: The dorsal distal interphalangeal joint ganglion. Plast Reconstr Surg 53:313, 1974

177. Johnson WC, Graham JH, Helwig EB: Cutaneous myxoid cyst. JAMA 191:15, 1965

178. Lattanand A, Johnson WC, Graham JH: Mucous cyst (mucocele). Arch Dermatol 101:673, 1970

179. Johnson WC, Helwig EB: Cutaneous focal mucinosis. Arch Dermatol 93:13, 1966

180. Pinkus H: Alopecia mucinosa. Arch Dermatol 76:419, 1957

181. Emmerson RW: Follicular mucinosis. Br J Dermatol 81:395, 1969

182. Muller SA, Winkelmann RK, Brunsting LA: Calcinosis in dermatomyositis. Arch Dermatol 79:669, 1959

183. Golitz LE, Fields JP: Metastatic calcification with skin necrosis. Arch Dermatol 106:398, 1972

184. Kossard S, Winkelmann RK: Vascular calcification in dermatopathology. Am J Dermatopathol 1:27, 1979

185. Shmunes E, Wood MG: Subepidermal calcified nodules. Arch Dermatol 105:593, 1972

186. Shapiro L, Platt N, Torres-Rodriguez VM: Idiopathic calcinosis of the scrotum. Arch Dermatol 102:199, 1970

187. Swinehart JM, Golitz LE: Scrotal calcinosis: Dystrophic calcification in epidermoid cysts. Arch Dermatol 118:985, 1982

188. Lichtenstein L, Wayne Scott H, Levin MH: Pathologic changes in gout: Survey of eleven necropsied cases. Am J Pathol 32:871, 1956

189. Fleischmajer R, Dowlati Y, Reeves JRT: Familial hyperplipidemias: Diagnosis and treatment. Arch Dermatol 110:43, 1974

190. Schreiber MM, Shapiro SI: Secondary eruptive xanthoma. Type V hyperlipoproteinemia. Arch Dermatol 100:601, 1969

191. Moschella SL: Plane xanthomatosis associated with myelomatosis. Arch Dermatol 101:683, 1970

192. Winkelmann RK, Muller SA: Generalized eruptive histiocytoma. Arch Dermatol 88:586, 1963

193. Taunton OD, Yeshurun D, Jarratt M: Progressive nodular histiocytoma. Arch Dermatol 114:1505, 1978

194. Gordon H: Erythema nodosum: A review of one hundred and fifteen cases. Br J Dermatol 73:393, 1961

195. Perry HO, Winkelmann RK: Subacute nodular migratory panniculitis. Arch Dermatol 89:10, 1964

196. Fine RM, Meltzer HD: Chronic erythema nodosum. Arch Dermatol 100:33, 1969

197. Christian HA: Relapsing febrile nodular nonsuppurative panniculitis. Arch Intern Med 41:338, 1928

198. Milner RDG, Mitchinson MJ: Weber-Christian disease. J Clin Pathol 18:150, 1965

199. Anderson S la C: Erythema induratum (Bazin) treated with isoniazid. Acta Derm Venereol (Stockh) 50:65, 1970

200. Montgomery H, O'Leary PA, Barker NW: Nodular vascular diseases of the legs. JAMA 128:335, 1945

201. Weary PE, Graham GF, Selden RF Jr: Subcutaneous fat necrosis of the newborn. South Med J 59:960, 1966

202. Chen TH, Shewmake SW, Hansen DD, et al: Subcutaneous fat necrosis of the newborn. Arch Dermatol 117:36, 1981

203. Thompsen RJ: Subcutaneous fat necrosis of the newborn and idiopathic hypercalcemia. Arch Dermatol 116:1155, 1980

204. Kellum RE, Ray TL, Brown GR: Sclerema neonatorum: Report of case and analysis of subcutaneous and epidermal-dermal lipids by chromatographic methods. Arch Dermatol 97:372, 1968

205. Potts DE, Mass MF, Iseman MD: Syndrome of pancreatic disease, subcutaneous fat necrosis and polyserositis. Am J Med 58:417, 1975

206. Szymanski F, Bluefarb SM: Nodular fat necrosis and pancreatic disease. Arch Dermatol 83:224, 1961

207. Tuffanelli DL: Lupus erythematosus panniculitis (profundus): Clinical and immunological studies. Arch Dermatol 103:231, 1971

208. Christianson HB, Dorsey CS, O'Leary PA, et al: Localized scleroderma: A clinical study of two hundred and thirty-five cases. Arch Dermatol 74:629, 1956

209. Tuffanelli DL, Winkelmann RK: Systemic scleroderma. Arch Dermatol 84:359, 1961

210. Fleischmajer R, Damiano V, Nedwich A: Alteration of subcutaneous tissue in scleroderma. Arch Dermatol 105:59, 1972

211. Fleischmajer R, Nedwich A: Generalized morphea. I.

Histology of the dermis and subcutaneous tissue. Arch Dermatol 106:509, 1972

212. Förström L, Winkelmann RK: Factitial panniculitis. Arch Dermatol 110:747, 1974

213. Urbach F, Wine SS, Johnson WC, et al: Generalized paraffinoma (sclerosing lipogranuloma). Arch Dermatol 103:277, 1971

214. Ackerman AB, Mosher DT, Schwamm HA: Factitial Weber-Christian syndrome. JAMA 198:731, 1966

215. Golitz LE: Fasciitis with eosinophilia: The Shulman syndrome. Int J Dermatol 19:552, 1980

216. Botet MV, Sánchez JL: The fascia in systemic scleroderma. J Am Acad Dermatol 3:36, 1980

217. Weedon D, Searle J, Kerr JF: Apoptosis: Its nature and implications for dermatopathology. Am J Dermatopathol 1:133, 1979

9

Neoplasms of the Skin

Richard J. Reed

Tumors of the skin are histologically and histogenetically diverse. The general category includes hyperplasias, heterotopias, hamartomas, congenital dysplasias, premalignant dysplasias, carcinomas, and sarcomas. The epithelial structures of the skin include the epidermis and the skin appendages. For the native epithelial structures, classification of the related tumors is complicated by the varied populations of cells of which these structures are composed. The morphologic expressions of physiologic modulations in these epithelial structures are remarkably preserved in many neoplasms of the skin.

The histogenesis of some epithelial neoplasms, particularly in regard to the expression of either eccrine and apocrine qualities, is controversial. In some examples, the histochemical findings conflict with clearly defined histologic patterns of differentiation. For example, the histologic evidence strongly favors apocrine differentiation for syringocystadenoma papilliferum. These features are contradicted by some of the histochemical findings. Similarly, the eccrine cylindroma occasionally has unmistakable markers for hair follicle differentiation. If it shows follicular and glandular patterns, the mixed patterns are more reasonably related to the multipotent blastema of both the pilosebaceous unit and the apocrine gland rather than the unipotent blastema of the eccrine gland. Thus, histochemistry is of questionable value in defining histogenesis and, in turn, in developing a classification of primary tumors of the skin.

Clinical concepts fundamental to a trained dermatologist may be misleading to a general pathologist. By historical precedence, however, the terminology for tumors of the skin is strongly weighted with clinical concepts. As an example, the concept of a nevus as a congenital blemish, distinct from a melanocytic hamartoma, is confusing.

Among the many possibilities, a nevus may be a local overgrowth of fibrous tissue, a local area of hyperelastosis, a local defect in formation and growth of pilosebaceous units, or a regional abnormality in the growth of the epidermis. For the general pathologist, hamartomas that are manifested by abnormal extracellular products may be a source of confusion.

The persnickety approach of dermatopathologists has complicated the classification of skin tumors. Minor histologic variants are commonly interpreted and reported as new entities.

In many genetic diseases, the skin is an accessible museum of significant markers. The diagnosis of disorders such as Cowden's disease, tuberous sclerosis, neurofibromatosis, and the mucosal neuroma syndrome is facilitated by the identification and study of cutaneous tumors and hamartomas.

The etiologic factors in the development of skin cancers are complex. The behavior of tumors of similar cell type may vary greatly depending on their etiologic backgrounds. The actinic squamous carcinoma may not have the same potential as its de novo counterpart. Lentigo maligna melanoma is a distinctive form of melanoma, but there is controversy regarding its malignant potential in comparison with other forms of cutaneous melanoma. Some observers have found this actinic variant to have a favorable prognosis in comparison with other variants at comparable depths of invasion. The manifestations of Kaposi's hemorrhagic sarcoma vary greatly depending upon the clinical setting and the immune status of the affected individual.

In this chapter, the classification of tumors is based primarily on histologic patterns with secondary attention to etiologic factors, if they have biologic significance.

GENERAL GROSS PATHOLOGY

Specimens that are the product of a punch biopsy are the mainstay of the dermatologist. For the common carcinomas of the skin, a punch biopsy provides a suitable specimen for the classification of a tumor and a general guide for subsequent therapeutic endeavors. If the specimen is less than 4 mm in diameter, it should not be bisected. Specimens with vesicular lesions also should be submitted intact.

From the examination of an incisional biopsy specimen that includes the interface between a lesion and the adjacent skin, it may be possible to provide additional information about the pattern of growth at the advancing margin of a tumor.

An excisional biopsy specimen provides all the preceding facets. From the examination of such a specimen, it is possible to evaluate the adequacy of the surgical margins, the relationships between tumor cells and nerves or blood vessels, and any regional variations in pattern.

A biopsy specimen is sectioned in a manner that best demonstrates the relationships between the tumor and the margins of excision. A permanent marker such as India ink simplifies the histologic interpretation of the surgical margins and eliminates errors related to improper embedding of the specimen or fragmentation of sections. For orientation of the specimen, the clinician should clearly identify the anatomic site (with the normal anatomic position as a model) and mark at least one margin in relation to significant boundaries of the body (anterior, posterior, inferior, superior, medial, lateral). Significant regional variations on the cut surface of the tumor should be represented on the histologic sections. The described gross features should be precisely identified by appropriate labels.

GENERAL MICROSCOPIC PATHOLOGY

The microscopic examination of a tumor of the skin includes an evaluation of the following features:

1. Overall contour and relationships between a tumor and normal anatomic boundaries
    In situ, expansile or infiltrative
    Uniformly symmetrical or irregular in outline
2. Stromal response
    Condensed, relatively acellular fibrous tissue at interface
    Infiltration of normal dermal connective tissue
    Infiltration of tumor stroma
    Infiltration of trophic structures (vessels or nerves)
3. Character of host immune response (if any)
4. Phenotypic expressions
5. Cytologic features

With these guidelines and some competence in general microscopy, many of the tumors of the skin are easily characterized. Epithelial hamartomas and hyperplasias generally respect the normal relationships between epithelium and stroma. Adenomas are generally expansile and symmetric. They usually compress the stroma at the interface with normal skin. There are exceptions such as dermal duct tumor, eccrine papillary adenoma or even eccrine cylindroma. Primary carcinomas are divisible into lesions with delicate reactive stromas (e.g., well differentiated basal cell carcinomas) and those with inflamed, reactive stromas. The latter stromal responses are not peculiar to neoplasms of the skin and are indistinguishable from those associated with a variety of carcinomas in other organ systems. Often the recognition of a reactive stroma is basic to the distinction between an in situ and an invasive lesion on small biopsy specimens. For many tumors of the skin, cytologic features may be deceptive and may not provide a distinction between carcinoma and hamartoma. As an example, cytologic features are of little importance in making the distinction between trichoepithelioma and a well differentiated basal cell carcinoma.

BENIGN EPIDERMAL HYPERPLASIAS

The epidermis is composed of a basal unit and a superficial unit. The basal unit is concerned with replication of cells, the pattern of rete ridges, and the integrity of the basement membrane. The superficial unit is concerned with the formation of keratinosomes, the closure of the interstitial spaces, and the formation of the keratin layer.[1] It is also concerned with the formation of an impervious barrier at the surface. The surface topography of an area of hyperplastic epidermis reflects the contributions of the superficial and basal units and the influence of the altered epidermis on the papillary dermis.[2] The morphologic expressions of a potential for follicular neogenesis may also contribute to the overall configuration.[3] Cutaneous epithelial hyperplasias with tumoral qualities are common; they are either verrucoid, inverted, invasive, or combinations of the three.

Verrucoid epidermal hyperplasia, as a nonspecific pattern, is a common cutaneous lesion. Some examples may represent old verrucae; others may represent a response to external trauma. In verrucoid epidermal hyperplasia, the epidermis adapts to a limited area by forming ridges and folds that are supported by delicate fronds from the papillary dermis (papillomatosis). In these lesions, a hyperplastic basal unit undergoes an orderly maturation to a superficial unit. The keratin layer is usually thickened and either anucleate (hyperkeratotic) or nucleated (parakeratotic).

The epidermis responds to external trauma with varying degrees of verrucoid hyperplasia. As an additional response, the dermis shows telangiectasia and fibrosis. These localized hyperplasias are classified as scratch papules (picker's nodules). They lack the lichenoid qualities and the inflammatory infiltrates of lichen simplex chronicus.

Virus-Induced Epidermal Hyperplasias

The effects of the papillomavirus are manifested in the common verrucae. There are correlations between anatomic sites and types of papillomavirus.[4]

Verruca Vulgaris

In verruca vulgaris, the cells in the basal unit contain small cytoplasmic vacuoles. In the superficial unit, the vacuoles are large and perinuclear.[5] The nuclei of infected cells are plump and central. In the superficial epidermal unit, they occasionally contain acidophilic inclusions and show marginated chromatin (Fig. 9-1). Keratohyaline granules are coarse, lavender, and angulated; they do not displace or compress the nucleus. The keratin layer is characteristically nucleated, particularly at the tips of the papillae. At the margins of such a lesion,

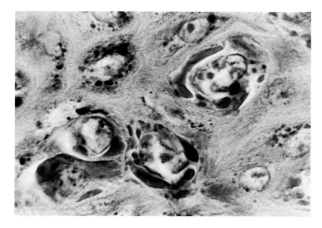

Fig. 9-1. Verruca vulgaris. Coarse keratohyaline granules in the cytoplasm adapt to the centrally placed nuclei. The nuclei are vacuolated. They contain nucleoli and poorly outlined inclusions.

elongated rete ridges are gently curved with their apices pointing toward the central axis of the lesion.[6]

The viral verrucae have a life history. Senescence is manifested by progressive disappearance of the most characteristic features. The vacuolated keratinocytes and the abnormal keratohyaline granules become less conspicuous. In transition phases, the zones of parakeratosis in verruca vulgaris may be confined to the tips of prominent papillae. Senescence with disappearance of characteristic histologic markers does not necessarily equate with restoration of a normal epidermal pattern. Viral verrucae, particularly condyloma acuminatum, may persist as nonspecific papillomas after the characteristic histologic markers have disappeared.

Occasionally, a lesion of verruca vulgaris is characterized by a dense infiltrate of lymphocytes, histiocytes, plasma cells, and neutrophils. Inflammatory cells also migrate into the hyperplastic epidermis. In the latter location, they produce lysis and coagulation of clusters of infected keratinocytes. This reaction shares features with inflammatory changes seen in some examples of molluscum contagiosum[3] and expresses immune-mediated regression of the virus-induced verruca.

Condyloma Acuminatum

Condyloma acuminatum is a virus-induced verruca, closely related to verruca vulgaris, but with the anogenical area as the predilected site. The virus of condyloma acuminatum is antigenically distinct from the virus of verruca vulgaris.[2,7] Condyloma acuminatum is characterized histologically by marked papillomatosis, focal parakeratosis, vacuolization of cells, and intraepithelial infiltrates of neutrophils (Fig. 9-2). Large keratohyaline granules, characteristic of an active lesion of verruca vulgaris, are not a prominent feature of condyloma acuminatum. The dermis beneath the area of papillary epithelial hyperplasia contains infiltrates of chronic inflammatory cells.

Condylomata may persist as squamous papillomas. Genital papillomas as a manifestation of senescence in the evolution of condyloma acuminatum are common. In occasional papillomas, the pattern overlaps with inverted follicular keratosis. Some condylomas are relatively flat; they qualify as flat warts but display the antigenic features of lesions of condyloma acuminatum. This feature is more characteristic of lesions on mucous membranes. Large genital condylomas are qualified as giant condylomas. If, in addition, such a lesion is invasive, it qualifies as a variant of verrucous carcinoma (invasive squamous carcinoma with minimal cytologic deviation). Recent studies implicate the condyloma virus in site-specific carcinogenesis, such as carcinoma in situ of the anogenital area and the uterine cervix.

cells in the upper stratum malpighii and in the granular layer have vacuolated, clear cytoplasm (Fig. 9-3). Inflamed (regressing) flat warts may not demonstrate the diagnostic epidermal changes. As a consequence, they may be lost in the default category of lichenoid keratosis.

Orf and Milker's Nodule

Other viral diseases may produce verrucoid epidermal hyperplasia.[5] The lesions of orf and milker's nodule share many histologic features. They are characterized by marked hyperkeratosis, parakeratosis, acanthosis, elongation of rete-ridges, and papillomatosis. The abnormal keratinocytes in the area of epidermal hyperplasia often have plump nuclei, and pale watery cytoplasm (show ballooning degeneration) (Fig. 9-4). Nuclear chromatin is marginated. Acidophilic intranuclear inclusions occasionally are identified on hematoxylin and eosin (H & E)-stained sections. Dense, band-like infiltrates of lymphoid cells accumulate in the upper portion of the dermis.[8] They hug the hyperplastic epidermis and, in many areas, migrate into it. The intermingling of lymphoid cells and kertinocytes obscures the boundaries between the rete ridges and the adjacent dermis. Many of the lymphoid cells have deeply basophilic cytoplasm and plump nuclei with prominent nucleoli and marginated chromatin. They are morphologic immunoblasts. If close attention is not given to the epidermis, the pleomorphic dermal infiltrate may be misinterpreted as lymphomatous.

Molluscum Contagiosum

The most characteristic example of a virus-induced, inverted epidermal hyperplasia is molluscum conta-

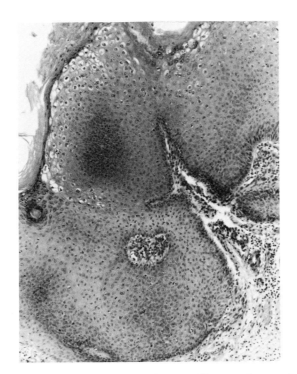

Fig. 9-2. Condyloma acuminatum. Papillomatosis, parakeratosis, and vacuolar changes in the superficial unit characterize the reaction.

Verruca Plana

Verruca plana (flat wart) is a variant of verruca vulgaris. It is distinguished by a loosely laminated, hyperkeratotic scale, a prominent granular layer, and acanthosis with mild papillomatosis. Many of the squamous

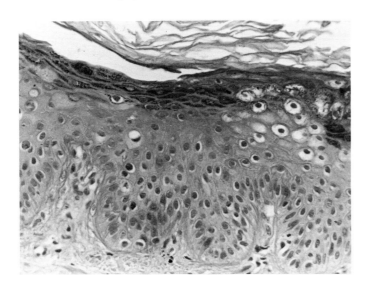

Fig. 9-3. Verruca plana. Hypergranulosis and vacuolar changes are prominent. Hyperplasia with papillomatosis is not as well developed as in verruca vulgaris.

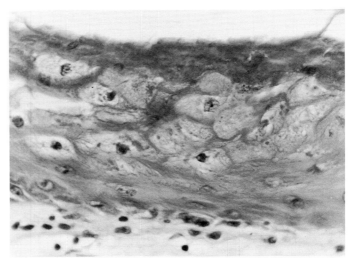

Fig. 9-4. Milker's nodule. The vacuolated cells in the superficial epidermal unit contain intranuclear and cytoplasmic inclusions.

NEOPLASMS OF THE SKIN

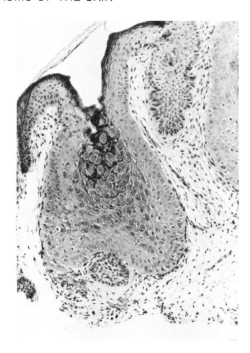

Fig. 9-5. Molluscum contagiosum. The epithelium of a newly formed follicle is hyperplastic. Molluscum bodies distort cells in the superficial unit and have been discharged into the lumen of the follicle. Basal cells with trichilemmal qualities form a bulb at the extremity of the altered follicle.

giosum. The lesion is composed of newly formed, bulbous follicles (Fig. 9-5). The morphologic features of the lesion express the capacity of the virus to induce follicular neogenesis.[3] The nuclei of infected individual follicular keratinocytes are compressed by particulate cytoplasmic inclusions. Condensed homogeneous inclusions and keratinized debris are discharged into the lumen of each affected follicle. The follicles are outlined by sheaths of fibrous tissue, which are an extension of the adventitial dermis (papillary dermis and perifollicular connective tissue sheath).

Invasive Epidermal Hyperplasia

Invasive (pseudoepitheliomatous) epidermal hyperplasia is a response to many inflammatory and infectious processes in the dermis.[9] The hyperplastic epithelium is poorly organized, and the columns of invasive cells are irregular in distribution. Invasive hyperplasia is commonly seen in deep fungal infections of the skin and in atypical acid-fast infections. It may be seen in halogen granulomas. The infiltrating nests generally are bulbous but occasionally are thin and angulated. The affected keratinocytes show bland cytologic features and display hypertrophy of individual cells and cytoplasmic pallor

(glycogen-rich cytoplasms). Pseudoepitheliomatous hyperplasia is basic to the phenomena of transepidermal elimination.

Symptomatic Keratoacanthomas

Keratoacanthomas are localized, spontaneous tumors. The group includes actinic, de novo, and symptomatic variants. The latter category gives recognition to peculiar epithelial hyperplasias in association with a common dermatitis. In the symptomatic variants, cytologically benign, invasive epidermal hyperplasias complicate a variety of inflammatory disorders including psoriasis, lichen planus, and lupus erythematosus. In the latter settings, the keratoacanthomas are usually multiple and, in many instances, are associated with defective or altered host immune responses.[10] In some examples, the lesions are well developed and, with the exception of cytologic dysplasia, share many features with actinic keratoacanthoma. In other examples, particularly in lesions of lupus erythematosus, the invading nests of cells are rather small and widely spaced. Such a pattern may be mistaken for early invasive squamous carcinoma.

PREMALIGNANT EPIDERMAL DYSPLASIAS (CLONAL KERATOSES)

In the premalignant epidermal dysplasias, keratinocytes have abnormal cytologic features, are aggregated in abnormal patterns, demonstrate defective contact inhibition, and elicit a host immune response. Remnants of a premalignant dysplasia, if preserved in the epidermis adjacent to an invasive carcinoma, implicate the dysplasia as a precursor for the carcinoma.

A *clonal keratosis* is characterized by (1) cytologically distinctive cells within the domain of the abnormal clone; (2) characteristic, sharp interfaces between the clone and the adjacent population of epidermal cells; (3) an abnormal keratinized product at the surface; and (4) abnormalities in the size and number of epidermal cells per unit area. In addition, it is characterized by (1) fibrosis and angioplasia in the stroma, and (2) cellular host immune response with focal lichenoid patterns.[11] In toto, the effects of these two processes find expression in patterns of regression. Included in the patterns of regression are altered rete ridges, fibrosis of the adventitial dermis, and an abnormal distribution of small vessels in the adventitial dermis (poikilodermatous qualities).

The cells of a premalignant clonal keratosis (epidermal dysplasia) are characterized by (1) variations in nuclear size and staining, (2) abnormal chromatin patterns, (3) abnormal nucleolar-nuclear-cytoplasmic ratios, (4) loss of nuclear polarity, (5) dyskeratosis, (6) varying degrees of acantholysis, and (7) increased mitotic rate with abnormal mitoses.

Actinic Keratosis

An actinic keratosis is an actinically induced epidermal dysplasia (clonal keratosis). The effects of actinic irradiation are best displayed in fair-skinned patients who have been subjected to long-term exposure. They are manifested clinically by alterations in the texture of the skin and by keratoses and carcinomas.

An actinic keratosis is characterized by a nucleated stratum corneum, by hyperplasia of the epidermis (acanthosis), and by cellular atypism, generally most prominent in the basal unit (Fig. 9-6). Rete ridges are partially effaced or irregularly elongated. Occasionally, the basal unit shows melanocytic hyperplasia and hyperpigmentation (pigmented actinic keratosis). The dysplastic cells form sharp interfaces with normal keratinocytes either in the adjacent epidermis or in those sites in which the abnormal population of cells abuts on the intraepidermal portions of skin appendages[12] (Fig. 9-6). The clones of atypical cells may extend for a short distance along the follicular epithelium. The underlying papillary dermis usually contains perivascular infiltrates of chronic inflammatory cells and ectatic vessels. Altered elastotic connective tissue (solar elastosis) forms a band in the upper portion of the reticular dermis.

The lymphocytes within an actinic keratosis are a morphologic expression of cellular host immune response.[11] In one or more sites, the lymphocytes may migrate into the dysplastic epithelium. In occasional examples, the infiltrates are dense and bandlike. They hug the hyperplastic epithelium and migrate into it. This interplay at the dermoepidermal interface produces a cellular, lichenoid reaction. The host immune response may be successful and may partially or completely destroy the abnormal population of keratinocytes. Lesions of this type are classified as *lichenoid actinic keratoses*[11] (Fig. 9-7). Similar lichenoid reactions may complicate solitary pigmented keratoses such as senile lentigines and seborrheic keratoses on nonexposed surfaces (lichenoid keratoses). The lichenoid reaction may alter and mask the underlying keratosis.

The atypism in an actinic keratosis is variable. It ranges from mild to severe. Severe dysplasias that involve the entire thickness of the viable epidermis qualify as actinic carcinoma in situ.

Bowen's Disease and Related Processes

The pattern of nonactinic keratinocytic dysplasias is often psoriasiform; the rete ridges are elongated and the basal unit is hyperplastic. The basal layer is often intact and cytologically bland. The suprabasal epithelium is

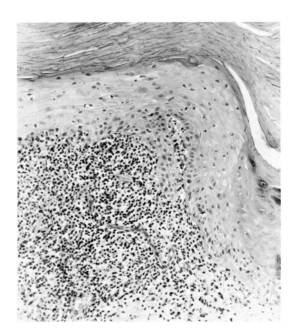

Fig. 9-7. Lichenoid actinic keratosis, moderate dysplasia. A band-like infiltrate of lymphoid cells hugs the epidermis. It produces lysis of dysplastic basal keratinocytes and effacement of rete ridges. A clonal interface on the right defines the junction between the dysplastic clone and follicular epithelium.

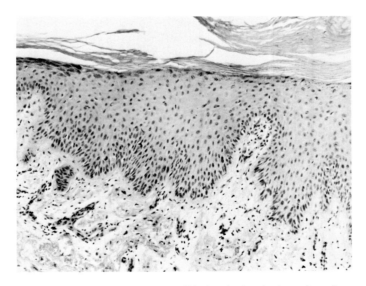

Fig. 9-6. Actinic keratosis, mild dysplasia. A sharp interface defines the junction of the dysplastic cells on the right with the normal epidermis on the left.

composed of basaloid cells, often with scant, basophilic cytoplasm. The nuclei are crowded and show loss of polarity.[11] In bowenoid carcinoma in situ, the atypical changes involve the entire thickness of the epidermis and are often associated with a parakeratotic cap. Dyskeratotic cells are numerous and some are atypical. Focally, the patterns in the nonactinic dysplasias (bowenoid dysplasias) are evidence of the spread of an abnormal clone of keratinocytes into the adjacent epithelium above the level of the basal cells. The dysplastic cells migrate more freely in the bowenoid dysplasias than in the actinic dysplasias. In this manner, nests of benign keratinocytes are often entrapped within the confines of the dysplasia. The clone also has a tendency to invade follicular epithelium. The latter feature has prompted some observers to classify bowenoid dysplasias in the category of follicular dysplasias.

In some examples, the atypical cells form compact nests or fascicles within an otherwise normal epidermis. This peculiar nesting pattern is seen in both benign hyperplasias and premalignant dysplasias; it is the pattern of the intraepithelial epithelioma. A special variant has been classified as hidroacanthoma simplex. It is additionally characterized by glycogen-rich cells.

Severe keratinocytic dysplasias on skin that is not sun-damaged have been given separate recognition as Bowen's disease. In spite of the general acceptance of Bowen's disease as a specific process, the histologic criteria do not clearly distinguish between keratinocytic dysplasias of actinic and nonactinic origin (Figs. 9-8 and 9-9). They fail to distinguish variants of bowenoid nonactinic dysplasias, such as Bowen's disease, arsenical keratoses, virus-related keratoses (koilocytotic variants), and erythroplasia of Queyrat. For lesions on the glabrous skin, an association between Bowen's disease and arsenical intoxication has been proposed. For the anogenital lesions, an association with viral verrucae seems likely.

Condyloma acuminatum commonly shows focal areas of mild or moderate keratinocytic dysplasia.[7,13] Carcinoma in situ of the anogenital area often is papillary. By inference, papillary carcinoma in situ of the anogenital area may express progressive neoplastic transformation of a viral papilloma.

Some lesions of condyloma acuminatum persist as slowly enlarging papillary growths.[13] They may exceed 5 or 6 cm in diameter (*giant condyloma acuminatum*). These chronic, virus-induced papillomas may be locally invasive (*verrucous carcinoma*).[13] They invade in an indolent, expansile manner but may extend into muscular vessels. They show mild keratinocytic atypia and rarely metastasize. Virus-related verrucous carcinomas also are found in other sites.[14]

Vulvar carcinomas in situ are relatively restricted in anatomic distribution but are often multifocal. They have

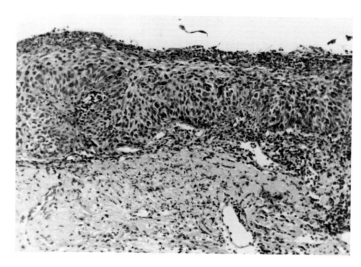

Fig. 9-8. Actinic carcinoma in situ. The dysplasia uniformly involves the epidermis. The dysplastic keratinocytes have scanty cytoplasm and atypical nuclei. Nuclear polarity is disturbed. The surface layer is parakeratotic and inflamed. The dermis shows solar elastosis.

a peculiar association with carcinoma in situ of the cervix that is manifested by neither actinic variants of carcinoma in situ nor variants on the glabrous skin.[15]

The recently described papular lesions of the anogenital area known as *bowenoid papulosis* are histologically bowenoid dysplasias or bowenoid carcinoma in situ, but clinically they resemble verrucae.[16–18] Their biologic potential has not been clearly defined. Their relationship to

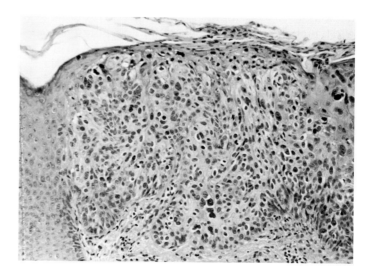

Fig. 9-9. Basaloid keratinocytic dysplasia, bowenoid variant. The entire epidermis within the lesion is dysplastic. The keratinocytes show nuclear atypism and crowding, loss of nuclear polarity, and cytoplasmic vacuoles. The surface layer is parakeratotic. A clonal interface is represented on the left.

erythroplasia of Queyrat has not been defined. Paradoxically, some examples of bowenoid papulosis in pregnant women have spontaneously regressed following the termination of pregnancy.

The association between the papilloma virus and carcinoma is best displayed in *epidermodysplasia verruciformis*.[19] In this genodermatosis, virus-induced papillomas (flat warts) are multiple and chronic. Viral particles have been demonstrated. With the passage of time, some of the lesions acquire the characteristics of a keratinocytic dysplasia, carcinoma in situ, or invasive carcinoma. Such transformations may be related to specific antigenic variants. Viral particles generally are not demonstrable in the dysplastic lesions or in the carcinomas. Viral DNA has been demonstrated in lesions of the latter type. It has been demonstrated in Bowen's disease of the anogenital areas, bowenoid papulosis, verrucous carcinoma of the anogenital areas, and cervical carcinomas.[4,13]

Keratinocytic and melanocytic dysplasias, including carcinoma in situ, invasive carcinoma, and melanoma, are a complication of *xeroderma pigmentosa*. In the latter disorder, a defect in the enzymatic repair of environmental or actinic, chromosomal damage finds expression in keratoses, lentigines, melanomas, and carcinomas.

Porokeratosis of Mibelli is a genetically determined clonal keratosis.[20] A related process is peculiar to sun-exposed surfaces (disseminated superficial actinic variant). It occurs most commonly in women and is classified as *disseminated superficial actinic porokeratosis*. In both variants, a sharply localized column of parakeratotic debris (cornoid lamella) is produced by an architecturally deranged superficial epidermal unit (Fig. 9-10). The latter locus contains dyskeratotic and vacuolated cells. The keratinocytes show loss of polarity and are intermingled with lymphocytes. Lymphoid infiltrates are present in the papillary dermis. In the actinic variant, some of the lesions show varying degrees of keratinocytic dysplasia. Within the actinic lesions, senescent lichenoid reactions are common. Carcinomas may complicate the actinic and Mibelli variants.[21] On the basis of clinical or histologic peculiarities, other variants of porokeratosis have been described.[22]

Paget's disease of the skin expresses the invasive growth of a clone of secretory cells in squamous epithelium.[23,24] Two disparate populations of epithelial cells, one of which is squamous and normal and the other glandular and neoplastic, occupy a limited epithelial domain. The neoplastic clone is relatively protected by its association with the squamous cells and by a relatively intact basement membrane. Contact inhibition does not influence the neoplastic cells; they spread freely in the epithelial domain. The active migration of cells in the epidermis may be away from zones of active inflammation (negative immunotaxis).

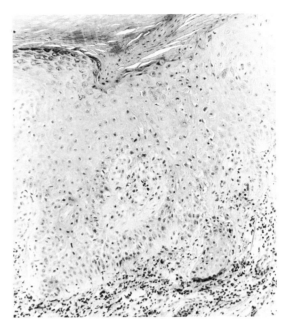

Fig. 9-10. Porokeratosis of Mibelli. A column of parakeratotic debris overlies an angulated indentation. Beneath the zone of parakeratosis, the granular layer is interrupted. The superficial unit shows individual cell dyskeratosis, vacuolar changes, and loss of nuclear polarity.

In Paget's disease of the nipple and in some examples of extramammary Paget's disease, the dysplastic clone spreads from a neighboring invasive or intraductal carcinoma. In rare examples of Paget's disease of the nipple and in most examples of extramammary Paget's disease, it is difficult to identify a site of origin other than the epidermis for the clone of dysplastic cells. The dysplastic clone may invade the dermis, and commonly the invasive foci are multiple. A mucicarmine stain is useful in identifying secretory cells in extramammary Paget's disease. Immunoperoxidase reactions for the demonstration of carcinoembryonic antigen (CEA), epithelial membrane antigen (EMA), and S-100 protein would be of value in the differential diagnosis of cutaneous Paget's disease, particularly if the differential includes melanoma or melanocytic dysplasia. CEA and EMA are marker for secretory cells and S-100 protein is a valuable marker for dysplastic and neoplastic melanocytes.

CARCINOMA OF THE SKIN

In the classification of carcinomas of the skin, attention is given to the basic type of cell and to specific patterns of differentiation.[25] Two types of cells, the basal cell and the squamous cell, are given recognition and are comparable

NEOPLASMS OF THE SKIN

to cell types displayed in the normal epidermis. The process of keratinization and the formation of an impervious barrier at the surface are functions of the superficial epidermal unit. The latter is composed of mature squamous cells. Replication of cells and maintenance of a stable interface with the papillary dermis are the functions of the basal unit and its basal cells. The potential for follicular neogenesis resides in the basal unit. The modulations and the distinctive cells in these two functioning units provide models for the classification of most cutaneous carcinomas.

In squamous carcinoma, the tumor cells recapitulate the cellular modulations of the superficial epidermal unit. The end product in a well differentiated variant is keratinized debris.

In some carcinomas, the tumor cells are basophilic and resemble cells of a hyperplastic basal unit. Keratinization is less prominent. These variants are classified as poorly differentiated squamous carcinoma, as metatypical carcinoma, or as basosquamous carcinoma. Some basosquamous carcinomas arise de novo and some are preceded by basosquamous keratinocytic dysplasias (bowenoid dysplasias). A third variant of basosquamous carcinoma is an expression of dedifferentiation in a basal cell carcinoma.

A large group of cutaneous carcinomas recapitulate patterns seen in the embryologic development of hair follicles or in postnatal follicular neogenesis. They are classified as basal cell carcinomas.[26]

Squamous carcinomas arise de novo, in areas of chronic inflammation and scarring, or most commonly in actinically damaged skin. Basal cell carcinomas arise in undamaged skin, in areas of chronic inflammation and scarring, or in actinically damaged skin. In the latter setting, they are seldom preceded by actinic keratoses. In undamaged skin, most basal cell carcinomas are neoplastic expressions of follicular dysplasias. Basal cell carcinomas in the first three decades of life generally belong in the category of nevoid lesions.

In the histologic evaluation of cutaneous carcinomas, three basic stromal patterns are recognized: (1) induced stroma, (2) immunologically reactive stroma, and (3) refractory stroma (11).

The induced stroma is a specialized fibromucinous matrix (Fig. 9-11) that is variably cellular and characteristically free of inflammatory cells. It is a specific expression of the inductive influence of tumor cells on stromal cells and is basic to the diagnosis of well differentiated basal cell carcinomas. The stromal changes of trichoepithelioma are even more characteristic. The character and organization of induced tumor stroma provide a differentiation between trichoepithelioma and basal cell carcinoma.

The immunologically reactive stroma is cellular, lami-

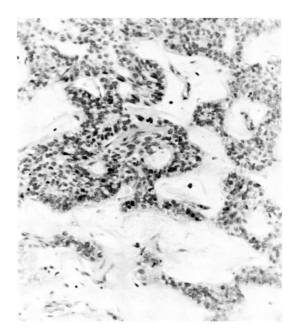

Fig. 9-11. Well differentiated basal cell carcinoma, induced stroma. The stroma is mucinous and not inflamed. Fibrocytes are small, widely spaced, and inconspicuous.

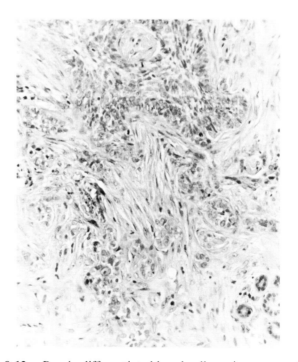

Fig. 9-12. Poorly differentiated basal cell carcinoma, reactive stroma. The stroma is fibrous, laminated, and cellular. In the large nest, the tumor cells are basosquamous.

nated fibrous tissue (Fig. 9-12). The lamellae parallel the contours of the nests of infiltrating tumor cells; they offer a rigid but not impenetrable barrier. The fibrous matrix invariably contains an infiltrate of lymphocytes, histiocytes, eosinophils, and plasma cells. A reactive stroma is the characteristic response in squamous and basosquamous carcinomas. Some basal cell carcinomas have a reactive stroma. They usually qualify as poorly differentiated variants and may acquire the characteristics of a basosquamous or squamous carcinoma.

In scattered sites, the inflammatory cells in a reactive stroma intermingle with neoplastic keratinocytes (target cells). They produce lysis and coagulation of target cells and lytic defects in nests of tumor cells (attritive phase of the lichenoid reaction)[11] (Fig. 9-13). The defects are inlaid with newly formed fibrous tissue (accretive phase of the lichenoid reaction).[11] The interplay between tumor cells and aggressive T-lymphocytes exerts a stabilizing influence on the growth of tumor cells. The target of an aggressive T-cell response (lichenoid reaction) includes melanocytes as well as keratinocytes. In occasional examples, the immune response may eradicate the evolving tumor, a phenomenon given recognition in the concepts of keratoacanthoma, halo nevus, and senescent li-

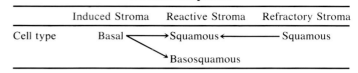

TABLE 9-1. Relationships Between Cell Types and Stromal Responses

	Induced Stroma	Reactive Stroma	Refractory Stroma
Cell type	Basal ⟶	Squamous ←	Squamous
		Basosquamous	

chenoid reaction. The lichenoid reaction at the advancing margin of a carcinoma of the skin satisfies Waksman's criteria for a cell-mediated immune reaction.[11] Plasma cells in the infiltrates provide a marker for the participation of B-lymphocytes.

The refractory stroma is peculiar to lesions that rapidly invade the dermis. The tumor cells break into the dermis; they disrupt connective fibers; and they trap the fragments in their interstices. The refractory stroma is also a basic reaction in processes that are classified as transepidermal elimination. The relationships between cell types and stromal responses are shown in Table 9-1. The refractory stroma is discussed in detail in the section on keratoacanthoma.

Squamous Carcinoma

Squamous carcinomas of the skin are divided into a transformed group, which is preceded by a keratinocytic dysplasia, and a de novo group, which is not sequentially related to a keratinocytic dysplasia. Most of the actinic squamous carcinomas are preceded by actinic keratoses, which persist as markers at the margin of infiltrating tumors.

Clinically, indentations in the surface contours with irregular accumulations of keratinized debris produce the roughened, irregular surface of cutaneous squamous carcinoma. Some of the tumors are crateriform. On cut surface, the nests and cords of tumor cells are opaque and white. The opaque areas correspond to zones of keratinization.

Squamous carcinomas are composed of acidophilic, polygonal cells. In the differentiated variants, the cells have cytoplasmic tonofibrils, and in keratinizing variants, some of the cells contain keratohyaline granules. The spaces between neighboring cells are bridged by desmosomes (intercellular bridges or prickles). These histologic characteristics are basic to the grading of squamous carcinomas.[27] The rationale for grading tumors is found in correlations between the grade of a tumor and its biologic aggressiveness. Well differentiated (grade I) tumors are characterized by bulbous columns and nests of squamous cells. Cytologic atypism is relatively confined to one or two cell layers at the periphery of each nest. The more

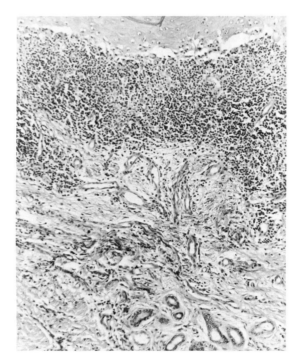

Fig. 9-13. Regressing keratocanthoma, lichenoid reaction. The base of the crater is outlined by hyperplastic squamous epithelium. A band-like infiltrate of lymphocytes hugs the epithelium and produces lytic defects in the epithelial domain. The fibrosis beneath the inflammatory infiltrate is a marker for the accretive (desmoplastic) phase of the lichenoid reaction.

centrally placed cells in each nest have uniform nuclear characteristics. They show progressive keratinization and are eventually converted to central aggregates of keratinized debris. In their progressive keratinization, they mimic the changes seen in the normal epidermis.

In grade II tumors, keratinization is less conspicuous. Atypism is evident throughout each nest rather than confined to two or three peripheral layers of cells (Fig. 9-14). The nests and cords of cells are less bulbous. At the advancing margin, the tumor cells form thin, elongated columns.

In grade III tumors, keratinization is not a significant feature. The tumor cells form thin columns and show uniform nuclear atypism throughout each nest of cells (Fig. 9-15).

In grade IV tumors, the cytologic characteristics of a squamous cell are lost. The tumor is undifferentiated.

Most of the actinic squamous carcinomas are small, superficially invasive, and usually confined to the dermis. In contrast, scar carcinomas or de novo carcinomas of the skin are often large and deeply invasive. In the category of actinic squamous carcinomas, metastases are exceptional. In scar and de novo carcinomas, metastases are relatively common. The parameters for predicting metastasis for squamous carcinomas of the skin are tumor grade, size, depth of invasion, and lymphatic or blood vascular invasion.[27] With comparable prognostic parameters, there is little or no evidence that the actinic carcinoma is the more favorable process.

The prognostic importance of the dermis as a defense against the spread of primary cutaneous carcinomas should be emphasized. Carcinomas that have infiltrated soft tissue beyond the dermis, or have invaded nerve sheaths and cutaneous vessels qualify as aggressive variants.

Scar carcinomas are related to chronic, fibrosing, inflammatory processes.[28] They arise in burn scars, radiodermatitis, or chronic infectious processes (e.g., lupus vulgaris). Some scar carcinomas transform into desmoplastic spindle cell carcinomas.[11] *Spindle cell carcinomas* are a special variant of grade IV squamous carcinomas. The spindle cells form compactly aggregated, interlacing fascicles near the epidermis (Fig. 9-16). In the deeper portions, tumor cells are isolated in a fibrous matrix. The desmoplastic portion of a spindle cell carcinoma shows a progressive reduction in cellularity at the advancing margin. It is often impossible histologically to define an interface between the tumor and reactive fibroplasia in the adjacent dermis. Immunologic markers for cytokeratins and vimentin may provide information regarding the nature of the neoplastic cells.

The *adenoid variant* of squamous carcinoma is common. It is characterized by mucin-filled acantholytic clefts (Fig. 9-14) in a suprabasal location. The clefts often

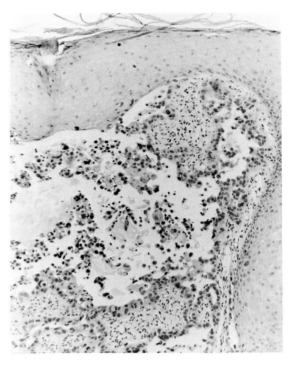

Fig. 9-14. Moderately differentiated squamous carcinoma, adenoid variant. Cords of atypical squamous cells extend from the epidermis into the dermis. The tumor shows suprabasal acantholysis and dyskeratosis. The clear matrix has mucinous qualities.

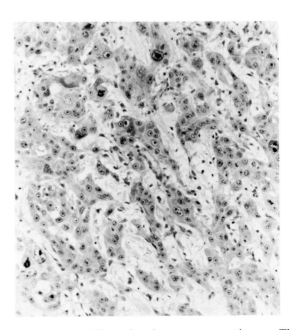

Fig. 9-15. Poorly differentiated squamous carcinoma. The tumor cells are polygonal. They form delicate, closely aggregated, interconnected cords.

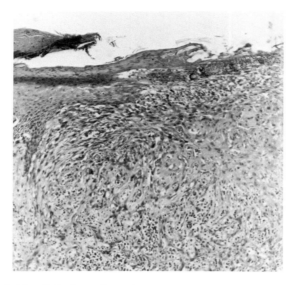

Fig. 9-16. Spindle cell carcinoma, lower lip. Atypical spindle cells are closely aggregated at the dermoepidermal interface. They form delicate fascicles that extend into an inflamed reactive stroma.

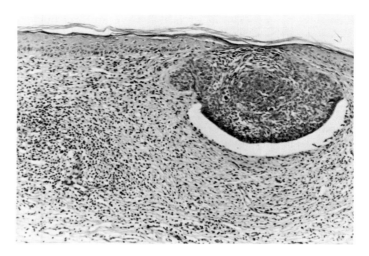

Fig. 9-17. Superficial basal cell carcinoma.

contain dyskeratotic tumor cells. A capacity for sarcomatoid transformation may reside in this histologic variant.[11]

Basal Cell Carcinomas

Most basal cell carcinomas have follicular qualities. The aggregates of tumor cells superficially resemble a developing hair bulb.[26] At the periphery of each nest, cells are palisaded (Fig. 9-12). The tumor cells often induce a specialized stroma.

At sites of origin, columns, cords, or nests of basal cells are attached to the basal unit of the epidermis (Fig. 9-17). The epidermis between adjacent nests of basal cells is not significantly disturbed. Some basal cell carcinomas arise from follicular epithelium rather than from the basal unit of the epidermis. Rarely, the follicles bordering a basal cell carcinoma are dysplastic. They are abnormal in outline and in degree of differentiation. These dysplastic follicles apparently are predisposed to malignant transformation. In the group with dysplastic follicles as precursors of basal cell carcinoma, the patients are younger than those in the group with actinic basal cell carcinomas. Basal cell carcinomas rarely have their origin in actinic keratoses.

In superficial basal cell carcinoma, the capacity for invasive growth is limited. Cords and plaques of basal cells are attached to the epidermis and bulge into the dermis (Fig. 9-17). They stimulate an immunologically reactive

stroma or a specialized induced stroma. Characteristically, in some areas, the nests of tumor cells are separated from the mucinous stroma by a cleft. In histologic sections, the tumor is represented by widely scattered nests that are attached to the epidermis. With appropriate sections, many of the isolated collections of cells prove to be tortuous cords of neoplastic cells which in cross section appear as nests. Superficial basal cell carcinoma should not be confused with the common follicular neogenesis that occurs over some dermatofibromas. Remnants of superficial basal cell carcinoma occasionally are preserved at the margin of an invasive component.

Basal cell carcinomas are divisible into well and poorly differentiated variants, but the division is somewhat arbitrary.[11] The distinction is based on cytologic features and on the character of the stroma. In well differentiated variants, the stroma is fibromucinous, loosely cellular, and only sparsely infiltrated with lymphocytes (see Fig. 9-11). In poorly differentiated basal cell carcinomas, the stroma is inflamed, laminated fibrous tissue (see Fig. 9-12). Stromal cells are spindle-shaped and tend to parallel the lamellae of fibrous tissue. In both variants, a thin band of relatively acellular mucinous matrix often separates the tumor cells from inflamed stroma. A cleft commonly separates the tumor cells from the mucinous matrix. In addition to the stromal changes, the cells in the well differentiated variants usually show small, uniform nuclei with delicately stippled chromatin. Nests of cells are often bulbous. In the poorly differentiated variants, the cells often form cords rather than bulbous nests. Nuclei in the tumor cells often are plump, vary in size, and show irregular clumping of chromatin. Mitoses are more common in the poorly differentiated variants.

Tumors that induce an abundant amount of mucinous matrix and are well differentiated are likely to produce a polypoid elevation of the surface of the skin. Tumors with trabecular qualities and poorly differentiated tumors are less likely to elevate the surface of the skin. Both variants commonly ulcerate. Clinically and histologically, the term *sclerosing basal cell carcinoma* is most appropriate for tumors that are composed of delicate, widely spaced trabeculae in a cellular fibrous matrix.

Well-differentiated basal cell carcinomas are usually confined to the dermis. Rarely, a well differentiated variant will invade the subcutis or skeletal muscle. Poorly differentiated variants are locally aggressive. They invade the subcutis or skeletal muscle and, occasionally, nerve sheaths (Fig. 9-18). Deeply invasive basal cell carcinomas and those with demonstrable nerve sheath or vascular invasion are appropriately qualified as aggressive. Some of the aggressive tumors are capable of metastasis. Occasionally, neglected basal cell carcinomas produce destruction of the midline structures of the face but maintain the pattern of a well differentiated lesion.

Melanocytes and their pigmentary products are a common feature of well differentiated basal cell carcinomas. Pigment is transferred from the melanocytes into the tumor cells and into dendritic melanophages in the stroma.

In many well differentiated basal cell carcinomas, amyloid deposits are found in the stroma.[11] These deposits resemble amyloid in other forms of primary cutaneous amyloidosis, such as macular or lichen amyloidosis. They are not a manifestation of systemic disease. They consist of aggregated globules, some of which are in direct contact with tumor cells. Melanocytes are commonly identified in amyloid-producing basal cell carcinomas. Pigmented melanophages or morphologically comparable amelanotic dendritic cells are found in the deposits of amyloid.

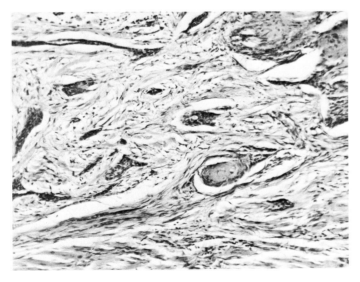

Fig. 9-18. Aggressive basosquamous carcinoma showing nerve sheath invasion.

Well differentiated basal cell carcinoma shares some properties with ameloblastic fibroma of the jaw bones. Both tumors express the properties of limited local growth and the induction of a specialized stroma. Poorly differentiated basal cell carcinoma is comparable to ameloblastoma. Both tumors are locally invasive and show variable admixtures of induced and reactive stromas. These cutaneous and odontogenic tumors recapitulate in an abortive fashion the formation of specialized structures during embryologic development. Basal cell carcinoma recapitulates the formation of pilosebaceous units and ameloblastoma the formation of the enamel organ. Neither tumor metastasizes with a predictable frequency.

Sebaceous epithelioma is a basal cell carcinoma in which individual cells or clusters of cells show sebaceous differentiation. An induced or reactive stroma supports the nests of tumor cells. Cells with multiple uniform cytoplasmic vacuoles and others with clear cytoplasm produce regional clear cell patterns in an otherwise typical basal cell carcinoma.

Basal cell carcinoma is one of the common postpubertal tumors complicating nevus sebaceus of Jadassohn.[29] In the setting of nevus sebaceus of Jadassohn, patterns of follicular neogenesis and follicular dysplasia are more common than basal cell carcinomas. It is important to recognize the distinctions.

Nevoid Basal Cell Carcinoma Syndrome

The nevoid basal cell carcinoma syndrome is a genetic follicular dysplasia manifested by basal cell carcinomas, skeletal defects, central nervous system (CNS) defects, and keratocysts of the jaws.[30] The basal cell nevi are indistinguishable from well differentiated basal cell carcinomas.[31] They are rather indolent lesions for variable periods but eventually may show clinical activity. Patterns of both well and poorly differentiated basal cell carcinoma are representative of basal cell nevi. The keratocysts are keratin-filled cysts lined by stratified squamous epithelium. They are derived from buds of basal cells, which project from the squamous epithelium of the gingiva. Peculiar palmar pits are an additional feature.[30,31] They show a local defect in the superficial epidermal unit and elongated rete ridges in an intact basal unit. Basal cell carcinomas may develop in the palmar pits. Rarely, the basal cell lesions may be systematized in the pattern of an epithelial nevus.

Fibroepithelioma of Pinkus

Fibroepithelioma of Pinkus is a well differentiated basal cell tumor with a florid induced stroma.[32] The tumor cells form interconnected delicate trabeculae (Fig. 9-19)

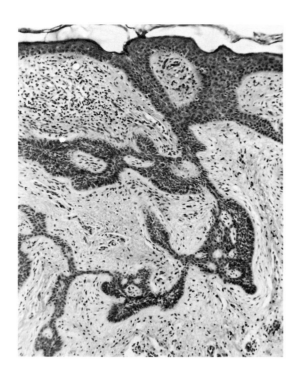

Fig. 9-19. Fibroepithelioma of Pinkus. Delicate elongated cords of basal cells extend from the epidermis into an induced stroma.

with variable admixtures of small squamous cells and basal cells. The trabeculae are supported by a uniformly cellular, myxomatous matrix. Some of the cords of cells may terminate in bulbous expansions which resemble hair bulbs. The tumor compresses the underlying dermis and produces a polypoid elevation of the surface of the skin. In some examples, the pattern of a fibroepithelioma is combined with an infiltrating basal cell carcinoma. Rarely, the pattern of fibroepithelioma is displayed as a regional variation in a seborrheic keratosis. There are overlaps between the epithelial patterns in fibroepithelioma of Pinkus and those in the tumor of the follicular infundibulum.

Basosquamous Carcinoma

Hyperplasia of the basal unit is a specific response of cells concerned with epidermal rather than follicular kinetics. Many of the basosquamous dysplasias and carcinomas are neoplastic expressions of the cellular kinetics observed in hyperplasia of the basal unit (with psoriasis as the prototype). The dysplastic cells show an increased nuclear to cytoplasmic ratio. Nuclei are crowded, and the cytoplasm has a distinct basophilia. This pattern expresses an increased turnover of cells; it is not anticipatory of follicular neogenesis. It is characteristic of bowenoid dysplasias.

In the invasive phase of a basaloid (bowenoid) keratinocytic dysplasia, the malignant cells retain most of the distinctive cytologic features of the dysplasia. They are basophilic and squamoid but poorly keratinized (metatypical or basosquamous). They form elongated columns that extend into the reticular dermis. In one or more foci, the tumor may acquire the characteristics of a keratinizing squamous carcinoma. In areas with a well developed lichenoid host response, the surviving target cells are likely to be acidophilic and keratinized.

As an expression of neoplasia, follicular neogenesis is manifested by a sharply localized group of basal cells that bulges from the epidermis into the papillary dermis. This pattern is characteristically displayed in superficial basal cell carcinoma. In poorly differentiated basal cell carcinomas, the histologic characteristics of the component cells are often basosquamous rather than basal. The cells are elongated with oval, plump nuclei and prominent nucleoli. Tonofilaments are a prominent cytologic feature. Palisading of peripheral cells becomes less conspicuous but is preserved as a marker. In recurrent or irradiated basal cell carcinomas, a basosquamous pattern is often dominant (Fig. 9-18). Basosquamous carcinoma as the expression of a dedifferentiated basal cell carcinoma is a locally aggressive tumor with a potential for metastasis.[33] Most often, basosquamous carcinomas (as an expression of poorly differentiated basal cell carcinomas) are associated with a reactive stroma.

Keratoacanthoma

With rare exceptions, keratoacanthomas are expressions of the same carcinogenic stimuli as actinic keratoses and actinic squamous carcinoma.[34] Although it is stated that keratoacanthomas do not evolve from actinic keratoses, prospective studies that document the nature of the skin in the precursory areas are not available. The changes of an actinic keratosis are common in the epidermis bordering a keratoacanthoma.

Keratoacanthoma is a rapidly evolving crateriform lesion. It briefly stabilizes and subsequently regresses, partially or completely. Rapid growth occurs over a period ranging from weeks to two or three months. The stable period persists for three or four months and is followed by slow regression over a period of several months. The concept of keratoacanthoma *implies* complete spontaneous regression as the natural and final evolution of an undisturbed tumor. Evidence in support of this concept is lacking. Partial central regression and lateral progression are common histologic findings in a mature keratoacanthoma (Fig. 9-20). Emphasis on the feature of clinical regression begs the issue of the pathogenesis of keratoacanthoma. The most characteristic histologic feature

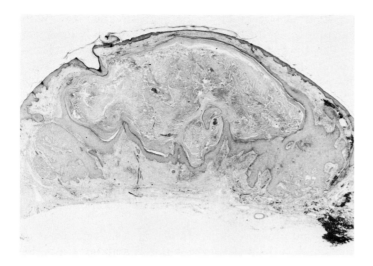

Fig. 9-20. Keratoacanthoma. The base of the lesion shows regression. Progression is manifested at both lateral margins.

of keratoacanthoma is invasion of unprepared dermal connective tissue.[35] Nests of pale, glycogen-rich, hypertrophied keratinocytes invade the reticular dermis. They flood the dermis and disrupt elastic and collagen fibers and elastotic material (Fig. 9-21). The connective tissue is entrapped in the interstices of the invading epithelium. In this initial phase, the tumor cells are not supported by a reactive or an induced stroma. The stroma is refractory but often is inflamed. The rapidly invading tumor cells exceed the capabilities of dermal cells, whose usual response is the formation of an immunoreactive stroma. Thus, an actinic keratoacanthoma is distinguished by (1) rapid invasive growth of a keratinocytic tumor, and (2)

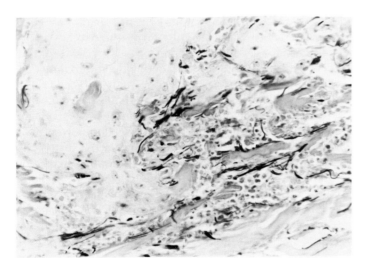

Fig. 9-21. Keratoacanthoma. Invasive squamous cells have disrupted connective tissue fibers. Elastic fibers and collagen bundles are trapped in the epithelial interstitium. (VVG stain.)

refractory stroma. Keratoacanthoma may express the immunostimulatory phase[36] of an evolving keratinocytic neoplasm.[35] Keratoacanthoma may be the expression of dyssynchronous activity by B-lymphocytes and T-lymphocytes.

During the period of stabilization and regression, the normal sequence in the host immune response to an invading tumor is established. The stable period expresses the mounting of an effective host immune response and is manifested histologically by a reactive stroma and a prominent lichenoid reaction[35] (see Fig. 9-13). The period of regression is an expression of a successful host immune response. It is the desmoplastic phase of the lichenoid reaction.[35]

Rarely, keratoacanthomas persist as chronic, slowly progressive tumors (squamous carcinomas or giant keratoacanthomas) or behave as locally aggressive, recurrent tumors.[37,38] These exceptional lesions demonstrate a sequence in which the host immune response is unsuccessful. Either the lymphoid response is inadequate or the tumor cells acquire the capacities to resist the effects of the lymphoid response.

The sequence of events can be summarized as follows:

Phase of rapid growth

1. Nests and cords of keratinocytes flood the dermis.
2. Keratinocytes have abundant, pale cytoplasm.
3. The pale cells are glycogen-rich.
4. Connective tissue (collagen fibers, elastic fibers, and elastotic debris) are entrapped in the epithelial interstitium.
5. Older generations of tumor cells are converted to keratinized debris.
6. The keratinized debris accumulates in a central crater.
7. Transition from epidermis to tumor is abrupt at the buttress outlining the crater.
8. Growth is usually confined to reticular dermis.
9. Growth extends to level of sweat glands.
10. Epidermis, follicular epithelium, and poral epithelium lose their identity in the tumor (field phenomenon).

Period of stable growth

1. Reactive stroma appears, outlining nests of cells, particularly at deep margin.
2. Lymphoid cells and eosinophils aggregate in reactive stroma.
3. Lymphoid cells migrate into nests of tumor cells.
4. Immune-mediated lysis and coagulation of tumor cells follows.
5. Lytic defects are produced in target organ (tumor).
6. Fibrous inlay of lytic defects (loss of tumor domain to the immune-mediated reactive stroma) follows.

7. Focal, partial, or complete regression of tumor is the end result.

Period of regression
1. Lymphoid cellular infiltrates become less conspicuous.
2. Prominent reactive stroma in various stages of organization becomes more conspicuous.
3. Keratinized debris and foreign body granulomas aggregate in the reactive stroma.
4. The identity of epidermis (thin lining of crater), sweat ducts, and hair follicles on or within the reactive stroma is re-established.

In this sequence, the cytologic character of the infiltrating keratinocytes has been ignored. In large series of keratoacanthomas, two thirds of tumors show moderate or marked dysplasia and are cytologically indistinguishable from squamous carcinomas.[34] In individual keratoacanthomas, the degree of cytologic atypism is variable. Some of the nests and cords of cells are clearly neoplastic, and neighboring nests are often cytologically benign. The neoplastic cells probably are derived from actinically induced clones in the epidermis. They are of the same order as clones in actinic keratoses or actinic squamous carcinomas. The cytologically benign nests probably are derived from adnexal epithelium.[35] They provide a marker for a field phenomenon affecting all the epithelial structures in the area of the tumor (immune stimulation?).[35] In the regressing phase, the identity of distinctive epithelial populations in the skin is re-established. The neoplastic population loses its identity.

At the end of the cytologic spectrum, the degree of cytologic atypism in a keratoacanthoma is severe. The infiltrating cells often form elongated, thin cords rather than broad, bulbous columns. These extreme expressions are often excluded from studies of keratoacanthomas and are arbitrarily assigned to the category of squamous carcinoma.[34] These patterns may be represented focally in an otherwise typical keratoacanthoma. Severe dysplasia is consistent with a diagnosis of keratoacanthoma. The degree of dysplasia should be noted in the diagnosis. Some of the atypical foci may be markers for evolving clones of malignant cells.

There is no evidence that invasion of nerve sheaths and blood vessels has prognostic significance,[11] but the identification of these features qualifies such a tumor as an aggressive variant. Keratoacanthomas that extend beyond the reticular dermis should be viewed with suspicion. They also qualify as aggressive keratocanthomas.

Conceptually, actinic keratoacanthoma might be defined as an expression of a brief immune dysfunction in the site of an actinically induced dysplasia. The delay in the expression of the immune response allows the neoplasm to enlarge rapidly in an aggressive manner. With the appearance of the full expression of the immune response, the growth of the tumor is modified, and on occasion the immune response may eradicate the lesion. This, however, is by no means the rule. The options include complete regression, partial regression but continued lateral growth, and transformation to a carcinoma. No clues in the histologic pattern during the period of rapid growth relate to the options. Rarely, an epidermoid carcinoma displays the rapid growth of a keratoacanthoma. Such lesions are associated with a reactive stroma that is more or less devoid of lymphoid infiltrates. These rare lesions lack the regionally variable patterns of keratoacanthomas.

In immunosuppressed patients or in association with inflammatory skin diseases, keratoacanthomas may be multiple.[10] They show little or no cytologic atypism and often lack the crateriform quality of the actinic keratoacanthoma. In this group of patients, the instability of the cutaneous epithelial layer is manifested in a variety of reactions. Reactive perforating collagenosis, Kyrle's disease, perforating folliculitis, perforating elastosis, and keratoacanthoma are clinical designations for epithelial instabilities commonly expressed in immunosuppressed patients. Rarely, reactive perforating collagenosis appears to be a peculiar expression of the tissue response in a neurotic excoriation. Keratoacanthomas are extremely rare on nonexposed surfaces and in dark-skinned patients.

BASAL CELL SKIN APPENDAGE TUMORS

Trichoepithelioma

In a trichoepithelioma (Brooke's tumor, epithelioma adenoides cysticum), the tumor cells are small, basaloid, and cytologically uniform. They form rounded nests, often with prominent adenoid patterns, or they form central nests with peripherally radiating, interconnected cords[39,40] (Fig. 9-22). The cords are usually two cell layers in thickness. The central nests often show squamous differentiation surrounding small keratin-filled cysts. The tumor cells are arranged in lobules, each supported by a uniform rim of cellular fibrous tissue. The stroma of neighboring lobules blends in areas of contact. In some of the lobules, one or more cords show a terminal, bulbous expansion with a row of palisaded basal cells (Fig. 9-23). Stromal cells with scanty cytoplasm are closely aggregated in a mucinous or fibrous matrix bordering the bulbous expansion of tumor cells. These specialized structures mimic hair bulbs and papillae as seen in early anagen phases of the hair cycle. They are basic to the diagnosis of trichoepithelioma but are no more important than the characteristic stroma.

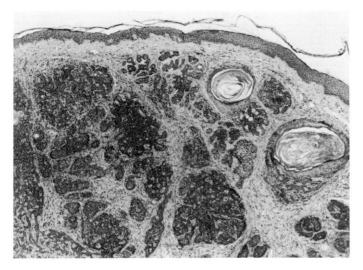

Fig. 9-22. Multiple trichoepithelioma. The lesion is lobulated and each lobule has a special cellular stroma. Delicate cords of basal cells radiate from a nidus. There are scattered keratin-filled cysts.

A trichoepithelioma is organoid. It induces a distinctive, cellular, fibrous stroma that usually has a sharp interface with the neighboring dermis. It rarely shows the mucin-filled clefts of a basal cell carcinoma.

Most trichoepitheliomas are composed of basal cells with keratinizing squamous epithelium surrounding the keratin-filled cysts. The so-called *desmoplastic trichoepithelioma* is composed preponderantly of small squamous cells.[41] The squamous cells form narrow, solid cords that resemble the angulated cords in a syringoma. In contrast to syringoma, the cords show prominent pe-

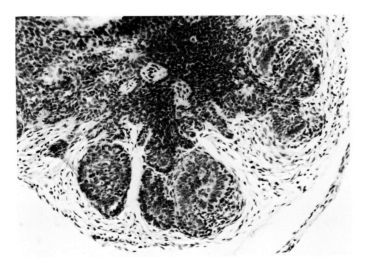

Fig. 9-23. Trichoepithelioma. Hair bulb differentiation and the specialized stroma are illustrated.

ripheral palisades of nuclei. Keratin-filled cysts, some of which are calcified, are a prominent feature. The stroma is not sharply defined at its interface with the adjacent dermis. The tumor is small and circumscribed. Hair bulb differentiation is not a feature of desmoplastic trichoepithelioma.[41] The collagen bundles of the reticular dermis in areas of infiltration are coarsened. The stroma of the tumor contains plump fibrocytes. It lacks the distinctive qualities of the common trichoepithelioma. Desmoplastic trichoepithelioma clinically is flat and indurated with ill defined margins. It often is less than a centimeter in diameter. In size, histologic differentiation, and behavior, desmoplastic trichoepithelioma is distinguished from a sclerosing basal cell carcinoma.

Giant solitary trichoepithelioma is large and circumscribed and bulges into the subcutaneous fat. It has an abundant induced fibrous stroma and contains multiple epithelial lobules. Hair-bulb differentiation is a prominent feature. These large solitary lesions have also been classified as trichoblastomas. If in such a lesion some of the nests of cells show pilar differentiation, the lesion qualifies as trichogenic trichoblastoma.[42]

The small, solitary trichoepithelioma and the lesions in the multiple trechoepithelioma syndrome have a low potential for malignant degeneration. Rarely, an infiltrating basal cell carcinoma blends with a solitary trichoepithelioma. These rare leisons may represent collision tumors but probably represent carcinoma arising in a trichoepithelioma. Carcinomas are rare complications of multiple trichoepitheliomas.

BASALOID SKIN APPENDAGE TUMORS
Basaloid Pilar Tumors

Pilomatrixoma

Pilomatrixoma (calcifying epithelioma of Malherbe) is a self-limited tumor of the skin whose most distinctive quality is a tendency for spontaneous necrosis.[43] In an early phase, the tumor is composed of columns and nests of basophilic cells whose cytologic qualities are identical to those of the hair bulb and the inner root sheath. Occasionally, continuity between a hair follicle and the tumor can be demonstrated. Pigmented melanocytes are an occasional component. The tumor cells have scanty, basophilic cytoplasm and plump, round nuclei with marginated chromatin. In some areas, they are vacuolated and contain trichohyalin. The transition from viable cells to aggregates of coagulated "ghost cells" is abrupt (Fig. 9-24). The conversion of tumor cells to keratinized debris occurs without the intermediary of a granular layer and without distortion of cell outlines. Focally, the popula-

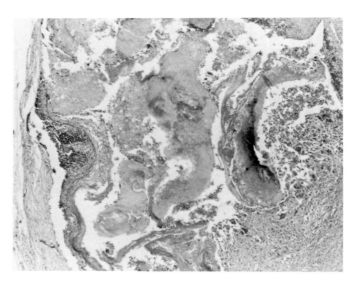

Fig. 9-24. Pilomatrixoma. Basophilic (hair matrix and hair sheath) cells are preserved focally on the left. Most of the tumor cells are necrotic and coagulated (ghost cells). On the right, the necrotic debris has been invaded and partially resorbed by inflamed granulation tissue.

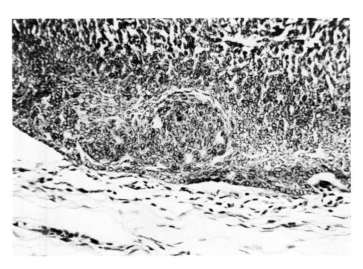

Fig. 9-25. Hair matrix adenoma. The tumor cells are uniform. They have marginated chromatin, scanty cytoplasm, prominent nucleoli, and indistinct cell membranes. Some of the tumor cells are arranged in whorls.

tion of ghost cells extends to the interface with the stroma. The coagulated cells stimulate a foreign body response. Aggregates of the necrotic cells are invaded by granulation tissue and partially resorbed by inflammatory cells, including foreign body giant cells. Some of the necrotic epithelium is calcified. The calcified debris may induce osseous metaplasia. Pilomatrixomas may be multiple. They are usually small lesions, less than a centimeter in diameter. Rarely, a variant qualifies as giant pilomatrixoma. A malignant variant has been described.

Hair Matrix Adenoma

Hair matrix adenoma is a relatively rare, benign skin appendage tumor, usually found on the scalp. It is a circumscribed, multilobulated tumor composed of basaloid cells. The tumor cells have basophilic cytoplasm and plump nuclei with prominent nucleoli (Fig. 9-25). The cells are similar to components in an active hair bulb. Focally, the cells are arranged in whorls and some of the whorls show keratinization. In some examples, lysis of tumor cells results in the formation of irregular clefts in the nests of tumor cells. Mucinous clefts at the interface between tumor and stroma are not a feature of the hair matrix adenoma. The tumors may exceed 5 cm in diameter. Abortive or dysplastic hair follicles are found in the adjacent dermis (Fig. 9-26). The stroma of the tumor is delicately fibrous. It is likely that this lesion also has been included in the category of trichoblastoma.[42]

Basaloid Carcinoma With Hair Sheath Differentiation

Basaloid carcinomas showing hair sheath differentiation are not well defined. One variant is composed of basaloid cells and small squamous cells in nests and cords. The tumor cells form prominent peripheral palisades. Lymphocytes intermingle with tumor cells within the nests (lymphoepithelial patterns). The tumor is supported by a fibrotic reactive stroma. It is indolent but

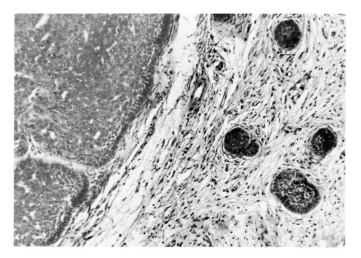

Fig. 9-26. Hair matrix adenoma. The tumor is lobulated and shows peripheral nuclear palisades. Condensed, delicate fibers outline the lobules. Abortive hair follicles are present in the adjacent dermis.

classified as a low-grade carcinoma on the basis of the reactive stroma. A rare variant of basaloid pilar carcinoma qualifies as a malignant hair matrix adenoma. It actively infiltrates the dermis and subcutis.

Basaloid Sebaceous Tumors

Sebaceous Adenoma

It is difficult to clearly define the histologic boundaries between *sebaceous gland hyperplasia* and sebaceous adenoma.[44] Sebaceous gland hyperplasia as a localized lesion is relatively common. It is characterized by a dilated follicle that contains keratinized debris and sebum. Sebaceous gland lobules, which are increased in size and number, surround the dilated follicle. In one variant of sebaceous adenoma, newly formed lobules are attached to a verrucoid hyperplastic epidermis. The verrucoid epidermis commonly shows histologic features of an inverted follicular keratosis.

In a sebaceous adenoma, follicular orientation of sebaceous gland lobules is not a consistent feature. The sebaceous gland lobules vary in size and form a circumscribed nodule. Hyperplasia of germinative, basaloid cells is a prominent feature at the periphery of each lobule. The germinative cells form two or more layers, peripheral to the differentiated sebaceous cells. A variant is characterized by a greatly expanded solitary lobule. Ghost sebaceous cells accumulate in the central portion of the lobule. Sebaceous adenomas and related tumors are multiple in Torre's syndrome and are associated with internal carcinomas.[45,46]

Sebaceous Carcinoma

Sebaceous carcinoma is an infiltrating basosquamous tumor.[44,47] The tumor cells form nests and columns, some of which are attached to the epidermis. The nests of cells are supported by a reactive stroma. Carcinoma in situ, often with an intraepithelial epitheliomatous pattern, is common in the epidermis adjacent to the infiltrating tumor. Sebaceous carcinoma should be distinguished from sebaceous adenoma and epithelioma, but the distinctions are not clearly defined.[44] *Sebaceous epithelioma* is rare. It is characterized by multifocal origin from the epidermis rather than a zone of carcinoma in situ. Peripheral palisading of nuclei and an induced stroma are additional features favoring a sebaceous epithelioma. Nucleoli are inconspicuous in sebaceous epithelioma; they are a conspicuous feature of the nuclei in sebaceous carcinomas. Sebaceous carcinomas occur most commonly on the face. A peculiar biologic aggressiveness has been proposed for facial sebaceous carcinomas as contrasted with the behavior of similar lesions in other sites.[44] This distinction has not been generally accepted.[47] In part, an inability to clearly distinguish between adenomas and carcinomas may account for the apparent relationship between anatomic site and biologic behavior.

Basaloid Sweat Gland Tumors

The basaloid sweat gland tumors include mixed tumors, spiradenomas (eccrine spiradenomas), and cylindrical and lobular adenomas (eccrine cylindromas). The term *cylindroma* is a source of confusion; adenoid cystic carcinoma is also recognized as cylindroma and occasionally involves the skin. The cylindrical and lobular variant corresponds to the so-called turban tumor of the scalp.

The patterns in basaloid sweat gland tumors are generally accepted as evidence of eccrine differentiation. The eccrine derivation of the lobular and cylindrical variant is questionable. It occasionally is possible to establish continuity between a nest of tumor cells and a sweat duct. Tumor lobules occasionally blend with hair follicles. Nests of basal cells showing abortive patterns of follicular differentiation are occasionally represented in the adjacent dermis. Tubular patterns are seldom well developed but are occasionally evident in some of the lobules. If the lobular and cylindrical variant occasionally expresses histologic patterns of sweat duct and hair follicle differentiation, it is a compound skin appendage tumor.

Basaloid adenomas of the skin are composed of two cell types: a basal cell and a small squamous cell. The basal cells form peripheral palisades. They have scanty cytoplasm and small nuclei with uniformly distributed chromatin. The squamous cells form aggregates that are outlined by basal cells. A lymphoid cell commonly intermingles with the basic tumor cells. Hyaline membranous material is associated with the basal cells.

The lobular and cylindrical variant (eccrine or dermal cylindroma) is found mainly on the scalp and face; the spiradenoma occurs more commonly on the trunk and extremities. In occasional patients with multiple basaloid sweat gland adenomas, some of the lesions have been lobular and cylindrical adenomas, and some have been spiradenomas. Occasionally, some of the lesions display the features of trichoepithelioma. The spiradenoma often is painful and may be confused clinically and histologically with glomus tumor.

The *basaloid spiradenoma (eccrine spiradenoma)* is a lobulated tumor. Within the lobules, there is a regular orientation of basal cells and squamous cells.[48] In cords or tubules, the basal cells define the limits of aggregates of squamous cells (Fig. 9-27). The squamous cells are arranged in three or four cell layers and form solid cords

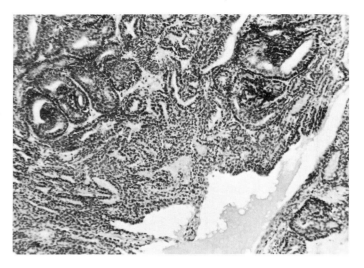

Fig. 9-27. Basaloid (eccrine) spiradenoma. Tubular and trabecular patterns are represented. The tubules are uniform in width. Most of the tubules are lined by two distinct layers of cells. The epithelial component is regularly spaced in the stroma.

or outline tubular lumina. The cords and tubules are supported by a delicate, edematous fibrous matrix that is cell poor but richly vascularized. Hyaline basement membrane material is focally prominent and outlines the cords and tubules. Regional variations are manifested by clear cell acinar patterns and nuclear atypism. Occasionally, the tumor shows extensive cystic degeneration, necrosis, and hemorrhage.

The *lobular* and *cylindrical variant (eccrine cylindroma)* may show cylindrical, lobular, or combined patterns. In the lobules, the cells are uniformly distributed with intermingling of basal and squamous cells (Fig. 9-28). Focally. the cells may form trabecular patterns. Basal cells form palisades at the periphery of the lobules. Tubular patterns are rarely prominent. Thick hyaline membranes outline the lobules.

The cylindrical pattern is characterized by tortuous cylinders (columns) of cells that appear to rest within and adapt to the interstices of the reticular dermis[49] (Fig. 9-29). They commonly extend into the subcutaneous tissue, where they are supported by the adipose tissue. They show a peripheral sheath of hyaline membranous material. Basal cells abut on the peripheral sheath. Basal cells and squamous cells intermingle within the cylinders of cells. Tubules and cords are only focally developed in the lobules or cylinders. In both patterns, rounded hyaline deposits are outlined by rosettes of basal cells.

The poorly defined margins of the cylindrical and tubular variant complicates the surgical management. The widely spaced nests in the dermis and the subcutis are difficult to detect during surgery and may serve as nidi for local recurrences.

The differentiation between the two variants of basaloid sweat gland tumors is based on the arrangement of the cells, the prominence of hyaline deposits and the anatomic distribution. Occasional patterns suggesting hair follicle differentiation are features of the lobular and cylindrical variant. Similar lesions in salivary glands are classified as dermal analogue tumors.[49,50] It would be equally appropriate to classify the cutaneous lesions as salivary gland analogue tumors.

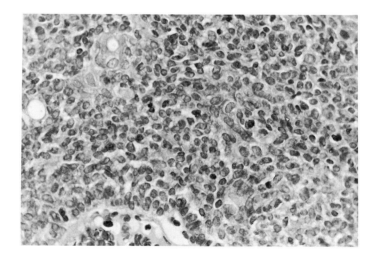

Fig. 9-28. Lobular and cylindrical basaloid adenoma. The lobular component is represented. The basal and squamous cells are haphazardly arranged. There are two areas of poral differentiation.

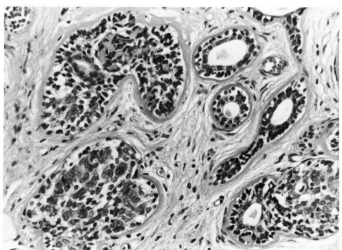

Fig. 9-29. Lobular and cylindrical basaloid adenoma. The cylindrical component is represented. Cords of basal and small squamous cells are outlined by hyaline membranes. Some of the aggregates of cells form tubular patterns.

NEOPLASMS OF THE SKIN

Basaloid Sweat Gland Carcinoma

Basaloid adenomas occasionally evolve into basaloid or basosquamous adenocarcinomas.[51-53] The relationship is best established by identifying a remnant of the benign adenoma in an infiltrating carcinoma. The carcinoma is generally basaloid with occasional patterns of glandular differentiation. The tumor cells in irregular nests and cords actively infiltrate a reactive stroma (Fig. 9-30). Basosquamous variants commonly are associated with a dense infiltrate of lymphoid cells in the stroma. In some examples, the lymphoid cells intermingle with tumor cells. Similar patterns may be seen in some basaloid carcinomas of salivary glands in which careful examination will occasionally reveal a remnant of a basal cell adenoma. The cutaneous basaloid carcinomas may be confused with metastatic lymphoepitheliomas of the nasopharynx. Low-grade or borderline basaloid adenocarcinomas are cellular tumors that are locally infiltrative (Fig. 9-31).

Basaloid sweat gland carcinomas of the skin may metastasize to regional lymph nodes, but their behavior is not as aggressive as their histologic features indicate. They are commonly misinterpreted as metastatic poorly differentiated squamous carcinoma or adenocarcinoma. They may also be confused with *trabecular carcinomas* of the skin. Trabecular carcinoma was originally described as a sweat gland tumor,[54] but emphasis has recently shifted to a neurocrine origin.[55,56] The trabecular carcinoma shares morphologic features, including cytoplasmic dense core vesicles, with oat cell carcinoma of the lung.[57,58]

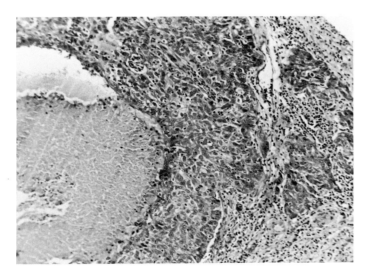

Fig. 9-30. Basaloid adenocarcinoma (malignant basaloid adenoma). The tumor has basaloid qualities. The cells form nests and cords and are supported by a reactive stroma. A cystic space contains cellular debris. A remnant of the basaloid adenoma was preserved within the carcinoma.

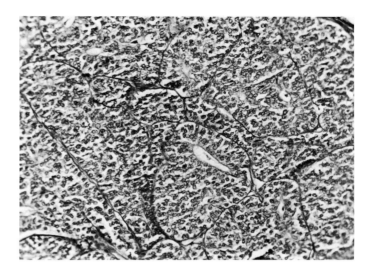

Fig. 9-31. Basaloid adenocarcinoma (malignant basaloid adenoma). In this low-grade, infiltrating tumor, the basic pattern is preserved. The cords and tubules are hypercellular and are compactly aggregated.

Mixed Tumors of Sweat Gland Origin

The mixed tumors of the skin *(chondroid syringoma)* are tubular and basaloid.[58,59] The tubules are tortuous but regularly spaced in a vascularized, delicate, fibrous matrix. They are usually composed of two cell layers. The luminal layers are squamoid or cuboidal; the peripheral layer is a single row of basal cells. In many areas, the basal cells are triangular and widely spaced in a clear or mucinous matrix; they are myoepithelial cells. Focally, some of the epithelial cells lining the tubules have apocrine qualities. In areas, myoepithelial cells proliferate and isolate themselves in a mucinous matrix. Some of the mucinous zones acquire chondroid characteristics. Adipose tissue is an occasional component of the stroma.

A variant of cutaneous mixed tumor has a uniform chondromyxoid matrix in which small acini are regularly spaced. The acini are outlined by cuboidal epithelial cells.

Mixed tumors are circumscribed and partially outlined by a condensation of fibrous tissue. In some examples, particularly in lesions from the perioral region, the basal cells focally may form bulbous expansions with striking nuclear palisades in the peripheral row of cells. These structures represent areas of hair follicle differentiation. Sebaceous differentiation may also be manifested. Tumors showing pilosebaceous and sweat duct differentiation qualify as compound mixed tumors. They may express apocrine qualities in which the potentials of the apocrine and follicular anlage are manifested.

Malignant mixed tumor of the skin is rare. The acral portions of the extremities are favored sites. The tumor cells are squamoid and epithelioid.[60] In focal areas, they isolate themselves in a mucinous or chondroid matrix. Epithelioid cells are most prominent in the mucinous or chondroid areas. They have hyperchromatic, plump, eccentric nuclei and acidophilic homogeneous or fibrillated cytoplasm. Malignant mixed tumors actively infiltrate the dermis and subcutaneous fat. Metastases and local recurrences are potential problems. Some examples of basaloid eccrine carcinoma[61] with fibromyxomatous stroma may represent a variant of malignant mixed tumor.[62]

Adenoid cystic carcinoma is a special variant of sweat gland carcinoma. It has basal cell qualities. In areas, the tumor cells produce a mucinous matrix that surrounds cords, tubules, and nests.[63,64] Deposits of mucin accumulate in the nests of cells to produce adenoid and cystic patterns. The tubules are composed of two layers of cells with a luminal row of squamoid cells. The peripheral row often has the qualities of triangular cells in a mucinous matrix, as commonly seen in mixed tumors. In slowly growing tumors, the mucinous matrix is often hyalinized. Some adenoid cystic carcinomas of the skin are well circumscribed, a feature which may have prognostic significance. Rare examples of adenoid cystic carcinoma are characterized by rather pure tubular patterns. The so-called *basaloid eccrine carcinoma* may be a tubular variant of adenoid cystic carcinoma (Fig. 9-32).

Adenoid cystic carcinoma in the skin is comparable to histologically identical tumors in other sites such as the salivary glands, the upper respiratory tract, and the breast. It is relatively common in the axilla and may be confused with an adenoid cystic carcinoma arising in the axillary extension of the breast. This tumor has a potential for local recurrence. Metastases seem to be less common from cutaneous variants than from salivary gland variants.

SQUAMOUS SKIN APPENDAGE TUMORS
Squamous Follicular Tumors

Included in this category are keratinous cysts. In classifying such cysts, comparisons are made between the epithelial lining of a cyst and the epithelium of a normal hair follicle. Hair follicles have three distinctive regions. The epithelium of the infundibular portion of follicles resembles the squamous epithelium of the epidermis. In the isthmic portion, the squamous epithelium keratinizes without an intermediate granular layer. The cells at the interface are rounded and bulge into the lumen of the follicle. The outer root sheath is outlined by a hyaline membrane. Its cells keratinize without an intermediate granular layer. Some of the cells are glycogen rich and vacuolated. The *epidermoid cyst* is lined by keratinizing epithelium with infundibular characteristics. The *pilar (trichilemmal) cyst* has an epithelial lining with isthmic qualities. There is no granular layer and the final layer of viable cells bulges into the lumen of the keratin-filled cyst.

The *steatocystoma* also has an epithelial lining that is devoid of a granular layer. The luminal surface is corrugated. The keratinized cells are flattened, wavy, and loosely laminated. Sebaceous gland lobules are attached to the wall of the cyst. Occasionally, the lining epithelium differentiates into abortive hair follicles. In the latter type, the lumen may contain vellus hairs (*vellus hair cyst*). Steatocystomas may be multiple.[65]

The *dermoid cyst* is a special variant in which skin appendages are attached to the lining epithelium. Hair follicles and sweat gland units are represented. The periorbital area is a common location.

Proliferating Pilar Tumor

A pilar cyst is occasionally transformed into a solid tumor. The transformation is accomplished by proliferation of the lining epithelium and by an ingrowth of granulation tissue into the keratin-filled cyst. The granulation tissue resorbs the keratinized debris and in multiple sites isolates nests of proliferating tumor cells. Neighboring nests of viable epithelium thus come to be separated by organizing granulation tissue in which aggregates of keratinized debris are embedded. In spite of the complex patterns, the contour of such a lesion is smoothly spheri-

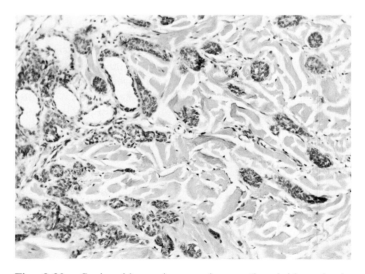

Fig. 9-32. Syringoid eccrine carcinoma (basaloid variant). Atypical small basaloid cells form cords and tubules in a relatively unaltered reticular dermis. Some of the tubules are lined by a double layer of epithelial cells. This tumor metastasized to regional lymph nodes.

A distinctive feature of this group of lesions is the ability of isolated squamous cells to form a single, cytoplasmic vacuole (Fig. 9-35), sometimes outlined by a condensation of cytoplasmic fibrils (cuticle). The vacuole may expand to form a small cyst containing inspissated material. The vacuolated tumor cells share features with cells in regenerating sweat duct (poral) epithelium. The vacuolar process recapitulates the formation of a lumen in the embryologic development of a sweat duct.

Squamous poroadenomas are subdivided into three variants, depending on the arrangement of tumor cells.[11] They may be lobular (eccrine acrospiroma), cylindrical or ductal (dermal duct tumor), or papular (eccrine poroma). Two or all of the variable patterns may be combined in a single lesion. The lobules may be solid or cystic. Squamous epithelium is basic to this group of lesions, but epithelial variations include glycogen-rich clear cells, mucus-secreting goblet cells, and pseudostratified columnar epithelium. In some examples, melanocytes and pigmented squamous cells are a feature. The papular and cylindrical variants are composed preponderantly of squamous cells with focal ductal patterns. The more complicated epithelial patterns are found in the lobular variants.

The *papular* variant *(eccrine poroma)* occurs frequently on the acral portions of the lower extremities. It is a clonal disease of the epidermis in which a cytologically distinctive population of squamous cells forms a sharp interface with the normal epidermis. Columns of cells extend into the dermis from the distinctive epidermal plaque (Fig. 9-36). The overall contour often is that of an inverted wedge with the base at the surface of the skin. The columns of cells may differentiate focally to form small cysts and tubules, particularly near the deep margin of the lesion. They partially converge to an apex in the dermis. Some of the columns communicate with dilated sweat ducts. They are supported by an edematous, papillary dermis containing tortuous, ectatic vessels.

The *cylindrical* variant *(dermal duct tumor)* is composed of coarse, tortuous cylinders of squamous cells in the dermis. Some of the aggregates of cells form tubules (see Fig. 9-35). The aggregates of cells are accommo-

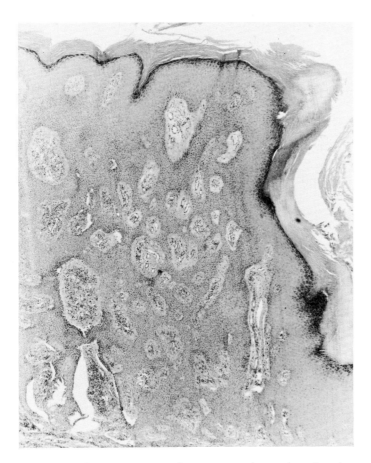

Fig. 9-36. Squamous poroadenoma, papular variant (eccrine poroma). Columns of small squamous cells extend from the epidermis into the dermis. There are focal areas of tubular differentiation.

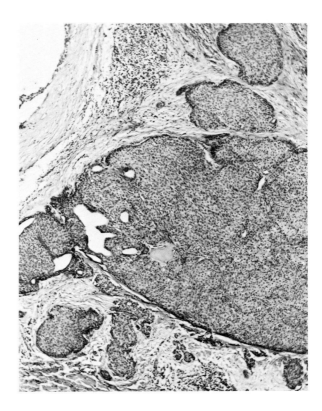

Fig. 9-37. Squamous poroadenoma, lobular variant (eccrine acrospiroma). Small squamous cells form a lobule in the reticular dermis. There are small cysts lined by cuboidal epithelium in the lobule. Irregular cords of tumor cells infiltrate a reactive stroma.

dated by collagen bundles of the reticular dermis; there is no specialized tumor stroma.

The *lobular* variant (*eccrine acrospiroma*) is characteristically multilobular within the dermis and subcutis.[59,71,72] Some of the lobules are solid and others are partially cystic. The lobules are composed of squamous cells. Focally, the squamous cells may have vacuolated (clear, glycogen-rich) cytoplasm. Individual cells may contain distinct cytoplasmic vacuoles (poral or syringeal differentiation). Occasionally, particularly on the scalp, some of the cells may contain melanin. Squamous, mucinous, or columnar cells may form the surface layer bordering the cysts. Small nests and cords of cells may extend into the adjacent dermis in an infiltrating pattern and stimulate a delicate reactive stroma (*infiltrating poroadenoma*) (Fig. 9-37). Occasionally, the separate small nests infiltrate lymphatic spaces in the dermis. Rarely, squamous poroadenomas of the lobular variety have metastasized without a significant change in histologic pattern. The metastases have involved the lymphatics and bloodstream, with lymph nodes, lungs, and bones as common sites.[72,73]

OTHER TUBULAR ADENOMAS OF SWEAT GLANDS

Rare *apocrine tubular adenomas* of sweat glands do not qualify as either squamous or basaloid variants. The tumor cells have granular, acidophilic cytoplasm and show decapitation secretion. Some tubular adenomas are characterized by uniform tubules lined by a double layer of small squamous cells. They are circumscribed and supported by a delicate fibrous matrix. They may represent *monomorphic* variants of *mixed tumors*. The tubules are better developed and more widely spaced than tubules in basaloid spiradenomas.

Papillary eccrine adenoma occurs most commonly on the lower extremities.[74] It is composed of tortuous, dilated ducts which are lined by a double layer of cuboidal cells. Irregular epithelial papillae are common. The tumor infiltrates the dermis and is supported by a delicate, reactive stroma. In spite of worrisome histologic features, it is apparently benign.

CARCINOMAS OF SWEAT GLAND ORIGIN

Carcinomas of sweat gland origin have not received serious consideration. Reported studies, in providing data on biologic behavior, have grouped tumors showing a variety of histologic patterns.[75] It is possible to recognize the following variants[73,75]:

1. Ductal carcinoma
   Sclerosing sweat duct carcinoma (syringomatous carcinoma, microcystic carcinoma)
   Porocarcioma
   Solid and ductal carcinoma (analogue of breast carcinoma)
   Papillary carcinoma
2. Malignant mixed tumor
3. Basaloid and basosquamous adenocarcinoma (malignant spiradenoma and lobular and cylindrical basaloid adenoma)
4. Apocrine adenocarcinoma
5. Adenoid cystic carcinoma
6. Mucinous carcinoma
7. Clear cell carcinoma

Sclerosing sweat duct carcinoma is composed of irregularly spaced cords and tubules. The tubules are composed of a double layer of small squamous cells and resemble sweat ducts.[76,77] The tubules and cords infiltrate the reticular dermis between collagen bundles or are supported by a dense fibrous matrix. As a regional variation, some of the nests of cells may show central areas of keratinization (microcystic pattern). The histologic pattern, especially on small biopsy specimens, is deceptively bland. The tumor infiltrates the dermis, nerve sheaths, and adjacent soft tissue. Clinically, the margins are difficult to define. This carcinoma may evolve into a destructive, local lesion. Rarely, it metastasizes.

A similar neoplasm involving the nipple has been designated *syringomatous adenoma*. Features which sets syringomatous adenoma apart from sclerosing sweat duct carcinoma have not been defined.

Basaloid eccrine carcinoma[73,78] has similar syringomatous qualities but the tumor cells are basaloid rather than squamoid. Regional variations include adenoid patterns. This carcinoma probably is a variant of adenoid cystic carcinoma.

Porocarcinoma is a relatively common variant. It is composed of minimally to moderately atypical basaloid and rounded squamous cells.[73,78] The cells commonly form tubular patterns with basaloid cells at the periphery and squamous cells outlining the lumens (Fig. 9-38). The neoplastic cells in nests actively infiltrate the dermis and subcutis. They are supported by a reactive stroma. Lymphatic invasion is a common feature. Carcinoma in situ in a pattern of intraepithelial epithelioma (malignant hidroacanthoma in situ) is a common feature in the overlying epidermis. Focal areas of dedifferentiation are characterized by cellular atypism and tumor giant cells. Occasionally, porocarcinomas arise in squamous lobular

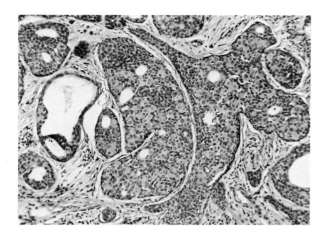

Fig. 9-38. Porocarcinoma. Atypical basaloid and rounded squamous cells form tubules and cords in an inflamed fibrous matrix. The small vacuoles are cytoplasmic and express sweat pore differentiation. The tumor metastasized to regional lymph nodes and to the lungs.

poroadenomas. Tumor cells with a single well defined cytoplasmic vacuole are a distinctive marker for poral differentiation.

The *solid* and *ductal variant* of carcinoma is a close histologic simulant of ductal carcinoma of the breast.[78] Occasionally, the cylindrical components show central areas of necrosis to produce a comedo pattern.

In the *papillary* variant, the tumor cells are cuboidal or columnar. They have basophilic cytoplasm and plump atypical nuclei. The cells form complex interconnected papillae in which nuclei are occasionally stratified. An acral variant of papillary sweat gland carcinoma has been recently described.[79] It is characterized by papillary and microglandular (cribriform) patterns.

Malignant mixed tumors, adenoid cystic carcinomas, and basosquamous adenocarcinomas have been discussed.

Apocrine carcinoma is composed of granular, acidophilic cells with atypical, hyperchromatic nuclei.[73] Decapitation secretion is usually a feature. The cells form glandular, papillary, and solid patterns. The axilla or genital areas are the usual sites of involvement. In the axilla, the tumor is commonly misdiagnosed as carcinoma of the breast.

Mucinous adenocarcinoma is composed of clusters of atypical epithelial cells in pools of extracellular mucins.[80,81] It is comparable to the mucinous (gelatinous or colloid) carcinoma of the breast or gastrointestinal tract. It is a low-grade carcinoma.

Rare *clear cell carcinomas* of the skin are difficult to classify. Some may represent glycogen-rich sweat gland carcinomas, possibly related to squamous lobular poroadenomas (eccrine acrospiromas). Others, which are uniformly composed of clear cells, may represent glycogen-rich hair sheath carcinomas or a clear cell variant of epidermoid carcinoma. Columnar patterns and peripheral palisading of nuclei are features favoring the diagnosis of trichilemmal (pilar) carcinoma. Hyaline deposits are in keeping with either sweat gland or trichilemmal differentiation. Sweat gland carcinomas are immunoreactive for CEA. If eccrine differentiation is a feature, the neoplastic cells also may react for S-100 protein.

METASTATIC CARCINOMAS

Metastatic carcinomas are common in the skin.[82,83] They are characteristically dermal or subcutaneous lesions without continuity with the overlying epidermis. They may, however, invade the epidermis. The invading tumor cells often form discrete nests in the epidermis; they may loosely infiltrate the epidermis in pagetoid patterns. Some carcinomas of skin appendages appear isolated in the dermis without an epidermal component. They may be mistakenly diagnosed as metastases.

Neuroendocrine carcinomas, including oat cell carcinoma of the lung and bronchial carcinoid tumors, metastasize to the skin.[84] When the differential diagnosis includes small cell undifferentiated carcinoma, *trabecular carcinoma* is a rare source of confusion.[56–58] Its cells contain neurosecretory granules.[85] The latter are often assumed to be markers for cells derived from the neural crest and for amine precursor uptake and decarboxylation (APUD) properties. Recent embryologic studies on the origin of islet cells have weakened the significance of dense core granules as neurocristic markers.[86] Trabecular carcinomas may show areas of squamous differentiation or pseudorosettes. Fragmentation of the nuclei of the neoplastic cells is an additional feature. Ultrastructurally, a juxtanuclear condensation of filaments (dotlike) is characteristic.[85]

Tumors that are commonly metastatic to the skin include carcinomas of the lung, kidney, breast, and GI tract. Squamous carcinomas and adenosquamous carcinomas most often prove to be metastatic from the lung. Carcinoma of the breast in its scirrhous (signet ring) pattern and as infiltrating lobular carcinoma has a distinct tendency to form Indian files. Clinically, clear cell carcinoma of the kidney is extremely protean in its metastatic features. Histologically, it is composed of trabeculae supported by a rich plexus of delicate vessels. Extravasated erythrocytes are common and may collect in gland-like spaces. The latter pattern is commonly mistaken for angiosarcoma. The gland-like spaces commonly contain colloid.

Epithelioid sarcoma is a special problem. This soft tissue tumor of fascia and aponeuroses produces cutaneous metastases (pattern of satellitosis) that often show central areas of necrosis. The metastases may be confused with a palisaded granuloma or with satellite lesions of amelanotic melanoma.[87,88]

Occasionally it is possible to predict the site of an occult carcinoma by the recognition of distinctive patterns in cutaneous lesions. Fat necrosis in the subcutis may be a feature of pancreatic carcinoma. Necrolytic migratory erythema may be a feature associated with glucagonoma.[89]

HAMARTOMAS (CONGENITAL AND ACQUIRED)

The hamartomas of the skin include a group of tumorous malformations that may be solitary or multiple. The multiple hamartomas commonly are an expression of a genetic disorder. In hamartomas, the affected tissues are native to the involved site. Choristomas are related malformations but contain extraneous as well as native components. Most hamartomas are small, self-limited lesions. Some have been discussed previously. Table 9-2 lists representative examples of solitary hamartomas and syndromes associated with multiple hamartomas.

Pilosebaceous Hamartomas

The outer root sheath has distinctive qualities, which include vacuolated glycogen-rich cells, palisaded basal cells, and a hyaline membrane. In *trichilemmoma,* these

features are expressed in a localized tumor, usually confined to the butterfly area of the face.[90] The lesion consists of a plaque of hyperplastic squamous cells, often exhibiting a verrucoid surface. Columns of squamous cells and basaloid cells extend from the plaque into a widened papillary dermis (Fig. 9-39). The height of the lesion (from the deep margin to the surface) is usually greater than the cross-sectional diameter (width). At the surface, the plaque of hyperplastic epidermis often has a prominent granular layer with vacuolated cells, features that are reminiscent of a viral verruca late in its evolution. At the deep margin, basaloid cells are often a prominent component. They may form a distinct row of palisaded basal cells with a peripheral, thick hyaline membrane.

The histologic limits between *inverted follicular keratosis* and trichilemmoma are not sharply defined. Both lesions have the same anatomic distribution, although the inverted follicular keratosis is more common in the periorbital areas, and the trichilemmoma tends to favor the nasal skin and the perioral areas. Patterns of trichilemmoma and inverted follicular keratosis are frequently combined, and the assignment of a given lesion to one or the other category is often arbitrary.

Inverted follicular keratosis is a vertically oriented hamartoma, commonly showing a verrucoid surface.[91] Columns of cells extend from the verrucoid hyperplastic epidermis into a widened papillary dermis. The preponderant cell is a small squamous cell, but there are prominent whorls of plump keratinizing squamous cells (Fig. 9-40). The whorls surround collections of keratinized debris. Pale or vacuolated glycogen-rich cells are often a

TABLE 9-2. Representative Types of Hamartomas and Hamartomal Syndromes

Solitary	Multiple
Trichoepithelioma	Multiple trichoepitheliomas
Syringoma	Multiple syringomas
Lobular and cylindrical basaloid adenoma	Turban tumor of the scalp
Tubular basaloid adenoma	Multiple eccrine spiradenomas
Melanocytic angiofibroma (fibrous papule)	Tuberous sclerosis complex
True neuroma	Multiple neuromata syndrome
Trichilemmoma	Multiple hamartoma syndrome (Cowden's syndrome)
Steatocystoma	Steatocystoma multiplex
Sebaceous adenoma	Multiple sebaceous adenomas (Torre's syndrome)
Seborrheic keratosis	Multiple seborrheic keratoses (Leser-Trelat syndrome)

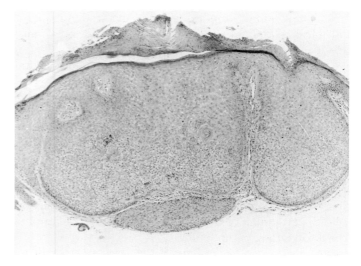

Fig. 9-39. Trichilemmoma. Bulbous columns of basaloid and squamous cells extend from the epidermis into a widened papillary dermis. The epithelium has trichilemmal qualities.

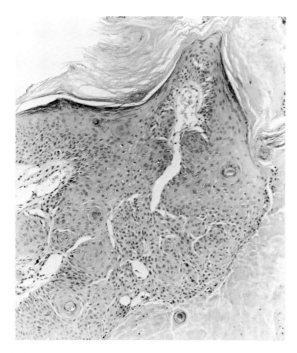

Fig. 9-40. Inverted follicular keratosis. The epidermis shows papillomatosis and hypergranulosis. Columns of squamous and basaloid cells extend into a widened papillary dermis. The squamous cells are arranged in whorls.

feature. Irregular clefts often separate the small basaloid cells from each other and from the whorls.

Giant inverted follicular keratoses are broad, plaque-like lesions with columns of squamous cells that infiltrate the dermis. Individually, the columns of cells have the histologic features of an inverted follicular keratosis. These lesions appear to be more common on the trunk or buttocks.

The pattern of inverted follicular keratosis is occasionally a regional variation in condyloma acuminatum. The pattern of inverted follicular keratosis is also recapitulated in irritated, acquired infundibular keratosis.

Trichilemmoma and inverted follicular keratosis have a tendency to degenerate in focal areas.[91] Cellular fibrous tissue invades the degenerating epithelium, producing a complex pseudoinvasive pattern in which interconnected cords of basaloid cells are supported by a cellular fibromucinous matrix (sclerosing entrapment). The pseudoinvasive pattern occurs within the confines of the hamartoma and does not produce irregular extensions into the adjacent dermis.

The lesions in *Cowden's syndrome* are verrucoid.[92,93] Some of the lesions show a nonspecific pattern of verrucoid hyperplasia. Lesions showing the histologic features of trichilemmoma also are common. Some of the lesions more closely resemble an inverted follicular keratosis.

In both trichilemmomas and inverted follicular kera-

toses, dilated keratin-filled ostia are present in the hyperplastic epidermis. In small lesions, it is sometimes possible to identify a single follicle that contributes epithelial cells to the lesion.

The *tumor of the follicular infundibulum* is a variant of a follicular hamartoma.[67] This plaque-like lesion consists of columns of pale squamous cells extending into a widened papillary dermis that interconnect with neighboring columns. In the lesion, specialized epithelium forms the ostia of hair follicles but this is also a feature of acquired infundibular keratoses.

Papillomas are common on the face, particularly the periorbital regions. They may be relatively pure, verrucoid epidermal hyperplasias or may be the surface expression of trichilemmomas or inverted follicular keratosis. They commonly show virus-like features, including a prominent granular layer and keratinocytes with vacuolated cytoplasm. Some papillomas are associated with abnormal sebaceous gland lobules. The lobules are attached to the verrucoid epidermis without an intervening follicle. They often show incomplete maturation with a prominent layer of germinative cells.

Trichofolliculoma[67] is a follicular hamartoma characterized by a dilated pore through which white lanugo hairs often project. The lesion is characterized histologically by an elongated, dilated follicle containing keratinized debris. The lining squamous epithelium has

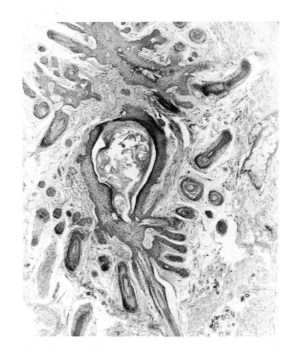

Fig. 9-41. Trichofolliculoma. An elongated keratin-filled follicle is lined by squamous epithelium. Multiple small hair follicles extend from the lining epithelium into a widened perifollicular sheath.

isthmic or infundibular qualities. Multiple abortive hair bulbs and their root sheaths project from the follicular lining into the adjacent perifollicular fibrous sheath (Fig. 9-41). Some of the abortive hair bulbs form the lanugo hairs.

Giant pore[67] is similar to a trichofolliculoma but is devoid of abortive hair bulbs. The pattern of a giant pore is commonly represented over an epidermoid cyst. The close association between the two is evidence that many epidermoid cysts are sequentially related to giant pores.

Some of the *congenital preauricular sinuses* (branchial cleft remnants) histologically resemble a trichofolliculoma. Hyaline cartilage may be found in the adjacent dermis (accessory tragus).

Multiple follicular hamartomas (dysplasias) that are composed of basal cells in abortive follicular patterns have been described. These lesions are occasionally associated with multiple basal cell carcinomas and in some examples, the hamartomas and carcinoma have been systematized.

Sweat Gland Hamartomas

Syringomas are sweat duct hamartomas. They are common on the face, particularly the periorbital regions, and may also involve the upper portion of the trunk. They may appear in eruptive fashion after puberty.

Syringomas are composed of small squamous cells. The cells form solid thin cords of two or three layers or tubules lined by a double layer of cells.[59] Some of the tubules are focally dilated (microcystic) and contain granular inspissated secretions. Cells bordering the dilated lumina commonly have clear cytoplasm. Occasionally, some of the nests of cells form keratin-filled cysts. Some of the cords of cells have a comma-like configuration. The nests of cells are supported by a dense fibrous matrix. A punch biopsy specimen often includes the entire lesion.

Hidrocystoma is a cystically dilated sweat gland or duct lined by a double layer of cuboidal cells or by a single layer of apocrine cells showing decapitation secretion. Focal papillary epithelial hyperplasia and squamous metaplasia are variant features. The epithelium is supported by a thin fibrous membrane. *Papillary cystadenoma* is a related lesion, but is also characterized by glandular components. Some epithelial cysts of the skin are lined by cilated columnar epithelium. They generally occur on the thighs of young women.

Connective Tissue Hamartomas

In some genetic disorders, the connective tissue is affected. If mesenchymal cells are affected, the end prod-

uct (the connective tissue) is likely to be abnormal. A variety of connective tissue hamartomas are manifested by abnormal fibrous or mucinous products. Some of these cutaneous hamartomas acquire diagnostic significance in the appropriate clinical settings.[94,95]

Angiofibroma (adenoma sebaceum, fibrous papule, perifollicular fibroma) is a peculiar dysplasia of connective tissue.[96–98] Solitary or multiple lesions occur on the butterfly area of the face. The solitary lesions are usually classified as fibrous papules or melanocytic angiofibromas. The multiple lesions are a marker for the *tuberous sclerosis complex* (*adenoma sebaceum* of Pringle).[94]

Angiofibroma is a fibrous hamartoma that widens the papillary dermis and the perifollicular sheaths. The matrix is densely fibrous and laminated or edematous. Plump spindle and stellate cells are distributed throughout the matrix but are most numerous near the epidermis. Some of the cells contain coarsely clumped melanin. Multinucleated cells that resemble nevus cells are occasionally a prominent feature. Vessels in the lesion are ectatic. Follicular neogenesis is a common feature. The epidermis shows hyperkeratosis, acanthosis, effacement of rete ridges, and melanocytic hyperplasia. Isolated, vacuolated keratinocytes are often a feature of the epidermis.

Solitary melanocytic angiofibroma (fibrous papule)[96] is a histologic simulant of adenoma sebaceum of the tuberous sclerosis complex. Other connective tissue hamartomas of the tuberous sclerosis complex are characterized by coarsened collagen bundles in the reticular dermis. The interwoven fiber pattern is preserved. Shagreen patch of the tuberous sclerosis complex is an example.[94,99,100] Not all connective tissue nevi of the collagenous type are associated with tuberous sclerosis.[95]

The most common connective tissue hamartoma is a polypoid overgrowth of the reticular dermis. Occasionally, adipose tissue also is represented. These acquired or congenital lesions are classified as *skin tags, acrochordons,* or *fibroepithelial polyps.* The congenital lesions are often plaque-like and commonly involve the buttocks. They are classified as *nevus lipomatosus superficialis.* The elastic fibers of skin tags (fibroepithelial polyps) are coarse and membranous; they have the characteristics of the elastica of the reticular dermis. The common dermal nevus is of the same order as skin tags.

Follicular mesenchymal hamartomas include *perifollicular fibroma, fibrofolliculoma,* and *trichodiscoma.*[101] The perifollicular fibroma is difficult to define as an entity separate from angiofibroma. Fibrofolliculoma is a hyperplasia of the perifollicular connective tissue sheath and lattice-like proliferation of outer sheath cells within the confines of the altered connective tissue sheath. Trichodiscoma is a localized hyperplasia of fibromyxomatous matrix in association with a follicle. Conceptually, it is a hamartoma of the tactile hair disc (which also is a site rich in Merkel cells). Vessels are focally clustered in the matrix. The lesion involves the upper portion of the dermis and presses on the epidermis. Trichodiscomas, fibrofolliculomas, and skin tags are occasionally multiple and familial.[101]

Some connective tissue hamartomas contain abnormal elastica *(nevus elasticus)*. The elastic fibers are coarsened and increased in number in the reticular dermis.[95] Occasionally, the fibers are structurally abnormal with a laminated structure in which the outer lamella is fibrinoid (yellow) with a Verhoeff-van Gieson stain.[102] Nevus elasticus may be associated with osteopoikilosis.

TUMOROUS DYSPLASIAS OF THE SKIN

Nevus sebaceus of Jadassohn (organoid nevus) is a congenital tumorous dysplasia.[29] The scalp is the common site, and the initial clinical manifestation is an area of alopecia. The lesion, with advancing age, slowly enlarges and becomes verrucoid. It has a life history, both clinically and histologically.

Nevus sebaceus is characterized by hyperplasia of the basal layer of the epidermis, abortive development of pilar units, hyperplasia and defective maturation of sebaceous units, and apocrine sweat glands (Fig. 9-42). With advancing age, the epidermis shows verrucoid hyperplasia and areas of follicular neogenesis. The follicles progressively enlarge and elongate, but the pilar units persist

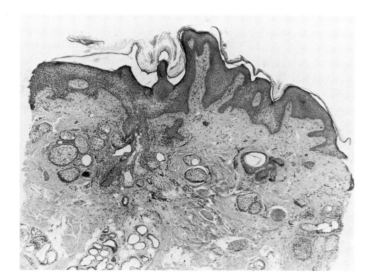

Fig. 9-42. Nevus sebaceus of Jadassohn. The three basic epithelial components are represented: (1) verrucoid epidermal hyperplasia, (2) hyperplasic sebaceous glands with an abortive hair follicle, and (3) apocrine sweat glands.

in an immature stage. Sebaceous lobules increase in number and size (but some show defective maturation) and may bud from earlier generations rather than from follicular epithelium. Vacuoles in some of the sebaceous lobules are a characteristic feature.

In the pre- or postpubertal phase, nevus sebaceus may be complicated by *syringocystadenoma papilliferum*. The latter tumor is characterized by cysts or papillae lined by a double layer of cuboidal epithelial cells or by squamous epithelium. The papillae may project through an epidermal defect to the surface of the skin. Lymphoid infiltrates with numerous plasma cells concentrate in the fibrous fronds supporting the epithelium. Syringocystadenoma papilliferum is a papillary tubular adenoma. It is a tumorous expression of a dysplasia of the apocrine apparatus. At its deep margin, it may be associated with an apocrine tubular adenoma.

Other tumors that are usually postpubertal complications include the following[29]:

1. Basal cell carcinomas
2. Keratoacanthomas
3. Squamous carcinomas
4. Apocrine tubular adenomas and carcinomas
5. Tubular adenocarcinomas
6. Sebaceous adenomas and carcinomas
7. Trichilemmomas

Epithelial nevi show a variety of patterns but some are characterized by verrucoid epidermal hyperplasia *(nevus verrucosis)*. The distinction between nevus verrucosis and nevus sebaceus can be made histologically only if the specimen includes pilosebaceous units.

Hidradenoma papilliferum is a benign, button-like tumor of apocrine glands, more or less peculiar to the external genitalia of women.[59] Histologically, it is composed of pseudostratified columnar epithelium in complex glandular and papillary patterns. The epithelial cells are supported by a scant fibrous matrix that is overshadowed by the glandular component. Ectopic breast may show proliferative patterns; in some examples, a distinction between hidradenoma papilliferum and ductal hyperplasia of ectopic breast may be difficult. Fibroadenomas of ectopic breast may involve the genital areas.

Comedo nevus is a tumorous follicular dysplasia.[67] The involved follicles are clustered and dilated. They are lined by flattened squamous epithelium and contain keratinized debris. They do not have a sebaceous component. Individually, they resemble comedones and collectively qualify as a tumorous dysplasia. Acquired comedones may be focally prominent, as in the Favre-Racouchot syndrome. In the latter syndrome, periorbital comedones are associated with actinically damaged dermal connective tissue.

Eccrine miliary nevus is a rare tumorous dysplasia. The milia are keratin-filled cysts lined by flattened epithelium. Each cyst communicates with altered sweat ducts in the dermis but shows no communication with the overlying epidermis. This rare dysplasia is a malformation of sweat ducts.

MELANOCYTIC DYSPLASIAS

Melanocytes reside in the basal epidermis, in the outer sheath and bulbs of hair follicles, and, occasionally, in the dermis. They are migrants to the skin[103] and first select the developing dermis as a residence. From the latter location, they migrate into the developing follicular epithelium and then into the epidermis. The conclusion seems inescapable that the neural crest derivatives contribute to the mesenchyme of the dermis.[104] In this concept, they are progressively incorporated into the fibrocytic population of the developing dermis. If the incorporation is defective, the neural crest derivatives are identified as abnormal populations of cells in the dermis (and the epidermis). On this basis, the congenital melanocytic nevus and the cellular blue nevus are neural crest dysplasias expressing an arrest in the development of the dermis.[104] The presence of cells in lentiginous and junctional patterns in the epidermis over a congenital melanocytic nevus should not be accepted as evidence that a population of nevus cells in the reticular dermis are recent migrants from the population of cells at the dermal-epidermal interface. In a congenital nevus, the population of cells that commonly resides at the interface between the reticular dermis and the papillary dermis[105,106] is a marker for a surplus of cells whose destiny was the cellular population of the dermis and which in turn affects the quality and quantity of the fibrous mat.

A nevus cell retains the phenotypic potential of its neurocristic precursor.[104] In benign dysplasias, it tends to relinquish its most recently acquired attributes and to revert to more primitive functions, namely fibrogenesis and neurosustentation. The significance of the patterns in common nevi has not been adequately defined.

A diffuse hyperplasia of melanocytes in the basal epidermal unit is qualified as lentiginous.[105] The distinctions between ephilides and lentigines are not as sharply defined at the level of the light microscope as the popular definitions indicate. Local hyperpigmentation of the epidermis is a feature of such diverse processes as Becker's nevus and café-au-lait spots. Mucosal lentigines are a feature of Peutz-Jeghers syndrome.[107] Cardiocutaneous syndromes are characterized by cutaneous pigmentations[108–110] and include the leopard syndrome and the LAMB syndrome. In the latter, cutaneous and cardiac myxomas are variously associated with endocrine abnormalities and with a distinctive sex cord tumor.

Nevus spilus is not clearly defined at a histologic or clinical level. It is macular and generally larger than a centimeter in diameter. Its other qualities are too variable to place any reliance on the term in defining a homogeneous category. It is likely that premalignant dysplasias have been included in this general category.

Clustering of melanocytes at the dermal-epidermal interface in nests or fascicles is a junctional quality. The migration of melanocytes from the epidermis into the dermis is often characterized by altered cytoplasmic functions; melanogenesis is decreased and cholinesterase activity is increased.

Benign Melanocytic Dysplasias

The *congenital nevus* (small or giant variant) is evident at or soon after birth.[105,106] It may be pigmented or amelanotic. In later years, it commonly is hairy. A variable pattern is characterized by nests of cells at the dermal-epidermal interface and nests and fascicles or cells in a widened papillary dermis. This component is usually indistinguishable from an acquired melanocytic nevus. The more characteristic pattern is seen in the reticular dermis. Melanocytes form nests and lentiginous patterns along the skin appendages. They form nests and cords in the reticular dermis between collagen bundles. Melanocytes in Indian files between collagen bundles are most characteristic (Fig. 9-43). Nevus cells may be found in nerve sheaths and in the subendothelial layer of muscular vessels. Occasionally, a congenital nevus is composed in part of spindle cells in patterns that resemble a blue nevus or a neurotized nevus. Clusters of nevus cells may be found in the capsules of regional lymph nodes.

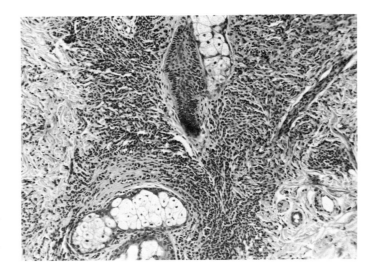

Fig. 9-43. Congenital nevus. Nevus cells are concentrated in the reticular dermis along a hair follicle. They extend in Indian files between collagen bundles of the reticular dermis.

Acquired melanocytic nevus is composed of nests and fascicles of nevus cells (small epithelioid cells). It has a life history characterized by nests of melanocytes at the dermal-epidermal interface early in its evolution. The nevus cells extend in fascicles into a progressively widened papillary dermis and form diffuse aggregates at the interface between the papillary and reticular dermis. Senescence is characterized by progressive incorporation of nevus cells in the fibrocytic population of the papillary dermis. The end result is a fibrous polyp, morphologically devoid of nevus cells. In the organization and maturation of a nevus, many of the older populations of nevus cells are isolated in a delicate fibrous matrix or are arranged in complex lamellar patterns that resemble tactile corpuscles *(neurotization)*. The initial phase of growth in which cells are arranged in nests at the dermal-epidermal interface is classified as a *junctional nevus*. If nests of nevus cells are in the epidermis and the dermis, the lesion is a *compound nevus*. If nests of nevus cells are confined to the dermis, the lesion is a *dermal nevus*.

Melanocytes manifest three cytologic patterns in the skin. In lentiginous processes and in junctional components, the melanocyte is usually a dendritic melanogenic cell. It may be epithelioid (rounded) or spindle-shaped. In its migratory phase, it is usually epithelioid and amelanotic. In some examples, it is spindle-shaped and either amelanotic or melanotic. The amelanotic spindle cell generally has more abundant cytoplasm than its melanotic counterpart. Melanogenic spindle cells usually migrate in concert. They tend to form closely aggregated fascicles. Amelanotic spindle cells tend to form fascicles but characteristically discharge individual cells from the fascicles into the reticular dermis.

The common *spindle cell nevus* (Spitz tumor, epithelioid nevus) is generally amelanotic.[111] Rigid fascicles of plump spindle melanocytes extend from the epidermis, through a widened, edematous papillary dermis into the reticular dermis[112,113] (Fig. 9-44). Individual cells that have acquired epithelioid qualities are discharged from the fascicles into the reticular dermis between the collagen bundles. There is a general reduction in the size of tumor cells from the surface to the deep margin. The fascicles are regularly spaced in the widened papillary dermis. The epidermis over a Spitz nevus is usually hyperplastic. Columns of squamous cells often accompany the fascicles of tumor cells into the papillary dermis. Some of the cells in these aggregates may degenerate to form acellular, acidophilic bodies (Kamino bodies). The latter are common in Spitz nevi but are not a diagnostic feature.

Unusual features of a spindle cell nevus include the following:

1. Focal cellular atypism
2. Focal abnormal aggregation of fascicles of cells
3. High mitotic rate
4. Relative confinement of tumor cells to widened papillary dermis
5. Prominent lymphoid infiltrates
6. Nerve sheath invasion
7. Lymphatic invasion
8. Desmoplasia

None of these features is a reliable indicator of metastases or progressive disease. The term juvenile melanoma has been discarded.

The differentiation of spindle cell nevus and melanoma is a common problem.[114] The concept of tumor symmetry is basic to an understanding of the spindle cell nevus. A spindle cell nevus has overall symmetry and intralesional, aggregate, and cytologic symmetry. Overall symmetry is manifested by uniform contours from side to side and top to bottom. The lesion often has the shape of an inverted wedge with the apex sometimes extending into the subcutaneous fat. Cytologic symmetry finds expression in uniform nuclear qualities at any level in the lesion. There may be cytologic variations in neighboring levels, as often expressed in the observation that spindle cell nevi undergo "maturation" in the deep component. Aggregate symmetry finds expression in uniformity in the size and the spacing of fascicles of tumor cells at comparable levels. Aggregate asymmetry is manifested by variations in size of fascicles of cells at comparable levels and by closely aggregated fascicles that displace or compress

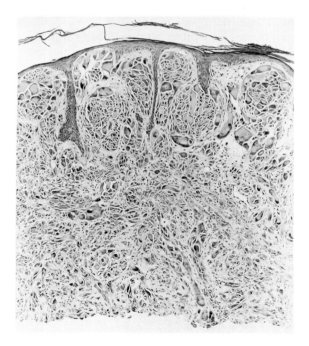

Fig. 9-44. Spindle cell nevus. Fascicles of spindle and epithelioid cells extend from the dermal-epidermal interface into the reticular dermis. Giant cells are prominent in this example.

their stroma. Melanomas are commonly asymmetrical in contours. Cytologic asymmetry (atypism) is a significant aid in diagnosis of a melanoma.

The *pigmented spindle cell nevus* is distinctly different from the Spitz variant.[111] It is less exclusively a disease of children and young adults. It is a pigmented lesion, often with a macular component that may be mistaken for the radial growth component of a melanoma. Histologically, the epidermis shows acanthosis and elongation of rete ridges. Pigmented spindle melanocytes with prominent dendrites form lentiginous patterns in the epidermis. They also form fascicles or oval nests at the dermoepidermal interface and within the hyperplastic epidermis (Fig. 9-45). The cells have oval nuclei with variable nucleoli. Some of the fascicles connect adjacent rete ridges. As the tumor progresses, fascicles of cells in a portion of the lesion form compact aggregates that fill the papillary dermis and infiltrate the reticular dermis. The infiltrating portion is a compactly organized, expansile nodule. Mitoses are common. The component in the epidermis commonly extends away from the nodule in the pattern of radial growth. The macular phase of the evolving lesion is commonly misdiagnosed as a superficial spreading malignant melanoma.

Cellular blue nevus is a congenital tumor commonly involving the buttocks, the scalp, or the dorsum of the foot.[111] It is composed of spindle melanocytes with variable pigmentation. Commonly, most of the cells are pigmented. They form fascicles that are compactly aggregated. Regional variations are common, and in areas spindle melanocytes and melanophages are individually isolated in a dense fibrous matrix (Fig. 9-46). Multinucleate melanocytes are often admixed with spindle cells. Occasionally, the tumor cells form neuroid fascicles cir-

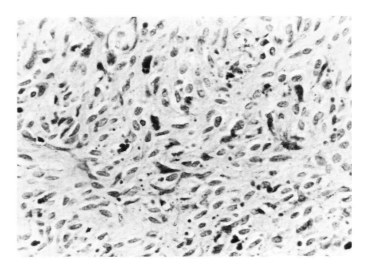

Fig. 9-46. Cellular blue nevus. Plump spindle melanocytes with vacuolated cytoplasm are supported by a fibrous matrix. The cells have oval nuclei with delicate chromatin.

cumscribed by concentric layers of tumor cells. Peripheral nerves are commonly infiltrated by tumor cells. The tumor bulges into the subcutaneous fat. Mitoses are not a feature of an uncomplicated cellular blue nevus. Cellular blue nevus may be associated with capsular inclusions of similar cells in regional lymph nodes.

The *acquired blue nevus* is a small pigmented tumor, relatively confined to the reticular dermis.[111] The overlying epidermis commonly shows elongated rete ridges with lentiginous melanocytic hyperplasia. The tumor has the configuration of an inverted wedge with the apex directed toward the subcutaneous fat and the base paralleling the epidermis. Spindle and dendritic melanocytes are embedded in a dense fibrous matrix. Regional variations in cellularity are common. Melanophages with coarsely clumped granules are interspersed between the melanocytes. The tumor cells tend to concentrate in perifollicular connective tissue sheaths. From this location, they form bulbous expansions into the subcutaneous fat. For some examples, the distinctions between an acquired and a cellular (congenital) blue nevus are arbitrary. For the problem lesions, the distinctions depend in part on history, size, and location.

Becker's hairy nevus qualifies as lentiginous melanocytic hyperplasia and as an epithelial nevus. The lesion is best distinguished by its clinical characteristics: it occurs on the trunk and most often affects adolescent boys. It is characteristically pigmented and hairy, but these features are variable. Histologically, the epidermis shows elongated rete ridges, variable papillomatosis, and mild to moderate lentiginous melanocytic hyperplasia. In the areas of hypertrichosis, the follicles are fully stimulated and extend their bulbs into the subcutis. The lesion is

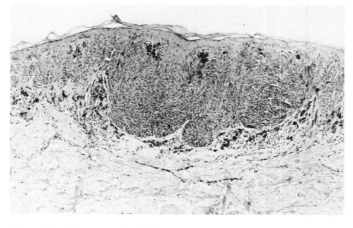

Fig. 9-45. Pigmented spindle cell nevus. Nests and fascicles of pigmented spindle melanocytes are compactly aggregated in the upper portion of the dermis. Lentiginous patterns are prominent in the adjacent epidermis.

benign but cosmetically disturbing. Arrector pili muscles are hyperplastic.

Premalignant Melanocytic Dysplasias

The concept of premalignant melanocytic dysplasia gives recognition to common precursors of cutaneous malignant melanoma. The premalignant dysplasias as precursors of the common malignant melanomas evolve at the dermoepidermal interface in lentiginous and junctional patterns.[115–118] They may be de novo or may take origin in remnants of a congenital or acquired nevus. They are characterized clinically by irregular contours and pigmentation. These clinical features are correlated with histologic features of cytologic atypism, eccentric distribution of the lentiginous and junctional components, and markers for host immune response. If a lesion on histologic examination exhibits the features of a dysplasia, in all likelihood other lesions from the same patient will display variations of the same pattern. Sporadic and familial cases have been identified. Atypism, characterized by scattered nevus cells with plump hyperchromatic nuclei, is a common feature of congenital and acquired nevi and is of questionable significance in the absence of some or all the following markers:

1. Lymphoid infiltrates with intermingling of inflammatory cells and melanocytes (Fig. 9-47)
2. Focal lamellar fibrosis of the papillary dermis, usually

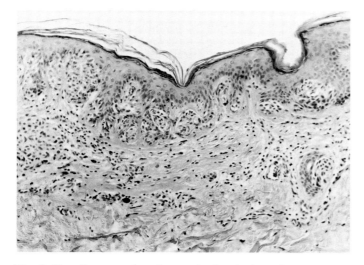

Fig. 9-47. Compound melanocytic dysplasia, mild dysplasia. Nests of atypical melanocytes at the dermal-epidermal interface are outlined by laminated fibrous tissue. There are scattered nests of dysplastic melanocytes in the fibrotic dermis. Perivascular infiltrates of lymphocytes express the host immune response.

associated with nests of cytologically atypical nevus cells (Fig. 9-47)
3. Asymmetry (irregular spacing of dysplastic cells in lentiginous patterns, and irregular spacing of junctional nests of dysplastic cells: eccentric spread in the epidermis away from a remnant of a pre-existing nevus)

These features define the common premalignant melanocytic dysplasias. The concept of melanocytic dysplasia is basic to the *atypical nevus-familial melanoma (dysplastic nevus) syndrome.*[116] In the latter disorder, nevi are numerous on the trunk. The atypical changes which, either simultaneously or over intervals of years, affect one or several nevi are manifested by discrete pigmented puncta, by irregularities in outline and pigmentation, and by growth and partial regression over a period of months and years. The atypical lesions often exceed 1 cm in diameter. Some of the atypical nevi may evolve into malignant melanomas, often in the pattern of superficial spreading melanoma. The affected melanocytic nevi display the characteristics of either congenital or acquired variants. Initially, the de novo lesions clinically and histologically resemble lentigo simplex.[118] The sequence in some of the lesions in the atypical nevus-familial melanoma syndrome provides insight into sporadic lesions showing similar histologic features. The role of melanocytic dysplasia as a precursor to malignant melanoma is significant.

Melanocytic dysplasias may be subdivided as follows:

1. Lentiginous dysplasias
2. Nevocytic dysplasias (characterized by small epithelioid cells)
   Junctional dysplasia
   Compound dysplasia
   Dermal dysplasia
3. Spindle cell dysplasias (in similar lentiginous, junctional, compound, and dermal patterns: as a manifestation of the common premalignant dysplasia or as a variation of the pattern seen in Spitz or pigmented spindle cell nevi)
4. Borderline melanomas

Lentiginous dysplasia is characterized by a diffuse distribution of atypical melanocytes in the basal epidermal unit.[117] It is the morphologic expression of a clone of melanocytes that is expanding within the confines of an epithelial domain. In one or more sites, atypical melanocytes may cluster in oval nests or fascicles at the dermal-epidermal interface; the aggregates of melanocytes herald a dermal migration and qualify as a junctional dysplasia. Nests of dysplastic cells that are widely spaced in the dermis qualify as dermal dysplasia. If junctional and dermal dysplasia coexist in a lesion, the combination is a compound dysplasia. By the nature of the process, junctional, dermal, or compound patterns are associated with a lentiginous component. The lentiginous pattern defines a property that is separate and distinct from those expressed in the nesting patterns.

A dysplasia is also qualified as to degree of atypism.[117] The degree of dysplasia is evaluated by the numerical representation of atypical cells at the dermal-epidermal interface and by the cytologic features of the dysplastic cells. At the mild end of the spectrum, the atypical changes are subtle and often the decision as to whether a significant dysplasia is represented must be judged a whim rather than an objective observation. At the opposite end of the spectrum, the pattern merges with the radial growth component of a fully evolved superficial spreading melanoma in vertical growth. The latter pattern in toto qualifies as the common final pathway.[119] A distinction between a severe lentiginous and compound dysplasia and so-called superficial spreading melanoma showing only level II invasion is arbitrary.

Melanocytic dysplasias often arise in pre-existing nevi. They are particularly common in small congenital nevi. Nests or clusters of cytologically benign nevus cells at the interface between the papillary dermis and the reticular dermis provide a marker for the pre-existing lesion. The dysplastic component is generally most prominent in the population of melanocytes near the dermoepidermal interface. It is characterized by nests of cells with plump, uniformly hyperchromatic nuclei. Some of the cells have prominent nucleoli. The nuclei within the nests show loss of polarity, and variations in size and intensity of nuclear staining. Loss of cellular cohesion in the nests is a variable feature. Neighboring nests of melanocytes often show varying degrees of atypism. Mitotic figures are found in some nests of melanocytes, and in general the mitotic rate is related to the degree of cytologic atypism. Aggregate asymmetry is manifested by irregular spacing of nests of melanocytes and by variation in the size of the nests at comparable levels (see Fig. 9-47).

The lymphoid response is variable and is related to the degree of the dysplasia. It has features of Waksman's invasive-destructive pattern of cell-mediated immunity.[11] In focal areas, nests or portions of nests of melanocytes are lysed or coagulated by the immune response. The lymphoid response is accompanied or followed by a desmoplastic response in which the final product is laminated fibrous tissue. A component of well developed laminated fibrous tissue is associated with focal loss of nests of melanocytes and a general reduction in the density of the lymphoid infiltrates. Scattered nests of dysplastic melanocytes trapped in the laminated fibrous tissue are outlined by concentric lamellae of fibrous tissue. There is provision for complete lysis of the dysplastic population of melanocytes, but, in most examples, scattered nests

survive. Halo nevus is a prototype for nevocytic dysplasias and may be junctional, compound, or dermal. It is distinguished by a dense, band-like infiltrate of lymphoid cells and intermingling of the nevus cells and lymphoid cells.[120] Varying degrees of cytologic atypism, ranging from mild to moderate, are displayed in halo nevi. Commonly the component at the dermoepidermal interface is composed of pigmented spindle cells. If the lentiginous and junctional component spreads in the epidermis away from the main portion of the lesion in the pattern of a premalignant dysplasia, the resulting lesion is an atypical *halo nevus*. It is implied in this terminology that on occasion halo nevi are premalignant lesions.

Spindle cell dysplasias as premalignant processes in which features of either the common Spitz nevus or the pigmented spindle cell nevus are represented are less easily defined.[120] Lymphoid infiltrates and lamellar fibrosis are variable features but occasionally are prominent. Cytologic changes include nuclear hyperchromatism, variation in nuclear size, and abnormal mitoses. At comparable levels in a lesion, fascicles of cells vary in size and outline and are irregularly spaced. Some spindle cell dysplasias are relatively confined to the papillary dermis and lack a component in the reticular dermis. Lentiginous and junctional components in the epidermis away from the main portion of the lesion and in association with markers for host immune response are basic to the diagnosis of atypical Spitz or atypical pigmented spindle cell nevi.

In general, the basic premise in the management of the premalignant dysplasias is conservative eradication. The offending cells are in the epidermal domain or widely and randomly spaced in the papillary dermis. A shave biopsy may be adequate for most examples (particularly in the category of mild to moderate dysplasia). If the margins are close by histologic criteria, a good guideline is the clinician's evaluation of the biopsy procedure. If, by clinical evaluation, the lesion has been eradicated, additional local surgery is not indicated. Perhaps a conservative reexcision of the biopsy site is indicated for moderately severe to marked dysplasias (pattern of common final pathway) if there are uncertainties regarding the adequacy of the biopsy procedure when evaluated by clinical criteria (i.e., has the visible lesion has been eradicated?).

The distinction between melanoma and premalignant dysplasia is best defined on the basis of patterns of cellular aggregation in the widened papillary dermis rather than on the basis of the degree of cytologic atypism in the component at the dermal-epidermal interface.[119–121] The distinction on any basis is arbitrary for lesions in the transition phase. Practically, the presence of four or five nests of at least moderately atypical cells which are regularly spaced in the widened papillary dermis is a marker for lesions in transition from dysplasia to melanoma. If the nests of cells are widely but regularly spaced, the resulting pattern qualifies as *variant* level III invasion. If the nests are closely spaced, the pattern qualifies as *typical* level III invasion. If a lesion showing level III invasion measures less than 1.00 mm in height, the lesion is properly qualified as borderline. For such lesions, the usual prognostic evaluations do not relate to prognosis in a predictable manner. For such lesions, it is unwise to provide therapeutic guidelines other than to recommend adequate, conservative local excision and careful follow-up.

MALIGNANT MELANOMA
Minimal Deviation Melanoma

In the category of nevocytic or lentiginous dysplasia, the appearance of an expansile nodule heralds the transformation to malignant melanoma.[119,120] If the dysplasia is transformed morphologically to an expansile tumor (melanoma) but cytologically qualifies as less than severe atypism, the transformed lesion is a minimal deviation melanoma[119-121] (Fig. 9-48) (If it also measures less than 1.00 mm in height, it is a borderline minimal deviation melanoma.). A similar melanoma may arise de novo without evidence of a preexisting dysplasia. If such a lesion arises in a dermal nevus, it evolves in the absence of an epidermal or junctional component. Some lesions of the latter type qualify as rare examples of melanoma arising in a dermal nevus (minimal deviation melanoma of the dermal type).[120]

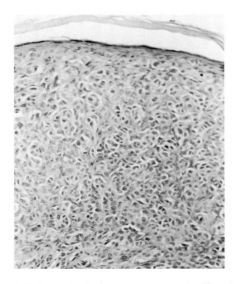

Fig. 9-48. Minimal deviation melanoma. Uniformly atypical small melanocytes in nests and fascicles form an expansile nodule.

An expansile nodule of uniformly and moderately atypical spindle cells in a cellular blue nevus qualifies as a minimal deviation spindle cell melanoma.[111,120] Mitoses are an additional marker of the dysplastic cells.

In spindle cell dysplasias, the appearance of closely aggregated fascicles of atypical spindle cells heralds a minimal deviation melanoma.[120] It is extremely difficult to document malignant transformation of a spindle cell dysplasia of the Spitz type by distant or regional metastases. Rare examples metastasize to a single node in a regional node group. The diagnosis of minimal deviation malignant spindle cell nevus of the Spitz type is mostly a histologic exercise. The diagnosis of the Spitz variant is an indication for an adequate local excision, but generally does not require a wide excision.

The difficulties in defining the limits between pigmented spindle cell dysplasias and pigmented spindle cell melanoma have been discussed. Minimal deviation pigmented spindle cell melanoma is an expansile nodule.[120] It is composed of moderately atypical, uniform spindle cells that form closely aggregated fascicles. It is a common expression of the vertical growth phase of lentigo maligna melanoma. Neurotropism is an option in the category of minimal deviation pigmented spindle cell melanoma.

Malignant Melanoma

Two basic cell types (spindle cells and epithelioid cells) and two patterns of epidermal melanocytic growth (dispersed or lentiginous, and aggregated or nevocytic) have been defined. To classify malignant melanomas, two additional properties require emphasis. Some melanomas evolve for a variable period of time at the dermal-epidermal interface.[122] The tumor cells migrate in the epidermis. In multiple foci, they seed the papillary dermis. This peculiar pattern expresses low biologic aggression on the part of the tumor cells and a strong immune response on the part of the host. It expresses host immune intolerance.[123] Clinically, it relates to macular or papular lesions that enlarge centrifugally and often show variations in surface colors. The surface variations in part express the degree of pigmentation, the rubor of an inflammatory response, and the depigmentation and altered vascularity of areas of spontaneous regression.[124] This macular or papular phase is the clinical expression of a premalignant dysplasia as a phase in the evolution of melanoma.[120]

After a period of interplay between tumor cells and the immune reaction, some of the tumor cells survive and multiply in the papillary dermis. They form a plaque or nodule that distorts the boundaries between the epidermis and the dermis and between the papillary and reticular dermis. This significant change in the relationship between tumor cells and host is the initial phase of immune tolerance.[123] It defines the histologic boundary between dysplasia and melanoma. Henceforth, any surviving remnant of the dysplastic precursor is characterized as the radial growth component, and the nodule or plaque is the vertical growth component. It is improper to speak of a radial growth component in the absence of a vertical growth component. In many melanomas, the tumor cells are relatively confined to the papillary dermis as an expanding nodule for months or years. A subsequent change in the host-tumor relationship permits the tumor cells to invade the reticular dermis actively between collagen bundles. This change is generally accompanied by a marked depression of the cellular component of the immune response.[123] It is the final phase of host immune tolerance. The expanding plaque or nodule that characterizes the phases of immune tolerance is the vertical growth phase.[123] Some melanomas evolve de novo as expanding plaques or nodules. They bypass a significant phase in the evolution of most melanomas. The de novo lesions are nodular melanomas.[123] With this background, the following variants of melanoma are recognized: (1) superficial spreading malenoma; (2) lentigo maligna melanoma; (3) acral lentiginous melanoma; (4) nodular melanoma; (5) heteromorphic melanoma (desmoplastic and neurotropic variants); and (6) unclassified melanoma.

Superficial Spreading Melanoma

Superficial spreading melanoma (Fig. 9-49) has the following characteristics[122,123]:

1. Vertical component arising within the confines of a premalignant dysplasia (so-called radial growth component), showing severe cytologic atypism and pagetoid invasion of the epidermis (common final pathway)
2. Nevocytic (nesting) patterns at dermal-epidermal interface
3. Severe melanocytic dysplasia (large epithelioid cells, generally pigmented)
4. Cellular host immune response in radial growth component
5. Usually shows distinct phases of immune tolerance (evolves at level III for sufficient period to produce a nodule at the surface of the skin)
6. Partial regression is common feature of radial and initial vertical growth components
7. Occasional, total, and spontaneous regression
8. Variable cytologic patterns in radial and vertical components (less atypical components are markers for an earlier stage in the evolving dysplasia)
9. Epidermis (superficial unit) usually hyperplastic
10. Active invasion of epidermis by individual tumor cells (pagetoid qualities)

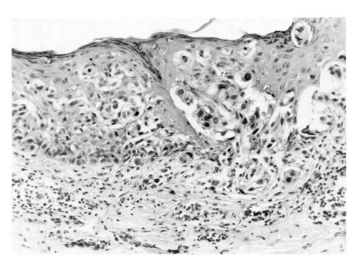

Fig. 9-49. Superficial spreading melanoma, radial growth. Atypical epithelioid melanocytes form nests and pagetoid patterns in the epidermis. The papillary dermis shows lamellar fibrosis and contains nests of atypical cells (thin level II invasion).

Lentigo Maligna Melanoma

Lentigo maligna melanoma (Fig. 9-50) has the following characteristics[123,125]:

1. Arises on sun-exposed surfaces of elderly, fair-skinned patients
2. Vertical component arising in remnant of lentiginous dysplasia (lentigo maligna)
3. Progression from radial to vertical phase is slow (measured in years)
4. Lentiginous patterns at dermal-epidermal interface (by definition, the radial component does not show the features of the common final pathway: the latter pattern is preferentially assigned to the category of superficial spreading melanoma regardless of the other clinical and histologic features)
5. Focal nests and fascicles at dermal-epidermal interface
6. In lentiginous component, cells melanocytic (well developed pigmented dendrites)
7. Marked cytologic variability in radial component (mild to severe dysplasia)
8. Lentiginous component involving skin appendages
9. Vertical component usually lacking two distinct phases: invasion of reticular dermis manifested in thin lesions
10. Invasion of reticular dermis that may occur in phase of premalignant dysplasia (in absence of vertical growth component)

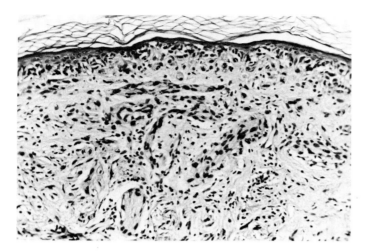

Fig. 9-50. Lentigo maligna melanoma, neurotropic variant. The lentiginous pattern in an atrophic epidermis is characteristic of lentigo maligna. The invasive component forms neuroid patterns in the dermis.

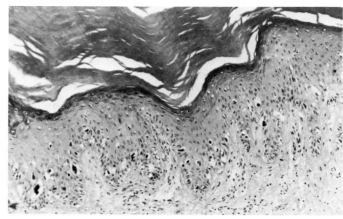

Fig. 9-51. Acral lentiginous melanoma, radial growth. Atypical melanocytes form lentiginous patterns in the hyperplastic epidermis.

11. Vertical component often showing cytologic qualities of minimal deviation spindle cell melanoma
12. Vertical component usually showing cytologic uniformity (monoclonism)
13. Cellular host immune response in radial component variable and often poorly developed
14. Epidermis (superficial unit) usually atrophic or thin
15. Vertical component occasionally desmoplastic

Acral Lentiginous Melanoma

Acral lentiginous melanoma (Fig. 9-51) has the following characteristics[123,126]:

1. Relative confinement to atrichic regions (palms, soles, subungual areas, and mucous membranes)
2. Vertical component arising in remnant of lentiginous melanocytic dysplasia
3. Lentiginous patterns at dermal-epidermal interface
4. Slow progression from radial to vertical component
5. Focal nests and fascicles at dermal-epidermal interface
6. In lentiginous component, cells melanocytic
7. Marked cytologic variation in radial component (least atypical cells usually represented at periphery of lesion)
8. Lentiginous component involving skin appendages
9. Vertical component usually showing cytologic uniformity (monoclonism)
10. If composed of spindle cells in vertical component (as is commonly the case), two distinct phases of immune tolerance rarely well developed

11. If composed of epithelioid cell in vertical component, two distinct phases often well developed
12. Host immune response usually well developed in radial component
13. Epidermis (basal and superficial units) usually hyperplastic (accentuation of rete pattern)
14. Individual cells often migrate into epidermis in radial component but are usually melanocytic with prominent dendrites
15. Vertical component occasionally desmoplastic and occasionally characterized by minimal cytologic deviation (in nevus cell-like patterns)

Nodular Melanoma

Nodular melanoma may not be a single, distinctive variant. In all likelihood, there are nodular (de novo) variants of acral lentiginous melanoma, lentigo maligna melanoma, and superficial spreading malignant melanoma.[123] These nodular variants have the characteristics outlined for the vertical growth of each of the recognized subtypes. Nodular melanomas of the atrichic areas generally are composed of spindle cells. Many nodular melanomas of actinically damaged skin are composed of spindle cells, and some show a minimal deviation pattern. Most nodular melanomas resemble the vertical growth phase of superficial spreading melanoma. They tend to show monomorphism rather than the polymorphism commonly displayed in the vertical growth component of superficial spreading melanoma.

The classification of a melanoma from an evaluation of the characteristics of its radial growth is occasionally a problem. In many of the problem lesions, the radial component shows admixtures of lentiginous and nevocytic patterns. Although these problem lesions qualify as malignant melanomas with mixed nevocytic and lentiginous radial components, usually they arbitrarily are assigned to the category of superficial spreading malignant melanoma. Occasionally, two distinctive patterns are combined in a radial growth component. The radial growth of acral lentiginous melanoma focally may have the characteristics of superficial spreading melanoma. Some of the problem melanomas have multiple vertical growth components. In lesions of the latter type, some of the nodules resemble the vertical growth phase of superficial spreading melanoma (epithelioid and polymorphic), and some resemble the vertical growth phase of a lentiginous melanoma (spindle cell, monomorphic, and, occasionally, focally desmoplastic). Rarely, the radial component of a melanoma is poorly developed and characterized by regularly spaced nests of minimally deviant melanocytes at the tips of rete ridges. In these lesions, the radial component is generally ignored and the tumor is classified as nodular melanoma. Practically, such lesions are better characterized as melanomas arising in premalignant dysplasias.

Heteromorphic Melanoma

The concept of heteromorphism gives recognition to the phenotypic pluripotency of neurocristic derivatives.[103,104] During embryologic development, migrants from the neural crest are phenotypically pluripotent. For migrants to the developing skin, the phenotypic options include melanogenesis, neurosustentation, and mesomorphogenesis. If the terminal (epigenic site) is the epidermis, the migrants differentiate as melanocytes. If the migrants settle in the vicinity of developing nerves, they differentiate into nerve sheath cells (Schwann cells and perineurial cells). There is indirect evidence that the developing dermis receives a contribution from the neural crest and that the migrants lose their identity in the population of dermal fibrocytes. Practically, the dermis is neuromesenchyme. From this perspective, lesions such as congenital nevocytic nevi and blue nevi are mesenchymal dysplasias in which the defect is expressed by phenotypic options. Thus, cells which during normal development function as fibrocytes revert to phenotypic alternatives in dysplasias. In the heteromorphic melanomas, the phenotypic diversity of neurocristic derivatives is convincingly displayed. In these variants during the process of neoplastic progression, cells of melanocytic lineage acquire the characteristics of fibroblasts or nerve sheath cells. The resulting neoplasms are desmoplastic melanomas and neurotropic melanomas, respectively.

Desmoplastic Melanoma

Desmoplastic melanoma comprises a heterogeneous group of melanomas, some of which are variants of lentigo maligna melanoma and others of acral lentiginous melanoma.[127] Rare variants are desmoplastic superficial spreading melanoma and desmoplastic minimal deviation melanoma. Desmoplasia is a peculiar property of neoplastic melanocytes. It does not express the same functions as does the process of neurotization during the "maturation" of a nevus. It may be comparable to desmoplastic patterns occasionally expressed in spindle cell nevi or to those commonly expressed in blue nevi and congenital nevi. In desmoplastic melanoma, the tumor cells are spindle-shaped and fibroblastic. Elongated cells, which are usually amelanotic, are isolated in a cellular, inflamed, fibrous matrix (Fig. 9-52). The tumor cells are deceptively bland, but occasional cells or nests of cells show diagnostic nuclear atypism. In areas in which the tumor has infiltrated fat, it is likely to be focally cellular and cytologically diagnostic. The tumor has a tendency to recur locally as a circumscribed fibrous nodule in the subcutaneous fat. Invasion of deep muscular vessels may be a feature. Desmoplastic melanomas are distinguished by a high rate of local recurrence.

Neurotropic Melanoma

Neurotropic melanoma demonstrates a peculiar affinity for peripheral nerves.[128] Neurotropism is usually manifested in the setting of either lentigo maligna or minimal deviation melanomas, and may be expressed as a variation in pattern in desmoplastic variants.[120] Some neuro-

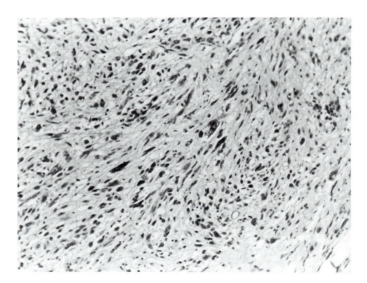

Fig. 9-52. Desmoplastic melanoma. Atypical spindle melanocytes are individually isolated in a fibrous matrix.

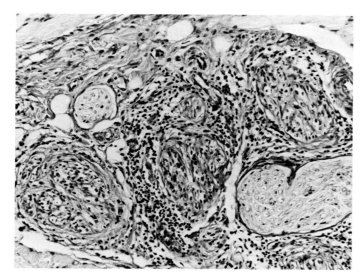

Fig. 9-53. Neurotropic malignant melanoma. Spindle melanocytes infiltrate small nerves in the subcutaneous fat.

tropic melanomas qualify as de novo variants and display a predilection for exposed surfaces such as the lower lip.[128] In neurotropic melanomas, the cells are spindle-shaped and have Schwann cell qualities. They form tortuous fascicles that blend with infiltrated peripheral nerves (Fig. 9-53). The fascicles are rigid, tortuous, and arborized (Fig. 9-50). The pattern resembles a traumatic neuroma but is differentiated from the latter by cellular atypism, clinical presentation, and ancillary findings such as remnants of a radial growth component of malignant melanoma. Neurotropic melanomas demonstrate a remarkable propensity for local recurrence and for local infiltration of soft tissue and peripheral nerves. After a period of years, often after multiple local recurrences, the tumor tends to dedifferentiate and metastasize. Some of the de novo neurotropic lesions may be primary malignant schwannomas rather than neurotropic melanomas.

Prognostic Criteria

Prognostic parameters have been developed for the histologic evaluation of malignant melanomas. *Clark's criteria*[119,121,122] are related to biologic phenomena in the evolution of melanomas and primarily relate to epithelioid nodular melanomas and superficial spreading malignant melanomas.

* *Level II invasion*—radial growth phase. It defines a period of immune intolerance and is characterized by an epidermal component and by widely spaced nests of cells in the papillary dermis (Fig. 9-49). By definition, nodular melanoma is excluded from the category of

lesions showing level II invasion. In the absence of a vertical growth component, it seems inappropriate to designate a premalignant dysplasia, regardless of the degree of cytologic atypism, as a radial growth component.
* *Level III invasion*—initial phase of host immune tolerance. It is characterized by an expanding plaque or nodule of tumor cells in the papillary dermis (Fig. 9-54). It is a significant phase in the evolution of many nodular melanomas and of most superficial spreading melanomas.
* *Level IV*—final phase of host immune tolerance. It is characterized by active invasion of the reticular dermis (Fig. 9-55). This phase may appear early in lentiginous melanomas, in which level III invasion is often a relatively brief or fleeting phase.
* *Level V*—simple expansion of tumor in space and is characterized by invasion of the subcutaneous fat.

In part, Clark's criteria find their value as a crude measure of increasing bulk with progressive levels of invasion. In spite of this criticism, Clark's levels are prognostically useful and are indispensable for an understanding of the biologic life history of the variants.

An alternate approach to prognostic evaluations is provided by a simple measurement from the granular layer of the epidermis to the deep margin of the lesion. Breslow[129] defined three categories: (1) less than 0.75 mm, (2) 0.75 to 1.50 mm, and (3) greater than 1.50 mm. These criteria do not have exact counterparts in Clark's levels of invasion. For lesions less than 1.5 mm in height,[130] there is little evidence that prophylactic lymph node dissections are of

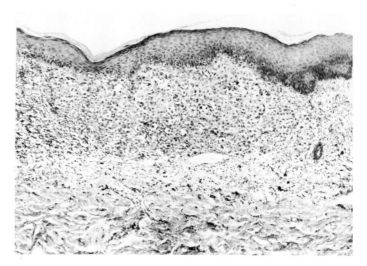

Fig. 9-54. Malignant melanoma, thin level III invasion. Tumor cells form a plaque in a widened papillary dermis.

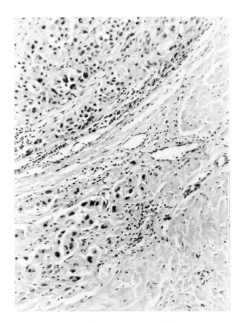

Fig. 9-55. Malignant melanoma, level IV invasion. At the top of the field, tumor cells form an expansile nodule (level III invasion). The tumor cells infiltrate the reticular dermis between collagen bundles.

value. For lesions less than 0.75 mm, metastases or local recurrences are unlikely if the margins of excision are free of involvement. Conservative excisions appear to be justified in the good prognostic range of less than 0.75 mm in height. Conceptually, lesions measuring less than 1.00 mm in height might be appropriately characterized as borderline malignancies. Conservative excisions with margins no greater than 2 cm also seem appropriate for most lesions in the range of 0.76 to 1.50 mm in height.[129]

For Clark's levels of invasion, local excisions are adequate therapy for premalignant dysplasias (level II lesions). At level III, particularly for superficial spreading and nodular melanomas, small, thin lesions and bulky, large lesions are included. For Clark's level III lesions, the correlations with prognosis are not a reliable guide to therapy. Breslow's criteria provide quantitative guidelines for good and poor prognosis lesions at Clark's level III invasion. The adjunctive value of Clark's criteria is found in the thin melanomas that have metastasized.[117,131] Some of the thin metastasizing melanomas show extensive regression at level II, and others show thin level III invasion. These findings confirm the biologic distinctions in the concepts of host immune tolerance and intolerance and in the distinctions between premalignant dysplasias and melanomas irrespective of the degree of cytologic atypism. A prognostic index has been offered as a refinement of Breslow's criteria.[132]

LYMPHOID HYPERPLASIAS AND LYMPHOMATOID PROCESSES

Benign cutaneous lymphoplasia (lymphocytoma cutis, Spengler-Fendt sarcoid) is common in the skin.[133] These benign lymphoid tumors form red-blue or brown nodules or plaques. They commonly affect the face and may be solitary, multiple and localized, or disseminated in the skin. Histologically, they are characterized by diffuse infiltrates in the reticular dermis and the subcutis (Fig. 9-56). The infiltrates are both perivascular and nodular and tend to spare the papillary dermis.[134,135] Occasionally, they extend into hair follicles. They are composed of small lymphocytes and pale, cytologically benign histiocytes. Variable components include clusters of epithelioid histiocytes, plasma cells, eosinophils, and germinal centers. The germinal centers may be small with ill defined margins, or they may be large and circumscribed. Tingible body macrophages are common in the large germinal centers. The lymphoid tissue is supported by a plexus of tortuous, thick-walled vessels with swollen endothelium. These vessels have the characteristics of postcapillary venules. Lymphoid cells commonly infiltrate the walls of small veins at the deep margin of the dermis. Usually, solitary lesions are easily managed. Rarely, a solitary lesion is histologically atypical. Some are locally aggressive. Disseminated lesions are occasionally a precursor of malignant lymphoma. Rarely, a

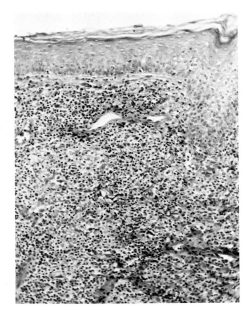

Fig. 9-56. Benign cutaneous lymphoplasia. A polymorphous infiltrate of small lymphocytes and pale histiocytes forms a tumor in the reticular dermis.

NEOPLASMS OF THE SKIN

transformation from benign cutaneous lymphoplasia to lymphoma has been documented.[136]

Studies with immunologic markers have produced conflicting results. Some of the studies have shown a mixture of peripheral T-lymphocytes and of polyclonal B-lymphocytes. In other studies, the preponderant cells have been T-lymphocytes. In practice, the immunologic markers on routine histologic material often are less than satisfactory and the interpretation of the nature of the lymphoid infiltrates is dependent on the skill of the pathologist and the quality of the routine sections.

Hematopathologists have recently demonstrated an interest in the lymphoid lesions of the skin.[137] In their studies, the problems in making a distinction between benign lymphoplasias and lymphomas appear minimal. It would appear that the hematopathologists bring a greater skill to the task than do the dermatopathologists, or at least the hematopathologists seem inclined to minimize the difficulties. In all likelihood, the hematopathologists are confronted with material that is heavily weighted with true lymphomas, and in addition they are asked to confirm an established diagnosis rather than interpret an isolated lesion. It is unlikely that their material consists of the products of a punch biopsy of a lesion from a patient who is essentially well. The problems related to the interpretation of material of the latter type remain considerable. Practically, if the infiltrate is not readily classified as one of the common lymphomas, it is probably a benign cutaneous lymphoplasia.

Self-Healing Lymphomatoid Vasculitides

The lymphomatoid lesions of the skin are cytologically atypical and are angiocentric and vasculitic. They often display the quality of self-healing. The best characterized example is *lymphomatoid papulosis*.[138] The original definition of lymphomatoid papulosis has proved to be too limited. With added experience, it is apparent that classic lymphomatoid papulosis may modulate on occasion as a somewhat different disorder in which the lesions tend to be fewer in number, nodular in character, and histologically polymorphic.[139] In addition, on occasion the lesions may modulate in patterns that are histologically and clinically indistinguishable from the T-cell dysplasias as seen in the clinical setting of cutaneous T-cell lymphoma (mycosis fungoides). The nodular, polymorphic variants have been recognized for years but have been variously classified as primary cutaneous Hodgkin's disease,[139] atypical regressing histiocytosis,[140] and polymorphic immunoblastic reticulosis. In recent attempts to bring the nodular, polymorphic variants into the spectrum of lymphomatoid papulosis, it has been proposed that the nodular lesions qualify as type A variant of lymphomatoid papulosis. In this classification, the classic variant is qualified as the type B variant. The term polymorphic reticulosis retains a descriptive quality. It gives recognition to the mixed character of the infiltrates and does not clearly identify the large atypical cells as lymphoid. The large cells often are histiocytoid but in recent studies have marked immunologically as T-lymphocytes.[141–143]

Polymorphic Immunoblastic Reticulosis (Lymphomatoid Papulosis Type A)

Some papular or nodular lesions of the skin have a self-healing quality but are histologically atypical. In some examples, the perivascular infiltrates consist of atypical "reticulum cells" and immunoblasts with admixtures of atypical lymphocytes and various nonspecific inflammatory cells (Fig. 9-57). Multinuclear tumor cells are a regular feature. Eosinophils are common components. The infiltrates may be diffuse or perivascular. The infiltrates often are vasocentric and vasodestructive. Some of the vessels show fibrinoid necrosis and thrombosis, and the lesion displays regions of infarction. If such a lesion clinically has self-healing qualities over a period of weeks and months, caution should be exercised in recommending aggressive treatment. In some cases, the monomorphic infiltrates are lymphomatous but the lesions are episodic, few in number, and display the quality of self-healing. Some of these processes are indolent, remittent diseases of the skin that have limited potential to disseminate. In regional lymph nodes, the pattern resembles Hodgkin's disease. Lesions of this type have been classified as primary Hodgkin's disease of the skin.[139] They qualify as polymorphic immunoblastic reticulosis.

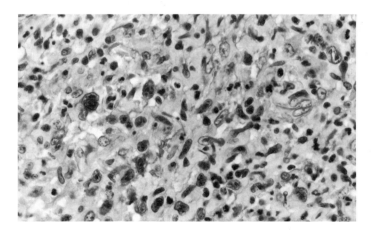

Fig. 9-57. Type A lymphomatoid papulosis (polymorphic immunoblastic reticulosis). A mixed infiltrate is composed of fibrocytes, atypical lymphoid cells, atypical histiocytoid cells, and bland histiocytes. One binucleate cell has features of a Reed-Sternberg cell.

Classic Hodgkin's disease[144] may involve the skin, but with few exceptions it does so as retrograde spread from involved regional lymph nodes or as direct extension from involved lymph nodes through soft tissue. Extensive mediastinal involvement may result in direct spread through the chest wall into the skin.

Polymorphic T-cell lymphomas may involve the skin and be difficult to distinguish from polymorphic immunoblastic reticulosis. The clinical evolution of the disease may be more informative than predictions based upon histologic interpretations. The lymphomas are more likely to be characterized by monotonous sheets of large cells. The cell types in peripheral T-cell lymphomas include small cells (poorly differentiated lymphocytes), large cells with pale cytoplasms, and cells with convoluted or hyperlobated nuclei.

Lymphomatoid Papulosis (Type B)

Pityriasis lichenoides is an expression of a T-cell reaction (lichenoid lymphocytic vasculitis). It has features of Waksman's invasive-destructive reaction of cellular immunity and may be complicated by a necrotizing vasculitis (a reaction also seen in the classic model of cellular immunity, the tuberculin reaction). Lesions that satisfy the clinical and most of the histologic criteria for the diagnosis of pityriasis lichenoides on occasion contain numerous transformed T-lymphocytes. Lesions of the latter type are generally classified as lymphomatoid papulosis.[138] The atypical cells mark immunologically as T-lymphocytes.[141,142] Clinically the lesions vary in number and display the quality of self-healing. The epidermal changes may resemble those of a lesion of pityriasis lichenoides but tend to be less severe. The dermal infiltrates are vasocentric and vasodestructive. They are polymorphic and consist of atypical lymphocytes and a high component of histiocytes. Some of the atypical cells have the characteristics of transformed T-lymphocytes with convoluted nuclear membranes. Other lymphoid cells have large, round nuclei with uniformly dense chromatin. Cells of the latter type are often individually isolated between the collagen bundles of the reticular dermis. The clinical course is chronic and rarely progressive.

Some observers have proposed that the distinction between lymphomatoid papulosis and pityriasis lichenoides should be based on a quantitation of the percentage of atypical lymphocytes in the infiltrates. If the number of atypical lymphocytes exceeds 10 percent, the lesion belongs in the category of lymphomatoid papulosis.

Lymphomatoid Granulomatosis

Lymphomatoid granulomatosis[145,146] is a peculiar lymphomatoid process with a predilection for the lungs. In the lungs, the lesions are multiple, more common in the lower lobes, and occasionally cavitated. There is a tendency for some pulmonary or cutaneous lesions to regress at a time when other lesions are progressing. The cutaneous lesions are perivascular or diffuse in the dermis. In the subcutis, they are diffuse. In the lungs, the infiltrates are diffuse, interstitial, and vasocentric. The infiltrates are lymphohistiocytic. Lymphocytes with plump, round, or cleaved nuclei are admixed with pale histiocytes. Occasionally, the infiltrates contain immature lymphohistiocytic cells and plasmacytoid cells. The nature of the atypical lymphoid cell has not been identified,[146] but the high component of histiocytes in the infiltrate is a feature of T-cell neoplasia. In the skin, the lesions may be anesthetic.[147] The high component of histiocytes may suggest the possibility of a peculiar granuloma or even Lennert's lymphoma. The vasocentric infiltrates are also vasodestructive. The term granulomatosis as defined by Leibow gives recognition to large areas of coagulation necrosis. Vessels bordering the necrotic tissue show fibrinoid necrosis and thrombosis.

The diagnosis is best reserved for minimally atypical infiltrates. Comparable lesions with markedly atypical cells qualify as malignant lymphoma, although there appear to be modulations in the character of the neoplastic cells in individual lesions that are not necessarily correlated with progressive disease. The infiltrates in lymphomatoid granulomatosis involve the viscera and the brain. Lymph node involvement is not common. Involvement of peripheral nerves may provide an explanation for clinically demonstrable anesthesia.

LYMPHOMAS OF THE SKIN

Cutaneous lymphomas are divisible into evolved and de novo variants.[135,148] With few exceptions, the evolved lesions are primary in the skin and represent T-cell processes. They are characterized by macular lesions that give way over a period of years to plaques and to tumors. The de novo lesions are tumorous and most examples are cutaneous manifestations of disseminated lymphomas; they usually represent B-cell processes. In the tumor stage, a clinical distinction between a B-cell and a T-cell lymphoma may not be possible unless remnants of a T-cell dysplasia are preserved in the form of plaques or poikilodermatous areas.

B-Cell Lymphomas

B-cell lymphomas are first manifested in the skin in the vascular adventitia of the reticular dermis and subcutis. The tumor cells move from the perivascular spaces into the reticular dermis, where they may form Indian files between collagen bundles. They form diffuse infiltrates that displace the collagen bundles of the reticular dermis, but they tend to spare the papillary dermis and may spare perifollicular connective tissue sheaths.[148,149] Leukemic infiltrates also show a similar pattern. The infiltrates of granulocytic leukemia contain eosinophilic myelocytes and show cytoplasmic staining with the chloroacetate esterase reaction.[150] The lesions of the leukemia-lymphoma group of disorders are characterized by dense infiltrates (crowding of nuclei), monotony of cell type, and destruction of skin appendages.[137] The latter feature, unfortunately, may not be evident in small, early lesions.

The skin may be involved by any of the histologic subtypes, including plasmacytic, lymphoblastic, immunoblastic, and nodular variants.[135,137,151,152] The well differentiated variants, which are relatively confined to vascular adventitia, are difficult to diagnose; they resemble the benign lymphocytic infiltrates of the dermis. When the infiltrates become diffuse, the monotony of the cellular pattern distinguishes a lymphoma from benign cutaneous lymphoplasia.[133-135,148,149,152] A distinctive lymphoid lesion of the skin has been characterized as a large cell lymphocytoma.[153] The lesion is composed of large lymphoid cells with elongated nuclei. The large cells are arranged in sheets and trabecular patterns in a background of small lymphocytes. The scalp is a commonly affected site. The lesion does not commonly disseminate but the histologic features are more in keeping with the diagnosis of lymphoma. This peculiar lymphomatoid lesion may represent a low-grade primary lymphoma of the skin.

In the diagnosis of cutaneous lymphoma, it is important to emphasize the identity of dermal infiltrates with nodal infiltrates of B-cell lymphomas.[154] If the dermal infiltrates deviate from lymphomatous patterns as seen in lymph nodes, caution should be observed in the diagnosis of cutaneous malignant lymphoma. In paraffin-embedded tissue, the clonality of the infiltrates can be evaluated with variable success by reactions for κ- and λ-light chains.

T-Cell Lymphomas

The T-lymphocyte has specific markers (e.g., lymphocyte transformation tests, rosette formation with erythrocytes.[155] A variety of immunologic markers have been identified. In part, they provide correlations between stages of embryologic differentiation and stages of neoplastic transformation (dedifferentiation). Differentiated cells mark as peripheral lymphocytes. In characterizing T-cell lymphomas, a peripheral T-cell lymphoma may also be interpreted as displaying blastoid qualities. Blastic transformation is not synonymous with dedifferentiation. The much sought-after marker for malignancy has

not been defined. As a marker for a T-cell lymphoma, monoclonality, with rare exceptions, is only relative. Phenotypic heterogeneity characterizes many peripheral T-cell lymphomas.

The T-lymphocyte is a migratory cell whose immune functions require close contact with the target cell or tissue.[156] One of the secretory products migration inhibition factor of the T-lymphocyte decreases the migratory functions of the macrophage: another attracts eosinophils.

Conceptually, the category of cutaneous T-cell lymphoma embraces premalignant dysplasias and fully evolved, rapidly fatal lymphomas. Morphologically the transformed T lymphocyte in the cutaneous T-cell lymphoma *(mycosis fungoides-Sézary syndrome)* has distinctive nuclear characteristics.[157] Its chromatin is uniformly dense (lymphoid), and its nuclear membrane is convoluted (Fig. 9-58). Cells with these characteristics have been classified as Lutzner's cells; dysplastic counterparts are known as mycosis cells or Sézary cells.

Of special interest is the identification of dysplastic T-lymphocytes in some premalignant cutaneous reticuloses.[157] With immunologic markers, the cells in most examples have expressed the characteristics of helper T-lymphocytes.[155] At the light microscopic (LM) level, the distinctive cytologic characteristics of the mycosis cell have been emphasized for years. The ultrastructural characteristics of the transformed T-lymphocyte are those of the mycosis cell and the Sézary cell. Immunologic studies have also confirmed the T-cell origin of the dysplastic cells in mycosis fungoides and in Sezary syndrome. The characteristic patterns of a lichenoid reaction are recapitulated in the *premalignant cutaneous T-cell dysplasias*.[157] The following patterns in T-cell dysplasias are recognized:

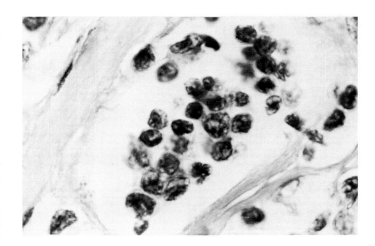

Fig. 9-58. T-cell dysplasia with leukemia (Sézary phenomenon). Atypical lymphocytes have plump nuclei, convoluted nuclear membranes, and dense chromatin.

1. Simulant of primary lichenoid reaction (Alibert type of mycosis fungoides)

> Band-like lymphoid infiltrate in papillary dermis (Fig. 9-59)
> Psoriasiform epidermal hyperplasia (defines epidermal response in primary lichenoid reaction)
> Migration of lymphoid cells into epidermis
> Intermingling of lymphoid cells and keratinocytes
> Lysis of keratinocytes at dermoepidermal interface and focally in epidermis
> Variable changes in superficial epidermal unit (i.e., focal parakeratosis)

2. Simulant of established lichenoid reaction with hyperplasia or no significant alteration in superficial unit (mycosis fungoides, parapsoriasis, Sézary syndrome)

> Band-like infiltrate in papillary dermis
> Atrophy of basal unit (single row of small basal cells with focal areas of lysis: defines epidermal response in established lichenoid reaction)
> Normal superficial unit (epidermis appears atrophic), or
> Hyperplastic superficial unit (epidermis appears hyperplastic with increased cytoplasmic acidophilia)
> Relative confinement of epidermal lymphoid infiltrates to areas of lysis (unless there is a significant degree of lymphoid dysplasia)

3. Simulant of senescent lichenoid reaction (mycosis fungoides, parapsoriasis, poikiloderma atrophicans vasculare)

> Widened fibrotic papillary dermis
> Atrophy of basal unit (effacement of rete ridges)
> Partial or complete resolution of lymphoid infiltrate (Fig. 9-60)

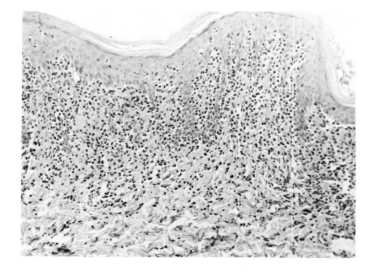

Fig. 9-59. T-cell dysplasia, psoriasiform pattern. Atypical lymphocytes form diffuse infiltrates in the papillary dermis and migrate into the epidermis in lichenoid patterns.

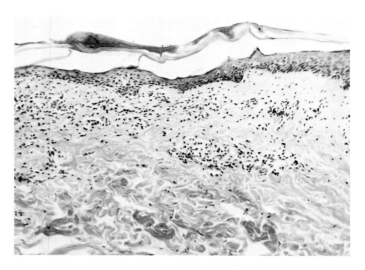

Fig. 9-60. T-cell dysplasia, senescent lichenoid reaction. The dysplasia is mild. The papillary dermis is widened, fibrotic, and sparsely cellular. The epidermis shows atrophy of the basal unit.

> Ectasia of vessels in papillary dermis
> Absence of epidermal lymphoid infiltrate (unless there is a significant degree of lymphoid dysplasia)
> The first four items define the senescent lichenoid response

In practice, the established lichenoid patterns in the clinical setting of parapsoriasis invariably overlap with the senescent patterns of poikiloderma. These two syndromes are properly united in the concept of the parapsoriasis-poikiloderma complex.[157] After years of controversy, the term *parapsoriasis* acquired some specificity with particular reference to a stage in the evolution of T-cell neoplasia. Unfortunately, the pendulum has swung and the concept has reverted to a controversy, somewhat comparable to the nature of the disorder when defined by Brocq at the turn of this century. In the current trend, the term embraces a hodgepodge of lesions.[158]

The lichenoid dysplasias contain dysplastic T-lymphocytes. The degree of dysplasia is evaluated on the basis of the number of dysplastic cells and on nuclear size and atypism.[157] Characteristically, the nucleus of a dysplastic T-lymphocyte is as large as or larger than the nucleus of a basal keratinocyte. The dysplastic cells are easiest to evaluate when there is a significant epidermal component. Some of the dysplastic cells have round nuclei with a prominent nucleolus and marginated chromatin (stem cell), but this nuclear configuration is less useful in distinguishing T-lymphocytes from B-lymphocytes. The dysplastic cells may be seen in association with primary, established or senescent lichenoid patterns. They may collect in lytic defects in the epidermis (Pautrier microabscesses). The dysplasia is qualified as mild, moderate, or severe. The dysplasia progresses in the papillary dermis by increasing numbers of atypical cells and depletion of nonspecific lymphoid cells. If, in toto, the epidermal and papillary dermal infiltrates are plaque-like and composed of uniform, dysplastic cells, the process qualifies as malignant T-cell lymphoma in situ. Eventually, if undisturbed, the dysplastic cells may form a tumor that infiltrates the reticular dermis. This tumor stage is a clinical and histologic marker for disseminated disease with visceral involvement (T-cell malignant lymphoma).[157,159,160]

Classically, mycosis fungoides is divided into three clinical stages corresponding to erythematous (psoriasiform) lesions, plaques, or tumors.[157] For clinical staging, it is implied that the potential for progression is variable and may be partially or completely interrupted by spontaneous regression. The accumulated data indicate that progression to the tumor stage also heralds dissemination to lymph nodes and viscera.[155] If concepts of tumor biology that have been gleaned from the study of malignant melanomas are applied to the T-cell dysplasias, there are remarkable similarities. In both disorders, some tumors evolve slowly through stages of progressive dysplasia. In the dysplastic phase, the tumor cells are relatively confined to the superficial functioning unit of the skin (the epidermis and the adventitial dermis). An interplay between tumor cells and host immune response determines the evolution of the dysplasia, including rate of progression, regression, and dissemination. In some lesions in both disorders, a phase of immune tolerance is manifested by the aggregation of tumor cells in an expansile nodule and by invasive growth into the reticular dermis. On this basis, the archaic classifications may be defined in terms of modern concepts of the neoplastic transformation of T-lymphocytes:

1. *Mycosis fungoides:* an evolving, cutaneous T-cell dysplasia that is multifocal, slowly progressive, and in its early phases psoriasiform and lichenoid. The dysplasia evolves in the adventitial dermis but may also evolve in the T-cell domain of regional lymph nodes.

2. *Parapsoriasis-poikiloderma complex:* an evolving cutaneous T-cell dysplasia that is multifocal, minimally dysplastic, and dominated by a lichenoid host immune response. The lichenoid qualities are expressed clinically and histologically. They are dominantly expressed as a senescent phase in which epidermal atrophy, papillary dermal fibrosis, and telangiectasia are combined clinically in the term poikiloderma.

3. *Sézary syndrome:* an evolving, diffuse T-cell dysplasia in which the dysplastic T-lymphocytes seed the peripheral blood (dermatopathic leukemia). The dysplastic cells initially do not colonize the viscera from the circulation.

The effects of the dysplasia on epidermal kinetics find expression in an erythroderma.

4. *Cutaneous T-cell lymphoma:* a malignant lymphoma derived from T-lymphocytes and manifested initially as a cutaneous disorder. The evolved variants are preceded by the clinical manifestations of a premalignant dysplasia (mycosis fungoides, the parapsoriasis-poikiloderma complex, or the Sézary syndrome). The *de novo (d'emblée)* variant is tumorous and lymphomatous from its inception. In either variant, cutaneous tumors are followed in short order by evidence of disseminated disease.[156,157]

In the T-cell dysplasias of the skin, the dysplastic lymphocyte retains some of the functions of a reactive T-lymphocyte.[157] It is a migratory cell with special affinity for the paracortical regions of lymph nodes, the splenic periarteriolar lymphoid sheath, and the adventitial portions of the dermis. The dysplasia may evolve in the skin or the paracortical tissue of a lymph node, separately or simultaneously. The dysplastic cell may also be identified in the circulation (Sézary cell). Circulating dysplastic lymphocytes and an erythroderma define the Sézary syndrome. The phenomenon of dermatopathic leukemia in Sézary syndrome is not simply related to the density or number of cells in the peripheral infiltrate. The circulating cells have distinguishing markers.

In the lymph nodes in early phases, the process is characterized by lymphoid hyperplasia and sheets of pale histiocytes (interdigitating reticulum cells) in the paracortical zones (*dermatopathic lymphadenitis*).[161] Occasional isolated, dysplastic lymphocytes are usually identified in the histiocytic infiltrates. They are of no more significance than occasional dysplastic lymphocytes in the dermal infiltrates. They should be evaluated by the same criteria as the dermal infiltrates (number, characteristics, and aggregation of dysplastic cells, and depletion of nonspecific cells). Occasionally, the nodal infiltrates will be lymphomatous at a time when the dermal infiltrates are dysplastic (confined to adventitial dermis and admixed with nonspecific lymphoid cells).

Attempts to relate the stage of dysplasia to immunologic markers have not produced significant improvements in the early diagnosis of mycosis fungoides.[162-164] Emphasis has been on specific markers and on ratios of helper to suppressor lymphocytes.

Pagetoid reticulosis of Woringer-Kolopp is a rare disorder characterized by a solitary plaque in which dysplastic T lymphocytes infiltrate the epidermis. The atypical cells preferentially collect in the epidermis and are inconspicuous in the underlying papillary dermis.[165]

There has been recent emphasis on a variant of T-cell lymphoma with cutaneous lesions, leukocytosis, and hypercalcemia with or without osteolytic lesions.[166-171] The disease affects adults with an acute or subacute onset. It is characterized by cutaneous eruptions, lymphadeno-pathy, hepatosplenomegaly, and pulmonary infiltrates. The mediastinum is often spared. The circulating cells have multilobated nuclei. In some examples, particularly in Asians, there is an association with HTLV I virus. In contrast with the lesions of the common cutaneous T-cell dysplasias, the infiltrates tend to be vasculitic as well as lichenoid (band-like in the papillary dermis). The cytologic features are variable and may overlap somewhat with those of lymphomatoid papulosis. Small cells, cells with convoluted nuclei (mycosis cells), and large atypical cells with pale cytoplasm are admixed with a high component of histiocytes and variable eosinophils in the infiltrates.

In the category of T-cell lymphomatoid lesions and lymphomas, there are occasional examples characterized by rapid clinical and cytologic progression. Over a period of months, the lesions enlarge and increase in number. If the clinical course is related to patterns in biopsy material, it is often possible to document transformation from a bland lymphohistiocytic infiltrate to a polymorphic, large cell lymphoma that is vasocentric and vasodestructive. In the latter phase, there are overlaps with lesions of type A lymphomatoid papulosis. These lesions qualify as rapidly progressive T-cell cutaneous lymphomas. Their relationship to the HTLV I-related lymphoma has not been defined. Some examples of rapidly progressive cutaneous T-cell lymphoma share features clinically and histologically with lymphomatoid granulomatosis.

Reticuloses

The Langerhans cell of the epidermis and the interdigitating reticulum cell of the T-cell domain of a lymph node are part of a sustentacular system, which is concerned with antigen presentation to T lymphocytes. They are basic to patterns of cell-mediated immunity in the skin. They are prominently displayed in lesions of the cutaneous T-cell dysplasias. They are incidentally displayed as residents in a variety of epithelial and mesenchymal neoplasms of the skin. The neoplastic cells in histiocytosis X have the characteristics of Langerhans cells.

Histiocytosis X

Histiocytosis X is a proliferative disorder of Langerhans cells. Cutaneous lesions are common. Classically, clinicopathologic syndromes were defined as independent processes. *Eosinophilic granuloma, Hand-Schüller-Christian disease,* and *Letterer-Siwe disease* are examples. These disorders were united in the concept of histiocytosis X with a distinctive histiocyte as the common factor. The validity of this unified concept was reinforced with the characterization of the Langerhans cell

and the demonstration of similar qualities in the neoplastic cells of histiocytosis X.

The variants include

1. Chronic localized forms (eosinophilic granuloma)
2. Chronic disseminated forms (Hand-Schüller-Christian disease)
3. Acute disseminated forms (Letterer-Siwe disease)

There are inconsistencies in the manifestations of lesions in the various categories that limit the usefulness of the definition of the classic syndromes. The age of onset (e.g., infancy) and the number of cutaneous lesions (e.g., multiple) are not invariable markers for a widespread, rapidly progressive disorder. Such features may be in keeping with a relatively benign course. It is uncommon for a lesion of histiocytosis X to be congenital (evident at the time of birth).

Self-Healing Congenital Reticulohistiocytoma

Self-healing congenital reticulohistiocytoma is a proliferative disease of distinctive histiocytes generally affecting the skin of infants.[172] The lesions tend to be few in number and nodular. They may be crusted and partially necrotic. The disease is benign and usually self-limited. Two cytologic variants of histiocytes are clustered in the lesions. Near the epidermis, the preponderant cell has the features of the cells of histiocytosis X, both cytologically and immunologically (immunoreactive for S-100 protein). The second population tends to cluster in the deeper portions of a lesion. They are smaller and do not display the deep nuclear grooves of the superficial cells (and of the cells in histiocytosis X). They do not immunoreact for S-100 protein. Nonspecific infiltrates of lymphocytes and eosinophils are clustered among the tumor cells.

MESENCHYMAL TUMORS

The skin and subcutaneous tissue are affected by most of the tumors that involve the deep soft tissue. There are tumors whose manifestations in the skin and subcutis are peculiar. Only distinctive cutaneous tumors or tumors with peculiar cutaneous manifestations will be discussed. Other tumors will receive attention in the chapter on soft tissue tumors.

Fibrous Hamartoma of Infancy

Fibrous hamartoma of infancy is an infiltrating tumor that is more or less peculiar to the first 3 years of life.[173,174] It is composed of fibroblastic cells in a fibromyxomatous matrix. The tumor forms a plaque at the interface between dermis and subcutis. Complex, interconnected septa dissect lobules of adipose tissue and extend to the deep fascia. Variable cytologic patterns are displayed in the septa. In areas, the spindle cells are closely aggregated in a myxomatous matrix. In neighboring areas, the cells are widely spaced and compressed in a dense fibrous matrix. In some lesions, a tumor nodule forms in the subcutis. In the latter variant, the diagnosis is best established by identifying the characteristic cellular septa extending from the nodule into the adipose tissue. The life history of fibrous hamartoma of infancy has not been documented.

Nodular Fasciitis

Nodular fasciitis (pseudosarcomatous fasciitis) is most common in the subcutaneous fat, but it also occurs in the deep soft tissue.[175,176] It is a benign proliferative process involving myofibroid cells in fascia and adipose tissue. It begins as a plaque-like thickening of a fibrous septum or fascia. Plump spindle and stellate cells are supported by a mucinous matrix and by rigid capillaries that extend into the lesion at right angles to the fascial membrane. The tumor enlarges as an expansile nodule that replaces adipose tissue and blends with fascia at points of contact. The mature lesion is characterized by:

1. Circumscription, occasionally with a peripheral condensation of fibrous tissue
2. Close attachments to fascia
3. Rigid peripheral capillaries
4. Regional variations in pattern
    Myxomatous
    Fibromyxomatous
    Fibrous
5. Mitoses
6. Plump nuclei but uniform nuclear characteristics
7. Angulated mucin-filled clefts
8. Focal lymphoid infiltrates
9. Focal stromal hemorrhages
10. Focal collections of foreign body giant cells

The life history of nodular fasciitis has not been clearly defined but the process is self-limited. Occasionally, a lesion of nodular fasciitis recurs locally, although this has been disputed. In some early lesions, focal areas of coagulated adipose tissue may provide a marker for the initial insult. Some mature lesions show central areas of cystic degeneration. In mature lesions, focal areas with fibrohistiocytic qualities (interlacing fascicles in starburst patterns) are a feature. Some lesions of the soft tissue (benign fibrous histiocytomas) may represent maturation in nodular fasciitis. Perhaps this variant accounts for some

of the recurrences and has been selectively deleted from some studies.

Dermatofibrosarcoma Protuberans

Dermatofibrosarcoma protuberans is peculiar to the skin and subcutaneous fat.[177,178] It characteristically has two phases of growth evolving from a plaque into a nodule. The histologic pattern is most characteristic in the plaque stage. The tumor is composed of fibroblastic spindle and stellate cells. The spindle cells are thin and elongated. Tumor cells are supported by a fibromyxomatous matrix. They form fascicles that produce starburst patterns at points of intersection (Fig. 9-61). In the plaque stage, the tumor infiltrates the dermis and forms a plaque between the reticular dermis and subcutaneous fat. It extends as irregular septa into the subcutaneous fat to the level of the deep fascia. After a variable period, usually years, one or more expanding nodules develop in the plaque. Within the nodules, the starburst pattern is usually preserved, but a regional variation is characterized by plump stellate cells in a myxomatous matrix. Melanocytes are a component of some examples.[179]

In the evaluation of dermatofibrosarcoma protuberans, mitoses are not a useful prognostic indicator. In large tumors, focal areas may show a herringbone pattern that is indistinguishable from fibrosarcoma of the deep soft tissues. These patterns are of questionable prognostic significance. Dermatofibrosarcoma protuberans rarely metastasizes, but local recurrences are common. Infiltrative growth at the periphery of the tumor is clinically imperceptible. Wide local excisions including the superficial layer of the deep fascia are indicated. Careful atten-

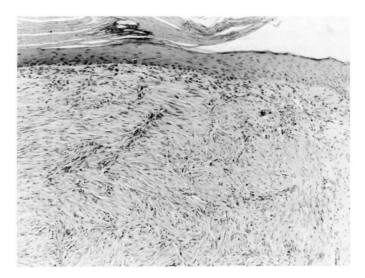

Fig. 9-61. Dermatofibrosarcoma protuberans. Fibroblastic spindle cells form fascicles that intersect in starburst patterns.

tion should be given to the margins in evaluating adequacy of a local excision.

Smooth Muscle Tumors

Leiomyomas in the skin are derived from blood vessels, from arrector muscles of hair follicles, or from leiomyomatous fascia (dartos fascia). Leiomyomas derived from arrector muscles are not encapsulated. Fascicles of tumor cells extend between collagen bundles of the reticular dermis. Some lesions in this category are nevoid: they are plaque-like and multinodular.

The vascular leiomyomas are circumscribed and encapsulated. They are composed of compactly aggregated fascicles of tumor cells. Muscular vessels are uniformly distributed throughout the tumor.

Leiomyosarcomas that are primary in the skin may be derived from arrector muscles or from the smooth muscle of blood vessels.[180-182] Some are apparently derived from preexisting smooth muscle tumors. Leiomyosarcomas are circumscribed or infiltrating tumors. Mitoses are prognostically significant but clearly defined relationships between mitotic figures and behavior are not available. Aggressive local growth and metastases are more common from smooth muscle tumors involving the subcutaneous fat than from those confined to the dermis. Many leiomyosarcomas of the skin or subcutaneous fat represent metastases from a deep soft tissue sarcoma.

Glomus Tumors

Glomus tumors are derived from specialized epithelioid cells in the wall of a myoarterial glomus.[183]

The solitary, subungual glomus tumor is a circumscribed small lesion that is composed of uniform, acidophilic, epithelioid cells in a myxomatous matrix. The cells form interconnected trabeculae and nests. Most of the cells are outlined by reticulum fibers. Blood vessels and nerves are present in the adjacent soft tissue. Axons are numerous within the tumor. In rare examples, the background matrix is densely fibrous. In these sclerosing variants, the cells form widely spaced clusters and much of the lesion is paucicellular.

In the soft tissue in sites other than the subungual areas, glomus tumors are circumscribed and encapsulated. They are more uniformly cellular and have less matrix than do subungual lesions (Fig. 9-62). Sinusoidal and muscular vessels are prominent in the lesions. In some vessels, epithelioid glomus cells are intermingled with smooth muscle cells. The lesions may be multiple.

Glomus tumors, particularly in the subungual area, are painful. Pain is a less characteristic feature of glomus

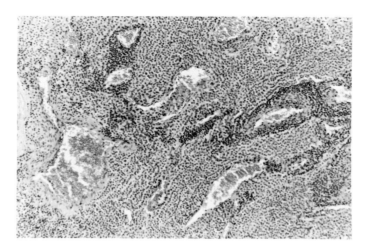

Fig. 9-62. Glomus tumor (glomangioma). Small uniform epithelioid cells form cuffs around blood vessels and compact aggregates. The tumor is surrounded by a fibrous capsule (not seen here).

tumors in other sites. Pain is not a unique feature of a glomus tumor. Eccrine spiradenoma (basaloid spiradenoma) and leiomyoma are other painful tumors of the skin.

Occasionally, glomus tumors are infiltrative rather than expansile. They show mitotic activity and may infiltrate blood vessels. Periarticular glomus tumors have a tendency to infiltrate soft tissues. Rare examples in the skin are composed of large atypical cells and qualify as *glomangiosarcomas*.[184]

Dermatofibroma

A group of cutaneous lesions with variable histologic patterns are grouped generically in the category of dermatofibromas (i.e., fibrous histiocytomas, sclerosing hemangiomas, nodulus cutaneus). Dermatofibromas are often paucicelluar and fibrous. These small lesions are not polypoid and measure 1.5 cm or less in diameter. Histologically, lesions larger than 1.5 cm in diameter tend to be cellular and to display storiform patterns. They are composed of plump fibrocytes, histiocytes, and blood vessels. Multinucleated giant cells and hemosiderin deposits are a variable component. Atypical giant cells are an occasional feature. In cellular areas, the cells form interlacing fascicles in starburst patterns. The tumor infiltrates the dermis between collagen bundles. It bulges into the subcutis but does not infiltrate widely in the manner of dermatofibrosarcoma protuberans. Some examples have prominent aneurysmal spaces (aneurysmal sclerosing hemangiomas).[185] The epidermis over a dermatofibroma is hyperplastic and may show areas of follicular neogenesis.

There is no evidence of a sequential relationship between dermatofibroma and dermatofibrosarcoma protuberans. Dermatofibromas, particularly the cellular or atypical variants, occasionally recur locally.

Digital Fibroma

The digital fibroma is a rare tumor of infancy with a predilection for the digits and a propensity for local recurrence. It is a noncapsulated, fibroblastic tumor of the dermis. Some of the fibroblastic spindle cells contain peculiar cytoplasmic inclusions.[186] Digital fibroma is characterized as a lesion of infancy but similar lesions may be discovered in adults. Rarely, a similar lesion involves a site other than a digit.

Atypical Fibroxanthoma

Atypical fibroxanthoma (AFX) is a generic designation for a group of pleomorphic fibrous tumors of damaged skin. It characteristically arises in skin showing elastosis and fibrosis as a consequence of actinic damage, thermal damage, or x-irradiation. The lesion grows rapidly and is usually ulcerated and polypoid.[187-189]

The tumor is composed of pleomorphic, fibroblastic spindle and epithelioid cells and tumor giant cells. It presses on the epidermis and in one or more sites, if the epidermis is intact, blends with the basal layer (Fig. 9-63). The neoplastic cells are diffusely arranged in a fibromyxomatous matrix; in some areas, they form interlacing fascicles. Mitoses, some of which are atypical, are common. In many examples, with a reticulum or PAS stain, the

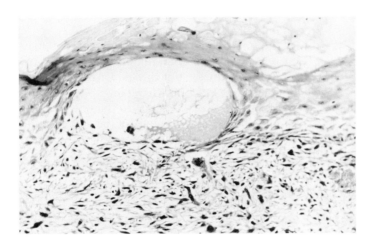

Fig. 9-63. Atypical fibroxanthoma. A tumor in the dermis presses on the epidermis. It is composed of atypical spindle and stellate cells in a loose fibrous matrix. There are scattered tumor giant cells.

basal membrane of the epidermis is focally interrupted by rigid, thin fascicles of tumor cells that are outlined by silver- and PAS-positive rigid membranes. The membranous material may be found throughout the tumor and has tinctorial qualities of a basement membrane. Occasionally, nests of atypical squamous cells showing a peripheral adenoid pattern may be identified in an atypical fibroxanthoma. Most examples show regional variations in pattern, with focal areas of fibrosis in which cellular atypism is less prominent. In general, atypism is more prominent near the epidermis. The changes of an actinic keratosis are common in the adjacent epidermis. A mesenchymal origin was implied in the original description of AFX.

The problems are such that the diagnosis of AFX must be qualified as a generic term for a variety of polymorphic neoplasms arising in damaged skin. The differential diagnosis includes melanoma and spindle cell carcinoma. Melanomas are occasionally pleomorphic. If fine melanin granules are identified in the cytoplasm of an occasional tumor cell or if the epidermis shows the pattern of lentigo maligna, the tumor is probably a polymorphic desmoplastic melanoma. The demonstration of immunoreactivity for S-100 protein in tumor cells is strong evidence favoring the diagnosis of polymorphic melanoma. The prognostic implications of a melanoma masquerading as a mesenchymal neoplasm of low-grade malignancy are such that it becomes imperative to consider melanoma in the differential diagnosis for this group of pleomorphic lesions.

Some examples of AFX are special variants of spindle cell carcinoma.[11,190] They are circumscribed variants that occasionally recur but rarely metastasize. Immunoreactivity for cytokeratins favors the interpretation that a so-called atypical fibroxanthoma is in fact a spindle cell carcinoma. Immunoreactivity for vimentin is cited as evidence in favor of a mesenchymal origin, but there are no studies defining the exclusivity of immunoreactions in cells that are expressing unusual phenotypes or undergoing phenotypic transformations. It would be a disservice to imply that immunoreactions will simplify the precise characterization of lesions in this generic category. Too often the reactions are unsatisfactory (conflicting immunoreactions or confusing background staining).

Clinicians commonly display a nonchalant approach to the treatment of AFX. The concept of pseudomalignancy as applied to a variety of processes, and to AFX in particular, has fostered the concept that the lesion is invariably benign. The malignant potential of the lesion has been documented.[191] Occasionally, an AFX will be managed conservatively in the face of multiple local recurrences. AFX that infiltrate aggressively and that have invaded the subcutaneous fat should be viewed with caution. They qualify as aggressive variants.

For the proponents of the mesenchymal derivation of atypical fibroxanthoma, the distinctions between AFX and *malignant fibrous histiocytoma* (MFH) are found in biologic behavior rather than in histologic or histogenetic features. Pleomorphic MFH is not a disorder of the dermis. It arises in the fascia or adipose tissue and involves the dermis secondarily, if at all. It is multinodular and fibrous or myxomatous. Its tumor cells are epithelioid and spindle-shaped. They show variations in nuclear size and staining. Tumor giant cells are a characteristic feature. Malignant fibrous histiocytoma (or xanthoma) commonly recurs locally and may metastasize. The biologic distinctions between AFX and MFH should give pause to those who view the two as histogenetic and histologic clones.

Other soft tissue tumors of importance in the practice of dermatopathology include infantile myofibromatosis,[192] giant cell fibroblastoma,[193] pleomorphic lipoma,[194] and lipoblastomatosis.[196] Congenital hemangiopericytoma[195] should be considered in the differential diagnosis of infantile myofibromatosis. It may simply represent a variant of the latter disorder.

Vascular Tumors and Proliferations

Lymphangiomas are simple ectasias (lymphangioma circumscriptum superficialis) or tumorous malformations. The vascular spaces are dilated, lined by flattened endothelial cells, and contain a pink coagulum (lymph) and lymphocytes.

Hemangiomas of the skin are lobulated and expansile. They may be circumscribed or infiltrating.

Hemangioma of infancy appears shortly after birth and may show an alarming period of growth. It eventually stabilizes over a period of months and years and partially or completely regresses. Some persist as localized tumors. They may be multiple, disseminated, or infiltrating. Large hemangiomas are occasionally associated with thrombocytopenia (Kassenbach-Merritt syndrome).

Angiodysplasias appear in childhood or adolescence as soft tissue tumors with or without dermal components.[197] The lesions in the deep soft tissue may be associated with arteriovenous fistulas and with localized skeletal overgrowth. The dermal components may be telangiectatic or tumorous. They may be associated with a verrucoid surface (verrucous hemangioma).

Acquired hemangiomas of adults are generally small polypoid lesions, but some are multiple and compressible *(blue rubber bleb nevus syndrome)*.[198] If multiple, they may be associated with angiomas of the gastrointestinal tract (Bean's syndrome).

Pyogenic granuloma is the most common acquired hemangioma. It is polypoid and is composed of lobular ag-

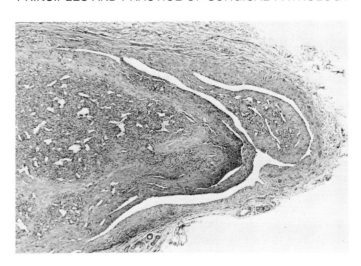

Fig. 9-64. Intravascular pyogenic granuloma. Lobules of newly formed vessels are supported by a fibrous matrix. The tumor is polypoid. It is attached to the wall of the involved vessel.

gregates of newly formed vessels. Rarely, a similar lesion is intravascular[199] (Fig. 9-64).

Microscopically, hemangiomas are immature or mature, a distinction based on the character of the endothelial cells. In immature hemangiomas, the lobules are composed of plump endothelial cells arranged in solid cords or tubules. The cords and tubules are supported by basement membranes that do not encircle individual endothelial cells. Mitoses are common. Capillary hemangiomas of infancy and pyogenic granulomas qualify as immature hemangiomas.

Mature hemangiomas are also lobular. They may show focal immature areas, but maturation is characterized by dilatation of the lumina of the abnormal vessels (cavernous spaces) and flattening of the endothelial cells.

In addition to cavernous spaces, angiodysplasias may contain lymphangiomatous components and aggregates of smooth muscle. Mature hemangiomas are unlikely to regress spontaneously. Phleboliths and metaplastic ossification are variable features. The diffuse nature of many of these lesions must be appreciated by the surgeon and should serve to temper the zeal for extensive surgical procedures.

The *angiokeratomas* are composed of superficial, ectatic vessels. Some of the vessels may press upon or appear to be within the confines of the epidermis. Thrombosis is a common feature. The only significant variant is a manifestation of Fabry's disease.

Angiosarcomas include hemangiosarcomas and lymphangiosarcomas.[200-203] It is not possible to clearly distinguish the two in all cases. *Hemangiosarcomas* have blood-filled spaces and may have well developed tubular patterns. Lymphangiosarcomas are characterized by anastomosing angulated vessels. Lymphoid infiltrates are often a prominent feature. In many cases, a problem lesion is simply qualified as angiosarcoma.

Angiosarcomas are associated with several distinctive clinical settings:

1. Postmastectomy lymphangiosarcoma (Stewart-Treves syndrome)
2. Angiosarcoma of the elderly (face and scalp)
3. Lymphedematous angiosarcomas (of which postmastectomy lymphangiosarcoma is a special variant)[201]
4. Malignant transformation of congenital angiodysplasia (often a complication of x-irradiation)
5. De novo angiosarcomas

Histologically, the neoplastic cells form cords or tubules that extend between and are supported by collagen bundles (Fig. 9-65).[200–202] They may be well or poorly differentiated and repeated biopsies may document sequential changes ("dedifferentiation"). Well differentiated lesions are composed of widely spaced vessels with plump uniform endothelial cells. Nuclei are pale with marginated chromatin and prominent nucleoli. Focally, the endothelial cells may form complex intraluminal papillae. Papillary hemangioendothelioma of childhood is a low grade, well differentiated angiosarcoma.[204] In the poorly differentiated variants, the endothelial cells are plump and have hyperchromatic nuclei. Regional variations are common. In areas, the widely spaced ectatic vessels are difficult to distinguish from localized lymphangiectasia. In other areas, the large, solid aggregates of cells may be confused with metastatic carcinoma or undifferentiated sarcoma. The tumor cells form scattered nodules in the dermis. Adjacent nodules are connected by anastomosing neoplastic vessels. The vessels widely infiltrate the skin and adequate surgical margins are extremely difficult to define. A reticulum stain will demonstrate the endothelial quality of the tumor cells, which is better confirmed by electron microscopy, immunoperoxidase reactions for factor VIII (if positive), or an affinity for lectins. Endothelial cells of lymphatic vessels generally are not immunoreactive for factor VIII.[202]

Angiosarcomas have a poor prognosis. Well differentiated lesions are difficult to control locally but are unlikely to metastasize. Poorly differentiated lesions are aggressive locally and metastasize to lymph nodes and through the bloodstream.[203]

Angioblastomas

Angioblasts are the precursors of endothelial cells.[205] They form interconnected cords rather than tubules. In essence, the angioblast is a proliferating vasoformative cell in the stage prior to channelization. The concept of the angioblast finds application to a group of vascular neoplasms.[206–210] In this group, there is often evidence of an origin of the neoplasm from a single pre-existing muscular vessel. In contrast, most hemangiomas and angiosarcomas do not have a clearly defined relationship with a preexisting vessel. Many lesions in this general category are also characterized by zonal patterns of maturation. For these examples, the most immature cells (angioblasts) are found near the vessel of origin and more differentiated cells with endothelial qualities are found at the periphery of such a lesion. There is an additional quality of cytophilia (with a particular attraction for lymphocytes and eosinophils). The association of distinctive vessels and a background of lymphocytes produces a pattern reminiscent of the paracortical zones of lymph nodes. In these areas, the vessels display the characteristics of postcapillary venules and may function in a similar manner.

The angioblastomas can be divided into the following categories:

1. Cytophilic differentiating variants
   Cutaneous (solitary or pattern of satellitosis)
   Subcutaneous (solitary and angiocentric)
   Subcutaneous and deep (solitary or disseminated);
   the disseminated lesions may also involve the skin
2. Angiocentric variants
   Infiltrating
   Infiltrating with myxoid stroma

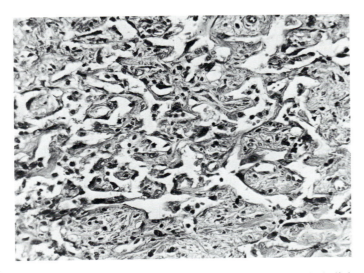

Fig. 9-65. Lymphangiosarcoma of scalp. Atypical endothelial cells from angulated vessels between collagen bundles of the dermis.

Angioblastomas as a group are vasoproliferative and vasoformative disorders. In the angioblastic zones the cells are plump and spindle-shaped or epithelioid. The latter qualities have been offered as a basis for the classification of this group of disorders. Characteristic deeply cleaved nuclei are emphasized in this approach.[208] In the differentiated areas, well formed vessels are lined by a single row of plump endothelial cells. In the angioblastic zones, the cells have hyperchromatic nuclei and a moderate amount of acidophilic cytoplasm (Fig. 9-66). The endothelial cells bulge into the lumen of the involved vessel to produce an irregular or cobblestone surface.

Examples of this general group have been characterized as atypical pyogenic granuloma, Kimura's disease, angiolymphoid hyperplasia with eosinophilia, histiocytoid hemangioma, epithelioid hemangioma, malignant myxoid angioblastoma, epithelioid hemangioendothelioma, and even as intravascular bronchoalveolar tumor of the lung or cholangiolar carcinoma of the liver.

When the endothelial changes are associated with the feature of cytophilia, the resulting lesion qualifies as *angiolymphoid hyperplasia with eosinophilia*.[206] Evidence that similar endothelial lesions which are not cytophilic constitute a separate clinicopathologic entity is lacking. In the absence of lymphoid infiltrates and eosinophilia, some of these endothelial lesions have been classified as *atypical intravascular angioendotheliomas.*

Atypical pyogenic granuloma has usually been defined on the basis of clinical characteristics.[207] It is a polypoid lesion which tends to recur locally with multiple satellite lesions. On a histologic basis, many atypical pyogenic

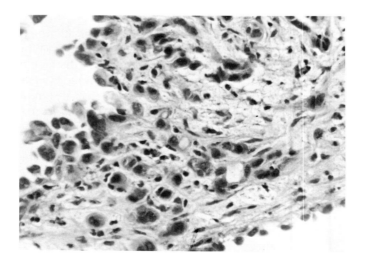

Fig. 9-66. Subcutaneous cytophilic angioblastoma (angiolymphoid hyperplasia with eosinophilia). A portion of a feeder vessel is represented. Atypical endothelial cells outline the lumen of the dilated vessel. Similar cells in cords and tubules extend into the wall of the altered vessel.

granulomas lack the lobular quality of a true pyogenic granuloma. They are composed of tortuous vessels with laminated fibrous walls. Plump atypical endothelial cells line the vessels. The vessels are supported by dense fibrous tissue containing perivascular infiltrates of lymphocytes, eosinophils, plasma cells, and histiocytes. In some lesions, lymphoid nodules with germinal centers are a feature. The infiltrates may surround and extend into hair follicles. They are associated with mucinous degeneration of the involved follicular epithelium (follicular mucinosis). In some examples, the atypical endothelial changes are focal alterations in an otherwise characteristic pyogenic granuloma.

The cutaneous localized variant is indistinguishable histologically from the polypoid variant. It is a localized plaque with surface irregularities and lacks the quality of separate, isolated, polypoid lesions. Some of the involved muscular vessels apparently represent feeder vessels. In both the polypoid and the localized variants, the changes in the epidermis and the papillary dermis are lichenoid. They often resemble a severe form of lichen simplex chronicus.

The subcutaneous localized variant is circumscribed and easily enucleated. It has most of the features of the cutaneous variants but has remarkable organoid qualities. Usually, a muscular arterial vessel is included in the tumor. It shows a localized area of atypical angioblastic hyperplasia and aneurysmal dilatation. Cords and tubules of atypical angioblasts extend through a mucinous defect in the arterial wall (Fig. 9-66). They form compact aggregates near the vessel wall but become widely spaced in delicate, inflamed fibrous tissue near the periphery of the lesion. There is a progressive reduction in nuclear atypism of the endothelial cells (maturation) and an increased prominence of the process of channelization as the distance increases from the site of origin in the altered artery.

In the disseminated variant *(Kimura's disease)* the histologic features are similar to those of cutaneous lesions, but the deep soft tissues are involved. The lesions have ill defined margins and may involve skeletal muscle. Endothelial cells are less characteristic in the disseminated lesions.

These peculiar atypical endothelial dysplasias are not confined to soft tissue. The low-grade hemangioendothelioma of bone qualifies as a localized cytophilic variant.[208] In the soft tissue and skin, the lesions have a tendency to recur locally, with the exception of the circumscribed subcutaneous variant. Angioblastomas should not be confused with *vegetative intravascular hemangioendothelioma*.[211] The latter lesion is a peculiar proliferative process usually associated with intravascular thrombi. Endothelial cells form complex, delicate fronds.

Angioendotheliomatosis is a rare disorder characterized by disseminated lesions involving small vessels. Benign and malignant variants are recognized.[212-216] The former is often associated with infectious processes, such as bacterial endocarditis. In this variant, bland endothelial cells proliferate and occlude the lumina of the involved vessels.

In the malignant variant, the evidence favors the interpretation that most cases are a peculiar angiotropic variant of a large cell lymphoma rather than a distinctive process of endothelial origin.[214] There are conflicting data.[215] Often the endothelial cells of the involved vessels appear intact and unaltered. Atypical cells with plump, hyperchromatic nuclei cluster in the lumens of the involved vessels. The aggregates of abnormal cells are often associated with thrombi and with areas of necrosis. The lesions are disseminated and the clinical manifestations are protean, depending on the most affected organs.

Kaposi's hemorrhagic sarcoma is clearly defined on the basis of clinicopathologic features, but its cell of origin is disputed. Until recently, it has been a disease primarily of the elderly in the United States, but in certain regions of Africa during the same period, children and adults were affected. It is basically a cutaneous disease, but visceral lesions may complicate the clinical course. In the skin, lesions of Kaposi's sarcoma are multifocal. In contrast to angiosarcomas of the skin, neoplastic vessels do not extend in the intervening skin between adjacent nodules. Multifocality may also account for lymph node and visceral involvement.

In the classic expression of the disorder, the lesions are papular or polypoid and favored sites are the lower extremities.[217] Often the involved extremities are lymphedematous. The disease is usually chronic and localized, but in occasional examples, is fulminant and widely disseminated. Visceral involvement is variable, but the submucosa of the intestinal tract is a favored site.[217] Lymph nodes are occasionally involved. The disorder has a peculiar association with malignant lymphomas.

The prevalence and the clinical manifestations have been modified by the current epidemic of virus-related (HIV) AIDS. In this syndrome, Kaposi's sarcoma is a common complication, as are a variety of opportunistic infections. In AIDS, the lesions of Kaposi's sarcoma are commonly disseminated in the skin and viscera.[218]

The histogenesis of Kaposi's sarcoma is controversial, and proposed origins include perithelial cells and reticuloendothelial cells.[217] On simple morphologic features, the lesion qualifies as a dysplasia of vascular mesenchyme variously expressed in patterns of lymphatic differentiation in the reticular dermis. Vasoformative mesenchyme with convergent lymphatic and blood vascular differentiation has been proposed as an explanation for the peculiar histologic patterns.[219] Reticulum stains produce patterns that strongly favor an endothelial origin.

The histologic patterns in the skin include the following:

1. Fibrotic variant (generally small macular lesions)
2. Angiomatous variant (macular, papular, or polypoid lesions)
3. Solid variant (papular or polypoid)
4. Angiosarcomatous variant (tumoral with extension into the soft tissue)

Histologically, the minimal fibrotic lesion is vasoformative, desmoplastic and focal in the reticular dermis. Generally, the process is not pandermal in the area of involvement. Tortuous vessels form small clusters irregularly at the periphery of the zone of sclerosis. The tortuous vessels are associated with infiltrates of lymphoid cells and thin sheaths of elongated spindle cells with pale cytoplasm (Fig. 9-67). The spindle cell component is variable and often is inconspicuous. The lymphoid infiltrates contain plasma cells. In the zone of sclerosis, the pattern of collagen bundles is preserved but the collagen bundles are coarsened. Elongated spindle cells form traceries between the collagen bundles. They tend to pull away from the collagen bundles on one side to form slit-like spaces. In a few areas, they appear to form thin anastomosing channels between the collagen bundles. The resulting pattern and the open-ended quality of some of the spaces is reminiscent of the relationships between collagen of the reticular dermis and dermal lymphatic vessels.

The angiomatous pattern is a variation on the basic fibrotic pattern. In this pattern, the clustered, tortuous blood vessels form larger aggregates and acquire angiomatous qualities. The lumens are dilated, and the vessels form lobular aggregates. The remnants of the fibrotic patterns may be inconspicuous, and the resulting lesion diffi-

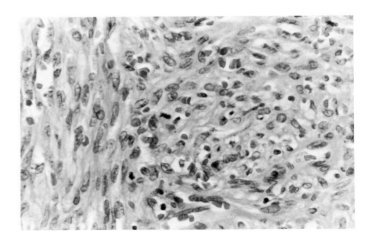

Fig. 9-67. Kaposi's sarcoma (solid variant). Plump spindle cells are compactly aggregated. They outline small slit-like spaces that contain red blood cells.

cult to distinguish from an angioma. Clues to the diagnosis are found in the spindle cell component (if a remnant is preserved), in the clinical presentation, in the location (reticular dermis in contrast to most acquired angiomas which are polypoid in the papillary dermis), and in the associated lymphoid infiltrates with plasmocytosis.

In the solid variants, the spindle cell components of the perivascular sheaths progressive enlarge and become confluent. They form richly vascularized, expansile tumors composed of plump spindle cells. The spindle cells are arranged in interlacing fascicles. Perivascular lymphoplasmacytic infiltrates and hemosiderin deposits in the adjacent dermis are additional features. In individual lesions, there may be variations in the degree of nuclear atypism in the spindle cell component. Mitoses are common. Colloid droplets in the cytoplasm of some of the tumor cells have been emphasized as a diagnostic feature but are an aid only if they can be identified. The tumors may be confined to the dermis or may produce polypoid elevations at the surface that clinically resemble pyogenic granulomas.

In the spindle cell component, the cells are outlined by rigid reticulum fibers. The relationship between reticulum fibers and tumor cells resembles the pattern in tumors of endothelial origin. In cross section, some of the cells appear to have cytoplasmic vacuoles. In longitudinal sections, some of the red blood cells are found in spaces between tumor cells. Hemosiderin deposits are common in the tumor and in the adjacent inflammatory infiltrates. Rarely, Kaposi's sarcoma of an extremity loses its multifocal quality to become a diffusely infiltrating angiosarcoma.

Spindle cell hemangioendothelioma is an organoid hemangioma with spindle-shaped endothelial cells. The vascular spaces tend to be elliptical in outline. Lesions of this type may recur locally. They may be confused with solid lesions of Kaposi's hemorrhagic sarcoma.[220] They are found mainly in the subcutis.

Acquired progressive lymphangioma is a macular lesion commonly affecting the skin of the neck. Histologically, thin-walled dilated lymphatic vessels anastomose between collagen bundles of the reticular dermis. The endothelial cells are flattened and cytologically bland. The lesion is benign but may be confused with the endothelioma patterns manifested in some early lesions of Kaposi's sarcoma.[221] *Acquired tufted angioma*[222,223] should also be considered in the differential diagnosis of Kaposi's sarcoma.

Nerve Sheath Tumors

The peripheral nerves are composed of axons and a sustentacular system.[223–225] Included in the latter are Schwann cell fascicles, the endoneurium, and the peri-

neurium. The Schwann cells and perineurial cells are functional variants of a line of cells derived from the neural crest. An evaluation of the representation of the component cells or cell processes forms the basis for the classification of tumors and tumorous dysplasias of peripheral nerves. These are discussed in greater detail in Chapter 49.

A *true neuroma* is a tumorous hyperplasia of axons and reactive hyperplasia of the associated sustentacular system.[224,226] It may be solitary or multiple. In the *multiple neuroma syndrome*, lesions are prominent at mucocutaneous junctions. Pheochromocytomas and medullary carcinomas of the thyroid are associated lesions.

Traumatic neuroma is an acquired lesion.[223] In contrast to the encapsulated true neuroma, the acquired neuroma extends into mesenchyme through a defect in the perineurium. It is a hyperplasia of both axons and Schwann cells in relative normal porportions.

Schwannoma (neurilemoma) is an expansile tumor of Schwann cells that is confined by the perineurium.[227] The Schwann cells, the endoneurium, and the perineurium contribute. Schwannomas are uncommon in the skin, and in this location tend to be primarily confined to the subcutis.

The *solitary neurofibroma* is an inlay of neuromesenchyme in a defect in the dermis.[104,224] It is a variant of a diffuse neurofibroma and is axon poor. In essence, it is a local extraneural proliferation of neurosustentacular cells and their matrix. Skin appendages are regularly spaced in the tumor.

Plexiform neurofibromas may involve the skin and subcutaneous fat.[223,224] They are stigmata of von Recklinghausen's disease. Rarely, a superficial plexiform neurofibroma may transform into a malignant schwannoma. A pure plexiform neurofibroma is an intraneural dysplasia. The perineurium, the endoneurium, and the Schwann cell fascicles all contribute, but the contributions are variable when comparisons are made of several lesions or even of different regions of a single lesion. Some plexiform neurofibromas are associated with an extraneural diffuse component (paraneurofibroma).[224] Tactoid bodies and melanocytes are common features of the extraneural component. Neurofibromatosis is not a single disorder.[228]

Perineurial myxoma (nerve sheath myxoma) is a rare tumor of the dermis.[229–232] It is lobulated and fasciculated. Stellate or spindle cells are supported by a mucinous matrix (Fig. 9-68). In areas, the cells may be compactly aggregated. Mucinous changes are occasionally identified in the perineurium of adjacent small nerves. Mitoses are variable. The lesion is benign but may recur locally.

Palisaded perineurial fibroma is an uncommon variant of cutaneous nerve sheath tumor.[224] It is symmetrically expansile in the dermis but is not encapsulated. Collagen bundles in the lesion are broad, rigid and laminated. They

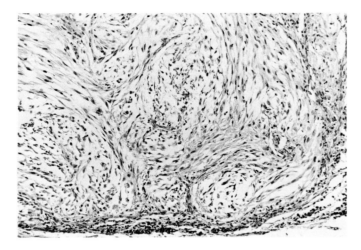

Fig. 9-68. Nerve sheath (perineurial) myxoma. The tumor is multinodular and fasciculated. Tumor cells are supported by a myxomatous matrix.

often appear to radiate from the walls of the vascular plexus in the lesion. Rarely, such a lesion also contains clusters of melanocytes. Focally, some examples are myxomatous.

REFERENCES

1. Reed RJ, Meek T, Ichinose H: Lichen striatus: A model for the histologic spectrum of lichenoid reactions. J Cutan Pathol 2:1, 1975
2. Mitrani E: Possible role of connective tissue in epidermal neoplasia. Br J Dermatol 99:233, 1978
3. Reed RJ, Parkinson RP: The histogenesis of molluscum contagiosum. Am J Surg Pathol 1:161, 1977
4. Zur Hausen H: Papillomaviruses in human cancer. Cancer 59:1692, 1987
5. Steigleder GK: Histology of benign virus induced tumors of the skin. J Cutan Pathol 5:45, 1978
6. Pinkus H, Mehregan AH: A Guide to Dermatohistopathology. 2nd Ed. Appleton & Lange, East Norwalk, CT, 1976, pp 428–429
7. Powell LC Jr: Condyloma acuminatum: Recent advances in development, carcinogenesis, and treatment. Clin Obstet Gynecol 21:1061, 1978
8. Leavell UW, McNamara, MJ, Muelling R, et al: Orf: Report of 19 human cases with clinical and pathological observations. JAMA 204:657, 1968
9. Civatte J: Pseudo-carcinomatous hyperplasia. J Cutan Pathol 12:214, 1985
10. Marshall V: Premalignant and malignant skin tumours in immunosuppressed patients. Transplantation 17:272, 1974
11. Reed RJ: New Concepts in Surgical Pathology of the Skin. pp. 33, 42, 53, 58. Wiley Medical, New York, 1976
12. Pinkus H: The borderline between cancer and noncancer.

p. 5. In Kopf AW, Andrade R (eds): Year Book Medical Publishers, Chicago, 1966
13. Syrjanen KJ: Human papillomavirus (HPV) infections of the female genital tract and their associations with intraepithelial neoplasia and squamous carcinoma. Pathol Annu 21(1):53, 1986
14. Brownstein MH, Shapiro L: Verrucous carcinoma of the skin: Epithelioma cuniculatum plantare. Cancer 38:1710, 1976
15. Okagaki T: Female genital tumors associated with human papillomavirus infection, and the concept of genital neoplasm-papilloma syndrome (GENPS). Pathol Annu 19(2):31, 1984
16. Wade TR, Kopf AW, Ackerman AB: Bowenoid papulosis of the penis. Cancer 42:1890, 1978
17. Gross G, Hagedorn M, Ikenberg H, et al: Bowenoid papulosis. Arch Dermatol 121:858, 1985
18. Patterson JW, Kao GF, Graham JH, Helwig EB: Bowenoid papulosis: A clinicopathologic study with ultrastructural observations. Cancer 57:823, 1986
19. Jablonska S, Dabrowski J, Jakubowicz K: Epidermodysplasia verruciformis as a model and studies on the role of the papova virus in oncogenesis. Cancer Res 32:583, 1972
20. Reed RJ, Leone P: Porokeratosis—A mutant clonal keratosis of the epidermis. Arch Dermatol 101:304, 1970
21. Manfredi G, Bordi C, Allegra F: Porokeratose de Mibelli et keratoses actiniques: Considérations cliniques, histologiques, et ultrastructurales à propos d'un cas avec degénérescence. Ann Dermatol Venereol 105:741, 1978
22. Chernosky M: Porokeratosis. Arch Dermatol 122:869, 1986
23. Jones RE Jr, Austin C, Ackerman AB: Extramammary Paget's disease: A critical reexamination. Am J Dermatol 1:101, 1979
24. Ordonez NG, Awalt H, Mackay B: Mammary and extramammary Paget's disease. Cancer 59:1173, 1987
25. McGibbon DH: Malignant epidermal tumours. J Cutan Pathol 12:224, 1985
26. Kumakiri M, Hashimoto K: Ultrastructural resemblance of basal cell epithelioma to primary epithelial germ. J Cutan Pathol 5:53, 1978
27. Kabulski Z, Frankman O: Histologic malignancy grading in invasive squamous cell carcinoma of the vulva. Int J Gynaecol Obstet 16:233, 1978
28. Stromberg BV, Keiter JE, Wray RC, et al: Scar carcinoma: Prognosis and treatment. South Med J 70:821, 1977
29. Domingo J, Helwig EB: Malignant neoplasms associated with nevus sebaceus of Jadassohn. J Am Acad Dermatol 1:545, 1979
30. Southwick GJ, Schwartz RA: The basal cell nevus syndrome: Disasters occurring among a series of 36 patients. Cancer 44:2294, 1979
31. Howell JB: Nevoid basal cell carcinoma syndrome. J Am Acad Dermatol 11:98, 1984
32. Pinkus H, Mehregan AH: A Guide to Dermatopathology. 2nd Ed. Appleton & Lange, East Norwalk, CT, 1976, p. 570
33. von Domarus H, Stevens PJ: Metastatic basal cell carcinomas J Am Acad Dermatol 10:1043, 1984

34. Reed RJ: Actinic keratoacacthoma. Arch Dermatol 106:858, 1972

35. Clark WH, Reed RJ, Richfield DF: Case 9. p. 30. In Budinger JM (ed): Proceedings of the Forty-First Annual Anatomic Pathology Slide Seminar, American Society of Clinical Pathologists, Chicago, 1977

36. Prehn RT: Immunostimulation of the lymphodependent phase of neoplastic growth. J Natl Cancer Inst 59:1043, 1977

37. Sullivan JJ, Colditz GA: Keratoacanthoma in a sub-tropical climate. Aust J Dermatol 20:34, 1979

38. Janecka IP, Wolff M, Crikelair GF, et al: Aggressive histological features of keratoacanthoma. J Cutan Pathol 4:342, 1978

39. Mehregan AH: Hair follicle tumors of the skin. J Cutan Pathol 12:189, 1985

40. Gray HR, Helwig EB: Epithelioma adenoides cysticum and solitary trichoepithelioma. Arch Dermatol 87:102, 1963

41. Brownstein MH, Shapiro L: Desmoplastic trichoepithelioma. Cancer 40:2979, 1977

42. Headington JT: Tumors of hair follicle. Am J Pathol 85:480, 1976

43. Hashimoto K, Nelson RG, Lever WF: Calcifying epithelioma of Malherbe: Histochemical and electron microscopic studies. J Invest Dermatol 46:391, 1966

44. Roulon D, Helwig EB: Cutaneous sebaceous neoplasms. Cancer 33:82, 1974

45. Schwartz RA, Flieger DN, Saied NK: The Torre syndrome with gastrointestinal polyposis. Arch Dermatol 116:312, 1980

46. Banse-Kupin L, Morales A, Barlow M: Torre's syndrome: Report of two cases and review of literature. J Am Acad Dermatol 10:803, 1984

47. Wick MR, Goellner JR, Wolfe JT, Su WPD: Adnexal carcinomas of the skin. II. Extraocular sebaceous carcinomas. Cancer 56:1163, 1985

48. Hashimoto K, Gross BG, Nelson RG, et al: Eccrine spiradenoma: Histochemical and electron microscopic studies. J Invest Dermatol 46:347, 1966

49. Headington JT, Batsakis JG, Beals TF, et al: Membranous basal cell adenoma of the parotid gland, dermal cylindromas, and trichoepitheliomas: Comparative histochemistry and ultrastructure. Cancer 39:2460, 1977

50. Luna M, Tortoledo ME, Allen M: Salivary dermal analogue tumors arising in lymph nodes. Cancer 59:1165, 1987

51. Evans HL, Su WPD, Smith JL, et al: Carcinoma arising in eccrine spiradenoma. Cancer 43:1881, 1979

52. Galadari E, Mehregan AH, Lee KC: Malignant transformation of eccrine tumors. J Cutan Pathol 14:15, 1987

53. Cooper PH, Frierson HF Jr, Morrison AG: Malignant transformation of eccrine spiradenoma. Arch Dermatol 121:1445, 1985

54. Tang CK, Toker C: Trabecular carcinoma of the skin: An ultrastructural study. Cancer 42:2311, 1978

55. Hall PA, I'Ardenne AJ, Butler MG, et al: Cytokeratin and laminin immunostaining in the diagnosis of cutaneous neuro-endocrine (Merkel cell) tumours. Histopathology 10:1179, 1986

56. Sibley RK, Dehner LP, and Rosai J: Primary neuroendocrine (Merkel cell?) carcinoma of the skin. Am J Surg Pathol 9:95, 1985

57. Sibley RK, Dahl D: Primary neuroendocrine (Merkel cell?) carcinoma of the skin. Am J Surg Pathol 9:109, 1985

58. Varela-Duran J, Diaz-Flores L, Varela-Nunez R: Ultrastructure of chondroid syringoma: Role of the myoepithelial cell in the development of the mixed tumor of the skin and soft tissues. Cancer 44:148, 1979

59. Massa MC, Medenica M: Cutaneous adnexal tumors and cysts: A review. Pathol Annu 22(1):225, 1987

60. Hilton JMW, Blackwell JB: Metastasizing chondroid syringoma. J Pathol 109:167, 1973

61. Sanchez NP, Winkelmann RK: Basal cell tumor with eccrine differentiation. J Am Acad Dermatol 6:514, 1982

62. Swanson PE, Cherwitz DL, Neumann MP, Wick MR: Eccrine sweat gland carcinoma: An histologic and immunohistochemical study of 32 cases. J Cutan Pathol 14:65, 1987

63. Headington JT, Teears R, Niederhuber JE, et al: Primary adenoid cystic carcinoma of skin. Arch Dermatol 114:421, 1978

64. Seab JA, Graham JH: Primary cutaneous adenoid cystic carcinoma. J Am Acad Dermatol 17:113, 1987

65. Egbert BM, Price NM, Segal RJ: Steatocystoma multiplex: Report of a florid case and a review. Arch Dermatol 115:334, 1979

66. Reed RJ, Lamar LM: Invasive hair matrix tumors of the scalp. Arch Dermatol 94:310, 1966

67. Massa MC, Medenica M: Cutaneous adnexal tumors and cysts: A review. Part I. Tumors with hair follicle differentiation and cysts related to different parts of the hair follicle. Pathol Annu 20(2):189, 1985

68. Holmes EJ: Tumors of the lower hair sheath. The common histogenesis of certain so-called "sebaceous cysts", adenomas, and "sebaceous carcinomas." Cancer 21:234, 1968

69. Kossard S, Berman A, Winkelmann RK: Seborrheic keratosis and trichostasis spinulosa. J Cutan Pathol 6:492, 1979

70. Rahbari H, Mehregan A, Pinkus H: Trichoadenoma of Nikolowski. J Cutan Pathol 4:90, 1977

71. Johnson BL, Helwig EB: Eccrine acrospiroma: A clinicopathologic study. Cancer 23:641, 1969

72. Kersting DW: Clear cell hidradenoma and hidradenocarcinoma. Arch Dermatol 87:323, 1963

73. Cooper PH: Carcinomas of sweat glands. Pathol Annu 22(1):83, 1987

74. Roulon DB, Helwig EB: Papillary eccrine adenoma. Arch Dermatol 113:596, 1977

75. Berg JW, McDivitt RW: Pathology of sweat gland carcinoma. Pathol Annu 3:123, 1968

76. Cooper PH, Mills SE, Leonard D, et al: Sclerosing sweat duct (syringomatous) carcinoma. Am J Surg Pathol 9:422, 1985

77. Cooper PH: Sclerosing carcinoma of sweat ducts (microcystic adnexal carcinoma). Arch Dermatol 122:261, 1986

78. Wick R, Goellner JR, Wolfe JT, Su WPD: Adnexal carcinomas of the skin: I. Eccrine carcinomas. Cancer 56:1147, 1985

79. Kao GF, Helwig EB, Graham JH: Aggressive digital papillary adenoma and adenocarcinoma. J Cutan Pathol 14:129, 1987

80. Wright JD, Font RL: Mucinous sweat gland adenocarcinoma of eyelid: A clinicopathologic study of 21 cases with histochemical and electron microscopic observations. Cancer 44:1757, 1979

81. Headington JT: Primary mucinous carcinoma of the skin: Histochemistry and electron microscopy. Cancer 39:1055, 1977

82. Brownstein MH, Helwig EB: Patterns of cutaneous metastasis. Arch Dermatol 105:862, 1972

83. McKee PH: Cutaneous metastases. J Cutan Pathol 12:239, 1985

84. Wick M, Millns JL, Sibley RK, et al: Secondary neurocrine carcinomas of the skin. J Am Acad Dermatol 13:134, 1985

85. Silva EG, Mackay B, Goepfert H, et al: Endocrine carcinoma of the skin (Merkel cell carcinoma). Pathol Annu 19(2):1, 1984

86. Fontaine J, Lelievre C, LeDouarin NM: What is the developmental fate of the neural crest cells which migrate into the pancreas in the avian embryo? Gen Comp Endocrinol 33:394, 1977

87. Clark WH, Reed RJ, Richfield DF: Case 15. p. 68. In Budinger JM (ed): Proceedings of the Forty-First Annual Anatomic Pathology Slide Seminar, Chicago, American Society of Clinical Pathology, 1977

88. Heenan PJ, Quirk CJ, Papadimitriou JM: Epithelioid sarcoma: A diagnostic problem. Am J Dermatopathol 8:95, 1986

89. Kheir SM, Omura EF, Grizzle WE, et al: Histologic variation in the skin lesions of the glucagonoma syndrome. Am J Surg Pathol 10:445, 1986

90. Ingrish F, Reed RJ: Tricholemmoma. Dermatol Int 7:182, 1968

91. Pulitzer DR, Reed RJ: Inverted follicular keratosis and human papillomaviruses. Am J Dermatol 5:453, 1983

92. Weary PE, Gorlin RJ, Gentry WC Jr, et al: Multiple hamartoma syndrome (Cowden's disease). Arch Dermatol 106:682, 1972

93. Starnik ThM: Cowden's disease: Analysis of 14 new cases. J Am Acad Dermatol 11:1127, 1984

94. Reed RJ: Cutaneous manifestations of neural crest disorders (neurocristopathies). J Int Dermatol 16:807, 1977

95. Uitto J, Santa Cruz DJ, Eisen AZ: Connective tissue nevi of the skin. J Am Acad Dermatol 3:441, 1980

96. Reed RJ, Hairston MA, Palomeque FE: The histologic identity of adenoma sebaceum and solitary melanocytic angiofibroma. Dermatol Int 5:3, 1966

97. Meigel MN, Ackerman AB: Fibrous papule of the face. Am J Dermatopathol 1:329, 1979

98. Belaich S, Civatte J, Bonvalet D, et al: Fibromes perifolliculaires multiples du visage et du cou posant le problème des adenomes sebaces symétiques blanc et fibreux. Ann Dermatol Venereol 105:959, 1978

99. Reed RJ, Clark WH, Mihm MC: The cutaneous collagenoses. Hum Pathol 4:165, 1973

100. Raque CJ, Wood MG: Connective tissue nevus. Arch Dermatol 102:390, 1970

101. Balus L, Crovato F, Breathnach AS: Familial multiple trichodiscomas. J Am Acad Dermatol 15:603, 1986

102. Reed RJ, Clark WC, Mihm MC: The cutaneous elastoses. Hum Pathol 4:187, 1973

103. Weston RP: The migration and differentiation of neural crest cells. Adv Morphogenol 8:41, 1971

104. Reed RJ: Neuromesenchyme: The concept of a neurocristic effector cell for dermal mesenchyme. Am J Dermatopathol 5:385, 1983

105. Reed RJ: Melanocytic Nevi and Related Tumors of the Skin: An Atlas of Dermatopathology. American Society of Clinical Pathologists, Chicago, 1975

106. Mark GJ, Mihm MC, Liteplo MG, et al: Congenital melanocytic nevi of the small and garment type. Hum Pathol 4:395, 1973

107. Marita T, Eto T, Ito T: Peutz-Jeghers syndrome with adenomas and adenocarcinomas in colonic polyps. Am J Surg Pathol 11:76, 1987

108. Peterson LL, Serrill WS: Lentiginosis associated with a left atrial myxoma. J Am Acad Dermatol 10:337, 1984

109. Rhodes AR, Silverman RA, Harrist TJ, Perez-Atayde AR: Mucocutaneous lentigines, cardiomucocutaneous myxomas, and multiple blue nevi: The "LAMB" syndrome. J Am Acad Dermatol 10:72, 1984

110. Carney JA, Headington JT, Su WPD: Cutaneous myxomas. Arch Dermatol 122:790, 1986

111. Reed RJ, Ichinose H, Clark WH Jr, et al: Common and uncommon melanocytic nevi and borderline melanomas. Semin Oncol 2:119, 1975

112. Paniago-Pereira C, Maize JC, Ackerman AB: Nevus of large spindle and/or epithelioid cells (Spitz's nevus). Arch Dermatol 114:1811, 1978

113. Weedon D, Little JH: Spindle and epithelioid cell nevi in children and adults: A review of 211 cases of the Spitz nevus. Cancer 40:217, 1977

114. Peters MS, Goellner JR: Spitz naevi and malignant melanomas of childhood and adolescence. Histopathology 10:1289, 1986

115. Clark WH Jr, Reimer RR, Greene M, et al: Origin of familial malignant melanomas from heritable melanocytic lesions. Arch Dermatol 114:732, 1978

116. Kelly JW, Crutcher WA, Sagebiel RW: Clinical diagnosis of dysplastic melanocytic nevi. J Am Acad Dermatol 14:1044, 1986

117. Reed RJ, Clark WH, Mihm MC: Premalignant melanocytic dysplasias. p. 159. In Ackerman AB, (ed): Melanoma. Masson, New York, 1981

118. Elder DE: The dysplastic nevus. Pathology 17:291, 1985

119. Reed RJ: The histological variance of malignant melanoma: the interrelationship of histological subtype, neoplastic progression, and biological behavior. Pathology 17:301, 1985

120. Reed RJ: Minimal deviation melanoma. p. 110. In Murphy GF, Mihm MC, Kaufman N (eds): IAP Monograph: Pathobiology and Recognition of Malignant Melanoma. Williams & Wilkins, Baltimore, 1988

121. Reed RJ: Consultation case. Am J Surg Pathol 2:215, 1978

122. Clark WH Jr, From L, Bernadino EA, et al: The histogenesis and biologic behavior of primary human malignant melanomas of the skin. Cancer Res 29:705, 1969

123. Reed RJ: The pathology of malignant melanoma. p. 85. In Costanzi JJ (ed): Malignant Melanoma. Vol. I. Martinus Nijhoff, The Hague, 1983

124. Sober AJ, Fitzpatrick TB, Mihm MC Jr: Primary melanoma of the skin: Recognition and management. J Am Acad Dermatol 2:179, 1980

125. Clark WH Jr, Mihm MC Jr: Lentigo maligna and lentigo malignant melanoma. Am J Pathol 55:39,1969

126. Arrington JJ III, Reed RJ, Ichinose I, et al: Plantar lentiginous melanoma: A distinctive variant of human cutaneous malignant melanoma. Am J Surg Pathol 1:131, 1977

127. Conley J, Lattes R, Orr W: Desmoplastic malignant melanoma (a rare variant of spindle cell melanoma). Cancer 28:914, 1971

128. Reed RJ, Leonard DD: Neurotropic melanoma: A variant of desmoplastic melanoma. Am J Surg Pathol 3:301, 1979

129. Breslow A: Prognostic factors in the treatment of cutaneous melanoma. J Cutan Pathol 6:208, 1979

130. Balch CM, Murad TM, Soong S, et al: Tumor thickness as a guide to surgical management of clinical stage I melanoma patients. Cancer 43:883,1979

131. Gromet MA, Epstein WL, Blois MS: The regressing thin malignant melanoma: A distinctive lesion with metastatic potential. Cancer 42:2282, 1978

132. Kopf AW, Gross DF, Rogers GS, et al: Prognostic index for malignant melanoma. Cancer 59:1236, 1987

133. Cerio R, MacDonald DM: Benign cutaneous lymphoid infiltrates. J Cutan Pathol 12:442, 1985

134. Evans HL, Winkelmann RK, Banks PM: Differential diagnosis of malignant and benign cutaneous lymphoid infiltrates: A study of 57 cases in which malignant lymphoma had been diagnosed or suspected in the skin. Cancer 44:699, 1979

135. Murphy GF, Mihm MC Jr: Benign, dysplastic, and malignant lymphoid infiltrates of the skin: An approach based on pattern analysis. p. 123. In Murphy GF, Mihm MC Jr (eds): Lymphoproliferative Disorders of the Skin. Buttersworth, Boston, 1986

136. Shelly WB, Wood MG: Observations on occult malignant lymphomas in the skin. Cancer 38:1757, 1976

137. Burke JS, Hoppe RT, Cibull ML, Dorfman RF: Cutaneous malignant lymphoma: A pathologic study of 50 cases with clinical analysis of 37. Cancer 47:300, 1981

138. Macaulay WL: Lymphomatoid papulosis—Review. Int J Dermatol 17:204, 1978

139. Willemze R, Meyer CJLM, van Vloten WA, Scheffer E: The clinical and histological spectrum of lymphomatoid papulosis. Br J Dermatol 107:131, 1982

140. Rilke F, Giardini R, Lombardi L: Recurrent atypical cutaneous histiocytosis. Pathol Annu 20(2):29, 1985

141. Kadin ME: Characteristic immunologic profile of large atypical cells in lymphomatoid papulosis. Arch Dermatol 122:1388, 1986

142. Wood GS, Strickler JG, Deneau DG, et al: Lymphomatoid papulosis expresses immunophenotypes associated with T cell lymphoma but not inflammation. J Am Acad Dermatol 15:444, 1986

143. Ralfkiaer E, Stein H, Wantzin GL, et al: Lymphomatoid papulosis. Am J Clin Pathol 84:587, 1985

144. Rubins J: Cutaneous Hodgkin's disease: Indolent course and control with chemotherapy. Cancer 42:1219, 1978

145. Leibow AA, Carrington CRB, Friedman PJ: Lymphomatoid granulomatosis. Hum Pathol 3:457, 1972

146. Katzenstein AA, Carrington CB, Liebow AA: Lymphomatoid granulomatosis: A clinicopathologic study of 152 cases. Cancer 43:360, 1979

147. Brodell RT, Miller CW, Eisen AZ: Cutaneous lesions of lymphomatoid granulomatosis. Arch Dermatol 122:303, 1986

148. Saxe N, Kahn LB, King H: Lymphoma of the skin: A comparative clinicopathologic study of 50 cases including mycosis fungoides and primary and secondary cutaneous lymphoma. J Cutan Pathol 4:111, 1977

149. Long JC, Mihm MC, Qaze R: Malignant lymphoma of the skin: A clinicopathologic study of lymphoma other than mycosis fungoides diagnosed by skin biopsy. Cancer 38:1282, 1976

150. Long JC, Mihm MC: Multiple granulocytic tumors of the skin: Report of six cases of myelogenous leukemia with initial manifestations in the skin. Cancer 39:2004, 1977

151. Buechner SA, Li C-H, Su WPD: Leukemis cutis: a histopathologic study of 42 cases. Am J Dermatopathol 7:109, 1985

152. Zaatari GS, Chan WC, Kim TH, Williams DL, Kletzel M: Malignant lymphoma of the skin in children. Cancer 59:1040, 1987

153. Duncan SC, Evans HL, Winkelmann RK: Large cell lymphocytoma. Arch Dermatol 116:1142, 1980

154. Mann RB, Jaffe ES, Berard CW: Malignant lymphomas— A conceptual understanding of morphologic diversity. Am J Pathol 94:105, 1979

155. Berger CL, Warburton D, Raafat J, et al: Cutaneous T-cell lymphoma: Neoplasm of T cells with helper activity. Blood 53:642, 1979

156. Streilein JW: Lymphocyte traffic, T-cell malignancies and the skin. J Invest Dermatol 71:167, 1978

157. Reed RJ: Mycosis fungoides. Cancer 27:322, 1977

158. Lambert C, Everett MA: The nosology of parapsoriasis. J Am Acad Dermatol 5:373, 1981

159. Long JC, Mihm MC: Mycosis fungoides with extracutaneous dissemination: A distinct clinicopathologic entity. Cancer 34:1745, 1974

160. Rappaport H, Thomas LB: Mycosis fungoides: The pathology of extracutaneous involvement. Cancer 34:1198, 1974

161. Scheffer E, Meijer CJLM, van Vloten WA: Dermatopathic lymphoadenopathy and lymph node involvement in mycosis fungoides. Cancer 45:137, 1980

162. Tosca AD, Varelzides AG, Economidou J, Stratigos JD: Mycosis fungoides: evaluation of immunohistochemical

criteria for the early diagnosis of the disease and differentiation between stages. J Am Acad Dermatol 15:237, 1986

163. McMillan EM: Monoclonal antibodies and cutaneous T cell lymphomas. J Am Acad Dermatol 12:102, 1985

164. Vonderheid EC, Tan E, Sobel E, et al: Clinical implications of immunologic phenotyping in cutaneous T cell lymphoma. J Am Acad Dermatol 17:40, 1987

165. Mandojana RM, Helwig EB: Localized epidermotropic reticulosis (Woringer-Kolopp disease). J Am Acad Dermatol 8:813, 1983

166. Whitcomb CC, Olivella JE, Byrne GE Jr: T-cell lymphoma-leukemia: Pathologic observations in three cases. Cancer 52:1202, 1983

167. Grogan TM, Fielder K, Rangel C, et al: Peripheral T-cell lymphoma: Aggressive disease with heterogeneous immunotype. Am J Clin Pathol 83:279, 1985

168. Chan H-L, Su I-J, Kuo T-T, et al: Cutaneous manifestations of adult T cell leukemia-lymphoma. J Am Acad Dermatol 13:213, 1985

169. Yamamura T, Aozasa K, Sano S: The cutaneous lymphomas with convoluted nucleus. J Am Acad Dermatol 10:796, 1984

170. Su I-J, Shih L-Y, Kadin ME, et al: Pathologic and immunologic characterization of malignant lymphoma in Taiwan. Am J Clin Pathol 84:715, 1985

171. Kiyokawa T, Yamaguchi K, Takeya M, et al: Hypercalcemia and osteoblast proliferation in adult T cell leukemia. Cancer 59:1187, 1987

172. Hashimoto K, Bale GF, Hawkins HK, et al: Congenital self-healing reticulohistiocytosis (Hashimoto-Pritzker type). Int J Dermatol 25:516, 1986

173. Enzinger FM: Fibrous hamartoma of infancy. Cancer 18:241, 1965

174. Chung EB: Pitfalls in diagnosing benign soft tissue tumors in infancy and childhood. Pathol Annu 20(2):321, 1985

175. Allen PW: Nodular fasciitis. Pathology 4:9, 1972

176. Bernstein KE, Lattes R: Nodular (pseudosarcomatous) fasciitis, a nonrecurrent lesion. Cancer 49:1668, 1982

177. Alguacil-Garcia A, Unni KK, Goellner JR: Histogenesis of dermatofibrosarcoma protuberans: An ultrastructural study. Am J Clin Pathol 69:427, 1983

178. Fletcher CDM, Evans BJ, Macartney JC, et al: Dermatofibrosarcoma protuberans: A clinicopathological and immunohistochemical study with a review of the literature. Histopathology 9:921, 1985

179. Depree WB, Langloss JM, Weiss SW: Pigmented dermatofibrosarcoma protuberans (Bednar tumor). Am J Surg Pathol 9:630, 1985

180. Headington JT, Beals TF, Niederhuber JE: Primary leiomyosarcoma of skin: A report and critical appraisal. J Cutan Pathol 4:308, 1977

181. Dahl I, Angervall L: Cutaneous and subcutaneous leiomyosarcoma: A clinicopathologic study of 47 patients. Pathol Eur 9:307, 1974

182. Fields JP, Helwig EB: Leiomyosarcoma of the skin and subcutaneous tissue. Cancer 47:156, 1981

183. Pepper MC, Laubenheimer R, Cripps DJ: Multiple glomus tumors. J Cutan Pathol 4:244, 1977

184. Enzinger FM, Weiss SW: Glomus tumors. p. 461. In Enzinger FM, Weiss SW (eds): Soft Tissue Tumors. CV Mosby, St Louis, 1983

185. Hairston MA, Reed RJ: Aneurysmal sclerosing hemangioma of skin. Arch Dermatol 93:439, 1966

186. Santa Cruz DJ, Reiner CB: Recurrent digital fibroma of childhood. J Cutan Pathol 5:339, 1978

187. Dahl L: Atypical fibroxanthoma of the skin: a clinicopathological study of 57 cases. Acta Pathol Microbiol Scand 84:183, 1976

188. Fretzin DF, Helwig EB: Atypical fibroxanthoma of the skin: A clinicopathologic study of 140 cases. Cancer 31:1541, 1973

189. Leong ASY, Milios J: Atypical fibroxanthoma of the skin: A clinicopathological and immunochemical study and a discussion of its histogenesis. Histopathology 11:463, 1987

190. Woyke S, Domagala W, Olszewski W, et al: Pseudosarcoma of the skin: An electron microscopic study and comparison with the fine structure of the spindle-cell variant of squamous carcinoma. Cancer 33:970, 1974

191. Helwig EB, May D: Atypical fibroxanthoma with metastasis. Cancer 57:368, 1986

192. Chung EB, Enzinger FM: Infantile myofibromatosis. Cancer 48:738, 1981

193. Dymock RB, Allen PW, Stirling JW, et al: Giant cell fibroblastoma: A distinctive recurrent tumor of childhood. Am J Surg Pathol 11:263, 1987

194. Shmookler BM, Enzinger FM: Pleomorphic lipoma: A benign tumor simulating liposarcoma. Cancer 47:126, 1981

195. Hanada M, Tokuda R. Ohnishi Y, et al: Benign lipoblastoma and liposarcoma in children. Acta Pathol Jpn 36:605, 1986

196. Hayes MMM, Dietrich BE, Uys CJ: Congenital hemangiopericytomas of the skin. Am J Dermatopathol 8:142, 1986

197. Clark WH, Reed RJ, Richfield DF: Case 11. p. 43. In Budinger JM (ed): Proceedings of the Forty-First Annual Anatomic Pathology Slide Seminar, American Society of Clinical Pathology, Chicago, 1977

198. Laugier P: Blue rubber bleb naevus. Ann Dermatol Venereol 105:729, 1978

199. Cooper PH, McAllister HA, Helwig EB: Intravenous pyogenic granuloma: A study of 18 cases. Am J Surg Pathol 3:221, 1979

200. Rosai J, Sumcer HW, Kostianovsky M, et al: Angiosarcoma of the skin: A clinicopathologic and fine structural study. Hum Pathol 7:83, 1976

201. Alessi E, Sala F, Berti E: Angiosarcomas in lymphedematous limbs. Am J Dermatopathol 8:371, 1986

202. Holden CA, Spaull J, Das AK, McKee PH, Wilson Jones E: The histogenesis of angiosarcoma of the face and scalp: An immunohistochemical and ultrastructural study. Histopathology 11:37, 1987

203. Holden CA, Spittle MF, Wilson Jones E: Angiosarcoma of the face and scalp, prognosis and treatment. Cancer 59:1046, 1987

204. Dabska M: Malignant endovascular papillary angioendothelioma of the skin in childhood. Cancer 24:503, 1969

205. Reed RJ: Consultation case (malignant myxoid angioblastoma). Am J Surg Pathol 6:159, 1982

206. Reed RJ, Terezakis N: Subcutaneous angioblastic lymphoid hyperplasia with eosinophilia (Kimura's disease). Cancer 29:489, 1972

207. Wilson-Jones E, Bleehen SS: Inflammatory angiomatous nodules with abnormal blood vessels occurring about the ears and scalp (pseudo or atypical pyogenic granuloma). Br J Dermatol 81:804, 1969

208. Rosai J, Gold J, Landry R: The histiocytoid hemangiomas: A unifying concept embracing several previously described entities of skin, soft tissue, large vessels, bone, and heart. Hum Pathol 10:707, 1979

209. Olsen TG, Helwig EB: Angiolymphoid hyperplasia with eosinophilia. J Am Acad Dermatol 12:781, 1985

210. Enzinger FM, Weiss SH: Epithelioid hemangioendothelioma: A vascular tumor often mistaken for a carcinoma. Cancer 50:970, 1982

211. Kuo TT, Sayers CP, Rosai J: Masson's "vegetant intravascular hemangioendothelioma": A lesion often mistaken for angiosarcoma: Study of seventeen cases located in the skin and soft tissues. Cancer 38:1227, 1976

212. Pasyk K, Depowski M: Proliferating systematized angioendotheliomatosis of a 5-month-old infant. Arch Dermatol 1512, 1978

213. Kurrein F: Systemic angioendotheliomatosis with metastases. J Clin Pathol 29:347, 1976

214. Theaker JM, Gatter KC, Esire MM, Easterbrook P: Neoplastic angioendotheliosis—Further evidence supporting a lymphoid origin. Histopathology 10:1261, 1986

215. Kitagawa M, Matsubara O, Song S-Y, et al: Neoplastic angioendotheliosis. Cancer 56:1134, 1985

216. Wicks MR, Mills SE, Scheithauer BW, et al: Reassessment of malignant angioendotheliomatosis. Am J Surg Pathol 10:112, 1986

217. Reed WB, Kamath HM, Weiss L: Kaposi's sarcoma, with emphasis on the internal manifestations. Arch Dermatol 110:115, 1974

218. Dorfman RF: Kaposi's sarcoma. Am J Surg Pathol 10(suppl I):68, 1986

219. Dictor M: Kaposi's sarcoma: Origin and significance of lymphaticovenous connections. Virchows Arch [A] 409:23, 1986

220. Weiss SW, Enzinger FM: Spindle cell hemangioendothelioma. Am J Surg Pathol 10:521, 1986

221. Watanabe M, Kishiyama K, Ohkawara A: Acquired progressive lymphangioma. J Am Acad Dermatol 8:663, 1983

222. Alessi E, Bertani E, Sala F: Acquired tufted angioma. Am J Dermatopathol 8:426, 1986

223. Harkin JC, Reed RJ: Tumors of the peripheral nervous system. pp. 1, 19, 67. Atlas of Tumor Pathology. Ser. 2, fasc. 3. Armed Forces Institute of Pathology, Washington, DC, 1969

224. Reed RJ, Harkin JC: Tumors of the peripheral nervous system. In Hartman WT (ed.): Atlas of Tumor Pathology. Ser. 2, fasc. 3, (suppl.). Armed Forces Institute of Pathology, Washington, DC, 1982

225. Reed RJ: The neural crest, its migrants, and cutaneous malignant neoplasms related to neurocristic derivatives. p. 171. In Lynch HT, Fusaro RM (eds.): Cancer-Associated Genodermatoses. Van Nostrand Reinhold, New York, 1982

226. Reed RJ, Fine RM, Meltzer HD: Palisaded and encapsulated neuromas of the skin. Arch Dermatol 106:865, 1972

227. Shishiba T, Niimura M, Ohtsuka F, Tsuree N: Multiple cutaneous neurilemmomas as a skin manifestation of neurilemmomatosis. J Am Acad Dermatol 10:744, 1984

228. Riccardi VM: Neurofibromatosis: The importance of localized or otherwise atypical forms. Arch Dermatol 123:882, 1987

229. Pultizer DR, Reed RJ: Nerve sheath myxoma (perineurial myxoma). Am J Dermatopathol 7:409, 1985

230. Fletcher CDM, Chan JK-C, McKee PH: Dermal nerve sheath myxoma: A study of three cases. Histopathology 10:135, 1986

231. MacDonald DM, Wilson-Jones E: Pacinian neurofibroma. Histopathology 1:247, 1977

232. King DT, Barr RJ: Bizarre cutaneous neurofibromas. J Cutan Pathol 7:21, 1980

10

Soft Tissue Tumors

Jorge Albores-Saavedra
Azorides R. Morales

Soft tissue tumors constitute a heterogeneous group of neoplasms in terms of clinical presentation, morphologic features, and clinical behavior. They arise from the extraskeletal mesenchymal tissues, which lie between the epidermis and the parenchymal organs. Tumors arising from the lymphoid system and from the supporting tissues of specific organs and viscera are not included in this group. Neuroectodermally derived peripheral nerve tumors, however, have been included traditionally among the soft tissue tumors because they present similar problems in regard to diagnosis and treatment[1] (these are discussed in detail in Ch. 49).

CLINICAL ASPECTS

Symptomatology

A soft tissue tumor is usually manifested as a mass that interferes with the function and/or cosmetic well-being of the patient. Very few soft tissue tumors are associated with the production of biologically active substances.[2] Among the rare systemic manifestations, the hypoglycemic and osteomalacia-rickets syndromes have been studied most extensively.[2–4]

Symptoms may not reflect the biologic behavior of the tumor. Both benign and malignant soft tissue tumors can present as painless masses. In general, however, rapidly growing soft tissue neoplasms that are fixed to surrounding tissues or that invade or destroy adjacent structures must be considered malignant neoplasms until proved otherwise.

Soft tissue tumors of the abdominal cavity and retroperitoneum frequently produce signs and symptoms by means of displacement, compression, or obstruction. Most benign soft tissue neoplasms tend to be confined to their anatomic compartments. However, some benign tumors and pseudotumors may mimic sarcomas because of their infiltrative growth patterns. The stimulus for the growth of soft tissue hamartomas may originate early in embryonic and fetal development, before definitive tissue and organ boundaries are established; therefore, these tumors may involve many structures, mimicking the insinuative growth of sarcomas. Hemangiomas and lymphangiomas of childhood are conspicuous examples of this type of growth pattern.

Several soft tissue tumors, some of which are hamartomas or hyperplastic lesions, are components of heritable syndromes.[5–9] Renal angiomyolipomas and pulmonary lymphangiomyomas are associated with tuberous sclerosis.[10–12] Gardner's syndrome, the association of fibromatosis with familial polyposis, may sometimes manifest the symptoms of the soft tissue tumors before the intestinal polyposis becomes apparent.[13] The multiple symmetric lipomatoses, including familial cervical lipodysplasia, are associated with metabolic disorders,[5] while the multiple cutaneous leiomyomata of pilar origin[14] and neurofibromatosis (von Recklinghausen's disease) may be complicated by the development of sarcomas.[15] A small percentage of angiolipomas are multiple and genetically determined but do not become malignant. Patients with Werner's syndrome, a rare autosomal-recessive disorder characterized by shortness of stature and premature aging, often develop a variety of soft tissue sarcomas.[16]

Diagnostic Procedures

The images of soft tissue tumors on routine radiologic examination are often too vague to permit precise definition of the lesion. Lipomatous tumors, however, can be recognized in plane radiography because of their low density. The presence of calcifications in a clinically malignant soft tissue tumor reduces the diagnostic possibilities. Calcifications are more often seen in synovial sarcomas, chondrosarcomas, and osteosarcomas than in any other type of soft part sarcoma. Computed tomography (CT),[17,18] ultrasonography, and magnetic resonance imaging (MRI) define clearly the anatomy, extent, and outline of the tumor and its effects on the surrounding tissue.[19] In fact, tumors previously undetectable without surgical exploration can now be visualized readily and staged with these techniques. Moreover, identification of the specific tissue type is sometimes possible.[20] Angiography adds information concerning invasion and compression or destruction of local blood vessels. Thus, angiography further defines the extent of disease and aids the surgeon in demonstrating the source(s) and patterns of the vascular supply to the tumor as well as the status and pattern of the blood supply to the limb or region in which the tumor resides.[21] Likewise, the angiographic vascular pattern may help differentiate between benign and malignant fibrous tumors[22] and between hemangiopericytoma and other neoplasms with prominent vascular components.[23,24] Clinical assessment of certain hemangiomas and vascular malformations[8,9] requires angiographic study; this procedure can also be used to delineate heavily vascularized segments of the sarcoma, which should be biopsied because they contain the most anaplastic portions.[22]

The true biologic nature of a soft tissue mass can be determined only by histologic examination of representative portions or all of the mass. In small tumors, the entire specimen should be removed for morphologic assessment. Total removal of the tumor is frequently cosmetically and psychologically gratifying to the patient who has a benign soft tissue tumor. This approach is usually necessary to ensure that the disturbing lump does not harbor any malignancy. If the surgeon plans an excisional biopsy of a tumor mass, a rim of surrounding normal tissue should be included, whenever possible. However, the surgeon should try to maintain the cosmetic and/or functional integrity of the affected area until the histologic diagnosis is made. Therapeutic wide excision of a soft tissue sarcoma usually necessitates removal of at least a 3 to 5 cm rim of grossly normal tissue around the apparent neoplasm. If the surgeon decides to use that approach, it behooves the pathologist to exercise judgment in the morphologic evaluation of the biopsy specimen. The gross and microscopic examination should always include specific observations regarding the relationship of the tumor to surrounding tissues and the relationship of the tumor to resection margins. If the mass is a sarcoma or a biologically aggressive lesion such as a desmoid tumor, the therapeutic surgical approach will be greatly influenced by the pathologist's report of how much of the tumor was left behind and where any remnants may have been located. Drawings, photographs, and detailed identification of the anatomic sources of specific representative histologic sections are essential for proper evaluation of the surgical margins. If the malignant tumor is found at a resection margin, the surgeon can then complete management of the case. The pathologist must request that the surgeon orient the specimen anatomically to ensure the best outcome for the patient.

When soft tissue tumors are too large for diagnostic excision, incisional biopsy is indicated. Whether that is done with a cutting needle, punch, or scalpel, the sample taken must be representative of the tumor. Multiple incisional biopsies of the edges and center of the tumor may be necessary to establish the diagnosis. Soft tissue tumors frequently elicit inflammatory and/or fibrous host responses and nonspecific degenerative changes at their edges. Biopsies of these areas may lead to erroneous diagnoses. Ischemic degenerative changes and fibrosis, hemorrhage, and/or necrosis in the centers of large tumors can obscure the basic pathologic process. Large, ulcerated soft tissue tumors are usually inflamed, and incisional superficial biopsies of the ulcer are generally useless in regard to diagnosis.

Although exfoliative cytology has not proved useful in establishing the diagnosis of soft tissue tumors, fine needle aspiration has reawakened the interest of pathologists in this rapid and relatively risk-free type of diagnostic procedure.[25,26] In fact, cytologic criteria are now available for many of these neoplasms.[27–34] The major obstacle to the cytologic study of soft tissue tumors is the entrapment of cells in the fibrous network intrinsic to most of the masses. Multiple aspirations may be required to obtain adequate numbers of neoplastic cells, but in most cases, the pathologist is forced to work with a scanty specimen when evaluating the cytologic material obtained from soft tissue tumors. Although the precise identification of many soft tissue tumors by fine needle aspiration biopsy is difficult and requires considerable experience, the pathologist can usually separate soft tissue sarcomas from malignant lymphomas and carcinomas by this means.[35] For the Papanicolaou (Pap) stain, the cytologic specimen should be fixed immediately in alcohol; for the hemtoxylin and eosin (H&E) stain, it should be fixed in 10% formalin; and for the Wright-Giemsa stain, it should be air-dried.

Frozen section diagnosis of soft tissue tumors is a routine procedure that may be followed by definitive surgery. To avoid serious mistakes, the pathologist should have broad experience not only with these tumors and with the technique, but with the complete clinical information regarding each case as well. Otherwise, it is preferable not to undertake definitive treatment on the basis of that diagnostic procedure. However, frozen sections should still be encouraged in order to determine adequacy of the tissue for definitive diagnosis and in preparation for other diagnostic techniques, such as immunohistochemistry and electron microscopy.

THE PATHOLOGIST'S APPROACH TO THE STUDY OF SOFT TISSUE TUMORS

The pathologic assessment of soft tissue tumors should yield the information required to prognosticate biologic behavior and to plan the course of treatment. Histologic classification, extent of the tumor, adequacy of surgical excision, and histologic grading are the important parameters to keep in mind when studying these surgical specimens. In addition to the routine H&E preparation, other stains and/or histologic techniques may be required to demonstrate the cellular constituents necessary to establish the correct diagnosis. Accordingly, samples of tissue should be fixed in the most appropriate solutions.

Traditionally, pathologists have used a variety of special stains to assist in establishing tumor histogenesis.[36] Unfortunately, the substances demonstrated by these techniques are nonspecific and are almost universally present in any tumor, regardless of its histogenesis. However, in spite of these obvious limitations, the techniques may provide significant additional information in some instances. Reticulin stains may be of help in differentiating mesenchymal from epithelial neoplasms by showing groups of tumor cells in the latter, while in the former, tumor cells are often individualized by a network of reticulin fibers. The parallel arrangement of reticulin fibers to the long axis of tumor cells in neurogenic and smooth muscle tumors may assist in the diagnosis of these lesions, and an otherwise inconspicuous vascular pattern can be made apparent with this stain.

The importance of fat stains is often overemphasized. The cells of virtually every line may contain globules of lipid. However, few small globules of fat with a tendency to coalesce, hence forming large globules displacing the nucleus eccentrically, are helpful in establishing the diagnosis of liposarcoma. Fibrous histiocytic tumors typically contain intracytoplasmic fat but do not have aggregates of lipid large enough to displace the nucleus.

Collagen stains such as Masson trichrome are commonly used in the microscopic assessment of soft tissue

tumors. However, their value is rather limited, since a greater or lesser amount of collagen may be seen in any of these lesions, regardless of their histogenesis. However, these stains may accentuate the intracytoplasmic filaments of smooth muscle tumors as well as the cross-striations of rhabdomyoblasts. The phosphotungstic acid hematoxylin (PTAH) stain is also used quite often with the same purpose in mind, but it is doubtful at best whether either of these stains (i.e., trichrome or PTAH) may add significant information to that obtained with routine H&E stains. Mesenchymal tumors contain variable amounts of interstitial and often intracytoplasmic polysaccharides that can be demonstrated with periodic acid-Schiff (PAS), colloidal iron, Alcian blue, and other stains. Treatment of the tissue with diastase or hyaluronic acid preceding the appropriate staining may be quite valuable, the former in identifying glycogen as an aid in the differential diagnosis of look-alike tumors such as rhabdomyosarcoma, Ewing's sarcoma, lymphoma, and neuroblastoma. Hyaluronic acid digestion of polysaccharides can help in instances of suspected mesothelioma and extraskeletal chrondrosarcoma.

Enzyme histochemistry is of limited help in the differential diagnosis of soft tissue tumors because of its lack of specificity. Oxidative enzymes, for example, are present in many tumors regardless of their histogenesis. The need to use fresh frozen sections further discourages the use of this group of procedures.

Likewise, tissue culture, because of its requirement for an assortment of facilities and expertise and its limited yield, is not generally considered a practical diagnostic tool in surgical pathology. In some laboratories, however, it is considered valuable in establishing the histogenesis of a number of soft tissue tumors.[37–39]

Ultrastructural evaluation of soft tissue tumors permits resolution of a number of problems in differential diagnosis.[40–43] It is particularly helpful in determining the mesenchymal, epithelial, or lymphoreticular nature of undifferentiated tumors. The interrelationship between neighboring cells is well established in normal and neoplastic epithelial cells because of the presence of desmosomes and other junctional complexes. With rare exception, these structures are absent in sarcomas and lymphomas.

Electron microscopic studies may also permit the pathologist to establish the diagnosis of rhabdomyosarcoma, leiomyosarcoma, neuroblastoma, and neurogenic sarcoma; these studies are helpful in distinguishing liposarcoma from malignant fibrous histiocytoma and in establishing the diagnosis of tumors that present an undifferentiated small cell pattern (i.e., carcinoma, melanoma, rhabdomyosarcoma, Ewing's sarcoma, malignant glomus tumor, neuroblastoma, and malignant lymphoma).

A hexagonal array of actin and myosin filaments is specific for skeletal muscle. Demonstration of these fila-

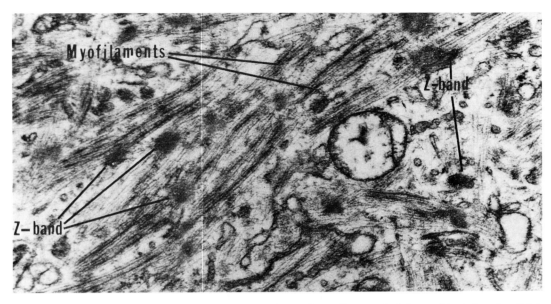

Fig. 10-1. Rhabdomyosarcoma. Portion of the cytoplasm of a malignant rhabdomyoblast showing thick and thin filaments and Z-band material.

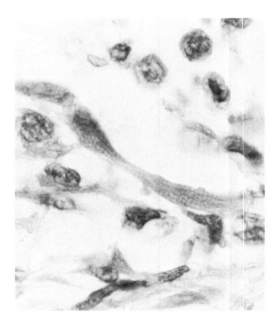

Fig. 10-2. Embryonal rhabdomyosarcoma. Well differentiated rhabdomyoblast showing cross-striations of the cytoplasm.

ments in a malignant tumor with or without Z-band material establishes the diagnosis of rhabdomyosarcoma (Fig. 10-1). The number and arrangement of these proteins depend on the stage of development of the rhabdomyoblasts and are in direct relationship to the degree of differentiation of the tumor. Only in the most mature rhabdomyoblasts are they present in sufficient number and

aligned in a manner so as to replicate mature skeletal muscle, forming the cross-striations of light microscopy (Fig. 10-2).

The longitudinally striated rod-shaped bodies described by Weibel and Palade[44] are also intracytoplasmic components specific for a cell line (i.e., endothelial cells) (Fig. 10-3). Therefore, the demonstration of these bodies in neoplastic cells permits identification of that cell line. However, Weibel-Palade bodies are rarely seen in sarcomas.[45]

Ultrastructurally, smooth muscle contains thin filaments in association with dense bodies similar to the Z-band material of skeletal muscle, condensation plaques on the cytoplasmic side of the plasma membrane, and pinocytotic vesicles.[40,46] These elements are diagnostic when demonstrated in neoplastic lesions (Fig. 10-4), and their development is related to the degree of differentiation of the tumor.

Bundles of microtubules associated with neurosecretory granules in a tumor of small round cells joined by occasional desmosomes are characteristic of neuroblastomas. By contrast, the discovery of longitudinally arranged microtubules and elongated cytoplasmic processes in a spindle cell sarcoma establishes the neurogenic nature of the tumor (Fig. 10-5).

Intracytoplasmic fat is almost always present in relatively large amounts in liposarcomas and fibrous histiocytomas, adding to the difficulties in the differential diagnosis of these two lesions, which may mimic each other at the light microscopic (LM) level. By electron microscopy it is possible to show that neoplastic lipoblasts have ul-

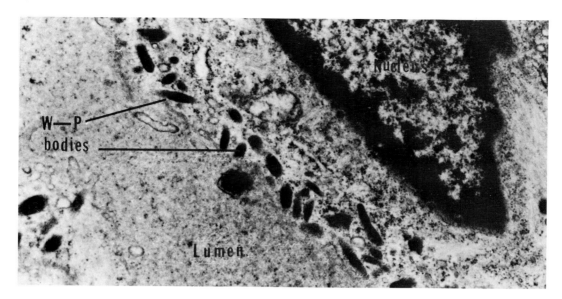

Fig. 10-3. Normal endothelial cells and capillary lumen. Distinct elongated electron-dense formations, the Weibel-Palade bodies, are specifically found in vascular endothelial cells.

trastructural appearances that replicate the embryonic stages of development of adipose tissue[47–49] and that the intracytoplasmic fat globules are associated with the cellular organelles responsible for the elaboration of fat (Fig. 10-6). These organelles are not developed to the same extent in fibrous histiocytomas, where fat often accumulates in cells having abundant rough endoplasmic reticulum (fibroblast-like) (Fig. 10-7). In addition, these tumors often show abundant intracytoplasmic filaments, lysosomes, and filopodial processes of the cellular membrane. A frequent problem in surgical pathology is the differential diagnosis of undifferentiated small round cell tumors, as epithelial, mesenchymal, and lymphoreticular neoplasms may adopt that morphology. The patient's age as well as the location of the tumor, its size, distribution of metastases, and other clinical information may help

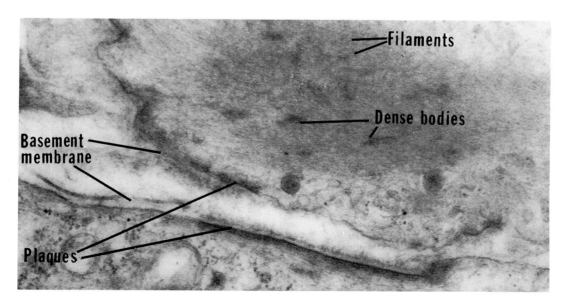

Fig. 10-4. Leiomyosarcoma. Ultrastructural characterization of this type of neoplasm is based on the findings of orderly arranged filaments with interspersed dense bodies and condensation plaques in the cytoplasmic portion of the plasma membrane, as exemplified by these two malignant cells.

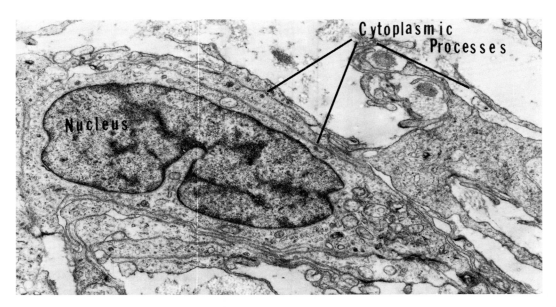

Fig. 10-5. Malignant peripheral nerve sheath tumor. Numerous elongated cytoplasmic processes are the main ultrastructural feature of this type of tumor.

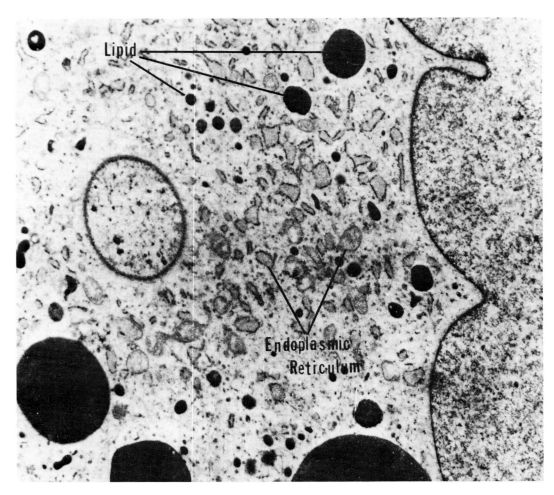

Fig. 10-6. Liposarcoma. Numerous variable-sized lipid droplets in close association with endoplasmic reticulum are indicative of the lipogenic nature of this neoplastic cell.

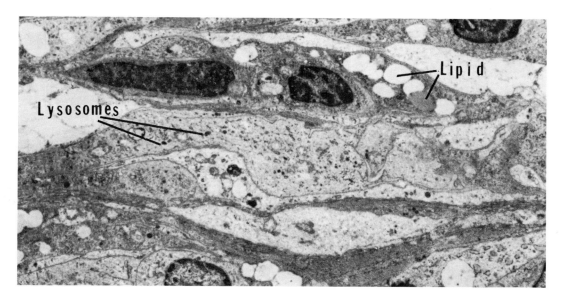

Fig. 10-7. Malignant fibrous histiocytoma. In contrast to lipoblasts, these lipid-containing cells lack those organelles known to participate in the elaboration of adipose tissue. Lysosomes are present in a number of cells.

establish the diagnosis, but on occasion it may depend entirely on pathologic studies. This is one situation in which electron microscopy has proved useful in establishing the diagnosis by demonstrating cellular junctions in carcinomas, with keratofilaments in those derived from squamous epithelium; cellular junctions, primitive neurofibrils, and neurosecretory granules in neuroblastomas; melanosomes in melanomas; actin and myosin filaments and Z-band material in rhabdomyosarcomas; and absence of junctional attachments, pseudopodial projections of the cytoplasm, and abundant RNA in malignant lymphomas.

Electron microscopic examination of soft tissue tumors presents many disadvantages,[50] including the requirement for proper fixation, availability of instrumentation, and technical and professional expertise, in addition to the attendant expense. Immunologic techniques, and particularly the immunoperoxidase procedures, are very helpful in the study of soft tissue tumors, sometimes obviating the need for ultrastructural studies because they demonstrate specific cell and tissue antigens.

Immunocytochemical markers for tumors of muscle, endothelial, Schwann, and histiocytic cells are now used widely as diagnostic tools in surgical pathology,[51-61] although the specificity and sensitivity of these markers vary considerably (Figs. 10-8 to 10-10). Antigens associated with melanocytes, lymphoid cells, and epithelial cells can also be demonstrated by immunohistochemistry and, in selected cases, help distinguish melanomas, lymphomas, and carcinomas from different types of sarcomas.

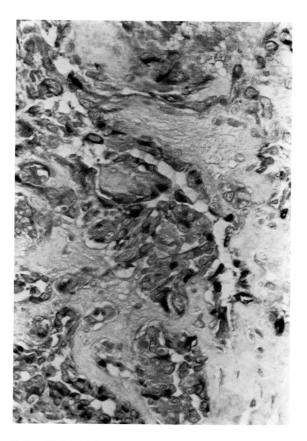

Fig. 10-8. Epithelioid angiosarcoma showing factor-VIII-positive cells.

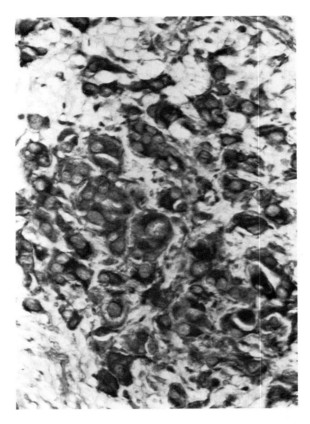

Fig. 10-9. Epithelioid sarcoma. Tumor cells are keratin-positive.

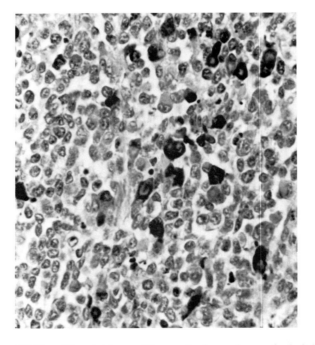

Fig. 10-10. Myoglobin-positive cells in embryonal rhabdomyosarcoma.

STAGING, CLASSIFICATION, GRADING, AND MORPHOLOGIC AND BIOLOGIC CHARACTERISTICS OF SOFT TISSUE TUMORS

Several staging systems for soft tissue sarcomas were designed in the recent past, but their prognostic power was considered insufficient when tested in a series of soft tissue sarcomas excised with wide surgical margins.[62] A new model with four risk factors has been developed and found useful for prognostic purposes. According to this system, the key risk factors for death due to tumor are male sex, grade III to IV malignancy, tumor necrosis, and tumor size over 10 cm.[63]

The diverse morphologic and overlapping histologic patterns of soft tissue tumors have led to multiple, often empirical, classifications. Grouping these tumors into spindle cell, round cell, and pleomorphic sarcomas, as was done in the past, is meaningless. Any type of sarcoma can present with areas of various histologic patterns; therefore, a classification based purely on descriptive morphology has virtually no value in predicting biologic behavior and in deciding what constitutes appropriate therapy. As our diagnostic tools continue to proliferate, become more sophisticated, and are more readily available, it has become possible to phenotype soft tissue tumors in most cases. This permits classification of these lesions into homogeneous groups, although morphologic dissimilarities are often apparent within any given group of tumors. Accordingly, as recommended by the World Health Organization (WHO),[1] we currently group these neoplasms on the basis of their cellular line of differentiation (fibrous tissue, adipose tissue, muscle tissue, blood vessels, lymph vessels, and synovial tissue) and, as a separate group, soft tissue tumors with distinct clinicopathologic manifestations but uncertain phenotype. Likewise, we describe fibrous histiocytic tumors as a single group because of their frequency, clinicopathologic relevance, and disputed histogenesis. Other histogenetically different tumors that can be included in this discussion, particularly tumors of peripheral nerves and also mesotheliomas, are described in Chapters 49, 25, and 26, respectively.

The basis for histopathologic diagnosis of sarcomas resides in the discovery of a gradation in maturation from primitive mesenchymal cells to those cellular elements mimicking mature mesenchymal tissue. This general principle is based on the belief that sarcomas originate not from dedifferentiation of mature cells but from primitive mesenchymal tissue, which, in its neoplastic growth and differentiation, replicates embryologic stages of development of the various normal mesenchymal tissues, as has been shown in rhabdomyosarcomas, leiomyosarcomas, and liposarcomas. This common ancestry (primitive mesenchymal cell) may explain the histologic similarities among these different types of tumors. In addition, the histologic type, patient age, grade, stage, and anatomic location of the tumor are also important parameters in determining prognosis of, and therapy for, soft tissue sarcomas. According to the degree of cellularity, cellular pleomorphism, mitotic activity, and necrosis, sarcomas can be divided into three histologic grades that correlate well with prognosis.[63-65] While this grading system can be applied to most sarcomas (fibrosarcoma, leiomyosarcoma, extraskeletal chondrosarcoma), it is apparent that some histologic types are almost always high grade (grade III). Such is the case with alveolar rhabdomyosarcoma, Ewing's sarcoma, and most angiosarcomas.

TUMORS AND DISORDERS OF FIBROUS TISSUE

Fibroma

Fibromas—benign neoplasms consisting of untransformed fibroblasts—are, like the unicorn, described frequently in the literature but not found in real life. It is true that many soft tissue tumor masses do contain fibroblasts and their secretory products (collagen, reticulin, elastin, and ground substances), but many of these lesions may be the result of exuberant reparative or inflammatory reactions rather than neoplasia. In some cases, etiologic factors such as trauma, infection, antigen-antibody immune complex formation, drugs, and local hemorrhage have been implicated in the pathogenesis of fibrous tumor masses.

Hypertrophic Scars and Keloids

Wound healing with controlled proliferation of fibroblasts and blood vessels and the production of a fibrous scar can apparently go awry in some people, with the formation of hypertrophic scars and keloids.[66] Keloid formation is found predominantly, but not exclusively, in blacks. Deep wounds, incisions, and burns that damage the lowermost layers of the dermis are thought to contribute to keloid formation. The precise pathogenetic mechanism, however, is unknown; an autoimmune response to trapped sebum produced by sebaceous cells pushed deep into the dermis has been postulated by Osman et al.,[67] who claimed that their hypothesis was substantiated by the anatomic distribution of these lesions around the head, neck, and upper trunk and in the inguinal and pubic areas. In fact, keloids can be found anywhere in the skin

except on the vermilion of the lips and the palms and soles—areas that contain no sebaceous glands. Autoimmune responses have been suggested as pathogenetic factors in the formation of nonkeloid hypertrophic scars.

Elastofibroma

The rare elastofibroma is usually found in the infrascapular region. It has also been described adjacent to the greater trochanter and the ischial tuberosity. Although these lesions have been thought to be reactive and the result of mechanical stress, their precise pathogenesis has not been determined.[68-69]

Cicatricial Fibrosis

Cicatricial fibrosis secondary to irradiation can appear as invasive or compressive tumor masses, sometimes leading to severe functional and/or cosmetic impairment.[70] Microscopically, it may be highly cellular, resulting in its confusion with fibrosarcoma.

Retroperitoneal and Mediastinal Fibrosis, Mesenteric Panniculitis

Retroperitoneal and mediastinal fibrosis and mesenteric panniculitis are related entities capable of producing large fibrous masses. Careful evaluation of the clinical and epidemiologic histories of patients with these diseases has demonstrated a myriad of possible etiologic factors.[71-75] Intra-abdominal and visceral infections and inflammations, surgical and blunt trauma, hemorrhage, and aortic aneurysm have been associated with retroperitoneal and mediastinal fibrosis. Serotonin, produced by carcinoid tumors, and the ergot derivative, methysergide, have been associated with retroperitoneal fibrosis. Withdrawal of these substances may be followed by regression of the fibrosis.[76] An autoimmune pathogenetic mechanism has been suggested for those cases of retroperitoneal fibrosis apparently not associated with obvious causes. Some investigators have proposed that the prominent vasculitis and perivasculitis present in the lesions may be related to antigen-antibody complex-induced vascular damage. Methysergide and the few other drugs associated with this disease are thought to act as haptens or initiate the immune response. Idiopathic retroperitoneal fibrosis has been reported in fetuses, infants, and children.[77] Probably the closest relationship these lesions have with neoplasia is their similarity to certain retroperitoneal, mesenteric, and mediastinal cancers that can elicit an abundant desmoplastic reaction in the host. The correct diagnosis of cancer may elude the surgeon and pathologist, unless many deep biopsy specimens of the fibrous tumor mass are obtained.[73]

Penile, Palmar, and Plantar Fibromatosis

Penile fibromatosis (Peyronie's disease),[78–81] palmar fibromatosis (Dupuytren's contracture),[82,83] and plantar fibromatosis (Ledderhose's disease)[84,85] form cellular tumor nodules and plaques and areas of relatively less cellular fibrosis that infiltrate tissue surrounding the aponeurotic (palmar and plantar) and fascial (penile) structures from which they arise. Severe contractures of the fibrous masses can lead to distressing dysfunction best treated surgically by partial or complete excision of the tumors and release of the engulfed tendons and fascia. Palmar fibromatosis may occur in patients who have Peyronie's disease,[78] and both palmar and plantar fibromatoses have been found to occur in the same person. While trauma has often been associated with these conditions, it has not been proved an etiologic factor.[78,79] By contrast, genitourinary tract infections and administration of the use of β-adrenergic blocking agents[86] have been cited as etiologic factors in the development of Peyronie's disease.

Juvenile Nasopharyngeal Angiofibroma

Juvenile nasopharyngeal angiofibroma is a highly vascular fibrous tumor that occurs almost exclusively in adolescent boys. It arises in the posterior superior nasal cavity and usually involves the nasal septum, the nasopharynx, and the pterygoid region by the time it produces symptoms of unilateral nasal obstruction and hemorrhage.[87–89] The tumor is locally expansive, growing into the soft tissues of the retropharyngeal area through the openings between the bones of the posterior face and the base of the skull and eroding the bone to break into the regional sinuses, the orbit and, in some advanced cases, the base of the cranium. This pattern of growth produces characteristic radiographic changes.[90] Histologically, it is composed of a fibrous stroma with varying amounts of collagenous fibrous tissue arranged in irregular interwoven or myxomatous patterns. Stellate and elongate fibrocytes and myofibroblasts are the predominant stomal cells. The tumor is richly endowed with small and large endothelium-lined vascular channels whose walls contain no elastic fibers and few irregularly arranged smooth muscle cells. The relative rigidity of the fibrous stroma and the lack of vascular mural contractile elements are thought to be important factors in the pathogenesis of the sometimes massive, uncontrollable hemorrhages.

Trauma to these lesions, including that of biopsies, has been associated with life-threatening hemorrhages; therefore, if necessary, biopsies of suspicious posterior polypoid nasal masses in young men are best done in the operating room with blood available for transfusion.

Recurrences after surgery are frequent because of the insinuative growth of the tumor into inaccessible places in the head. Surgery is the most successful treatment; irradiation is reserved for residual and recurrent tumor beyond the reach of the surgeon's knife. Because these lesions tend to occur predominantly in the hormonally turbulent environment of the adolescent boy, attempts have been made to relate either their pathogenesis or treatment, or both, to sex hormones.[91] Treatment with estrogens has succeeded in reducing tumor size in some, but not all, patients. Significant numbers of testosterone receptors, but not estradiol or progesterone receptors, have been demonstrated in juvenile nasopharyngeal angiofibromas. Abnormal sexual maturity and serum hormone levels have not been found in the few isolated cases studied specifically. The tumor regresses as the patient gets older, but treatment is necessary for the adolescent boy for whom one cannot risk the morbidity of invasive growth or the possibility of massive hemorrhage from the tumor.

Aggressive Fibromatosis (Desmoid)

Aggressive fibromatosis of the abdominal wall (desmoid)[92,93] and other sites[94–97] is a relentless, locally infiltrative tumor akin to sarcomas in its growth but lacking the capability to metastasize (Fig. 10-11). Arising from musculoaponeurotic structures, they can be differentiated from fibrosarcomas despite having a common cellu-

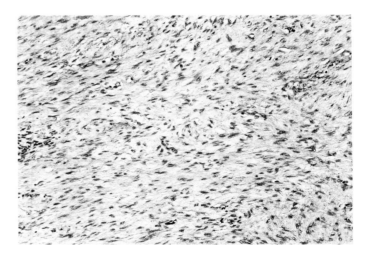

Fig. 10-11. Aggressive fibromatosis. Bundles of fibroblasts with collagen fibers between them.

lar denominator, the fibroblast, which forms bundles of cells laying down variable amounts of collagen and collagen precursors. Both desmoids and fibrosarcomas may form bulky masses that irregularly infiltrate adjacent tissues, and in both, local recurrence is usually the rule, particularly following a too conservative surgical excision. Fibrosarcomas are more cellular and exhibit a more advanced degree of cellular anaplasia. Moreover, mitotic figures are more frequent and collagen bundles less abundant in fibrosarcomas, which also present a herringbone pattern.[98] There is a definite prevalence of abdominal desmoids in young women, sometimes following pregnancies, whereas extraabdominal desmoids have no sex predilection. As is the case with most soft tissue tumors, their etiology is unknown, although trauma, scar, and other factors have been implicated in their development. The presence of desmoid in the abdominal wall, mesentery, or retroperitoneum in association with intestinal adenomas constitutes part of *Gardner's syndrome,* which is inherited as a dominant trait.[99–101] Mesenteric and retroperitoneal fibromatosis may grow rapidly and form large masses that compress and sometimes infiltrate the intestinal wall leading to obstruction. Pelvic fibromatosis, on the other hand, may be confused with an ovarian tumor or infiltrate the urinary bladder, vagina or rectum. Desmoid tumors of children are histologically similar to those of adults, although they are more common in boys than in girls and are usually located in the extremities or head and neck.[102,103]

Juvenile Hyaline Fibromatosis

Juvenile hyaline fibromatosis is an exceedingly rare hereditary disorder characterized by fibroblastic proliferation and the production of hyalinized collagen.[103–106] The basic abnormality appears to be a metabolic disturbance in the formation of collagen, probably caused by incomplete alignment of precollagen or protocollagen. These patients are usually children under 5 years of age with multiple cutaneous painless nodules about the head and neck and in the extremities. Some of these patients have bone involvement.

Congenital Fibromatoses

Congenital fibromatoses are rare, multiple fibrous tumors affecting the soft tissues, bones, and viscera of newborns.[107–109] The condition is almost always fatal in infants who have visceral involvement, especially when the lungs are affected. Infants with congenital fibromatosis without visceral involvement have a good prognosis, for their tumors will regress spontaneously over a few

months.[110] The viscera involved in congenital generalized fibromatosis include the gastrointestinal (GI) tract, lungs, heart, kidneys, and many other organs. The central nervous system (CNS) is affected only by invasion from osseous or dural lesions.

Congenital fibromatosis can also be distinguished from the even more rare case of *congenital fibrosarcoma.* The latter is usually a single large mass with the gross and histologic features of an aggressive, locally invasive neoplasm and, in some instances, cytologic atypicality.[111–113]

Congenital fibromatoses and fibrosarcomas have not been associated with familial syndromes, except in one family in which four siblings had congenital generalized fibromatosis.

Fibromatosis Colli

Fibromatosis colli is a tumorous, sometimes locally infiltrative, fibromatosis of the sternocleidomastoid muscle of infants that disappears within 3 to 4 months, either producing little or no deformity of the muscle or forming fibrous scar tissue, which can eventuate in torticollis (wry neck) by contracture.[108] The lesion rarely appears before 2 weeks of age, and it is in the early tumor stage that the infiltrative fibroblastic growth characteristic of fibromatosis is seen. Intrauterine factors, including trauma, have been suggested as causes of fibromatosis colli. Birth trauma such as breech delivery, previously thought to be a primary cause, may be actually secondary to intrauterine development of the lesion that subsequently interferes with the proper movement and placement of the head before delivery.

Idiopathic Gingival Fibromatosis

Idiopathic gingival fibromatosis, a benign fibrous tumor of the gingiva that appears first in childhood, is an autosomal-dominant heritable tumor with no other associated lesion.[114] Cure is accomplished easily by surgical removal of this slowly growing tumor, which is confined to the gingiva of the alveolar ridges of the maxilla and mandible. If not removed, the tumor may enlarge to fill the oral cavity and oropharynx, resulting in death by starvation.

Fibrous Hamartoma of Infancy

Enzinger designated as fibrous hamartoma of infancy[115,116] a lesion occurring during the first 2 years of life, affecting the deep dermis and subcutaneous tissue, usually of the axilla, shoulder, or upper arm. Despite its benign nature, it may be confused with sarcomas or aggressive fibromatosis or with other benign lesions such as

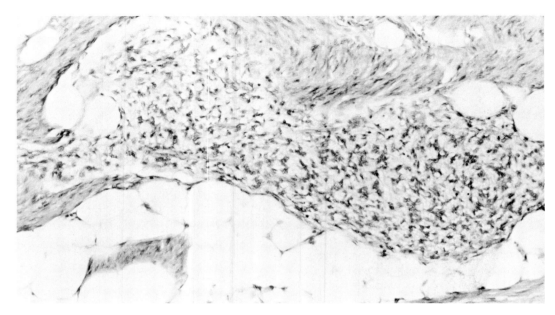

Fig. 10-12. Fibrous hamartoma of infancy. Characteristic histologic pattern showing primitive mesenchyme, fibrous connective tissue, and mature adipose tissue.

aponeurotic fibroma, dermatofibroma, or nodular fasciitis. Fibrous hamartoma of infancy can be distinguished, however, by its distinctive histology, consisting of an admixture of mature adipose tissue, interlacing bundles of fibrous connective tissue, and islands of primitive mesenchyme composed of loosely arranged spindle or stellate cells (Fig. 10-12). This organoid configuration is interrupted in areas of some lesions by dense, wavy bands of collagen with interspersed fibrocytes.

Juvenile Aponeurotic Fibroma

Juvenile aponeurotic fibroma (calcifying fibroma) is a rare infiltrating fibroblastic proliferation that affects the hands and feet of children and often recurs following local excision. The tumor is densely cellular, and consists of plump fibroblasts and dense collagen fibers (Fig. 10-13). The presence of islands of chondroid tissue with foci of calcification is a characteristic feature that distinguishes this lesion from palmar and plantar fibromatosis. Mature bone trabeculae are seen in a few cases. Aponeurotic fibromas have also been reported in adults, in sites other than the palms and soles.[117–119]

Infantile Digital Fibromatosis

Infantile digital fibromatosis (recurrent digital fibroma of childhood) is an infiltrative cellular fibrous tumor that almost always involves the toes and fingers of infants and

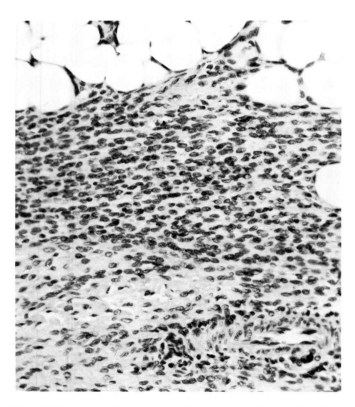

Fig. 10-13. Juvenile aponeurotic fibroma. Plump fibroblasts infiltrating adipose tissue.

rarely young children.[120–123] These red or tan subcutaneous tumors usually arise on the dorsa of the tips of the digits and can infiltrate deeply into the periosteum. Lesions outside the digits have also been reported.[124] They may be multiple and may recur frequently following incomplete excision. Curiously, they have not been reported in the great toes or thumbs. Histologically, these tumors are composed of myofibroblasts that contain diagnostic round eosinophilic cytoplasmic inclusions usually located at one pole of the elongate nucleus (Fig. 10-14). Ultrastructurally, these inclusions have been found to be composed of amorphous granular material and numerous filaments. The nature of the inclusions, however, is still a matter of controversy.[125]

Fibroma of Tendon Sheath

Fibromas of tendon sheaths are circumscribed lobulated tumors attached to tendon and tendon sheaths, which occur in the fingers, hands, and wrists of children and adults.[126,127] Microscopically, they are predominantly hypocellular dense hyalinized collagenous nodules containing numerous small vascular channels. More cellular areas, found in some tumors, contain spindled and stellate fibroblasts arranged in a vaguely storiform pattern; this cellular phase may represent an earlier stage of tumor development, which then progresses to the more common hyalinized fibrous form. Recurrences occur following incomplete excision.

Giant Cell Fibroblastoma

Giant cell fibroblastoma is a rare and distinctive fibrous tumor of childhood and adolescence that often recurs following local excision but does not metastasize.[128,129] Grossly, it is well circumscribed and involves the superficial soft tissues. Microscopically, there are varying proportions of cellular solid areas and cystic or angiectoid areas, both containing fibroblastic cells as well as multinucleated floret-like cells.

Intramuscular Myxoma

Intramuscular myxoma, an uncommon benign fibroblastic tumor, must be distinguished from other myxoid neoplasms, notably liposarcoma and aggressive angiomyxoma. Most myxomas arise in the large muscles of the thigh, pelvic girdle, and shoulder and on gross examination appear as well circumscribed gelatinous nodules; few are completely encapsulated.[130–132] Fewer than 10 percent of myxomas are multiple and associated with fibrous dysplasia of adjacent bones.[133] The tumor cells are spindle-shaped or stellate, having drawn-out cytoplasmic

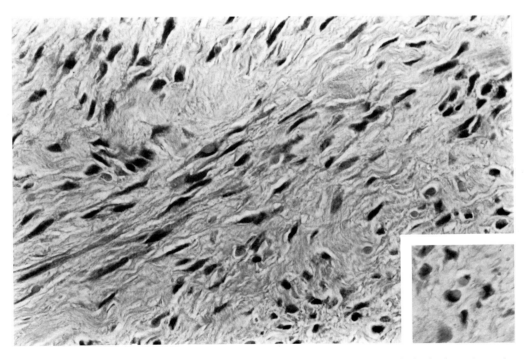

Fig. 10-14. Infantile digital fibroma. Some fibroblasts contain large eosinophilic inclusions (seen in cross-section in inset).

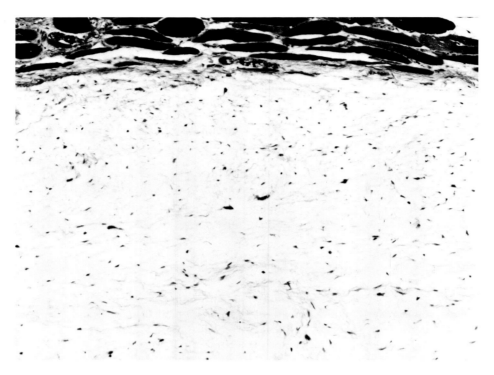

Fig. 10-15. Intramuscular myxoma. A well circumscribed intramuscular nodule composed of fibroblast-like cells lying in a myxoid stroma.

processes and lying in an abundant mucoid matrix (Fig. 10-15). The degree of cellularity and vascularization varies from tumor to tumor but most of them appear hypocellular and poorly vascularized. Electron microscopic studies have shown that the principal cell of intramuscular myxomas is similar to a fibroblast.[134]

Fibrosarcoma

Although once considered frequent neoplasms, increasing awareness of the existence of other fibrosarcomatoid neoplasms and pseudoneoplasms has made it apparent that fibrosarcomas are relatively uncommon. This

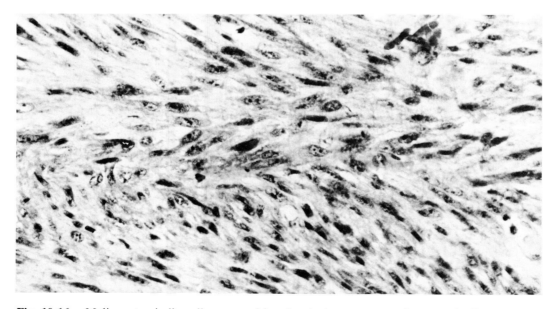

Fig. 10-16. Malignant spindle cells arranged in a herringbone pattern often seen in fibrosarcoma.

is particularly the case if the histologic diagnosis of this neoplasm is restricted to tumors composed of spindle cells exhibiting a herringbone pattern (Fig. 10-16). Using this criterion, it is possible to separate fibrosarcomas from fibromatosis, fibrous histiocytic tumors, nodular fasciitis, proliferative myositis, and the myriad other neoplastic and nonneoplastic cellular proliferations with similar histologic features. It is therefore likely that a number of reported cases of fibrosarcoma may have included other neoplasms and that a true assessment of its biologic behavior is possible only through review of the slides of those who have followed rigid histologic criteria. On this basis, the following statements can be made: (1) the largest number of fibrosarcomas appear in superficial soft tissues; (2) the tumor is less aggressive in children than in adults[112,113]; (3) its behavior is related to the degree of anaplasia; and (4) marked cellular pleomorphism is not a feature of fibrosarcoma. While lymph node metastases do occur, fibrosarcomas spread almost exclusively through vascular channels, and metastases appear most often in the lungs.

FIBROUS HISTIOCYTIC TUMORS

Practically unknown a few years ago, fibrous histiocytic tumors are now recognized as a heterogeneous group of neoplasms with well established clinicopathologic manifestations. Unquestionably, the broad spectrum of their histologic features has led to the inclusion of these tumors in other groups of look-alike but histogenetically different neoplasms, such as fibrosarcoma, rhabdomyosarcoma, and liposarcoma. They continue to be confused with these and other tumors. Moreover, whether some neoplasms, such as epithelioid sarcoma and dermatofibrosarcoma protuberans, are derived from histiocytes has not yet been determined.[135,136] In fact, the histogenesis of fibrous histiocytic tumors is still uncertain. The usual mixture of different cellular elements and growth patterns in these tumors raises the question of whether they all originate from one common ancestry, a primitive mesenchymal cell, that gives rise to fibroblastic and histiocytic elements,[137,138] or from a tissue histiocyte that acts as a facultative fibroblast.

Malignant Fibrous Histiocytoma

Malignant fibrous histiocytomas are primarily tumors of adults, having a peak incidence during the seventh decade of life.[138–145] They are most common in the extremities, trunk, and retroperitoneum and are rare in the head, neck, and viscera. Tumors of the extremities and trunk become apparent as painless masses, whereas the retroperitoneal tumors are often associated with fever, fatigue, loss of weight, and GI symptoms. Lymphoproliferative disorders, including leukemia, Hodgkin's disease, malignant lymphoma, multiple myeloma, and malignant histiocytosis, occur in association with malignant fibrous histiocytomas.[138] In common with other mesenchymal tumors, particularly hemangiopericytoma, episodic hypoglycemia may also appear in association with these lesions but is extremely rare.[138]

Malignant fibrous histiocytomas are perhaps the most common radiation-induced soft tissue sarcomas.[146,147] Likewise, these tumors may originate at sites of surgical scars.[148,149] Since the process of repair and scarring involves histiocytes, fibroblasts, and primitive mesenchymal cells, it has been postulated that on rare occasions such a process may predispose to malignant transformation.[149]

While grossly these neoplasms are usually well circumscribed, they present no evidence of encapsulation and may infiltrate between muscle fascicles or along fascial planes. The bulkiest masses may exhibit foci of hemorrhage and necrosis. Malignant fibrous histiocytomas typically present a wide spectrum of cellular constituents and pleomorphism, with an admixture of spindle-shaped fibroblastic cells focally arranged in cartwheel-like formations around slit-like vessels (storiform pattern), rounded histiocytoid cells, pleomorphic giant cells, foam cells, and inflammatory cells (mainly lymphocytes and plasma cells and sometimes numerous neutrophils) (Fig. 10-17). As in every other soft tissue tumor, myxoid areas are not uncommon. Based on the relative predominance of these various cellular forms and interstitial constituents, at least five subtypes can be recognized: storiform-pleomorphic, myxoid, giant cell, inflammatory, and angiomatoid. Tumors with overlapping histologic features are not uncommon, and conversion from one type to another has been well documented.[142]

The most significant prognostic parameter of malignant fibrous histiocytoma is not the histologic type but the depth of the tumor.[140,141] Retroperitoneal lesions are almost invariably fatal because they are rarely amenable to surgical excision; death occurs as the result of local invasion and less frequently, pulmonary metastasis. In more superficial locations, it has been found that the deeper the tumor, the greater the incidence of metastasis.[140] Thus, tumors located entirely within subcutaneous tissue (about one third of superficial fibrous histiocytomas) have the best prognosis. By contrast, superficial tumors have a high recurrence rate, which has been attributed to longer survival of the patients, more conservative treatment, and easier detection prior to death from metastasis.[140–142]

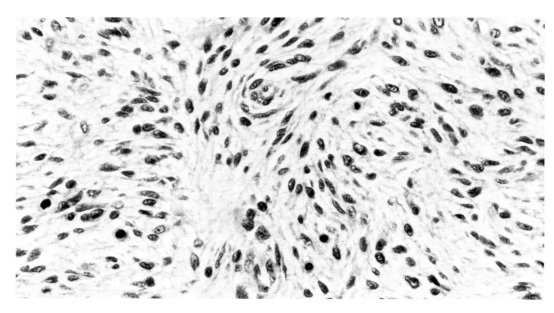

Fig. 10-17. Malignant fibrous histiocytoma. Spindle cells forming a storiform pattern characteristic of malignant fibrous histiocytoma.

Storiform-Pleomorphic Type

The storiform pleomorphic type contains, in addition to histiocytes and fibroblasts arranged in a storiform pattern, multinucleated giant cells and strap cells with abundant eosinophilic cytoplasm resembling rhabdomyoblasts.[139,140,144] These cells have large pleomorphic and hyperchromatic nuclei and may contain cytoplasmic lipid droplets. Mitotic figures are common. Inflammatory cells, mainly lymphocytes and plasma cells, are always present in this tumor. Occasionally, polymorphonuclear leukocytes, eosinophils and even lipid-laden histiocytes may also be present.

Myxoid Type

As its name implies, the myxoid type of malignant fibrous histiocytoma is characterized by extensive myxoid areas merging with cellular areas in which the storiform pattern is apparent.[149,150] The myxoid areas show prominent curvilinear blood vessels and cells with cytoplasmic vacuoles, features that may lead to confusion of this tumor with liposarcoma. However, the vacuoles contain acid mucopolysaccharides instead of fat, and the blood vessels do not form the delicate plexiform network seen in liposarcoma. Some myxoid malignant fibrous histiocytomas contain a moderate number of inflammatory cells. The cellular areas, on the other hand, may show nuclear polymorphism sometimes approaching that seen in the pleomorphic type of the tumor. However, the myxoid type should be separated from the pleomorphic malignant

fibrous histiocytoma because of the better prognosis of the former as compared to that of the latter.

Inflammatory Type

The inflammatory malignant fibrous histiocytoma, described originally in the retroperitoneum as xanthogranuloma, consists of a mixed population of inflammatory cells, chiefly xanthoma cells, polymorphonuclear leukocytes, lymphocytes, and plasma cells. For this reason, it may be confused with xanthogranulomatous inflammation.[145] However, the cytologic atypia present in some of the histiocytic cells permits separation. Multinucleated giant cells with inflammatory cells in their cytoplasm are usually present. Some of the histiocytic cells may have multilobed nuclei with prominent nucleoli, thus resembling Reed-Sternberg cells (Figs. 10-18 and 10-19). This tumor occurs most often in the retroperitoneum but may also be found in the extremities. Despite its deceptively benign microscopic appearance, local recurrence has been reported in about one half the patients and distant metastasis in one third.

Giant Cell Type

The giant cell type, with a histologic appearance resembling that of a giant cell tumor of bone, has been described in the superficial and deep soft tissues of the extremities, head, and neck.[151–154] The neoplastic giant and mononuclear cells are arranged in different sized

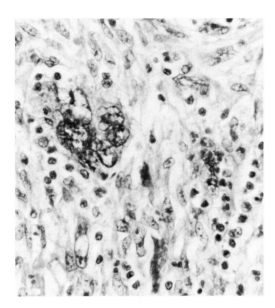

Fig. 10-18. Malignant fibrous histiocytoma. Multinucleated giant cell in malignant fibrous histiocytoma.

nodules, which on occasion contain osteoid and mature bone trabeculae (Fig. 10-20). The superficial neoplasms arise in the subcutaneous tissue, fascia, or dermis and may appear as skin tumors,[155] while the deep-seated tumors involve skeletal muscle, fascia, and tendons. Their size and anatomic location correlate well with prognosis. Superficial giant cell tumors are smaller than the deep ones and may recur after limited local excision, but in

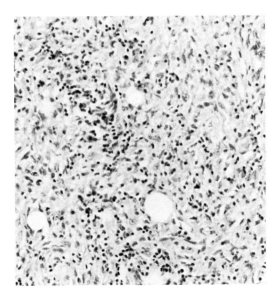

Fig. 10-19. Malignant fibrous histiocytoma, inflammatory variant. Numerous inflammatory cells are found in this tumor composed of fibroblast-like spindle cells.

general they are less aggressive than the larger, deep-seated ones, which often metastasize and may lead to the death of the patient.

Angiomatoid Type

The angiomatoid malignant fibrous histiocytoma is characterized by three different components: nodules and sheets of histiocytes, vascular-like spaces containing erythrocytes, and a prominent lymphoplasmacytic infiltrate (Fig. 10-21). The vascular-like spaces seem to be the result of hemorrhage and lack an endothelial lining.[156–158] Some of these blood-filled spaces have a thick and fibrotic wall. The neoplastic cells show little nuclear atypia; they are α_1-antichymotrypsin positive and factor VIII antigen negative. A cutaneous and a deep form of the tumor have been recognized. Clinically, the cutaneous tumors are often confused with hemangiomas, hematomas, or melanocytic lesions. Most of these patients are children, adolescents, or young adults who, in addition to the soft tissue tumor, may develop systemic symptoms such as fever, anemia, and weight loss. Local recurrence has been documented in about two thirds of patients and metastasis in about 20 percent.

Dermatofibrosarcoma Protuberans

No other tumor can better exhibit the formation of a storiform pattern than dermatofibrosarcoma protuberans.[136,159] While some include it in the group of histiocytic lesions, its biologic behavior is different from malignant fibrous histiocytoma. This slow-growing dermal and sometimes subcutaneous tumor has a tendency to recur following local excision. It is seen most often in the chest wall, extremities, and head and neck of young adults and adolescents, but it may occur at any age and in other anatomic sites. Metastases are exceptional. Microscopically, the diagnostic areas show plump fibroblasts arranged in a prominent storiform pattern. This tumor lacks the admixture of other cellular components present in malignant fibrous histiocytomas. Focal myxoid changes are sometimes seen, more often in local recurrences than in the primary tumors. Rarely these tumors contain melanin-bearing cells with dendritic processes; this is the so-called *Bednar tumor*[160] (Fig. 10-22).

Giant Cell Tumor of Tendon Sheath (Localized Nodular Tenosynovitis)

These are relatively small (2 to 3 cm) nodules most commonly seen in the hands of young adults, although they do occur in other anatomic sites.[161,162] These slow

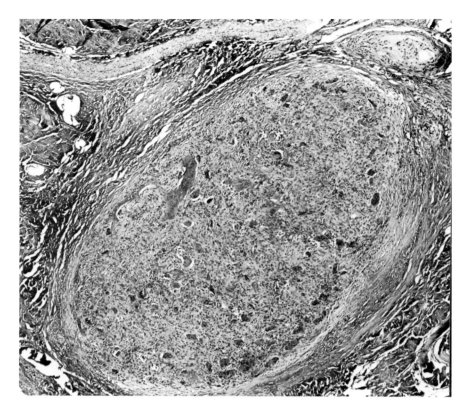

Fig. 10-20. Giant cell type of malignant fibrous histiocytoma, or malignant giant cell tumor of soft tissues. Well defined nodule composed of mononuclear cells and multinucleated giant cells. A bone trabecula is present at the periphery of the nodule.

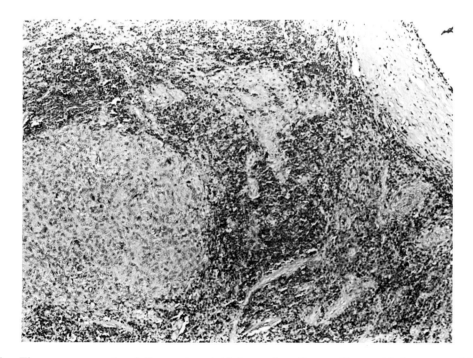

Fig. 10-21. Three components of the angiomatoid type of malignant fibrous histiocytoma. Nodules of histiocytes, a lymphoplasmacytic infiltrate, and vascular-like spaces.

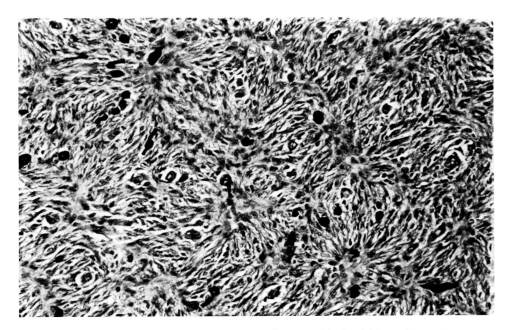

Fig. 10-22. Dermatofibrosarcoma protuberans with dendritic melanocytes.

growing, well circumscribed, lobulated, yellow nodules are associated with tendons and are not attached to the skin. A rare diffuse infiltrating variant has also been described. About 10 percent of them produce cortical erosion of the underlying bone.[163] Microscopically, they contain variable numbers of histiocyte-like mononuclear cells, multinucleated giant cells and lipid-laden histiocytes (Fig. 10-23). Recent immunohistochemical observations indicate that both the mononuclear cells and the multinucleated giant cells are of histiocytic derivation.[164] Some of these tumors are densely cellular, while others are predominantly fibrotic and hyalinized. Mitotic figures and blood vessel invasion are rare and do not correlate with malignant clinical behavior. Local recurrence is seen in about 15 percent of cases. We are unable to separate the malignant giant cell tumor of tendon sheath from the malignant fibrous histiocytoma, giant cell type.[165,166]

Others

It is now recognized that a number of benign neoplasms and tumor-like lesions are probably of histiocytic origin. These include fibrous xanthoma, atypical fibrous xanthoma, dermatofibroma, and juvenile xanthogranuloma.[119] These lesions are discussed in more detail in Chapter 9.

TUMORS OF ADIPOSE TISSUE

Lipoma

Benign tumors composed entirely of adult adipose tissue occur at all ages and are the most common soft tissue tumors in man. They are slow growing, relatively small,

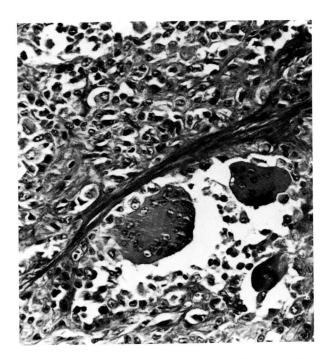

Fig. 10-23. Mononuclear and multinucleated giant cells in a giant cell tumor of tendon sheath.

and often located in the subcutaneous tissue. By contrast, intramuscular, mesenteric, mediastinal, and retroperitoneal lipomas are less common and are larger than those located in the subcutis. Moreover, these deep-seated tumors often extend to adjacent tissues and may recur following local excision.[167–171] Although most lipomas are separated from surrounding tissues by thin fibrous capsules, some have an infiltrative growth pattern, for example, in intramuscular lipomas, in which skeletal muscle fibers are separated and flattened by the tumor.[172–175] The presence of a tumor mass and absence of a clinical history of muscle disease helps distinguish intramuscular lipoma from muscle replacement by fat in severe muscle atrophy. Focal myxoid changes in lipomas may lead to confusion of this tumor with liposarcoma.

Familial lipomas are multiple, sometimes symmetric, and not infrequently associated with metabolic disorders, especially hypercholesterolemia.[5,6,172] Regional lipomatosis of the extremities has been associated with gigantism.[173]

Excessive growth of mature adipose tissue having infiltrative properties and involving extensive portions of the trunk or extremities is known as *diffuse lipomatosis*. Although clinically this condition may simulate liposarcoma, microscopically it resembles an ordinary lipoma.

Lipoma Arborescens

Adipose tissue tumors of the joints associated with synovia (lipoma arborescens) and tendon sheaths are thought to represent reactive inflammatory lesions because of their relatively frequent association with trauma, chronic tenosynovitis or arthritis.

Angiolipoma

Angiolipomas are solitary or multiple asymptomatic or painful subcutaneous nodules.[174] Some, especially the multiple ones, are genetically determined and inherited as an autosomal dominant trait.[175] Microscopically, the focal angiomatous component consists of small vessels lined by prominent endothelial cells and often containing erythrocytes and fibrin thrombi. Infiltrating angiolipomas are found in skeletal muscle and may form large masses in the extremities or paravertebral region.[176]

Angiomyolipoma

Angiomyolipomas are composed of mature fat, blood vessels, and smooth muscle. Thought to be hamartomas, they are found most frequently in the kidney and have been described in association with tuberous sclerosis and pulmonary lymphangiomyomatosis.[177,178] Angiomyolipomas are usually single except in patients with tuberous sclerosis, in which these renal tumors may be multiple and bilateral. Histologically, angiomyolipomas may be quite cellular and show marked cytologic atypia, but these features do not indicate aggressive clinical behavior. Eight well documented examples of renal angiomyolipomas with lymph node involvement interpreted as multicentric foci rather than metastases have been reported.[179–181] One case with distant metastases and another with renal vein invasion have also been observed.[182,183]

Myelolipoma

Myelolipoma, a tumor-like lesion composed of a mixture of mature fat and bone marrow, is most often seen in the adrenal glands, although it has been reported rarely in the soft tissues.[184–185] Most patients with myelolipomas are asymptomatic. The tumors vary in size from microscopic foci to large masses.[187] A few myelolipomas have been reported in association with endocrine abnormalities such as Cushing's syndrome or Addison's disease.[188] Few of these tumors have had features of both myelolipoma and adrenocortical adenoma.[189]

Spindle Cell Lipoma

Subcutaneous lipomas that contain a variable proportion of atypical cells and simulate liposarcoma include spindle cell lipomas, pleomorphic lipomas, and atypical lipomas. Spindle cell lipomas occur predominantly in the posterior aspect of the neck and shoulders of adult male patients. Grossly, they are encapsulated and indistinguishable from an ordinary lipoma. Microscopically, in addition to mature adipose tissue, they contain bundles of spindle cells and collagen fibers.[190–193] In most cases, mature adipose tissue predominates and the spindle cells, which are indistinguishable from fibroblasts and which show little nuclear atypia, represent a minor component of the tumor. Myxoid changes and prominent vascular proliferation are noted in some spindle cell lipomas.[194]

Pleomorphic Lipoma

Pleomorphic lipomas are also well circumscribed subcutaneous lipomatous tumors that histologically display a number of atypical spindle-shaped cells as well as bizarre pleomorphic giant cells with multiple nuclei arranged in a floret-like pattern (Fig. 10-24). In spite of their disturbing

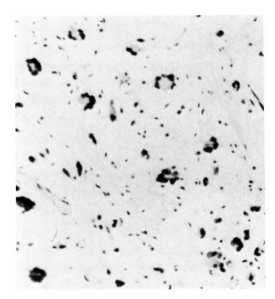

Fig. 10-24. Pleomorphic lipoma. Numerous floret-like cells are characteristic of this histologic variant of lipoma.

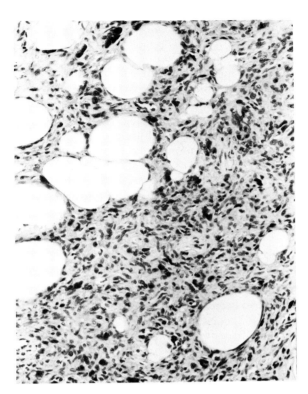

Fig. 10-25. Atypical lipoma with features of both spindle cell lipoma and pleomorphic lipoma.

histologic features, these tumors follow a benign clinical course.[195,196] Although they may recur following incomplete removal, no distant metastases have been reported. Because of the overlapping features of spindle cell lipomas and pleomorphic lipomas, the term *atypical lipomas* has been suggested for these two tumors[197-199] (Fig. 10-25). It is important to recognize that retroperitoneal tumors similar to atypical lipomas behave as locally aggressive neoplasms that may extend into neighboring organs and cause death. Therefore, they should be considered to be well differentiated liposarcomas.

Lipoblastomatosis

Lipoblastomatosis, a benign adipose tissue tumor of children, is characterized by lobules containing a variable proportion of mature fat cells and lipoblasts in different stages of development (Fig. 10-26). Myxoid changes and a prominent capillary network are commonly included.[200-205] A circumscribed form (benign lipoblastoma) is confined to the subcutaneous tissue, while the diffuse form (diffuse lipoblastomatosis) tends to infiltrate muscle and may recur following local excision.

Hibernoma

Hibernomas are uncommon benign adipose tissue tumors composed of cells that biochemically and histologically resemble brown fat.[206-208] A few examples of the malignant counterpart of hibernoma have been re-

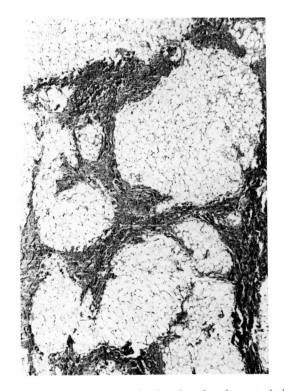

Fig. 10-26. Lipoblastomatosis showing the characteristic lobulation of the fetal type of adipose tissue.

corded.[209,210] Brown adipose tissue is present in relatively large amounts in certain animals that hibernate, is metabolically quite different from white adipose tissue, and is thought to be an important tissue in the production of nonshivering thermogenesis in some animals.[206] It is found in various locations in the adult human but is more abundant in fetuses and infants. Hibernomas have a unique, easily identifiable light microscopic appearance; they consist of round to polygonal, multivacuolated cells with centrally located nuclei (Fig. 10-27). These cells are clustered in a lobular pattern around the numerous blood vessels of the tumor. Ultrastructurally, numerous mitochondria are present in the cytoplasm of brown fat and hibernoma cells, even those cells with large unilocular fat vacuoles, which at the LM level resemble the lipocytes of white adipose tissue. Scanty endoplasmic reticulum and small Golgi apparatus further distinguish the cells of the hibernoma and brown fat from those of fetal or adult white adipose tissue.[207] Biochemically, the same types of lipids are found in hibernomas and lipomas but are present in different proportions. This is interpreted to reflect the relatively large number of mitochondria in the hibernoma cell as compared with those of the white adipose cells constituting the lipoma.[211,212]

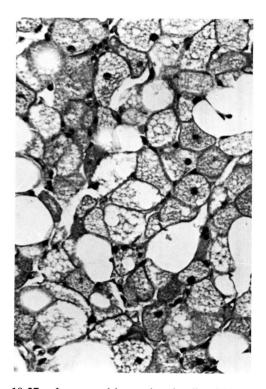

Fig. 10-27. Large multivacuolated cells of hibernoma.

Liposarcoma

Liposarcomas are the second most common soft tissue sarcomas, surpassed in frequency only by malignant fibrous histiocytomas. They affect adults almost exclusively and are practically nonexistent in the first decade of life.[213] These tumors usually originate in deep tissues, frequently of the extremities, particularly the thigh and retroperitoneum.[199,214–217]

Because of the variety of histologic patterns and biologic behavior, it is possible to distinguish four different subtypes of liposarcoma: the *myxoid, well differentiated, round cell,* and *pleomorphic.*[214] In some liposarcomas, these various histologic types appear together. The existence of the round cell liposarcoma as an independent subtype has been questioned recently.[199,215] In fact, it has been shown that round cell liposarcoma does not occur in a pure form but usually appears as a component of myxoid liposarcomas. However, the presence of round cells connotes a more aggressive biologic behavior. The well differentiated and myxoid liposarcomas sometimes attain enormous size but seldom metastasize. Therefore, they are usually associated with a good prognosis. By contrast, more than 50 percent of tumors that have a predominant round cell component and of the pleomorphic type develop metastases within 5 years.[218] Recurrence is frequent in any histologic type. Metastases are almost always hematogenous and appear primarily in the lung. Some consider the occurrence of multiple liposarcomas of the myxoid variety within different soft tissue sites as multicentric tumors, while others interpret these as being metastatic.[215]

Liposarcomas are usually lobulated and pseudoencapsulated. The well differentiated and myxoid varieties are usually yellow, while the pleomorphic and those with a predominant round cell component are gray due to the scant amount of fat. Necrosis, hemorrhage, and cystic degeneration are not uncommon.

Microscopically, the myxoid type contains a number of lipoblasts in a stroma with abundant acid mucopolysaccharides and a prominent capillary vascular network (Fig. 10-28). A round cell component of variable extent is present in some of the tumors (Fig. 10-29). The well differentiated liposarcomas are composed predominantly of mature adipose tissue traversed by broad fibrous bands containing atypical lipoblasts and pleomorphic cells. Some well differentiated liposarcomas show little or no sclerosis, but the mature adipocytes exhibit hyperchromatic nuclei or the fatty tissue contains a variable number of atypical lipoblasts (Fig. 10-30). In the pleomorphic liposarcoma, plump spindle-shaped cells and multinucleated giant cells predominate. At least some of these cells have vacuolated cytoplasm. Mitotic

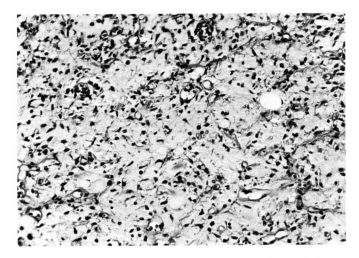

Fig. 10-28. Myxoid liposarcoma. Numerous stellate lipoblasts lying in a myxoid stroma rich in capillaries characterize this tumor.

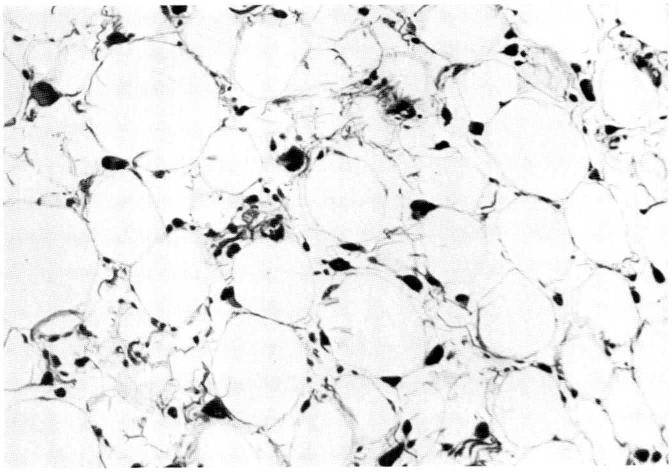

figures are common in this type of liposarcoma. This type can be recognized readily when it occurs in association with well differentiated or myxoid liposarcoma; however, it is almost impossible to distinguish it from malignant fibrous histiocytoma when these elements are not present. Fortunately, this distinction is not clinically significant, since both tumors are high-grade sarcomas, treated in the same fashion.

Ultrastructurally, the malignant lipoblasts replicate the various embryonic stages of development of white adipose tissue.[49,219] As the primitive (fibroblast-like) mesen-

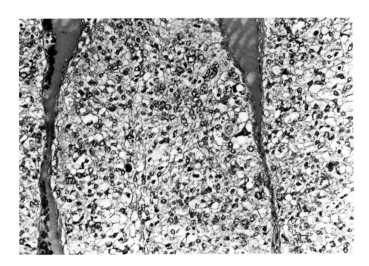

Fig. 10-29. Round cell component of a mixed type of liposarcoma is seen. The cells are cohesive and have a vacuolated cytoplasm.

Fig. 10-30. Well differentiated liposarcoma. Atypical lipoblasts are present among mature adipocytes.

chymal cell begins lipoblastic differentiation, the rough endoplasmic reticulum becomes less apparent and smooth endoplasmic reticulum more prominent. Lipid appears as fine droplets dispersed in the cytoplasm (see Fig. 10-6), later aggregating into large globules, which distort the nuclei, leading to scalloping of the nuclear outline in multivacuolated lipoblasts and eventually displacing the nucleus to the periphery of the cell in signet ring forms.

TUMORS OF SMOOTH MUSCLE

The most frequent sites of smooth muscle tumors are the uterus, the GI tract, and, to a lesser extent, the retroperitoneum, muscles of the skin and the walls of small and large blood vessels.

Leiomyoma

Cutaneous leiomyomas are small, often painful, dermal or subcutaneous nodules that usually measure less than 2 cm. They can be single or multiple.[220–223] They arise most frequently from the arrectores pilorum muscles of the extremities and have been reported to be familial. The patients are usually adolescent or young adults but affected children have also been reported.[224] Recurrence after excision may be due to incomplete removal of the lesion. Solitary lesions of the nipple, vulva, and scrotum arise from the smooth muscle around the areola and the dartos.[225] Other solitary leiomyomas originate from the smooth muscle of blood vessel walls. In the latter case, these lesions have a prominent vascular component and should be considered *angiomyomas* or *angioleiomyomas*.[226] They are more common in the extremities of adult females and have been divided into three histologic subtypes: capillary, cavernous, and venous type.

Leiomyomas are exceedingly rare in deep soft tissues.[227–229] These smooth muscle tumors are larger than the superficial ones; they may become calcified, and their sites of origin may be obscure. Cellularity, cytologic atypia, and mitotic activity are the best parameters to use in separating leiomyomas from leiomyosarcomas of soft tissues. In some cases, however, these features may not be as reliable as in other anatomic locations. Moreover, some of these leiomyomas may contain bizarre cells with large hyperchromatic nuclei and multinucleated giant cells; these features have been interpreted as being of degenerative nature. Most of the *leiomyoblastomas* or *epithelioid leiomyomas* occur in the GI tract and the uterus. They are exceedingly rare in the soft tissues.

Leiomyosarcoma

According to anatomic site, leiomyosarcomas are divided into three groups: deep, superficial or cutaneous, and those arising from the walls of large blood vessels.

Most deep leiomyosarcomas occur in the retroperitoneum, omentum, or mesentery.[230,231] They are more common in females between forty and sixty years of age and can be quite large. Retroperitoneal tumors may infiltrate the kidney, colon and other viscera, making surgical resection impossible.

Cutaneous leiomyosarcomas are less common and smaller than the deep ones and of low-grade malignancy. Most of these tumors are solitary, painful nodules that may appear at any age and at any anatomic site but occur preferentially in the lower extremities.[232] They are seen more often on the extensor than the flexor aspects of the extremities.

Rarely, leiomyosarcomas arise from the walls of the blood vessels, especially the large veins of the extremities.[233] Most of these tumors exhibit intraluminal growth with invasion of the vessel wall and adjacent soft tissues. For this reason, venography, arteriography, and computed tomography (CT) are important tools in preoperative diagnosis and planning of surgical treatment.

Despite the fact that leiomyosarcomas show several growth patterns and variable degrees of differentiation, the histologic diagnosis is not difficult because most of these tumors contain well differentiated areas in which smooth muscle cells forming fascicles can be easily identified (Fig. 10-31). Distinction of cellular leiomyomas

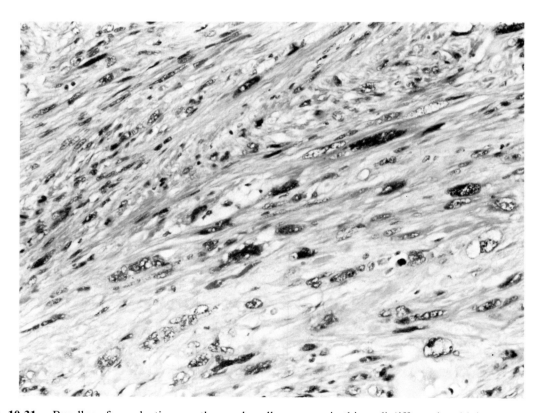

Fig. 10-31. Bundles of neoplastic smooth muscle cells are seen in this well differentiated leiomyosarcoma.

from well differentiated leiomyosarcomas is a much more difficult task. The mitotic index is not always a reliable diagnostic criterion and other features such as size, anatomic location, cellularity, and cytologic atypia must be taken into account.

Most of these tumors are composed of fascicles of well differentiated smooth muscle cells. However, leiomyosarcomas with extensive myxoid features, a hemangiopericytic pattern (vascular leiomyosarcoma),[234] and pleomorphic giant cells resembling pleomorphic rhabdomyosarcoma or malignant fibrous histiocytoma have been described. Not infrequently, leiomyosarcomas show more than one histologic growth pattern. Ultrastructural studies are helpful in demonstrating cytoplasmic features akin to those present in normal smooth muscle (see Fig. 10-4). Myofilaments, however, are scanty and not universally present and are seen only in a small percentage of the neoplastic cells.[235] The recognition of leiomyosarcoma can now be assisted by the demonstration of smooth muscle antigens such as desmin and muscle-specific actin by immunohistochemistry. Like synovial sarcoma and epithelioid sarcoma, leiomyosarcoma can also express cytokeratin and epithelial membrane antigen.[236-239]

Prognosis correlates well with the size and anatomic location of the leiomyosarcoma. Most patients with tumors of the retroperitoneum and veins of the extremities have large tumors and die as a result of metastases. By contrast, cutaneous leiomyosarcomas are relatively small and often recur following local excision, but rarely metastasize.

TUMORS OF STRIATED MUSCLE

Rhabdomyoma

If the relative bulk and ubiquity of a tissue were the major determinants in the prevalence of soft tissue tumors, rhabdomyomas would be among the most common benign soft tissue tumors. In fact, however, rhabdomyomas are among the rarest benign soft tissue tumors and are to be found not in the bulky muscles of the trunk and extremities, but almost exclusively in the head and neck, vagina, vulva, and anus.[240-243] Rhabdomyomas rarely occur as multiple lesions and occasionally recur after incomplete resection.[242-244] They are polypoid or nodular, well circumscribed, solid red, gray, or light tan tumor masses that grow very slowly, seldom measure more than 2 to 3 cm in diameter, and sometimes have been present for years before excision.[242]

Two distinctive histologic types are recognized: the adult and the fetal. The adult rhabdomyoma is composed of large, round to polygonal cells with conspicuous pe-

ripherally arranged vacuoles surrounding centrally located granular eosinophilic cytoplasm (Fig. 10-32). In some cells, thin strands of cytoplasm extend between the vacuoles to the distinct cell boundaries, producing the characteristic spider cell appearance. The fetal type of rhabdomyoma is composed of elongate spindle cells resembling the various developmental stages of striated skeletal muscle. Unlike those of the adult rhabdomyosarcoma, the nuclei of the fetal type are small and uniform and mitoses are sparse. In some tumors, the cells are dispersed in a myxoid stroma, in others (the cellular variant), the cells are densely packed, forming interlacing fascicles.[240]

The adult type is more common and occurs almost exclusively about the head and neck of adult men,[240-244] whereas fetal rhabdomyomas have a broader anatomic distribution and occur in men, women, and children. The vaginal and vulvar rhabdomyomas are mainly myxoid fetal rhabdomyomas.[245-247] The cellular variant of the fetal rhabdomyomas is confined, for the most part, to the head and neck in adult men. The latter tumors have been misdiagnosed as sarcomas because of their cellular pleomorphism, but the paucity of mitoses and the circumscribed growth of these tumors distinguish them from sarcomas.[248]

Rhabdomyomas contain large accumulations of intracytoplasmic glycogen dissolved during routine tissue processing, resulting in the vacuolated appearance of the tumor cells. These vacuoles are less prominent in the spindle cells of the fetal variant than in the large polygonal cells of the adult type. Longitudinal and cross-striations in the eosinophilic cytoplasm can be demonstrated with a variety of histochemical stains, and the organization of myofibrils into highly organized sarcomeres is observed readily with electron microscopy.[245,248] Eosinophilic crystalline structures arranged in haphazard

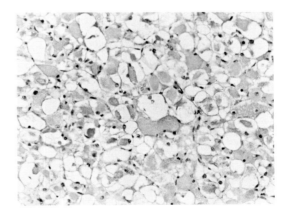

Fig. 10-32. Adult rhabdomyoma. This tumor consists of cells with small uniform nuclei and voluminous granular eosinophilic cytoplasm. Cytoplasmic vacuolization is prominent.

fashion in the cytoplasm of rhabdomyomas, first described by Moran and Enterline,[243] are hypertrophied, densely packed Z bands.[242,249]

Cardiac rhabdomyomas, most likely hamartomas rather than neoplasms of the myocardium, are usually multiple, affect infants and small children, and are frequently associated with tuberous sclerosis. They are composed of cardiocytes bearing a large accumulation of glycogen, which also imparts a spidery appearance to involved cells.[250]

Rhabdomyosarcoma

In contrast to liposarcomas, rhabdomyosarcomas are more frequent in children under 10 years of age. Regardless of their histologic appearance, rhabdomyosarcomas are high-grade malignant tumors. They grow rapidly and develop early hematogenous spread to the lungs and other viscera. Lymph node metastases are also common, especially in the alveolar type, reaching an incidence at autopsy as high as 74 percent of patients dying of the disease.[251] In spite of this aggressive biologic behavior, modern multimodal therapy has considerably improved the survival rate of patients with these tumors.[252] On the basis of their microscopic features, three histologic types have been described: embryonal, alveolar, and pleomorphic.[253,254]

Embryonal

The embryonal rhabdomyosarcoma, the most common variant, occurs most often about the head and neck and especially in the orbit in children.[255–258] Few congenital rhabdomyosarcomas of the orbit have been reported.[259,260] Other common sites are the deep soft tissues of the extremities and the urogenital tract. In hollow organs—urinary bladder, vagina, biliary tract—they form characteristic edematous, polypoid masses *(sarcoma botryoides)*. The histologic appearance varies from one tumor to another and in different fields of the same tumor, from round cells with hyperchromatic nuclei and scanty cytoplasm to elongate cells displaying centrally placed vesicular or hyperchromatic nuclei and abundant acidophilic cytoplasm (Fig. 10-33). Myxoid areas are common and may predominate in some tumors.

Alveolar

Alveolar rhabdomyosarcomas appear predominantly in adolescents and young adults, are more common in the extremities than in the head and neck, and comprise the most aggressive variant.[251,253] They are composed primarily of round cells with scanty cytoplasm, vesicular or

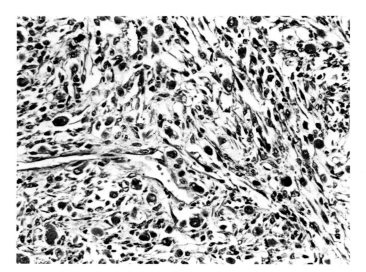

Fig. 10-33. Embryonal rhabdomyosarcoma. Round and spindle cells mixed with numerous rhabdomyoblasts having abundant eosinophilic cytoplasm.

hyperchromatic nuclei and prominent nucleoli; occasional cells exhibit abundant cytoplasm, and multinucleated giant cells may be seen in some tumors. The cellular elements are characteristically separated by strands of fibrous connective tissue forming lobules in an alveolar pattern (Fig. 10-34).

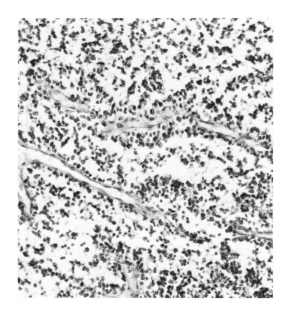

Fig. 10-34. Alveolar rhabdomyosarcoma. The fibrovascular septa provide the characteristic alveolar pattern of this variant of rhabdomyosarcoma.

Pleomorphic

The pleomorphic variant of rhabdomyosarcoma is usually described as being composed of spindle cells and numerous multinucleated giant cells with abundant acidophilic cytoplasm. It is a rare variant, and probably the great majority of reported instances of pleomorphic rhabdomyosarcomas correspond to other histogenetically different sarcomas, primarily malignant fibrous histiocytoma or pleomorphic liposarcoma.[261] In fact, immunoperoxidase studies of muscle antigens are now essential in establishing the diagnosis of this rare variant of rhabdomyosarcoma.[262]

The diagnosis of rhabdomyosarcoma is based on the identification of tumor cells constituting the neoplastic counterpart of the cellular elements present during the various embryonic stages of development of skeletal muscle. Only the best differentiated, certainly a minority, of rhabdomyosarcomas contain cells with cross-striations visible at the light microscopic level (see Fig. 10-2). The histologic pattern of either embryonal or alveolar variants and the presence of cells with deeply acidophilic and fibrillar cytoplasm raise strong suspicion of their rhabdomyoblastic nature. The ultrastructural observation of myofilaments (actin and myosin) and, more often than not, associated Z-band material, establishes the rhabdomyosarcomatous nature of a malignant tumor (see Fig. 10-1). However, in addition to the problems common in every ultrastructural study, the electron microscopic search for myofilaments is not an easy task, particularly in poorly differentiated tumors.[263] These problems are circumvented by immunohistologic assays. Immunoperoxidase demonstration of antigenic substances (myoglobin) specific for skeletal muscle (see Fig. 10-10) is useful in the diagnosis of these tumors.[264–266]

TUMORS OF BLOOD VESSELS

Hemangioma

Most benign vascular tumors arise in the skin and subcutaneous tissues, but no organ or tissue is exempt.[267–273] Hemangiomas are primarily tumors of infancy and childhood. Some are evident at birth; relatively few become manifest after the age of 30 years. Females are afflicted slightly more frequently than males, but males can predominate in some of the clinical syndromes that include vascular tumors.[8,9] Certain types of benign vascular tumors are associated with familial disease.[273]

Benign vascular tumors of the mucosal surfaces, including hemangiomas, hereditary hemorrhagic telangiectasia (Rendu-Osler-Weber disease), and arteriovenous malformations, frequently produce acute and chronic hemorrhage and, sometimes, resultant anemia. The association of giant cavernous hemangiomas with thrombocytopenia and extensive purpura, the Kasabach-Merritt syndrome, was first described in 1940 in an infant boy whose purpura disappeared when sclerosis of the hemangioma was accomplished by means of radiation therapy.[274] More recent studies have shown this syndrome to be a consumptive coagulopathy with reactive fibrinolysis and traumatic intravascular hemolysis.[275] The precise mechanism of the coagulopathy is unknown. Platelet sequestration has been demonstrated in the tumor, but other coagulation abnormalities seem to be operative.[268] Treatment includes heparinization, but the ultimate cure is achieved by means of irradiation of the tumor.

Skeletal and soft tissue gigantism associated with vascular tumors seems to depend on the presence of arteriovenus fistula in the tumor mass.[276] The most extreme clinical manifestations of these problems are exemplified by the Klippel-Trenaunay and Parkes-Weber syndromes, which include extensive cutaneous capillary hemangiomas of the extremities, usually the legs, with superficial varicose veins and hypertrophy of the bones of the affected part. Angiography can sometimes demonstrates arteriovenous fistulas that can be ligated to control the gigantism. Unlike the continuing gigantism which occurs sometimes with lipomatosis or neurofibromatosis, the growth of the soft tissues, bones, and sometimes the hemangiomas arrests when the patient reaches the third decade of life.

Capillary Hemangioma

Capillary hemangiomas are the most common vascular tumors. They are found most frequently in infants and children, especially in the head and neck. These tumors are multilobular and are composed of capillary channels each lined by a single layer of endothelial cells. In some, the vascular channels are obliterated by plump endothelial cells. This histologic pattern has led to the designation benign "juvenile" hemangioendothelioma.[277] The tumor may grow rapidly, and mitoses and papillary tufts may be present, features that sometimes lead to confusion of these lesions with malignant vascular tumors. The lack of anastomosing channels is helpful in distinguishing the hemangiomas from angiosarcomas, as is the patient's age, since angiosarcomas are very rare in children.[278] Most of the cellular capillary hemangiomas regress spontaneously.

Cavernous Hemangioma

Cavernous hemangiomas are composed of dilated channels lined by endothelial cells. Their walls may contain pericytes, fibroblasts, and collagen, but not in the regular arrangement seen in normal venules and arterioles. Capillary and cavernous hemangiomas of the skin are components of several clinical syndromes, as described previously.

Venous and Racemose Hemangioma

These lesions best reflect the evidence for an anomalous rather than neoplastic nature of hemangiomas.[268,273] Smooth muscle, pericytes, collagen, and irregular elastic fibers are arranged to form venules in the former, whereas racemose hemangiomas are composed of vascular channels with tortuous thick walls resembling arteries and veins. Not infrequently, these lesions are associated with other mesenchymal elements, such as adipose tissue, smooth muscle, and fibrous connective tissue, strongly supporting their hamartomatous origin. Differentiation of the hemangiomas from angiolipomas and angiomyolipomas is based primarily on the predominance of the dysplastic vascular component in the lesions.

Intramuscular Hemangioma

Intramuscular hemangiomas can be predominantly capillary, cavernous, arteriovenous, or a mixture of these types.[279,280] They are found most frequently in children and young adults and can be circumscribed, but frequently infiltrate into adjacent muscle, nerves, and vascular walls (Fig. 10-35). Those that invade through fascia into adjacent muscles, periosteum, and subcutaneous tissue must be distinguished from extensive regional hemangiomatosis. Careful physical examination and angiography are invaluable diagnostic tools in these situations. Intramuscular hemangiomas are common in the extremities but have been found in the skeletal muscles of the chest wall with surprising frequency.

Hemangiomatosis

Hemangiomatosis with or without congenital arteriovenous fistulas includes a large spectrum of vascular lesions usually affecting the upper and lower extremities. The diffuse or regional capillary and cavernous hemangiomas and hemolymphangiomas characteristic of these lesions are associated with many types of vascular dysplastic lesions including arteriovenous fistulas and capillary-venous, arteriocavernous, and arteriovenous vascular malformations. Venous and arterial ectasia, sometimes with aneurysmal dilatation of large vessels, may be due to dysplasia of the vessel wall or to secondary effects of abnormal blood flow or pressure. Blood vessel hypoplasia or atresia can be associated with the hemangiomatosis. Limb and regional gigantism of soft tissues and bone have been thought to be related to the presence of arteriovenous fistulas within the vascular lesions. Experimentally induced arteriovenous fistulas can produce

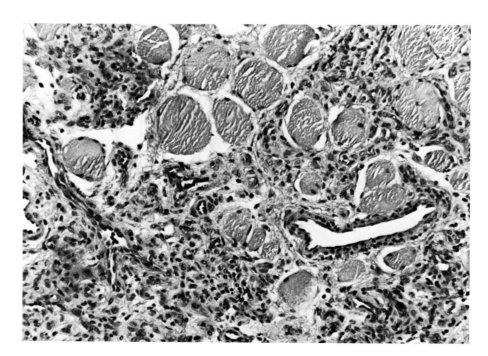

Fig. 10-35. Capillaries lined by prominent endothelial cells infiltrate skeletal muscle fibers. Intramuscular hemangioma.

growth in long bones in the affected limbs of chicken embryos[8] and puppies.[281] Conversely, gigantism has been controlled by ligation of the arteriovenous components of vascular lesions.[9] Gigantism is not necessarily related to the size, number, or anatomy of the arteriovenous fistulas but rather to their mere presence. Although arteriography has been quite useful in the demonstration and localization of arteriovenous fistulas, some are so small as to escape radiologic detection. Phlebosclerosis and ischemic ulcers may be prominent factors in the ultimate progression of these diseases. Congestive heart failure can be a significant complication of arteriovenous fistulas, but cardiac decompensation occurs mostly in older patients.[9]

Systemic hemangiomatoses are not distinct histologic lesions but are diseases and syndromes in which multiple organs and/or tissues are distorted by diffuse or multiple hemangiomas.[8,9]

Pyogenic Granuloma

Pyogenic granulomas, first thought to be reactive granulation tissue formed as a result of pyogenic infection, are now recognized as a variant of capillary hemangioma. When they occur on a cutaneous or mucosal surface, they can be distorted by secondary ulceration and granulation tissue formation. Histologically, the capillaries are arranged in lobules separated by fibrous connective tissue containing small veins and arteries.[282] Each lobule is fed by a large vessel, often with a muscular wall. Infiltrates of inflammatory cells are most dense adjacent to areas of ulceration and granulation tissue. A collarette of acanthotic epithelium may surround the base of the pyogenic granuloma, especially in lesions of the lip and oral mucosa. Classically, these lesions have been described as polypoid, but sessile nodules and more deep-seated lesions have also been reported. Pyogenic granulomas occur on the skin, especially that of the extremities and external genitalia, and the mucosal surfaces of the oral cavity and nose. *Intravenous pyogenic granulomas* involving medium-sized and small veins of the head and neck and upper extremity are small painless nodules.[283,284] They seem to arise out of the venous wall, perhaps from the vasa vasorum in the larger vessels.[284] Pyogenic granulomas are benign lesions but recurrences with satellite lesions have occurred after surgical removal and cauterization.[285]

Epithelioid Hemangioma

The epithelioid hemangioma, also known as *angiolymphoid hyperplasia with eosinophilia,* is a distinctive benign vascular tumor seen most often in the face and scalp of young persons.[286–289] The lesion appears as small papular or nodular dermal or subcutaneous lesions measuring less than 2 cm in diameter. Occasionally it may arise within a blood vessel, especially a vein. Microscopically, one sees proliferation of small blood vessels, each lined by large epithelioid endothelial cells. An inflammatory infiltrate of variable extent, containing lymphocytes and eosinophils, is usually present. This tumor can be separated from *Kimura's disease* on morphologic grounds.[289] A vascular proliferation similar to that of epithelioid hemangioma but containing Gram-negative rods has recently been reported in acquired immunodeficiency syndrome (AIDS) patients.[290]

Glomus Tumor

The glomus tumor was originally described as a tumorous caricature of the glomus apparatus, a specialized arteriovenous shunt that functions to regulate local blood flow in response to local neural mediators.[291] These tumors are composed of organoid lobules and trabeculae of clear, polygonal epithelioid cells surrounding open vascular channels (Fig. 10-36). Dilated unmyelinated axons course through the connective tissue between the groups of glomus cells. Axons, which are relatively easily demonstrated in cutaneous lesions, are not seen in visceral glomus tumors.[292] Mast cells are scattered throughout the lesions and may participate in the regulation of blood flow by their production of vasoactive amines.[293] The connective tissue stroma of these tumors frequently is hyalinized or myxoid. The glomus cells has been de-

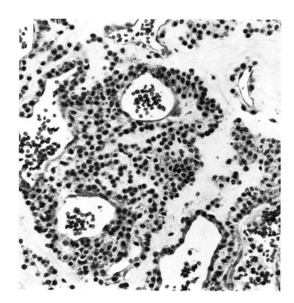

Fig. 10-36. Numerous blood vessels surrounded by round epithelioid cells. The stroma is hyalinized. Glomus tumor.

scribed as having many tissue culture and ultrastructural features in common with the pericyte of Zimmerman,[293–295] but others have emphasized the similarity of the glomus cell to smooth muscle cells[296–301] (Fig. 10-37).

Glomus tumors are most frequent in the skin, especially in the subungual parts of the fingers, but they occur also in the deep soft tissues and bone[290,298] and rarely in the viscera where, unlike the cutaneous lesions, they are seldom associated with pain.[302,303] The stomach is the most frequent site of visceral involvement. Patients with the lesion experience ulceration and hemorrhage.[303] The glomus tumor is well circumscribed in adults but may be large and infiltrative both in children[304] and in adults.[302,305,306] It is usually solitary; however, instances of multiple glomus tumors have been reported.[289]

Glomangiosarcoma

Glomangiosarcoma, a malignant variety of glomus tumor, has been described.[306,307] It is highly cellular with numerous mitotic figures; it invades surrounding tissues but rarely metastasizes. The lesion may grow to be as much as 12 cm in diameter. The histologic diagnosis of glomangiosarcoma can be made by the demonstration of the malignant component as well as areas of conventional glomus tumor. Glomangiosarcoma may be confused with

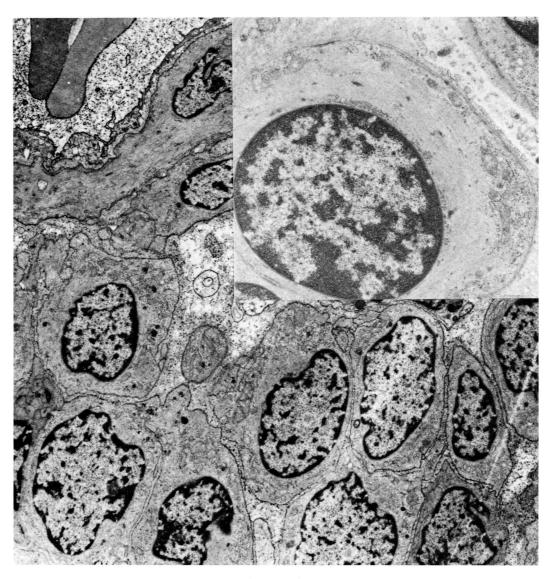

Fig. 10-37. Glomangioma. Ultrastructurally, this tumor is composed of round cells with cytoplasmic features of smooth muscle. Insert clearly shows elements of smooth muscle, particularly the orderly arranged filaments with dense bodies.

other malignant round cell sarcomas such as Ewing's sarcoma and rhabdomyosarcoma.

Epithelioid Hemangioendothelioma

Epithelioid hemangioendothelioma, a distinctive low-grade malignant neoplasm, first described in the lung as "intravascular bronchioloalveolar tumor",[308] is composed of large epithelioid vacuolated endothelial cells that grow predominantly in anastomosing cords and nests; for this reason, it is often confused with metastatic carcinoma[309] (Fig. 10-38). However, at least in some areas, the tumor cells are vasoformative and line small vascular channels. The hyalinized stroma usually contains myxoid foci superficially resembling chondroid matrix.[310] The endothelial nature of the tumor has been well documented both by immunohistochemical methods and by electron microscopy. Tumor cells are factor VIII positive and contain Weibel-Palade granules. Superficial and deep tumors have been recognized in the extremities, head and neck, and chest wall of adult patients. Superficial tumors involve the subcutis and may appear as skin tumors.[311] The deep ones infiltrate skeletal muscle. Approximately one half of these tumors appear to arise from the walls of blood vessels, especially veins, and exhibit angiocentric features. About 20 percent of epithelioid hemangioendotheliomas give rise to metastases in lungs, bones, and lymph nodes.

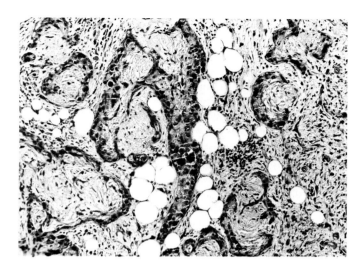

Fig. 10-38. Anastomosing cords of large epithelioid cells characterize this epithelioid hemangioendothelioma.

neoplastic, cytologically atypical endothelial cells (Fig. 10-39). These neoplastic channels freely infiltrate surrounding structures, usually following perivascular and perineural spaces. In the skin, they infiltrate around skin adnexa and between individual collagen fibers.[34] On occasion, tumor cells may form solid cords of epithelioid cells closely resembling carcinoma. Undifferentiated

Spindle Cell Hemangioendothelioma

Another recently recognized vascular tumor of low-grade malignancy is the spindle cell hemangioendothelioma. It combines the features of cavernous hemangioma and Kaposi's sarcoma.[312] Although local recurrence is common, metastases are rare. It is important to distinguish it from Kaposi's sarcoma because it has not been found in association with the acquired immunodeficiency syndrome.

Angiosarcoma

Angiosarcoma is a highly malignant tumor, most commonly located in the breast of young women[313] and in the head and neck, trunk, and extremities of elderly patients.[45,314] The liver is the viscus most often the site of primary angiosarcoma. Most of these neoplasms are multicentric and appear as dark red nodular elevations of the skin.

Microscopically, they are characterized by interconnecting, often deceptively benign channels lined by the

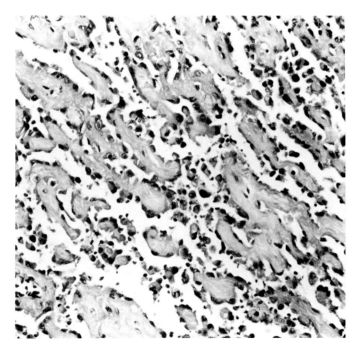

Fig. 10-39. Angiosarcoma. Interbranching vascular channels lined by hyperchromatic endothelial cells.

spindle-shaped cells may predominate in some areas. Besides the extensive local growth, metastases develop primarily in the lungs, with a relatively high incidence of lymphatic spread. In the rare instances when the endothelial nature of the lesion is difficult to ascertain, electron microscopy may be of some help. Immunoperoxidase stains for endothelial markers are particularly valuable in demonstrating the histologic nature of these tumors with a predominantly solid pattern.[315] A number of cases of radiation-induced angiosarcomas have been reported.[316,317]

Kaposi's Sarcoma

Kaposi's sarcoma is particularly common in African countries.[318] It was relatively rare in the United States until the advent of the epidemic of AIDS.[316] It has also been reported to occur in association with other immunodeficiency states. In organ transplant recipients, Kaposi's sarcoma may account for 5 percent of all malignancies in the post-transplantation period.[318] In 30 to 40 percent of AIDS patients, Kaposi's sarcoma develops; this figure is even higher in patients who die of AIDS.[319] In addition to skin lesions, involvement of the GI tract, lymph nodes and lungs is common in these patients. However, AIDS patients rarely die as a result of Kaposi's sarcoma.

Clinically, Kaposi's sarcoma is manifested by multiple purpuric plaques in the distal portions of the extremities, later becoming darker, more nodular, and eventually ulcerated. In about 15 percent of cases, the lesion is solitary and may be confused with pyogenic granuloma. Some patients with the sporadic type of Kaposi's sarcoma also develop lesions in lymph nodes, mucous membranes, and viscera.[320]

Microscopically, the lesion is characterized by spindle-shaped fibroblast-like tumor cells in a fascicular arrangement with intervening clefts or vascular channels (Fig. 10-40). The early patch and plaque stages have been well documented in AIDS patients. In some cases, however, the histologic features may be indistinguishable from the conventional angiosarcoma. A number of cells have been implicated in the histogenesis of Kaposi's sarcoma.[320] Immunoperoxidase studies have demonstrated the presence of factor-VIII-related antigen, an endothelial marker, in both the endothelial and spindle-shaped cells of Kaposi's sarcoma.[321,322] Although these studies would seem to establish the endothelial nature of this neoplasm, they do not permit us to know whether the cells in question derive from vascular or lymphatic vessels.[323]

The association of multicentric Castleman's disease and Kaposi's sarcoma has been documented in recent years.[324,325] These two rare lesions may appear simultaneously and may even coexist in the same lymph node.[325]

Hemangiopericytoma

Hemangiopericytomas are composed of a branching networks of capillaries surrounded by clumps, trabeculae, or sheets of polygonal and spindle cells (Fig. 10-41),

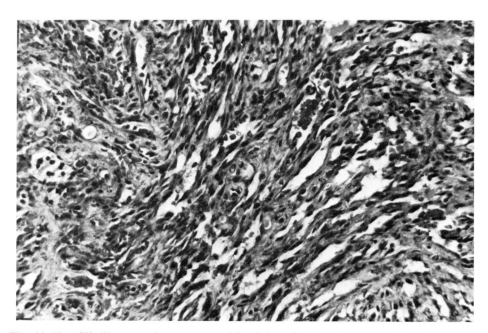

Fig. 10-40. Slit-like vascular spaces and fascicles of spindle cells in Kaposi's sarcoma.

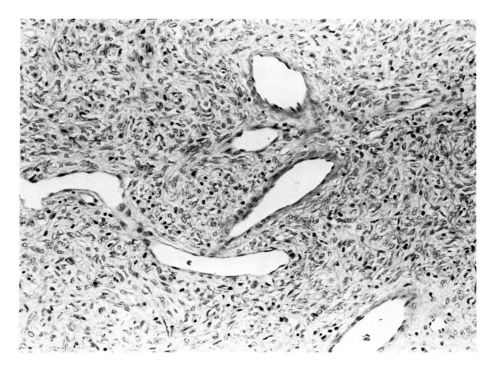

Fig. 10-41. Spindle cells proliferate between capillaries in this hemangiopericytoma.

thought to be derived from the vascular pericyte.[325,326] They are differentiated from hemangioendotheliomas by the demonstration of proliferating cells outside the capillary basement membrane, as revealed by silver reticulin stains. More important in the differential diagnosis is the fact that many soft tissue tumors may show hemangiopericytic areas, which can confuse the pathologist. However, adequate sampling usually solves that diagnostic dilemma. Ultrastructural and organ culture studies have not clarified the histogenesis of hemangiopericytomas conclusively. This may be due to the great variation of histologic and cytologic features seen among, and sometimes within, hemangiopericytomas at the LM and electron microscopic level. Ultrastructural study of one tumor showed that it was composed of large, nondescript cells with some intercellular spaces containing material that resembled basement membrane.[290] Others have been shown to be composed of a variety of cells, some of which contain cytoplasmic fibrillar bundles like those found in smooth muscle and glomus tumor cells, pinocytic vesicles similar to those in endothelial and smooth muscle cells, and long cytoplasmic projections as in the pericytes surrounding capillaries.[327] The tumor cells are usually surrounded by varying amounts of basement membrane material, a feature seen also in light microscopy with silver reticulin stains. None of these ultrastructural features is distinctive, nor does any of them unequivocally identify the proliferating cell as a pericyte;

however, they have been useful in confirming the diagnosis.[327,328] It is possible that the cytologic variation of hemangiopericytomas is a reflection of the property of the pericyte to act as a precursor cell for the formation of fibroblasts, endothelial cells, and histiocytes.[2,286]

Hemangiopericytomas are primarily tumors of adults that occur anywhere in the body, including the meninges and viscera, but are most common in the deep tissues of the lower extremities.[2,329–331] In infants and very young children, hemangiopericytomas tend to occur more frequently in subcutaneous tissues, where they exhibit an almost uniform benign behavior.[332–335] Familial hemangiopericytomas have been described.[336]

Hemangiopericytomas have a high incidence of recurrence and metastasis.[2,329] Not uncommonly, recurrences and metastases appear for the first time 5 to 10 years after the initial treatment. Long-term survival, even in the presence of metastasis, is not unusual. In contrast, some patients succumb soon after diagnosis because of extensive local and metastatic growth of the neoplasm. For some time, the morphologic features of the lesion were not considered helpful in differentiating between benign and malignant hemangiopericytoma, and they were all thought to have a malignant potential regardless of their histologic appearance. Recent studies, with long-term follow-up, suggest that large (6.5 cm) tumors, tumors with foci of necrosis and hemorrhage, and those with increased mitotic rate, cellularity, and anaplasia are more likely to exhibit malignant biologic behavior.[2,325] Metastases are primarily hematogenous, but lymph node metastasis has been reported.

TUMORS OF LYMPHATIC VESSELS

Lymphangioma

In comparison with tumors of blood vessels, the frequency of benign and malignant neoplasms of lymphatic vessels is very low. Most lymphangiomas are found in newborns, infants, and small children.[267,337,338] Frequently, they are responsible for significant disease because they form large deforming masses that impinge on vital structures or are widely infiltrative. The lumens of the cavernous and cystic lymphangiomas are filled with fluid resembling extracellular fluid, lymph, or chylous lymph. These fluids provide excellent nutrition for bacteria, so that superimposed infection can be a serious problem.

The anatomic location and infiltrative growth pattern may impede total surgical excision of lymphangiomas. Irradiation, including x-rays and placement of radioactive metallic seeds within the lesion, is no longer acceptable treatment for these biologically benign lesions. As much tumor as possible should be surgically excised when it is not possible to remove all of the infiltrative lesion.[337] Surgical excision has been shown to provide significant relief of symptoms for many patients. Injection of sclerosing agents (to reduce tumor size) has been modestly successful and with the advent of improved surgical techniques, especially in the realm of plastic surgery, it has become apparent that sclerosing therapy is best avoided. However, in women with diffuse, inoperable mediastinal and pulmonary lymphangiomyomas, intracavitary installation of sclerosing agents is used to control the sometimes massive pleural effusions in these patients.

Capillary Lymphangioma

The histologic classification of lymphangiomas proposed by Wegner in 1877 is used widely.[337] The pure, simple, or capillary lymphangioma is uncommon and is found in the skin or subcutaneous tissue of the head and neck. These lesions are composed of small, sometimes compressed, vascular channels lined by endothelial cells. They are difficult to distinguish from capillary hemangiomas. Ultrastructurally, the endothelium of lymphangiomas differs from that of hemangiomas by a relative lack of fenestrations and tight junctions, and the presence of fragmented, scanty basal lamina.[338,339]

Cavernous Lymphangioma

The cavernous lymphangioma is the most common type. It is found in varying sizes and shapes in the skin; portions of the head including the mouth, tongue, and cheek; the neck; the mesentery; the retroperitoeum[267,337,339–341]; and the mediastinum.[270] These lesions, whether small and localized or extensively infiltrative, are composed of dilated, communicating channels lined by endothelium and surrounded by small amounts of smooth muscle. The vascular lumens are filled with clear or chylous fluid, depending on the anatomic and embryologic relationship of the tumor to the mesentery of the small intestine or the thoracic duct. Direct communication with normal lymphatic vessels has been difficult to demonstrate. Grossly, the tumors are variably firm, rubbery, and sometimes spongy. They are rarely circumscribed; in the more diffuse, infiltrative lesions, gross examination may reveal only multiple holes, like those in a sponge, in otherwise normal muscle or fibroadipose tissue.

Cystic Lymphangioma

Cystic lymphangiomas (cystic hygromas) occur most commonly in the neck and upper mediastinum but can form large tumor masses in the axillary and inguinal areas, retroperitoneum, omentum, mesentery, liver, and spleen.[338,342,343] They are seen most frequently in the young pediatric age group (60 percent under the age of 5 years).[270,338] Cystic hygromas may be a manifestation of Turner's syndrome.[340] Those of the neck occur predominantly in newborns and infants, while cystic lymphangiomas located elsewhere can present at any age.[343,344] Most frequently, cystic lymphangiomas are multilocular. As in cavernous lymphangiomas, the cysts contain clear or chylous fluid. Hemorrhage, inflammation secondary to rupture of the cysts, and infection can change the character of the fluid. The cysts are lined with attenuated endothelial cells and the walls are composed of fibrous connective tissue containing scattered, irregularly arranged thin layers of smooth muscle.

Systemic Lymphangiomatosis

Extensive involvement of a region of a portion of the body by lymphangioma is known as systemic lymphangiomatosis. This condition may affect the extremities, the trunk, or the viscera.[270,342] Capillary, cavernous, and sometimes cystic components are found in these lesions.

Lymphangiomas are generally accepted as congenital lymphatic vascular malformations.[338] Most cystic lymphangiomas occur in the head and neck and adjacent axilla, the mediastinum, posterior abdominal structures and retroperitoneum, and the inguinal areas. At these sites, they seem to correspond with the earliest embryonic vestiges of the lymph vascular system, the lymph sacs.[345]

Lymphangiomyoma

Lymphangiomyomas are distinctive hamartomatous lesions[346,347] found almost exclusively in women of the childbearing age.[347] Some have suggested that this lesion is a component of the tuberous sclerosis syndrome. The lesions involve the thoracic duct, pulmonary lymphatics, and mediastinal and retroperitoneal lymph nodes and lymphatic vessels. Grossly, the single or multiple lesions are nodular or cylindrical masses that can be spongy, cystic, or rubbery. They may measure up to 10 cm in diameter but are usually smaller, measuring up to only a few centimeters. No actual masses are found in some patients, and the diagnosis is established by microscopic examination of paraortic lymph nodes or the thoracic duct and adjacent tissues.

The lesion is histologically distinctive, characterized by the presence of narrow and broad trabeculae of smooth muscle derived from the walls of anastomosing lymphatic channels, which are lined by a single layer of endothelial cells. Foci of lymphoid tissue, sometimes containing germinal centers, can be seen in many of these lesions. Affected patients suffer from chylothorax and/or chylous ascites, and pulmonary lymphangiomyomatosis can produce pneumothorax and pulmonary hemorrhage, leading to significant respiratory insufficiency. The pulmonary lesions consist of lymphangiectasia, pulmonary parenchymal honeycombing with proliferation of smooth muscle, and atypical lipid pneumonia.[348,349] Death may occur as the result of pulmonary insufficiency secondary to the pulmonary parenchymal disease rather than the chylous effusions. Abdominal lymphangiomyomas are differentiated histologically from other forms of abdominal chylous cysts by the prominent smooth muscle component and the presence of lymphoid tissue.[343] Chylous ascites is a common complication of retroperitoneal lymphangiomyomas. The high incidence of these lesions in young women suggests an etiologic relationship with ovarian function and, more specifically, with estrogens. With this in mind, castration[350] and pharmacologic doses of progesterone[351] have been used, with some success, to diminish the size of the pulmonary and abdominal lesions and to control the formation of effusions. Dietary fat manipulation[352] and surgical bypass procedures[350] have also been used to treat the ascites that so often complicates the lives of the women with this disease.

Lymphangiosarcoma

Lymphangiosarcomas are very rare lesions; nearly all of them have been found in patients who suffered severe lymphedema after radical mastectomy[353,354] or in extremities with primary or secondary lymphedema.[355,356] Some of these tumors appear to be preceded by the development of dermal lymphangiomatosis, a nodular proliferation of small lymphatic channels lined by normal-appearing endothelial cells. The tumor usually appears as a single or multiple cutaneous nodules covered by purple skin.

Histologically, this lesion is often indistinguishable from the conventional angiosarcoma. Like angiosarcomas, these tumors may contain solid nests or cords of epithelioid endothelial cells that mimic carcinoma (Fig. 10-42). They can be distinguished from carcinoma by means of immunostaining of endothelial cell markers such as factor-VIII-related antigen.[55,357]

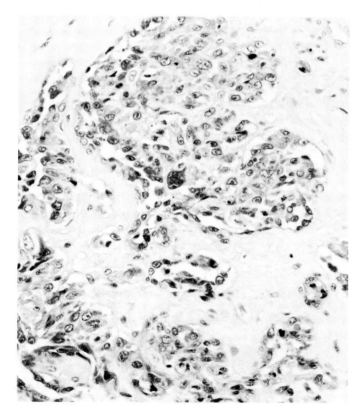

Fig. 10-42. Postmastectomy epithelioid angiosarcoma. The vascular spaces are filled with epithelioid endothelial cells.

TUMORS OF SYNOVIAL TISSUES

Synovial Sarcoma

The existence of benign neoplasms of synovial tissue is controversial. In fact, synovial sarcomas do not arise from synovial membranes, but they are formed by two types of cells that resemble normal synovial cells. These tumors are most commonly found in the lower extremities of young adults, but they have also been reported in children and elderly patients.[358–360] Likewise, they have been described in many other anatomic sites, including the head and neck, chest wall, mediastinum, and retroperitoneum. Microscopically, synovial sarcomas exhibit a biphasic morphology with a variable proportion of spindle-shaped and epithelial cells (Fig. 10-43). The spindle-shaped cells usually predominate and are arranged in fascicles, while the epithelial cells form glands, cords, nests, or papillary structures. The existence of monophasic synovial sarcomas, composed entirely of spindle cells or epithelial cells, is now widely accepted.[361] Extensive calcification is seen in some tumors. In terms of immunohistochemistry, both cell types show epithelial markers and are keratin- and epithelial membrane antigen positive.[362–364] Carcinoembryonic antigen has also been identified in some of these tumors. Electron microscopic studies tend to give credence to the existence of monophasic, fibrosarcoma-like synovial sarcomas, since the monophasic tumors are ultrastructurally identical to the spindle cell component of biphasic synovial sarcomas.[365,366] Patients having predominantly glandular biphasic tumors with a low mitotic index have a longer disease-free interval than do those with highly mitotic or purely monophasic tumors. The 5-year survival rate for the former tumors is more than 90 percent and about 40 percent for the latter group.[367] Patients with densely calcified synovial sarcomas have a better prognosis than those with noncalcified tumors.[368]

TUMORS OF PLURIPOTENTIAL MESENCHYME

Mesenchymoma

The term mesenchymoma is reserved for tumors containing two or more distinct types of mesenchyme-derived tissues ordinarily not associated with each other, and found in regions of the body not usually associated with those tissues.[369] In some cases, more descriptive terms such as angiolipoma enjoy more common usage than the equally correct term, benign mesenchymoma, because the descriptive term is more informative. Mixed tumors composed of both epithelial and stromal elements, most frequently found in the genitourinary tract, skin, breast, and salivary glands, and the benign and malignant Triton tumors (see Ch. 49), are not included among the mesenchymomas of the soft tissues.

Benign mesenchymomas contain various combinations of mature mesenchymal tissues, including adipose tissue, smooth and striated muscle, blood vessels, cartilage, myxomatous tissue, and lymphoid and hemopoetic tissues, in addition to fibrous connective tissue.[370] The proposal that benign mesenchymomas are hamartomas rather than true neoplasms is debated.[371]

Malignant mesenchymomas are composed of two or more sarcomas. Fibrosarcomatous elements are not considered separate components of malignant mesenchymomas; however, in children, one of the components can be an undifferentiated mesenchymal sarcoma.[372]

Both benign and malignant mesenchymomas are found in infants, children, and adults.[370,372–376] In children, benign mesenchymomas most frequently involve the kidney and upper and lower extremities. Renal lesions may be components of the tuberous sclerosis syndrome. Tumors of the extremities can be quite large and may involve an entire limb, necessitating amputation.[27] Both malignant and benign mesenchymomas can be congenital and can interfere, because of their size, with normal delivery.[371,373]

Ectomesenchymoma

An exceedingly rare malignant soft tissue tumor termed ectomesenchymoma has recently been described. It is characterized by the admixture of ganglion cells, neuroblasts, and mesenchymal elements, usually rhabdomyoblasts.[377–380]

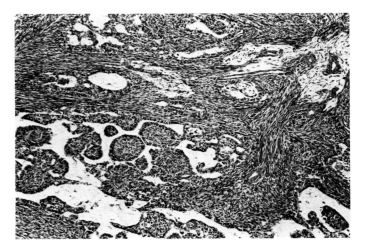

Fig. 10-43. Both the fibrosarcomatous and the epithelial components of this synovial sarcoma are clearly seen.

TUMORS OF UNCERTAIN HISTOGENESIS

A number of benign and malignant soft tissue tumors, despite their fairly well defined pathologic features and biologic behavior, still defy histogenetic characterization.

Granular Cell Tumor

Granular cell tumors are yellow or yellow-tan indistinct tumor nodules found in the skin, tongue, oral cavity, GI and respiratory tracts, biliary tree, genitourinary tract, central and peripheral nervous systems, uterus, vulva, and breast.[381–387] The round to polygonal cells have a distinctive, uniformly finely granular eosinophilic cytoplasm, and indistinct cytoplasmic borders (Fig. 10-44). The cytoplasmic granules are associated with histochemical reactions characteristic of lysosomes; when viewed through the electron microscope, the cytoplasm is crowded with numerous secondary lysosomes packed with various kinds of material and cytoplasmic debris.[388] The granular cells of granular cell tumors can be distinguished from reactive histiocytes, fibroblasts, and smooth muscle cells distorted by inflammation.[389]

The histogenesis and pathogenesis of the granular cell tumor are still debated. In the past, the granular cell was thought to resemble a myoblast and to be derived from muscle cells, hence its older but now less favored name, granular cell myoblastoma.[390] The anatomic relationship and frequent association of granular cells with peripheral nerves and many ultrastructural and histochemical features of the cells are used to support the argument that these lesions are of Schwann cell origin.[388] However, other electron microscopic features suggest that the precursor cell is an undifferentiated mesenchymal cell.[384,391]

Granular cell tumors rarely measure more than 1 to 2 cm in diameter but can be multiple and multifocal.[390] Pseudoepitheliomatous hyperplasia may be prominent in the epithelium overlying these tumors.

Malignant Granular Cell Tumor

Rare cases of malignant granular cell tumors have been described.[391,392–395] Some appear both histologically and biologically malignant, whereas others that follow a malignant biologic course are histologically similar to benign granular cell tumors.[395] Malignant granular cells tumors tend to be larger, more rapidly growing, and located predominantly in the extremities as compared to the smaller benign granular cell tumors that appear more frequently in the head, neck, and trunk. Widespread lymphatic and hematogenous metastases have been major factors in causing the deaths of these patients, occurring usually within 4 years of the diagnosis.

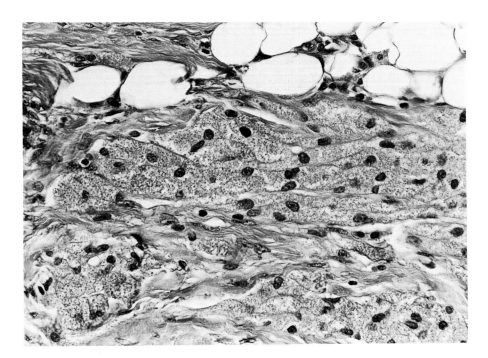

Fig. 10-44. Granular cell tumor. Large granular cells are infiltrating adipose tissue.

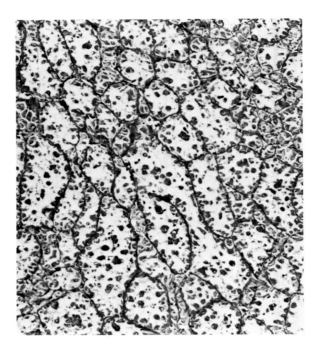

Fig. 10-45. Characteristic alveolar pattern and cell composition of alveolar soft part sarcoma are clearly shown.

Alveolar Soft Part Sarcoma

The term *alveolar soft part sarcoma,* coined by Christopherson et al.,[396] emphasizes the characteristic histologic appearance of a tumor consisting of groups of tumor cells in an organoid or alveolar pattern resulting from septation of the mass by thin bands of fibrovascular tissue (Fig. 10-45). This tumor has been subjected to many ultrastructural and immunohistochemical studies, yet histogenesis remains unknown.[397-399] The tumor cells have abundant eosinophilic cytoplasm, and some contain characteristic PAS-positive intracytoplasmic crystals readily defined with the electron microscope[400] (Fig. 10-46). Most tumors appear in the thighs of young adults. In children, they are more frequent in the head and neck.[401,402] Although these tumors exhibit a fairly uniform histologic pattern and few mitoses, they are very malignant. Metastases develop early and extend via the hematogenous route. About 50 percent of patients die within 5 years as a result of the disease.

Epithelioid Sarcoma

In 1970, Enzinger[403] described a morphologically distinct soft tissue neoplasm, epithelioid sarcoma, frequently confused with granulomatous inflammation or some other malignant tumor such as carcinoma or synovial sarcoma. This tumor is most frequently located in the extremities of adolescents and young adult men.

The neoplasm usually appears as single or multiple nodules in the dermis; these nodules enlarge rapidly and ulcerate the skin, thus mimicking abscesses, granulomas, or nonspecific ulcers clinically. Deeper lesions form larger nodules that infiltrate tendons and aponeuroses.

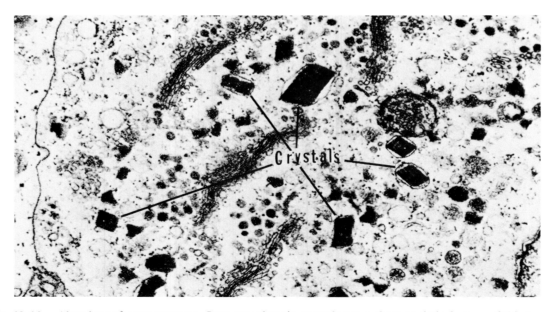

Fig. 10-46. Alveolar soft part sarcoma. Intracytoplasmic crystals are a characteristic feature of this tumor. (Courtesy of Dr. Philip H. Lieberman.) (×12,000)

Tumor cells are polygonal or fusiform with dense aci-dophilic cytoplasm and are grouped in nodules with central necrosis or hyalinization (Figs. 10-47 and 10-48). Spindle-shaped cells sometimes cluster at the periphery of the nodules; when they become numerous, the histologic appearance of the lesion may be confused with that of a fibrosarcoma.[404] Multinucleated giant cells are occasionally present. Moreover, tumor cells may form cords or nests in the midst of a dense desmoplastic reaction, enhancing the epithelioid appearance.[405] Epithelioid sarcomas usually follow a protracted course. Local recurrences are common and metastases are most often blood-borne to the lungs, although lymph node metastases are relatively frequent. A more rapid clinical course is associated with proximal or axial tumor locations, increased size and depth of the tumor, hemorrhage, many mitotic figures, necrosis, or vascular invasion.[406] Ultrastructural studies[407,408] have suggested either a synovial or fibrohistiocytic derivation for these tumors.[409] More recently, however, a number of immunohistochemical assays have demonstrated epithelial markers in most of them.[410–414]

An aggressive round cell tumor similar to the *rhabdoid tumor* of the kidney was recently reported in soft tis-

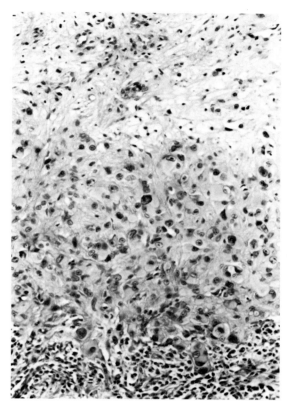

Fig. 10-48. Higher magnification of nodule of epithelioid sarcoma showing malignant histiocytic cells surrounded by inflammatory cells.

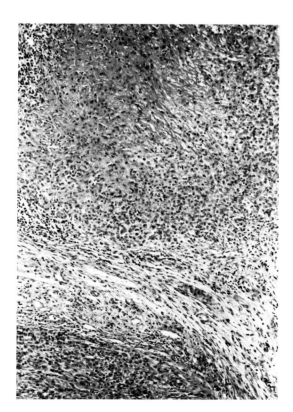

Fig. 10-47. Epithelioid sarcoma. Two nodules surrounded by lymphocytes and separated by a band of connective tissue. One of the nodules shows central necrosis.

sues.[415,416] The neoplastic cells have characteristic keratin-positive acidophilic inclusions in their cytoplasm.

Clear Cell Sarcoma of Tendons and Aponeuroses

Clear cell sarcoma of tendons and aponeuroses (or *malignant melanoma of soft parts*) is a rare neoplasm, primarily of the foot and knee of young adults, where it attaches firmly to tendons and aponeuroses.[417] It is formed by groups and fascicles of predominantly round and spindle cells with clear cytoplasm. About 70 percent of these tumors contain melanin. Most are S-100 protein-positive and also contain other melanoma antigens, indicating that they are malignant melanomas of soft tissue.[418,419] However, unlike the garden varieties of malignant melanoma, clear cell sarcomas are deep, are always associated with tendon or aponeuroses, and lack epidermal involvement. About 50 percent of patients die of their metastatic disease.[419]

BONE NEOPLASMS AS PRIMARY EXTRASKELETAL SOFT TISSUE TUMORS

A number of histogenetically different tumors ordinarily affect bone but may appear as primary neoplasms of soft tissue. These are benign chondromatous tumors, chondrosarcoma, osteogenic sarcoma, and Ewing's sarcoma.

Chondroma

Chondromas of soft tissues are uncommon and more often seen in the hand and feet of young adults.[420,421] Some are associated with tendons, tendon sheaths, or joint capsules. Most are solitary and small (less than 3 cm in diameter), but multiple chondromas have also been reported. Microscopically, they are lobulated and densely cellular and may show considerable cytologic atypia.[422–424] Because of these features, they have been confused with chondrosarcomas. However, these tumors follow a benign clinical course. Some may recur following local excision, but so far metastases have not been recorded.

Chondrosarcoma

Several distinct clinicopathologic types of extraskeletal chondrosarcomas are recognized in the soft tissues, myxoid and mesenchymal chondrosarcomas being the most common.

Myxoid Chondrosarcoma

Myxoid chondrosarcomas are usually of low-grade malignancy, occurring mainly in the deep tissues of the extremities of adults.[425,426] Occasionally these tumors may arise in other anatomic locations.[427] They are well circumscribed and multinodular, with a lobulated microscopic pattern; lobules are separated by connective tissue bands of variable thickness. Tumor cells usually have hyperchromatic or vesicular nuclei with scanty acidophilic cytoplasm and often form interconnecting cords (Fig. 10-49). The stroma is rich in sulfated mucopolysaccharides resistant to hyaluronidase digestion, a feature that permits separation from other myxoid mesenchymal tumors such as liposarcoma.[428] Electron microscopic studies have confirmed the cartilaginous nature of these tumors, as well as those referred to as *chordoid sarcomas*.[429,430]

Mesenchymal Chondrosarcoma

Mesenchymal chondrosarcoma is a considerably more aggressive, high-grade malignant tumor, with frequent hematogenous dissemination.[431–433] The most common site is the head and neck, most often in young adults. These tumors are usually lobulated and exhibit hemorrhage, necrosis, and cystic degeneration. This type of

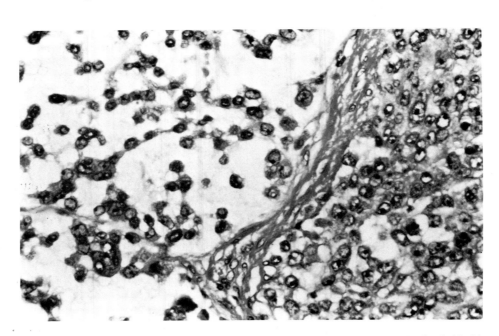

Fig. 10-49. Myxoid chondrosarcoma. Small round cells, some with prominent nucleoli, divided into lobules by bands of fibrous tissue. The stroma is myxoid in one of the lobules.

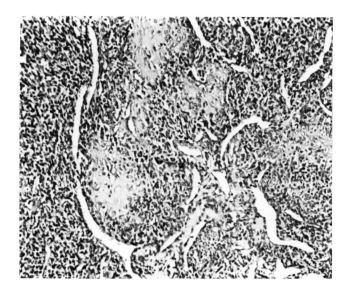

Fig. 10-50. Mesenchymal chondrosarcoma. Small undifferentiated cells, foci of hyaline cartilage and numerous capillaries are characteristic features.

tumor presents a rather characteristic microscopic appearance consisting of closely packed undifferentiated round to oval cells, numerous vascular channels, and islands of well differentiated cartilage (Fig. 10-50). Metastases may occur late in the course of the disease.

Other Chondrosarcomas

Well differentiated and clear cell chondrosarcomas are exceedingly rare in soft tissues; therefore, little is known about their natural history. The embryonal chondrosarcoma first described in the nasoethmoidal region of children is also very rare.[434] Only seven examples of this distinctive type of chondrosarcoma have been reported in soft tissues.[435,436]

Osteogenic Sarcoma

Extraskeletal osteogenic sarcomas are extremely rare. In contrast to those that are primary in bone, the extraskeletal lesions are more common in adults and practically nonexistent during the first two decades of life.[437] These tumors are more common in the extremities and retroperitoneum.[438–440] Like osteosarcoma of bone, the soft tissue osteosarcoma exhibits a broad morphologic spectrum, with areas resembling malignant fibrous histiocytoma, fibrosarcoma, and schwannoma. However, all contain varying amounts of neoplastic osteoid, bone, and cartilage, permitting their recognition. Nearly two thirds of patients die with lung and bone metastases.[440]

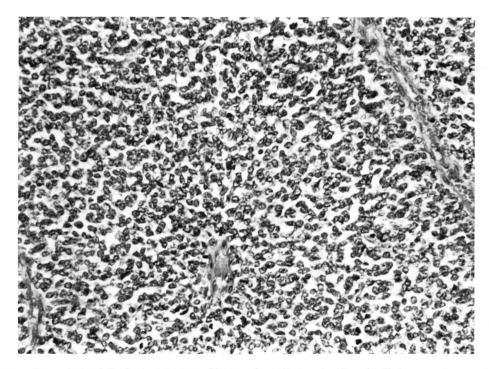

Fig. 10-51. Extraskeletal Ewing's sarcoma. Sheets of small round cells with little cytoplasm are present. The stroma is scant and contains some small blood vessels.

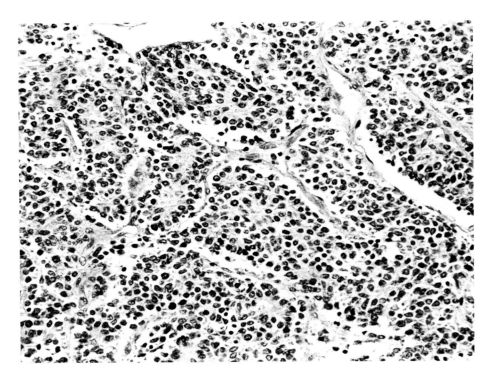

Fig. 10-52. Neuroblastoma of sciatic nerve. Organoid pattern in a small round cell neoplasm showing pseudorosettes and a fibrillary background. Compare with Ewing's sarcoma (Fig. 10-51).

Ewing's Sarcoma

A small round cell neoplasm similar to Ewing's sarcoma of bone has been recognized in the soft tissues.[441–445] Extraosseous Ewing's sarcoma originates preferentially in the extremities, trunk, and retroperitoneum of children, adolescents, and young adults. Microscopically, some of these tumors show rosettes, are neuron-specific enolase-positive, and contain neurosecretory-like granules by electron microscopy, suggesting neural derivation[446] (Figs. 10-51 and 10-52). Whether these cases represent primitive neuroectodermal tumors or an unusual variant of extraosseous Ewing's sarcoma is a matter of controversy. Survival rates of patients with Ewing's sarcoma of soft tissues are comparable to those with embryonal rhabdomyosarcoma, with which it can be confused.[446]

PSEUDOSARCOMAS

Not all soft tissue masses that look like sarcomas are malignant. Many benign soft tissue tumors, such as pleomorphic lipoma and fetal rhabdomyoma, closely simulate sarcoma. In addition, certain fleshy tan or white hard masses are the result of exuberant inflammatory, reac-

tive, or regenerative processes; however, because of their gross and microscopic resemblance to sarcomas, they have been designated pseudosarcomas. Trauma, hemorrhage, thrombosis, and infection have been implicated, but not proved, as etiologic factors in the development of these lesions. An exception is the *exuberant fibrohistiocytic reaction to silica* that closely resembles malignant fibrous histiocytoma.[447] Most of these lesions result from the injection of silica, which in the past was used for the treatment of hernias. These tumor-like masses are seen most often in the inguinal region or abdominal wall and occur many years after the injection of silica. Sheets of well differentiated histiocytes and a few multinucleated giant cells are recognized microscopically. The silica crystals can be identified under polarized light.

Nodular Fasciitis and Related Lesions

A common soft tissue pseudosarcoma is nodular fasciitis, a rapidly growing lesion arising in association with the deep cutaneous or muscle fascia of the trunk, proximal extremities, or head.[448–452] These lesions are usually small (about 2 cm in diameter), but they may measure up to 6 cm and have infiltrating borders. Microscopically, the plump fibroblasts, the proliferating endothelial cells,

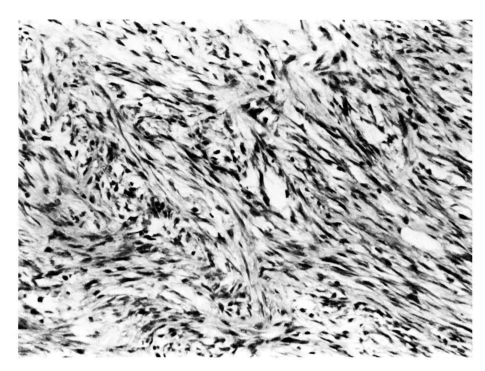

Fig. 10-53. Interlacing fascicles of young fibroblasts and microcystic degeneration are noted in this nodular fasciitis.

and sometimes the numerous, yet normal, mitoses in the tumor cause it to be confused with sarcoma. These biologically benign tumors can be correctly diagnosed by recognizing their characteristic combination of anatomic features: the usual anatomic locations; the radial arrangement of the numerous vascular channels in the mass, reflecting a reparative process; the admixture of lymphocytes, histiocytes, multinucleated giant cells, and occasional plasma cells; and the myxomatous stroma (Fig. 10-53). Nodular fasciitis may also develop within blood vessels, further suggesting a malignant behavior. However, these examples of intravascular fasciitis behave in the same manner as the conventional form.[453] Another type of nodular fasciitis, *cranial fasciitis,* occurs exclusively in the cranium of infants and children and usually produces a large defect in the outer table of the skull.[454] Subcutaneous lesions that have prominent populations of large fibroblasts have been separated from the general group of nodular fasciitis because of their resemblance to proliferative myositis, an inflammatory tumor thought to be related to trauma.[455] In *proliferative myositis,* bands of bizarre fibroblasts and ganglion-like cells separate but do not destroy groups of muscle fibers[456] (Fig. 10-54). The term *proliferative fasciitis* was proposed specifically for these subcutaneous lesions that resemble proliferative myositis.

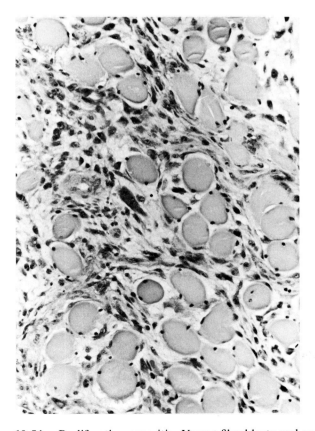

Fig. 10-54. Proliferative myositis. Young fibroblasts and ganglion-like cell dissociate skeletal muscle fibers.

Inflammatory Pseudotumor

Tumor-like masses composed of fascicles of myofibroblasts and a dense inflammatory infiltrate rich in plasma cells have occasionally been reported in the soft tissues.[457-460] The term inflammatory pseudotumor has been applied to these lesions, which are thought to be reparative phenomena in inflammatory processes. The lesion bears a close resemblance to the plasma cell granuloma of the lung and may be confused with malignant fibrous histiocytoma of the inflammatory type and plasmacytoma.[460]

Myositis Ossificans

Myositis ossificans is a lesion that closely simulates osteosarcoma.[461,462] About one half of patients have a history of trauma before the appearance of the mass. The muscles of the thigh are commonly affected, but the lesion may be seen in any muscle group. A periostial reaction is seen in many cases. Ossification can be demonstrated roentgenographically 4 to 6 weeks after trauma. Microscopically, three zones can be identified. The first, in the central portion of the mass, is composed of atypical spindle cells with mitotic figures. Osteoid and cartilage are seen in the middle zone and mature bone trabeculae at the periphery of the lesion. Myositis ossificans usually regresses spontaneously.[463]

Vascular Pseudosarcoma

Several vascular lesions may resemble angiosarcomas histologically. Most of the vascular pseudosarcomas occur in the skin, but they have been found elsewhere.

Pyogenic Granuloma

Pyogenic granulomas may occur in unusual locations, which can confuse the clinician and pathologist alike. They may occur deep in the dermis and subcutaneous tissue and within the lumens of large and small veins. When pyogenic granulomas recur as multiple satellite lesions, they may be clinically confused by the clinician with malignant melanoma.[285]

Organizing Thrombi

Organizing thrombi in which the endothelial cells grow in fascicles can mimic Kaposi's sarcoma. We have seen rare capillary hemangiomas composed of fascicles of spindle-shaped endothelial cells closely simulating Kaposi's sarcoma. The lobular pattern in these hemangiomas

helps one to distinguish them from Kaposi's sarcoma (Albores-Saavedra J: unpublished observations). Exuberant endothelial proliferations arranged in papillary patterns can occur in vascular thrombi and less frequently in hematomas and in hemangiomas.[464,465] This lesion, known as *Masson's hemangioma, vegetative intravascular hemangioendothelioma,* or *papillary endothelial hyperplasia,* is thought to represent organization of a thrombus or a hematoma with exuberant endothelial cell proliferation.[466,467] In its late stage, it may simulate an angiosarcoma (Fig. 10-55). Two forms of papillary endothelial hyperplasia have been described. The primary form is usually associated with a vascular thrombus and rarely with a hematoma, whereas the secondary type constitutes a component of another lesion such as hemangioma, pyogenic granuloma or lymphangioma.[467,468] Primary papillary endothelial hyperplasia occurs commonly in subcutaneous tissue and, less frequently, in the dermis. The most common locations are the fingers and the head and neck, followed by the extremities. The location of the secondary type is determined by the underlying disease process.

Carcinoma

A number of carcinomas can be composed of sheets of spindle or polygonal cells that may resemble the histologic patterns associated with sarcomas. Squamous cell

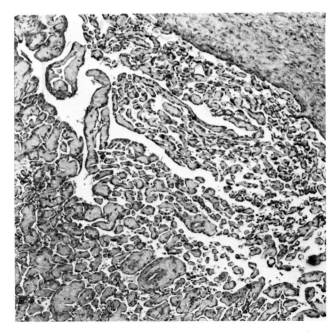

Fig. 10-55. Intravascular papillary endothelial hyperplasia. Fibrotic vein containing endothelium-covered papillary fronds. Part of the fibrotic wall of the vein is seen.

carcinomas of the head and neck[469,470] and esophagus,[471] renal cell carcinoma, anaplastic thyroid carcinoma, and malignant melanoma are notorious for mimicking sarcomas microscopically. Sometimes histochemical procedures and electron microscopy are necessary to demonstrate their epithelial nature.

REFERENCES

1. Enzinger FM, Lattes R, Torloni H: Histologic Typing of Soft Tissue Tumors. World Health Organization, Geneva, 1969
2. Enzinger F, Smith B: Hemangiopericytoma: An analysis of 106 cases. Hum Pathol 7:61, 1976
3. Evans DJ, Azzopardi JG: Distinctive tumors of bone and soft tissue causing acquired Vitamin-D-resistant osteomalacia. Lancet 1:353, 1972
4. Weidner N, Santa-Cruz D: Phosphaturic mesenchymal tumors. A polymorphous group causing osteomalacia or rickets. Cancer 59:1442, 1987
5. Gorlin RJ: Some soft tissue heritable tumors. Birth Defects 12:72, 1976
6. Stout AP, Lattes R: Tumors of the soft tissues. p. 38. In Atlas of Tumor Pathology, Ser. 2, Fasc. 1. Armed Forces Institute of Pathology, Washington, DC, 1967
7. Wells HG: Adipose tissue: A neglected subject. JAMA 114:2, 1940
8. Malan E, Puglionisi A: Congenital angiodysplasias of the extremities. Generalities and classifications. Venous dysplasias. J Cardiovasc Surg 5:87, 1964
9. Malan E, Puglionisi A: Congenital angiodysplasias of the extremities. Arterial, arterial and venous and hemolymphatic dysplasias. J Cardiovasc Surg 6:255, 1965
10. Bissada M, White JH, Sun CN, et al: Tuberous sclerosis complex and renal angiomyolipoma. Urology 6:105, 1975
11. Valensi QJ: Pulmonary lymphangiomyoma, a probable forme fruste of tuberlous sclerosis. Am Rev Respir Dis 108:1, 411, 1973
12. Jao J, Gilbert S, Messer R: Lymphangiomyoma and tuberous sclerosis. Cancer 29:1, 188, 1972
13. Simpson RD, Harrison EG Jr, Mayo CW: Mesenteric fibromatosis in familial polyposis. Cancer 17:526, 1964
14. Fisher WC, Helwig EB: Leiomyomas of the skin. Arch Dermatol 88:78, 1963
15. Ducatman BS, Scheithauer BW, Piepgras DR, Reiman HM: Malignant peripheral nerve sheath tumor: A clinicopathologic review of 120 cases. Cancer 57:2006, 1986
16. Usui M, Ishui S, Yamawaki S, Hirayama T: The occurrence of soft tissue sarcomas in three siblings with Werner's syndrome. Cancer 54:2580, 1984
17. de Santos AL, Ginaldi S, Wallace S: Computed tomography in liposarcoma. Cancer 47:46, 1981
18. Sartoris DJ, Resnick D: MR imaging of the musculoskeletal system: Current and future status. Am J Radiol 149:457, 1987
19. Martel W: Radiologic evaluation of soft tissue tumors. p. 865. In Proceedings of the Seventh National Cancer Conference. JB Lippincott, Philadelphia, 1973
20. Waligore MP, Stephens DH, Soule EH, et al: Lipomatous tumors of the abdominal cavity: CT appearance and pathologic correlation. AJR 137:539, 1981
21. Ekelund L, Laurin S, Lunderquist A: Comparison of a vasoconstrictor and a vasodilator in pharmacoangiography of bone and soft tissue tumors. Radiology 122:95, 1977
22. Yaghmai I: Angiographic features of fibromas and fibrosarcomas. Radiology 124:57, 1977
23. Yaghmai I: Angiographic manifestations of soft tissue and osseous hemangiopericytoma. Radiology 126:653, 1978
24. Angervall L, Kindbloom L-G, Nielsen JM, et al: Hemangiopericytoma: A clinicopathologic, angiographic and microangiographic study. Cancer 42:2, 412, 1978
25. Bottles K, Cohen MB, Sacks ST: Clinical perception of fine needle aspiration cytology. Diagn Cytopathol 1:249, 1985
26. Chess Q, Hajdu SI: The role of immunoperoxidase staining in diagnostic cytology. Acta Cytol (Baltimore) 30:1, 1986
27. Dahl I, Akerman M: Nodular fasciitis. A correlative cytologic and histologic study of 13 cases. Acta Cytol (Baltimore) 25:215, 1981
28. Rydholm A, Akerman M, Idvall I, et al: Aspiration of cytology of soft tissue tumors. A prospective study of its influence on choice of surgical procedures. Int Orthop 6:209, 1982
29. Akerman M, Rydholm A: Cytodiagnosis of intramuscular myxoma. A comparative clinical, cytologic and histologic study of ten cases. Acta Cytol (Baltimore) 5:505, 1983
30. Akerman M, Rydholm A, Persson BM: Aspiration cytology of soft tissue tumors. Acta Orthop Scand 56:407, 1985
31. Walaas L, Kindblom LG: Lipomatous tumors. Correlative cytologic and histologic study of 27 tumors examined by fine needle aspiration cytology. Hum Pathol 16:6, 1985
32. Walaas L, Angervall L, Hagmar B, et al: A correlative cytologic and histologic study of malignant fibrous histiocytoma: An analysis of 40 cases examined by fine needle aspiration cytology. Diagn Cytopathol 2:46, 1986
33. Hales M, Bottles K, Miller T, Donegar E, Ljung BM: Diagnosis of Kaposi's sarcoma by fine needle aspiration biopsy. Am J Clin Pathol 88:20, 1987
34. Ordonez NG, Hickey RC, Brooks TE: Alveolar soft part sarcoma. A cytologic and immunohistochemical study. Cancer 61:525, 1988
35. Angervall L, Kindblom LG, Rydholm A, Stener B: The diagnosis and prognosis of soft tissue tumors. Semin Diagn Pathol 3:240, 1986
36. Fine G, Horn RC: Soft tissue tumors: Aids in differential diagnosis. Pathol Annu 4:211, 1969
37. Murray MR, Stout AP: The classification and diagnosis of human tumors by tissue culture methods. Tex Rep Biol Med 12:898, 1954
38. Ozzello L, Stout AP, Murray MR: Cultural characteristics of malignant fibrous histiocytomas and fibrous xanthomas. Cancer 16:331, 1963

39. Escalona-Zapata J, Fernandez EA, Escuin FL: The fibro-blastic nature of dermatofibrosarcoma protuberans: A tissue culture and ultrastructural study. Virchows Arch 391:165, 1981

40. Morales AR: Electron microscopy of human tumors. Prog Surg Pathol 1:51, 1980

41. van Haelst U: General considerations on electron microscopy of tumors of soft tissues. Prog Surg Pathol 2:225, 1980

42. Alguacil-Garcia A, Unni KK, Goellner JR: Histogenesis of dermatofibrosarcoma protuberans: An ultrastructural study. Am J Clin Pathol 69:427, 1978

43. Hoffman MA, Dickersin GR: Malignant fibrous histiocytoma: An ultrastructural study of eleven cases. Hum Pathol 14:913, 1983

44. Weibel ER, Palade GE: New cytoplasmic components in arterial endothelia. J Cell Biol 23:101, 1964

45. Rosai J, Sumner HW, Kostianovsky M, et al: Angiosarcoma of the skin: A clinicopathologic and fine structural study. Hum Pathol 7:83, 1976

46. Ferenczy A, Richart RM, Okagaki T: A comparative ultrastructural study of leiomyosarcoma, cellular leiomyoma and leiomyoma of the uterus. Cancer 28:1004, 1971

47. Napolitano L: The differentiation of white adipose cells. J Cell Biol 8:663, 1963

48. Kalderon AE, Fethiere W: Fine structure of liposarcomas. Lab Invest 28:60, 1973

49. Rossouw DJ, Cinti S, Dickersin GR: Liposarcoma. An ultrastructural study of 15 cases. Am J Clin Pathol 85:649, 1986

50. Kaye GI: The futility of electron microscopy in determining the origin of poorly differentiated soft tissue tumors. Prog Surg Pathol 3:171, 1981

51. Nadji M, Gonzalez MS, Castro A, et al: Factor VIII-related antigen. An endothelial cell marker (abstract). Lab Invest 42:139, 1980

52. Mukai K, Rosai J, Hallaway BE: Localization of myoglobin in normal and neoplastic skeletal muscle cells using an immunoperoxidase method. Am J Surg Pathol 3:373, 1979

53. Corson JM, Pinkus GS: Intracellular myoglobin—A specific marker for skeletal muscle differentiation in soft tissue sarcomas. Am J Pathol 105:384, 1981

54. Ordonez NG, Batsakis FG: Comparison of Ulex europeus I lectin and factor VIII-related antigen in vascular lesions. Arch Pathol Lab Med 108:129, 1984

55. Capo V, Ozzelo L, Fenoglio CM, Lombardi L, Rilke F: Angiosarcomas arising in edematous extremities: Immunostaining for Factor VIII-related antigen and ultrastructural features. Hum Pathol 16:144, 1985

56. Miettinen M, Lehto VP, Badley RA, Virtanen I: Alveolar rhabdomyosarcoma—Demonstration of the muscle type of intermediate filament protein, desmin, as a diagnostic aid. Am J Pathol 108:246, 1982

57. de Jong ASH, Van Vark M, Albus-Lutter CE, et al: Myosin and myoglobin as tumor markers in the diagnosis of rhabdomyosarcoma. Am J Surg Pathol 8:521, 1984

58. Molenaar WM, Oosterhuis JW, Oosterhius AM, Ramaekers FCS: Mesenchymal and muscle-specific intermediate filaments (vimentin and desmin) in relation to differentia-tion in childhood rhabdomyosarcomas. Hum Pathol 16:838, 1985

59. Leader M, Collins JPM, Henry K: 1-antichymotripsin staining of 194 sarcomas, 38 carcinomas and 17 malignant melanomas. Its lack of specificity as a tumor marker. Am J Surg Pathol 11:133, 1987

60. Nakajima T, Watanabe S, Sato Y, et al: An immunoperoxidase study of S-100 protein distribution in normal and neoplastic tissues. Am J Surg Pathol 6:715, 1982

61. Strauchen JA, Dimitriu-Bona A: Malignant fibrous histiocytoma. Expression of monocyte/macrophage differentiation antigens detected with monoclonal antibodies. Am J Pathol 124:303, 1986

62. Rooser B, Attewell R, Rydholm A: The staging of soft tissue sarcoma. Int Orthop In Press.

63. Rooser B, Attewell R, Berg N, Rydholm A: Prognostication in soft tissue sarcoma. A model with four risk factors. Cancer 61:817, 1988

64. Costa J, Wesley RA, Glatstein E, Rosenberg SA: The grading of soft tissue sarcomas. Results of a clinico-pathologic correlation in a series of 163 cases. Cancer 53:530, 1984

65. Condre JM, Bui NB, Bonochon F, et al: Histopathologic grading in spindle cell soft tissue sarcomas. Cancer 61:2305, 1988

66. Crockett DJ: Regional keloid susceptibility. Br J Plast Surg 17:245, 1964

67. Osman AAA, Gumma KA, Satir AA: Highlights on the etiology of keloid. Int Surg 63:33, 1978

68. Barr JR: Elastofibroma. Am J Clin Pathol 45:679, 1966

69. Peters JL, Fisher CS: Elastofibroma. J Thorac Cardiovasc Surg 75:836, 1978

70. Fajardo LF, Berthrong M: Radiation injury in surgical pathology. Part I. Am J Surg Pathol 2:159, 1981

71. Ormand JK: Idiopathic retroperitoneal fibrosis. A discussion of the etiology. J Urol 94:385, 1965

72. Lepor H, Walsh PC: Idiopathic retroperitoneal fibrosis. J Urol 122:1, 1979

73. Webb AJ, Dawson-Edwards P: Malignant retroperitoneal fibrosis. Br J Surg 54:505, 1967

74. Webb AJ, Dawson-Edwards P: Non-malignant retroperitoneal fibrosis. Br J Surg 54:508, 1967

75. Clyne CH, Ambethrombe GF: Perianeurysmal retroperitoneal fibrosis. Two cases responding to steroids. Br J Urol 49:463, 1977

76. Drugs and retroperitoneal fibrosis (Editorial). Lancet 1:969, 1966

77. Chan SL, Jonson HW, McLoughlin MC: Idiopathic retroperitoneal fibrosis in children. J Urol 122:103, 1979

78. Smith BH: Peyronie's disease. Am J Clin Pathol 45:670, 1966

79. Billig R, Baker R, Immergut M, et al: Peyronie's disease. Urology 6:409, 1975

80. Chesney J: Peyronie's disease. Br J Urol 47:209, 1975

81. Bodner H: Peyronie's disease revisited. Int Surg 63:69, 1978

82. Luck JV: Dupuytren's contracture: A new concept of the pathogenesis correlated with surgical management. J Bone Joint Surg [Am] 41:635, 1959

83. Gabbiani G, Majno G: Dupuytren's contracture: Fibroblast contraction. Am J Pathol 66:131, 1972

84. Pickren JW, Smith AG, Stevenson TW, et al: Fibromatosis of the plantar fascia. Cancer 4:846, 1951

85. Aviles E, Arlen M, Miller T: Plantar fibromatosis. Surgery 69:117, 1971

86. Pryor JP, Khan O: Beta blockers and Peyronie's disease (letter). Lancet 1:331, 1979

87. Fu Y-S, Perzin KH: Nonepithelial tumors of the nasal cavity, paranasal sinus, and nasopharynx: A clinicopathologic study. I. General features and vascular tumors. Cancer 33:275, 1974

88. Neel HB III, Whicker JH, Devine KD, et al: Juvenile angiofibroma: Review of 120 cases. Am J Surg 126:547, 1973

89. Hicks JL, Nelson JF: Juvenile nasopharyngeal angiofibroma. Oral Surg 35:807, 1973

90. Gonsalves CG, Briant TDR: Radiologic findings in nasopharyngeal angiofibromas. J Can Assoc Radiol 29:209, 1978

91. Lee DA, Rao BR, Meyer JS, et al: Hormonal receptor determination in juvenile nasopharyngeal angiofibromas. Cancer 46:547, 1980

92. Mackenzie DH: The fibromatoses: A clinicopathologic concept. Br Med J 4:277, 1972

93. Allen PW: The fibromatoses: A clinicopathologic classification based on 140 cases. Parts 1 and 2. Am J Surg Pathol 1:255, 1977

94. Das Gupta TK, Brasfield RD, O'Hara J: Extra-abdominal desmoids. A clinicopathological study. Ann Surg 170:109, 1969

95. Conley JWVH, Stout AP: Fibromatosis of the head and neck. Am J Surg 112:609, 1966

96. Masson JK, Soule EH: Desmoid tumors of the head and neck. Am J Surg 112:615, 1966

97. Enzinger FM, Shiraki M: Musculo-aponeurotic fibromatosis of the shoulder girdle (extra-abdominal desmoid). Analysis of 30 cases followed up for 10 or more years. Cancer 21:1131, 1967

98. Pritchard DJ, Soule EH, Taylor WF, et al: Fibrosarcoma—A clinico-pathologic and statistical study of 199 tumors of the soft tissues of the extremities and trunk. Cancer 33:888, 1974

99. Weary PPE, Linthicum A, Cawley EP, et al: Gardner's syndrome. A family group and review. Arch Dermatol 90:20, 1964

100. Gardner EJ: Follow-up study of a family group exhibiting dominant inheritance for a syndrome including intestinal polyps, osteomas, fibromas and epidermal cysts. Am J Hum Genet 14:376, 1982

101. Simpson RD, Harrison EG, Mayo CW: Mesenteric fibromatosis in familial polyposis. Cancer 17:526, 1964

102. Ayala AG, Ro JY, Goepfert H, et al: Desmoid fibromatosis: A clinicopathologic study of 25 children. Semin Diagn Pathol 3:138, 1986

103. Rock MG, Pritchard DJ, Reiman HM, et al: Extraabdominal desmoid tumors. J Bone Joint Surg [Am] 66:1369, 1984

104. Woyke A, Domagala W, Olszuvski WW: Ultrastructure of a fibromatosis hyalinica multiplex juvenilis. Cancer 26:1157, 1970

105. Gutierrez G: Fibromatosis hialinica juvenil. A proposito de un caso. Med Cut 7:283, 1973

106. Kitano Y: Juvenile hyalin fibromatosis. Arch Dermatol 112:86, 1976

107. Stout AP: Juvenile fibromatosis. Cancer 7:953, 1954

108. Rosenberg HS, Stenback WA, Spjut HG: The fibromatoses of infancy and childhood. Persp Pediatric Pathol 4:269, 1978

109. Roggli VL, Kim H-S, Hawkins, E: Congenital generalized fibromatosis with visceral involvement. Cancer 45:954, 1980

110. Briselli MF, Soule EH, Gilchrist GS: Congenital fibromatosis. Report of 18 cases of solitary and 4 cases of multiple tumors. Mayo Clin Proc 55:554, 1980

111. Stout AP: Fibrosarcoma in infants and children. Cancer 15:1028, 1962

112. Balsaver AM, Butler JJ, Martin RG: Congenital fibrosarcoma. Cancer 20:1607, 1967

113. Chung EB, Enzinger FM: Infantile fibrosarcoma. Cancer 38:729, 1976

114. Yurosko JJ, Wall TM, Vopal JJ, et al: Idiopathic gingival fibromatosis. J Oral Surg 35:820, 1977

115. Enzinger FM: Fibrous hamartoma of infancy. Cancer 18:241, 1965

116. Greco MA, Schinella RA, Vuletin JC: Fibrous hamartoma of infancy. An ultrastructural study. Hum Pathol 15:517, 1984

117. Keasbey LF: Juvenile aponeurotic fibroma (calcifying fibroma). Cancer 6:338, 1953

118. Allen PW, Enzinger FM: Juvenile aponeurotic fibroma. Cancer 26:857, 1970

119. Goldman RL: The cartilage analogue of fibromatosis (aponeurotic fibroma). Further observations based on 7 new cases. Cancer 26:1325, 1970

120. Beckett JH, Jacobs AH: Recurring digital fibrous tumors of childhood. A review. Pediatrics 59:401, 1977

121. Santa Cruz DJ, Reiner CB: Recurrent digital fibroma of childhood. J Cutan Pathol 5:339, 1978

122. Finges B, Thais H, Bohm N, et al: Identification of actin microfilaments in the intracytoplasmic inclusions present in recurring infantile digital fibromatosis (Reye tumor). Pediatr Pathol 6:311, 1986

123. Iwasaki H, Kikuchi M, Ohtsuki I, et al: Infantile digital fibromatosis: Identification of actin filaments in cytoplasmic inclusions by heavy meromyosin binding. Cancer 52:1653, 1983

124. Purdy LJ, Colby TV: Infantile digital fibromatosis occurring outside the digit. Am J Surg Pathol 8:787, 1984

125. Yun K: Infantile digital fibromatosis. Immunohistochemical and ultrastructural observations of cytoplasmic inclusions. Cancer 61:500, 1988

126. Chung EB, Enzinger FM: Fibroma of tendon sheath. Cancer 44:1, 945, 1979

127. Lundgren LG, Kindblom LG: Fibroma of tendon sheath. A light and electron microscopic study of 6 cases. Acta Pathol Microbiol Immunol Scand 92:401, 1984

128. Dymock RB, Allen PW, Stirling JW, et al: Giant cell fi-

broblastoma. A distinctive, recurrent tumor of childhood. Am J Surg Pathol 11:263, 1987

129. Shmookler BM, Enzinger FM: Giant cell fibroblastoma: A peculiar childhood tumor. Lab Invest 46:76A, 1983

130. Enzinger FM: Intramuscular myxoma: A review and follow-up study of 34 cases. Am J Clin Pathol 43:104, 1965

131. Rosen RD: Intramuscular myxomas. Br J Surg 60:122, 1973

132. Kindblom LG, Sten B, Angervall L: Intramuscular myxoma. Cancer 34:1737, 1974

133. Ireland DCR, Soule EH, Irvins JC: Myxoma of somatic soft tissues: A report of 58 patients, 3 with multiple tumor and fibrous dysplasia of bone. Mayo Clin Proc 48:401, 1973

134. Feldman PS: A comparative study of intramuscular myxoma and myxoid liposarcoma. Cancer 43:512, 1979

135. Soule EH, Enriquez P: Atypical fibrous histiocytoma, malignant fibrous histiocytoma, malignant histiocytoma and epithelioid sarcoma: A comparative study of 65 cases. Cancer 30:128, 1973

136. Fletcher CDM, McKee PH: Sarcomas—A clinicopathological guide with particular reference to cutaneous manifestation. I. Dermatofibrosarcoma protuberans, malignant fibrous histiocytoma and the epithelioid sarcoma of Enzinger. Clin Exp Dermatol 9:451, 1984

137. Fu YS, Gabbianai G, Kaye GI, et al: Malignant soft tissue tumors of probable histiocyte origin (malignant fibrous histiocytoma). General considerations and electron microscope and tissue culture studies. Cancer 35:176, 1975

138. Weiss SW, Enzinger FM: Malignant fibrous histiocytoma: An analysis of 200 cases. Cancer 41:250, 1978

139. Kempson RL, Kyriakos M: Fibroxanthosarcoma of the soft tissues: A type of malignant fibrous histiocytoma. Cancer 29:961, 1972

140. Kearney MM, Soule EH, Ivins JC: Malignant fibrous histiocytoma. A retrospective study of 167 cases. Cancer 45:167, 1980

141. Bertoni F, Cappana R, Biagini R, et al: Malignant fibrous histiocytoma of soft tissue. An analysis of 78 cases located and deeply seated in the extremities. Cancer 56:356, 1985

142. Hashimoto H, Enjoji M: Recurrent malignant fibrous histiocytoma. A histologic analysis of 50 cases. Am J Surg Pathol 5:753, 1981

143. Raney RB Jr, Allen A, O'Neill J, et al: Malignant fibrous histiocytoma of soft tissue in childhood. Cancer 57:2198, 1986

144. Taxy JB, Battifora H: Malignant fibrous histiocytoma. An electron microscopic study. Cancer 40:254, 1977

145. Kyriakos M, Kempson RL: Inflammatory fibrous histiocytoma: An aggressive and lethal lesion. Cancer 37:1584, 1976

146. Harcy TJ, An T, Brown PW, Terz JJ: Post-irradiation sarcoma (malignant fibrous histiocytoma) of axilla. Cancer 42:118, 1978

147. Kin JH, Chu FC, Woodard HQ, et al: Radiation-induced soft tissue and bone sarcoma. Radiology 129:501, 1979

148. Weinberg DS, Maini BS: Primary sarcoma of the aorta associated with a vascular prosthesis. A case report. Cancer 46:398, 1980

149. Inoshita T, Youngberg GA: Malignant fibrous histiocytoma in previous surgical sites. Report of two cases. Cancer 53:176, 1984

150. Weiss SW, Enzinger FM: Myxoid variant of malignant fibrous histiocytoma. Cancer 39:1672, 1977

151. Guccion JG, Enzinger FM: Malignant giant cell tumor of soft parts. An analysis of 32 cases. Cancer 29:1518, 1972

152. Salm R, Sissons HA: Giant cell tumors of soft tissues. J Pathol 107:27, 1972

153. Alguacil-Garcia A, Unni K, Goellner J: Malignant giant cell tumor of soft parts. An ultrastructural study of four cases. Cancer 40:244, 1977

154. Angerwall L, Hagmar B, Kindblom LG, Merck C: Malignant giant cell tumor of soft tissues. A clinicopathologic, cytologic, ultrastructural, angiographic and microangiographic study. Cancer 47:736, 1981

155. Gould E, Albores-Saavedra J, Roth M, et al: Malignant giant cell tumor of soft parts presenting as a skin tumor. Am J Dermatopathol, in press

156. Enzinger FM: Angiomatoid malignant fibrous histiocytoma. A distinct fibrohistiocytic tumor of children and young adults simulating a vacular neoplasm. Cancer 44:147, 1979

157. Wegmann W, Heitz PU: Angiomatoid malignant fibrous histiocytoma. Evidence for the histiocytic origin of tumor cells. Virchows Arch 406:59, 1985

158. Kay S: Angiomatoid malignant fibrous histiocytoma. Report of two cases with ultrastructural observations of one case. Arch Pathol Lab Med 109:934, 1985

159. Taylor HB, Helwig EB: Dermatofibrosarcoma protuberans, a study of 114 cases. Cancer 15:717, 1962

160. Dupree WB, Langloss JN, Weiss SW: Pigmented dermatofibrous sarcoma protuberance (Bednar tumor). A pathologic ultrastructural and immunohistochemical study. Am J Surg Pathol 9:630, 1985

161. Jones FE, Soule EH, Coventry MB: Fibrous histiocytoma of synovium (giant cell tumor of tendon sheath, pigmented nodular synovitis). J Bone Joint Surg [Am] 51:76, 1969

162. Ushijima M, Hashimoto H, Tsuneyoshi M, Enjoji M: Giant cell tumor of the tendon sheath (nodular tenosynovitis). A study of 207 cases to compare the large joint group with the common digit group. Cancer 57:875, 1986

163. Kindblom LG, Gunterberg B: Pigmented villonodular synovitis involving bone. J Bone Joint Surg [Am] 60:830, 1978

164. Wood GS, Beckstead JH, Medeiros JL, et al: The cells of giant cell tumor of tendon sheath resemble osteoclasts. Am J Surg Pathol 12:444, 1988

165. Kahn LB: Malignant cell tumor of the tendon sheath. Arch Pathol Lab Med 95:203, 1973

166. Carstens PHB, Howell RS: Malignant giant cell tumor of tendon sheath. Virchows Arch 382:237, 1979

167. Signen RD, Bregman D, Klausner S: Giant lipoma of the mesentery: Report of an unusual case and review of the literature. Am Surg 42:595, 1976

168. Bennhoff DF, Wood JW: Infiltrating lipomata of the head and neck. Laryngoscope 88:839, 1978

159. Politis J, Funchashi A, Gehlsen JA, et al: Intrathoracic

lipomas: Report of three cases and review of the literature with emphasis on endobronchial lipoma. J Thorac Cardiovasc Surg 77:550, 1979

170. Weitzner S, Blumenthal BI, Moynihan PC: Retroperitoneal lipoma in children. J Pediatr Surg 14:88, 1979

171. Banny JM, Bilbao MK, Hodges CV: Pelvic lipomatosis: A rare cause of suprapubic mass. J Urol 109:592, 1973

172. Kauffman SL, Stout AP: Lipoblastic tumors of children. Cancer 12:912, 1959

173. Yaghmai I, Mickouwne F, Alizadeh A: Macrodactilya: Fibrolipomatosis. South Med J 69:1565, 1976

174. Howard WR, Helwig ER: Angiolipoma. Arch Dermatol 82:924, 1960

175. Belcher RW, Czarnetzki BM, Carney JF: Multiple (subcutaneous) angiolipomas. Clinical, pathologic and pharmacologic studies. Arch Dermatol 110:583, 1974

176. Lin JJ, Lin F: Two entities in angliolipoma: A study of 459 cases of lipoma with review of the literature on infiltrating angiolipoma. Cancer 34:720, 1974

177. Hajdu SI, Foote FW Jr: Angiomyolipoma of the kidney: Report of 27 cases and review of the literature. J Urol 102:396, 1969

178. Farrow GM, Harrison EG Jr, Utz DC, et al: Angiomyolipoma. A clinicopathologic study of 32 cases. Cancer 22:564, 1968

179. Busch FM, Bark JC, Clyde HR: Benign renal angiomyolipoma with regional lymph node involvement. J Urol 116:715, 1976

180. Bloom DA, Scardino PT, Ehrlich RM, et al: The significance of lymph nodal involvement in renal angiomyolipoma. J Urol 128:1292, 1982

181. Brecher ME, Gill WB, Strauss FH: Angiomyolipoma with regional lymph node involvement and long-term follow-up study. Hum Pathol 17:962, 1986

182. Hartveit F, Halleraker B: A report of three angiolipomyomata and one angiolipomyosarcoma. Acta Pathol Microbiol Scand 49:329, 1960

183. Berg JW: Angiomyoliposarcoma (malignant hamartomatous angiomyolipoma) in a case with solitary metastasis from bronchogenic carcinoma. Cancer 8:759, 1955

184. Benson PA, Janko AB: Pelvic myelolipoma (rare presacral tumor). Am J Obstet Gynecol 92:884, 1965

185. Dodge OG, Evans DMD: Haemopoiesis in a presacral fatty tumor (myelolipoma). J Pathol 72:313, 1956

186. Burrows S, Drake WM Jr, Singley TL: Large retroperitoneal myelolipoma associated with acute myelogenous leukemia. Am J Clin Pathol 52:733, 1969

187. Wilhelmus JL, Schrodt GR, Alberhasky MT, Alcorn MO: Giant adrenal myelolipoma. Arch Pathol Lab Med 105:532, 1981

188. Bennett BD, McKenna TJ, Hough AJ et al: Adrenal myelolipoma associated with Cushing's disease. Am J Clin Pathol 73:443, 1980

189. Vyberg M, Sestoft L: Combined adrenal myelolipoma and adenoma associated with Cushing's syndrome. Am J Clin Pathol 86:541, 1986

190. Enziner FM, Harvey DA: Spindle cell lipoma. Cancer 36:1, 852, 1975

191. Kitano M, Enjoji M, Iwasaki H: Spindle cell lipoma. A clinico-pathologic analysis of twelve cases. Acta Pathol Jpn 29:891, 1979

192. Fletcher CD, Martin-Bates E: Spindle cell lipoma. A clinico-pathological study with some original observations. Histopathology 11:803, 1987

193. Bolen JW, Thorning D: Spindle cell lipoma. A clinical, light and electron microscopic study. Am J Surg Pathol 5:435, 1981

194. Warkel RL, Rehme CG, Thompson WH: Vascular spindle cell lipoma. J Cutan Pathol 9:113, 1982

195. Shnookler BM, Enzinger FM: Pleomorphic lipoma: A benign tumor simulating liposarcoma. A clinico-pathologic analysis of 48 cases. Cancer 47:126, 1981

196. Azzopardi JG, Iocco J, Salm R: Pleomorphic lipoma: A tumor simulating liposarcoma. Histopathology 7:511, 1983

197. Evans HL, Soule EH, Winklemann RK: Atypical lipoma, atypical intramuscular lipoma, and well differentiated retroperitoneal liposarcoma. Cancer 43:574, 1979

198. Kindblom LG, Angerwall L, Fassina AS: Atypical lipoma. Acta Pathol Microbiol Immunol Scand 90:27, 1982

199. Azumi V, Curtis J, Kempson RL, Hendrickson MR: A typical and malignant neoplasms showing lipomatous differentiation. A study of 111 cases. Am J Surg Pathol 11:161, 1987

200. Vellios F, Baez J, Shumacker HB: Lipoblastomatosis: A tumor of fetal fat different from hibernoma. Am J Pathol 34:1149, 1958

201. Chung EB, Enzinger FM: Benign lipoblastomatosis: An analysis of 35 cases. Cancer 32:482, 1973

202. Greco MA, Garcia RL, Vuletin JC: Benign lipoblastomatosis: Ultrastructure and histogenesis. Cancer 45:5100, 1980

203. Hanada M, Tokuda R, Ohnishi Y, et al: Benign lipoblastoma and liposarcoma in children. Acta Pathol Jpn 36:605, 1986

204. Gaffney EF, Vellios F, Hargreaves HK: Lipoblastomatosis: Ultrastructure of two cases and relationship to human fetal white adipose tissue. Pediatr Pathol 5:207, 1986

205. Jimenez JF: Lipoblastoma in infancy and childhood. J Surg Oncol 32:238, 1986

206. Dardik IU: Hibernoma: A possible model of brown fat histogenesis. Hum Pathol 9:321, 1978

207. Levine GD: Hibernoma: An electron microscopic study. Hum Pathol 3:351, 1972

208. Seemayer TA, Knaak J, Wang N-S, et al: On the ultrastructure of hibernoma. Cancer 36:785, 1975

209. Albores-Saavedra J, Alonso-Viveros P, Larraza O: Hibernoma maligno con metastasis pulmonares. Patologia 6:240, 1980

210. Enterline HT, Lowry LD, Richman AV: Does malignant hibernoma exist? Am J Surg Pathol 3:265, 1979

211. Angervall L, Bjorntorp P, Stener B: The lipid composition of hibernoma as compared to that of lipoma and of mouse brown fat. Cancer Res 25:408, 1965

212. Jeanrenaud B: Lipid components of adipose tissue. p. 169. In Handbook of Physiology. American Physiological Society, Washington DC, 1965

213. Shmookler BM, Enzinger FM: Liposarcoma occurring in

children. An analysis of 17 cases and review of the literature. Cancer 52:567, 1983

214. Enzinger FM, Winslow DJ: Liposarcoma: A study of 103 cases. Virchows Arch 335:367, 1962

215. Evans HL: Liposarcoma. A study of 55 cases with a reassessment of its classification. Am J Surg Pathol 3:507, 1979

216. Kimbrough RF, Soule EB: Liposarcoma of the extremities. Clin Orthop 19:40, 1971

217. Reszel PA, Soule EH, Coventry MB: Liposarcomas of extremities and limb girdles. Study of 222 cases. J Bone Joint Surg [Am] 48:229, 1966

218. Enterline HT, Culberson JD, Rochlin DB, et al: Liposarcoma: A clinical and pathological study of 53 cases. Cancer 13:392, 1960

219. Kindblom LG, Save-Soderbergh J: The ultrastructure of liposarcoma. A study of 10 cases. Acta Pathol Microbiol Scand 87:109, 1979

220. Klopfer HW, Krafchuk J, Dubes V, et al: Hereditary multiple leiomyoma of the skin. Am J Hum Genet 10:48, 1958

221. Jansen LH, Driessen FML: Leiomyoma Cutis. Br J Dermatol 70:446, 1958

222. Fisher WC, Helwig EB: Leiomyomas of the skin. Arch Dermatol 88:510, 1963

223. Smith LJ Jr: Tumors of the corium. p. 533. In Helwig EB, Mostofi FK (eds): The Skin. International Academy of Pathology Monograph. Williams & Wilkins, Baltimore, 1971

224. Botting AJ, Soule EH, Brown AL Jr: Smooth muscle tumors in children. Cancer 18:711, 1965

225. Nascimenta AG, Karas M, Rosen PP, et al: Leiomyoma of the nipple. Am J Surg Pathol 3:151, 1979

226. Hachisuga T, Hashimoto H, Enjoji M: Angioleiomyoma. A clinico-pathologic reappraisal of 562 cases. Cancer 54:126, 1984

227. Goodman AH, Briggs RC: Deep leiomyoma in an extremity. J Bone Joint Surg [Am] 47:529, 1965

228. Bulmer JH: Smooth muscle tumors of the limbs. J Bone Joint Surg [Br] 49:52, 1967

229. Ledesma-Medina J, Oh KS, Girdany BR: Calcifications in childhood leiomyoma. Radiology 135:339, 1980

230. Shmookler BM, Lauer DH: Retroperitoneal leiomyosarcoma. A clinico-pathologic analysis of 36 cases. Am J Surg Pathol 7:269, 1983

231. Wile AG, Evans HL, Romsdahl MM: Leiomyosarcoma of soft tissue. A clinico-pathologic study. Cancer 48:1022, 1981

232. Fields JP, Helwig EB: Leiomyosarcomas of the skin and subcutaneous tissue. Cancer 47:156, 1981

233. Berlin O, Stener B, Lars-Gunner K, Angervall L: Leiomyosarcoma of venous origin in the extremities. Cancer 54:2147, 1984

234. Varela-Duran J, Oliva H, Rosai J: Vascular leiomyosarcoma. The malignant counterpart of vascular leiomyoma. Cancer 44:1684, 1979

235. Seo IS, Warner TFCS, Glant MD: Retroperitoneal leiomyosarcoma: A light and electron microscopic study. Histopathology 4:53, 1980

236. Tsukada T, Tippens D, Gordon D, et al: HHF 35, a muscle actin-specific monoclonal antibody: I. Immunocytochemical and biochemical characterization. Am J Pathol 126:51, 1984

237. Miettinen M: Immunoreactivity for cytokeratin and epithelial membrane antigen in leiomyosarcoma. Arch Pathol Lab Med 112:637, 1988

238. Brown DC, Theaker JM, Banks PM, et al: Cytokeratin expression in smooth muscle tumors. Histopathology 11:477, 1987

239. Norton AJ, Thomas AJ, Isaacson PG: Cytokeratin-specific monoclonal antibodies are reactive with tumors of smooth muscle derivation: An immunocytochemical and biochemical study using antibodies to intermediate filament cytoskeletal proteins. Histopathology 11:487, 1987

240. Di Sant'Agnese PA, Knowles DM II: Extracardiac rhabdomyoma: A clinico-pathologic study and review of the literature. Cancer 46:780, 1980

241. Solomon MP, Tolete-Velcek F: Lingual rhabdomyoma (adult variant) in a child. J Pediatr Surg 14:91, 1979

242. Scrivner D, Meyer JS: Multifocal recurrent adult rhabdomyoma. Cancer 46:790, 1980

243. Moran JJ, Enterline HT: Benign rhabdomyoma of the pharynx: A case report, review of the literature and comparison with cardiac rhabdomyosarcoma. Am J Clin Pathol 42:174, 1964

244. Goldman RL: Multicentric benign rhabdomyoma of skeletal muscle. Cancer 16:1609, 1963

245. Leone PG, Taylor HB: Ultrastructure of a benign polypoid rhabdomyoma of the vagina. Cancer 31:414, 1973

246. Gold JH, Bossen EH: Benign vaginal rhabdomyoma: A light and electron microscopic study. Cancer 37:283, 1976

247. Czernobilsky B, Cornog JL Jr, Enterline HT: Rhabdomyoma: Report of a case with ultrastructural and histochemical studies. Am J Clin Pathol 49:782, 1968

248. Dehner LP, Enzinger FM, Font RL: Fetal rhabdomyoma. Cancer 30:160, 1972

249. Cornog JL, Gonatas NK: Ultrastructure of rhabdomyoma. J Ultrastruct Res 20:433, 1967

250. Bruni C, Prioleau PG, Ivey HH, et al: New fine structural features of cardiac rhabdomyoma: Report of a case. Cancer 46:2068, 1980

251. Enzinger FM, Siraki M: Alveolar rhabdomyosarcoma. An analysis of 110 cases. 24:18, 1969

252. Bale PM, Parsons RE, Stevens MM: Diagnosis and behavior of juvenile rhabdomyosarcoma. Hum Pathol 14:596, 1983

253. Albores-Saavedra J, Martin RG, Smith JL: Rhabdomyosarcoma: A study of 35 cases. Ann Surg 157:186, 1963

254. Horn RC, Enterline HT: Rhabdomyosarcoma. Clinicopathological study and classification of 39 cases. Cancer 11:181, 1958

255. Gonzalez-Crussi F, Black-Schaffer S: Rhabdomyosarcoma of infancy and childhood. Problems of morphologic classification. Ann J Surg Pathol 3:157, 1979

256. Albores-Saavedra J, Butler JJ, Martin RG: Rhabdomyosarcoma. Clinicopathologic considerations and report of 85 cases. p. 349. In MD Anderson Hospital and Tumor Institute: Tumors of Bone and Soft Tissue. Year Book Medical Publishers, Chicago, 1965

257. Porterfield JF, Zimmerman LE: Rhabdomyosarcoma of the orbit. A clinicopathologic study of 55 cases. Virchow Arch 335:329, 1962

258. Masson JK, Soule EH: Embryonal rhabdomyosarcoma of head and neck: Report of 88 cases. Am J Surg 110:585, 1965

259. Ellenbogen E, Lasky MA: Rhabdomyosarcoma of the orbit in the newborn. Am J Ophthalmol 80:1024, 1975

260. Harlow PJ, Kaufman FR, Siegel SE, Quevedo E: Orbital rhabdomyosarcoma in a neonate. Med Pediatr Oncol 7:123, 1979

261. Molenaar WM, Oosterhuis AM, Ramaekers FCS: The rarity of rhabdomyosarcoma in the adult. A morphologic and immunohistochemical study. Pathol Res Pract 180:400, 1985

262. De Jong ASH, van Kessel-van Vark M, Albus-Lutter ChE: Pleomorphic rhabdomyosarcoma. Immunohistochemistry as a tool for its diagnosis. Hum Pathol 18:298, 1987

263. Morales AR, Fine G, Horn RC: Rhabdomyosarcoma: An ultrastructural appraisal. Pathol Annu 7:81, 1972

264. De Jong ASH, van Vark M, Albus-Lutter CE, et al: Myosin and myoglobin as tumor markers in the diagnosis of rhabdomyosarcoma. A comparative study. Am J Surg Pathol 8:521, 1984

265. De Jong ASH, van Kessel-van Vark M, Albus-Lutter ChE, et al: Skeletal muscle actin as tumor marker in the diagnosis of rhabdomyosarcoma in childhood. Am J Surg Pathol 9:467, 1985

266. Mukai M, Iri H, Torikata C et al: Immunoperoxidase demonstration of a new muscle protein (Z-protein) in myogenic tumors as a diagnostic aid. Am J Pathol 114:164, 1984

267. Watson WL, McCarthy WD: Blood and lymph vessel tumors. A report of 1,056 cases. Surg Gynecol Obstet 71:569, 1940

268. Bland KI, Abney HT, MacGregor AMC, et al: Hemangiomatosis of the colon and anorectum. Case report and a review of the literature. Am Surg 40:626, 1974

269. Hoehn JG, Farrow GM, Devine KD, et al: Invasive hemangioma of the head and neck. Am J Surg 120:495, 1970

270. Balbaa A, Chesterman JT: Neoplasms of vascular origin in the mediastinum. Br J Surg 44:540, 1957

271. Gindhart TD, Tucker W, Choy SH: Cavernous hemangioma of the superior mediastinum. Am J Surg Pathol 3:353, 1979

272. Johnson EW, Ghormley RK, Dockerty MB: Hemangioma of the extremities. Surg Gynecol Obstet 102:531, 1956

273. Johnson WC: Pathology of cutaneous vascular tumors. Int J Dermatol 15:239, 1976

274. Kasabach HH, Merritt KK: Capillary hemangioma with extensive purpura. Am J Dis Child 59:1,063, 1940

275. Rodriguez-Erdmann F, Button L, Murray JE, et al: Kasabach-Merritt syndrome: Coagulo-analytical observations. Am J Med Sci 261:9, 1971

276. Goidanick IF, Campanancci M: Vascular hamartomata and infantile angioectatic osteohyperplasia of the extremities. J Bone Joint Surg [Am] 44:815, 1962

277. Nagao K, Matsuzaki O, Shigematsu H et al: Histopathologic studies of benign infantile hemangioendothelioma of the parotid gland. Cancer 46:2250, 1980

278. Kauffman SL, Stout AP: Malignant hemangioendothelioma in infants and children. Cancer 14:1186, 1961

279. Scott JE: Hemangiomata in skeletal muscle. Br J Surg 44:496, 1957

280. Allen PW, Enzinger FM: Hemangioma of skeletal muscle. Cancer 29:8, 1972

281. Janes J, Musgrove JE: Effect of arteriovenous fistula on growth of bone: An experimental study. Surg Clin North Am 30:1191, 1950

282. Mills SE, Cooper PH, Fechner RE: Lobular capillary hemangioma: The underlying lesion of pyogenic granuloma: A study of 73 cases from the oral and nasal mucous membranes. Am J Surg Pathol 4:471, 1980

283. Cooper PH, McAllister HA, Helwig EB: Intravenous pyogenic granuloma: A study of 18 cases. Am J Surg Pathol 3:221, 1979

284. Ulbright TM, Santa Cruz DJ: Intravenous pyogenic granuloma: Case report with ultrastructural findings. Cancer 45:1646, 1980

285. Warner J, Wilson-Jones E: Pyogenic granuloma recurring with multiple satellites: A report of 11 cases. Br J Dermatol 80:218, 1968

286. Wells GC, Whimster IW: Subcutaneous angiolymphoid hyperplasia with eosinophilia. Br J Dermatol 81:1, 1969

287. Wilson-Jones E, Blehen SS: Inflammatory angiomatous nodules with abnormal blood vessels occurring about the ears and scalp (pseudo or atypical pyogenic granuloma). Br J Dermatol 81:804, 1969

288. Olsen TG, Helwig EB: Angiolymphoid hyperplasia with eosinophilia: A clinico-pathologic study of 116 patients. J Am Acad Dermatol 12:781, 1985

289. Atsumichi U, Tsuneyoshi M, Enjoji M: Epithelioid hemangioma versus Kimura's disease. A comparative clinico-pathologic study. Am J Surg Pathol 11:758, 1987

290. Leboit P, Egbert BM, Stoler MH, et al: Epithelioid hemangioma-like vascular proliferation in AIDS. Manifestation of Cat-Scratch disease bacillus infection. Lancet 111:960, 1988

291. Stout AP: Tumors featuring pericytes: Glomus tumor and hemangiopericytoma. Lab Invest 5:217, 1956

292. Bailey OT: The cutaneous glomus and its tumors, glomangiomas. Am J Pathol 1:915, 1935

293. Murray MR, Stout AP: The glomus tumor: Investigation of its distribution and behavior and the identity of its "epithelioid cell". Am J Pathol 18:183, 1942

294. Kuhn C III, Rosai J: Tumors arising from pericytes: Ultrastructure and organ culture of a case. Arch Pathol Lab Med 88:653, 1969

295. Murad TM, vom Haam E, Narasimha-Murthy MS: Ultrastructure of a hemangiopericytoma and a glomus tumor. Cancer 22:1239, 1968

296. Venkatachalam MA, Greally JG: Fine structure of glomus tumor: Similarity of glomus cells to smooth muscle. Cancer 23:1, 176, 1969

297. Toker C: Glomangioma: An ultrastructural study. Cancer 23:487, 1969

298. Stout AP: Tumors of the neuromyoarterial glomus. Am J Cancer 24:255, 1935

299. Miettinen M, Lehto V-P, Virtanen I: Glomus tumor cells. Evaluation of smooth muscle and endothelial cell properties. Virchows Arch 43:139, 1983

300. Tsuneyoshi M, Enjoji M: Glomus tumor: A clinicopathological and electron microscopic study. Cancer 50:1601, 1982

301. Morales AR, Fine G, Pardo V, et al: The ultrastructure of smooth muscle tumors with a consideration of the possible relationship of glomangioma, hemangiopericytomas, and cardiac myxomas. Pathol Annu 10:65, 1975

302. Shugart RR, Soule EH, Johnson EW Jr: Glomus tumor. Surg Gynecol Obstet 117:340, 1963

303. Almagro UA, Schulte WJ, Norback DH, et al: Glomus tumor of the stomach: Histologic and ultrastructural features. Am J Clin Pathol 75:415, 1981

304. Kohout E, Stout AP: The glomus tumor in children. Cancer 14:555, 1961

305. Lumley JSP, Stansfeld AG: Infiltrating glomus tumor of lower limb. Br Med J 1:484, 1972

306. Gould E, Albores-Saavedra J, Manivel C, Monforte H: Malignant glomus tumor. Submitted.

307. Aiba M, Hirayama A, Kuramochi S: Glomangiosarcoma in a glomus tumor. An immunohistochemical and ultrastructural study. Cancer 61:1467, 1988

308. Dail D, Liebow AA: Intravascular bronchiolo-alveolar tumor. Am J Pathol 78:6, 1975

309. Weiss SW, Enzinger FM: Epithelioid hemangioendothelioma. A vascular tumor often mistaken for a carcinoma. Cancer 50:970, 1982

310. Weiss SW, Ishak KG, Dail GH, et al: Epithelioid hemangioendothelioma and related lesions. Semin Diagn Pathol 3:259, 1986

311. Rosai J, Gold J, Landy R: The histiocytoid hemangiomas. A unifying concept embracing several previously described entities of skin, soft tissue, large vessels, bone and heart. Hum Pathol 10:707, 1979

312. Weiss SW, Enzinger FM: Spindle cell hemangioendothelioma. A low grade angiosarcoma resembling cavernous hemangioma and Kaposi's sarcoma. Am J Surg Pathol 10:521, 1986

313. Donnell RM, Rosen PP, Lieberman PH, et al: Angiosarcoma and other vascular tumors of the breast. Pathologic analysis as a guide to prognosis. Am J Surg Pathol 5:629, 1981

314. Maddox J, Evans HL: Angiosarcoma of skin and soft tissue: A study of forty-four cases. Cancer 48:1907, 1981

315. Roholl PJM, de Jong ASH, Ramaekers FCS: Application of markers in the diagnosis of soft tissue tumors. Histopathology 9:1019, 1985

316. Goette DK, Detlefs RL: Post irradiation angiosarcoma. J Am Acad Dermatol 12:922, 1985

317. Lo TCM, Silverman ML, Edelstein A: Postirradiation hemangiosarcoma of the chest wall. Acta Radiol Oncol 24:237, 1985

318. Penn I: Kaposi's sarcoma in organ transplant recipients: Report of 20 cases. Transplantation 27:8, 1979

319. Niedt GW, Schinella RA: Acquired immunodeficiency syndrome: Clinicopathologic study of 56 autopsies. Arch Pathol Lab Med 109:727, 1985

320. Anthony CW, Koneman EW: Visceral Kaposi's sarcoma. Arch Pathol Lab Med 70:108, 1960

321. Nadji M, Morales AR, Ziegles-Weissman J, et al: Kaposi's sarcoma. Immunologic evidence for an endothelial origin. Arch Pathol Lab Med 105:274, 1981

322. Beckstead JH, Wood GS, Fletcher V: Evidence for the origin of Kaposi's sarcoma from lymphatic endothelium. Am J Pathol 119:294, 1985

323. Rywlin AA, Rosen L, Cabello B: Coexistence of Castleman's disease and Kaposi's sarcoma. Report of a case and a speculation. Am J Dermatopathol 5:277, 1983

324. Frizzera G, Banks PM, Massaulki G, Rosai J: A systemic lymphoproliferative disorder with morphologic features of Castleman's disease. Am J Surg Pathol 7:211, 1983

325. McMaster MJ, Soule EH, Ivins JC: Hemangiopericytoma: A clinicopathologic study and long term follow-up of 60 patients. Cancer 36:2232, 1975

326. Stout AP, Murray MR: Hemangiopericytoma: A vascular tumor featuring Zimmerman's pericytes. Ann Surg 116:26, 1942

327. Battifora H: Hemangiopericytoma: Ultrastructural study of five cases. Cancer 31:1418, 1973

328. Nunnery EW, Kahn LB, Reddick RL, et al: Hemangiopericytoma: A light microscopic and ultrastructural study. Cancer 47:906, 1981

329. Backwinkel KD, Diddans JA: Hemangiopericytoma. Report of a case and comprehensive review of the literature. Cancer 25:896, 1969

330. Pitluk HC, Conn J Jr: Hemangiopericytoma: Literature review and clinical presentations. Am J Surg 137:413, 1979

331. Kauffman SL, Stout AP: Hemangiopericytoma in children. Cancer 13:695, 1960

332. Alpers CE, Rosenau W, Finkfeiner WE, et al: Congenital (infantile) hemangiopericytoma of the tongue and sublingual region. Am J Clin Pathol 81:377, 1984

333. Seibert JJ, Seibert RW, Weisenberg DS, et al: Multiple congenital hemangiopericytomas of the head and neck. Laryngoscope 88:1006, 1978

334. Hayes MMM, Dietrich BE, Uys CJ: Congenital hemangiopericytomas of skin. Am J Dermatopathol 8:148, 1986

335. Chen K, Kassel S, Medrano V: Congenital hemangiopericytoma. J Surg Oncol 31:127, 1986

336. Plukker J, Koops HS, Molenaar I, et al: Malignant hemangiopericytoma in three kindred members of one family. Cancer 61:841, 1988

337. Galifer RB, Pous JP, Juskiewenski S, et al: Intra-abdominal cystic lymphangiomas in childhood. Prog Pediatr Surg 11:173, 1978

338. Waldo ED, Vuletin JC, Kaye GI: The ultrastructure of vascular tumors. Additional observations and a review of the literature. Pathol Annu 12:279, 1977

339. Goetsch E: Hygroma colli cysticum and hygroma axillare. Arch Surg 36:394, 1938

340. Carr RF, Ochs RH, Ritter DA, et al: Fetal cystic hygroma and Turner's syndrome. Am J Dis Child 140:580, 1986

341. Mennemeyer R, Smith M: Multicystic peritoneal mesothelioma. Cancer 44:692, 1979

342. Avigad S, Jaffe R, Frand M, et al: Lymphangiomatosis with splenic involvement. JAMA 236:2315, 1976

343. Engel S, Clagett OT, Harrison EG Jr: Chylous cysts of the abdomen. Surgery 50:593, 1961

344. Kalish M, Dorr R, Hoskins P: Retroperitoneal cystic lymphangioma. Urology 6:503, 1975

345. Hamilton WJ, Mossman HW: Human Embryology. 4th ed. Williams & Wilkins, Baltimore, 1973

346. Cornog JL Jr, Enterline HT: Lymphangiomyoma: A benign lesion of chyliferous lymphatics synonymous with lymphangiopericytoma. Cancer 19:1909, 1966

347. Wolff M: Lymphangiomyomas: Clinicopathologic study and ultrastructural confirmation of its histogenesis. Cancer 31:988, 1973

348. Bush JK, McLean R, Sieker HO: Diffuse lung disease due to lymphangiomyoma. Am J Med 46:645, 1969

349. Corrin B, Liebow AA, Friedman PJ: Pulmonary lymphangiomyomatosis. Am J Pathol 79:348, 1975

350. Kitzsteiner KA, Mallen RG: Pulmonary lymphangiomyomatosis: Treatment with castration. Cancer 46:2248, 1980

351. McCarty KS Jr, Mossler JA, McLeland R, et al: Pulmonary lymphangiomyomatosis responsive to progesterone. N Engl J Med 303:1, 461, 1980

352. Calabrese PR, Frank HD, Taubin HL: Lymphangiomyomatosis with chylous ascites: Treatment with dietary fat restriction and medium chain triglycerides. Cancer 40:895, 1977

353. Stewart FW, Treves N: Lymphangiosarcoma in postmastectomy lymphedema. Cancer 1:64, 1948

354. Woodward AH, Ivings JJ, Soule EH: Lymphangiosarcoma arising in chronic lymphedematous extremities. Cancer 30:562, 1972

355. Eby CS, Brennan MJ, Fine G: Lymphangiosarcoma: A lethal complication of chronic lymphedema. Arch Surg 94:223, 1967

356. Sordillo EM, Sordillo PP, Hadju SI, Good RA: Lymphangiosarcoma after filarial infection. J Dermat Surg Oncol 7:235, 1981

357. Miettinen M, Lehto V, Virtanen I: Postmastectomy angiosarcoma (Stewart Treves syndrome) light microscopic, immunohistological and ultrastructural characteristics of two cases. Am J Surg Pathol 7:329, 1983

358. Cadman NL, Soule EH, Kelly PJ: Synovial sarcoma. An analysis of 134 tumors. Cancer 18:613, 1965

359. Wright PH, Sim EH, Soule EH, et al: Synovial sarcoma. J Bone Joint Surg [Am] 64:112, 1982

360. Crocker SW, Stout AP: Synovial sarcoma in children. Cancer 12:1123, 1959

361. Krall R, Kostianovsky M, Patchefsky A: Synovial sarcoma. A clinical, pathological and structural study of 26 cases supporting the recognition of a monophasic variant. Am J Surg Pathol 5:137, 1980

362. Corson JM, Weiss LM, Banks-Schlegel SP, Pinkus G: Keratin proteins and carcinoembryonic antigen in synovial sarcomas: An immunohistochemical study of 24 cases. Hum Pathol 15:615, 1984

363. Fisher C: Synovial sarcoma. Ultrastructural and immunohistochemical features of epithelial differentiation in monophasic and biphasic tumors. Hum Pathol 17:996, 1986

364. Abenoza P, Manivel C, Swanson PE, Wick MR: Synovial sarcoma. Hum Pathol 17:1107, 1986

365. Gabbiani G, Kaye G, Lattes R, et al: Synovial sarcoma: Electron microscopic study of a typical case. Cancer 28:103, 1971

366. Mickelson MR, Brown GA, Maynard JA, et al: Synovial sarcoma: An electron microscopic study of monophasic and biphasic forms. Cancer 45:2109, 1980

367. Cagle LA, Mirra JM, Storm K, et al: Histologic features relating to prognosis in synovial sarcoma. Cancer 59:1810, 1987

368. Varela-Duran J, Enzinger FM: Calcifying synovial sarcoma. Cancer 50:345, 1982

369. Stout AP: Mesenchymoma, the mixed tumor of mesenchymal derivatives. Ann Surg 127:278, 1948

370. Le Ber MS, Stout AP: Benign mesenchymomas in children. Cancer 15:598, 1962

371. Becker SN: Dystocia, consumptive coagulopathy, and cardiac failure as complications of a congenital benign mesenchymoma. Am J Surg Pathol 4:401, 1980

372. Nash A, Stout AP: Malignant mesenchymomas in children. Cancer 14:524, 1961

373. Kaufman S, Stout AP: Congenital mesenchymal tumors. Cancer 18:460, 1965

374. Bures C, Barnes L: Benign mesenchymomas of the head and neck. Arch Pathol Lab Med 102:237, 1978

375. Bugg EI, Mathews RS: Benign mesenchymoma. South Med J 63:268, 1970

376. Januska J, Leban SG, Mashberg A: Mesenchymoma: A review of the literature and report of two cases. J Surg Oncol 8:229, 1976

377. Kawamoto EH, Weidner N, Agostini RM, Jaffe R: Malignant ectomesenchymoma of soft tissue. Report of two cases and review of the literature. Cancer 59:1791, 1987

378. Karcioglu Z, Someren A, Mates SJ: Ectomesenchymoma: A malignant tumor of migratory neural crest (ectomesenchyme) remnants showing ganglionic, Schwannian, melanocytic and rhabdomyoblastic differentiation. Cancer 39:2486, 1977

379. Cozzutto C, Cormelli A, Bandelloni R: Ectomesenchymoma: Report of two cases. Virchows Arch 398:185, 1982

380. Kodet R, Kashuri N, Marsden HB, et al: Gangliorhabdomyosarcoma: A histopathological and immunohistochemical study of three cases. Histopathology 10:181, 1986

381. Vance SF, Hudson RP Jr: Granular cell myoblastoma: Clinico-pathologic study of forty-two patients. Am J Clin Pathol 52:208, 1969

382. Compagno J, Hyams VJ, Ste-Maire P: Benign granular cell tumors of the larynx: A review of 36 cases with clinicopathologic data. Ann Otol 84:308, 1975

383. Farris KB, Faust BF: Granular cell tumors of biliary ducts. Report of two cases and review of the literature. Arch Pathol Lab Med 103:510, 1979

384. Regezi JA, Batsakis JG, Courtney RM: Granular cell tumors of the head and neck. J Oral Surg 37:402, 1979

385. Valenstein SL, Thurer RJ: Granular cell myoblastoma of the bronchus. J Thorac Cardiovasc Surg 76:465, 1978

386. Dgani R, Czernobilsky B, Borenstein R, et al: Granular cell myoblastoma of the vulva: Report of 4 cases. Acta Obstet Gynecol Surg 57:385, 1978

387. Strong W, McDivitt RW, Brasfield RD: Granular cell myoblastoma. Cancer 25:415, 1970

388. Sobel HJ, Marquet E, Avrin E, et al: Granular cell myoblastoma: An electron microscopic and cytochemical study illustrating the genesis of granules and aging of myoblastoma cells. Am J Pathol 65:54, 1971

389. Sobel HJ, Avrin E, Marquet E, et al: Reactive granular cells in sites of trauma. A cytochemical and ultrastructural study. Am J Clin Pathol 61:223, 1974

390. Lack EE, Worsham GF, Calihan MD, et al: Granular cell tumor: A clinicopathologic study of 110 patients. J Surg Oncol 13:301, 1980

391. Al-Sarraf M, Loud AV, Vaitkevicius VK: Malignant granular cell tumor: Histochemical and electron microscopic study. Arch Pathol Lab Med 91:550, 1971

392. Usui M, Ishii S, Yamawaki S, et al: Malignant granular cell tumor of the radial nerve. An autopsy observation with electron microscopic and tissue culture studies. Cancer 39:1547, 1977

393. Cadotte M: Malignant granular cell myoblastoma. Cancer 33:1417, 1974

394. Mackenzie DH: Malignant granular cell myoblastoma. J Clin Pathol 20:739, 1967

395. Gamboa LG: Malignant granular cell myoblastoma. Arch Pathol Lab Med 60:663, 1955

396. Christopherson WM, Foote FW, Stewart FW: Alveolar soft part sarcomas. Structurally characteristic tumors of uncertain histogenesis. Cancer 5:100, 1952

397. Skipkey FH, Lieberman PH, Foote FH, et al: Ultrastructure of alveolar soft part sarcoma. Cancer 17:821, 1964

398. Mukai M, Torikata C, Iri H, et al: Histogenesis of alveolar soft part sarcoma: An immunohistochemical and biological study. Am J Surg Pathol 10:212, 1986

399. Ordonez HG, Hickey RC, Brooks TE: Alveolar soft part sarcoma. A cytologic and immunohistochemical study. Cancer 61:525, 1988

400. Mukai M, Torikata C, Iri H, et al: Alveolar soft part sarcoma: An elaboration of a three-dimensional configuration of the crystalloids by digital image processing. Am J Pathol 116:398, 1984

401. Lieberman PH, Foote FW, Stewart FW, et al: Alveolar soft part sarcoma. JAMA 198:1047, 1966

402. Evans H: Alveolar soft part sarcoma: A study of 13 typical examples and one with a histologically atypical component. Cancer 55:912, 1985

403. Enzinger FM: Epithelioid sarcoma. A sarcoma simulating granuloma. Cancer 26:1029, 1970

404. Bryan RS, Soule EH, Dobyns JH, et al: Primary epithelioid sarcoma of the hand and forearm. A review of thirteen cases. J Bone Joint Surg [Am] 56:458, 1974

405. Santiago H, Feinerman LK, Lattes R: Epithelioid sarcoma. Hum Pathol 3:133, 1972

406. Chase DR, Enzinger FM: Epithelioid sarcoma: Diagnosis, prognostic indicator and treatment. Am J Surg Pathol 9:241, 1985

407. Gabbiani G, Fu Y-S, Kaye GI, et al: Epithelioid sarcoma: A light and electron microscope study suggesting a synovial origin. Cancer 30:486, 1972

408. Frable WJ, Kay S, Lawrence W, et al: Epithelioid sarcoma. An electron microscopic study. Arch Pathol Lab Med 95:8, 1973

409. Lombardi L, Rilke F: Ultrastructural similarities and differences of synovial sarcoma, and clear cell sarcoma of the tendons and aponeuroses. Ultrastruct Pathol 6:209, 1984

410. Chase DR, Weiss SW, Enzinger FM, et al: Keratin in epithelioid sarcoma. An immunohistochemical study. Am J Surg Pathol 8:435, 1984

411. Daimaru Y, Hashimoto H, Tsuneyoshi M, et al: Epithelial profile of epithelioid sarcoma: An immunohistochemical analysis of eight cases. Cancer 59:134, 1987

412. Manivel JC, Wick MR, Dehner LP, Sibley RK: Epithelioid sarcoma. An immunohistochemical study. Am J Clin Pathol 87:319, 1987

413. Fisher C: Epithelioid sarcoma. The spectrum of ultrastructural differentiation in seven immunohistochemically defined cases. Hum Pathol 19:265, 1988

414. Mukai M, Torikata C, Iri H, et al: Cellular differentiation of epithelioid sarcoma; an electron microscopic, enzyme histochemical and immunohistochemical study. Am J Pathol 119:44, 1985

415. Tsuneyoshi M, Daimaru Y, Hashimoto H, et al: Malignant soft tissue neoplasms with the histologic features of renal rhabdoid tumors: An ultrastructural and immunohistochemical study. Hum Pathol 16:1235, 1985

416. Sotelo-Avila C, Gonzalez-Crussi F, deMello D, et al: Renal and extrarenal rhabdoid tumors in children: A clinicopathologic study of 14 patients. Semin Diagn Pathol 3:151, 1986

417. Enzinger FM: Clear cell sarcoma of tendons and aponeurosis. An analysis of 21 cases. Cancer 18:1163, 1965

418. Kindblom LG, Lodding P, Angervall L: Clear cell sarcoma of tendons and aponeuroses; an immunohistochemical and electron microscopic analysis indicating neural crest origin. Virchows Arch (A) 401:109, 1983

419. Chung EB, Enzinger FM: Malignant melanoma of soft parts. A reassessment of clear cell sarcoma. Am J Surg Pathol 7:405, 1983

420. Lichtestein L, Goldman RL: Cartilage tumors in soft tissues, particularly in the hand and food. Cancer 17:1203, 1964

421. Dahlin DC, Salvador AH: Cartilaginous tumors of the soft tissues of the hands and feet. Mayo Clin Proc 49:721, 1974

422. Chung EB, Enzinger FM: Chondroma of soft parts. Cancer 41:1414, 1978

423. Humphreys S, Pambakian H, McKee PH, Fletcher CDM: Soft tissue chondroma—A study of 15 tumors. Histopathology 10:147, 1986

424. Reiman HM, Dahlin DC: Cartilage and bone-forming tumors of the soft tissues. Semin Diagn Pathol 3:288, 1986

425. Enzinger FM, Shiraki M: Extraskeletal myxoid chondrosarcoma. An analysis of 34 cases. Hum Pathol 3:421, 1972

426. Stout AP, Verner EW: Chondrosarcoma of the extraskeletal soft tissues. Cancer 6:581, 1953

427. Fukuda T, Ishikawa H, Ohnishi Y, et al: Extraskeletal myxoid chondrosarcoma arising from the retroperitoneum. Am J Clin Pathol 85:514, 1986

428. Winslow DJ, Enzinger FM: Hyaluronidase-sensitive acid mucopolysaccharides in liposarcomas. Am J Pathol 37:497, 1960

429. Martin RF, Melmick PJ, Warner NE, et al: Chordoid sarcoma. Am J Clin Pathol 59:623, 1973

430. Tsuneyoshi M, Enjoji M, Iwasaki H, Shinohara N: Extraskeletal myxoid chondrosarcoma. A clinicopathologic and electron microscopic study. Acta Pathol Jpn 31:439, 1981

431. Salvador AH, Beabout JW, Dahlin DC: Mesenchymal chondrosarcoma. Observations in 30 new cases. Cancer 28:605, 1971

432. Guccion JG, Font RL, Enzinger FM, et al: Extraskeletal mesenchymal chondrosarcoma. Arch Pathol Lab Med 95:336, 1973

433. Nakashima Y, Unni KK, Shives TC, et al: Mesenchymal chondrosarcoma of bone and soft tissue. A review of 111 cases. Cancer 57:2444, 1986

434. Albores-Saavedra J, Angeles-Angeles A, Ridaura C, Brandt H: Embryonal chondrosarcoma in children. Patologia 15:153, 1977

435. Jessurun J, Rojas ME, Albores-Saavedra J: Congenital extraskeletal embryonal chondrosarcoma. J Bone Joint Surg [Am] 64:293, 1982

436. Hachitanda Y, Tsuneyoshi M, Daimaru Y, et al: Extraskeletal myxoid chondrosarcoma in young children. Cancer 61:2521, 1988

437. Allan CS, Soule EH: Osteogenic sarcoma of the somatic soft tissues. Cancer 27:1121, 1971

438. Huvos AG: Osteogenic sarcoma of bones and soft tissues in older persons: A clinicopathologic analysis of 117 patients older than 60 years. Cancer 57:1442, 1986

439. Sordillo PP, Hajdu SI, Magill GB, Golbey RB: Extraosseous osteogenic sarcoma: A review of 48 patients. Cancer 51:727, 1983

440. Chung EB, Enzinger FM: Extraskeletal osteosarcoma. Cancer 60:1132, 1987

441. Angervall L, Enzinger FM: Extraskeletal neoplasm resembling Ewing's sarcoma. Cancer 36:240, 1975

442. Soule EH, Newton W, Moon TE, et al: Extraskeletal Ewing's sarcoma. A preliminary review of 26 cases encountered in the intergroup rhabdomyosarcoma study. Cancer 42:259, 1978

443. Gillespie JJ, Einhorn LH, Roth LM, et al: Extraskeletal Ewing's sarcoma. Histologic and ultrastructural observations in three cases. Am J Surg Pathol 3:99, 1979

444. Hashimoto H, Tsuneyoshi M, Daimaru Y, et al: Extraskeletal Ewing's sarcoma: A clinicopathological and electron microscopic analysis of 8 cases. Acta Pathol Jpn 35:1087, 1985

445. Dickman PS, Triche TJ: Extraosseous Ewing's sarcoma versus primitive rhabdomyosarcoma: Diagnostic criteria and clinical correlation. Hum Pathol 17:881, 1986

446. Shimada H, Newton WA, Soule EH, et al: Pathologic features of extraosseous Ewing's sarcoma. A report from the intergroup rhabdomyosarcoma study. Hum Pathol 19:442, 1988

447. Weiss SW, Enzinger FM, Johnson FB: Silica reaction simulating fibrous histiocytoma. Cancer 42:2738, 1978

448. Konwaler BE, Keasbey L, Kaplan L: Subcutaneous pseudosarcomatous fibromatosis (fasciitis). Am J Clin Pathol 25:241, 1955

449. Price EB Jr, Silliphant WM, Shuman R: Nodular fasciitis: A clinicopathologic analysis of 65 cases. Am J Clin Pathol 35:122, 1961

450. Stout AP: Pseudosarcomatous fasciitis in children. Cancer 14:1,216, 1961

451. Bunstein KE, Lattes R: Nodular (pseudosarcomatous) fasciitis, a non-recurrent lesion: Clinico-pathologic study of 134 cases. Cancer 49:1668, 1982

452. Shimizu S, Hashimmoto H, Enjoji M: Nodular fasciitis: An analysis of 250 patients. Pathology 16:161, 1984

453. Patchefsky A, Enzinger FM: Intravascular fasciitis. Am J Surg Pathol 5:29, 1981

454. Lauer DH, Enzinger FM: Cranial fasciitis of childhood. Cancer 45:401, 1980

455. Chung EB, Enzinger FM: Proliferative fasciitis. Cancer 36:1450, 1975

456. Enzinger FM, Dulcey F: Proliferative myositis: Report of thirty-three cases. Cancer 20:2213, 1967

457. Wu JP, Yunis EJ, Fetterman G, et al: Inflammatory pseudotumor of the abdomen: plasma cell granulomas. J Clin Pathol 26:943, 1973

458. Keen PE, Weitzner S: Inflammatory pseudotumor of mesentery: A complication of ventriculoperitoneal shunt. J Neurosurg 38:371, 1973

459. Dehner LP: Extrapulmonary inflammatory myofibroblastic tumor. The inflammatory pseudotumor as another expression of the fibrohistiocytic complex. Lab Invest 54:115A, 1986

460. Pettinato G, Manivel C, Insabato L, et al: Plasma cell granuloma (inflammatory pseudotumor) of the breast. Am J Clin Pathol, in press

461. Ackerman LV: Extraosseous localized non-neoplastic bone and cartilage formation (so-called myositis ossificans). Clinical and pathological confusion with malignant neoplasms. J Bone Joint Surg [Am] 40:279, 1958

462. Dahl I, Angervall L: Pseudosarcomatous proliferative lesions of soft tissue with or without bone formation. Acta Pathol Microbiol Scand (A) 85:577, 1977

463. Coblentz CL, Cockshott WP, Martin RF: Resolution of myositis ossificans in a hemophiliac. J Can Assoc Radiol 36:161, 1985

464. Salyer WR, Salyer DC: Intravascular angiomatosis. Development and distinction from angiosarcoma. Cancer 36:995, 1975

465. Kuo T-T, Sayers P, Rosai J: Masson's vegetant intravascular hemangioendothelioma: A lesion often mistaken for angiosarcoma. Cancer 38:1227, 1976

466. Cleackin KP, Enzinger FM: Intravascular papillary endothelial hyperplasia. Arch Pathol Lab Med 100:441, 1976

467. Hashimoto H, Daimaru Y, Enjoji M: Intravascular papillary endothelial hyperplasia: A clinicopathologic study of 91 cases. Am J Dermatopathol 5:539, 1983

468. Kuo T, Gomez LG: Papillary endothelial proliferation in cystic lymphangiomas. Arch Pathol Lab Med 103:306, 1979

469. Friedel W, Chambers RG, Atkins JP: Pseudosarcomas of the pharynx and larynx. Arch Otolaryngol 102:286, 1976

470. Lasser KH, Naeim F, Higgins J, et al: Pseudosarcoma of the larynx. Am J Surg Pathol 3:397, 1979

471. Martin MR, Kahn LB: So-called pseudosarcoma of the esophagus: Nodal metastases of the spindle cell element. Arch Pathol Lab Med 101:604, 1977

11

The Breast

Claude Gompel
Daniel Faverly
Steven G. Silverberg

Lesions of the mammary gland, by virtue of their incidence, constitute one of the most important chapters in a text on human pathology, and the major topic of mammary pathology is the diagnosis of malignant tumors. In several regions of the world, malignant breast tumors constitute the most common group of cancers among women, and men are by no means exempt from them. In the United States, for example, approximately 18 percent of all malignant tumors are breast cancers, representing the most important cause of death by cancer in women; in absolute figures, this means approximately 42,000 deaths per year.[1]

It is nonetheless important to understand the benign lesions, whether they are tumoral or not. These lesions manifest their own specific characteristics and require equally specific treatments. Furthermore, an intimate knowledge of benign breast lesions facilitates the differential diagnosis between them and malignant lesions. Consequently, the discussion in this chapter will cover both the benign and the malignant morphologic alterations of the human breast.

The signs, symptoms, and sometimes even the morphologic manifestations of an intraparenchymal mass are often discrete, requiring a multidisciplinary approach for their proper interpretation. The information provided by pathologists, based on the study of histologic and cytologic specimens, is of maximum value only when integrated with both radiologic and clinical findings.[2] Only in this manner can we ensure efficient and precise diagnosis and rule out possible recurrences or metastases. As an

example, let us remind both the clinician and the pathologist that it is the responsibility of the latter to determine whether a specimen sent to him by the clinician is an adequate and representative one, or whether it is necessary to obtain another. The requirement for well preserved, high-quality specimens is one about which the pathologist must be intransigent, since such a requirement will prove considerably less blameworthy than an erroneous diagnosis.

EMBRYOLOGY AND HISTOLOGY

The understanding and correct interpretation of the morphologic lesions of mammary tissue require a knowledge of the normal histologic structures and their embryologic origins.

The early embryo produces a ventral, linear, ectodermal thickening extending from the axillary region to the inguinal region, along both sides of the midsagittal plane. These thickenings are the milk ridges. By the ninth week of embryonic development, these ridges persist only in the pectoral region, where the ectoderm undergoes further thickening and produces solid cords of cells that burrow into the underlying mesenchyme[3] (Fig. 11-1).

Near the end of the embryonic period, these cords become hollow and thus constitute the future mammary gland parenchyma: the lactiferous sinuses, the lactiferous ducts, and the secretory alveoli.[4] The stroma of the fu-

311

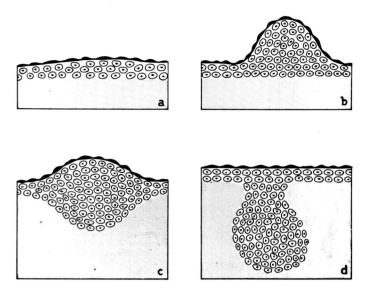

Fig. 11-1. Embryonic development of the mammary gland. **(A)** Ectoderm. **(B, C)** Thickening of ectoderm. **(D)** Solid ectodermal cord invading the underlying mesenchyme.

ture mammary gland includes tissue situated around the lobar glandular formations; this is the intralobar connective tissue. Beyond the limits of the intralobar connective tissue, the stroma is denser and constitutes the interlobar connective tissue. The resting gland consists of approximately 20 to 25 lobes separated by the dense interlobar fibrous septa. Each lobe is subdivided into lobules that represent the functional units of the mammary parenchyma. A surface ectodermal thickening, pushed anteriorly by the mesenchyme, constitutes the nipple, which is surrounded by a pigmented ectodermal zone called the areola. Ultrastructurally, the walls of the glandular system consist of a basal lamina, a discontinuous layer of

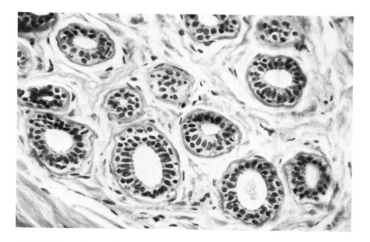

Fig. 11-2. Normal mammary gland. Lactiferous ducts and the surrounding connective tissue are shown.

myoepithelial cells, and two layers of columnar cells. The columnar cells possess numerous microvilli on the luminal surface as well as between the cells,[5-7] and the myoepithelial cells are characterized by an abundant contractile fibrillar cytoplasmic apparatus.[8]

During gestation, the fetal mammary gland undergoes hormonal stimulation of maternal origin, producing signs of secretory activity that regress at birth.[9] At puberty, under the influence of sexual hormones, the female mammary gland acquires its ultimate maturation: the development of the lactiferous duct system and the process of lobulation occur simultaneously with a proliferation of the surrounding connective and adipose tissues (Fig. 11-2).

During the period of sexual activity, the mammary gland reacts to the influences of the hormonal cycle, and the glandular system thus undergoes a cellular proliferation during the estrogenic phase, followed by discrete secretory activity at the end of the cycle.[10] Concomitant with these changes, the intralobular connective tissue increases its capacity to bind water, particularly near the end of the cycle. This phenomenon explains the impression of heaviness and fullness experienced by certain women in the premenstrual period.

During periods of lactation, under the action of different hormones (estrogens, progesterone, prolactin, and others such as cortisol and insulin), the acinar cells undergo a marked secretory differentiation and the lobules become hyperplastic and crowded (Fig. 11-3). The interlobular septa are markedly thinned. Colostrum production and subsequently milk production occur at the distal part of the glandular system, the cellular activities of which thus comprise protein and lipid synthesis. Proteins are elaborated along the membranes of the rough endoplasmic reticulum and are packaged in granules, 400 nm in diameter, which are concentrated within the Golgi zone.[10] These granules are expelled from the luminal surface of the cells by merocrine secretion. Lipids appear as cytoplasmic droplets surrounded by a membrane and are expelled by apocrine secretion (reversed pinocytosis). Once secreted, ejection of the milk requires sucking, oxytocin secretion, and myoepithelial cell contraction. After menopause, the lobules become atrophic and the excretory ducts undergo cystic degenerative dilatation. The surrounding stroma manifests a loss of cellularity accompanied by fibrosis.[11]

MACROSCOPIC ANATOMY

The mammary gland is a glandular system surrounded by fibroadipose tissue that rests on a musculoconnective tissue bed. The gland is covered by the epidermis. Centrally located is the nipple, a cylindrical excrescence,

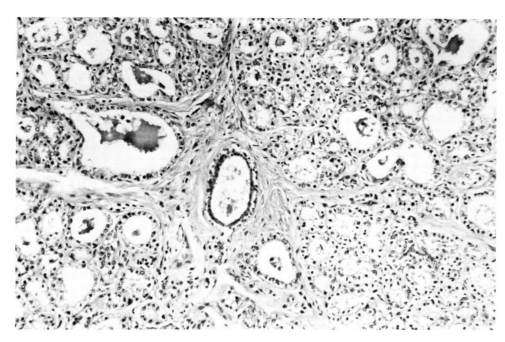

Fig. 11-3. Lactating mammary gland, secretory differentiation of acinar cells. Note the structural difference between the secretory acini and the lactiferous ducts.

which is surrounded by a circular, pigmented area called the areola; the tubercles of Montgomery[12] are specialized sebaceous glands of the areola that enlarge during pregnancy and lactation. The arteries of the mammary gland are branches of the internal mammary, external mammary, and intercostal arteries. The veins are the axillary, internal mammary, and intercostal veins.

The structure of the lymphatic system has a direct influence on the mode of dissemination of tumors (Fig. 11-4). The cutaneous lymphatics and some of the perilobular, perialveolar, and ductal lymphatic pathways drain into the areolar plexus.[13,14] Three main lymphatic groups arise from this plexus: the external, internal, and inferior

groups. The majority of the deep lymphatics bypass the areolar plexus and drain into these groups. The external mammary lymphatics terminate in the external mammary nodes. These nodes are in continuity with the different axillary groups: the scapular nodes, the central nodes, the axillary vein nodes, and the subclavicular nodes. From there, large lymphatic trunks drain into the jugular-subclavian venous system. The interpectoral nodes described by Rotter are of little significance and are usually not dissected unless the pectoralis major muscle is removed. The internal mammary lymphatics drain into the internal mammary nodes between the costal cartilages. These nodes surround the internal mammary vessels and are usually small. They receive some drainage from the lateral half of the breast. Connecting lymphatics between the left and right lymphatic chains exist at the level of the first costal interspace. The inferior mammary lymphatics empty into the anterior pectoral, axillary, and subclavicular nodes. When the lymphatic drainage is blocked by metastases, retrograde lymphatic spread develops, explaining various metastatic locations such as the opposite axilla and the liver.

CONGENITAL ANOMALIES

Like other organs, the mammary gland can present congenital anomalies resulting from improper embryonic development:

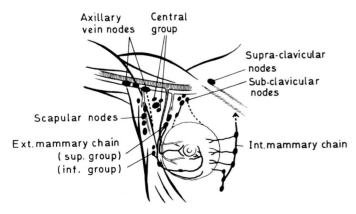

Fig. 11-4. Structure of the lymphatic system of the mammary gland.

Athelia: lack of nipple; generally occurs with amastia, both rare

Amastia: absence of the mammary gland; can be uni- or bilateral

Polythelia: the presence of supernumerary nipples

Polymastia: presence of supernumerary mammary glands (polymastia and polythelia result from the persistence of portions of the milk ridge that normally undergo involution)

NEUROENDOCRINE ANOMALIES

The normal development of the mammary gland is under the influence of the neuroendocrine system. When this stimulation is absent or disturbed, abnormalities occur:

Precocious development of the breasts occurs as part of the clinical presentation of premature—although normal—adolescence. Rarely, it is associated with estrogen-producing ovarian tumors, lutein cysts, or tumors of the adrenal cortex.

Micromastia is insufficient development of the gland at puberty. Failure of development can be due to ovarian insufficiency or congenital adrenal hyperplasia, or the development may be simply delayed because of late menarche.

Macromastia is hypertrophy of the mammary gland.[15,16] When it occurs, it is generally at puberty and may result in markedly voluminous breasts. This hypertrophy is due to an abnormal sensitivity to estrogenic hormones and is sometimes symmetric. The microscopic structure reveals a remarkable growth of the connective and adipose tissues. A few cases of massive breast hypertrophy have been reported during pregnancy.

Gynecomastia is the unilateral or bilateral development of the mammary gland in the male. When it occurs, it is usually at puberty or in old age. This anomaly is discussed in detail later in the section on pathologic conditions of the male breast.

BASIC TECHNIQUES OF HANDLING BREAST SPECIMENS

The main types of specimens submitted to the pathologist in various breast disorders are from needle aspirations, from incisional and excisional biopsies, from the different techniques of mastectomy, and from therapeutic local excisions or re-excisions.

An accurate description of the gross appearance of the specimen is a primordial step in the evaluation of breast disease, because it can be made only once, while the specimen is fresh. A good description must be sufficiently detailed so anyone familiar with pathology can visualize the specimen on the basis of the report alone. Careful palpation of the specimen is of great importance for detection of any malignant lesion.

The examination includes the gathering of the following information: the weight, the dimensions, the number of fragments, and the description of each fragment. More specifically, this description gives the following details: color, consistency, infiltration of the surrounding tissues, and aspect of the different slices obtained through the specimen. Any pathologic condition, such as cysts, fibrosis, inflammation or hemorrhagic foci, necrosis, firm areas, and granular degeneration with chalky streaks, should be noted. The presence of microcalcifications detected by mammography should be confirmed by specimen radiography. If the presence of an intraductal papilloma is suspected, the main lactiferous ducts should be opened lengthwise and a careful excision of the papilloma with surrounding tissues performed. If the search for papilloma is negative, transverse sections should be made and totally embedded.

Imprints of the lesion are made to obtain fine details of the cytologic structures. Needle aspiration biopsies are studied similarly. Two methods can be used: the air-dried smear stained with Giemsa stain or the wet-smear technique with fixation in 95 percent alcohol. Both methods are satisfactory, but the second technique gives better nuclear detail and allows comparison with tissue biopsy specimens. These imprints provide information that is complementary to histologic slides.

When an immediate frozen section examination is requested, the most suspicious area of the specimen is carefully selected. The fragments must be thin (less than 0.5 cm in thickness) in order to obtain readable frozen sections. After freezing and sectioning, the fragment is placed in fixative. The number of blocks of tissue taken from a given specimen depends on the circumstances, diffuse or ill defined lesions requiring more sections for accuracy.

The detection of asymptomatic anomalies such as in situ lobular carcinoma depends on the number of blocks examined, but the chance of correctly diagnosing lobular carcinoma in situ is low, about 18 percent.[17] If the lesion has been detected by clinical mammography, the selection of a suitable block is made by the use of specimen mammography[18] (see under Mammography). In most cases, a frozen section of good technical quality will allow the pathologist to give a valid diagnosis. However, difficulties will be encountered with certain lesions, such as in situ lobular carcinoma, intraductal papilloma, and well differentiated papillary carcinoma. In many of these cases, intraoperative smears or imprints may be easier to interpret than frozen sections[19]; in other instances, it is wiser to wait for paraffin-embedded permanent sections in order to avoid a false positive or a false negative result.

Mastectomy Specimens

When dealing with a simple mastectomy specimen, the description must include the appearance of the nipple and skin and the localization and description of pathologic foci. The biopsy incision, when present, should be opened, and any residual tumor should be sought. The following fragments should be sampled: the nipple, the region beneath the nipple, the tumor and any abnormal macroscopic lesion, as well as the presumably normal parenchyma.

The frequency of nipple involvement by breast cancer varies according to the number of sections taken from the area. Taking a cylindrical block 1 cm deep containing the nipple and the areola, and performing 14 horizontal sections has demonstrated that the percentage of nipple involvement increases significantly and may attain 50 percent. Therefore, the risk of leaving a malignant focus in the nipple area can be important when subcutaneous mastectomy techniques are used.

The dissection of the axillary tail is important because lymph nodes may be found even if there had been no formal dissection of the axilla. The remaining fragments of the specimen can then be fixed and retained for possible further examination.

Sectioning of fresh breast tissue is not easy, particularly when there is marked fatty infiltration. Different methods have been proposed to overcome this difficulty, among which are partial freezing or fixation until the tissues are firm enough to be sliced. These techniques are particularly useful when large sections of breast parenchyma are needed (e.g., for comparison with mammography results).

In radical mastectomy (a less frequently performed procedure in recent years), the examination of the mammary gland is followed by a careful dissection of the axillary fat. The nodes are usually divided into three groups: those lateral to and below the pectoralis minor, those behind and within the borders of the muscle, and those above or medial to the muscle. The most medial nodes are near the apex of the axilla. Sometimes nodes are found between the pectoralis minor and the excised fragment of the pectoralis major (Fig. 11-5). Lymph nodes that are dissected out without their respective muscles should be identified with respect to their position and should be so labeled by the surgeon.

The most widely used method for detection of metastases is based on careful palpation and removal of lymph nodes present in the axillary fat tissue. This is preferred to the more time consuming and perhaps more sophisti-

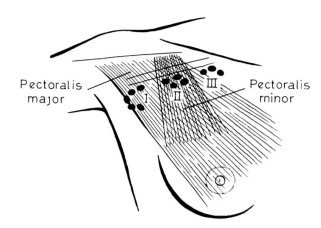

Fig. 11-5. Dissection of axillary nodes. The nodes are divided into three groups according to anatomic location with respect to the pectoralis muscles.

cated method that uses benzol derivatives to clear the adipose tissue. Extended radical mastectomy may include, along the medial border, fragments of costal cartilage, sternum, and internal mammary lymph nodes. All the nodes should be dissected, measured, labeled and embedded.

The number of nodes recovered from the axillary region of a radical or modified radical mastectomy varies from 0 to 81. These variations are due to anatomic differences. It is important to remember that approximately 30 to 40 percent of clinically normal nodes exhibit metastases histologically. Also, enlarged, suspicious lymph nodes may reveal merely a massive fatty infiltration or lymphoid hyperplasia.

Clinical staging is based partially on the presence of palpable lymph nodes. The American and International Classifications of clinical staging are presented in Table 11-1. A few minor discrepancies exist between the two, but both demonstrate the prognostic value of clinical staging. There is, in fact, a direct relationship between the pathologic lymph node status and the histologic grade of the tumor.

Mastectomy scars often become the site of tumor recurrence; any suspicious modification of a scar should be removed and examined microscopically, because granulomatous reaction to suture material may simulate carcinoma.

Local Excision (Lumpectomy, Tylectomy, Quadrantectomy) Specimens

In many centers in North America and Europe, many if not most patients with primary operable breast cancer are now treated by a breast-conserving local excision with or without radiation therapy. The choice of such therapy

**TABLE 11-1. American and International
Classifications of Clinical Staging: TNM System**

International Classification

T1	Tumor less than 2 cm in greatest diameter without skin involvement
T2	Tumor more than 2 cm in diameter or with skin involvement or nipple retraction
T3	Tumor of any size with skin infiltration, ulceration, or edema or pectoral muscle attachment
N0	No palpable axillary lymph nodes
N1	Palpable but movable ipsilateral axillary nodes
N2	Palpable and fixed ipsilateral axillary or infraclavicular nodes
M0	No evidence of distant metastases
M1	Clinical and radiographic evidence of distant metastases
Stage I	T1 or 2; N0; M0
Stage II	T1 or 2; N1; M0
Stage III	T1 or 2; N2; M0
	T3; N0, 1, or 2; M0
Stage IV	All M1

American Classification

T—Primary tumor

T1	Tumor of 2 cm or less in its greatest dimension; skin not involved, or involved locally with Paget's disease
T2	Tumor over 2 cm in size, or with skin attachment (dimpling of skin), or nipple retraction (in subaraeolar tumors); no pectoral muscle or chest wall attachment
T3	Tumor of any size with any of the following: skin infiltration, ulceration, peau d'orange, skin edema, pectoral muscle or chest wall attachment

N—Regional lymph nodes

N0	No clinically palpable axillary lymph node(s) (metastasis not suspected)
N1	Clinically palpable axillary lymph nodes that are not fixed (metastasis suspected)
N2	Clinically palpable homolateral axillary or infraclavicular lymph node(s) that are fixed to one another or to other structures (metastasis suspected)

M—Distant metastasis

M0	No distant metastasis
M1	Clinical and radiographic evidence of metastasis except those to homolateral axillary or infraclavicular lymph nodes

over mastectomy depends in part on the evaluation by the pathologist of the initial excision specimen.[20] It is crucial in these cases to (1) record the gross dimensions of the tumor before removing any of it for special studies, such as hormone receptor assays or flow cytometry; (2) carefully note the gross relationship of the tumor to the resection margins; and (3) mark the surface of the specimen with some type of ink, which must be dried before the specimen is incised. We have found the resection margins in these cases to be often extremely difficult to evaluate microscopically, despite the employment of one of the suggested techniques of cutting and embedding[20]; nevertheless, surgeons usually request that a statement appear in the final pathology report describing the adequacy of resection. The tumor differentiation (grade), ex-

tent of intraductal carcinoma within and/or adjacent to an infiltrating carcinoma, and presence or absence of lymphatic invasion adjacent to or distant from the primary tumor are also important determinations that will influence subsequent management. Even if the initial excision is not intended as the final operative treatment, many patients will obtain a second opinion after this excision, and some will decide not to have further surgery. Therefore, the information specified above[20] should be supplied in every case.

METHODS OF DIAGNOSIS

Clinical Method

The medical history and physical examination of the breast are essential steps in diagnosis. The clinical signs of primary breast neoplasms are few. In the overwhelming majority of cases, there is painless breast mass and, less frequently, nipple discharge or erosion, skin retraction, or the presence of an axillary mass. The differential diagnosis between borderline and malignant lesions relies on more elaborate diagnostic methods such as mammography, thermography, and echography, but most of all on tissue examination. Education of the public about the fundamental facts of cancer and self-examination of the breast also represents an important factor in the early detection of breast diseases.

Mammography

Mammography is basically a soft tissue radiologic examination of the breast that is now an indispensable part of the workup of breast lesions.[21] Perhaps its main asset is its ability to detect clinically impalpable malignant lesions.[22,23] This new technology has modified the way in which surgical specimens should be handled. Stereotactic localization of the radiographic abnormalities is followed by pathologic examination of the identified areas. This procedure correlates the radiographic abnormalities with the histologic images: microcalcifications and epithelial and stromal alterations. When the lesion is small and not grossly malignant, frozen section examination should not be performed, in order to obtain good quality permanent sections. A radiogram of the surgical specimen enables the pathologist to identify with certainty that the lesion present in the preoperative mammogram was localized and properly processed for microscopic examination.[23–25]

The recognition of microcalcifications is important. Table 11-2 summarizes the sources of interpretative error in the evaluation of biopsies directed by microcalcifications. In the absence of microcalcifications, soft tissue densities may be more difficult to localize and interpret pathologi-

TABLE 11-2. Problems and Solutions in Evaluation of Mammographically Directed Biopsies

No confirmation of microcalcifications in the specimen radiograph
   Mammographic abnormalities inadequately localized or surgical sample misdirected
   Definite absence of microcalcifications in the preoperative mammograms
   Microcalcifications located in the dermis; ellipse of skin should be embedded
   Inadequate x-ray equipment does not reveal microcalcifications in the specimen radiograph
Presence of noncorresponding microcalcifications in the specimen radiograph
   Microcalcifications do not correspond to those detected preoperatively: mammogram review or rebiopsy if calcifications are still present.
   Microcalcifications have not been excised entirely: additional biopsy
   Microcalcifications seen in specimen represent talc or other radioopaque contaminant.
Specimen radiograph demonstrates the presence of a lesion, but microcalcifications not identified in microscopic sections
   Microcalcifications are composed of oxalate crystals: use polarization lenses
   Microcalcifications have not been removed by the biopsy: x-ray paraffin blocks and remaining fixed tissue (if any)
   Microcalcifications lie deeper in block: cut deeper, x-ray block
   Microcalcifications have been leached by acidic fixative or shattered out of section: check pH of fixative and with the histotechnologist for knife chatter

(Data from Lagios.[534])

cally. Careful comparison of pre- and postoperative radiograms will contribute to solve the problem.

The efficiency of mammography to detect in situ carcinomas, both intralobular and intraductal, is well demonstrated and is responsible for the higher percentage of detection of these lesions in biopsies performed because mammograms are interpreted as suspicious or positive.[26,27]

Thermography

Thermography measures temperature differences between normal breast tissue and pathologic tissues. The results should always be verified by morphologic techniques, as this method is not highly specific or sensitive. Thermography cannot be used as a sole modality in a screening program. Interesting to mention is the fact that thermographic positivity is related to the aggressive characteristics of the tumor cells and may represent a quantitative evaluation of the clinical prognosis.[28]

Ultrasonography

Ultrasonography does not replace mammography for the detection of subclinical malignant tumors. It is useful in the characterization of lesions in dense mammary parenchyma and in the differential diagnosis between cystic and solid masses.[29]

Galactography

Galactography is another diagnostic radiologic procedure. A radiopaque medium is injected into the main lactiferous ducts, and mammograms are taken. It is a useful technique for detection of any tumor lesion in the main ducts.[30]

Fine Needle Aspiration (Aspiration Cytology)

Obtaining a preoperative diagnosis benefits the patient, the surgeon, and the pathologist. Fine needle aspiration, which permits such precocious diagnosis, proves to be an easy, rapid, and efficient modality in the workup of breast cancer.[31–35] This relatively low cost, sensitive technique offers simplicity of fixation and staining and provides fine cytologic details. In addition, it does not require the use of anesthesia or other special patient preparation. It may not supplant frozen section examination of a biopsy specimen, but its results are accurate enough to help shorten the period of psychologic anxiety of every woman faced with the possible diagnosis of a malignant breast tumor. Furthermore, the rare false positive results reported in the literature can be eliminated if the morphologic criteria provided by cytologic study are correlated with the clinical and radiologic data.

Needle aspiration of a benign cystic lesion combines diagnosis and therapy. The study of the desquamated cells present in the fluid and the disappearance of the lesion after aspiration confirm the benign nature of this condition.[36]

Needle aspiration specimens of fibrocystic disease, fibroadenoma, or any kind of adenoma will reveal an abundance of various types of benign-looking cells[37] (Fig. 11-6). Cytologic examination of nipple secretions will reveal the existence of intraductal papillomatous lesions.[38] Malignant tumors will be characterized by various amounts of cellular clusters exhibiting all the criteria of malignancy: anisonucleosis, hyperchromatism, hypertrophy of the nucleolus, increased nuclear-cytoplasmic ratio, anisocytosis, and disorderly cellular clumps (Fig. 11-7). With some experience, even the degree of differentiation of the tumor can be evaluated on a smear.[39,40]

Differential diagnosis becomes difficult when benign alterations are very atypical or when neoplastic changes are discrete or present only in a small number of cells. One must remember that each domain in clinical cytology requires specific knowledge of the precise type of cells in question.

318

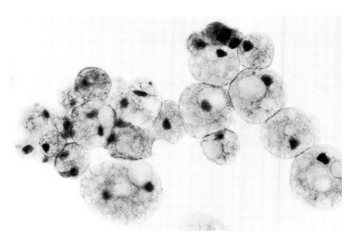

Fig. 11-6. Breast needle aspiration, mammary benign cyst. Note the desquamated foamy cells.

Aspiration cytology is also a valuable method for detecting subcutaneous tumors and mastectomy scar tumor recurrences. Also, postradiation treatment follow-up using cytologic rather than histologic examination avoids damaging tissue biopsies. However, one must remember that cytologic study offers no means of detecting certain histologic anomalies such as epithelial hyperplasia and in situ carcinoma. The following rules should be strictly observed by those who use the cytologic method:

1. A negative result is valueless, particularly when clinical findings and mammography are suspicious.

2. A positive result should usually be confirmed by frozen section examination of a biopsy specimen before any major surgical or radiation therapy is considered.

We repeat and re-emphasize that the rare cytologic false-positive results reported in the literature can be eliminated if the morphologic data are correlated with the clinical and radiologic evaluations.

Imprint cytologic examination performed concomitantly with a frozen section examination of a biopsy specimen is another useful adaptation of the technique.[19,41] Staining with a 1 percent aqueous solution of toluidine blue after rapid fixation in 70 percent alcohol is a very practical method. The metachromatic properties of this stain procure very fine details of the cellular structures. There is a close correlation between frozen section results and the results of imprint cytologic studies.[19,42] Also, in certain borderline lesions, the imprint slides provide further valuable structural details that help to define the benign or malignant nature of the disease (Fig. 11-8). False positive and false negative results are negligible in well trained hands. Thus, cytologic diagnosis is an extremely valuable part of breast lesion diagnostic armament.

Needle Biopsy

Needle biopsy techniques such as the Tru-Cut needle and the speed drill biopsy procedures produce a core of tissue and are preferred by some pathologists to the aspiration cytology method, which, according to them, gives greater numbers of false negative and false positive diagnoses. However, this opinion is not shared by all investigators.[43,44]

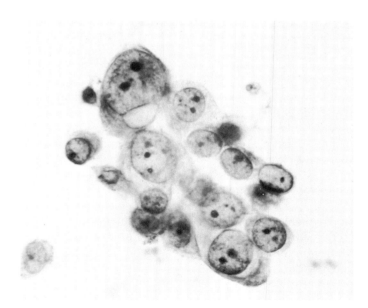

Fig. 11-7. Breast needle aspiration, infiltrating duct carcinoma. Cluster of neoplastic cells showing moderate hyperchromatism, nucleolar hypertrophy, and anisonucleosis.

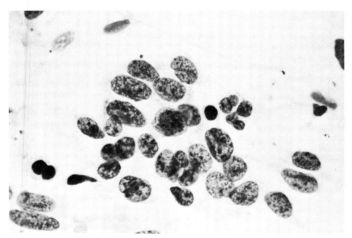

Fig. 11-8. Imprint cytology of infiltrating duct carcinoma. Note the irregular hyperchromatic nuclei and partial lysis of the cytoplasm.

Excisional Biopsy

Biopsy is the most appropriate and definitive diagnostic method for most breast lesions. The reliability of the frozen section examination is indeed excellent in the hands of well trained and experienced pathologists, the accuracy being above 95 percent in published series.[45-47] However, since breast biopsies today are generally not followed immediately by definitive therapy, and since a higher proportion of cancers are impalpable and often noninvasive, many pathologists are performing progressively fewer frozen section examinations on these specimens. In most of these cases, it is more appropriate to wait for the results of the examination of good paraffin-embedded sections of the biopsy specimen than to depend on the results of frozen section examination.

The danger of tumor dissemination initiated by a biopsy procedure or enhanced by a delay between diagnosis and treatment has been extensively discussed.[48] To avoid any risk, an excisional biopsy of all suspicious lesions should be performed, and adequate treatment should be started without delay after the pathologic report has been obtained. If these recommendations are followed, the prognosis is comparable in series of patients who have immediate major surgery and patients who undergo major surgery after a few days delay.

INFLAMMATORY LESIONS

Acute Mastitis

Acute mastitis generally occurs during periods of lactation. Predisposing factors include fissures of the nipple and hypertrophy of either the functional components or the lymphatics of the mammary gland. *Staphylococcus aureus* and *Streptococcus* are the most common etiologic agents, and thus the prognosis of this disease has considerably improved with the development of antibiotic therapy.

Clinically, acute mastitis manifests as usual inflammation: the breast is edematous, painfully swollen, and red. There may be a discharge from the nipple. Microscopically, we observe neutrophilic and histiocytic inflammatory infiltration, as well as vascular congestion and edema of the lactiferous ducts and surrounding stroma. There also may be zones of necrosis, which lead to abscess formation.[49,50]

Chronic Mastitis

Chronic mastitis with abscess formation is a complication of the acute form. We observe highly vascularized inflammatory granulomas, rich in polynuclear cells and histiocytes and enclosed in a dense fibrous capsule (Fig. 11-9). Foreign body giant cells and epithelioid cells may

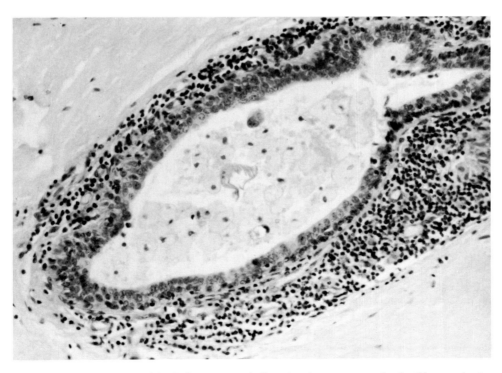

Fig. 11-9. Chronic mastitis. Inflammatory infiltration is seen around a lactiferous duct.

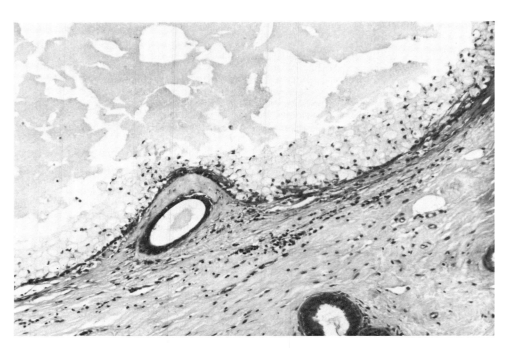

Fig. 11-10. Galactocele. Note the cystic degeneration of a duct with the presence of desquamated foamy cells.

be present in granulomatous lesions. Mammary duct fistula is a lesion associated with a duct lined with metaplastic squamous epithelium. The presence of lymphocytes, plasma cells, and foamy cells is a constant finding around ductal cysts, ruptured or not. It is a manifestation of structural modifications and it is not related to any infection.[51]

Galactocele

Galactocele, which occurs during lactation, is a slowly evolving cystic degeneration of a duct with secondary inflammation and necrosis.[52] Lymphocytes are abundant in the surrounding stroma (Fig. 11-10). It has been observed in women taking oral contraceptives.[53]

Specific Chronic Mastitides

In certain cases, the lesions of chronic mastitis can be specific to the agent involved. *Tuberculous mastitis* is rare and is a complication of a primary pulmonary or lymph node tuberculosis spreading by vascular dissemination.[54,55] Macroscopically, soft, yellowish nodules scattered in the breast tissue are observed. Abscedation of converging nodules and external fistula formation may occur. If these lesions undergo secondary fibrosis, they may macroscopically resemble tumoral lesions. Microscopically, tuberculoid granulomas with Langhans cells

and central caseation indicate the nature of the lesions; the histologic diagnosis is of course confirmed by the presence of acid-fast bacilli in culture. Regional lymph nodes may reveal the presence of solitary tubercles without caseation.

Syphilitic involvement of the mammary gland is extremely rare. Those cases reported in the older literature resulted from contamination during lactation by newborns suffering from congenital syphilis. Rare cases of secondary and tertiary syphilis have been reported.[56]

Mammary gland *actinomycosis* is an infrequent disease resulting from a primary pulmonary infection. Diagnosis is made by observation of the organism within the inflammatory granulomas.[57]

Rare cases of mammary sarcoidosis have been reported. One should remember that sarcoidlike pictures can be observed in lymph nodes draining breast carcinoma. Other rare diseases include filariasis,[58] scleroderma,[59] blastomycosis,[60,61] cryptococcosis, and histoplasmosis.

Fat Necrosis

Fat necrosis can occur in large breasts secondary to trauma or may be associated with carcinoma or any lesion provoking suppurative or necrotic degeneration.[62] It is also seen following the trauma of biopsy and may be difficult to distinguish grossly from residual tumor at the biopsy site. The clinical manifestations of fat necrosis may mimic a malignant tumor and, in the past, these nodular, solid lesions were, in fact, frequently misinterpreted as carcinoma.

A history of pain and tenderness, ecchymosis, and retraction of the skin are the most common clinical features. Even the macroscopic granulomatous, nodular, yellow appearance of the lesion is suggestive of a malignant tumor.[63] Histologically, however, the diagnosis of this benign lesion presents no problem. It is a typical inflammatory granuloma of the fat tissue with areas of fibrosis and necrosis. Large fat vacuoles are surrounded by histiocytes. Multinucleated giant cells are present, as well as blood pigment and lipid crystals (Fig. 11-11). At a later stage, more and more fibrous tissue gradually replaces the active granulomatous process. Typical calcified formations, which represent the walls of cysts, are often observed on mammograms.

The description of fat necrosis illustrates rather well the necessity of performing a biopsy of every suspicious lesion before major surgery. The skin retraction, the suspicious macroscopic aspect, and the calcifications are all misleadingly suggestive of malignancy, and, without histologic proof, such lesions could be misinterpreted and unnecessary mastectomy could be performed.[64]

Plasma Cell Mastitis (Mammary Duct Ectasia)

Plasma cell mastitis was described in 1923 by Bloodgood, who called it varicocoele tumor, and subsequently by Adair, who called it plasma cell mastitis.[65] Haagensen suggested the term *mammary duct ectasia*. Although plasma cell mastitis is not a frequent lesion, its correct interpretation by the pathologist is extremely important, as its clinical and macroscopic manifestations can closely resemble those of carcinomas. The formation of a firm lump and possibly a retraction of the nipple may erroneously suggest the diagnosis of tumor. A serous, purulent, or blood discharge from the nipple can be observed. Plasma cell mastitis occurs at menopause in multiparous women. Its etiology is not known, but this seems to be a lesion of the aging breast. Its high incidence has been confirmed by studies of autopsy material in which 25 percent of supposedly normal breasts in fact showed plasma cell mastitis. The treatment is local surgical excision.

Grossly, there is a firm, poorly defined mass measuring up to 5 cm in diameter. The cut surface reveals a yellow or white granular tissue with dilated ducts that contain brown granular or creamy necrotic material. Compression of the dilated ducts expels this material.

Histologically, this lesion represents a progressive dilation of the main lactiferous ducts with chronic inflammatory lesions and foreign body granuloma formation. The granulomas occur around the necrotic cellular debris and lipids released by the damaged and ruptured ducts (Fig. 11-12). The dilated ducts are lined by flattened cells and contain foamy macrophages, neutrophils, lymphocytes, and sometimes numerous plasma cells. Neutral fat and crystalline lipid bodies are found in this material. There is marked periductal fibrosis often accompanied by a surrounding lymphocytic or plasma cell infiltration. A

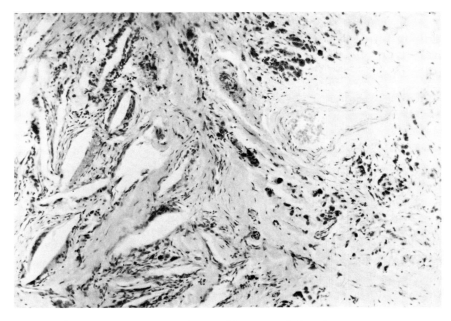

Fig. 11-11. Fat necrosis. Inflammatory granuloma with areas of fibrosis and lipid crystals surrounded by multinucleated giant cells.

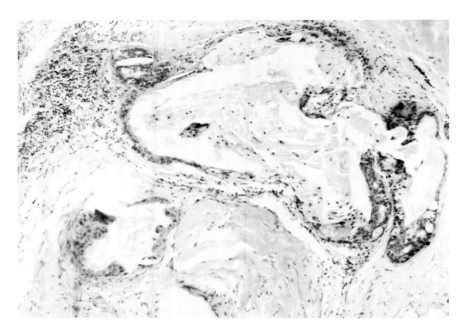

Fig. 11-12. Plasma cell mastisis. Dilated lactiferous ducts with inflammatory infiltrate and giant cell granuloma around cellular debris and lipids.

sarcoid reaction has been described in a few cases. Microscopically, there is no difficulty diagnosing this lesion and thus ruling out the clinical suspicion of malignancy.

Recurrent Subareolar Granuloma

Recurrent subareolar granuloma is a particular form of chronic mastitis associated with lactation. It consists of an inflammatory alteration of the subareolar ducts with recurrent abscess formation and possibly secondary skin fistula. The cystic lesion is lined by stratified squamous epithelium. Careful removal of the involved area is adequate treatment.

Mammary Subcutaneous Phlebitis

Mammary subcutaneous phlebitis (Mondor's disease) is characterized by superficial thoracic vein thrombophlebitis.[66] The cause is unknown and it occurs more frequently in women. Clinically, it occurs as a painful superficial cord beneath the skin of the mammary region. Microscopically, there is a thrombosis of the subcutaneous veins with secondary fibrosis of the vein wall. Strictly speaking, Mondor's disease is not a mastitis but is included in this chapter because it may represent a problem in differential diagnosis.

Cosmetic Mammary Injections

For cosmetic reasons, various materials (oil, paraffin wax, epoxy resin, silicone compounds) have been injected or otherwise introduced into human breasts.[67,68] These substances are in general well tolerated, but they may also provoke the formation of an inflammatory reaction with chronic abscesses, giant cell foreign body granulomas, necrosis, and cutaneous fistulas.

The existence of a tender, firm nodule combined with the clinical history will suggest the diagnosis. The histologic examination shows a foreign body granuloma surrounded by more or less pronounced inflammatory reaction. Involvement of the thoracic wall and even the pleural cavity by the inflammatory process has been reported.

Infarction

Infarction can be related to different clinical conditions. It may appear during pregnancy and lactation. The lesion is usually small with well defined borders and arises in the parenchyma or in benign tumors (fibroadenomas). The pathogenesis is not clear; since there is no evidence of vascular anomaly or history of trauma, an abnormally elevated metabolic activity of the mammary parenchyma has been suggested. In older women, it can be associated with thromboembolic diseases, with cases of Wegener's granulomatosis, and with anticoagulant therapy.[69,70] Massive necrosis of the parenchyma has been described, particularly with use of dicoumarol derivatives.

The histologic appearance is characterized by ischemic necrosis with or without hemorrhage. The lesion is of practical importance because it can grossly mimic carcinoma, and the pathologist must therefore be aware of this differential diagnosis.[71,72]

FIBROCYSTIC MASTOPATHY

The wide variety of terms (cystic hyperplasia, Reclus' disease, Schimmelbusch's disease, mammary dysplasia, sclerosing adenosis, mastodynia, fibroadenosis, Brodie's cystic disease, fibrous dysplasia, chronic cystic mastitis, fibrous mastopathia) found in the literature describing fibrocystic change reflects its extreme polymorphism and the difficulty of integrating so many varied lesions under one simple heading. This is why various attempts at precise pathologic classification have been made.[73–75]

The etiology of fibrocystic mastopathy—the most common lesion of the breast—remains only partially understood. All we can say at present is that the histologic structures of the mammary tissue are submitted to different influences and factors that may permanently modify them. Genetic background, hormonal balance, age, parity, lactation history, and possibly viruses and psychosomatic illnesses can all influence the morphology of the mammary glands.[76–79] The existence of hormonal factors is suggested by various clinical and experimental findings; for example, the lesion develops at an age when the mammary gland has already been exposed to a long estrogenic stimulation, and experimental estrogen injections induce the development of cysts in the mammary gland of the rhesus monkey.

Fibrocystic mastopathy is a common condition among young women and the incidence rate increases with age, reaching a peak at about 40 to 45 years of age. Clinically, the patient reports the presence of a poorly defined mass often accompanied by discomfort and tenderness and aggravated during the premenstrual period. The lesion may appear in a localized or a diffuse form, and frequently, both mammary glands are involved. Clinical examination reveals the beads on a string sign, that is, one or several fine nodules of different sizes. Mammography reveals microcalcifications and other pathologic radiologic findings.

Macroscopically, the lesion is characterized by the dense, often glistening appearance of the involved tissue, with the presence of a variable number of blue or yellow cysts of different sizes. Sclerosing adenosis appears as a moderately firm, lobular, circumscribed mass; the section reveals lobulated gray-white granular tissue. A careful search for any area suggestive of cancer must be performed; more specifically, the presence of fine, granular, dense tissue with chalky yellow streaks is highly suspicious.

It is time to reconsider histologically the old concept of fibrocystic "disease," described by Reclus and Schimmelbusch almost a century ago, and to separate definite benign lesions from a spectrum of proliferative epithelial lesions, some of which are related to neoplasia.[80–85] The benign lesions, which could be named *functional mastopathies*, are very common. They represent physiologic alterations due to cyclic or unbalanced hormonal stimulations or mammary tissue hypersensitive to normal hormonal activity. Therefore, the term *disease* should be abandoned to qualify these alterations, which include cysts of various sizes, duct ectasia, stromal fibrosis, sclerosing and blunt duct adenosis, and apocrine change.

When proliferative epithelial changes are present, we are dealing with the *proliferative form of fibrocystic mastopathy*. The proliferative changes are seen in the ductal system, the lobules or both, and current classifications rely on a system of grading of the different degrees of proliferative changes or hyperplasias[86–92] (Table 11-3). The grading goes from mild to severe in terms of epithelial proliferation, loss of cell polarity, number of cell layers and cellular atypias, and is further subdivided by the unit(s) (ducts, lobules) involved. It is important to evaluate the presence and the severity of the hyperplasia because they enable the assignment of the patient to a specific risk category for the development of carcinoma. From the abundant literature available on benign mastopathy and its relationship to breast cancer risk, it is now imperative that the pathologist grade the severity of the hyperplasia and discuss the findings with the surgeon to arrive at the optimal treatment.

A few rules should be followed to adopt a coherent attitude toward the management of this frequent breast pathology. The breast biopsy material should be totally

TABLE 11-3. Classifications of Proliferative Mastopathy

Black et al.[90]	Wellings et al.[91]	Page et al.[92]
1: Normal	Grade I	Normal
2: Hyperplasia	Grade II	Hyperplasia without atypia
3: Distinct but minimal atypia	Grade III	Atypical hyperplasia (mild, moderate, or severe)
4: Atypia suggestive of in situ carcinoma	Grade IV	DCIS or LCIS
5: Atypia consistent with in situ carcinoma	Grade V (DCIS or LCIS)	

DCIS, ductal carcinoma in situ; LCIS, lobular carcinoma in situ.

examined and the precise location of mammographic anomalies identified, usually by specimen radiography. The pathologist and the clinician should carefully discuss the therapeutic program and agree on the significance of the terms adopted to describe the lesions.

Lactiferous Cysts

Lactiferous cysts represent the most minimal changes observed in fibrocystic mastopathy.[93] They are small and disseminated in the parenchyma, and their number and size vary greatly. These cysts develop as the result of the dilatation of ducts or as the multiplication of terminal ductules (blunt duct adenosis of Foote and Stewart) (Fig. 11-13). They are lined by a flattened, cuboidal, or columnar epithelium, which may reveal degenerative cellular alterations. The desquamated cells in the cystic fluid exhibit a characteristic, finely vacuolar, abundant pale cytoplasm and small, round, regular nuclei.[94] Abundant lipids can be detected in the cytoplasm. Necrosis with accumulation of cellular debris may result in cholesterol crystal formation with secondary fibrosis. Necrosis and secondary calcifications may be observed in the cyst epithelium.

Stromal Fibrosis

Fibrosis is a constant feature of fibrocystic disease. The modified epithelial structures are surrounded by variable amounts of dense and poorly cellular stroma;

collagen fibers are abundant (Fig. 11-13). Epithelial proliferation seems to stimulate this stromal growth.

Adenosis

Adenosis is a proliferation of ductules and acini with the persistence of structures suggesting the lobular disposition observed in the normal gland. This proliferation may be accompanied by variable degrees of myoepithelial hyperplasia and fibrosis. There may be an increased number of cellular layers above the basal lamina; cellular atypias are very discrete, a characteristic that helps differentiate this from more severe lesions such as atypical hyperplasia and in situ or infiltrating carcinoma. Apocrine metaplasia may be present.

Some subclassifications have been proposed to qualify particular images. *Sclerosing adenosis*, the most common type, is discussed in detail below. In *florid adenosis*, the ductal proliferation is particularly evident and is associated with myoepithelial proliferation and fibrosis. Multiple foci of the lesions are commonly observed and they are rather well circumscribed. *Blunt duct adenosis* is characterized by lobular dilatation with varying degrees of cellular proliferation. The term *nodular adenosis* has been proposed to describe a lesion consisting of a nodular proliferation of tubules of relatively uniform size and the absence of the whorled arrangement usually provoked by the marked fibrosis. Nodular adenosis should not be confused with tubular carcinoma. The absence of a double-layered epithelium with myoepithelial cells and the presence of cellular atypia and intraductal epithelial bridging

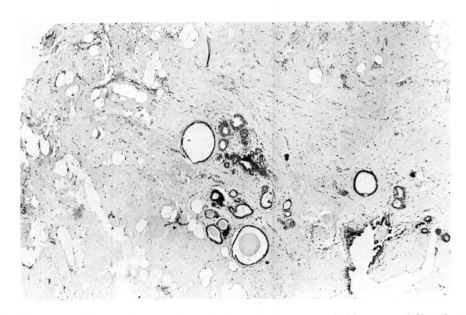

Fig. 11-13. Fibrocystic disease. Rare cystic ductal structures surrounded by stromal fibrosis are shown.

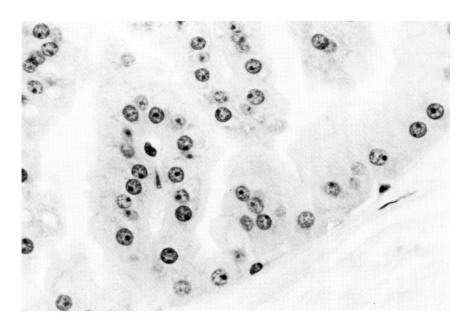

Fig. 11-18. Apocrine metaplasia: large eosinophilic cells with bulging apical poles.

The lesion consists of a central area of sclerosis with engulfed haphazardly arranged ducts around this central core. The central area has a radial disposition and may be surrounded by adenosis, intraductal papillary proliferations, and epithelial hyperplasia (Fig. 11-19). The central scar contains collagen and elastic fibers.[111] The ductal structures maintain their two cell layers, except when epithelial cells are altered by sclerosis and elastosis. Multiple and bilateral locations have been observed.

The distorted and irregular disposition of the glandular structures explains our concern when a diagnostic decision has to be made. The main difficulty lies in the confusion with tubular carcinoma. The absence of cellular atypia and mitoses, the persistence of a double-layered epithelium and the characteristic circumscription of the lesion are in favor of benignity. The histogenesis of this lesion is a matter of controversy; some investigators have suggested that it represents a proliferation of terminal ducts and lobules accompanied by occlusive fibrosis of ductal laminae. Radial scar is usually associated with fibrocystic changes. Divergent views on the significance of scar lesions have been expressed in the literature, but opinions are generally in favor of their benign evolution.[112]

Epithelial Proliferation or Hyperplasia

Under this heading we gather all degrees of ductal epithelial proliferation that can be observed in fibrocystic mastopathy. It includes the lesions mentioned as duct,

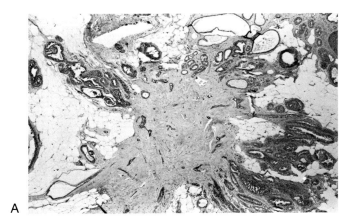

A

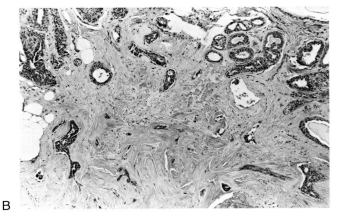

B

Fig. 11-19. Radial sclerosing lesion. **(A)** Central sclerosis surrounded by radially arranged ducts, many of which are hyperplastic. **(B)** Sclerotic center of lesion at higher magnification contains entrapped pseudoinfiltrative ducts.

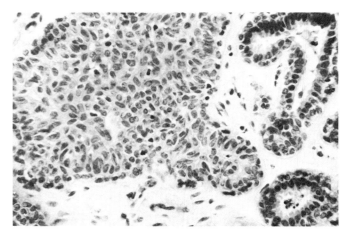

Fig. 11-20. Ductal cell hyperplasia. Note the solid cellular growth without marked cellular atypia; partial obliteration of the ductular lumen by cellular proliferation; and absence of cellular atypia and mitoses (high magnification).

lobular, and papillomatoid hyperplasia, adenomatosis, and epitheliosis (the term used by British pathologists).[113] When the proliferation is moderate and not accompanied by cellular atypia, the benign character of the lesion is evident. The recognition of an atypical hyperplasia is important, as we now have pertinent data showing that these patients are subject to a greater risk of developing cancer, ranging from 1.5 to 5 times that of the general population. The variety of terms proposed to characterize these proliferations is a source of confusion among pathologists; therefore, it is to be desired that a clear definition of every term used should be expressed.

All variations of epithelial proliferation can be observed from the benign type with preservation of normal cellular structure to in situ carcinoma (Figs. 11-20 to 11-22). In evaluating the character of these lesions, the pathologist should investigate the following criteria: the composition of the epithelium, which is normally lined by two cellular layers[92]; cellular structure; obliteration of the ductular lumen by the epithelial proliferation; and ductal dilation. The absence of cellular and architectural atypia indicates a lesion that should be designated *epithelial* (ductal or lobular) *proliferations* or *hyperplasia without atypia*. By contrast, epithelial proliferation with atypia or atypical hyperplasia reveals the presence of cellular anomalies and alterations of the ductal disposition. The most severe of these lesions can be distinguished from in situ carcinoma only with difficulty.

A schematic representation of these modifications is provided in Figure 11-23; Table 11-3 summarizes some of the different classifications proposed in the literature. Electron microscopic studies have been quite disappointing in terms of differential diagnosis between hyperplastic fibrocystic mastopathy and carcinoma, as the cellular changes prove to be more quantitative than qualitative.[97,102] This underscores the difficulties of differentiating morphologically benign and malignant cells in borderline lesions. Experimental and clinical data suggest that atypical lobular and ductal hyperplasias represent precursors of carcinoma.

The relationship between fibrocystic mastopathy and

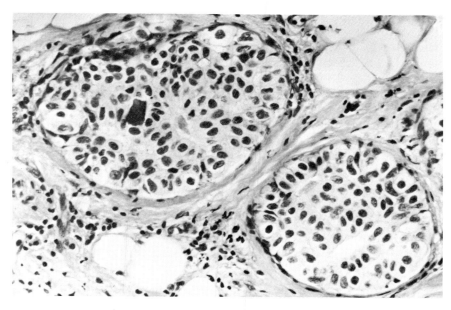

Fig. 11-21. Atypical epithelial proliferation. The persistence of small glandular lumina indicates benignity. Note the presence of cellular atypia and macrocalcifications.

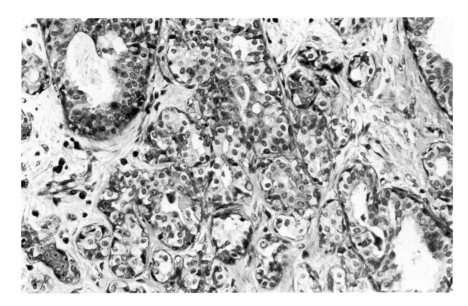

Fig. 11-22. Florid epithelial proliferation. Note the presence of cellular atypia but persistence of glandular lumina.

an increased risk of breast cancer has been a matter of discussion for some time.[72,86,114,115] While the coexistence of both diseases is established, this could conceivably represent only two unrelated disorders linked to a common cause, and not different steps in the evolution of one disease process. In a study of 1,000 breast carcinomas,

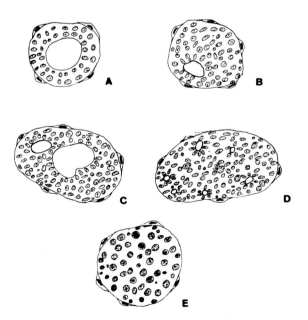

Fig. 11-23. Schema of the various degrees of ductular hyperplasia. **(A)** Normal lactiferous duct. **(B)** Moderate proliferation of the cellular layers. **(C)** Proliferation with cribriform pattern. **(D)** Proliferation with obliteration of the lumen and cellular atypia. **(E)** Carcinoma in situ.

this association was present in 34.9 percent of the cases.[116]

The arguments in favor of the relation include the frequently noted association in surgical specimens of fibrocystic mastopathy in the vicinity of mammary cancer, the incidence of fibrocystic changes in previous biopsies from patients whose breasts have been removed for cancer, and prospective studies of patients with fibrocystic mastopathy who later develop carcinoma.[81,82] However, the lack of adequate control groups, improper mortality statistics, and insufficient follow-up explain why this possible relationship cannot presently be definitively evaluated. Moreover, it is hazardous to rely only on anatomic associations to conclude that atypical hyperplasia and carcinoma are causally related.[74] However, we know that fibrocystic mastopathy shares certain immunologic, epidemiologic, and biochemical characteristics with breast carcinoma.

Epidemiologic studies on fibrocystic mastopathy in oral contraceptive users, for example, have produced evidence that there are in fact two types of fibrocystic mastopathy: one with minimal epithelial atypia and one with marked epithelial atypia.[117,118] Long-term use of oral contraceptives is associated with a decreased incidence of fibrocystic mastopathy with minimal epithelial changes but not of the forms showing marked epithelial changes.[118,119]

As discussed above, fibrocystic mastopathy can be separated into a proliferative and a nonproliferative form: the nonproliferative type includes fibrosis, cysts, sclerosing adenosis, blunt duct adenosis, and apocrine changes; the proliferative type includes intraductal and lobular hyperplasias. It is only the proliferative lesions that must be considered as a potential precancerous tissue alteration. It has been estimated that patients with atypical hyperplasia increase their risk of developing an invasive carcinoma by four- to fivefold. The mean interval between the diagnosis of atypical hyperplasia and invasive carcinoma is 8.2 years with extreme limits between 1 and 24 years.[88,120,121] Atypical hyperplasia is found in about 3 percent of all mammary biopsies. If we exclude the lesions of atypical epithelial hyperplasia, the evidence for a link between mastopathy and an increased risk of breast cancer is exceedingly weak.

BENIGN NEOPLASMS

Fibroadenoma

The fibroadenoma is the most frequent benign tumor of the breast. Rare before puberty, it usually appears in the 15- to 35-year age group, the greatest frequency being in the 20s. It is a slowly growing, estrogen-dependent, fibroepithelial neoplasm. Dysmenorrhea, premenstrual tension, and irregular menses are often mentioned in the clinical history of the patient, suggesting a hormonal disturbance. Clinical and pathologic studies of fibroadenomas in patients receiving oral contraceptives have been published.[122]

The fibroadenoma usually manifests as a single mass, but it may be multifocal and may occur in both breasts simultaneously. Clinically it is a circumscribed, movable mass with a firm, elastic consistency. The tumor does not adhere to adjacent tissues or the overlying skin.

There is still some debate over whether the fibroadenoma is a true neoplasm or represents hyperplastic change of both the stromal and epithelial components. Fibroadenoma and certain foci of fibrocystic mastopathy sometimes exhibit identical structures, which suggests etiologic and morphologic relationships between the two lesions.[123]

Macroscopically, the lesion is a well encapsulated, firm rubbery mass, measuring 0.5 to 5 cm in diameter. The cut section reveals a gray or pink lobulated, bulging tissue; the lobules are bordered by fibrous septa. When the epithelial elements are abundant, the color tends to be more pink or light tan. The mass is encapsulated by a thin fibrous surface (Fig. 11-24).

Microscopically, the fibroadenoma is a benign, localized proliferation of epithelial cells and fibroblasts, occurring in a voluminous and misshapen lobule. Classically, we distinguish two histologic types, which may occur alone or in combination. The *pericanalicular* form exhibits well preserved glandular structures with normal bistratified epithelium, embedded in a loose connective

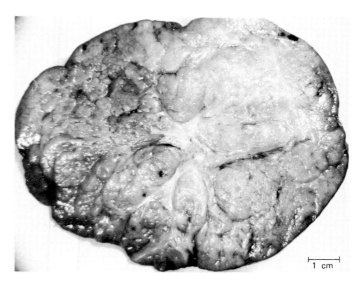

Fig. 11-24. Giant fibroadenoma, macroscopic aspect.

tissue stroma whose cells tend to adopt a concentric arrangement about the glands. While collagen and reticulin are abundant, the number of elastic fibers is not significantly increased. Capillary vascularization is discrete. Glandular proliferation with moderate cytologic atypia can be observed, but these lesions raise no suspicion of malignancy. Hyalinization, edema, and myxoid degeneration can be observed. Neutral mucopolysaccharides have been identified in the ground substance of the connective tissue proliferation. Squamous metaplasia with keratinized cyst formation is possible, but rare.[124] In the *intracanalicular* form, the glandular structures are enveloped and tightly compressed by a hyperplastic fibrous stroma arranged in irregular nodules (Fig. 11-25). The epithelial structures thus appear stretched out, distorted, or atrophic. The stroma may be densely or poorly cellular and rich in collagen, or it may be calcified. Acid mucopolysaccharides are present in the ground substance. Squamous, bony, and cartilaginous metaplasia as well as the presence of smooth muscle fibers have been reported.[125,126]

Ultrastructural studies demonstrate that the stromal proliferation is responsible for the tumor growth.[127,128] Secretory cells generally constitute a single cell layer; the presence of occasional cilia has been reported. Myoepithelial cells whose long axis runs parallel to the basement membrane lie beneath the epithelial cells. Multilayered basal lamina may be present. These multiple layers of basal lamina may result from successive episodes of cell death and new proliferation, each new generation of cells laying down a new membrane parallel to the last.

This phenomenon is often observed in benign proliferations in general, the fibroadenoma being one example.

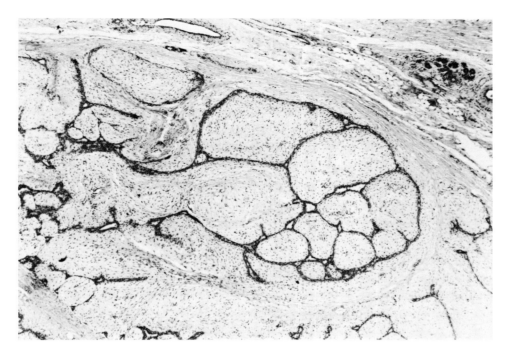

Fig. 11-25. Fibroadenoma, intracanalicular type.

Surrounding the cellular structures are bundles of collagen fibers and aggregates of microfibrils. Myoepithelial cells retain their usual relationship to the basement membrane.[129]

Evolution and Prognosis

The growth of fibroadenoma is slow; it may take years before these lesions reach a palpable size. At menopause, fibroadenomas stabilize or regress; growth may be rapid during pregnancy, and signs of secretion have been observed during lactation.[130]

Infarction of fibroadenoma is an uncommon complication that may occur during pregnancy or lactation.[131] The possible etiologic mechanisms are thrombosis of the feeding vessel or a relative vascular insufficiency with respect to increased metabolic activity. This complication should be borne in mind since the infarcted benign lesion may grossly simulate carcinoma.[131,132]

The possibility of malignant transformation of fibroadenoma has given rise to much controversy.[133–137] A few cases have been reported in the literature, the most frequent type of associated carcinoma described being lobular in situ carcinoma. The exact incidence of malignant transformation is difficult to evaluate because some carcinomas may totally replace a pre-existent fibroadenoma. Since fibroadenoma is a common lesion, one can expect to observe the coincidental and simultaneous presence of fibroadenoma and carcinoma in the same breast, espe-cially in older patients. The development of sarcoma is discussed with cytosarcoma phyllodes.

Juvenile Fibroadenoma

The juvenile fibroadenoma is a rapidly growing, often bilateral tumor of young patients. Histologically, this lesion manifests an active proliferation of the epithelial and connective tissue elements. Essentially, it is the age of the patient and the rapid growth of the lesion that characterize this type of fibroadenoma.[138–140]

Adenoma

The adenoma (tubular adenoma, pure adenoma, fetal adenoma) is a well demarcated pure adenomatous proliferation of the breast tissue with a very sparse stroma.[141] This rare, benign lesion appears in young, nonpregnant women and seems to be unrelated to contraceptive hormonal therapy.

Other histologic types have been described. The *lactating adenoma* appears during pregnancy or lactation.[142,143] The closely packed cells show mitoses and cytoplasmic vacuoles. The *tubular adenoma* shows tubular structures that are very regular in size and shape and are lined by a single layer of epithelial cells. The *pleomorphic adenoma* resembles the benign mixed tumor of salivary gland.[144]

Nipple Adenoma

The nipple adenoma[145–147] (subareolar papillomatosis, florid papillomatosis, papillary adenoma) is an uncommon entity observed in a wide range of age groups. It consists of a nodule localized immediately beneath the nipple, which is often clinically misdiagnosed as carcinoma or Paget's disease. The nipple can be crusted or ulcerated. A serous or bloody discharge is frequently observed. The macroscopic appearance is that of a circumscribed, solitary, solid mass.

The cut section reveals a gray or tan, soft to firm tissue. Microscopically, we observe a proliferation of ducts of variable sizes with characteristic papillary structures (Fig. 11-26A,B). The intensity of the papillary proliferation varies from one case to another: sometimes this proliferation is very abundant and plugs the ducts, and sometimes it is absent. The ductal structures are lined by a double-layered epithelium. The nuclei may be moderately enlarged but are uniform and normochromatic. Mi-

totic figures are rare. Apocrine metaplasia and squamous cysts are common. Dense fibrosis may occur between the ducts, resembling the pseudoinvasive pattern encountered in sclerosing adenosis.

Despite the occasional clinical and even pathologic mimicking of a malignant tumor, and the fact that nipple adenomas are sometimes incidental findings in breasts removed for carcinoma, the risk of progression to malignancy is minimal, and this is a benign lesion that may be treated by local excision in uncomplicated cases.

The nipple adenoma is histologically identical to hidradenoma papilliferum of the vulva and may arise in the modified sweat glands of the areolar region. *Syringomatous adenoma* occurs beneath the areolar region.[148] This lesion is more infiltrative and more likely to recur locally but also is benign.

Adenomyoepithelioma

In this uncommon tumor, there is a biphasic proliferation of ducts lined by epithelial cells and surrounding polygonal to spindled myoepithelial cells, which make up the most conspicuous element (Fig. 11-27). Local recurrences have been reported, but distant metastases have not occurred to date.[149] Rare pure myoepithelial cell tumors, both benign and malignant, have also been observed.

Intraductal Papilloma

The intraductal papilloma is a benign papilliform proliferation of the ductal epithelium.[150,151] It is not a frequent lesion, and care must be taken to avoid misinterpreting it as carcinoma. Papillomas may be solitary or multiple; in

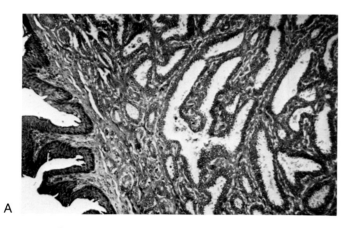
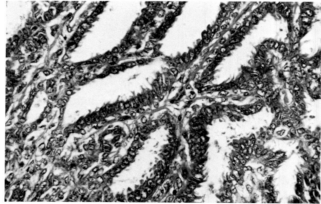

Fig. 11-26. Nipple adenoma. **(A)** Low magnification. Ductal proliferation is localized beneath the mammary skin (seen at left). **(B)** High magnification. The glandular structures are lined by columnar epithelium underlain by myoepithelium. The nuclei are regular and mitoses are absent.

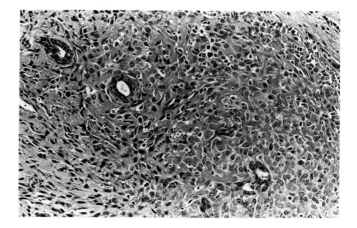

Fig. 11-27. Adenomyoepithelioma. Locally recurrent tumor contains small ductal structures engulfed by polygonal myoepithelial cells becoming spindled at periphery of nodule.

THE BREAST

the latter case, we speak of papillomatosis. Solitary papillomas are more frequent, and they develop in the terminal portion of a main duct. A third type of papilloma, the nipple adenoma, has been discussed previously.

Intraductal papilloma may appear at any age but is more common between 30 and 50 years. The main clinical features include spontaneous or induced serous or bloody nipple discharge, the presence of a small subareolar tumor and, more rarely, nipple retraction.

Mammography following intraductal injection of contrast medium helps to identify and localize intraductal papillomas. Cytologic study of the discharge reveals the presence of clusters of benign-looking epithelial cells. Gross examination of the surgical specimen, including a careful dissection of the ducts, reveals a soft, friable, yellow or red papilliform structure attached to the inner wall of a duct. The size varies from a few millimeters to a few centimeters in diameter. Cystic changes are occasionally produced by obstruction of the duct harboring the papilloma. Dissection of the lesion should be carefully performed by gently opening the duct with scissors; proper fixation and embedding of the specimen are essential to obtain an easily readable slide. Frozen section should be avoided if at all possible; the distinction of these lesions from intraductal carcinomas may be difficult, and tissue should be fixed properly and submitted in its entirety for permanent section examination.

Microscopic examination reveals delicate branching of papillary structures, consisting of connective tissue covered by epithelial cells (Fig. 11-28). These cells are arranged in two layers, which include myoepithelial cells (Fig. 11-29). The presence of a double row of cells is one of the morphologic criteria proposed by Kraus and Neubecker[152] to distinguish a papilloma from a papillary carcinoma. The myoepithelial cells may require immunohistochemical techniques for their demonstration.[153] The epithelial cells may also proliferate to form solid masses. These masses may surround empty spaces, but these are usually variable in size and shape and compressed into flattened slits by the cells, unlike the uniform round spaces in a cribriform type of intraductal carcinoma. The papillae are located in enlarged ducts, which are sometimes filled by these florid structures. When the tension within the cystic duct is high, the superficial cellular layers are flattened or exhibit small foci of erosion.

The epithelial cells resemble those of a normal duct; mitoses are rare and the nuclei are regularly oriented parallel to the long axis of the cells. Sometimes, these cells exhibit hyperplastic changes. They may be larger than normal duct cells, and the nuclei are discretely irregular and hyperchromatic. Apocrine cells may be present. In some cases, the proliferating myoepithelial cells invade and distend the connective tissue of the papillary processes. These pictures are quite similar to those of

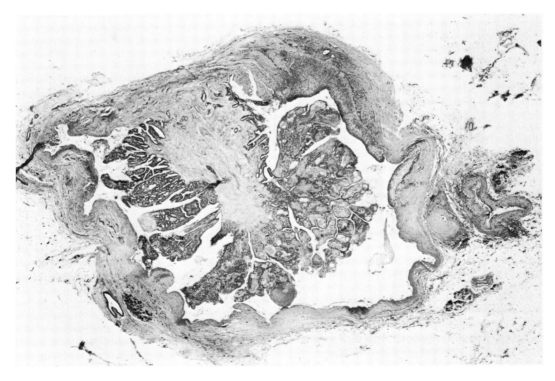

Fig. 11-28. Intraductal papilloma.

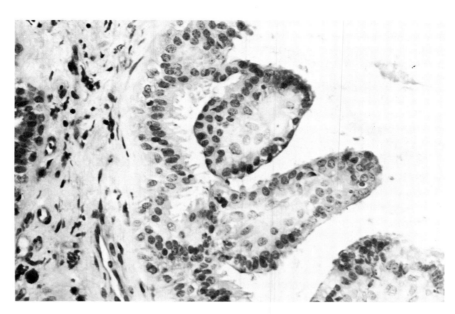

Fig. 11-29. Intraductal papilloma, detail of a papillary structure.

sclerosing adenosis and can be confused with a carcinomatous infiltration.[106]

The differential diagnosis between a florid atypical papilloma and an intraductal papillary carcinoma is sometimes extremely difficult. Generally, when a diagnostic error is made, it is a false positive one rather than a false negative one, benign lesions being taken for malignant ones. Papillary carcinomas exhibit the presence of multilayered epithelial papillae without central connective tissue cores, often with loss of nuclear polarity and cytologic atypia. The presence of a true cribriform pattern, that is, cell strands bridging the duct lumen and forming uniform round spaces, is also characteristic of malignancy. Very thin stromal formations may sometimes separate the epithelial components. Large solid proliferations favor benignity, since solid intraductal carcinomas tend to develop central necrosis (comedocarcinoma). Foci of apocrine metaplasia also favor benignity.

There is much diversity of opinion about the malignant potential of intraductal papillomas. While Cutler[154] maintains that patients with intraductal papilloma have a greater chance of developing cancer later, most authors question this malignant potential. Most diagnostic errors probably concern lesions in which malignant changes are minimal, as is the rule in these well differentiated tumors. Ashikari et al.[155] showed in a retrospective study of a series of papillary carcinomas, that the prior biopsies of these patients reported as benign papillomas were in reality already malignant papillary lesions. In these cases, one should be very cautious about making a diagnosis on a frozen section. Even careful study of well fixed, paraffin-embedded material does not always completely solve the problem. Ultrastructural and histochemical studies show similarities that confirm the relationship between benign and malignant lesions and the existence of borderline cases.

Generally speaking, the evolution of these lesions is benign in most cases; thus, the pathologist must avoid overdiagnosing benign papillary lesions in fear of missing differentiated carcinoma. In any case, excision of these lesions must be complete to avoid any risk of local recurrence. Multiple papillomas probably have a greater cancer risk than solitary ones.[153,156]

It has been reported that florid papillomatosis occurs with greater frequency in association with carcinoma even if there is no evidence to suggest that the lesion is itself malignant.[157] This association can be compared with the previously mentioned relation between atypical hyperplasia and cancer.

Juvenile Papillomatosis

In 1980, Rosen et al.[158] recognized juvenile papillomatosis as a clinicopathologic entity. The lesion is more frequent in adolescents and young women but occasionally occurs in women up to the age of menopause. Clinically, it is characterized by a painless, movable, circumscribed mass that is often interpreted as fibroadenoma. Macroscopically, juvenile papillomatosis is composed of nonencapsulated multinodular masses. Microscopically, there is cystic duct dilation with intraductal solid or papillary epithelial proliferation, often associated with fibrosis, sclerosing adenosis, apocrine metaplasia, and intraductal foamy histiocytes. When the epithelial proliferation is quite marked, it should not be confused with an intraductal carcinoma. The premalignant potential of juvenile papillomatosis is not yet determined; therefore, wide excision followed by a careful follow-up is suggested.[159]

Benign Tumors of Connective Tissue

Benign tumors of the connective tissue may arise in the mammary gland. *Leiomyomas* may develop deep in the breast from the vessels or in the areola from the smooth muscle fibers present in this region. They occur in women in their fifth and sixth decades and have a slow rate of growth.[160,161] *Lipomas* are well encapsulated, palpable, soft masses that are seen in women aged 40 to 60 years.[162] Fibromas and osteomas are exceptionally rare. Myofibroblastoma has been described as more common in the male than in the female breast.[163]

Granular cell "myoblastoma" has been described in the mammary gland.[164,165] Grossly, it is a firm, round mass that adheres to adjacent tissue and may simulate a carcinoma. Microscopically, characteristic large clear cells with a granular, PAS positive, eosinophilic cytoplasm and small round nuclei are arranged in clumps or nests surrounded by large collagenous and reticular bundles. Ultrastructural studies reveal that these granules correspond to lyosomes. Recent electron microscopic and immunohistochemical investigations tend to support a neurogenic origin for these tumors.[166]

Adenolipoma is a hamartoma containing typical mammary lobules included in the fatty tissue.[162]

Hemangiomas, previously thought to be rare, have been described recently in 1.2 percent of mastectomy specimens, usually as incidental microscopic findings. They must be distinguished from well differentiated angiosarcomas.[167–171]

CYSTOSARCOMA PHYLLODES

A giant type of fibroadenoma was described in 1838 by Müller[172] who used the name cystosarcoma phyllodes to qualify the leaflike and fleshy gross appearance of this tumor. This term has since been consecrated by use, although it is confusing. It is essentially a fibroepithelial tumor in which the stroma or mesenchymal component shows a marked proliferation. Cystosarcoma phyllodes (pseudosarcomatous fibroadenoma, giant intracanalicular fibroadenoma, Brodie's serocystic disease) is a rare type of mammary neoplasm. It appears most frequently in middle-aged women, an older age group than those

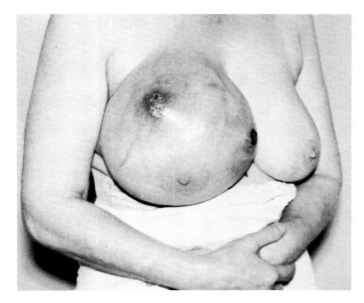

Figure 11-30. Cystosarcoma phyllodes in a 52-year-old woman.

with fibroadenoma, and represents approximately 1 percent of all fibroepithelial tumors of the breast. It has been reported more rarely in younger women[173] and in the elderly.[174]

Clinically, it is usually a rapidly growing, bulky tumor that may attain a diameter of 15 cm or more (Fig. 11-30). In spite of its large size and rapid growth, it does not infiltrate adjacent tissues or the overlying skin. Skin ulceration may occur, however, resulting from the pressure exerted by the underlying tumor. Thus, the presence of a rapidly growing mass and skin alterations may produce a clinical condition that mimics carcinoma.

The macroscopic appearance is that of a firm, nodular, well-circumscribed, displaceable tumor. Sections of the tumor reveal numerous, gray-white to yellow nodules surrounded by fibrous septa that evoke a leaf-like appearance. In large tumors, hemorrhagic and cystic areas and necrosis may be present. Smaller tumors may also be encountered.

Microscopic examination reveals an intense proliferation of the stromal cells with overgrown epithelial formations (Fig. 11-31A,B). The stromal cells are large and elongated and reveal different degrees of cellular atypia. Foci of hyalinized or densely collagenous tissue and deposits of intercellular mucoid material are observed.[175]

Some tumors are classified as histologically benign, while others are considered histologically malignant. In the first group, the general pattern of the tumors resembles the fibroadenoma except for increased stromal cellularity. Mitoses are rare and cellular atypias are very discrete. In the second group, the stroma is markedly cellular, and there is a haphazard arrangement of the

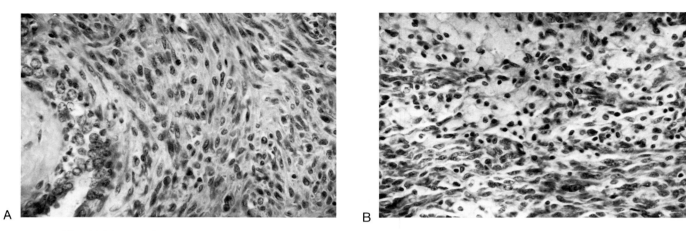

Fig. 11-31. Benign cystosarcoma phyllodes. **(A)** The stroma is very cellular but exhibits no marked atypia. **(B)** Note the presence of cells with fatty cytoplasm.

cells. All degrees of nuclear atypia and nuclear hypertrophy are present.[176] The sarcoma-like foci reproduce the aspect of a differentiated fibrosarcoma or liposarcoma[177,178] or, in the most undifferentiated cases, the structure of an anaplastic and pleomorphic sarcoma. There is increased mitotic activity. The ductal formations are distorted by the marked stromal overgrowth but exhibit no signs of malignancy. Some cases may show an intense proliferative activity of the epithelial structures and even squamous metaplasia. The atypical stromal overgrowth is evident at the periphery of the tumor, where secondary infiltration of the adjacent tissues is observed. Some tumors have a mucinous matrix, which makes them resemble myxoliposarcomas.[177] Chondroid and osteoid metaplasia are also observed. Finally, there is a borderline group that shows intermediate alterations that are difficult to classify.

Some investigators advocate this subdivision into his-

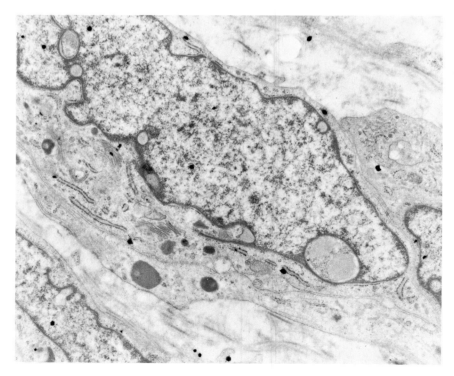

Fig. 11-32. Cystosarcoma phyllodes. Electron micrograph shows a stromal cell with intranuclear vacuoles and abundant cytoplasmic organelles.

tologically benign and malignant categories based on criteria such as cellular atypia, mitotic activity, the type of margin (pushing or infiltrating) and the ratio of mesenchymal over epithelial tissue,[178-180] Others have challenged the validity of this practice. Since the histologic grading of cystosarcomas has not proved to be a totally reliable prediction of the clinical behavior, all these lesions should be considered potentially aggressive tumors. Those with marked cellularity, cytologic anaplasia, and high mitotic activity pose no diagnostic problem.[181,182]

Local recurrences are seen in approximately 20 percent of the benign variant,[183] but metastases are infrequent (approximately 10 percent), even in the histologically malignant group, and should not occur in the benign group. In some cases, recurrences of initially benign lesions present obviously malignant features. Metastases consist of poorly differentiated mesenchymal elements whose most common site is pulmonary tissue. A few cases of metastases to axillary lymph nodes have been reported. Wide local excision is adequate treatment for the histologically benign lesions, and mastectomy is required for voluminous or histologically malignant tumors.

Electron microscopic observations (Fig. 11-32) of malignant cystosarcoma phyllodes are suggestive of the mesenchymal origin of this tumor.[184,185] Estrogen and progesterone receptors are present or absent according to different authors; these findings may reflect the relative amounts[186,187] of epithelial and stromal components. Malignant cystosarcoma should not be confused with fibrosarcoma. Ductal elements, which represent an integral portion of cystosarcoma phyllodes, are absent in fibrosarcoma. Carcinosarcoma is a very rare lesion exhibiting both epithelial and mesenchymal malignant elements.[188]

MALIGNANT TUMORS

In spite of the apparent progress made in surgery, radiotherapy, and chemotherapy, the percentage of deaths caused by breast cancer has varied little over the past 30 years. What little improvement we have made in diagnosis and treatment seems counterbalanced by an increased incidence of the disease. In the United States, it is estimated that one woman in about 15 will develop breast cancer at some time in her life, and that approximately 40,000 women will die of it each year. Thus, we can understand the importance of improving our knowledge of the etiologic risk factors, as well as of the biological behavior of breast malignancies.

The combination of modern and often sophisticated diagnostic procedures, including mammography, thermography, ultrasonography, and xerography, allows ear-

lier diagnosis of early lesions.[189,190] Mammography is an indispensible technique in the detection of nonpalpable lesions. Thermography has a less clearly defined value because of its nonspecificity and the frequency of false positive and false negative results.[191] Therefore, while it is true that borderline lesions and in situ cancers are currently more frequently diagnosed, many tumors have nevertheless advanced beyond the local stage at the time of diagnosis. The ignorance of the public, the fear of consulting the doctor, the clinical impossibility of detecting all lesions at a very early stage, and the skeptical attitude of some doctors about the value of early diagnosis partially explain the delay in diagnosis and therapy.[192]

As a rule, when a tumor has attained its clinical stage, it has already been quietly evolving over a long period, during which the tumor's own biological behavior and the host's defense mechanisms must come to terms. Variations of these two factors explain the differences in prognosis from individual to individual. In any case, it is acceptable that the smallest and most slowly evolving tumors generally afford the best clinical prognosis.[193-195]

It is important to point out that the diagnosis of breast cancer is, in the final analysis, the responsibility of the pathologist, and that the anatomic and histologic data he can provide are essential criteria of the cancer's evolution; for example, the size of the tumor and the evaluation of lymph node metastases represent simple and accurate information about the clinical prognosis.

Etiology and Risk Factors

The etiology of breast cancer remains unknown, but the large volume of information gathered in recent years, including experimental, epidemiologic, and clinical data, is progressively bringing us to a more accurate approach to the problem.[196-200] However, the factors that will be discussed should be interpreted with caution because they are not particularly strong determinants of risk, they do not have the same importance in different populations, and their effects are not additive and can seemingly be cancelled out by favorable factors.[201] For example, environmental factors rather than genetic ones seem to explain certain geographic and ethnic differences such as the low incidence of breast cancer in Japanese women; also, increased parity lowers the survival rate even in patients whose first pregnancy took place at an early age, a factor that in itself is generally considered favorable.[202] The following factors will be discussed in the succeeding sections: incidence with respect to age, age at menarche, age at menopause, age at first childbirth, premenopausal ovarian status, breast feeding, nutrition, family history, previous breast disease, ethnic group, endogenous and exogenous hormonal status, immunologic factors, viruses, and ionizing radiation.

Incidence and Age

The risk of developing carcinoma increases with every year of life. The effect of age is reflected by the rising incidence up to age 50 and by another steep increase after a period of constant incidence between the ages of 50 and 55. Increased interest in early diagnosis has in effect shown that cancer of the breast in women under the age of 30 is not rare.[203–206]

Age and Other Factors

Late age at menarche and early artificial or natural menopause are considered to be favorable factors. These facts should be interpreted as clinical expressions of hormonal climates: late menarche and early menopause reduce the period of ovarian hormonal activity.[207]

Nutrition

Dietary fats and obesity seem to be related to breast carcinoma, particularly after 50 years of age, because they are associated with endogenous hormonal modifications. In obese, menopausal patients, estrogen production occurs by the conversion of androstenedione to estrone, primarily in adipose tissue. The difference in rates of breast carcinoma between American and Japanese women thus could be related to higher fat consumption in the United States.[208,209] Dietary factors are not the only explanation, however, as second generation Japanese living in the United States have a lower frequency of breast cancer than the Caucasian population.[209,210] This suggests the existence of some genetic differences and illustrates the interaction of different risk factors. A recent report minimizes the role of dietary fats.[211]

Endogenous Hormones

There are strong suggestions, including experimental, epidemiologic, and clinical data, that endogenous ovarian hormones play a role in the genesis of breast cancer.[212] For example, estrogens have been shown to be cocarcinogens in rodents. Also, breast cancer is essentially a disease of women; it is very rare before puberty, and patients who undergo ovariectomy before the age of 40 rarely develop it. However, the mechanisms by which these hormones act are not fully understood.[213] For example, the differences in hormonal excretion of estrogen metabolites and certain androgens noted in patients with

breast cancer may represent factors secondary to unknown modifications due to cancer growth and induction.

Family History

A family history of breast cancer is known to increase the risk of developing this lesion (Paul Broca, in 1866, observed his own family, in which 24 women died of cancer of the breast). Recent studies have shown that a positive family history correlates not only with increased risk but also with the development of the disease at an earlier age and frequently bilaterally. Of special interest is the indication in family histories that the disease has developed at a younger age in patients from successive generations. This is a common observation in diseases related to a genetic factor.[214–217] No definite association between histology and a family history of breast cancer has been clearly demonstrated.[218]

Breast Feeding

The concept of a protective effect of breast feeding against cancer has recently been challenged by different authors; the difference between women with cancer of the breast and those unaffected by the disease is not significant if we keep in mind that patients with cancer have fewer pregnancies.[219–222]

The possibility of a favorable modulating effect of estriol with respect to estradiol and estrone on breast growth—an effect that could be of practical importance in the prevention of breast cancer—has not been confirmed by all investigators treating this subject.[223] During pregnancy, the increase in estriol production, which constitutes an alleged protection against breast cancer, is matched by a similar elevation of other estrogens, making it difficult to relate diminished incidence of breast cancer to estriol alone.[224]

Other hormones such as progesterone, prolactin, androgens, thyroid hormones, corticoids, and pituitary hormones may also have an influence on carcinogenesis in the human breast, either inducing or maintaining the tumor growth.[225,226] A few examples can illustrate how debatable these data still are. Inhibition of tumor growth by progesterone has been observed in mice but on the contrary, stimulation was observed in rats. An adrenal dependence is illustrated by the regression of metastases after adrenalectomy, and hypophysectomy or destruction of the pituitary gland by radioactive implants can cause regression of metastases.

Generally speaking, prolactin levels are within normal limits in women with breast cancer. In experimental model systems, however, prolactin stimulates breast tumor growth, and breast cancer incidence has been observed to be greater in women with elevated prolactin levels specifically related to hypothyroidism. On the contrary, prolonged breast feeding and child bearing at a young age, considered as protective factors, are two conditions in which there is prolonged stimulation of the mammary tissue by prolactin.[227] These examples demonstrate that unanswered questions remain despite intensive investigations into the relationship between endogenous hormones and breast cancer.[228,229]

Exogenous Hormones

Exogenous hormones have been investigated, notably oral contraceptives and estrogens used at menopause; thus far, little evidence exists that these hormones have a carcinogenic effect. Histologic investigations have failed to demonstrate any specific change that could be attributed to exogenous hormones.[230–234] In fact, epidemiologic studies have tended to show a decrease in benign disease in users of oral contraceptives. These results should be interpreted with some caution, however, since a long latent period may be involved. The administration of hormones, and particularly estrogens, should be considered with caution in patients belonging to high-risk groups.[235,236]

Immunologic Factors

The well documented clinical evidence of spontaneous regressions of histologically proved cancer illustrates the existence of immune mechanisms against human tumors, including breast carcinomas. Also, the high incidence of bilateral and multicentric foci of in situ lobular carcinoma without clinical expression of the disease suggests the control of these lesions by immune mechanisms. Immunity may partially explain why some patients survive despite the presence of disseminated foci of tumor. The regression of lymph node metastases after mastectomy is another example of the immune phenomenon.[237–239]

Viruses

Various studies have suggested that viruses cause cancer or that they represent cofactors that must be associated with hormonal changes. The isolation of different oncogenic viruses, such as the murine mammary tumor virus and the Mason-Pfizer virus of the rhesus monkey, and the evidence of some identity between these viruses and human mammary virus, are strong arguments in favor of viruses as possible agents.[240–242] The route of viral transmission in humans is still a matter of debate. One suggested route is breast feeding. If breast feeding is an important route of transmission, one could reasonably ask why the marked reduction in breast feeding in the Western world has not been accompanied by a decrease in the incidence of breast cancer.[243] Viral transmission through the sperm has also been suggested. Whatever the means of transmission, the definite demonstration of a viral origin of cancer could drastically modify our concepts of breast cancer prophylaxis.

Ionizing Radiation

Ionizing radiation also has a role in the genesis of breast cancer, as illustrated by the high incidence among patients who received multiple fluoroscopic examinations in the course of treatment for pulmonary tuberculosis.[244]

Classification of Malignant Neoplasms

The continual development of more and more sophisticated methods of breast tissue retrieval and evaluation has significantly increased the possibility of the recognition and interpretation of very early, morphologically discrete cancerous lesions. Thus, whatever system is used to describe and classify breast cancers must be adapted to the requirements of the small and difficult borderline lesions. Various classifications of breast cancers have been devised, and each of them is subject to criticism in one way or another. A perfect classification system would ideally correlate both clinical manifestation and histologic features with prognosis.[245] Unfortunately, no perfect classification system has yet been elaborated— either by the ''lumpers'' or ''splitters.'' Therefore, we propose the use of the World Health Organization (WHO) system,[246] which has the definite advantages of worldwide distribution and which, with minor modifications, represents a decent compromise among different opinions (Table 11-4). Table 11-5 divides breast carcinomas into three groups according to prognosis. It is worth remembering that most breast cancers (65 to 75 percent) are infiltrating duct carcinomas of no specific subtype.

Lobular Carcinoma In Situ

Lobular carcinoma is an uncommon variant of mammary cancer, representing approximately 10 percent of all malignant tumors of the breast. It arises in the distal portion of the ductules of the lobular system, usually in the upper-outer quadrant of the breast. Two stages of the disease, seen with about equal frequency, can be observed: the *in situ* type and the *infiltrating* type. The infiltrating type will be described later.

TABLE 11-4. World Health Organization Histologic Classification of Proliferative and Tumoral Lesions of the Breast

A. Benign mammary dysplasias
  I.   Cysts
     a. Simple cyst
     b. Papillary cyst
  II. Adenosis
  III. Typical, regular epithelial proliferation of the lactiferous ducts or the lobules
  IV. Duct ectasia
  V. Fibrosis
  VI. Gynecomastia
  VII. Other noncancerous proliferative lesions
B. Benign or apparently benign tumors
  I.   Breast adenoma
  II. Nipple adenoma
  III. Lactiferous duct papilloma
  IV. Fibroadenoma
     a. Pericanalicular fibroadenoma
     b. Intracanalicular fibroadenoma
       1) Simple type
       2) Cellular type (cystosarcoma phyllodes)
  V. Benign soft tissue tumors
C. Carcinomas
  I.   Intracanalicular and noninfiltrating intralobular carcinoma
  II. Infiltrating carcinoma
  III. Specific histologic types of carcinoma
     a. Medullary carcinoma
     b. Papillary carcinoma
     c. Adenoid cystic (cribriform) carcinoma
     d. Mucoid carcinoma
     e. Lobular carcinoma
     f. Squamous carcinoma
     g. Paget's disease
     h. Carcinoma arising from cystosarcoma phyllodes
D. Sarcomas
  I.   Sarcoma arising in cystosarcoma phyllodes
  II. Other sarcomas
E. Carcinosarcoma
F. Unclassified tumors

(From World Health Organization,[535] with permission.)

Lobular carcinoma in situ (LCIS) was first thoroughly described by Foote and Stewart in 1941,[247] who recognized the lesion as a special type of breast carcinoma. They pointed out the multicentricity of the lesion and its association with invasive carcinoma. Since this first de-

TABLE 11-5. Prognosis of Breast Carcinoma Related to Histologic Type

Favorable	Intermediate	Unfavorable
Noninvasive carcinoma (DCIS, LCIS)	Infiltrating duct carcinoma	Inflammatory carcinoma
Cribriform carcinoma	Infiltrating lobular carcinoma	Signet ring carcinoma
Mucinous carcinoma		Lipid-rich carcinoma
Medullary carcinoma	Apocrine carcinoma	Metaplastic carcinoma
Papillary carcinoma		
Tubular carcinoma		
Adenoid cystic carcinoma		
Secretory carcinoma		
Paget's disease		

scription, a large number of cases have been reported.[248–256]

Lobular carcinoma in situ is associated with 0.8 to 3.6 percent of all benign epithelial lesions of the breast.[253,255] It is classically observed more or less fortuitously in biopsy specimens of mammary parenchyma removed for various other reasons, such as fibrocystic mastopathy. In recent years, more cases have been detected by mammography. As the chance of discovering a focus of LCIS by blind biopsy is very low, it would not be advisable to advocate routine large excision of apparently normal breast tissue merely to look for such foci. The disease is usually seen in premenopausal women.

Since the first description of this lesion, ideas about its malignant potential have varied. More recent and comprehensive data indicate that LCIS does, in fact, represent a precursor of invasive malignancy: subsequent ipsilateral invasive carcinoma arises in approximately 15 percent of cases, with contralateral breast involvement in approximately 9 percent.[257] The relatively high percentage (36 percent) of subsequent invasive carcinoma of lobular type[256,258] is a good indication of the relationship that exists between in situ and invasive forms. A clear distinction should be made between LCIS and intraductal carcinoma, since we know that the risk of subsequent invasive carcinoma is greater in the intraductal lesion.[259,260] The interval between the diagnosis of LCIS and the development of ipsilateral or contralateral carcinoma varies in published series from less than 5 years to more than 30 years. The frequency of subsequent carcinoma in breasts not treated with mastectomy ranges from 10 to 25 percent in ipsilateral breasts and from 10 to 20 percent in contralateral breasts.

Microscopically, the lesion is characterized by intralobular proliferation of the cells lining the acini; the lumen becomes packed with cells and progressively disappears as the lobule becomes more and more distended. Some lumina may persist.[261,262] Two types of cells are observed: cells with small oval or round hyperchromatic nuclei, no apparent nucleoli, and pale cytoplasm and cells with large, hyperchromatic nuclei, and prominent nucleoli.[263] Both cell types are found in the same acini (Fig. 11-33). Pleomorphism, however, is usually minimal, necrosis is absent, and mitoses are extremely rare. Cohesion between cells is minimal. Intracytoplasmic vacuoles of mucinous material are observed frequently. The lesion is usually limited to the acini, but terminal ducts are sometimes involved by the cellular proliferation. This is known as pagetoid extension. The ductal cells are replaced by larger cells having a prominent round nucleus and pale cytoplasm (Fig. 11-34).

The number of lobules involved is variable. In some cases, the proliferation may be limited to a single lobule, but multicentric foci often occur, and it is necessary to

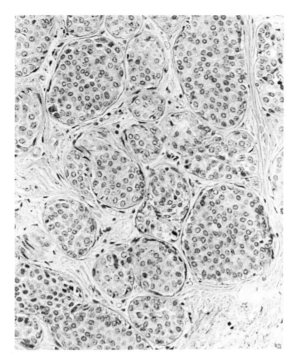

Fig. 11-33. LCIS. Enlarged acini are filled with uniform cells lacking pleomorphism or mitotic activity.

evaluate multiple tissue blocks. According to Rosen,[260] at least 75 percent of a lobule should be involved in order to recognize the lesion as LCIS. A valid evaluation of the extent of this disease is in fact dependent on the tissue sample obtained from the surgeon. This is an excellent example of the necessity of obtaining enough representative breast parenchyma to make a meaningful diagnosis. Silver stains display the presence of a reticulum network surrounding the lobule, confirming the noninvasive nature of the lesion. No reticular fibers are noted amid the epithelial cells present within the lobules.

Tentative studies have been made to correlate the histologic structure with the subsequent development of invasive carcinoma.[264] These investigations have failed to demonstrate the existence of a reliable, specific predictive factor. The lesion may represent a marker of risk rather than a precancerous lesion that will itself transform into a carcinoma.

Prognosis is good, even if we take into consideration the previous comments on the potential risk of invasion. In our series, 81 percent of patients with LCIS are alive after 5 years, as compared with 51 percent of those with infiltrating types of carcinoma. The remaining 19 percent died within 3 years after the diagnosis, a fact that suggests that these lesions were accompanied by invasive lesions.

The characteristics of the disease make it difficult to recommend a definite type of treatment for LCIS.[265,266] The potential risk of the coexistence or subsequent development of invasive carcinoma suggests to some investigators the most cautious attitude: total mastectomy with low axillary dissection. Subcutaneous mastectomy cannot eliminate the risk of leaving some breast tissue, especially if the nipple is not removed. Another possibility is a careful, lifetime follow-up program with regular clinical and radiologic examination.[253] The patient must be fully informed of the risks of this choice, however, since we know it cannot be totally safe until effective methods of early detection of invasive transformation of LCIS become available. However, clinical experience has shown that this choice is more helpful to the patient. As we have mentioned earlier, contralateral carcinoma represents a definite risk.[255,257] Therefore, it has been suggested that a substantial contralateral biopsy or even a mastectomy be performed. The specimen should include approximately 25 percent of the parenchyma, in order to eliminate the possible presence of invasive carcinoma.[267] If the results of biopsy are negative, lifetime follow-up is mandatory. An alternative to blind contralateral biopsy is careful mammographic study with biopsy of suspicious lesions. It is important that the patient participate in the therapeutic decision, as it is still a controversial problem.

Differential Diagnosis

Lobular carcinoma in situ should not be confused with atypical lobular hyperplasia, papillomatosis of small ducts, or intraductal carcinoma with extension into the acini.[268] The lobules of atypical lobular hyperplasia usually have open lumina, which are filled with cells in LCIS. Intracytoplasmic mucin vacuoles are less frequent in hyperplastic lesions than in LCIS.[269] Papillomatosis shows typical ramifying papillary structures with fibrous

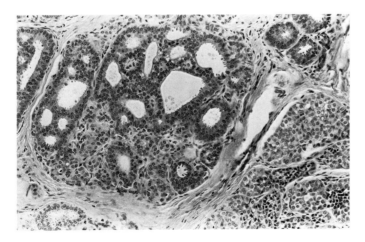

Fig. 11-34. LCIS intermingling in pagetoid fashion with cribriform type of intraductal carcinoma.

cores. Intraductal carcinoma in lobules shows marked cellular atypia and frequent foci of necrosis, both of which are lacking in LCIS.

Intraductal Carcinoma

Contrary to LCIS, it is possible to distinguish two types of intraductal carcinoma. One is clinically evident and is characterized by a palpable tumor, a form of Paget's disease or a bloody discharge without palpable mass; the other is a microscopic disease observed as a fortuitous finding in breast tissue removed because of the presence of a mass or detected by an abnormal mammogram.[270,271]

The relatively small number of existing studies dealing with intraductal carcinoma (DCIS) relates to poor detection in previous times.[272–277] This is confirmed by autopsy studies, which reveal only few cases of DCIS. It appears most frequently in the fifth decade, and the reported clinical signs are the presence of a mass, nipple discharge, and local pain. The lesion is often identified by mammography because of the frequent presence of calcification. It is occasionally bilateral.

Grossly, the tumor is often multicentric and measures from microscopic size to a few centimeters in diameter. The ill defined mass reveals cystic cavities filled with a creamy exudate. Microscopically, intraductal carcinoma is characterized by a neoplastic growth within the mammary ducts.[276,277] Different histologic variants have been described and include solid, comedo, cribriform, papillary, cystic hypersecretory, and mixed types. The ductal epithelium in the more florid cases exhibits chaotically arranged polyhedral, sometimes anaplastic, cells with enlarged and hyperchromatic nuclei; mitoses are conspicuous. The solid type of tumor shows enlarged ducts filled with these malignant cells. The comedo type, which is usually admixed with the solid type (Fig. 11-35), is characterized by central necrosis of the involved ducts. The cribriform type (Figs. 11-34 and 11-36) reveals a glandular arrangement consisting of cuboidal cells oriented around small regular round lumina. Atypia is often minimal in the latter type (Figs. 11-36 and 11-37). In the papillary type (Fig. 11-38), papillae without central fibrovascular connective tissue cores are lined by atypical cells and project into one or more ducts. In the cystic hypersecretory type,[278] the malignant ducts are greatly dilated and filled with luminal dense colloid-like material (Fig. 11-39).

Secondary calcification of necrotic foci is common; it is a diagnostic criterion of considerable significance in mammography, yet in itself is certainly not diagnostic. Also typically seen are stromal condensation and lymphoid infiltrates around the involved ducts. Myoepithelial cells can be demonstrated in the different histologic types,[279] but are usually less prominent than in benign intraductal papilloma (for other differentiating features of these two lesions, refer to the section above on intraductal papilloma).

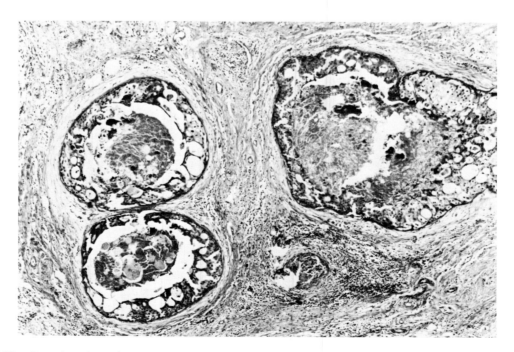

Fig. 11-35. Intraductal carcinoma, comedo type. Large ducts are lined by malignant cells growing in solid and cribriform patterns with extensive central necrosis.

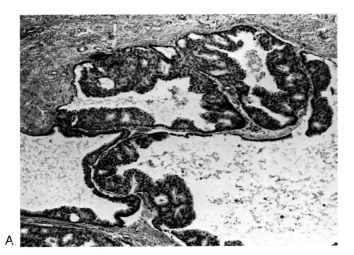

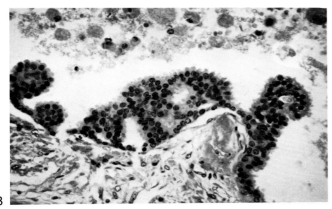

Fig. 11-36. Intraductal carcinoma, cribriform type. **(A)** Ducts contain heaped-up epithelium with round spaces of uniform size and shape. (In a benign papilloma, many of these spaces would be compressed and flattened by solid proliferations of cells.) **(B)** Higher magnification of one area showing regularity of spaces, lack of fibrous stroma within the cellular masses, and lack of cytologic atypia.

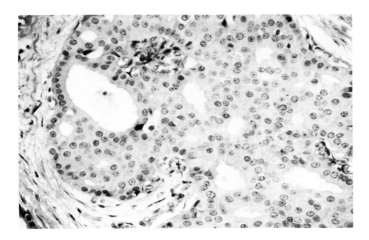

Fig. 11-37. Intraductal carcinoma, cribriform type. Note the regular cribriform pattern and minimal cellular atypia.

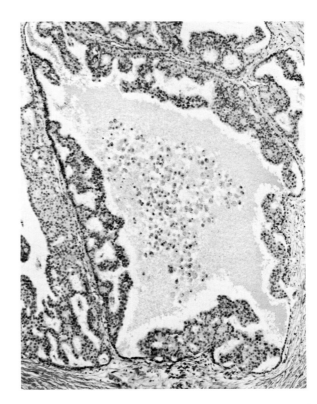

Fig. 11-38. Intraductal carcinoma, mixed papillary and cribriform type. In addition to forming cribriform spaces, tumor cells project into duct lumina as papillae without central fibrovascular connective tissue cores.

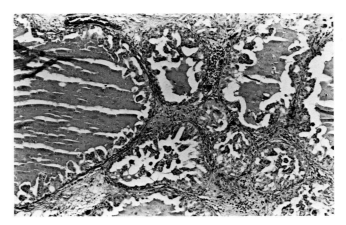

Fig. 11-39. Cystic hypersecretory duct carcinoma. Dilated ducts contain colloid-like secretory material and are lined by malignant papillae.

Ultrastructural studies have shown a great heterogeneity of the cells.[280] The main type is a voluminous cell with a large irregular nucleus and often two nucleoli. The endoplasmic reticulum is well developed, and ribosomes are abundant. Semithin sections have revealed the presence of light and dark cells whose differences are explained by variations in cytoplasmic organelle density. Stromal invasion was present in ultrastructural studies in the majority of cases that showed no infiltration by light microscopic examination.[281] This finding demonstrates that light microscopy is not an accurate method for defining intraductal carcinoma, and that pure intraductal lesions represent a minority of the cases originally believed to be preinvasive. The basement membrane is altered or disrupted and epithelial elements are present in the stroma.

The prognosis is good and supports the view that this type of tumor does not exhibit aggressive behavior; lymph node metastases have rarely been reported,[275,282,283] and probably signify that a small focus of invasion was missed by inadequate sectioning. Local excision would be adequate therapy for an intraductal carcinoma confirmed as such by multiple permanent sections, were it not for the risk of multifocal disease. The lesion should not be diagnosed definitively by frozen section examination, because of confusion with benign intraductal papilloma on the one hand and focal stromal infiltration on the other. When the latter occurs, the potential for metastatic dissemination exists.[276,284] Promising results have been reported with excision and radiation therapy.[285]

Infiltrating Duct Carcinoma

Infiltrating duct carcinoma is the most frequent type of breast carcinoma and is thus a very common tumor. The histologic characteristics of infiltrating duct carcinoma within a given lesion can be so diversified that careful examination may reveal almost all the different types—present in different proportions—described in the morphologic classifications of the lesion. The existence of a preinvasive phase is suggested by certain cases in which intraductal malignant proliferations coexist with the infiltrating malignant structures.

Grossly, infiltrating duct carcinoma is characterized by a very firm, poorly defined nodule measuring from a few millimeters to a few centimeters in diameter. Cut sections reveal a gray-white, slightly retracted granular tissue with small white or yellow streaks disposed in a radial fashion around the center of the nodule. (These yellow streaks are due to elastosis rather than to tumor necrosis.) The firmness, the granularity of the nodule, and its gritty consistency are constant and typical features of this tumor (Fig. 11-40). The dense and retracted aspect of the tumor is related to the abundance of the fibrous and elastic tissue. The nodule margins are irregular and adhere to the peripheral fibroadipose tissue. Mammographic studies have shown two types of tumoral outgrowth into the surrounding tissues: pushing and infiltrating. Multiple tumor nodules can sometimes be observed grossly and are very frequent in whole-organ sections.

Bilateral development occurs and represents either two independent tumors or metastatic involvement of the contralateral breast.[286,287] Skin involvement is characterized by thickening and induration.

Microscopically, the diagnosis is best made architecturally at low-power magnification (Fig. 11-41). The neoplastic cells are arranged in single files, small solid clus-

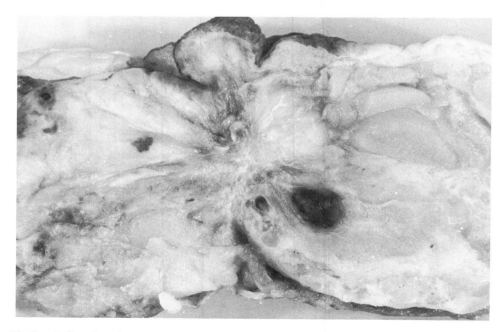

Fig. 11-40. Infiltrating duct carcinoma. Typical gross appearance of a firm, stellate, scar-like process.

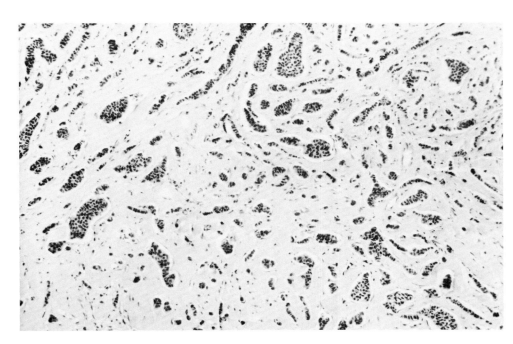

Fig. 11-41. Infiltrating duct carcinoma, scirrhous type. Abundant dense stroma compresses the epithelial structures.

ters, tubes, long cords, large sheets, syncytia, glandular or anastomosing structures, and mixtures of all these types. The masses are irregular in size and shape and infiltrate and deform the intervening stroma, in which collagen and reticulin fibers are present. The number of elastic fibers is increased and represents an intense stromal reaction (elastosis).[100]

The malignant cells exhibit different degrees of polymorphism. Any type of cellular structure can be found, from the small regular element with a round, slightly hyperchromatic nucleus and a relatively normal nuclear-to-cytoplasmic ratio to the anaplastic, large irregular cell with a voluminous, hyperchromatic nucleus, a hypertrophied nucleolus, and a markedly reduced cytoplasm. Mi-

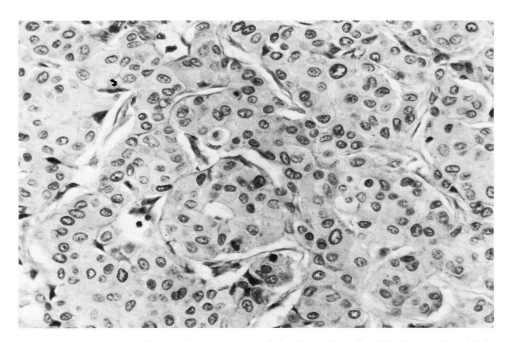

Fig. 11-42. Infiltrating duct carcinoma. Numerous glandular formations lined by large cells with hyperchromatic but relatively uniform nuclei are seen. Minimal stroma is present.

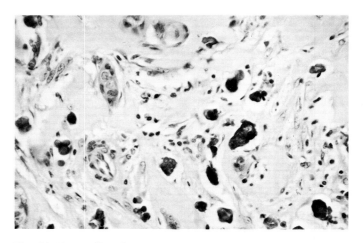

Fig. 11-43. Infiltrating duct carcinoma. Note the presence of diffuse fibrosis and numerous microcalcifications.

toses are present in variable numbers. Stromal fibrosis varies greatly in intensity. Some carcinomas reveal few neoplastic cells dispersed in abundant fibrous tissue, while others exhibit only fine fibrous strands around numerous epithelial structures (Fig. 11-42). The *scirrhous type* is defined by the abundance of the dense fibrous stroma in which the epithelial cells are engulfed and compressed (Fig. 11-41).

Electron microscopy shows that the neoplastic cords are always surrounded by a basal lamina. The presence of myoepithelial cells can be identified in some cases. Cartilaginous and bony metaplastic changes may occur.[288,289] Foci of necrosis, myxoid degeneration, and calcifications are common findings (Fig. 11-43). The presence of benign stromal multinucleated giant cells which are phenotypically related to osteoclastic cells is another manifestation of osseous metaplasia.[290] When necrosis is marked, granulomatous inflammatory changes may be present, with foreign-body giant cells around the necrotic tissular material. Lipid degeneration with large foamy cells may occur. Infiltration of lymphatics should be carefully searched for, since this finding worsens the clinical prognosis.

The multicentric cancers which are undetected clinically or grossly are by no means rare and may represent more than 10 percent of carcinomas.[287,291] However, the occurrence of two dominant primary lesions in the same breast is a rarity. The multicentric lesions are usually of the noninvasive type (LCIS or intraductal carcinoma). This eventuality occurs more frequently in the presence of large (more than 5 cm in diameter) uncircumscribed primary lesions with nipple and skin involvement. The multicentricity of carcinoma is well established and explains why the treatment of this disease is still a matter of

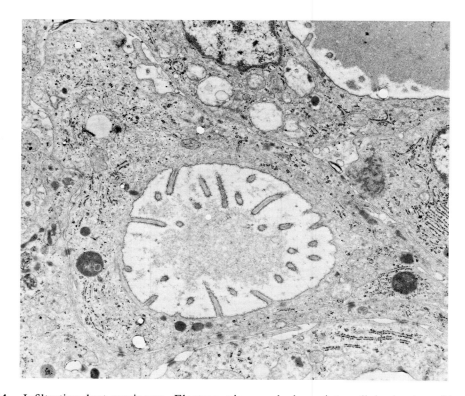

Fig. 11-44. Infiltrating duct carcinoma. Electron micrograph shows intracellular lumina with microvilli.

discussion. There is a discrepancy between the relatively low rate of local recurrence in the remaining breast tissue following segmental resection and the high percentage of tumor multifocality in mastectomy specimens. Absence of correlation between pathologic and clinical studies, the relatively benign evolution of occult lesions considered to be histologically malignant, and the eradication of tumor foci left in the remaining tissue by postoperative radiotherapy are some of the proposed explanations found in the literature.[287]

While the ultrastructure of all types of malignant cells is characterized by prominent organelles, none of the modifications is absolutely specific.[99,280] For example, intracytoplasmic lumina (Fig. 11-44) have been described in all types of carcinomas but are more abundant in the infiltrating lobular type.[292] They appear as spherical cavities of variable size and are lined by microvilli. The lumina contain electron-dense material, some of which corresponds to mucin. The presence of cilia is not frequent (Fig. 11-45). More specific alterations are mentioned in the discussion of each histologic type of tumor. Finally, it should be remembered that qualitative ultrastructural features distinguishing ducts from lobules in normal resting breasts have not been identified. This indicates that

an ultrastructural differentiation between lobular and ductular carcinomas is not realistic.

Differential Diagnosis

Difficulties of differential diagnosis reside more in the distinction between benign hyperplastic epithelial lesions and carcinoma than in the recognition of the different types of malignancy. This problem becomes even more complicated in frozen section examinations. A highly cellular adenosis, for example, can mimic an infiltrating duct carcinoma. Needless to say, if doubt exists in the mind of the pathologist, he should resist the surgeon's impatience and defer diagnosis until adequate permanent sections can be prepared and studied.

Prognostic Factors

Prognosis is determined by the interval to recurrence and the length of survival; therefore, treatments that delay but do not reduce the frequency of recurrence may increase the length of survival without reducing the mortality of the disease. Any information gathered by the pathologist about the prognosis of a breast cancer will

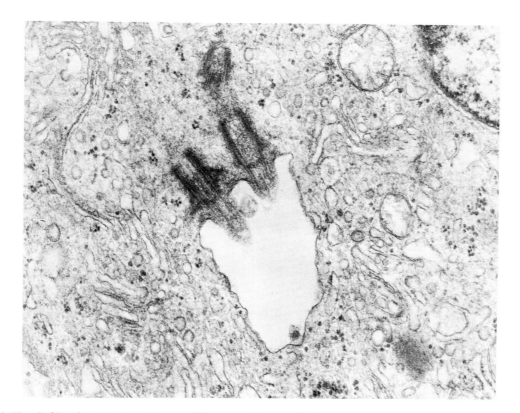

Fig. 11-45. Infiltrating duct carcinoma. Electron micrograph shows presence of cilia in an intracellular lumen.

help the clinician treat and follow the patient.[293] Accurate collection, interpretation, and reporting of such information are clearly essential. Several factors are considered to have some prognostic value. The two most consistent factors that reflect the extent of the disease at the time of diagnosis and treatment are the size of the tumor and lymph node involvement.

Tumor Size

The size of the tumor is a good, although rudimentary, criterion for evaluating the duration of the disease and the survival time.[294] However, size is not always related to the age of the lesion; growth rates may vary considerably, and doubling times from less than 30 to more than 300 days have been reported. Nonetheless, the larger tumors are associated with more positive nodes, blood vessel and lymphatic dissemination, multicentricity, and short-term treatment failures. In general, this information can be safely translated in terms of poorer prognosis, but it does not provide any specific indication of rates of recurrences and mortality differences. Current data show that the percentage of small tumors (less than 2 cm in diameter) has increased in recent years, compared with the percentage of medium-sized tumors (2 to 5 cm in diameter). This finding suggests that breast tumors are being clinically diagnosed earlier.[295]

Lymph Node Involvement

Lymph node involvement is an important prognostic factor in mammary cancer.[296–303] Approximately 25 percent of clinically negative axillary nodes are in fact microscopically invaded by metastases. Furthermore, the number of lymph nodes detected depends on how meticulous a dissection is done on surgical specimens. More specifically, the following procedures will increase the percentage of nodal metastases found: dissection after treatment of the axillary fat with a clearing agent, histologic examination of all the nodes dissected, and sectioning of all nodes at different levels. For purposes of classification, the axilla has been commonly divided into three levels. Level I is the tissue inferior and lateral to the lower border of the pectoralis minor muscle, level II is the tissue located beneath the pectoralis minor, and level III corresponds to the tissue superior and medial to the pectoralis minor. This classification is now largely of historical interest since radical mastectomy is rarely performed in most institutions. It has been shown that, with respect to prognosis, it is more important to evaluate the absolute number of invaded nodes than the percentage of positive nodes.[304] Patients with fewer than four involved nodes have almost as good a prognosis as those with a negative axillary dissection, whereas four or more involved nodes indicates a poor prognosis.[299]

These data suggest that careful dissection of macroscopically detectable nodes and a reasonable number of tissue sections of all suspicious nodes will procure sufficient information for evaluation of tumor evolution and, possibly, prospective epidemiologic studies.[305–307] Some workers recommend the use of a hilar section alone, which permits a better identification of tumor-bearing nodes than random sections.[308] Immunohistochemical studies using monoclonal antibodies against epithelial antigens are able to detect micrometastases otherwise difficult to locate.[309]

Histologic Grading

Histologic grading methods have been discussed extensively, and their relative values have been confirmed by various studies. One may wonder then why so few laboratories use them routinely.[310–314] Perhaps it is because histologic grading is a relatively time-consuming procedure and requires a daily experience with breast carcinoma. In 1925, Greenough[312] proposed the histologic criteria that have since been used by various investigators. These criteria are the degree of tubule formation, the size of cells and nuclei, the degree of hyperchromatism, and the number of mitoses.

Fisher et al.[313] showed that the tumors with the most differentiated nuclei are associated with older age groups, with the absence of nodal involvement, and with histologic types associated with good prognosis. Anaplastic tumors are associated with a greater frequency of nodal extension. Medullary carcinoma, however, is one example of an exception to the value of such grading; the poorly differentiated nuclei of medullary carcinoma are, in fact, associated with a rather good prognosis. In this case, the grading is contradicted by the biological behavior of the tumor, and this shows that the value of isolated, independently considered prognostic factors can be quite relative.

Nonetheless, careful histologic grading generally proves to be a valuable method, and its daily application

---

TABLE 11-6. Histologic Grading Method for Malignant Breast Tumors

1. Histologic factors
   Degree of structural dedifferentiation as shown by the loss of tubular arrangement of the cells
   Variations in size, shape, and staining of the nuclei
   Frequency of hyperchromasia and mitotic figures
2. Points awarded according to whether each of the three histologic factors is present in slight (1), moderate (2), or marked (3) degree
3. Points added together, making a possible total of 3 to 9, the smallest number representing the lowest degree of malignancy
   3–5 points: low malignancy (grade I)
   6, 7 points: intermediate malignancy (grade II)
   8, 9 points: high malignancy (grade III)

(From Bloom and Richardson,[310] with permission.)

is recommended. The method proposed by Bloom and Richardson,[310] which adopts and refines these criteria, is the most widely accepted one (Table 11-6).

Tumor Immunity

The interrelationship between tumoral tissue and normal breast tissue varies with the quality of the individual's immunologic response, which may in some manner determine clinical prognosis. Different morphologic aspects of the axillary nodes have been considered to be histologic expressions of these immunologic characteristics. The histologic patterns that have been evaluated include sinus histiocytosis, lymphocyte predominance or depletion, germinal center predominance, and absence of nodal stimulation.

Sinus histiocytosis is characterized by the presence, in the distended nodal sinusoids, of large histiocytes that resemble macrophages but do not contain phagocytosed material. Certain authors have tried to correlate the prognosis with sinus histiocytosis of the lymph nodes draining the tumor.[315–319] These findings are at least partially open to question because the value of this prognostic factor seems to be counterbalanced by other tumor characteristics. Yet, in series of carcinomas showing identical characteristics, sinus histiocytosis may prove to be of some prognostic value. For example, sinus histiocytosis is related to better survival in cases of moderately or poorly differentiated carcinomas or in cases with a moderate number of nodal metastases; on the other hand, in well differentiated tumors or when nodal metastases are absent, the prognosis is good regardless of the presence or absence of sinus histiocytosis. The absence of any difference in the prevalence of the other patterns mentioned previously (lymphocytic predominance or depletion, germinal center predominance, and absence of nodal stimulation) in patients with positive or negative nodes fails to indicate any value of these factors as individual prognostic determinants

Type of Tumor Border

The type of tumor border (the microscopic malignant structures either push the surrounding tissues aside or frankly infiltrate them) has been considered as a prognostic factor, but it provides inconclusive results that again are explained by other interfering factors,[320–323] such as the histologic type.

Tumor in the Contralateral Breast

The risk of developing a tumor in the contralateral breast in patients with carcinoma is significantly higher than the risk of developing a first primary in the general population.[324–333]

Local Skin Involvement

Involvement of the skin overlying the primary tumor is a factor of poor prognosis. It has been shown that a significant proportion of carcinomatous cells that invade the epidermis are colonized by melanocytes migrating downward. Melanin pigment is found dispersed in fine granules in the cytoplasm of malignant cells.[334]

Nipple Involvement

Nipple involvement is another factor that worsens prognosis.[335,336]

Tumor Necrosis

There is some correlation between tumor necrosis and other factors that influence treatment failure or survival such as tumor size, histologic grade, clinical stage, histologic tumor type, and nipple involvement.[337]

Blood Vessel Invasion

Blood vessel invasion occurs in approximately 5 percent of all breast carcinomas[338,339] and is a bad prognostic sign. Special histochemical techniques that selectively stain elastic tissue improve the detection of vascular walls.

Perineural Space Invasion

Invasion of perineural spaces by neoplastic cells is not uncommon and is associated with tumors showing lymphatic invasion and nodal metastases. It has also been described in sclerosing adenosis.[340]

Presence of Estrogen and Progesterone Receptors

The demonstration of the presence of specific estrogen (ER) and progesterone (PR) receptors in breast cancer tissue indicates at least some sort of association between breast cancer and the endocrine system.[341–343] The practical use of receptor assay techniques can thus provide an approach to the prognostic significance of the hormonal sensitivity of breast cancer and also may help predict the response to endocrine treatments.[344–347]

New immunohistochemical techniques based on the direct recognition of the specific receptor protein by monoclonal antibodies have modified our concept of receptor pathophysiology. For example, it has been possible to demonstrate that receptors are localized in the nucleus and not in the cytoplasm, as first thought. Results of ER measurements evaluated by biochemical and immunoenzymatic methods can be compared with immunohistochemical results, with a good approximation. These techniques have also permitted the use of histochemical analyses using fine needle aspirations and will contribute to the selection of patients with potentially hormone-responsive tumors.[348–350]

Heterogeneity of the tumor cell population in terms of ER is a frequent finding that is not fully understood. Estrogen receptors have been localized in benign conditions such as fibrocystic mastopathy, fibroadenoma, and even normal breast tissue. Therefore, identification of ER is not a specific identification of malignancy.

Quantitative evaluation of PR, like that of ER, can be used for prediction of clinical prognosis and choice of the proper treatment of breast cancers. It has been shown that a positive statistical correlation exists between progesterone receptors and the disease-free interval.

The group of patients whose lesions contain both ER and PR have a higher probability of remission following hormonal therapy than the group of patients whose lesions contain only ER or only very low levels of the receptors.[351] Therefore, it is important that both types of receptors should be investigated. ER and PR positivity are strongly correlated with nuclear grade, better differentiated tumors being more frequently receptor-rich. However, this correlation is far from automatic, so fresh tumor tissue should be submitted for receptor analysis in every case in which this is feasible.

Tumor Markers

Different tumor markers have been evaluated and correlated with clinical prognosis. Although some studies tend to relate the presence of carcinoembryonic antigen (CEA) with the capability to metastasize in some tumors, recent investigations do not confirm these findings. Moreover, other markers such as human chorionic gonadotrophin (hCG), placental lactogen, lactalbumin, pregnancy-specific β_1-glycoprotein, and ABH isoantigens are also described, but no definite prognostic conclusions can be drawn.[352,353]

Oncogenes

Oncogenes and receptors of growth factors are currently being investigated with the purpose of demonstrating their value as prognostic factors. Although some oncogenes such as protein p21 or *ras* oncogene are not found exclusively in malignant mammary tissues, and thus have a moderate value in terms of clinical prediction, others such as epithelial growth factors seem to provide valuable data. Recent studies have suggested that the expression of certain oncogenes may be associated with a higher likelihood of metastatic disease.[354]

Flow Cytometry

In recent years, the prognostic value of DNA analysis of cancers of the breast by flow cytometry has been the subject of several reports.[355–357] Most studies have found that a diploid histogram is associated with a lower rate of axillary lymph nodal metastases and a higher survival rate, compared with aneuploid tumors. However, the ploidy values are also correlated with such better established indices of prognosis as tumor grade and steroid hormone receptor status, so the independent significance of flow cytometry remains to be established.

Evolution

Local Tumor Extension

Local extension of the tumor, which can be multifocal, takes place both within and along the lactiferous ducts, in the stroma, and in the surrounding adipose tissue. The rate of local extension of the primary lesion varies from one case to another and has little influence on the probability of metastatic dissemination. Ductal carcinomas progress from in situ to invasive more rapidly than do lobular ones. The frequency of nipple involvement varies from 8 percent to 50 percent, depending on the study. This discrepancy is due to differences in the nipple specimen examined.

Lymphatic Dissemination

Neoplastic cells enter the lymphatic system around the tumor nodules and adjacent ducts and from there spread to the subareolar plexus; the external, central, and apical axillary nodes; and the internal mammary lymphatics of the inner portion of the breast.[13,14] Later, supraclavicular nodes are infiltrated. More distant lymphatic dissemination includes the cervical, mediastinal, and inguinal nodes. The invasion of the internal mammary chain occurs in approximately one-third of all breast cancers and is more probable in large tumors and in those with a central or medial location and axillary metastases.[358]

Hematogenous Metastases

Blood-borne metastases are common in bones, lungs, liver, ovaries, adrenals, pleura, peritoneum, pituitary and other sites.[359–361] The most frequently involved bones are the vertebrae, pelvis, femur, humerus, skull, ribs, and clavicle.[362] Bone metastases are usually of the osteolytic type, but in about 10 percent of cases the osteoblastic type is encountered. Hypercalcemia is a frequent clinical finding in cases of bony metastases. Pulmonary metastases are usually nodular, but lymphatic dissemination can occur with carcinomatous lymphangitis. Pleural involvement with recurrent pleural effusion frequently accompanies the pulmonary infiltration.

Recurrences

Local recurrences may appear near the mastectomy scar within a few years after treatment and may involve large areas of the thoracic wall. Late recurrences are

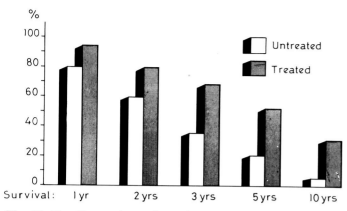

Fig. 11-46. Comparison of survival in treated and untreated cases of breast carcinoma (Institut Jules Bordet).

typical of breast cancer. It is not rare to diagnose recurrences or metastases 10 or even 20 years after the initial treatment. They may appear anywhere but are common in the contralateral breast,[286,363] possibly representing new primary foci. The explanation of this histologic behavior is not known; immunologic defense mechanisms can be suggested although there are as yet no substantial data to prove this idea. The existence of periods of survival exceeding 10 years without any treatment (Fig. 11-46) is another argument suggesting immunologic defense mechanisms.[364]

Apocrine Carcinoma

Apocrine carcinoma is a rare type of carcinoma.[365] The tumor consists of glandular structures lined by large cells with an abundant, bright, eosinophilic cytoplasm, resembling the apocrine cells of sweat glands (Fig. 11-47). The cytoplasm may be homogeneous or granular. These cells arise by a metaplastic process from the ductal epithelium.

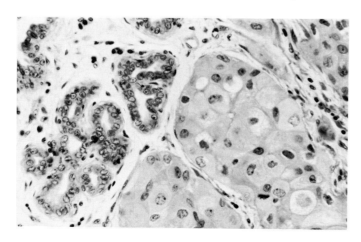

Fig. 11-47. Apocrine carcinoma. Glandular structures lined by large cells with an abundant eosinophilic cytoplasm are shown on the right. Compare these structures with the normal lactiferous ducts on the left.

Electron microscopic studies have not confirmed that these cells are truly apocrine in nature.[366]

Since the clinical history and the prognosis are similar to those of other infiltrating duct carcinomas, it has been proposed that we include these cases among the latter.[365] This tumor should not be confused with true sweat gland carcinoma, which may arise from sweat glands of the skin overlying the mammary gland. The exact frequency of this type of carcinoma is uncertain.

Infiltrating Lobular Carcinoma

Infiltrating lobular carcinoma (ILC), or small cell carcinoma, is a relatively rare form of breast cancer, accounting for approximately 5 percent of all breast tumors.[367–371] The peak incidence rate occurs around 50 years of age. In about 50 percent of the cases, it appears in association with LCIS.[372] It is frequently multifocal and bilateral.

Macroscopically, infiltrating lobular carcinoma is a firm, rubbery, poorly circumscribed, gray-white mass, which is indistinguishable from the much more common infiltrating duct carcinoma. Microscopically, it is characterized by threadlike strands of small to medium-sized epithelial cells that diffusely infiltrate a dense, fibrous matrix. The tumor cells secrete intracellular mucosubstances, which are PAS-positive after diastase digestion.[373] The single-file cellular arrangement, also called Indian file, is characteristic of this tumor (Fig. 11-48). Sometimes the cells form concentric rings around an apparently normal dilated duct; this is called the bullseye pattern. Care must be taken not to misinterpret this arrangement as chronic mastitis, especially on a frozen section.

Another histologic pattern that has been recognized recently is the *confluent* variant, in which infiltrating tumor cells (still typically small and uniform) maintain

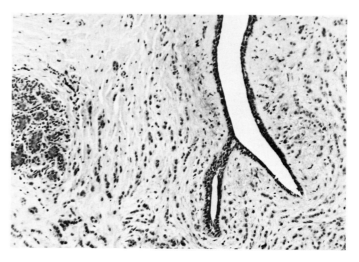

Fig. 11-48. Infiltrating lobular carcinoma. Note the Indian-file arrangement and swirling around normal duct.

somewhat of a lobular pattern.[374] This is currently separated into the *solid* and *alveolar* variants,[370,371] which are said by Dixon et al.[368] to have a less favorable prognosis than the classical type. These variants must also be distinguished from *carcinoid tumors*[375,376] of the breast.

Ultrastructural study of ILC shows the cells to be rich in organelles. The Golgi apparatus and rough endoplasmic reticulum are well developed. Ribosomes and mitochondria are abundant. The nuclei are lobulated and contain large nucleoli. Intracytoplasmic lumina are numerous and are seen at the light microscopic level as signet ring cells.

It is important to note that ILC cells have a distinctive biochemical characteristic: compared with other breast tumors, ILC cells have a higher percentage of positive estrogen receptors. However, this has not been confirmed in all studies.[377] Nodal metastases of this tumor usually exhibit a loose arrangement of small cells with a dense infiltration of the peripheral sinus (Fig. 11-49). This sinus catarrh pattern can thus simulate malignant lymphoma or even benign sinus histiocytosis. Study of the primary tumor will eliminate this error. Distant metastases are found with a predilection in the ovaries and uterus and the gastrointestinal (GI) tract, and particularly in the stomach, where the similarity with a primary carcinoma may lead to diagnostic difficulty. In some metastases, tumor cells resemble histiocytes. Mucin stains and immunohistochemical techniques (epithelial membrane antigen and cytokeratin) may help to solve the difficulty. Generally speaking, ILC is as lethal as the average infiltrating breast carcinoma.

Fig. 11-49. Sinus catarrh-like pattern of lymph node metastasis in infiltrating lobular carcinoma.

Metaplastic Carcinoma

Different types of metaplasia can be seen in mammary carcinoma.[378] All are very rare. Squamous metaplasia is the most common. The foci of metaplasia vary in size and are located in the tumor cords. Squamous cells reveal intercellular bridges, keratinization, and pearl formation. Squamous metaplasia is often associated with the presence of glycogen-laden tumor cells. Macroscopically, tumors ranging from 1 cm to more than 10 cm in diameter have been described.

Cartilaginous and *bony metaplasia* are very common. They consist of well differentiated osteoid and chondroid foci. Fibroblastic metaplasia has been described. *Myxoid foci* should be considered degenerative alterations and not as metaplasia. In all cases, even when the foci of metaplasia are very disseminated, areas of unquestionable carcinoma must be found to make the diagnosis.

Ultrastructural studies tend to show that metaplasia originates in altered and modified epithelial cells.[379] Immunohistochemistry may also help distinguish these lesions from sarcomas.[380] Flow cytometry confirms the malignant nature of both the ductal and the metaplastic components.[381] Carcinomas with squamous metaplasia do not show any particular clinical characteristics, but the cases with pseudosarcomatous, cartilaginous, and bony metaplasia seem to be more malignant.[289,381–383] These sometimes bizarre tumors should not be interpreted as carcinosarcomas (Fig. 11-50). Very rare cases of pure squamous carcinoma have been reported in the literature.[384]

Medullary Carcinoma

Medullary carcinoma (encephaloid carcinoma, circumscribed carcinoma, medullary carcinoma with lymphoid stroma) represents less than 5 percent of mammary malignant tumors and shows a significantly higher survival rate at 10 years than infiltrating duct carcinoma.[385–389] It usually occurs in patients in their 50s. Some investigators have questioned the favorable prognosis generally assigned to this particular type of carcinoma but, if the lesion closely fits the strictly defined morphologic criteria, there is no doubt that the prognosis is significantly more favorable. Table 11-7 summarizes the distinct morphologic criteria of typical medullary carcinoma. The atypical type exhibits some but not all features of the typical form and can probably be eliminated as a specific diagnosis if the strict criteria are applied.[386] Bilaterality has been reported.

Grossly, medullary carcinoma is characterized by a soft, sometimes bulky, circumscribed mass deeply situated in the mammary gland. The cut sections reveal dif-

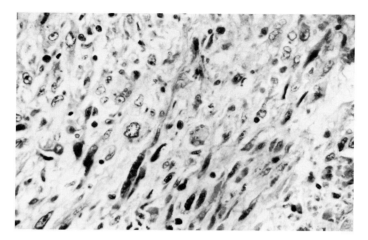

Fig. 11-50. Metaplastic carcinoma. Markedly pleomorphic lesion formed essentially of spindle cells. Nuclei are hyperchromatic and very irregular.

fuse, gray-tan, homogeneous tissue with hemorrhagic and sometimes necrotic foci. There is no skin attachment and no superficial ulceration even if the tumor is voluminous.

Microscopically, the tumor is characterized by a predominantly syncytial growth pattern of large, polymorphic cells with round or cleaved, vesicular nuclei and prominent nucleoli (Fig. 11-51A,B). Squamous metaplasia is seen in approximately 15 percent of cases. Cytoplasm is abundant and basophilic. Mitoses are quite frequent. Marked or moderate cellular pleomorphism is present; multinucleated cells and bizarre giant cell reactions can be observed. Calcifications are practically never encountered. No intraductal or microglandular neoplastic component should be present in the typical case. The stroma usually reveals a marked lymphocytic infiltration. The infiltrate is more or less abundant and may contain plasmacytes. The significance of the lymphocytic infiltrate has aroused much controversy; it has been suggested that it represents a host reaction to tumor cell antigens.[390,391]

The electron microscope reveals that myoepithelial cells and deposition of basal lamina are not frequent characteristics of medullary carcinoma.[392,393] These findings also apply to the tubular type of carcinoma, which has similarly a rather favorable clinical prognosis. Cytoplas-

TABLE 11-7. Typical Medullary Carcinoma

Predominantly syncytial growth pattern (>75%)
Microscopically completely circumscribed
No intraductal component
Moderate to marked diffuse mononuclear stromal infiltrate
Moderate to marked nuclear pleomorphism
Absence of microglandular features

(From Ridolfi et al.,[389] with permission.)

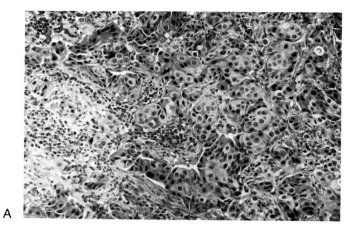

A

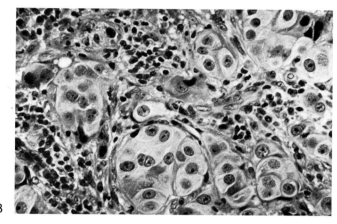

B

Fig. 11-51. Medullary carcinoma. Note the syncytial growth pattern of large cells with vesicular nuclei and prominent nucleoli. Cytoplasm is abundant and clear. Stroma is densely infiltrated by lymphocytes. **(A)** Low power view. **(B)** Detail.

mic fibrillar bundles and mitochondrial alterations have been described.[394]

The frequency of axillary lymph node metastases is similar to that calculated for infiltrating duct carcinomas, but the prognosis remains more favorable even if lymph node metastases are present.[386] The 10 year survival rate for this tumor exceeds 80 percent in typical cases.[395] The survival rate is even better if the primary lesion does not exceed 3 cm in diameter and is not accompanied by nodal metastases.[396] The enlargement of nodes in the absence of metastases is related to a follicular hyperplasia with sinus histiocytosis and lymphoplasmatic infiltration.[397]

Papillary Carcinoma

Infiltrating papillary adenocarcinoma constitutes less than 1 percent of all mammary tumors. It is more frequent in older patients, and the mean age of diagnosis varies from 63 to 67 years. It is characterized by the proliferation of papillary structures originating within the large lactiferous ducts and invading into the mammary stroma. A bloody or serous nipple discharge is a common finding.

Grossly, papillary carcinomas are usually large, rather well demarcated masses situated in the subareolar region with hemorrhagic and cystic foci. The softness of the specimen is due to the scarcity of stroma. Microscopically, the papillary structures are seen within a variable number of ducts (noninfiltrating type) and infiltrate the adjacent stroma. The infiltration of the stroma is usually associated with a loss of papillary differentiation.

Lymph node metastases appear late and reproduce the histologic pattern of the primary tumor. The prognosis is rather good and can be compared with the outcome of patients with mucinous and tubular carcinomas.[398]

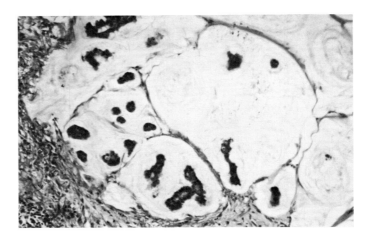

Fig. 11-52. Mucinous carcinoma. Well differentiated tumor cells in pools of abundant extracellular mucin.

Mucinous Carcinoma

Mucin production is a frequently observed phenomenon in mammary carcinoma. Massive production of mucin, described more than a century ago by Larrey,[399] is rare and characterizes mucinous carcinoma (colloid carcinoma, gelatinous carcinoma.[400–402] The pure type appears at a later age, is associated with a longer duration of symptoms, and reveals a larger size compared with other types of carcinoma, including the mixed mucinous or colloid type. Together they represent 2 to 3 percent of all breast carcinomas.

Grossly, mucinous carcinoma is represented by a firm, irregular, well circumscribed, gelatinous or glairy mass, sometimes measuring 10 cm or more in diameter. The mucinous material is contained in numerous cystic formations, which have a translucent blue-green or gray color. When the mucinous foci are discrete, the mixed type may look like an infiltrating duct carcinoma.

Microscopically, the epithelial cells are arranged as clusters, cords, or individual cells separated from the stroma by abundant extracellular mucin (Fig. 11-52). The malignant cells exhibit the usual criteria of malignancy and reveal variable tubular differentiation; sometimes the epithelial elements are so rare that a careful search is necessary to find them. Mucicarmine, Alcian blue, and PAS reactions are positive.[403,404] The pure type is characterized by well differentiated cells occurring singly or in small groups and dispersed within pools of mucin which comprise at least 50 percent of the whole tumor. The mixed type shows the concomitant presence of mucinous and other (usually infiltrating duct) elements. Even if the nonmucinous elements are rare, the tumor should be classified as mixed. The level of histologic differentiation is high in the pure type and mucinous foci in

the mixed type. Argyrophilic granules which ultrastructurally resemble endocrine granules have been observed in the cytoplasm.[405] One report mentions the presence of serotonin in these granules.[406]

The origin of the mucinous substances has been debated. The absence of intracellular mucin in some cases suggests a stromal origin; nevertheless, ultrastructural studies and the presence of mucin in nodal metastases tend to demonstrate the epithelial origin of the mucinous material.[407,408] Mucin production is accompanied by dilated rough endoplasmic reticulum (RER), large Golgi apparatus, and mucin granules contained within smooth membranes.

The prognosis, which is good, is better for the pure mucinous type.[400,401,409,410] This has been explained by the presence of large amounts of extracellular mucin acting as a mechanical barrier between the neoplastic cells and blood vessels.[410] The incidence of regional nodal metastases is low, particularly in cases of pure mucinous carcinoma. Mucin cerebral emboli have been reported as an unusual fatal complication.[411]

Tubular Carcinoma

Tubular carcinoma was first described by Cornil and Ranvier in 1869.[412] Macroscopically, it is a rather hard tumor with stellate or ill defined margins; cut sections show a gray-white color. Tumor size ranges from 0.2cm to 4cm,[413] but most tumors are quite small. Tubular carcinoma is an infrequent form (1 to 10 percent) of breast carcinoma, characterized by the presence of well formed regular tubules lined by a single layer of cuboidal cells and separated by a hyalinized stroma[414–419] (Fig. 11-53). Elastosis occurs chiefly around the tubules and the vessels. Myoepithelial cells are not abundant. Calcifications are frequent: more than 50 percent of cases show intraductal calcified foci; intraductal carcinoma is also commonly present.

Different histologic types have been recognized. The pure type has been described above; the sclerosing type is a small lesion characterized by haphazardly arranged tubules infiltrating into fat and connective tissue.[420] This type could represent an earlier form of the classic tubular type. In the mixed type, at least 75 percent of the tumor is of the tubular type.

The frequency of tubular carcinoma is considerably higher (about 10 percent) in recent series that include larger proportions of smaller tumors detected by mammographic screening. The tumor is much rarer (1 percent) in series in which larger tumors detected by palpation predominate. The high incidence of associated LCIS or ILC suggests that lobular and tubular carcinomas are two divergent types of a specialized form of secretory casein-producing carcinoma.[421] Ultrastructural studies show that the tumor cells resemble those of normal lactiferous ducts. They contain numerous bundles of filaments and reveal alterations of the basal membrane.[422,423] Cytoplasmic protrusions are present in both apical and basal poles of the cells. Myoepithelial cells are very rare, and the basal lamina is often broken or incomplete. Numerous elastic fibers are present around the tubular structures. The prognosis for this slowly growing tumor is very good when tubular elements comprise 75 percent or more of the tumor.[413,419] Axillary lymph node metastases occur in up to 30 percent of cases, but distant metastases are rare.

Differential Diagnosis

Tubular carcinoma is a well differentiated tumor that should not be mistaken for benign lesions such as sclerosing or microglandular adenosis or radial sclerosing lesion. The disorganized arrangement of the epithelial structures and the infiltration of the parenchyma surrounding the tumor are features indicative of carcinoma. The tubules are generally more widely spaced, and their lumina more dilated, than in sclerosing adenosis. Prominent myoepithelial cells are not observed ultrastructurally in tubular carcinoma but are found in sclerosing adenosis. They are also absent in microglandular adenosis, but this condition lacks the reactive stroma of tubular carcinoma. The basal membranes surrounding the glands are preserved in sclerosing adenosis; histochemical and electron microscopic observations show that this is not the case in tubular carcinoma.[424]

Infiltrating Cribriform Carcinoma

Infiltrating cribriform carcinoma has been characterized recently by Page and his colleagues.[425] It comprises 3 to 5 percent of all invasive breast cancers and tends to be intermediate in size between the smaller tubular carci-

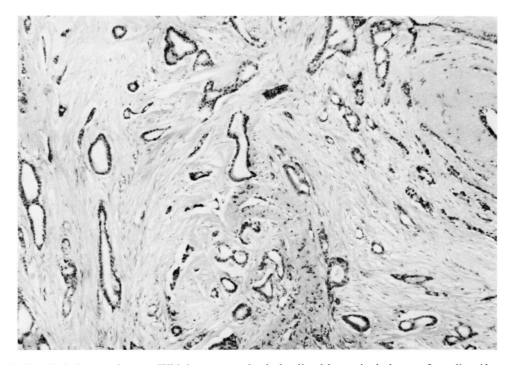

Fig. 11-53. Tubular carcinoma. Widely separated tubules lined by a single layer of small uniform cells.

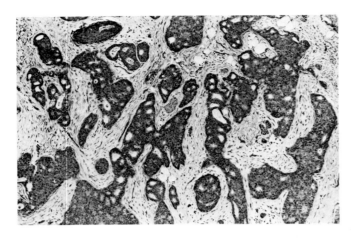

Fig. 11-54. Infiltrating cribriform carcinoma. Irregular nests of infiltrating duct carcinoma are punctuated by uniform punched-out spaces lined by well differentiated tumor cells.

noma and the larger infiltrating duct carcinoma.[426] Its gross appearance does not differ from that of these other two tumor types.

Histologically, this neoplasm displays islands of cells with punched-out spaces, identical to the picture of the cribriform pattern of intraductal carcinoma, but the irregular sizes and shapes of the islands, as well as a reactive stroma, indicate that this is an invasive tumor (Fig. 11-54). Some of the islands may be more solid, but all are characterized by a low or occasionally intermediate nuclear grade. Foci of intraductal carcinoma (often but not necessarily of cribriform type) and of tubular carcinoma are often intermixed.

Differential Diagnosis

The major differential diagnoses are with cribriform intraductal carcinoma and tubular or adenoid cystic carcinoma. Tubular carcinoma is distinguished by its lack of coalescence of tubules to form large islands with many lumina. The presence of basement membrane material within cystic spaces and of numerous myoepithelial cells is necessary for the diagnosis of adenoid cystic carcinoma; this tumor is considerably rarer than infiltrating cribriform carcinoma, and electron microscopy or immunohistochemistry may be required for its diagnosis.

Prognosis

The prognosis of infiltrating cribriform carcinoma is excellent as long as this pattern comprises more than 50 percent of the invasive component of a breast cancer.[425–427] Axillary lymph node metastases (almost always

to fewer than four nodes) are not uncommon, but distant metastases and death resulting from this tumor type are exceedingly rare.

Adenoid Cystic Carcinoma

The pure type of adenoid cystic carcinoma (cylindroma), described by Foote and Stewart,[428] is a very rare, slow-growing variant of duct carcinoma accounting for less than 1 percent of all breast tumors.[429–432] It is histologically identical to certain tumors of the salivary glands, bronchi, cervix, and Bartholin's gland (Fig. 11-55).

Most of these tumors appear in middle-aged women.[433] Grossly, it is usually a firm, small tumor that does not exhibit any specific characteristic. Microscopically, the tumor shows typical glandular, round, and regular honeycombed structures lined by small cuboidal cells with round and hyperchromatic nuclei.[434] The intraluminal material is mucicarmine positive. Electron microscopy characteristically displays the presence of true glandular structures and pseudocysts, which are extracellular compartments enclosed by tumor cells and lined by a basement membrane.[435,436] Myoepithelial cells are prominent in the tumor. Adenoid cystic carcinoma should not be confused with the cribriform type of ductal carcinoma. Electron microscopy is helpful in making this distinction.

The prognosis is excellent compared with the survival rate of the same type of tumor in other anatomic locations[437] and with that of other breast cancers. Regional lymph nodal metastases have been described, as well as recurrences in the mastectomy scar, but both are rare.[438]

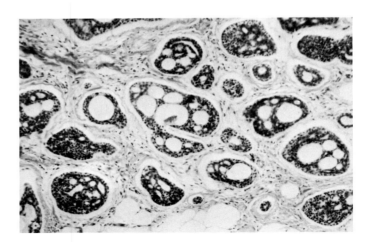

Fig. 11-55. Adenoid cystic carcinoma. Note the cylindromatous pattern with honeycombed cystic spaces.

Paget's Disease

The first clinical description of Paget's disease was published by Velpeau,[439] but it was Paget who first observed the association of the skin lesion with breast cancer.[440] Paget did not recognize the cancerous nature of the skin involvement, and this finding should be credited to Jacobeus.[441] Paget's disease is a particular form of ductal carcinoma accompanied by early invasion of the nipple[442] (Fig. 11-56). The major argument for considering this disease as a special form of intraductal carcinoma is the rather constant presence of a carcinoma in the depths of the gland. The clinical manifestation includes crusting and erosion of the nipple, pruritus, and bloody discharge. These characteristics explain why the lesion was initially considered to be a skin tumor. Paget's disease accompanies less than 5 percent of all breast cancers; the peak incidence rate occurs around 50 years of age. It rarely occurs in men.[443]

Microscopically, the nipple epidermis is infiltrated by large ovoid or round cells with a round nucleus and abundant clear cytoplasm (Fig. 11-57A,B). These cells (Paget cells) may exhibit hyperchromatic irregular nuclei and mitoses. They are isolated or constitute small masses or clumps, usually located in the deeper layers of the epithelium. When the cells occur in nests, this arrangement may recall the junctional component of an amelanotic melanoma; compounding the difficulty is the fact that

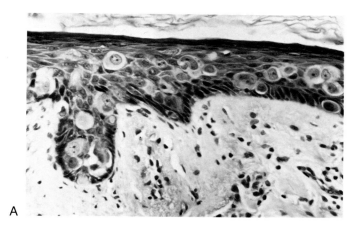

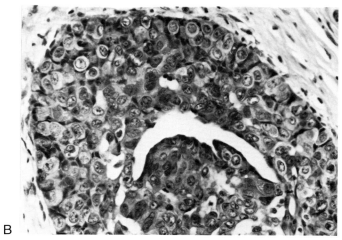

Fig. 11-57. Paget's disease. **(A)** The nipple epidermis is infiltrated by large round cells with a round nucleus and abundant clear cytoplasm. **(B)** An underlying lactiferous duct is infiltrated by the same type of neoplastic cells.

Paget cells may occasionally contain melanin granules.[444,445] However, melanoma of the nipple virtually never occurs.

The histogenesis of the disease is controversial. Neither histochemical techniques nor electron microscopy has definitively settled the matter. In most cases, if numerous serial sections of the underlying mammary parenchyma are made, the primary breast carcinoma will appear (always with an intraductal component). Also, ultrastructural studies generally confirm the great similarity between Paget cells and elements of the inner layer of the mammary ducts.[446] Thus, there is thought to be an extension of the malignant cells upward in the duct system with final infiltration of the overlying cutaneous epithelium. This theory is not unanimously accepted, and

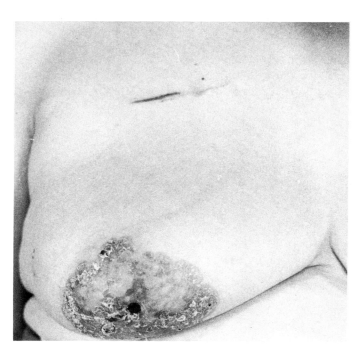

Fig. 11-56. Paget's disease, clinical aspect.

different arguments favor other sources of Paget's cells, such as malignant cells originating de novo within the epithelium of the nipple.[447,448] Even in the absence of microscopic evidence of the parenchymal tumor, there is a possibility that a very small focus of malignant ductal transformation is present but has escaped even a careful search. A field effect, with simultaneous primary tumors in epidermis and lactiferous ducts, is difficult to rule out, however.

The prognosis depends on the extension of the underlying mammary tumor and on the presence of metastatic regional nodes.[449] Treatment is the same as that of intraductal and/or infiltrating duct carcinoma.

Primary carcinoma of the nipple is a rarity and should not be misinterpreted as Paget's disease; both basal cell and squamous carcinoma of the nipple epithelium have been described.[450]

Inflammatory Carcinoma

Inflammatory carcinoma represents the gravest and most rapidly fatal type of all mammary cancers. Luckily, it is rare.[451–454] The average duration of symptoms does not exceed a few months before the lesion becomes clinically evident. The diagnosis of inflammatory carcinoma is suggested by the clinical appearance: a large portion of the breast presents fullness, enlargement, and edema. Except for the findings encountered in Tunisia,[455] this type of carcinoma is not statistically related to pregnancy or lactation.[456] Mammography reveals an overall increased density of the gland and generalized skin thickening.

Microscopically, all the histologic varieties of carcinoma are represented in inflammatory carcinoma; the specific morphologic feature is dermal lymphatic neoplastic infiltrates accompanied by edema of the dermis and vascular dilatation. The clinical features of inflammatory carcinoma are not always correlated with the presence of vascular tumor emboli[452,457] and lymphatic emboli have been reported in the absence of the clinical findings of inflammatory carcinoma.[457] Since any surgical procedure is contraindicated because of the diffuse tumoral infiltration, the diagnosis is better obtained by the less traumatic needle biopsy.

The prognosis is very poor; the 5-year survival rate does not exceed 5 percent. Information on the frequency and prognostic importance of ER and PR is limited, but ER−PR− tumors seem to be more frequent than ER+PR+ tumors.[458] Supravoltage irradiation is the palliative treatment. Chemotherapy has not been proved to modify the evolution of this type of carcinoma.[459]

Recurrent inflammatory carcinoma may present dermal lymphatic tumor emboli with or without inflamma-

tory clinical features.[450] Inflammatory carcinoma should not be confused with inflamed cysts, chronic subareolar disease, any true inflammatory diseases of the breast, or diffuse edema and skin-thickening resulting from congestive heart failure.

Lipid-Rich Carcinoma

Lipid-rich carcinoma has rarely been mentioned in the literature.[461,462] Grossly, these tumors are less firm than the usual infiltrating duct carcinoma, and there is no retraction of the surrounding tissues. Microscopically, they are characterized by poorly differentiated masses of large cells with irregular nuclei and sometimes clear cytoplasm containing neutral lipids. Two other features characterize lipid rich carcinoma; lymph node metastases may mimic a reticuloendotheliosis, and ocular metastases involve the orbital soft tissues and not the retina, the usual site of ocular metastasis in breast carcinoma. The prognosis is poor. Some authorities deny that this particular morphologic condition is a distinctive entity; they mention the presence of vacuolated cells in various conditions such as benign lesions and different types of carcinoma.[463]

Signet Ring Cell Carcinoma

Signet ring carcinoma is a rare type of tumor accounting for under 1 percent of breast carcinomas.[464–466] It is characterized by sheets, cords, and clusters of large round cells with nuclei compressed and displaced by large clear cytoplasmic vacuoles laden with mucin (Fig. 11-58). Compared with typical mucinous carcinoma, mucin-staining reactions in this tumor are only weakly posi-

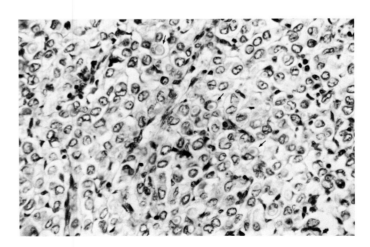

Fig. 11-58. Signet ring cell carcinoma. Some signet cells are indicated by arrows.

tive, and the mucin is intracellular rather than extracellular. Rarely mentioned in classifications of breast cancer, it has been considered by some authorities to be variant of lobular carcinoma. Ultrastructurally, the mucin is seen in intracellular lumina.[465] The presence of ER confirms the mammary origin of these tumors. Their clinical prognosis is poor. They should not be misinterpreted as rare examples of metastatic carcinoma to the breast originating in the digestive tract.

Secretory Carcinoma

This rare tumor has also been known as *juvenile carcinoma,* but recent series have included some cases in adults.[467–469] As the name suggests, the main histologic feature is the presence of voluminous intracellular and extracellular secretory material (predominantly sulfated acid mucopolysaccharide). The tumor, which is frequently grossly circumscribed, has a gray or yellow cut surface. Microscopically, the cells exhibit abundant clear or amphophilic cytoplasm and are arranged in papillary, lobular, or solid structures. Axillary nodal metastases, when they occur, contain the same secretory material. Distant metastases are rare, and the prognosis is excellent.

Carcinoid Tumor

Primary and secondary carcinoid tumors of the mammary gland have been described.[375,405,406] Microscopically, they consist of solid columns or masses of small, fairly uniform cells with round or oval nuclei and homogeneous granular cytoplasm. The presence of occasional microlumina in the cellular masses has been reported. It should be noted, however, that neuroendocrine granules and argyrophilia are observed in 3.3 to 50 percent of mammary tumors.[470] They are considered by some observers as a particular differentiation appearing with more frequency in certain types of carcinoma, such as lobular and mucinous. Some investigators have suggested that the granules represent a prelactional rather than a neuroendocrine secretion, but recent immunohistochemical observations tend to confirm that true neuroendocrine granules are present in tubular, lobular, and infiltrating duct carcinomas as well as in normal lactiferous ducts.[471] Despite these conflicting observations, there are probably rare primary tumors of the breast that both satisfy the diagnostic criteria for carcinoid tumor at the routine light microscopic level and contain neurosecretory granules histochemically and ultrastructurally. These tumors have no major clinical or prognostic differences from typical infiltrating duct carcinomas.[375,472]

Sarcomas

Sarcomas are very uncommon cancers of the breast, representing about 0.5 percent of mammary tumors.[473–475] They include all tumors originating in the mesenchymal stroma of the mammary gland. They occur in relatively elderly women and have great tendency to undergo various types of metaplasia, which include bony and cartilaginous metaplasia and their malignant counterparts.

Fibrosarcomas are rapidly growing, poorly demarcated firm tumors.[476] They represent the most common mammary sarcoma unassociated with cystosarcoma phyllodes[474] and must be distinguished from benign fibromatosis.[477] Microscopically, they are characterized by large bundles of fusiform cells with elongated or anaplastic hyperchromatic nuclei. Bizarre mitoses are common. Hematogenous metastases are frequent. Postradiation fibrosarcoma of the chest wall after mastectomy has been reported.[478] Isolated cases of *leiomyosarcoma* and *rhabdomyosarcoma* have been mentioned in the literature.[479,480] *Osteosarcoma* and *chondrosarcoma* are occasionally encountered and appear to be of relatively low-grade malignancy.[481,482] *Malignant fibrous histiocytoma* has been reported after irradiation.[483]

Malignant Cystosarcoma Phyllodes

Malignant cystosarcoma phyllodes has been described previously.

Liposarcoma

Liposarcoma is a very unusual tumor of the breast.[484–486] The reported cases are large, lobulated, soft yellow tumors often characterized by large, bizarre adipocytes and myxoid degeneration. Lymphatic and hematogenous metastases are frequent. Multiple local recurrences are observed in some cases.

Angiosarcoma

Angiosarcoma (malignant hemangioendothelioma, hemangiosarcoma) is an infrequent tumor that manifests as a rapidly growing breast mass with a blue-red discoloration of the overlying skin. It may appear in women of all ages. Microscopically, it consists of numerous irregular blood vessels in which the endothelial cells show nuclear and cytoplasmic anomalies, often separated by spindle cells. Reticulum and immunohistochemical staining confirm the endothelial location and nature of the neoplastic elements. Thromboses as well as necrotic and hemorrhagic zones are common. Hematogenous metastases are the rule. The prognosis is very poor in the high-grade

360

PRINCIPLES AND PRACTICE OF SURGICAL PATHOLOGY

sarcomas but may be more favorable in the better differentiated ones.[487–489] Angiosarcoma should not be mistaken for highly vascular carcinoma. Although deceptively benign-appearing angiosarcomas do occur, so do truly benign hemangiomas[168–170] and *hemangiopericytomas*.[490]

Postmastectomy Lymphangiosarcoma

Lymphangiosarcoma may develop in tissue that, after radical mastectomy, is the site of chronic lymphedema. It was first described by Stewart and Treves,[491] and more than 100 cases have since been reported.[492–495] Although some authors have believed that this tumor represents a metaplastic variant of the breast carcinoma altered by edema,[492] many publications emphasize the individuality of the lesion.[493–496] Clinically, the lesion first appears as rapidly growing ecchymotic nodules and progresses into a marked generalized edema of the whole arm. When it occurs, this disease usually appears within 10 years after mastectomy.

Microscopically, the tumor consists of numerous lymphatic spaces lined by large polyhedral endothelial cells with hyperchromatic nuclei. In some areas, the tumor cells form solid nests. Ultrastructural observations suggest a mesenchymal and vascular origin of the tumor. Lymphangiosarcoma must be distinguished from retrograde metastasis of breast carcinoma or extension of a primary epidermoid carcinoma of the arm. (Fig. 11-59). The prognosis is very poor.

Postirradiation Sarcoma

Approximately 40 cases of sarcomas complicating radiotherapy for breast cancer have been reported in the literature.[497,498] Most of these sarcomas occur in bones. Some criteria must be fulfilled to accept the postirradiation origin of the bone sarcoma: (1) localization of the tumor in the irradiated area; (2) clear distinction between the histology of the breast and the bone tumors; (3) a latent interval of at least several years; and (4) absence of bone lesion when the breast tumor was diagnosed.

Microscopically, the most common tumors are osteosarcoma, fibrosarcoma, chondrosarcoma, mixed mesenchymal sarcoma, malignant fibrous histiocytoma, and liposarcoma. These sarcomas must be distinguished from postirradiation fibrosis and radiation osteitis.[486]

Malignant Lymphomas

Different types of lymphomas and leukemic infiltrates may be observed as primary tumors of the breast. Most cases, however, represent part of the spectrum of a disseminated disease. Primary localizations manifest as a single nodule or as a diffuse infiltrative process. Microscopically, Hodgkin's disease, multiple myeloma, and various non-Hodgkin's lymphomas have been described.[499–504] The infiltrating cells extend around the ducts and lobules and infiltrate the adjacent stroma and fatty tissue.

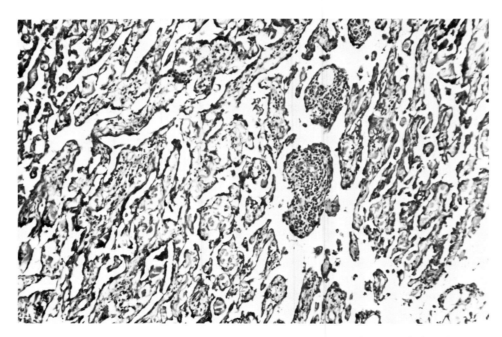

Fig. 11-59. Postmastectomy lymphangiosarcoma. Anastomosing lymphatic channels in subcutaneous tissue of arm.

Lymphoid pseudotumor, or *pseudolymphoma,* is sometimes encountered in the breast. It is characterized microscopically by the presence of follicular germinal centers showing phagocytosis and surrounded by a lymphoid infiltrate. The follicular cells do not exhibit any cytologic alterations suspicious of malignancy.[505]

The association of acute leukemia and breast cancer has been reported.[506] This may be understood by considering the fact that any individual with a given primary tumor is at an increased risk of developing a second, seemingly unrelated, neoplasm, or it may be related to the use of ratiotherapy and/or chemotherapy.

Carcinosarcoma

Carcinosarcoma is a very rare breast neoplasm characterized by the existence of both malignant epithelial and mesenchymal elements. These mixed malignant tumors raise many difficulties in interpretation. For example, their mesenchymal elements may represent a neoplastic proliferation or may merely be metaplastic elements (see discussion of metaplastic carcinomas above). They are quite common in canine and feline mammary glands. Metastases reveal both malignant components. Carcinosarcoma must be distinguished from carcinoma with pseudo-sarcomatous stroma, stromal sarcoma, or malignant cystosarcoma phyllodes, in which only one tissue component is malignant.

Metastatic Tumors

Metastatic tumors to the breast are rare.[507–511] Clinically, the lesion is indistinguishable from a primary tumor. The most frequent neoplasms reported (after carcinoma of the opposite breast) are melanomas,[509] lymphomas, carcinoma of the stomach, carcinoma of the ovary, and tumors of the nasopharyngeal region. The recognition of the metastatic nature of such lesions is important to avoid unnecessary radical surgical procedures. Usually metastatic nodules exhibit a sharp transition at the periphery with the normal breast tissue and do not reveal any in situ component.

PATHOLOGIC CONDITIONS OF THE MALE BREAST

Gynecomastia

Enlargement of the male breast can occur at any time during life. During adolescence, such enlargements are generally bilateral and temporary. This temporary hypertrophy may be due to some hormonal stimulation, which usually regresses spontaneously after a few months. An increase in the plasma estradiol level has been reported in these cases.

In adults, gynecomastia is associated with various clinical conditions that will be mentioned only briefly: Cushing's syndrome; Klinefelter's syndrome[512]; chronic liver disease; thyrotoxicosis[513]; hypogonadism; feminizing adrenal tumors; various testicular tumors with or without steroid production[514]; estrogen therapy; and other iatrogenic causes, such as digitalis,[515] chemotherapic agents (busulfan, vincristine), and phenothiazine or other tranquilizers. It has been reported in heroin addicts and in cannabis smokers. An idiopathic origin has also been reported.[516–520] Cystosarcoma phyllodes has been reported in a case of gynecomastia,[521] as have sclerosing adenosis[522] and many cases of carcinoma. Microscopically, the hypertrophy consists of a dense stromal proliferation accompanied by a variable hyperplasia of the lactiferous ducts.

Differential Diagnosis

Gynecomastia should not be mistaken for pseudogynecomastia, which is observed in obese patients and which consists of an adipose infiltration of the gland without epithelial or stromal proliferation.

Senescent gynecomastia appears in men over age 60; it has a unilateral or bilateral development. Spontaneous regression usually occurs within a few months. A unilateral lesion should not be confused with carcinoma. Microscopically, the lesion is characterized by dense fibrous proliferation with a few scattered remaining ducts.

Carcinoma of the Male Breast

Rare in those under 30 years of age, carcinoma of the breast in men arises at a later age than in women and is approximately 100 times less frequent than carcinoma of the female breast. It is more frequent in certain parts of the world such as Egypt, where it is related to chronic liver disease secondary to schistosomiasis. The epidemiologic and etiologic factors have been discussed previously. The association of carcinoma and gynecomastia has been mentioned. A few cases have been reported in patients who have received prolonged estrogen therapy, usually for prostatic carcinoma.[523,524] In this situation, an important differential diagnosis is with a metastasis from the prostate. Patients with Klinefelter's syndrome (chromosomes XXY) have a higher risk of developing breast cancer, approaching the risk for female patients.[512,525] All the histologic types of carcinoma encountered in the female breast may be seen in the male breast, but they

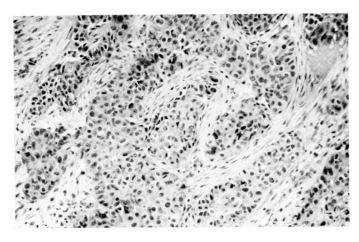

Fig. 11-60. Infiltrating duct carcinoma in a male breast.

usually exhibit poorer differentiation.[526–529] Familial cases have been reported.[530]

Infiltrating duct carcinoma is the most common type, but all types of carcinoma have been reported (Fig. 11-60). Paget's disease has been described.[531] Grossly, the tumor infiltrates the small mammary gland, as well as the skin and the pectoral fascia. Ulceration of the overlying skin is common. The prognosis is poor. ER and PR are present in an even higher percentage than in female patients.[532] Treatment in most reported series has been radical mastectomy with adjuvant radiotherapy and chemotherapy.[533]

REFERENCES

1. Silverberg E, Lubera JA: Cancer Stat 38:5, 1988
2. McLelland R: Mammography in detection, diagnosis and management of carcinoma of breast. Surg Gynecol Obstet 146:735, 1978
3. Propper A: Etude expérimentale des premiers stades de la morphogénèse mammaire. Ann Biol 9:267, 1970
4. Dawson EK: A histological study of the normal mamma in relation to tumor growth. I. Early development to maturity. Edinb Med J 41:653, 1934
5. Ozzello L: Ultrastructure of the human mammary gland. Pathol Ann 6:1, 1971
6. Stirling JW, Chandler JA: The fine structure of ducts and subareolar ducts in the resting gland of the female breast. Virchows Arch [A] 373:119, 1977
7. Tannenbaum M, Weiss M, Marx AJ: Ultrastructure of the human mammary ductule. Cancer 23:958, 1969
8. Linzell JL: The silver staining of myoepithelial cells, particularly in the mammary gland, and their relation to the ejection of milk. J Anat 86:49, 1952
9. Dawson EK: A histologic study of the normal mamma in relation to tumor growth. II. The mature gland in pregnancy and lactation. Edinb Med J 42:633, 1935

10. Fanger H, Ree HJ: Cyclic changes of human mammary gland epithelium in relation to the menstrual cycle. An ultrastructural study. Cancer 34:574, 1974
11. Kramer WM, Rush BF Jr: Mammary duct proliferation in the elderly. A histopathologic study. Cancer 31:130, 1973
12. Montagna W, Yun JS: The glands of Montgomery. Br J Dermatol 86:126, 1972
13. Servelle M, Boudin JS, Zafari I, et al: Les lymphatiques du sein et des muscles pectoraux. Semin Hop Paris 48:121, 1972
14. Turner-Warwick RT: The lymphatics of the breast. Br J Surg 46:574, 1979
15. Fisher W, Smith JW: Macromastia during puberty. Plast Reconstr Surg, 47:445, 1971
16. Strombeck JO: Macromastia in women and its surgical treatment. A clinical study based on 1042 cases. Acta Chir Scand 341(suppl):1, 1964
17. Ashikari R, Huvos AG, Snyder RE: Prospective study of noninfiltrating carcinoma of the breast. Cancer 39:435, 1977
18. Rosen PP: Specimen radiography and the diagnosis of clinically occult mammary carcinoma. Pathol Annu 15(pt 1):225, 1980
19. Esteran JM, Zaloudek C, Silverberg SG: Intraoperative diagnosis of breast lesions. Comparison of cytologic with frozen section technics. Am J Clin Pathol 88:681, 1987
20. Connolly JL, Schnitt SJ: Evaluation of breast biopsy specimens in patients considered for treatment by conservative surgery and radiation therapy for early breast cancer. Pathol Annu 23(pt 1):1, 1988
21. Gold RH: Mammography and related methods of breast cancer detection. In Hoogstraten B, McDivitt RW (eds): Breast Cancer. CRC Press, Boca Raton, FL, 1981
22. Frank HA, Hall FM, Steer ML: Preoperative localization of nonpalpable breast lesions demonstrated by mammography. N Engl J Med 295:259, 1976
23. Gallager HS: Breast specimen radiography. Obligatory, adjuvant and investigative. Am J Clin Pathol 64:749, 1975
24. Beahrs OH, McDivitt RW, Shapiro S, et al: Report of the working group to review the National Cancer Institute/American Cancer Society Breast Cancer Detection Demonstration Projects. J Natl Cancer Inst 62:647, 1979
25. Rosen PP, Snyder RE, Foote FW, Wallace T: Detection of occult carcinoma in the apparently benign breast biopsy through specimen radiography. Cancer 26:944, 1970
26. Hutter RV, Snyder RE, Lucas JC et al: Clinical and pathologic correlations with mammographic findings in lobular carcinoma in situ. Cancer 23:826, 1969
27. Margolin FM, Lagios MD: Mammographic detection of early breast cancer. 10 Years experience in a community hospital. West J Med 144:46, 1986
28. Moskowitz M, Milbrath J, Gartside P, et al: Lack of efficacy of thermography as a screening tool for minimal and Stage I breast cancer. N Engl J Med 295:249, 1976
29. Kobayashi T: Grey-scale echography for breast cancer. Radiology 122:207, 1977
30. Tabar L, Marton Z, Kadas I: Galactography in the examination of secretory breasts. Am J Surg 127:282, 1974
31. Franzen F, Zajicek J: Aspiration biopsy in diagnosis of

palpable lesions of the breast. Critical review of 3479 consecutive biopsies. Acta Radiol 7:241, 1968

32. Gompel C: Atlas of Diagnostic Cytology. Churchill Livingstone, New York, 1978

33. Koss LG, Woyke S, Oszewski W: Aspiration Biopsy. Cytologic Interpretation and Histologic Bases. Igaku-Shoin, New York, 1984

34. Hammond S, Keyhani-Rofagha S, O'Toole RV: Statistical analysis of fine needle aspiration cytology of the breast. A review of 678 cases plus 4265 cases from the literature. Acta Cytol 31:276, 1987

35. Lee KR, Foster RS, Papillo JL: Fine needle aspiration of the breast. Importance of the aspirator. Acta Cytol 31:281, 1987

36. Russ JE, Winchester DP, Scanlon EF, et al: Cytologic findings of aspiration of tumors of the breast. Surg Gynecol Obstet 46:407, 1978

37. Oertel YC: Fine Needle Aspiration of the Breast. Butterworths, Boston, 1987

38. King EB, Barrett D, Petrakis NL: Cellular composition of the nipple aspirate specimen of breast fluid. II. Abnormal findings. Am J Clin Pathol 64:739, 1975

39. Wilson SL, Ehrmann, RL: The cytologic diagnosis of breast aspirations. Acta Cytol 22:470, 1978

40. Mouriquand J, Pasquier D: Fine needle aspiration of breast carcinoma. Acta Cytol 24:153, 1980

41. Bloustein PA, Silverberg, SG: Rapid cytologic examination of surgical specimens. Pathol Annu 12(2):251, 1977

42. Tribe CR: A comparison of rapid methods including imprint cytodiagnosis for the diagnosis of breast tumors. J Clin Pathol 26:273, 1971

43. Minkowitz M, Moskowitz R, Khafif RA, Alderete MN: Tru-cut needle biopsy of the breast. An analysis of its specificity and sensitivity. Cancer 57:320, 1986

44. Elston CW, Cotton RE, Davies CJ, et al: A comparison of the use of the ''Tru-Cut'' needle and fine needle aspiration cytology in the pre-operative diagnosis of carcinoma of the breast. Histopathology 2:239, 1978

45. Rosen PP: Frozen section diagnosis of breast lesions. Recent experience with 556 consecutive biopsies. Ann Surg 187:17, 1978

46. Agnantis NJ, Apostolikas N, Christodoulou I, et al: The reliability of frozen-section diagnosis in various breast lesions: A study based on 3451 biopsies. Recent Results. Cancer Res 90:205, 1984

47. Fessia L, Ghiringhello R, Arisio R, et al: Accuracy of frozen section diagnosis in breast cancer detection. A review of 4436 biopsies and comparison with cytodiagnosis. Pathol Res Pract 179:61, 1984

48. Robbins GF, Bros ST: The significance of delay in relation to prognosis of patients with primary operable breast cancer. Cancer 10:338, 1957

49. Ekland DA, Zeigler MG: Abscess in the nonlactating breast. Arch Surg 107:398, 1973

50. Tedeschi LG, Ahari S, Byrne JJ: Involutional mammary duct ectasia and periductal mastitis. Am J Surg 106:517, 1963

51. Patey DH, Thackray AC: Pathology and treatment of mammary duct fistula. Lancet 2:871, 1958

52. Winker JM: Galactocele of the breast. Am J Surg 108:357, 1964

53. Rosen SW, Gahres EE: Nonpuerperal galactorrhea and the contraception pill. Obstet Gynecol 29:730, 1967

54. Mukerjee PK, Niden AH, Cohen RV: Tuberculosis of breast. Am Rev Respir Dis 104:661, 1971

55. Wilson TS, MacGregor JS: The diagnosis and treatment of tuberculosis of the breast. Can Med Assoc J 89:1118, 1963

56. Whitaker HT, Moore RM: Gumma of the breast. Surg Gynecol Obstet 98:473, 1954

57. Trempe F: Actinomycose mammaire primitive. Can J Surg 1:210, 1958

58. Miller MJ, Moore S: Nodular breast lesion caused by Bancroft's filariasis. Can Med Assoc J 93:711, 1965

59. Coleman M: Scleroderma simulating carcinoma of the breast. Br J Surg 25:61, 1937

60. Salfelder K, Schwartz J: Mycotic ''pseudotumors'' of the breast. Report of four cases. Arch Surg 110:751, 1975

61. Walia HS, Abraham TK, Shaikh H: Fungal mastitis. Case report. Acta Clin Scand. 153:133, 1987

62. Adair FE, Munzer JT: Fat necrosis of the female breast. Report of one hundred ten cases. Am J Surg 74:117, 1947

63. Kessler E, Wolloch Y: Granulomatous mastitis: A lesion clinically simulating carcinoma. Am J Clin Pathol 58:642, 1972

64. Meyer JE, Silverman P, Gandbhir L: Fat necrosis of breast. Arch Surg 113:801, 1978

65. Adair FE: Plasma cell mastitis; a lesion simulating mammary carcinoma; a clinical and pathologic study with a report of ten cases. Arch Surg 26:735, 1933

66. Hogan GF: Mondor's disease. Arch Intern Med 113:881, 1964

67. Nosanchuk JS: Silicone granuloma in breast. Arch Surg 97:583, 1968

68. Winer LH, Sternberg TH, Lehman R, et al: Tissue reaction to injected silicone liquids. A report of three cases. Arch Dermatol 90:588, 1964

69. Kipen CS: Gangrene of the breast. A complication of anticoagulant therapy. Report of two cases. N Engl J Med 265:638, 1961

70. Martin BF, Phillips JD: Gangrene of the female breast with anticoagulant therapy. Report of two cases. Am J Clin Pathol 53:622, 1970

71. Robitaille Y, Seemayer TA, Thelmo WL, et al: Infarction of the mammary region mimicking carcinoma of the breast. Cancer 33:1183, 1974

72. Wilkinson K, Green WO: Infarction of breast lesions during pregnancy and lactation. Cancer 17:1567, 1964

73. Donnelly PK, Baker KW, Carney JA, et al: Benign breast lesions and subsequent breast carcinoma in Rochester, Minnesota. Mayo Clin Proc 50:650, 1975

74. Gullino PM: Considerations on the preneoplastic lesions of the mammary gland. Am J Pathol 89:413, 1977

75. Page DL, Vander Zwaag R, Rogers LW, et al: Relation between component parts of fibrocystic disease complex and breast cancer. J Natl Cancer Inst 61:1055, 1978

76. Frantz VK, Pickren JW, Melcher GW, et al: Incidence of chronic cystic disease in so-called ''normal breasts'': A

study based on 225 post mortem examinations. Cancer 4:762, 1951

77. Fischer ER, Paulson JD: Karyotypic abnormalities in precursor lesions of human cancer of the breast. Am J Clin Pathol 69:284, 1978

78. Fechner RE: Influence of oral contraceptives on breast diseases. Cancer 39:2764, 1977

79. Nomura A, Comstock GW, Tonascia JA: Epidemiologic characteristics of benign breast disease. Am J Epidemiol 105:505, 1977

80. Hutter RVP: Goodbye to "fibrocystic disease." N Engl J Med 312:179, 1985

81. Donnelly PK, Baker KW, Carney JA, et al: Benign breast lesions and subsequent breast carcinoma in Rochester, Minnesota. Mayo Clin Proc 50:650, 1975

82. Haagensen CD: The relationship of gross cystic disease of the breast and carcinoma. Ann Surg 185:375, 1977

83. Page DL, Vander Zwaag R, Rogers LW, et al: Relation between component parts of fibrocystic disease complex and breast cancer. J Natl Cancer Inst 61:1055, 1978

84. Consensus meeting: Is "fibrocystic disease" of the breast precancerous? Arch Pathol Lab Med 110:171, 1986

85. McLaughlin CW Jr, Schenken JR, Tamisie AJ: A study of precancerous epithelial hyperplasia and non-invasive papillary carcinoma of the breast. Ann Surg 15:735, 1961

86. Deschamps M, Hislop TG, Band PR: Study of benign breast disease in a population screened for breast cancer. Cancer Detect Prev 9:151, 1986

87. Dixon JM, Lumsden AM: Miller WR: The relationship of cyst type to risk factors for breast cancer and the subsequent development of breast cancer in patients with breast cystic disease. Eur J Cancer Clin Oncol 21:1047, 1985

88. Dupont WD, Page DL: Risk factors for breast cancer in women with proliferative breast disease. N Engl J Med 312:146, 1985

89. Lagios MD: Human breast precancer: Current status. Cancer Surv 2:383, 1977

90. Black MM, Barclay TH, Cutler SJ, et al: Association of atypical characteristics of benign breast lesions with subsequent risk of breast cancer. Cancer 29:338, 1972

91. Wellings SR, Jensen HM, Marcum RG: An atlas of subgross pathology of the human breast with special reference to possible precancerous lesions. J Natl Cancer Inst 55:231, 1975

92. Page DL, Dupont WD, Rogers LW, et al: Atypical hyperplastic lesions of the female breast: A long-term follow-up study. Cancer 55:2698, 1985

93. Dixon JM, Anderson TJ, Lumsden AB, et al: Mammary duct ectasia. Br J Surg 70:601, 1983

94. McSwain GR, Valicenti JF, O'Brien PH: Cytologic evaluation of breast cysts. Surg Gynecol Obstet 146:921, 1978

95. Tavassoli FA, Norris HJ: Microglandular adenosis of the breast: A clinicopathologic study of 11 cases with ultrastructural observations. Am J Surg Pathol 7:731 1983

96. Rosenblum MK, Purrazella R, Rosen PP: Is microglandular adenosis a precancerous disease? A study of carcinoma arising therein. Am J Surg Pathol 10:237, 1986

97. Fisher ER, Palekar AS, Kotwal N, et al: Nonencapsulated sclerosing lesion of the breast. Am J Clin Pathol 71:240, 1979

98. Oberman HA: Benign breast lesions confused with carcinoma. p. 1. In: McDivitt RW, Oberman HA, Ozzello L, Kaufman N (eds): The Breast. Williams & Wilkins, Baltimore, 1984

99. Jao W, Recant W, Swerdlow MA: Comparative ultrastructure of tubular carcinoma and sclerosing adenosis of the breast. Cancer 38:180, 1976

100. Rickert RR, Kalisher L, Hutter RVP: Indurative mastopathy: A benign sclerosing lesion of breast with elastosis which may simulate carcinoma. Cancer 47:561, 1981

101. Wellings SR, Roberts P: Electron microscopy of sclerosing adenosis and infiltrating carcinoma of the human mammary gland. J Natl Cancer Inst 30:269, 1963

102. Martinez-Hernandez A, Francis DJ, Silverberg SG: Elastosis and other stromal reactions in benign and malignant breast tissue. An ultrastructural study. Cancer 40:700, 1977

103. Taylor HB, Norris HJ: Epithelial invasion of nerves in benign diseases of the breast. Cancer 20:2245, 1967

104. Murad TM, von Haam E: The ultrastructure of fibrocystic disease of the breast. Cancer 22:587, 1968

105. Wellings SR, Alpers CE: Apocrine cystic metaplasia: Subgross pathology and prevalence in cancer-associated versus random autopsy breasts. Hum Pathol 18:381, 1987

106. Fenoglio C, Lattes R: Sclerosing papillary proliferations in the female breast. Cancer 33:691, 1974

107. Eusebi V, Grassigh A, Grosso F: Lesioni focali sclero-elastotiche mammarie simulanti il carcinoma infiltrante. Pathologica 68:507, 1976

108. Fisher ER, Palekar AS, Kotwall N, Lapana N: A nonencapsulated sclerosing lesion of the breast. Am J Clin Pathol 71:240, 1979

109. Andersen JA, Gram JB: Radial scar in the female breast. A long term follow up study of 32 cases. Cancer 53:2557, 1984

110. Anderson TJ, Battersby S: Radial scars of benign and malignant breasts: Comparative features and significance. J Pathol 147:23, 1985

111. Tremblay G, Buell RH, Seemayer TA: Elastosis in benign sclerosing ductal proliferation of the female breast. Am J Surg Pathol 1:1155, 1977

112. Nielsen M, Christensen L, Andersen JA: Radial scars in women with breast cancer. Cancer 59:1010, 1987

113. Azzopardi JG: Problems in Breast Pathology. WB Saunders, Philadelphia, 1979

114. Roberts MM, Jones V, Elton RA, et al: Risk of breast cancer in women with history of benign disease of the breast. Br Med J 288:275, 1984

115. Silverberg SG, Chitale AR, Levitt SH: Prognostic implications of fibrocystic dysplasia in breasts removed for mammary carcinoma. Cancer 29:574, 1972

116. Fisher ER, Gregorio RM, Fisher B, et al: The pathology of invasive breast cancer. A syllabus derived from findings of the National Adjuvant Breast Project (Protocol No. 4). Cancer 36:1, 1975

117. Fechner RE: Fibrocystic disease in women receiving oral contraceptive hormones. Cancer 25:1332, 1970

118. Livolsi VA, Stadel BV, Kelsey JL, et al: Fibrocystic breast disease in oral contraceptive-users: Histo-patholog-

ical evaluation of epithelial atypia. N Engl J Med 299:381, 1978

119. Ory H, Cole P, MacMahon B, et al: Oral contraceptives and reduced risk of benign breast diseases. N Engl J Med 294:419, 1976

120. Page DL, Vander Zwagg R, Rogers LW, et al: Relation between component parts of fibrocystic disease complex and breast cancer. J Natl Cancer Inst 61:1055, 1978

121. Kodlin D, Winger EE, Morgenstern NL, et al: Chronic mastopathy and breast cancer: A follow up study. Cancer 39:2603, 1977

122. Fechner RE: Fibroadenomas in patients receiving oral contraceptives. A clinical and pathologic study. Am J Clin Pathol 53:857, 1970

123. Demetrakopoulos NJ: These dimensional reconstruction of a human mammary fibroadenoma. Q Bull Northwest U Med School 32:221, 1958

124. Crile G, Chatty EM: Squamous metaplasia of lactiferous ducts. Arch Surg 102:533, 1971

125. Lawler RG: Cartilaginous metaplasia in a breast tumour. J Pathol 97:385, 1969

126. Goodman ZD, Taxy JB: Fibroadenomas of the breast with prominent smooth muscle. Am J Surg Pathol 5:99, 1981

127. Murad TM, Greider MH, Scarpelli DG: The ultrastructure of human mammary fibroadenoma. Am J Pathol 51:663, 1967

128. Yeh IT, Francis DI, Orenstein JM, Silverberg SG: Ultrastructure of cystosarcoma phyllodes and fibroadenoma. A comparative study. Am J Clin Pathol 84:131, 1985

129. Jao W, Vasquez LT, Keh PC, et al: Myoepithelial differentiation and basal lamina deposition in fibroadenoma and adenosis of the breast. J Pathol 126:107, 1978

130. O'Hara MF, Page DL: Adenomas of the breast and ectopic breast under lactational influences. Hum Pathol 16:707, 1985

131. Rickert RR, Rajan S: Localized breast infarcts associated with pregnancy. Arch Pathol 97:159, 1974

132. Newman J, Kahn LB: Infarction of fibro-adenoma of the breast. Br J Surg 60:738, 1973

133. Eusebi V, Azzopardi JG: Lobular endocrine neoplasia in fibroadenoma of the breast. Histopathology 4:413, 1986

134. Buzanowski-Konakry K, Harrison EG Jr, Payne WS: Lobular carcinoma arising in fibroadenoma of the breast. Cancer 35:450, 1975

135. Fondo Y, Rosen PP, Fracchia AA, Urban JA: The problem of carcinoma developing in a fibroadenoma. Cancer 43:50, 1979

136. Moore IAR, Sandison AT: Triple carcinoma of the breast, one arising within a fibroadenoma. J Pathol 109:263, 1973

137. McDivitt RW, Stewart FW, Farrow JH: Breast carcinoma arising in solitary fibroadenoma. Surg Gynecol Obstet 125:572, 1967

138. Pike AM, Oberman HA: Juvenile cellular adenofibromas. A clinico-pathologic study. Am J Surg Pathol 9:730, 1985

139. Mies C, Rosen PP: Juvenile fibroadenoma: A study of 49 patients. Lab Invest 54:42A, 1986

140. Mies C, Rosen PP: Juvenile fibroadenoma with atypical epithelial hyperplasia. Am J Surg Pathol 11:184, 1987

141. Hertel BF, Zaloudek C, Kempson RL: Breast adenomas. Cancer 37:2891, 1976

142. O'Hara MF, Page DL: Adenomas of the breast and ectopic breast under lactation influences. Hum Pathol 16:707, 1985

143. Hogeman KE, Ostberg G: Three cases of post-lactational breast tumor of a peculiar type. Acta Pathol Microbiol Immunol Scand [A] 73:169, 1968

144. Willen R, Uvelius B, Camaron R: Pleomorphic adenoma in the breast of a human female. Aspiration biopsy findings and receptor determination. Case report. Acta Clin Scand 152:709, 1986

145. Nichols FC, Dockerty MB, Judd ES: Florid papillomatosis of the nipple. Surg Gynecol Obstet 107:474, 1958

146. Perzin KH, Lattes R: Papillary adenoma of the nipple (florid papillomatosis, adenoma, adenomatosis). A clinico-pathologic study. Cancer 29:996, 1972

147. Jones DB: Florid papillomatosis of the nipple ducts. Cancer 8:315, 1955

148. Rosen PP: Syringomatous adenoma of the nipple. Am J Surg Pathol 7:739, 1983

149. Rosen PP: Adenomyoepithelioma of the breast. Hum Pathol 18:1232, 1987

150. Hendrick JW: Intraductal papilloma of the breast. Surg Gynecol Obstet 105:215, 1957

151. Murad TM, Contesso G, Mouriesse H: Papillary tumors of the large lactiferous ducts. Cancer 48:122, 1981

152. Kraus FT, Neubecker RD: The differential diagnosis of papillary tumors of the breast. Cancer 15:444, 1962

153. Papotti M, Gugliotta P, Ghiringello B, Bussolati G: Association of breast carcinoma and multiple intraductal papillomas: An histological and immunohistochemical investigation. Histopathology 8:963, 1984

154. Cutler M: Tumors of the Breast, Their Pathology, Symptoms, Diagnosis and Treatment. JB Lippincott, Philadelphia, 1961

155. Ashikari P, Huvos AG, Snyder RE, et al: A clinicopathologic study of atypical lesions of the breast. Cancer 33:310, 1974

156. Carter D: Intraductal papillary tumors of the breast. Cancer 39:1689, 1977

157. Murad TM, Pritchett P: Malignant and benign papillary lesions of the breast. Hum Pathol 8:379, 1977

158. Rosen PP, Cantrell B, Mullen DL, et al: Juvenile papillomatosis (swiss cheese disease) of the breast. Am J Surg Pathol 4:3, 1980

159. Rosen PP, Holmes G, Lesser ML, et al: Juvenile papillomatosis and breast carcinoma. Cancer 55:1345, 1985

160. Craig JM: Leiomyoma of female breast. Arch Pathol 44:314, 1947

161. Daroca PJ Jr, Reed RJ, Love GL, Kraus SD: Myoid hamartomas of the breast. Hum Pathol 16:212, 1985

162. Spalding JE: Adeno-lipoma of the breast. Guy's Hosp Rep 94:80, 1945

163. Wargotz ES, Weiss SW, Norris HJ: Myofibroblastoma of the breast: Sixteen cases of a distinctive benign mesenchymal tumor. Am J Surg Pathol 11:493, 1987

164. Umansky C, Bullock WK: Granular cell myoblastoma of the breast. Ann Surg 168:810, 1968

165. Demay RM, Kay S: Granular cell tumors of the breast. Pathol Annu 18(2):121, 1984

166. Ingram DL, Mossler JA, Snowhite J, et al: Granular cell

tumors of the breast. Steroid receptor analysis and localisation of carcinoembryonic antigen, myoglobin and S100 protein. Arch Pathol Lab Med 108:897, 1984

167. Altermatt HJ, Gebbers JO, Laissue JA: Das Hamartom der Mamma. Schweiz Med Wochenschr 117:365, 1987

168. Rosen PP, Ridolfi RL: The perilobular hemangioma. A benign microscopic vascular lesion of the breast. Am J Clin Pathol 68:21, 1977

169. Rosen PP: Vascular tumors of the breast. III. Angiomatosis. Am J Surg Pathol 9:652, 1985

170. Rosen PP: Vascular tumors of the breast. IV. The venous hemangioma. Am J Surg Pathol 9:659, 1985

171. Merino MJ, Carter D: Angiosarcoma of the breast. Am J Surg Pathol 7:53, 1983

172. Müller J: Uber den feinern Ban und die Formen der krankhaften Geschwülste. G Reiner, Berlin, 1838

173. Stromberg BV, Golladay ES: Cystosarcoma phylloides in the adolescent female. J Pediatr Surg 13:423, 1978

174. Treves N, Sunderland DA: Cystosarcoma phyllodes of the breast. A malignant and a benign tumor. Cancer 4:1286, 1951

175. Mottot C, Poulique NX, Bastien H, et al: Fibro-adénomes et tumeurs phyllodes. Approche cyto-pathologique. Ann Anat Pathol 23:233, 1978

176. Kessinger A, Foley JF, Lemon HM, et al: Metastatic cystosarcoma phyllodes: A case report and review of the literature. J Surg Oncol 4:131, 1972

177. Qizilbash AH: Cystosarcoma phyllodes with liposarcomatous stroma. Am J Clin Pathol 65:321, 1976

178. Norris HJ, Taylor HB: Relationship of histologic features to behavior of cystosarcoma phyllodes. Analysis of ninety-four cases. Cancer 20:2090, 1967

179. Pietruszka M, Barnes L: Cystosarcoma phyllodes. A clinico-pathologic analysis of 42 cases. Cancer 41:1974, 1978

180. Hajdu S, Espinosa MH, Robbins GF: Recurrent cystosarcoma phyllodes. A clinico-pathologic study of 32 cases. Cancer 38:1402, 1976

181. Hart WR, Bauer RC, Oberman HA: Cystosarcoma phyllodes. A clinicopathologic study of 26 hypercellular periductal stromal tumors of the breast. Am J Clin Pathol 70:211, 1978

182. Ward RM, Evans HL: Cystosarcoma phyllodes: A clinicopathologic study of 26 cases. Cancer 58:2282, 1986

183. Grigoni WF, Santini D, Grassigli A, et al: A clinico-pathologic study of cystosarcoma phyllodes. Twenty case reports. Arch Anat Cytol Pathol 30:303, 1982

184. Kay S: Light and electron microscopic studies of a malignant cystosarcoma phyllodes featuring stromal cartilage and bone. Am J Clin Pathol 55:770, 1971

185. Fernandez BB, Hernandez FJ, Spindler W: Metastatic cystosarcoma phyllodes: A light and electron microscopic study. Cancer 37:1737, 1976

186. Kesterton GHD, Gorgiade N, Seigler HF, et al: Cystosarcoma phyllodes. A steroid receptor and ultrastructure analysis. Ann Surg 190:640, 1979

187. Porton WM, Poortman J: Estrogen receptors in cystosarcoma phyllodes of the breast. Eur J Cancer Clin Oncol 17:1147, 1981

188. Azzopardi JG: Sarcomas of the breast. p. 346. In Azzopardi JG (ed): Problems in Breast Pathology. Major Problems in Pathology. Vol. II. WB Saunders, Philadelphia, 1979

189. Tabar L, Gad A, Holmberg LH, et al: Reduction in mortality from breast cancer after mass screening with mammography. Lancet 1:829, 1985

190. Sayler C, Egan JF, Ranies JR, et al: Mammographic screening. Value in diagnosis of early breast cancer. JAMA 238:872, 1977

191. Gautherie M, Gros CM: Breast thermography and cancer risk prediction. Cancer 45:51, 1980

192. Blom HJG: The influence of delay on the natural history and prognosis of breast cancer. Br J Cancer 19:228, 1965

193. Ackerman LV, Katzenstein AL: The concept of minimal breast cancer and the pathologist's role in the diagnosis of "early carcinoma." Cancer 39:2755, 1977

194. Fisher B, Slack NH, Bross ID, et al: Cancer of the breast: Size of neoplasm and prognosis. Cancer 24:1071, 1969

195. Say CC, Donegan WL: Invasive carcinoma of the breast: Prognostic significance of tumor size and involved axillary lymph nodes. Cancer 34:468, 1974

196. Wynder EL, MacCormack FA, Stellman SD: The epidemiology of breast cancer in 785 United States Caucasian women. Cancer 41:2341, 1978

197. Choi NW, Howe GR, Miller AB, et al: An epidemiologic study of breast cancer. Am J Epidemiol 107:510, 1978

198. Alderson MR, Hamlin I, Stanton MD: The relative significance of prognostic factors in breast carcinoma. Br J Cancer 25:646, 1971

199. Papaioannou AN: Etiologic factors in cancer of breast in humans. Surg Gynecol Obstet 138:257, 1974

200. Miller AB, Bulbrook RD: Special report: The epidemiology and etiology of breast cancer. N Engl J Med 303:1246, 1980

201. De Bono AM, Pillers EMK: Carcinoma of the breast in East Anglia 1960–1975: A changing pattern of presentation? J Epidemiol Br Commonwealth 32:178, 1978

202. Waterhouse J, Muir C, Shanmugaratnam K, et al (eds): Cancer Incidence in Five Continents. Vol. 4. IARC Scientific Publication No. 42. International Agency for Research on Cancer, Lyons, 1982

203. Logan CJH: Carcinoma of the breast in women under the age of 30. Br Med J 2:1023, 1978

204. Stavraky K, Emmons S: Breast cancer in premenopausal and postmenopausal women. J Natl Cancer Inst 53:647, 1974

205. de Waard F, de Laive JWJ, Baanders-van Haliwijn EA: On the bimodal age distribution of mammary carcinoma. Br J Cancer 14:437, 1960

206. Backhouse CM, Lloyd-Davies ER, Shousha S, Burn JI: Carcinoma of the breast in women aged 35 or less. Br J Surg 74:591, 1987

207. Staszewski J: Age at menarche and breast cancer. J Natl Cancer Inst 47:935, 1971

208. de Waard F, Cornelis JP, Aoki K, et al: Breast cancer incidence according to weight and height in two cities of the Netherlands and Aichi Prefecture Japan. Cancer 40:1269, 1977

209. Buell P: Changing incidence of breast cancer in Japanese-American women. J Natl Cancer Inst 51:1479, 1973
210. Graham S, Marshall J, Mettlin C, et al: Diet in the epidemiology of breast cancer. Am J Epidemiol 116:68, 1982
211. Willett WC, Meir J, Stampfer MJ, et al: Dietary fat and the risk of breast cancer. N Engl J Med 316:22, 1987
212. Kirschner MA: The role of hormones in the etiology of human breast cancer. Cancer 39:2716, 1977
213. Henderson BE, Ross RK, Judd HL, et al: Do regular ovulatory cycles increase breast cancer risk? Cancer 56:1206, 1985
214. Anderson DE: Genetic study of breast cancer: Identification of a high risk group. Cancer 34:1090, 1974
215. Anderson DE, Badzioch MD: Risk of familial breast cancer. Cancer 56:383, 1985
216. Lynch HT, Guirgis H, Brodkey F, et al: Early age of onset in familial breast cancer. Arch Surg 111:126, 1976
217. Harris RE, Lynch HT, Guirgis H: Familial breast cancer: Risk to the contralateral breast. J Natl Cancer Inst 60:955, 1978
218. Adami HO, Jung B, Lindgren A, et al: Histopathological malignancy grading and familiality in an unselected series of 1303 women with breast carcinoma. Ann Clin Res 14:76, 1982
219. Robinson DW: Breast carcinoma associated with pregnancy. Am J Obstet Gynecol 92:658, 1965
220. Erwald R: Mammary carcinoma and pregnancy. Acta Obstet Gynecol Scand 46:316, 1967
221. Nugent P, O'Connell TX: Breast cancer and pregnancy. Arch Surg 120:1221, 1985
222. King RM, Welch JS, Martin JK, et al: Carcinoma of the breast associated with pregnancy. Surg Gynecol Obstet 160:228, 1985
223. Lemon HM: Endocrine influences on human mammary cancer formation. Cancer 23:781, 1969
224. Zumoff B, Fishman J, Bradlow HL, et al: Hormone profiles in hormone-dependent cancers. Cancer Res 35:3365, 1975
225. Bennett A, MacDonald AM, Simpson JS, et al: Breast cancer, prostaglandins and bone metastases. Lancet 1:1218, 1975
226. Wagner S, Mantel N: Breast cancer at a psychiatric hospital before and after the introduction of neuroleptic agents. Cancer Res 38:2703, 1978
227. MacMahon B, Liu JM, Lowe CR, et al: Lactation and cancer of the breast. A summary of an international study. Bull WHO 42:1249, 1969
228. Rissanen PM: Carcinoma of the breast during pregnancy and lactation. Br J Cancer 22:663, 1968
229. Wallack MK, Wolf JA Jr, Bedwinek J, et al: Gestational carcinoma of the female breast. Curr Probl Cancer 7:1, 1983
230. Taylor HB: Oral contraceptives and pathologic changes in the breast. Cancer 28:1388, 1971
231. Harris NV, Weiss NS, Francis AM, et al: Breast cancer in relation to patterns of oral contraceptive use. Am J Epidemiol 116:643, 1982
232. The Centers for Disease Control Cancer and Steroid Hormone Study: Long-term oral contraceptive use and risk of breast cancer. JAMA 249:1591, 1983
233. Rosenberg L, Miller DR, Kaufman DW, et al: Breast cancer and oral contraceptive use. Am J Epidemiol 119:167, 1984
234. Hulka BS, Chambless LE, Deubner DC, et al: Breast cancer and estrogen replacement therapy. Am J Obstet Gynecol 143:638, 1982
235. Brinton LA, Hoover RN, Szklo M, et al: Menopausal estrogen use and risk of breast cancer. Cancer 47:2517, 1981
236. Hunt K, Vessey M, McPherson K, Coleman M: Long-term surveillance of mortality and cancer incidence in women receiving hormone replacement therapy. Br J Obstet Gynaecol 94:620, 1987
237. Ellis RJ, Wernick G, Zabriskie JB, et al: Immunologic competence of regional lymph nodes in patients with breast cancer. Cancer 35:655, 1975
238. Anastassiades OT, Pryce DM: Immunological significance of the morphological changes in lymph nodes draining breast cancer. Br J Cancer 20:239, 1966
239. Crile G Jr: Possible role of uninvolved regional nodes in preventing metastasis from breast cancer. Cancer 24:1283, 1969
240. Bittner JJ: Some possible effects of nursing on the mammary gland tumor incidence in mice. Science 84:162, 1936
241. Moore DH, Charney J, Kramarsky B, et al: Search for a human breast cancer virus. Nature (Lond) 229:611, 1971
242. Bentvelzen P, Daams JH, Hageman P, et al: Intersections between viral and genetic factors in the origin of mammary tumors in mice. J Natl Cancer Inst 48:1089, 1972
243. Macklin MT: Comparison of the number of breast cancer deaths observed in relatives of breast cancer patients and the number expected on the basis of mortality rates. J Natl Cancer Inst 22:927, 1959
244. Land CE, Boice JD Jr, Shore RE, et al: Breast cancer risk from low-dose exposure to ionizing radiation. Results of parallel analysis of three exposed populations of women. J Natl Cancer Inst 65:353, 1980
245. Rosen PP: The pathological classification of human mammary carcinoma. Past, present and future. Ann Clin Lab Sci 9:144, 1979
246. Scarff RW, Torloni H: Histological Typing of Breast Tumours. World Health Organization, Geneva, 1968
247. Foote FW Jr, Stewart FW: Lobular carcinoma in situ. A rare form of mammary cancer. Am J Pathol 17:491, 1941
248. Andersen JA: Lobular carcinoma in situ. A long-term follow-up in 52 cases. Acta Pathol Microbiol Scand [A] 82:519, 1974
249. Andersen JA: Multicentric and bilateral appearance of lobular carcinoma in situ of the breast. Acta Pathol Microbiol Scand [A] 82:730, 1974
250. Newman W: Lobular carcinoma of the female breast. Report of 73 cases. Ann Surg 164:305, 1966
251. Lewison EF, Finney GG: Lobular carcinoma in situ of the breast. Surg Gynecol Obstet 126:1280, 1968
252. Black MM, Chabon AB: In situ carcinoma of the breast. Pathol Ann 4:185, 1969
253. Haagensen CD, Lane N, Lattes R, et al: Lobular neopla-

sia (so-called lobular carcinoma in situ) of the breast. Cancer 42:737, 1978

254. Frykberg ER, Santiago F, Betsill WL Jr, O'Brien PH: Lobular carcinoma in situ of the breast. Surg Gynecol Obstet 164:285, 1987

255. Wheeler JF, Enterline HT, Roseman JM, et al: Lobular carcinoma in situ of the breast: Long-term follow up. Cancer 34:554, 1974

256. Rosen PP, Lieberman DH, Braun DW, et al: Lobular carcinoma in situ of the breast: Detailed analysis of 99 patients with average follow up of 24 years. Am J Surg Pathol 2:225, 1978

257. Webber BL, Heise H, Neifeld JP, et al: Risk of subsequent contralateral breast carcinoma in a population of patients with in situ breast carcinoma. Cancer 47:2928, 1981

258. Fisher ER, Fisher B: Lobular carcinoma of the breast: An overview. Ann Surg 185:377, 1977

259. Betsill W, Rosen PP, Lieberman P, et al: Intraductal carcinoma. Long-term follow-up after treatment by biopsy alone. JAMA 239:1863, 1978

260. Rosen PP: Lobular carcinoma in situ and intraductal carcinoma of the breast. p. 59. In McDivitt RW, Oberman HA, Ozzello L, et al (eds): The Breast. Williams & Wilkins, Baltimore, 1984

261. Carter D, Yardley JH, Shelley WM: Lobular carcinoma of the breast. An ultrastructural comparison with certain duct carcinomas and benign lesions. Johns Hopkins Med J 125:25, 1969

262. Henson D, Tarone R: A study of lobular carcinoma of the breast based on the Third National Cancer Survey in the United States of America. Tumori 65:133, 1979

263. Ludwig AS, Okagaki T, Richart RM, et al: Nuclear DNA content of lobular carcinoma in situ of the breast. Cancer 31:1553, 1973

264. Andersen JA, Vendelboe ML: Cytoplasmic mucous globules in lobular carcinoma in situ. Diagnosis and prognosis. Am J Surg Pathol 5:251, 1981

265. McDivitt RW, Hutter RVP, Foote FW Jr, et al: In situ lobular carcinoma. A prospective follow up study indicating cumulative patient risks. JAMA 201:82, 1967

266. Frykberg ER, Santiago F, Betsill WL Jr, O'Brien PH: Lobular carcinoma in situ of the breast. Surg Gynecol Obstet 164:285, 1987

267. Donegan WL, Perez-Mesa CM: Lobular carcinoma. An indication for elective biopsy of the second breast. Ann Surg 176:178, 1972

268. Fechner RE: Ductal carcinoma involving the lobule of the breast: A source of confusion with lobular carcinoma in situ. Cancer 28:274, 1971

269. Breslow A, Brancaccio ME: Intracellular mucin production by lobular breast carcinoma cells. Arch Pathol Lab Med 100:620, 1976

270. von Rueden DG, Wilson RE: Intraductal carcinoma of the breast. Surg Gynecol Obstet 158:105, 1984

271. Gibbons CP: Intraductal breast cancer. Lancet 2:462, 1984

272. Ashikari R, Hajdu SI, Robbins GF: Intraductal carcinoma of the breast (1960–1969). Cancer 28:1182, 1971

273. Brown PW, Silverman J, Owens E, et al: Intraductal "non

274. Gillis DA, Dockerty MB, Clagett OT: Preinvasive intraductal cancer. Surg Gynecol Obstet 110:555, 1960

275. Millis RR, Thynne GSJ: In situ intraduct carcinoma of the breast: A long-term follow-up study. Br J Surg 62:957, 1975

276. Silverberg SG, Chitale AR: Assessment of significance of proportions of intraductal and infiltrating tumor growth in ductal carcinoma of the breast. Cancer 32:830, 1973

277. Fisher ER, Sass R, Fisher B, et al: Pathologic findings from the National Surgical Adjuvant Breast Project (Protocol 6). I. Intraductal Carcinoma (DCIS) Cancer 57:197, 1986

278. Guerry P, Erlandson RA, Rosen PP: Cystic hypersecretory hyperplasia and cystic hypersecretory duct carcinoma of the breast. Pathology, therapy, and follow-up of 39 patients. Cancer 61:1611, 1988

279. Gould VE, Miller J, Jao W: Ultrastructure of medullary, intraductal, tubular and adenocystic breast carcinomas. Comparative patterns of myoepithelial differentiation and basal lamina deposition. Am J Pathol 78:401, 1975

280. Ozzello L: Ultrastructure of human mammary carcinoma cells in vivo and in vitro. J Natl Cancer Inst 48:1043, 1972

281. Ozzello L: The behavior of basement membranes in intraductal carcinoma of the breast. Am J Pathol 35:887, 1959

282. Silverstein MI, Rosser RJ, Gierson ED, et al: Axillary lymph node dissection for intraductal carcinoma—Is it indicated? Cancer 59:1819, 1987

283. Rosen PP: Axillary lymph node metastases in patients with occult noninvasive breast carcinoma. Cancer 46:1298, 1980

284. Page DL, Dupont WD, Rogers LW, Laudenberger M: Intraductal carcinoma of the breast: Follow-up after biopsy only. Cancer 49:75, 1982

285. Recht A, Danoff BS, Salin LJ, et al: Intraductal carcinoma of the breast: results of treatment with excisional biopsy and irradiation. J Clin Oncol 3:1339, 1985

286. Moertel CG, Soule EM: The problem of the second breast: A study of 118 patients with bilateral carcinoma of the breast. Ann Surg 146:764, 1957

287. Holland R, Veling SHJ, Mravunac M, et al: Histologic multifocality of Tis, T1–2 breast carcinomas. Implications for clinical trials of breast-conserving surgery. Cancer 56:979, 1985

288. Smith BH, Taylor HB: The occurrence of bone and cartilage in mammary tumors. Am J Clin Pathol 51:610, 1969

289. Gonzalez-Licea A, Yardley JH, Hartmann WH: Malignant tumor of the breast with bone formation. Studies by light and electron microscopy. Cancer 20:1234, 1967

290. Chiloso M, Bonetti F, Menestrina F, et al: Breast carcinoma with stromal multinucleated giant cells. J Pathol 152:55, 1987

291. Lagios MD, Westdahl PR, Rose MR: The concept and implications of multicentricity in breast carcinoma. Pathol Annu 16:83, 1981

292. Battifora H: Intracytoplasmic lumina in breast carcinoma: A helpful histopathologic feature. Arch Pathol 99:614, 1975

293. Contesso G, Rouesse J, Petit JY, et al: Les facteurs anatomopathologiques du pronostic des cancers du sein. Bull Cancer 64:525, 1977

294. Fisher B, Slack NH, Bross ID, et al: Cancer of the breast: Size of neoplasm and prognosis. Cancer 24:1071, 1969

295. Bedwani R, Vani J, Rosner D, et al: Management and survival of female patients with "minimal" breast cancer. Cancer 47:2769, 1981

296. Black MM, Kerpe S, Speer FD: Lymph node structure in patients with cancer of the breast. Am J Pathol 29:505, 1953

297. Fisher ER, Gregorio R, Redmond C, et al: Pathologic findings from the National Surgical Adjuvant Breast Project (protocol no 4). II. The significance of regional node histology other than sinus histiocytosis in invasive mammary cancer. Am J Clin Pathol 65:21, 1976

298. Fisher ER, Reidbord H, Fisher B: Studies concerning the regional lymph node in cancer. V. Histologic and ultrastructural findings in regional and non-regional nodes. Lab Invest 28:126, 1973

299. Fisher B, Bauer M, Wickerham DL, et al: Relation of number of positive axillary nodes to the prognosis of patients with primary breast cancer. Cancer 52:1551, 1983

300. Kouchoukos NT, Ackerman LV, Butcher HR: Prediction of axillary nodal metastases from the morphology of mammary carcinomas: A guide to operative therapy. Cancer 20:948, 1967

301. Veronesi U, Rilke F, Luini A, et al: Distribution of axillary node metastases by level of invasion. Cancer 59:682, 1987

302. McLaughlin CW Jr, Coe JD, Adwers JR: A thirty year study of breast cancer in a consecutive series of private patients. Is axillary nodal study a valuable index in prognosis? Am J Surg 136:250, 1978

303. Weigand RA, Isenberg WM, Russo J, et al: Blood vessel invasion and axillary lymph node involvement as prognostic indicators for human breast cancer. Cancer 50:962, 1982

304. Say CC, Donegan WL: Invasive carcinoma of the breast: Prognostic significance of tumor size and involved axillary lymph nodes. Cancer 34:468, 1974

305. Morrow M, Evans J, Rosen PP, Kinne DW: Does clearing of axillary lymph nodes contribute to accurate staging of breast carcinoma? Cancer 53:1329, 1984

306. Nemoto T, Vana J, Bedwani RN, et al: Management and survival of female breast cancer: Results of a national survey by the American College of Surgeons. Cancer 45:2917, 1980

307. Fisher B, Slack NH: Number of lymph nodes examined and the prognosis of breast carcinoma. Surg Gynecol Obstet 131:79, 1970

308. Hartveit F: The routine histological investigation of axillary lymph nodes for metastatic breast cancer. J Pathol 143:187, 1984

309. Trojani M, De Mascarel I, Bonichou F, et al: Micrometastases to axillary lymph nodes from carcinoma of breast: Detection by immunohistochemistry and prognostic significance. Br J Cancer 55:303, 1987

310. Bloom HJG, Richardson WW: Histological grading and prognosis in breast cancer. A study of 1409 cases of which 359 have been followed for 15 years. Br J Cancer 11:359, 1957

311. Tough ICK, Carter DC, Fraser J, et al: Histological grading in breast cancer. Br J Cancer 23:294, 1969

312. Greenough RB: Varying degrees of malignancy in cancer of the breast. J Cancer Res 9:453, 1925

313. Fisher ER, Gregorio RM, Fisher B: The pathology of invasive breast cancer. A syllabus derived from findings of the National Surgical Adjuvant Breast Project (protocol no. 4). Cancer 36:1, 1975

314. Black MM, Barclay THC, Hankey BF: Prognosis in breast cancer utilizing histologic characteristics of the primary tumor. Cancer 36:2048, 1975

315. Fisher ER, Kotwal N, Hermann C, et al: Types of tumor lymphoid response and sinus histiocytosis. Arch Pathol Lab Med 107:222, 1983

316. Black MM, Speer FD: Sinus histiocytosis of lymph nodes in cancer. Surg Gynecol Obstet 106:163, 1958

317. DiRe JJ, Lane W: The relation of sinus histiocytosis in axillary lymph nodes to surgical curability of carcinoma of the breast. Am J Clin Pathol 40:508, 1963

318. Kister SJ, Sommers SC, Haagensen CD, et al: Nuclear grade and sinus histiocytosis in cancer of the breast. Cancer 23:570, 1969

319. Silverberg SG, Chitale AR, Hind AD, et al: Sinus histiocytosis and mammary carcinoma. Cancer 26:1177, 1970

320. Horst H-A, Horny H-P: Characterization and frequency distribution of lymphoreticular infiltrates in axillary lymph node metastases of invasive ductal carcinoma of the breast. Cancer 60:3001, 1987

321. Schiødt T: Breast Carcinoma. A Histologic and Prognostic Study of 650 Followed-up Cases. Copenhagen, Munksgaard, 1966

322. Silverberg SG, Chitale AR, Levitt SH: Prognostic significance of tumor margins in mammary carcinoma. Arch Surg 102:450, 1971

323. Van Bogaert LJ, Mazy G, Jeanmart L, et al: Etude anatomo-radiohistologique du cancer mammaire spiculaire. Senologia 2:63, 1977

324. Andersen JA: Multicentric and bilateral appearance of lobular carcinoma in situ of the breast. Acta Pathol Microbiol Scand [A] 82:730, 1974

325. Breslow, A.: Occult carcinoma of second breast following mastectomy. JAMA 226:1000, 1973

326. Hubbard TB Jr: Nonsimultaneous bilateral carcinoma of breast. Surgery 34:706, 1953

327. Lewison EF, Neto AS: Bilateral breast cancer at the Johns Hopkins Hospital. A discussion of the dilemma of contralateral breast cancer. Cancer 28:1297, 1971

328. Wanebo HJ, Senofsky GM, Fechner RE, et al: Bilateral breast cancer. Risk reduction by contralateral biopsy. Am Surg 201:667, 1985

329. Mueller CB, Ames F: Bilateral carcinoma of the breast: Frequency and mortality. Can J Surg 21:459, 1978

330. Prior P, Waterhouse JAH: Incidence of bilateral tumours in a population based series of breast cancer patients. I. Two approaches to an epidemiological analysis. Br J Cancer 37:620, 1978

331. Robbins GF, Berg JW: Bilateral primary breast cancers. A prospective clinicopathologic study. Cancer 17:1501, 1964

332. Urban JA: Bilaterality of cancer of the breast. Biopsy of the opposite breast. Cancer 20:1867, 1967

333. Lesser ML, Rosen PP, Kinne DW: Multicentricity and bilaterality in invasive breast carcinoma. Surgery 91:234, 1982

334. Azzopardi JG, Eusebi V: Melanocyte colonization and pigmentation of breast carcinoma. Histopathology 1:21, 1977

335. Andersen JA, Pallesen RM: Spread to the nipple and areola in carcinoma of the breast. Ann Surg 189:367, 1979

336. Congdon GH, Dockerty MB: Malignant lesions of the nipple exclusive of Paget's disease. Surg Gynecol Obstet 103:185, 1956

337. Fisher ER, Palekar AS, Gregorio RM, et al: Pathological findings from the national Surgical Adjuvant Breast Project (protocol no 4). IV. Significance of tumor necrosis. Hum Pathol 9:523, 1978

338. Friedell GH, Betts A, Sommers SC: The prognostic value of blood vessel invasion and lymphocytic infiltrates in breast carcinoma. Cancer 18:164, 1965

339. Gollinger RC, Gregorio R, Fisher ER: Tumor cells in venous blood draining mammary carcinomas. Arch Surg 112:707, 1977

340. Taylor HB, Norris HJ: Epithelial invasion of nerves in benign diseases of the breast. Cancer 20:2245, 1967

341. Silfverswärd C, Gustafsson J, Gustafsson S, et al: Estrogen receptor concentrations in 269 cases of histologically classified human breast cancer. Cancer 45:2001, 1980

342. DeSombre ER, Greene GL, King WJ, Jensen EV: Estrogen receptors, antibodies and hormone dependent cancer. p. 1. In Gurpide E, Calandra R, Levy C, Soto RJ (eds): Hormones and Cancer. Alan R Liss, New York, 1981

343. Jonat W, Maass H, Stegner HE: Immunohistochemical measurement of estrogen receptors in breast cancer tissue samples. Cancer Res 46:4296s, 1986

344. Alanko A, Scheinin T, Tolppanen EM, Vihko R: Significance of estrogen and progesterone receptors, disease-free interval, and site of first metastasis on survival of breast cancer patients. Cancer 56:1696, 1985

345. McClelland RA, Berger U, Miller LS, et al: Immunocytochemical assay for estrogen receptor in patients with breast cancer: Relationship to a biochemical assay and to outcome of therapy. J Clin Oncol 4:1171, 1986

346. McCarty KS, Miller LS, Cox EB, et al: Estrogen receptor analyses. Correlation of biochemical and immunohistochemical methods using monoclonal antireceptor antibodies. Arch Pathol Lab Med 109:716, 1985

347. Leclercq G, Bojar H, Goussard J, et al: Abbott monoclonal enzyme immunoassay for the measurement of estrogen receptors in human breast cancer: A European multicenter study. Cancer Res 46:4233s, 1986

348. Benyahia B, Magdelenat H, Zajdela A, Vilcoq JR: Ponction-aspiration à l'aiguille fine et dosage des récepteurs d'oestrogènes dans le cancer du sein. Bull Cancer 69:456, 1982

349. Flowers JL, Burton GV, Cox EB, et al: Use of monoclonal antiestrogen receptor antibody to evaluate estrogen receptor content in fine needle aspiration breast biopsies. Ann Surg 203:250, 1986

350. Tosi P, Baak JPA, Luzi P, et al: Correlation between immunohistochemically determined oestrogen receptor content, using monoclonal antibodies, and qualitative and quantitative tissue features in ductal breast cancer. Histopathology 11:741, 1987

351. Mason BH, Holdaway IM, Mullins PR, et al: Progesterone and estrogen receptors as prognostic variables in breast cancer. Cancer Res 43:2985, 1983

352. Lee AK, Rosen PP, Delellis RA, et al: Tumor marker expression in breast carcinomas and relationship to prognosis. An immunohistochemical study. Am J Clin Pathol 84:687, 1985

353. Cohen C, Sharkey FE, Shulman G, et al: Tumor-associated antigens in breast carcinomas. Prognostic significance. Cancer 60:1294, 1987

354. Lidereau R, Callahan R, Dickson C, et al: Amplification of the int-2 gene in primary human breast tumors. Oncogene Res 2:285, 1988

355. Coulson PB, Thornthwaite JT, Wooley TW, et al: Prognostic indicators including DNA histogram type, receptor content, and staging related to human breast cancer patient survival. Cancer Res 44:4187, 1984

356. Thorud E, Fussa SD, Vaaje S, et al: Primary breast cancer: Flow cytometric pattern in relation to clinical and histopathologic characteristics. Cancer 57:808, 1986

357. Berryman IL, Harvey JM, Sterrett GF, Papadimitriou JM: The nuclear DNA content of human breast carcinoma. Associations with clinical stage, axillary lymph node status, estrogen receptor status and outcome. Anal Quant Cytol Histol 9:429, 1987

358. Wyatt JP, Sugarbaker ED, Stanton MF: Involvement of internal mammary lymph nodes in carcinoma of breast. Am J Pathol 31:143, 1955

359. Lumb G, Mackenzie DH: The incidence of metastases in adrenal glands and ovaries removed for carcinoma of the breast. Cancer 12:521, 1959

360. de la Monte SM, Hutchins GM, Moore GW: Influence of age on the metastatic behavior of breast carcinoma. Hum Pathol 19:529, 1988

361. Ceci G, Franciosi V, Nizzoli R, et al: The value of bone marrow biopsy in breast cancer at time of diagnosis. A prospective study. Cancer 61:96, 1988

362. Viadana E, Bross IDJ, Pickren JW: An autopsy study of some routes of dissemination of cancer of the breast. Br J Cancer 27:336, 1973

363. Fenig J, Arlen M, Livingston SF, et al: The potential for carcinoma existing synchronously on a microscopic level within the second breast. Surg Gynecol Obstet 141:394, 1975

364. Everson TC: Spontaneous regression of cancer. Ann NY Acad Sci 114:721, 1964

365. Frable WJ, Kay S: Carcinoma of the breast. Histologic and clinical features of apocrine tumors. Cancer 21:756, 1968

366. Roddy HJ, Silverberg SG: Ultrastructural analysis of apocrine carcinoma of the human breast. Ultrastruct Pathol 1:385, 1980

367. Fisher ER, Fisher B: Lobular carcinoma of the breast: An overview. Ann Surg 185:377, 1977

368. Dixon JM, Anderson TJ, Page DL, et al: Infiltrating lobular carcinoma of the breast. Histopathology 6:149, 1982

369. Wheeler JE, Enterline HT: Lobular carcinoma of the breast in situ and infiltrating. Pathol Annu 14:161, 1979

370. Martinez V, Azzopardi JG: Invasive lobular carcinoma of the breast: Incidence and variants. Histopathology 3:467, 1979

371. Shousha S, Backhous CM, Alaghband-Zadeh J, Burn I: Alveolar variant of invasive lobular carcinoma of the breast. Am J Clin Pathol 85:1, 1986

372. Haagensen CD, Lane N, Lattes R, et al: Lobular neoplasia (so-called lobular carcinoma in situ) of the breast. Cancer 42:737, 1978

373. Gad A, Azzopardi JG: Lobular carcinoma of the breast: A special variant of mucin-secreting carcinoma. J Clin Pathol 28:711, 1975

374. Fechner RE: Histologic variants of infiltrating lobular carcinoma of the breast. Hum Pathol 6:373, 1975

375. Cubilla AL, Woodruff JM: Primary carcinoid tumor of the breast: A report of eight patients. Am J Surg Pathol 1:283, 1977

376. Gould VE, Chejfec G: The value of electron microscopy in diagnostic pathology. Case 13. Ultrastruct Pathol 1:151, 1980

377. Lesser ML, Rosen PP, Senie RT, et al: Estrogen and progesterone receptors in breast carcinoma: Correlations with epidemiology and pathology. Cancer 48:299, 1981

378. Huvos, AG, Lucas JC Jr, Foote FW Jr: Metaplastic breast carcinoma: Rare form of mammary cancer. NY State J Med 73:1078, 1973

379. An T, Grathwohl M, Frable WJ: Breast carcinoma with osseous metaplasia: An electron microscopic study. Am J Clin Pathol 81:127, 1983

380. Gersell DJ, Katzenstein ALA: Spindle cell carcinoma of the breast. A clinicopathologic and ultrastructural study. Hum Pathol 12:550, 1981

381. Flint A, Oberman HA, Davenport RD: Cytophotometric measurements of metaplastic carcinoma of the breast: Correlation with pathologic features and clinical behavior. Mod Pathol 1:193, 1988

382. Oberman HA: Metaplastic carcinoma of the breast. A clinicopathologic study of 29 patients. Am J Surg Pathol 11:918, 1987

383. Kaufman MW, Marti JR, Gallager HS, et al: Carcinoma of the breast with pseudosarcomatous metaplasia. Cancer 53:1908, 1984

384. Hasleton PS, Misch KA, Vasudev KS, et al: Squamous carcinoma of the breast. J Clin Pathol 34:116, 1978

385. Bloom HJG, Richardson WW, Field JR: Host resistance and survival in carcinoma of the breast. A study of 104 cases of medullary carcinoma in a series of 1411 cases of breast cancer followed for 20 years. Br Med J 3:181, 1970

386. Wargotz ES, Silverberg SG: Medullary carcinoma of the breast: A clinicopathologic study with appraisal of current diagnostic criteria. Hum Pathol 19:1340, 1988

387. Markovits P, Contesso G, Sarrazin D, et al: Le carcinome medullaire du sein. Etude clinique et anatomo-radiologique à propos de 56 observations. Bull Cancer 57:517, 1970

388. Richardson WW: Medullary carcinoma of the breast. A distinctive tumour type with a relatively good prognosis following radical mastectomy. Br J Cancer 10:415, 1956

389. Ridolfi RL, Rosen PP, Port A et al: Medullary carcinoma of the breast. A clinicopathologic study with 10 years follow-up. Cancer 40:1365, 1977

390. Flores L, Arlen M, Elguezabal A, et al: Host-tumor relationships in medullary carcinoma of the breast. Surg Gynecol Obstet 139:683, 1974

391. Ben-Ezra J, Sheibani K: Antigenic phenotype of the lymphocytic component of medullary carcinoma of the breast. Cancer 59:2037, 1987

392. Gould VE, Miller J, Jao W: Ultrastructure of medullary, intraductal, tubular and adenocystic breast carcinomas. Am J Pathol 78:401, 1975

393. Michaud J, Morin J: Ultrastructure d'un épithélioma médullaire de la glande mammaire. Laval Médical 42:496, 1971

394. Ahmed A: The ultrastructure of medullary carcinoma of the breast. Virchows Arch [A] 388:175, 1980

395. Maier WP, Rosemond GP, Goldman LI, et al: A ten year study of medullary carcinoma of the breast. Surg Gynecol Obstet 144:695, 1977

396. Rosen PP, Lesser ML, Kinne DW: Breast carcinoma of the extremes of age: A comparison of patients younger than 35 years and older than 75 years. J Surg Oncol 28:90, 1985

397. Schwartz GF: Solid circumscribed carcinoma of the breast. Ann Surg 169:165, 1969

398. Fisher ER, Palekar AS, Redmond C, et al: Pathologic findings from the National Surgical Adjuvant Breast Project (Protocol no. 4) VI. Invasive papillary cancer. Am J Clin Pathol 73:313, 1980

399. Larrey M: Tumeur gelatiniforme ou colloïde de la mamelle. Bull Soc Chir Paris 3:545, 1853

400. Rasmussen BB, Rose C, Christensen I: Prognostic factors in primary mucinous breast carcinoma. Am J Clin Pathol 87:155, 1987

401. Silverberg SG, Kay S, Chitale AR, et al: Colloid carcinoma of the breast. Am J Clin Pathol 55:355, 1971

402. Komaki K, Sakamoto G, Sugano H, et al: Mucinous carcinoma of the breast in Japan. A prognostic analysis based on morphologic features. Cancer 61:989, 1988

403. Cooper DJ: Mucin histochemistry of mucous carcinomas of the breast and colon and non-neoplastic breast epithelium. J Clin Pathol 27:311–314, 1974

404. Tellem M, Nedwich A, Amenta PS, et al: Mucin-producing carcinoma of the breast. Tissue culture, histochemical and electron microscopic study. Cancer 19:573, 1966

405. Rasmussen BB, Rose C, Thorpe SM, et al: Argyrophilic cells in 202 human mucinous breast carcinomas. Relation to histopathologic and clinical factors. Am J Clin Pathol 84:737, 1985

406. Feyrter F, Hartmann G: Uber die carcinoide Wuchsform des carcinoma mammae, ins besondere das carcinoma solidum (gelatinosum) mammae. Frankfurt Z Pathol 73:24, 1963

407. Harris M, Vasudev KS, Anfield C, et al: Mucin-producing carcinomas of the breast: Ultrastructural observations. Histopathology 2:177, 1978

408. Jao W, Lao IO, Chowdhury LN, et al: Ultrastructural aspects of mucinous (colloid) breast carcinoma. Diagn Gynecol Obstet 2:83, 1980

409. Clayton F: Pure mucinous carcinomas of breast. Hum Pathol 17:34, 1986

410. Norris HJ, Taylor HB: Prognosis of mucinous (gelatinous) carcinoma of the breast. Cancer 18:879, 1965

411. Towfighi J, Simmonds MA, Davidson EA: Mucin fat emboli in mucinous carcinomas causing hemorrhagic cerebral infarcts. Arch Pathol Lab Med 107:646, 1983

412. Cornil V, Ranvier L: Manuel d'histologie pathologique. G Baillière, Paris, 1869

413. Carstens PHB, Greenberg RA, Francis D, et al: Tubular carcinoma of the breast. A long-term follow-up. Histopathology 9:271, 1985

414. Carstens PHB: Tubular carcinoma of the breast. A study of frequency. Am J Clin Pathol 70:204, 1978

415. Carstens PHB, Huvos AG, Foote FW Jr, et al: Tubular carcinoma of the breast. A clinico-pathologic study of 35 cases. Am J Clin Pathol 58:231, 1972

416. Cooper HS, Patchefsky AS, Krall RA: Tubular carcinoma of the breast. Cancer 42:2334, 1978

417. Oberman HA, Fidler WJ: Tubular carcinoma of the breast. Am J Surg Pathol 3:387, 1979

418. Tobon H, Salazar H: Tubular carcinoma of the breast. Arch Pathol Lab Med 101:310, 1977

419. McDivitt RW, Boyce W, Gersell D: Tubular carcinoma of the breast. Clinical and pathological observations concerning 135 cases. Am J Surg Pathol 6:401, 1982

420. Andersson I: Radiographic screening for breast carcinoma. II. Prognostic considerations on the basis of a short-term follow-up. Acta Radiol [Diagn] (Stockh) 22:227, 1981

421. Fisher ER, Gregorio RM, Redmond C, Fisher B: Tubulo-lobular invasive breast cancer: A variant of lobular invasive cancer. Hum Pathol 8:679, 1977

422. Erlandson RA, Carstens PHB: Ultrastructure of tubular carcinoma of the breast. Cancer 29:987, 1972

423. Harris M, Ahmed A: The ultrastructure of tubular carcinoma of the breast. J Pathol 123:79, 1979

424. Flotte TJ, Bell DA, Greco MA: Tubular carcinoma and sclerosing adenosis. The use of basal lamina as a differential feature. Am J Surg Pathol 4:75, 1980

425. Page DL, Dixon JM, Anderson TJ, et al: Invasive cribriform carcinoma of the breast. Histopathology 7:525, 1983

426. Dawson PJ, Karrison T, Ferguson DJ: Histologic features associated with long-term survival in breast cancer. Hum Pathol 17:1015, 1986

427. Venable J, Oertel Y, Orenstein JM, et al: Infiltrating cribriform carcinoma of the breast. Lab Invest 58:98A, 1988

428. Foote FW Jr, Stewart FW: A histologic classification of carcinoma of the breast. Surgery 19:74, 1946

429. Anthony PP, James PD: Adenoid cystic carcinoma of the breast: Prevalence, diagnostic criteria, and histogenesis. J Clin Pathol 28:647, 1975

430. Cavanzo FJ, Taylor HB: Adenoid cystic carcinoma of the breast. An analysis of 21 cases. Cancer 24:740, 1969

431. Friedman BA, Oberman HA: Adenoid cystic carcinoma of the breast. Am J Clin Pathol 54:1, 1970

432. Ro JY, Silva EG, Gallager HS: Adenoid cystic carcinoma of the breast. Hum Pathol 18:1276, 1987

433. Qizilbash AH, Patterson MC, Oliveira KF: Adenoid cystic carcinoma of the breast. Light and electron microscopy and a brief review of the literature. Arch Pathol Lab Med 101:302, 1977

434. Lusted D: Structural and growth patterns of adenoid cystic carcinoma of breast. Am J Clin Pathol 54:419, 1970

435. Koss LG, Brannan CD, Ashikari R: Histologic and ultrastructural features of adenoid cystic carcinoma of the breast. Cancer 26:1271, 1970

436. Zaloudek C, Oertel YC, Orenstein JM: Adenoid cystic carcinoma of the breast. Am J Clin Pathol 81:297, 1984

437. Galloway JR, Woolner LB, Clagett OT: Adenoid cystic carcinoma of the breast. Surg Gynecol Obstet 122:1289, 1966

438. Peters GN, Wolff M: Adenoid cystic carcinoma of the breast: Report of 11 new cases. Cancer 52:680, 1982

439. Velpeau A: Traité des maladies du sein et de la région mammaire. Paris, Masson, 1858

440. Paget J: Disease of the mammary areola preceding cancer of the mammary gland. St Barth Hosp Rep 10:87, 1874

441. Jacobeus HC: Paget's disease und sein Verhältnis zum Milchdrüsen Karzinom. Virchows Arch 178:124, 1904

442. Helman P, Kliman M: Paget's disease of the nipple: A clinical review of 27 cases. Br J Surg 43:481, 1956

443. Lancer HA, Moschell SL: Paget's disease of the male breast. J Ann Acad Dermatol 7:393, 1982

444. Neubecker RD, Bradshaw RP: Mucin, melanin and glycogen in Paget's disease of the breast. Am J Clin Pathol 36:40, 1961

445. Toker C: Some observations on Paget's disease of the nipple. Cancer 14:653, 1961

446. Nadji M, Morales AR, Girtanner RE, et al: Paget's disease of the skin. Cancer 50:2203, 1982

447. Lagios MD, Westdahl PR, Rose MR, et al: Paget's disease of the nipple. Cancer 54:545, 1984

448. Toker C: Clear cells of the nipple epidermis. Cancer 25:601, 1970

449. Paone JF, Baker R: Pathogenesis and treatment of Paget's disease of the breast. Cancer 48:825, 1981

450. Congdon GH, Dockerty MB: Malignant lesions of the nipple exclusive of Paget's disease. Surg Gynecol Obstet 103:185, 1956

451. Droulias CA, Sewell CW, McSweeney MB, et al: Inflammatory carcinoma of the breast: a correlation of clinical, radiologic and pathologic findings. Ann Surg 184:217–222, 1976

452. Ellis DL, Teitelbaum SL: Inflammatory carcinoma of the breast: A pathologic definition. Cancer 33:1045, 1974

453. Lucas FV, Perez-Mesa C: Inflammatory carcinoma of the breast. Cancer 41:1595, 1978

454. Stocks LH, Patterson FMS: Inflammatory carcinoma of the breast. Surg Gynecol Obstet 143:885, 1976

455. Mourali N, Muenz LR, Tabbane F, et al: Epidemiologic features of rapidly progressing breast cancer in Tunisia. Cancer 46:2741, 1980

456. Levine PH, Steinhorn SC, Ries LGV, et al: Inflammatory breast cancer. The experience of the Surveillance, Epidemiology and End Results (SEER) Program. J Natl Cancer Inst 74:291, 1985

457. Saltzstein SL: Clinically occult inflammatory carcinoma of the breast. Cancer 34:382, 1974

458. Harvey HA, Lipton A, Lawrence BV, et al: Estrogen receptor status in inflammatory breast carcinoma. J Surg Oncol 21:42, 1982

459. Schaake-Koning C, van der Linden EH, Hart G, et al: Adjuvant chemo- and hormonal therapy in locally advanced breast cancer: A randomized clinical study. Int J Radiat Oncol Biol Phys 11:1759, 1985

460. Robbins GF, Shah J, Rosen P, et al: Inflammatory carcinoma of the breast. Surg Clin North Am 54:801, 1974

461. Ramos CV, Taylor HB: Lipid-rich carcinoma of the breast. A clinicopathologic analysis of 13 examples. Cancer 33:812, 1974

462. Lim-Co RY, Gisser SD: Unusual variant of lipid-rich mammary carcinoma. Arch Pathol Lab Med 102:193, 1978

463. Barwick KW, Kashgarian M, Rosen PP: Clear-cell change within duct and lobular epithelium of the human breast. Pathol Annu 17:319, 1982

464. Harris M, Wells S, Vasudev KS: Primary signet ring cell carcinoma of the breast. Histopathology 2:171, 1978

465. Steinbrecher JS, Silverberg SG: Signet-ring cell carcinoma of the breast. The mucinous variant of infiltrating lobular carcinoma? Cancer 37:828, 1976

466. Merino MJ, LiVolsi VA: Signet ring carcinoma of the female breast: A clinicopathologic analysis of 24 cases. Cancer 48:1830, 1981

467. Oberman HJ: Secretory carcinoma of the breast in adults. Am J Surg Pathol 4:465, 1980

468. Tavassoli FA, Norris HJ: Secretory carcinoma of the breast. Cancer 45:2404, 1980

469. Akhtar M, Robinson C, Ali MA, et al: Secretory carcinoma of the breast in adults. Light and electron microscopic study of three cases with review of the literature. Cancer 51:2245, 1983

470. McCutcheon J, Walker RA: The significance of argyrophilia in human breast carcinomas. Virchows Arch [A] 410:369, 1987

471. Bussolati G, Papotti M, Sapino A, et al: Endocrine markers in argyrophilic carcinomas of the breast. Am J Surg Pathol 11:248, 1987

472. Nesland JM, Menoli VA, Holm R, et al: Breast carcinomas with neuroendocrine differentiation. Ultrastruct Pathol 8:225, 1985

473. Oberman HA: Sarcomas of the breast. Cancer 18:1233, 1965

474. Norris HJ, Taylor HB: Sarcomas and related mesenchymal tumors of the breast. Cancer 22:22, 1968

475. Callery CD, Rosen PP, Kinne DW: Sarcoma of the breast—A study of 32 patients with reappraisal of classification and therapy. Ann Surg 201:527, 1985

476. Lerner HJ: Fibrosarcoma of the breast. Case report and literature review. Am Surg 31:196, 1965

477. Wargotz ES, Norris HJ, Austin RM, Enzinger FM: Fibromatosis of the breast. A clinical and pathological study of 28 cases. Am J Surg Pathol 11:38, 1987

478. Iwasaki K, Nagamitsu S, Tsuneyoshi M: Postirradiation fibrosarcoma following radical mastectomy. Jpn J Surg 8:73, 1978

479. Barnes L, Pietruszka M: Rhabdomyosarcoma arising within a cystosarcoma phyllodes. Case report and review of the literature. Am J Surg Pathol 2:423, 1978

480. Chen KTK, Kuo T, Hoffman KD: Leiomyosarcoma of the breast. Cancer 47:1883, 1981

481. Beltaos E, Banerjee TK: Chondrosarcoma of the breast. Report of two cases. Am J Clin Pathol 71:345, 1979

482. Going JJ, Lumsden AB, Anderson TJ: A classical osteogenic sarcoma of the breast: Histology, immunohistochemistry and ultrastructure. Histopathology 10:631, 1986

483. Luzzatto R, Grossmann S, Scholl JG, Recktenvald M: Postradiation pleomorphic malignant fibrous histiocytoma of the breast. Acta Cytol 30:48, 1986

484. Menon M, van Velthoven PLM: Liposarcoma of the breast. A case report. Arch Pathol 98:370, 1974

485. Kristensen PB, Kryger H: Liposarcoma of the breast. A case report. Acta Chir Scand 144:193, 1978

486. Arbari L, Warhol MJ: Pleomorphic liposarcoma following radiotherapy for breast carcinoma. Cancer 49:878, 1982

487. Donnell RM, Rosen PP, Lieberman PH, et al: Angiosarcoma and other vascular tumours of the breast. Pathologic analysis as a guide to prognosis. Am J Surg Pathol 5:629, 1981

488. Merino MJ, Carter D, Berman M: Angiosarcoma of the breast. Am J Surg Pathol 7:53, 1983

489. Rainwater LM, Martin JK, Gaffey TA, van Heerden JA: Angiosarcoma of the breast. Arch Surg 121:669, 1986

490. Arias-Stella J Jr, Rosen PP: Hemangiopericytoma of the breast. Mod Pathol 1:98, 1988

491. Stewart FW, Treves N: Lymphangiosarcoma in postmastectomy lymphedema. Cancer 1:64, 1948

492. Schafler K, McKenzie CG, Salm R: Postmastectomy lymphangiosarcoma: A reappraisal of the concept. A critical review and report of an illustrative case. Histopathology 3:131, 1979

493. Silverberg SG, Kay S, Koss LG: Postmastectomy lymphangiosarcoma: Ultrastructural observations. Cancer 27:100, 1971

494. Miettinen M, Lehto VP, Virtanen I: Postmastectomy angiosarcoma (Stewart-Treves syndrome): Light-microscopic, immunohistological and ultrastructural characteristics of two cases. Am J Surg Pathol 7:329, 1983

495. Capo V, Ozzello L, Fenoglio CM, et al: Angiosarcoma arising in edematous extremities: Immunostaining for Factor VIII-related antigen and ultrastructural features. Hum Pathol 16:144, 1985

496. Hashimoto K, Matsumoto M, Eto H, et al: Differentiation of metastatic breast carcinoma from Stewart-Treves angiosarcoma. Arch Dermatol 121:742, 1985

497. Huvos AG, Woodard HQ, Cahan WG, et al: Postradiation

osteogenic sarcoma of bone and soft tissues: A clinico-pathologic study of 66 patients. Cancer 55:1244, 1985

498. Kuten A, Sapir D, Cohen Y, et al: Postirradiation soft tissue sarcoma occuring in breast cancer patients: Report of seven cases and results of combination chemotherapy. J Surg Oncol 26:168, 1985

499. Tulesinghe PU, Anthony PP: Primary lymphoma of the breast. Histopathology 9:297, 1985

500. Mambo NC, Burke JS, Butler JJ: Primary malignant lymphomas of the breast. Cancer 39:2033, 1977

501. Proctor NSF, Rippey JJ, Schulman G, et al: Extramedullary plasmacytoma of the breast. J Pathol 116:97, 1975

502. Smith MR, Brustein S, Straus DJ: Localized non-Hodgkin's lymphoma of the breast. Cancer 59:351, 1987

503. Navas JJ, Battifora H: Primary lymphoma of the breast: Ultrastructural study of two cases. Cancer 39:2025, 1977

504. Sears HF, Reid J: Granulocytic sarcoma. Cancer 37:1808, 1976

505. Lin JJ, Farha GJ, Taylor RJ: Pseudolymphoma of the breast. I. In a study of 8654 consecutive tylectomies and mastectomies. Cancer 45:973, 1980

506. Rosner F, Carey RW, Zarrabim H: Breast cancer and acute leukemia. Report of 24 cases and review of the literature. Am J Hematol 4:151, 1978

507. Hajdu S, Urban JA: Cancers metastatic to the breast. Cancer 29:1691, 1972

508. Silverman EM, Oberman HA: Metastatic neoplasms in the breast. Surg Gynecol Obstet 138:26, 1974

509. Pressman PI: Malignant melanoma and the breast. Cancer 31:784, 1973

510. Nielsen M, Andersen JA, Henriksen FW, et al: Metastases to the breast from extramammary carcinomas. Acta Pathol Microbiol Scand [A] 89;251, 1981

511. McCrea ES, Johnston C, Haney DJ: Metastases to the breast. AJR 141:685, 1983

512. Dodge OG, Jackson AW, Muldal S: Breast cancer and interstitial cell tumor in a patient with Klinefelter's syndrome. Cancer 24:1027, 1969

513. Becker KL, Matthews MJ, Higgins GA Jr, et al: Histologic evidence of gynecomastia in hyperthyroidism. Arch Pathol 98:257, 1974

514. Gilbert JB: Studies in malignant testis tumors. Syndrome of choriogenic gynecomastia; report of 6 cases and review of 129. J Urol 44:345, 1940

515. Le Winn EB: Gynecomastia during digitalis therapy; report of 8 additional cases with liver function studies. N Engl J Med 248:316, 1953

516. Bannayan GA, Hajdu SI: Gynecomastia: Clinicopathologic study of 351 cases. Am J Clin Pathol 57:431, 1972

517. Carlson HE: Gynecomastia. N Engl J Med 303:795, 1980

518. Lee PA: The relationship of concentrations of serum hormones to pubertal gynecomastia. J Pediatr 86:212, 1975

519. Fagan TC, Johnson DG, Grosso DS: Metronidazole-induced gynecomastia. JAMA 254:3217, 1985

520. Harmon J, Aliapoulios MA: Gynecomastia in marijuana users. N Engl J Med 287:936, 1972

521. Pantoja EL, Lobert RE, Lopez E: Gigantic cystosarcoma phyllodes in a man with gynecomastia. Arch Surg 111:611, 1976

522. Bigotti G, Kasznica J: Sclerosing adenosis in the breast of a man with pulmonary oat cell carcinoma. Hum Pathol 17:861, 1986

523. Sobin LH, Sherif M: Relation between male breast cancer and prostate cancer. Br J Cancer 42:787, 1980

524. Benson WR: Carcinoma of the prostate with metastases to breasts and testis: Critical review of the literature and report of a case. Cancer 10:1235, 1957

525. Jackson AW, Muldal S, Ockey C, et al: Carcinoma of the breast associated with the Klinefelter syndrome. Br Med J 1:223, 1965

526. Heller KS, Rosen PP, Schottenfeld D, et al: Male breast cancer: A clinicopathologic study of 97 cases. Ann Surg 118:60, 1978

527. Liechty R, Davis J, Gleysteen J: Cancer of the male breast. Forty cases. Cancer 20:1617, 1967

528. Norris HJ, Taylor HB: Carcinoma of the male breast. Cancer 23:1428, 1969

529. Wolff MA, Rienis MS: Breast cancer in the male: clinicopathologic study of 40 patients and review of the literature. Progr Surg Pathol 3:77, 1981

530. Kozak FK, Hall JG, Baird PA: Familial breast cancer in males: A case report and review of the literature. Cancer 58:2736, 1986

531. Satiani B, Powell RW, Mathews WH: Paget disease of the male breast. Arch Surg 112:587, 1977

532. Pegoraro RJ, Nirmul D, Joubert SM: Cytoplasmic and nuclear estrogen and progesterone receptors in male breast cancer. Cancer Res 42:4812, 1982

533. Greene MH, Goedert JJ, Bech Hansen NT, et al: Radiogenic male breast cancer with in vitro sensitivity to ionizing radiation and bleomycin. Cancer Invest 1:379, 1983

534. Lagios MD: Pathologic examination and tissue processing for the mammographically directed biopsy. California Society of Pathologists, San Francisco December 3, 1987

535. World Health Organization: Histological Typing of Breast Tumours. 2nd Ed. International Histological Classification of Tumours. No. 2. WHO, Geneva, 1981

12

Lymph Nodes and Spleen

Ian Carr
Pamela J. Murari
Norman M. Pettigrew

The major problems encountered in lymph node examination are (1) diagnosis of a systemic disease from the examination of an enlarged lymph node, and (2) identification of the extent of disease, usually neoplastic, from the examination of an organ and its draining lymph nodes. In the former case, the question is usually: Is it reactive or neoplastic? and in the latter case: Is it primary or secondary? If a tumor and its draining sites are being examined, the problem is usually whether and to what extent metastasis has occurred. When dealing with a spleen, the most common diagnostic problem is whether lymphomatous infiltration is present in a patient with known lymphoma. Needle biopsy of lymphoreticular tissue is of limited value, except at a few centers. Lymphomas should not be classified on the basis of a frozen section. Fuller treatments of the subject are available elsewhere.[1-3]

The surgical pathologist dealing with the common problem of diagnosis of an enlarged lymph node or the less common problem of an excised spleen should interpret histologic appearances only in the light of full clinical information. A purely technical interpretation of a histologic section is fraught with danger. This clinical information must specifically include hematologic and immunologic data. The surgical pathology report should not be signed unless this information is available.

Greater care than usual is necessary in the preparation of these tissues.[4] If the lymph nodes or spleen can reliably reach the laboratory within 5 minutes of removal from the patient, it is best that they be sent dry (without

fixative). If not, they should be transported in fresh 10 percent buffered formalin.

On receipt, the specimen should be examined personally by a pathologist. A lymph node should be cut across, with a fresh scalpel or razor blade, in one stroke while it is held lightly with the gloved hand. At this stage a thin (1 mm) slice should be removed and immersed in 3 percent buffered glutaraldehyde for 30 minutes in case electron microscopy is needed. This is then chopped into small (less than 1 mm) blocks and postfixed for 3 hours. A thin slice should be placed in B5 fixative, and the remainder should be placed in 10 percent neutral formalin for 1 hour to harden a little, and definitive blocks then taken. The new cut face will show mechanical deformation. The definitive block should include all or a large part of a node. This will be fixed overnight in a tissue processor, in a cassette with the new face uppermost to ensure optimum flow of fixative over the side to be cut. These precautions should minimize crush artifact and increase the chance that the sections finally examined will be well fixed and devoid of zonal poor fixation. The paraffin wax should have a melting point below 58°C to avoid drying artifacts; the cut sections should be stood vertically to drain off excess and then dried horizontally at 30°C. If necessary, the sections can be dried for 2 to 3 hours at 50°C.

The initial sections should be stained with hematoxylin and eosin (H&E), reticulin-Van Gieson, and periodic acid-Schiff (PAS) stains by standard techniques. Methyl green-pyronin may be useful; acid phosphatase, esterase, and lipid stains on frozen sections are occasionally use-

375

ful. Immunoperoxidase staining for a wide variety of antigens is of use in the diagnosis of secondary carcinoma and to a lesser degree in the classification of lymphomas. An incomplete list of antisera in common use includes those against IgG, IgA, IgM, κ- and λ-light chains, lysozyme, prostate-specific antigen, factor VIII, epithelial membrane antigen, carcinoembryonic antigen (CEA), keratin, actin, α_1-antitrypsin, α-fetoprotein (AFP), serotonin, nonspecific esterase, S-100 protein, desmin, vimentin, leukocyte common antigen, and human chorionic gonadotrophin.

Many pathologists use touch preparations made by touching a fresh cut surface on a glass slide, with subsequent fixation and Giemsa or H&E staining. The examination of plastic-embedded sections may be valuable, whether small blocks processed for electron microscopy, or larger plastic blocks. Where appropriate, material should be taken for bacteriologic examination before tissue is immersed in fixative. The cornerstone of diagnosis remains the good H&E section.

The spleen should be weighed, measured, and cut in its long axis; in the absence of a gross lesion, it should be cut into slices 1 cm thick. After appropriate prefixation, 6 to 12 blocks should be taken, preferably from regions where the white pulp is prominent. A gross excess of fixative should be used. A lymph node is usually present in the hilum; this should be examined histologically. The weight of the spleen varies with body weight and the degree of venous congestion. A spleen weighing more than 250 g is probably abnormal, and one more than 300 g is almost certainly abnormal.

CELLS OF LYMPHORETICULAR TISSUES

Like other lymphoreticular organs, lymph nodes and spleen consist of a connective tissue framework in which some cells reside and through which others migrate, some in an ordered pattern of actual circulation. Running through these organs are a blood vascular system and a lymph vascular system, through which these fluids circulate. It is not always possible to be certain whether individual cells or cell groups are moving or static. The following cells are found in lymphoreticular organs: lymphocytes, immunoblasts, plasma cells, macrophages, endothelial cells, fibroblasts, other vascular cells and nerves, and a group of cells variously described as dendritic or reticular cells.

Lymphocyte

Lymphocytes (Figs. 12-1 and 12-2) range in size from 6 to 12 μm; the term *lymphoblast* refers to an immature

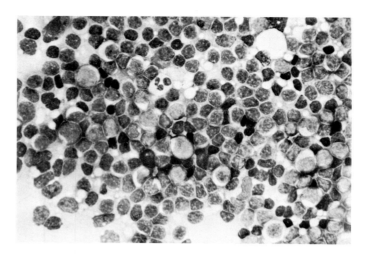

Fig. 12-1. Touch imprint of a normal lymph node. Note the polymorphic cell population of small and large lymphocytes, macrophages, and occasional neutrophils.

proliferating large lymphocyte. The small lymphocyte has a densely staining nucleus and scanty cytoplasm with a few small mitochondria, a centriole, and some ribosomes; there are few cytomembranes. There are relatively few small cytoplasmic processes. Lymphocytes

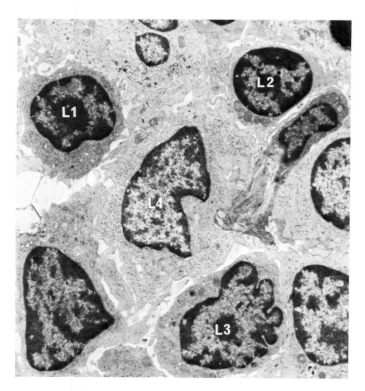

Fig. 12-2. Lymphocytes in a lymph node. Three small lymphocytes contain nuclei with condensed chromatin and relatively scanty cytoplasm (L1, L2, L3). The large lymphocyte in the center of the field (L4) has less condensation of nuclear chromatin. The cytoplasm contains numerous polyribosomes. ($\times$10,500)

are freely mobile and trail a projecting handlelike process behind them.

The large lymphocyte or lymphoblast has a nucleus with less dense chromatin in an open meshwork, and bulky cytoplasm with a basophilic staining reaction on light microscopy, due to the presence of numerous polyribosomes. Large lymphocytes take up tritiated thymidine and show mitosis; the immunocyte or *immunoblast* is often described as a separate cell type; it is in fact merely an immunologically reacting large lymphocyte, usually with amphophilic and pyroninophilic cytoplasm, but not fitting the classical description of a plasma cell.

Thymic (T)-lymphocytes derive originally from the bone marrow but immediately from the thymus. Their life span may be fairly long (months or years). Many lymphocytes recirculate round the body, leaving the bloodstream through the postcapillary venules to enter peripheral lymphoid organs and draining with the lymph back into the venous circulation. The major part of the recirculating pool is composed of T-lymphocytes. T-lymphocytes are found in the deep cortical and interfollicular areas in lymph nodes, in the periarteriolar regions of the spleen, and in the perifollicular areas in Peyer's patches. T-lymphocytes enlarge and divide in vitro when treated with phytohemagglutinin (PHA). T-lymphocytes are responsible for cell-mediated immunity and cooperate with B-lymphocytes in the humoral immune response to some antigens, although they are not responsible for the actual synthesis of antibody. T-lymphocytes produce a wide range of biologically active soluble factors (lymphokines) that mediate delayed hypersensitivity, amplifying the effects of the reaction of antigen with a very few sensitized lymphocytes into a well marked mononuclear cell response. Such effects include activation, chemotaxis, and immobilization of macrophages; resorption of bone; destruction of cells; inhibition of viral growth; sensitization of nonsensitized lymphocytes; and transfer of cellular immunity. *Bursa-dependent* (or *B*)-*lymphocytes* derive ultimately from the marrow, and have a shorter life span—days or weeks rather than months—and are a less important component of the recirculating pool. B-lym-

phocytes are found in the subcapsular and medullary areas of lymph nodes and in the germinal centers. The small round B-lymphocyte is thought to move into the follicle from the periphery. As it does so, the round nucleus becomes irregular in shape with an indentation or cleavage (the small cleaved cell). The cell enlarges (the large cleaved cell), the nucleus loses its cleavage, and nucleoli appear and enlarge (the large noncleaved cell). The latter cell is the main dividing form (Fig. 12-3). B-cells are also found in the peripheral white pulp and red pulp of the spleen and in the central follicles of Peyer's patches. B-lymphocytes interact with T-lymphocytes in the induction of many humoral immune responses, although other responses are T-cell independent. B-lymphocytes carry a prominent and easily recognizable surface immunoglobulin component (of the order of 100,000 molecules per cell) and mature into plasma cells, producing immunoglobulin at various stages during maturation. B-lymphocytes also carry surface receptors for complement, enabling them to bind antigen-antibody complexes.

Some lymphocytes have pronounced cytotoxic properties for other cells (killer or K-cells); some bear no evidence of T- or B-cell markers: so-called N- or U-cells. Some of the properties of T- and B-lymphocytes are summarized in Table 12-1.

T- and B-cells cannot be clearly distinguished from each other by morphologic features or physical properties. This may be achieved by surface-marker studies performed on viable cell suspensions and on frozen tissue specimens.

B-cells have plentiful surface Ig markers and C' receptors, which are scarce on T-cells. An EAC rosette assay is used for detecting C' receptors on B cells. Rosettes form with sheep red blood cells (SRBC) pretreated with antibody and complement. Eighty to 100 percent of human T-lymphocytes, when treated with normal (nonimmunized) SRBC, will form E rosettes (Fig. 12-4).

B-cell surface immunoglobin G (IgG) and Fc receptors are determined by immunofluorescence using fluorescein-conjugated antisera specific for the heavy chains of IgG, IgA, IgM, IgD, and IgE and for κ- and λ-light chains.

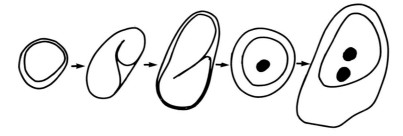

Fig. 12-3. Schema of transformation of follicular center cells. (Modified from Lukes RJ, Collins RD: A functional classification of malignant lymphomas. p. 213. In Rebuck JW, Berard CW, Abell MR (eds): The Reticuloendothelial System. Williams & Wilkins, Baltimore, 1975)

TABLE 12-1. Characteristics of B- and T-Lymphocytes

	B	T
Origin		
Ultimate	Marrow	Marrow
Proximate	? Gut-associated lymphoid tissue	Thymus
Recirculation	Less important	Important
Longevity	Fewer long-lived	More long-lived
Site		
Lymph node	Subcapsular Medullary Germinal centers	Interfollicular
Spleen	Peripheral white pulp Red pulp	Periarteriolar
Peyer's patch	Follicular	Perifollicular
Response to mitogens		
Phytohemagglutinin	Less marked	Marked
Pokeweed	Marked	Less marked
Function		
Cell-mediated immunity	Trivial	Important
Humoral immunity		
Induction	Important	Important
Antibody synthesis	Important	Uninvolved
Memory	Important	Important
Production of lymphokines	Unimportant	Important
Surface characteristics	Prominent surface Ig	Less prominent surface Ig

B-cells have intracellular IgG, which may be detected in thin formalin-fixed, paraffin-embedded tissue by an immunoperoxidase technique.

Another marker for T-cells is the detection of the nuclear enzyme, terminal deoxynucleotidyltransferase (TdT), a distinct DNA polymerase of immature thymic-related lymphocytes. TdT may be detected by an indirect immunofluorescence assay or by biochemical assay. There is a dual assay for E-rosette formation and TdT. An antiserum against T-cell determinants is now available.

Plasma Cell

The mature plasma cell (Fig. 12-5) is characterized by a nucleus with prominent peripheral speckles of chromatin and cytoplasm with a marked affinity for basic dyes due to the presence of very well developed granular endoplasmic reticulum. Ig is demonstrable within the cisterns of the endoplasmic reticulum. Antibody production is most active in young plasma cells (plasmablasts). The older plasma cells often contain crystalline aggregates of Ig within the endoplasmic reticulum. These may be stainable and visible with light microscopy as eosinophilic masses (Russell bodies).

Macrophage

Macrophages are avidly phagocytic medium to large cells (12 to 30 μm in diameter). They have irregular surfaces because of the presence of cytoplasmic processes; mature cells show a moderate content of mitochondria, and often well developed prominent granular endoplasmic reticulum (Fig. 12-6). Mature macrophages carry on their surfaces a receptor that specifically recognizes certain classes of Ig, the Fc receptor. They contain numerous lysosomal dense bodies, some small and homogeneous in structure (probably primary lysosomes composed of newly formed lysosomal enzymes), and others larger and more heterogeneous, containing ingested foreign material, RBC debris, lipid, and so forth. The lysosomes contain a wide variety of hydrolytic enzymes capable of breaking down proteins to the level of small peptides or amino acids. Characteristically, the cytoplasm contains numerous 6 nm microfibrils, probably actin.

Macrophages are responsible for the phagocytosis of bacteria and viruses and are the histologic hallmark of granulomata. They take up antigen, but their precise role in the immune response is not clear. They may break up large particulate antigens into a form that can be dealt with by the lymphocyte. Alternatively, antigen may be retained on the surface of the macrophage to interact there with the lymphocyte. They may mop up excess antigen, inhibiting immunologic tolerance. Macrophages have a role in lipid metabolism, phagocytosing particulate lipid and being able to esterify and to solubilize lip-

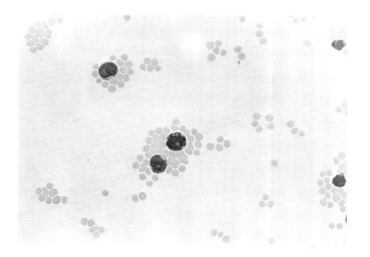

Fig. 12-4. T-lymphocytes exhibiting E rosettes with sheep red blood cells.

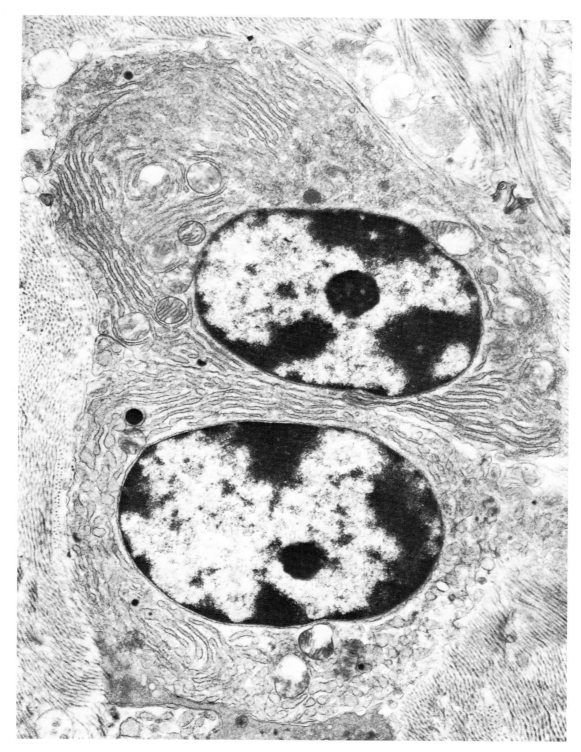

Fig. 12-5. Normal plasma cells showing massively developed granular endoplasmic reticulum. (×5,900)

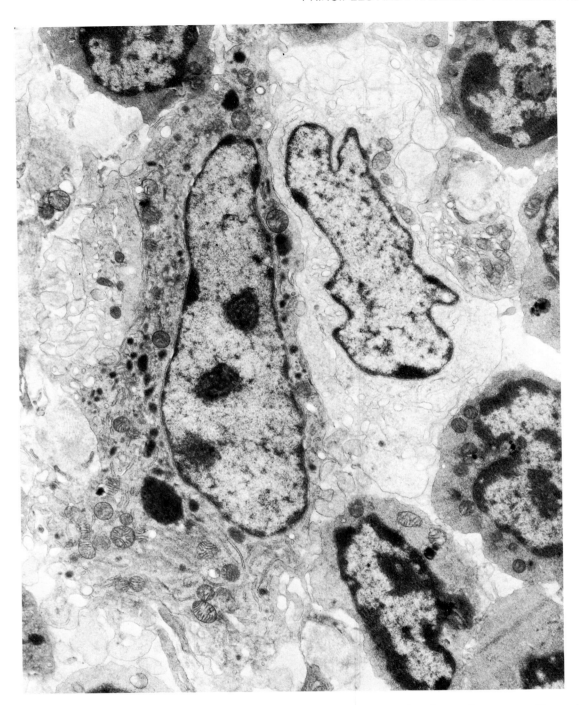

Fig. 12-6. Elongated macrophage in lymph node showing numerous cytoplasmic membranous profiles and many lysosomes, primary and secondary. The elongated pale cell adjacent with voluminous cytoplasm and few lysosomes is of the type sometimes described as a dendritic cell. (×12,650)

ids. They phagocytose effete erythrocytes and store the iron derived therefrom. Many have secretory properties, being able to produce notably pyrogen, interferon (IFN), lysozyme, and the third component of complement. Macrophages in inflammatory lesions and in many other sites derive from blood monocytes and ultimately from a rapidly dividing marrow precursor, justifying the use of the term *mononuclear phagocyte system*. Local division in many sites takes place, and macrophages long resident in peripheral sites become cytochemically distinct.

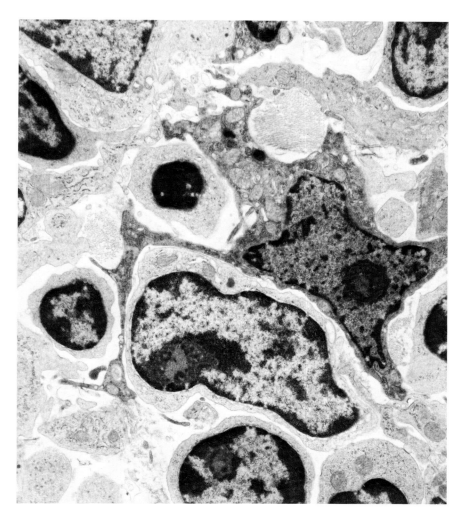

Fig. 12-7. Dendritic reticular cell from germinal center of lymph node. Elongated cytoplasmic processes project out between the surrounding lymphocytes. (×13,000)

The macrophages in a granuloma are large and mature, derived in the main from circulating monocytes that are immobilized in the site by factors produced by the interaction of sensitized lymphocytes with antigen. The mature macrophages divide and also coalesce with recently emigrated monocytes to form *giant cells* or macrophage polykaryons of variable, usually low, phagocytic activity. Some macrophages enlarge, come to contain numerous large, moderately electron-lucent vacuoles, and are known as *epithelioid cells*. These cells are poorly phagocytic and are probably secretory.

Dendritic Cells

Other cells in lymphoreticular tissues do not fit the above categories. These were called reticular or reticulum cells, terms now less used. Many of these cells are poorly phagocytic, and have long processes extending in several directions (Fig. 12-7). They fall into several poorly defined subclasses. Follicular dendritic cells are identified by electron microscopy in sections of lymphoid follicles and are able to trap and retain antigen-antibody complexes on their surfaces. Lymphoid dendritic cells were identified in cell suspensions of lymphoid tissues, are rich in Ia antigen but lack Fc and C3 receptors and are potent stimulators of certain immunologically related cellular reactions, such as the mixed leucocyte reaction. Interdigitating dendritic cells are found by electron microscopy in T-dependent areas of lymphoid tissues, interlock with adjacent lymphocytes, and may be important in their maturation. Langerhans cells may be very similar to interdigitating dendritic cells; they are identified in skin by general morphology rather similar to that of a macrophage. Their characteristic feature is the presence of a granule, the Birbeck granule, about 42 nm in external diameter, with a core 11 nm in diameter and a repeating density.

Identification of Lymphoreticular Cells

Attempts are being made to identify the sub-types of lymphoreticular cells in great detail, using monoclonal antibodies, which are becoming increasingly commercially available. The aim is to be able to compare the clinical course of a lymphoma with its histology and immunophenotype. This may lead to improved prediction of prognosis, but there is not yet a consensus on what is useful in practice. Such attempts depend on the hypothesis that each type of neoplasm derives from a distinct normal cell precursor, whose characteristics are not lost in neoplasia. This may not be so, but it may yet be possible to define immunophenotypes which on an empirical basis correlate with malignancy.[5]

Role of Flow Cytometry in Lymphoma Diagnosis

The development of monoclonal antibodies to detect cell surface markers has provided new parameters in the diagnosis and classification of lymphoma. The use of these reagents in conjunction with flow cytometry has provided a powerful technique that is now being applied in diagnosis.[6,7]

The principle of flow cytometry was first applied to hematology as the Coulter technique for counting and sizing blood cells. Using this technique, a flow of particles is created by passing cells in suspension through a small orifice and past an electronic measuring device. The limited parameters of number and size have been expanded in the laser-powered flow cytometer to include the texture of cells and also the detection of any fluorescent substance within the cell or nucleus or attached to the cell surface. In addition, by using a differential electric charge, cells can be sorted according to chosen parameters, enabling an individual population of cells to be both isolated and concentrated. This latter technique, however, has more applications in the research environment, and straightforward flow cytometry of labeled cells has remained the most immediately useful. Flow cytometry is relatively rapid and simple, and can be done on small samples of cells (one million or less). It can detect small numbers of cells, obviating complex purification procedures.

Flow cytometry can be applied to the diagnosis of solid tumors, including lymphomas. It can be used in the differential diagnosis between lymphomas and benign or pseudolymphomatous lymphoproliferative lesions,[8] but

the problem is that normal lymphocytes are usually found in lymph nodes despite the presence of a lymphomatous infiltrate. For this reason, in B-cell lymphomas a true monoclonal population may not be recognized, while in T-cell lymphomas there is still no true marker for a neoplastic proliferation. It is therefore important to use flow cytometry in conjunction with routine morphology and in situ cell marker studies. Most of the monoclonal antibodies used in flow cytometry can also be applied by the immunoperoxidase technique to stain frozen sections.[9]

It is usually possible, using a panel of monoclonal antibodies, to separate B-cell from T-cell proliferations, but the absence of monoclonal proliferation does not exclude lymphoma. This failure may be due to sampling error or to a high proportion of reactive cells infiltrating the neoplasm. The expression of Calla (J5) antigen may raise the suspicion of a neoplastic proliferation when no true monoclonal pattern is obtained.

An adjunct to cell marker analysis is the measurement of DNA ploidy by flow cytometry. If the instrument is properly standardized, this may be performed by staining of DNA by ethidium bromide on fresh cells. This method is both reliable and reproducible.[10] The ploidy measurement may also be applied to paraffin-embedded tissue; this is, however, less sensitive and more difficult to standardize. While many lymphomas are diploid, the presence of aneuploidy correlates with the grade of the lymphoma.[11,12] Studies of normal and reactive lymphoid tissues have shown a normal diploid DNA content.[13]

Thus, a combination of cell marker and DNA ploidy studies may help delineate neoplastic proliferation. The stage of differentiation of the neoplastic cell population is also demonstrated; this is useful in classifying the tumor and in monitoring any dedifferentiation of the tumor cells in response to treatment. The appearance of an aneuploid population in a previously diploid tumor may be an important prognostic sign. Since flow cytometry is applicable to aspiration biopsies of lymph nodes as well as examination of cellular effusions and the detection of small populations within the peripheral blood, it is useful in follow-up as well as in the initial diagnosis.

In Situ Labeling

Flow cytometry should be performed in conjunction with in situ labeling. Until recently this was limited to frozen section and cytospin preparations. However, the recent availability of monoclonal antibodies reactive with leukocyte subsets in paraffin-embedded tissue greatly increases the scope of this diagnostic procedure[14]; with five new monoclonal antibodies, optimal results were obtained by Poppema et al.[14] on B5-fixed tissues, although good staining was also found with other fixatives. The staining results on reactive lymphoid tissues demonstrated that these reagents could distinguish between T-cells, B-cells and macrophages and also between maturation stages of B-cells and T-cells. Poppema et al.[14] also state that a study of a series of well defined lymphomas shows that a combination of two of the antisera can identify all hematopoietic neoplasms except plasmacytomas. It is probable that the reagents react with members of the so-called leukocyte common antigen (LCA) family. The further application of these reagents and the development of future antisera should permit better correlation of cell markers with morphology than has been possible with frozen section techniques. It will also permit retrospective analysis of lymph nodes from archival material. If these antibodies are used as a panel, they may permit the separation of B-cells and T-cells in paraffin sections.[15]

Genotypic Analysis

Genotypic analysis of DNA extracted from frozen tissue biopsy specimens or peripheral blood leukocytes can be used to look for the genes that control Ig synthesis. The presence of consistent rearrangements of genes in a manner deviating from the normal is evidence for the presence of neoplastic clones. This technique may have important applications not only in the delineation of T-cell, B-cell, and true histiocytic lesions, but also in the separation of florid hyperplasias from neoplasias.[16,17]

NORMAL LYMPH NODE AND ITS TISSUE RESPONSES

The structure of normal lymph nodes (Figs. 12-8 and 12-9) varies with site and age. A normal cervical lymph node from a young adult is bean shaped and measures 1 to 2 cm in maximum diameter. The capsule is composed of two or three layers of fibroblasts and the collagen that they lay down. Below the capsule lies a subcapsular sinus lined peripherally by endothelial cells and elsewhere by macrophages with gaps between them. Across the sinus run strands of collagen, covered by the cytoplasm of endothelial cells. Macrophages lining the inner layer of the sinusoid lie on a layer of collagen in which are a few fibroblasts. The subcapsular sinus is continuous with radial sinuses, and these with anastomosing medullary sinuses, which in turn join to form the efferent ducts of the node. The structure of the wall of all the sinuses is similar. Macrophages form a particularly prominent part of the wall of the medullary sinus.

The parenchyma of the lymph node outside the sinuses is built on a framework of elongated fibroblasts with nu-

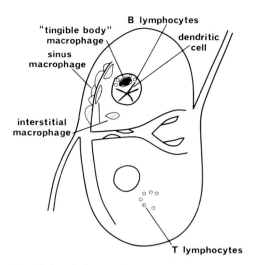

Fig. 12-8. Schema of a normal lymph node.

merous long spidery processes, each lying on and surrounding a trabeculum of collagen. This is often described as the reticulin framework of the node. In between, there are packed lymphocytes and other lymphoreticular cells in varying proportions; the areas of the

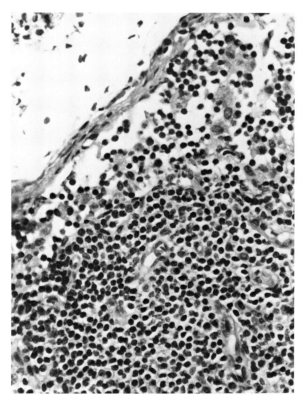

Fig. 12-9. Normal lymph node showing subcapsular sinus and underlying lymphoid tissue.

parenchyma are conveniently divided into the outer cortex; germinal centers and lymphocytic follicles; inner cortex or paracortex; and medullary cords.[18]

The *outer cortex* is composed of undifferentiated areas that contain predominantly small lymphocytes with a few plasma cells.

The *germinal center* is spherical and surrounded by small lymphocytes. It is composed of large lymphocytes and blast cells. Sometimes a lighter-staining superficial zone is less densely packed and may show a few plasma cells, while in a darker-staining deep zone mitosis is very evident. The background framework contains dendritic reticular cells and conventional macrophages, often with prominent ingested dead cells (the tingible body macrophages of Flemming). Germinal centers vary in structure, showing cyclical activity. After stimulation of the node, mitosis may be very prominent. Later, mitosis is less prominent, but there may be numerous macrophages containing cell debris. Sometimes, the center may be largely replaced by epithelioid macrophages. Lastly, a center may have a very dense thick peripheral cuff of lymphocytes but show little central activity. Dense aggregates of small lymphocytes, so-called primary lymphoid follicles, may represent an extremely inactive form of germinal center. Germinal centers have a light and a dark zone classified on the staining qualities of the cells, and the light zone has a peripheral cap of dark-staining lymphocytes. This cap points to the direction from which the lymph flows, and thus by implication, that from which the antigenic stimulus is coming. It is thought, although by no means proved, that B-lymphocytes migrate into the follicle. At first, the nuclei are not indented (or cleaved). The nuclei then become cleaved and the cells enlarge. The nuclei then lose their cleaved appearance. The large noncleaved cell is the main dividing cell in the follicle. Lymphocytes may ultimately leave the follicle as immature plasma cells.

The deeper part of the cortex, called the *inner cortex* or *paracortex*, is composed of rather more loosely arranged lymphoid tissue; most of the lymphocytes in this area are thymus derived, at least in experimental animals, and there is a moderate number of macrophages. When scanty, these produce a starry sky effect and, when plentiful, nodular aggregates. These nodular aggregates do not contain plasma cells and are found in reactive lesions, notably in dermatopathic lymphadenitis. They are more common in superficial nodes. Postcapillary venules are found in this area; the thick walls usually show numerous emigrating T-lymphocytes. During a cell-mediated immune response, this area becomes edematous due to blockage of the sinusoids; numerous lymphocytes migrate through the walls of the postcapillary venules into the paracortex and there proliferate.

The *medullary cords* are the areas of lymphoid tissue that lie between the medullary sinusoids. They are packed with plasma cells during an immune response.

Several basic variations in structure may occur during lymph node reactions.

1. Stimulation of germinal center activity
2. Plasma cell proliferation and maturation
3. Maturation, enlargement, and division of sinus and interstitial macrophages
4. Increased cell traffic through the node seen as
   Increased passage of monocytes and lymphocytes in the afferent lymph
   Increased migration and maturation of T-lymphocytes
   Banal acute inflammatory reaction
   Increased monocyte immigration, macrophage maturation, and formation of granulomata, often with epithelioid cells

Variations in normal lymph node structure also occur under physiologic circumstances; nodes vary with site, age, and antigenic stimulation.

Substantial variations occur in lymph node structure between different sites in the body. As compared with cervical nodes, nodes derived from sites draining the alimentary tract tend to have prominent sinusoids and active germinal centers. Nodes from the groin may show a considerable amount of fibrous tissue, often arranged in trabeculae intersecting the node; germinal centers in this site may be few. DNA synthesis varies considerably with site. There is a considerable traffic of cells even through a normal node in resting conditions.

Substantial variations also occur with age. The lymph node of the child, like all juvenile tissues, contains little fibrous tissue. Immunologic reactions occurring in juvenile lymphoid tissue are particularly vigorous, and the degree of cellular pleomorphism may be marked. With age, there is generalized atrophy of lymphoid tissues; lymph nodes shrink in size, and few or no germinal centers may be present. Nodes become infiltrated with adipose tissue and a variable degree of fine fibrosis occurs. This atrophy occurs more markedly in the cervical, axillary, and inguinal nodes. In extreme old age, lymph nodes may be very hard to find.

The histologic differences between a lymph node undergoing a humoral immune reaction and a lymph node undergoing a cellular immune reaction may thus be summarized as follows. In the former, germinal centers are prominent and contain many dividing immunoblasts; the medullary cords contain many plasma cells. In the latter, the paracortical areas fill with newly arrived immunoblasts that proliferate and block the sinusoids but do not mature into plasma cells. Most natural immune responses contain both components, and in most cases most lymph nodes are engaged in responding to one or several antigens.

The degree of response varies from site to site; moreover, antigens encountered in the daily course of life are not purified, and their portals of entry may vary. Even the same antigen given under different conditions may produce humoral or cellular immunity; therefore, in the human a rather mixed histologic picture occurs. Many antigens affecting the human are bacterial or viral in origin, and these will be self-replicating in the body. Therefore, if they are not eliminated rapidly, the primary and secondary responses will merge as the organism continues to produce antigen over a period of time, with consequent blurring of the morphologic changes. If the antigen is organismal in nature, its presence in the node may elicit an inflammatory as well as an immunologic reaction, rendering the distinction between reactive hyperplasia and lymphadenitis less precise. It is worth noting that in practice a normal resting human lymph node is rarely encountered.

DIFFERENTIAL DIAGNOSIS OF THE DIFFICULT LYMPH NODE

The diagnosis of most lymph node sections is fairly easy; some are difficult, a few very difficult, and a very few quite impossible. The diagnostic process involves, as usual, several questions: Is this normal tissue? Is there a congenital abnormality? Is there inflammation? and what kind? And, as a related question, is there reactive hyperplasia, and what kind? Is there neoplasia? Is it secondary? and from where? Or primary? Is it lymphoma? Hodgkin's disease? or non-Hodgkin's lymphoma? Is it histiocytosis? Or leukemia?

The following steps may be useful in difficult cases:

1. Full clinical information, including hematologic and immunologic details, should always be obtained.
2. Step sections should be obtained at several levels of the available blocks, as well as single PAS- and Van Gieson-reticulin-stained sections.
3. The usual first question to be asked is: Hyperplasia or a neoplasm? The major features of hyperplasia are retention of tissue architecture and some banal evidence of inflammation such as the presence of a few neutrophils. Cellular pleomorphism, while of course characteristic of neoplasm, may be evident in reactive lesions. The same is true for a high mitotic rate. If the lesion is reactive or hyperplastic, then full bacteriologic and immunologic investigation of the patient is required. A search for organ-

isms (*e.g.,* acid-fast bacilli or fungi) should be conducted in the tissues submitted. The major difficulty here is distinguishing a follicular reaction from a nodular follicular lymphoma. A reactive nodule retains normal architecture and cell composition, notably tingible-body macrophages, and a normal peripheral rim of reticulin, and does not spill into the pericapsular surrounding tissue. Neoplastic follicles have abnormal cells, although mitosis may be paradoxically less evident than in the reactive follicle. The neoplastic follicles may spill into the surrounding tissue. A node may be partly involved by tumor and may contain both reactive and neoplastic follicles.
4. If the lesion is neoplastic, the next question is: Is it primary or secondary? A lesion is more likely to be secondary if there is demarcation between tumor cells and the normal structures of the node and if large numbers of tumor cells exist in the sinusoids. If the lesion is primary, the next question is: Is it Hodgkin's disease or non-Hodgkin's lymphoma? If the lesion looks like Hodgkin's disease, then two decisions must be made. Is this one of the lesions that closely mimics Hodgkin's disease, such as Dilantin adenopathy or angiofollicular hyperplasia? If it is not, then into which subtype of Hodgkin's disease does it fall? If it is a malignant lymphoproliferative disease but does not fit into the above categories, then in which group (e.g., malignant histiocytosis) does it fit?
5. Because of the major side effects of modern treatment of lymphoma, unless a lymphoma is an obvious classical lesion, sections should always be examined by two histopathologists, one of whom should preferably have a special interest in lymphoreticular disease. If there is serious suspicion of lymphoma, but the appearance in a node is not diagnostic, the pathologist should not hesitate to request a biopsy of another node, preferably of the largest available node.

HISTOPATHOLOGY OF LYMPH NODES
Congenital Abnormalities

Congenital abnormalities of lymph nodes are uncommon. In this category fall two major types of lesions: the congenital or acquired hypoplasias and the presence in lymph node tissue of abnormal or heterotopic epithelium.

Congenital Immunodeficiency Syndromes

The congenital immunodeficiency syndromes fall into three essential groups: deficiencies of B-cell maturation with defective antibody formation, deficiencies of T-cell maturation with defective cellular immunity, and combined immunodeficiency. The tissue pathologist is rarely called on to make a diagnosis from examination of nodes from such patients. The histologic appearances are pre-dictable.

In antibody deficiency syndromes, the lymph nodes show failure of cortical development with absence of follicles and germinal centers. Plasma cell maturation is deficient. In cellular deficiency syndromes, there is a failure of development of paracortical areas. Follicles and germinal centers are normal, as is plasma cell maturation. In combined immunodeficiency syndromes, the changes in lymph nodes vary with the severity of the syndrome. In severe combined immunodeficiency (Swiss-type agammaglobulinemia), the lymph nodes may be very hard to identify. The capsule is fibrotic; the subcapsular sinus is partly obliterated; and the fibrous stroma of the node is increased. Follicular development is absent and plasma cells are not evident. In immunodeficiency with ataxia-telangiectasia, the atrophy is similar but less well marked, while in immunodeficiency with eczema and thrombocytopenia (Wiskott-Aldrich syndrome), the lymph nodes in young children may be almost normal or show only slight lymphoid depletion of paracortical areas. In older patients, however, the depletion of cortical and paracortical areas may become more marked, and germinal centers may be absent.

Changes occur in lymph nodes in patients with dysphagocytosis syndromes such as chronic granulomatous disease of childhood. These consist largely of reactive hyperplasia with macrophage granulomata, juxtaposed to suppurative lesions. The macrophages contain prominent yellow pigment.[19]

The primary aplasias of the lymphoreticular system are less common than the secondary aplasias, which result from treatment with cytotoxic and immunosuppressive drugs. The lymphocytes and germinal centers of nodes may be entirely wiped out, leaving only the fibrous framework, with a varying edema and fibrosis.

Congenital Heterotopias

Congenital heterotopias[20–24] are rare rests of several types of tissue, notably squamous epithelium, columnar epithelium, glandular epithelium, melanocytes, and thyroid epithelium. Rests of nevus cells are perhaps the most common, usually occurring in the axilla and always in nodes associated with the skin; such rests are most common in the capsule but may be found elsewhere in the node. As a result of ultrastructural studies, it has been suggested that these are in fact glomus cells. Discrimination from secondary neoplasm rests chiefly on the differentiation of the cells and the absence of pleomorphism and mitoses. The problem may be particularly difficult in the case of rests of melanocytes in a node draining a

malignant melanoma and in rests of aberrant thyroid epithelium (so-called lateral aberrant thyroid). The general current opinion is that the latter usually represent metastasis from an occult thyroid primary; rarely, however, genuine heterotopia may occur. Very rarely, benign inclusions have undoubtedly given rise to carcinoma primary in that site.

Reactive and Inflammatory Lymphadenopathy

Two concomitant changes can occur in a lymph node. First, the node may react to a stimulus; the changes seen are known as reactive hyperplasia. Second, the organism or other causative substances may elicit an active inflammatory reaction in the lymph node with migration into the node of the cells characteristic of an inflammatory reaction, notably polymorphs and macrophages. Three different reactions can occur in reactive lymphadenopathy, often simultaneously: (1) sinus hyperplasia, (2) proliferation of reactive follicles, and (3) proliferation of pulp elements. In sinus hyperplasia, the sinus macrophages increase in size and number, often solidly packing the sinuses. In addition, there may be an increase in traffic of monocytes and macrophages through the node. In follicular hyperplasia, numerous large reactive follicles are scattered throughout the node (Fig. 12-10). The overall reticulin pattern of the node is retained. The follicles may vary widely in size and form, sometimes dumbbell shaped. There is usually a rim of small lymphocytes clearly demarcating the periphery. Within the follicle are seen the usual cellular components. Mitosis is common, and there may be large tingible-body macrophages containing cellular debris. There may be well marked nuclear pleomorphism. Rarely, macrophages may show epithelioid cell transformation. The interfollicular pulp is compressed. Proliferation of pulp elements as the main reaction is best seen in cell-mediated immune reactions, when the interfollicular tissue becomes packed with immunoblasts. Postcapillary venules in the paracortical areas may be prominent, packed with emigrating lymphocytes and surrounded by maturing immunoblasts. All combinations of these forms of hyperplasia may occur and may be compounded by inflammatory changes.

The changes of inflammation as seen in a lymph node are similar to those seen elsewhere. In acute inflammation, the sinusoids are packed with polymorphs and suppuration may occur; in chronic inflammation there is accumulation of macrophages, often of epithelioid pattern, with giant cell and granuloma formation.

It may be very difficult to distinguish reactive conditions from neoplasia. Occasionally, a lymph node that subsequently proves to be reactive shows profound hy-

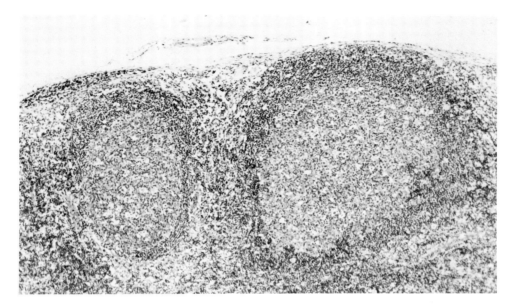

Fig. 12-10. Lymph node showing prominent reactive germinal centers (nonspecific follicular hyperplasia). The follicular structure is normal.

perplasia, cellular atypia, and obliteration of normal architecture. The critical diagnostic distinction is between reactive follicular hyperplasia and follicular lymphoma. In the reactive node, the follicles vary widely in size and shape but are distinct and rarely coalesce; they have a clear peripheral mantle of small lymphocytes and contain numerous mitotic figures and tingible-body macrophages; they do not spill out into or excessively compress the intervening interfollicular pulp. In the neoplastic node, the nodules are of uniform size and distribution throughout the node, spill into and compress adjacent tissue, and contain abnormal cells; gross pleomorphism may be seen but mitoses are paradoxically often less frequent. Tingible-body macrophages are uncommon. The reactive and inflammatory lesions occurring in lymph nodes will now be considered individually.

Nonspecific Lymphadenopathy

It is not uncommon to examine lymph nodes removed either because of enlargement or as part of a pathologic specimen removed for other reasons and to identify to a varying degree the reactions described above without finding an obvious cause. The presence of a few polymorphs in the sinusoids may suggest inflammation, and this may lead to fibrosis. Infective foci in the drainage area of the node should be sought, and serologic tests for such conditions as mononucleosis, toxoplasmosis, and rheumatoid disease should be performed. Sometimes, no good cause for the adenopathy will be found. Some of these patients later develop lymphoma, and it seems

likely that the node initially examined lay peripheral to a lymphomatous focus. For this reason, a surgeon carrying out lymph node biopsy should always remove not the most accessible but the largest and most obviously abnormal node.

The term *atypical hyperplasia* has been used to describe cases in which the pathologist expresses concern about neoplasia but is unable to diagnose lymphoma. Up to a third of such cases may subsequently develop lymphoma.

Tuberculous Lymphadenitis

Lymphadenopathy is a fairly common manifestation of tuberculosis, accounting for 40 percent of cases of nonrespiratory infection. The classic appearance of caseating giant cell granulomas containing acid-fast bacilli presents little diagnostic problem. In so-called nonreactive tuberculosis, there may be extensive necrosis with scanty granulomatous reaction; numerous acid-fast bacilli are demonstrable. This lack of reaction may be seen in patients with a hematologic abnormality that depresses immunity or in patients under treatment with cytotoxic, immunosuppressive or steroid drugs. Infection with atypical mycobacteria may lead to lymphadenopathy in which giant cells are scanty and suppuration is present.[25,26,27,28]

Lymphadenopathy in Leprosy

The role of the immune response in the formation of granulomas is clearly seen in the response to infection with *Mycobacterium leprae*. The response varies from a tuberculoid form (in patients with well developed cell-mediated immunity and a positive lepromin reaction) to the lepromatous reaction. Intermediate cases are described as borderline leprosy. Lymph nodes from patients with tuberculoid leprosy show only reactive changes, even though granulomatous lesions are present in the tissues of the draining area. Such nodes may show hyperplasia of the paracortical areas with dividing immunoblasts. Borderline cases show less ability to inhibit the spread of the organism, and sarcoid-like granulomas develop in and may almost replace the paracortical areas. Acid-fast bacilli are either absent or are seen only in small numbers.

In the lepromatous form, the lymph nodes are commonly enlarged; the paracortical areas show extensive lymphoid depletion and are infiltrated with large numbers of foamy macrophages containing acid-fast bacilli. The macrophages may tend to coalesce into syncytial clumps and giant cells may be seen, but no true granulomas are formed. The cortex of the node may show a follicular reaction with germinal center formation and abundant plasma cells. These patients have defective cellular and normal humoral immunity; this, however, is clearly insufficient in itself to eliminate the infection. In leprosy, necrosis is rarely seen in the lymph nodes, but an acute necrotizing lymphadenitis may be seen in some patients with lepromatous leprosy and erythema nodosum leprosum. This may be a manifestation of an acute vasculitis and is probably immunologically mediated.[29,30]

Sarcoidosis and Sarcoid-like Reactions

Sarcoidosis is a systemic granulomatous disease of unknown etiology which affects adults most commonly between the ages of 20 and 40. Blacks are affected approximately 10 times more frequently than whites and females are affected twice as often as males. Lesions are widespread and involve many organs. Lymph nodes are very commonly involved. The lymph node architecture is partially or wholly replaced by noncaseating granulomas containing occasional multinucleated giant cells of the Langhans type (Fig. 12-11). Occasional granulomas may show small central foci of fibrinoid necrosis. Three kinds of inclusions may be found within the giant cells or may be extruded into the extracellular space. Birefringent crystals (3 to 10 mm) of calcium carbonate are common, as are larger concentrically laminated basophil bodies consisting of protein containing calcium carbonate and iron (Schaumann bodies). Acidophilic star-shaped inclusions (asteroid bodies) are less common. Hamazaki-Wesenberg bodies are believed to represent giant lysosomes. These are usually present extracellularly and on silver stains have the appearance of budding yeast, for

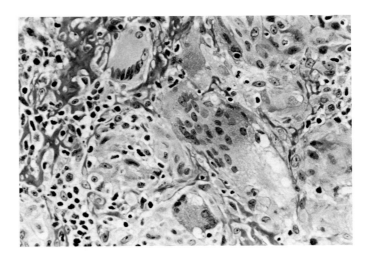

Fig. 12-11. Sarcoidosis in a lymph node showing characteristic large sarcoid giant cells.

which they have often been mistaken.[31-33] Sarcoid-like granulomas may be found in the lymph nodes draining neoplasms in Hodgkin's and non-Hodgkin's lymphomas and in other unrelated disorders, such as berylliosis, Crohn's disease and Whipple's disease.[34] In Whipple's disease, the node shows a patchy infiltration of large macrophages with a strikingly PAS-positive reaction. The diagnosis can be clinched by electron microscopic demonstration of numerous bacilli: these are well preserved even in material reclaimed from paraffin blocks.

A definitive diagnosis of sarcoidosis can only be made after all other causes have been reasonably excluded. Supporting clinical data, a positive skin test (Kveim test), and an elevated serum angiotensin-converting enzyme level help establish the diagnosis.

Syphilitic (Luetic) Lymphadenitis

Lymphadenitis may be regional or generalized and is common in the primary and secondary stages and rare in the tertiary stage. Occasionally the enlarged nodes constitute the initial manifestation and a diagnostic lymph node biopsy is undertaken.

Histopathologic features include marked follicular hyperplasia and capsular fibrosis accompanied by vascular proliferation (Fig. 12-12). Vessels show marked hyperplasia of lining endothelium, which may sometimes obliterate the lumen. Perivascular cuffs of lymphocytes and plasma cells, and occasionally intramural lymphocytes, are noted. Interfollicular areas show vascular proliferation and a proliferation of plasma cells, which sometimes may occur in sheets. Occasionally, aggregates of epithelioid histiocytes or small noncaseating granulomas may be present. Rarely, necrotizing granulomas may be present,

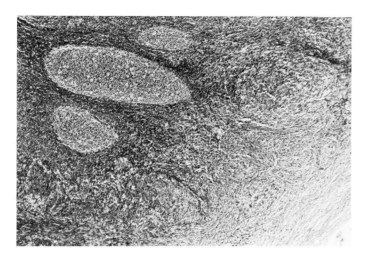

Fig. 12-12. Lymph node in syphilis showing combination of follicular hyperplasia and marked fibrosis.

resembling chlamydial, mycobacterial, or fungal infection. Spirochetes have been demonstrated in these areas of necrosis. However, spirochetes are usually demonstrable by silver stain in the walls of postcapillary venules. Diagnosis should be confirmed serologically.[35,36]

Brucellosis

In the few recorded cases of brucellosis in which lymph nodes have been examined histologically, the nodes show areas of granulomatous inflammation resembling tuberculosis but with scanty caseation and occasional giant cell formation. The changes are not diagnostic.[37,38]

Chlamydial Infections

The chlamydiae (formerly *Bedsonia*) are the causative agents of psittacosis, trachoma, and lymphogranuloma venereum. In *lymphogranuloma* the regional lymph nodes are often enlarged. Initially, there may be ill-defined infiltration with immunoblasts, neutrophils, plasma cells, and small epithelioid cell granulomas lying near the point of entry of afferent lymphatics to the node. The peripheral sinuses are filled with inflammatory cells, and the follicles are enlarged with reactive germinal centers. Later, characteristic stellate microabscesses with a core of polymorphs form first in the cortex, then in the medulla. At the edge of the abscess, epithelioid and giant cells are found. Giemsa staining may show inclusion bodies. The abscesses may coalesce and extend outside the node. The diagnosis can be confirmed serologically in lymphogranuloma.

Cat-Scratch Disease

Cat-scratch disease[39] is caused by an infectious agent introduced through the skin following a scratch by a cat or, less commonly, by a dog. A skin lesion may be present. Within 3 weeks, regional lymph nodes become enlarged. Lymphadenopathy is usually unilateral. Nodes initially show reactive follicular hyperplasia with increased numbers of macrophages and immunoblasts in interfollicular areas and sinuses. Subsequently, granulomas appear that develop central necrosis. In advanced lesions, the entire node may be replaced by stellate granulomas with central microabscesses (Fig. 12-13).

Histopathologic examination of lymph nodes has demonstrated delicate pleomorphic Gram-negative bacilli.[40] They are best seen with a Warthin-Starry silver impregnation stain performed at a pH of 3.8 to 4.0. Bacilli are commonly observed in walls of capillaries, in macrophages lining sinuses or near germinal centers, and in areas of necrosis. Bacilli occur singly, in chains or clumps. The organism has not been successfully cultured to date; growth requirements may be difficult to define, or they may be obligate intracellular parasites with host specificity. The etiologic relationship of the organism to the disease has not been totally proved. A cat-scratch skin test is available to assist in the diagnosis. Differential diagnoses would include mycobacterial and fungal infection and lymphogranuloma venereum.

Yersinial Infections

The lymph nodes draining the ileocecal region infected with *Yersinia enterocolitica* (formerly *Pasteurella pseudotuberculosis*) initially show nonspecific sinus and

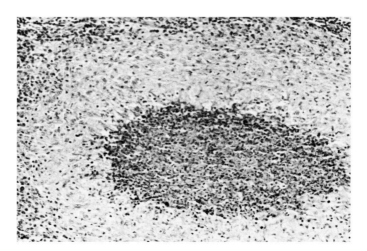

Fig. 12-13. Lymph node showing changes of cat-scratch disease. A palisaded rim of macrophages surrounds a central core of neutrophils.

follicular hyperplasia, and later an accumulation of neutrophils in the germinal centers of the follicles. These accumulations eventually enlarge to form round microabscesses surrounded by palisaded histiocytes but without giant cells. Gram-negative acid-fast diplobacilli may be seen in the lesions. Similar changes may be noted in the appendix when it is removed.[41]

Pneumocystis Infection

Pneumocystis pneumonia is a pulmonary infection caused by a protozoal organism *(Pneumocystis carinii)*. It is seen most commonly today in patients with acquired immune deficiency syndrome (AIDS). Lymph nodes are rarely involved, but cases of lymphadenitis with granulomatous lesions containing the organism have been reported.[42]

Fungal Infection

Fungal infections seldom present initially in lymph nodes but rather usually form part of an infection primarily involving other organs. A wide variety of fungi have been described as occasionally causing lymphadenitis. The lymph nodes show an equally wide variety of reactions ranging from acute suppuration to chronic granulomatous inflammation. There may be necrotic areas in which fungi can be readily demonstrated. The diagnosis depends on demonstration of the organism by PAS, Gridley, or Grocott methenamine silver stains.

Kikuchi's Disease

Kikuchi's disease is also called necrotizing lymphadenitis or histiocytic necrotizing lymphadenitis without granulocytic infiltration. It was first described in the Japanese literature in 1972[43] and more recently in the American literature.[44] Kikuchi's disease characteristically affects young women, with the cervical lymph nodes being most commonly involved. The nodes may be tender. Histologically, there is a roughly circumscribed necrotizing process in the paracortical area. Rarely, the entire lymph node may be necrotic. The necrotic area contains numerous histiocytes, karyorrhectic nuclear debris, and immunoblasts. Neutrophils are absent. The sheets of histiocytes and immunoblasts may lead to a misdiagnosis of a large cell lymphoma or malignant histiocytosis. The disease is usually self-limited and subsides in 1 to 4 months. In a few cases, serologic studies have demonstrated increased viral titers to such viruses as the Epstein-Barr virus (EBV) and cytomegalovirus (CMV). Differential diagnosis would include lupus erythematosus; serologic

studies to exclude this possibility may be indicated. The differential diagnosis from some of the specific infections discussed earlier is largely based on the absence of abscesses containing neutrophils and of granulomata.

Toxoplasmic Lymphadenopathy

Toxoplasmic lymphadenopathy, due to infection with the protozoon *Toxoplasma gondii*, may range from the enlargement of a solitary node to a generalized lymphadenopathy with pyrexia, resembling glandular fever.[45–47] An involved lymph node shows preservation of the architecture and follicular hyperplasia with germinal centers in which tingible body macrophages are prominent. Small aggregates of large epithelioid macrophages are prominent in the interfollicular cortex and germinal centers (Fig. 12-14 and 12-15); neither giant cells nor caseation is seen. The sinusoids are densely packed with macrophages and epithelioid histiocytes. Many plasma cells are present throughout the node and in the capsule. Organisms are rarely seen, although *Toxoplasma* cysts have occasionally been found. A positive histologic diagnosis should not be made in the absence of a positive dye test or hemagglutination or complement-fixation tests. The presence of well marked germinal centers with large tingible body macrophages coupled with the presence of numerous epithelioid histiocytes is sufficient for a provisional diagnosis of toxoplasmosis, pending the result of the dye test or other serologic tests. Infectious mononucleosis may produce similar appearance and may be excluded serologically.

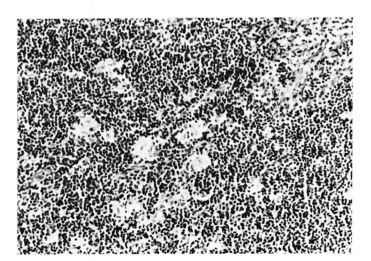

Fig. 12-14. Toxoplasmic lymphadenopathy. Clusters of pale macrophages are scattered throughout the node, notably in the medulla.

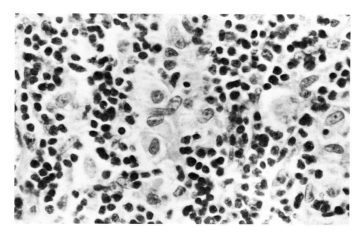

Fig. 12-15. Toxoplasmic lymphadenopathy. Detail of clusters of macrophages, which often contain cellular debris.

Rheumatoid Disease

While more than 50 percent of patients with rheumatoid disease have enlargement of lymph nodes, the nodes are rarely excised. In cases in which this has been done, the nodes show extreme follicular hyperplasia with follicles in both the cortex and medulla and even outside the capsule.[48–50] The follicles may be rather vascular. Germinal centers are well marked and show tingible body macrophages. Numerous plasma cells are present in the interfollicular pulp, and occasional histiocytes, neutrophils, and eosinophils may be seen. The vascular endothelial cells are hypertrophied, and there may be formation of new connective tissue in the node. Periadenitis may be seen, and occasional nodes show a little sinus reaction. In a small number of cases, amyloid deposition can be demonstrated. The differential diagnosis is mainly with the follicular forms of lymphoma.

Systemic Lupus Erythematosus

Lymphadenopathy is commonly observed in systemic lupus erythematosus. The nodes are usually enlarged and soft, and on cut section may show focal areas of necrosis. Microscopically, nodal architecture is partially or totally destroyed, and necrosis, initially subcapsular, may be focal or involve the whole node, usually unaccompanied by significant inflammation. Clumps of intense blue-staining material (H&E stain) representing nuclear debris may be seen. These so-called hematoxylin bodies also stain positively with PAS and Feulgen stains. The cellular component includes lymphocytes, plasma cells, immunoblasts, and macrophages. Vessels are lined by plump endothelium. Fibrinoid necrosis of vessel walls may be present.

Larger vessels may show a perivascular collagen degeneration and deposition of Ig. The diagnosis should be confirmed serologically.

Viral Infections

Little is known about the detailed histologic structure of the response of lymph nodes to viruses. Many such infections may be associated with general or regional lymphadenopathy, but this forms part of a general febrile illness, and since the diagnosis can be made by other means, lymph node biopsy is rarely indicated. The pattern of reaction has been defined in several instances (e.g., vaccinia, measles, and infectious mononucleosis).

Postvaccinial Lymphadenopathy

The nodes show considerable hyperplasia, follicular or diffuse, with preservation of the basic architecture. Numerous immunoblasts are present (Fig. 12-16), often in mitosis, and the sinusoids contain a mixed population of lymphocytes, plasma cells, and eosinophils. Focal collections of eosinophils may be present in the nodal parenchyma, but no Reed-Sternberg cells are identifiable. Pericapsular involvement is also seen. Sinus histiocytosis may occur. Plasma cells are present in abundance in cases in which a biopsy is done more than 10 days after vaccination, and follicular hyperplasia is not in evidence after 15 days. Similar changes are seen in herpes zoster. The histologic appearance may mimic Hodgkin's disease, which may be excluded on the basis of the history, the retention of normal architecture, and the absence of Reed-Sternberg cells.[51]

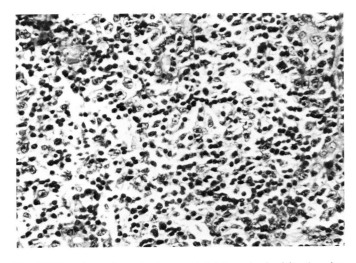

Fig. 12-16. Lymph node in vaccinial lymphadenitis showing infiltrate of large atypical lymphoid cells.

Measles

Enlarged lymph nodes in measles characteristically show syncytial giant cells with up to 100 nuclei in a grape-like cluster in the center of the cell. Such Warthin-Finkeldey cells are also seen in the tonsils and in the lymphoid tissue of the gut, especially the appendix.[52,53] Similar changes occur in the draining lymph nodes after measles immunization.[54]

Infectious Mononucleosis

Since the diagnosis can be made by hematologic and serologic means, lymph node biopsy is rarely undertaken. Biopsy is more likely to be performed in the atypical case, and mistakes in diagnosis can occur. The histologic features have been described by several investigators.[55–59] The appearance varies with the stage of the disease. Initially, the architecture of the node is normal. There is follicular hyperplasia, and the prominent germinal centers contain tingible body macrophages and show mitotic activity. The interfollicular cortex shows immunoblastic hyperplasia and collections of epithelioid histiocytes. The sinus pattern is maintained, but some sinuses may contain lymphocytes and larger cells apparently identical to the circulating atypical mononuclear cells. The sinus-lining cells undergo hyperplasia, and the medullary cords show a proliferation of lymphocytes and atypical mononuclear cells, although few plasma cells are seen. Lymphocytes may infiltrate the capsule and pericapsular tissues.

At this stage, the node looks similar to that seen in toxoplasmosis but contains fewer plasma cells in the medulla. The condition may now regress, in which case the lymph node reverts to normal. However, some nodes may show a continuing hyperplasia with enlargement and fusion of the germinal centers distorting the architecture and producing solid areas of tissue where the follicular structure is indistinct or altogether absent. The capsule is often infiltrated. At the same time, there is hyperplasia of immunoblasts with abundant mitotic activity. At this stage, there may be a considerable resemblance to malignant lymphoma (Fig. 12-17). The diagnosis is rendered more difficult by the occasional presence of cells resembling Reed-Sternberg cells. However, although the architecture of the node is distorted, it is not destroyed; while atypical immunoblasts may be present, no abnormal mitoses are seen. There may be scanty necrosis. A histologic diagnosis of infectious mononucleosis always requires serologic confirmation. EBV antigen may be demonstrated immunohistochemically in the node. Very rarely, lymphoma may follow infectious mononucleosis, and in difficult cases, careful follow-up and repeated biopsy may be required.

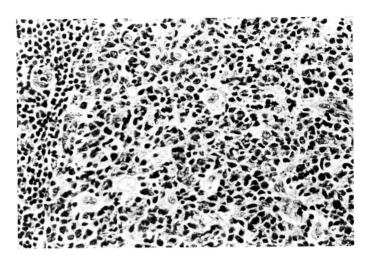

Fig. 12-17. Infectious mononucleosis. At the edge of a large germinal center, there is gross pleomorphism of nuclei. Numerous large macrophages contain cellular debris. The patient had grossly enlarged nodes and serologic evidence of infectious mononucleosis and was well four years later.

Lymph Nodes in AIDS and AIDS-Related Complex

AIDS is thought to be caused by a lymphotropic retrovirus belonging to the human T-cell leukemia virus group referred to as the human immunodeficiency virus (HIV) (previously HTLV-III). The virus infects and kills T-helper lymphocytes, resulting in inversion of the T-helper/T-suppressor cytotoxic ratio. AIDS is usually fatal and is the severest form of what is considered a broad-spectrum disease. It is characterized by opportunistic infections and/or malignant tumors, including Kaposi's sarcoma and malignant lymphoma. A more common and perhaps prodromal phase of the disease is referred to as persistent generalized lymphadenopathy (PGL) and is considered part of the AIDS-related complex (ARC), which might be predictive of AIDS.[60–62]

ARC is diagnosed in the presence of any two of the clinical features listed in Table 12-2 plus any two abnormal laboratory tests. Some patients with ARC have progressed rapidly to AIDS, whereas others have not progressed over several years.

Enlarged lymph nodes in ARC may show different histologic patterns, which have been variously designated type I, or reactive follicular hyperplasia; type II, or selective paracortical lymphoid depletion; and type III, or severe lymphoid depletion, or burnout. Much of this reaction is nonspecific and can be seen in patients with neither ARC nor AIDS (see Ch. 4 for illustrations of these histologic patterns).

TABLE 12-2. Clinical Features Useful in Diagnosing AIDS-Related Complex

Clinical	Laboratory
Fever (>38°C) for >3 months	Decreased T-helper cells (fewer than 400/mm³; normal = 518–1,650/mm³);
Weight loss (>10% of total body weight)	Decreased T-helper/T-suppressor ratio (<1.0)
Diarrhea for >3 months	Depressed lymphocyte blastogenesis (phytohemag-glutinin);
Fatigue	Anergy to skin tests
Night sweats	

Reactive Follicular Hyperplasia (Type I Pattern)

Lymph nodes show florid reactive follicular hyperplasia and contain numerous follicles with large, mitotically active germinal centers. Abnormal and sometimes bizarre-shaped germinal centers may be seen. Mantle zones are attenuated and there is accompanying vascular proliferation with venules lined by plump endothelium. Sinuses contain histiocytes, neutrophils, lymphocytes and erythrocytes. Histiocytes may reveal phagocytosis. Interfollicular areas contain neutrophils and plasma cells, which may be prominent. Occasional multinucleated cells resembling Warthin-Finkeldey cells may be present.

Selective Paracortical Lymphoid Depletion (Type II Pattern)

Germinal centers are atrophic or absent and are often replaced by scars. Nodal architecture may be partially effaced. Lymphocytes, plasma cells, and immunoblasts are present, and many of the lymphocytes may have clear cytoplasm. Vascular proliferation is present. Other features described in the type I pattern are present to a varying degree. Patients with the type II pattern often progress to AIDS.

Severe Lymphoid Depletion or Burn-out (Type III Pattern)

The nodes are usually small and lack germinal centers. There is marked depletion of lymphocytes. Vascular proliferation is noted. Sinuses are prominent and sinus histiocytosis is usually present, with erythrophagocytosis noted in more than 50 percent of cases. Plasma cells are increased and occasional large atypical forms may be seen. Multinucleated cells, including bizarre forms, are often seen. This pattern is usually seen in patients with AIDS and results from overwhelming destruction of T-helper lymphocytes by the virus.

Other processes may be seen in the nodes of AIDS patients, including mycobacterial, fungal and viral infections, Kaposi's sarcoma, and malignant lymphoma. These are rarely seen in lymph nodes showing the type I pattern and are commonest in patients with AIDS exhibiting the type III nodal pattern.

Immunologic confirmation is necessary to confirm the diagnosis of AIDS. These include T-helper/T-suppressor cell ratios and serum antibody to HIV.

Lymphadenopathy Due to Anticonvulsant Drugs

Lymphadenopathy rarely complicates the use of the anticonvulsant phenytoin (diphenylhydantoin).[63–66] The lymph nodes show variably distorted architecture with a proliferation of atypical immunoblasts, often dividing, and infiltration with plasma cells, eosinophils, and immature lymphoid cells (Fig. 12-18). There may be focal necrosis, capsular infiltration with cells, and variable follicular hyperplasia. The simulation of Hodgkin's disease may be close, but true Reed-Sternberg cells are not seen, blood vessels are not invaded, and the lymph node architecture is distorted rather than destroyed. Systemic clinical manifestations such as favor, eosinophilia, and hepatosplenomegaly may make it more difficult to avoid confusion with lymphoma. Lymphadenopathy usually regresses when the drug is discontinued. Sometimes, however, the adenopathy does not regress and, rarely, Hodgkin's disease, "histiocytic" lymphoma or lymphocytic lymphoma may occur. Similar reactions may occur

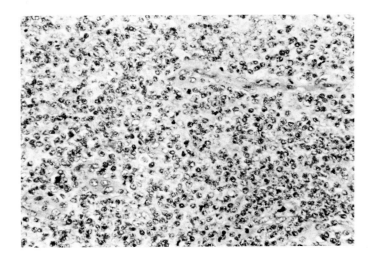

Fig. 12-18. Lymph node showing loss of normal structure and atypical hyperplasia of small and large lymphocytes. The patient was being treated with Dilantin (diphenylhydantoin), and the lymphadenopathy regressed on cessation of treatment.

to other drugs (*e.g.*, para-aminosalicylic acid and phenyl-butazone), and similar appearance may be seen in serum sickness.

Reaction of Lymph Nodes to Lipid

Injected lipid passes to the local lymph nodes and is taken up by sinusoidal macrophages and later induces a granulomatous response; this produces a foamy appearance in paraffin sections. Endogenous lipid may also be taken up by the lymph node.

Exogenous lipid may derive from lymphangiography, bronchography, inhalation lipoid pneumonia, injection of hemorrhoids with lipid-based material, or injection of Freund's adjuvant in animals and, rarely, in humans. Most commonly seen is the lymph node response to lymphangiography, in which contrast medium in an oily base is injected directly into a lymphatic vessel and passes to the lymph node, forming large droplets up to 100 μm in diameter in the subcapsular and medullary sinuses; after about 4 days, a reaction is seen around the oil droplets, with prominent giant cell formation (Fig. 12-19). The nodes may eventually return to normal, though only after a prolonged period.[67]

Lipogranulomatosis[68,69] refers to the reaction in lymph node or spleen to any lipid material arising from such endogenous sources as hematomas, tumors, cholesterol deposits, xanthomatous lesions, fat embolism, and fat necrosis. Lipogranulomatosis is commonly seen in the nodes draining the biliary system, notably the cholecystic lymph node, in cholelithiasis. Lipid accumulation may cause formation of giant cell granulomata and ultimate fibrosis. This lesion is twice as frequent in men. Similar lesions of unknown origin occur in the spleen.

Dermatopathic Lymphadenopathy

Dermatopathic lymphadenopathy is a nonspecific lymph node reaction to skin lesions, characterized by the accumulation of lipid material, melanin, and occasionally hemosiderin. It may be caused by the skin condition itself or by associated scratching, and usually resolves as the primary skin condition heals.

The affected node shows some follicular reaction and prominent accumulation of pale macrophages in the outer medulla or in the cortex, wisely separating the follicles. These macrophages contain lipid, usually cholesterol, melanin, and sometimes hemosiderin. There is some sinus hyperplasia and sometimes infiltration with plasma cells and eosinophils.[70]

Angiofollicular Lymph Node Hyperplasia

Angiofollicular lymph node hyperplasia has been reported under several synonyms since 1921[71] and manifests lymphadenopathy, which may be either mediastinal, cervical, or disseminated.[72,73] It has also been reported in various viscera. The lesion has been variously interpreted as reactive or neoplastic. It is benign.

Approximately 10 percent of affected patients have systemic symptoms that are cured by surgical removal of the lesion. They include fever with a raised erythrocyte sedimentation rate (ESR), sweating, and fatigue; hematologic abnormalities, including thrombocytopenia and ane-

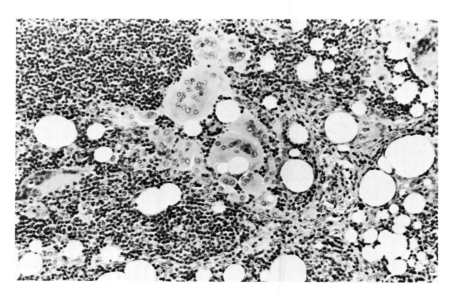

Fig. 12-19. Postlymphangiography granuloma. Lymph node showing a granulomatous reaction to lipid. Numerous multinucleate giant cells are related to oil vacuoles.

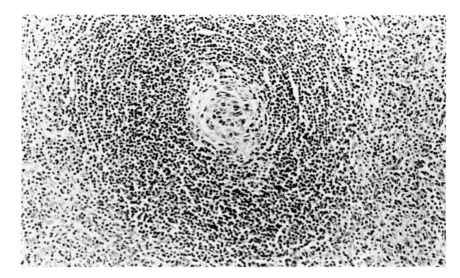

Fig. 12-20. Angiofollicular hyperplasia. In the core of a nodule of small lymphocytes lies a mass of hyaline connective tissue with a blood vessel.

mia[74]; and immunologic disorders, including hyperglobulinemia[75] and even myasthenia gravis.[76] The condition has been divided into two groups: the hyaline vascular type and the rarer plasma cell type.[73,77] In the hyaline vascular type, systemic symptoms are rare, whereas in the plasma cell type, they are common.

Hyaline Vascular Type

Follicular masses of lymphocytes are evenly distributed throughout the lesion, but germinal centers are small in the hyaline vascular type. In the center of each follicle lies a capillary blood vessel with plump endothelial cells (Figs. 12-20 and 12-21). The surrounding cells may be flattened; thus, the structure comes to resemble a Hassall's corpuscle. There is a considerable amount of hyaline fibrous tissue both around the central blood vessel and in the interfollicular tissue, with occasional areas of calcification. The lymphocytes in the centers of the follicles are arranged in a concentrically laminated fashion. Between the follicles there is an abundance of small capillaries and a mixed infiltrate of lymphocytes, plasma cells, eosinophils, and immunoblasts. In many cases, areas of normal lymph node structure can be identified, although in the lesion itself no sinusoids are present. Sometimes, sections of adjacent lymph nodes show plasma cell accumulation or hyaline follicles.

Plasma Cell Type

In the plasma cell type, the interfollicular tissue contains sheets of mature plasma cells. Other cells are few, except for occasional immunoblasts. Occasional sinusoids are present. The follicles contain germinal centers, often large, with mitotic figures, nuclear debris, and histiocytes; no central blood vessel is seen, and there is no hyalinization. Remnants of lymph node architecture may be present, and some follicles may be of the hyaline vascular type. The clinical mass is usually a collection of discrete lymph nodes.

Some cases show a mixture of plasma cell and hyaline vascular reactions; the former may be an earlier phase of the latter.

Differential diagnosis is from follicular lymphoma, Hodgkin's disease, thymoma, and reactive conditions with numerous plasma cells, such as rheumatoid disease. A reticulin stain is often valuable to emphasize the vascularity of the lesion.

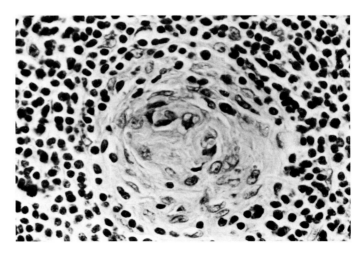

Fig. 12-21. Detail of center of nodule in angiofollicular hyperplasia showing collagenous core with a small blood vessel.

Multicentric Angiofollicular Lymph Node Hyperplasia

Multicentric angiofollicular lymph node hyperplasia has been recently described.[78,79] This multicentric lymphoproliferative disorder is associated with systemic manifestations and resembles angiofollicular lymph node hyperplasia histologically. In many of these patients, the disease has an aggressive course with a fatal outcome. There is multicentric lymph node enlargement, and splenomegaly is common. Patients are usually anemic and have polyclonal hypergammaglobulinemia. The bone marrow often shows plasmacytosis. Histologically, the nodes resemble the plasma cell variant of angiofollicular lymph node hyperplasia. Non-Hodgkin's lymphoma and, rarely, Kaposi's sarcoma may ensue.

Although multicentric lymph node hyperplasia appears to be a variant of classic angiofollicular lymph node hyperplasia, patients have higher morbidity and mortality and are at risk for the development of malignant tumors. It has been suggested that multicentric lymph node hyperplasia is a disease entity, distinct from the classic form. The differential diagnosis includes angioimmunoblastic lymphadenopathy, T-cell lymphoma resembling angioimmunoblastic lymphadenopathy, and the lymph node hyperplasia associated with AIDS.

Angioimmunoblastic Lymphadenopathy

Angioimmunoblastic lymphadenopathy with dysproteinemia is a disorder of uncertain pathogenesis that occurs in the elderly. Patients present with generalized lymphadenopathy, hepatosplenomegaly, hypergammaglobulinemia, and often autoimmune hemolytic anemia. This is usually accompanied by severe constitutional symptoms, such as fever, night sweats, and malaise.[80–82]

The lymph node is effaced by a proliferation of lymphocytes, plasma cells and immunoblasts; the latter may be binucleate and may resemble Reed-Sternberg cells. Eosinophils and neutrophils may be present, and occasionally eosinophils may be prominent. Scattered epithelioid histiocytes may also be present, although well formed granulomas are rare. An occasional small burnt-out germinal center may be present. There is a proliferation of small blood vessels resembling postcapillary venules, lined by reactive endothelium which may actually obliterate the lumen. There may be a precipitate of intercellular PAS-positive eosinophilic material (Figs. 12-22 and 12-23). Extranodal sites that may also be involved include the liver, spleen, bone marrow, and skin.

Response to therapy, including chemotherapy and steroids, is unpredictable and may actually worsen the prognosis. Many patients succumb to severe infections.

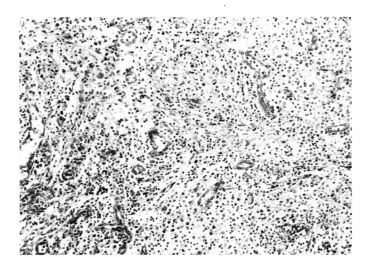

Fig. 12-22. Angioimmunoblastic lymphadenopathy. Lymph node showing prominent vascularity and structureless interstitial material.

Angioimmunoblastic lymphadenopathy may represent a progressive proliferation within the B-cell system that may terminate fatally without neoplastic transformation. In a small number of patients, the syndrome has terminated as immunoblastic sarcoma.

Criteria used for the diagnosis of angioimmunoblastic lymphadenopathy with immunoblastic lymphoma[83] include the histologic features described for angioimmunoblastic lymphadenopathy together with well defined aggregates of large transformed lymphocytes with or without plasmacytoid features. These large cells may form clusters or islands or may occur in diffuse sheets, depleting the small lymphocytes. Immunoblastic lymphoma is considered a high-grade malignant lymphoma in

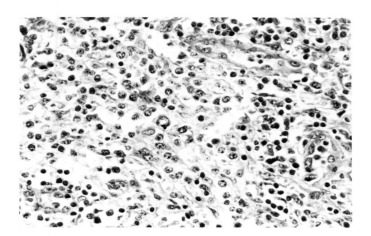

Fig. 12-23. Detail of Figure 12-22 showing infiltrate of lymphocytes and immunoblasts and prominent structureless interstitial material.

the working formulation for the classification of lymphoma.

Sinus Histiocytosis with Massive Lymphadenopathy

Sinus histiocytosis with massive lymphadenopathy is a benign condition of unknown etiology first described by Rosai and Dorfman.[84] It most commonly affects children and usually manifests as massive cervical lymphadenopathy. Other groups of nodes are less commonly affected; occasionally, there is involvement of other tissues such as tonsil, testis, orbit, and skin.

The enlarged nodes are painless, and constitutional symptoms are not prominent, although fever and a raised ESR do occur. Anemia and leukocytosis have been reported, and there is a significant degree of hyperglobulinemia (usually IgG).[85] The disease runs a benign course with eventual resolution after several months or years.

Lymph nodes are large, fibrotic, and matted together. Microscopically, there is marked dilation of the sinuses, which contain numerous histiocytes and fewer lymphocytes, erythrocytes, and plasma cells, and occasional neutrophils. Histiocytes are large, with abundant eosinophilic cytoplasm and nuclei with prominent nucleoli. The histiocytes are actively phagocytic and ingest a variety of cells, including lymphocytes, neutrophils, plasma cells, and erythrocytes. Initially, the phagocytosed cells are well preserved, but they are eventually broken down; the histiocytes then contain cell debris and lipid material (Fig. 12-24). The phagocytosed lymphocytes are viable (emperipolesis). The medullary portion of the node contains numerous plasma cells and occasional histiocytes. Immunohistochemical stains using the peroxidase-antiperoxidase technique reveal the histiocytes to stain positively for S-100 protein.[86] An infectious agent has not been identified in these lymph nodes. This relatively rare condition must be distinguished from malignant lymphoma and malignant histiocytosis.

Hyaline Sclerosis of Lymph Nodes

Lymph nodes are occasionally seen infiltrated with hyaline eosinophilic material arranged in trabeculae, which are often concentric, with obliterated blood vessels and focal infiltration of lymphocytes and plasma cells. This may be true amyloid and may be the initial manifestation of systemic amyloidosis[87,88] or it may be nonamyloid, amorphous material when seen electron microscopically[89] but accompanied by hypergammaglobulinemia. Similar sclerosis may be seen in nodes in malignant lymphoma.

Secondary Neoplasms in Lymph Nodes

Reaction to Neoplasm

Lymph nodes react to tumors in their drainage area in a number of ways: (1) enlargement of lymphoid follicles and formation of prominent germinal centers (a B-cell response), (2) increase in size of paracortical areas due to entry and proliferation of lymphocytes (a T-cell response), and (3) sinus histiocytosis, an increase in prominence of sinus macrophages (a macrophage response) involving probably both local proliferation and entry of peripherally derived macrophages. This last reaction is probably a complex response to the shedding of tumor antigens and to cell death in the tumor with consequent inflammation (Fig. 12-25). It is widely believed, and as

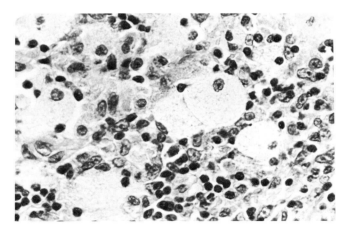

Fig. 12-24. Grossly enlarged macrophages in lymph node sinusoids in sinus histiocytosis with massive lymphadenopathy.

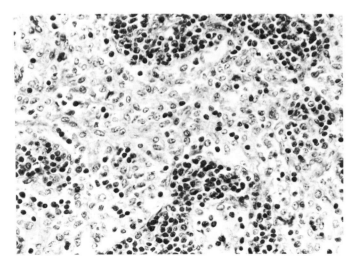

Fig. 12-25. Sinus histiocytosis. Note the prominent but normal-sized sinus histiocytes lining sinusoids in lymph node draining a neoplasm.

widely doubted, that sinus histiocytosis is associated with an improved prognosis, especially in carcinoma of the breast. Careful analysis of the relationship between changes in the lymph nodes draining a tumor and the prognosis of the tumor suggests that the key factor may be changes in the lymphocyte population of the node, rather than the macrophages.[90–92] Four patterns have been described: (1) lymphocytic predominance, in which the extrafollicular parts of the node are stuffed with lymphocytes; (2) follicular reaction; (3) an intermediate (average) state; and (4) lymphocytic depletion, often with hyaline fibrosis. Thus, in endometrial, cervical, breast, and upper respiratory carcinomas, lymphocyte predominance is associated with a good prognosis and lymphocyte depletion with a poor prognosis. Lymph nodes with metastatic deposits contain fewer T-lymphocytes. This may be true also of cancer of the cervix and bronchus, but in colonic carcinoma no clear relationship between reactive changes and prognosis has been established. Sarcoid-like reactions in nodes draining tumors are rare and their significance is not certain. A practical conclusion would be that the histopathologist should report histologic changes in lymph nodes draining a cancer, along with the degree of lymphocyte reaction in the tumor itself. However, except for such well known lesions as medullary carcinoma of the breast and seminoma of the testis, it is not certain what these findings mean for the individual patient. In general, it is likely that the presence of a florid lymphocytic reaction in a tumor, along with marked lymphocytic predominance in a node that does not contain metastasis, may imply a better prognosis.

Reactive hyperplasia may be mistaken for neoplasm, usually for a primary lymphoreticular neoplasm. Reactive hyperplasia may be present in one pole of a lymph node that contains metastasis. Active tumor cell destruction is rarely seen in a human lymph node, but necrotic debris, keratin, or psammoma bodies may be present. Confusion between metastatic carcinoma and reactive hyperplasia may occur; in secondary anaplastic carcinoma of the cervical lymph nodes from a nasopharyngeal primary (so-called lymphoepithelioma), the metastasis, like the primary lesion, may be so smothered in lymphocytes as to render it almost unrecognizable (Fig. 12-26). In this situation, immunohistochemical stains for epithelial cell markers are usually helpful (see Ch. 7).

Metastatic Tumor in Lymph Nodes

The problem of metastatic tumor in lymph nodes may present either as the identification of metastatic neoplasm in an isolated lymph node or as the detection of metastatic neoplasm in lymph nodes submitted with the primary tumor. This can be crucial in staging a tumor.

Accurate staging of cancer is dependent on careful

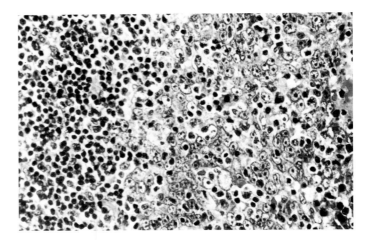

Fig. 12-26. Secondary carcinoma in a lymph node draining a primary upper respiratory carcinoma. Tumor cells are mixed with lymphocytes. Elsewhere in this tumor the tumor cells were almost completely obscured by lymphocytes.

pathologic examination of a specimen submitted by a surgeon who has adequately identified the specimen and its component parts. The palpable lymph nodes should be removed for histologic examination and their sites recorded. If examination of single sections does not show metastasis, step sections of the paraffin blocks at a minimum of five levels per block must be examined. The pathologic report should note the degree of reaction in each node and the extent of metastasis.

The histologic changes in a lymph node containing metastatic tumor vary. There may be obvious replacement with secondary neoplasm of evident type. Amelanotic melanoma may be confused with secondary carcinoma, and when the sinusoids are packed with melanoma or carcinoma cells, there may be a danger of confusion with malignant (or even benign) histiocytosis. In this situation, immunohistochemical or ultrastructural studies may reveal the correct diagnosis (see Ch. 7). Small foci of neoplastic cells in a subcapsular sinus may readily be missed. Rarely, such foci may appear degenerate. Even more rarely, clusters of neoplastic cells may be seen in the blood vessels, leading to invasion of the lymph node in patients with hematogenous dissemination of cancer. Carcinoma cells may mingle diffusely with lymphocytes in secondary deposits from lymphoepithelioma of the nasopharynx; this may be difficult to identify as metastasis. Similarly, infiltration with small round or oat-shaped cells derived from a bronchial primary tumor may be hard to discriminate from small cell lymphoma. Occasionally, infiltration with large carcinoma cells with some fibrosis may be difficult to distinguish from atypical Hodgkin's disease. Tumor cells can sometimes be seen in the extracapsular lymphatics of the node and may block these, forming an extracapsular mass. Within the node, tumor cells sometimes can be found only in the subcapsular sinus, free or adhering to the wall. Thereafter, they move down the sinusoids, distending them as they go, and later invading and destroying the adjacent lymph node parenchyma. Ultimately, the node may be completely replaced by tumor. Tumor cells may sometimes be seen in the efferent sinusoids. The tumor may stimulate the formation of stroma similar to that seen in the primary, such as dense fibrous tissue or a prominent blood capillary plexus. The nodal metastasis, however, may be quite different from the primary, notably in the amount of stroma evoked and in the resultant compression of the tumor cells. There may be extensive degenerative changes in the tumor, for example, mucinous change in an adenocarcinoma or frank necrosis, presumably ischemic. In differentiated adenocarcinomas, tumor may seed down the sinusoids as single cells, maturing into acinar elements later, and inducing a characteristic stroma. The reaction in a node may include neutrophils and giant cells. A node containing a small metastasis may show any of the forms of reaction just noted. Occasionally, a node grossly enlarged by reaction may contain a small metastasis.

Identification of the primary site whence the neoplasm has arisen is usually obvious when a primary tumor and its draining nodes are examined, and is obviously more difficult when only a node is submitted. The solitary node with metastatic tumor can pose difficult diagnostic problems (see Ch. 7). Cervical lymph node metastases manifesting in this way usually originate from an upper alimentary or respiratory tract primary site, or from the thyroid.[93] Axillary metastases from an unknown primary site are most often of mammary origin but may derive from such varied sites as lung, skin, stomach, or pharynx, or from melanoma or sarcoma of the upper extremity.[94] In one large series of inguinal lymph node deposits, not only carcinoma and melanoma, but other tumors such as neuroblastoma, retinoblastoma, various sarcomas, and choriocarcinoma, were also represented.[95] For the most part, these tumors are derived from such obvious sites as the skin of the lower limbs or trunk, ovary, cervix, vulva, penis, anus, and rectum, but rarely from such remote sites as nasopharynx, respiratory tract, eye, salivary gland, urinary tract, or bone. Rarely, in disseminated carcinomatosis, tumor cells may enter a lymph node from the blood. Usually, a combination of clinical information and histologic experience can identify the primary tumor in most cases, but occasionally the primary is not identified during life, or even after careful necropsy.

In specimens of a primary tumor and attached tissues, the more carefully lymph nodes are sought, the more will be found, especially if the specimen is chilled to solidify the fat and a very sharp knife is used.[96] If lymph nodes are sought before fixing the tissue, they are pinker and more evident. A further refinement is to clear the gross surgical specimen in graded alcohols and cedar oil. More lymph nodes can be found this way, but the procedure is time-consuming and expensive, and the additional nodes identified are usually negative for tumor. When lymph nodes are identified, it is essential to cut several nodes that grossly do not contain neoplasm. In a series of 51 radical mastectomy specimens, Pickren[97] found occult metastasis in 22 percent of cases by step-sectioning the lymph node blocks at three levels. While gross nodal metastasis is of obvious importance in prognosis, the presence of such occult metastases is less important.

It is classically held that carcinoma tends to metastasize by the lymphatics and sarcoma by the bloodstream. Melanoma also metastasizes by the lymphatic system as well as the bloodstream. Sarcomas, however, metastasize by lymphatics more often than was thought, particularly in patients who have survived for considerable periods because of anticancer treatment.[98] Antisera against marker antigens are useful to trace the origin of metastatic neoplasms, but unfortunately anaplastic tumors tend to lose antigenicity.

An unusual and complex set of changes is seen in lymph nodes in *Kaposi's sarcoma*. There may be a follicular hyperplasia, sometimes of striking vascularity, accompanied by plasma cell infiltration of the medullary cords. The node may also show an angiomatous pattern and spindle cell proliferation in the sinusoids, presumably representing metastasis (Fig. 12-27). The lymphadenopathy may be accompanied by hepatosplenomegaly, anemia, and hyperglobulinemia.[99] Patients with Kaposi's sarcoma also have an increased incidence of malignant lymphoma.

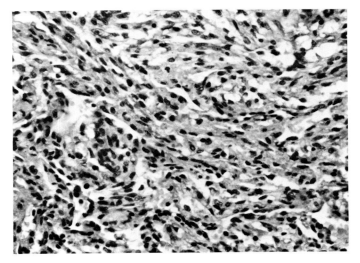

Fig. 12-27. Kaposi's sarcoma. Lymph node showing replacement by sinusoidal spaces with fibrosis.

Vascular Lesions of Lymph Nodes

Infarction of lymph nodes is rare. In a series of five cases,[100] patients had swelling of a superficial lymph node chain. A central extensive area of necrosis was surrounded by a rim of surviving tissue in which reactive granulation tissue appeared (Fig. 12-28). The lesions were attributable to thrombosis of veins within and at the hila of the nodes. Such lesions may be accompanied by a systemic febrile reaction.[101] *Necrosis* is seen in tuberculosis and other granulomatous inflammation, in acute suppurative lymphadenitis (where it is distinguished by the greater extent of the inflammation), in hypersensitivity states, and in Kikuchi's disease.

The result of *venous obstruction*[102] is that the lymph node sinusoids are transformed into structures that resemble blood capillaries and contain many RBC. The initial access of blood to the lymphatic sinusoids occurs presumably through the normal lymphaticovenous connections. There is considerable associated fibrosis. *Nodal angiomatosis*—benign proliferation of blood vessels in nodes—is different.[103] Nodes removed incidentally are partly replaced by cords of proliferating endothelial cells with slitlike, round, or oval lumina containing red blood cells. Fibrosis is scanty; the rest of the node shows normal structure.

Malignant Lymphoma

Hodgkin's Disease

If a lymph node shows malignant lymphoma, the first decision is: Is this Hodgkin's disease? Thomas Hodgkin in 1832 reported seven cases in which gross enlargement

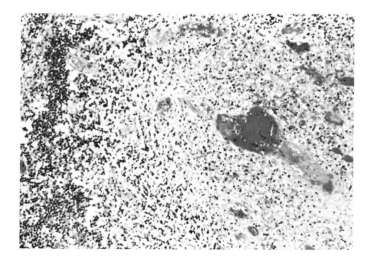

Fig. 12-28. Infarcted lymph node. There is a rim of peripheral surviving lymph node. In the necrotic center, the vessels are grossly distended with blood. The specimen came from an obstructed inguinal hernia.

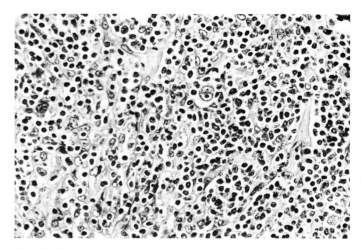

Fig. 12-29. Lymph node showing the changes of classical (mixed) Hodgkin's disease—fibrosis, malignant cells, binucleate Reed-Sternberg cells, and an infiltrate of lymphocytes and eosinophils.

of lymph nodes and, with one exception, spleen was found at autopsy. The classic histologic appearance of the lesion in a lymph node includes fibrosis, large mononuclear malignant (Hodgkin) cells, binucleate malignant (Reed-Sternberg) cells, and variable infiltration with lymphocytes and eosinophils (Figs. 12-29 and 12-30).

Since 1965, the Rye classification of Hodgkin's disease has been widely accepted. This divides Hodgkin's disease into four histologic types: lymphocyte predominance (LP), nodular sclerosis (NS), mixed cellularity (MC), and lymphocyte depletion (LD). The diagnostic reproducibility and clinical usefulness of this classification has been well established.[104–107] Occasional problems may be encountered in classification of atypical cases.

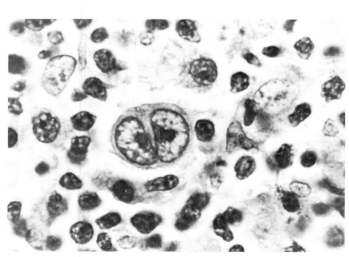

Fig. 12-30. Binucleate Reed-Sternberg cell with large nucleoli and mirror-image nuclei.

Reed and Sternberg described the classic Reed-Sternberg cell as a large cell with multilobed nucleus, often "owl-eye" with two mirror-image nuclei, each containing a single large inclusion-like eosinophilic nucleolus; the cytoplasm is abundant and eosinophilic. This classic Reed-Sternberg cell (Fig. 12-30), in association with the proper background, is essential for a definitive diagnosis of Hodgkin's disease. Many variants of neoplastic cells are recognized; these may be useful in subclassification of the disease, but cannot be used for establishing a definitive diagnosis. In addition to the classic Reed-Sternberg cell, mononuclear variants and lacunar cells may be present. Mononuclear variants have a single nucleus and large eosinophilic nucleoli. Lacunar cells have multilobed nuclei, ample cytoplasm and nucleoli, which are not as prominent as those of the classic Reed-Sternberg cells or mononuclear equivalents (Fig. 12-31). These cells are associated with NS Hodgkin's disease and are surrounded by spaces or lacunae, which represent an artifact of fixation. Another variant—the lymphocyte/histiocyte (L/H) variant—is seen in LP Hodgkin's disease and in the so-called lymphohistiocytic type. L/H variants are polyploid cells. They are large cells with large vesicular nuclei, irregular or folded nuclear membranes, and rather inconspicuous nuclei. These cells are seen in LP Hodgkin's disease and the so-called lymphohistiocytic type.[108]

Another feature of Hodgkin's disease is a cellular polymorphous infiltration of variable numbers of lymphocytes, eosinophils, plasma cells, histiocytes, and less often, neutrophils. Prognosis relates to the degree of lymphocytic infiltration and to the initial peripheral lymphocyte count.

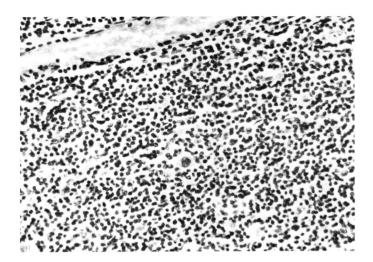

Fig. 12-32. Lymph node showing the changes of lymphocyte predominant Hodgkin's disease. The lymph node structure is lost due to diffuse infiltration with lymphocytes. A single malignant cell lies in the middle of the field.

Lymphocyte Predominance Hodgkin's Disease

Hodgkin cells and Reed-Sternberg cells are scanty, mature small lymphocytes and/or histiocytes are plentiful, and eosinophils and neutrophils are absent. The malignant cells may be very hard to find. In the lymphocytic/histiocytic variant, histiocytes are common, and there are numerous characteristic lymphocytic/histiocytic variant neoplastic cells. The prognosis is very favorable (Figs. 12-32 and 12-33).

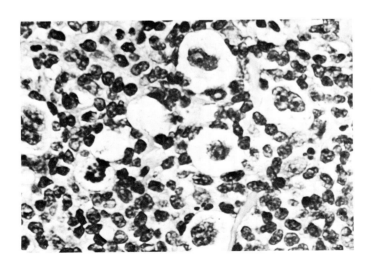

Fig. 12-31. Group of lacunar cells from a lymph node in nodular sclerosing Hodgkin's disease. The characteristic cytoplasmic vacuolation is probably artifactual.

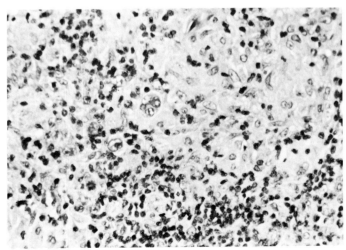

Fig. 12-33. Lymph node showing the changes of the histiocytic variant of lymphocytic predominant Hodgkin's disease (lymphocytic-histiocytic). Two malignant cells and a considerable infiltrate of reactive non-neoplastic histiocytes are present.

Nodular Variant. More recently, a nodular variant of lymphocyte predominance Hodgkin's disease (also referred to as nodular lymphocytic and histiocytic Hodgkin's disease) has been described.[109,110] Difficulties in diagnosis have arisen because it is an uncommon lesion, nodes may be only partially involved and Reed-Sternberg cells are not prominent. Indeed, further confusion arises because of the association between this type of Hodgkin's disease and what has been termed progressive transformation of germinal centers (PTGC).[111]

Progressive Transformation of Germinal Centers. In PTGC, small lymphocytes from the mantle zone grow into and distort and obscure the germinal centers of follicles. The pathogenesis is obscure, and PTGC may be seen in chronic reactive lymphadenitis including viral lymphadenitis and the lymphadenopathy associated with ARC (see Ch. 4). Lymph nodes involved with the nodular variant of lymphocyte predominance Hodgkin's disease present a nodular appearance. Lymphocytic and histiocytic cells are rather easily identified and may occur in small clusters. Reed-Sternberg cells are not prominent and often are extremely hard to find. Immunoperoxidase studies show the nodules to contain many dendritic reticulum cells and polyclonal B-lymphocytes. A few T-lymphocytes, mostly of the T-helper/inducer phenotype, are also present. It has been suggested that this form of lymphocyte-predominant Hodgkin's disease is immunophenotypically distinct from the histologically diffuse form and from the other types of Hodgkin's disease.[112]

Nodular Sclerosing Hodgkin's Disease

Nodular sclerosis may be defined by a histologic triad of sclerosis, lacunar cells, and diagnostic Reed-Sternberg cells. Coarse or fine bands of birefringent collagen divide the node into nodules (Fig. 12-34). Lacunar cells are prominent and frequently occur in clusters or sheets (Fig. 12-31). The term syncytial variant is used to describe cases of NS Hodgkin's disease in which large numbers of these atypical Reed-Sternberg variants are present.[113]

Nodular sclerosing Hodgkin's disease is further subclassified by some as LP, MC, and LD types. All subtypes contain variable numbers of Reed-Sternberg cells, which are few in LP, more readily identified in MC, and predominate in the LD type. It is not universally accepted that this subdivision is useful, but we are currently utilizing it.

Mixed Cellularity Hodgkin's Disease

This form of Hodgkin's disease is intermediate in histologic appearance and prognosis between the LP and LD forms. Reed-Sternberg cells and mononuclear equiva-

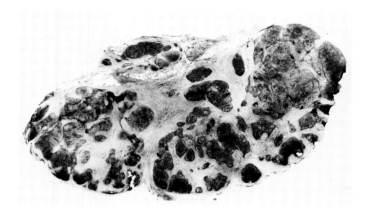

Fig. 12-34. Lymph node showing the gross intersecting bands of fibrous tissue and cellular nodules characteristic of nodular sclerosing Hodgkin's disease.

lents are readily identified. The mixed cellular background contains plasma cells, lymphocytes, eosinophils, and histiocytes. Although this background has been considered the hallmark of MC disease, it need not be present to establish the diagnosis. Hitherto, borderline cases difficult to subclassify have been included in the wastebasket of MC Hodgkin's disease. A more precise method of subclassification that helps in borderline cases is based on strict quantification of Reed-Sternberg cells. MC Hodgkin's disease has been defined as having between 5 and 15 classic Reed-Sternberg cells and mononuclear equivalents per high power field. The LP type has fewer than 5 per high-power field (hpf) and LD has more than 15 per hpf. This criterion has proved very useful in some hands in classifying borderline cases.[114]

Lymphocyte Depletion Hodgkin's Disease

In this form, Reed-Sternberg cells predominate. They are often highly pleomorphic; the overall picture resembles sarcoma. Fibrosis is commonly observed (Fig. 12-35). Two morphologic subtypes have been identified. In the *reticular subtype,* diagnostic Reed-Sternberg cells predominate, which may be of the classic multilobed form or pleomorphic and sarcomatous. There is a definite decrease of lymphocytes, and the polymorphous cellular background is absent. Focal necrosis is commonly observed. There may be varying degrees of fibrosis. In the *diffuse fibrosis subtype,* the prominent feature is disorderly fibrosis. The numbers of Reed-Sternberg cells vary, and often diagnostic Reed-Sternberg cells are rare. Focal necrosis is common. The fibrous tissue is nonbirefringent, in contrast to the fibrosis of NS Hodgkin's disease, which is birefringent.

Some cases of Hodgkin's disease are considered unclassifiable because they do not fit the criteria established

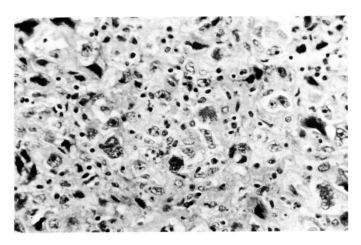

Fig. 12-35. Lymph node showing the changes of lymphocyte depletion Hodgkin's disease. There are numerous pleomorphic malignant cells, fibrosis, and a few scattered lymphocytes.

for classification as LP, NS, MC, or LD types. It may be better to diagnose Hodgkin's disease, not otherwise sub-classified, rather than to include them within the MC category. Cases of so-called interfollicular Hodgkin's disease or focal lymph node involvement can also be included within this category.[107]

Extranodal Hodgkin's disease is also often unclassifiable histologically and may be classified as Hodgkin's disease, not otherwise specified. The surgeon should be encouraged to biopsy a lymph node, if available, in order to establish the diagnosis.

Histogenesis of the Reed-Sternberg Cell

Despite extensive study over many years, the true nature of the Reed-Sternberg cell still remains in doubt. The neoplastic cell has been variously thought to represent a macrophage, B-cell, T-cell, dendritic, or interdigitating reticulum cell. Various attractive theories have been put forward by supporters of the various views. However, to date, the precise nature of the neoplastic cell characteristic of Hodgkin's disease remains elusive.

Differential Diagnosis

The LP form of Hodgkin's disease may show such an intense proliferation of lymphocytes as to resemble small lymphocytic lymphoma (well differentiated lymphocytic lymphoma of Rappaport) or chronic lymphocytic leukemia. The latter can be excluded by hematologic examination. The constant presence of epithelioid histiocytes, either singly or in small groups, is often a pointer to Hodgkin's disease and should initiate a search for Reed-Sternberg cells.

Lymph nodes associated with infectious mononucleo-

sis may contain cells which fit the histologic criteria for so-called classic Reed-Sternberg cells. A detailed clinical history, peripheral blood examination and serology are essential to establish the diagnosis.

Reed-Sternberg-like cells in malignant melanoma may lead to an erroneous diagnosis of Hodgkin's disease. Immunohistochemical and ultrastructural investigation may be necessary to establish a diagnosis.

Carcinoma metastatic to lymph nodes and associated with sclerosis may sometimes be confused with NS Hodgkin's disease. Notable among these is nasopharyngeal carcinoma. Immunohistochemical analysis will demonstrate keratin in the neoplastic cells and ultrastructural evaluation will reveal cell junctions and tonofibrils in the neoplastic cells.

Epithelioid histiocytes are commonly observed in LP and MC Hodgkin's disease. These are also noted in non-Hodgkin's lymphomas including B- and T-cell lymphomas in the low-grade, intermediate-grade, and high-grade categories. Epithelioid histiocytes are also seen in benign lymphadenopathies, including toxoplasmosis, tuberculosis and fungal infections. Adherence to the strict histologic criteria for LP and MC Hodgkin's disease should establish the diagnosis. However, occasional cases will present a true diagnostic problem. Immunohistochemical analysis often proves helpful.[115]

The monoclonal antibody Leu-M1 is particularly useful in the diagnosis of Hodgkin's disease. Reed-Sternberg cells and mononuclear equivalents stain for Leu-M1. This stain can be performed on paraffin sections.

The reticular variant of LD Hodgkin's disease may resemble a sarcoma. Immunohistochemical and ultrastructural studies should establish the diagnosis.

Occasionally, histologic distinction between LD Hodgkin's disease and immunoblastic polymorphous lymphoma (high-grade malignant lymphoma by the working formulation) may be very difficult. This non-Hodgkin's lymphoma may contain many cells fitting the description of classic Reed-Sternberg cells and mononuclear equivalents. These lymphomas may be of B- or T-cell lineage; thus, immunohistologic analysis may be helpful. However, a small proportion of immunoblastic lymphomas may be negative for some of the commonly used monoclonal antibodies, which may confound the picture. Also, Reed-Sternberg cells in Hodgkin's disease may phagocytose immunoglobulin, which may suggest a non-Hodgkin's lymphoma of B-cell lineage. The presence of immunoglobulin in malignant lymphomas is of significance only if determined to be monoclonal. On rare occasions, it may be impossible to distinguish between immunoblastic polymorphous lymphoma and LD Hodgkin's disease. In such cases, it is entirely acceptable to report a case as large cell lymphoreticular malignant neoplasm, either Hodgkin's disease or immunoblastic lymphoma, or comment to the effect that histologic differentiation between the two is impossible.

Relationship Between Subclassification and Prognosis

The LP form and NS (subclassified as LP) carry the best prognosis and LD (including the LD subcategory of NS) the worst prognosis. Average 5-year survival rates for the LP type (including NS with LP subtype) are 47 to 55 percent; MC, 3 to 18 percent; and LD, 0 to 8 percent. Patients with the LD form rarely survive for 10 years. Prognosis in both Hodgkin's disease and non-Hodgkin's lymphomas is also related to clinical staging, and treatment is certainly influenced more by clinical stage than by histologic subtype. The difference in the prognosis of the subtypes of Hodgkin's disease has been reduced by the effectiveness of modern therapy.

Clinical Staging

The universally used Ann Arbor classification[116] is as follows:

> *Stage I:* Involvement of a single lymph node region or involvement of a single extralymphatic organ or site (Ie)
>
> *Stage II:* Involvement of two or more lymph node regions on the same side of the diaphragm or with involvement of limited contiguous extralymphatic organs or tissues (IIe)
>
> *Stage III:* Involvement of lymph node regions on both sides of the diaphragm (III), which may include the spleen (IIIs) and/or limited contiguous extralymphatic organs or sites (IIIe, IIIes)
>
> *Stage IV:* Multiple or disseminated foci of involvement of one or more extralymphatic organs or tissues, with or without lymphatic involvement

All stages are further divided on the basis of the absence (A) or presence (B) of systemic symptoms, that is, fever, night sweats, and/or weight loss of more than 10 percent of normal body weight. As would be expected, the prognosis is better with low stage and A disease.

Laparotomy Staging

The role of laparotomy for pathologic (as opposed to purely clinical) staging of Hodgkin's and non-Hodgkin's lymphomas is disputed. Some authorities believe that clinical staging is still unreliable and that the risk involved in a routine laparotomy is minimal, while others believe that laparotomy should be undertaken only when clinical staging is equivocal or when positive findings at laparotomy will change the stage of the disease sufficiently to alter the therapy.

In most series, the preoperative stage is changed (usually, but not always, to a higher stage) as a result of laparotomy in 30 to 40 percent of cases.

What exactly constitutes a staging laparotomy? The staging procedure has not been standardized throughout the world but entails variations of the following: splenectomy, bone marrow (bilateral iliac crest) and liver biopsies, and biopsies of specified node groups, which include splenic, porta hepatis, paraortic, iliac, and mesenteric.

Postoperative complications appear to be both more frequent and more serious in non-Hodgkin's lymphoma than in Hodgkin's disease, in clinical stage III or IV than in stage I or II disease, and in children than adults. Thus, many authors recommend a less extensive procedure, such as laparotomy without splenectomy or laparoscopy and splenic biopsy, in the higher risk groups.

It is important for the surgical pathologist to process the specimens received from these procedures in a manner that will yield maximal diagnostic information. Lymph nodes should be identified separately as to site and should be processed as described earlier in this chapter. Each liver biopsy specimen should be sectioned at several levels; the spleen should be "bread-loafed" and examined carefully grossly, followed by submission of sections from any suspicious lesions seen, or multiple random sections if gross inspection is negative.

Histologic examination should always be carried out with reference to the initial diagnostic biopsy. For example, a periportal infiltrate of small lymphocytes in the liver is probably of no significance in lymphocyte depletion Hodgkin's disease but should lead to a careful search for malignant cells if the original diagnosis was lymphocyte predominance or nodular sclerosis. Most pathologists do not demand the presence of classic Reed-Sternberg cells in laparotomy material to diagnose Hodgkin's disease if a previous biopsy specimen confirming this diagnosis is available for review and if current material is otherwise consistent with the diagnosis. However, it should be remembered that nonspecific granulomata, lymphoid infiltrates, or foci of fibrosis alone should not be overdiagnosed as tumor, since this may lead to overly aggressive therapy and the complications thereof. Similarly, histologic subtyping can often be performed in nonnodal material if the volume and preservation of tumor are adequate, but subtyping should certainly not be attempted if the diagnostic tumor nodule is minute or largely necrotic.

Non-Hodgkin's Lymphoma

Once the diagnosis of malignant lymphoma has been made, the first decision is whether it is Hodgkin's disease. If it is not, then the overall label is non-Hodgkin's lymphoma. The next step is to decide whether the lesion

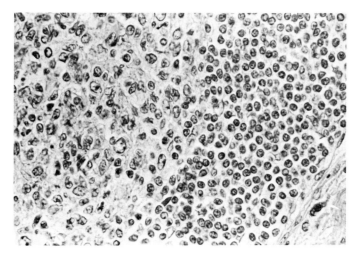

Fig. 12-36. Lymph node showing reactive follicular hyperplasia. Note the clear delineation of the follicle by a rim of small lymphocytes. Within the follicle (left) are seen pleomorphism, nuclear debris, and mitotic activity.

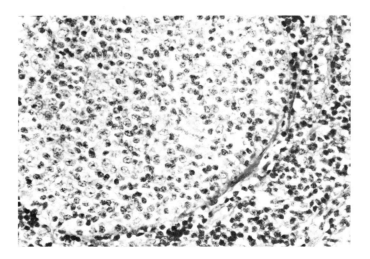

Fig. 12-37. Lymph node showing follicular lymphoma, small cleaved cell type. The nodule illustrated (left) is poorly delineated from internodular cells, and all cells are uniform in appearance.

is follicular (nodular) or diffuse in pattern. Follicular lesions have a better, and diffuse lesions a worse prognosis. Differentiation between follicular lesions and reactive hyperplasia can be very difficult (Figs. 12-36 and 12-37). Some important differential points are listed in Table 12-3.

The next decision is whether the cells are small or large. Nuclear size is used as a major criterion in classification. Lymphoma cells with nuclei smaller than those of nonneoplastic histiocytes or endothelial cells are considered to be of the small cell type and those equal in size to or larger than the nuclei of histiocytes or endothelial cells are considered to be of the large cell type.

A classification of non-Hodgkin's lymphoma devised by Rappaport in 1966[117] was based on morphology, principally on whether the pattern was nodular or diffuse (Table 12-4).

Further subclassification was based on cell types. The term *well differentiated* was used to describe cells that resembled mature lymphocytes. Larger cells were called histiocytes, in the belief that these cells were of histiocytic origin. Cells in between the well differentiated lymphocytic and histiocytic were referred to as undifferentiated. Mixed lymphocytic-histiocytic lymphomas were composed of an admixture of the two cell types. This classification gained wide acceptance.[118]

It was subsequently modified to accommodate such entities as lymphocytic lymphoma of intermediate differentiation and lymphoblastic lymphoma (Table 12-5).

This classification gained in popularity and was widely accepted as being very useful in determining a clinical approach. It is still used as the basic diagnostic language for the communication of therapeutic results among clinicians.

During the 1960s, with advances in knowledge of the immune system came controversy and criticism of the Rappaport classification; in 1974, a new classification emerged, immunologically based, largely on the newly discovered B- and T-cell systems, and hypotheses on lymphocyte transformation in follicles (Table 12-6).[119]

TABLE 12-3. Differential Diagnosis of Follicular Hyperplasia Versus Nodular Lymphoma

Histologic Criteria	Hyperplasia	Lymphoma
Nodal architecture	Retained	Obliterated (partially or totally)
Follicles/nodules	Mainly cortical and variable in size and shape; cells variable in size, with large phagocytic cells (tingible bodies) and mitotic activity	Nodules distributed throughout the node and relatively uniform in size; nodules composed of generally uniform neoplastic cells
Interfollicular/nodular areas	Predominantly lymphocytes with scattered macrophages, plasma cells, eosinophils, and neutrophils	Cells similar to those in the nodules (except in very early disease limited to nodules)
Follicle/nodule boundaries	Well delineated by a rim of small lymphocytes	Boundaries not well defined; cells within nodules often appear to spill out into surrounding tissue
Capsule	Usually not infiltrated (but moderate degrees of infiltration may be present)	Often infiltrated

**TABLE 12-4. Malignant
Non-Hodgkin's Lymphomas:
Classification of Rappaport**

Nodular or Diffuse
Lymphocytic, well differentiated
Lymphocytic, poorly differentiated
Mixed lymphocytic-histiocytic
Histiocytic
Undifferentiated

**TABLE 12-5. Malignant
Non-Hodgkin's Lymphomas:
Modified Rappaport Classification**

Nodular
    Lymphocytic, poorly differentiated
    Mixed lymphohistiocytic-histiocytic
    Histiocytic

Diffuse
    Lymphocytic, well differentiated
    Lymphocytic, intermediate differentiation
    Lymphocytic, poorly differentiated
    Mixed lymphocytic-histiocytic
    Lymphoblastic
        Convoluted
        Nonconvoluted
    Undifferentiated, Burkitt's type
    Undifferentiated non-Burkitt's type
    Histiocytic
    Lymphocytic

**TABLE 12-6. Malignant Non-Hodgkin's Lymphomas:
Lukes and Collins Classification**

Undefined cell types

T-cell types
    Small lymphocytic
    Mycosis fungoides/Sézary syndrome (cerebriform)
    Convoluted lymphocytic
    Immunoblastic sarcoma (T-cell)

B-cell types
    Small lymphocytic (CLL)
    Plasmacytoid lymphocytic
    Follicular center cell (FCC) types (follicular, diffuse, follicular and
        diffuse, and sclerotic)
        Small cleaved
        Large cleaved
        Small noncleaved
        Large noncleaved
        Immunoblastic sarcoma (B-cell)

Histiocytic type

Unclassifiable

Numerous classifications, different in approach and nomenclature, have since appeared, causing considerable confusion. In September 1976, an international multi-institutional clinical-pathologic study was sponsored by the National Cancer Institute in Bethesda, Maryland, to compare the value of the six major classifications. On the basis of this study a new Working Formulation of non-Hodgkin's lymphoma for clinical usage was introduced.[120,121]

This is not to be considered as an entirely new classification, but rather as a common language of communication, by which all previous classifications can be translated from one scheme to another. The working formulation is based on prognostic significance, and non-Hodgkin's lymphomas are subdivided into three prognostic groups: (1) low grade, with a median survival of 6.0 years; (2) intermediate grade, with a median survival of 3.5 years; and (3) high grade, with a median survival of 1.4 years (Table 12-7). It should be emphasized that these prognostic figures relate to the first diagnostic lymph node biopsy of an untreated patient.

Low-Grade Lymphomas

Malignant Lymphoma, Small Lymphocytic. This low-grade malignant lymphoma (Rappaport equivalent: malignant lymphoma, diffuse, well differentiated lymphocytic), is usually seen in adults over age 40, with a peak in the sixth decade. Lymph nodes, bone marrow, blood, spleen and liver may be involved. Lymphadenopathy is usually generalized. Most small lymphocytic neoplasms are of the B-cell type. Confusion in terminology may arise in the small lymphocytic lymphomas when there is bone marrow and blood involvement. Often it is not clear whether a process should be called chronic lymphocytic leukemia (CLL) or small lymphocytic lymphoma with involvement of the bone marrow and peripheralization of lymphocytes. For practical purposes, lymph node and bone marrow involvement without peripheral blood lymphocytosis should be referred to as malignant lymphoma, small lymphocytic, and when there is peripheral blood involvement (absolute lymphocyte count greater than 4,000 per mm) the diagnosis should be malignant lymphoma, small lymphocytic, with CLL.

The lymph node is effaced by a diffuse monotonous proliferation of small lymphocytes. The nuclei are round and cytoplasm is scanty. Chromatin is clumped and occasional small nucleoli may be seen. Mitotic activity is low. Infiltration of the capsule and perinodal tissues, when present, is a helpful diagnostic clue. Occasional larger lymphocytes (prolymphocytes) with more prominent nucleoli are usually seen. Occasional immature cells with the appearance of blasts may also be noted. These larger cells may be scattered and few in number or may form

**TABLE 12-7. Malignant Non-Hodgkin's Lymphomas:
The New Working Formulation**

Working Formulation	Rappaport Equivalent
Low grade	
Malignant lymphoma (small lymphocytic)	Well differentiated lymphocytic
Consistent with CLL	
Plasmacytoid	
Malignant lymphoma, follicular (predominantly small cleaved cell)	Nodular poorly differentiated lymphocytic
Diffuse areas	
Sclerosis	
Malignant lymphoma, follicular (mixed small cleaved and large cell)	Nodular mixed cell
Diffuse areas	
Sclerosis	
Intermediate Grade	
Malignant lymphoma, follicular (predominantly large cell)	Nodular histiocytic
Diffuse areas	
Sclerosis	
Malignant lymphoma, diffuse (small cleaved cell)	Diffuse poorly differentiated lymphocytic
Sclerosis	
Malignant lymphoma, diffuse (mixed small and large cell)	Diffuse mixed cell (lymphocytic-histiocytic)
Sclerosis	
Epithelioid cell component	
Malignant lymphoma, diffuse (large cell)	Diffuse histiocytic
Cleaved cell	
Noncleaved cell	
Sclerosis	
High grade	
Malignant lymphoma (large cell, immunoblastic)	Diffuse histiocytic
Plasmacytoid	
Clear cell	
Polymorphous	
Epithelioid cell component	
Malignant lymphoma (lymphoblastic)	Lymphoblastic
Convoluted cell	
Nonconvoluted cell	
Malignant lymphoma (small noncleaved cell)	Diffuse undifferentiated
Burkitt's	Burkitt's
Follicular areas	Non-Burkitt's

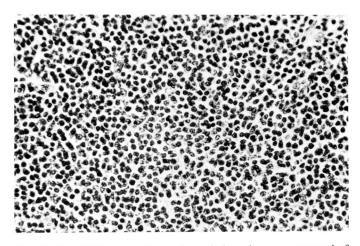

Fig. 12-38. Diffuse small lymphocytic lymphoma composed of small lymphocytes of monomorphic appearance.

Malignant Lymphoma, Small Lymphocytic, Plasmacytoid. The node is effaced by a population of small lymphocytes, lymphocytes with a plasmacytoid appearance, and plasma cells. Plasmacytoid cells have increased cytoplasm. The nucleus may be somewhat eccentric and the nuclear chromatin is usually that of a small lymphocyte. These cells and plasma cells are pyroninophilic and frequently demonstrate PAS-positive cytoplasmic (Russell body) and nuclear (Dutcher body) inclusions. Serum protein studies frequently reveal a monoclonal gammopathy. Lymph nodes involved in *Waldenstrom's macroglobulinemia* will show a similar appearance (Fig. 12-39).

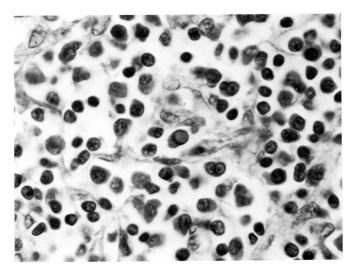

Fig. 12-39. Malignant lymphoma, small lymphocytic, plasmacytoid. Note eccentrically situated lymphocyte-like nuclei, some of which (center) contain inclusions (Dutcher bodies).

focal aggregates imparting to the node a follicular appearance. These aggregates have been referred to as immature foci or pseudofollicular proliferation centers or growth centers. They should not be interpreted as follicular lymphoma or mixed small and large cell lymphoma. When bone marrow is involved, the lymphocytic infiltrate is diffuse. A marrow lymphocytosis of greater than 40 percent in a cellular bone marrow is considered diagnostic of involvement (Fig. 12-38).

The spleen is commonly involved in malignant lymphoma, small lymphocytic. Small lymphocytes usually involve the white pulp and expand into the red pulp. The cords and sinuses of the red pulp will also show lymphocytosis.

When the liver is involved, the infiltrate is predominantly portal. However, when there is peripheral blood involvement, sinusoidal infiltration will also be present.

Proliferation of epithelioid histiocytes, singly or in small aggregates, is not unusual in small lymphocytic lymphomas and is of no prognostic significance.

Large cell lymphomas have been described as occurring in patients who have had malignant lymphoma, small lymphocytic, or CLL for a long time. When accompanied by B symptoms, such as fever and weight loss, this is referred to as *Richter's syndrome*. It is uncertain whether the large cell lymphomas arise as a result of transformation of the small lymphocytic tumor or whether they arise de novo. However, the former is considered more likely.

Malignant Lymphoma, Follicular, Small Cleaved. This is also a low-grade malignant lymphoma (Rappaport equivalent: malignant lymphoma, nodular, poorly differentiated lymphocytic), which characteristically occurs in the middle and older age groups. The disease is characterized by a protracted clinical course, and most patients have evidence of widespread disease at the time of initial diagnosis. In spite of this, the prognosis is favorable. These lymphomas are of follicular center cell origin and have a unique nodular or follicular growth pattern. This growth characteristic and protracted clinical course led to considerable controversy as to whether this was truly a lymphoma. Sometimes distinguishing between reactive follicular hyperplasia and follicular lymphoma can be difficult (Table 12-3).

The statistical analysis of certain morphologic parameters, including architectural and cytologic features, may distinguish between follicular lymphoma and follicular hyperplasia.[122]

Normal lymph node architecture is altered by the presence of numerous nodules that are fairly uniform in size. These involve the cortex and medulla and often extend into perinodal fibroadipose tissue. Lymph nodes may be partially involved; often coalescence of nodules may present the appearance of a diffuse peripheral cuff of lymphocytes. Intervening tissue between nodules is compressed and often the nodules appear to be back-to-back with negligible intervening tissue. The cells comprising the nodules are monotonous and consist predominantly of small cleaved lymphocytes that are slightly larger than normal lymphocytes. Nuclei have irregular to cleaved margins and small nucleoli. The cytoplasm is scanty. A few larger cells are usually present, but these account for less than 20 percent of the neoplastic cells. There is a paucity of mitotic figures and phagocytosis within the neoplastic nodules. In a majority of involved lymph nodes, neoplastic cells are observed outside the nodules.

The bone marrow is involved in approximately 50 to 60 percent of cases at diagnosis. Characteristically, the neoplastic infiltrates are focal, paratrabecular in distribution and may be associated with an increase in reticulin fibers. Peripheralization of neoplastic cells results in what has been referred to as lymphosarcoma cell leukemia. The neoplastic cells appear as indented to deeply cleaved lymphocytes.

Malignant Lymphoma, Follicular, Mixed, Small Cleaved and Large Cell Type. The nodules are composed of an admixture of small cleaved lymphocytes and large cells (Rappaport: nodular, mixed lymphocytic-histiocytic lymphoma) (Fig. 12-40). The small cleaved lymphocytes are identical to those described in follicular lymphoma, small cleaved cell type. The large cells are at least twice the size of a small lymphocyte, with round vesicular nuclei and one to three prominent nucleoli. Mitoses are fairly frequent. At times, a pathologist may experience difficulty in classifying a follicular lymphoma as follicular small cleaved or mixed. It is recommended that in the mixed lymphoma, large cells within the follicle should account for greater than 20 percent but less than 50 percent of the neoplastic population. This is a rather imprecise method of subclassification and often has had poor reproducibility among reviewers. Although both are considered low grade malignant lymphomas, it is important to be able to diagnose the mixed category, as at this time these are treated more aggressively by clinicians.

Bone marrow involvement varies from approximately 20 to 40 percent and is also focal and paratrabecular in distribution.

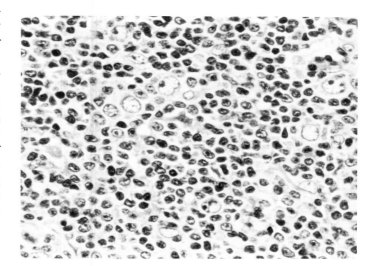

Fig. 12-40. Follicular mixed cell lymphoma. The lesion is composed of a mixture of small cleaved and large cells.

The low grade follicular lymphomas may have diffuse areas and may be accompanied by sclerosis. Focal areas of diffuse involvement do not alter the prognosis, which is still considered favorable in terms of survival. Some authors believe that prominent sclerosis is associated with a better prognosis, while others are unable to demonstrate improved survival in cases with sclerosis.

Intermediate Grade Lymphoma

Malignant Lymphoma, Follicular, Large Cell Type. This lymphoma (Rappaport equivalent: malignant lymphoma, nodular, histiocytic) is relatively rare. Large cells predominate and may be cleaved or noncleaved (Fig. 12-41). These large cells are two to three times the size of a small lymphocyte and have irregular to cleaved nuclear margins, small nucleoli and scanty cytoplasm. The large noncleaved cells have round vesicular nuclei and one to three prominent nucleoli. Mitoses are frequent and often numerous, indicating a higher cell turnover rate. Bone marrow involvement is rare.

The white pulp of the spleen is involved in approximately 50 percent of follicular lymphomas. The cells are similar to those described for lymph node involvement.

Malignant Lymphoma, Diffuse, Small Cleaved Cell Type. This B-cell lymphoma arises from follicular center cells of the germinal center and represents the diffuse counterpart of the follicular lymphoma, small cleaved cell type (Rappaport equivalent: malignant lymphoma, diffuse, poorly differentiated lymphocytic) (Figs. 12-42 and 12-43).

Malignant Lymphoma, Diffuse, Mixed, Small Cleaved and Large Cell Type. These lymphomas are aggressive and may be of B- or T-cell type (Rappaport equivalent:

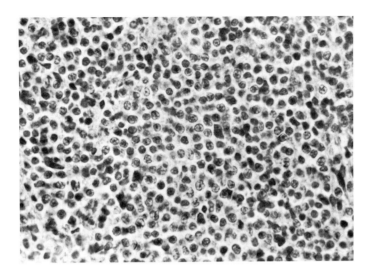

Fig. 12-42. Diffuse small cleaved cell lymphoma. The component cells are small and large lymphocytes with nuclei varying in size and shape.

malignant lymphoma, diffuse, lymphocytic-histiocytic). They are composed of an admixture of small cleaved and large cells similar to those described for the follicular mixed lymphoma.

Malignant Lymphoma, Diffuse, Large Cell Type. Large cell lymphomas represent approximately 30 percent of adult and childhood aggressive non-Hodgkin's lymphomas and may be of B- or T-cell origin (Rappaport equivalent: malignant lymphoma, diffuse, histiocytic). Approximately 40 percent are considered to be of T-cell origin.

Neoplastic cells may be either large cleaved or non-cleaved cells (Fig. 12-44). Necrosis is fairly common, and there may be accompanying sclerosis.

Lymphocytic Lymphoma of Intermediate Differentiation. This is a relatively rare lymphoma that occurs predominantly in the older age group. It is not yet accepted by all as a separate entity, distinct from lymphocytic lymphoma, poorly differentiated.[123] The term is used to describe cases intermediate between the small lymphocytic and small cleaved cell types of malignant lymphoma. The node is effaced by a population of small, round lymphocytes, small cleaved lymphocytes and cells intermediate between these two, with slightly irregular nuclear margins and coarse chromatin. Occasional large lymphoid cells may occur singly or in clusters imparting a pseudo-follicular appearance. An occasional germinal center-like structure may also be present. The bone marrow is involved in most cases at the time of presentation.

High Grade Lymphomas

Malignant Lymphoma, Diffuse, Large Cell, Immunoblastic. This is a highly aggressive high-grade malignant lym-

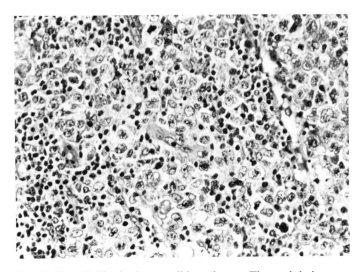

Fig. 12-41. Follicular large cell lymphoma. The nodule is composed predominantly of large cleaved cells.

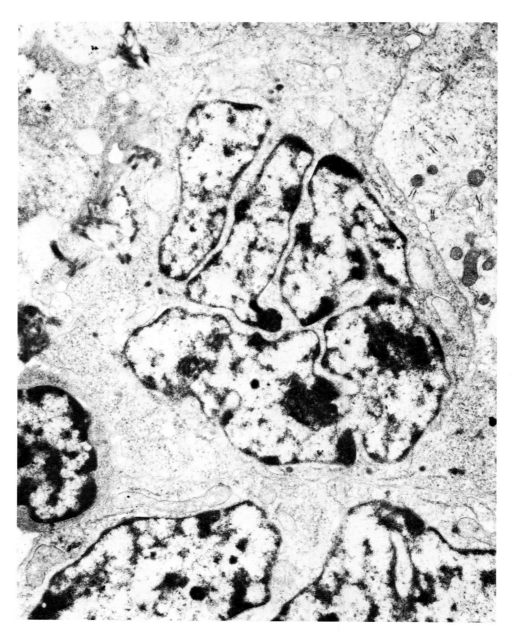

Fig. 12-43. Electron micrograph of small cleaved cell lymphoma showing deeply indented nucleus, characteristic of follicular origin. (×13,400)

phoma that may be of B- or T-cell origin (Rappaport equivalent: malignant lymphoma, diffuse, histiocytic). The node is effaced by a monotonous population of large lymphoid cells that have the appearance of transformed lymphocytes. The cells have round, vesicular nuclei with prominent central nucleoli. The cytoplasm exhibits pyroninophilia. Some cells may exhibit plasmacytoid features and these are usually of B-cell origin.

A polymorphous variant of immunoblastic lymphoma, in addition to the cells described above, also has multinucleated and pleomorphic cells with prominent nucleoli,

which may be indistinguishable from lymphocyte-depleted Hodgkin's disease.

All the malignant lymphomas described so far, irrespective of whether they are of B- or T-cell origin, may be associated with a proliferation of epithelioid cells. This does not in any way alter the behavior or prognosis of the lymphoma.

Lymphoblastic Lymphoma. This high-grade, very aggressive malignant lymphoma (Rappaport equivalent: lymphoblastic lymphoma) occurs most frequently in ado-

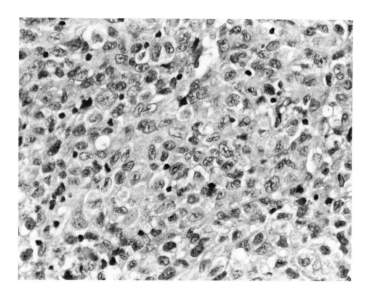

Fig. 12-44. Diffuse large cell lymphoma showing replacement of lymph node by large cells, predominantly noncleaved, as large as or larger than a histiocyte.

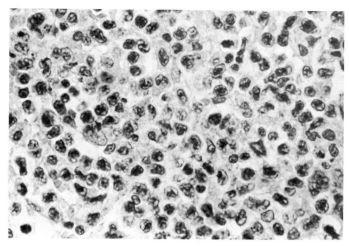

Fig. 12-45. Malignant lymphoblastic lymphoma of childhood. The node is diffusely infiltrated with immature convoluted lymphocytes. This tumor was of thymic origin.

lescents with a male preponderance. It constitutes approximately 30 percent of all childhood lymphomas and less than 5 percent of all adult lymphomas. Involvement of mediastinal lymph nodes and bone marrow is common, as is central nervous system involvement. When the peripheral blood is involved, it is difficult to determine whether the process represents acute lymphoblastic leukemia or lymphoblastic lymphoma. The majority of these lymphomas (approximately 70 percent) are of T-cell origin, as is the acute lymphoblastic leukemia in cases in which there is peripheralization.

Lymph nodes may show localization of the neoplastic cells to the T-zone areas, or the node may be entirely effaced. The cells are monotonous, noncohesive, and small with round nuclei and fine dusty chromatin. Nucleoli are inconspicuous, and cytoplasmic margins are indistinct. Frequent mitoses are noted. Necrosis is common, as is a proliferation of histiocytes that may impart a starry-sky appearance and lead to an erroneous diagnosis of Burkitt's lymphoma. Occasionally, the nuclei may appear convoluted. Thus, the neoplastic cells in lymphoblastic lymphoma may be convoluted or nonconvoluted (Fig. 12-45).

Malignant Lymphoma, Small, Noncleaved, Burkitt's Type. Burkitt's lymphoma (Rappaport equivalent: malignant lymphoma, undifferentiated, Burkitt's type) was first described in Uganda by Burkitt, a surgeon, in 1958. He reported that round cell sarcomas occurred with great frequency in the jaws of children in East Africa.[124] These children presented with facial tumors and rarely with abdominal tumors.

In 1964, Epstein, Achong and Barr first observed the DNA herpes virus now known as the Epstein-Barr virus (EBV) in a cultured Burkitt's cell line. In 1965, O'Conor and Dorfman independently reported similar cases in retrospective reviews of childhood lymphomas in the United States.[125,126] In both the endemic (African) and nonendemic (North American and other) forms, the disease occurs over a wide age range, but it is most common in children, with the African variety being commonest between the ages of 6 and 8 years and the American variety between the ages of 10 and 12 years.

Jaw tumors predominate in the African variety, while abdominal and pelvic (particularly ovarian) tumors predominate in the North American variety. Notable in both is the lack of prominence of peripheral lymphadenopathy. The clinical and pathologic features of the American patients have been well defined.[127,128] Burkitt's lymphoma comprises approximately one third of all childhood non-Hodgkin's lymphomas in the United States.

Burkitt's lymphoma is a tumor of B-cell origin. Histologically, there is a diffuse infiltrate of closely packed small noncleaved lymphoid cells (Figs. 12-46 and 12-47). Usually, there are interspersed large macrophages containing cellular debris, imparting to the node the so-called starry-sky appearance. The tumor cells are monotonous and approximate the size of the macrophage nuclei. They have coarse nuclear chromatin and two to five small basophilic nucleoli, and the cytoplasm contains fat vacuoles which can be demonstrated by an oil red O stain on frozen section, by air-dried imprints of fresh tissue, or by electron microscopy. In addition, the cytoplasm is intensely pyroninophilic. Necrosis is common, and the mi-

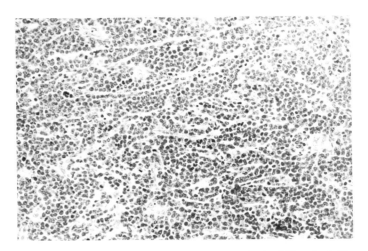

Fig. 12-46. Burkitt's lymphoma. The node is diffusely infiltrated with lymphocytes; scattered throughout are numerous pale histiocytes, giving a starry-sky appearance.

totic index is high. Occasionally, Burkitt's lymphoma may involve germinal centers (follicular), sparing other portions of the node. Specific cytogenic abnormalities have been identified that correlate with the B-cell phenotype of this neoplasm.[129]

Antibodies to the Epstein-Barr virus and EBV genome within the neoplastic cells can be demonstrated in nearly all the African cases and much more variably in the American cases. In addition, higher antibody titers are found in younger patients.

Malignant Lymphoma, Small, Noncleaved (non-Burkitt's). This is a very aggressive lymphoma (Rappaport equivalent: malignant lymphoma, undifferentiated, non-Burkitt's) that normally occurs in adults in the third and fourth decades. Tumors are composed of cells which often resemble Burkitt's lymphoma. However, the cell population is not as monotonous as in Burkitt's lymphoma. The cell size approximates that of a macrophage nucleus. However, there is much more variation in nuclear size and shape than is seen in Burkitt's lymphoma. Occasional multinucleated cells are noted. Nuclear chromatin is delicate, and cells often have a prominent centrally situated nucleolus.

Diffuse Lymphoma With High Content of Epithelioid Histiocytes. This lymphoma, also called lymphoepithelioid cell lymphoma or Lennert's lymphoma, was first described by Lennert and Mestdagh.[130] Although it has since been reviewed by many authors, it remains an ill defined clinical and morphologic entity.[131] It was suggested that it may represent a variant of Hodgkin's disease, although now it is believed that Lennert's lymphoma is a non-Hodgkin's lymphoma. The patients are usually elderly and present with generalized lymphadenopathy and B symptoms. Nodes are effaced by a population of small cleaved and large cells accompanied by diffuse proliferation of epithelioid histiocytes (Fig. 12-48). Occasional cells with the appearance of immunoblasts and cells resembling Reed-Sternberg cells may be present. Most of these cases have proved to be of T-cell origin. This is considered to be a high-grade malignant lymphoma.

Lymph Nodes in Cutaneous T-Cell Lymphoma

Mycoses fungoides and the Sézary syndrome are referred to as cutaneous T-cell lymphomas. These lymphoproliferative disorders are characterized by cutaneous infiltration of atypical or frankly neoplastic T-lymphocytes that have a special affinity for the epidermis and superfi-

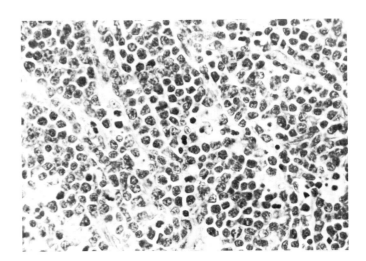

Fig. 12-47. Burkitt's lymphoma. Detail of Figure 12-46. Lymphocytes are monomorphic, small, and noncleaved.

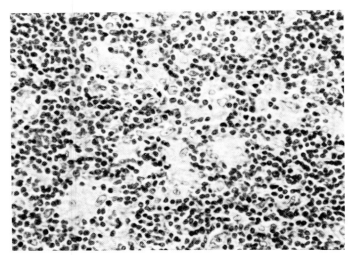

Fig. 12-48. Lennert's lymphoma. Lymph node showing an infiltrate of clusters of large pale epithelioid histiocytes.

cial dermis. In Sézary syndrome, the abnormal cells circulate in the peripheral blood and are always of the small convoluted or cerebriform type.

Lymphadenopathy reflects involvement secondary to drainage from diseased cutaneous sites. Axillary and inguinal nodes are most commonly involved. Involved nodes usually show nonspecific hyperplasia and/or focal fibrosis. Dermatopathic lymphadenitis is a prominent feature. Histologically, there is a proliferation of abnormal lymphoid cells which fall into two distinct categories: (1) small cells with deeply indented, cleaved, or cerebriform nuclei; and (2) large cells with hyperchromatic nuclei with or without nuclear indentations, referred to as MF cells.

Nodes involved by mycoses fungoides may be partially or totally effaced by an infiltrate of neoplastic cells which may occur in small clusters, larger aggregates, or in sheets which may totally replace the node (Fig. 12-49).

In an attempt to evaluate the significance of atypical lymphocytes in lymph nodes showing dermatopathic lymphadenitis in cases of mycoses fungoides, a histologic classification scheme was suggested. Lymph nodes are designated LN-0 through LN-4, with LN-0 representing lymph nodes with no atypical lymphocytes and LN-4 representing partial or complete replacement of nodal architecture by atypical or frankly neoplastic cells.[132–134]

Composite and Other Rare Lymphomas

It is not rare for a patient to have two distinct lymphomatous lesions at different sites. Usually the term composite lymphoma is reserved for the occurrence of two distinctly different types of non-Hodgkin's lymphoma (e.g., small cleaved and large cell type), occurring in the same tissue or anatomic site. The rare occurrence of Hodgkin's disease and non-Hodgkin's lymphoma in the

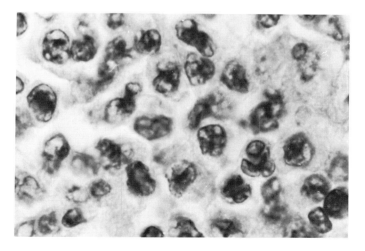

Fig. 12-49. Mycosis fungoides showing cells with large indented to cerebriform nuclei.

same tissue or anatomic site is considered by most to represent the chance occurrence of two different disease processes rather than a composite lymphoma. The behavior and prognosis are those of the most aggressive component.

A number of lymphomas do not fit neatly into any of the above classifications, and new entities gradually become known. For example, there is a rare lymphoma (*signet ring cell lymphoma*) composed of cells resembling signet ring cells, which proves on immunohistochemical analysis to contain immunoglobulin, not mucin.[135] Another lesion or group of lesions is characterized by the presence of numerous long filiform process (*filiform large cell lymphoma*[136]). Diagnosis in each case requires electron microscopic and immunohistochemical analysis. The prognosis of such lesions, until further elucidated, should be regarded as that of large cell lymphoma.

Malignant Histiocytosis and True Histiocytic Lymphoma

Malignant histiocytosis was described by Rappaport as "a systemic progressive invasive proliferation of morphologically atypical histiocytes and their precursors."[137]

True histiocytic lymphomas are usually localized tumors which may or may not progress to disseminated disease. There is some dispute as to the genuine incidence of true histiocytic lymphoma, and there may be genuine geographic variations.

Both are considered to represent malignant tumors of true histiocytes or macrophages. Lymph nodes are enlarged in about 50 percent of the cases. There is a proliferation of cytologically atypical histiocytes showing evidence of phagocytosis. The histiocytes may contain red blood cells, leukocytes, hemosiderin, cholesterol and sudanophilic lipid.

Neoplastic cells are large, with nuclei that are usually lobulated, with finely granular chromatin and one or two eosinophilic nucleoli. The cytoplasm may be vacuolated. Variable numbers of plasma cells are usually present. Pleomorphism may be marked, and cells that resemble Reed-Sternberg cells may occur (Fig. 12-50).

Ultrastructural examination (Fig. 12-51) and immunologic and cytochemical marker studies are necessary to establish the histiocytic origin of the malignant cells. Cells are usually positive for α_1-antitrypsin, which can be demonstrated in paraffin sections. Special stains are best performed on touch imprints, air-dried smears, or frozen sections. The malignant cells show diffuse reactivity for nonspecific esterase using the α-naphtholbutyrate esterase reaction. Activity is usually inhibited by fluoride. Cells also show diffuse positivity for acid phosphatase, β-glucuronidase, and α_1-antitrypsin. Lysozyme is present inconsistently in the malignant histiocytes and often may

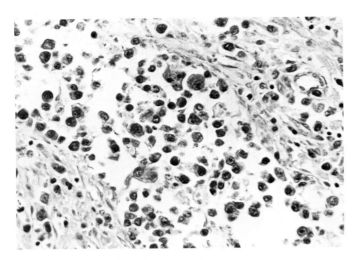

Fig. 12-50. Lymph node sinusoid containing numerous pleomorphic malignant cells, some evidently phagocytic, in malignant histiocytosis.

not be demonstrable. Immunologic markers show the cells to have the phenotype of mononuclear phagocytes.[138,139]

A characteristic pattern of involvement of reticuloendothelial tissues is noted. In the lymph nodes, the sinuses are involved, as are the sinusoids of the liver and the red pulp of the spleen. Bone involvement is often extensive and results in lytic lesions. Skin and GI tract are commonly involved in malignant histiocytosis.

Malignant histiocytosis and true histiocytic lymphoma occur most commonly in adults. Hepatosplenomegaly is common in malignant histiocytosis and is rare in true histiocytic lymphoma.

The condition *histiocytic medullary reticulosis,* described by Scott and Robb-Smith[140] and characterized by the syndrome of pancytopenia, fever, hepatosplenomegaly and jaundice, is considered by some to be a variant of malignant histiocytosis. This syndrome is rarely seen in association with malignant histiocytosis and true histiocytic lymphoma, and histiocytic medullary reticulosis is often considered to be associated more with the erythrophagocytic syndromes, which are reactive conditions related to viral infections.

Hemophagocytic Syndromes

Familial erythrophagocytic lymphohistiocytosis is a rare, rapidly fatal disorder that occurs in children, usually under the age of five years.[141] It is characterized by fever, hepatosplenomegaly with abnormal liver function tests, pancytopenia and lymphadenopathy. The mode of inheritance of the disease is autosomal recessive. Familial erythrophagocytic lymphohistiocytosis is thought to

represent an infection (usually virus)-associated hemophagocytic syndrome in immunodeficient children. Both cellular and humoral immunity are impaired. The reticuloendothelial organs, including the lymph nodes, liver, spleen and bone marrow, are extensively infiltrated by histiocytes with prominent erythrophagocytosis. The histiocytes appear morphologically benign, and immunoperoxidase studies identify the histiocytes as belonging to the mononuclear phagocytic system with a phenotype of sinus histiocytes.

Risdall et al.[142] described a *virus-associated hemophagocytic syndrome* in 1979. Viruses incriminated were the herpes and adenoviruses.[142] Many other infections have since been associated with the syndrome, including viral infection with CMV, EBV, and the parainfluenza virus, and bacterial, fungal and parasitic infections.

Patients present with peripheral blood cytopenias that may be profound, with abnormal coagulation parameters, and with hepatosplenomegaly with abnormal liver-function tests. There is striking histiocytic proliferation in the bone marrow, splenic red pulp, hepatic sinusoids and lymph node sinuses. This is associated with marked erythrophagocytosis and sometimes with leukophagocytosis. The histiocytes appear morphologically benign. Patients at risk to develop this disorder appear to be those with some degree of immunodeficiency. If a cause of immunodeficiency can be identified and removed, or if an infection can be identified and expeditiously treated, most patients will recover with supportive care. The failure to diagnosis this essentially benign disorder, and thus the lack of supportive care, has led to its being associated with a high mortality rate. Hemophagocytic syndromes have also been reported in association with malignant lymphomas and leukemias, most often of T-cell phenotype.

Leukemic Infiltration of Lymph Nodes

In several other lymphoreticular lesions, the lymph nodes, while commonly affected, rarely present as a problem to the surgical pathologist. In *chronic leukemic reticuloendotheliosis* (*hairy cell leukemia*), cells with long processes containing tartrate-resistant acid phosphatase infiltrate the node. In *myeloid* leukemia, the node is infiltrated by myeloid cells of varying degrees of maturity, distinguishable by a positive naphthol-ASD-esterase reaction. In disseminated *mastocytosis*, the node is infiltrated by cells that stain metachromatically with toluidine blue. In *lymphocytic leukemia,* the histologic appearance may mimic closely that of malignant lymphoma. In *Waldenstrom's macroglobulinemia,* infiltrates of atypical plasmacytoid cells are seen. In all these situations, diagnosis must be based on hematologic and clinical as well

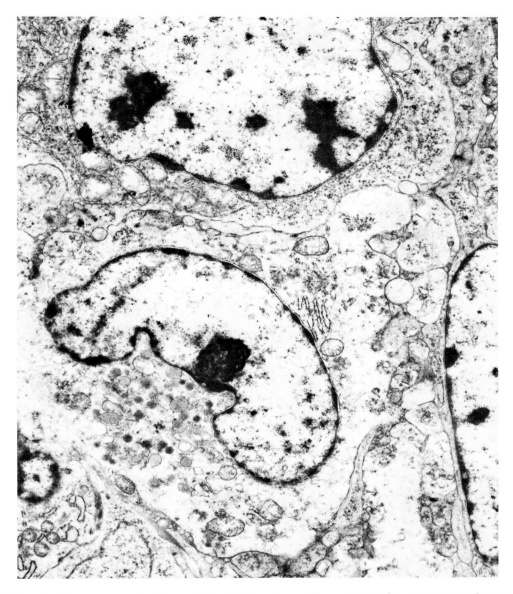

Fig. 12-51. Electron micrograph of true histiocytic lymphoma. The numerous lysosomes near the concavity of the nucleus indicate histiocytic origin. The large nucleolus suggests that the cell is part of the neoplastic cell population. (×12,500)

as histologic data. *Extramedullary hemopoiesis* in lymph nodes is rare and can only be absolutely distinguished morphologically from leukemic infiltration by the presence of megakaryocytes.

Lipid Histiocytoses

In a number of disorders, the macrophages of the reticuloendothelial system may store excessive amounts of various lipids. For instance, in *Hand-Schüller-Christian disease*—a systemic, often febrile, slowly progressive,

but not always fatal, disorder of childhood—granulomatous lesions are found in skull, bones, lungs, skin, and reticuloendothelial system. The lymph node lesion is an infiltrate of eosinophils and large macrophages containing cholesterol and granules similar to those of Langerhans cells. Rarely, *eosinophilic granuloma* may manifest as a lymph node lesion.[143] The overall structure of the node is retained, with normal lymphoid follicles; there is a florid sinus histiocytosis and a heavy infiltrate with eosinophils, sometimes forming abscesses. In a group of rare congenital disorders due to enzyme defects, sphingolipids accumulate in the reticuloendothelial system. The best known

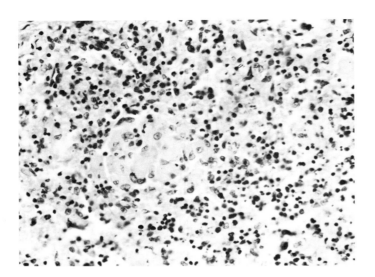

Fig. 12-52. Lymph node infiltrated with large pale histiocytic cells in Gaucher's disease.

of these is *Gaucher's disease,* in which large histiocytes contain PAS-positive and Sudan black B-positive fibrils, granules, and at the ultrastructural level, elongated rod-shaped inclusions. These histiocytes can be found infiltrating the lymph nodes (Fig. 12-52), although this is not a presenting feature. Similarly, In *Niemann-Pick disease,* foamy histiocytes are found in lymph nodes; these stain positively with PAS and acid hematin but poorly with Sudan IV.

HISTOPATHOLOGY OF THE SPLEEN

Examination of the Spleen

The histologic examination of the spleen is a problem that presents itself less often to the pathologist than does the examination of lymph nodes.[144–148] Spleens are removed because of splenomegaly, often in the presence of an obscure hemolytic anemia; because of rupture, often in the presence of acute splenic enlargement; as a diagnostic staging procedure in lymphoma; and as a matter of surgical convenience during gastrectomy. The histology of the spleen at necropsy frequently presents problems, partly due to autolysis.

The hilar fibrous and fatty tissues and lymph nodes should be dissected off, and the splenic vein opened. The organ should be measured, weighed and gently palpated, and then sliced with a long sharp knife, in a consistent axis (usually the short axis) into slices 5 mm to 1 cm thick. Each section should be inspected. Depending upon the indication for removal, from six to 12 blocks should

be taken, preferably from regions where the white pulp is prominent, but including normal areas. A lymph node protocol should be followed. A lymph node is usually present in the hilum; this should be examined histologically. The weight of the spleen varies very widely with body weight, and (in autopsy specimens) with the manner of dying and the degree of terminal venous congestion. A spleen weighing more than 250 g is probably abnormal, and one weighing more than 300 g is almost certainly abnormal.

A discussion of the histopathology of the spleen falls into an analysis of the tissue reactions and the specific lesions.

Normal Histology

The structure of the spleen may be best understood by reference to the pathway of blood through it (Figs. 12-53 to 12-55). The branches of the splenic artery run in fibrous trabeculae that are continuous with the splenic capsule. Branches emerge from the trabeculae into masses of lymphoreticular tissue, the white pulp. Each mass of white pulp has an eccentric artery; some of its blood is distributed by capillary branches in the white pulp or into the marginal sinusoids at the edge of the white pulp. Other small arteries run directly from the white pulp into the red pulp and branch into small straight (penicilliary) arterioles with little smooth muscle in their walls, sometimes ending in capillaries with a sheath of macrophages. These open into venous sinusoids, either directly or via the interstitial tissue of the red pulp, and thence into trabecular veins; the circulation is at least partly open.

Fig. 12-53. Normal spleen showing white pulp with eccentric artery and adjacent red pulp.

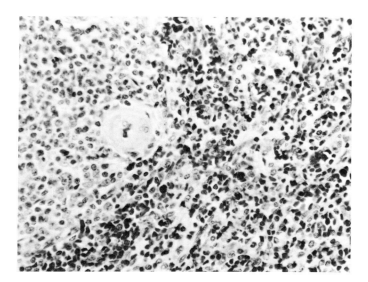

Fig. 12-54. Detail of normal spleen showing white pulp and adjacent red pulp.

The proportion of white pulp to red pulp is normally within the range of 1 : 3 to 1 : 6. The white pulp is composed of lymphoreticular tissue densely packed with small lymphocytes. The area around the small arteries (the periarteriolar lymphocytic sheath) contains interdigitating cells, macrophages on which T-cells hone and within which they are thought to mature. Elsewhere in the white pulp lie germinal centers similar to those seen in lymph nodes and similarly containing antigen-retaining dendritic reticular cells. Germinal centers in the spleen often contain trabeculae of hyaline eosinophilic, largely

collagenous material and may show similar changes to those described as occurring in lymph nodes.

The red pulp is composed of sinusoids lined by poorly phagocytic endothelial cells containing clusters of prominent microfilaments, which suggest their (known) contractility. Red cells leak readily between these endothelial cells. The interstitial area of the red pulp is composed of cords of irregularly arranged macrophages showing good evidence of phagocytosis of erythrocytes and other cells. Lying among these are erythrocytes and leukocytes in transit. Normally scattered polymorphs in small clusters of not more than two or three are seen; eosinophils are present in the spleens of those who have died suddenly, although they are often absent when death is protracted. The normal spleen contains some iron, as shown by the Prussian blue reaction.

After intravenous administration of antigens, the spleen shows morphologic changes similar to those occurring in lymph nodes after local administration. Antigen is retained on dendritic reticular cells in germinal centers, and there is a proliferation of lymphoid cells that mature into plasma cells and migrate first to the edge of the red pulp and then into it. The spleen of an animal or human undergoing an active humoral immune response will therefore show much white pulp with many germinal centers and numerous plasma cells. Similarly, if an active systemic delayed hypersensitivity response is in progress, the spleen will show prominent white pulp with cellular proliferation outside the germinal centers.

The major morphologic change occurring with age is traditionally held to be inactivity and then atrophy of white pulp. Germinal centers are infrequent over the age of 30, and white pulp is often reduced in old age.

Tissue Responses of the Spleen

The histology of the spleen represents the sum of the interaction between focal pathologic lesions and the general tissue response. The latter can be considered under the following headings; lesions may involve red and/or white pulp partially or completely.

Hypertrophy of the White Pulp

In follicular hypertrophy, the white pulp may enlarge (the normal ratio of white to red pulp is between 1 : 3 and 1 : 6), often with the development of active germinal centers similar to those of lymph nodes. This is accompanied by the appearance of foci of lymphocytes and plasma cells in the red pulp and represents a humoral immune response. In parafollicular hypertrophy, the appearance of proliferating lymphocytes and blast cells in the paravascular areas of the white pulp is related to a cellu-

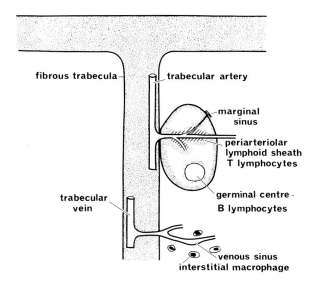

Fig. 12-55. Schema of normal spleen.

fibrous trabecula

trabecular artery

marginal sinus

periarteriolar lymphoid sheath T lymphocytes

trabecular vein

germinal centre B lymphocytes

venous sinus
interstitial macrophage

lar immune reaction. Lukes[147] discriminates between different types of activation. In graft rejection, infections, mononucleosis, herpes simplex infections, and after irradiation or bone marrow damage, the white pulp contains lymphocytes and large basophilic stem cells. In acute sepsis, measles, pertussis, typhoid, and a number of chronic conditions like idiopathic thrombocytopenic purpura, acquired hemolytic anemia, and rheumatoid disease, there is a prominent follicular reaction with perivascular plasma cells.

Reduction of White Pulp

In patients dying of severe generalized shock and toxemia, the white pulp may be grossly reduced; similar appearances may be induced by massive doses of corticosteroids and cytotoxic or immunosuppressive drugs. Similarly, in patients dying after prolonged chemotherapy for malignant lymphoma the white pulp disappears. Inactive white pulp composed only of small lymphocytes is found in the fetus, the unstimulated, the senescent, and in patients with agammaglobulinemia. An infiltrate of plasmacytoid cells with hypertrophy is found in dysproteinemias such as macroglobulinemia. Benign red pulp lesions do not infiltrate the red pulp; malignant red pulp lesions may.

Hypertrophy of Splenic Macrophages

In prolonged systemic infections, the spleen comes to contain numerous large swollen macrophages rich in acid phosphatase and often iron pigment. This process is essentially a process of macrophage maturation, induced mainly by phagocytosis and similar to that occurring during the maturation of monocytes into macrophages. Hypertrophy of macrophages is often accompanied by hypertrophy of splenic sinus endothelial cells.

Sinus Hyperplasia

Sinus endothelial cells also may enlarge and come to contain excess iron, indicating increased phagocytic capacity. This occurs when there is severe erythrocytic abnormality, such as in spherocytic anemia, and in severe venous congestion.

Congestion of Pulp Cords

The extravascular compartment of the red pulp may become stuffed with RBC. This is accompanied secondarily by a moderate degree of hypertrophy of splenic macrophages with a high iron content.

Variation in the Polymorph Content of the Spleen

The most common example of this is the depletion of eosinophils due to corticosteroid excess, occurring in the spleens of people dying of protracted diseases; the spleen of someone killed suddenly in an accident normally contains numerous eosinophils. Less commonly, in patients dying of severe sepsis, the spleen will be stuffed with large numbers of neutrophils. In severe infections, this change is commonly accompanied by hypertrophy of the white pulp.

Splenic lesions may be classified as follows.

1. Splenic rupture
2. Circulatory disorders
   Chronic venous congestion
   Portal hypertension
   Infarction
3. Degenerative disorders—amyloidosis
4. Infective and inflammatory disorders
   Acute pyogenic systemic infections—the septic spleen
   Subacute systemic infections, notably subacute bacterial endocarditis
   Viral infections, notably infectious mononucleosis
   Focal granulomatous lesions
   Rheumatoid disease, lupus erythematosus, and other collagen vascular diseases
5. Lipidoses
   Diabetes mellitus
   Gaucher's disease, Niemann-Pick disease
6. Blood disorders
   Idiopathic thrombocytopenic purpura
   Hemolytic anemia
   Leukemia
   Myelofibrosis
7. Tumors
   Lymphoma, malignant histiocytosis
   Secondary carcinomatosis
   Angiomata
   Cysts
8. The spleen in hypersplenism
9. Splenic atrophy

If this list seems incomplete, it should be noted that almost any lesion that occurs in a lymph node can occur in the spleen.

Rupture

Rupture is a common reason for splenectomy. A normal spleen does not rupture except under the influence of considerable external trauma. An enlarged spleen, on the other hand, requires little trauma to cause rupture and may indeed rupture spontaneously.[149] There may or may not be massive intraperitoneal hemorrhage; the peritoneal cavity may therefore be seeded with nodules or splenic tissue *(splenosis)*.[150] The important determination for the surgical pathologist is the presence or absence of underlying disease.

Circulatory Disorders

Portal Hypertension

In portal hypertension, due to hepatic cirrhosis or less commonly to portal venous thrombosis with cavernous transformation of the portal vein, the spleen is commonly grossly enlarged.[151] The spleen is firm and the cut surface dark red with scattered brown spots, which represent scars at the site of small hemorrhages. Histologically, the white pulp is atrophic; the red pulp shows congestion, although not so obviously as in many other conditions, and an increase in deposition of fine collagen (reticulin) fibers (Fig. 12-56). Scattered throughout are small scars consisting of fibrous tissue containing iron and sometimes calcium—the site of organization of small hemorrhages (Gamna-Gandy bodies). It is striking that after portocaval anastomosis, there is little reduction in the size of the spleen. The pathologic changes in the spleen in portal hypertension can be summarized as those of venous congestion, generalized reactive fine fibrosis, focal hemorrhage, and focal reactive fibrosis.

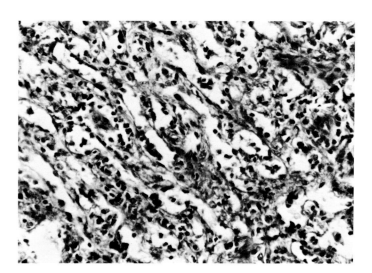

Fig. 12-56. Spleen in portal hypertension. There is an increase in interstitial collagen with apparent thickening of the walls of sinusoids.

Chronic Venous Congestion

In generalized chronic venous congestion, due, for instance, to long-standing cardiac failure, the changes are similar but less well marked. The spleen is slightly enlarged (200 to 300 g), firm, and dark. Histologically, the sinuses are congested with blood; there is slight fibrosis, and white pulp may be atrophic.

Infarction

Infarction of areas of the spleen, or even of almost the whole spleen, may be due either to emboli from mural thrombi on the left side of the heart (as after myocardial infarction) or to local thrombosis. Local thrombosis may be due to such generalized arterial lesions as polyarteritis nodosa or to a local inflammatory lesion. Local thrombosis may also occur in the abnormal spleens of patients with leukemia, lymphoma, sickle cell anemia, and malaria. Infarcts may be single or multiple wedge-shaped necrotic areas that heal by peripheral fibrosis, leaving a yellow inert center. In *polyarteritis nodosa,* there may be multiple small, usually central infarcts. Healed infarcts are usually evident on the splenic surface by the presence of a white, fibrotic "sugar-iced" area. Fibrotic thickening of the splenic capsule, focal or diffuse *(hyaline perisplenitis)*, is common in the absence of infarction. While it may be the residue of an acute perisplenitis or occur in long-standing ascites, most such cases are of unknown cause.

Degenerative Changes

The most common degenerative change is *hyaline change* seen in splenic arterioles. The arteriolar wall is deeply eosinophilic, thickened, and structureless, due to the insudation of plasmatic contents including fibrin (Fig. 12-57). Elsewhere in the body, such a lesion would indicate hypertension, but in this site it is a normal phenomenon over the age of 30 years. Trabeculae of hyaline material are less commonly seen in the white pulp of the normal spleen. The normal spleen contains a moderate diffusely scattered amount of sudanophilic lipid. Focal lipid globules in the white pulp have no particular significance.

Amyloid disease frequently affects the spleen, producing a moderate enlargement, usually up to 500 g. Amyloidosis occurs in patients with chronically elevated Ig levels due to chronic infection or multiple myeloma and involves the deposition of a carbohydrate-protein complex containing immunoglobulin fragments.[152] The material is laid down initially in a subendothelial position,

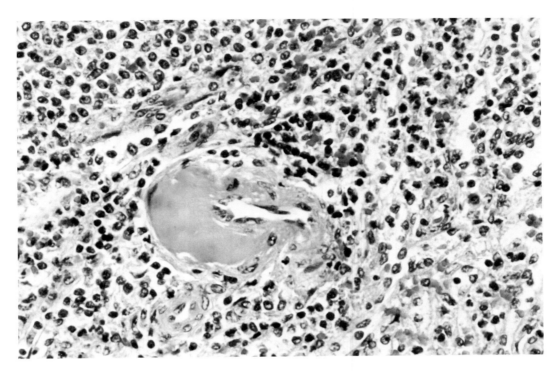

Fig. 12-57. Hyaline sclerosis of the wall of a splenic arteriole. This occurrence is normal over the age of 30.

either focally in the white pulp or diffusely (Fig. 12-58). The spleen in amyloid disease may show infiltrates of plasma cells, typical or atypical.

Infectious and Inflammatory Conditions

Acute Generalized Infections

In severe acute generalized infections, especially in children, the spleen is moderately enlarged (up to 500 g in an adult), pale, and soft. The white pulp may be enlarged with prominent reactive germinal centers, and the red pulp contains numerous polymorphs and plasma cells. In overwhelming infections, the lymphoid tissue may be greatly depleted due to prolonged high output of glucocorticoids, which cause degeneration of lymphocytes.

Subacute or Chronic Infections

In more chronic infections, the above-mentioned changes are seen to a lesser degree and are accompanied by increased numbers and size of macrophages in the red pulp. In typhoid fever, there is a diffuse mononuclear cell infiltrate.

Viral Infection—Infectious Mononucleosis

In infectious mononucleosis, the spleen is enlarged in at least 50 percent of cases to usually two to three times its normal size. It is usually soft, bulky, and congested. Spontaneous rupture is not uncommon.

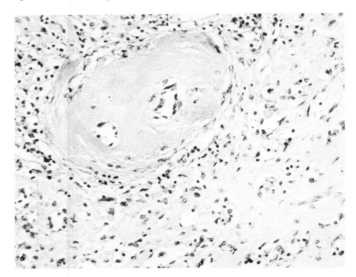

Fig. 12-58. Amyloidosis of spleen. Note amyloid deposition in the pulp and wall of a medium-sized vessel.

Histologically, the normal architecture is obscured by a diffuse infiltrate of lymphocytes into the capsules and trabeculae. Many of these are atypical large lymphocytes, or immunoblasts (see Fig. 12-17). There may also be plasma cells and eosinophils, and occasional cells resembling Reed-Sternberg cells, with large nucleoli, which, however, tend to be basophilic rather than the eosinophilic nucleoli of Hodgkin's disease.

Other Infections and Inflammations

In *rheumatoid disease,* the white pulp is very prominent with large germinal centers. In *protozoal* infections the spleen is enlarged. In acute *malaria,* there is gross hyperemia with some macrophage proliferation, while in more chronic malaria there is gross splenomegaly due to proliferation of pulp macrophages, which are packed with blood pigment, and to fibrosis. The hard, friable spleen is apt to rupture. In *kala-azar,* the spleen is similarly enlarged due to proliferation of macrophages, which are packed with *Leishmania donovani,* followed by stasis of blood and phagocytosis of RBC. There is subsequent fibrosis and dilation of sinusoids.[153]

Focal Granulomatous Lesions

Focal granulomatous lesions are found in the spleen in a wide variety of systemic disorders: tuberculosis, atypical mycobacterial infections, brucellosis, syphilis, and *Pneumocystis* and fungal infections. The granulomas range from merely small aggregates of lymphocytes and macrophages to fully formed caseating giant cell granulomas with fibrosis. The nature of the granuloma may point to the diagnosis but often does not. In 20 patients with multiple splenic granulomas, organisms were isolated from only three: atypical mycobacteria, *Histoplasma capsulatum,* and *Sporotrichum schenkii.*[154] Small granulomas are frequently found, often containing lipid, in spleens removed as a staging procedure in lymphoma, but are not diagnostic thereof.[155] Such lesions occur in spleens removed for many reasons and are unexplained. The spleen is commonly involved in miliary tuberculosis.

Lipidoses

In untreated *diabetes mellitus,* while the spleen is not grossly enlarged, an excess of cholesterol and sometimes sudanophilic lipid may be found in macrophages. In *Gaucher's disease,* the spleen is often grossly enlarged and pale gray, weighing up to 6 kg, and shows diffuse infiltration of the red pulp with large (up to 80 μm), often multinucleate macrophages. The cytoplasm may appear clear or vacuolated but often has a characteristic fibrillar appearance due to the presence of cytoplasmic glucocerebrosides (Fig. 12-52). Ultrastructural studies show that the irregular fibrillar configuration is produced by large cytoplasmic bodies containing tubular elements. The cytoplasmic bodies are massively dilated lysosomes, and the tubular elements are thought to be complexes of glucocerebrosides. The cells are rich in acid phosphatase, which can be demonstrated by histochemical staining.

In *Niemann-Pick disease,* accumulation of sphingomyelin with small amounts of cholesterol and other phosphatides occurs in the cytoplasm of large mononuclear cells. This imparts a fine reticular foamy appearance to the cytoplasm. The cells stain positively with PAS and Sudan IV.[158]

Sea-blue Histiocyte Syndrome

The sea-blue histiocyte syndrome occurs throughout life in a variety of races. The mean age of incidence is 21 years; most patients have an enlarged liver and spleen and, less often, mild or moderate lymphadenopathy. It seems[156,157] that it comprises a range of clinical conditions characterized by infiltration of lymphoreticular tissues by cells that stain sea-blue with Romanowsky stains. Thrombocytopenia is nearly universal, purpura common and massive gastrointestinal bleeding less common. In most patients, the disease runs a benign course; far less often, particularly in children and young adults, there is progressive pulmonary and hepatic involvement and sometimes a progressive neurological disorder. The condition is clearly familial, probably inherited as an autosomal recessive.

The diagnosis is made by identifying large histiocytes or macrophages in the marrow. These cells have a nucleus with fairly dense chromatin and a recognizable nucleolus, and the cytoplasm is packed with granules that stain sea-blue (or blue-green) with Wright-Giemsa stain; other macrophages have fewer smaller granules in a foamy cytoplasm. The cells do not label in vitro with ³H-thymidine; they stain positively with PAS and Sudan Black B, are autofluorescent, and probably contain sphingomyelin and glycosphingolipids.

The spleen is large (over 1000g) and shows foamy histiocytes through the red pulp, both between and lining sinusoids. Lesions have also been identified in lymph nodes, usually in medullary sinuses, and in the liver.

The syndrome may be a primary entity or may be a nonspecific manifestation of other diseases such as Tay-Sachs disease, Niemann-Pick disease, Gaucher's disease, chronic granulocytic leukemia, idiopathic thrombocytopenic purpura, sickle cell anemia and malabsorption syndromes. It now seems likely that the phenomenon is much more often secondary than primary.

Blood Disorders

Idiopathic Thrombocytopenic Purpura

In idiopathic thrombocytopenic purpura, the spleen is of normal size or only slightly enlarged. The germinal centers are rather prominent and active, and there may be evidence of phagocytosis of platelet masses by macrophages. These cells are large and have foamy, finely granular cytoplasm, containing much phospholipid (Figs. 12-59 and 12-60). Rather similar changes may occur in secondary thrombocytopenia. In idiopathic thrombocytopenic purpura splenomegaly may be associated with an excess of platelets in the splenic cords.[159,160]

Hemolytic Anemias

In the hemolytic anemias, the spleen is moderately enlarged (300 to 600 g), although it may be much larger, particularly in the acquired hemolytic anemias. The cords are intensely congested with red cells, and the sinus-lining cells are hyperplastic. There is marked phagocytosis by the enlarged red pulp macrophages, which contain an excess of iron.

In addition to the general pattern seen in hemolytic anemia, the spleen in *sickle cell anemia* shows some additional changes. There is marked focal pooling of blood around the white pulp, with episodes of infarction and fibrosis. The spleen may ultimately become small, shrunken, and fibrotic. In the acquired hemolytic anemias, the white pulp germinal centers are prominent, presumably because of an immunologic response. In hemolytic anemia with hemoglobinuria, there is only slight splenomegaly, with some congestion of the medulla but little evidence of excess erythrophagocytosis or hemosiderin deposition.

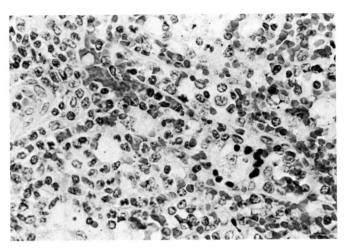

Fig. 12-60. Spleen in idiopathic thrombocytopenic purpura. High-power detail of the aggregates of foamy macrophages.

Leukemias

Splenic enlargement is found in all forms of leukemia, reaching an extreme degree in the chronic leukemias, notably chronic myeloid leukemia.[161] Treatment will modify the histologic appearance. In lymphocytic leukemia, the cellular infiltrate is confined at least initially to the white pulp. In myeloid leukemia, there is greater cellular pleomorphism, at least a few immature myeloid cells may be seen, and the infiltrate at least initially is confined to the red pulp, with compression atrophy of the white pulp (Fig. 12-61). Chloroacetate esterase staining is useful for distinguishing granulocyte precursors. The changes in monocytic leukemia are not extensively documented but appear to be similar to those in myeloid leukemia. The mast cell infiltration in systemic mastocytosis is recognizable in sections staining with metachromatic stains.

Hairy Cell Leukemia

Hairy cell leukemia (leukemic reticuloendotheliosis) affects men predominantly over the age of 30.[162] Examination of the blood shows pancytopenia and hairy cells, which are slightly larger than large lymphocytes and have delicate nuclear chromatin with occasional nucleoli. The spleen, liver, lymph nodes, and bone marrow are diffusely infiltrated by mononuclear cells that on phase-con-

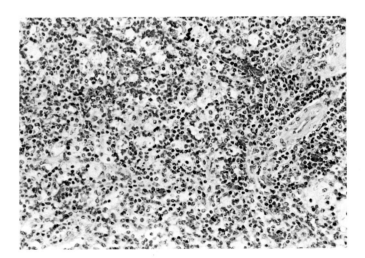

Fig. 12-59. Spleen in idiopathic thrombocytopenic purpura showing aggregates of large foamy macrophages.

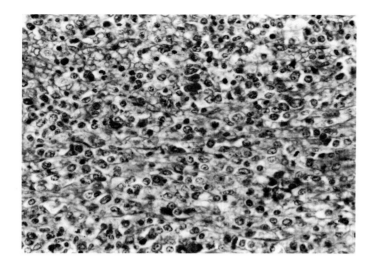

Fig. 12-61. Spleen in patient with chronic myeloid leukemia showing diffuse infiltration with immature hemopoietic cells, some of evident myeloid origin.

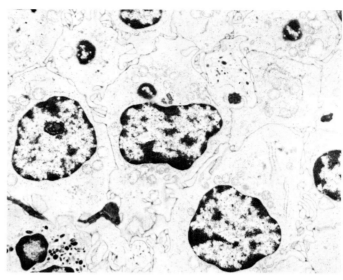

Fig. 12-63. Spleen in hairy cell leukemia showing diffuse infiltrate of large lymphoid cells with prominent interdigitating cytoplasmic processes and without evidence of phagocytosis. (×6,000) (Courtesy of Dr. L. F. Skinnider.)

trast microscopy show fine cytoplasmic "hairy" processes. They are probably of B-cell origin.[163]

The splenic red pulp is diffusely infiltrated and expanded by mononuclear cells with folded, irregular or indented nuclei and indistinct cytoplasmic margins. The infiltrate may extend into and often obliterates the white pulp (Fig. 12-62). The hairy nature of the cells is not visible in histologic sections by light microscopy but is readily evident on scanning or transmission electron microscopy (Fig. 12-63). Histochemical staining is helpful to demonstrate the presence of tartrate-resistant acid phosphatase isoenzyme in the neoplastic cells.

Extramedullary Hematopoiesis—Myeloid Metaplasia

When the marrow is replaced by fibrous tissue (myelofibrosis), myeloid metaplasia is found in the spleen, which may be massively enlarged. All the constituents of normal hematopoietic marrow can be recognized, and the easiest to identify are megakaryocytes (Fig. 12-64). The formation of megakaryocytes and RBC tends to predomi-

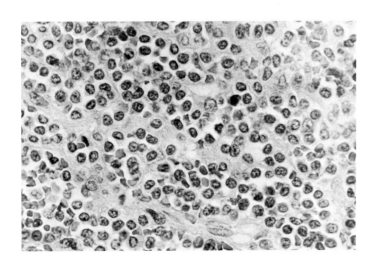

Fig. 12-62. Hairy cell leukemia showing diffuse infiltration of spleen with small cells with round or elongated nuclei.

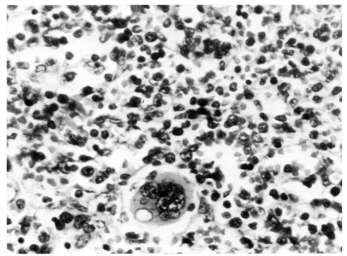

Fig. 12-64. Spleen showing myeloid metaplasia in a patient with myelofibrosis. A megakaryocyte is illustrated.

424

nate in the sinusoids and granulocyte production in the cords. There also may be excessive RBC breakdown.

Similar changes may be found in the spleen when hemopoietic marrow is replaced by a process such as secondary carcinoma (myelophthisis). Patients with myeloid metaplasia may eventually develop myeloid leukemia.

Tumors

Lymphoma

The spleen is often affected in malignant lymphoma, usually secondarily, very rarely as the primary site of disease. In terminal untreated lymphoma, the spleen may be very large (2,000 to 3,000 g), showing either nodular or diffuse infiltration with gray to white neoplasm.

In early Hodgkin's disease, as seen in staging splenectomy specimens, there is commonly hyperplasia of the white pulp with prominent germinal center formation. Often, no abnormal cells can be seen. The earliest deposits are usually seen in the white pulp in a paravascular position. The walls of veins may be invaded. There may be small lipid granulomata or sarcoid-like granulomatous reaction, which are not diagnostic of Hodgkin's disease. However, in about 50 percent of cases subjected to staging laparotomy, overt Hodgkin's lesions are present. Lymphocyte predominant Hodgkin's disease is rarely identified in the spleen. Subclassification of Hodgkin's disease on the basis of the splenic lesion alone is difficult.

In non-Hodgkin's lymphoma, the earliest lesions are also usually in the white pulp. It may be difficult or impossible to discern whether a lymphoma is nodular from examination of the splenic lesions alone. In nodular lymphomas, there may be multiple, fairly large lesions restricted to the white pulp, but these ultimately become confluent to form masses 2 cm or more in diameter, indistinguishable from diffuse lymphoma. Diffuse splenic infiltration occurs characteristically in malignant histiocytosis; the cords are primarily affected.

Primary lymphoma of the spleen is rare. Of 49 patients in whom the lesion appeared to start in the spleen, 8 had tumor in the spleen only, and another 9 had tumor in the spleen and splenic hilar node only.[164] Hodgkin's disease was less common than other lymphomas, and lesions varied from homogeneous infiltration through small miliary and multiple larger nodules to single nodules. The rare nodular or follicular lymphomas occurring primarily in the spleen have a good prognosis after splenectomy.[165,166]

The lesion of *angioimmunoblastic lymphadenopathy* appears in the white pulp in a paravascular position. Infiltration may occur in myeloma and in macroglobulinemia.

In the spleen, as in lymph nodes, lymphomas present diagnostic problems. The following points are useful to note. (1) Diffuse well differentiated lymphocytic lymphoma and all the follicular lymphomas usually involve all the malpighian bodies, and this is evident both on gross and microscopic examination. (2) Diffuse lymphomas rarely involve the spleen at staging laparotomy; however, when this occurs one sees grossly discrete large white nodules, which on closer inspection are composed of closely packed smaller nodules. (3) These lymphomas involve the entire malpighian body; Hodgkin's disease often does not.

Secondary Carcinomatosis

While the spleen is not a characteristic site for secondary carcinoma, scattered carcinoma cells may be found in 5 percent or more of patients dying of carcinomatosis and nodules of tumor in about 5 percent. The more careful the histologic examination, the more often tumor cells are found. The periarterial lymphatics may be distended with carcinoma cells.

Vascular Tumors

Angiomata are usually *hemangiomas*, are less often lymphangiomas, and are usually cavernous rather than capillary in structure. The usual cavernous hemangioma may be single or multiple and may involve a large part of the spleen. The demarcation from the surrounding spleen may or may not be discrete. Occasionally, such lesions result in massive hemorrhage. Such lesions shade into the *hamartomas* of the spleen—congenital tumors composed mainly of red pulp, with a variable amount of white pulp.

Hemangiosarcoma of spleen is very rare and is identified by the usual histologic criteria of anaplasia and pleomorphism (Fig. 12-65). Its histologic appearance is dis-

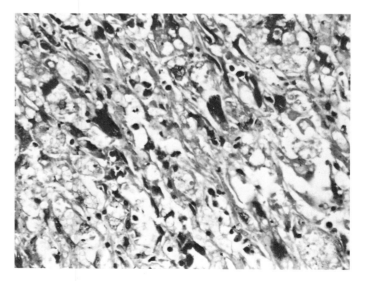

Fig. 12-65. Hemangiosarcoma of spleen. Note the pleomorphic anaplastic cells lining sinusoids.

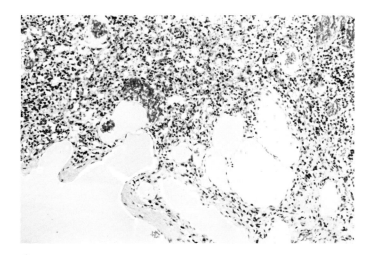

Fig. 12-66. Benign cavernous lymphangioma of spleen. The thin-walled sinusoids are widely dilated, lined by flattened endothelium, and contain eosinophilic lymph.

cussed in more detail in Chapter 32, since it is more common (although still rare) in the liver.

Lymphangiomas are rare. They are usually small and subcapsular. The vessel walls are lined by flattened endothelial cells and contain only coagulated protein (Fig. 12-66).

Cysts

Cysts of the spleen are rare. They may be (1) congenital—either mesothelial, usually just below the capsule, or dermoid, sometimes with hair follicles and sebaceous glands; (2) degenerative, following liquefaction necrosis or infarcts of thrombosed angiomata; or (3) parasitic, usually due to *Taenia echinococcus*.

The Spleen in Hypersplenism

The term hypersplenism means functional hyperactivity of the spleen and is commonly applied to a clinical syndrome in which there is massive splenomegaly and anemia. The hematologic findings include reticulocytosis, neutropenia, and thrombocytopenia. There are usually no immature red or white blood cells in the circulation, and the bone marrow shows no gross abnormality.

Many patients with hypersplenism have a malignant lymphoma, a lipidosis (notably Gaucher's disease), or persistent chronic infection (e.g., tuberculosis, brucellosis, kala-azar, or malaria). The spleens from these patients show, in addition to the primary lesion, a hyperplasia of red pulp macrophages with erythrophagocytosis and increase in iron deposition. Hypersplenism may also occur in rheumatoid disease, where again there is some hyperplasia of red pulp macrophages, but the prominent feature is the germinal center hyperplasia. Hypersplenism occurs occasionally in diffuse carcinomatosis with splenic involvement.

Hypersplenism also occurs in the absence of demonstrable primary lesions, usually in tropical countries, such as New Guinea.[167] The spleens in this report were grossly enlarged (mean weight: 3,200 g) and showed inconspicuous white pulp; the red pulp showed distension of venous sinuses with swollen endothelial cells showing active phagocytosis. Red pulp macrophages were prominent, showing evidence of phagocytosis of cell debris and iron and moderate fibrosis. There was some evidence of myeloid metaplasia. Many if not all such patients have malaria.

A similar syndrome occurs in temperate climates—*nontropical idiopathic splenomegaly* (primary hypersplenism).[168] The spleens are grossly enlarged (mean weight 2,400 g). About one half show white pulp hyperplasia. There is usually dilatation of venous sinuses and increased macrophage activity in the red pulp with erythrophagocytosis. There are small lymphocytic foci but no myeloid metaplasia. Two of the 10 patients in this report subsequently developed lymphoma.

Splenic Atrophy

Splenic atrophy is rare.[169] As an exceptional occurrence, the spleen may be congenitally absent or small, sometimes associated with marrow hypoplasia. Acquired atrophy may be due to autodestruction by numerous small infarcts in sickle cell anemia, after irradiation, or, rarely, in thrombocytopenic purpura. A diffuse atrophy may uncommonly occur in celiac disease and other malabsorption states, and even less often in alcoholism, hypopituitarism, hyperthyroidism and, rarely, without evident cause. The normal reserve of splenic function is great, but when splenic mass sinks below about 20 g, a failure of hemophagocytic functions results in the appearance of excessively thin RBC in peripheral films (leptocytes). These often contain abnormal inclusions, notably nuclear fragments (Howell-Jolly bodies) and denatured hemoglobin (Heinz bodies). Impaired splenic function may be detected in malabsorption states in life by impaired clearance of chromium-labeled RBC and by reduction of splenic size as seen radiographically.[170,171] In a series of 14 patients with splenic atrophy diagnosed clinically by RBC survival studies and radiographically, 8 had intestinal malabsorption and the remainder had a high incidence of autoimmune disease.[172] There seems to be some correlation between autoantibody formation and splenic atrophy. Hyposplenism has been demonstrated in ulcerative colitis and there is some evidence that these patients may be prone to severe bacterial infection.[173]

Infections, often fulminating septicemias, may occasionally follow removal of the spleen, sometimes many weeks or months later.[174] Patients having splenectomy for traumatic rupture rarely suffer such complications, and those having the operation for idiopathic thrombocytopenia purpura, hereditary spherocytosis, local tumor or aplastic anemia run only a small hazard. In contrast, the risks with thalassemia major, portal hypertension, and malignant lymphoma may be greater. Such infections are more common in children and in immunosuppressed patients and are often pneumococcal. The risk of infection may be related to the fall in serum IgM observed after splenectomy.

ACKNOWLEDGMENTS

As in the first edition, we would like to thank the following for providing photographs: photographic unit, Department of Pathology, University of Saskatchewan; A. Sylvester, Weston Park Hospital, Sheffield; Howard Mitchell, University of Colorado School of Medicine, Denver; and Dr. L. Skinnider for an illustration. In addition, we thank Blackwell Scientific Publications for permission to reuse material from the text *Lymphoreticular Disease* (I. Carr, B. W. Hancock, L. Henry, and A. M. Ward). Finally, we would like to acknowledge the secretarial assistance of Mavis Hopewell and Jeanne Gousseau, as well as the critical help of Dr. G. Vadas and Dr. C. Littman.

REFERENCES

1. Jaffe ES: Surgical Pathology of the Lymph Nodes and Related Organs. Major Problems in Pathology, Vol. 16. WB Saunders, Philadelphia, 1985
2. Robb-Smith AHT, Taylor CR: Lymph Node Biopsy: A Diagnostic Atlas. Oxford University Press, New York, 1981
3. Carr I, Hancock BW, Henry L, et al: Lymphoreticular Disease. Blackwell, Oxford, 1984
4. Banks PM, Long JC, Howard CA: Preparation of lymph node biopsy specimens. Hum Pathol 1:617, 1979
5. Mason DY: A new look at lymphoma immunohistology. (Editorial.) Am J Pathol 128:1, 1987
6. Barlogie B, Raber MN, Schumann TS, et al: Flow cytometry in clinical cancer research. Cancer Res 43:3982, 1983
7. Ault KA: Clinical applications of fluorescence-activated cell sorting techniques. Diagn Immunol 1:2, 1983
8. Lovett EJ III, Schnitzer B, Keren DF, et al: Application of flow cytometry to diagnostic pathology. Lab Invest 50:115, 1984
9. Harris NL, Bhan AK: B-cell neoplasms of the lymphocytic lymphoplasmacytoid, and plasma cell types: Immunohistologic analysis and clinical correlation. Hum Pathol 16:829, 1986
10. Petersen SE: Accuracy and reliability of flow cytometric DNA analysis using a simple one-step ethidium bromide straining protocol. Cytometry 7:301, 1986
11. Shackney SE, Skromstrad RE, Cunningham DJ, et al: Dual parameter flow cytometry studies in human lymphomas. J Clin Invest 66:1281, 1980
12. Costa A, Mazzini G, Delbino G, et al: DNA content and proliferative characteristics of non-Hodgkin's lymphoma: Determined by flow cytometry and autoradiography. Cytometry 2:185, 1981
13. Barlogie B, Drewinko J, Schumann J, et al: Cellular DNA content as a marker of neoplasia in man. Am J Med 69:195, 1980
14. Poppema S, Hollema H, Visser LM, et al: Monoclonal antibodies (MT, MT2, MB1, MB2, MB3) reactive with leukocyte subsets in paraffin-embedded tissue sections. Am J Pathol 127:418, 1987
15. Hall PA, D'Ardenne MG, Butler JR, et al: New marker of B lymphocytes, MB2: Comparison with other lymphocyte subset markers active in conventionally processed tissue sections. J Clin Pathol 40:151, 1987
16. Arnold A, Cossman J, Bakhshi A, et al: Immunoglobulin-gene rearrangements as unique clonal markers in human lymphoid neoplasms. N Engl J Med 309:1593, 1983
17. O'Connor NTJ, Gatter KC, Wainscoat JS, et al: Practical value of genotypic analysis for diagnosing lymphoproliferative disorders. J Clin Pathol 40:147, 1987
18. Cottier H, Turk J, Sobin C: A proposal for a standardized system of reporting human lymph morphology in relation to immunological function. J Clin Pathol 26:317, 1973
19. Symchych PS, Wanstrup J, Andersen V: Chronic granulomatous disease of childhood. A morphologic study. Acta Pathol Microbiol Scand 74:179, 1965
20. Edlow DW, Carter D: Heterotopic epithelium in axillary lymph node. Report of a case and review of the literature. Am J Clin Pathol 59:666, 1973
21. Hart WR: Primary nevus of a lymph node. Am J Clin Pathol 55:88, 1971
22. McCarthy SW, Palmer AA, Bale PM, et al: Naevus cells in lymph node. Pathology 6:351, 1974
23. Meyer JS, Steinberg LS: Microscopically benign thyroid follicles in cervical lymph nodes. Cancer 24:302, 1969
24. Osmond R, Kalinovsky P: Epithelial inclusion cysts in axillary nodes associated with malignant disease. Med J Aust 2:834, 1972
25. Hooper AA: Tuberculous peripheral lymphadenitis. Br J Surg 59:353, 1972
26. O'Brien JR: Non-reactive tuberculosis. J Clin Pathol 7:216, 1954
27. MacKellar A, Hilton HB, Masters PL: Mycobacterial lymphadenitis in childhood. Arch Dis Child 42:70, 1967
28. Reid JD, Wolinsky E: Histopathology of lymphadenitis caused by atypical mycobacteria. Am Rev Respir Dis 99:8, 1969
29. Turk JL, Waters MFR: Immunological significance of

changes in the lymph nodes across the leprosy spectrum. Clin Exp Immunol 8:363, 1971

30. Karat AB, Karat S, Job CK, et al: Acute necrotizing lepromatous lymphadenitis. An erythema nodosum-like reaction in lymph nodes. Br Med J 4:223, 1968

31. Citron KM: Sarcoidosis. Medicine (Baltimore) 14:896, 1972

32. Jones Williams W, Williams D: The properties and development of conchoidal bodies in sarcoid and sarcoid-like granulomas. J Pathol 96:491, 1968

33. Jones Williams W, Erasmus DA, James EMV, et al: The fine structure of sarcoid and tuberculous granulomas. Postgrad Med J 46:496, 1970

34. Cook MG: The size and histological appearances of mesenteric lymph nodes in Crohn's disease. Gut 13:970, 1972

35. Hartsock FJ, Halling LW, King FM: Luetic lymphadenitis: A clinical and histological study of 20 cases. Am J Clin Pathol 53:304, 1970

36. Turner DR, Wright DJM: Lymphadenopathy in early syphilis. J Pathol 110:305, 1973

37. Sharp WB: Pathology of undulant fever. Arch Pathol Lab Med 18:72, 1934

38. Sprunt H, McBryde A: Morbid anatomic changes in cases of Brucella infection in man with report of necropsy. Arch Pathol Lab Med 21:217, 1936

39. Winship T: Pathological changes in so-called cat-scratch fever. Am J Clin Pathol 23:1012, 1953

40. Wear DJ, et al: Cat scratch disease: A bacterial infection. Science 221:1403, 1983

41. Carlsson MG, Ryd H, Sternby NH: A case of human infection with pasteurella pseudotuberculosis X. Acta Pathol Microbiol Scand 62:128, 1964

42. Barnett RN, Hull JG, Vortel V: Pneumocystis carinii in lymph nodes and spleen. Arch Pathol Lab Med 88:175, 1969

43. Kikuchi M: Lymphadenitis showing focal reticular cell hyperplasia with nuclear debris and phagocytes: A clinicopathological study. Acta Haematol Jpn 35:379, 1972

44. Turner FR, Martin J, Dorfman RF: Necrotizing lymphadenitis: A study of 30 cases. Am J Surg Pathol 7:115, 1983

45. Saxen E, Saxen L: The histological diagnosis of glandular toxoplasmosis. Lab Invest 8:386, 1959

46. Stansfeld AG: The histological diagnosis of toxoplasmic lymphadenitis. J Clin Pathol 14:565, 1961

47. Stanton MF, Pinkerton H: Benign acquired toxoplasmosis with subsequent pregnancy. Am J Clin Pathol 23:1199, 1953

48. Motulsky AG, Weinberg S, Saphir O, et al: Lymph nodes in rheumatoid arthritis. Arch Intern Med 90:660, 1952

49. Cruickshank B: Lesions of lymph nodes in rheumatoid disease and in disseminated lupus erythematosus. Scott Med J 3:110, 1958

50. Nosanchuk JS, Schnitzer B: Follicular hyperplasia in lymph nodes from patients with rheumatoid arthritis. A clinicopathologic study. Cancer 24:243, 1969

51. Hartsock RJ: Postvaccinial lymphadenitis. Hyperplasia of lymphoid tissue that simulates malignant lymphomas. Cancer 21:632,1968

52. Warthin AS: Occurrence of numerous large giant cells in the tonsils and pharyngeal mucosa in the prodromal stage of measles. Report of 4 cases. Arch Pathol Lab Med 11:864, 1931

53. Finkeldey W: Uber Riesenzellbefunde in den Gaumenmandeln, zugleich ein Beitrag zur Histopathologie der Mandel Veränderungen in maserninkubations-Stadium. Virchows Arch 281:323, 1931

54. Allen MS, Talbot WH, McDonald RM: Atypical lymph node hyperplasia after administration of attenuated live measles vaccine. N Engl J Med 274:677, 1966

55. Downey M, Stasney J: The pathology of the lymph nodes in infectious mononucleosis. Folia Haematol (Leipz) 54:417, 1936

56. Gall EA, Stout HA: The histological lesion in the lymph nodes in infectious mononucleosis. Am J Pathol 16:433, 1940

57. Custer RP, Smith EB: Pathology of infectious mononucleosis. Blood 3:830, 1948

58. Beswick IP: The spleen in glandular fever. J Pathol 70:407, 1955

59. Carter RL, Penman HG: Infectious Mononucleosis. Blackwell, Oxford, 1969

60. Laurence J: AIDS: Definition, Epidemiology and Etiology: Symposium on AIDS. Lab Med 17:659, 1986

61. Ewing EP Jr, Chandler FW, Spira TJ, et al: Primary lymph node pathology in AIDS and AIDS-related lymphadenopathy. Arch Pathol Lab Med 109:977, 1985

62. Jaffe ES, Clark J, Steis R, et al: Lymph node pathology of HTLV-associated neoplasms. Cancer Res. 45(suppl):4662, 1985

63. Saltzstein SL, Ackerman LV: Lymphadenopathy induced by anticonvulsant drugs and mimicking clinically and pathologically malignant lymphomas. Cancer 12:164, 1959

64. Saltzstein SL: Lymphoma or drug reaction occurring during hydantoin therapy for epilepsy. Am J Med 32:286, 1962

65. Hyman GA, Sommers SC: The development of Hodgkin's disease and lymphoma during anticonvulsant therapy. Blood 28:416, 1966

66. Krasznai G, Gyory G: Hydantoin lymphadenopathy. J Pathol 95:314, 1968

67. Harrison CV: In Harrison CV (ed): Recent Advances in Pathology. 8th Ed. Churchill, London, 1966

68. Warner NE, Friedman NB: Lipogranulomatous pseudosarcoid. Ann Intern Med 45:662, 1956

69. Spain DM: Sex differences in incidence and severity of lymph node lipogranulomatosis. Arch Pathol Lab Med 64:54, 1957

70. Nairn RC, Anderson TE: Erythrodermia with lipomelanic reticulum cell hyperplasia of lymph nodes (dermatopathic lymphadenitis). Br Med J 1:820, 1955

71. Symmers D: Primary haemangiolymphoma of the haemal nodes. An unusual variety of malignant tumour. Arch Intern Med 28:467, 1921

72. Castleman B, Iverson L, Pardo Menendez V: Localized Mediastinal lymph node hyperplasia resembling thymoma. Cancer 9:822, 1956

73. Anagnostou D, Harrison CV: Angiofollicular lymph node hyperplasia (Castleman). J Clin Pathol 25:306, 1972
74. Kahn LB, Ranchod M, Stables DP, et al: Giant lymph node hyperplasia with haematological abnormalities. S Afr Med J 47:811, 1973
75. Ballow M, Park BH, Dupont B, et al: Benign giant lymphoid hyperplasia of mediastinum with associated abnormalities of the immune system. J Pediatr 84:418, 1974
76. Emson HE: Extrathoracic angiofollicular lymphoid hyperplasia with coincidental myasthenia gravis. Cancer 31:241, 1973
77. Keller AR, Hochholzer L, Castleman B: Hyaline vascular and plasma cell types of giant lymph node hyperplasia of the mediastinum and other locations. Cancer 29:670, 1972
78. Frizzera G, Banks PM, Massarelli G, et al: A systemic lymphoproliferative disorder with morphologic features of Castleman's disease. Pathologic findings in 15 patients. Am J Surg Pathol 7:211, 1983
79. Weisenburger D, Nathwani B, Winberg C, Rappaport H: Multicentric angiofollicular lymph node hyperplasia. A clinicopathologic study of 16 cases. Hum Pathol 16:162, 1985
80. Bluming AZ, Cohen HG, Saxon A: Angioimmunoblastic lymphadenopathy with dysproteinaemia. Am J Med 67:421, 1979
81. Lukes RJ, Tindle BM: Immunoblastic lymphadenopathy: A hyperimmune entity resembling Hodgkin's disease. N Engl J Med 292:1, 1975
82. Frizzera G, Moran EM, Rappaport H: Angioimmunoblastic lymphadenopathy with dysproteinaemia. Lancet 1:1070, 1974
83. Nathwani BN, Rappaport H, Moran EM, et al: Malignant lymphoma arising in angioimmunoblastic lymphadenopathy. Cancer 41:578, 1978
84. Rosai J, Dorfman RF: Sinus histiocytosis with massive lymphadenopathy. A newly recognized benign clinicopathological entity. Arch Pathol Lab Med 87:63, 1969
85. Foucar E, Rosai J, Dorfman RF, Eyman JM: Immunologic abnormalities and their significance in sinus histiocytosis with massive lymphadenopathy. Am J Clin Pathol 92:515, 1984
86. Miettinen M, Paljakka P, Haveri P, Saxen E: Sinus histiocytosis with massive lymphadenopathy. A nodal and extranodal proliferation of S-100 protein-positive histiocytes. Am J Clin Pathol 88:270, 1987
87. Mackenzie DH: Amyloidosis presenting as lymphadenopathy. Br Med J 2:1449, 1963
88. Ko HS, Davidson JW, Pruzanski W: Amyloid lymphadenopathy. Ann Intern Med 85:763, 1976
89. Osborne BM, Butler JJ, MacKay B: Proteinaceous lymphadenopathy with hypergammaglobulinaemia. Am J Surg Pathol 3:137, 1979
90. Tsakraklides V, Olson P, Kersey JH, et al: Prognostic significance of the regional lymph node histology in cancer of the breast. Cancer 34:1259, 1974
91. Tsakraklides E, Tsakraklides V, Ashikarai H, et al: In vitro studies of axillary lymph node cells in patients with breast cancer. J Natl Cancer Inst 54:549, 1975
92. Tsakraklides V, Wanebo HJ, Sternberg SS, et al: Prognos-

tic evaluation of regional lymph node morphology in colorectal cancer. Am J Surg 129:174, 1975
93. Jesse RH, Perez CA, Fletcher G: Cervical lymph node metastasis; unknown primary cancer. Cancer 31:854, 1973
94. Copeland EM, McBride CM: Axillary metastasis from an unknown primary site. Ann Surg 178:25, 1973
95. Zaren HA, Copeland EM: Inguinal node metastases. Cancer 41:919, 1978
96. Haagensen CD, Feind CR, Herter FP, et al: Lymphatics in Cancer. WB Saunders, London, 1972
97. Pickren JW: Significance of occult metastases. Cancer 14:1266, 1961
98. Lee Y-TNM: p. 410. In Weiss L, Gilberg HA, Ballon S (eds): Lymphatic System Metastasis. GK Hall, Boston, 1980
99. Lubin J, Rywlin AM: Lymphoma-like lymph node changes in Kaposi's sarcoma. Arch Pathol Dermatol 93:554, 1971
100. Davies JD, Stansfeld AG: Spontaneous infarction of superficial lymph nodes. J Clin Pathol 25:689, 1972
101. Benisch BM, Howard RG: Lymph node infarction in two young men. Am J Clin Pathol 673:818, 1975
102. Haferhamp O, Rosenau W, Lennert K: Vascular transformation of lymph node sinuses due to venous obstruction. Arch Pathol Lab Med 92:81, 1971
103. Fayemi AO, Toker C: Nodal angiomatosis. Arch Pathol Lab Med 99:170, 1975
104. Kaplan MS: Hodgkin's Disease. Harvard University Press, Cambridge, MA, 1972
105. Smithers DW: Modes of spread of Hodgkin's disease. p. 107. In Smithers DW (ed): Hodgkin's disease. Churchill Livingstone, Edinburgh, 1973
106. Butler JJ: Natural history of Hodgkin's disease and its classification. p. 184. In Rebuck JW, Berard CW, Abell MR (eds): The Reticuloendothelial System. Williams & Wilkins, Baltimore, 1975
107. Grogan TM: Hodgkin's disease. p. 86. In Jaffe ES (ed): Major Problems in Pathology, Vol. 16: Surgical Pathology of the Lymph Nodes and Related Organs. WB Saunders, Philadelphia, 1985
108. Lukes RJ, Butler JJ: The pathology and nomenclature of Hodgkin's disease. Cancer Res 26:1063, 1966
109. Burns BF, Colby TV, Dorfman RF: Differential diagnostic features of nodular L & H Hodgkin's disease, including progressive transformation of germinal centers. Am J Surg Pathol 8:253, 1984
110. Pinkus GS, Said JW: Hodgkin's disease, lymphocyte predominance type, nodular—A distinct entity? Am J Pathol 118:1, 1985
111. Rappaport H, Harris NL (eds): Controversies in Hodgkin's disease. Am J Surg Pathol 11:148, 1987
112. Regula DP Jr, Hoppe RT, Weiss LM: Nodular and diffuse types of lymphocyte predominance Hodgkin's disease. N Engl J Med 318:214, 1988
113. Strickler, Michie SA, Warnke RA, Dorfman RF: The "syncytial variant" of nodular sclerosing Hodgkin's disease. Am J Surg Pathol 10:470, 1986
114. Correa P, O'Conor GT, Berard CW, et al: International comparability and reproducibility in histologic subclassifi-

cation of Hodgkin's disease. J Natl Cancer Inst. 50:1429, 1973

115. Martin SE, et al: Immunologic methods in cytology: Definitive diagnosis of non-Hodgkin's lymphomas using immunologic markers for T and B cells. Am J Clin Pathol 82:666, 1984

116. Carbone PT, Rappaport H, Rosenberg SA, et al: Symposium (Ann Arbor): Staging in Hodgkin's disease. Cancer Res 31:1707, 1971

117. Rappaport H: Tumors of the hematopoietic system. p. 8. Atlas of Tumor Pathology. Section 3. Armed Forces Institute of Pathology, 1966

118. Berard CW, Dorfman EF: Histopathology of malignant lymphomas. Clin Hematol 3:39, 1974

119. Lukes RJ, Collins RD: Immunological characterization of human malignant lymphomas. Cancer 34:1488, 1974

120. Rosenberg SA, et al: National Cancer Institute-sponsored study of classification of non-Hodgkin's lymphomas: Summary and description of a working formulation for clinical usage. Cancer 49:2112, 1982

121. Sommers SC, Rosen PP (eds): Malignant lymphomas. Appleton & Lange, E. Norwalk, CT, 1983

122. Nathwani BN, Winberg CD, Diamond LW, et al: Morphologic criteria for the differentiation of follicular lymphoma from florid reactive follicular hyperplasia: A study of 80 cases. Cancer 48:1794, 1981

123. Weisenburger DD, Nathwani BN, Diamond LW, et al: Malignant lymphoma, intermediate lymphocytic type; a clinicopathologic study of 42 cases. Cancer 48:1415, 1981

124. Burkitt D: A sarcoma involving the jaws in African children. Br J Surg 46:218, 1958

125. O'Conor GT, Rappaport H, Smith EB: Childhood lymphoma resembling Burkitt's tumor in the U.S. Cancer 18:411, 1965

126. Dorfman RF: Childhood lymphosarcoma in St. Louis, Missouri, clinically and histologically resembling Burkitt's tumor. Cancer 18:418, 1965

127. Arsenean JC, Carellos GP, Banks PM, et al: American Burkitt's lymphoma: a clinico-pathologic study of 30 cases. I. Clinical factors relating to prolonged survival. Am J Med 58:314, 1975

128. Arsenean JC, Carellos GP, Banks PM, et al: American Burkitt's lymphoma: A clinico-pathologic study of 30 cases. II. Pathologic correlations. Am J Med 58:322, 1975

129. Taub R, Kirsch I, Morton C, et al: Translocation of the C-myc gene into the immunoglobulin heavy chain locus in human Burkitt's lymphoma and plasmacytoma cells. Proc Natl Acad Sci USA 79:7837, 1982

130. Lennert K, Mestdagh J: Lymphogranulomatosen mit konstant hohem epithelioid-Zellgehalt. Virchows Arch 344:1, 1968

131. Kim H, Nathwani BN, Rappaport H: So-called "Lennert's lymphoma." Is it a clinicopathologic entity? Cancer 45:1379, 1980

132. Edelson RL: Cutaneous T cell lymphomas. Perspective Ann Intern Med 83:548, 1975

133. Clendenning WE, Rappaport HW: Report of the Committee of Pathology on cutaneous T cell lymphomas. Cancer Treatm Rep 63:719–721, 1979

134. Rappaport H, Thomas LB: Mycosis fungoides. The pathology of extracutaneous involvement. Cancer 34:1198, 1974

135. Kim H, Dorfman RF, Rappaport H: Signet ring lymphoma. A rare morphologic and functional expression of nodular (follicular) lymphoma. Am J Surg Pathol 2:119, 1978

136. Bernier V, Azar HA: Filiform large-cell lymphoma. An ultrastructural and immunohistochemical study. Am J Surg Pathol 11:387, 1987

137. Rappaport H: Atlas of Tumor Pathology. Section III Fascicle 8. Tumors of the Hematopoietic System. Wash. D.C., A.F.I.P., 1966

138. Isaacson P, Wright DH, Jones DB: Malignant lymphoma of true histiocytic (monocyte-macrophage) origin. Cancer 51:80, 1983

139. Furth RB, Raeburn JA, Van Zwet T: Characteristics of human mononuclear phagocytes. Blood 54:485, 1979

140. Scott RB, Robb-Smith AH: Histocytic medullary reticulosis. Lancet 2:194, 1939

141. Wieczorek R, Greco MA, et al: Familial erythrophagocytic lymphohistiocytosis: Immunophenotypic, immunohistochemical and ultrastructural demonstration of the relation to sinus histiocytes. Hum Pathol 17:55, 1986

142. Risdall RJ, McKenna RW, Nesbit ME, et al: Virus-associated hemophagocytic syndrome: A benign histiocytic proliferation distinct from malignant histiocytosis. Cancer 44:993, 1979

143. Reid H, Fox H, Whittaker JS: Eosinophilic granuloma of lymph nodes. Histopathology 1:31, 1977

144. MacPherson AIS, Richmond J, Stuart AE: The Spleen. Charles C Thomas, Springfield, IL, 1973, pp. 83–151

145. Klemperer P: The pathological anatomy of splenomegaly. Am J Clin Pathol 6:99, 1936

146. Rappaport H: The pathologic anatomy of the splenic red pulp. In Lennert K, Harris D (eds): The Spleen. Springer-Verlag, Berlin, 1970

147. Lukes RJ: The pathology of the white pulp of the spleen. In Lennert K, Harris D (eds): The Spleen. Springer-Verlag, Berlin, 1970

148. Robb-Smith AHT: Pathological lesions in surgically removed spleens. Br J Hosp Med 3:19, 1970

149. Stites TB, Ultmann JE: Spontaneous rupture of the spleen in chronic lymphatic leukaemia. Cancer 19:1587, 1966

150. Szabo A de K: Splenosis. The autotransplantation of splenic tissue. Am J Surg 101:208, 1961

151. McMichael J: The pathology of hepatolienal fibrosis. J Pathol Bacteriol 39:481, 1934

152. Stirling GA: Amyloidosis. p. 249. In Harrison CV, Weinbren K (eds): Recent Advances in Pathology. Vol. 9. Churchill Livingstone, Edinburgh, 1975

153. Kirk R: The pathogenesis of some tropical splenomegalies. Ann Trop Med Parasitol 51:225, 1957

154. Kuo T, Rosai J: Granulomatous inflammation in splenectomy specimens. Clinico-pathologic study of 20 cases. Arch Pathol 98:261, 1974

155. Kadin ME, Donaldson SS, Dorfman RF: Isolated granulomas in Hodgkin's disease. N Engl J Med 283:859, 1970

156. Silverstein MN, Ellefstein RD: The syndrome of the sea-blue histiocyte. Semin Hematol 9:299, 1972

157. Varela-Duvan J, Roholt PC, Ratcliff NB: Sea blue histiocyte syndrome. A secondary degenerative process of macrophages. Arch Pathol Lab Med 104:30, 1980

158. Volk BW, Adaehi M, Schneck L: The pathology of sphingolipidoses. Semin Hematol 9:317, 1972

159. Firkin BG, Wright R, Miller S, et al: Splenic macrophages in thrombocytopenia. Blood 33:240, 1969

160. Saltzstein SL: Phospholipid accumulation in histiocytes of splenic pulp associated with thrombocytopenic purpura. Blood 18:73, 1961

161. Kostich ND, Rappaport H: Diagnostic significance of the histologic changes in the liver and spleen in leukemia and malignant lymphoma. Cancer 18:1214, 1965

162. Burke JS, Byrne GE, Rappaport H: Hairy cell leukaemia (leukaemic reticulo-endotheliosis). I. A clinical-pathologic study of 21 patients. Cancer 33:1399, 1974

163. Zidar BL, Winkelstein A, Whiteside TL, et al: Hairy cell leukemia. 7 Cases with probable B lymphocytic origin. Br J Haematol 37:455, 1977

164. Ahmann DL, Kiely JM, Harrison EG, et al: Malignant lymphoma of the spleen. A review of 49 cases in which the diagnosis was made at splenectomy. Cancer 19:461, 1966

165. Hickling RA: Giant follicle lymphoma of the spleen; recovery after splenectomy. Br Med J 1:1464, 1960

166. Hickling RA: Giant follicle lymphoma of the spleen: A condition closely related to lymphatic leukaemia but apparently curable by splenectomy. Br Med J 1:787, 1964

167. Pitney WR, Pryor DS, Tait-Smith AL: Morphological observations on livers and spleens of patients with tropical splenomegaly in New Guinea. J Pathol 95:417, 1968

168. Dacie JV, Brain MC, Harrison CV, et al: Non-tropical idiopathic splenomegaly (primary hypersplenism): A review of ten cases and their relationship to malignant lymphomas. Br J Haematol 17:317, 1969

169. Crosby WH: Hyposplenism: An enquiry into normal functions of the spleen. Annu Rev Med 14:349, 1963

170. McCarthy CF, Fraser ID, Evans KT, et al: Lymphoreticular dysfunction in idiopathic steatorrhoea. Gut 7:140, 1966

171. Marsh GW, Stewart JS: Splenic function in adult coeliac disease. Br J Haematol 19:445, 1970

172. Wardrop CA, Dagg JH, Lee FD, et al: Immunological abnormalities in splenic atrophy. Lancet 2:4, 1975

173. Ryan FP, Preston FE, Smart RC, et al: Abnormalities of splenic function in ulcerative colitis and Crohn's disease. Gut 16:834, 1975

174. Desser RK, Ultmann JE: Risk of severe infection in patients with Hodgkin's disease or lymphoma after diagnostic laparotomy and splenectomy. Ann Intern Med 77:143, 1972

13

Bone Marrow

Nora C.J. Sun

Bone marrow examination is a well established procedure in the study of hematologic disorders, in the evaluation of fever of unknown origin,[1] in the evaluation of other systemic diseases,[2-4] and for the staging of malignant lymphoma.[5,6] However, the controversial question has been whether aspiration (traditionally studied by hematologists) or surgical trephine biopsy (traditionally studied by pathologists) is superior. Recent improvements in bone marrow biopsy instruments[7,8] and methods of processing specimens,[9,10] a realization of the importance of biopsy in the evaluation of marrow architecture and cellular distribution,[11-14] and advances in the correlation of the morphology of the bone marrow with that of other tissues have led to widespread adoption of the histologic examination of bone marrow biopsies and of the use of such examinations to supplement the information gained from the study of aspiration smears.

HANDLING AND PROCESSING OF SPECIMENS

The conventional approach to the study of the bone marrow includes: (1) a pertinent clinical history and physical examination, (2) complete blood cell and white cell differential counts, (3) sections of bone marrow aspiration (clot) and/or bone marrow biopsy, (4) smears of bone marrow aspirations or touch preparations of bone marrow biopsy, and (5) other tests.[15-17] Bilateral or multiple bone marrow biopsies have been advocated[3,18] in the staging of malignant lymphomas and in the search for other malignant tumors or granulomas.

The choice of a site for bone marrow aspiration and/or biopsy depends on the age of the patient, the previous history of irradiation, the presence of local skin conditions, and the preference of the examiner. In general, anterior or posterior iliac crest is the choice for adults and anterior tibia is the choice for children. The density and content of hematopoietic elements, fat, and bony trabeculae are different in different parts of bone. An aspiration of bone marrow particles usually precedes the bone marrow biopsy. Proper selection of marrow particles for smears or electron microscopic study is an art learned by practice and experience. Some investigators advocate aspiration only, followed by concentration of particles for section preparation.[19] Others feel that sections of bone marrow biopsies have the added advantage of permitting the examination of the bony architecture to identify diseases affecting the bone and to study the distribution of hematopoietic elements and their relationship to bony trabeculae, and to study the effect of intramedullary disease on bone.[14,20] Touch preparations should be made from the bone biopsy, especially when there is a "dry tap." The air-dried smears and touch preparations may be used for Romanowsky's stain, special cytochemical stains, and terminal deoxynucleotidyl transferase (TdT) immunocytochemical stain. Cytologic study is most useful in classifying leukemia and myelodysplastic syndrome and in identifying dyspoiesis by examining the Romanowsky-stained smears. It is a valuable adjunct to the study of histologic sections. Extra slides may be fixed in acetone or alcohol for other monoclonal or polyclonal antibody studies. The collected particles or the biopsy specimen are then fixed in Zenker's or B5 solutions. Specimens that have been well fixed in 10 percent buffered formalin and properly processed can also give satisfactory preparations for interpretation.

Decalcification of bone biopsy specimens frequently causes leaching of iron from the tissue, resulting in inaccurate assessment of body iron stores,[21] and it also interferes with histochemical and immunohistochemical stains.[14] Thus, these special studies are preferentially performed on smears or on bone marrow particle or clot sections. Routine stains for bone marrow examination include hematoxylin and eosin (H&E) and periodic acid–Schiff (PAS) stains. The latter highlights myeloid cells and megakaryocytes because these cells contain glycogen. Reticulin stain is particularly helpful in the study of myeloproliferative disorders and for delineation of the marrow meshwork. The specific (α-naphthol chloroacetate) esterase (Leder) stain may be used on formalin-fixed, paraffin-embedded sections and is a useful marker for neutrophils and tissue mast cells.[17]

Recent studies indicate that enzyme cytochemistry, immunocytochemistry, flow cytometry, DNA restriction enzyme analysis, and cytogenetic examinations are invaluable tools in classifying hematopoietic and lymphoreticular malignancies and in predicting the prognosis for these patients.[22–32] However, some of these techniques are rather sophisticated, requiring special and expensive equipment and trained and experienced personnel. If collaborative studies can be arranged, fresh specimens should be collected in tissue culture media for transportation. In most of the surgical pathology labora-

tories in daily practice, a panel of polyclonal and monoclonal antibodies may be applied to formalin-fixed or B5-fixed, paraffin-embedded sections by using an immunoperoxidase or an immunoalkaline phosphatase technique for identification and classification of hematologic disorders[33–38] (Table 13-1).

NORMAL BONE MARROW

The hematopoietic marrow is red (red marrow), and the nonhematopoietic marrow is yellow and fatty (yellow marrow). The distribution of red and yellow marrow in the bones is usually constant. Whenever there is an increased level of hematopoiesis, hematopoietic marrow rapidly expands into the yellow marrow. This replacement may occur within 24 to 48 hours after a massive hemorrhage.

The marrow is traversed by bony trabeculae, consists of vascular and hematopoietic compartments, and is organized about blood vessels. The vascular sinuses play an important role in many of the marrow's functions. The adventitial cells of the vascular sinuses are capable of becoming voluminous, forming gelatinous or fat cells; if such change is extensive, the marrow may become grossly gelatinous or fatty. The proportion of fatty to hematopoietic marrow varies in different bones and in different age groups under normal condition,[39] although the relationship in a given age group and anatomic site is usually quite constant. Hartsock et al.,[40] on the basis of a study of bone marrow from the anterior iliac crest, concluded that the amount of hematopoietic tissue in the first decade was 80 percent, which diminished to about 50 percent at the age of 30 and remained relatively constant until the age of 70, at which time the mean value became 30 percent. Similar trends may be seen in bone marrow obtained from the ribs, sternum, and vertebrae.

The hematopoietic elements include erythrocytes, granulocytes, megakaryocytes, lymphocytes, plasma cells, macrophages, mast cells, and their precursors. They are located in the marrow spaces in the extravascular compartments in a certain topographic distribution.[41] Erythropoietic islands and megakaryocytes are associated with the sinusoids in the central regions of the marrow cavities. Early myeloid precursors lie close to the endosteal surfaces and to the arterioles. As the myeloid cells mature, they are found in the central part of the marrow cavity. The myeloid-to-erythroid ratio is usually 3:1 or 4:1 but may range from 2:1 to 6:1 under physiologic conditions. This paradox of more myeloid elements in marrow despite more red cells in the peripheral blood is due to the much shorter life span of granulocytes (the time from myeloblast to death is 9 to 10 days, in compari-

TABLE 13-1. Common Antibodies Used for Antigen Detection in Histologic Sections of Bone Marrow

Antibodies	Reactive Cells
HbA	Majority of NRBCs and RBCs
HbF	Minority of NRBCs and RBCs
Lysozyme	Granulocytes, mono/histiocytes
Leu M₁	Most granulocytes and monocytes, some Reed-Sternberg cells
Leukocyte common antigen	Lymphocytes, monocytes, and mast cells; some histiocytes, plasma cells, and polymorphonuclear leukocytes
LN1	Germinal center B-cells, NRBCs, peripheral B-cells
LN2	B-cells in germinal center and mantle zone, interdigitating histiocytes, and Reed-Sternberg cells
LN3	HLA-DR antigen: B-cells, mono-histiocytes, and activated T-cells
Immunoglobulin (individual heavy or light chain)	B-immunoblasts and plasma cells; some large and small noncleaved follicular center cells
UCHL-1	Thymocytes, activated T-cells, and a proportion of resting T-cells
Factor VIII–related antigen	Megakaryocytes, platelets, endothelial cells

Abbreviation: NRBC, nucleated red blood cells.

son with the 120-day life span of a red cell). A marked derangement in myeloid to erythroid ratio indicates hematologic disorders.

Erythropoiesis

Islands of erythropoiesis are easily identified on histologic sections or smears. They are characterized by perfectly round nuclei, evenly distributed chromatin, and a moderate amount of cytoplasm, which is often intensely basophilic in proerythroblasts and basophilic normoblasts by the Giemsa stain and bright red with the methyl green–pyronine stain. The more mature forms (polychromatophilic and orthochromatophilic normoblasts) have more condensed or pyknotic nuclei (Fig. 13-1). The former have a clear cytoplasm and the latter have eosinophilic cytoplasm as hemoglobinization of the cytoplasm becomes more evident. The nucleated red blood cells (NRBCs) may be easily differentiated from myeloid precursors by their PAS-negative cytoplasm (except in erythroleukemia and a few disease entities in which the cytoplasm of erythroblasts may contain PAS-positive granules or may be diffusely stained by the PAS method). Lymphocytes or lymphoid aggregates may at times be confused with NRBCs. However, foci of erythropoiesis usually contain a spectrum of NRBCs, indicating subsequent maturation, while small lymphocytes in lymphoid aggregates tend to be monomorphic. In addition, the nuclei of lymphoid cells are usually slightly irregular, the nuclear membranes are thickened, and the chromatin is more clumped. Plasma cells, blood vessels, immunoblasts, and mast cells are often found in lymphoid

aggregates. Erythropoiesis tends to be present in the vicinity of sinusoids. Hemosiderin-laden macrophages (Ferrata cells or nurse cells), which are found in the center of an erythroblastic island, may be easily identified by a Prussian blue (iron) stain.

Body iron stores are best assessed by an iron stain on the bone marrow smear or clot section. Although serum ferritin correlates well with the bone marrow iron stain under normal conditions, an increased serum ferritin concentration may be found in a variety of pathologic conditions unrelated to body iron stores.[42] Normally, iron is present in the histiocytes. A few (up to four) Prussian blue–positive (siderotic) granules may be normally seen in erythroid precursors (sideroblasts). Under pathologic conditions the NRBCs contain iron-laden mitochondria (sideromitochondria), which are distributed perinuclearly in humans, thus appearing as "ring sideroblasts" by iron stain. Sideroblastic anemia is defined as a refractory dyserythropoietic anemia with marked erythroid hyperplasia and an excess of iron and many ring sideroblasts in the marrow. It is a syndrome with diverse etiologies.

Myelopoiesis

The earlier myeloid precursors, myeloblasts and promyelocytes, have an oval vesicular nucleus, small but distinct nucleoli, and a moderate amount of eosinophilic cytoplasm (Fig. 13-2). As the cells become more mature, the nuclear-to-cytoplasmic ratio decreases and specific (neutrophilic, basophilic, and eosinophilic) granules appear in the cytoplasm starting from the myelocytic stage. However, neutrophilic granules are often difficult to see on H&E-stained sections, and basophilic granules dis-

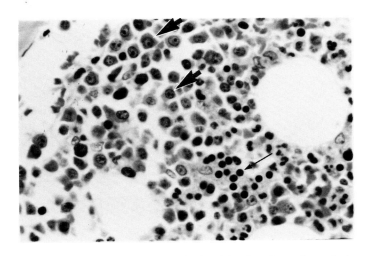

Fig. 13-1. Normal hematopoiesis. Islands of erythropoiesis are easily seen. The earlier erythroid precursors have round nuclei, prominent nucleoli, and fine chromatin (arrow heads). As the cells mature, the nuclei become pyknotic and are surrounded by clear cytoplasm (arrow). (H&E stain, ×200.)

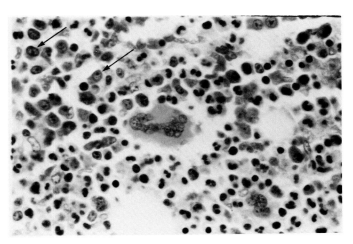

Fig. 13-2. Normal hematopoiesis. The earlier myeloid cells usually have an oval nucleus, lacy chromatin pattern, and one or more distinct nucleoli (arrows). Megakaryocytes are also present. (H&E stain, ×200.)

solve during tissue processing. As mentioned early, PAS and specific esterase (Leder) stains are helpful in recognizing granulocytes.

Megakaryopoiesis

The more primitive cells—megakaryoblasts and pro-megakaryocytes—are difficult to identify on H&E-stained sections, although they are readily recognized on Romanowsky-stained smears. Their number is increased in acute megakaryocytic myelosis or other acute myelo-proliferative disorders. Electron microscopic examination or specific monoclonal antibodies (such as glycoprotein IIB/IIIA or HP1-1D) are used to confirm their presence.[43,44] Following subsequent maturation, the cells are enlarged, the nuclei have become lobulated, and the cytoplasm is voluminous and contains numerous granules on Romanowsky-stained smear or contains PAS-positive cytoplasm on histologic section (Fig. 13-2). Margination of intensely PAS-positive granules may be seen on sections, which indicates platelet production. Occasionally polymorphonuclear leukocytes or red cells are seen in the cytoplasm of megakaryocytes (emperipolesis).[45] Megakaryocytes are easily differentiated from osteoclasts, which are multinucleated cells in which each nucleus is identical, with an evenly distributed chromatin pattern and a small nucleolus. Osteoclasts are present along the bony trabeculae and are considered to be generated from the same hematopoietic stem cell as megakaryocytes. They are important in bony remodeling.[41]

Other Cells

Monocytes originate from the same stem cells as myeloblasts, but they are difficult to find in bone marrow sections. *Histiocytes* with phagocytosis (phagocytes, macrophages), epithelioid cells, foamy cells, or other variations are seen in physiologic or pathologic conditions. *Lymphocytes* are present in an appreciable number in very young and very old individuals. Aggregates of lymphocytes in association with capillaries, histiocytes, plasma cells, and mast cells are seen in increased frequency in elderly individuals.[46] Very few *plasma cells* (less than 2 percent) are normally seen in the bone marrow[47]; they are usually scattered in the marrow cavity. A perivascular cuffing of plasma cells is seen in alcoholic liver disease, cirrhosis, collagen vascular disease, and other chronic conditions. *Osteoblasts*, cells that produce bone matrix, should be differentiated from plasma cells on bone marrow smears. These cells are often in clusters, with each cell containing one oval nucleus, evenly distributed smooth chromatin, and one small nucleolus. A

hof is present away from the nucleus. Osteoblasts frequently line bony trabeculae in young children, as seen on sections. *Mast cells* lie adjacent to the endothelial cells of sinusoids, at the endosteal surface of the trabecular bone, and frequently at the edges of lymphoid nodules or aggregates. They are difficult to recognize in H&E-stained sections of bone marrow but are readily identifiable by PAS or Leder stains. Increased numbers of lymphocytes, plasma cells, and mast cells are frequently noted in hypoplastic or aplastic bone marrow.

PRACTICAL APPROACH TO BONE MARROW EXAMINATION

As stated earlier, knowledge of the clinical history, the peripheral blood cell count, and the white cell differential count and of other important laboratory test results (serum and urine protein studies, serum levels of lactate dehydrogenase, iron, etc.) is essential prior to examination and interpretation of peripheral blood smears, bone marrow biopsy and clot sections, and bone marrow smears. Since this book is for surgical pathologists, a checklist for evaluation of bone marrow biopsy sections is given in Table 13-2.

A bone marrow report includes description, diagnosis, and comment. Needless to say, all pertinent findings should be described. A systemic approach is always helpful. For example, I usually read the clinical history first and then examine the peripheral blood smear, bone marrow biopsy, bone marrow clot section, bone marrow smear and the results of other special studies. On each of these preparations I routinely examine the red cell series first and then the myeloid and megakaryocytic series and other cells. It is important to remember the patient's age (bony remodeling and cellularity) and sex (especially in considering anemia) when you do the examination, and it is important to know the patient's ethnic background (for instance, hemoglobinopathy is common in certain ethnic groups). Sometimes a definitive diagnosis may not be made; then a summation of pertinent findings is listed, followed by comments, which include a list of differential diagnoses and, frequently, suggestions for additional studies.

PATHOLOGY OF BONE MARROW

The pathology of bone marrow may be classified according to etiology (infectious disease, iron deficiency anemia, etc.), type of cell involved, (red cell disorders, white cell disorders, etc.), and pathologic changes. I have chosen to discuss the marrow abnormalities according to the predominant pathologic changes in the following or-

TABLE 13-2. Evaluation of the Bone Marrow Biopsy Sections—A Checklist

Quality of the specimen
  Satisfactory
  Inadequate

Bony architecture and content
  Evidence of remodeling
    Yes (increased, decreased)
    No
  Trabecular bone
    Normal
    Abnormal (osteoporosis, osteomalacia, osteosclerosis)
  Pagetoid change

Marrow space
  Hematopoietic elements
    Fat to cell ratio
    Cellularity (normal, increased, decreased)
    Erythropoiesis and maturation sequence
    Granulopoiesis and maturation sequence
    Myeloid to erythroid ratio
    Megakaryopoiesis and maturation sequence
    Marrow necrosis
  Stroma
    Fat
      Normal, increased, decreased
      Gelatinous degeneration
      Necrosis, edema, hemorrhage
    Blood vessels
      Normal
      Abnormal (vasculitis, arteriosclerosis, amyloid deposition, intravascular fibrin or platelet thrombi, vascular proliferation or tumor, dilation of sinuses, intrasinusoidal hematopoiesis)
    Reticulin meshwork
      Normal
      Abnormal (reticulin fibrosis or collagen fibrosis; focal or diffuse; collapsed reticulin meshwork)
  Other cells
    Histiocytes (phagocytes, foamy cells, epithelioid cells, giant cells, granulomas)
    Lymphocytes (small aggregates, nodules, follicles. Pattern of infiltration: interstitial, nodular, or paratrabecular; focal or diffuse)
    Plasma cells
      Increased (perivascular or intramedullary infiltration)
    Mast cells
    Foreign cells

TABLE 13-3. Common Causes or Clinical Conditions Associated with Hypocellular Bone Marrow

Normal aging process

Nutritional (anorexia nervosa)

Infectious (e.g., viral hepatitis or miliary tuberculosis)

Marrow toxicity (drugs, chemicals, or ionizing radiation)

Some leukemias

Some refractory anemias

Paroxysmal nocturnal hemoglobinuria

Congenital (Fanconi's syndrome or constitutional hypoplastic anemia)

Idiopathic (aplastic anemia)

Normal or Hypocellular Bone Marrow

Hypocellular bone marrow is defined by a decrease in volume of hematopoietic elements in relation to fat, with the patient's age taken into consideration. The cellular components of a hypocellular marrow must be studied carefully, because the different cell series may not be affected to the same degree and because an increased number of blasts (acute leukemia) may be observed in hypocellular marrow (discussed later). Lymphocytes, plasma cells, histiocytes, and mast cells are usually quite prominent in such specimens. The common causes or clinical conditions associated with hypocellular bone marrow are listed in Table 13-3. Intramedullary hemorrhage following bone marrow aspiration should not be confused with hypocellular marrow. Likewise, the marrow cavities in the subcortical region are usually more hypoplastic (especially in old age) and should not be relied on for diagnosis. Selective hypoplasia in the iliac crest has also been observed in certain conditions, such as autoimmune states.[48]

Serous (Mucinous, Gelatinous) Degeneration of the Marrow

Serous marrow degeneration is characterized by multifocal gelatinous transformation of the non-hematopoietic marrow and is associated with malnutrition, emaciation, anorexia nervosa, and a variety of chronic disorders, including malignant disease, tuberculosis, and chronic renal disease.[49] Microscopic examination reveals the fat cells to be decreased in size, with pink amorphous material in the interstitium (Fig. 13-3). They have a granular or fibrillary appearance on higher magnification and stain pale pink with the PAS stain (Fig. 13-4). Histochemical studies show that the extracellular substance consists primarily of hyaluronic acid.[50] The adjacent marrow is usually hypoplastic, but the total amount of hematopoietic material is usually not decreased. Serous atrophy may be found in the adipose tissue in other parts of the body.

der: (1) cellularity, (2) fibrosis, (3) lymphocytic infiltrates, (4) granulomatous changes, (5) histiocytic proliferative disorders, (6) metastatic tumors, (7) bone marrow necrosis and infarction, and (8) vascular lesions in marrow.

Cellularity

The hematopoietic elements may become hypocellular or hypercellular in physiologic or pathologic conditions. A hypocellular bone marrow is often associated with peripheral cytopenia, while hypercellular bone marrow may be manifested as polycythemia, leukocytosis, thrombocytosis, or one or more cytopenias in the peripheral blood.

Aplastic Anemia

Aplastic anemia may be classified as constitutional (congenital or hereditary) or acquired and is usually characterized by peripheral blood pancytopenia and marrow panhypoplasia.[51] Isolated single cell-line deficiency may also occur. The congenital form is uncommon. The acquired form is frequently related to drugs, chemicals, ionizing radiation, or viral infections. Sometimes the episode may be transient, and the marrow may recover after removal of the insulting agent(s).[52] Aplastic anemia may be a manifestation of preleukemia[53] and has been observed in patients with paroxysmal nocturnal hemoglobinuria[54]; thus, it may be a stem cell defect. Bone marrow examination reveals moderately hypocellular (hypoplastic) or severely hypocellular (aplastic) marrow with an increased amount of adipose tissue with scattered lymphocytes, plasma cells, mast cells, and hemosiderin-laden macrophages. Small collections of erythroid, myeloid, or megakaryocytic precursors may be observed in hypoplastic anemia. Bone marrow transplantation is a treatment of choice in selected patients.

Pure Red Cell Aplasia

Pure red cell aplasia may be congenital (Diamond-Blackfan anemia) or acquired (associated with spindle cell thymoma or other types of malignancy, aplastic crisis in hemolytic anemia, drugs, or other causes).[55,56] Vacuolated erythroblasts are seen in chloramphenicol-associated aplasia, erythroleukemia, alcoholism (in which vacuolated myeloid precursors may also be present), and hyperosmolar coma.[57,58] PAS-positive granules are usu-

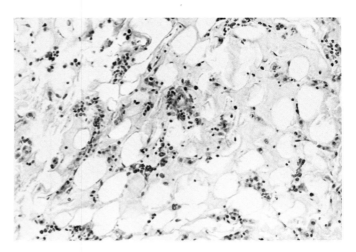

Fig. 13-4. Hypocellular bone marrow with gelatinous degeneration of fat cells. (H&E stain, ×70.)

ally demonstrated in erythroblasts of erythroleukemia. The marrow is normocellular or hypercellular.

Agranulocytosis

Agranulocytosis is a severe degree of neutropenia, which is often drug-related.[59] Neutropenia may be caused by underproduction, excessive destruction, or abnormal distribution of neutrophils. Thus, while granulocytic hypoplasia in the bone marrow is always associated with neutropenia in the peripheral blood, not all neutropenias are associated with granulocytic hypoplasia in the marrow. Congenital abnormalities of granulopoiesis are rare. Some patients with autoimmune disorders or viral infections may have selective granulocytic hypoplasia.[60,61]

Isolated or selective megakaryocytic hypoplasia or aplasia is very rare,[62] although thrombocytopenia is not uncommon clinically.

Paroxysmal Nocturnal Hemoglobinuria

Paroxysmal nocturnal hemoglobinuria is a stem cell disorder characterized by the formation of defective hematopoietic cells. The etiology of this acquired disorder is unknown. The clinical manifestations of pancytopenia and reticulocytosis are due to increased sensitivity of erythrocyte membranes to complement-mediated lysis. Sucrose hemolysis and Ham acid hemolysis tests are useful for the diagnosis. The marrow cellularity is quite variable.[63]

Hypoplastic Acute Leukemia

Although acute leukemia is usually characterized by hypercellular bone marrow, some patients, mostly elderly men, may present with hypocellular marrow and other morphologic features indicative of acute leukemia

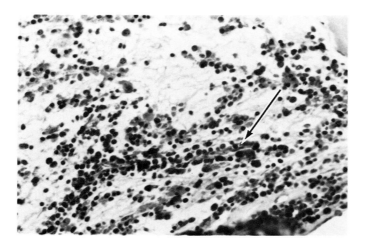

Fig. 13-3. Bone marrow biopsy from a patient with acquired immune deficiency syndrome (AIDS). Note mucinous degeneration of fat (the fat cells become very small and poorly outlined). The plasma cells are markedly increased with perivascular cuffing (arrow). Note that the overall marrow cellularity is not decreased. (H&E stain, ×100.)

(increased number of blasts, presence of Auer rods, dyserythropoiesis, and chromosomal abnormalities).[64,65] Hypoplastic acute leukemia was defined as occurring when the hematopoietic elements occupied a volume equal to or less than 40 percent in one series,[64] and equal to or less than 50 percent in another series.[65] The incidence of this form of acute leukemia was said to be 7.7 percent[65] to 10.7 percent.[64] Most of these patients had acute nonlymphocytic leukemia, and many of them responded to aggressive chemotherapy. However, a number of patients in both studies[64,65] do not fulfill the diagnostic criteria of acute leukemia as delineated by the French-American-British (FAB) cooperative group,[66–68] although hypocellular acute leukemia does exist when the marrow is hypocellular but the blast count in the peripheral blood or bone marrow exceeds 30 percent of all nucleated cells.[68] Recently, Gladson and Naeim collected 20 patients who had hypocellular bone marrow and increased blasts.[69] They found that a history of alcohol abuse (30 percent), potential exposure to toxic chemicals (20 percent), second malignancies (20 percent), and aplastic anemia (25 percent) were common in this group of patients, and they also found that overall mortality was high, especially in patients undergoing chemotherapy. More study is apparently needed for the characterization of hypocellular acute leukemia, which should be differentiated from myelodysplastic syndrome (MDS). "Smoldering acute leukemia" is a poorly defined entity,[70] and the term should be abandoned.

Transient pancytopenia has been occasionally noted preceding the onset of acute leukemia in children (2 percent).[71] These patients have had peripheral pancytopenia and a hypocellular bone marrow aspirate, have responded rapidly to steroid therapy, and have later developed acute lymphoblastic leukemia (ALL). The patients developed overt leukemia within 5 to 38 weeks of first presentation with features of marrow failure. Immunologic study revealed that blasts with ALL possessed the phenotype of common ALL. This phenomenon has not been widely recognized and has been described as a "preleukemic state" in the literature.[72] It should be differentiated from preleukemia in adults (which is discussed later).

Postchemotherapy Bone Marrow Aplasia

Sequential evaluation of bone marrow changes following administration of chemotherapeutic agents for acute leukemias frequently reveals marrow necrosis and aplasia in the immediate stage, with deposition of eosinophilic amorphous material in the interstitium, edema, and marked dilatation of sinuses (Fig. 13-5). Erythroid cell regeneration usually appears at first, followed by the granulocytic and megakaryocytic precursors in successfully treated patients. A similar process is observed in

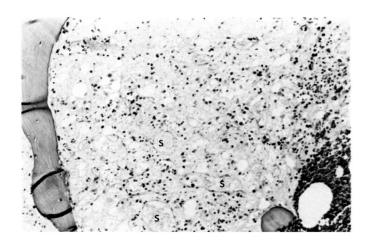

Fig. 13-5. Postchemotherapeutic effect. Note markedly hypocellular bone marrow, with edema and deposition of eosinophilic granular material in the interstitium and sinusoids (s). (H&E stain, ×40.)

bone marrow necrosis of other etiologies (Fig. 13-6). Wittels[73] described two phases of marrow response to effective chemotherapy in acute leukemia: (1) cellular depletion characterized by progressive emptying of the initially packed marrow to leave an essentially vacant fibrillary reticulin stroma punctuated by dilated sinusoids containing fibrin; and (2) marrow reconstitution, during which the intertrabecular space is refilled by proliferation of hematopoietic cells and generation of fat cells, collagen, or bone. In my experience, leukemic cells seen in relapse of leukemia or residual leukemic cells are often focally clustered; thus, histologic section provides a better mean for assessment than aspirated smears.

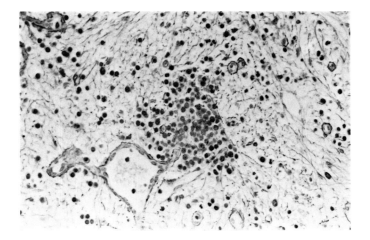

Fig. 13-6. Bone marrow biopsy from a patient who had SS disease (sickle cell anemia) in aplastic crisis. Note that the reticulin meshwork is maintained, although the cellularity is markedly decreased. An island of erythropoiesis is seen in the center of the field. (Snook's reticulin stain, ×100.)

TABLE 13-4. Common Causes or Clinical Conditions Associated with Hypercellular Bone Marrow

Newborn

Compensatory increase in hematopoiesis
  Erythroid hyperplasia in hemolytic anemia, pernicious anemia, hypoxia, and others
  Leukemoid reaction to infections, neoplasia, or others
  Megakaryocytic hyperplasia in immune thrombocytopenia purpura
  Panhyperplasia in hypersplenism

Congenital dyserythropoietic anemia

Neoplastic conditions (polycythemia vera, leukemias, myelodysplastic syndrome, and chronic myeloproliferative disorders)

Hypercellular Bone Marrow

Hypercellular bone marrow may be broadly classified as nonneoplastic or neoplastic hyperplasia (Table 13-4).

Nonneoplastic Hyperplasia

Reactive hyperplasia is a compensatory mechanism responding to peripheral destruction or utilization of blood elements; the production and maturation of these elements are usually normal. Sometimes nonneoplastic hyperplasia may occur under nonphysiologic conditions.

Erythroid Hyperplasia. Erythroid hyperplasia may be normoblastic, megaloblastic, or megaloblastoid.

Normoblastic Hyperplasia. Normoblastic hyperplasia may be manifested as peripheral erythrocytosis or anemia. *Erythrocytosis* (secondary polycythemia) results from increased erythropoiesis due to increased production of erythropoietin. Chronic tissue hypoxia of various etiologies (such as living in high altitude or cardiopulmonary disease resulting in a right-to-left cardiac shunt) and hemoglobinopathy with increased oxygen affinity are more common than is inappropriate secretion of erythropoietin by a tumor (such as hypernephroma or cerebellar hemangioblastoma). The bone marrow shows erythroid hyperplasia without accompanying myeloid or megakaryocytic hyperplasia. Anemia of hereditary red cell abnormalities (red cell membrane defect, enzymopathy, or hemoglobinopathy) or of acquired disorders (iron deficiency anemia, hemolytic anemia, some forms of refractory anemias, or some forms of sideroblastic anemias) is often associated with erythroid hyperplasia. Erythroid hyperplasia also is observed a few days after acute massive hemorrhage or bleeding and in patients with congenital dyserythropoietic anemia.[74]

Hypochromic anemia, the most common form of anemia, is characterized by normocytic or microcytic, hypochromic red cell morphology. It includes a variety of clinical conditions (such as iron deficiency anemia, thalassemia, sideroblastic anemia, and anemia of chronic disease), all of which are related to impaired hemoglobin synthesis. Of the disease entities listed above, all but iron deficiency anemia are associated with iron overload.

A normal individual absorbs 5 to 10 percent of the total iron ingested, the rest being lost with sloughed mucosal cells of the small intestine. All body iron is combined (chelated) with one or another protein. For instance, plasma iron is transported bound to transferrin. By far the greatest amount of iron in the body is present within cells as heme iron (iron chelated to the porphyrin ring), which is then combined with globins and becomes hemoglobin (for oxygen transport), myoglobin (for oxygen storage), and cytochrome C (an enzyme responsible for oxygen activation in biologic oxidation).

Iron is stored equally as ferritin (ferric hydroxyphosphate micelles attached to apoferritin, a globulin) and hemosiderin (aggregates of ferritin particles) in the reticuloendothelial cells of the liver, spleen, and bone marrow and the parenchymal cells of the liver. Ferritin is finely dispersed within the cytoplasm, is water-soluble, and is invisible with the light microscope, although it is readily seen with the electron microscope. Hemosiderin is visible as yellow to brown granules by light microscopy but is best demonstrated by the Prussian blue stain. Only intracellular granules should be considered in the evaluation of iron stores. The iron not utilized for the red cell pool is shifted to the stores. Prolonged intravascular hemolysis is associated with hemosiderinuria and depletion of iron stores. In extravascular hemolytic processes, including ineffective erythropoiesis (as in thalassemia), and also in patients who have received multiple blood transfusions for chronic anemias, increased marrow hemosiderin is seen (hemosiderosis). A subgroup of sideroblastic anemias will be discussed in connection with myelodysplastic syndrome. Ring sideroblasts may be found in megaloblastic anemia, thalassemia, alcoholism, lead intoxication, drug reactions (to chloramphenicol or isoniazid), and in certain hereditary anemias.

Clinically, iron deficiency anemia may be divided into three stages: (1) iron depletion, (2) iron-deficient erythropoiesis, and (3) iron-deficient anemia. Although decreased levels of serum ferritin and marrow iron stores are noted in the earliest stage, it is not until the third stage that microcytic hypochromic anemia becomes evident.

Megaloblastic Hyperplasia. Megaloblastic anemia includes a group of disorders characterized by one or more peripheral cytopenias, oval macrocytosis, iron overload, and megaloblastic erythroid hyperplasia. It is commonly caused by a vitamin B_{12} or folate deficiency, resulting in impairment of DNA synthesis. A megaloblastic erythroid cell is larger than a corresponding normoblastic cell, with a high cytoplasmic-to-nuclear area ratio and an open, lacy chromatin pattern (dyssynchrony in nuclear and cytoplasmic maturation). Multinuclearity, nuclear fragments

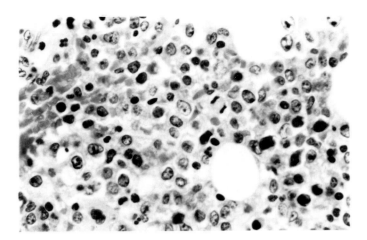

Fig. 13-7. Hypercellular bone marrow from a patient with megaloblastic anemia. Note marked erythroid hyperplasia, which is distinctly different from normoblastic erythropoiesis (Fig. 13-1). Mitotic figures are also seen. (H&E stain, ×200.)

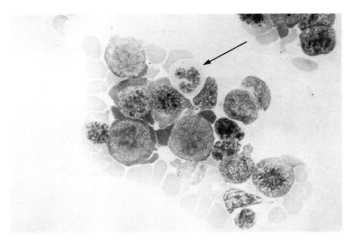

Fig. 13-9. Bone marrow aspiration smear from a patient with megaloblastic anemia. Note megaloblastic change involving entire erythroid cell line. A monocytoid band is also present (arrow). (Wright-Giemsa stain, ×400.)

or Howell-Jolly bodies (dyserythropoiesis), and mitoses are seen. Megaloblastic change affects all dividing cells. Giant bands, monocytoid bands, hypersegmented neutrophils, and hyperlobulated megakaryocytes are all present. Ineffective erythropoiesis (premature death of erythroid cells during the maturation sequence in the marrow) is increased. Megaloblastic hyperplasia may be so florid as to be confused with acute leukemia (Fig. 13-7). Identification of intracytoplasmic HbA or HbF by an immunoperoxidase method may be helpful in recognizing that these immature cells are megaloblastic erythroblasts (Fig. 13-8). Megaloblastic change is most evident on bone marrow smears. Figures 13-9 and 13-10 are used to compare megaloblastic with normoblastic erythropoiesis.

Pernicious anemia is a form of megaloblastic anemia, caused by atrophic gastritis with circulating antiparietal cell and/or intrinsic factor antibody in the blood, resulting in vitamin B_{12} deficiency. The most significant clinical manifestations are neurologic symptoms due to subacute combined degeneration of the spinal cord. It affects middle-aged or elderly women with a familial and racial disposition. A juvenile form has also been recognized.[75]

Megaloblastoid Hyperplasia. Megaloblastoid erythropoiesis display morphologic features intermediate between those of megaloblastic and normoblastic erythropoiesis. It has been called ''intermediate megaloblastic,'' ''macronormoblastic,'' or ''transitional megaloblastic''

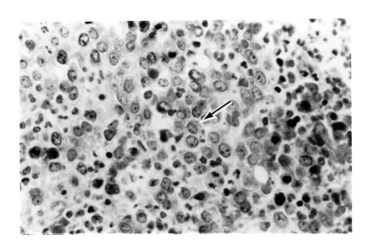

Fig. 13-8. Megaloblastic anemia. Note that many immature cells are weakly stained by anti-hemoglobin A (arrow). (Immunoperoxidase stain, ×200.)

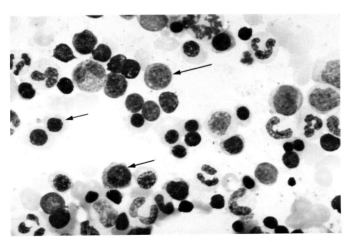

Fig. 13-10. Normoblastic erythropoiesis. Note that the size of the cells and the chromatin pattern of the immature erythrons (arrows) are different from those in megaloblastic anemia (see Fig. 13-9). (H&E stain, ×400.)

erythropoiesis. A megaloblastoid erythroid cell is larger than the corresponding erythrons of the normoblastic series, with evidence of dissociation in nuclear/cytoplasmic maturation. However, the chromatin pattern is punctate and clumping, and the chromatin strands are coarser than in megaloblastic maturation. Thus, there are more parachromatin spaces. Multinuclearity and nuclear fragmentation are common. Both megaloblastic and megaloblastoid erythropoiesis are dyserythropoiesis, but the megaloblastoid change is more common clinically. It may be observed in acute and chronic myeloproliferative disorders (CMPDs), myeloplastic syndrome (MDS), pregnancy, and alcoholic liver disease and in patients undergoing chemotherapy. Lewis and VerWilghen preferred to reserve the term *dyserythropoietic anemia* for congenital (and acquired primary) cases only.[76]

Myeloid Hyperplasia. Myeloid hyperplasia with peripheral leukocytosis (in excess of 50×10^9 leukocytes per liter) is called *leukemoid reaction*. Leukemoid reaction may be seen in other white cells. Reactive myeloid hyperplasia secondary to severe sepsis may occasionally be associated with leukopenia. Leukemoid reaction may be elicited by bacterial (neutrophilic), viral (lymphoid), allergic (eosinophilic), or inflammatory diseases, necrosis, burns, drugs, toxins, and neoplasms. Myeloid hyperplasia or granulocytic hyperplasia may display normal maturation with a marked increase in the myeloid to erythroid ratio. It can also exhibit a "shift to the left" (an increased number of the more immature granulocytic cells). The term *maturation arrest* of the granulocytic series is used to describe granulocytic hyperplasia with a shift to the left and very rare segmented neutrophils and bands. It may be associated with leukemia, or it may reflect granulocytic hyperplasia associated with an increased delivery of more mature granulocytes to the peripheral blood. Histologic differentiation between a leukemoid reaction and chronic granulocytic leukemia (CGL) in the marrow may not be possible, but the following guidelines may be helpful:

1. Granulocytic proliferation in CGL is most evident along the paratrabecular region.
2. Increased eosinophils and basophils are more commonly seen with CGL.
3. Megakaryocytic hyperplasia with abnormal forms is common in CGL.
4. Increased reticulin fibers are more frequently seen in CGL.
5. The marrow fat cells are relatively well preserved in leukemoid reaction but not in CGL.
6. The presence of Philadelphia chromosome [Ph¹ : t(9;22)] and decreased leukocyte alkaline phosphatase score confirm the diagnosis of CGL.

Megakaryocytic Hyperplasia. Increased numbers of normal megakaryocytes are typically seen in immune thrombocytopenic purpura or other clinical conditions associated with increased destruction of platelets (thrombotic thrombocytopenic purpura, consumption coagulopathy, etc.) or with peripheral thrombocytosis. Increased megakaryocytes with abnormal morphology are seen in myeloproliferative disorders.

Neoplastic Hyperplasia

Included as forms of neoplastic hyperplasia are a group of acute leukemias, CMPDs, and MDS. Chronic lymphocytic leukemia and non-Hodgkin's lymphoma will be discussed in connection with lymphocytic infiltrate.

Acute Leukemia. Acute leukemia is defined as uncontrolled clonal proliferation of immature white cells in the blood-forming organs, which chiefly affects the bone marrow and eventually replaces the normal hematopoietic cell lines, resulting in peripheral cytopenias. In clinical practice, acute leukemia is diagnosed when there are more than 30 percent of blasts in the bone marrow,[68] although the reported percentage of blasts required for diagnosing acute leukemia varies from 30 to 50 percent in the literature.

The classification of acute leukemia is based on morphologic examination of Romanowsky-stained bone marrow smears, supplemented by a few cytochemical stains.[77,78] According to the criteria proposed by the French-American-British (FAB) cooperative group,[66–68,79] acute leukemias may be broadly classified into acute nonlymphocytic leukemia (ANLL) and acute lymphocytic leukemia (ALL) based on the presence (ANLL) or absence (ALL) of 3 percent or more blasts containing myeloperoxidase- or Sudan black B-positive granules. It should be re-emphasized, however, that immunologic study is important in classifying ALL, and that nonrandomized chromosomal changes are seen in specific types of acute leukemias, which makes chromosomal studies recommended whenever possible in acute leukemia and MDS. It should be pointed out that blasts in M7 (megakaryoblasts) do not contain myeloperoxidase- or Sudan black B-positive granules; therefore, other studies (electron microscopy or immunocytochemistry) should be made to confirm the diagnosis.[43,44,80]

Acute Nonlymphocytic Leukemias. The FAB group now proposes to establish the percentage of erythroblasts as the first step in classifying ANLLs. If erythroblasts comprise fewer than 50 percent of all nucleated bone marrow cells (ANC) and there are 30 percent or more blasts of ANC, then the leukemia may be classified as M1 to M5. If erythroblasts account for more than 50 percent of ANC and blasts represent 30 percent or more of nonerythroid cells (NEC), a diagnosis of erythroleukemia (M6) may be made. If erythroblasts account for more than 50 percent of ANC but blasts account for less than 30 percent of NEC, a diagnosis of MDS may be considered. The FAB classification of ANLLs is listed as follows:

M1—myeloblastic leukemia without maturation. At least 3 percent of the blasts are myeloperoxidase- or Sudan black B-positive. Blasts contain a few azurophilic granules and/or Auer rods and make up at least 90 percent of nonerythroid cells (NEC).

M2—myeloblastic leukemia with maturation. Blasts make up 30 percent or more of NEC and monocytic cells less than 20 percent. Promyelocytes to mature neutrophils account for more than 10 percent.

M3—promyelocytic leukemia. Most marrow cells are abnormal hypergranular promyelocytes; some may contain bundles of Auer rods. The nuclei vary in size and shape and may be reniform or bilobed.

M4—myelomonocytic leukemia. Blasts make up 30 percent or more and granulocytic elements make up more than 20 percent of NEC, and 20 percent or more of NEC are of monocytic lineage; or there are 5×10^9 or more monocytic elements per liter of peripheral blood. A significant monocytic component is confirmed either by cytochemical stain or by a serum or urine lysozyme level more than three times normal.

M5—monocytic leukemia. At least 80 percent of NEC are monoblasts, promonocytes, or monocytes. This type is subdivided into MSa, in which 80 percent or more of all monocytic cells are monoblasts, and MSb, in which less than 80 percent of all monocytic cells are monoblasts.

M6—erythroleukemia. At least 50 percent of all nucleated marrow cells are erythroblasts, and at least 30 percent of the remaining nonerythroid cells are blasts.

M7—megakaryocytic leukemia. Megakaryoblasts, which should be confirmed by platelet peroxidase on electron microscopy or immunocytochemistry with antibodies to platelet glycoprotein or factor VIII–related antigen, make up 30 percent or more of all nucleated marrow cells. If there is a "dry tap," a bone marrow biopsy must show excess blasts with increased numbers of maturing megakaryocytes plus circulating megakaryoblasts.

Most forms of ANLL exhibit a hypercellular marrow with few fat cells seen; however, hypocellular ANLL is not uncommon (Fig. 13-11). Megakaryocytes and erythroid precursors are generally sparse, with the exception of M7 and M6, respectively. The blasts are usually large, with increased nuclear to cytoplasmic ratio, round to oval or folded nuclei, finely dispersed chromatin, and small but distinct nucleoli. Auer rods, which appear as

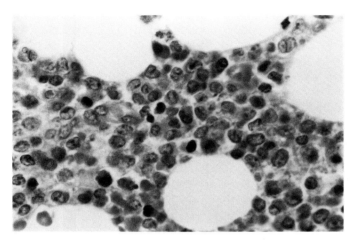

Fig. 13-11. Hypocellular acute leukemia of nonlymphocytic type (M1). Note that the vast majority of cells are immature with little differentiation. (H&E stain, ×250.)

eosinophilic rodlike structures, may be identified (Fig. 13-12). They are usually positively stained by PAS and Leder stains. A combination of Leder stain and immunocytochemical stain for lysozyme (muramidase) can differentiate a myelocytic component (positive with both stains) from a monocytic component (positive with lysozyme only). Maturing granulocytic cells may be seen interspersed among blasts, in contrast to ALL, in which Leder-positive maturing granulocytes are decreased and pushed aside to the periphery of the leukemic foci. Reticulin fibers are often slightly increased.

The incidence of various subgroups is somewhat different from report to report.[30,81–83] In general, M2 is the most common (about 30 percent incidence), followed by M1

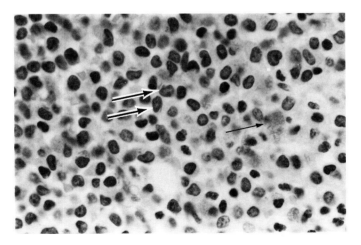

Fig. 13-12. Acute promyelocytic leukemia (M3). Bundles of Auer rods (small arrow) and leukemic cells containing a single Auer rod (large arrows) can be found. (H&E stain, ×400.)

(20 percent), M4 (20 percent), M5 (15 percent), M3 (10 percent), and M6 (5 percent). A greater proportion of ANLLs secondary to chemotherapy and/or radiotherapy were unclassifiable according to the FAB classification in comparison with de novo ANLLs. M3 is frequently associated with disseminated intravascular coagulation,[84] and a nonrandomized chromosomal anomaly [t(15;17)(q22;q21)] is seen in 40 to 50 percent of M3 patients. The M5 and M4 subgroups are commonly associated with leukemic tissue infiltration.[85] M6 should be differentiated from megaloblastic anemia and acute myelogenous leukemia (AML) with dyserythropoiesis. Although dyserythropoiesis is seen in all three conditions, vacuolated proerythroblasts and giant erythroblasts with multinuclearity are only seen in erythroleukemia. Intracytoplasmic PAS-positive granules and PAS-positive cytoplasm are also seen in erythroleukemia. The erythroblasts in M6 are stained by nonspecific esterase or chloroacetate esterase.[86] In addition, a therapeutic trial of vitamin B_{12} and folic acid or blood transfusion often corrects the morphologic abnormalities in megaloblastic anemia and AML with dyserythropoiesis. It should be pointed out that PAS-positive normoblasts have been reported in thalassemia[87] and in chronic renal disease,[88] and vacuolated proerythroblasts are seen in a variety of clinical conditions, such as alcoholism, chloramphenicol therapy, copper deficiency, riboflavin deficiency, galactoflavin ingestion, and erythroleukemias.[58]

Dameshek defined the *DiGuglielmo syndrome* as a self-perpetuating, highly variable, but generalized myeloproliferative disorder in which erythremic myelosis, erythroleukemia, and myeloblastic leukemia may all appear, either sequentially or in a "mix" that is difficult to classify.[89] Although the criteria defined by the FAB group generally separate ALL from ANLL, lineage infidelity of blasts in acute leukemias has been described.[32,90]

Acute Lymphocytic Leukemia. ALL is more common in children than in adults. The FAB group classifies this entity into three morphologic groups: L1, L2, and L3.[66] The L1 subgroup is characterized by a homogeneous population of small cells having up to twice the diameter of a small lymphocyte. The nucleus is large and round, with occasional clefting or indentation. The amount of cytoplasm is scanty, with slight or moderate basophilia. The nucleoli are invisible or small and inconspicuous. L2 cells are large with considerable heterogeneity in size. Nuclear clefting, indentation and folding are characteristic. Nucleoli are always present, and often large. The amount of cytoplasm varies but is often abundant. Cytoplasmic basophilia may be marked. L3 cells (Burkitt type) are large and characteristically homogeneous. The nucleus is oval to round and regular. The chromatin is finely stippled. One or more prominent vesicular nucleoli

are seen in the majority of cells. The cytoplasm is voluminous and intensely basophilic. Prominent cytoplasmic vacuolization is often present.

L1 morphology has been associated with a better prognosis and is more common in children,[91] but it is nevertheless difficult to separate L1 from L2 at times. The FAB group has therefore modified its criteria and developed a score system for L1 and L2,[92] which is based on four features: (1) nuclear/cytoplasmic ratio, (2) presence, prominence, and frequency of nucleoli, (3) regularity of nuclear membrane outline, and (4) cell size. It has been stated that the overall concordance among observers is improved by using this score system.

With the exception of L3 (a B-cell tumor), there is no correlation between morphologic and immunologic classification.[78,92,93] L2, which is more common in adults, has to be differentiated from ANLL (M1). Scattered rare azurophilic granules may be seen in L2, but these granules do not react with myeloperoxidase. The FAB group claims that the presence of up to 3 percent of peroxidase-positive blasts is still considered compatible with L2.[66]

Unlike ANLL, in which tissue infiltration (granulocytic sarcoma, chloroma) is uncommon, ALL frequently presents with lymphadenopathy and/or hepatosplenomegaly (lymphoma). These cases have been classified as lymphoma/leukemia. The L1 or L1/L2 ALL is frequently associated with lymphoblastic lymphoma (convoluted cell lymphoma), and the L3 is associated with Burkitt's lymphoma. Histologic examination of ALL in bone marrow is almost identical to that of the corresponding non-Hodgkin's lymphoma (NHL) in lymph nodes or other tissues (Figs. 13-13 and 13-14). The marrow is markedly hypercellular with absence of fat cells. Hematopoietic

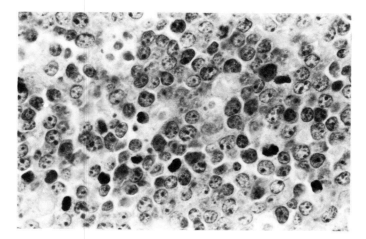

Fig. 13-13. Burkitt's lymphoma involving bone marrow. The nuclei of acute lymphocytic leukemia (L3) may be round to oval, the chromatin is stippled, and each nucleus contain one or more nucleoli. Note the mitotic figures and nuclear fragments. (H&E stain, ×400.)

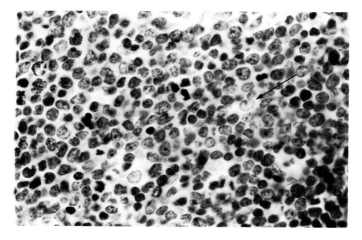

Fig. 13-14. Convoluted cell lymphoma involving bone marrow. The neoplastic cells range in size from that of a small lymphocyte to several times larger than a small lymphocyte. The nuclei have irregular outlines with a coarse chromatin pattern and indistinct nucleoli. Mitotic figures are frequently seen. The nucleus of a histiocyte (arrow) is illustrated for comparison. (H&E stain, ×250.)

elements are markedly depleted. A few lymphocytes and plasma cells may be present, and mitoses may be numerous. Necrosis is not uncommon, but fibrosis is rarer than in ANLL.

Cytogenetic abnormalities are seen in ALL. The most important anomalies are: (1) positive Philadelphia chromosome, usually corresponding to a worse prognosis than that of patients who do not have the marker chromosome; and (2) a translocation involving chromosome 8 and 14 [t(8q−;14q+)], characteristically seen in Burkitt's lymphoma and its corresponding leukemia (L3). These cells are TdT negative. TdT is a DNA polymerase, characteristically present in stem cells, pre-T-cells, cortical thymocytes, and some pre-B-cells. There are fewer than 2 percent of TdT-positive cells in normal bone marrow. TdT positivity is found in 95 percent of patients with untreated ALL and in 30 to 60 percent of blasts in patients with CGL in blast crisis.[78] L3 cells also carry membrane surface immunoglobulin or intracytoplasmic immunoglobin (frequently IgM kappa). The vacuoles in blasts react with Oil Red O or Sudan IV (neutral lipid). These patients frequently present with abdominal lymphomas, especially small bowel lymphomas, which run an aggressive course.

Convoluted cell lymphoma characteristically involves adolescent boys. These patients tend to have a higher peripheral white cell count and blast count, with blasts displaying L1 (in the majority of cases) or L2 morphology. The blasts are TdT-positive, exhibiting focal globular paranuclear acid phosphatase positivity, and spontaneously forming rosettes with sheep erythrocytes. These patients frequently present with a mediastinal mass. Although they may initially respond to chemotherapy, remission duration is short, and testicular or central nervous system relapse is common.

Myeloproliferative Disorders. The term *myeloproliferative syndrome* was introduced by Dameshek to include a heterogeneous group of disorders characterized by proliferation of any or all cell lines originating from the marrow simultaneously during the course of the disease.[94] Dameshek divided the syndrome into acute and chronic types. The acute type includes acute granulocytic leukemia, erythroleukemia, and acute myelosclerosis with myeloid metaplasia, while the chronic type encompasses CGL, thrombocythemia, myelosclerosis with myeloid metaplasia, and polycythemia. Histologic recognition and classification of chronic myeloproliferative disorders (CMPDs) depend on (1) the predominant proliferative cell line, (2) the degree of its differentiation, and (3) the fibrotic reaction. It should be emphasized that subgroups of CMPD often overlap. Polycythemia vera, agnogenic myeloid metaplasia (AMM), and CGL may evolve to acute leukemia.

Acute Malignant Myelosclerosis. Acute malignant myelosclerosis (AMF) is a rare but rapidly fatal disease, characterized by pancytopenia and minimal or no splenomegaly.[95,96] Teardrop cells, characteristically seen in AMM (or myelosclerosis with myeloid metaplasia), are rare, and there is little anisopoikilocytosis on the peripheral blood smear. The bone marrow examination often yields a "dry tap." Histologic examination of bone marrow biopsy specimens shows replacement of normal hematopoietic elements and fat by fibrous tissue interspersed with sheets of blasts, dysplastic megakaryocytes, and residual dyspoietic hematopoietic cells. Recent cytogenetic studies support the concept that AMF is a primary malignancy of hematopoietic cells associated with secondary nonneoplastic fibrosis.[97,98] Chemotherapy is ineffective, but marrow transplantation may offer a cure.[99] Some patients terminate in acute leukemia.[100,101]

Polycythemia vera. Polycythemia vera (PV) is a slowly progressive myeloproliferative disorder characterized by an absolute erythrocytosis, hypervolemia, and panhyperplasia of the bone marrow (Fig.13-15). Megakaryocytic hyperplasia may be striking, with abnormal forms present (variably sized and shaped nuclei and variable cytoplasmic density). In addition, they frequently cluster together. Increased reticulin fibers may be demonstrated by special stains (Fig. 13-16). Irregularly dilated and expanded sinusoids are seen, some of which contain islands of nucleated red cells and megakaryocytes. Occasionally, bilinear type hyperplasia consisting of erythrocytic and megakaryocytic lines only or erythrocytic and granulo-

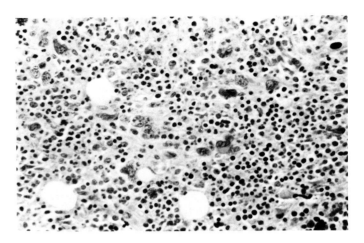

Fig. 13-15. Spent phase of polycythemia vera. Panhyperplasia of marrow is noted with aggregates of megakaryocytes. (H&E stain, ×100.)

cytic lines only may be seen. Occasionally, patients with PV will have a normal marrow.[102] Even in those, close observation will reveal clustering of enlarged and atypical megakaryocytes. The diagnostic laboratory abnormalities include an increase in the red cell mass; mild to moderate leukocytosis with neutrophilia, eosinophilia, and basophilia; and thrombocytosis. The leukocyte alkaline phosphatase (LAP) score is typically increased. Absent iron stores are characteristic, and may be secondary to repeated phlebotomies. The diagnostic criteria have been established by the Polycythemia Study Group.[103] Among those patients who lived more than 8 years, about 10 to 25 percent developed postpolycythemic myeloid metaplasia[104] and another 5 to 10 percent developed AML.[105,106] Barosi and associates reported polycythemia

following splenectomy in myelofibrosis with myeloid metaplasia.[107] The differential diagnosis includes: (1) secondary erythrocytosis (in which megakaryocytes are normal in number and in morphology, with preservation of fat cells and reticulin structure); (2) CGL (in which megakaryocytes are usually normal in quantity and quality and in addition, the LAP score is decreased and Philadelphia chromosome is demonstrated in most cases); and (3) AMM. The last cannot be differentiated from postpolycythemic myeloid metaplasia.[104]

Idiopathic Thrombocythemia. Idiopathic (or essential) thrombocythemia is characterized by a sustained increase in the platelet count at a level of $1,000 \times 10^9$ per liter or higher. Bone marrow cellularity is variable, but there is definitive hyperplasia of megakaryocytes. These cells frequently form clusters of polymorphic cells of variable size and shape, which contain polymorphic nuclei. Megakaryocytes are found not only at the walls of the sinusoids but also projecting into their lumina. Progression into myelofibrosis is seen. The topic has recently been reviewed.[108]

Chronic Granulocytic Leukemia. In CGL the bone marrow is extremely hypercellular, with marked granulocytic hyperplasia. Although granulopoiesis appears to be normal in maturation, there is a marked increase in eosinophils and basophils. Mast cells are usually normal. Erythropoiesis is appreciably decreased, with a myeloid to erythroid ratio of 15:1 to 20:1 or even higher (Fig. 13-17). Megakaryocytes may be increased, in which case they may display abnormal morphology. Histiocytes containing crystalloid structures (Gaucher-like cells) are seen. Reticulin fibers may be increased. As stated earlier, a marker chromosome, the Philadelphia chromosome

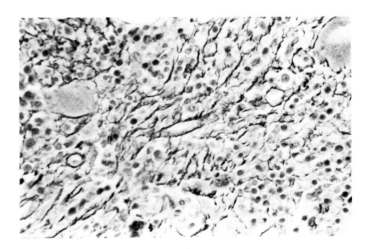

Fig. 13-16. Agnogenic myeloid metaplasia. Snook's reticulin stain displays increased reticulin fibers, which are coarser than usual and surround megakaryocytes. (Snook's reticulin stain, ×160.)

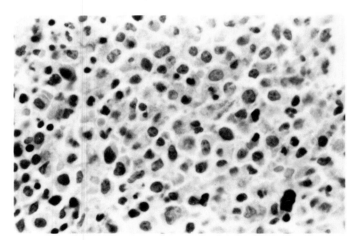

Fig. 13-17. Chronic granulocytic leukemia. Note marked granulocytic hyperplasia with a predominance of myelocytes and metamyelocytes. Only a few nucleated red cells and one megakaryocyte are identified. (H&E stain, ×250.)

(Ph¹), is demonstrated in 80 to 90 percent of cases. Ph¹-negative CML is more commonly seen in infants and in older adults.

It has been said that *blast crisis* (in which the proportion of blasts exceeds 30 percent) is commonly seen in the pure granulocytic type of CGL, while cases with mixed proliferation of granulocytes and megakaryocytes have a greater tendency to develop into AMM.[109] The morphology of the blasts may be myeloid, lymphoid, megakaryocytic, or mixed.[110] The histopathology of the bone marrow may be indistinguishable from that of acute leukemias, except that an increase of eosinophils and basophils is more common in CGL in blast crisis than in acute leukemias.

Agnogenic Myeloid Metaplasia. AMM is characterized by a leukoerythroblastic blood picture, hepatospleno-megaly, hyperuricemia, and bone marrow fibrosis. Radiographic evidence of osteosclerosis has been reported in 30 to 70 percent of patients. Bone marrow aspiration is usually unsuccessful (dry tap). Bone biopsy is necessary for diagnosis, and the following patterns have been described[111]:

1. Panhyperplasia. The marrow is hypercellular with effacement of normal architecture and compartmentalization of hematopoiesis. Aggregates of dysplastic megakaryocytes frequently surrounded by reticulin fibers are seen. The sinusoids are irregular in shape, often dilated, with sclerosis of sinusoidal walls. Intrasinusoidal hematopoiesis is evident.
2. Myeloid atrophy and fibrosis. Alternating areas of fibrosis and hematopoiesis are seen.
3. Myelofibrosis and sclerosis. This is characterized by replacement of the marrow cavity with broad, irregular, twisted trabeculae (without the regular lamellar appearance) and fibrotic marrow. Normal hematopoietic elements are markedly decreased.

These different patterns may be found simultaneously in different parts of the skeleton or even of the same section. However, as the disease progresses, reticulin fibrosis is often replaced with collagen fibrosis (Fig. 13-18). The topic of myelofibrosis has been recently reviewed by Varki and associates.[112]

The pathogenesis of the reticulin and collagen myelofibrosis in the myeloproliferative disorders is not clear. It has been shown that megakaryocytes and platelets are capable of producing a growth factor (which is mitogenic for fibroblasts) and platelet factor IV (which inhibits collagenase).[113] It has been postulated that ineffective megakaryopoiesis leads to disintegration of large number of megakaryocytes and platelets, the result of which is fibroblast proliferation and fibrillogenesis.

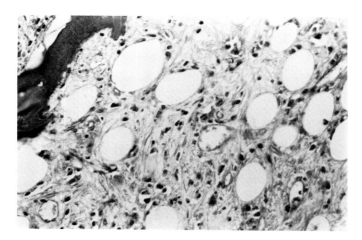

Fig. 13-18. Fibrotic bone marrow with marked decrease in hematopoietic elements. Snook's reticulin stain did not show increased reticulin. Trichrome stain displays increased collagen fibers. (Snook's reticulin stain, ×100.)

Fibrosis of the bone marrow will be discussed further in a later section.

Preleukemia and Myelodysplastic Syndromes. *Preleukemia syndromes, myelodysplastic syndromes, hemopoietic dysplasias,* and *dysmyelopoietic syndromes* are some of the terms used to describe a group of clinically recognizable hematologic disorders in which 15 to 25 percent of patients having the disease finally develop acute leukemia. The affected patients are usually in their sixth or seventh decade, with an insidious onset and slowly progressive course. Cytopenias with refractory anemia and dyspoiesis of marrow cell lines are pertinent laboratory findings. The morphologic, biochemical, and functional changes of the hematopoietic cell lines have been well described.[114] The term *preleukemia syndromes* should not be used to designate any congenital or hereditary disorders known to be associated with an increased incidence of acute leukemia, or to designate those well defined myeloproliferative disorders in which the terminal event is often acute leukemia.

The diagnostic criteria for preleukemia syndromes are listed in Table 13-5. The FAB cooperative group subclassifies the preleukemia syndromes, or MDS, into five groups[67]: (1) refractory anemia (RA); (2) RA with ring sideroblasts (RARS); (3) RA with excess of blasts (RAEB); (4) chronic myelomonocytic leukemia (CMML); and (5) RAEB in transformation (RAEBIT). The characteristics of the various subtypes are listed in Table 13-6. The FAB states that, when the percentage of blasts present in the bone marrow is in excess of 30 percent, a diagnosis of acute leukemia is made. The number of blasts present in the bone marrow of patients with preleukemia can range from normal to 30 percent.

TABLE 13-5. Diagnostic Criteria for Preleukemia Syndrome

Prerequisites
  Peripheral blood:
    Anemia with oval macrocytosis
  Bone marrow
    Megaloblastoid erythropoiesis with or without ring sideroblasts
    Abnormal megakaryocytes and/or disorderly granulopoiesis (e.g., a maturation "bulge" at the myelocyte stage)
    Absence of overt leukemia (less than 5% myeloblasts or promyelocytes, no Auer bodies)
  Others
    No evidence of vitamin B_{12} or folate deficiency
    No history of cytotoxic therapy in past 6 months

Corroborative findings
  Peripheral blood
    Leukoerythroblastic picture
    Bizarre platelet size and granulation
    Thrombocytopenia
    Neutropenia
    Monocytosis or atypical monocytoid cells
    Qualitative granulocytopathy, such as Pelger-Huetlike anomaly, coarse granulation, or degranulation
    Hypochromia
  Bone marrow
    Erythrocytic hyperplasia
    Megakaryocytic hyperplasia
    Adequate or increased iron stores

(From Sun NCJ: Hematology: An Atlas and Diagnostic Guide. WB Saunders, Philadelphia, 1983, with permission.)

The cellularity of marrow may be variable, although hypercellular marrow is most common. All hematopoietic cell lines may exhibit dysplastic changes, with increased precursors. In addition, the normal topographic distribution of erythropoiesis, myelopoiesis, and megakaryopoiesis may be disrupted. Increased reticulin fibers are seen more commonly than in acute leukemia. Monocytes, mast cells, eosinophils, and plasma cells may be prominent, and lymphoid nodules may be present.[115] Interstitial edema, dilation of sinusoids with thickened walls, and increased numbers of iron-laden macrophages are also seen. Tricot and associates noted that clustered myeloblasts may be present in the central part of the marrow prior to the increased blast count by aspiration.[116] These investigators observed that patients with this abnormal localization of immature precursors had a more rapid progression to acute leukemia than patients with MDS without this abnormal pattern. Riccardi and colleagues found that a hypocellular bone marrow appeared to be a favorable prognostic factor in MDS. Patients with refractory cytopenias, especially those with a hypocellular bone marrow, may respond to androgens.[117]

Cytogenetic abnormalities are common in MDS, their incidence ranging from 20 to 90 percent of cases in the literature.[118] Most studies report that the bone marrows of 40 to 60 percent of patients contain nonrandom chromosomal abnormalities, the most common of which affect chromosomes 5 and 7.[26] A new entity, 5q− anomaly, has been described.[119] It appears that patients who have monosomy 7 tend to have a markedly shortened survival, although patients with multiple chromosomal abnormalities in a marrow clone have a high chance of developing acute leukemia or other complications of hemopoietic dysfunction.[120] Preleukemia syndrome has also been described in children.[121]

Fibrosis

Fibrosis of the bone marrow, or myelofibrosis, may be primary (idiopathic) or secondary. The peripheral blood in both conditions is characterized by a leukoerythroblastic picture (presence of immature myeloid and erythroid series in the peripheral blood, accompanied by giant and bizarre thrombocytes) with circulating teardrop erythrocytes. The number of circulation nucleated RBCs is often excessive compared with the degree of anemia. Reticulocytosis is *not* seen in most cases. This peripheral blood picture is specific for myelophthisic anemia (a normocytic, normochromic anemia with leukoerythroblastosis due to replacement of normal bone marrow by nonmarrow elements).

TABLE 13-6. Comparison of Morphologic Features in Subgroups of Myelodysplastic Syndrome According to FAB Classification

Subgroups	Percent of Blasts		Marrow Cellularity	Dyspoiesis Seen in Bone Marrow			Other
	PB	BM		Erythroid	Myeloid	Megakaryocytic	
RA	<1	<5	Hyper-, normo-, or hypo-	Yes	No	No	
RARS	<1	<5	Same as above	Yes	Some	Some	15% ring sideroblasts
RAEB	<5	5–20	Same as above	Yes	Yes	Some	No Auer rods
CMML	<5	<20	Hypercellular	Some	Yes	Variable	Absolute monocytosis and 20% monocytic cells in marrow
RAEBIT	>5	20–30	Hypercellular	Yes	Yes	Some	Auer rods may be present

Abbreviations: PB, peripheral blood; BM, bone marrow.

Primary Myelofibrosis

The clinical presentation of primary myelofibrosis may be acute or chronic. Acute myelosclerosis is uncommon, and morphologic change in peripheral blood is often minimal. Chronic myelofibrosis, or agnogenic myeloid metaplasia, is a form of chronic myeloproliferative disorder (CMPD). Both entities have been discussed earlier.

Secondary Myelofibrosis

Secondary myelofibrosis may be caused by chemicals, radiation exposure, occlusive vascular disease, metastatic carcinomas, and malignant lymphomas. It is also common in CMPDs, such as chronic myelogenous leukemia or polycythemia vera. Focal myelofibrosis may be seen in areas of inflammatory reaction to an infectious agent (such as tuberculosis) or sarcoidosis, or in areas adjacent to bone marrow necrosis and fracture of bone. The hematopoietic elements are normal or decreased in most of these disorders (with the exception of fibrosis associated with CMPDs), and the morphology of megakaryocytes is normal. The primary cause of fibrosis (such as metastatic carcinoma) may be identified on the same bone marrow section or on deeper sections.

Primary osseous, renal, or endocrine diseases, such as osteitis fibrosa cystica, fibrous dysplasia, and osteopetrosis, are also associated with marrow fibrosis and osteosclerosis. Microcystic resorption of bone, marrow fibrosis, and increased osteoclastic activity are seen in the recently recognized and studied adult T-cell leukemia/lymphoma.

Lymphocytic Infiltration

Lymphocytic infiltrates may be broadly separated into (1) benign lymphocytic infiltrate, which may be physiologic (in young children) or reactive (infectious lymphocytosis, infectious mononucleosis, tuberculosis, etc.); and (2) malignant lymphoproliferative disorders, including chronic lymphocytic leukemia (CLL) and related disorders, the leukemic phase of NHL, and multiple myeloma and related disorders.

Nonneoplastic Lymphocytic Infiltration

Lymphocytes, a normal component of the bone marrow, may constitute up to 50 percent of all nucleated cells in marrow in a child 1 month to 1 year old and about 20 percent of all nucleated cells from 1 year old and onward.[122] Lymphoid nodules or lymphoid aggregates are a relatively common finding in routine bone marrow examination; their reported incidence varies from 1 to 9 percent in antemortem specimens and from 21 to 62 percent in

autopsy material. Prevalences of 17.9 and 47 percent, respectively, were cited in two large series.[46,123] These nodules are more commonly seen in older women and are frequently present around the blood vessels, associated with plasmacytosis and lipid granulomas. They are composed of small lymphocytes, a few plasma cells, histiocytes, and occasionally eosinophils and mast cells, organized around a capillary or arteriole within a reticulin fiber network. Rywlin and associates divided *lymphoid nodules* into lymphoid infiltrates and lymphoid follicles, which measured from 0.08 to 0.6 mm in greatest dimension.[46] These authors defined *nodular lymphoid hyperplasia* (NLH) of the bone marrow as present when (1) four or more normal lymphoid nodules are seen in any low-power (80 mm^2) field or (2) a lymphoid nodule exceeds 0.6 mm in greatest dimension. The nodules in NLH may consist of both lymphoid follicles or lymphoid infiltrates, although the former type is more common. The clinical significance of this differentiation is unclear. Some patients have associated infections or autoimmune disorders; others may be immunodeficient. Identification of lymphoid nodules or NLH in a patient with a history of lymphoma of small lymphocytes often creates diagnostic difficulty. Irregularity, asymmetry, great variability in size and shape, tendency to fragmentation of the nodules, and abnormal cytology with increased number of large "blastic" lymphocytes are criteria for malignant lymphoma.

Lymphoproliferative Disorders

Chronic Lymphocytic Leukemia and Related Disorders

Included under disorders related to CLL are a variety of diseases that have an insidious or chronic onset with circulating neoplastic lymphoid cells and are not generally considered as leukemic conversion of malignant lymphoma.

Chronic Lymphocytic Leukemia. CLL is a disease of elderly men. It accounts for approximately 25 percent of all cases of leukemia and about 75 percent of all cases of chronic leukemia in Western countries. The clinical presentations are variable, but the general criterion for the diagnosis of CLL is a sustained and absolute lymphocytosis in peripheral blood and bone marrow not attributable to any other cause. Currently, the Cancer and Leukemia Group B uses an absolute blood lymphocyte count of 15×10^9 per liter or more in the peripheral blood and 40 percent in the bone marrow.[124,125] Most of the neoplastic small lymphocytes (in more than 95 percent of cases) possess weak monoclonal surface immunoglobulins (usually IgM or IgD) on their cell membranes, and they also carry weak complement- and Fc-receptors as well as receptors for mouse erythrocytes. In addition, CLL cells react with monoclonal antibodies against HLA-DR locus (Ia-like antigen), B1, B2, B4, BA-1, and Leu1 (OKT$_1$, T101, T1).[126]

A clinical staging system for CLL was introduced by Rai and colleagues to assess the tumor burden.[125] Later, Binet and associates proposed a new system[127] consisting of three stages (simpler than Rai's five stages). However, neither system can predict for the large majority of patients in the low and intermediate risk groups. In 1987 Rai and Montserrat suggested combining the bone marrow histology, the lymphocyte doubling time, and the threshold values of blood lymphocyte counts with the clinical staging system to distinguish between indolent and aggressive clinical courses on a prospective basis within a given clinical stage.[128]

Histopathologic findings in the bone marrow that were capable of predicting prognosis in patients with CLL were first noted by Rozman and associates.[129] These authors described four different histologic patterns: (1) interstitial lymphoid infiltration without displacement of fat cells (Fig. 13-19); (2) nodular (abnormal lymphoid nodule without interstitial infiltration) (Fig. 13-20); (3) mixed (combination of interstitial and nodular patterns); and (4) diffuse (replacement of both hematopoietic cells and fat cells by lymphoid infiltration). The difference between normal and neoplastic nodules has been described earlier. Cytologically the neoplastic lymphocytes are small and contain round or slightly irregular nuclei, clumped chromatin, and an indiscernible amount of cytoplasm. A small nucleolus may be observed in some cells (Fig. 13-21). Some intermediate lymphocytes and lymphoblasts may also be present. The reticulin framework is moderately accentuated in the majority of cases. Kubic and

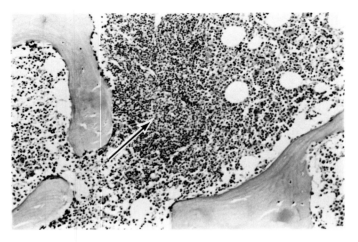

Fig. 13-20. Nodular infiltrate of CLL. This pattern of CLL infiltrate (arrow) is difficult to differentiate from benign lymphoid nodules. (H&E stain, ×40.)

Brunning found that in 13 percent of cases (1 of 8) of CLL there was a reaction with monoclonal antibody against LN1, in comparison with 77 percent of cases (10 of 13) of benign lymphoid aggregates. However, reaction with anti-LN2 was found in all cases of CLL and benign lymphoid aggregates.[130]

The pattern of bone marrow histology (diffuse or nondiffuse) in B-CLL patients has been proved to be a better single prognostic parameter than any one of the clinical or laboratory variables employed in current clinical staging systems.[131,132] The diffuse pattern of bone marrow histology is considered the best criterion for initiation of therapy in these patients.[132] Pangalis and associates also observed that bone marrow involvement in patients with malignant lymphoma of small lymphocytes always dis-

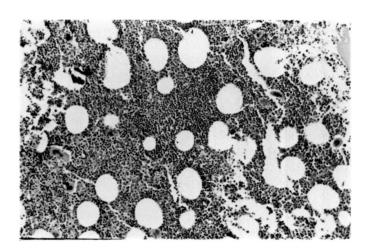

Fig. 13-19. Interstitial infiltration in CLL. Note that megakaryocytes are present at the periphery. (H&E stain, ×40.)

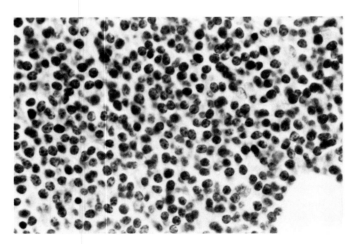

Fig. 13-21. The leukemic cells in CLL contain round nuclei with thickened nuclear membranes, clumped chromatin, and indistinct nucleoli. (H&E stain, ×160.)

played nodular patterns even though these patients had advanced disease.[133]

T-CLL is uncommon, accounting for about 2 percent of CLL in Western countries. Many of these patients have splenomegaly and skin involvement, and they tend to have a worse prognosis than patients with B-CLL.[134,135] The bone marrow cellularity is variable. Lymphocytic infiltration also varies and frequently occurs in an interstitial pattern, but it may be diffuse. Cytologically, the neoplastic cells may be indistinguishable from those of B-CLL. Immunologically they marked as post-thymic T-cells (OKT3+) and may carry helper/inducer or suppressor/cytotoxic cell marker. T-CLL should be differentiated from Sézary syndrome and Tγ-lymphoproliferative disease.[135–139]

Although blast crisis is very uncommon in patients with CLL when compared with its frequency in CGL, occasional case reports are noted in the literature.[140–142] The reported morphology of the blasts varies from "prolymphocytes" to "granulocytic or reticulum cell series" to "stem cells." Enno and associates suggested differentiating prolymphocytoid transformation of CLL, acute leukemia occurring in CLL, and Richter's syndrome[142] because of different clinicopathologic presentations and clinical outcomes.

Prolymphocytoid transformation may represent an accelerated phase of CLL in which the disease undergoes an insidious, although aggressive, change in character, with increasing refractoriness to treatment. These patients not only have a previous history of CLL but also have a double population of lymphocytes (prolymphocytes and "mature" small lymphocytes) that retain most of the marker characteristics of B-CLL. Melo and associates have recently studied the relationship of CLL and prolymphocytic leukemia in detail.[143–146] Prolymphocytoid transformation should be differentiated from Galton's prolymphocytic leukemia.[147]

Richter's syndrome is characterized by fever, weight loss, localized lymphadenopathy, dysglobulinemia, and a pleomorphic malignant lymphoma occurring terminally in patients with a previous history of CLL.[148–151] Immunohistopathologic study has revealed that the malignant lymphoma was a B-cell immunoblastic sarcoma in most instances. An incidence of 3 percent has been cited.[150] A similar evolution has been described in other lymphoproliferative disorders of small B-cell type, including multiple myeloma.[152–153]

Prolymphocytic Leukemia of Galton. Prolymphocytic leukemia (PLL), as defined by Galton and associates, is an uncommon variant of CLL,[147] although Catovsky claimed that PLL occupied an intermediate position between CLL and acute lymphosarcoma cell leukemia of poorly differentiated type.[154] Patients with PLL are often elderly men, with massive splenomegaly, absent or minimal lymphadenopathy, striking lymphocytosis (average lymphocyte count 355×10^9 per liter), resistance to conventional therapy for CLL, and a poor prognosis. Histologically PLL may be differentiated from CLL by the characteristic cytology of the neoplastic cells (a larger cell than CLL, with an immature-appearing round nucleus containing one prominent nucleolus and an abundant amount of cytoplasm).[155] Phenotypically the neoplastic cells marked as B-cells in the majority of cases, but T-PLLs have been reported.[126,154,156] Histologic examination shows a nodular or diffuse pattern. Some of the nodules are paratrabecular in location.

Hairy Cell Leukemia. Hairy cell leukemia (HCL) is a chronic lymphoproliferative disorder, chiefly affecting middle-aged or elderly men. The neoplastic cell is a mononuclear cell of intermediate to large size. The eccentrically located nucleus often contain lacy chromatin and a small and inconspicuous nucleolus. The light blue cytoplasm displays typical fine filamentous ("hairy") projections on peripheral blood smear. The nature of the hairy cell has yet to be determined, and there are numerous hypotheses, attested to by a long list of synonyms. Most investigators now accept that hairy cells are most probably of B-cell origin.[157] The leukemic cells are characteristically stained with acid phosphatase (multiple paranuclear granules), and this positive reaction is resistant to tartaric acid inhibition.[158] One or more ribosome-lamellar complexes may be demonstrated intracytoplasmically by electron microscopy.[159] However, none of these characteristics are pathognomonic, and hairy cell leukemia may simulate a variety of myeloid and lymphoid proliferative disorders.[157]

In a typical case the disease is characterized by an insidious onset, marked splenomegaly, pancytopenia, and circulating hairy cells. The bone marrow aspiration often yields a dry tap. The marrow cellularity is variable in biopsy specimens. The neoplastic infiltrate may be focal, patchy, or diffuse[160] and is composed of uniform mononuclear cells with a distinct cell membrane, giving a "mosaic" pattern (Fig. 13-22). The nucleus may be round, ovoid, indented, or coffee-bean in shape, surrounded by a "halo" of pale cytoplasm; the nuclear chromatin is finely stippled, and the nucleolus is indistinct (Fig. 13-23). Mitoses and nuclear pleomorphism are usually absent. Similar morphologic features may be observed in other involved organs. This loose network of monomorphic cells is in contrast to the tightly packed, paratrabecular arrangement of lymphomatous involvement of the marrow. Increased reticulin fibers are seen in the infiltrated areas.

Although peripheral lymphadenopathy is usually minimal, significantly enlarged mediastinal, retroperitoneal,

450

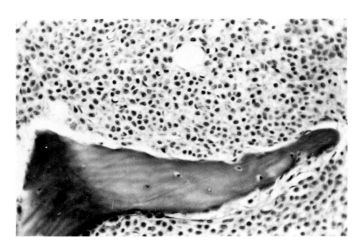

Fig. 13-22. Hairy cell leukemia, with diffuse infiltrate of bone marrow. Note clear spaces between cells. (H&E stain, ×100.)

and abdominal lymph nodes were seen in 15 of 22 patients in one series.[161] The changes in the spleen are characteristic and distinct from those of other lymphoproliferative disorders.[162,163] An accurate diagnosis of HCL is most important because the vast majority of these patients respond to splenectomy.[164] Recently, α-interferons have been found to be very effective in treating patients with HCL in all clinical stages of the disease.[165]

Sézary Syndrome. Sézary syndrome is characterized by generalized erythroderma, pruritis, peripheral lymphadenopathy, hepatomegaly, and the presence of Sézary (Lutzner) cells in the skin and peripheral blood.[135] Lutzner and associates proposed the term *cutaneous T-cell lymphomas* to include both the Sézary syndrome and *mycosis fungoides* (MF).[166] The neoplastic cells of both

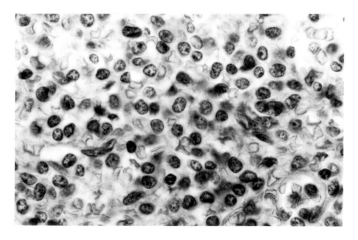

Fig. 13-23. Hairy cell leukemia. Higher magnification reveals round, oval, or coffee-bean-shaped nuclei, evenly distributed chromatin, and indistinct nucleoli. (H&E stain, ×250.)

diseases possess similar morphologic findings (cerebriform nuclei), carry T-cell (helper cell) markers, and have a predilection for the skin. Circulating atypical lymphoid (Sézary) cells are classically present in Sézary syndrome but much rarer in MF. Histopathologic examination of bone marrow biopsy samples reveals limited involvement.[135,167] The cellularity is usually normal, with a heterogeneous population of cells. The hematopoietic elements are not decreased, although small aggregates or collections of mononucleated cells are noted. These cells have a very high nuclear-to-cytoplasmic ratio and contain a hyperchromatic nucleus with irregular nuclear contour. Nuclear indentation or convolution may be appreciated under oil immersion with fine adjustment.

Adult T-Cell Leukemia/Lymphoma. Adult T-cell leukemia/lymphoma (ATL), or subacute leukemia of Japan, is linked to human T-cell leukemia virus.[168] This disorder was first described by Japanese investigators and was found in an endemic area in southwest Japan.[169] Later, it was reported from the West Indies and Africa and in blacks in the southeastern United States.[170–172] Patients with ATL characteristically present with subacute leukemia, hypercalcemia, lytic lesions in bones, generalized lymphadenopathy, hepatosplenomegaly, and cutaneous lesions. Although the disease has a insidious or subacute onset, it frequently runs an aggressive course, leading to death in a few months to a year. The malignant cell is a small to intermediate T-cell, with a markedly irregular ("knobby") nucleus. Polymorphism is characteristic of ATL. These cells frequently mark as T-helper/inducer cells, but they generally do not have detectable helper function. They may function as suppressor/cytotoxic T-cells. Variation in the clinical manifestations has been described.[173]

Bone marrow biopsies show microcystic resorption with focal fibrosis and increased osteoclastic activity in some patients. Of those patients who had lymphomatous involvement in the marrow, the degree of marrow replacement was not prominent. The infiltrate is patchy or interstitial but not paratrabecular. Some patients who had circulating leukemic cells did not have evidence of bone marrow involvement.[172] Histopathology of involved lymph nodes exhibits a spectrum of morphology, and there is no correlation between clinical course and histologic type.[172]

The human T-cell leukemias have been recently thoroughly reviewed by Knowles.[174]

Leukemic Phase of Non-Hodgkin's Lymphoma

Bone marrow involvement is quite common in NHL. However, the incidence varies among different series of studies (from 36 to 63 percent), different histologic types, and different methods of obtaining the specimens. As a rule, histologic examination of a bone marrow clot section or biopsy specimen is better than that of Wright-Giemsa-stained bone marrow smears,[13] bilateral bone marrow biopsy is better than unilateral biopsy,[18] and open bone marrow biopsy is better than needle biopsy.[6] However, bilateral needle biopsies are adequate for staging purpose. Bone marrow involvement is more frequently seen in patients with lymphocytic lymphomas than in those with ''histiocytic'' lymphomas,[6,175-178] although lymphocytic lymphomas often have a more indolent clinical course. The initial histologic diagnosis of malignant lymphoma was established by bone marrow biopsy in 36 percent of the positive cases in one series.[178] Bone marrow examination frequently changes clinical staging from a more localized form of disease to a disseminated form (stage IV).[179-180] A positive bone marrow examination is frequently obtained in patients with a normal complete blood cell count and without evidence of a leukoerythroblastic picture. The absolute blood lymphocyte count is considered to be an important diagnostic criterion in differentiating malignant lymphomas from leukemic infiltration of the bone marrow.

Histopathologic examination of a bone marrow biopsy reveals the following patterns: (1) interstitial, (2) nodular, (3) paratrabecular, or (4) packed marrow.[178] Combinations of one or more of the above patterns are also seen. The neoplastic lymphocytes are seen infiltrating between fat cells and replacing normal hematopoietic elements in the interstitial pattern. The focal or nodular involvement in poorly differentiated lymphocytic lymphoma, or small cleaved follicular center cell (FCC) lymphoma, is characterized by a paratrabecular distribution (Fig. 13-24). The nodular pattern of infiltration is unrelated to the histologic finding of nodular or diffuse poorly differentiated lymphocytic lymphoma in the lymph node biopsy. Cyto-

logically, lymphomatous infiltration in the marrow shows morphologic features similar to those observed in lymph node biopsies from the same patients.

Foucar et al. found that 53 percent of their 176 patients with non-Hodgkin's lymphoma—51 percent of B-cell types and 65 percent of T-cell types—had bone marrow involvement.[181] Of patients with small B-lymphocyte lymphomas, 89 percent (16 out of 18) had bone marrow involvement, as did 60 percent of patients with convoluted lymphocyte lymphomas and 55 percent of patients with small cleaved FCC lymphoma. In contrast, only 27 percent of patients with noncleaved FCC lymphoma displayed bone marrow involvement. The convoluted lymphocyte lymphomas frequently showed diffuse involvement, whereas 64 percent of small cleaved FCC lymphomas exhibited a paratrabecular distribution, and 69 percent of small B-lymphocyte lymphomas displayed a focal, although nontrabecular, pattern. Extensive blood involvement was noted most frequently in small cleaved FCC lymphomas, and the term *lymphosarcoma cell leukemia,* has been used widely in the literature.[78]

This term, however, is confusing and may have different meanings to different people, as it may describe (1) a variant of CLL, (2) a leukemic phase of poorly differentiated lymphocytic lymphoma, or (3) a leukemic phase of any non-Hodgkin's lymphoma. Strictly speaking, the term should be reserved for the leukemic phase of small cleaved FCC lymphoma (poorly differentiated lymphocytic lymphoma).

Multiple Myeloma and Related Diseases

The plasma cell is an end cell of B-cell lineage, and a small number of plasma cells are normally present in the marrow. Plasmacytic disorders may also be divided into nonneoplastic and neoplastic diseases. A mixed proliferation of lymphocytes and plasma cells is seen sometimes.

Nonneoplastic Plasma Cell Disorders. *Reactive Plasmacytosis.* Reactive plasmacytosis is a common feature of several clinical disorders, including carcinomatosis, chronic granulomatous infections, hepatic diseases, and autoimmune disorders. The prevalence of plasmacytosis (defined as 2 percent or more of plasma cells in the differential count of the bone marrow cells) was found to be 29 percent in a series of consecutive studies of 1,000 bone marrow aspirates.[47] The morphology of the plasma cells is often mature, and they cluster around (cuffing) the blood vessels on histologic sections (Fig. 13-3). Reactive plasmacytosis should be differentiated from plasma cell myeloma.

Benign Monoclonal Gammopathy. Bone marrow examination in patients with benign monoclonal gammopathy often reveals normal marrow, although a mild or moderate

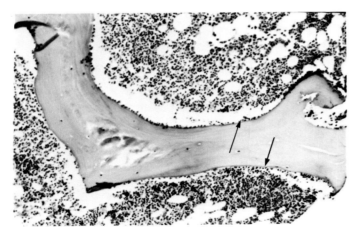

Fig. 13-24. Paratrabecular infiltrate (arrows) of small cleaved cell lymphoma (poorly differentiated lymphocytic lymphoma). (H&E stain, ×40.)

degree of plasmacytosis may be observed. These patients lack other clinical and/or laboratory findings seen in multiple myeloma. However, continuous follow-up should be undertaken.

Neoplastic Proliferation of Plasma Cells. *Multiple Myeloma.* Multiple myeloma (plasma cell myeloma) is a neoplastic proliferation of plasma cells in the bone marrow, which accounts for slightly more than 10 percent of hematologic malignancies. The disease commonly affects elderly men. The usual presentation includes bone pain, anemia, renal insufficiency, and hypercalcemia. Multiple osteolytic lesions or diffuse osteoporosis, clonal proliferation of plasma cells in the bone marrow, serum monoclonal paraprotein (M protein), and/or Bence-Jones proteinuria are frequent laboratory findings.[182–183] Several subtypes, such as localized myeloma, indolent myeloma, smouldering myeloma, nonsecretory myeloma, light chain myeloma, and multiple myeloma with osteosclerotic lesions have been described.[183]

The histologic pattern of myelomatous involvement of the bone marrow is variable, ranging from nodular or patchy to diffuse. In most instances solid sheets of plasma cells infiltrate the fat and replace the normal elements of the marrow; occasionally an "interstitial" pattern may be observed, with preservation of fat cells but replacement of the normal hematopoietic elements. The cytology of myeloma cells may be poorly differentiated, resembling an immunoblastic sarcoma of B-cells (Fig. 13-25), or may be well differentiated, displaying characteristics of normal plasma cells with little cellular pleomorphism or atypism. However, a spectrum of plasma cells may be observed in the latter instance, and monoclonal immunoglobin is demonstrated in the neoplastic plasma cells by an immunoperoxidase method.[188] Recent studies have indicated that the morphology of the neoplastic cells

and the tumor burden assessed by bone marrow biopsy are important predictors of survival duration in patients with multiple myeloma.[184,185]

Bone destruction is the usual manifestation of multiple myeloma, frequently demonstrated by radiology and histology. Pathologic fractures are common. Occasionally, myeloma may be associated with osteosclerotic lesions, as mentioned above.[183] Bone marrow biopsy is also useful for the study of primary amyloidosis.[186]

Plasma cell leukemia is uncommon. It may occur as a terminal event of multiple myeloma or may be the initial presentation in some patients with IgD or IgE myeloma. Plasma cell leukemia has also been observed in light chain disease, and occasionally in IgA myeloma.

Waldenström's Macroglobulinemia. Waldenström's macroglobulinemia (WMG) is a neoplastic clonal proliferation of B-lymphocytes that secrete monoclonal IgM. Clinically, these patients resemble those having malignant lymphoma, with generalized lymphadenopathy and splenomegaly. The bone marrow may be partially or largely replaced by lymphocytes, plasmacytoid lymphocytes (or lymphocytoid plasma cells), and plasma cells (Fig. 13-26). Intranuclear or intracytoplasmic PAS-positive inclusions (Dutcher bodies) may be identified.

Heavy Chain Diseases. *Gamma heavy chain disease* has more of the features of a malignant lymphoma than of multiple myeloma.[187] *Alpha chain disease* predominantly involves the gastrointestinal tract, although there is also a respiratory variant. These cases are also more like a malignant lymphoma.[188] *Mu chain disease* is characterized by the presence of vacuolated plasma cells, small lymphocytes, and plasmacytoid lymphocytes in the bone marrow, with a prolonged antecedent history of CLL.[189] Serum protein study reveals hypogammaglobulinemia

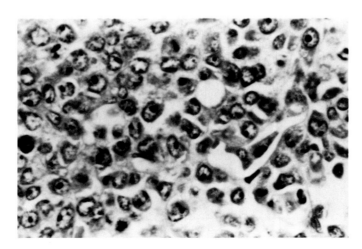

Fig. 13-25. Anaplastic myeloma with plasma cell leukemia. (H&E stain, ×250.)

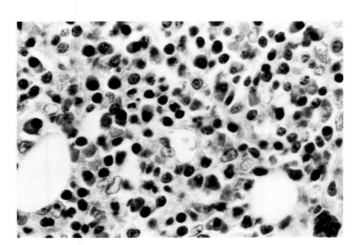

Fig. 13-26. Waldenström's macroglobulinemia. There is a mixed infiltration of plasma cells, plasmacytoid lymphocytes, and lymphocytes. (H&E stain, ×250.)

with the presence of a mu chain. Light chain (kappa) may be detected in the urine.

Granulomatous Changes

A *granuloma* is defined as a host chronic inflammatory reaction with a predominance of cells of the macrophage series. A granulomatous reaction may be elicited by a wide variety of stimuli mediated by immunologic or chemical mechanisms, but the etiology may be difficult to establish from a tissue examination alone. A list of possible causes that may produce a granulomatous response in the bone marrow is listed in Table 13-7.[190] The reason for including some lymphoproliferative disorders under the heading of "granulomatous changes" is to emphasize that histiocytic proliferation and granuloma formation are integral features of their pathology.

A granulomatous lesion may be classified as proliferative, necrotic, or suppurative. The latter two types are most commonly seen in infectious diseases as a form of systemic reaction. Proliferative granuloma is characterized by a focal aggregation of epithelioid cells with or without Langhans giant cells and may be seen in a variety of conditions, including sarcoidosis, infectious mononucleosis, tuberculosis, Hodgkin's disease, NHL, multiple myeloma, liver disease, and drug reactions (Fig. 13-27). It has been speculated that proliferative or epithelioid granuloma may be a manifestation of host immune response to overload of antigens or defective lymphocyte-macrophage function[191]; others have demonstrated non-immune mechanisms for granuloma formation.[192] A

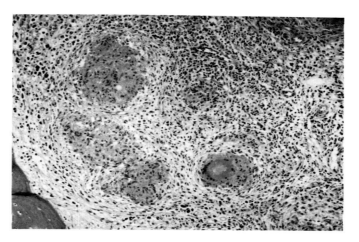

Fig. 13-27. Noncaseating granuloma of the marrow with marrow fibrosis and chronic inflammatory cell infiltrate. Langhans' giant cells are seen. The patient was later found to have sarcoidosis. (H&E stain, ×40.)

1983 study disclosed that the most common cause of granulomatous lesions in bone marrow is infection (38 percent), followed by malignancy (21 percent), drug reaction (12 percent), allergic or autoimmune disease (9 percent), and sarcoidosis (7 percent).[193] However, the etiology of granulomatous disease in marrow was unknown in 13 percent of patients in the same study.

Benign Nonhematologic Conditions

Infectious Granulomata and Acquired Immune Deficiency Syndrome

The morphology of the granuloma in some infectious diseases is quite characteristic and is similar to that in other parts of the body. Microorganisms may be demonstrated on H&E-stained or special-stained sections. Serial sections or step sections are sometimes needed to localize the granuloma or to identify the Reed-Sternberg cells in the case of Hodgkin's disease (specific lesions). A "doughnut" granuloma, which is characterized by a central empty space surrounded by polymorphonuclear leukocytes, epithelioid cells, and/or eosinophils, has been observed in Q fever (Fig. 13-28).[194] Similar lesions have been described in typhoid fever and Hodgkin's disease.[190]

Acquired immune deficiency syndrome (AIDS) is an infectious disease caused by a retrovirus, human immunodeficiency virus (HIV).[195] Other synonyms for the virus include human T-cell lymphotropic virus type III/lymphadenopathy-associated virus (HTLV-III/LAV) and AIDS-related virus (ARV).[196–198] The development of an antibody test against this virus has broadened the recognition of the spectrum of HIV infection.[199,200] A new classification system for this viral infection has been rec-

TABLE 13-7. Possible Causes of Granulomatous Lesions in the Marrow

Nonspecific: lipid granuloma

Infectious
  Mycobacteria: tuberculosis, leprosy, and atypical mycobacteria
  Fungi: coccidioidomycosis, histoplasmosis, cryptococcosis, and others
  Viruses; infectious mononucleosis
  Bacteria: typhoid fever, brucellosis, and others
  Rickettsial disease: Q fever
  Spirochetes: syphilis (secondary stage)

Associated with malignant lymphoma or histiocytosis
  Specific lesion: Hodgkin's disease, Lennert's lymphoma, eosinophilic granuloma, Hand-Schüller-Christian disease, and others
  Nonspecific lesion: Sarcoid-like granuloma (associated with Hodgkin's disease, non-Hodgkin's lymphoma, and multiple myeloma)

Lesions resembling granuloma: Systemic mastocytosis, eosinophilic fibrohistiocytic lesion of the bone marrow, metastatic carcinoma

Miscellaneous: Sarcoidosis, polyarteritis nodosa, foreign body granuloma, and others

(From Sun NCJ: Hematology: An Atlas and Diagnostic Guide. WB Saunders, Philadelphia, 1983, with permission.)

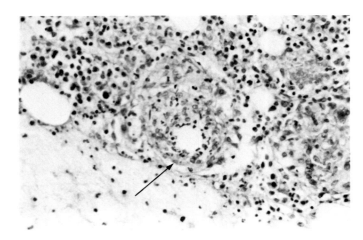

Fig. 13-28. "Doughnut" granuloma is characterized by a central clear space surrounded by a rim of polymorphonuclear leukocytes, fibrinoid material, and epithelioid cells (arrow). Epithelioid cells are also seen in the right side of the photomicrograph. The material is taken from a patient with Q fever. (H&E stain, ×100.)

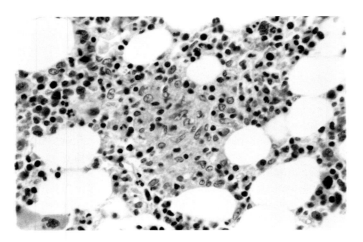

Fig. 13-29. Epithelioid granuloma from a patient with AIDS and disseminated histoplasmosis. *Histoplasma capsulatum* was demonstrated by PAS and methenamine-silver stain. (H&E stain ×160.)

ommended.[201] Identification of a systemic opportunistic infection, such as *Mycobacterium avium-intracellulare,* in an HIV antibody-positive patient will fulfill the definition of AIDS. Thus, accurate diagnosis and identification of opportunistic infection is important.

Most patients develop one or more cytopenias during the course of the disease.[202–207] Bone marrow examinations often reveal normal or decreased fat cells, with hematopoietic elements occupying the rest of the marrow spaces (normocellular or hypercellular bone marrow). Serous or mucinous degeneration of fat cells may be observed in the late stage of the disease, and the density of hematopoietic cells is often decreased, with deposition of eosinophilic granular or fibrillary material in the interstitium. This material may or may not be stained by PAS and is usually unstained by reticulin. It is similar to that observed in patients after radiation or chemotherapy and may represent disintegrated cellular elements. The myeloid to erythroid ratio is usually increased, with a normal or increased number of megakaryocytes. Marrow plasma cells and lymphocytes (including immunoblasts and transformed lymphocytes) are increased, with cuffing of plasma cells around the blood vessels. Lymphoid infiltrates may also be present. Increased iron stores are usually demonstrable by Prussian blue stain, and focal increase in reticulin fibers is also noted with the reticulin stain.

Granulomas (usually small, epithelioid, and without necrosis) may be present (Fig. 13-29), and special stains are required to demonstrate the microorganisms within them. It should be pointed out that the methenamine-silver stain appears to be superior to PAS in demonstrat-

ing fungi on bone marrow biopsy. As a matter of fact, special stains for mycobacteria and fungi should be routinely used in bone marrow specimens from these patients. Foamy cells in the marrow of these patients should alert the observers to the possibility of *M. avium-intracellulare* infection (Figs. 13-30 and 13-31). None of these findings are pathognomonic for AIDS. However, a decreased number of fat cells with low-density hematopoietic elements interspersed by eosinophilic granular or fibrillary material in a young man should alert the observer to the possibility of AIDS or AIDS-related complex.

The mechanism of peripheral cytopenias in an AIDS patient with normal or hypercellular marrow is unclear.

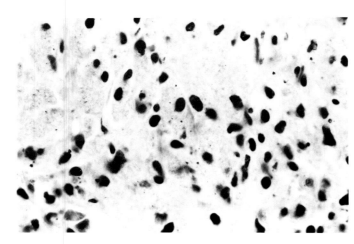

Fig. 13-30. Foamy histiocytes from a patient with AIDS. Note that the cytoplasm contains granular material. (H&E stain, ×250.)

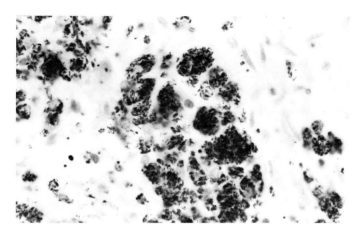

Fig. 13-31. Fite-Faraco stain reveals clumps of acid-fast bacteria in the cytoplasm of the foamy cells (same case as Fig. 13-30). (Fite-Faraco stain, ×250.)

Hypotheses include: (1) peripheral destruction secondary to hypersplenism; (2) immune complex–mediated autoimmune phenomenon; (3) drug reactions to trimethoprim-sulfamethoxazole for presumed *Pneumocystis* pneumonia; and (4) stimulation of the reticuloendothelial system due to multiple viral infections. It is most likely that several factors are contributing to the pancytopenia.

Lipid Granuloma

Lipid granuloma is a relatively common finding in elderly patients and patients with diabetes mellitus.[208] The morphology is similar to that found in the liver or spleen. Lipid granuloma consists of a collection of macrophages containing vacuoles of various sizes, which are, however, always smaller than the single vacuole in normal fat cells. Plasma cells, lymphocytes, and sometimes eosinophils and mast cells are all seen in the lipid granuloma. Microcysts lined by compressed histiocytes and multinucleated giant cells may also be present. Lipid granulomas associated with hyperlipidemia often contain foam cells and Touton-type giant cells. Foamy cells may be seen in a variety of clinical conditions (Table 13-8)[190] (Figs. 13-30 to 13-32). It is important to differentiate the nonspecific lesion of lipid granuloma from other granulomatous lesions.

Granulomatous Changes Associated with Hematologic Disorders

Lymphomas or lymphomalike lesions may contain granulomas or display granulomatous changes.[190] These include Hodgkin's disease, Lennert's lymphoma (lymphoepithelioid cell lymphoma), and angioimmunoblastic

TABLE 13-8. Clinical Conditions with Foamy Cells in the Marrow

Common conditions: lipophages associated with
  Alcoholic liver disease
  Fat necrosis secondary to bony fracture, infarction, and pancreatitis

Less common conditions
  Infections: Leprosy, Whipple's disease, *M. avium intracellulare*, leishmaniasis, histoplasmosis, and others
  Metastatic tumors: Metastatic renal cell carcinoma and others
  Hyperlipoproteinemias: Niemann-Pick disease, Gaucher's disease, Fabry's disease, Farber's disease, Wolman's disease, some mucopolysaccharidoses, mucolipidoses, glycogen storage disease, and others
  Histiocytosis X: Eosinophilic granuloma, Hand-Schüller-Christian disease, and others

(From Sun NCJ: Hematology: An Atlas and Diagnostic Guide. WB Saunders, Philadelphia, 1983, with permission.)

lymphadenopathy. Other lesions, such as eosinophilic fibrohistiocytic lesion of the bone marrow, systemic mastocytosis, and histiocytosis X, may produce lesions simulating granulomas. Histiocytosis X will be discussed under histiocytic proliferative disorders. The diagnostic criteria for these lesions in the bone marrow are the same as those in other parts of the body.

Hodgkin's Disease

Hodgkin's disease is a lymphoreticular malignancy characterized by a neoplastic proliferation of malignant cells (Reed-Sternberg cells) associated with an impaired host immune response.[209] Identification of the classic Reed-Sternberg cell is necessary for the diagnosis of Hodgkin's disease, although the mere presence of such a cell is not sufficient for this diagnosis. A classic Reed-Sternberg cell has a lobulated nucleus or is multinucle-

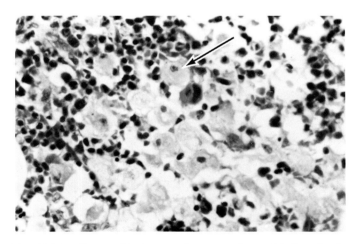

Fig. 13-32. Foamy histiocytes from a patient with Gaucher's disease. Note crystalloid structures in the cytoplasm (arrow). (H&E stain, ×160.)

ated. Each lobe or individual nucleus contains a large, homogeneous, eosinophilic, inclusionlike nucleolus, which often reaches the size of a red cell or the nucleus of a small lymphocyte. The cytoplasm contains a large quantity of ribonucleic acid and is strongly pyroninophilic when stained by methyl green–pyronine. Several types of Reed-Sternberg variants have been described and are very useful in the subclassification of the disease.

The nature of Reed-Sternberg cells is unclear. However, they are known to be reactive with monoclonal or polyclonal antibodies directed against the following antigens: LeuM1, LN2, HLA-DR, Peanut agglutinin, Ki-1, LCA, and both lambda and kappa light chains.[38,210]

Bone marrow involvement is not uncommon in certain subtypes of Hodgkin's disease, although the overall frequency of bone marrow involvement reported in the literature ranges from 5 to 22 percent.[5,211–213] Bartl and associates noted that bone marrow involvement was found in 10 percent of untreated and 25 percent of treated patients with Hodgkin's disease.[214] The most frequent type of Hodgkin's disease involving bone marrow is the diffuse fibrosis of the lymphocytic depletion type, with a reported incidence varying from 40 to 79 percent.[215–217] Bone marrow involvement also occurs in patients with the mixed cellularity or nodular sclerosis type of Hodgkin's disease. It appears that bone marrow involvement does not have an adverse effect on the patient's response to treatment, ability to achieve complete remission, or overall prognosis.[212,213] Furthermore, marrow fibrosis due to increased collagen or reticulin in the pretreatment specimens was found to have completely disappeared in many patients, with a reversion to normal marrow, after therapy.[213] Peripheral complete blood cell counts generally appear to be unreliable indicators of bone marrow involvement.

The histopathologic diagnosis of Hodgkin's disease of the marrow is not difficult to make when the normal marrow architecture is disrupted and is focally or diffusely replaced by a polymorphic cellular infiltrate consisting of lymphocytes, plasma cells, eosinophils, fibroblasts, and classic Reed-Sternberg cells, especially when the diagnosis of Hodgkin's disease has been previously established by lymph node biopsy (Fig. 13-33). The general rule of thumb is. that if a tissue diagnosis has not been established by a previous lymph node biopsy, the criteria should be more rigid, and diagnostic or classic Reed-Sternberg cells must be identified in the lesion; otherwise, polyploid cells that contain at least one huge nucleolus or Reed-Sternberg variants in a proper cellular background are adequate for the diagnosis of Hodgkin's disease involving the marrow[218,219] (Figs. 13-34 and 13-35). The frequency of Hodgkin's disease involvement of marrow apparently depends on the size or volume of the specimen, the method of examination, and the histologic

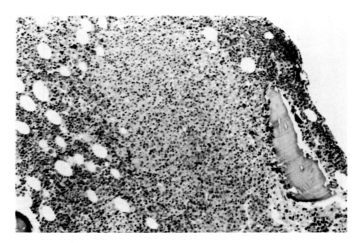

Fig. 13-33. Hodgkin's disease. A solitary lesion is seen in the marrow. This pattern of infiltrate is common for Hodgkin's disease, T-cell immunoblastic sarcoma, Lennert's lesion, and others. (H&E stain, ×40.)

type (i.e., an open biopsy is better than a bilateral needle biopsy, a histologic examination is superior to an aspiration smear, and patients with diffuse fibrosis, nodular sclerosis, and mixed cellularity have a higher incidence of marrow involvement). Osseous changes may also be noted in the area adjacent to the lesion.

Sarcoidlike granulomas may be found in the bone marrow of patients with Hodgkin's disease[220,221] and should not be confused with the specific lesions of this disease. It has been said, however, that survival and relapse-free survival are significantly more favorable for those patients who have noncaseating granulomas in the material

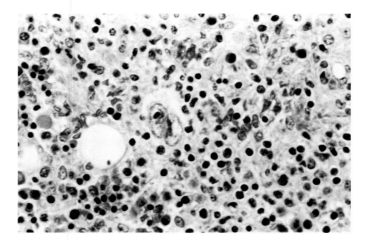

Fig. 13-34. Hodgkin's disease. A binucleated giant cell is seen in the center of this photomicrograph. Note that the size of the nucleolus reaches that of a small lymphocyte. The morphology is that of a Reed-Sternberg cell. Note also polymorphic cellular background. (H&E stain, ×250.)

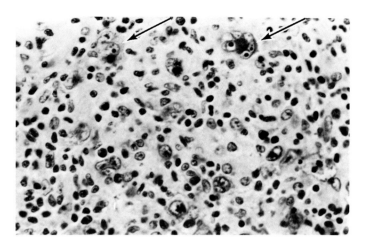

Fig. 13-35. Same case as above. Paranuclear and diffuse intra-cytoplasmic stain with anti-Leu M1 (arrows) is demonstrated in the Reed-Sternberg cells and their variants by an immuno-peroxidase stain with 3,3'-diaminobenzidine (DAB) as chromogen. Cytoplasmic-membranous staining may also be seen. (×160.)

obtained at initial staging procedures than for those who do not.[221] Benign lymphoid aggregates are also occasionally seen in involved or uninvolved marrow from patients with Hodgkin's disease.

Angioimmunoblastic (Immunoblastic) Lymphadenopathy

Angioimmunoblastic lymphadenopathy is a distinct clinicopathologic entity characterized by an acute clinical onset with fever, sweats, weight loss, and generalized lymphadenopathy. Skin rash, pruritus, hepatosplenomegaly, hypergammaglobulinemia, and Coombs-positive hemolytic anemia are other common features. A history of hypersensitivity reaction to drugs or other substances immediately preceding the onset of symptoms may be obtained in some patients. The disease is generally considered to be an abnormal immune response involving a deficiency of T-cell regulatory function or an exaggeration of lymphocyte transformation of the B-cell system.[222–224]

Bone marrow involvement occurred in approximately 70 percent of patients who underwent bone marrow examination.[225] The lesions are usually hypocellular, focal, and paratrabecular in distribution. Cells with fibroblast-like spindle-shaped nuclei are often prominent. In addition, lymphocytes, transformed lymphocytes, histiocytes, plasma cells, and eosinophils are present in the lesion. Increased numbers of reticulin fibers are frequently demonstrated. The involvement of bone marrow does not correlate with the clinical course and prognosis.[225]

Lennert's Lymphoma (Lymphoepithelioid Cell Lymphoma)

The lesion of Lennert's lymphoma is histologically characterized by diffuse malignant lymphocytic infiltration interspersed with clusters of epithelioid histiocytes. Other terms have been applied.[226–230]

The lesion primarily involves lymph nodes, but extranodal tissues are commonly involved. In addition to tonsils, the nasopharynx, spleen, liver, skin, and lung may be involved. Bone marrow was infiltrated in 17 percent of cases in one study and 53 percent in another.[229] Histologically, the lesion consists of atypical small and large lymphoid cells in varying proportions. Clusters of ill defined epithelioid cells are seen scattered throughout the stroma. The vascularity is generally not prominent. Foci of necrosis and giant cells are occasionally seen. A slight infiltrate of eosinophils and plasma cells is also present. Immunologic study has revealed that this is a malignant lymphoma of T-cells.

T-Cell Immunoblastic Sarcoma and Peripheral T-Cell Lymphoma

T-cell immunoblastic sarcoma may evolve from other types of T-cell lymphoma or arise de novo. It encompasses a variety of lesions known under different terminologies,[231–234] in which the presence of large transformed lymphocytes (T-immunoblasts) is the cardinal feature. Based on the composition of T-immunoblasts and background lymphocytes, various terms have been applied. A spectrum of atypical lymphocytes with highly folded nuclei and variable cell sizes is frequently seen in the background. Reed-Sternberglike cells may also be identified. Reactive histiocytes, plasma cells, and eosinophils may be present in considerable number. T-cell immunoblastic sarcoma usually presents as a disease of lymph nodes, but bone marrow involvement occurs in approximately one-third of patients.[234] The bone marrow in limited cases that I have seen revealed focal involvement. The morphologic features are the same as those observed in the lymph nodes. Hodgkin's disease is a frequent diagnostic consideration.

Hanson and associates recently collected bone marrow specimens from 30 patients with *peripheral T-cell lymphoma*.[235] They found that 80 percent of patients had marrow involvement with the lymphoma in trephine biopsies at the time of initial diagnosis. The pattern of infiltration may be diffuse or focal (nonparatrabecular). The neoplastic lesion is composed of a polymorphic cellular infiltrate consisting of a heteromorphous population of lymphocytes, plasma cells, eosinophils, and histiocytes. Prominent vascularity with endothelial cell proliferation and reticulin fibrosis are also noted. The histopathology is not pathognomonic and has to be differentiated from that of other diseases.

Eosinophilic Fibrohistiocytic Lesion of Bone Marrow

This unusual lesion of bone marrow, first described by Rywlin et al.,[236] was characterized histologically by a collection of cells having oval to spindle-shaped nuclei, measuring 12 to 14 μm in length and 4 to 6 μm in width. Numerous eosinophils were interspersed among the spindle-shaped cells, together with some plasma cells and occasional mast cells. The lesion often occurred in close proximity to a blood vessel, lymphoid follicle, and/or sinusoidal space. All five patients in Rywlin's series were over 55 years old (median age, 66 years) and presented with symptoms of chest pain, bony fracture, back pain, cataract requiring surgery, and other findings related to advanced age. Four of the patients had mild to moderate anemia, and four had absolute eosinophilia. A drug history was obtained in each patient, and the lesions were found to have completely or almost completely disappeared after the withdrawal of the incriminated drug in some patients. Ampicillin was the drug thought to be most likely involved; others included propranolol, procainamide, allopurinol, erythromycin, and minocycline.

More recently, te Velde et al. noted that similar lesions were found on nondecalcified plastic-prepared marrow sections from seven patients with bony disease (six patients with severe osteoporosis and one with osteogenesis imperfecta).[237] The elongated "fibrohistiocytes" of Rywlin were found to be elongated mast cells. The infiltrate also consisted of other cellular components, such as eosinophils, lymphocytes, and plasma cells. These authors wondered whether this peculiar lesion might represent an unusual form of mast cell disease in which other features of mastocytosis were absent.

Systemic Mastocytosis

Systemic mastocytosis may be manifested clinically in two ways.[238,239] (1) An infiltrative process is characterized by osteoporosis or osteosclerosis, hepatosplenomegaly, lymphadenopathy, and/or mast cell infiltration in the skin (urticaria pigmentosa), gastrointestinal tract, heart, and lungs. Anemia, leukocytosis, leukopenia, eosinophilia, basophilia, or hypocholesterolemia may occur. (2) Pharmacologic effects may occur secondary to release of chemicals following degranulation of mast cells. These are characterized by flushing, pounding headache, bronchospasm, hypotension, diarrhea, rhinorrhea, urticaria, palpitation, dyspnea, peptic ulcer, and gastrointestinal bleeding. Various combinations and clinical syndromes are seen.

Mast cell disease is most commonly manifested as skin involvement only (urticaria pigmentosa). It may also present as a combination of skin and bone disease. The other, less common syndromes include systemic mastocytosis in association with leukemia and systemic mastocytosis without skin involvement.[240] Systemic mastocytosis almost always involves both the bone and marrow and produces small "granulomalike" lesions characterized by slight increase in fibrous tissue and inflammatory cells. The normal hematopoietic elements and fat cells are often replaced by the lesion, and there is an increase in reticulin fibrosis. Eosinophilia may also be noted.[241] Osteosclerosis, resorption of bone, or a combination of both may be present. With appropriate processing and staining techniques, increased numbers of mast cells are easily seen in the granulomalike areas, which are often found in a perivascular location.

Histiocytic Proliferative Disorders

Histiocytic proliferative disorders may be classified as (1) reactive, (2) associated with genetic disorders, and (3) neoplastic or malignant proliferations.[242] Reactive histiocytic proliferation is usually transient and is caused by an infectious process or increased cell death. Granulomatous lesions described above are examples of histiocytic reaction. The various genetic disorders that result in excessive accumulation of biologic products in the histiocytes, such as Gaucher's disease and Niemann-Pick disease, are beyond the scope of this chapter. It is important to recognize that the presence of "sea blue histiocytes" or "Gaucher cells" may be due to either genetic disorders or reactive proliferation.[243,244] The neoplastic proliferation of histiocytes is uncommon, and the nature of some entities, such as Hand-Schüller-Christian syndrome, eosinophilic granuloma, and sinus histiocytosis with massive lymphadenopathy, is uncertain. It has been postulated that they may represent a reactive histiocytic proliferation in response to an unidentified microorganism.

Muller-Hermelink and Lennert classified histiocytes (reticulum cells) into four groups: (1) histiocytic reticulum cells; (2) fibroblastic reticulum cells; (3) dendritic reticulum cells; and (4) interdigitating reticulum cells.[245] Cells in each group have their specific function, anatomic location, enzyme content, and reaction to different monoclonal or polyclonal antibodies.[246] The histiocytic reticulum cells of Muller-Hermelink and Lennert are equivalent to our sinus histiocytes; they are present in the sinuses and possess phagocytic activity. The hemophagocytic syndrome caused by a variety of pathogens is associated with proliferation of these cells.[247-249] In 1986 Wieczorek and associates reported that the proliferative cells in familial erythrophagocytic lymphohistiocytosis also originate from sinus histiocytes.[250] Both disease entities display hypercellular bone marrow infiltrated by numerous histiocytes with prominent erythrophagocytosis. Multinucleated giant cells may be found, but cytologic atypia is distinctly absent. Differential diagnosis between these two entities rests on clinical grounds.[157] Erythrophagocytosis by itself is not diagnostic for any diseases. It indicates a stimulated reticuloendothelial system and may be observed in a variety of clinical conditions associated with infections or malignant diseases.[251,252] Hemophagocytic syndrome of infectious etiology should be differentiated from sinus histiocytosis with massive lymphadenopathy,[253] erythrophagocytic T-gamma lymphoma,[136] and histiocytic medullary reticulosis[254] or malignant histiocytosis.[255]

The spectrum of clinicopathologic findings in malignant histiocytosis has been well illustrated by Ducatman and associates.[256] The malignant process in the marrow is either focal or diffuse and may be mistaken for Hodgkin's disease, large cell lymphoma, or virus-associated hemophagocytic syndrome. Neoplastic cells exhibit varying degrees of cytologic atypia and phagocytosis. In one case, atypical histiocytes were scattered in a myxoid stroma, resembling those seen in malignant fibrous histiocytoma.[256] Robb-Smith and Taylor cautioned that the term *malignant histiocytosis* used by Byrne and Rappaport[257] embraces a whole range of conditions involving abnormal histiocytes, including histiocytic lymphoma, whereas "histiocytic medullary reticulosis" was used to describe a clinicopathologic entity characterized by a proliferation of atypical and phagocytic histiocytes in the sinuses of the reticuloendothelial system, which leads to a rapidly downhill course for the patients.[258]

The widely used term *histiocytosis X* is believed to be related to Langerhans cells of the skin (equivalent to interdigitating reticulum cells in other parts of the body). This term, initially proposed by Lichtenstein,[259] has now received challenges by several authors who consider Hand-Schüller-Christian disease to be a multifocal or generalized variant of eosinophilic granuloma unrelated to Letterer-Siwe disease.[260–262] The bone marrow findings in *Hand Schüller-Christian disease* and *eosinophilic granuloma* are identical. Sheets and islands of histiocytes containing an abundant amount of eosinophilic cytoplasm and a bland, twisted nucleus are intermingled with a variable number of eosinophils. Foamy histiocytes and multinucleated giant cells may also be present. The lesion in *Letterer-Siwe syndrome,* also called *disseminated visceral histiocytosis,*[262] consists of proliferation of well differentiated histiocytes with or without foamy cells.

Metastatic Tumors

The frequency of metastatic carcinoma in bone marrow from all patients who have had marrow examinations has varied from 1 to 2 to 2.7 percent.[263,264] A routine bone

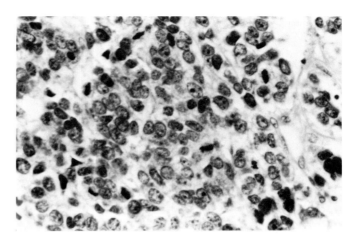

Fig. 13-36. Metastatic undifferentiated small cell (oat cell) carcinoma. Note the coherence of neoplastic cells, with numerous mitoses. (H&E stain, ×200.)

marrow examination of patients with nonhematopoietic malignant tumors revealed metastatic carcinoma in 9.1 percent.[265] Metastasis was most frequent in patients with neuroblastoma (48 percent), Ewing's sarcoma (36 percent), oat cell carcinoma (21 percent), prostatic carcinoma (20 percent), and breast carcinoma (20 percent).[265] The frequency of positive bone marrow pathology in patients suspected of having or showing evidence of metastatic carcinomas was even higher (37 to 44 percent).[18,266] The incidence of metastatic lesions in bone marrow varies from series to series, depending on the purpose of the study, the histopathologic type of tumor, the stage of the disease, and the method of bone marrow examination.[267] Generally speaking, both biopsy and aspiration should be

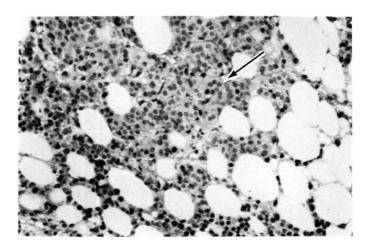

Fig. 13-37. Metastatic breast carcinoma. Islands of well differentiated adenocarcinoma (arrow) are illustrated. Compare these cells with normal erythropoietic islands. (H&E stain, ×100.)

performed when evaluating metastatic disease of the marrow.[268]

Histopathologic examination of bone marrow reveals necrosis, fibrosis, increased osteoblastic activity (most notably in carcinomas of the prostate and breast but also in other tumors), osteoclastic activity (as in metastatic oat cell carcinoma), or a combination of both (most common form of bone reaction), and replacement of normal fat cells and hematopoietic elements by metastatic carcinoma (Figs. 13-36 and 13-37). Oat cell carcinoma and neuroblastoma may produce a picture simulating malignant lymphoma, but metastatic tumor cells are often larger than lymphoma cells, the neoplastic cells are more coherent than lymphoma cells, and immunoperoxidase study or electron microscopy can differentiate these entities in a majority of difficult cases. The surrounding hematopoietic elements may show dyspoiesis. In addition, increased numbers of plasma cells, eosinophils, and sometimes lymphocytes are seen.

Bone Marrow Necrosis and Infarction

Bone marrow necrosis is very uncommon, with a prevalence of 0.15 percent,[269] although another retrospective study revealed that approximately one-third of 368 bone marrow biopsy specimens displayed focal necrosis and degenerative changes.[270] The most commonly associated clinical conditions are sickle cell disease, myeloproliferative disorder, acute leukemia, malignant lymphoma, and metastatic carcinomas. Bone marrow necrosis may also occur in patients with sepsis, vasculitis, or disseminated intravascular coagulation.[271] In 1981 osteonecrosis of either the femoral or humeral head secondary to the administration of steroid-containing combined chemotherapy for malignant lymphomas was reported.[272]

Histopathologic examination may reveal a spectrum of morphologies ranging from total necrosis and infarction to individual cell necrosis (Fig. 13-38). In foci of bone marrow necrosis, the fatty and hematopoietic marrow are replaced by granular eosinophilic debris. It is important to identify the underlying disease, such as acute leukemia or metastatic carcinoma. Deep sections or step sections may be needed to search for viable cells or tissues. Occasionally, repeated biopsy is indicated.

Fat necrosis of bone marrow is identical with that seen in other adipose tissue. The causes include fracture of bone and infarct. During the healing process, lipophages (foamy cells) and lipid granulomas are seen.

Vascular Lesions in Marrow

Vascular lesions, either localized[273] or systemic (such as thrombotic thrombocytopenic purpura, collagen vascular disease, or amyloidosis) may be diagnosed on histologic sections of bone marrow.[274,275] Cholesterol emboli can be recognized with ease and may be a manifestation of a multisystem illness.[276] Kaposi's sarcoma is very uncommon in the bone marrow even in this era of the worldwide endemic spread of AIDS, although in 1986 Conran and associates reported a case[273] (Fig. 13-39). The lesion should be differentiated from a variety of disorders associated with primary or secondary myelofibrosis and vascular proliferation.

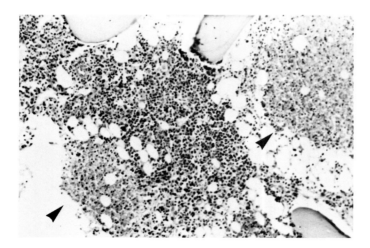

Fig. 13-38. Malignant lymphoma with bone marrow necrosis. Foci of eosinophic granular material admixed with pyknotic nuclei and cellular debris are seen in the upper and lower corners (arrowheads), in this specimen from a patient with malignant lymphoma. (H&E stain, ×40.)

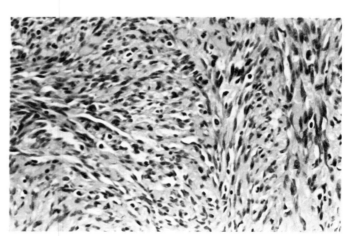

Fig. 13-39. Kaposi's sarcoma of bone marrow. Note the interlacing spindle cells, which form slits and spaces. Mitotic figures are seen. (H&E stain, ×100.) (Courtesy of Dr. Richard Conran and associates).

REFERENCES

1. Petersdorf RG, Beeson PB: Fever of un-explained origin: Report on 100 cases. Medicine (Baltimore) 40:1, 1961
2. Contreras E, Ellis LD, Lee RE: Value of the bone marrow biopsy in the diagnosis of metastic carcinoma. Cancer 29:788, 1972
3. Ellman L: Bone marrow biopsy in the evaluation of lymphoma, carcinoma and granulomatous disorders. Am J Med 60:1, 1976
4. Pease GL: Granulomatous lesions in bone marrow. Blood 11:720, 1956
5. O'Carroll DI, McKenna RW, Brunning RD: Bone marrow manifestations of Hodgkin's disease. Cancer 38:1717, 1976
6. Rosenberg SA: Bone marrow involvement in the non-Hodgkins lymphomata. Br J Cancer 31:suppl II, 261, 1975
7. Jamshidi K, Swaim WR: Bone marrow biopsy with unaltered architecture: A new biopsy device. J Lab Clin Med 77:335, 1971
8. Islam A: A new bone marrow biopsy needle with core securing device. J Clin Pathol 35:359, 1982
9. Bartl R, Frisch B, Burkhardt R: Bone Marrow Biopsies, Revisited. A New Dimension for Hematologic Malignancies. S Karger AG, Basel, 1982
10. Rywlin AM: Histopathology of the Bone Marrow. p. 1. Little, Brown, Boston, 1976
11. Brynes RK, McKenna RW, Sundberg RD: Bone marrow aspiration and trephine biopsy. An approach to a thorough study. Am J Clin Pathol 70:753, 1978
12. Gruppo RA, Lampkin BC, Granger S: Bone marrow cellularity determination: Comparison of the biopsy, aspirate and buffy coat. Blood 49:29, 1977
13. Liao KT: The superiority of histologic sections of aspirated bone marrow in malignant lymphomas: A review of 1,124 examinations. Cancer 27:618, 1971
14. Westerman MP: Bone marrow needle biopsy: An evaluation and critique. Semin Hematol 18:293, 1981
15. Bain NT, Pickett JP: Glycol methacrylate for routine, special stains, histochemistry, enzyme histochemistry and immunohistochemistry. A simplified method for surgical biopsy tissue. J Histotechnol 2:125, 1979
16. Beckstead JH, Bainton DF: Enzyme histochemistry on bone marrow biopsies: Reactions useful in the differential diagnosis of leukemia and lymphoma applied to 2-micron plastic sections. Blood 55:386, 1980
17. Sun NCJ: Hematology: An Atlas and Diagnostic guide. p. 23. WB Saunders, Philadelphia, 1983
18. Brunning RD, Bloomfield CD, McKenna RW, et al: Bilateral trephine bone marrow biopsies in lymphoma and other neoplastic diseases. Ann Intern Med 82:365, 1975
19. Ioannides K, Rywlin AM: A comparative study of histologic sections of bone marrow obtained by aspiration and by needle biopsy. Am J Clin Pathol 65:267, 1976
20. Gruber HE, Stauffer ME, Thompson ER, et al: Diagnosis of bone disease by core biopsies. Semin Hematol 18:258, 1981
21. Fong TP, Okafor LA, Thomas W Jr, et al: Stainable iron in aspirated and needle-biopsy specimens of marrow: A source of error. Am J Hematol 2:47, 1977
22. Ribeiro RC, Abromowitch M, Raimondi SC, et al: Clinical and biologic hallmarks of the Philadelphia chromosome in childhood acute lymphoblastic leukemia. Blood 70:948, 1987
23. Korsmeyer SJ: Antigen receptor genes as molecular markers of lymphoid neoplasms. J Clin Invest 79:1291, 1987
24. Parker JW: Flow cytometry in the diagnosis in hematologic diseases. Ann Clin Lab Sci 16:427, 1986
25. Christensson B, Tribukait E, Linder I-L, et al: Cell proliferation and DNA content in non-Hodgkin's lymphoma: flow cytometry in relation to lymphoma classification. Cancer 58:1295, 1986
26. Bitter MA, LeBeau MM, Rowley JD, et al: Associations between morphology, karyotype, and clinical features in myeloid leukemias. Hum Pathol 18:211, 1987
27. Sandberg AA: The chromosomes in human leukemia. Semin Hematol 23:201, 1986
28. Foon KA, Gale RP, Todd RF III: Recent advances in the immunologic classification of leukemia. Semin Hematol 23:257, 1986
29. Waldmann TA (moderator): Molecular genetic analysis of human lymphoid neoplasms. Immunoglobulin genes and the c-myc oncogene. Ann Intern Med 102:497, 1985
30. Groupe Français de Morphologie Hématologique: French registry of acute leukemia and myelodysplastic syndromes: Age distribution and hemogram analysis of the 4496 cases recorded during 1982–1983 and classified according to FAB criteria. Cancer 60:1385, 1987
31. Sobol RE, Mick R, Royston I, et al: Clinical importance of myeloid antigen expression in adult acute lymphoblastic leukemia. N Engl J Med 316:1111, 1987
32. Pui C-H, Behm FG, Kalwinsky DK, et al: Clinical significance of low levels of myeloperoxidase positivity in childhood acute nonlymphoblastic leukemia. Blood 70:51, 1987
33. Pinkus GS, Said JW: Intracellular hemoglobin—a specific marker for erythroid cells in paraffin sections. Am J Pathol 102:308, 1981
34. Hanyan SNS, Kearney JF, Cooper MD: A monoclonal antibody (MMA) that identifies a differentiated antigen on human myelomonocytic cells. Clin Immunol Immunopathol 23:172, 1982
35. Epstein AL, Marder RJ, Winter JN, et al: The new monoclonal antibodies (LN-1, LN-2) reactive in B5, formalin-fixed, paraffin-embedded tissues with follicular center and mantle zone human B lymphocytes and derived tumor. J Immunol 133:1028, 1984
36. Kurtin PJ, Pinkus GS: Leukocyte common antigen—a diagnostic discriminant between hematopoietic and nonhematopoietic neoplasms in paraffin sections using monoclonal antibodies: Correlation with immunologic studies and ultrastructural localization. Hum Pathol 16:353, 1985
37. Linder J, Ye Y, Harrington DS, et al: Monoclonal antibodies marking T lymphocytes in paraffin-embedded tissue. Am J Pathol 127:1, 1987

38. Taylor CR: Immunomicroscopy: A Diagnostic Tool for the Surgical Pathologist. pp. 70, 116, 142. WB Saunders, Philadelphia, 1986

39. Custer, RP: An Atlas of the Blood and Bone Marrow. p. 33. WB Saunders, Philadelphia, 1974

40. Hartsock RJ, Smith EB, Petty CS: Normal variations with aging of the amount of hematopoietic tissue in bone marrow from the anterior iliac crest. A study made from 177 cases of sudden death examined by necropsy. Am J Clin Pathol 43:326, 1965

41. Frisch B, Lewis SM, Burkhardt R, et al: Biopsy Pathology of Bone and Bone Marrow. p. 28. Raven Press, New York, 1985

42. Brittenham GM, Danish EH, Harris JW: Assessment of bone marrow and body iron stores: Old techniques and new technologies. Semin Hematol 18:194, 1981

43. Huang B-J, Li C-Y, Nichols WL, et al: Acute leukemia with megakaryocytic differentiation: A study of 12 cases identified immunocytochemically. Blood 64:427, 1984

44. Ruiz-Arguelles GJ, Marin-Lopez A, Lobato-Mendizabal E, et al: Acute megakaryoblastic leukemia: A prospective study of its identification and treatment. Br J Haematol 62:55, 1986

45. Larsen TE: Emperipolesis of granular leukocytes within megakaryocytes in human hematopoietic bone marrow. Am J Clin Pathol 53:485, 1970

46. Rywlin AM, Ortega RS, Dominguez CJ: Lymphoid nodules of the bone marrow: Normal and abnormal. Blood 43:389, 1974

47. Hyun BH, Kwa D, Gabaldon H, et al: Reactive plasmacytic lesions of the bone marrow. Am J Clin Pathol 65:921, 1976

48. Farrant A, Rodham J, Cordier A, et al: Selective hypoplasia of pelvic bone marrow. Scand J Haematol 25:12, 1980

49. Seaman JP, Kjeldsberg CR, Linker A: Gelatinous transformation of the bone marrow. Hum Pathol 9:685, 1978

50. Amrein PC, Friedman R, Kosinsku K, et al: Hematologic changes in anorexia nervosa. JAMA 241:2190, 1979

51. Alter BP, Potter NU, Li FP: Classification and aetiology of the aplastic anemia. Clin Haematol 7:431, 1978

52. Mir MA, Geary CG: Aplastic anaemia: An analysis of 174 patients. Postgrad Med J 56:322, 1980

53. Pierre RV: Preleukemia states. Semin Hematol 11:73, 1974

54. Rosse WF: Paroxysmal nocturnal hemoglobinuria in aplastic anemia. Clin Haematol 7:541, 1978

55. Diamond LK, Blackfan KD: Hypoplastic anemia. Am J Dis Child 56:464, 1938

56. Slater WM, Schultz MJ, Armentrout SA: Remission of pure red cell aplasia associated with nonthymic malignancy. Cancer 44:1879, 1979

57. LeHane DE: Vacuolated erythroblasts in hyperosmolar coma. Arch Intern Med 134:763, 1974

58. McCurdy R, Rath CE: Vacuolated nucleated bone marrow cells in alcoholism. Semin Hematol 17:100, 1980

59. The international agranulocytosis and aplastic anemia study: Risks of agranulocytosis and aplastic anemia—a first report of their relation to drug use with special reference to analgesics. JAMA 256:1749, 1986

60. Levitt LJ, Ries CA, Greenberg PL: Pure white cell aplasia. Antibody mediated autoimmune inhibition of granulopoiesis. N Engl J Med 308:1141, 1983

61. Carmel R: An unusual case of autoimmune agranulocytosis with total absence of myeloid precursors. Am J Clin Pathol 79:611, 1983

62. Stoll DB, Blum S, Pasquale D, et al: Thrombocytopenia and decreased megakaryocytes. Evaluation and prognosis. Ann Intern Med 94:170, 1981

63. Beal RW, Kronenberg H, Firkin BG: The syndrome of paroxysmal nocturnal hemoglobinuria. Am J Med 37:899, 1964

64. Howe RB, Bloomfield CD, McKenna RW: Hypocellular acute leukemia. Am J Med 72:391, 1982

65. Needleman S, Burns CP, Dick FR, et al: Hypoplastic acute leukemia. Cancer 48:1410, 1981

66. Bennett JM, Catovsky D, Daniel M-T, et al: Proposals for the classification of the acute leukemias. Br J Haematol 33:451, 1976

67. Bennett JM, Catovsky D, Daniel MT, et al: Proposals for the classification of the myelodysplastic syndrome. Br J Haematol 51:189, 1982

68. Bennett JM, Catovsky D, Daniel M-T, et al: Proposed revised criteria for the classification of acute myeloid leukemia: A report of the French-American-British Cooperative Group. Ann Intern Med 103:626, 1985

69. Gladson CL, Naeim F: Hypocellular bone marrow with increased blasts. Am J Hematol 21:15, 1986

70. Rheingold JJ, Kaufman R, Adelson E, et al: Smoldering acute leukemia. N Engl J Med 268:812, 1963

71. Breatnach F, Chessells JM, Greaves MF: The aplastic presentation of childhood leukemia: A feature of common ALL. Br J Haematol 49:387, 1981

72. Sills RH, Stockman JA III: Preleukemic states in children with acute lymphoblastic leukemia. Cancer 48:110, 1981

73. Wittels B: Bone marrow biopsy change following chemotherapy for acute leukemia. Am J Surg Pathol 4:135, 1980

74. Sun NCJ: Hematology: An atlas and diagnostic guide. p. 113. WB Saunders, Philadelphia, 1983

75. Spector JL: Juvenile achlorhydric pernicious anemia with IgA deficiencies: A family study. JAMA 228:334, 1974

76. Lewis SM, Verwilghen RL: Dyserythropoiesis and dyserythropoietic anemia. Prog Hematol 8:99, 1973

77. Bennett JM, Reed CE: Acute leukemia cytochemical profile: Diagnostic and clinical implications. Blood Cells 1:101, 1975

78. Sun NCJ: Hematology: An atlas and diagnostic guide. pp. 173, 228, 288, WB Saunders, Philadelphia, 1983

79. Bennet JM, Catovsky D, Daniel M-T, et al: Criteria for the diagnosis of acute leukemia of megakaryocyte lineage (M$_7$): A report of the French-American-British Cooperative Group. Ann Intern Med 103:460, 1985

80. Sun NCJ: Diagnosing leukemias with granulated leukemic cells (excluding eosinophilic leukemia) (editorial). Mayo Clin Proc 62:1059, 1987

81. Head DR, Cerezo L, Savage RA, et al: Institutional performance in application of the FAB classification of acute leukemia: The Southwest Oncology Group experience. Cancer 55:1979, 1985

82. Stanley M, McKenna RW, Ellinger G, et al: Classification of 358 cases of acute myeloid leukemia by FAB criteria: Analysis of clinical and morphologic features. p. 147. In Bloomfield C (ed): Chronic and Acute Leukemias in Adults. Martinus Nijhoff, Boston, 1985

83. Mertelsmann R, Thaler HT, To L, et al: Morphological classification, response to therapy and survival in 263 adult patients with acute nonlymphoblastic leukemia. Blood 56:773, 1980

84. Jones ME, Saleem A: Acute promyelocytic leukemia. Am J Med 65:673, 1978

85. Shaw MT: Monocytic leukemias. Hum Pathol 2:215, 1980

86. Kass L: Bone marrow interpretation. p. 43. JB Lippincott, Philadelphia, 1979

87. Quaglino D, Hayhoe FG: Periodic-acid-Schiff positivity in erythroblasts with special reference to di Guglielmo's disease. Br J Haematol 6:26, 1960

88. Klein HO, Heller A: PAS-positive erythroblasts in kidney disease. Acta Haematol (Basel) 37:225, 1967

89. Dameshek W: The di Guglielmo syndrome revisited. Blood 34:567, 1969

90. Smith LJ, Curtis JE, Messner HA, et al: Lineage infidelity in acute leukemia. Blood 61:1138, 1983

91. Miller DR: Acute lymphoblastic leukemia. Pediatr Clin North Am 27:269, 1980

92. Bennett JM, Catovsky D, Daniel MT, et al: The morphological classification of acute lymphoblastic leukemia: Concordance among observers and clinical correlations. Br J Haematol 47:553, 1981

93. McKenna RW, Brynes RK, Nesbit ME, et al: Cytochemical profiles in acute lymphoblastic leukemia. Am J Pediat Hematol Oncol 1:263, 1979

94. Dameshek W: Some speculations on the myeloproliferative syndromes. Blood 6:392, 1951

95. Lewis SM, Szur L: Malignant myelosclerosis. Br Med J 2:472, 1963

96. Bearman RM, Pangalis GA, Rappaport H: Acute (malignant) myelosclerosis. Cancer 43:279, 1979

97. Shah I, Mayeda K, Koppitch F, et al: Karyotypic polymorphism in acute myelofibrosis. Blood 60:841, 1982

98. Clare N, Elson D, Manhoff L: Case report: Cytogenetic studies of peripheral myeloblasts and bone marrow fibroblasts in acute myelofibrosis. Am J Clin Pathol 77:762, 1982

99. Rozman C, Granena A, Hernandez-Nieto, et al: Bone marrow transplantation for acute myelofibrosis. Lancet 1:618, 1982

100. Puckett JB, Cooper MR: Acute myelofibrosis evolving into acute myeloblastic leukemia. Ann Intern Med 94:545, 1981

101. Tada T, Nitta M, Kishimoto H: Acute myelofibrosis terminating in erythroleukemia state. Am J Clin Pathol 78:102, 1982

102. Ellis JT, Peterson P: The bone marrow in polycythemia vera. Pathol Annu 14 (pt. 1):383, 1979

103. Berlin NI: Polycythemia. I. Semin Hematol 12:335, 1975

104. Silverstein MN: Postpolycythemia myeloid metaplasia. Arch Intern Med 134:113, 1974

105. Rosenthal DS, Molony WC: Occurrence of acute leukemia in myeloproliferative disorders. Br J Haematol 36:373, 1977

106. Berlin NI: Polycythemia. II. Semin Hematol 13:1, 1976

107. Barosi G, Baraldi A, Calolla M, et al: Polycythemia following splenectomy in myelofibrosis with myeloid metaplasia. A reorganization of erythropoiesis. Scand J Haematol 32:12, 1984

108. Bellucci S, Janvier M, Tobelem G, et al: Essential thrombocythemias: Clinical evolutionary and biological data. Cancer 58:2440, 1986

109. Frisch B, Bartl R, Burkhardt R, et al: Histologic criteria for classification and differential diagnosis in the chronic myeloproliferative disorders. Haematologia (Budap) 17:209, 1984

110. Korostoff NR, Sun NCJ, Okun DB: Atypical blast crisis in chronic myelogenous leukemia. JAMA 245:1245, 1981

111. Ward HP, Block MH: The natural history of agnogenic myeloid metaplasia (AMM) and a critical evaluation of its relationship with the myeloproliferative syndrome. Medicine (Baltimore) 50:357, 1971

112. Varki A, Lottenberg R, Griffith R, et al: The syndrome of idiopathic myelofibrosis. A clinicopathologic review with emphasis on the prognostic variables predicting survival. Medicine (Baltimore) 62:353, 1983

113. Moore MAS: Bone marrow culture: Leucopoiesis and stem cells. p. 110. In Hoffbrand AV (ed): Recent Advances in Haematology. Churchill Livingstone, Edinburgh, 1982

114. Sun NCJ: Hematology: An Atlas and Diagnostic Guide. p. 140. WB Saunders, Philadelphia, 1983

115. Frisch B, Schlag R, Bartl R, et al: Histologic characteristics of myelodysplasia. Verh Dtsch Ges Pathol 67:132, 1983

116. Tricot G, de Wolf-Peeters C, Vlietinck R, et al: The importance of bone marrow biopsies in myelodysplastic disorders. Bibl Haematol 50:31, 1984

117. Riccardi A, Geordano M, Girino M, et al: Refractory cytopenias: Clinical course according to bone marrow cytology and cellularity. Blut 54:153, 1987

118. Koeffler HP: Myelodysplastic syndrome (preleukemia). Semin Hematol 23:284, 1986

119. Sokal G, Michaux J, Berghe VD, et al: A new hematologic syndrome with a distinct karyotype: The 5 q- chromosome. Blood 46:519, 1975

120. Nowell PC, Besa EC, Stelmach T, et al: Chromosome studies in preleukemic states. V. Prognostic significance of single versus multiple abnormalities. Cancer 58:2571, 1986

121. Sarrinen UM, Wegelius R: Preleukemia syndrome in children: Report of four cases and review of literature. Am J Pediatr Hematol Oncol 6:137, 1984

122. Wintrobe MM, Lee GR, Boggs DR, et al: Clinical Hematology. p. 66. Lea & Febiger, Philadelphia, 1981

123. Maeda K, Hyun BH, Rebuck JW: Lymphoid follicles in bone marrow aspirates. Am J Clin Pathol 67:41, 1977

124. Silver RT, Sawitsky A, Rai K, et al: Guidelines for proto-

col studies in chronic lymphocytic leukemia. Am J Hematol 4:343, 1978

125. Rai KR, Sawitsky A, Cronkite EP, et al: Clinical staging of chronic lymphocytic leukemia. Blood 46:219, 1975

126. Foon KA, Todd RF III: Immunologic classification of leukemia and lymphoma. Blood 68:1, 1986

127. Binet J, Auquier A, Dighiero G, et al: A new prognostic classification of chronic lymphocytic leukemia derived from a multivariate analysis. Cancer 48:198, 1981

128. Rai KR, Montserrat E: Prognostic factors in chronic lymphocytic leukemia. Semin Hematol 24:252, 1987

129. Rozman C, Hernandez-Nieto L, Montserrat E, et al: Prognostic significance of bone-marrow patterns in chronic lymphocytic leukemia. Br J Haematol 47:529, 1981

130. Kubic VL, Brunning RD: Immunohistochemical evaluation of neoplasms in bone marrow biopsy using the monoclonal antibodies (MoAbs) LN1, LN2 and LeuM₁. Lab Invest 56(1):40A, 1987

131. Rozman C, Montserrat E, Rodriguez-Fernandez JM, et al: Bone marrow histologic pattern—the best single prognostic parameter in chronic lymphocytic leukemia: A multivariate survival analysis of 329 cases. Blood 64:642, 1984

132. Pangalis GA, Roussou PA, Kittas C, et al: B-chronic lymphocytic leukemia. Prognostic implication of bone marrow histology in 120 patients: Experience from a single hematology unit. Cancer 59:767, 1987

133. Pangalis GA, Roussou PA, Kittas C, et al: Patterns of bone marrow involvement in chronic lymphocytic leukemia and small lymphocytic (well differentiated) non-Hodgkin's lymphoma. Its clinical significance in relation to their differential diagnosis and prognosis. Cancer 54:702, 1984

134. Brouet JC, Flandrin G, Sasportes M, et al: Chronic lymphocytic leukemia of T-cell origin. Immunologic and clinical evaluation in eleven patients. Lancet 2:890, 1975

135. Sun, NCJ: Hematology: An Atlas and Diagnostic Guide. p. 323. WB Saunders, Philadelphia, 1983

136. Kadin ME, Kamoun N, Lamberg J: Erythrophagocytic Tγ lymphoma. A clinical pathologic entity resembling malignant histiocytosis. N Engl J Med 304:648, 1981

137. Reynolds CW, Foon KA: Tγ-lymphoproliferative disease and related disorders in man and experimental animals: A review of the clinical, cellular and functional characteristics. Blood 64:1146, 1984

138. Newland AC, Catovsky D, Linch D, et al: Chronic T cell lymphocytosis. A review of 21 cases. Br J Haematol 58:433, 1984

139. Laughran TP, Kadin ME, Starkbaum G, et al: Leukemia of large granular lymphocytes: Association with clonal chromosomal abnormalities and autoimmune neutropenia, thrombocytopenia, and hemolytic anemia. Ann Intern Med 102:169, 1985

140. McPhedran P, Heath CW Jr: Acute leukemia occurring during chronic lymphocytic leukemia. Blood 35:7, 1970

141. Dighiero G, Follezou JY, Roisin JP, et al: Comparison of normal and chronic lymphocytic leukemia lymphocyte surface Ig determinants using peroxidase-labeled antibodies. II. Quantification of light chain determinants in atypical lymphocytic leukemia. Blood 48:449, 1976

142. Enno A, Catovsky D, O'Brien M, et al: "Prolymphocytoid" transformation of chronic lymphocytic leukemia. Br J Haematol 41:9, 1979

143. Melo JV, Catovsky D, Galton DAG: The relationship between chronic lymphocytic leukaemia and prolymphocytic leukaemia. I. Clinical and laboratory features of 300 patients and characterizations of an intermediate group. Br J Haematol 63:377, 1986

144. Melo JV, Catovsky D, Galton DAG: The relationship between chronic lymphocytic leukaemia and prolymphocytic leukaemia. II. Patterns of evolution of "prolymphocytoid" transformation. Br J Haematol 67:77, 1986

145. Melo FV, Wardle J, Chetty M, et al: The relationship between chronic lymphocytic leukaemia and prolymphocytic leukaemia. III. Evaluation of cell size by morphology and volume measurements. Br J Haematol 64:469, 1986

146. Melo JV, Catovsky D, Gregory WM, et al: The relationship between chronic lymphocytic leukaemia and prolymphocytic leukaemia. IV. Analysis of survival and prognostic features. Br J Haematol 65:23, 1987

147. Galton DAG, Goldman JM, Wiltshaw E, et al: Prolymphocytic leukaemia. Br J Haematol 27:7, 1974

148. Richter MN: Generalized reticular cell sarcoma of lymph nodes associated with lymphocytic leukemia. Am J Pathol 4:285, 1928

149. Long JC, Aisenberg AC: Richter's syndrome. A terminal complication of chronic lymphocytic leukemia with distinct clinicopathologic features. Am J Clin Pathol 63:786, 1975

150. Armitage JO, Dick FR, Corder MP: Diffuse histocytic lymphoma complicating chronic lymphocytic leukemia. Cancer 41:422, 1978

151. Foucar K, Rydell RE: Richter's syndrome in chronic lymphocytic leukemia. Cancer 46:118, 1980

152. Sun NCJ, Fishkin BG, Nies KM, et al: Lymphoplasmacytic myeloma. An immunological, immunohistochemical and electron microscopic study. Cancer 43:2268, 1979

153. Choi YJ, Yeh G, Reiner L, et al: Immunoblastic sarcoma following Waldenstrom's macroglobulinemia. Am J Clin Pathol 71:121, 1979

154. Catovsky D: Hairy cell leukemia and prolymphocytic leukemia. Clin Haematol 6:245, 1977

155. Bearman RM, Pangalis GA, Rappaport H: Prolymphocytic leukemia. Clinical, histological and cytochemical observations. Cancer 42:2360, 1978

156. Catovsky D, Okos A, Wiltshar F, et al: Prolymphocytic leukemia of B and T cell type. Lancet 2:232, 1973

157. Sun NCJ: Hematology: An Atlas and Disgnostic Guide. p. 348. WB Saunders, Philadelphia, 1983

158. Yam LT, Li CY, Lam KW: Tartrate-resistant acid phosphatase isoenzyme in the reticulum cells of leukemic reticuloendotheliosis. N Engl J Med 284:357, 1971

159. Katayama I, Li CY, Yam LT: Ultrastructural characteristics of the "hairy cells" of leukemic reticuloendotheliosis. Am J Pathol 67:361, 1972

160. Burke JS: The value of the bone marrow biopsy in the diagnosis of hairy cell leukemia. Am J Clin Pathol 70:876, 1978

161. Vardiman JW, Colomb HM: Autopsy findings in hairy cell leukemia. Semin Oncol 11:370, 1984

162. Neiman RS, Sullivan AL, Jaffe R: Malignant lymphoma simulating leukemic reticuloendotheliosis. A clinicopathologic study of ten cases. Cancer 43:329, 1979

163. Palutke M, Tabaczka P, Mirchandani I, et al: Lymphocytic lymphoma simulating hairy cell leukemia: A consideration of reliable and unreliable diagnostic features. Cancer 48:2047, 1981

164. VanNorman AS, Nagorney DM, Martin K, et al: Splenectomy of hairy cell leukemia. A clinical review of 63 patients. Cancer 57:644, 1986

165. Quesada JR, Gutterman JU, Hersh EM: Treatment of hairy cell leukemia with alpha interferons. Cancer 57:1678, 1986

166. Lutzner M, Edelson R, Schein P, et al: Cutaneous T-cell lymphoma: The Sezary syndrome, mycosis fungoides, and related disorders. Ann Intern Med 83:534, 1975

167. Edelson RL, Lutzner MA, Kirkpatrick CH, et al: Morphologic and functional properties of the atypical T lymphocytes of the Sezary syndrome. Mayo Clin Proc 49:558, 1974

168. Blattner WA, Takatsuki K, Gallo RC: Human T-cell leukemia-lymphoma virus and adult T-cell leukemia. JAMA 250:1074, 1983

169. Uchiyama T, Yodoi J, Sagawa K, et al: Adult T-cell leukemia: Clinical and hematologic features of 16 cases. Blood 50:481, 1977

170. Catovsky D, Greaves MF, Rose M, et al: Adult T-cell lymphoma-leukaemia in blacks from the West Indies. Lancet 1:639, 1982

171. Blayney DW, Jaffe ES, Blattner WA, et al: The human T-cell leukemia/lymphoma virus associated with American adult T-cell leukemia/lymphoma. Blood 62:401, 1983

172. Broder S (moderator): T-cell lymphoproliferative syndrome associated with human T-cell leukemia/lymphoma virus. Ann Intern Med 100:543, 1984

173. Kawano F, Yamaguchi K, Nishimura H, et al: Variation in the clinical courses of adult T-cell leukemia. Cancer 55:851, 1985

174. Knowles DM II: The human T-cell leukemias: Clinical, cytomorphologic, immunophenotypic, and genotypic characteristics. Hum Pathol 17:14, 1986

175. Stein RS, Ultmann JE, Byrne GE Jr, et al: Bone marrow involvement in non-Hodgkin's lymphoma. Implications for staging and therapy. Cancer 37:629, 1976

176. Brunning RD: Bone marrow and peripheral blood involvement in non-Hodgkin's lymphomas. Geriatrics 30:75, 1975

177. Chabner BA, Fisher RI, Young RC, et al: Staging of non-Hodgkin's lymphoma. Semin Oncol 7:285, 1980

178. Bartl R, Frisch B, Burkhardt R, et al: Assessment of bone marrow histology in the malignant lymphomas (non-Hodgkin's): Correlation with clinical factors for diagnosis, prognosis, classification and staging. Br J Haematol 51:511, 1982

179. Rosenberg SA, Dorfman RF, Kaplan HS: The value of sequential bone marrow biopsy and laparotomy and splenectomy in a series of 127 consecutive untreated patients with non-Hodgkin's lymphoma. Br J Cancer 31:suppl 2, 221, 1975

180. Viniciguerra V, Silver RT: The importance of bone marrow biopsy in the staging of patients with lymphosarcoma. Blood 41:913, 1973

181. Foucar K, McKenna RW, Frizzera G, et al: Incidence and patterns of bone marrow and blood involvement by lymphoma in relationship to the Lukes-Collins classifications. Blood 54:1417, 1979

182. Kyle RA: Multiple myeloma. Review of 869 cases. Mayo Clin Proc 50:29, 1975

183. Sun NCJ: Hematology: An Atlas and Diagnostic Guide. p. 259. WB Saunders, Philadelphia, 1983

184. Carter A, Hocherman I, Linn S, et al: Prognostic significance of plasma cell morphology in multiple myeloma. Cancer 60:1060, 1987

185. Bartl R, Frisch B, Fateh-Moghadam A, et al: Histologic classification and staging of multiple myeloma. A retrospective and prospective study of 674 cases. Am J Clin Pathol 87:342, 1987

186. Wolf BC, Kumar A, Vera JC, et al: Bone marrow morphology and immunology in systemic amyloidosis. Am J Clin Pathol 86:84, 1986

187. Bloch KJ, Lee L, Mills JA, et al: Gamma heavy chain disease—expanding clinical and laboratory spectrum. Am J Med 55:61, 1973

188. Seligmann M: Immunochemical, clinical and pathological features of α-chain disease. Arch Intern Med 135:78, 1975

189. Franklin EC: Mu-chain disease. Arch Intern Med 135:71, 1975

190. Sun NCJ: Hematology: An Atlas and Diagnostic Guide. p. 398. WB Saunders, Philadelphia, 1983

191. Choe JK, Hyun BH, Salazar GH, et al: Epithelioid granulomas of the bone marrow in non-Hodgkin's lymphoproliferative malignancies. Am J Clin Pathol 80:19, 1983

192. Jagadha V, Andavolu RH, Huang CT: Granulomatous inflammation in the acquired immune deficiency syndrome. Am J Clin Pathol 84:598, 1985

193. Bodem CR, Hamory BH, Taylor HM, et al: Granulomatous bone marrow disease. A review of the literature and clinicopathologic analysis of 58 cases. Medicine (Baltimore) 62:372, 1983

194. Okun DB, Sun NCJ, Tanaka KR: Bone marrow granulomas in Q fever. Am J Clin Pathol 71:117, 1979

195. Coffin J, Haase A, Levy JA, et al: Human immunodeficiency viruses (letter). Science 232:697, 1986

196. Barr-Sinoussi F, Chermann JC, Rey F, et al: Isolation of a T-lymphotropic retrovirus from a patient at risk for acquired immunodeficiency syndrome (AIDS). Science 220:868, 1983

197. Gallo RC, Salahuddin SZ, Popovic M, et al: Frequent detection and isolation of cytopathic retroviruses (HTLV-III) from patients with AIDS and at risk for AIDS. Science 224:500, 1984

198. Levy JA, Hoffman AD, Kramer SM et al: Isolation of lymphocytopathic retroviruses from San Francisco patients with AIDS. Science 225:840, 1984

199. Sarngadharan MG, Popvic M, Bruch L, et al: Antibodies reactive with human T-lymphotropic retroviruses (HTLV-III) in the serum of patients with AIDS. Science, 224:506, 1984

200. Centers for Disease Control: Antibodies to a retrovirus

etiologically associated with acquired immunodeficiency syndrome (AIDS) in populations with increased incidences of the syndrome. MMWR 33:377, 1984

201. Centers for Disease Control: Classification system for human T-lymphotropic virus type III/lymphadenopathy-associated virus infections. MMWR 35:334, 1986

202. Farhi DC, Mason UG III, Horsburgh CR: The bone marrow in disseminated *Mycobacterium avium-intracellulare* infection. Am J Clin Pathol 83:463, 1985

203. Castella A, Croxson TS, Mildvan D, et al: The bone marrow in AIDS: A histologic, hematologic, and microbiologic study. Am J Clin Pathol 84:425, 1985

204. Greene JB, Sidhu GS, Lewin S, et al: *Mycobacterium avium-intracellulare:* A cause of disseminated life-threatening infection in homosexuals and drug abusers. Ann Intern Med 97:539, 1982

205. Abrams DI, Chinn EK, Lewis BJ, et al: Hematologic manifestations in homosexual men with Kaposi's sarcoma. Am J Clin Pathol 81:13, 1984

206. Sun NCJ, Leung L, Lachant N, et al: Hematologic abnormalities in patients with acquired immune deficiency syndrome (AIDS). Blood 62:suppl. 1, 117a, 1983

207. Walsh C, Krigel R, Lennett E, et al: Thrombocytopenia in homosexual patients: Prognosis, response to therapy, and prevalence of antibody to the retrovirus associated with the acquired immunodeficiency syndrome. Ann Intern Med 103:542, 1985

208. Rywlin AM, Ortega R: Lipid granulomas of the bone marrow. Am J Clin Pathol 57:457, 1972

209. Kaplan HS: Hodgkin's disease: Biology, treatment, prognosis (review). Blood 57:813, 1981

210. Hsu S-M, Yang K, Jaffe ES: Phenotypic expression of Hodgkin's and Reed-Sternberg cells in Hodgkin's disease. Am J Pathol 118:209, 1985

211. Webb DI, Urogy G, Silver RT: Importance of bone marrow biopsy in the clinical staging of Hodgkin's disease. Cancer 26:313, 1970

212. Rosenberg SA: Hodgkin's disease of the bone marrow. Cancer Res 31:1733, 1971

213. Myers CE, Chabner BA, De Vita VT, et al: Bone marrow involvement in Hodgkin's disease: Pathology and response to MOPP chemotherapy. Blood 44:197, 1974

214. Bartl R, Frisch B, Burkhardt R, et al: Assessment of bone marrow histology in Hodgkin's disease. Correlation with clinical factors. Br J Haematol 51:345, 1982

215. Kinney NC, Greer JP, Stein RS, et al: Lymphocyte-depletion Hodgkin's disease. Histopathologic diagnosis of marrow involvement. Am J Surg Pathol 10:219, 1986

216. Bearman RM, Pangalis GA, Rappaport H: Hodgkin's disease, lymphocytic depletion type. A clinicopathologic study of 39 patients. Cancer 41:293, 1978

217. Neiman RS, Rosen PJ, Lukes RJ: Lymphocyte depletion Hodgkin's disease: A clinicopathologic entity. N Engl J Med 288, 1973

218. Lukes RJ: Criteria for involvement of lymph node, bone marrow, spleen and liver in Hodgkin's disease. Cancer Res 31:1755, 1971

219. Rappaport H, Berard CW, Butler JJ, et al: Report of the committee on histopathological criteria contributing to staging of Hodgkin's disease. Cancer Res 31:1864, 1971

220. Kadin ME, Donaldson SS, Dorfman RF: Isolated granulomas in Hodgkin's disease. N Engl J Med 283:859, 1970

221. Sacks EL, Donaldson SS, Gordon J, et al: Epithelioid granulomas associated with Hodgkin's disease. Cancer 41:562, 1978

222. Lukes RJ, Tindle BH: Immunoblastic lymphadenopathy. A hyperimmune entity resembling Hodgkin's disease. N Engl J Med 292:1, 1975

223. Frizzera G, Moran EM, Rappaport H: Angioimmunoblastic lymphadenopathy: Diagnosis and clinical course. Am J Med 59:803, 1975

224. Neiman RS, Dervan P, Haudenschild C, et al: Angioimmunoblsatic lymphadenopathy: An ultrastructural and immunologic study with review of the literature. Cancer 41:507, 1978

225. Pangalis GA, Moran EM, Rappaport H: Blood and bone marrow findings in angioimmunoblastic lymphadenopathy. Blood 51:71, 1978

226. Lennert K, Mestdagh J: Lymphogranulomatosen mit konstant hohem Epitheloidzellgehalt. Virchows Arch [Pathol Anat] 344:1, 1968

227. Lukes RJ, Parker JW, Taylor CR, et al: Immunologic approach to non-Hodgkin lymphomas and related leukemias. Analysis of the results of multiparameter studies of 424 cases. Semin Hematol 15:322, 1978

228. Burke JS, Butler JJ: Malignant lymphoma with a high content of epithelioid histiocytes (Lennert's lymphoma). Am J Clin Pathol 66:1, 1976

229. Kim H, Jacobs C, Warnke RA, et al: Malignant lymphoma with a high content of epithelioid histiocytes. A distinct clinicopathologic entity and a form of so-called "Lennert's lymphoma." Cancer 41:620, 1978

230. Lennert K, Mohri N, Stein H, et al: The histopathology of malignant lymphoma. Br J Haematol [Suppl] 31:193, 1975

231. Neiman RS: Immunoblastic sarcoma. Am J Surg Pathol 6:755, 1982

232. Schneider DR, Taylor CR, Parker JW, et al: Immunoblastic sarcoma of T- and B-cell types: Morphologic description and comparison. Hum Pathol 16:885, 1985

233. Waldron JA, Leech JH, Glick AD, et al: Malignant lymphoma of peripheral T-lymphocyte origin. Cancer 40:1604, 1977

234. Levine AM, Taylor CR, Schneider DR, et al: Immunoblastic sarcoma of T-cell versus B-cell origin: I. Clinical features. Blood 58:52, 1981

235. Hanson CA, Brunning RD, Gajl-Peczalska KJ, et al: Bone marrow manifestations of peripheral T-cell lymphoma. A study of 30 cases. Am J Clin Pathol 86:449, 1986

236. Rywlin AM, Hoffman EP, Ortega RS: Eosinophilic fibrohistiocytic lesion of bone marrow: A distinct new morphologic finding, probably related to drug hypersensitivity. Blood 40:464, 1972

237. Te Velde J, Vismans FJFE, Leenheers-Binnendijk L, et al: The eosinophilic fibrohistiocytic lesion of the bone marrow: A mastocellular lesion in bone disease. Virchows Arch [Pathol Anat] 377:277, 1978

238. Cryer PE, Kissane JM: Clinicopathologic conference: Systemic mastocytosis. Am J Med 61:671, 1976

239. Lennert K, Parwaresch MR: Mast cells and mast cell neoplasia: A review. Histopathology 3:349, 1979

240. Travis WD, Li C-Y, Hoagland HC, et al: Mast cell leukemia: Report of a case and review of the literature. Mayo Clin Proc 61:957, 1986

241. Yam LT, Yam CF, Li C-Y: Eosinophilia in systemic mastocytosis. J Clin Pathol 73:48, 1980

242. Sun NCJ: Hematology: An Atlas and Diagnostic Guide. WB Saunders, Philadelphia, 1983

243. Sawitsky A, Rosner F, Chodsky S: The sea-blue histiocyte syndrome, a review: Genetic and biochemical studies. Semin Hematol 9:285, 1972

244. Dosik H, Rosner F, Sawitsky A: Acquired lipidosis: Gaucher-like cells and "blue cells" in chronic granulocytic leukemia. Semin Hematol 9:309, 1972

245. Muller-Hermelink H-K, Lennert K: The cytologic, histologic, and functional bases for a modern classification of lymphomas. p. 52. In Lennert K, Stein H, Mohri N, et al (eds): Malignant Lymphomas Other Than Hodgkin's Disease. Histology, Cytology, Ultrastructure, Immunology. Springer-Verlag, New York, 1978

246. Turner RR, Colby TV, Wood GS, et al: Histocytic malignancies. Morphologic, immunologic, and enzyme heterogeneity. Am J Surg Pathol 8:485, 1984

247. Risdall RJ, McKenna RW, Nesbit ME, et al: Virus-associated hemophagocytic syndrome: A benign histiocytic proliferation distinct from malignant histiocytosis. Cancer 44:993, 1979

248. Mroczek EC, Weisenburger DD, Grierson L, et al: Fatal infectious mononucleosis and virus-associated hemophagocytic syndrome. Arch Pathol Lab Med 111:530, 1987

249. Campo E, Condom E, Miro M-J, et al: Tuberculosis-associated hemophagocytic syndrome. A systemic process. Cancer 58:2640, 1986

250. Wieczorek R, Greco MA, McCarthy K, et al: Familial erythrophagocytic lymphohistiocytosis: Immunophenotypic, immunohistochemical, and ultrastructural demonstration of the relation to sinus histiocytes. Hum Pathol 17:55, 1986

251. James JP, Stass SS, Peterson V, et al: Abnormalities of bone marrow simulating histiocytic medullary reticulosis in a patient with gastric carcinomas. Am J Clin Pathol 71:600, 1979

252. Monoharan A, Catovsky D, Lampert I, et al: Histiocytic medullary reticulosis complicating chronic lymphocytic leukemia: Malignant or reactive: Scand J Haematol 26:5, 1981

253. Walker PD, Rosai J, Dorfman RF: The osseous manifestations of sinus histiocytosis with massive lymphadenopathy. Am J Clin Pathol 75:131, 1981

254. Scott RB, Robb-Smith AHT: Histiocytic medullary reticulosis. Lancet 2:194, 1939

255. Rappaport H: Tumors of the hematopoietic system. p. 49. In Atlas of Tumor Pathology, Section III. Fasc. 8. Armed Forces Institute of Pathology, Washington, 1966

256. Ducatman BS, Wick MR, Morgan TW, et al: Malignant histiocytosis: A clinical, histologic, and immunohistochemical study of 20 cases. Hum Pathol 15:368, 1984

257. Byrne GE, Rappaport H: Malignant histiocytosis. Gann Monogr 15:145, 1973

258. Robb-Smith AHT, Taylor CR: Lymph Node Biopsy. p. 137. Oxford University Press, New York, 1981

259. Lichentein L: Histiocytosis X: Integration of eosinophilic granuloma of bone marrow. Letterer-Siwe disease and Schüller-Christian disease as related manifestations of a single nosologic entity. Arch Pathol 56:84, 1953

260. Lieberman PH, Jones CR, Dargeon HWK, et al: A reappraisal of eosinophilic granuloma of bone, Hand-Schüller-Christian syndrome and Letterer-Siwe syndrome. Medicine (Baltimore) 48:375, 1969

261. Vogel JM, Vogel P: Idiopathic histiocytosis: A discussion of eosinophilic granuloma, the Hand-Schüller-Christian syndrome, and the Letterer-Siwe syndrome. Semin Hematol 9:349, 1972

262. Daneshbod K, Kissane JM: Idiopathic differentiated histiocytosis. Am J Clin Pathol 70:381, 1978

263. Pittman G, Tung KSK, Hoffman GC: Metastatic cells in bone marrow: study of 83 cases. Cleve Clin Q 38:55, 1971

264. Contreras E, Ellis LD, Lee RE: Value of the bone marrow biopsy in the diagnosis of metastatic carcinoma. Cancer 29:778, 1972

265. Anner RM, Drewinko B: Frequency and significance of bone marrow involvement by metastatic solid tumors. Cancer 39:1337, 1977

266. Leland J, MacPherson B: Hematologic findings in cases of mammary cancer metastatic to bone marrow. Am J Clin Pathol 71:31, 1979

267. Sun NCJ: Hematology: An Atlas and Diagnostic Guide. p. 158. WB Saunders, Philadelphia, 1983

268. Bearden JD, Ratkin GA, Coltman CA: Comparison of the diagnostic value of bone marrow biopsy and bone marrow aspiration in neoplastic disease. J Clin Pathol 27:738, 1974

269. Kiraly JF, III, Wheby MS: bone marrow necrosis. Am J Med 60:361, 1976

270. Norgard MJ, Carpenter JT, Conrad ME: Bone marrow necrosis and degeneration. Ann Intern Med 139:905, 1979

271. Brown CH: Bone marrow necrosis in a study of seventy cases. Johns Hopkins Med J 131:189, 1972

272. Engel IA, Straus DJ, Lacher M, et al: Osteonecrosis in patients with malignant lymphoma: a review of twenty-five cases. Cancer 48:1245, 1981

273. Conran RM, Granger E, Reddy VB: Kaposi's sarcoma of the bone marrow. Arch Pathol Lab Med 110:1083, 1986

274. Krause JR: Value of bone marrow biopsy in the diagnosis of amyloidosis. South Med J 70:1072, 1977

275. Kwaan HC: Clinicopathologic features of thrombotic thrombocytopenic purpura. Semin Hematol 24:71, 1987

276. Pierce JR, Wren MV, Cousar JB: Cholesterol embolism: Diagnosis antemortem by bone marrow biopsy. Ann Intern Med 89:937, 1978

14

Non-neoplastic Diseases of Bones and Joints

Peter G. Bullough

This chapter will discuss both the special problems that relate to the interpretation of bone lesions and, briefly, the more common orthopaedic diseases that may come across the surgical pathologist's desk.

METHODS OF EXAMINATION

A major problem in dealing with bone specimens is the preparation of reasonable histologic sections. In many laboratories is bone tissue either overdecalcified or the acid is inadequately removed; in both cases poor staining results. In our laboratory, after sectioning of the bone into slices 3 to 5 mm thick and adequate fixation with buffered formalin, decalcification is achieved with 5 percent nitric acid. The volume of acid should be at least 10 times that of the tissue, and since the acid is neutralized as the calcium is removed from the tissue, the acid must be changed twice a day. To ensure access of the acid to the tissue, gentle agitation is provided by means of a shaker. By using this technique, most bones are decalcified in 1 or 2 days. After decalcification adequate washing is essential; otherwise good differentiation of the hematoxylin and eosin (H&E) stain is not possible. We have found that better sections of bone are obtained after vacuum embedding. This is very simply arranged and well worth the effort involved.

Gross

Bone specimens received by the surgical pathologist often consist only of fragments, the anatomic site of which cannot be recognized. On the other hand, when a larger piece of bone is submitted, anatomic landmarks should be carefully sought. Large specimens should be cut into parallel slices 4 or 5 mm thick with a band saw, so the interior appearance of the bone may be examined.

On occasion, the color of the bone may be particularly helpful; for example, necrotic bone is an opaque yellow, in contrast to the rather translucent and pink appearance of living bone. A generalized or localized increase in porosity or sclerosis should be sought. When multiple pieces are received, the pieces chosen for embedding should be preferably those that appear to show the most departure from normal.

A particularly useful adjunct to gross examination is the preparation of radiographs of the surgical specimens with low-voltage x-rays (Faxitron x-ray machine) and industrial film (Kodalith Ortho film, type 3). These radiographs not only help in choosing the areas to section but also are frequently helpful in the interpretation of histologic material, for example, in bone-forming tumors, finding a nidus in osteoid osteoma, or defining an infarct (Fig. 14-1). Because bone and cartilage are somewhat translucent, it is frequently difficult to get acceptable black and white photographs. This problem can be overcome by using a monochromatic short wave light source, such as ultraviolet.[1]

Microscopic

The histologist uses various staining techniques to demonstrate the components of the matrix.

The collagen may be demonstrated by a trichrome stain or van Gieson's stain and also by the use of polarized light. This latter technique is particularly useful because

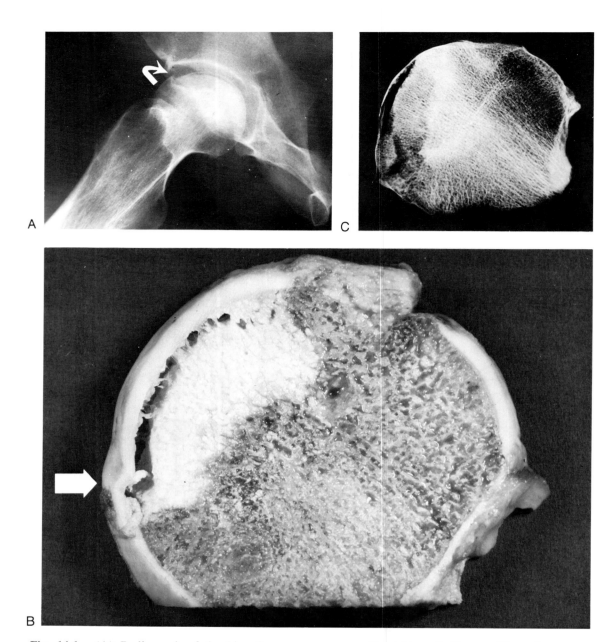

Fig. 14-1. **(A)** Radiograph of the hip of a young person with sickle cell disease. There is segmental infarction of the superior portion of the femoral head recognized radiologically by the presence of a small step-fracture at the lateral margin of the femoral head (arrow) and a radiolucent crescent on the superior surface of the femoral head just beneath the articular surface. **(B)** Photograph of the femoral head resected in this case. The infarcted area is clearly differentiated from the surrounding bone by its opaque yellowish white appearance. At the margin of the infarct there is hyperemia, and the subchondral crescent is seen as a defect beneath the articular cartilage. At the margin of the infarct a fracture through the articular surface with wrinkling of the articular cartilage is clearly seen (arrow). **(C)** A radiograph of the specimen shown in Fig. B demonstrates that the margin of the infarct is sclerotic. This sclerosis is the result of reparative bone formation. (See also Figs. 14-9, 14-10.)

it not only clearly shows the collagen fibers but also allows us to determine the orientation of the collagen and to study the microarchitecture of the tissue.[2,3]

The proteoglycans can be demonstrated by the use of safranin O or alcian blue stains and less specifically by toluidine blue and periodic acid–Schiff (PAS) stains.[4]

Mineral components can only be demonstrated in undemineralized tissue. It is possible, by embedding the tissue in plastic and using specially hardened knives, to cut histologic sections that still contain the minerals within the bone matrix. The mineral may be stained by two techniques: alizarin red, which will stain the calcium components of the hydroxyapatite, and the von Kossa method, which will stain the phosphate component. The distribution of mineral in the tissue may also be studied by the technique of microradiology.[5] By using low-kilovoltage x-rays from an x-ray tube with a very fine focal spot, radiographs are made from thin slices of bone, which have been cut with a diamond saw at approximately 100 μm. Undecalcified sections are particularly important in the assessment of metabolic disturbances.

An essential component in interpretation of bone and joint histology is careful correlation with the clinical radiographs and history.

BONES AND BONE TISSUE

Bones

Bone structure[6,7] may be briefly summarized as follows. Each bone has a delimiting shell or cortex, which varies in thickness from bone to bone and from area to area within a given bone. The interior of a bone is occupied by a varying amount of porous, cancellous bone tissue. The proportion of cortical to cancellous bone reflects the mechanical requirements of the bone as a whole. In the spaces between the plates and rods of cancellous bone are blood vessels, nerve fibers, fat, and hematopoietic tissue. In the adult most of the hematopoietic tissue is confined to the axial skeleton (spine, pelvis, and shoulder girdles). However, occasionally hematopoietic tissue may be seen in the femoral head or humeral head. On the other hand, in the infant the entire skeleton contains hematopoietic tissue. During growth the hematopoietic tissue in the appendicular skeleton (arms and legs) is slowly replaced by fat advancing proximally until the adult state is reached.

Except for the insertion of the tendons and the articular ends of the bone, the cortex is covered by a thin layer of dense fibrous tissue, the periosteum. The periosteal layer adjacent to the bone, the cambium layer, has bone-forming potential. This potential becomes apparent after trauma and infection and in association with certain tumors. In the child the periosteum is only loosely attached to the underlying bone, whereas in the adult it is firmly attached; this accounts for the more extensive periosteal reaction seen in children as compared with adults.

The terms epiphysis, metaphysis, and diaphysis are used to designate regions of bones. The epiphysis is the portion of the bone that lies between the joint and the site of the growth plate; the metaphysis is the region of bone adjacent to the growing side of the growth plate; and the diaphysis is the portion of the bone between the growth plates.

Bone Tissue

In studying and interpreting bone connective tissues,[8,9] it is important to realize that unlike parenchymal organs, the bulk of which is formed of cells, the bulk of connective tissue is made up largely of an extracellular matrix, and the cells represent only a small percentage of the tissue bulk. Bone, cartilage, and fibrous connective tissues differ not only grossly and microscopically but also in their mechanical properties. This variation reflects the variable composition of their extracellular matrices; for example, tendons, whose function is to resist tension, are formed mainly of well oriented parallel bundles of collagen. On the other hand, cartilage and bone, which are subject to compression, have in addition to collagen either large molecules of proteoglycan (cartilage) or hydroxyapatite crystals (bone). These substances, restrained by the collagen running between them, resist compressive forces and provide rigidity to the tissue.

Microscopic examination reveals two possible appearances of bone tissue:

In lamellar bone, the type found in normal individuals, the collagen is in sheets of parallel fibers, stacked one upon another, giving rise in cross section to a striped appearance, which can be heightened by polarized light. The bone cells (osteocytes) are widely separated from each other, and the osteocytic lacunae are flattened (Fig. 14-2).

In the fetus and in conditions in which the metabolism of the skeleton is accelerated, such as fracture repair, periosteal reactions, parathyroid dysfunction, and tumors, the collagen is arranged haphazardly, again made more apparent by examination with polarized light. The osteocytes are more closely packed together, and the lacunae are larger and rounder than those seen in lamellar bone. This type of bone is called woven bone, fiber bone, or immature bone (Fig. 14-3). (It is incorrect to refer to this type of bone as *osteoid*, as is often done.)

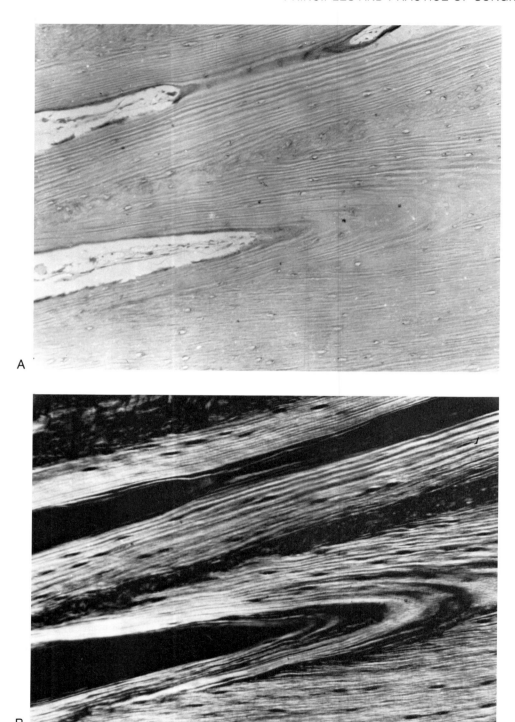

Fig. 14-2. **(A)** Photomicrograph of lamellar bone. Note the distribution of the osteocytes in the orientation of the lamellae. **(B)** The same field as that illustrated in Fig. A but examined under polarized light. (Fig. 14-2 continues.)

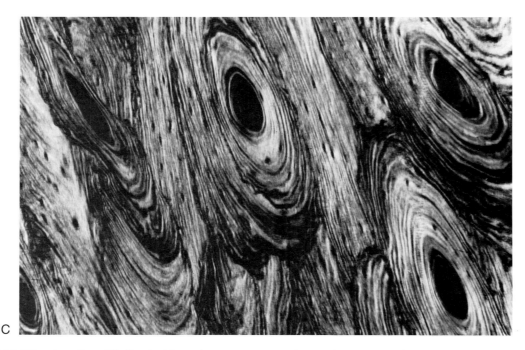

Fig. 14-2 (*Continued*).   (**C**) Cortical bone in transverse section to demonstrate the osteons. Polarized light microscopy.

Recognition of these two types of bone tissue is very important to the surgical pathologist in the interpretation of bone disease.

Bone Cells

The skeleton is not merely an inanimate structure serving a mechanical need—it is composed of living, constantly changing tissue involved in mineral homeostasis

and with the capability of growth and repair. These processes are effected through the bone cells, which include the osteoblasts, the osteocytes, and the osteoclasts.[8,9]

Osteoblasts

Osteoblasts are the cells responsible for the synthesis of bone matrix. They form a continuous covering over the bone tissue, and at any particular time they may be either actively forming bone or inactive. The active cells

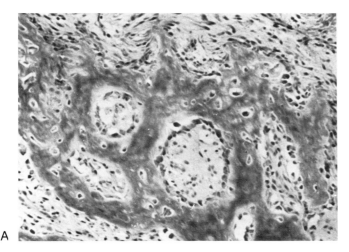
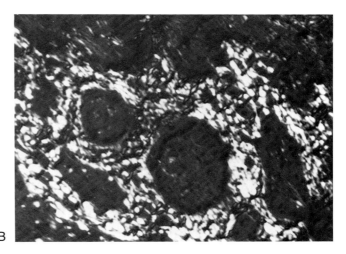

Fig. 14-3. Photomicrograph of a section taken from fracture callus to demonstrate the appearance of woven bone. Note the irregularity of the bone trabeculae that are being formed, the prominent osteoblasts and osteocytes, and the collagen fibers arranged in a basket-weave pattern. (**A**) Transmitted light. (**B**) Polarized light. (H&E)

are plump and crowded along the bone surface, whereas inactive osteoblasts are flat and inconspicuous. In those areas where bone is actively being made, the cells lie on a thin, smooth layer of unmineralized bone matrix called osteoid. The junction between the mineralized bone and the unmineralized osteoid at the surface is often marked in H&E-stained sections by a basophilic line indicating the mineralization front.

Osteocytes

Osteoblasts, when incorporated into the bone after the process of matrix formation, are called *osteocytes*. The osteocytes are connected with one another and also with the surface of the bone by an intricate network of canals, the *osteocytic canaliculi*. Through these canaliculi cytoplasmic processes extend from osteocyte to osteocyte and also to the osteoblasts on the surface, making tight junctions with one another. The elaborate structure of the osteocytic network strongly suggests a metabolic function, probably for mineral homeostasis.

Osteoclasts

Those portions of the bone surface undergoing resorption have an irregular, gnawed-out appearance. Covering this irregular surface are mononuclear and sometimes multinucleate osteoclasts. By electron microscopy these cells are seen to have ruffled borders on the surface facing the bone, numerous cytoplasmic vesicles, lysosomal bodies, and mitochondria, but unlike osteoblasts, little endoplasmic reticulum. In sections of normal bone, multinucleate osteoclasts are rarely seen, although irregular resorbing surfaces are apparent over about 7 to 20 percent of the total bone surface. The absence of multinucleate osteoclasts from normal bone may simply reflect the fact that giant cells are obvious only when resorption is proceeding at an extraordinary or pathologic rate.

Bone Physiology

As already indicated, the bones have two quite different basic functions: (1) mechanical, providing for movement and protection, and (2) maintenance of the "milieu intérieur," especially with respect to plasma calcium, phosphorus, and magnesium. As a consequence, the bone and bone tissue are a compromise in both form and structure.

The formation and resorption of bone continue throughout life, and in normal bone these processes are more or less in balance. Microscopic examination will often show one surface of a trabeculum to be smooth with

a layer of active osteoblasts, while the other shows irregular resorption (Fig. 14-4). In this way, spatial reorganization of the cancellous and cortical bone to accommodate the mechanical requirements is constantly taking place. Resorbing surfaces that have become inactive later become the site for active bone deposition, and evidence of this process is seen in the form of cement lines (reversal lines), dense basophilic lines separating distinct areas of bone matrix. The chemical composition of the cement line is not known, but examination by polarized light will show that no collagen fibers cross it.[10] In processes in which there is accelerated remodeling of bone (e.g., Paget's disease), the cement lines may become very prominent (Fig. 14-5).

The density of the bone in healthy people depends on several factors, including race, sex, and occupation. On the whole, blacks have heavier and denser bones than whites, men have denser bones than women, and manual workers have denser bones than sedentary workers. With advancing age, there is a steady loss of bone tissue, which occurs in everyone but is more likely to give rise to clinical problems (e.g., osteoporosis) in a white woman than in a black man, because the white woman starts with so much less bone.[11] (*Osteoporosis* is a clinical term, which indicates an absolute loss of bone tissue sufficient to lead to fracture, whereas *osteopenia* indicates a decrease in bone mass and is often used by radiologists to indicate a decrease in radiodensity on rad. While such a decrease in radiodensity may be due to osteoporosis, it may also result from a decrease in the

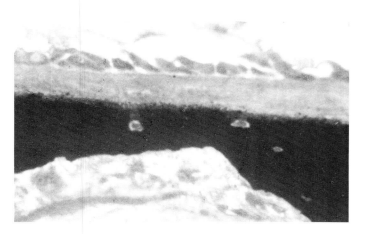

Fig. 14-4. Photomicrograph of an individual trabeculum from a patient with a metabolic disturbance, showing on the upper surface bone formation with active osteoblasts and on the lower surface the irregular gnawed-out appearance of resorption. This section of undecalcified bone was stained by the von Kossa stain. Mineralized bone is black, whereas the unmineralized osteoid is a smooth gray zone between the osteoblastic cell layer on the surface and the fully mineralized bone beneath.

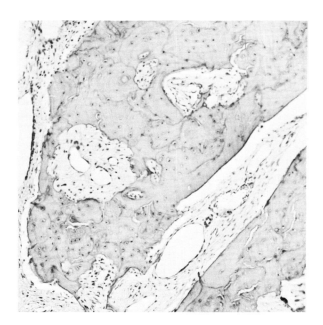

Fig. 14-5. Photomicrograph of a section taken from pagetoid bone. The cement lines are seen as irregular wavy gray lines coursing through the matrix of the bone. In many areas clefts are seen in the region of these lines. These clefts represent a cracking artifact at the time of sectioning. They indicate the ease with which this bone will fracture. The marrow spaces are fibrotic, and large dilated vessels are present.

amount of mineralized bone tissue, as in rickets or osteomalacia.)

Skeletal Development

Developmental disease is rarely seen by the surgical pathologist, with the exception of certain hamartomatous malformations, such as bone islands or fibrous dysplasia, and developmental aberrations, such as the common osteochondroma, all of which are described in Chapter 15. However, the surgical pathologist should know the basics of bone growth and development since they are helpful to the understanding of bone disease in general.

The majority of bones are preformed in a cartilage model, which, in the course of development, undergoes calcification followed by vascular invasion and the laying down of osseous tissue on the remnants of calcified cartilage matrix. This process is known as *endochondral ossification.* The viable cartilage continues to grow and subsequently calcifies, thus providing for the growth of the skeletal elements. During most of childhood the principal source of cartilage growth and subsequent endochondral ossification is found in the growth plate. Disturbances in cell maturation in the growth plate, such as those that

occur in achondroplasia and may also occur in hormonal disturbances such as hypothyroidism or hypopituitarism, result in decreased cartilage proliferation and decreased endochondral ossification, the ultimate effect being dwarfing of the child. Hyperpituitarism results in giantism and in adult acromegaly because of stimulation of cartilage growth and subsequently increased endochondral ossification. (Interpretation of the changes in the growth plate require familiarity with the appearance of the normal growth plate at the various stages of growth up to adolescence, and such considerations are outside the scope of the chapter.)

The bone that is first laid down on the calcified cartilage is referred to as the primary spongiosa (Fig. 14-6). This mixture of bone and calcified cartilage is remodeled by osteoclastic activity and eventually the bone trabeculae are formed only of bone tissue, referred to as the secondary spongiosa. A rare disease results from a failure of the normal remodeling of primary to secondary spongiosa. In this condition, osteopetrosis,[12] most of the skeletal tissue is formed of primary spongiosa. This bone is extremely dense, and pieces of bone from osteopetrotic subjects will be found to be unduly heavy and difficult to decalcify and section (Fig. 14-7).

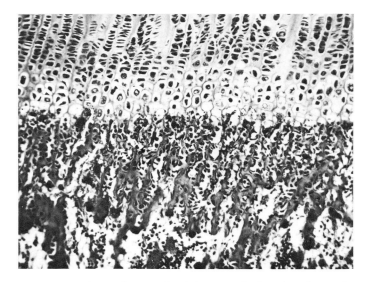

Fig. 14-6. Photomicrograph of the growth plate in a 2-month-old pig. In the upper part of the photograph one can see the columnar arrangement of the hypertrophic zone of the growth plate, which then goes into the degenerative and calcified zone of the growth plate. The calcified zone is invaded by capillaries, which deposit the first bone onto the surface of calcified cartilage matrix. The bone trabeculae of the metaphysis are therefore characterized by a central core of calcified cartilage and a thin layer of bone matrix on the surface. This bone is called the *primary spongiosa.*

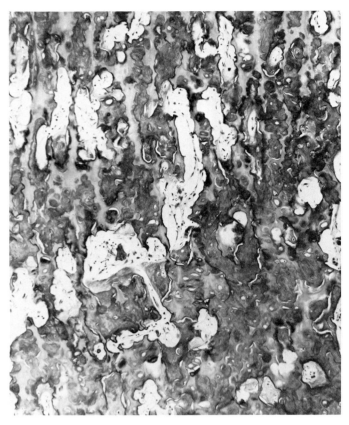

Fig. 14-7. Photomicrograph of a section of the cancellous bone from a patient with osteopetrosis. Note the increased amount of bone, the loss of the normal trabecular architecture, and the residual calcified cartilage within the bone. In this condition the osteoclasts, though present, do not appear to resorb the bone.

SKELETAL DISEASE

The clinical symptoms of disease in the skeletal tissues, whether we are speaking of bones or joints, are most likely to result from mechanical failure.

Fracture Healing

A broken bone results from either a violent force or significant weakening (pathologic fracture). The latter may occur because of either a localized replacement by tumor or a generalized disturbance (e.g., senile osteoporosis, osteomalacia, Paget's disease, osteogenesis imperfecta).

The reparative response[13] depends on the site of injury and the bone involved; in general, it corresponds to the richness of the vascular bed. For example, a fracture

through the midshaft of the tibia in a poorly vascularized area is notorious for both delayed healing and nonunion.[14]

A fracture inevitably results in some degree of necrosis. We tend to speak of bone necrosis, but remember, only cells can necrose. The extracellular matrix is nonviable to begin with. In favorable circumstances, the necrosis of the cellular elements (i.e., bone cells and bone marrow cells) extends for only a short distance on each side of the fracture line, but, depending on local factors, large fragments may become necrotic and significantly interfere with the healing process. In the process of bone healing the necrotic bone will be resorbed by osteoclasts.

The periosteum is an extremely important source of repair tissue (callus) following fracture. At the time of the initial injury the periosteum may be elevated from the underlying bone by hemorrhage, and the osteogenic cells of the cambium layer may rapidly become activated and begin to lay down woven bone. This immature subperiosteal bone eventually bridges the fracture site and renders the fractured bone stable. In the medullary cavity, the osteoblasts lining the trabeculae on either side of the fracture site also become very active and lay down new bone on the existing bone trabeculae.

In the face of extensive soft tissue damage, a large amount of callus may be seen in the surrounding soft tissues. This takes the form of irregular trabeculae of *woven bone,* and in fractures that are particularly unstable, this extraosseous callus may be quite immature and contain a high proportion of cellular cartilage, giving rise to a pseudosarcomatous appearance (Fig. 14-8).

After stabilization of the fracture, remodeling takes place, with restoration to an anatomic state similar to that present before fracture. Stabilization of the fracture usually takes place in 4 to 8 weeks, but anatomic restitution takes many months or even years. Since the callus serves to immobilize the fracture, it should be obvious that the amount of callus is in general proportional to the stability of the fracture, and therefore, in a fracture that has been immobilized surgically by internal fixation, little or no callus may form.

It is important for the surgical pathologist to know that fracture can occur in a bone without the patient being aware of it. These fractures classically occur in healthy young athletic adults and are termed *stress fractures;* they are common in the metatarsals and tibia. In such a case the patient may complain of pain and swelling over a bone, and radiographs may show localized exuberant new bone. Biopsy will show a very proliferative osseous and cartilaginous tissue, which because of its deranged pattern and cellularity may be mistaken for osteogenic sarcoma (Fig. 14-8). Obviously, this is a most important differential diagnosis and requires careful correlation of the clinical history, radiographs, and pathologic findings.

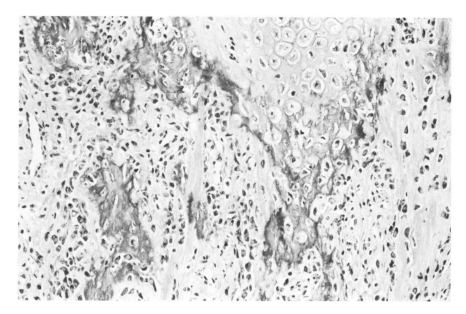

Fig. 14-8. Photomicrograph of a section taken from a fracture approximately 10 days old. The irregularity of the bone and cartilage being formed, together with the crowded and varying appearance of the stromal cells, imparts a pseudosarcomatous appearance.

Bone Infarction (Osteonecrosis)

Localized bone and bone marrow death (osteonecrosis)[15] is a common complication of osteomyelitis and conditions in which the bone marrow is replaced by massive cellular infiltrates, such as Gaucher's disease, lymphoma, or primary or metastatic tumor. Osteonecrosis may also occur as a result of the "bends" in deep sea divers or hemoglobinopathies such as sickle cell disease and is frequently seen in association with cortisone therapy and alcoholism. In clinical practice, osteonecrosis is most commonly seen in the juxta-articular area, usually the hip, and gives rise to articular symptoms, as will be described below.

Grossly, dead bone is generally yellow and chalky in appearance (Fig. 14-1B). The recognition of dead bone microscopically is not difficult: the marrow cells are necrotic and ghostlike, the walls of the fat cells break down to form irregular fat cysts, and sometimes calcification of the fat occurs. The bone matrix is usually palely stained and the osteocytic lacunae enlarged and empty. As occurs with infarcts in other organs, the necrotic tissue is invaded by granulation tissue, removed, and replaced by scar. However, in the case of bone, the scar tissue is organized as osseous tissue (Fig. 14-9).

In revascularized bone, the bone marrow space is filled with granulation tissue, and it is common to see a layer of new living bone being deposited on a core of dead bone tissue, a process that is often referred to as "creeping substitution" (Fig. 14-10).

Infarcts in the shafts of long bones are likely to be asymptomatic.[16] They may be found as an incidental finding on radiographic films, in which case they are frequently misinterpreted as tumors, particularly cartilaginous tumors.

Clinically, infarction is usually seen adjacent to a joint, particularly the femoral head, although it may occur in other joints. In the femoral head it commonly complicates fracture[17] but is also frequently seen without fracture, in which case there is frequently a clinical history of either cortisone therapy or alcoholism. In alcoholics the systemic nature of the disease is apparent by the presence of multiple bone infarcts in almost 50 percent of the patients.

The radiologic features of infarction of the femoral head are increased bone density and a change in joint contour. The increased density is the result of reparative new bone and trabecular thickening at the edge of the infarct. The change in the contour of the articular surface is due to a failure of repair and central collapse of the infarcted area with the overlying articular cartilage.

Gross examination of the femoral head resected because of early stage osteonecrosis is likely to reveal fairly intact articular cartilage, although there will probably be wrinkling of the surface marking the edge of the necrotic area (Fig. 14-1). On vertical sectioning, the infarcted

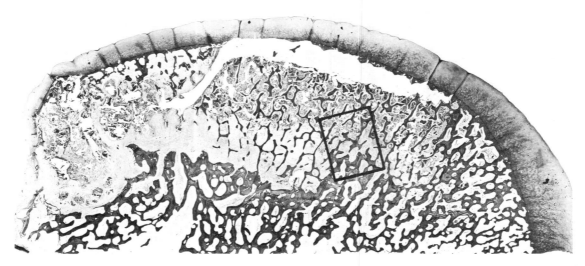

Fig. 14-9. Photomicrograph of a histologic preparation of the specimen shown in Fig. 14-1. An enlarged view of the outlined area is shown in Fig. 14-10.

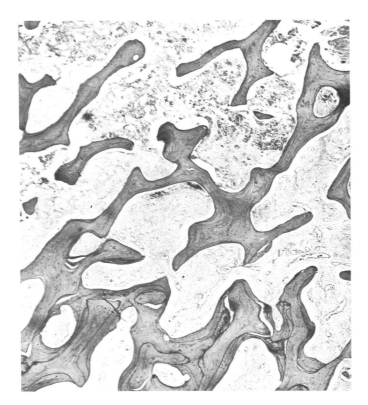

Fig. 14-10. Photomicrograph of area outlined in Fig. 14-8. In the upper part, the fatty marrow is necrotic. The amorphous granular material seen within the fat is calcium soap. In this area the bone trabeculae have an abnormal outline, but a close view would show that the osteocytic lacunae are empty. In the lower part of the picture, a layer of new bone is seen covering the original bone trabeculae. This is evidence of healing and is known as *creeping substitution*. The bone marrow in this area is hyperemic and, together with the new bone formation, represents the repairing margin of the infarct.

zone exhibits a characteristic bright yellow, opaque appearance. At its margin there is a hyperemic zone or a band of fibrous scar tissue. In the later stages of the disease, the articular cartilage becomes detached over the infarcted area, the underlying bone gradually fragments and erodes, and secondary osteoarthritis ensues (Fig. 14-11). There have been several reports of sarcomas, usually malignant fibrous histiocytoma, developing as a complication of long-standing infarcts in long bones.[18]

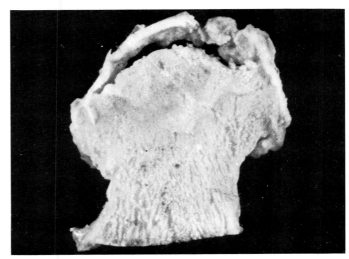

Fig. 14-11. A photograph of a coronal section through the femoral head of a patient with more advanced osteonecrosis than that shown in Fig. 14-1. The articular cartilage is almost entirely detached. Once the cartilage detaches, the necrotic bone beneath will rapidly be eroded away, and secondary osteoarthritis will ensue.

Heterotopic Calcification and Bone Formation

The distinction between calcification in soft tissue and ossification in soft tissue is an important one. Extensive calcification of soft tissue may result from disturbed calcium metabolism, as in hyperparathyroidism, metastatic carcinoma, myeloma, and hypervitaminosis D, or may complicate systemic connective tissue diseases such as scleroderma. Localized diffuse calcification may be seen in fat necrosis, old tuberculous cavities, phlebolithiasis, or synovioma (Fig. 14-12).

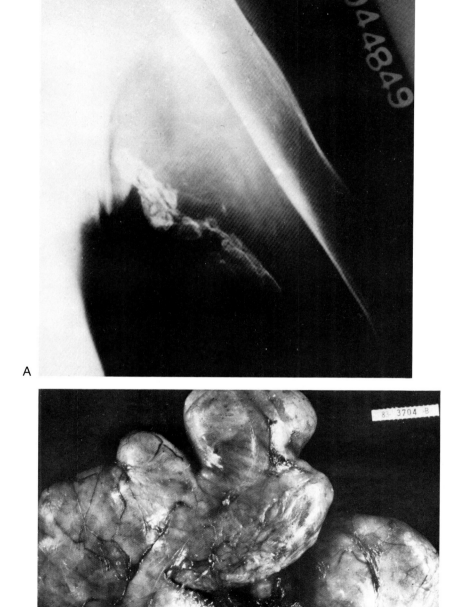

A

B

Fig. 14-12. **(A)** A radiograph of the upper arm of a 50-year-old man complaining of a swelling on the inner aspect of the left arm. A heavily calcified mass is apparent. **(B)** A photograph of the calcified lipoma removed from this patient.

The most common sites of heterotopic bone are in calcified laryngeal or tracheal cartilage and in the media of calcified arteries. In these situations bone is formed by vascular invasion of calcified tissue, similar to endochondral ossification of the growth plate (see earlier). However, any tissue that has calcified may later ossify.

Myositis Ossificans

Two entirely separate conditions are included under the diagnosis of myositis ossificans. First is a congenital progressive disease in which groups of tendons and muscle, usually around major joints, become progressively ossified, producing severe functional disability.[19] Microscopic examination will reveal poorly organized bone, both lamellar and woven, and dense fibrous scar tissue. Occasionally, one may observe islands of poorly formed cartilage.

Second is myositis ossificans circumscripta, in which the patient usually has a lump in a muscle, which has been present for some weeks and may have been somewhat painful.[20] A history of trauma can usually be elicited but is often of a trivial nature and occasionally may be absent. A radiograph taken soon after the onset of symptoms may not show an opacity, but within 1 or 2 weeks a poorly defined shadow will appear, and over the following weeks the periphery will become increasingly well delineated from the surrounding soft tissue.

On gross examination, a focus of myositis ossificans circumscripta present for a few months shows a shell of bony tissue with a more or less soft reddish brown central area. It is usually 2 to 5 cm in diameter and adherent to the surrounding muscle.

Microscopic examination reveals, in the central part of the lesion, an irregular mass of active mesenchymal cells with foci of interstitial microhemorrhage that are rarely extensive (Fig. 14-13A). Occasionally, hemosiderin-filled macrophages and degenerative muscle fibers are encountered. The whole lesion is intensely vascular, the vessels being dilated channels lined by endothelium but without any formed media or adventitia. At some distance from the center of the lesion, depending on the age of the lesion in question, one finds small foci of osteoid production and, rarely, even cartilage production; this tissue may be disorganized and hypercellular. As one approaches the periphery there are more and more clearly defined trabeculae (Fig. 14-13B). The bone is usually of the primitive woven type with large, round, and crowded osteocytes; however, in cases of long standing the bone is mature and has a lamellar pattern.

Histologically it may be difficult to differentiate a focus of myositis, especially in its acute and active stage, from a sarcoma. A careful correlation of the clinical and radio-

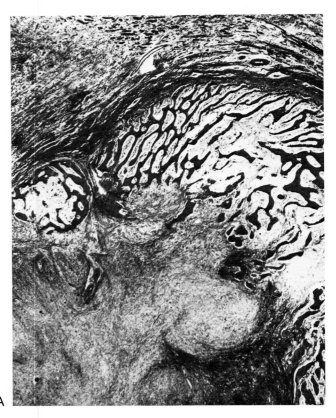

A

Fig. 14-13. **(A)** Photomicrograph to show a portion of a specimen of myositis ossificans circumscripta. In the upper part of the photograph, there is scar tissue with compressed muscle fibers. The lesion itself shows trabecular bone at the periphery and at the center a cellular tissue. (Fig. 14-13 continues.)

graphic findings is therefore essential. An important distinction that must be emphasized is that whereas myositis ossificans is most mature at its periphery and least mature at its center (Fig. 14-13C), the opposite is true of osteosarcoma.

Metabolic Disease

Skeletal disease secondary to disturbed metabolism can be considered under three headings of disturbance or disease, which are discussed below.

Disturbances in the Formation or Breakdown of the Matrix Components

Skeletal disease due to matrix component disturbances may involve the collagen, proteoglycan, or mineral components of the matrix.

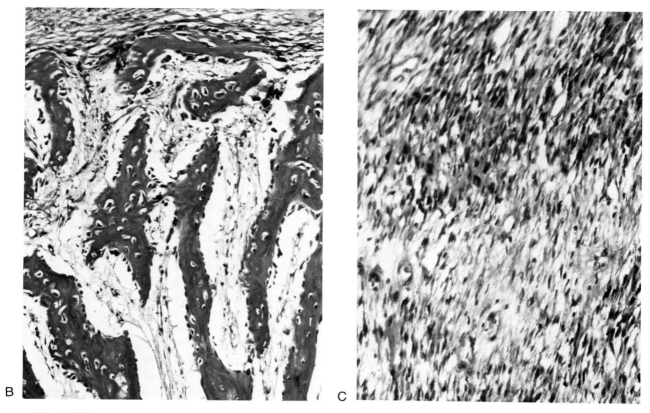

Fig. 14-13 (*Continued*). **(B)** Photomicrograph to show detail of periphery of lesion shown in Fig. A. Note the trabeculae of woven bone with crowded osteocytes and prominent osteoblasts on the surface of the trabeculae. Between the trabeculae there is innocuous fibrous tissue. **(C)** Photomicrograph to show detail of center of lesion in Fig. A. Note the crowded spindle cells, which give a pseudosarcomatous appearance to the lesion.

Collagen

An abnormality in collagen synthesis may result from an inborn error such as occurs with osteogenesis imperfecta or the Ehlers-Danlos syndrome (diseases characterized histologically by severe osteoporosis, often a hypercellular immature bone tissue, and deficient fibrous connective tissue throughout the body)[21] or from extrinsic disturbances such as vitamin C deficiency and lathyrism, in which the intracellular formation of the collagen molecule is disturbed.

Proteoglycan

Most disturbances of proteoglycan metabolism are the result of overproduction of one or another type of glycosaminoglycan (mucopolysaccharide), most commonly dermatan sulfate and heparan sulfate. Accumulation of glycosaminoglycan occurs within the reticuloendothelial cells of many organs, and this may or may not be associated with excess excretion in the urine of these substances. These disorders, which are collectively known as the mucopolysaccharidoses, may exhibit marked skeletal abnormalities.[22] One of these diseases, Morquio's disease, probably specifically involves a defect in the proteoglycan metabolism of cartilage.

Minerals

Disturbances in the mineral component of the matrix may result from inborn errors in metabolism in which there is either a relative absence or excess of the enzyme alkaline phosphatase. *Hypophosphatasemia*[23] is characterized by an extremely osteopenic skeleton, which radiologically mimics rickets. Microscopically the bone tissue is disorganized and poorly mineralized, with an excess of unmineralized osteoid tissue. *Hyperphosphatasemia*,[24] on the other hand, results in a dense and irregularly formed skeleton. Histologically the bone tissue resembles that of Paget's disease. Hyperphosphatasemia is often referred to as *juvenile Paget's disease*.

A number of metallic elements may also deposit in the bone, resulting in interference with the normal process of mineralization. These include lead, iron, and aluminum. Aluminum toxicity has recently been recognized as a major complication of the administration of phosphate bindings in the management of renal dialysis patients. Not only does aluminum result in an encephalopathy, eventually leading to an irreversible psychosis, but it also deposits at the mineralization fronts in the bone, effectively blocking further mineralization and leading to an osteomalacialike picture. In undecalcified sections the aluminum in the bone can be demonstrated by using the aurinetricarboxylic acid stain, which stains the aluminum red.[25] Fluoride in excessive amounts, either endemic or iatrogenic, results in increased bone formation, the matrix of the newly formed bone showing a patchy and abnormal mineralization.[26]

Osteoporosis

Osteoporosis is a decrease in mass of normally mineralized bone, which results in thinning of the bone cortices and in thin, widely spaced trabeculae in the cancellous bone (Fig. 14-14). It is the result of a relative decrease in osteoblastic (bone-forming) activity as compared with osteoclastic (bone-resorbing) activity, usually with an increase in osteoclastic activity.

Osteoporosis may be localized or generalized. Localized osteoporosis occurs after immobilization, for example, in a plaster cast. It may also be seen in the region of a joint associated with localized pain and hyperemia—*Sudeck's atrophy*. This type of localized patchy osteoporosis occasionally seems to involve several joints, usually in the lower limbs, in a transient fashion—so-called idiopathic transient osteoporosis.[27] In one form of localized osteoporosis, *disappearing bone disease,* the bone may eventually entirely disappear on the radiograph.[28] In all these forms of localized osteoporosis, no specific microscopic appearance other than the obvious loss of bone tissue has been identified, although it has been suggested that there is an increased vascularity of the bone.

Clinical generalized osteoporosis as a factor of age is most common in white women for the reasons discussed earlier. It may also occur in a severe form after meno-

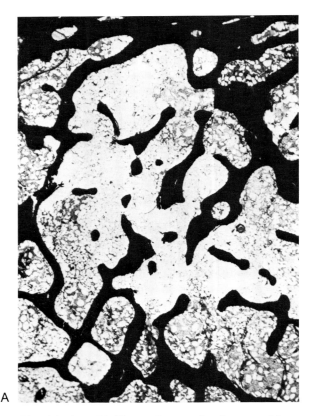 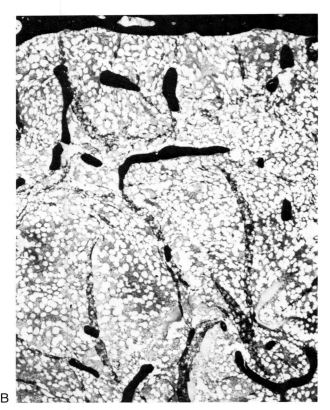

A B

Fig. 14-14. **(A)** Photomicrograph of a core biopsy specimen of the iliac crest in a normal 35-year-old woman. Note that for the most part the trabeculae are connected with one another and to the cortex, a portion of which is seen in the upper part of the picture. Compare this appearance with that in **(B),** which is from an osteoporotic 65-year-old woman. In Fig. B not only are the trabeculae much thinner and sparser, but they are not connected with one another or with the cortical bone at the surface.

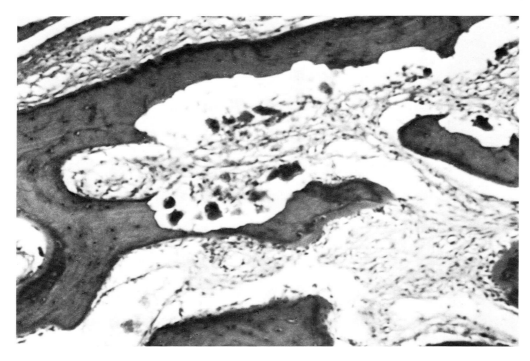

Fig. 14-15. Photomicrograph of section taken from a patient with hyperparathyroidism. Note the way the resorbing surfaces dissect into the bone trabeculae, resulting in a tunneling effect characteristic of hyperparathyroidism.

pause, presumably as a result of endocrine imbalance, and it also complicates hypercortisonism.

Proper evaluation of osteoporosis, as of the other metabolic disturbances of bone, requires quantitative histology, the parameters to measure are the percentage of tissue occupied by bone tissue as opposed to marrow, and the percentage of the bone surface that is actively laying down bone or that is actually resorbing bone as compared with the inactive surfaces. (For a full discussion, see Rasmussen and Bordier.[29])

Disturbances in Calcium Homeostasis

Disturbances in calcium homeostasis result in osteitis fibrosa (hyperparathyroidism) and/or osteomalacia (rickets).

Hyperparathyroidism

Hyperparathyroidism may be either primary, due to a functioning adenoma, primary hyperplasia, or, rarely, a carcinoma of the parathyroid glands[30] or secondary, due to renal disease.[31] With the advent of renal dialysis the latter form of disease (secondary hyperparathyroidism) has become much more frequent. In hyperparathyroid bone disease the characteristic microscopic change is localized osteoclastic resorption of the bone tissue, which

characteristically and frequently shows a dissecting pattern (Fig. 14-15). Associated with the foci of osteoclastic resorption, localized fibrosis of the marrow adjacent to the bone is seen. (The localization of the fibrosis against the bone trabeculae distinguishes this type of fibrosis from that seen in myelofibrosis.) The increased bone resorption results in a secondary increase in bone deposition, and the result is an increased turnover rate that is generalized throughout the skeleton, although it is more apparent in sections of cancellous bone than in sections of dense cortical bone.

Occasionally, the proliferation of osteoclasts and fibrous tissue is associated with hemorrhage and a giant-cell reaction. This results in the so-called brown tumor of hyperparathyroidism, which may be confused with a giant cell tumor. This error may be avoided by careful correlation of the microscopic appearance with the clinical chemistry findings and radiographs.

Osteomalacia

Although childhood rickets is now an uncommon condition, this is not the case with adult rickets, or osteomalacia. Osteomalacia may result from malabsorption syndrome, after intestinal surgery or poor diet, or from a disturbance in vitamin D metabolism.[32] One current cause of disturbance in vitamin D metabolism is treat-

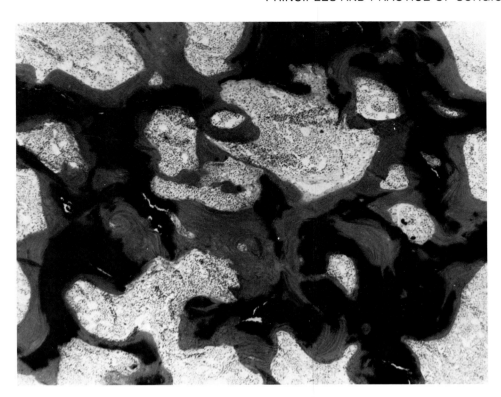

Fig. 14-16. Photomicrograph of a section taken from a patient with osteomalacia. The section has been prepared from undecalcified bone and stained by the von Kossa method. The area stained black represents mineralized bone. On the surface, there is a thick layer of nonmineralized bone matrix (osteoid). This osteoid seam, which is characteristic of osteomalacia, cannot be appreciated on decalcified sections.

ment with anticonvulsive drugs such as diphenylhydantoin (Dilantin). However, whatever the cause of the disturbance in vitamin D metabolism or calcium absorption, the effects are similar. The bone that is laid down fails to be calcified. As a result the osteoblasts tend to be overactive, laying down even more bone, which in turn remains unmineralized. It is not possible to appreciate the extent of unmineralized bone tissue unless undecalcified sections are prepared (Fig. 14-16). When this is done, most of the bone trabeculae are covered by a prominent layer of unmineralized bone or osteoid, and this can be best appreciated by the use of the von Kossa stain. In osteomalacia not only is upward of 40 percent of the bone unmineralized, but it will also be apparent that the mineralization front is very irregular and fuzzy in appearance.

Disease Resulting From Deposition of Abnormal Extrinsic Metabolic Products

The last group of metabolic disturbances commonly seen by the surgical pathologist are the conditions in which an abnormal extrinsic metabolic product is deposited in the skeleton. Such conditions include the so-called lipid histiocytoses (Gaucher's, Niemann-Pick, and Tay-Sachs diseases), ochronosis,[33] cystinosis, and oxalosis,[34] but the two most common diseases are calcium pyrophosphate dihydrate crystal deposition disease and gout.

Calcium Pyrophosphate Dihydrate Deposition Disease (Pseudogout)

Calcium pyrophosphate dihydrate is a chalky white material often found in the synovial membrane, articular cartilage, and/or fibrocartilaginous menisci of old people, and it does not usually result in clinically significant disease.[35] However, some cases of inflammatory joint disease and secondary osteoarthritis may be the result of deposition of calcium pyrophosphate, and occasional patients are seen who develop clinically significant pseudogout before the age of 35. These individuals have an autosomal dominant pattern of inheritance.

The histologic appearance of these deposits is similar enough to that of gout to have given rise to the term *pseudogout* to describe the clinical syndrome. In histologic sections the material is usually crystalline, the crystals being small and rectangular and exhibiting a weak positive birefringence. On occasion, noncrystalline deposits that do not polarize may also be seen. These crystalline deposits are sometimes surrounded by giant cells and occasional histiocytes and chronic inflammatory cells (Fig. 14-17).

Gout

Gout[36] results from the precipitation of monosodium urate monohydrate in the synovial fluid and other tissues after prolonged hyperuricemia. It is most commonly seen in the kidney and the large joints, especially the first metatarsophalangeal joint. There are three stages of involvement to the joint by gout: (1) acute gouty synovitis; (2) the deposition of sodium urate in the form of chalky concretions or tophi in the synovium, bone, bursae, and subcutaneous tissues; and (3) chronic gouty arthritis. In patients with acute gouty arthritis, the synovial fluid invariably contains crystals that are usually needle-shaped and when examined with polarized light demonstrate strong negative birefringence. The crystals may be free in the synovial fluid or may be engulfed within polymorphonuclear leukocytes. The ingested crystals result in the release of lysosomal enzymes, which in turn perpetuate the acute inflammatory reaction. After a number of years, chalky deposits of sodium urate, known as tophi, may develop in the articular and periarticular tissues. These deposits are surrounded by chronic inflammatory cells, foreign body giant cells, and dense fibrous scar. Destruction of the bone and capsular tissues results in chronic arthritis with disabling deformities.

Gaucher's Disease

Gaucher's disease[37] is a lipid histiocytosis resulting from an accumulation of glycocerebrosides within the histiocytes of the reticuloendothelial system, particularly in bones and spleen. It is mostly seen in Ashkenazic Jews and is transmitted as an autosomal recessive trait. The bone marrow shows more or less replacement by sheets of large pale cells, with a distinctive crumpled appearance to the cytoplasm. Because the disease is inherited, the bone marrow replacement may result in developmental deformities in the more rapidly growing parts of the skeleton, that is, the lower end of the femur, the upper tibia, and the upper end of the humerus. This takes the form of widening of the metaphyseal portion of bone, resulting in a deformity known as the "Erlenmeyer flask deformity." Radiographically, the affected bones are frequently osteoporotic and may show a lytic or soap bubble appearance. The extending mass of lipid-laden histiocytes may interfere with the blood supply to the bone and cause infarction. Unilateral or bilateral avascular necrosis of the femoral head is a common complication of Gaucher's disease and may be the presenting clinical sign. Because of the relative ischemia of the affected bone, biopsy is attended by a high incidence of secondary infection.

Paget's Disease

Paget's disease[38] is a localized disturbance in bone cell activity, the cause of which is unknown, although recently there have been reports of viral inclusions in the osteoclasts.[39] It is a fairly common disease, occurring in about 4 percent of the northern European male population over the age of 40. However, in the majority of instances the disease is not clinically significant, usually being confined to only one vertebral body or one other focus in the skeleton. Generalized clinical Paget's disease is much less common.

The microscopic appearance of Paget's disease is variable and depends on the state of activity. In active disease, the histologic appearance is difficult to distinguish from that of hyperparathyroidism (Fig. 14-18). There is very active osteoclastic resorption and, associated with this, increased osteoblastic activity. These changes result in an increased number of reversal lines (cement lines), which are apparent even in the early or active stage of the disease. The marrow spaces are fibrosed, but the dissecting type of resorption, which typifies hyperparathyroidism, is not usually seen. In the later, quiescent stages of the disease, the bone becomes very dense, and the previous overactivity is represented by multiple cement lines, giving rise to the descriptive mosaic appearance (Fig. 14-5). The bone marrow will be noted to have many dilated vascular channels, which is consistent with the clinical observation that these patients frequently have a high output type of failure. In a small percentage of patients sarcoma may develop[40] (see Ch. 15).

Infection

Before the advent of antibiotics, infection[41,42] was among the most common indications for inpatient treatment in orthopedic hospitals, and in developing countries bone infection is still the most common cause of bone and joint disease. In the United States, however, it is now rare and for this reason may give rise to problems in differential diagnosis.

Infection of the bones and joints may result from either hematogenous spread or direct implantation. In the latter case, the infection usually complicates either a compound fracture or surgery, nowadays particularly prosthetic replacement of joints.

Hematogenous osteomyelitis is most commonly seen in children and is usually due to *Staphylococcus aureus*

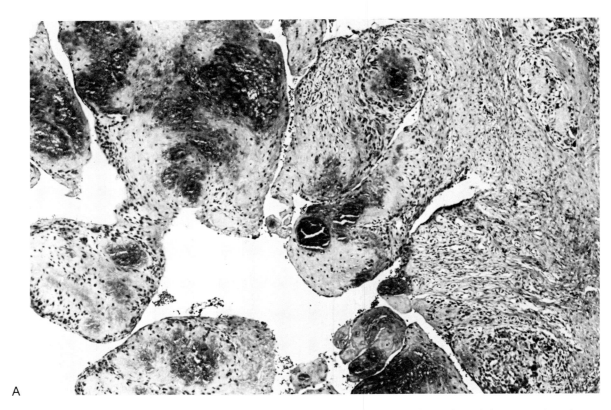

A

Fig. 14-17. **(A)** Photomicrograph of a section of synovium taken from a patient with calcium pyrophosphate dihydrate deposition disease. The deposits of calcium pyrophosphate are often crystalline and surrounded in some areas by histiocytes, giant cells, and a mild chronic inflammatory infiltrate. (Fig. 14-17 continues.)

infection. Bacteremia alone is probably not sufficient to cause osteomyelitis, and generally a history of trauma will be elicited from the patient, the trauma presumably giving rise to local blood stasis or thrombosis, thereby providing a site for bacterial growth. Infection is most commonly seen in children in the metaphyseal region of long bones and particularly around the knee joint. Usually, the patient has a high fever, pain, and local tenderness, and during the first week or so of the disease radiographs will not show any bony change. (Nowadays, since patients with fever are frequently treated with antibiotics without further diagnosis, osteomyelitis in children may present as a chronic problem.)

In adults, hematogenous osteomyelitis is less common. When it is seen, it is more common in the vertebral column. It has been described recently as occurring in heroin addicts and may also complicate urinary tract infection, presumably via Batson's plexus. An unusual form of osteomyelitis is the multiple bony involvement seen in patients with sickle cell disease, in which the causative organism is often *Salmonella*.

In osteomyelitis, the inflammatory exudate usually results in widespread bone and bone marrow necrosis.

This results from the increased pressure within the closed cavity of the cancellous bone, which rapidly leads to vascular occlusion. The inflammatory exudate tracks through the haversian systems of the cortex to elevate the overlying periosteum, which in turn is activated to form a sleeve of new bone (the *involucrum*) around the necrotic infected bone (the *sequestrum*) beneath. This classic sequence is aborted by the use of adequate antibiotic therapy. However, unless the disease is treated with adequate doses of antibiotics, it may become chronic and in this case is likely to continue for many years with recurrent episodes of local infection, which may be accompanied by sinus formation. Rare long-term complications of osteomyelitis include secondary amyloidosis and the formation of squamous cell carcinoma in the sinus tract.[43]

Occasional adult patients with hematogenous osteomyelitis may present without significant systemic signs. As likely as not, the radiologic diagnosis on these patients will be that of a tumor, possibly a malignant round cell tumor. A biopsy specimen revealing small, round inflammatory cells may also be misinterpreted by the pathologist as a round cell tumor, and on occasion this differen-

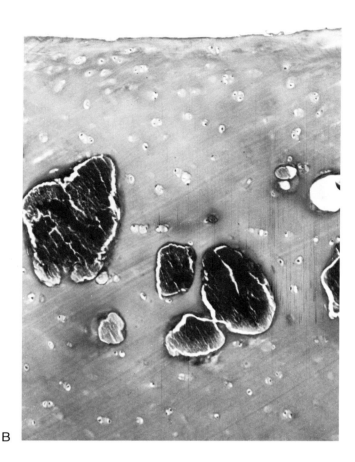

B

Fig. 14-17 (*Continued*). **(B)** Photomicrograph of section of articular cartilage from the same case demonstrated in Fig. A. Large irregular noncrystalline deposits of calcified material are present. Undecalcified frozen section stained by the von Kossa method.

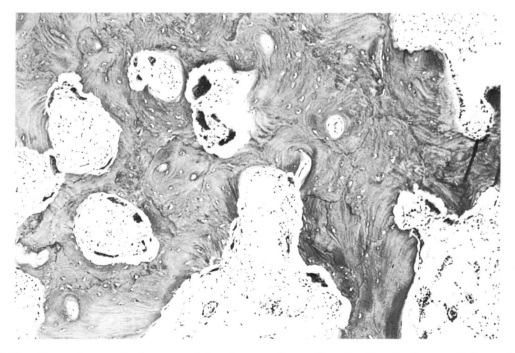

Fig. 14-18. Photomicrograph of a section taken from a patient with active Paget's disease. At the surface of the bone there is considerable osteoclastic activity. Some of these osteoclasts have many nuclei. Giant osteoclasts tend to be characteristic of Paget's disease. In other areas, abundant osteoblastic activity can be discerned.

487

tial diagnosis may be problematic. In this regard it also should be noted that occasional children with Ewing's tumor may have an elevated temperature, increased sedimentation rate, and leukocytosis.

Granulomatous infection is usually due to *Mycobacterium tuberculosis,* but occasionally to blastomycosis, cryptococcosis, coccidioidomycosis, or sporotrichosis; rarely, it results from sarcoidosis. These infections are most commonly seen either in the spine or in the large joints (the hip and the knee). Histologically, typical granulomas with giant cells, epithelioid cells, and chronic inflammatory cells are seen. Organisms may be difficult to demonstrate in bony tissue. Often, granulomatous infection, because of its rarity, is not suspected clinically, and the diagnosis does not become apparent until the pathologist has examined the tissue. For this reason cultures may not have been taken, and the causative organism may be difficult to establish.

The Histiocytoses

The histiocytoses are characterized by the proliferation of histiocytes in the bone and/or soft tissues.[44] Depending on the presentation, they are classified as eosinophilic granuloma, Hand-Schüller-Christian disease, or Letterer-Siwe disease.

In the skeleton, *eosinophilic granuloma* is usually unifocal but occasionally may be multifocal. The majority of patients are under age 10. It may occur anywhere in any bones, but the most common sites are the skull, the shafts of the long bones (particularly the femur and tibia), and the ilium. The patient usually has localized aching pain and, less commonly, a low-grade fever and an elevated erythrocyte sedimentation rate. In radiographs the lesions are osteolytic and generally round to oval, but they may show considerable periosteal reaction and a ragged appearance suggestive of a malignant tumor. Involvement of the vertebral body frequently leads to collapse and flattening (so-called Calve's disease). On gross examination, the curetted material is usually scant and pinkish gray. Microscopic examination will reveal masses of histiocytes and focal or diffuse collections of eosinophils (Fig. 14-19). Occasionally, lymphocytes and plasma cells may also be present. During the healing phase, scar tissue and lipid-laden macrophages may become predominant.

Overdecalcification of the tissue may result in the eosinophilic granules not being apparent, and the lesion may be mistaken for osteomyelitis. The numerous histiocytes, occasionally with large nuclei and even occasionally binucleate forms, can lead to the erroneous impression of Hodgkin's disease.

The histopathology of *Hand-Schüller-Christian disease* is similar to that of eosinophilic granuloma, but the clinical involvement is more widespread. In addition to multiple osteolytic lesions, the patient may have hepatosplenomegaly, lymphadenopathy, and diabetes insipidus.

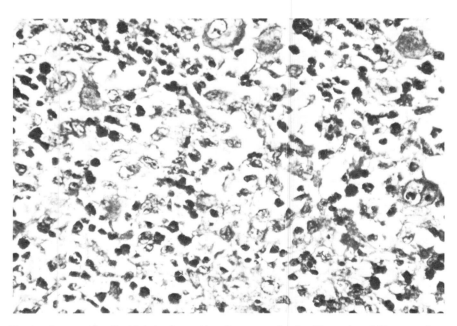

Fig. 14-19. Photomicrograph of a histologic section from a patient with eosinophilic granuloma. There is a background of pale-staining histiocytic cells with abundant loose cytoplasm, which vary considerably in size and shape. The small dark cells are mostly eosinophils, but there are a few plasma cells and lymphocytes present. This microscopic appearance can be confused on occasion with Hodgkin's disease or with infection.

Because of the lymphadenopathy and hepatosplenomegaly, the lesion may be mistaken for a malignant lymphoma, particularly Hodgkin's disease.

Letterer-Siwe disease is a rare condition affecting infants less than 2 years of age and is characterized by an acute onset of hepatosplenomegaly, lymphadenopathy, and sometimes bone lesions. In the past, this has been considered a form of histiocytosis, but Lieberman et al.[44] have suggested that the cases can be separated into two groups. In one group anaplastic histiocytes predominate, and this lesion would appear to be a form of malignant lymphoma. In the other group the histiocytes have a benign cytology, and this lesion may well be an infantile form of multifocal eosinophilic granuloma.

JOINT TISSUES

The joints[44a] provide for motion and stability. These functions are achieved through the anatomy of the joint—its shape and the cartilage and bone of which it is made—and through the neuromuscular control of the joint. Dysfunction of the joint, which is generally called arthritis, occurs because of an alteration in the anatomy or its neuromuscular control. Obviously, such changes may result from congenital disease, metabolic disturbances, infection, or mechanical trauma.

The diarthrodial joints are composed of the articulating cartilages, synovial membrane, bone ends, and surrounding ligaments, tendons, and muscles.[45] Disease may begin in any of these structures, but by the time it comes to the attention of a physician, most or all of them are involved.

The synovial membrane, which lines the inner surface of the joint capsule and all other intra-articular structures with the exception of the articular cartilage, is composed of a smooth moist intimal layer and either a fibrous or a fatty subsynovial (or subintimal) supportive or backing layer that is. Microscopic examination shows at the surface a layer of closely packed cells with elliptical nuclei and abundant cytoplasm.

The articular cartilage is largely composed of collagen, proteoglycan, and water, and it distributes the load through the joint onto the underlying subchondral bone. To achieve this, the collagen fibers are distributed in a very precise way, as is the proteoglycan.[9] The cells on the surface of the cartilage are flat with their long axes parallel to the surface. The cells that are lower down in the cartilage are rounded and lie in well-defined lacunae. Other forms of cartilage in the body (epiphyseal cartilage, fibrocartilage, and elastic cartilage) do not function in the same way as articular cartilage and therefore have a different chemical composition and a different organization of the extracellular matrix.[46]

JOINT DISEASE

The most important therapeutic advance since the 1960s has been the development of artificial articulations to replace joints affected by various diseases. On most orthopedic services, endoprosthetic replacements probably account for about one third of all operations. For the surgical pathologist this means a considerable increase in the amount of orthopedically related tissue to be studied and reported on.

The most common pathologic diagnoses following total hip replacement in our experience are osteoarthritis (about 65 percent), avascular necrosis (about 20 percent), and rheumatoid arthritis (about 15 percent). (It should be emphasized that these diagnoses are not completely objective and that end-stage hip disease, like end-stage kidney disease or end-stage liver disease, looks very much the same regardless of its etiology.)

The arthritides that are the result of metabolic disturbances and infection have been referred to earlier and will not be further discussed here.

Osteoarthritis

Osteoarthritis[47] (degenerative joint disease, osteoarthrosis) is generally regarded as a noninflammatory condition that begins as a disruption of the bearing surfaces of the articular cartilage and ends with disintegration of the mechanical joint. In about one fifth of the cases, an antecedent condition causally related to the osteoarthritis is evident to the clinician. These conditions include Perthe's disease, slipped epiphysis, previous infection, and osteonecrosis.

A patient with clinical osteoarthritis complains of pain and disability, and movement of the affected joint may be very limited. Examination of a joint removed at surgery or autopsy shows the most obvious features of an osteoarthritic joint to be a change in the shape of the articular surfaces and damage of the cartilage. In the weight-bearing areas of a joint, the cartilage may be entirely absent, and the exposed subchondral bone has a dense polished appearance like marble (eburnation) (Fig. 14-20). In these areas of absent cartilage, the bone trabeculae are markedly thickened (sclerotic), and, adjacent to the surface in the subchondral bone there may be cystic defects filled by loose fibromyxoid tissue or sometimes by a thick fluid. In the eburnated areas the superficial bone may be necrotic, presumably from the excessive pressure. In some specimens the weight-bearing surface may be covered by few or many tufts of fibrocartilage, and this seems to be a reparative phenomenon. In the areas of the joint that are not weight-bearing and around the margins, there are bony and cartilaginous overgrowths (osteophytes or ex-

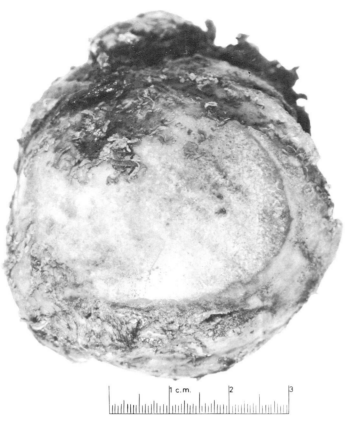

Fig. 14-20. Photograph of a femoral head removed from a patient with osteoarthritis of the hip joint. The superior articular surface has a shiny appearance where the articular cartilage has been worn away and the underlying polished bone exposed. The cartilage that remains around the periphery is irregular and roughened.

ostoses), which on the medial and inferior aspect of the femoral head may be in the form of large, flat plaques of bone and cartilage.

The cartilage that remains on the joint surface may have many clefts in its substance, most, but by no means all, being vertical in disposition. The cartilage cells may show considerable proliferation, with the formation of prominent cell nests (Fig. 14-21). Generally, basophilic staining of the matrix with hematoxylin stain will be found to be diminished. The synovial membrane shows some villous proliferation and mild hyperplasia of the intima. There may be a mild chronic inflammation (Fig. 14-22). Small osteochondral loose bodies are not unusual both in the synovium and also free in the joint. In Charcot joints, which are very severe examples of osteoarthritis, the synovium is generally full of bone and cartilage fragments, and there are many loose bodies.

On the basis of anatomic features, Nichols and Richardson[48] in 1909 distinguished the two forms of chronic arthritis that we would call, respectively, inflam-

matory arthritis and degenerative arthritis—most of the former comprising the clinical syndrome of rheumatoid arthritis and the latter that of osteoarthritis.

How well are we able to distinguish rheumatoid arthritis and osteoarthritis of the hip using histopathologic criteria? This is a summary of my own experience:

1. Histologically, there is more inflammation in association with the clinical diagnosis of rheumatoid arthritis than with the clinical diagnosis of degenerative joint disease. However, there is considerable overlap, and in 40 percent of the cases, no clear distinction can be made on the basis of the inflammatory infiltrate.
2. Pannus, a fibrous or inflammatory covering of the cartilage, often regarded as a hallmark of rheumatoid arthritis, is not uncommon in osteoarthritis.

Salvati et al.[49] reported on the specific activity of cathepsin D in synovial membrane and a histologic quantification of inflammation on synovial tissue obtained from 36 patients undergoing total hip replacement. Among patients with degenerative hip disease, two groups could be

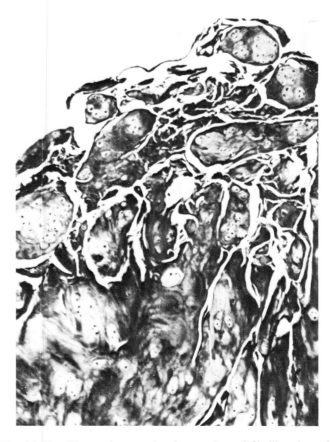

Fig. 14-21. Photomicrograph of a section of fibrillated cartilage from a patient with osteoarthritis. Note the proliferating nests of chondrycytes particularly evident towards the surface.

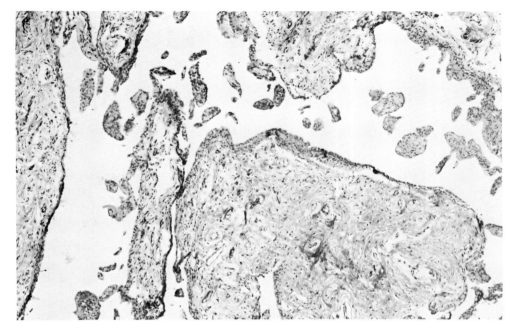

Fig. 14-22. Photomicrograph of a section of synovium taken from a patient with osteoarthritis of the hip joint. The synovial membrane is hypertrophied, hyperplastic, and thrown up into fine microvilli. In the subsynovial tissue there is a mild chronic inflammatory infiltrate.

identified. In the first, which accounted for 20 percent of the cases, there were high enzyme levels and high histologic scores. In the rest low enzyme levels were accompanied by low histologic scores. It would seem, therefore, that there are a significant number of patients who have an inflammatory arthritis by all pathologic criteria even though clinically they have been diagnosed as having osteoarthritis.

Some patients with osteoarthritis have a spontaneous tendency to improve symptomatically and radiologically.[50] This may be explained by the histologic finding that in advanced stages of disease, eburnated areas tend to resurface with fibrocartilage. It suggests that osteoarthritis is not necessarily a progressive and continually degenerative process, but rather that there are two opposing processes occurring in a joint, namely breakdown and repair.

Rheumatoid Arthritis

Rheumatoid arthritis[51] is a chronic systemic disease frequently involving peripheral joints, two to three times more common in females, and characterized by spontaneous remission and exacerbation.[52] Of all affected patients, 70 to 80 percent have histocompatibility antigen Dw4, which implies a strong hereditary component.[53]

Clinically, the acutely affected joint is hot, swollen, and tender. The synovial effusion is milky and turbid and contains 20,000 to 50,000 inflammatory cells, about 50 percent of which are polymorphonuclear leukocytes (compared with septic arthritis, in which the count is in excess of 100,000 with 75 percent polymorphonuclear leukocytes). No causative organism has been identified.

The principal morphologic feature of rheumatoid disease is joint destruction. Unlike osteoarthritis, there is little reparative activity, and osteophytes and new bone formation are not prominent.

The earliest histologic finding (Fig. 14-23) is a nonsuppurative chronic inflammation of the synovium characterized by:

1. Hypertrophy and hyperplasia of the synovial cells, resulting in a papillary and villous pattern at the surface of the synovium
2. An infiltrate of lymphocytes and plasma cells, the latter often containing eosinophilic inclusions (Russell bodies, evidence of γ-globulin production); neutrophils are common in the synovial exudate but much less so in the synovial membrane
3. Lymphoid follicles (Allison-Ghormley bodies)
4. Fibrinous exudation both at the surface of the synovium and within the synovial tissue

Although these histologic changes are very typical of rheumatoid arthritis, similar changes may also be seen in patients with *systemic lupus erythematosus, psoriasis, and other inflammatory arthritides.* For this reason a de-

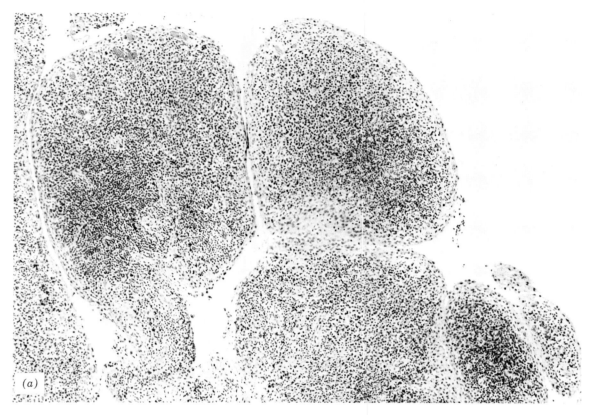

Fig. 14-23. (A) Photomicrograph of a histologic section of synovium from a patient with rheumatoid arthritis. There is prominent villous proliferation, with a heavy subsynovial inflammatory infiltrate and marked hyperplasia of the synovial lining cells. (Fig. 14-23 continues.)

finitive diagnosis of rheumatoid arthritis cannot be made on histologic examination of the synovium alone.

The hypertrophied, inflamed synovium often extends over the articular surface (pannus) and destroys the underlying cartilage by enzymatic degradation of the matrix (Fig. 14-24). The end result of this inflammatory destruction of the articular surfaces may be fusion of the joint (ankylosis), either by fibrous granulation tissue or by bone. (Note: Ankylosis is *not* a feature of osteoarthritis.)

As well as destroying the cartilaginous surfaces of the joint, the rheumatoid synovium may invade the bone at the articular margin, the joint capsule, and other periarticular supportive tissues, resulting in marked instability of the joint and, frequently, subluxation or complete dislocation. Extra-articular synovitis may lead to carpal tunnel syndrome in which there is compression of the median nerve, or trigger finger, and on occasion these clinical syndromes may be heralds of rheumatoid arthritis.

One histologic feature that is not usually commented on is considerable chronic inflammation and lymphoid follicle formation in the subchondral bone. In some cases this inflammatory tissue may destroy the articular cartilage from below.

Radiographs of affected joints will usually show osteopenia of the juxta-articular bone ends. This may be due to either inflammation of the subchondral bone or hyperemia secondary to inflammation of the synovium.

About 25 percent of patients with rheumatoid arthritis have subcutaneous nodules, most commonly over the extensor surfaces of the elbow and forearm. The nodules may also occur in synovial membrane and in the gastrointestinal tract, lung, and heart. The nodules may be present before any other sign of rheumatoid disease. The rheumatoid nodule is characterized histologically by an irregular shape and a central zone of necrotic fibrinoid material surrounded by histiocytes and some chronic inflammatory cells. The long axes of these histiocytes are frequently radially disposed or palisaded. The fact that generalized vasculitis is much more common in patients with rheumatoid nodules is consistent with the belief that the nodules result from vascular damage[54] (Fig. 14-25).

Although the ultimate cause of rheumatoid disease is unknown, there are two important contributory factors: an immunologic reaction and increased degradative enzymes. Patients with rheumatoid arthritis have a number of immunoglobulins in their serum and synovial fluid,

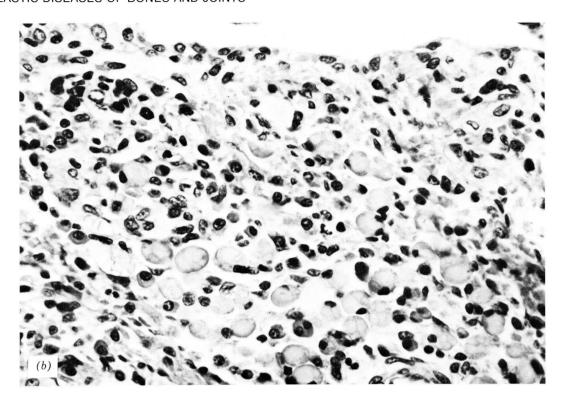

Fig. 14-23 (*Continued*). **(B)** A high-power view of this synovium showing the plasma cell and lymphocyte infiltrate. Many of the plasma cells contain cytoplasmic inclusions (Russell bodies).

most commonly IgM. These immunoglobulins are known as *rheumatoid factors* and, as can be demonstrated by immunofluorescence, are made by plasma cells in the synovium and lymphoid system. They can be seen microscopically in H&E-stained sections, both intracellularly and extracellularly as dense homogeneous eosinophilic globules (Russell bodies).

As already noted, in the late stages of rheumatoid arthritis the affected joint may show very little in the way of inflammation and may be anatomically indistinguishable from osteoarthritis.

Synovitis and Other Tissue Responses to Implanted Artificial Joints

A small percentage of total joint replacements fail either because of mechanical loosening or breakage, or, less commonly, because of infection. In these cases the prosthesis is usually removed.[55]

In patients who have had a prosthesis in which metal articulates on metal, it is not uncommon to see a distinct gray-black discoloration at the synovial surface.[55] Microscopic examination of removed tissue shows irregular metal fragments measuring between 1 and 3 μm, mostly within histiocytes. The metallic nature of these particles has been confirmed by various techniques.[56]

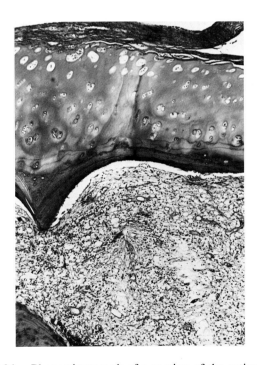

Fig. 14-24. Photomicrograph of a section of the articular surface of a joint involved by rheumatoid arthritis. Covering the articular cartilage is a layer of inflamed synovium (pannus). Underlying the pannus the chondrocytic lacunae are markedly enlarged. A heavy inflammatory infiltrate is also seen in the subchondral bone.

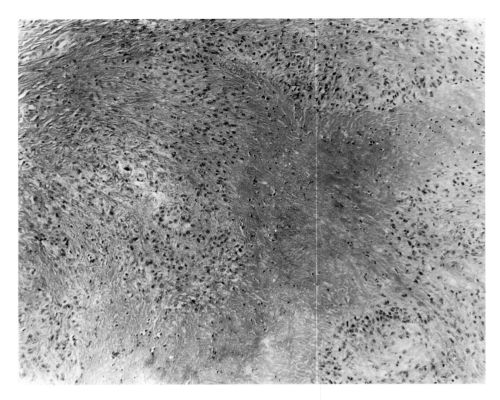

Fig. 14-25. Photomicrograph of a portion of a rheumatoid nodule. Note the geographic central fibrinoid necrosis with the surrounding palisaded histiocytes and scattered chronic inflammatory cells.

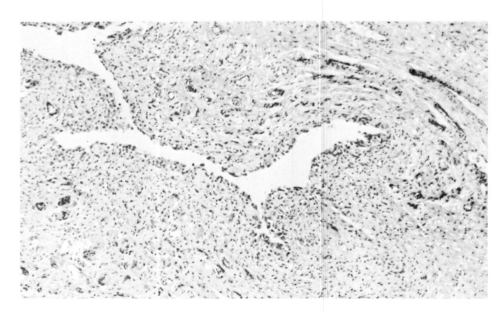

Fig. 14-26. Photomicrograph of a histologic section taken from a patient with a failed total knee replacement. The synovial membrane shows hyperplasia of the synovial lining and foreign body giant cell reaction. Irregular fragments of plastic can be demonstrated in these giant cells by polarized light. Proliferative synovium such as this may result in periarticular erosion of the bone. (H&E, polarized light.)

Wear particles from the plastic, polyethylene components of artificial joints are only visible when the tissue is examined by polarized light. Mostly, they are intracellular and threadlike and measure about 1 μm across and 4 to 10 μm in length. A severe histiocytic response in the synovium is frequently observed, and foreign body giant cells are common. Occasionally, the fragments of polyethylene result in a tumorlike mass developing in the joint capsular tissue, and occasionally erosion of the periarticular bone has been observed (Fig. 14-26).

Both the polyethylene and the metallic components of the artificial joint are usually keyed to the underlying bone by an interposed layer of methyl methacrylate cement.

Abraded particles of cement produce in the capsular tissues a foreign-body giant cell reaction. Often the particles are fairly small (10 to 30 μm), in which case they are surrounded by recognizable giant cells. Sometimes the pieces are very large (100 μm or more), and in this case histologic sections reveal large irregular spaces surrounded by flattened giant cells (Fig. 14-27). In the routine preparation of histologic sections, any cement in the tissue will be dissolved out by the solvents used in the processing, and microscopic examination will reveal only spaces where the cement was. However, it usually leaves behind a marker in the form of the insoluble barium sulfate that is put into the cement to render it radiopaque.

In all the removed prostheses we have examined, wear debris from one or all of these three sources was present histologically. This debris may be found also in draining lymph nodes. The long-term effects on the body are not known.

Pigmented Villonodular Synovitis and Tenosynovitis

Pigmented villonodular synovitis and tenosynovitis[57] is characterized by a nodular or diffuse proliferation of mononuclear cells, resembling synoviocytes, in tendon sheath or a joint. Frequently, these cells coalesce to form multinucleate giant cells, and for this reason the lesion is sometimes called a *giant cell tumor of tendon sheath*. In addition to the mononuclear histiocytic-type cells, one may also see some admixed chronic inflammatory cells (Fig. 14-28). A varying degree of collagen will be observed in the lesion; this may be minimal in amount or may be so extensive as to obliterate most of the cellular elements. The more cellular the tumor, the more likely one is to see mitotic figures and occasional bizarre cells.

Although grossly these lesions most often show some brown-tan staining, despite the name *pigmented* villonodular synovitis hemosiderin pigment is not abundant microscopically. It is probably an incidental finding secondary to hemorrhage rather than an etiologic factor.

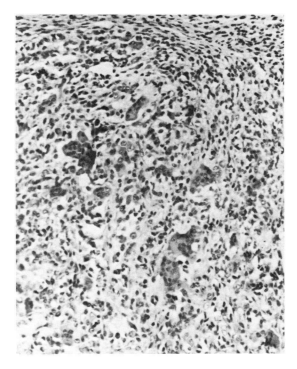

Fig. 14-28. Photomicrograph of a section taken from a patient with pigmented villonodular synovitis. The tissue is composed of sheets of mononuclear cells, some of which are forming multinucleate giant cells. An admixture of chronic inflammatory cells is also present.

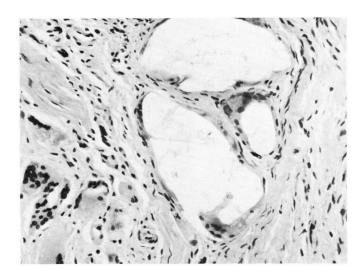

Fig. 14-27. Photomicrograph of a section of synovial tissue taken from a patient with a failed knee prosthesis. The large irregular spaces surrounded by flattened giant cells originally contained methyl methacrylate cement, dissolved out during processing. The finely granular material seen in these spaces is barium sulfate, which is used as a clinical radiopaque marker.

This lesion is most commonly seen in the fingers, where it has been called by various names, including giant cell tumor of tendon sheath, benign synovioma, and fibroxanthoma. It usually occurs in the flexor tendon sheath and is rarely seen on the extensor surface of the finger. In most instances of major joint involvement, it is the knee that is involved, although occasionally one may see involvement of the hip or other joints. It is grossly nodular and slowly growing. In rare instances, multiple sites may be involved in the form of multiple nodules or a diffuse involvement of the synovium. In the latter case total removal may be impossible. Often the bone underlying the lesion is eroded, which may give rise to the erroneous impression on a radiograph that one is dealing with an osseous tumor that has broken out of the bone into the soft tissue. In such a case, multiple giant cells could lead to the incorrect diagnosis of a giant cell tumor of bone.

Although most patients with pigmented villonodular synovitis are middle-aged at the time the disease manifests, it may occur at any age. There is a high rate of recurrence after surgery, particularly when the lesion involves a large joint. Metastasis does not occur.

Synovial Chondromatosis

Foci of metaplastic cartilage within the synovial tissues are not an uncommon finding in patients with various types of underlying arthritis, and often the cartilaginous nodules in the synovium may become detached and grow independently within the synovial fluid, where they may attain very large sizes.[58] In the majority of instances, synovial chondromatosis is secondary to some underlying joint condition, and frequently one can find at the centers of the loose bodies small fragments of bone or necrotic articular cartilage or fibrin that acted as seeds on which the cartilaginous loose body grew, rather like pearl formation inside an oyster. When such a loose body is sectioned, one will find evenly spaced chondrocytes of uniform size, although the cartilage will be excessively cellular (Fig. 14-29). When the cartilage nodules are in the form of loose bodies, they will undergo recurrent calcification as they get larger, leaving rings of calcium rather like the rings in a tree trunk. If the cartilage nodule is within the synovial membrane, then it may become invaded by blood vessels and endochondral ossification may occur.

Primary chondromatosis, on the other hand, is a very uncommon disease and is not preceded by any recognizable underlying arthritis. Histologically, the lesions in primary synovial chondromatosis or chondrometaplasia are much more bizarre. The chondrocytes are cloned into

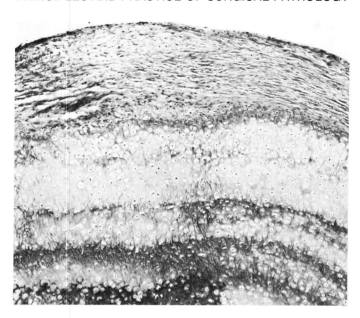

Fig. 14-29. Photomicrograph of a loose body that formed secondary to a detached portion of the articular surface of a knee. The proliferating cartilage is very cellular but with regularly spaced chondrocytes. Concentric rings of calcification are apparent. Compare this photograph with Fig. 14-30.

very cellular atypical nests of chondrocytes, calcification occurs in a haphazard and diffuse manner, and the lesional tissue could easily be mistaken for chondrosarcoma (Fig. 14-30). After excision, the rate of recurrence is high. The lesions may occur both in large joints and also in the synovial sheaths of tendons, particularly in the fingers.

Torn Meniscus

A very common orthopaedic lesion that frequently follows trauma is a tear of one or another of the menisci of the knee.[59] The tear is usually in the posterior horn and usually runs for some distance within the substance of the meniscus before turning medially to extend onto the medial edge, consequently giving rise to a tag or on occasion a "bucket handle" type of tear. If these lesions have been present for a long time, the edges become very rounded, and occasionally a tag of the posterior meniscus may become detached into the joint, giving rise to a fibrocartilaginous loose body. Histologically, the meniscus is formed of a relatively avascular, highly collagenized tissue, in which the blood vessels are confined to the outer third. Cystic degeneration with mucoid-filled microcysts is fairly common. Occasionally, large cysts may form, particularly in the lateral meniscus.

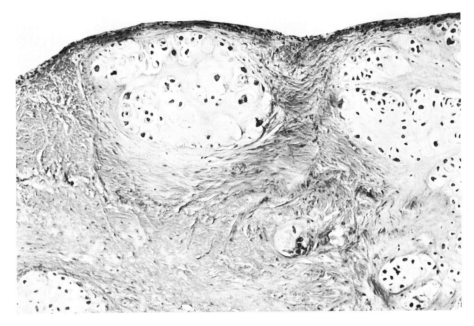

Fig. 14-30. Photomicrograph of a section taken from the synovium of a patient with primary synovial chondromatosis. The islands of cartilage, which form metaplastically within the synovium, are very irregular. The chondrocytes are crowded and vary considerably in size and shape.

MISCELLANEOUS DISEASES OF CONNECTIVE TISSUE

Ganglion

A ganglion is a fibrous walled cyst filled by clear mucinous fluid and usually without a recognizable cyst lining. Ganglia occur in the soft tissues, usually around the hands and feet, and particularly on the extensor surfaces near joints. They may arise as herniations of the synovium or from mucinous degeneration within dense fibrous connective tissue, possibly secondary to trauma. On occasion, they may erode the adjacent bone and even become totally intraosseous; the most common site for such an intraosseous ganglion is the medial malleolus of the tibia.[60]

Trigger Finger, de Quervain's Disease, and Carpal Tunnel Syndrome

In both trigger finger and de Quervain's disease,[61] a thickening of the tendon sheath gives rise to clinical problems with movement of the tendon through the sheath. In carpal tunnel syndrome[61] there is compression of the median nerve by thickening of the tissue forming the transverse carpal ligament. These conditions may precede or accompany some systemic disease of the connective tissues such as rheumatoid arthritis. Histologic examination of the resected thickened tendon sheath will generally show a rather clear-cut cartilaginous or fibrocartilaginous metaplasia of the otherwise delicate tendon sheath (Fig. 14-31). In some cases of carpal tunnel syndrome, amyloid deposits have been recognized as the causative agent.[62]

Morton's Neuroma

Morton's neuroma[63] is a lesion characterized by thickening of the interdigital nerve as it runs between the third and fourth metatarsal heads. Clinically, the patient, who is usually a woman, experiences sharp shooting pains in the sole of the foot extending onto the extensor surface. The resected specimen usually includes the neurovascular bundle and the bifurcation to the third and fourth toe. Just proximal to the bifurcation a fusiform thickening of the neurovascular bundle can usually be observed. Histologic sections will generally show two characteristic features: (1) an occlusion of the digital artery and (2) extensive fibrosis both around and within the nerve, giving rise to a marked depletion of axons within the digital nerve (Fig. 14-32). The term *neuroma* is a misnomer, since there is no evidence in the vast majority of cases of either a traumatic type of neuroma or a neurilemoma.

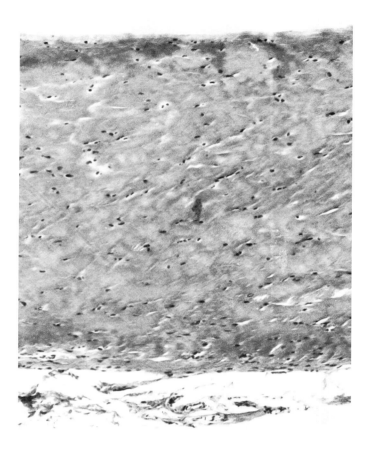

Fig. 14-31. Photomicrograph of a section taken from a patient with a trigger finger. The wall of the tendon sheath, which is normally a very delicate structure, shows a localized thickening by densely collagenized tissue with cells resembling cartilage cells (i.e., fibrocartilage).

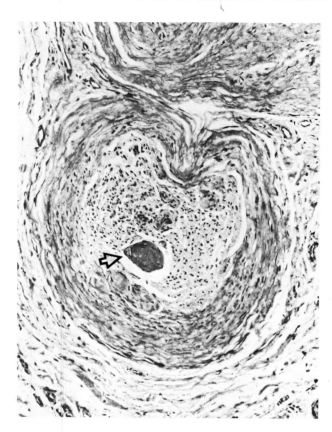

Fig. 14-32. Photomicrograph of a histologic section taken from a patient with Morton's neuroma. The nerve bundles show considerable fibrous proliferation and collagen deposition in the perineurium, as well as within the endoneurium. There is a marked diminution in the number of axons present, and on occasion focal deposits of homogeneous pink material (Renaut bodies—arrow.)

Prolapsed Intervertebral Disc

Curettage of prolapsed intervertebral disc tissue[64] is an operation commonly undertaken by either the orthopaedic surgeon or the neurosurgeon. It usually provides multiple gelatinous pieces of tissue, which on histologic examination will be seen to be composed of portions of fibrous tissue, fibrocartilage, and cartilaginous tissue, the latter with a considerable amount of myxoid material in the matrix. Often, the chondrocytes are necrotic, but in other areas the chondrocytes may be seen to be proliferating, and large clones of cells may be observed. Just as cartilage loose in the joint may give rise to cartilage proliferation, growth, and loose bodies, it is entirely possible that prolapsed intervertebral disc tissue may also, when removed from the constraints of the annulus fibrosa, undergo cellular proliferation and growth and result in secondary nerve root compression.

ACKNOWLEDGMENT

I am extremely grateful to Dr. E. DiCarlo for his help in the preparation of this chapter.

REFERENCES

1. Drury DJ, Bullough PG: Improved photographic reproduction of bone and cartilage specimens using ultraviolet illumination. Med Biol Illus. January 1970
2. Bullough PG, Goodfellow J: The significance of the fine structure of articular cartilage. J Bone Joint Surg 50B:852, 1968
3. Minns RJ, Steven FS: The collagen fibril organization in human articular cartilage. J Anat 123:437, 1977
4. Scott JE: The histochemistry of cartilage proteoglycans in light and electron microscopy. In Ali SY, Elves MW,

Leaback DH (eds): Normal and Osteoarthrotic Articular Cartilage. Institute of Orthopaedics (University of London), London, 1974

5. Jowsey J: The Bone Biopsy. Plenum Medical Books, New York, 1977

6. Enlow DH: Principles of Bone Remodeling. An Account of Postnatal Growth and Remodeling Processes in Long Bones and the Mandible. Charles C Thomas, Springfield, IL, 1963

7. Jaffe HL: Metabolic, Degenerative and Inflammatory Disease of Bones and Joints. Lea & Febiger, Philadelphia, 1972

8. Bourne GH (ed): The Biochemistry and Physiology of Bone. Vols. 1–4. Academic Press, Orlando, FL, 1971–1976

9. Ham AW: Bone and bones. Ch. 15. In Histology. 8th Ed. JB Lippincott, Philadelphia, 1979

10. Sokoloff L: Note on the histology of cement lines. p. 135. In Kenedi RM (ed): Perspectives in Biomedical Engineering. MacMillan, London, 1973

11. Avioli LV: Senile and postmenopausal osteoporosis. Adv Intern Med 21:391, 1976

12. Johnston CC, Lavy N, Lord T, et al: Osteopetrosis: A clinical, genetic, metabolic and morphologic study of the dominantly inherited, benign form. Medicine (Baltimore) 47:149, 1968

13. Ham AW, Harris WR: Repair and transplantation of bone. Ch. 10. In Bourne GH (ed): Biochemistry and Physiology of Bone. 2nd Ed. Academic Press, Orlando FL, 1971

14. Cruess R, Dumont J: Healing of bone, tendon and ligament. p. 97. In Rockwood CA Jr, Green DP (eds): Fractures. JB Lippincott, Philadelphia, 1975

15. Davidson JK: Aseptic Necrosis of Bone. American Elsevier, New York, 1976

16. Bullough PG, Kambolis CP, Marcove RC, et al: Bone infarctions not associated with caisson disease. J Bone Joint Surg [Am] 47:477, 1965

17. Catto M: A histological study of avascular necrosis of the femoral head after transcervical fracture. J Bone Joint Surg [Br] 47:749, 1965

18. Mirra JM, Bullough PG, Marcove RC, et al: Malignant fibrous histiocytoma and osteosarcoma in association with bone infarcts: Report of four cases, two in caisson workers. J Bone Joint Surg [Am] 56:937, 1974

19. Smith R, Russell RGG, Woods CG: Myositis ossificans progressiva. J Bone Joint Surg [Br] 58:48, 1976

20. Paterson DC: Myositis ossificans circumscripta. J Bone Joint Surg [Br] 52:296, 1970

21. Trelstad RL, Rubin D, Gross J: Osteogenesis imperfecta congenita. Lab Invest 36:501, 1977

22. McKusick VA, Neufeld EF, Kelly TE: The mucopolysaccharide storage diseases. p. 1282. In Stanbury JB, Wyngaarden JB, Fredrickson DS (eds): The Metabolic Basis of Inherited Disease. 4th Ed. McGraw-Hill, New York, 1978

23. Teitelbaum SL, Rosenberg EM, Bates M, et al: The effects of phosphate and vitamin D therapy on osteopenic, hypophosphatemic osteomalacia of childhood. Clin Orthop 116:38, 1976

24. Whalen JP, Horwith M, Krook L, et al: Calcitonin treatment in hereditary bone dysplasia with hyperphosphatase-

mia: A radiographic and histologic study of bone. AJR 129:29, 1977

25. Malluche HH, Faugere MC, Smith AJ, Friedler RM: Aluminum intoxication of bone in renal failure—fact or fiction? Kidney Int 29:S70, 1986

26. Epker BN: A quantitative microscopic study of bone-remodelling and balance in a human with skeletal fluorosis. Clin Orthop 5:87, 1967

27. Langloh ND, Hunder GG, Riggs LB, et al: Transient painful osteoporosis of the lower extremities. J Bone Joint Surg [Am] 55:1188, 1973

28. Bullough PG: Massive osteolysis. NY State J Med 71:2267, 1971

29. Rasmussen H, Bordier P: The Physiological and Cellular Basis of Metabolic Bone Disease. Williams & Wilkins, Baltimore, 1974

30. Wilde CD, Jaworski ZF, Villaneuva AR, et al: Quantitative histological measurements of bone turnover in primary hyperparathyroidism. Calcif Tissue Int 12:137, 1973

31. Teitelbaum SL, Bullough PG: The pathophysiology of bone and joint disease. Am J Pathol 96:283, 1979

32. DeLuca HF: Recent advances in our understanding of the vitamin D endocrine system. J Lab Clin Med 87:7, 1976

33. O'Brien WM, Banfield WG, Sokoloff L: Studies on the pathogenesis of ochronotic arthropathy. Arthritis Rheum 4:137, 1961

34. Kinnett JG, Bullough PG: Identification of calcium oxalate deposits in bone by electron diffraction. Arch Pathol Lab Med 100:656, 1976

35. McCarty DJ (ed): Conference on pseudogout and pyrophosphate metabolism. Arthritis Rheum 19:275, 1976

36. Wyngaarden JB, Holmes EW: Clinical gout and the pathogenesis of hyperuricemia. p. 1193. In McCarty DG (ed): Arthritis and Allied Conditions, a Textbook of Rheumatology. 9th Ed. Lea & Febiger, Philadelphia, 1979

37. Brady RO: Glucosyl ceramide lipidosis (Gaucher's disease). p. 731. In Stanbury JB, Wyngaarden JB, Fredrickson DS (eds): Metabolic Basis of Inherited Disease. 4th Ed. New York, McGraw-Hill, 1978

38. Barry H: Paget's Disease of Bone. Williams & Wilkins, Baltimore, 1969

39. Rebel A, Malkain K, Basel M, et al: Osteoclast ultrastructure in Paget's disease. Calcif Tissue Res 20:187, 1976

40. Price CHG, Goldie W: Paget's sarcoma of bone. A study of 80 cases. J Bone Joint Surg [Br] 51:205, 1969

41. Kelly PJ, Fitzgerald RH (eds): Symposium on infections in orthopedics. Orthop Clin North Am, 6(4):915, 1975

42. Miller J (ed): Bone infections symposium. Clin Orthop 96:2, 1973

43. Spjut HJ, Dorfman HD, Fechner RE, et al: Tumors of bone and cartilage. p. 387. In Atlas of Tumor Pathology, Series 2. Fasc. 5. Armed Forces Institute of Pathology, Washington, 1970

44. Lieberman PH, Jones CR, Dargeon HWK, et al: A reappraisal of eosinophilic granuloma of bone, Hand-Schüller-Christian syndrome and Letterer-Siwe syndrome. Medicine (Baltimore) 48:375, 1969

44a. Ham AW: Joints. Ch. 16. In Histology. 8th Ed. JB Lippincott, Philadelphia, 1979

45. Hamerman D, Rosenberg LC, Schubert M: Diarthrodial joints revisited. J Bone Joint Surg [Am] 52:725, 1970
46. Muir IHM: Biochemistry. p. 145. In Adult Articular Cartilage. 2nd Ed. Kent, MAR Freeman Pittman Medical Publishers, 1979
47. Meisel AD, Bullough PG: Atlas of Osteoarthritis. Lea & Febiger, Philadelphia, 1984
48. Nichols EH, Richardson FL: Arthritis deformans. J Med Res 21:149,1909
49. Salvati EA, Granda JL, Mirra J, et al: Clinical, enzymatic and histologic study of synovium in coxarthrosis. Int Orthop 1:39, 1977
50. Perry GH, Smith JG, Whiteside CG: Spontaneous recovery of the joint space in degenerative hip disease. Ann Rheum Dis 31:440, 1972
51. Sokoloff L: Pathology of rheumatoid arthritis and allied disorders. p. 429. In McCarty, DJ (ed): Arthritis and Allied Conditions, a Textbook of Rheumatology. 9th Ed. Lea & Febiger, Philadelphia, 1979
52. Rodnan GP (ed): Primer on the Rheumatic Diseases. 8th Ed. The Arthritis Foundation, New York, 1980
53. Winchester RJ: B Lymphocyte alloantigens, cellular expression, and disease significance with special reference to rheumatoid arthritis. In Arthritis Rheum 20:S159, 1977
54. Sokoloff L: Pathophysiology of peripheral blood vessels in collagen diseases. In Orbison JL, Smith DE (eds): The Peripheral Blood Vessels. Williams & Wilkins, Baltimore, 1963
55. Bullough PG: Some considerations of chronic hip disease and its treatment. J Irish Coll Phys Surg 8:43, 1978
56. Semlitsch M, Willert HG: Gewebsveränderungen im Bereiche metallischer Hüftgelenke; mikroanalytische Untersuchungen mittels Spektralphotometrie, Elektronemikroscopie und der Elektronenstrahlmikrosonde. VI Internat Symp für Mikrochemie, Vol C, p. 70, 1970
57. Byers PD, Cotton RE, Deacon OW, et al: The diagnosis and treatment of pigmented villonodular synovitis. J Bone Joint Surg [Br] 50:290, 1968
58. Villacin AB, Brigham LN, Bullough PG: Primary and secondary synovial chondrometaplasia. Hum Pathol 10:439, 1979
59. Smillie IS: Surgical pathology of the menisci. In Injuries of the Knee Joint. Churchill Livingstone, Edinburgh, 1978
60. Kambolis C, Bullough PG, Jaffe HL: Ganglionic cystic defects of bone. J Bone Joint Surg [Am] 55:496, 1973
61. Phalen GS: The carpal-tunnel syndrome. J Bone Joint Surg [Am] 48:211, 1966
62. Massachusetts General Hospital: Case records. Weekly clinicopathological exercises. Case 10. N Engl J Med 286:534, 1972
63. Asbury AK, Johnson PC: Morton's neuroma. p. 204. In Pathology of Peripheral Nerve. WB Saunders, Philadelphia, 1978
64. Schmorl G: The displacement of intervertebral disc tissue in the human spine. p. 158. In Junghanns H (ed): Besemann EF (trans-ed): Health and Disease. 5th German Ed., 2nd American Ed. Grune & Stratton, Orlando, FL, 1971

15

Neoplasms and Tumor-like Lesions of Bone

Harlan J. Spjut
Alberto G. Ayala

Neoplasms of bone are often a diagnostic problem, since they are uncommon and represent a rather small part of the diagnostic experience of most pathologists. Even so, the pathologist may enhance the diagnosis of neoplasms of bone by knowledge of the clinical presentation, the biologic behavior, and their radiologic features. In addition, close cooperation with the orthopaedic surgeon and the radiologist is essential for arriving at an accurate diagnosis. Admittedly, the clinical manifestation of most neoplasms of bone is rather nonspecific, in that the patient has pain, tenderness, or swelling of the affected part. Nevertheless, if the pathologist is aware of a few bits of clinical information, such as localization of the lesion, radiologic features, and age of the patient, reasonable differential diagnostic possibilities can be considered. For example, it is distinctly uncommon for giant cell tumors to occur before the age of 15. Thus, a pathologist insisting on a diagnosis of giant cell tumor in a child aged 10 or 11 years must give strong consideration to some other lesion that contains many multinucleated giant cells. By contrast, chondrosarcomas are most likely to occur beyond the age of 20, whereas a Ewing's sarcoma is common before age 20. Similar observations can be applied to localization in long bone; for example, a giant cell tumor is epiphyseal and metaphyseal in location, thus given a lesion that histologically contains numerous multinucleated giant cells and does not have an epiphyseal component radiologically, one must strongly consider some other lesion. The same holds true for chondroblastomas, which are recognized to be epiphyseal lesions, but commonly have a metaphyseal component. Osteosarcomas of the long bones are likely to be metaphyseal, whereas Ewing's sarcoma or malignant lymphomas may involve the diaphysis, the metaphysis, or both. The latter three tumors are unlikely to be epiphyseal only. Thus, if the pathologist takes care to review the clinical and radiologic information, the differential diagnosis of neoplasms of bone can be more practical.

Radiologic findings, including computed tomography (CT), magnetic resonance imaging (MRI), and skeletal radionuclide scanning, of skeletal tumors are an integral part of the examination and diagnosis of these lesions. Many times, the radiologic features represent the only opportunity that the pathologist has of seeing the tumor intact, since many benign lesions are curetted, depriving the pathologist of an intact lesion. In effect, radiologic findings represent the gross findings for many neoplasms as far as the pathologist is concerned. Therefore, the pathologist must be familiar with the radiologic features of neoplasms and lesions that simulate neoplasms of bone to better interpret histologic material. Obviously, detailed interpretation of the radiographs must be done by the radiologist, with whom the pathologist should have a consultative working relation. There are tumors that are almost specifically diagnosable radiologically, such as the nonossifying fibroma, the osteoid osteoma, and some of the chondrosarcomas. In some instances, the radiologic diagnosis is more easily made or suggested than is the pathologic diagnosis, emphasizing the importance of the radiologic features as an aid to the pathologist.

In the same light, an understanding of the anatomic and histologic features of bone is essential in the diagnosis of skeletal tumors. The histologic features of normal bone have been discussed in Chapter 14. Awareness of the

501

epiphysis, the growth plate, the metaphysis, and diaphysis is important in regard to a differential diagnosis of neoplasms of long bones. It is of interest to remember that there are ossification centers in the pelvis and the vertebra that serve as sites of tumors that are generally considered to arise from an epiphysis (e.g., chondroblastoma and giant cell tumor).

The decision for biopsy may depend on the differential diagnostic possibilities. For example, it may not be necessary to do a biopsy on a lesion that is entirely characteristic of a nonossifying fibroma and does not seem to present high risk of pathologic fracture. The same might be said for characteristic lesions of fibrous dysplasia. However, if it is not possible to suggest a specific radiologic diagnosis or if the findings strongly point to a malignant lesion, there is a need for a biopsy. It should be kept in mind that some malignant tumors may appear to be benign, and that benign lesions such as osteomyelitis or eosinophilic granuloma will mimic malignant lesions. After the need for biopsy has been determined, the site from which the biopsy is to be taken becomes important. Radiographic features are of great importance in this decision; areas that are radiographically progressive and actively destructive should be chosen, since they should contain diagnosable rather than reactive tissue.

Densely sclerotic sites may not be diagnostic, consisting of bone, calcium, or calcified necrotic tissue. Tumors such as parosteal osteosarcomas are uniformly dense, leaving little choice as to biopsy site. Many malignant tumors of bone frequently have an extracortical component that is ideal for biopsy and frozen section examination.

The type of biopsy must be considered. For lesions that are benign and radiologically strongly suggestive of tumors, such as chondroblastoma, osteoid osteoma, aneurysmal bone cyst, enchondroma, and fibrous dysplasia, the biopsy may be excisional or a curettage, which will serve also as definitive treatment. Skeletal location leads to modification of the biopsy technique; for example, an aneurysmal bone cyst of a vertebra is not likely to be excised, whereas one of the fibula may be resected en bloc. Incisional biopsy should be considered for large lesions that might require a major surgical procedure for their extirpation (e.g., chondrosarcoma of the upper end of the femur or of the pelvic bones). If incisional biopsy is decided on, a deep wedge is suggested to avoid the possibility of only including the reactive tissues around an expanding neoplasm. Reactive tissues have been mistaken for neoplasm both by the surgeon and the pathologist. Thus, in nearly all instances, we advise the orthopaedic surgeon to obtain a frozen section examination of the material removed for biopsy. It is not always possible to select tissue that can be cut on frozen section, but in most cases, small particles of tissue free of bone or containing osteoid can be summitted for frozen section. Even though a specific diagnosis may not be made or the surgeon may not be willing to accept the diagnosis, the frozen section serves the purpose of demonstrating that lesional tissue has been obtained. This is important to avoid a second biopsy, should only reactive tissue be included in the biopsy material.

We have had considerable experience with needle biopsies in the diagnosis of neoplasms of bone.[1] The site for needle biopsy is carefully determined after thorough roentgenographic examination of the lesion. Usually, a core of tissue 2 mm in diameter is obtained and lends itself to frozen section examination if requested. In the majority of cases, a specific diagnosis has been made from the needle biopsy.[1] The needle biopsy has the advantage of usually not requiring general anesthesia, thus saving the patient the risk, however minor, and the expense of an operating room. We are conservative in the interpretation of needle biopsy specimens. If a diagnosis cannot be made or is equivocal, open biopsy is done. The liquid material from the aspiration is submitted for cytologic examination. This, at times, enhances the histologic interpretation.

Regardless of the type of biopsy, tissue should be saved for electron microscopic examination. In most cases, it is not necessary to examine the tissue electron microscopically for a diagnosis, but in some, it is an important part of the diagnosis. This is particularly true of the undifferentiated malignant tumors such as Ewing's sarcoma, malignant lymphomas, and metastatic tumors such as neuroblastoma and undifferentiated carcinoma.

The affinity of tetracycline for osteoid, reactive or malignant, can be utilized in diagnosis. At the M. D. Anderson Hospital, for example, tetracycline is extremely helpful in the identification of the nidus in osteoid osteoma. A patient suspected of having an osteoid osteoma receives therapeutic doses of tetracycline 2 days before resection. The bone resected at surgery is then subjected to ultraviolet (UV) light. The nidus, if present, will give a golden fluorescence. Tetracycline labeling has also been recommended in osteosarcomas to evaluate skip metastasis.

When possible, it is recommended that the pathologist go into the operating room and view the biopsy procedure. This serves the dual purpose of aiding the surgeon to determine whether adequate tissue has been obtained and enabling the pathologist to see the gross aspects of the lesion.

As with any surgical specimen, proper fixation, appropriate choice, and thickness of blocks is key to obtaining adequate histologic sections. In addition, when bone or calcific areas are present, decalcification must be carried out. Many solutions are available for decalcification, all of which serve the purpose well. The pathologist must be careful that the tissues are not overdecalcified, as this will distort the osseous and soft tissue components. Since decalcified tissues seem to take up eosin rather avidly, in the staining process less time in eosin is advisable.

Intact, locally excised lesions and amputation specimens deserve special attention. In addition to adequate descriptions and measurements, radiologic examination of the intact and sliced specimen may be useful. Also, the radiologic studies may point out areas that may be of interest for histologic examination. For the smaller specimens, the slicing may be done with a sharp hand saw or a power band saw. Amputation specimens may be examined in two ways.[1] The specimen may be deep frozen and then cut sagitally or crosswise with a hand saw or power band saw with the soft tissues intact. This has the advantage of maintaining the relations of the soft tissues, particularly muscles and the neurovascular bundles, to the neoplasm. It has a disadvantage of resulting in freezing artifact in the subsequent histologic examinations. To circumvent freezing artifacts, it is suggested that blocks of the tumor be removed before the specimen is frozen. This ordinarily does not distort the specimen greatly, as a biopsy site is usually present.[2] The soft tissues are removed after careful notation of their relationship to the tumor; the specimen can be either fixed or cut fresh with a hand saw or a power band saw. After fixation of the slices, the blocks are selected. It may be desirable to indicate the site of the blocks diagrammatically in the event that careful radiologic and gross correlations are to be undertaken (Fig. 15-1). With amputation specimens, it is desirable to obtain marrow specimens proximal to the tumor to determine whether there are intramedullary sites of the neoplasm that were not detectable radiologically. In addi-tion, the amputation site should be examined histologically for the possibility of spread to this area. If there is transection of a bone rather than disarticulation, the proximal end of the bone is curetted by the orthopaedic surgeon at the time of the amputation and submitted as a separate specimen; frozen section may be done. If the amputation specimen includes lymph-node-bearing areas, the nodes, of course, should be isolated and examined. In all instances, photographic documentation of the gross specimen is helpful.

CLASSIFICATION OF BONE TUMORS

The classification of neoplasms of bone is and has been based on histologic patterns and on tissue or cell or origin, which in turn have, in general, correlated with the biologic behavior of the tumor.[2] Although this type of classification is not ideal, it has served a purpose in grouping lesions according to histologic patterns, representing a means of communication between and among physicians caring for patients and reporting in medical journals. There have been suggestions that classification be based on skeletal localization of the tumor or lesion. This has some merit in that many tumors have reasonably well defined localizations; for example, a large number of chondrosarcomas occur in the pelvic bones, and giant cell tumors appear to be epiphyseal and metaphyseal in location. However, there is considerable overlapping of locations, rendering this type of classification cumber-

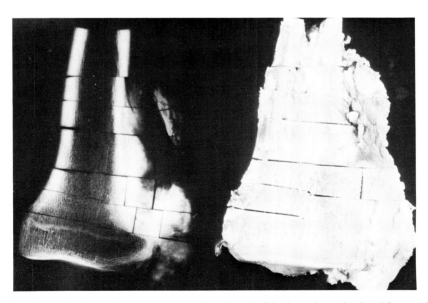

Fig. 15-1. Hemisection of a femoral osteosarcoma showing the blocks to be submitted for sectioning. A film of the specimen is to the left.

some. A classification based on etiologic factors would be meaningful, but in most instances, the etiology remains unknown. Even though classification based on histologic patterns is, at the moment, the most acceptable, there are weaknesses to be pointed out. The major one is that of the presence of a mixture of tissues in many tumors. For example, it is common to find malignant cartilage, malignant stroma, and malignant osteoid in an osteosarcoma, and one finds osteoid and cartilage in Ewing's sarcoma. The mixture of the histologic types that may be seen in any given neoplasm make the precise classification hazardous at times. Another weakness is the difficulty in always being able to define histologically osteoid versus collagen or chondroid material versus cartilage or in separating reactive lesions from true neoplasms. Experience resolves some but not all of the problems.

We have modified the WHO classification, which follows.

    I. Bone-forming tumors
      A. Benign
        1. Osteoma
        2. Osteoid osteoma and osteoblastoma (benign osteoblastoma)
      B. Indeterminate
        1. Aggressive osteoblastoma
      C. Malignant
        1. Osteosarcoma (osteogenic sarcoma)
        2. Juxtacortical osteosarcoma (parosteal osteosarcoma)
        3. Periosteal osteosarcoma
    II. Cartilage-forming tumors
      A. Benign
        1. Chondroma (enchondroma)
        2. Osteochondroma (osteocartilaginous exostosis)
        3. Periosteal chondroma
        4. Chondroblastoma (benign chondroblastoma, epiphyseal chondroblastoma)
        5. Chondromyxoid fibroma
      B. Malignant
        1. Chondrosarcoma
        2. Mesenchymal chondrosarcoma
        3. Dedifferentiated chondrosarcoma
        4. Clear cell chondrosarcoma
   III. Giant cell tumor
   IV. Marrow tumors
      1. Ewing's sarcoma
      2. Malignant lymphoma
      3. Myeloma
    V. Vascular tumors
      A. Benign
        1. Hemangioma
        2. Lymphangioma
        3. Glomus tumor (glomangioma)
      B. Intermediate or indeterminate
        1. Hemangiopericytoma
      C. Malignant
        1. Angiosarcoma (hemangioendothelioma)
   VI. Other connective tissue tumors
      A. Benign
        1. Desmoplastic fibroma
        2. Lipoma
      B. Malignant
        1. Fibrosarcoma
        2. Malignant fibrous histiocytoma
        3. Liposarcoma
        4. Malignant mesenchymoma
        5. Undifferentiated sarcoma
  VII. Other tumors
      1. Chordoma
      2. Adamantinoma of long bones
      3. Neurilemoma (schwannoma, neurinoma)
      4. Neurofibroma
      5. Parachordoma
      6. Primary neuroendocrine tumor
 VIII. Unclassified tumors
  IX. Tumor-like lesions
      1. Solitary bone cyst (simple or unicameral bone cyst)
      2. Aneurysmal bone cyst
      3. Juxta-articular bone cyst (intraosseous ganglion)
      4. Metaphyseal fibrous defect (nonossifying fibroma)
      5. Eosinophilic granuloma
      6. Fibrous dysplasia and ossifying fibroma
      7. Myositis ossificans
      8. Brown tumor of hyperparathyroidism
      9. Giant cell reaction
    10. Invasive benign lesions, e.g., pigmented villonodular synovitis
   X. Metastatic malignant neoplasms

BONE-FORMING TUMORS

Osteoma

Osteomas are uncommon bony lesions that are predominantly found in the paranasal sinuses, particularly the frontal sinus.[3] They may be seen at any age. Osteomas are uncommon in bone other than the paranasal sinuses; Dahlin and Unni[4] described two osteomas (tibia and rib) involving extracranial bones. Grossly, the lesions are rock hard and nodular, correlating with the radiologic findings of a radiodense, somewhat lobulated lesion. Cut surfaces of an osteoma demonstrate bone that is extremely dense and hard, similar to normal cortical bone. Histologically, the lesion consists of cortical bone with Haversian systems and broad bony trabeculae. The marrow space is consequently sparse. Osteoblasts are usually inconspicuous. Probably the osteoma does not have a malignant counterpart. It has been suggested that osteomas represent an end stage of fibrous dysplasia or of ossifying fibroma, especially those of the skull and jaws.

The lesions most likely to be confused with osteoma are bony spurs and osteochondromas. The bony spur is radiologically not as dense as the osteoma, nor is it lobular in pattern. The same holds true for the osteochondroma, which generally involves the metaphysis of long bones and has a pedicle that melds with the cortex. Histologically, a bony spur is likely to exhibit osteoblastic activity and does not have the extreme thickness of the bony trabeculae seen in osteoma. Osteochondromas are identified by a cartilaginous cap, but in the absence of a cartilaginous cap, islands of cartilage may be found in the bony trabeculae; the trabeculae are not as broad or dense as those of an osteoma.

Osteoid Osteoma

Osteoid osteoma is considered a benign neoplasm occurring predominantly in males in the pediatric age group. The majority (85 percent) occur between the ages of 5 and 24, and rarely before 5 or after 50 years. It is most commonly seen in the long bones, particularly the tibia and femur, although a wide variety of skeletal locations have been described. This is a lesion that may be diagnosed quite readily radiologically and often clinically.[5] The clinical presentation is classically that of pain in the affected part, for example, the thigh, with the pain being more severe during the night and relieved by aspirin. However, this clinical presentation represents the minority of patients having osteoid osteoma. Osteoid osteomas of the vertebra may produce pain that simulates intervertebral disc disease.[6] At times, scoliosis may be due to osteoid osteoma, which is said to be the most common cause of painful scoliosis in children.[7] Osteoid osteomas located near an articular surface, particularly the hip, may be associated with early onset of degenerative joint disease.[8]

Radiologically, one sees a zone of bony sclerosis, particularly if the osteoid osteoma involves the cortex of a long bone. Within the zone of sclerosis there is a radiolucency representing the nidus (Fig. 15-2). The amount of sclerosis surrounding the nidus is somewhat dependent on its location, with less seen in the periosteal and intramedullary localizations of the nidus. An abscess of bone may exhibit a similar radiologic picture.

Grossly, the nidus is hyperemic, round, and surrounded by a zone of sclerotic bone. The nidus usually measures 10 mm or less in diameter. Radiologic studies

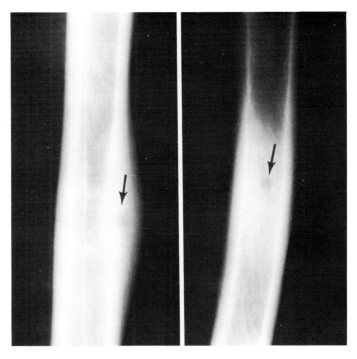

Fig. 15-2. Anteroposterior and lateral views of an osteoid osteoma of the femur. It is cortical in location and has resulted in bony sclerosis. Arrows indicate the nidus.

of the gross specimen may be helpful in locating the nidus, should it be inconspicuous. Histologically, there are poorly oriented bony trabeculae, some of which are heavily calcified and others which show less to no calcification. The irregular arrangement of the bony trabeculae serves to set the nidus off from the surrounding medullary or compact bone, which may be near normal (Fig. 15-3). Osteoblasts are abundant lining the trabeculae of the nidus (Fig. 15-4). Although large, they are uniform and do not show nuclear pleomorphism. Osteoclasts are quite frequent and of normal configuration. The intertrabecular stroma is loose areolar tissue and is vascular. There are no inflammatory cells. Only rarely have nerve fibers been demonstrated in the nidus.[9]

The differential diagnosis of osteoid osteoma includes osteomyelitis, osteoblastoma, and osteosarcoma. Bone abscesses may simulate osteoid osteoma radiologically. However, with a bone abscess, one expects to see an acute or chronic inflammatory infiltrate, but inflammation is not part of an osteoid osteoma. To be sure, osteoblasts are prominent in healing of osteomyelitis, but the trabeculae are not as irregularly arranged as in a nidus, and again evidence of inflammation is present. Osteoblastoma has an identical histologic pattern to that of osteoid osteoma and is therefore indistinguishable. The lesion is distinguished from osteoid osteoma on the basis of size, with the nidus of the osteoblastoma exceeding 2 cm in greatest dimensions. Radiologically, osteoblastoma

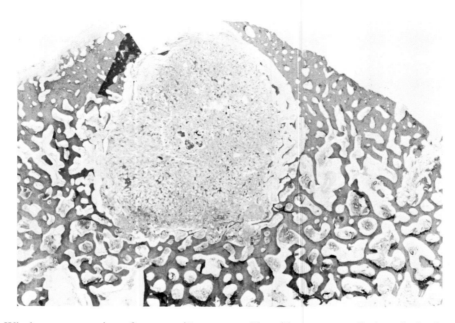

Fig. 15-3. Whole-mount section of an osteoid osteoma. The nidus seems to lie loosely in the surrounding sclerotic bone.

causes considerable less bony sclerosis than does osteoid osteoma.

Osteoid osteoma is only a problem, in relation to a diagnosis of osteosarcoma, when the nidus is curetted and the pathologist is unaware of the radiologic or clinical findings. Because of the numerous osteoblasts, the pathologist may be led into considering osteosarcoma. However, the osteoblasts of the nidus, although numerous, are not anaplastic and are orderly in their arrange-

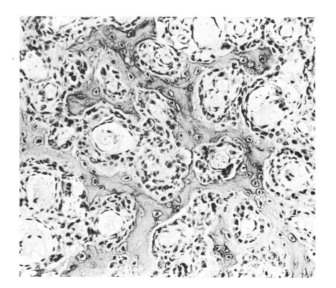

Fig. 15-4. Osteoid osteoma. Irregular partially mineralized bone, abundant osteoblasts, and numerous small blood vessels comprise the nidus.

ment about the bony trabeculae. The stroma is benign in contrast to that of osteosarcoma. Attention to the radiologic findings will alleviate any possibility of mistaking these two lesions.

Uninterrupted biologic behavior of the osteoid osteoma is obscure; there is evidence that they may regress occasionally.[9]

If the nidus is not completely removed, symptoms may persist or recur. It is possible that some "recurrences" are due to multicentric nidi.[10] There apparently is no malignant counterpart of osteoid osteoma.

Benign Osteoblastoma

Benign osteoblastoma occurs predominantly in males and in the pediatric age group, with most of the lesions diagnosed in the first three decades of life. The age range is 5 to 78 years.[11] Benign osteoblastoma is mostly localized to long bones and the vertebrae.[9] Osteoblastoma is less likely to provoke the outstanding bony sclerosis typical of osteoid osteoma. Radiologically, it is a lucent defect surrounded by a narrow zone of bony sclerosis. At times, the sclerosis may be as marked as that of osteoid osteoma. The nidus of an osteoblastoma measures 2 cm or more and may be as large as 10 cm. Because the lesion may be large and radiolucent, it may be mistaken for a more serious lesion radiologically, such as osteosarcoma.

Grossly, the nidus is hyperemic and often is loosely attached to the surrounding bone. It surfaces are somewhat nodular. The cut surfaces are red to reddish brown and gritty. Bone is evident. Histologically, it is similar to

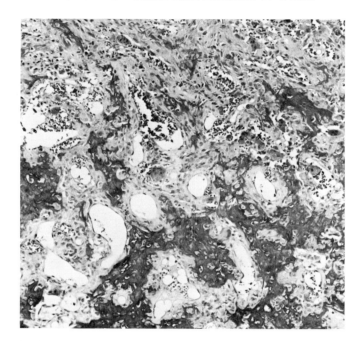

Fig. 15-5. Osteoblastoma. The similarity with osteoid osteoma is apparent. At higher magnification osteoblasts and osteoclasts are readily seen.

if not indistinguishable from osteoid osteoma (Fig. 15-5). It has been stated that the bony trabeculae of osteoblastoma are slightly wider than those of osteoid osteoma, and that there is less irregularity in their arrangement. The major histologic problem is differentiation between benign osteoblastoma and osteosarcoma and aggressive osteoblastoma. The problem arises only in those osteosarcomas that are osteoblastic (bone productive), since those with obviously malignant cartilage or stroma would not be problems. In osteosarcoma, the osteoblasts and osteocytes are pleomorphic. In addition, rather than the loose areolar connective tissue stroma seen in osteoblastoma, the stroma is malignant. The difficulty lies in the osteoblastomas in which there is more compactness to the bone and stroma, leading to increased cellularity. Radiographic studies may be an important aid in the difficult case.

Equally difficult to determine is the distinction between benign osteoblastoma and aggressive osteoblastoma.[11,12] In the latter lesion, the findings are those that suggest the possibility of osteosarcoma rather than an obviously benign lesion. In other words, the stroma rather than being loose areolar tissue may be compact and cellular, and there may be some osteoblastic pleomorphism and mitotic figures. If these findings are present, then one would consider the possibility of aggressive osteoblastoma or of osteosarcoma. In contrast to osteoid osteoma, a few acceptable cases of osteosarcoma arising either in association with or from an os-

teoblastoma have been reported, but this is a rare occurence.[12]

Aggressive osteoblastoma is designated as such partly on the basis of its clinical behavior and partly on the basis of its histologic features. Histologically, this tumor is not always easily defined, but Dorfman and Weiss[13] pointed out the feature of plump epithelioid osteoblasts that are helpful in distinguishing aggressive osteoblastoma from other osteoblastic tumors. In addition, it has been noted that the clinical behavior of these lesions is aggressive, in that recurrence is common, often with extension into adjacent tissues; recurrence may be massive. Differentiation of this lesion from osteosarcoma is difficult, if not impossible at times.

Osteosarcoma

Under the term osteosarcoma, several different malignant bone-producing tumors are identified. These lesions have as a common denominator the production of malignant osteoid, bone and/or cartilage and each has a distinct natural behavior. Until recently we have utilized the classification of osteosarcoma proposed by Dahlin and Unni[4]; however, based on Dahlin's concepts, Raymond et al.[14] have proposed a new classification that incorporates new developments and reorganizes existing concepts. In this classification, four major groups are considered: (1) conventional osteosarcoma, (2) osteosarcoma arising in special clinical settings, (3) osteosarcoma defined by histologic parameters, and (4) osteosarcoma arising on the surface of a bone (see Table 15-1). Conventional osteosarcoma is composed of a malignant, undif-

TABLE 15-1. Osteosarcoma Classification

Conventional
  Osteoblastic
  Chondroblastic
  Fibroblastic

Clinical variants
  Osteosarcoma of the jaws
  Postradiation osteosarcoma
  Osteosarcoma in Paget's disease of bone
  Multifocal osteosarcoma
  Osteosarcoma arising in benign conditions

Morphologic Variants
  Intraosseous well differentiated osteosarcoma
  Osteosarcoma resembling osteoblastoma
  Telangiectatic osteosarcoma
  Small cell osteosarcoma
  ? Dedifferentiated chondrosarcoma
  ? Malignant fibrous histiocytoma

Surface Variants
  Parosteal osteosarcoma
  Dedifferentiated parosteal osteosarcoma
  Periosteal osteosarcoma
  High-grade surface osteosarcoma

ferentiated stroma that produces osteoid and bone. Osteoblasts with pleomorphic, often bizarre nuclei and frequent mitoses are associated with the neoplastic osteoid and bone.

The osteocytes show similar cytologic features. In addition to these components, cytologically malignant cartilage and a stroma often resembling that of fibrosarcoma or malignant fibrous histiocytoma may be seen in osteosarcoma. Osteosarcoma has a peak occurrence in the second decade of life and occurs more frequently in males than in females. The lesion may be detected in any decade of life, but less frequently arising de novo in the older adult.[4,15]

Generally, the signs and symptoms caused by an osteosarcoma are nonspecific. The patient frequently complains of pain (which usually awakens the patient at night) and/or swelling in the affected part, commonly near the knee. Depending on the size of the mass, the swelling may be slight or marked. At times there may be heat and redness of the overlying skin. Often, there is a history of recent trauma that is considered to be a factor that calls the attention of the patient to a pre-existing lesion. Laboratory data are often noncontributory, although a few patients may have an elevated alkaline phosphatase level.

The major prebiopsy diagnostic procedure is the radiologic study (Fig. 15-6). A careful radiologic examination is important since it is often the first indication as to whether the lesion in question is benign or malignant and its probability of being an osteosarcoma. In addition, radiographs show the extent of the lesion, the presence or absence of a soft tissue component, the degree of destruction, and the degree of sclerosis, all of which may have a bearing on determining a biopsy site and perhaps on the site of resection or amputation. Arteriographic studies and skeletal scans are of help in determining whether or not there are skip areas of tumor within the medullary cavity. CT, MRI, and arteriography often add information about the extent of the neoplasm.

Either an incisional or needle biopsy will provide satisfactory tissue in a suspected osteosarcoma. However, a biopsy should not be done indiscriminately, since contamination of the soft tissues along with a poorly placed incision may handicap a limb salvage procedure.[1] In our hands, a needle biopsy often yields satisfactory results, in that an osteosarcoma can be identified.[1] Should there by any question about the diagnosis, an incisional biopsy is recommended. If an incisional biopsy is performed, then we recommend that a frozen section examination be done on a portion of the specimen to determine with certainty that lesional tissue has been obtained. In addition, as is our practice, we save a fragment of tissue for electron microscopic study, should it be needed and save tissue for flow cytometry. In addition to determining ade-

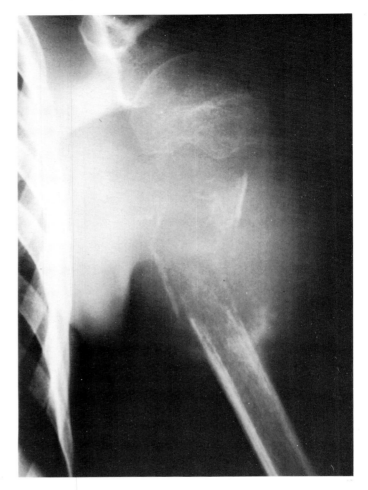

Fig. 15-6. Humeral osteosarcoma with a pathologic fracture. The lesion permeates the humerus and destroys cortex. The extraosseous component is evident.

quacy of the tissue, the frozen section examination will yield a specific diagnosis of osteosarcoma in many cases, and should an immediate amputation be advisable, this can be done on this basis. However, presently many of the treatment protocols for osteosarcoma call for preliminary dosages of a chemotherapeutic agent with delayed amputation or resection. Thus, a specific diagnosis of osteosarcoma from a frozen section may not be critical and should not be attempted if the pathologist is not familiar with the appearance of this tumor on frozen section.

The gross features of an osteosarcoma are somewhat varied, but there is destruction of the cortex and replacement of the medullary cavity by tumor that varies from gray-white to yellow-red. The firmness is also variable. Evidence of necrosis is frequent (Fig. 15-7). If a cartilaginous element is dominant, the lesion will have a shiny gray appearance. Often, the osteosarcomas are hyper-

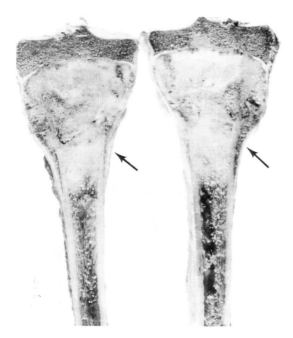

Fig. 15-7. Hemisection of a tibial osteosarcoma. The tumor is the gray-white area in the metaphysis. It has reached the growth plate. Periosteal reaction and extension of tumor are indicated by the arrows.

vascular, and there may be extensive areas of hemorrhagic necrosis and even cystic alteration. If this is a dominant pattern, then the tumor is probably a telangiectatic osteosarcoma. Periosteal reaction may be identified with evidence of bone production and spiculation. Destruction and permeation of the cortex lead to an extraosseous component of the osteosarcoma. If the growth plate has not closed, it serves as a barrier to the advance of the osteosarcoma into the epiphysis. In rare circumstances, osteosarcoma may penetrate the growth plate and even the articular cartilage. The interface of tumor and medullary bone is often quite distinct but may show slight sclerosis or evidence of fibrosis; tumor permeation may be subtle.

Histologically, the two outstanding and important features are the identification of a malignant stroma and malignant osteoblasts associated with osteoid and bone (Fig. 15-8). The stroma is usually undifferentiated or differentiated toward a fibrosarcomatous appearance. Foci of necrosis are common. In some osteosarcomas with abundant osteoid, the pattern of the osteoid is complex (filigreed) and is itself suggestive of osteosarcoma. At times, the osteoid is sparse and requires many blocks or step sections to identify neoplastic osteoid. It is not always easy to be certain of the presence of osteoid; special stains are not helpful. Only the rimming of the spicule by neoplastic osteoblasts serves to identify osteoid.

Conventional osteosarcoma has been subclassified based on the dominant tissue identified. There are three types: osteoblastic, chondroblastic, and fibroblastic.[4] In the latter two, even though malignant cartilage or a malignant fibrous stroma is dominant, malignant osteoid and bone are identifiable somewhere in the sections. Even though the malignant osteoid or bone is a minor element, the tumor is still designated as an osteosarcoma rather than chondrosarcoma or fibrosarcoma. Whether this subclassification will remain pertinent in the prognosis in relation to chemotherapy remains to be determined.

Morphologic variants of osteosarcoma include essentially three subgroups of lesions: high-grade, low-grade, and lesions that share some features with osteosarcoma.[14] The first group is represented by *telangiectatic osteosarcoma*[16,17] and *small cell osteosarcoma*.[14] Telangiectatic osteosarcoma includes in its definition the radiologic findings, which should be those of a totally lytic destructive lesion of the affected bone (Fig. 15-9). Grossly, these tumors are hemorrhagic, destructive, and often partly cystic and, since they contain large vascular channels (Fig. 15-10), they may be mistaken for aneurysmal bone cysts. Histologically, they are osteoblastic osteosarcomas, and with ample sampling malignant osteoid and stroma will be identified to distinguish the tumor from aneurysmal bone cyst. As with other tumors of bone, the radiologic features are an important aid in this regard. Just like telangiectatic osteosarcoma, small cell osteosarcoma occurs in the same age group and bone

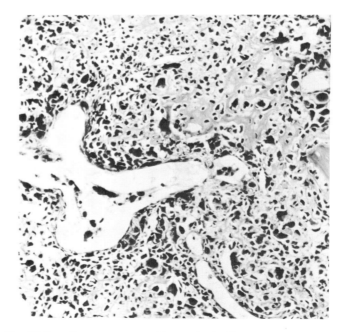

Fig. 15-8. Osteosarcoma with cytologically malignant osteoid and an undifferentiated stroma. The pleomorphism of the osteoblasts is evident.

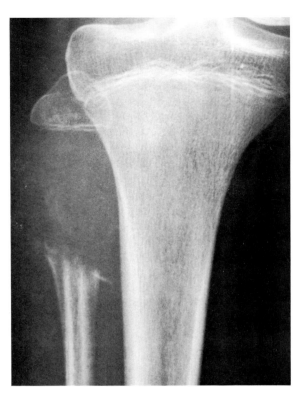

Fig. 15-9. Telangiectatic osteosarcoma of the fibula shows destruction of the metaphysis. At the lower end of the tumor, Codman's triangle represents periosteal reaction to tumor.

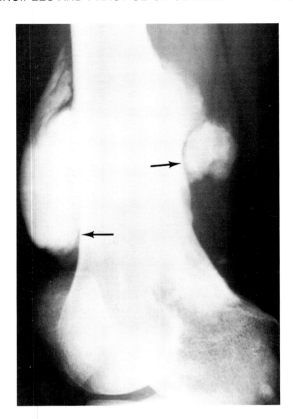

Fig. 15-11. Lobular radiodensity of parosteal osteosarcoma. Note zone of radiolucency, fairly characteristic of parosteal sarcoma (arrows). This lesion was recurrent in a 30-year-old woman.

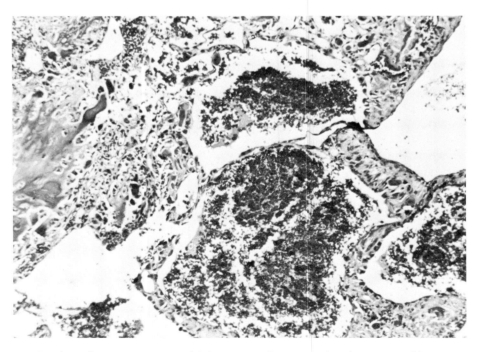

Fig. 15-10. Telangiectatic osteosarcoma with large vascular spaces bearing a resemblance to aneurysmal bone cyst.

location as conventional osteosarcoma. Radiologically, most lesions are mixed blastic and lytic, but occasionally a lesion may be entirely lytic. Histologically small cell osteosarcoma is composed of small round cells that can form three patterns: Ewing's-like, lymphoma-like, and spindle cell. Although these patterns simulate the histology of nonosteosarcoma entities, all cases show evidence of osteoid formation.[14]

Osteosarcoma resembling osteoblastoma and *well differentiated medullary osteosarcoma* are low-grade osteosarcomas.[18] The former lesion has histologic features that closely mimic osteoblastoma, but the neoplastic cells are much more atypical, with some mitotic activity, and the matrix is more complex than that of an osteoblastoma.[11] Well differentiated medullary osteosarcoma is more likely to be mistaken for a benign neoplasm or tumor-like lesion of bone than a malignant one. In the reported cases, the most frequent benign diagnosis made from a biopsy specimen was fibrous dysplasia, indicating the well differentiated pattern of the lesion. Histologically, it is the medullary counterpart of parosteal osteosarcoma. In contrast to telangiectatic osteosarcoma, which is particularly aggressive, well differentiated medullary osteosarcoma behaves in a rather indolent fashion and has a low rate of distant metastases.

Surface osteosarcomas include high-grade osteosarcoma,[14] parosteal osteosarcoma,[19,20] dedifferentiated parosteal osteosarcoma,[21] and periosteal osteosarcoma.[22,23] High-grade osteosarcoma on the surface is identical in morphology to conventional (medullary) osteosarcoma.[24] It is extremely rare and behaves as conventional osteosarcoma. *Parosteal osteosarcoma* is a low-grade osteosarcoma that occurs predominantly at the posterior distal end of the femur but may develop in other locations, and is more common in females. It affects patients in the third, fourth, and fifth decades of life. Radiologically, the lesions may be small, but if they develop, undiagnosed, for many years, they become large in bulk.

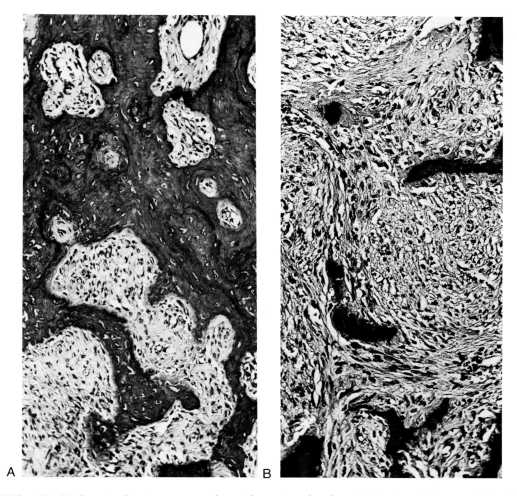

Fig. 15-12. (A, B) Parosteal osteosarcoma shows the mature but irregularly shaped bone and the slightly hypercellular stroma.

It is not unusual to see a tumor arising from the cortex of a bone showing extension around the entire shaft (Fig. 15-11). This lesions hould not have an intramedullary portion.

Histologically, the parosteal osteosarcoma has well differentiated bone and stroma that may vary little from normal.[19,20] The bony trabeculae may be poorly oriented and broad, but osteoblasts are not prominent. The stroma is fibrous and at least focally hypercellular (Fig. 15-12A,B). Cartilage may be present and rarely may form a cap. These tumors are often mistaken histologically for fibrous dysplasia and, because of the cartilage, for osteochondroma (Fig. 15-13). Occasionally, areas characteristic of conventional osteosarcoma may be present. When they occur, the tumor has dedifferentiated toward a high-grade tumor. Radiologically, the presence of large lytic areas, usually vascular angiographically, in a parosteal osteosarcoma make it suspect of dedifferention. Dedifferentiated parosteal osteosarcomas are more aggressive than parosteal osteosarcoma.[21]

Periosteal osteosarcoma also arises on the surface of a bone but, unlike parosteal osteosarcoma, occurs in a younger age group. The prognosis is similar to or better than that of conventional osteosarcoma, but worse than that of parosteal osteosarcoma. Histologically, it is composed of a malignant chondroblastic proliferation with minimal osteoid formation (Fig. 15-13).[22,23]

The *clinical* variants of osteosarcoma include those associated with Paget's disease or infarct of bone. In addition, it is well known that osteosarcoma complicates radiation therapy. Histologically, the osteosarcomas arising in these situations are similar to conventional osteosarcoma. Other variants include osteosarcoma of the jaws, multifocal osteosarcoma, and osteosarcoma associated with other benign conditions.

Conventional osteosarcoma frequently metastasizes to the lungs, massive metastases being a cause of death. Metastases to other visceral organs and bones are less common; metastases to regional lymph nodes occur in approximately 5 percent of patients. The five year survival rate for patients with osteosarcoma before chemotherapy was 15 to 20 percent. Since institution of the various treatment protocols, the prognosis has changed in regard to the 2 year and 5 year survival, although this may not be entirely attributable to chemotherapy.[24] Five year survival rate for patients with osteosarcoma is close

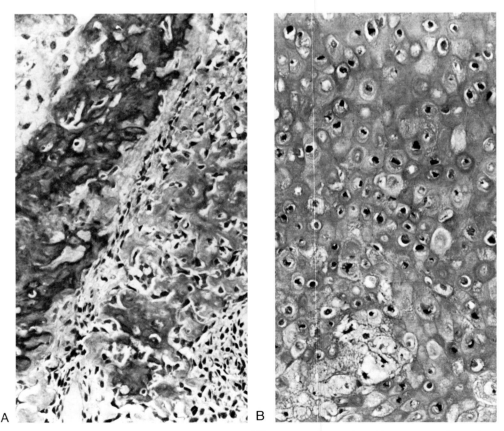

Fig. 15-13. (A, B) Periosteal osteosarcoma shows different patterns of malignant osteoid and a field of malignant cartilage.

to 65 percent. Tumor necrosis due to chemotherapy has been found to be an excellent prognostic factor in patients with conventional osteosarcoma who have been treated with intra-arterial infusion of cisplatin and systemic Adriamycin.[14] Approximately two thirds of patients with well differentiated osteosarcoma will survive 5 years or more. At least 50 percent of patients treated for parosteal osteosarcoma survived 5 or more years, even before the chemotherapeutic era, similar to expectations for patient treated for periosteal osteosarcoma.

CARTILAGINOUS TUMORS

Interpretation of cartilaginous tumors of the skeleton presents some of the most difficult histologic problems related to neoplasms of bone. This is especially true of the well differentiated chondrosarcomas that closely resemble the hyaline cartilage of osteochondromas and chondromas. By contrast, these two lesions may have chondrocytes that have nuclear atypicalities that correspond to the criteria accepted for chondrosarcoma. The proper histologic interpretation of cartilaginous tumors must include, in addition to adequate biopsy and well prepared slides, the clinical data, age of the patient, location of the tumor, its size, and a review of the radiographs of the tumor.[25]

Osteochondroma

Osteochondromas are the most common of the benign neoplasms of bone, representing approximately 45 percent of benign tumors.[25] They are cartilaginous-capped bony projections, often from the metaphyseal end of a tubular bone. The majority are discovered in patients less than 21 years of age, but they may be observed at almost any age. There seems to be a predominance in males.

Radiologically, an osteochondroma is a bony projection that seems to be an extension of the cortex. Often, the lesion has a readily visible pedicle topped by a lobular radiodense mass. The density varies with the amount of cartilage and with the degree of calcification of the cartilaginous component (Fig. 15-14). At the base of the osteochondroma, there is a continuation or sweeping up of the cortex into the pedicle of the osteochondroma. This feature serves to distinguish it from other lesions such as the parosteal osteosarcoma and localized myositis ossifcans.

Grossly, the anatomy of osteochondromas corresponds well to the radiologic appearance. The pedicle is bony, cortical, and cancellous, and the head consists of a combination of cartilage and bone. The cartilaginous cap varies to some degree in thickness, related to the age of

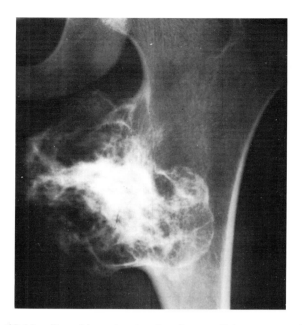

Fig. 15-14. Broad-based osteochondroma of the upper end of the femur. It is shown en face with the lobular nature and ossification evident. The sweep of the cortex into the pedicle is also seen at the top.

the patient; the younger the patient the thicker the cap may be. It may measured from 1 mm to 1 cm or more (Fig. 15-15). The cartilaginous surfaces are shiny, lobulated, gray-white, resembling hyaline cartilage. If calcification is present, it exhibits a yellow-white to dead-white coloration.

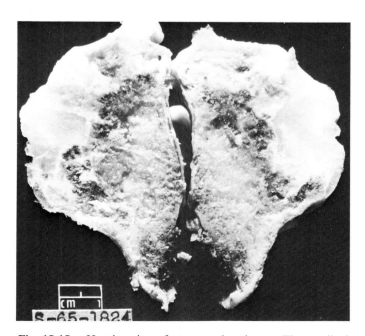

Fig. 15-15. Hemisection of an osteochondroma. The cartilaginous cap varies in thickness and is somewhat lobular.

Histologically, the cartilage is hyaline cartilage, which retains a normal organization of the chondrocytes. The nuclei of the chondrocytes tend to be small and without irregularity. Occasionally, one may encounter slightly enlarged abnormal nuclei. One histologic feature frequently seen in osteochondromas is evidence of enchondral bone formation, resembling an epiphyseal growth plate. Even in mature osteochondromas small islands of cartilage may be retained in the bony trabeculae. At times, it is difficult to distinguish large osteochondromas, up to 6 cm in greatest dimension, from a well differentiated peripheral chondrosarcoma. In such cases, the radiologic features, including the dimensions of the lesion, are helpful in arriving at a proper interpretation (those larger than 6 cm are suggestive of chondrosarcoma). Many blocks have to be taken of the cartilaginous component and have to be studied for nuclear atypia, enlarged nuclei, and binucleate cells. Because of the gross configuration of an osteochondroma, it is frequently considered that the peripheral type of chondrosarcomas arise from osteochondromas. This is difficult to prove, in that the larger lesions may no longer contain a benign component. However, it is accepted that patients having multiple hereditary exostoses have a higher risk of developing chondrosarcoma from one of their lesions.

Osteochondromas that are asymtomatic and solitary probably require no treatment, but those that become painful or have a protruding mass that is unsightly are properly treated by excision. For patients having multiple osteochondromas, it is impractical to excise each of the lesions. Thus, excision is reserved for those that apparently increase in size or otherwise become symptomatic.

Enchondroma

The enchondroma (chondroma) is a common tumor, but less so than osteochondroma. It occurs about equally in males and females and is commonly located in the small bones of the hand.[4] However, it may be seen in almost any of the bones, tubular or flat. It occurs at all ages, but most often before the fourth decade. It is usually asymptomatic, but it may occasionally cause pain. Frequently it is detected on routine radiologic examination done for some other reason. Occasionally, pathologic fractures may occur. Enchondromas may occur as multiple lesions and cause deformity of the affected bones. A person having multiple enchondromas (*Ollier's disease*) has a high risk of chondrosarcoma.

Radiologically, enchondromas of the bones of the hands are radiolucent and have a multilobular appearance with some slight deformity of the bone and thinning of the cortex. At times, evidence of calcification is noted, and this has a fluffy radiodense appearance; it may be semilunar or circular in contour, reflecting the lobular nature of the cartilaginous tumor. In the long bones, for example, the upper end of the humerus or the upper end of the femur, the calcification may be so dense that it resembles infarction of bone. Enchondromas may be large, measuring several centimeters in length, and have a somewhat lobular appearance, resulting in scalloping of the internal cortical surface.

Grossly, enchondromas are gray shiny cartilage with white or yellow-white areas that represent calcification. Enchondromas resected intact may show scalloping of the inner cortex. Most enchondromas are treated by curettage, thus only fragments of hyaline cartilage are available for gross examination.

Histologically, the neoplastic cartilage maintains, to some extent, the normal hyaline cartilage pattern of the chondrocytes. In many specimens, there may be evidence of mucoid degeneration of the matrix and nuclear abnormalities that raise the possibility of a malignancy (Fig. 15-16). Even though the small enchondromas may have histologic alterations to suggest malignancy, they should be considered as benign. Many of the larger lesions have fewer atypicalities of the nuclei than do the smaller ones. With the larger lesions, one considers more strongly the possibility of malignancy when nuclear atypicalities become more abundant and the patient has symptoms, particularly pain. The distinction from grade I chondrosarcoma may be difficult, if not impossible. Biopsy specimens of multiple enchondromas and solitary enchondromas are histologically similar.

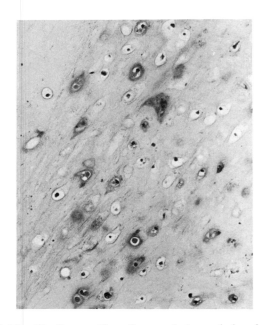

Fig. 15-16. Hyaline cartilage from a phalangeal chondroma. A few large nuclei are evident but do not signify malignancy.

Chondromyxoid Fibroma

Chondromyxoid fibroma (CMF) is a benign tumor of bone that combines connective tissue and chondroid and myxoid components. The lesion is most commonly found in metaphyses of the tubular bones, being quite uncommon in the flat bones such as the ribs, skull, sternum, and the pelvic bones.[26] The two bones most commonly involved are the femur and tibia. There is a slight predominance of the lesion in males, and it has a wide age range, but the lesion is most commonly seen in patients younger than 40 with a peak before 20 years. The patients often seek medical aid because of pain and swelling over the affected part. This may be of several weeks' or months' duration. At times, the patient may seek medical aid because of a pathologic fracture through the lesion.

Radiologically, CMF is metaphyseal, eccentrically located, well circumscribed, and radiolucent and appears to be multilobulated. The margins show a thin rim of bony sclerosis, but there may be destruction of the cortex. In some lesions, bony sclerosis may dominate much of the pattern. In the smaller bones, the bony contours will be deformed.

Excised specimens are grossly lobulated, solid, somewhat firm, and gray-white with tan areas. The tumor has a cartilaginous texture but usually lacks the slimyness that one might expect from the myxoid component. The cortex is often expanded and may be eroded. The periosteum serves to confine the tumor.

The microscopic pattern reflects the gross pattern in that a lobular outline is often maintained by thin fibrous trabeculae traversing the lesion. Chondromyxoid fibromas are quite varied, being predominantly myxoid with small chondroid areas intermingled with fibrous or collagenized zones. The lobules are outlined by peripheral congregation of spindled cells and occasional multinucleated giant cells. From the periphery toward the center of the lobules (Fig. 15-17), there is decreasing cellularity. In the central areas, the myxoid features are identified by the elongation of cytoplasmic processes that give somewhat of a stellate pattern to many cells (Fig. 15-18). Often, the nuclei are somewhat enlarged, perhaps hyperchromatic, and slightly irregular in outline. Because of this, the lesion may be mistaken for a chondrosarcoma. Focally, calcification may be seen.

These lesions are best treated by curettage, particularly when located in bones in which it is important to preserve the function of the bone or nearby joint. In small bones or flat bones where local en bloc excision is possible, this should be undertaken. There is a risk of local recurrence estimated to be approximately 25 percent.[27] For all practical purposes, the lesion is benign, with only rare cases recorded that presumably have undergone a

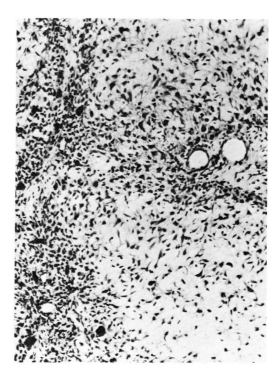

Fig. 15-17. Chondromyxoid fibroma. The lobular pattern is outlined by congregation of cells with few cells in the center.

malignant transformation.[21] These cases are open to question as one may wonder whether the original diagnosis of CMF was correct. In other words, the lesion may have been a chondrosarcoma originally and at the second examination.

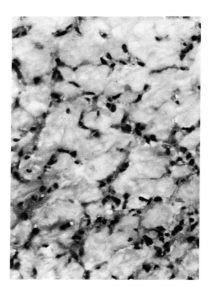

Fig. 15-18. Chondromyxoid fibroma. Cells in the myxoid center of a lobule.

Benign Chondroblastoma

Chondroblastoma is a cartilaginous tumor with a predilection for an epiphyseal localization in long bones, with a predominance in the upper end of the humerus and tibia and the lower end of the femur. Flat bones such as the sternum, ribs and pelvis are involved rarely.[28] It is seen most commonly in the male and in the second decade of life.[4] Clinically, chondroblastoma causes pain near or in the affected joint. Often, the pain seems more severe than would be expected from the size of the lesion. There may be evidence of swelling, but this is not especially common; pathologic fractures are infrequent.

Radiologically, a benign chondroblastoma should be suspected in any teenager who has a radiolucent lesion involving the epiphyseal end of a long bone (Fig. 15-19). Chondroblastomas are often multilobular with well defined sclerotic margins. They may be small, measuring 1 or 2 cm in greatest dimension, or so large as to involve the entire epiphyseal-metaphyseal portion of a long bone. The large lesions may be destructive of cortex and may alter the gross form of the bone. Some chondroblastomas are lightly to heavily calcified. Because of the calcification, chondroblastomas originally had been named calcifying epiphyseal giant cell tumor.

Grossly, the intact lesions are well demarcated from the surrounding bone. They may be ovoid to rounded and have a lobular pattern, as do most cartilaginous tumors. The cut surfaces are shiny gray to blue-gray to gray-yellow and suggest cartilage. Calcium deposits are seen as white to yellow-white material. If considerable calcium is present, the cut surfaces are gritty. Occasionally, a benign chondroblastoma is partially cystic, and rare lesions may be predominantly cystic. In the latter situation, a small nubbin of chondroblastoma may persist on one wall of the cyst.

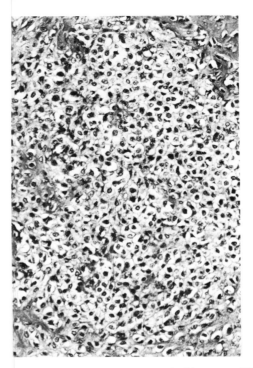

Fig. 15-20. Cellular pattern of a chondroblastoma. The chondroblasts are rounded with almost colorless to colorless cytoplasm. The cell outlines are frequently distinct.

Histologically, benign chondroblastoma is often richly cellular and therefore is mistaken for malignant tumors, especially chondrosarcoma. Multinucleate giant cells may be common, and for this reason a pathologist may diagnose giant cell tumor. However, the basic cells of the lesion are round with round to ovoid nuclei (Fig. 15-20). The cell boundaries are often quite distinct, and the cytoplasm varies from acidophilic to almost colorless. There

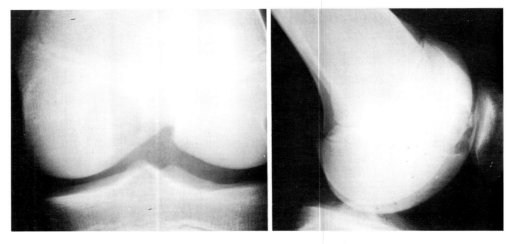

Fig. 15-19. Chondroblastoma of the femoral epiphysis. Note the open growth plate.

NEOPLASMS AND TUMOR-LIKE LESIONS OF BONE

are variations of this cell, even to the extent of being spindled. Small amounts of chondroid material may be identified, and in some lesions, it may be a major component. Calcification is frequently seen in undecalcified sections. The typical pattern of calcification is the outlining of individual chondroblasts to form a delicate network. Fibrosis, cystic alteration, and areas that resemble aneurysmal bone cyst may be found in chondroblastomas. Electron microscopic studies have demonstrated that the basic cell of this lesion is compatible with a chondroblast.[29]

Most chondroblastomas are treated by curettage. The recurrence rate may be as high as 40 percent.[29]

Chondroblastoma is generally considered a benign tumor, but there have been individual cases reported of pulmonary metastases.[30] The pulmonary metastases maintain the histologic appearance of the primary benign chondroblastoma. Most of the metastases followed multiple attempts at resection of the chondroblastoma; it is possible that the metastases were the result of the surgical procedures. At any rate, the risk of malignant transformation of benign chondroblastoma must be small.

Periosteal Chondroma

A periosteal chondroma is a benign cartilaginous tumor that apparently arises from the periosteum.[31] It erodes the underlying cortical bone to form a cup-shaped or saucer-like alteration of the cortex. The surrounding cortical bone becomes sclerotized. The most common sites are the phalanges and long bones.

Grossly, periosteal chondroma is a well circumscribed lesion that is confined to the cortex with its outer surface being covered by periosteum. The margins are well demarcated from the surrounding cortex, and the cut surfaces demonstrate a somewhat lobular cartilaginous tumor that is blue-gray to gray-white with evidence of calcification. Histologically, the lesion is composed of hyaline cartilage, and often one finds atypical nuclei that suggest the possibility of a chondrosarcoma. However, it has been demonstrated that these lesions do not metastasize despite atypical histologic findings. The ideal form of therapy is en bloc excision; local recurrence has been reported.[31] Periosteal chondrosarcoma may mimic periosteal chondroma radiologically and histologically. The former is more aggressive radiologically; histologically, it often invades the soft tissues.[32]

Chondrosarcoma

Chondrosarcoma is the second most common primary malignant tumor of bone—osteosarcoma is the most common.[25] In contrast to osteosarcoma, chondrosarcoma occurs at a later age, being more frequently seen in the fourth, fifth, and sixth decades. It is found predominantly in males.[4,25,33] Chondrosarcoma may occur at any site in the skeleton, with a preference for the pelvis and upper end of the femur; the ribs represent the next most common single site.

Most patients with chondrosarcoma will seek medical aid because of a mass or swelling at the site of the lesion. Frequently, there is associated discomfort or pain.

Radiologically and grossly, chondrosarcoma may be divided into two types: (1) a peripheral type that arises from the surface of a bone and grows into the surrounding tissues and (2) a central type that arises in the medullary cavity of the bone.[34] Radiologically, the peripheral form is quite characteristic and is often specifically diagnosable. It is a cauliflower-shaped mass that varies in its degree of calcification (Fig. 15-21). The shape is due to its lobulation, and calcification around and within the lobules accounts for the semilunar- and ring-shaped calcifications that are quite specific for cartilaginous tumors. Often with proper imaging studies an attachment of a chondrosarcomatous mass can be seen to the underlying bone; this aids in planning the surgical procedure.

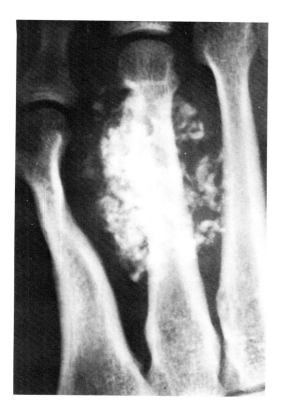

Fig. 15-21. Peripheral chondrosarcoma of a metatarsal. The fluffy calcification and the ring forms of calcification are prominent.

Central chondrosarcomas have radiologic features similar to those of enchondromas. They may be heavily calcified and may mimic infarcts of bone. Different degrees of cortical erosion are present, and if the cortex is penetrated, this would be an important sign of underlying chondrosarcoma. At times an extraosseous component may be large and mask the fact that the lesion began as a central chondrosarcoma.

Grossly, chondrosarcoma is a lobular mass of cartilage that on cut surface is shiny gray to gray-white (Fig. 15-22). Variable amounts of bone and calcium may be visible grossly. The central chondrosarcomas reside in the medullary cavity of bone, causing varied degrees of erosion of the inner surfaces of the cortex. The margins may be infiltrative, isolating fragments of cancellous bones. Yellow-white to white areas of calcium deposition may be seen and palpated throughout the lesion. Chondrosarcomas are variable in size, with peripheral chondrosarcomas generally measuring more than 5 cm in greatest dimension and occasionally exceeding 20 or 25 cm. Central chondrosarcomas likewise vary in size, measuring up to 8 or 10 cm. They are often elongated because of their location within the medullary cavity.

Histologically, the diagnosis of chondrosarcoma may be difficult, particularly when dealing with the well differentiated lesions. In such cases, the hyaline cartilage of the tumor closely resembles normal. In a case of well differentiated chondrosarcoma, the radiologic features often may be more helpful than the histologic examination in arriving at a diagnosis. Nevertheless, histologic examination is important and requires that many blocks be taken. Among the slides, one is searching for nuclear changes, which comprise binucleate cells and enlarged nuclei of the chondrocytes. If these are found, with the proper radiologic and gross features, then one can diagnose well differentiated chondrosarcoma. Chondrosarcomas have been graded according to the degree of nuclear alteration (Fig. 15-23). Grade I lesions are characterized by a marked preponderance of small densely staining nuclei, absence of cellular areas, and lack of mitoses. Grade II tumors are those in which evidence of malignancy is more easily found. The nuclei are medium sized, occasionally large, with visible intranuclear detail, and cellular areas are evident. Rarely, one may find mitoses; when present, fewer than two mitoses per 10 high-power fields (HPF) should be found. Histologically, grade III tumors are obviously malignant with cellular areas that contain two or more mitoses per 10 HPF.[33]

Grading is related to survival. Grade I chondrosarcomas are locally aggressive tumors with potential for recurrence and absence of metastases, while grade III lesions have high potential for metastases. Grade II lesions rarely metastasize. In addition to grading, it is important to note the matrix. In well differentiated lesions, the matrix is often densely hyaline, whereas in the lesions that become less well differentiated, one is more likely to encounter mucoid alteration of the matrix, giving it a less dense appearance. The histologic findings of peripheral and central chondrosarcomas are similar. One may encounter bone within the chondrosarcomas; this is not an indication of osteosarcoma. This bone does not have the cytologic features of malignancy, even though it is part of the neoplasm. Should bone or osteoid be encountered that have features of malignancy, then the lesion should be classified as a chondroblastic osteosarcoma. Most chondrosarcomas fall into grades I and II; approximately 20 percent are poorly differentiated.[33,34] In general, the recurrences and metastases reflect the grade of the original lesion. Occasionally, after repeated recurrences, the chondrosarcoma may take on a higher degree of malignancy.

The ideal form of therapy for chondrosarcoma is complete ablation of the lesion. This, however, means sacrifice of a limb or even a greater portion of the body in many instances. Recognizing the fact that the major problem is local recurrence for well-differentiated lesions (grade I), one should consider procedures that will preserve the function of a part or a limb. Thus, well planned en bloc resections of either peripheral or central chondrosarcomas are often undertaken. In the case of chondrosarcomas localized to the bony pelvis, a hemipelvectomy may be considered the only means of ablating the tumor, but for many smaller lesions, lesser procedures can be

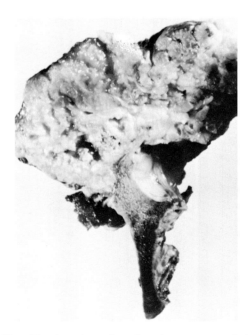

Fig. 15-22. Hemisection of a chondrosarcoma of the ilium. The lobular features are prominent.

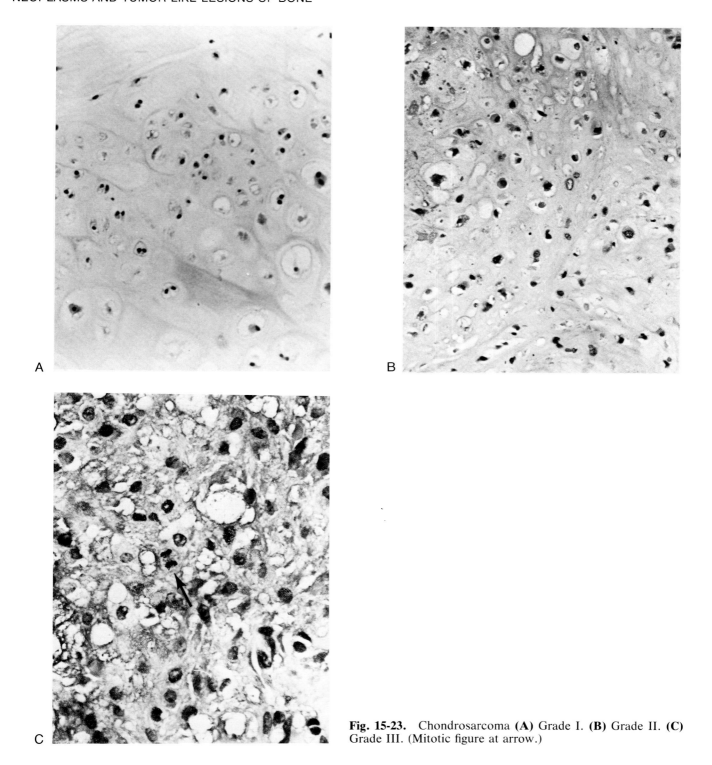

Fig. 15-23. Chondrosarcoma **(A)** Grade I. **(B)** Grade II. **(C)** Grade III. (Mitotic figure at arrow.)

accomplished with success. The same holds true for central chondrosarcomas in which amputation may be necessary to ablate the lesion. However, it is possible to resect portions of the femur or of the tibia, for example, and replace them with a prosthesis or a homograft.

Chondrosarcomas are slowly evolving tumors that in many instances have been present for years before having become clinically apparent. This is reflected in the behavior of the chondrosarcomas after therapy, in that a major problem with well differentiated lesions is local recurrence.[33] Some patients may have multiple excisions over a number of years before the recurrences become so massive as to make their resection impossible. The poorly differentiated chondrosarcomas are more aggressive and more likely to metastasize. Factors related to prognosis include location, size of tumor, histologic grade, and the DNA content of the chondrocytes.[25] The overall 5 year survival rate for patients with chondrosarcoma is 28 to 53 percent; but for those accepting treatment, it may be as high as 76 percent. Likewise, the overall 10 year survival rate is near 39 percent; but for those patients accepting treatment, it may be as high as 69 percent.[36]

Variants of chondrosarcoma are mesenchymal chondrosarcoma, dedifferentiated chondrosarcoma, and clear cell chondrosarcoma. *Mesenchymal chondrosarcoma* resembles ordinary chondrosarcoma both radiologically and grossly. An interesting feature is that about one third of cases arise in nonskeletal sites, such as meninges or thigh. Histologically, it is composed of malignant cartilage associated with an undifferentiated stromal component (Fig. 15-24). These tumors have a high risk of local recurrence and seem to metastasize more widely than do other chondrosarcomas to unusual sites such as liver, lymph nodes, kidneys, and brain. The lungs are the most common site of metastases, however. Although survival

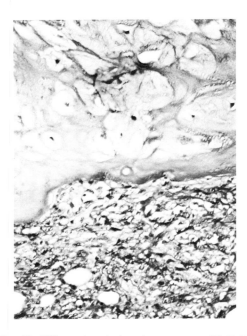

Fig. 15-25. Dedifferentiated chondrosarcoma. Well differentiated chondrosarcoma in the upper half of the field, undifferentiated sarcoma in the lower half.

may be prolonged, the long-term survival is poor, reported as 27 percent at 10 years.[37]

Dedifferentiated chondrosarcoma consists of malignant cartilage and an undifferentiated sarcomatous component. The tumor may occur in a patient previously treated for a well differentiated chondrosarcoma. During the follow-up period, a rather rapidly progressing recurrence appears. Other dedifferentiated chondrosarcomas are discovered as such without a known intervening chondrosarcoma. Radiographically, the tumor may simulate a central chondrosarcoma, but often there is considerable expansion and destruction indicative of a malignancy. Grossly, the cartilaginous portion may be identified, but the undifferentiated portion may be dominant and suggestive of a sarcoma other than chondrosarcoma. Histologically, it is identifiable by portions of well differentiated chondrosarcoma associated with a component that may have characteristics of fibrosarcoma, osteosarcoma, or anaplastic sarcoma (Fig. 15-25). The prognosis is poor, with most patients (about 90 percent) dying within 5 years.[38]

Clear cell chondrosarcoma varies radiologically from ordinary chondrosarcoma in that it may involve the epiphysis of a long bone, thus simulating a chondroblastoma.[39] Calcification in this tumor is not as common as in ordinary chondrosarcoma. It frequently expands a bone and is predominantly lytic radiologically. Grossly, it is not always recognized as being cartilaginous, since some

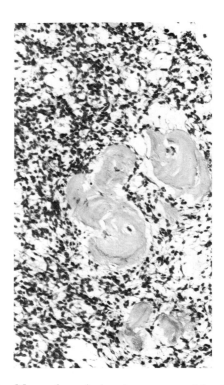

Fig. 15-24. Mesenchymal chondrosarcoma. Islands of cartilage in an undifferentiated stroma.

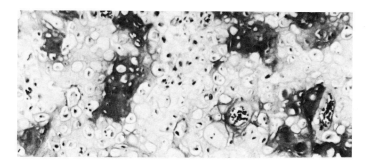

Fig. 15-26. Clear cell chondrosarcoma. Large clear cells and nuclear aberrations are apparent. The resemblance to chondroblastomatous cells can be seen (see Fig. 15-20).

clear cell chondrosarcomas are cystic and have been mistaken for aneurysmal bone cysts. Histologically, the tumor is made up of large cells that have colorless to faintly acidophilic to densely acidophilic cytoplasm (Fig. 15-26). It is because of the cells that have the colorless cytoplasm that the tumor has been given its name. In some lesions, the more conventional form of well differentiated chondrosarcoma may be seen. There may be patterns of calcification that resemble that seen in chondroblastoma. This, along with the cell pattern and the radiologic involvement of an epiphyseal end of bone, has suggested the possibility that clear cell chondrosarcomas are related to chondroblastoma. However, about one third of these patients have died of their disease.

Another form of chondrosarcoma is the *extraosseous chondrosarcoma*. This lesion apparently arises in the soft tissues and is radiologically, grossly, and histologically similar to conventional chondrosarcoma. To date, data on the biologic behavior of the lesion are sparse. Extraskeletal myxoid chondrosarcoma is similar but has myxoid areas that in themselves may be mistaken for carcinoma. It has a tendency for local recurrence and may metastasize to lymph nodes.[40]

GIANT CELL TUMOR

Giant cell tumor is a neoplasm that develops from mesenchymal cells with differentiation toward fibroblast-like stroma, multinucleate giant cells, and a mixture of other cells, predominantly inflammatory. It is a tumor of bone that can be suspected on the basis of the radiologic and clinical features. It rarely occurs in the pediatric age group or after the age of 50. The peak incidence is within the third and fourth decades of life, and it occurs more frequently in females than in males. Giant cell tumor has been reported as occurring in most bones, with a predominance in the distal end of the femur and in the proximal end of the tibia.[4,41] Only rarely has giant cell tumor occurred in multiple skeletal sites.[42] Thus, a patient in the late teens or in the third or fourth decade with swelling around the knee and with indicative radiologic findings should be strongly suspected of having a giant cell tumor.

Radiologically, the characteristic giant cell tumor has a metaphyseal and epiphyseal component. Without an epiphyseal component, the lesion is not readily diagnosable. The features of the lesion are those of a radiolucent expanding lesion, often with indistinct margins but at times with quite distinct and sclerotic margins. The cortex becomes attenuated and almost imperceptible. In the large tubular bones, the entire width of the bone may be involved. In the small tubular bones, the entire bone may be involved and in effect may be destroyed. An important radiologic feature is extension of the tumor to abut on the articular cartilage (Fig. 15-27). At times, the giant cell tumor will penetrate the cortex and have an extraosseous component.

Grossly, giant cell tumors are gray-white to gray-red to red-brown and well circumscribed and, as would be expected from the radiologic findings, extend to and abut on the articular cartilage. They are often hemorrhagic (sometimes predominantly) and may be partly cystic. Occasionally, there will be areas of fibrosis, which may be extensive. Because of the presence of histiocytes, which in some cases may be numerous, yellow areas may be distinguished.

Histologically, giant cell tumor is identifiable by the myriad multinucleate giant cells that are usually dispersed throughout the tumor (Fig. 15-28) except in areas of degeneration or fibrosis. The intervening stroma is somewhat variable, composed of rounded to spindle-shaped cells; often the rounded cells predominate. Foamy macrophages, scattered inflammatory cells such as lymphocytes and plasma cells, and hemosiderin are often present. Giant cell tumors have been and are graded histologically, but recent studies indicate that the grade does not necessarily correspond to the aggressiveness. For this reason, there is a tendency among pathologists to discard grading. The degree of aggressiveness displayed by giant cell tumor radiologically more closely relates to its behavior than does histologic grading.[43] Electron microscopic studies[44,45] suggest that the basic cell of giant cell tumor is the mononuclear stromal cell. These may be of fibroblastic origin, or perhaps histiocytic. The multinucleate giant cells are considered to be the result of fusion of stromal cells. This is borne out by immunohistochemical studies that indicate that the multinucleated giant cell originates from mononuclear phagocytes.[46]

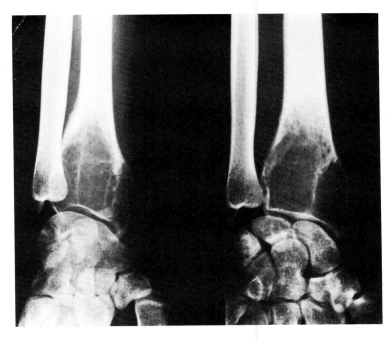

Fig. 15-27. Giant cell tumor of a metacarpal from a 22-year-old woman. The bone is expanded, and about two thirds of the length of the bone is involved by the radiolucent tumor. The lobulated character of the tumor is responsible for the bubbled effect.

Metastases from giant cell tumors are identical to the primary lesion. For the most part, metastases from giant cell tumors have occurred only after surgical intervention, the implication being that they are iatrogenic. Metastases are overwhelmingly pulmonary.

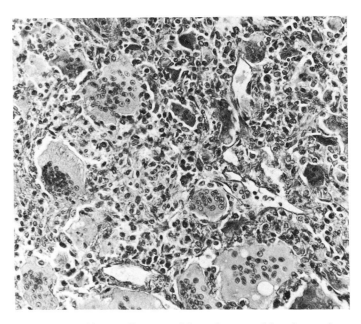

Fig. 15-28. Giant cell tumor. Many large multinucleate giant cells are seen in a vascular stroma in which the cells are rounded to spindle-shaped.

The ideal form of therapy for a giant cell tumor is ablation of the lesion. However, this is not always practical since the majority occur near a major joint. Thus, the decision to sacrifice the function of a major joint for a lesion that in most instances behaves as a benign tumor is difficult. Because of this, curettage of giant cell tumor has been a common means of treatment. However, the local recurrence rate is high, exceeding 50 percent[43]; from this standpoint, it is unacceptable, and other means of treatment have been devised. These include cryosurgery, radiation therapy, and resection of the tumor with replacement of the bone and joint with an allograft or a prosthetic joint. Resection has resulted in a decrease in local recurrence.[25,43]

Histologically, giant cell tumor presents a wide range of differential diagnostic possibilities, as almost any disease of bone may exhibit multinucleate giant cells. A lesion commonly mistaken for giant cell tumor is the fibrous cortical defect or nonossifying fibroma. However, this lesion is diagnosable radiologically, as has been described previously. The pathologist confronted with a lesion with many multinucleate giant cells should review the radiographs to determine the precise site of the lesion. Aside from the characteristic radiologic findings, most nonossifying fibromas will have a storiform stromal pattern reminiscent of fibrous histiocytoma. This histologic pattern is also seen in giant cell tumors but is not dominant.

Brown tumors secondary to hyperparathyroidism are

indistinguishable histologically from giant cell tumor, but again the radiologic findings and a serum calcium and phosphorus study should serve to differentiate the two lesions without difficulty.

Giant cell reparative granuloma occurs mainly in the jaws, but a number have been described in other bones, particularly of the hands and feet.[47,48] Histologically, they may be indistinguishable from giant cell tumor. Usually they have fewer and smaller multinucleate giant cells and considerably more stroma, which is more likely to be fibrous. The giant cells have a tendency to congregate around areas of hemorrhage, in contrast to the usually more diffuse distribution seen in giant cell tumors. In addition, there may be evidence of bone production, although osteoid and cartilage may also be found in the genuine giant cell tumor. Multinucleate giant cells will be found in a wide variety of lesions, including chronic osteomyelitis, Paget's disease of bone, eosinophilic granuloma, healing fracture, benign chondroblastoma, osteosarcoma, and nodular tenosynovitis or pigmented villonodular synovitis that invades bone. If close attention is paid to the pathologic, clinical, and radiologic findings, the pathologist is not likely to mistake these lesions for a genuine giant cell tumor.

Malignant giant cell tumors may arise from nontreated benign giant cell tumors, but most patients have had previous surgical treatment with added irradiation.[49] To confirm this transformation, one should endeavor to demonstrate histologically benign areas in an otherwise malignant tumor. Malignant giant cell tumors are rare and occur at a slightly older age than the usual giant cell tumor. They are most commonly seen at the distal end of the femur or at the proximal end of the tibia. Radiologically, there is evidence of a malignant lesion in that there is widespread destruction of bone, appearing diffusely radiolucent. Most malignant giant cell tumors are fibrosarcomas; a few are osteosarcomas. Survival is poor, with a death rate of 68 percent.[49]

MARROW TUMORS

Ewing's Sarcoma

Ewing's sarcoma, comprising approximately 5 to 6 percent of all malignant bone tumors, is basically an undifferentiated malignant neoplasm that apparently has its origin in the primitive mesenchyme. Recent studies indicate that these cells may differentiate into cells with mesenchymal, epithelial, or, at times, neural features.[50] Other studies using cell cultures from Ewing's sarcoma and immunohistochemical techniques indicate that Ewing's sarcoma may be of neural origin.[51] Almost all skeletal sites have been the source of Ewing's sarcoma.

In addition, a Ewing's sarcoma-like lesion has been identified in the extraskeletal soft tissues. The femur, humerus, and tibia are the most common locations of Ewing's sarcoma of the long bones, and the ilium and ribs are the most frequently involved flat bones.[4,25]

Ewing's sarcoma is mainly a disease of childhood and adolescence, with at least 80 percent of the lesions occurring before the age of 30 and the majority between the ages of 10 and 20 years. Females are less frequently affected than males.[4,25]

The majority of patients complain of pain and swelling in the area of the tumor. There may be altered function of adjacent joints. Fever, anemia, elevated sedimentation rate (ESR), and occasionally leukocytosis may be present. Pathologic fractures are infrequent.

Radiologically, Ewing's sarcoma has a variety of patterns. It may cause considerable sclerosis or may be radiolucent with sclerotic areas (Fig. 15-29). Often it expands and deforms the bone to some degree. Ewing's sarcoma provokes considerable periosteal reaction (immature) in most cases. It is a permeative lesion, thus having indistinct boundaries. The periosteal layering (onion skin effect) is said to be characteristic, but not necessarily specific for Ewing's sarcoma. Although the radiologic features are not specific, they nearly always suggest a malignant tumor. In fact, a young person having a radiologically malignant lesion of a flat bone has a strong possibility of Ewing's sarcoma. Eosinophilic granuloma and osteomyelitis are two non-neoplastic diseases that may closely mimic Ewing's sarcoma.

It is not often that intact gross specimens are available for examination. Usually, only a biopsy is done of the tumor, and the surgeon encounters a soft, somewhat hemorrhagic, gray-pink to gray-red tissue that resembles lymphoid tissue. In those few specimens that are resected, there is evidence of permeation by the sarcoma of the medullary cavity, with extension through the cortex into the surrounding soft tissues. The cut surfaces are homogeneous, gray-white to pink-gray, and the softness and homogeneity, aside from the areas of necrosis, correlate with the rich cellularity of Ewing's sarcoma.

Histologically, Ewing's sarcoma exhibits a highly cellular, rather monotonous pattern of round to ovoid nuclei. The cell boundaries are often indistinct, and the cytoplasm appears to be somewhat scanty. Necrosis is often present. The stroma is ordinarily scant but vascular. The tumor nuclei are fairly uniform in size, shape, and stainability with little pleomorphism (Fig. 15-30). The chromatin is usually not dense, but occasionally there are cellular foci in which the nuclear chromatin is dense, representing perhaps a second cell population. Possibly the cells with increased nuclear density represent degenerating cells. Nucleoli are present but generally are small and inconspicuous. Stains for reticulin demonstrate retic-

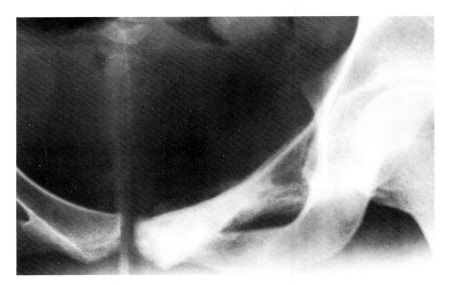

Fig. 15-29. Ewing's sarcoma of the pubis and ischium with sclerotic and lytic areas.

ulum to be sparse and seldom related to individual cells; it is more likely related to blood vessels or fibrous septa. In recent years, it has been common to use PAS stain with and without diastase to differentiate Ewing's sarcoma from other round cell tumors, particularly malignant lymphoma, leukemia, neuroblastoma, and embryonal rhabdomyosarcoma. Approximately 80 percent of

Ewing's sarcomas will show PAS-positive and diastase-digested material within the cytoplasm. By contrast, PAS-positive granules are rarely if ever found in the cytoplasm of malignant lymphomas and only on rare occasions in the cytoplasm of neuroblastomas but are expected in rhabdomyosarcomas. The presence of glycogen (PAS-positive) or its absence does not mean that the tumor is or is not a Ewing's sarcoma. The stain should be considered an aid in the diagnosis. PAS-positive material may be seen in the cytoplasm of leukocytes, but this material is diastase resistant.

Electron microscopic studies are often essential in the differentiation of the round cell tumors that involve the skeleton.[52,53] Electron microscopically (Fig. 15-31), the cells of Ewing's sarcomas have few cytoplasmic organelles and round to ovoid nuclei. There may be a few tight junctions and a few cytoplasmic filaments. An important feature is the presence of glycogen granules in the cytoplasm, correlating with the histologic finding of PAS positivity. By contrast, lymphomas do not have cytoplasmic glycogen and tight junctions. Neuroblastomas are identified by processes with secretory granules. Embryonal rhabdomyosarcomas are identified by Z-bands.

Metastases from this tumor may be widespread, with other bones involved commonly; although anywhere from 40 to 75 percent of patients will have involvement of other bones, the lungs are usually the first metastatic site. Metastases to lymph nodes and other viscera are frequent.[54]

The treatment of Ewing's sarcoma at the moment is dominated by radiation therapy and adjuvant chemotherapy. Because of the high incidence of postradiation sarcomas, there appears to be a shift toward chemotherapy

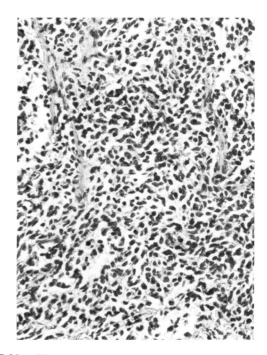

Fig. 15-30. The uniform cellularity of Ewing's sarcoma is apparent. The nuclei are quite uniform in size and shape, and the cytoplasmic boundaries are indistinct.

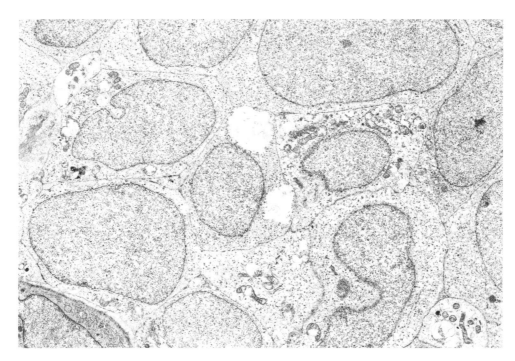

Fig. 15-31. Ewing's sarcoma, ultrastructure. The cells show round to oval nuclei with smooth contours. The chromatin is evenly and finely dispersed, and there are rare small nucleoli. The cytoplasm contains no significant number of organelles. In the center, there is a cell showing two irregular electron-lucent areas, which represent glycogen. The cytoplasmic membranes show occasional junctions. (×4,900)

followed by amputation or resection when applicable, and less radiotherapy. Amputation or resection has not been a popular part of the treatment. The prognosis of Ewing's sarcomas has improved with the institution of adequate radiation therapy and chemotherapy. Local control is good (90 to 95 percent). The expected 5 year survival rate before chemotherapy was 0 to 10 percent. The expected 5 year survival rate is 30 to 50 percent with chemotherapy.[55]

Malignant Lymphoma of Bone

Primary lymphoma of bone is uncommon, comprising approximately 4 percent of primary malignant tumors of bone. It has arisen in most bones, predominantly those of the lower extremity and the flat bones. It occurs predominantly in males with a ratio of 2:1 to 3:2.[56,57] In contrast to Ewing's sarcoma, malignant lymphoma of bone occurs usually after the second decade of life and is thus an uncommon tumor in the pediatric age group.

As with most malignant tumors of bone, pain and swelling are common complaints. The pain becomes more severe and distressing at night. Local tenderness and heat may be associated with the swelling but, in contrast with Ewing's sarcoma, fever is uncommon. Patho-

logic fractures occur quite frequently, with as many as 20 percent of the patients having this complication. Laboratory examinations generally are unrewarding.

Radiologically, malignant lymphoma of bone frequently is an extensively destructive lesion of the medulla and cortex (Fig. 15-32). Even though destruction is usually a prominent feature, there may be areas with patchy sclerosis and rarely some lesions may be mostly sclerotic. Periosteal reaction, although present, is not as noteworthy as that seen in Ewing's sarcoma. An extraosseous component is common. In the older patient, the findings of a primary lymphoma may mimic those of metastatic carcinoma, an important consideration in the differential diagnosis.

The gross features of primary lymphoma of bone are not distinctive. It may be difficult to distinguish from metastatic carcinoma, Ewing's sarcoma, or some other primary sarcoma of bone. The findings correspond well with the radiologic findings in that there is destruction and permeation of the marrow cavity and erosion and penetration of the cortex, and nearly always an extraosseous component. Necrosis and hemorrhage into the tumor are frequent. The cut surfaces are homogeneous, vary from light red to pink-gray, and, because of their homogeneity and friability, suggest rich cellularity. Aside from the fact that the lesion is located in bone, the gross

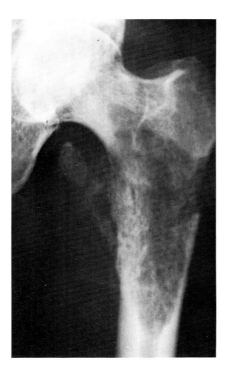

Fig. 15-32. Malignant lymphoma of the upper end of the femur in a 50-year-old woman. The tumor is permeative and destructive of cancellous and cortical bone.

features are similar to those of a malignant lymphoma of a lymph node.

Histologically, primary malignant lymphomas of bone resemble those of lymph nodes (see Ch. 12). Generally, they most closely resemble the large cell ("histiocytic") lymphoma. The cells have indistinct cell boundaries with faintly acidophilic or basophilic cytoplasm. The nuclei are approximately the same size as those of a Ewing's sarcoma, but the nucleus is often indented and nucleoli are commonly prominent. Most primary lymphomas of bone have a mixed cell population. Rarely has Hodgkin's disease of bone been reported. Aside from the lymphomatous component, there are varied quantities of a fibrous stroma, and the lesions are often notably vascular. Areas of necrosis and hemorrhage and occasionally granulomatous lesions may be seen. In contrast with Ewing's sarcoma, reticulin stains often demonstrate fibers related to individual cells. Another helpful stain is the methyl green pyronine, which stains cytoplasmic RNA of the transformed lymphocytes. In addition, PAS stains of malignant lymphoma are negative. Electron microscopic and immunohistochemical examinations are also helpful in distinguishing this tumor from other round cell tumors of bone.

Primary malignant lymphoma of bone in all likelihood will be indistinguishable from secondary lymphomatous involvement of bone. Thus, it is important in diagnosing

skeletal lymphoma that the clinician be alerted to the possibility that the lesion may be secondary. Only careful clinical and hematologic evaluation and follow-up will firmly establish the diagnosis of a primary lymphoma of bone.

Metastases to visceral organs and other bones are common; metastases to regional lymph nodes occur in approximately one-fifth of the cases. Widespread metastases may occur.

The treatment of primary lymphoma of bone is irradiation accompanied by chemotherapy. The 5 year survival rate is between 40 and 45 percent, and the 10 year survival rate is close to 35 percent.[56,57]

Plasma Cell Myeloma

Plasma cell myeloma is a neoplastic proliferation of plasma cells presenting as clinically localized osseous lesions or as part of a systemic disease. Skeletal involvement is almost universal and therefore myeloma is one of the most common of malignant tumors of bone. There is a wide age range, with myeloma being rare in the pediatric age group and more common in persons beyond the age of 40 years. The male to female ratio is approximately 2 : 1.[4] In patients having apparently solitary myeloma, the male dominance is approximately 4 : 1. The clinical manifestations of myeloma are many and are often related to the overproduction of immunoglobulins. Pathologic fractures are frequent and are often the presenting complaint of otherwise asymptomatic patients. The laboratory data, which are important in the diagnosis and evaluation of patients with myeloma, are described in Chapter 13.

Radiologically, myeloma is commonly a destructive lesion of bone; only occasionally is it sclerotic. Considering the patient's age and the radiologic findings of a malignant tumor, the major differential diagnostic possibility is metastatic carcinoma. This is stated to highlight the importance of myeloma in the differential diagnosis of destructive lesions of bone in the adult. The manifestations in the skeleton vary from site to site: skull lesions often have well circumscribed, punched-out, lucent areas, while in the long bones or pelvis, myeloma may appear as a purely radiolucent area with maintenance of the contours of the bone. Myeloma may be a multiloculated lesion. The most common sites of involvement are the vertebral column, ribs, skull, pelvis, and long bones.

Grossly, myeloma is red-gray, soft, and fairly homogeneous. There is destruction of the cancellous bone and, if involved, the cortex. It is difficult to distinguish it from other cellular lesions, such as malignant lymphoma or some metastases. Myeloma might present as diffuse involvement of an area of bone or as a multinodular lesion, having the same features described above.

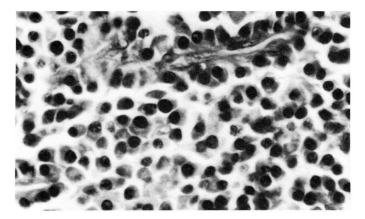

Fig. 15-33. Well differentiated plasma cells in multiple myeloma.

The histologic features of myeloma cells are described in Chapter 13. Differentiation of myeloma varies from cases in which the plasma cells appear normal (Fig. 15-33) to those in which the plasma cells are poorly differentiated and histologically may mimic poorly differentiated lymphomas or undifferentiated carcinomas. If these three cannot be distinguished by careful histologic examination, immunopathologic procedures will be helpful. The common leukocyte antigen will separate myeloma and lymphoma from carcinoma. Chronic osteomyelitis has been confused with myeloma, but the two can usually be identified properly. Chronic osteomyelitis may present numerous plasma cells, but there will be other cells such as lymphocytes, neutrophils, occasional eosinophils, and histiocytes. Evidence of bone repair is commonly present. Myelomas are infrequently associated with as much fibrous tissue as is seen in most instances of chronic osteomyelitis. In poorly differentiated forms of myeloma, the problem may be more difficult, and one must search for cells that morphologically resemble plasma cells. If these are lacking and myeloma is suspected on the basis of the clinical and radiologic features, the methyl green-pyronine stain may be an aid, as the cytoplasm of plasma cells take a reddish stain. If this fails, electron microscopic studies serve as the means by which histologic confirmation of myeloma can be made.

Nearly all apparently solitary plasma cell myelomas of the skeleton will eventually disseminate. As far as therapy is concerned, irradiation remains the choice for myelomas that are localized. For those that are disseminated, a combination of radiation therapy and chemotherapy will serve to prolong life. With chemotherapy the average survival has been remarkably improved.[58] There is some correlation between differentiation and survival. It has been demonstrated that when the myeloma is well differentiated the average life span is 3.5 years, but when

it is poorly differentiated the life span is 2 years or less. Aside from the complications of dissemination, patients with myeloma die of infections, cardiopulmonary disease, uremia, and hemorrhage.

Mastocytosis

Mastocytosis is mentioned merely as a means of differential diagnosis in regard to its radiologic and histologic findings. About 15 percent of the patients with mastocytosis will have radiologic changes in the skeleton.[25] A presumptive diagnosis can be made on the bony abnormalities when the typical skin lesions are present and are confirmed by histologic examination. It is rare for a patient to have skeletal involvement without the dermal lesions. Radiologically, the lesion may appear to be permeative and occasionally sclerotic, and in a child it may be mistaken for a Ewing's sarcoma. However, the lesions are often multiple and extensive. Histologically, mastocytosis may closely mimic a malignant lymphoma or histiocytosis. The granules may be demonstrated with Wright and Giemsa stains. Electron microscopic studies will demonstrate the classic features of mastocytes.

TUMORS OF VASCULAR ORIGIN
Hemangioma

Hemangiomas or vascular malformations are common skeletal lesions, particularly of the vertebral bodies, but those associated with symptoms such as mass, pain, or pathologic fracture are uncommon.[59] Among those that are clinically significant, there is a slight predominance in the female. Hemangiomas are seen in different age groups with a peak in the third to the seventh decades.

Radiologically, the lesions are usually solitary and may mimic other neoplasms. Frequently, they are well circumscribed and radiolucent, but they may produce considerable bony sclerosis with a so-called sunburst pattern (Fig. 15-34). At times hemangiomas may cause sclerotic streaking and linear radiolucency that mimic osteomyelitis or a malignant lesion, such as lymphoma or Ewing's sarcoma. The most common sites of hemangiomas are the skull, ribs, long bones, vertebra, mandible, and facial bones.[25]

Grossly, hemangiomas are bluish red to dark red. The cut surfaces may have a spongy appearance due to the bony trabeculation. The histologic pattern of most hemangiomas of bone is that of a cavernous hemangioma. Capillary hemangiomas are rare. The treatment varies with the location of the lesion, but generally surgical excision is recommended. For inaccessible lesions, radiation therapy may be effective in relieving symptoms.

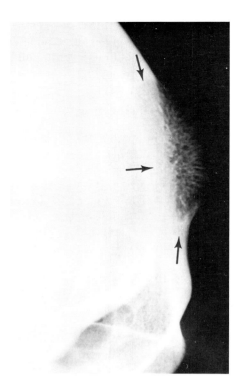

Fig. 15-34. Hemangioma of the skull of a 2-year-old boy. The bony defect and the spiculation are evident.

Lymphangioma

Lymphangioma is a rare lesion of bone that has histologic features similar to lymphangiomas of skin and soft tissues.[60] Whether there are lymphatics within the medullary portion of bone has been questioned, but lymphangiographic studies in patients with lymphedema have confirmed the presence of intraosseous lymphatic channels.

Radiologically, the lesions are similar to hemangioma, often being well outlined and with a soap-bubble appearance. Although rare, the reported examples of lymphangioma have all involved multiple bones.

Skeletal Angiomatosis

Skeletal angiomatosis is characterized by multicentric vascular tumors of the skeleton. The lesion is chiefly discovered in children, with a predominance in males.[61] Approximately 50 percent of the patients have associated skin, soft tissue, and visceral angiomas. Usually, medical aid is sought because the skeletal lesions have lead to vertebral compression and neurologic symptoms. Any and all bones have been reported as being involved, with the most common sites being the skull, ribs, pelvis, scapula, humerus, tibia, and femur.

Radiologically, the lesion has multiple bubbly appearing defects of the skeleton, often associated with bony sclerosis. The multiplicity of lesions is the key to the radiologic diagnosis. The gross examination of intact specimens is similar to that of hemangiomas. In most cases, only a biopsy specimen is submitted, and it is not particularly characteristic of any lesion. Histologically, skeletal angiomatosis is similar to localized hemangiomas. The lesions are generally combinations of cavernous and capillary formations.

For patients with lesions confined to the skeleton, the prognosis is good and, in most instances, the lesions tend to stabilize, but there may be progression. Patients with skeletal and visceral lesions may succumb to angiomatosis, since the disease may be complicated by heart failure, hemolytic anemia, microangiopathic anemia, and thrombocytopenia.[61]

Massive Osteolysis

Massive osteolysis is a rare, destructive lesion of bone also known as *disappearing bone disease* or *Gorham's disease*. It affects young people, usually under the age of 30 and is widely destructive of a bone or several bones.[62] This results in pathologic fractures, and, at times, death, particularly if bones of the thorax and/or the vertebrae are involved. Radiologically, the lesions may resemble hemangiomas, but they may often show destruction of a bone to the point where the bone or bones are imperceptible. Histologically, the lesion appears to be angiomatous. Thus, the disease is defined by its clinical manifestation, its radiologic features, and to a lesser degree the histologic findings. A possible variant of massive osteolysis has similar clinical features; histologically, however, it is not vascular but exhibits extensive bone resorption with abundant osteoclasts.[63]

Angiosarcoma

Malignant tumors of vascular origin arising in the skeleton are rare. These lesions may be seen at almost any age but are more common in adults. There does not appear to be a skeletal site of predilection, as they are seen in both flat bones and long bones. The clinical manifestation is not specific, usually being that of pain and/or swelling of the affected part. The laboratory findings are not contributory. Radiologically, angiosarcomas are ordinarily radiolucent, appearing as areas of destruction; they may appear well circumscribed or permeative. Often, they have a soap-bubble appearance (Fig. 15-35). Periosteal reaction may or may not be present. About one third of angiosarcomas are multifocal within one bone or

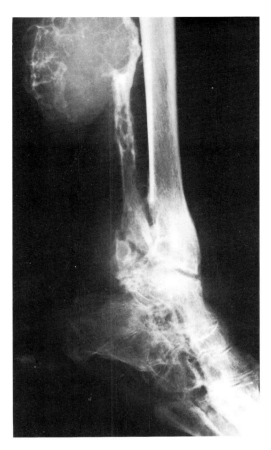

Fig. 15-35. Angiosarcoma of the fibula in a 65-year-old woman. Note the enlarged multiloculated mass and multiple lucent areas elsewhere in the fibula, tibia, and bones of the foot.

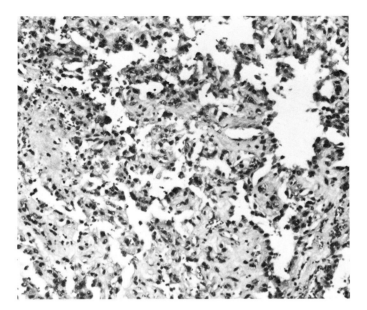

Fig. 15-36. Intricate vascular pattern of an angiosarcoma. Papillary structures lined by anaplastic endothelial cells are present.

involve adjacent bones. This finding in itself suggests a tumor of vascular origin.

Grossly, the tumors are bloody, dark red to bluish red, soft, and may appear to be spongy. There is often evidence of bony destruction and permeation of the cortical and medullary bone.

Histologically, the major feature to seek is enlarged cytologically malignant endothelial cells (Fig. 15-36). These are identified by enlarged nuclei, with chromatin-clumping and large nucleoli. In addition to the cytologic changes, the configuration of the vessels suggests an angiosarcoma, that is, the vessels are varied in size and shape, often with irregular ramifications and anastomoses (Fig. 15-36). In addition, there are papillary infoldings of the endothelium, at times forming thin bridges. If the vessels are small and the endothelial cells are unusually plump, the lesion may simulate carcinoma. It is this pattern that has been designated hemangioendothelioma (well differentiated angiosarcoma). The tumor is characterized by proliferation of small vessels lined by plump endothelial cells, which often obliterate the lumen (Fig.

15-37). Mitoses may be seen. At the periphery of the lesion, the vascular proliferation is usually less compact. Lymphocytes and eosinophils may be present. The lesion has a strong resemblance to Kimura's disease of the skin (angioendothelial hyperplasia with eosinophilia). It is im-

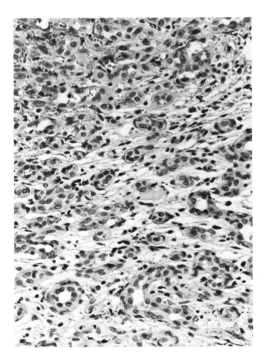

Fig. 15-37. Well differentiated angiosarcoma (hemangioendothelioma).

portant to separate this lesion from the higher grade angiosarcoma, since the latter has a propensity for metastasis, while hemangioendothelioma is essentially a locally aggressive lesion that may metastasize. Both hemangioendothelioma and angiosarcoma may be confused with metastatic carcinoma, especially with metastatic renal cell carcinoma, which can be extremely vascular. A review and an attempt to unify these lesions has been made by Rosai et al.[64]

Vascular proliferation associated with fractures or chronic inflammation may simulate angiosarcomas. In this circumstance, one must pay particular attention to the details of the nuclei of the endothelial cells and the morphologic features of the vessels. In most proliferative lesions, the vessels do not ramify nor is there evidence of the bridging and papillary in-foldings seen in angiosarcomas. The endothelial cells also lack criteria that satisfy those of malignancy. Angiosarcomas may metastasize widely with the most common sites being lungs, brain, liver, pleura, and occasionally lymph nodes.

Treatment has generally been local excision, amputation, irradiation, or a combination of these. Occasional survivors who have been treated by irradiation only have been recorded. Because of the relatively few cases reported, good follow-up data are not available. In general, those patients with well differentiated lesions have a better survival rate than those with poorly differentiated angiosarcomas.[65]

Hemangiopericytoma

Hemangiopericytoma is an extremely rare lesion of the skeleton. Histologically, it presents the same pattern as when found in the soft tissues. As with other hemangiopericytomas, the malignant potential of skeletal hemangiopericytomas may be difficult to predict from the histologic findings. Of the 10 cases reported, three have developed metastases, two known to be pulmonary.[66]

OTHER CONNECTIVE TISSUE TUMORS

Desmoplastic Fibroma

Desmoplastic fibroma, an uncommon benign tumor of bone, is formed by fibrous tissue and collagen (Fig. 15-38). The lesion probably belongs to the family of fibromatosis. Most patients are less than 30 years of age.[67] There is a prevalence for involvement of long bones. Radiologically, desmoplastic fibroma is radiolucent, and, because of this, it may be mistaken for a malignancy or for lesions

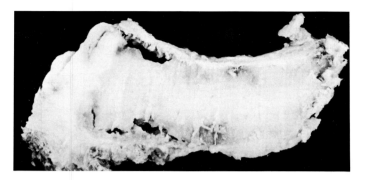

Fig. 15-38. Desmoplastic fibroma of pubic bone. There is fibrous replacement of the cancellous bone.

such as aneurysmal bone cyst, solitary cyst, or chondromyxoid fibroma. Occasionally a pathologic fracture may occur through the tumor. Histologically, desmoplastic fibroma is fibroblastic with evidence of collagenization, resembling fibromatoses of the soft tissues (Fig. 15-39). Ultrastructurally, myofibroblasts are common and are mixed with fibroblasts and primitive mesenchymal cells.[68] It may be difficult to differentiate from well differentiated fibrosarcoma. The evidence of collagenization and the bundles of collagen fibers seen in desmoplastic fibroma are an aid in differentiating it from a fibrosarcoma. When the lesion occurs in the jaws, especially in children, it appears to be more aggressive than in long bones, extending into the adjacent soft tissue and showing multiple recurrences.

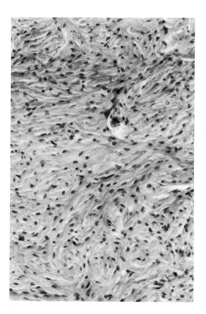

Fig. 15-39. Desmoplastic fibroma. The mature fibrous nature of the lesion can be seen.

Periosteal Desmoid

Periosteal desmoid is an uncommon lesion that has a predilection for the distal end of the femur, apparently arising in the periosteum. Radiologically, it causes what appears to be a scooped-out defect of the cortex.[25] Histologically, it is densely fibrous with evidence of considerable collagenization. Because of the maturity of the lesion, it is not easily mistaken for a fibrosarcoma. Periosteal desmoid is best treated by bloc excision, although curettage may be done with expectancy of success.

Fibrosarcoma

Fibrosarcoma is a rare primary malignant tumor of bone that apparently arises from the fibrous elements and histologically resembles fibrosarcoma of the soft tissues. Perhaps one fifth of fibrosarcomas of bone arise on the basis of a pre-existing lesion such as Paget's disease, fibrous dysplasias, infarcts of bone, or irradiation.[69] In contrast to osteosarcoma, fibrosarcoma is more likely to be diagnosed in the second, third, and fourth decades and beyond. Fibrosarcoma is slightly more common in females than in males. The tumor has a widespread localization in the skeleton with a predominance in the lower end of the femur and upper end of the tibia.[4,69] Radiologically in long bones, fibrosarcoma is predominantly metaphyseal with evidence of destruction that is mostly radiolucent (Fig. 15-40). There may be patches of radiodensity, and the lesion is often fairly well circum-

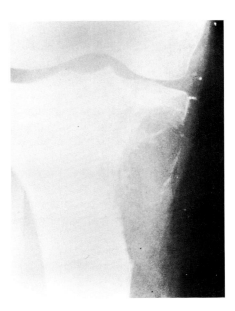

Fig. 15-40. Destructive fibrosarcoma of the tibia. The inner margin is fairly distinct.

scribed by is pure destructiveness. Periosteal reaction is identifiable but often is not as outstanding as that seen with osteosarcoma.

Grossly, fibrosarcoma is well circumscribed and varies from gray-white to pink-white with areas of necrosis and degeneration. Penetration of the cortex is almost invariably present. The better differentiated lesions may have a whorled and slightly lobulated appearance.

Histologically, fibrosarcoma has features of its soft tissue counterpart. Degrees of differentiation are based on nuclear pleomorphism and the presence of mitotic figures. One must be careful in the diagnosis of fibrosarcoma in that osteosarcomas may have a dominant fibrous component with little evidence of malignant osteoid or bone. Therefore, it is important that multiple blocks be taken of the lesion, searching for evidence of an osteosarcoma. In light of the prominence of malignant fibrous histiocytoma (MFH) in present-day histologic diagnoses, it is possible, if not probable, that many of the lesions designated poorly differentiated fibrosarcomas in the past represent MFH. Thus, MFH forms an important differential diagnostic consideration for the primary spindle cell tumors of the skeleton. The histologic features of fibrosarcoma and MFH are discussed in more detail in Chapter 10. Fibrosarcoma with an MFH component is quite common but apparently does not alter the prognosis according to a study done by Taconis and van Rijssel.[70]

The treatment for fibrosarcoma is ablative surgery, which generally means an amputation or, if located in pelvic bones or upper end of the femur, a hemipelvectomy. The effects of chemotherapy remain to be determined.

The overall 5 year survival rate for fibrosarcoma is 25 to 28 percent. This overall 5 year survival rate is slightly better than that for osteosarcoma before chemotherapy and represents a practical point for the distinction of fibrosarcoma from osteosarcoma. It is of interest that the mortality of patients having fibrosarcoma of the jaws is relatively low, with a 5 year survival rate of 71 percent.[71]

The differential diagnosis of fibrosarcoma includes benign tumors such as fibrous dysplasia, ossifying fibroma, desmoplastic fibroma, and periosteal desmoid. Fibrous dysplasia causes bony deformities and radiolucent areas in bones, although radiologically the findings are often diagnosable by the radiologist. Histologically, fibrous dysplasia may have broad zones of fibrous tissue, which may be fairly cellular and thus may be mistaken for fibrosarcoma. However, the osseous component is an integral part of fibrous dysplasia, and the osseous component usually shows bizarre bony forms such as circles, semicircles, and other configurations. In addition, the bony component often lacks osteoblastic activity. Ossifying fibroma has a fibrous stromal component, but the bony component is important to the diagnosis. In contrast to fibrous dysplasia, the bony component does not have a bizarre configuration but more likely resembles normal bony trabeculae with evidence of osteoblastic activity. The desmoplastic fibroma and periosteal desmoid histologically show features that are comparable with those seen in soft tissue desmoids or fibromatoses. There may be bundles or nodules in which the stroma is cellular, but in other areas there will be evidences of collagenization and maturation. A bony component will not be present.

Malignant Fibrous Histiocytoma of Bone

Malignant fibrous histiocytoma (MFH), a common malignant tumor of soft tissues, also arises primarily in bone. Although recently described, it is not a new lesion but was formerly included among other tumors of bone such as fibrosarcomas and osteosarcomas.[72]

The lesion predominates in the male and has a wide age range, with most patients being in the third decade and beyond.[72-74] Patients often have pain in the affected part and a slowly enlarging mass. Symptoms may have been present for a short period of time or for several months to 1 or 2 years. Pathologic fractures are apparently rare. MFH has wide skeletal distribution, but about 75 percent arise in the lower extremity and pelvis.[75] Occasionally, MFH has been noted in the jaws. MFH may arise secondary to irradiation, infarcts of bone and fibrous dyspla-

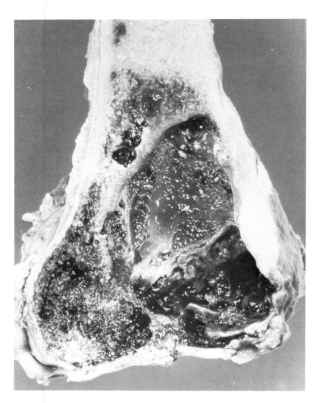

Fig. 15-42. Malignant fibrous histiocytoma of the femur. The tumor is partly cystic and hemorrhagic.

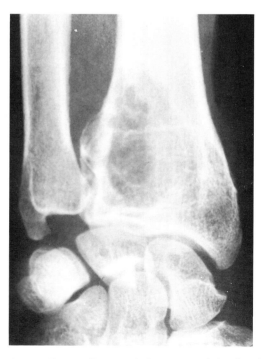

Fig. 15-41. Malignant fibrous histiocytoma of the distal radius, simulating a giant cell tumor.

sia.[75,76] Radiologically, MFH is permeative and generally an osteolytic lesion.[73] Occasionally, there may be dense mottling and slight sclerosis at the margin of the lesion (Fig. 15-41). There is destruction of the cortex and periosteal reaction is frequent, although not always present. A soft tissue component may be identified. Radiologically, the features add up to those of a malignant disease, and the differential diagnosis would include osteosarcoma, fibrosarcoma, and a malignant lymphoma.

Grossly, malignant fibrous histiocytoma is a fairly well circumscribed tumor because of its consistency and color (Fig. 15-42). It destroys the medullary portion of bone, often extending beyond the confines of the bone. The cut surfaces are yellow to gray-white to tan or brown, often with focal necrosis. Bony trabeculae may be identified in the tumor. The findings are not specific and could be those of a fibrosarcoma or an osteosarcoma, for example.

Histologically, MFH has features identical to those arising in the soft tissues (Fig. 15-43A,B) (see also Ch. 10). The storiform pattern of the stroma is present, but not in all fields. Pleomorphism of the nuclei is common, and there may be foamy cells that have the appearance of Touton giant cells. Bizarre mitotic figures, clusters of foamy cells, and a sprinkling of inflammatory cells are frequent. In many areas, the stroma is identical to a fibro-

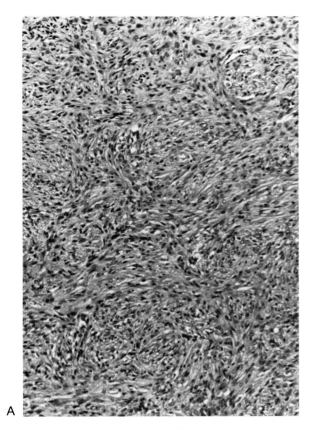

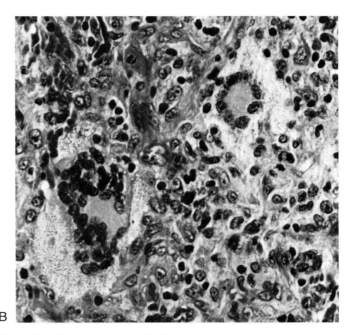

Fig. 15-43. Malignant fibrous histiocytoma. **(A)** Storiform fibroblastic pattern. **(B)** Histiocytes and Touton giant cells.

sarcoma. Special stains are not helpful in the diagnosis of this lesion, although stains for lipids will be positive. Huvos[75] noted that different histological variants of MHF do not exhibit differing behaviors.

Electron microscopic studies[74] suggested a variety of origins for this lesion, including fibroblastic or histiocytic. It would appear that the lesson is of fibroblastic origin with transformation of fibroblasts into histiocytic-appearing cells.

Malignant fibrous histiocytoma frequently metastasizes to other bones, to the lungs, and occasionally to lymph nodes.[73]

Surgical therapy seems to be the most effective; adjuvant radiotherapy and chemotherapy have an, as yet, undetermined effect. Survival from treatment of malignant fibrous histiocytomas is somewhat variable, but as many as one third of patients may survive beyond 5 years.

Rare Lesions

Three rare lesions of bone—*lipoma, liposarcoma,* and *leiomyosarcoma*—should be mentioned.[77–79] The first manifests as a radiolucent defect of bone and is histologi-

cally identical to lipomas of the soft tissues. Its importance lies mainly in the differential diagnosis of the roentgenograms in regard to radiolucent defects of bone. Liposarcoma and leiomyosarcoma manifest radiologically as malignant lesions, without specific changes to suggest the underlying tumor. Both are histologically identical to the soft tissue counterpart. Another rare tumor is parachordoma; it is slow growing with a potential for recurrence. It shares histologic features with chordoma and extraskeletal myxoid chondrosarcoma.[80,81]

OTHER TUMORS

Adamentinoma of Long Bones

Adamantinoma of the long bones is a rare lesion of the skeleton of unknown histogenesis.[82,83] The name derives from its histologic resemblance to adamantinoma of the jaw bones. There has been considerable discussion in the literature about its histogenesis, with a vascular or epithelial origin most prominently mentioned. Histologically, there are areas in most of the tumors that have a vascular appearance, and in many, there are areas with epithelial differentiation. Ultrastructurally, support has been advanced for both histogenetic theories. Immunohistochemical studies indicate an epithelial component if not histogenesis of adamantinoma.[84,85] Nevertheless, adamantinoma does represent a distinctive tumor of the skeleton.

The lesion occurs in young adults and slightly more frequently in males than in females.[82,83] Clinical manifestations are not specific—often a mass or slight discomfort over the lesion. Approximately 90 percent of adamantinomas occur in the tibia. Only occasional adamantinomas have been reported in the femur and in the long bones of the upper extremity. Occasionally, multiple adamantinomas may occur in the same patient.

Radiologically, the lesion is fairly distinctive, particularly if the tibia is involved. It presents with sharply outlined margins and signs of trabeculation that impart a lobulated or bubbly effect to the tumor. There may be multiple small, lucent zones in the vicinity of the larger one. Often, there is sclerosis of the cortex around the tumor.[82]

Grossly, adamantinoma is well circumscribed with adjacent bony sclerosis. The cut surfaces are often shiny gray-white. There may be multiple separate foci of gray-white tissue. In some lesions, there may be broad areas of fibrous tissue, which correspond histologically to sites that resemble fibrous dysplasia.

Histologically, adamantinomas exhibit a variable pattern.[82,83] There may be strands of small dark cells embedded in fibrous tissue, and there may be spaces that resemble blood vessels (Fig. 15-44) and other sites with an epithelial appearance (Fig. 15-45). In fact, the epithelial

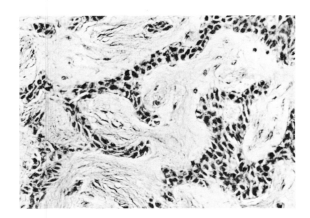

Fig. 15-45. Adamantioma exhibiting an epithelial appearance.

areas occasionally show evidence of keratinization. In some of the epithelial areas, there is reticulation of the cells, which imparts an appearance similar to that of adamantinoma of the jaws. Campanacci et al.[86] classified the histologic patterns into four types: spindle, basaloid, squamoid, and tubular. Apparently, these have no prognostic implications but do contribute to differential diagnostic difficulties.

In some areas, the epithelial components and those that appear to be vascular may be large enough to present as small cysts. The stroma between the more cellular elements is fibrous and does not have malignant features. On occasion, the stroma may predominate, giving a fibrous dysplasia-like appearance.

Histologically, a prominent differential diagnostic problem with adamantinoma is metastatic carcinoma, most commonly metastatic squamous or transitional cell carcinoma. In addition, primary angiosarcoma must be ruled out. Attention to the variety of patterns frequently present in the adamantinoma will help solve the histologic dilemma. If the radiograms are studied in concert with the histologic features, the proper diagnosis can usually be made.

Adamantinomas are malignant, even though they have a slow evolution. In carefully selected cases, bloc excision of the lesion with restitution of the tibia is possible. Many of the lesions are curetted initially because of their benign radiologic appearance; this results in local recurrence. When curettage fails, local en bloc excision, or even amputation, may have to be considered.

Patients may survive a number of years with adamantinoma, even though it is recurrent. Data in regard to precise survival are difficult to obtain, since there are relatively few cases. Adamantinoma metastasizes to the lungs and occasionally to other bones and to lymph nodes.[83]

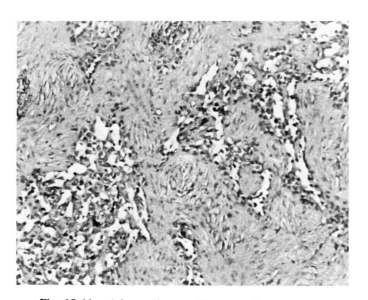

Fig. 15-44. Adamantioma with a vascular appearance.

Neurogenic Tumors of the Skeleton

Neurilemmoma arises from the nerve sheath and is rarely primary in bone. Radiologically, it is a radiolucent area that has benign but not distinctive characteristics. Most intraosseous neurilemmomas have occurred in the mandible, with others in the femur, humerus, small bones of the hand, scapula, sacrum, and maxilla.[4] Grossly, the few that have been removed intact show features similar to those of the soft tissues, that is, cystic degeneration of a well defined gray-white to gray-yellow nodule. Histologically, the lesion is identical to neurilemmoma in the soft tissues. Treatment of these lesions is curettage or bloc excision, where feasible.

Among the patients with neurofibromatosis are many who have skeletal involvement and deformities. One of the common skeletal deformities is kyphoscoliosis,[87] which occurs in 10 to 41 percent of the patients with neurofibromatosis. Any part of the vertebral column may be involved, with the thoracic being the most common site. Other bony lesions include localized overgrowth (a form of focal giantism that may involve any part of the skeleton), bowing deformity of the long bones, pseudoarthrosis, and erosive lesions due to neurofibroma.[88] The latter often have sclerotic zones radiologically and may appear as grooves or as subperiosteal blisters. Neurofibromas are not necessarily seen in the lesions described above. Several, such as kyphoscoliosis, are considered a dysplastic change of bone related to neurofibromatosis.

A rare neurogenic lesion is ganglioneuroma, which presents as a radiolucent defect in bone. Histologically, the lesion has the identical features of ganglioneuroma occurring in extraosseous sites.[89] (See Ch. 49 for a fuller discussion of the neurogenic tumors.)

Intraosseous Ganglion

Intraosseous ganglion is a cystic benign lesion of bone that radiologically is well defined and osteolytic. The lesion should be considered as a possibility in any well defined radiolucent radiologic lesion seen near a joint. Most of the patients are adolescents or adults with an almost equal number being male and female. Intraosseous ganglion is most commonly seen at the ends of long tubular bones, but it has been described in flat and small bones and in a periosteal location.[90]

Grossly, the lesions have characteristics similar to those of ganglion of the soft tissues. They have a fibrous wall and contain a thick viscous fluid. Histologically, the wall is fibrous with evidence of collagenization. Only occasionally may synovial tissue be identified. The lining

may be similar to that of a solitary cyst, but the fluid is viscid rather than watery as in the solitary cyst. Because intraosseous ganglion occurs at distal ends of long bones, a chondroblastoma may be considered in the differential diagnosis radiologically. Those that are metaphyseal and eccentric raise the possibility of nonossifying fibroma, chondromyxoid fibroma, or aneurysmal bone cyst.[91]

TUMOR-LIKE LESIONS

Aneurysmal Bone Cyst

Aneurysmal bone cyst (ABC) is a benign expansile lesion of bone. Its pathogenesis is somewhat controversial. There has always been some question as to whether ABC represents a neoplasm or a reaction to injury. Recently, it has been considered that many aneurysmal bone cysts arise on the background of a pre-existing benign lesion such as chondroblastoma, fibrous dysplasia, or giant cell tumor.[4,25] Since ABCs are composed of blood-filled spaces, a relation to hemangioma has frequently been suggested. ABC may occur at any age but is most common in the pediatric and adolescent age groups.[4,92] There appears to be a predominance in the female. Pain, swelling, and tenderness are common signs and symptoms related to ABC. Since many of the lesions are located near the distal end of long bones, there may be associated limitation of motion of the nearby joint. A number of ABCs may involve the vertebrae and in their expansion impinge on nerves, causing pain and paresthesias.

Radiologically, ABC is a benign expansile lesion that in long bones is often eccentric (Fig. 15-46). However, it may be widely destructive and may simulate a malignant tumor, particularly osteosarcoma. Many ABCs have a bubbly appearance radiologically, correlating with multicystic features seen grossly. Some ABCs are centrally located and do not cause the typical blow-out radiologic pattern. Those located near the distal end of long bones are often mistaken for giant cell tumors, solitary bone cysts, osteosarcomas, hemangiomas, and even Ewing's sarcoma. This merely reflects the wide variety of patterns that an ABC may assume.

The long bones of the limbs are the most common sites of the lesion. Approximately 10 percent of ABCs involve the vertebral column; few involve that flat bones.[4,25] The gross features of intact specimens are those of a spongy, bloody, somewhat lobulated mass (Fig. 15-47). The cortex is often attenuated or destroyed. On the outer surfaces, the periosteum is intact and thickened. The cut surfaces are dark red to brown, with cystic spaces of varied sizes containing blood and clotted blood. In some

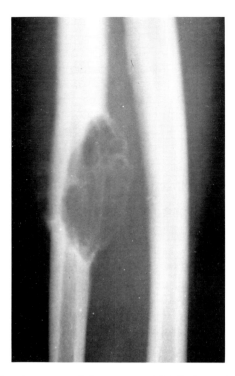

Fig. 15-46. Aneurysmal bone cyst (ABC) in a 20-year-old woman. Eccentric, expansile, lucent lesion of the midshaft of the ulna. The borders are well defined.

lesions, there may be solid fibrous areas; bone is commonly palpable.

Histologically, ABCs are composed of blood-filled spaces with walls formed by fibrous tissue and, in many instances, osteoid and bone (Fig. 15-48). In some areas, the walls of the blood spaces may be lined by multinucleate giant cells (Fig. 15-49). Evidence of an endothelial

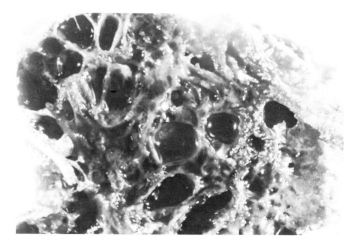

Fig. 15-47. Multicystic hemorrhagic cut surface of an aneurysmal bone cyst.

lining is infrequent. In some of the cellular areas, the stroma may be spindled and raise the possibility of a malignant neoplasm, and in other areas, multinucleate giant cells may be abundant, raising the consideration of a giant cell tumor. Osteoid formation raises the possibility of osteosarcoma (Fig. 15-50). To rule out other lesions, as mentioned earlier, one must pay careful attention to the radiologic features, and numerous blocks of the lesion should be taken to determine whether the aneurysmal bone cyst is actually part of a giant cell tumor or whether, for example, one is examining an aneurysmal component of fibrosarcoma or osteosarcoma. In the case of either of the latter two lesions, the stroma should have histologically malignant characteristics, and in the case of an osteosarcoma histologically malignant osteoid and bone would be identifiable.

Surgical removal of the aneurysmal bone cyst is the most effective means of treatment. For those located at sites that do not permit surgical resection, radiation therapy has been useful. Smaller lesions may be curetted, although bleeding may be encountered. Recurrence, particularly after curettage, has been reported in as many as one third of patients.[92]

Solitary Simple Bone Cyst

A solitary bone cyst is a benign, often unicameral, fluid-containing lesion of unknown etiology. Approximately three fourths are located in the upper end of a humerus or the upper end of a femur and frequently lie near or abut on the epiphyseal plate. Solitary bone cyst is seen most commonly in children and adolescents but may occur in people as old as 72 years of age. There is a predominance in the male, with the male to female ratio being approximately 3 : 1.[25]

Clinically, solitary cysts are often asymptomatic, being diagnosed only as a result of a pathologic fracture. Uncommonly, patients have pain or swelling caused by the lesion. Solitary cysts involving flat bones are usually asymptomatic.

Radiologically solitary cysts are radiolucent and, unless complicated by fracture or previous treatment, do not deform the contours of the bone. Characteristically, in a young person, the lesion is cone shaped, abutting on the epiphyseal growth plate (Fig. 15-51). The cortex is attenuated although intact. The cyst may appear to be loculated due to bony trabeculation of the wall. The boundaries of the lesion are often fairly distinct, being slightly sclerotized. The cysts that abut on the growth plate are known as active cysts, and those that have "grown" away are inactive cysts.

Grossly, the contents shine through a thin cortex and impart a bluish discoloration. The fluid in an uncompli-

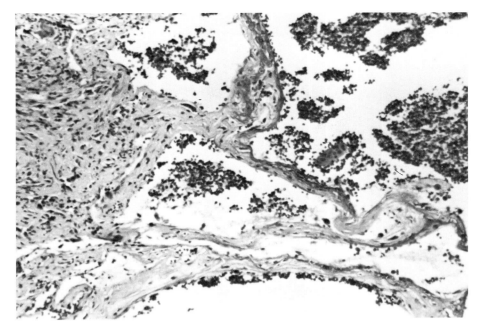

Fig. 15-48. Low-power view of an aneurysmal bone cyst. The irregularly shaped blood spaces are formed by fibrous tissue and osteoid.

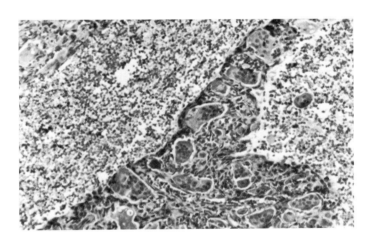

Fig. 15-49. Aneurysmal bone cyst. Blood spaces partly lined by multinucleate cells. The trabeculae are formed by a cellular stroma in which many multinucleate cells are seen.

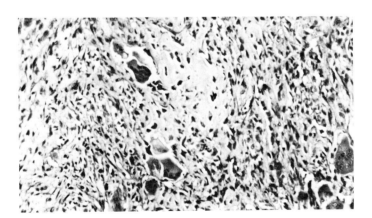

Fig. 15-50. Osteoid and multinucleate cells in a solid area of an aneurysmal bone cyst.

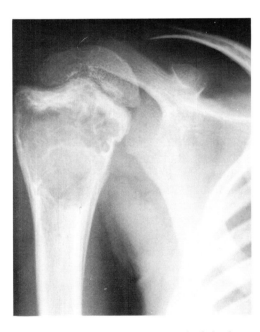

Fig. 15-51. Simple cyst of the upper end of the humerus of a 4-year-old boy. The cyst abuts on the epiphyseal growth plate. Mature periosteal reaction is seen on the medial humeral surface; it reflects previous trauma.

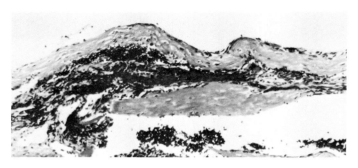

Fig. 15-52. Solitary bone cyst. Lining consists of a collagenous membrane.

cated cyst is clear yellow and sometimes blood-tinged. It may be bloody if fracture has occurred previously. Examination of fluid indicates it to be similar to serum. The cysts are usually composed of one compartment with bony trabeculation. The lining membrane may be thickened and red-brown.

Histologically, the lining membrane is somewhat nondescript in that it is composed of partly hyalinized connective tissue (Fig. 15-52). There may be evidence of osteoid formation and vascular proliferation. In lesions complicated by trauma, there may be areas of inflammation, multinucleate giant cells, and evidence of fracture repair. Because of the latter, the curettings from a cyst may be mistaken for fibrous dysplasia or giant cell tumor, for example. Therefore, review of the roentgenograms by the pathologist is important.

Most solitary bone cysts are treated by curettage and packing with bone chips; some have advocated subtotal resection.[93] Those that lie adjacent to the epiphyseal plate are most likely to recur, since curettage of the epiphyseal plate would retard bone growth. The likelihood of recurrence varies from 18 to 41 percent. Since there is a tendency for cysts in the long bones to migrate from the epiphyseal plate, it is often advisable to delay treatment until this has occurred.

There is interest in a simple form of treatment, the injection of steroids into the cyst without further surgical intervention. In preliminary studies, this approach appears to have promise.[94]

Nonossifying Fibroma

Nonossifying fibroma and its companion, fibrous cortical defect, are common, being seen in an estimated 50 percent of children who have radiographs taken of their knees. Nonossifying fibroma is readily diagnosable radiologically.[95] Most of the patients are asymptomatic, and if symptoms appear, they usually follow a pathologic fracture. The most common sites are the metaphyses of the

lower end of the femur and upper end of the tibia.[25] Distal ends of tibia and fibula are also fairly common sites.

Radiologically, the lesion is well circumscribed, eccentric, and usually radiolucent. The margins are sclerotic and exhibit a lobular pattern. The cortex may be thin. As the lesion matures, it becomes increasingly sclerotic, as it has been demonstrated that the nonossifying fibroma heals by bony sclerosis.

Grossly, the lesions are usually seen as curettings, and these fragments of tissue vary from light brown to dark brown with yellow areas. Occasionally, an intact nonossifying fibroma is seen in conjunction with an amputation (Fig. 15-53). These lesions correlate perfectly with the radiologic findings, that is, there is sclerosis of the margins of an eccentrically located metaphyseal lesion that on cut surface is yellow-brown to brown.

Histologically, the lesions have a pattern of a fibrous histiocytoma, that is, there is a storiform pattern to the spindled stroma (Fig. 15-54A). In contrast to a genuine giant cell tumor, the multinucleate giant cells, although present, are scattered and may be clustered. Hemosiderin and numerous histiocytes are frequently identified (Fig. 15-54B). Specimens from patients in the late teens or early 20s may show evidence of bone formation. In the immature and in the nontraumatized nonossifying fibroma, bone and osteoid are not seen. Histologically, nonossifying fibroma and *fibrous cortical defect* are identical and are generally considered one and the same lesion, except the latter is smaller and likely to be confined to the cortex. Bosch et al.[96] in 1974 suggested a histo-

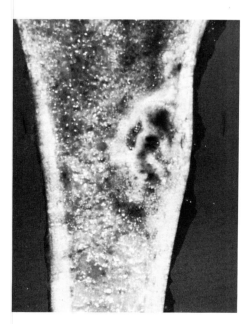

Fig. 15-53. Intact nonossifying fibroma. The lobular pattern and sclerotized margins are identical to the radiologic picture. (Courtesy of S. Saltzstein, M.D., San Diego.)

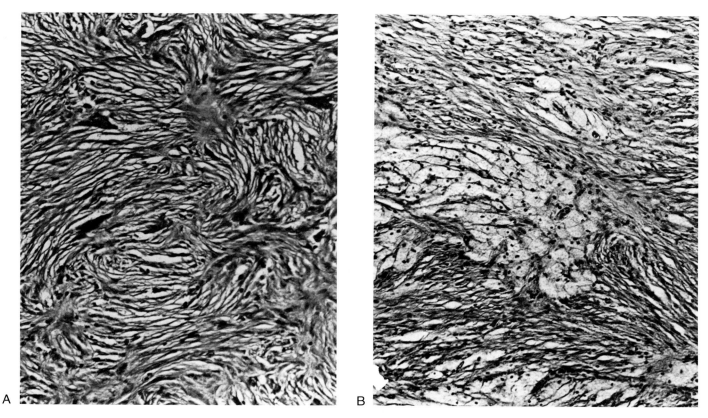

Fig. 15-54. Nonossifying fibroma. **(A)** Fibrous storiform stromal pattern. **(B)** Note clusters of foamy histiocytes and scattered multinucleate cells.

chemical difference between the two. Basically, the lesion is a self-limited one, and a major reason for surgical intervention is danger of fracture in large lesions.[95]

Ossifying Fibroma

Ossifying fibroma is a fibro-osseous lesion that most commonly involves the jaws and rather uncommonly the long bones.[97] It is important because it is frequently mistaken histologically for fibrous dysplasia. However, it differs from fibrous dysplasia in that it is seldom, if ever, a polyostotic lesion. In the jaws, it manifests as a radiolucent or radiodense lesion that is often well circumscribed. In the long bones, it often appears to be a multifocal radiolucent lesion with sclerotic borders. The overlying cortex is attenuated, and there may be slight bowing of the bone. In the long bones, its clinical behavior differs somewhat from fibrous dysplasia in that it has a high propensity to recur after treatment. Thus, in the treatment of these lesions, it is often necessary to do an en bloc resection that includes periosteum. There are case reports, however, that suggest that the lesion may gradually undergo spontaneous regression.[98]

Histologically, ossifying fibroma resembles fibrous dysplasia, but there are two important differences: (1) most of the bony trabeculae will exhibit osteoblasts (osteoblastic rimming) and (2) the bony trabeculae are better oriented than are those of fibrous dysplasia, in which there are many bizarre forms (Fig. 15-55). The stroma of the two lesions is essentially identical. With polarized light, it is possible to accentuate the difference in the type of bone present in the two lesions.[25] The bone of ossifying fibroma is dominantly lamellar bone with areas that are woven bone (immature). The reverse is true in most examples of fibrous dysplasia. However, there are many exceptions to these rules (see Ch. 22).

Fibrous Dysplasia

Fibrous dysplasia is a benign fibro-osseous lesion of bone that may be monostotic or polyostotic. About one third of patients will have polyostotic involvement.[20] Polyostotic fibrous dysplasia is more likely to be symptomatic and to present with bone pain or bone deformities. It is much more common in girls than in boys; girls may present with precocious menarche. Other manifestations

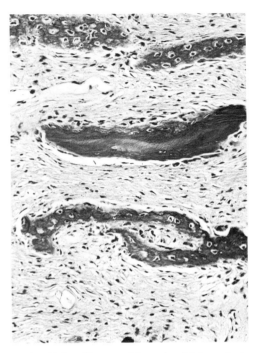

Fig. 15-55. Ossifying fibroma. Note the fairly orderly orientation of bony trabeculae. The stroma is only moderately cellular, and osteoblasts are associated with the bony trabeculae.

such as hyperthyroidism, hypophosphatemia, and hearing loss may occur.[99] The monostotic form is usually asymptomatic, coming to the attention of the patient because of the presence of a mass or pathologic fracture. Fractures and repeated fractures are frequent in patients with polyostotic disease. The lesion may involve almost any bone, with the skull, ribs, femur, and tibia being common sites.[97] The polyostotic form is more likely to be associated with focal skin pigmentation than is monostotic fibrous dysplasia.

Radiologically, fibrous dysplasia exhibits a variety of alterations (Fig. 15-56). Typically, it is a fairly well circumscribed lesion that expands a bone. The lesion is faintly osteosclerotic, imparting the so-called ground-glass appearance. Some may appear cystic. At times, the picture may be dominated by osteosclerosis, and in patients with polyostotic fibrous dysplasia, bony deformities are fairly frequent and may be severe.

Grossly, the cut surface imparts a gritty sensation to palpation (Fig. 15-57). The surfaces are gray-white to yellow-white to light brown. Occasionally, fibrous dysplasia exhibits microcysts or is mainly cystic. The margins are

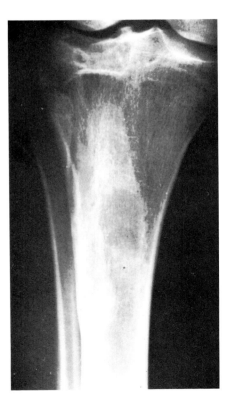

Fig. 15-56. Admixture of sclerotic and lucent areas in tibial fibrous dysplasia. The boundaries of the lesion are vague. There is little deformity of the tibia.

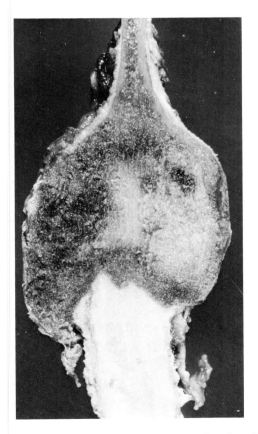

Fig. 15-57. Hemisection of fibrous dysplasia of a rib at the costochondral junction. The rib is enlarged, and the lesion gives the impression of grittiness.

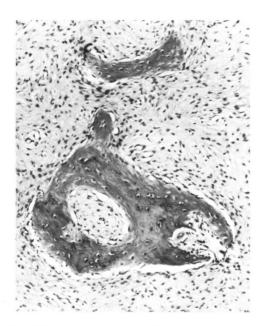

Fig. 15-58. Fibrous dysplasia. Oddly shaped bony trabeculae are evident. Osteoblasts are sparse, if present.

not cleanly defined, with the lesion appearing to blend with the surrounding bone.[4]

Histologically, fibrous dysplasia is composed of bony trabeculae and a fibrous stroma, which mingle intimately. The bony trabeculae often form numerous bizarre shapes such as Os and Cs (Fig. 15-58). The bone in most portions of the specimen will be woven or immature bone (Fig. 15-59), readily demonstrable by polarized light. For the most

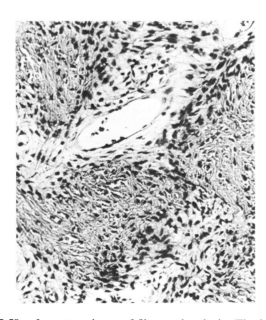

Fig. 15-59. Immature bone of fibrous dysplasia. The bone almost appears to spring from the proliferative stroma.

part, osteoblasts around the bony trabeculae are uncommon (Fig. 15-58). If there has been previous fracture, osteoblasts may be prominent. The paucity or lack of osteoblasts about the trabeculae serves as a means of differentiating fibrous dysplasia from ossifying fibroma, in which osteoblasts are usually common. The stroma varies in cellularity and is fibrous. Quite commonly, the stroma has foci that resemble a fibrous histiocytoma. In some areas, vascularity may be prominent; occasionally, clusters of multinucleate giant cells are seen.

Treatment of monostotic fibrous dysplasia is excision or curettage, depending on the location of the lesion. In most instances, this is successful, although recurrence may be observed after curettage. The recurrences usually maintain the histologic pattern of the original lesion. In polyostotic fibrous dysplasia, orthopaedic correction may be required because of bony deformities, and some lesions may have to be resected because of symptoms due to compression, for example, large rib lesions compressing the lungs. A rare complication of either polyostotic or monostotic fibrous dysplasia is transformation into a malignant tumor, most of which are osteosarcomas, although chondrosarcomas and fibrosarcomas have been noted.[100]

Localized Myositis Ossificans

Localized myositis ossificans (LMO), heterotopic bone and cartilage formation, is mentioned briefly, since it enters into the differential diagnosis of extraskeletal osteosarcoma, parosteal osteosarcoma, periosteal osteosarcoma, and osteochondroma. (See Ch. 14 for further discussion.) LMO may be localized entirely in the soft tissues, but when it is juxtacortical or periosteal, it raises questions in the differential diagnosis.[25] The lesion is not always associated with a known incident of trauma, but when it is and a series of films are available, its development and maturation are most helpful in ruling out malignant neoplasms. An osteosarcoma, for example, would not be expected to mature. The juxtacortical mature LMO may be quite difficult to distinguish radiologically from parosteal osteosarcoma. Usually, the latter is lobulated, whereas LMO ordinarily has a smooth outline.

Histologically, the problems are evident by the names *pseudomalignant* and *pseudosarcomatous* that have been applied to LMO.[101,102] With a deep wedge biopsy or excisional biopsy of a developing lesion of LMO, it can be seen that the interior is highly proliferative and taken in itself appears malignant. However, toward the periphery of the lesion, there is maturation of bone and stroma, which is most helpful in interpreting these reactive lesions. Because cartilage may be present, osteochondroma or chondrosarcoma have been mistakenly considered. All in all, the zoning phenomenon, maturation from interior to periphery of the mass, is an important key to the diagnosis. Small biopsy specimens, however, are easily misinterpreted as being from some other lesion. As with skeletal neoplasms, radiologic studies are an integral part in the proper interpretation of LMO and the tumors that it simulates.[25]

METASTATIC AND SECONDARILY INVASIVE TUMORS

In the differential diagnosis of neoplasms of bone, secondary involvement should be given at least a passing thought and in certain situations prime consideration. Benign or malignant extraosseous tumors may invade adjacent bone. Examples of benign lesions that may secondarily involve bone are nodular tenosynovitis, pigmented villonodular synovitis, glomus tumors, epidermal cysts, and fibromatoses. Soft tissue sarcomas may invade bone. In some of the lesions, such as pigmented villonodular synovitis, bony destruction may be extensive enough to suggest malignancy radiologically. Many of the lesions, both benign and malignant, cause alterations that are at least suggestive of an extraosseous lesion. Radiologically, the bone is often saucerized, probably the result of long-continued pressure. The defect is smooth and not necessarily indicative of malignancy. By contrast, carcinoma invading bone (e.g., gingival carcinoma invading the mandible) is destructive and generally interpreted as being malignant.

Metastatic cancer is the most common malignancy to involve bone. When encountering a lesion of bone that is radiologically malignant in a person over 40 years of age, one should first rule out the possibility of a metastasis. Plasma cell myeloma must also receive top consideration in the same circumstance. Radiologically, most metastases are destructive (radiolucent), many exhibit destruction and bone formation, and others are predominantly productive of bone (such as metastases from adenocarcinoma of the prostate).

Aside from radiologic and radionuclide studies, marrow aspirations and biopsies from iliac crest have been an aid in the diagnosis of metastases. The latter yield cancer cells, even though a lesion is not demonstrable at the aspiration site.[103] Fine-needle aspiration will yield diagnostic material from metastatic lesions, particularly those that are destructive. This procedure may forestall the need for open biopsy.

Patients having known cancer and adults who incur what appear to be pathologic fractures should have tissue submitted for pathologic examination if open fixation is carried out. In fact, a biopsy should be taken of any frac-

ture site, particularly in an elderly person, if open reduction and fixation are required.

Treatment of bony metastases incorporates all modalities. Satisfactory response may occur with irradiation, chemotherapy, or hormonal manipulation. For the cancer patient who develops a pathologic fracture, internal fixation has proved successful in reducing pain and reestablishing function. The latter is important to facilitate mobilization.[104]

REFERENCES

1. Ayala AG, Zornoza J: Primary bone tumors: Percutaneous needle biopsy. Radiologic-pathologic study of 222 biopsies. Radiol 149:675, 1983
2. Spjut HJ: Histologic classification of primary tumors of bone. p. 57. In Management of Primary Bone and Soft Tissue Tumors. Year Book Medical Publishers, Chicago, 1977
3. Childrey JH: Osteoma of sinuses, the frontal and the sphenoid bone. Report of fifteen cases. Arch Otolaryngol 30:63, 1939
4. Dahlin DC, Unni, KK: Bone Tumors. 4th Ed. Charles C Thomas, Springfield, IL, 1986
5. Swee RG, McLeod RA, Beabout JW: Osteoid osteoma. Detection, diagnosis, and localization. Radiology 130:117, 1979
6. Mehta MH, Murray RO: Scoliosis provoked by painful vertebral lesions. Skel Radiol 1:223, 1977
7. Pettine KA, Klassen RA: Osteoid-osteoma and osteoblastoma of the spine. J Bone Joint Dis 68A:354, 1986
8. Norman A, Abdelwahab IF, Buyon J, Matzkin E: Osteoid osteoma of the hip stimulating an early onset of osteoarthritis. Radiology 158:417, 1986
9. Byers PD: Solitary benign osteoblastic lesions of bone. Cancer 22:43, 1968
10. Glynn JJ, Lichtenstein L: Osteoid-osteoma with multicentric nidus. J Bone Joint Surg 55A:855, 1973
11. Marsh BW, Bonfiglio M, Brady LP, et al: Benign osteoblastoma: Range of manifestations. J Bone Joint Surg [Am] 57:1, 1975
12. Schajowicz F, Lemos C: Malignant osteoblastoma. J Bone Joint Surg [Br] 58:202, 1976
13. Dorfman HD, Weiss SW: Borderline osteoblastic tumors: Problems in the differential diagnosis of aggressive osteoblastoma and low-grade osteosarcoma. Semin Diagn Pathol 1:215, 1984
14. Raymond AK, Chawla S, Carrasco CH, et al: Osteosarcoma chemotherapy effect: A prognostic factor. Semin Diagn Pathol 4:212, 1987
15. Uribe-Botero G, Russel WO, Sutow WW, et al: Primary osteosarcoma of bone. A clinicopathologic investigation of 243 cases, with necropsy studies in 54. Am J Clin Pathol 67:427, 1977
16. Matsuno T, Unni KK, McLeod RA, et al: Telangiectatic osteogenic sarcoma. Cancer 38:2538, 1976

17. Farr GH, Huvos AG, Marcove RC et al: Telangiectatic osteogenic sarcoma. A review of twenty-eight cases. Cancer 34:1150, 1974
18. Unni KK, Dahlin DC, McLeod RA, et al: Intraosseous well differentiated osteosarcoma. Cancer 40:1337, 1977
19. Unni KK, Dahlin DC, Beabout JW, et al: Parosteal osteogenic sarcoma. Cancer 37:2466, 1976
20. Vander Heul RO, von Ronnen JR: Juxtacortical osteosarcomas. J Bone Joint Surg 49A:415, 1967
21. Raymond AK, Ayala AG, Carrasco HC, et al: Parosteal osteosarcoma vs dedifferentiated: Preoperative identification (abstract). Lab Invest 54:53A, 1986
22. Unni KK, Dahlin DC, Beabout JW: Periosteal osteogenic sarcoma. Cancer 37:2476, 1976
23. Spjut HJ, Ayala AG, deSantos LA, et al: Periosteal osteosarcoma. p. 79. In Management of Primary Bone and Soft Tissue Tumors. Year Book Medical Publishers, Chicago, 1977
24. Taylor WF, Ivins JC, Dahlin DC, et al: Trends and variability in survival from osteosarcoma. Mayo Clin Proc 53:695, 1978
25. Spjut HJ, Dorfman HD, Fechner RE, et al: Tumors of Bone and Cartilage. Atlas of Tumor Pathology. Second Series. Armed Forces Institute of Pathology, Washington, DC, 1970
26. Gherlinzoni F, Rock M, Picci P: Chondromyxoid fibroma. The experience at the Instituto Orthopedico Rizzoli. J Bone Joint Surg [Am] 65:198, 1983
27. Rahmi A, Beabout JW, Ivins JC, et al: Chondromyxoid fibroma: A clinicopathologic study of 76 cases. Cancer 30:726, 1972
28. Bloem JL, Mulder JD: Chondroblastoma: A clinical and radiological study of 104 cases. Skel Radiol 14:1, 1985
29. Huvos AG, Marcove RC, Erlandson RA, et al: Chondroblastoma of bone. A clinicopathologic and electron microscopic study. Cancer 29:760, 1972
30. Reyes CV, Kathuria S: Recurrent and aggressive chondroblastoma of the pelvis with late malignant neoplastic changes. Am J Surg Pathol 3:449, 1979
31. Fornasier VL, McGonigal D: Periosteal chondroma. Clin Orthop 124:133, 1977
32. Nojima T, Unni KK, McLeod RA, Pritchard DJ: Periosteal chondroma and periosteal chondrosarcoma. Am J Surg Pathol 9:666, 1985
33. Evans HL, Ayala AG, Rhomsdahl MM: Prognostic factors in chondrosarcoma of bone. A clinicopathologic analysis with emphasis on histologic grading. Cancer 40:818, 1977
34. Campanacci M, Guerrelli N, Leonessa C, et al: Chondrosarcoma. A study of 133 cases, 8 with long-term follow-up. Ital J Orthoped Traumatol 1:388, 1975
35. Kreicsbergs A, Boquist L, Borssen B, Larsson S-E: Prognostic factors in chondrosarcoma. Cancer 50:577, 1982
36. Spjut HJ: Cartilaginous malignant tumors arising in the skeleton. p. 921. In Seventh National Center Conference Proceedings of American Cancer Society, New York, 1973
37. Nakashima Y, Unni KK, Shives CS, et al: Mesenchymal chondrosarcoma of bone and soft tissue. A review of 111 cases. Cancer 57:2444, 1986
38. Frassica FJ, Unni KK, Beabout JW, Sim FH: Dedifferentiated chondrosarcoma. J Bone Joint Surg [Am] 68:1197, 1986
39. Unni KK, Dahlin DC, Beabout JW, et al: Chondrosarcoma: Clear-cell variant. J Bone Joint Surg [Am] 58:676, 1976
40. Luger AM, Ansbacher L, Farrell C, et al: Extraskeletal myxoid chondrosarcoma. Skel Radiol 6:291, 1981
41. Goldenberg RR, Campbell CJ, Bonfiglio M: Giant-cell tumor of bone. Analysis of two hundred and eighteen cases. J Bone Joint Surg [Am] 52:619, 1970
42. Singson R, Feldman F: Multiple (multicentric) giant cell tumors of bone. Skel Radiol 9:276, 1983
43. Campanacci M, Baldini N, Boriani S, Sudanese A: Giant-cell tumor of bone. J Bone Joint Surg [Am] 69:106, 1987
44. Hanaoka H, Friedman B, Mack RP: Ultrastructure and histogenesis of giant-cell tumor of bone. Cancer 25:1408, 1970
45. Steiner GC, Ghosh L, Dorfman HD: Ultrastructure of giant cell tumors of bone. Hum Pathol 3:569, 1972
46. Brecher ME, Franklin WA, Simon MA: Immunohistochemical study of mononuclear phagocyte antigens in giant cell tumor of bone. Am J Pathol 125:252, 1986
47. Picci P, Baldini N, Sudanese A, et al: Giant cell reparative granuloma and other giant cell lesions of the bones of the hands and feet. Skel Radiol 15:415, 1986
48. Lorenzo JC, Dorfman HD: Giant cell reparative granuloma of short tubular bones of the hands and feet. Am J Surg Pathol 4:551, 1980
49. Rock MG, Sim FH, Unni KK, et al: Secondary malignant giant cell tumor of bone. J Bone Joint Surg [Am] 68:1073, 1986
50. Moll R, Lee I, Gould VE, et al: Immunocytochemical analysis of Ewing's tumors. Am J Pathol 127:288, 1987
51. Cavazzana AO, Miser JS, Jefferson J, Triche TJ: Experimental evidence for neural origin of Ewing's sarcoma of bone. Am J Pathol 127:507, 1987
52. Ayala A, Mackay B: Ewing's sarcoma: An ultrastructural study. p. 179. In Management of Primary Bone and Soft Tissue Tumors. Year Book Medical Publishers, Chicago, 1977
53. Mahoney JP, Alexander RW: Ewing's sarcoma. A light and electromicroscopic study of 21 cases. Am J Surg Pathol 2:283, 1978
54. Telles NC, Rabson AS, Pomeroy TC: Ewing's sarcoma: An autopsy study. Cancer 41:2321, 1978
55. Sutow WW: Chemotherapy of Ewing's sarcoma. p. 97. In Jaffe N (ed): Bone Tumors in Children. PSG Publishing Co., Littleton, MA, 1979
56. Shoji H, Miller TR: Primary reticulum cell sarcoma of bone. Cancer 28:1234, 1971
57. Boston HC Jr, Dahlin DC, Ivins JC, et al: Malignant lymphoma (so-called reticulum cell sarcoma) of bone. Cancer 34:1131, 1974
58. Kyle RA, Elveback LR: Management and prognosis of multiple myeloma. Mayo Clin Proc 51:751, 1976
59. Baker ND, Greenspan A, Neuwirth M: Symptomatic vertebral hemangiomas: A report of four cases. Skel Radiol 15:458, 1986

60. Falkner S, Tilling G: Primary lymphangioma of bone. Acta Orthop Scand 26:99, 1956

61. Gutierrez R, Spjut HJ: Skeletal angiomatosis. Clin Orthop 85:82, 1972

62. Halliday DR, Dahlin DC, Pugh DG, et al: Massive osteolysis and angiomatosis. Radiology 82:636, 1964

63. Pastakia B, Horvath K, Lack EE: Seventeen year follow-up and autopsy findings in a case of massive osteolysis. Skel Radiol 16:291, 1987

64. Rosai J, Gold J, Landy R: The histiocytoid hemangiomas. Hum Pathol 10:707, 1979

65. Wold LE, Unni KK, Beabout JW, et al: Hemangioendothelial sarcoma of bone. Am J Surg Pathol 6:59, 1982

66. Kahn LB, Nunnery EW, Lipper S, Reddick RL: Case report 144. Primary hemangiopericytoma of the right radius. Skeletal Radiol 6:139, 1981

67. Specchiulli F, Florio U: Desmoplastic fibroma of bone. Ital J Orthop Traumatol 2:141, 1976

68. Legacé R, Bouchard H-L, Delage C, et al: Desmoplastic fibroma of bone. An ultrastructural study. Am J Surg Pathol 3:423, 1979

69. Campanacci M, Olmi R: Fibrosarcoma of bone. A study of 114 cases. Ital J Orthop Traumatol 3:199, 1977

70. Taconis WK, van Rijssel TG: Fibrosarcoma of long bones. A study of the significance of areas of malignant fibrous histiocytoma. J Bone Joint Surg [Br] 67:11, 1985

71. Taconis WK, van Rijssel TG: Fibrosarcoma of the jaws. Skeletal Radiol 15:10, 1986

72. Dahlin DC, Unni KK, Matsuno T: Malignant fibrous histiocytoma of bone—Fact or fancy? Cancer 39:1508, 1977

73. Feldman F, Lattes R: Primary malignant fibrous histiocytoma (fibrous xanthoma) of bone. Skeletal Radiol 1:145, 1977

74. McCarthy EF, Matsuno T, Dorfman HD: Malignant fibrous histiocytoma of bone: A study of 35 cases. Hum Pathol 10:57, 1979

75. Huvos AG, Heilweil M, Bretsky SS: The pathology of malignant fibrous histiocytoma of bone. A study of 130 patients. Am J Surg Pathol 9:853, 1985

76. Abrahams TG, Huyll M: Malignant fibrous histiocytoma (MFH) arising in an infarct of bone. Skeletal Radiol 15:578, 1986

77. Fornasier VL, Paley D: Leiomyosarcoma in bone: Primary or secondary? A case report and review of the literature. Skeletal Radiol. 10:147, 1983

78. Larsson SE, Lorentzon R, Boquist L: Primary liposarcoma of bone Acta Orthop Scand 46:869, 1975

79. Moorefield WG, Urbaniak JR, Gonzalvo AAA: Intramedullary lipoma of the distal femur. South Med J 69:1210, 1976

80. Dabska M: Parachordoma. A new clinicopathologic entity. Cancer 40:1586, 1977

81. Ayala AG, Spjut HJ: Parachordoma. Report of two cases. Submitted for publication

82. Weiss SW, Dorfman HD: Adamantinoma of long bone. Hum Pathol 8:141, 1977

83. Moon HF: Adamantinoma of the appendicular skeleton— A statistical review of reported cases and inclusion of 10 new cases. Clin Orthop 43:189, 1965

84. Perez-Atayde AR, Kozakewich HPW, Vawter GF: Adamantinoma of the tibia. An ultrastructural and immunohistochemical study. Cancer 55:1015, 1985

85. Eisenstein W, Pitcock JA: Adamantinoma of the tibia. Arch Pathol Lab Med 108:246, 1984

86. Campanacci M, Giunti A, Bertoi F, et al: Adamantinoma of the long bones. Am J Surg Pathol. 5:533, 1981

87. Winter RB, Moe JH, Bradford DS, et al: Spine deformity in neurofibromatosis. A review of one hundred and two patients. J Bone Joint Surg [Am] 61:677, 1977

88. Holt JF: Neurofibromatosis in children. AJR 130:615, 1978

89. Wilber MC, Woodcock JA: Ganglioneuromata in bone. J Bone Joint Surg [Am] 39:1385, 1957

90. McCarthy EF, Matz F, Steiner GC, Dorfman HD: Periosteal ganglion: A cause of cervical bone erosion. Skeletal Radiol 10:243, 1983

91. Yaghmai I, Foster WC: Case report 404. Intraosseous ganglion of the distal end of the ulna with a pathological fracture. Skeletal Radiol 16:153, 1987

92. Ruiter DJ, van Rijssel TG, van der Velde EA: Aneurysmal bone cysts. A clinicopathological study of 105 cases. Cancer 39:2231, 1977

93. McKay DW, Nason SS: Treatment of unicameral bone cysts by subtotal resection without grafts. J Bone Joint Surg [Am] 59:515, 1977

94. Scaglietti O, Bartolozzi P: The effects of methylprednisolone acetate in the treatment of bone cysts. J Bone Joint Surg [Br] 61:200, 1979

95. Caffey J: On fibrous defects in cortical walls of growing tubular bones. Adv Pediatr 7:13, 1955

96. Bosch AL, Olaya AP, Fernandez AL: Non-ossifying fibroma of bone. A histochemical and ultrastructural characterization. Virchows Arch [A] 362:13, 1974

97. Dehner LP: Fibro-osseous lesions of bone. p. 209. In Ackerman LV, Spjut HJ (eds): Bones and Joints. International Academy of Pathology Monograph. Williams & Wilkins, Baltimore, 1976

98. Campanacci M: Osteofibrous dysplasia of long bones. A new clinical entity. Ital J Orthop Traumatol 2:221, 1976

99. Lee PA, Van Dop C, Migeon CJ: McCune-Albright syndrome. Long-term follow-up. JAMA 256:2980, 1986

100. Halawa M, Aziz AA: Chondrosarcoma in fibrous dysplasia of the pelvis. J Bone Joint Surg [Br] 66:760, 1984

101. Lagier R, Cox JN: Pseudomalignant myositis ossificans. Hum Pathol 6:653, 1975

102. Dahl I, Angervall L: Pseudosarcomatous proliferative lesions of soft tissue with or without bone formation. Acta Pathol Microbiol Immunol Scand [A] 85:577, 1977

103. Savage RA, Hoffman GC, Shaker K: Diagnostic problems involved in detection of metastatic neoplasms by bone-marrow aspirate compared with needle biopsy. Am J Clin Pathol 70:623, 1978

104. Vaughn PB, Bindley HH: Pathologic fractures of long bones. South Med J 72:788, 1979

16

Skeletal Muscle

Umberto DeGirolami
Thomas W. Smith
David Chad
Vernon W. Armbrustmacher

Muscle diseases can be classified into eight broad categories on the basis of genetic, clinical, and pathologic characteristics:

Neurogenic atrophy (hereditary and acquired)
Dystrophies (hereditary)
Inflammatory myopathies (acquired)
Ischemia
Trauma
Congenital myopathies (hereditary)
Metabolic myopathies (hereditary and acquired)
Diseases of neuromuscular junction (acquired)

The diagnosis of a muscle disorder in clinical practice is facilitated by the joint assessment of the patient's medical history, physical examination, clinical laboratory values, electromyogram (EMG)/nerve conduction studies, and the muscle biopsy. The surgical pathologist whose responsibility is to evaluate the muscle biopsy must consider in concert all the clinical and laboratory data obtained. In addition, knowledge of the techniques of and indications for the biopsy and a familiarity with the range of morphologic appearance in normal and diseased muscle is necessary for proper evaluation of the biopsy.

In the account of the pathology of skeletal muscle diseases that follows we consider in turn biopsy techniques and indications, normal muscle, basic pathologic reactions of muscle, and the eight broad categories of muscle mentioned above. The reader interested in a more extensive discussion will be rewarded by finding several outstanding treatises on the subject.[1-4]

MUSCLE BIOPSY: INDICATIONS AND TECHNIQUES

The evaluation of a skeletal muscle biopsy specimen is dependent on careful selection of patients and on equally careful selection of the individual muscle for biopsy. Often, the physician who decides that a biopsy is necessary is not the person who actually does it. In these circumstances, communication between the two is essential. In addition, there must be previous communication with the pathology laboratory so that preparations for the proper handling of the biopsy specimen can be made beforehand.

Several considerations are important in choosing the muscle for biopsy. Usually, neuromuscular diseases are of a generalized nature, and it is possible to demonstrate pathologic changes if one confines the biopsy site to one or two muscles. The advantage in limiting biopsies to the same muscle from case to case is that the normal pattern, especially when dealing with histochemical stains, may vary considerably from muscle to muscle. In our experience, biopsies either from the belly of the quadriceps

545

femoris or from the biceps brachii are optimal for most generalized neuromuscular diseases. Some processes are focal or regional, however, and modifications must be made in these circumstances. A biopsy of a minimally but definitely involved muscle is also to be considered. Muscles with end-stage weakness or atrophy reveal end-stage pathologic changes that are nonspecific (Fig. 16-1). The earliest changes of neuromuscular disease are the most informative in terms of understanding its pathophysiology. When choosing the biopsy site, the site of a tendon insertion should be avoided, since the histology of the muscle normally varies in this area. Myotendinous areas normally contain internal nuclei and have a pronounced endomysial pattern of collagenous connective tissue with fiber splitting (Fig. 16-2). These changes would be considered abnormal in the belly of a muscle.

Once the biopsy site has been chosen and the pathology laboratory has been informed beforehand, the procedure can begin. Two pieces of muscle should be obtained ordinarily. One is isometrically clamped and fixed in formalin for paraffin embedding and light microscopy; portions of it are fixed in glutaraldehyde and embedded in epon for electron microscopic examination. The second is neither clamped nor fixed and is submitted directly to the laboratory, wrapped in a saline-moistened gauze to

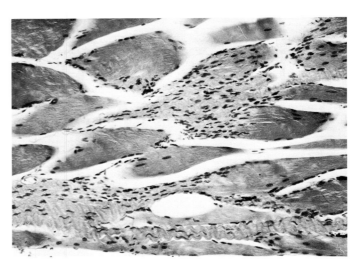

Fig. 16-2. Section of skeletal muscle fibers at a point of tendon insertion. Note the extensive fibrous tissue surrounding some of the fibers and the numerous internal nuclei. These changes may be mistaken for pathologic alterations. (Courtesy of AFIP.)

avoid drying, for snap-freezing and histochemical studies. Under special circumstances, when biochemical studies are needed, a third, unclamped specimen is snap-frozen and stored in the −80°C freezer until arrangements can be made for its transport to a laboratory that is equipped to perform the studies. Many types of clamps are now available for isometric fixation. We use the Price clamp, which has been very satisfactory.

In performing the biopsy, the skin is anesthetized and the incision over the biopsy site is made down to the fascia. The fascia is opened longitudinally, in parallel with the muscle fibers. A cylinder of skeletal muscle approximately the diameter of a pencil is gently dissected free. The isometric clamp is applied in situ, and the muscle cylinder is cut along the outside of the clamp. The isometrically clamped cylinder of muscle is placed in a fixative for approximately 30 minutes. The clamp may then be removed, with the muscle remaining in the fixative. Placing skeletal muscle directly into a fixative in an unclamped state causes a violent contraction and considerable disruption of the architecture of the muscle fibers, resulting in what is called contraction artifact (Fig. 16-3).

The unfixed piece of muscle must be snap-frozen to avoid artifactual disruption of the fibers due to the formation of ice crystals. The essence of the procedure is to cause the temperature of the specimen to drop from room temperature to below freezing as quickly as possible, causing the water more or less to freeze in situ, thereby preventing nidus formation of ice crystals that would otherwise grow into large crystals and disrupt the shape of the fiber (Fig. 16-4). Liquid nitrogen is used to cool iso-

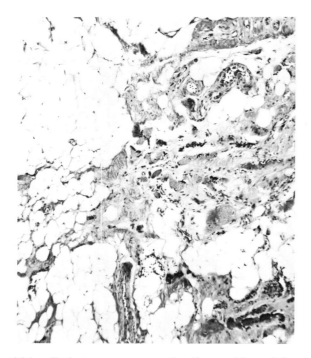

Fig. 16-1. End-stage neuromuscular disease. Most of the muscle has been replaced by fibrofatty tissue. The few remaining fibers are surrounded by collagen fibers. This pattern may be the end result of many neuromuscular diseases, either neuropathic or myopathic. (Courtesy of the Armed Forces Institute of Pathology [AFIP].)

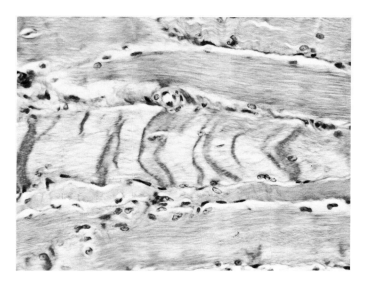

Fig. 16-3. Contraction artifact. Note the alternating dark (overly contracted) bands and pale areas. The myofibrils have been physically disrupted and have contracted into dense regions in the fiber. This artifact precludes meaningful evaluation of the architecture of the fiber and can be prevented by isometric fixation. (From Armbrustmacher.[174])

pentane (2-methylbutane), a substance that does not penetrate the muscle, has a very low freezing point, and will transmit heat efficiently. Isopentane is poured into a Pyrex container, immersed in the liquid nitrogen until the temperature of the isopentane is about −155°C. The muscle biopsy specimen, which has been mounted on a chuck in 7 percent gum tragacanth, is plunged into the cold isopentane. The biopsy specimen is mounted so that

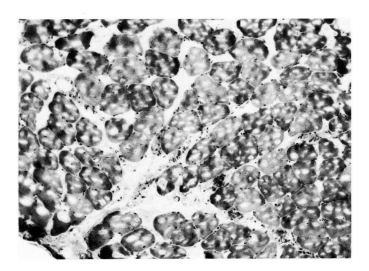

Fig. 16-4. Frozen section artifact. The fibers contain numerous "holes" caused by the development of large ice crystals due to slow freezing. (Courtesy of AFIP.)

cross sections will be obtained. Longitudinal sections can also be prepared if enough muscle is available. After 12 to 15 seconds, the chuck with the biopsy specimen is removed to prevent cracking of the mounting medium and put quickly and directly into a cryostat. Cryostat sections of the muscle biopsy are prepared, and the histochemical stains are performed.

If this biopsy specimen is to be shipped to another center for histochemical or biochemical studies, we have found that it is not necessary to mount the specimen on a chuck. In this case, the muscle can be placed directly in the cold isopentane. Once frozen, the specimen should be transferred to a precooled, sealable vial in an insulated styrofoam container filled with dry ice. We have found that an insulated styrofoam container with the capacity for approximately 1 cu ft of dry ice will keep a biopsy specimen frozen for 3 to 5 days, depending on external temperature conditions and the thickness of the insulation. The specimen should then be shipped air freight to the receiving center. It is wise to avoid holidays and weekends in the scheduling of this procedure.

If a biopsy specimen is studied by histochemical techniques, electron microscopy, and light microscopy of paraffin sections, a considerable expense is incurred. Often, it is possible to establish a definite diagnosis based on a single hematoxylin and eosin (H&E)-stained section from a paraffin-embedded block of tissue. To avoid unnecessary expense but still maintain the capacity for the complete study of the biopsy specimen, it is wise to obtain the two pieces of tissue as described. The frozen tissue may be stored in a deep freeze at −70°C indefinitely. The glutaraldehyde-fixed tissue may be minced, postfixed in osmium, and stored in unpolymerized epon indefinitely. If the problem is not solved with the examination of the paraffin-embedded tissue, the frozen and glutaraldehyde-fixed portions of the specimen may be either studied further or sent to a center at which appropriate studies can be performed.

NORMAL MUSCLE
Motor Unit

The functional unit of the neuromuscular system is the motor unit. Each motor unit consists of (1) the neuron located in the anterior horn of the spinal cord, or motor nucleus in the brainstem; (2) the axon of that neuron leaving the cord or stem, traversing the subarachnoid space via the anterior root, continuing peripherally via the motor (or mixed) nerve, terminating at the motor end plate, and (3) the muscle fibers it innervates. Motor neurons within the anterior horns are arranged somatotopically, so that those that supply the proximal limb muscles are located medially and those that supply the distal musculature are arranged laterally. The number of muscle fibers within a motor unit (i.e., those innervated by the axon of a single anterior horn cell) vary from a few to many hundreds. Muscles with highly refined movements, like the extrinsic muscles of the eye, have a high neuron to muscle fiber ratio (1 : 10); those with relatively coarse and stereotyped movements, like the calf muscles, have a much lower ratio (1 : 2,000). These autonomous units can be called upon to fire with increasing voluntary effort, thus explaining the gradation of power of a particular muscle. Histochemically, the muscle fibers of any given motor unit all react as either type I or II fibers (see the later section on histochemistry). It has been postulated that there are type-specific motor neurons in each motor unit that correspond to the two major histochemical types of muscle fibers.[5] The motor neuron in the anterior horn cell, in turn, determines the metabolic and physiological property of the muscle fibers in its domain. The neurons and axons of type I slow twitch units are relatively smaller than those of type II units. In man the muscle fibers within the purview of these units are intermingled within a particular muscle, giving the histochemical appearance of a checkerboard of alternating darkly and lightly stained fibers.

Development

Before discussing the histologic and histochemical characteristics of the normal adult muscle in detail, we briefly review the embryogenesis of skeletal muscle, since its understanding may be of value in the interpretation of morphologic changes in certain muscle diseases.[6,7]

The earliest cell that is recognized as committed to developing into skeletal muscle is called a myoblast. This cell is postmitotic and can be recognized by the presence of filaments of myosin and actin in its cytoplasm. Soon after the development of those identifying features, myoblasts acquire the unusual and unique capacity to fuse with other myoblasts, forming the myotube, the next stage in the embryogenesis of skeletal muscle. The myotube is a multinucleate cell with a roughly cylindrical configuration, in which there is very rapid accumulation of the filamentous proteins myosin and actin. These become arrayed in a very specific fashion causing the formation of myofibrils, which have a repeated cross-banded pattern. When these myofibrils line up in register, the entire myotube has a cross-striated configuration. The late stage of the myotube is then a cylindrical muscle fiber in which the nuclei are arranged in a clear central zone. The periphery becomes more and more packed with myofibrils (Fig. 16-5). There is no further development until the muscle fiber becomes innervated by a terminus of a lower motor neuron. By the time

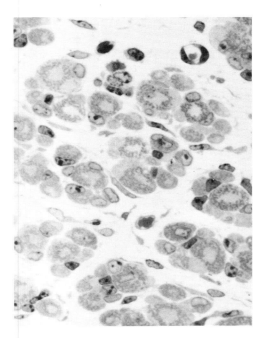

Fig. 16-5. Myotubes. Cross-section of developing skeletal muscle (mouse). Many of the fibers are at the myotube stage and are characterized by a pale homogeneous central zone or a single, central nucleus. The latter is relatively large and vesicular. The myofibrils are arranged around the periphery. (Courtesy of AFIP.)

the myotube is ready for innervation, the sarcolemma contains abundant, diffuse receptor protein for the neurotransmitter acetylcholine (ACh). This is the nicotinic acetylcholine receptor (AChR), and its presence seems necessary for the process of innervation. When the tip of the nerve fiber comes in contact with the muscle fiber, establishing a motor end-plate, the receptor protein becomes concentrated at the myoneural junction and disappears from the surface of the fiber elsewhere. It is possibly the disappearance of this extrajunctional receptor that prevents innervation of a fiber by more than one nerve terminal.

Once innervated, the fiber grows to maturity, apparently due to a complex and poorly understood trophic effect of the neuron on the muscle.[8,9] With this maturity, the muscle fiber becomes packed with myofibrils, and the nuclei arrange themselves in a specific pattern in a subsarcolemmal position according to nuclear territories.

Histology (Light and Electron Microscopy)

Mature striated muscle is composed of groups of fasciculi of longitudinally oriented muscle cells (fibers) (Figs. 16-6 and 16-7). Individual fibers run the length of the muscle from origin to insertion. Muscle fibers vary

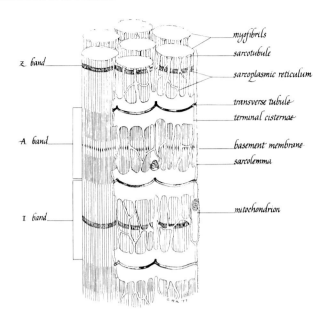

Fig. 16-6. Diagram of a portion of a skeletal muscle fiber. Note the arrangement of the sarcoplasmic reticulum and mitochondria (the membranous organelles) that surround the myofibrils. This network stains red with the modified Gomori trichrome stain, blue with Harris hematoxylin, and dark blue with the NADH-TR technique. The transverse tubular network, a continuation of the sarcolemma, is closely related to the dilated portion (cistern) of the sarcoplasmic reticulum. When isometrically fixed, the bands of the individual myofibrils are in register giving the entire muscle fiber its striated pattern. (From Armbrustmacher.[174])

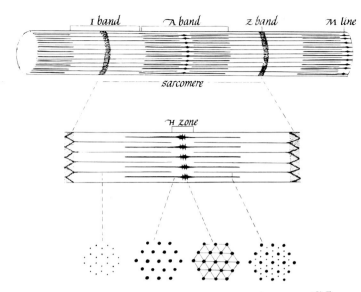

Fig. 16-7. Diagram of a sarcomere. The Z disc is the most dense band and apparently is a continuation of the actin filaments. It bisects the lighter (isotropic) I band, which is mainly composed of actin filaments arranged in a hexagonal array. The dark A band (anisotropic) is composed of overlapping actin and myosin filaments, the latter situated within the hexagonal space formed by the former. In the central region of the A band, where there are no overlapping filaments, there is a lighter zone (H zone). In the center of the H zone, the myosin filaments are thickened, and there is apparent intermolecular bridging, which is a thin dark line called the M line. A sarcomere, the functional and structural unit of the myofibril, extends from one Z disc to the next. (From Armbrustmacher.[174])

considerably in length and diameter, depending on the position and function of the muscle, age, skill, and the state of exercise (e.g., extrinsic eye muscles 17.5 to 20 μm, gluteus 87.5 μm in diameter). Males tend to have larger fibers than females. The cross-sectional shape of the adult muscle fiber is described as polygonal or multifaceted rather than round. Infant and fetal muscles and extrinsic eye muscles are normally round. The histologic structure of striated muscle is known to all students of biology and is best appreciated in longitudinal section. Muscle fibers are multinucleated cells bounded by a plasma membrane (sarcolemma) and a basement membrane and containing strategically arranged contractile proteins, a complex system of invaginating membranes, as well as the usual cellular organelles (e.g., mitochondria, Golgi apparatus, lysosomes). The nuclei are slender oval structures positioned beneath the sarcolemma and spaced about 10 to 50 μm apart. The chromatin is finely distributed and nucleoli are relatively inconspicuous except during active regeneration. Internalized nuclei occur in no more than about 3 percent of normal adult fibers. Satellite cells occur between the basement and plasma membranes and comprise about 4 to 10 percent of all the nuclei seen.

The familiar striations of skeletal muscle, seen as alternating dark and light regions with phase contrast, polarized light or interference microscopy, are imparted by repeating units of interlaced, longitudinally directed, thin myofilaments (actin) and thick, dark myofilaments (myosin). The dark regions do not permit light to pass through them and are referred to as anisotropic, while the light regions do and are isotropic. The anisotropic region or A zone is composed of myosin filaments alternating with actin filaments, whilst the isotropic region or I zone contains all actin filaments. A narrow dark band, the Z band, bisects the I zone and a narrow region of intermediate density, the H zone, composed of myosin filaments, bisects the A zone. A sarcomere is the distance between two Z bands; a myofibril is a longitudinally oriented cord of sarcomeres that runs the length of a fiber. The number of myofibrils in each fiber will vary considerably with the size of the fiber but on the average runs in the hundreds. At the tendinous insertion, myofibrils tend to fuse with the connective tissue and nuclei are often internalized and more numerous.

Electron microscopy has greatly advanced the understanding of the structural organization of skeletal muscle. Only through ultrastructural examination can the fine de-

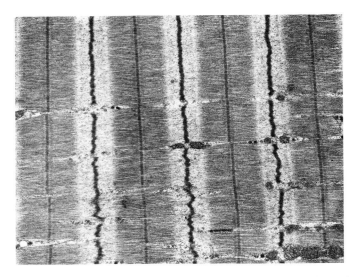

Fig. 16-8. Electron micrograph of a longitudinal section of skeletal muscle. Note the parallel arrangement of the myofibrils, so that the Z lines (dark) and A and I bands are in register. (×11,830) (From DeGirolami and Smith.[175])

tail of the sarcomere, the intracellular organelles and the specialized membranes be appreciated (Fig. 16-8). The plasma membrane is smooth and of even density (300 to 400 nm). It is uninterrupted except at invaginations of the tubular (T) system. The basement membrane overlies the sarcolemma and is separated from it by a space ranging from 1,000 to 3,000 nm. Variability in thickness and regularity of this membrane and redundance or reduplication of it are quite commonly seen both in the normal and in various disease states. Nuclei are in close proximity to the plasma membrane and separated from the underlying sarcomeres by mitochondria, fat globules, glycogen granules, smooth endoplasmic reticulum and the Golgi apparatus. The geometric beauty of the sarcomere is clearly evident. Each myofibril is 0.5 to 1.0 μm thick and separated from its neighbors by a loop of the T system, smooth endoplasmic (sarcoplasmic) reticulum, mitochondria, fat globules, and intervening unstructured myoglobin-containing cytoplasm. The T system is an invagination of the sarcolemmal membrane into the interior of the cell. In longitudinal sections it appears as a round or oval space bordered by a thick membrane. The T system runs parallel to the Z bands and is often seen beside the I band. It is accompanied by two cisterns of endoplasmic (sarcoplasmic) reticulum on either side. The profile of a centrally placed T tubule flanked by the two cysterns of sarcoplasmic reticulum is called a triad.

Histochemistry

Contraction (twitch), the muscle cells' main task, requires energy expenditure. Adenosine triophosphate

(ATP) is required for actin-myosin binding and for calcium reuptake by the sarcoplasmic reticulum. In man there are a variety of muscle cell types distinguished by their twitch speed and the way in which they derive their ATP. The type I fiber is concerned mainly with slow, sustained contractions and a slow twitch speed and is fatigue resistant. This type of fiber derives most of its energy from breakdown of lipid. Type I fibers are mitochondria- and oxidative enzyme-rich; glycogen- and glycolytic enzyme-poor. The type IIB fiber is concerned mainly with strong, short duration contractions; this type of fiber has a fast twitch speed, fatigues easily and derives most of its energy from glycogen breakdown. Type IIB fibers are rich in glycolytic but poor in oxidative enzymes. A third fiber type (type IIA) shares characteristics with both type I and type IIB fibers. This fast twitch fiber is relatively fatigue resistant; it is well endowed with both glycolytic and oxidative enzyme systems. A fourth fiber type (IIC) may represent undifferentiated fibers and is seen in fetal tissue. These functional properties are listed in Table 16-1. Histochemical reactions bring out these fiber types and are extremely important in the interpretation of muscle biopsies (Table 16-2).

Although in some animals, entire muscles are composed of one or another fiber type, in most human muscles both oxidative and glycolytic fibers are randomly distributed in a checkerboard pattern, with types I, IIA, and IIB each comprising about 30 percent of the total number of muscle fibers. Figure 16-9 demonstrates normal muscle fibers stained by the H&E method and Figure 16-10 with the alkaline ATPase technique. The latter is the basis for classifying fiber types.

Many other histochemical reactions are useful in certain situations. For example, in the reverse ATPase (RATPase) method, by preincubating the sections in an

TABLE 16-1. Muscle Fiber Types

Type I (37%)	Type II (63%)
Red	White
Sustained action	Sudden action
Weight-bearing	Purposeful motion
Slow-twitch	Fast-twitch
Soleus (pigeon)	Pectoral (pigeon)
Trichrome: red	Trichrome: green
High oxidative enzymes	Low oxidative enzymes
Low ATPase	High ATPase
Low phosphorylase	High phosphorylase
EM	EM
Many mitochondria	Few mitochondria
Abundant fat	Little fat
Wide Z band	Narrow Z band

TABLE 16-2. Histochemical Staining of Muscle Fibers

Stain	Fiber Type		
	I	IIA	IIB
H&E	+ +	+	+
Trichrome	+ + +	+ +	+ +
ATPase, pH 9.4	+	+ + +	+ + +
ATPase, pH 4.6	+ + +	0	+ +
ATPase, pH 4.3	+ + +	0	0
NADH-TR	+ + +	+ +	+
Oil-red O	+ +	+	+
PAS	+	+ + +	+ +
Phosphorylase	+	+ + +	+ + +

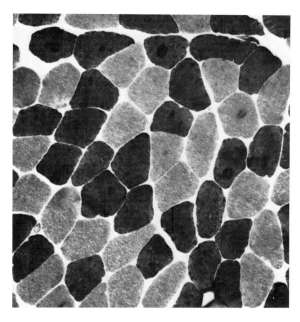

Fig. 16-10. Normal muscle fibers (frozen section, ATPase). The alkaline myosin myofibrillar ATPase stain is the basis for classifying fiber types. There is a crisp distinction between the dark (type 2) and light (type 1) fibers. This distinction is maintained even in advanced pathologic states of the fiber. The stain, done at an alkaline pH of 9.4, is deposited on the myofibrillar component of the fibers, in contrast to the NADH-TR reaction product, which is deposited on the membranous organelles. (Courtesy of AFIP.)

acid medium and then staining with the same technique as in Figure 16-10, a reversal of the pattern occurs. If the preincubation is at pH 4.3, the reversal is complete, with the type I fibers staining dark and type II fibers light. At pH 4.6, the reversal is partial, with a population of intermediate staining fibers. The dark fibers are type I, and the remaining fibers are type II. The latter are subdivided into type IIA fibers (those that are completely reversed

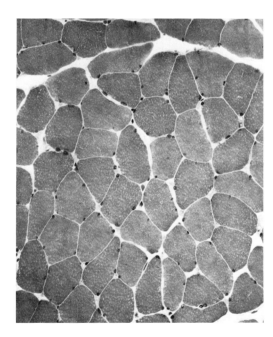

Fig. 16-9. Normal muscle fibers. (Frozen section, H&E) Note the complete absence of shrinkage artifact, which is unavoidable in paraffin-embedded tissue. This makes the assessment of atrophy or changes in fiber configuration more accurate. The endomysial connective tissue is not discernible. Nuclei are peripheral. The intermyofibrillar network (membranous organelles), which is barely perceptible, stains blue with Harris hematoxylin. The myofibrils are pink. (Courtesy of AFIP.)

and are light) and type IIB (the intermediate-staining fibers). Some pathologic changes selectively involve subtypes of type II fibers. For example, tubular aggregates, which may develop in periodic paralysis, occur only in type IIB fibers.

The reaction product in the nicotinamide adenine dinucleotide-tetrazolium reductase (NADH-TR) stain, the reduced tetrazolium—which is a formazan—is a dark precipitate that has an affinity for lipid membranes. The staining pattern thus reflects the distribution of the sarcoplasmic reticulum and mitochondria. Myofibrils are visible as unstained areas. Since type I fibers have more mitochondria, they appear darker with this stain. The distinction is not as clear as with the ATPase reaction, and many fibers of intermediate density are present. In addition, the fiber-type identity is often not maintained in pathologic situations. Fibers that are atrophic due to denervation are often excessively dark whether they are type I or type II. The value of this stain is its reflection of the architecture of the membranous organelles. Abnormal collections of mitochondria (as in "ragged red" fibers) and sarcoplasmic masses (aggregates of membranous material in degenerating fibers) are darkly stained. Target fibers (see Fig. 16-24) are best recognized with this stain.

Supporting Structures

Muscle fibers are supported by several layers of connective tissue sheaths. The epimysium envelops single muscles or large groups of fibers. Variable numbers of muscle fibers are grouped in primary and secondary bundles or fasciculi, enveloped by connective tissue, the perimysium, which is contiguous with the epimysium. The endomysium consists of a delicate network of connective tissue fibers, blood vessels, lymphatic tissue, and nerves, which surrounds the individual muscle fibers (Fig. 16-11). Detailed accounts of the microvascular supply of muscle are given by Kakulas and Adams[3] and the ultrastructural morphology of the vascular wall is discussed in standard textbooks of histology.[10]

Muscle spindles are found at the edge of a fasciculus or on the perimysium and away from the tendinous insertions. They are found in all muscles but are more numerous in certain muscles (lumbricals) and are difficult to find in others (eye). Each limb muscle might contain as many as 100 of these structures, although not necessarily evenly distributed throughout the muscle. Spindles are fusiform structures varying in length from 0.5 to 3.0 mm. They are oriented parallel to the direction of the muscle fibers and attach at the poles to the aponeuroses and connective tissue sheaths surrounding the muscle fasciculi. The normal muscle spindle has a very distinctive histologic appearance (Fig. 16-12). It is a rounded structure in cross section varying in diameter from 200 to 1,000 μm. The spindle contains easily distinguishable elements: a capsule, intrafusal muscle fibers, nerve fibers,

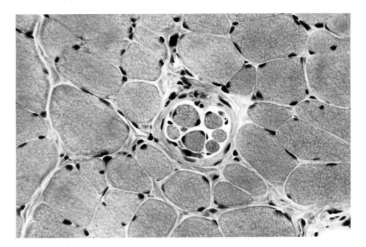

Fig. 16-12. Normal muscle spindle. (Frozen section, H&E) Note the prominent multilayered capsule. Six intrafusal fibers are well visualized. The extrafusal fibers show some variability in size. The biopsy specimen was taken from an 11-year-old girl with neurogenic muscular atrophy. (From DeGirolami and Smith.[175])

specialized nerve endings, and blood vessels. The intrafusal fibers contained within the capsule (between 4 and 16) are structurally similar but not identical to fibers outside the spindle (extrafusal fibers). The intrafusal fibers are either nuclear bag fibers (20 to 30 μm in diameter) or nuclear chain fibers (4 to 8 μm in diameter). Both fibers are generally round in cross-section and have unique histochemical reactions. The larger of the two, the nuclear

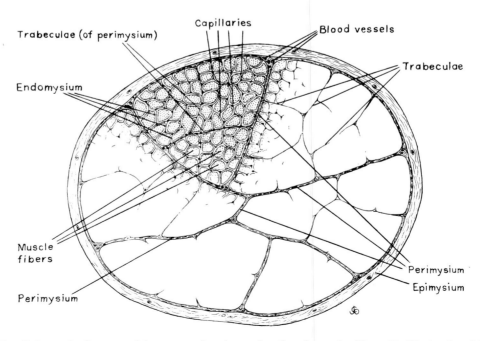

Fig. 16-11. Schematic diagram of the connective tissue sheaths of muscle. (From DeGirolami and Smith.[175])

bag fibers, contains a collection of nuclei at the equatorial zone of the fiber. Nuclear chain fibers have a row of internalized nuclei extending the length of the fiber. The muscle spindle capsule is a highly specialized structure containing several collagenous layers with intervening tight junctions that prevent the entrance of tracer substances applied to the surface of the spindle. The motor nerve supply is via the fusimotor system of efferents, and the afferent sensory fibers take origin from the primary (flower-spray) and secondary (annulospiral) endings. The function of spindles is sensory, responding to stretch in muscles and thus maintaining muscle tone.[11]

The junction of nerve and muscle (motor end plate, neuromuscular ending) is difficult to recognize in ordinary H&E-stained paraffin-embedded sections. It generally appears as an aggregate of nuclei and nerve fibers on the surface of the muscle fiber. Special techniques utilizing intravital dyes, metallic impregnation, histochemical reactions, or electron microscopy are required for their identification (Fig. 16-13). Motor nerves that leave the anterior horn of the spinal cord en route to skeletal muscles penetrate the connective tissue sheaths and subdivide into many branches until a single nerve fiber makes contact with a single muscle fiber. Occasionally, the same nerve fiber can be shown to give off two motor end plates to adjoining fibers. The connective tissue sheath of the nerve fiber fuses with that of the endomysium. The myelin sheath of the nerve terminates in a series of folds, after which a naked axon covered by connective tissue sheaths extends toward the muscle fiber for a distance of about 100 to 500 μm. At the surface of the muscle fiber, the nerve splits in an elaborate terminal arborization to make synaptic contact with the muscle. Each of the terminal branches has an expansion that lies in a relatively elevated portion of the muscle fiber, in which the surface membrane thickens into a series of folds. Beneath these folds are more than the usual complement of subsarcolemmal nuclei, mitochondria, glycogen, and other organelles. The end portion of the axon is the so-called axon terminal, containing synaptic vesicles and mitochondria. The space of the synaptic cleft is about 70 nm wide. The synaptic cleft is filled with fine granular material.[12]

Functional Relationships

It has been known since 1954 that muscle contracts because the actin filaments slide between the myosin filaments. During contraction, the sarcomere shortens. This results in narrowing of the I band, but the length of the A

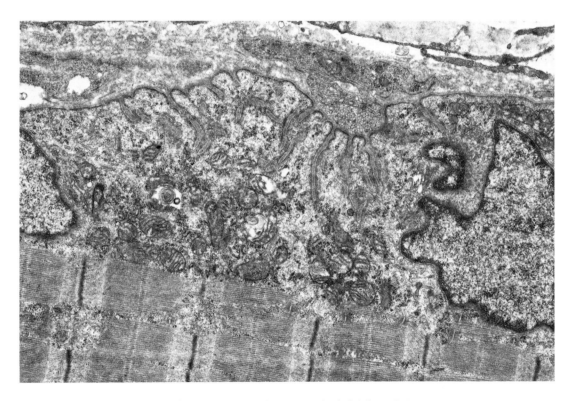

Fig. 16-13. Normal motor end plate (rat). ($\times$11,500) Note the infolding of the sarcoplasmic membrane and the adjacent axon terminal with synaptic vesicles and mitochondria. (Courtesy of Dr. Richard Evans, Department of Pathology [Neuropathology], University of Massachusetts Medical Center.)

band remains constant. A closer look at the filamentous proteins helps explain how muscle contraction occurs. Myosin and actin are involved in the process of contraction. Other proteins (tropomyosin and troponin) are concerned with the regulation of the myosin-actin interaction. Myosin, a complex, large protein capable of splitting ATP, is composed of two proteins: light meromyosin (LMM), a rod-shaped protein, and heavy meromyosin (HMM), which has two components: a short tail region that connects HMM to LMM, and a globular head region that projects upward from the rod-like protein backbone and forms attachments to actin. Thin filaments are made up of a double-strand helix of polymerized globular actin units. The regulatory proteins, tropomyosin and troponin, are attached to the actin. Tropomyosin is a fibrous protein and troponin is a globular one with three subunits. At rest, tropomyosin lies adjacent to actin in a potential myosin-binding site, sterically inhibiting myosin-actin interaction. When muscle is stimulated the intracellular concentration of calcium increases to a critical level at which a troponin subunit binds calcium and leads to a reorientation of the regulator proteins: tropomyosin moves into the groove between actin helices, and the myosin-binding site on the actin molecule is unmasked. Myosin heads then bind ATP, form cross-bridges with actin-binding sites, rotate (causing filament sliding and muscle shortening) and detach, releasing the products of ATP breakdown.

One property of sarcoplasmic reticulum is its ability to accumulate calcium and maintain very low intracellular concentrations of this ion. The wave of depolarization spreading down the T tubules appears to change sarcoplasmic reticulum calcium permeability, resulting in calcium release into the myofilamentous milieu. Contraction occurs and is followed a few milliseconds later by calcium reuptake by the sarcoplasmic reticulum, an ATP-consuming process. Return to low intracellular calcium concentration allows tropomyosin to slip back into the actin-myosin binding site; actin and myosin disengage and relaxation occurs.

GENERAL REACTIONS OF SKELETAL MUSCLE

The general reactions of skeletal muscle to injury are discussed in detail in the monographs by Engel and Banker[1] and Kakulas and Adams.[3]

Atrophy

Atrophy of muscle fibers refers to a reduction in cross-sectional girth that may be the result of abnormalities of innervation or myopathic disorders. The most commonly encountered type of atrophy is neurogenic. The end result of severance of the connection between nerve and muscle is atrophy of the muscle cell, broadly defined as a reduction in its size. Muscle fiber atrophy can also be observed as a result of immobilization, malnutrition in the broadest sense, compression, aging, vascular insufficiency, and other mechanisms. Most of the available information on muscle fiber atrophy comes from studies of atrophy caused by denervation and immobilization. In both forms of atrophy, the histopathologist is confronted with the interpretation of a dynamic process in which there may be gradations of injury and repair (reinnervation). The shape of the individual fiber that is volumetrically reduced in size, the distribution of such fibers in relation to normal ones, and the histochemical characteristics of the affected fibers become important considerations. Atrophic fibers are easily recognized histologically because they are smaller than normal in cross-section. The nucleus or nuclei tend to cluster together and seem more prominent than usual, and the shape of the fiber is distorted. The normal polygonal contour is lost, and the fiber assumes a roughly triangular (angulated) shape where the angles taper off acutely, sometimes partially encircling neighboring normal fibers and conforming to their shape (see Fig. 16-17). Within the first 3 weeks following experimental animal nerve section, there is about a two thirds reduction of the average cross-sectional area of the fiber. In the same period of time, the decrease in volume is less pronounced with immobilization (bed confinement, bone fracture, and splinting, experimental tenotomy, upper motor neuron paralysis). Many observers have demonstrated that the first fibers to atrophy in the early phases of immobilization and denervation are those fibers involved mainly in phasic movements (type II fibers histochemically). The structural events that attend shrinkage of the cell after immobilization and denervation are best seen with the electron microscope. The overwhelming change is the loss of myofibrils beginning at the periphery of the fiber and decreasing rapidly in number as the fiber atrophies. The nucleus is unremarkable, and sarcotubular profiles and mitochondria increase in density. The sarcolemma is intact, and reduplication of basement membrane material is often evident. In time, as the fiber shrinks, the normal myofibrillar organization is no longer recognizable: aggregates of haphazardly oriented "units" composed of thickened Z bands from which emanate filaments of variable thickness are seen streaming about, interspersed with loose myofilaments. The sarcoplasm continues to be fairly closely packed with contractile proteins, until the death of the cell. It is not clear how long the muscle fiber may remain in an atrophic state, but in humans, one may estimate in terms of months or years. As in other tissues, parenchymal cell death due to atrophy is followed by ingrowth of connective tissue and fat, presumably due to stimulation of pluripotential cells. This so-called end-stage muscle disease is common in the terminal phases of many muscle diseases. Recent work on muscle atrophy resulting from senescence shows little difference in the structure of aging atrophic muscle and that in denervation or immobilization. Lipofuscin pigment, although present, rarely fills more than one third of the cross-sectional area of the fiber and is generally not considered etiologically significant in the atrophy of senescence. A reduction in fiber size can also occur in congenital myopathies and dystrophies, perhaps because of faulty development or repeated cycles of necrosis and regeneration, respectively.

Hypertrophy

Hypertrophied fibers are larger than normal, although they are generally well proportioned in terms of shape and constituent organelles (Fig. 16-14). They may develop as a consequence of excessive work demands or possibly faulty reinnervation. Work hypertrophy of muscle is, of course, the basis for increase in muscle bulk in athletes. There seems to be little doubt that exercise-related muscular enlargement is related to hypertrophy and not hyperplasia of muscle fibers. Ultrastructural and biochemical studies of work-related hypertrophy of skeletal and cardiac muscle have shown the volumetric enlargement of the fiber to be due to an increase in the number of myofibrils and an increase of contractile protein. The stimulus for this work-induced hypertrophy is presumably neurogenic, because repetitive firing of motor units induces the muscle to do more work. Experimental studies on compensatory hypertrophy induced by tenotomizing the synergist of a muscle have demonstrated volumetric fiber enlargement following denerva-

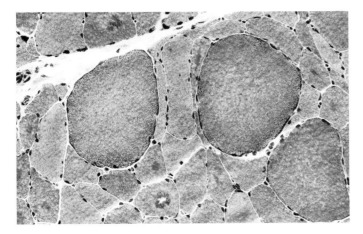

Fig. 16-14. Hypertrophy. (Frozen section, MGT) Note the presence of three very large fibers. (From DeGirolami and Smith.[175])

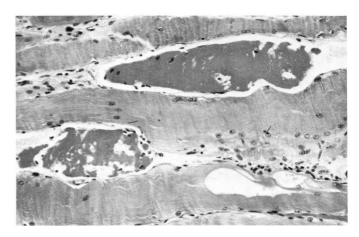

Fig. 16-15. Degeneration. (Paraffin section, H&E) Two fibers demonstrate hyaline degeneration, vacuolization, and fragmentation. (From DeGirolami and Smith.[175])

tion of the synergist. It is imperative in diagnostic work that one be familiar with the normal range of muscle fiber diameters for a given age, sex, muscle, and type of preparation. To this end, morphometric comparisons between normal and abnormal muscle are of great importance.[1]

Necrosis

An important general category of reactions of the muscle cell to injury includes those acute or subacute destructive changes that result in the death of the entire fiber, ultimately leading to phagocytosis by inflammatory cells (Fig. 16-15). The early phases of this type of injury can be distinguished histologically from the cellular atrophies just described. The severity of the insult and the efficacy of the regenerative response will determine the potential for functional restoration of the muscle. As in other tissues, the major stumbling blocks in the accurate identification of acute injury are the difficulties in distinguishing surgical, postmortem, or preparative artifact from disease. Indeed, the borderline between very acute injury and artifact may be blurred. Muscle fibers may be destroyed massively by trauma, ischemia, exposure to toxic chemicals, radiation, or invasion by microorganisms. The destroyed tissue during resolution of the process undergoes the sequence of inflammation and repair leading to a fibrous scar, as is typical of many other organs.

By contrast, the muscle fiber may be affected to a very slight extent, focally or segmentally, leaving the supporting tissues relatively intact. In general, this form of injury leads to a less marked inflammatory response and a more effective regenerative response. Segmental necrosis is found in a variety of experimental animal myopathies induced by vascular, traumatic, toxic, or immunologic mechanisms. In humans it is seen in idiopathic polymyositis, viral myositis, and partial ischemic lesions. It is typical to see focal loss of cross-striations for a relatively short segment along the length of a fiber. The otherwise normally organized myofiber may be replaced by a smudge of hyalinized or coagulated protein, in which the myofibrillar organization is lost. In the earliest stages of injury, the size of the necrotic lesions may vary considerably but ordinarily does not extend for more than 100 to 200 μm along the length of the fiber. Often, in small lesions, the subsarcolemmal myofibrils are damaged preferentially. The sarcolemma may rupture, and portions of the sarcoplasm may be seen extruding extracellularly. At the same time, neighboring nuclei become pyknotic or disappear. In the acute phase of injury, the changes are similar to those referred to as Zenker's waxy degeneration.

Regeneration

In spite of much literature on experimental models of skeletal muscle regeneration in mammalian and nonmammalian species, there has been considerable reticence on the part of pathologists to draw direct analogies from this work to human disease states. The regenerating fiber stained with H&E and examined under the light microscope has a number of distinctive features (Fig. 16-16). The cytoplasm is light blue, and cross-striations are difficult to see. The nuclei are more numerous in a given area and larger than normal, and one or more nucleoli may be

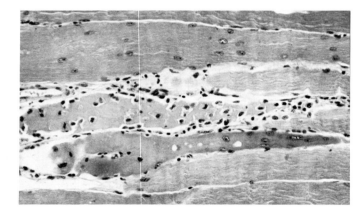

Fig. 16-16. Regenerating and degenerating muscle fibers. (Paraffin section, H&E) Note two abnormal fibers in the center of the field. The upper one is a degenerating fiber characterized by fragmentation and disintegration of the sarcoplasm and invasion by macrophages. The lower one is a regenerating fiber characterized by basophilic (darker staining) cytoplasm and large internalized nuclei with prominent nucleoli. Another regenerating fiber is seen at the top of the field. The biopsy was taken from a patient with polymyositis. (From DeGirolami and Smith.[175])

quite prominent. It is difficult to trace the fiber for any length because it tends to taper off or sometimes seemingly breaks off abruptly. Fibers tend to vary in size, some are thinner than normal, others about the normal size. Hypertrophic regenerating fibers are rare. Fibers sometimes take on the appearance of multinucleated cells or giant cells. Fusion between basophilic regenerating fibers and normal fibers is not infrequent. Regenerating fibers tend to occur in the vicinity of acute or ongoing muscle fiber injury.

Ultrastructurally, regenerating fibers can be recognized by their large nuclei and nucleoli, sometimes occupying an internal position within the fibers. The plasma and basement membranes are unremarkable, and the number of organelles is not especially different from normal, except perhaps for an increased number of free ribosomes. The most striking cellular alterations in regeneration are found in the contractile system. There may be large areas of the fiber in which the filaments are poorly organized into myofibrils, although they may be oriented in parallel. When Z bands are seen, the organization of the myofibrils seems much more normal. As in the atrophic fiber, clusters of short thick and thin filaments on each side of a thickened Z band may be strewn about haphazardly.

The mechanisms of regeneration in humans have not been fully clarified. Among the many postulated, there is evidence to support regeneration in the form of budding or sprouting of sarcoplasm from healthy ends of a severed, crushed, or otherwise segmentally injured muscle. The nuclei of the cell at the regenerating ends become prominent, and the nucleoli enlarge. New cells are formed (myoblasts, satellite cells), migrating in and out of the injured segment and eventually forming a new and usually thin muscle fiber. The term "fiber splitting" has been used by some workers to describe the light microscopic appearance of a muscle fiber in cross-section showing one or more lengthwise "cracks." The pathogenesis and significance of the change is controversial.

MUSCLE DISEASES

Table 16-3 presents our classification of muscle diseases. As the etiologic agent(s) of many of the conditions listed below are still unknown, the classification presented is tentative and will surely change many times in the years to come.

Neurogenic Atrophy

In this section, we shall use the term neurogenic atrophy to refer to those morphologic changes occurring in

TABLE 16-3. Classification of Muscle Diseases

Neurogenic atrophy

Muscular dystrophies
   X-linked muscular dystrophy
      Duchenne muscular dystrophy
      Becker muscular dystrophy
   Autosomal-dominant
      Facioscapulohumeral muscular dystrophy
      Oculopharyngeal dystrophy
      Myotonic dystrophy
   Other
      Limb girdle syndrome
      Congenital muscular dystrophy (and Fukuyama type)

Inflammatory myopathy
   Idiopathic polymyositis or dermatomyositis
   Granulomatous
   Infectious myositis

Ischemia

Trauma

"Congenital" myopathies
   Central core disease
   Nemaline myopathy
   Centronuclear (myotubular) myopathy
   Congenital fiber type disproportion

Metabolic myopathies
   Glycogenoses
   Myoadenylate deaminase deficiency (MDD)
   Mitochondrial myopathies
   Lipid myopathies
   Endocrine myopathies
   Periodic paralysis
   Myoglobulinuria

Disorders of the neuromuscular junction

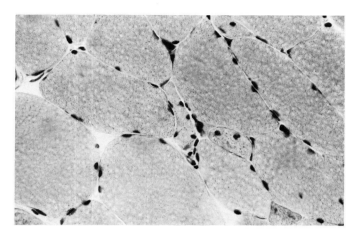

Fig. 16-17. Denervation atrophy. (Frozen section, H&E) Note the two small angulated fibers in the center of the field. (From DeGirolami and Smith.[175])

muscle which result from interruption of its normal innervation, i.e., denervation. These changes can be a reflection of disease affecting the lower motor neuron anywhere along its course, ranging from abnormalities affecting primarily the anterior horn cell, such as amyotrophic lateral sclerosis (ALS) or poliomyelitis, to disorders primarily affecting the axonal processes, as in anterior root disease and peripheral neuropathy.

Clinically, muscles involved by neurogenic disease are weaker and thinner than normal. Deep tendon reflexes gradually diminish as the disease progresses. In general, neurogenic atrophy tends to involve the distal musculature before the proximal, in contrast to many of the myopathic disorders, such as polymyositis or muscular dystrophy, in which the proximal muscles are more severely affected early in the disease. For the pathologist involved in the examination of a muscle biopsy from a patient with neurogenic disease, an important point to remember is that the histologic appearance of the muscle, while being highly characteristic, generally lacks sufficient specificity to allow determination of the precise etiology or ana-

tomic site of the disease process causing the denervation. For example, denervation atrophy observed in a muscle biopsy from a patient with ALS cannot be reliably distinguished from that seen in a peripheral neuropathy. Correlation of the histopathologic changes observed in the muscle with the clinical and laboratory findings is necessary in order to arrive at the most appropriate diagnosis in a given case.

The principal morphologic response of the muscle to denervation is atrophy of individual myofibers.[13] The involved fibers become progressively smaller and assume a characteristic angular, sharply contoured shape (Fig. 16-17). These configurational changes are thought to be largely the result of distortion of the atrophic fibers by the surrounding normal fibers. Although the presence of angulated fibers most often indicates a neurogenic disorder, they can also be observed in some myopathic conditions, including polymyositis, inclusion body myositis, facioscapulohumeral dystrophy, myotonic dystrophy, oculopharyngeal dystrophy, and Becker dystrophy. It is possible that the occurrence of the angulated atrophic fibers in these myopathic diseases may reflect a concomitant neurogenic component. As fiber atrophy progresses, the amount of cytoplasm shrinks to the point where only small aggregates or clumps of small pyknotic nuclei are visible by light microscopy. On electron microscopy, denervated fibers show loss of myofibrils beginning at the periphery of the fiber.[14] As atrophy progresses, there is gradual dissolution of both thick and thin myofilaments and smearing of the Z bands[15] (Fig. 16-18). The sarcolemma becomes wrinkled and the basement membrane is thrown into redundant folds.[16] In the early stages of denervation, when only a few anterior horn cells or axons may be involved by disease, the atrophic fibers are distributed more or less randomly throughout the muscle.

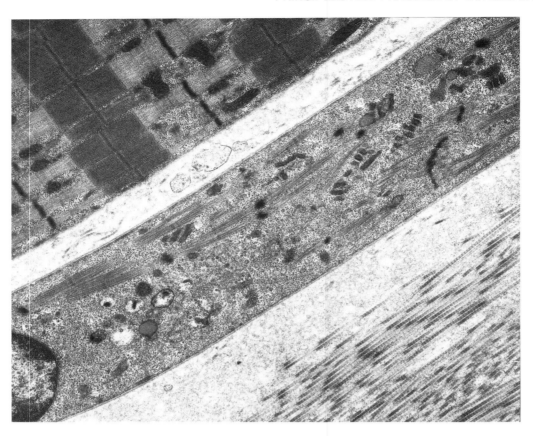

Fig. 16-18. Denervation atrophy. (×16,000) An atrophic fiber is next to a normal fiber. Note the loss of normal sarcomere structure. Disorganized myofibrils and organelles are present in the cytoplasm. The sarcolemmal and basement membranes are intact. (From DeGirolami and Smith.[175])

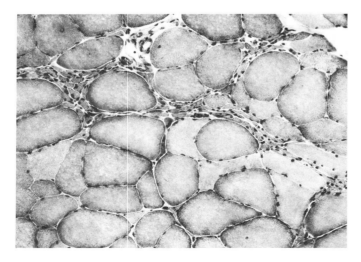

Fig. 16-19. Denervation atrophy. (Frozen section, H&E) As denervation progresses, the angular fibers appear in groups. There are pyknotic nuclear clumps among them, and many of the surrounding fibers have undergone hypertrophy. Some of the latter have internal nuclei. (Courtesy of AFIP.)

With progression of the disease, the atrophic fibers tend to cluster in small groups—a process sometimes referred to small group atrophy (Fig. 16-19). A characteristic feature of denervation is that, with histochemical staining using the myofibrillar ATPase reactions, the angular atrophic fibers are both type I and type II (Fig. 16-20). As yet, no known motor neuron diseases or neuropathies exclusively affect muscle fibers of only one histochemical type. Therefore, it follows that the finding of type-specific atrophy in a biopsy should suggest a process other than denervation. Another characteristic histochemical feature of denervation is that, with an oxidative enzyme stain such as NADH-TR or the nonspecific esterase reaction, virtually all the atrophic fibers tend to stain quite darkly regardless of their fiber type as determined by the myofibrillar ATPase stains[17] (Fig. 16-21). This phenomenon is most likely related to the relative increase in the concentration of various organelles, including mitochondria, secondary to loss of myofilaments and reduction in cytoplasmic volume.

Denervated fibers acquire the ability to synthesize extrajunctional ACh receptor along the sarcoplasmic membrane, analogous to the myotube stage of embryonic

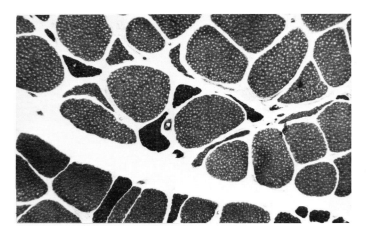

Fig. 16-20. Denervation atrophy. (Frozen section, ATPase pH 9.4) Both light (type 1) and dark (type 2) small angulated fibers are seen randomly dispersed throughout the field. (From DeGirolami and Smith.[175])

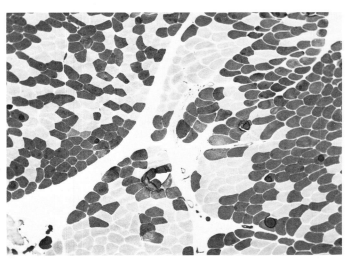

Fig. 16-22. Type-grouping. (Frozen section, ATPase) Note the loss of the normal checkerboard pattern. Groups of contiguous fibers are of the same histochemical type. This may be the only sign of a neuropathic process and represents reinnervation. (Courtesy of AFIP.)

muscle.[18] Coincident with this, adjacent intramuscular nerve twigs are stimulated to initiate collateral sprouting.[19] By this process, previously denervated fibers may become reinnervated. The reinnervated muscle fibers, however, will assume the fiber type of their new innervation. This will eventually lead to loss of the normal random histochemical checkerboard pattern, with the formation of small or large groups of contiguous fibers having the same histochemical fiber type. The process is referred to as fiber type grouping and is virtually pathognomonic of reinnervation, hence denervation[20,21]

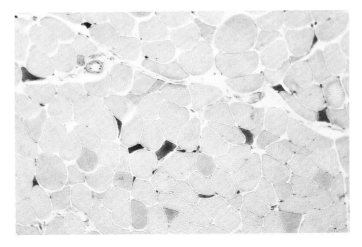

Fig. 16-21. Denervation atrophy. (Frozen section, esterase) The angular atrophic fibers are excessively stained, a feature suggestive of denervation atrophy. The small, dark, oval structures are pyknotic nuclear clumps, representing a late stage of atrophy. Pyknotic nuclear clumps are the end stage of fiber atrophy due to many causes and are not specific for denervation. (Courtesy of AFIP.)

(Fig. 16-22). We believe that at least 15 or more contiguous fibers of the same histochemical type should be present for the recognition of definitive fiber type grouping. Also, ideally, groups composed of both major types should be seen, so that type grouping due to reinnervation may be distinguished from fiber type predominance. In some chronic, slowly progressive denervating conditions (e.g., spinal muscular atrophy) or in patients who have suffered an acute episode of injury to the motor neurons in the remote past (e.g., in old poliomyelitis), reinnervation keeps close pace with denervation, resulting in a muscle that may appear essentially normal on H&E-stained sections. It follows that fiber type grouping (thus reinnervation) can only be reliably detected with histochemical techniques. If the denervating process is relentlessly progressive, the pace of denervation will exceed that of reinnervation, leading to atrophy of the enlarged previously reinnervated motor units with resultant type-specific group atrophy. This entire process is depicted schematically in Figure 16-23. Another morphologic change that may be observed in approximately 30 to 40 percent of cases of denervation is the target fiber.[22] This change affects predominantly—if not exclusively—type 1 fibers, and is best recognized in frozen sections stained for an oxidative enzyme such as NADH-TR. The affected fibers show a central area of diminished or absent enzyme activity surrounded by a narrow intermediate zone of increased activity, which is in turn surrounded by normally stained sarcoplasm. The combined effect of these zones of variable oxidative enzyme staining results in a characteristic bullseye appearance (Fig.

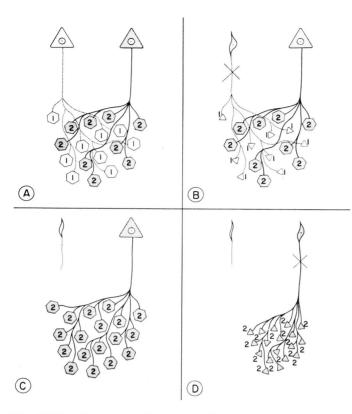

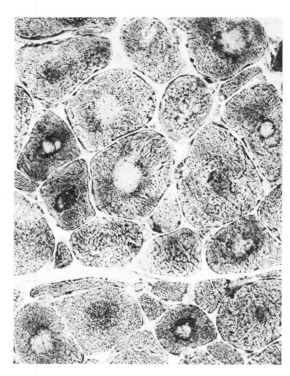

Fig. 16-24. Target fibers. (Frozen section, NADH-TR) These are characterized by a clearing of the membranous organelles from the central portion of the fibers. The NADH-TR stain will show the structure most consistently. They are characteristic of denervation and occur in type 1 fibers. (Courtesy of AFIP.)

Fig. 16-23. Schematic illustration of the process of denervation and reinnervation. **(A)** Normal. The light motor unit is composed of the anterior horn cell, nerve fibers, and the randomly distributed hexagonal muscle fibers labeled 1. The dark motor unit comprises the muscle fibers labeled 2. This accounts for the normal checkerboard pattern. **(B)** Random fiber atrophy. The muscle fibers of the light motor unit (triangles) have become atrophic because of interruption of their normal innervation. **(C)** Fiber type grouping. Through collateral sprouting, the previously denervated muscle fibers of the light motor unit are reinnervated by the dark motor unit. The atrophic fibers have regained their normal proportions but now have the histochemical properties of the dark motor unit. **(D)** Type-specific group atrophy. As the dark motor unit becomes affected by disease, all the fibers belonging to that unit (including those previously reinnervated) undergo atrophy. (From DeGirolami and Smith.[175])

16-24). On electron microscopy, the target fiber shows a central area of clearing of membranous organelles including mitochondria, surrounded by a ring of condensed sarcoplasmic reticulum and mitochondria.[23-27] In the central zone, the myofibrils may be preserved initially but will eventually degenerate. When the latter occurs, the target fiber may then be recognized by light microscopy with other staining methods (H&E, trichrome, ATPase). Target fibers are generally considered to be a manifestation of neurogenic disease, although their exact histogenesis is still unclear. Some investigators[24] regard them as a feature, possibly transient, of acute denervation,

whereas others[27] consider them a phase of reinnervation. Sometimes muscle fibers may be observed that have an appearance similar to that of target fibers but that lack the intermediate zone of increased oxidative enzymatic activity. These are known as targetoid or core-targetoid fibers, the latter referring to their apparent morphologic similarity to the fibers observed in central core disease, one of the congenital myopathies (see below). Targetoid fibers can also be seen in denervation but appear to be much less specific for neurogenic disease.[28]

In some long-standing denervative disorders, such as Charcot-Marie-Tooth disease, spinal muscular atrophy, and radiculopathies, the affected muscles may show, in addition to the typical histologic features of neurogenic atrophy, changes that may be described as myopathic in nature, such as increased numbers of internal nuclei, fiber splitting, focal necrosis, regeneration, and mild interstitial inflammation.[29-31] These so-called secondary myopathic changes may be reflected clinically by the presence of mild elevations of serum creatine kinase (CK). The precise mechanism for their formation is not known. Although they are generally mild compared with the neurogenic features seen in a given biopsy, it is important to be aware of them to avoid classifying a denervative disease as a primary myopathy. On the other hand, problems can occasionally arise in muscle biopsies obtained from patients with certain myopathic disorders, such as oculopharyngeal dystrophy, Becker muscular dystrophy, which may show small angulated fibers and apparent group atrophy in addition to the more typical myopathic changes. In these instances, one must rely on concomitant clinical and laboratory information for the correct diagnosis.

Although the histologic features of neurogenic atrophy generally do not permit recognition of the specific disease process that has given rise to the denervation, an exception to this is infantile (type I) spinal muscular atrophy (Werdnig-Hoffman disease). This disorder is inherited as an autosomal-recessive trait and is characterized by degeneration of lower motor neurons in the spinal cord and some cranial nerve nuclei. The disorder has its onset in early infancy and is characterized by generalized muscular weakness and hypotonia, with rapid progression to death usually before the age of two.[32,33] It is one of the causes of floppy infant syndrome. Muscle biopsies from affected individuals have a highly characteristic appearance, consisting of fascicles and large groups of extremely atrophic, rounded (rather than angulated) fibers of both fiber types; and clusters of markedly hypertrophic fibers that consistently stain as type I fibers as determined by ATPase reactions[2] (Figs. 16-25 and 16-26). One point of caution: this morphologic picture may not be seen in biopsies taken from infants in the early stages of

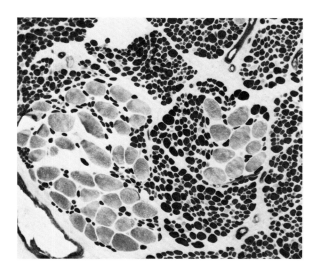

Fig. 16-26. Werdnig-Hoffmann disease. (Frozen section, ATPase) Same biopsy specimen as Figure 16-25. The normal and atrophic fibers are types 1 and 2. The hypertrophied fibers are characteristically type 1. (Courtesy of AFIP.)

the disease, when the biopsy may show only nonspecific variability in myofiber diameter and mild fiber atrophy.[34] Later-onset and more slowly progressive forms of spinal muscular atrophy are also recognized.[33] Childhood-onset cases are known as juvenile (type III) spinal muscular atrophy or Kugelberg-Welander disease. Muscle biopsies from these patients show the changes of chronic denervation and reinnervation as previously described, often associated with prominent secondary myopathic features.[2,35]

One condition that must be distinguished histologically from neurogenic atrophy on a muscle biopsy is atrophy that selectively involves only the type 2 fibers, that is, type II fiber atrophy. This rather common and nonspecific form of muscle atrophy is encountered in a variety of conditions, including disuse, cachexia, upper motor neuron disease, collagen-vascular disease, myasthenia gravis, Cushing's disease, and iatrogenic steroid myopathy.[2] On both paraffin-embedded and frozen sections stained with H&E, large numbers of angular atrophic fibers can be seen distributed randomly throughout the muscle. Although this appearance may superficially resemble denervation, the ATPase reactions will show that all the atrophic fibers are type II (Fig. 16-27). Also, in contrast to neurogenic atrophy, these small angulated fibers do not consistently stain darkly with the NADH-TR or nonspecific esterase reactions. The ATPase reaction performed at pH 4.6 indicates that the type IIB fibers are atrophic. The exact mechanism of type II fiber atrophy is not well understood. It is known that the volume of type II fibers is especially susceptible to trophic influences.

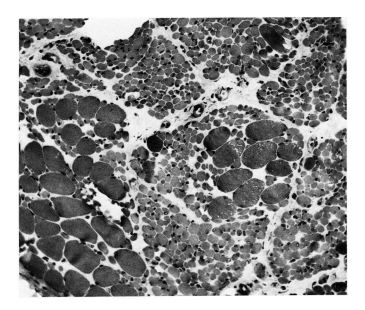

Fig. 16-25. Werdnig-Hoffmann disease. (Frozen section, MGT) There are groups of small, rounded atrophic fibers; normal-sized fibers; and clusters of fibers that are markedly hypertrophied. (Courtesy of AFIP.)

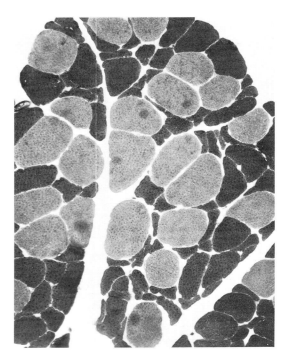

Fig. 16-27. Type 2 atrophy. (Frozen section, ATPase pH 9.4) Note that the type 1 fibers are not atrophic, and that all the small angular fibers are type 2. The atrophic fibers are not excessively dark with the NADH-TR and esterase reactions. This pattern, without histochemical studies, is often mistaken for denervation. (Courtesy of AFIP.)

Muscular Dystrophy

The muscular dystrophies are a heterogeneous group of inherited disorders of skeletal muscle in which there is an unknown factor that causes progressive destruction of muscle fibers without a prominent inflammatory reaction. They are characterized clinically by progressively severe muscular weakness and wasting, and often begin in childhood. Although a number of theories of pathogenesis have been proposed, the most widely accepted view holds that there is an abnormality of a gene or missing gene product which leads to destruction of the muscle fiber.[36] Some implicate a deficit in a muscle membrane protein as the primary site of the disorder in some dystrophies.[37,38] In Duchenne muscular dystrophy, dysfunction of membrane-associated enzymes has been demonstrated, and ultrastructural studies have shown gaps in the sarcolemmal membranes that permit the entry of large molecules such as horseradish peroxidase. Furthermore, there may be a systemic membrane abnormality in muscular dystrophy, as suggested by the finding of functional abnormalities in the membranes of erythrocytes, platelets and lymphocytes (defective capping phenomenon) in affected patients.[39]

X-Linked Muscular Dystrophy

Duchenne Muscular Dystrophy

Duchenne muscular dystrophy (DMD) is the most common and also the most severe of the muscular dystrophies, with a prevalence of about 1 per 10,000 males.[39] It is an X-linked recessive illness, although sporadic cases are common because of the high rate of spontaneous mutations. There have been rare reports of DMD in girls with Turner or Turner mosaic syndromes or X-autosomal translocations. The disorder becomes clinically manifest by the age of 5, progressing relentlessly until death in the early 20s. Boys with DMD are normal at birth and early motor milestones are met on time. Walking, however, is often delayed and the first indications of muscle weakness are clumsiness and inability to keep up with peers. Weakness begins in the pelvic girdle muscles and then extends to the shoulder girdle. Pseudohypertrophy of the calf muscles is an important clinical finding. The abnormally large muscle bulk is caused initially by an increase in the size of the muscle fibers and then, as the muscle atrophies, by an increase in fat and connective tissue. Myocardial involvement is common and characterized histologically by destruction of myocardial fibers and ingrowth of connective tissue. Some patients show mild mental retardation. Serum enzyme levels indicative of muscle destruction (e.g., CK) are elevated during the first decade of life but may be in the normal ranges in the later stages of the disease. Death results from respiratory insufficiency, pulmonary infection, and cardiac decompensation.

The histopathologic alterations in Duchenne muscular dystrophy are characteristic and generally representative of the changes seen in the muscles in the dystrophies as a group. Abnormalities (Figs. 16-28 and 16-29) include (1) a greater than normal size range in the cross-sectional fiber diameter (due to the presence of both small and giant fibers); (2) internalization of subsarcolemmal nuclei (beyond the normal range of 3 percent); (3) degeneration, necrosis, and phagocytosis of muscle fibers; (4) regeneration of muscle fibers; and (5) proliferation of endomysial connective tissue. One additional feature, which is said to be especially characteristic of the Duchenne form of dystrophy, is the presence of enlarged, rounded, hyaline fibers that have lost their normal cross-striations and are believed to be hypercontracted fibers. Fiber typing utilizing histochemical stains has been observed by most to show no alterations in the proportion and distribution of fiber types, so it is often not helpful from diagnostic point of view. Fibers sometimes cannot be typed. There is no selective fiber type involvement. Electron microscopic study shows muscle fibers in various stages of degeneration and regeneration but is generally of little diagnostic aid except in very early stages of the disease (Fig. 16-30).

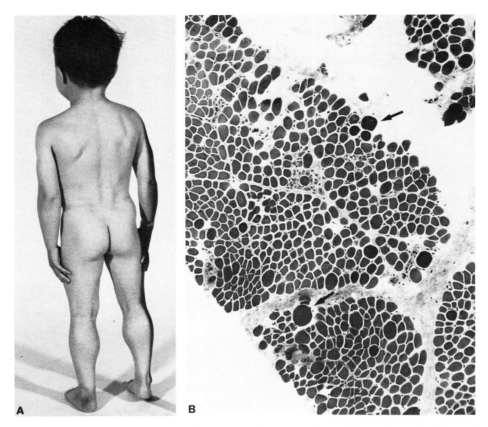

Fig. 16-28. **(A)** Duchenne muscular dystrophy. Note enlargement (pseudohypertrophy) of the calf muscles. **(B)** Duchenne muscular dystrophy. (Frozen section, H&E) Note variation in fiber size and enlarged round hyaline fibers (arrows). (From Chad et al.[176])

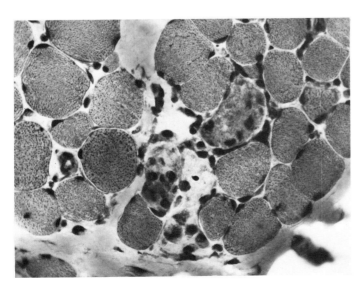

Fig. 16-29. Duchenne muscular dystrophy. (Frozen section, MGT) Several fibers are degenerating and undergoing phagocytosis. There is beginning endomysial fibrosis. (Courtesy of AFIP.)

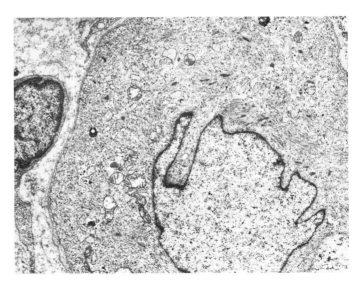

Fig. 16-30. Duchenne muscular dystrophy. (×6,300) Dystrophic fiber showing complete dissolution of the normal myofibrillar structure. The basement membrane and sarcolemmal membranes of this fiber are intact. (From DeGirolami and Smith.[175])

The plasma membrane defects (delta lesions) described by Engel and collaborators[39] are not easily demonstrable with certainty. In later stages of the disorder, the muscles eventually become almost totally replaced by fat and connective tissue. At this point, the histologic picture is indistinguishable from the end-stage of other severe myopathies, such as polymyositis, or neurogenic atrophy. Cardiac involvement, which may lead to arrhythmias and occasionally to congestive heart failure, consists of nonspecific interstitial fibrosis, more prominent in the subendocardial layers.

Definite female carriers are usually clinically asymptomatic but often have elevated serum CK (70 percent) and minimal myopathic histologic abnormalities on muscle biopsy. The advances in molecular genetics hold promise for a more definitive diagnostic test.

Becker Muscular Dystrophy

As in DMD, Becker muscular dystrophy is inherited as a sex-linked recessive or may occur sporadically. It is less common and much less severe than Duchenne dystrophy. The onset of the disease is later in childhood or in adolescence, and the rate of progression is slower and more variable, although there is considerable variation between pedigrees.[40] Many patients have a nearly normal life span. The morphologic changes in the muscle vary, but in general they are similar to but less severe than those seen in DMD. There are important differences, however. Histochemical staining generally shows better fiber type differentiation; type IIB fibers, which may not be demonstrable in DMD, are usually not deficient in the Becker type of dystrophy. The large hyalinized fibers seen in DMD are infrequent. Lastly, experienced investigators have stressed the concurrent appearance of striking neuropathic findings.[28]

Autosomal-Dominant Muscular Dystrophy

Facioscapulohumeral Muscular Dystrophy

Facioscapulohumeral (FSH) muscular dystrophy is inherited as an autosomal-dominant trait; therefore, both sexes may be affected. The age of onset is variable, but the more typical cases begin in the second or third decade. The muscles of the face, neck, and shoulder girdle are the first to be affected, and subsequently the disease may spread to the pelvic girdle. Deltoid muscles are uninvolved. The disorder, much milder than DMD, is slowly progressive. Patients may remain ambulatory even at advanced stages of the illness, but here again there is marked variability. Muscle hypertrophy and cardiac involvement are rare. The histologic findings on muscle biopsy are not specific, although most observers agree that the common findings are extreme variation in fiber size, with the presence of both markedly hypertrophied and severely atrophic, sometimes angular fibers, and relatively few degenerating myofibers. In some patients, the biopsy may show an unusually prominent mononuclear inflammatory response.[41]

Oculopharyngeal Muscular Dystrophy

Oculopharyngeal muscular dystrophy, which is frequently inherited as an autosomal-dominant trait, is characterized by ptosis and weakness of extraocular muscles, associated with difficulty in swallowing, occurring in mid-adult life.[42] Weakness of the face, jaw, and limb muscles may occur later in the disease. Most familial cases have been of French or French-Canadian origin. On microscopic examination, the skeletal muscle shows myopathic changes similar to those in the other dystrophies, with variation in fibers and scattered type I angular fibers. In addition, a distinct change—the so-called rimmed vacuole—may be seen in some of the muscle fibers. The central vacuoles contain granular material that stains red with Gomori trichrome and occur in type I fibers. Ultrastructural studies have demonstrated intranuclear filaments 7 to 9 μm in diameter[43] (Fig. 16-31).

Myotonic Dystrophy

Myotonic dystrophy stands apart from the previously described disorders because of its distinctive clinical and pathologic features.[44,45] Its inclusion with the other dystrophies has often been criticized for this reason. The disease, inherited as an autosomal-dominant trait with variable expressivity, has its onset between the ages of 20 and 40. The localization of the myotonic dystrophy gene is believed to be on chromosome 19. Cataracts, which are present in virtually every patient, may be detected early

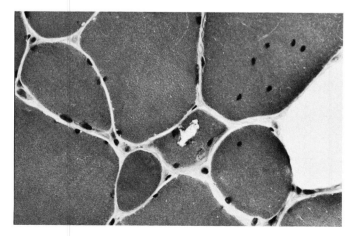

Fig. 16-31. Oculopharyngeal dystrophy. (Frozen section, H&E) Note variability in fiber size and internalized nuclei. The fiber in the center of the field contains a rimmed vacuole.

in the course of the disease with slit-lamp examination. Other associated abnormalities include frontal balding, gonadal atrophy, myocardiopathy, smooth muscle involvement, decreased plasma IgG, and an abnormal glucose tolerance test. Dementia has been reported in some cases. The disease begins in late childhood with gait difficulty secondary to weakness of foot dorsiflexors, then progressing to weakness of the hand intrinsic muscles and wrist extensors. Atrophy of muscles of the face (hatchet face) and ptosis ensue. Myotonia, or sustained involuntary contraction of a group of muscles, can be demonstrated in the tongue and thenar eminence upon percussion, vigorous contraction, or exposure to cold. The disease tends to increase in severity and to come on at a younger age in succeeding generations. The diagnosis can usually be confirmed by EMG, which shows characteristic myotonic discharges (the so-called dive-bomber effect acoustically). Congenital forms of the disease are recognized.

Pathologically, the skeletal muscles may show all the typical features of a dystrophy. In addition, there is a striking increase in the number of internal nuclei (Fig. 16-32). On longitudinal sections, these may form conspicuous chains. Another well recognized feature of myotonic dystrophy is the presence of ring fibers (Ringbinden, striated annulets). This is an abnormality of the muscle fiber in which there is a circumferential wrapping of a strip of the diseased fiber around itself. On cross-section, the abnormal fiber has a rim of sarcoplasm in which the myofibrils can be seen running tangentially in relation to the longitudinally oriented fibrils in the center of the fiber (Figs. 16-33 and 16-34). The ring fiber may be associated with an irregular mass of sarcoplasm (sarcoplasmic mass) extending outward from the ring. These sarcoplasmic masses stain blue with H&E, red with Gomori trichrome

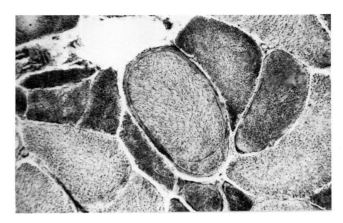

Fig. 16-33. Myotonic dystrophy. (Frozen section, NADH-TR) Ring fibers. A fiber in the center of the field demonstrates a thin circumferential strip of myofibrils running at right angles to the myofibrils in the rest of the fiber. (From DeGirolami and Smith.[175])

and intensely blue with the NADH histochemical reaction. Ultrastructurally, these masses are foci devoid of organized sarcoplasm and contain glycogen, mitochondria, ribosomes, and dense bodies. Although frequent in myotonic dystrophy, they can be seen in other neuromuscular disorders as well. The relation of the ring fiber to myotonia is not understood. Histochemical techniques have demonstrated a relative atrophy of type I fibers in some cases early in the course of the disease (Fig. 16-35).

A congenital form of myotonic dystrophy has been described in the neonate. Clinically, infants have severe hypotonia, facial diplegia, and respiratory difficulty. Pathologically the muscle may be normal or show atrophy of either type I or II fibers. Some fibers may be extremely small with internalized nuclei. Enzyme histochemistry fiber type differentiation may be impaired.

Other Muscular Dystrophies

Limb-Girdle Dystrophy

Limb-girdle dystrophy (syndrome) is a heterogeneous group of disorders that may be inherited as an autosomal-recessive trait or may occur sporadically.[46] The onset of the disease as well as its prognosis are extremely variable. It usually begins in the second or third decade of life, involving either the pelvic or shoulder girdle muscles with spread to others after a variable period of time. Cardiac involvement and pseudohypertrophy are rare. The disorder is generally slowly progressive, patients remaining ambulatory for 20 or more years. Pathologically, the muscle shows marked variation in fiber size with many extremely large fibers, pronounced fiber splitting, and many internalized nuclei. Degenerative and regenerative changes are also seen.

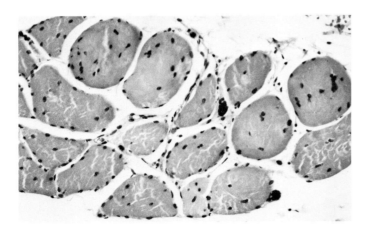

Fig. 16-32. Myotonic dystrophy. (Paraffin section, H&E) Note the striking increase in numbers of internalized nuclei and variation in fiber size. (From DeGirolami and Smith.[175])

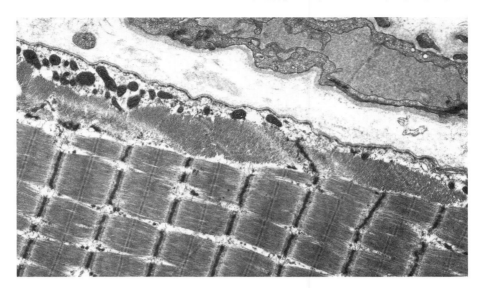

Fig. 16-34. Myotonic dystrophy. Electron micrograph of ring fiber. Disorganized myofibrils running perpendicular to the length of the fiber are observed beneath the sarcolemma. (From DeGirolami and Smith.[175])

Congenital Muscular Dystrophy

A heterogeneous group of hereditary neuromuscular diseases characterized by some degree of progressive hypotonia and muscle wasting evident at birth or in early infancy have been brought together for convenience under the heading congenital muscular dystrophy.[47] Although there has been considerable variability from case to case, most authorities agree that the histologic changes observed in skeletal muscle are similar in kind if not in

degree to those seen in the muscular dystrophies that occur at an older age. Endomysial fibrosis has been especially striking. These disorders are considered distinct from other myopathies that cause hypotonia in infancy, that is, the congenital myopathies. Too little is known about congenital muscular dystrophy to speculate on whether the primary defect is in the central nervous system (CNS), the peripheral nerves, or the skeletal muscle fiber itself. In the Fukuyama form described in Japan,[48] in addition to muscular weakness there are developmental abnormalities of the central nervous system.

Inflammatory Myopathies

Idiopathic

The most commonly encountered inflammatory myopathies are idiopathic. Immunologic mechanisms are presumed to play a major role in pathogenesis. These conditions are referred to as polymyositis (PM) when the muscle alone is affected and dermatomyositis (DM) when there is also cutaneous involvement. A convenient classification of these myopathies includes six forms: PM; DM; childhood DM; adult DM or adult PM associated with a malignancy; adult DM or adult PM associated with a collagenvascular disease; and inclusion body myositis (IBM).[49,50]

In general, these disorders are characterized by subacute, progressive proximal muscle weakness. The distal musculature tends to be affected in the later stages except in IBM, where early distal involvement is common. In all types cranial muscles are rarely affected. Dysphagia overall occurs in about one third of cases. In DM, the

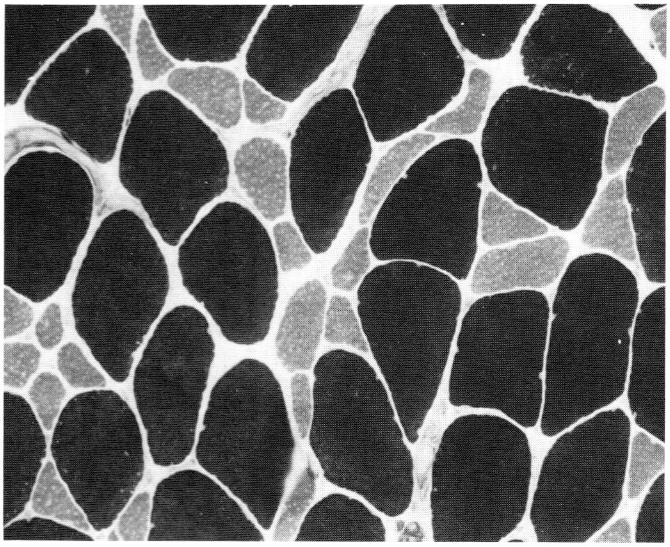

Fig. 16-35. Myotonic dystrophy. (Frozen section, ATPase pH 9.4) The type 1 fibers (light) are small and angulated, whereas the type 2 fibers (dark) are relatively unaffected. (Courtesy of AFIP.)

rash may precede, coincide with or follow the weakness. When the upper eyelids are involved, the pathognomonic heliotrope or blue discoloration is seen. In both PM and DM, electrocardiographic (ECG) abnormalities have been described.[51,52]

In childhood DM, subcutaneous calcification is frequent. PM and DM may be associated with well defined collagen-vascular diseases such as rheumatoid arthritis, scleroderma, polyarteritis nodosa, Sjögren's syndrome and lupus erythematosus. Neoplasia also occurs with increased frequency in adult PM and DM when compared with the normal population and the incidence increases with age.[49] One study suggested that the instance of malignancy in DM was five to seven times that of the general population.[53] Others have questioned whether a truly clinically significant relationship exists between malignancy and these myopathies.[54]

Laboratory studies show that the CK is elevated, and the EMG discloses short, polyphasic potentials with fibrillations, positive waves, and pseudomyotonic bursts. In general, the muscle biopsy discloses segmental fiber necrosis, fiber regeneration, and mononuclear cell infiltration around blood vessels, between fascicles and amongst muscle fibers (Figs. 16-36 and 16-37). Overall the muscle biopsy is abnormal in about 90 percent of patients who meet the clinical criteria for PM or DM.[55] Inflammatory cells are found in some 75 percent of patients. In large series, 10 to 20 percent of patients will show no evidence of inflammation.

Differences in pathologic features among the various types of inflammatory myopathy have been described. In childhood DM, Carpenter et al.[56] noted atrophic muscle fibers along the periphery of fascicles (perifascicular atrophy) (Fig. 16-38) and rarely muscle infarction associated

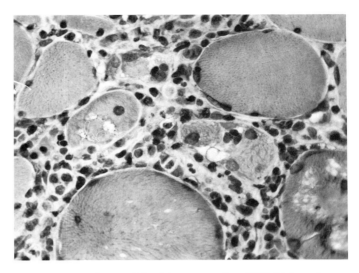

Fig. 16-37. Polymyositis. (Frozen section, H&E) Note degenerating fibers and extensive interstitial infiltrate of mononuclear inflammatory cells. The cluster of nuclei within the oval fiber in the center are probably phagocytes. (Courtesy of AFIP.)

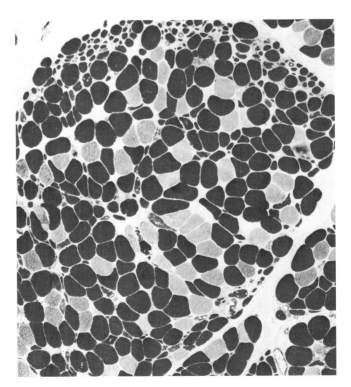

Fig. 16-38. Dermatomyositis. (Frozen section, ATPase) The atrophy and degeneration selectively involve the periphery of the fascicle. When this pattern is seen, there is usually minimal or no inflammation. The pattern is frequently present in childhood dermatomyositis and is rarely present in the adult form. (Courtesy of AFIP.)

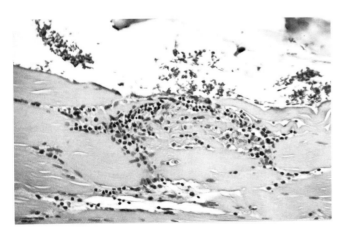

Fig. 16-36. Polymyositis. (Paraffin section, H&E) The muscle fiber in the center of the field is undergoing segmental necrosis, with focal destruction of the sarcoplasm and invasion by phagocytic inflammatory cells. (From DeGirolami and Smith.[175])

with loss of capillaries. Inflammatory cells are present in childhood DM but tend to be found mostly between fascicles with less mononuclear infiltration in the endomysium. In adult DM changes are similar except that perifascicular atrophy is less prominent. In adult PM, perifascicular atrophy is rare and there is little abnormality in muscle capillaries.[55] Inflammatory cells are present in the endomysium between and among muscle fibers. Necrosis and regeneration are scattered randomly throughout the fascicles. In IBM, a striking light microscopic feature is the presence of vacuoles containing basophilic granules (Fig. 16-39) (rimmed vacuoles).[57] As in PM, mononuclear inflammatory infiltration may be profuse, located mainly between fibers. A feature of IBM is the presence of clusters of atrophic fibers. No perifascicular atrophy is seen. Ultrastructural examination in IBM discloses abnormal intranuclear 18 nm filaments arranged in parallel or at random, oriented like bundles of sticks (Fig. 16-39). In PM or DM associated with an underlying neoplasm there are no characteristic muscle biopsy features. In PM or DM associated with a collagen-vascular disease, the pathology most closely resembles that seen in DM.[58]

Mechanisms of fiber damage in these diseases have yet to be completely defined, but there is much evidence to implicate immunologic factors. In DM, especially the childhood form, deposits of Ig and C3 have been found.[59] The complement system has been found to be deposited, bound, and activated to completion within the intramuscular microvasculature of patients with childhood DM (to a lesser extent, adult DM).[60] In childhood DM, necrosis and thrombosis of capillaries, small arteries, and venules has been found especially in those vessels at the periphery of muscle fascicles, accounting for perifascicular atrophy and microinfarction.

In PM and IBM the inflammatory cells consist largely of T-cells and macrophages.[55] Among the T-cells there is a T cytotoxic/suppressor predominance. There is focal invasion and destruction of nonnecrotic muscle fibers by T-cells and macrophages, suggesting previous sensitization to muscle fiber surface-associated antigen; cell-mediated immune damage seems to be of primary importance. In adult DM, humoral immunity appears to play an important part because the inflammatory infiltrate is composed mainly of B-cells and helper T-cells, although macrophages and cytotoxic/suppressor T-cells are also present.[55] In PM associated with the collagen-vascular disease scleroderma, an immunologic response mediated by T-cells appears to be directed against a connective tissue or vascular element, and not against the muscle fiber.

Granulomatous

Occasional patients with classic PM may have foci of granulomatous infiltrate in the muscle biopsy specimen.[61] If the granulomas are associated with active degeneration and regeneration of muscle fibers, they may well be a manifestation of PM. In these cases, however, it is important to search for such organisms as parasites, tubercle bacilli, and fungi.

If the granulomatous infiltrate is noncaseating, with striking clusters of epithelioid histiocytes and relatively few lymphocytes, and tends to infiltrate the connective tissue but not cause active myopathic changes, it may be a manifestation of *sarcoidosis*. This multisystem disease is characterized by the presence of granulomas in many different organs. Symptoms most commonly result from involvement of lung, eye and skin. Asymptomatic in-

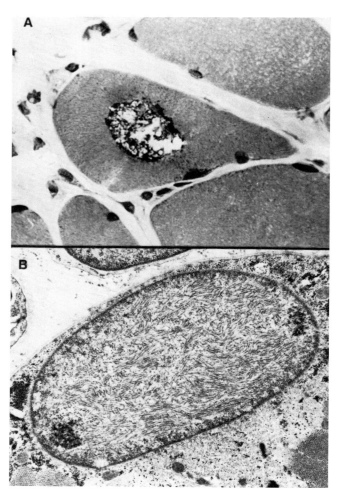

Fig. 16-39. **(A)** Inclusion body myositis. (Frozen section, H&E) A characteristic feature is the presence of vacuoles containing basophilic granules (rimmed vacuoles) within muscle fibers. **(B)** Inclusion body myositis. Electron microscopy discloses the presence of abnormal filaments within the cytoplasm or nuclei of muscle fibers. (From Chad et al.[177])

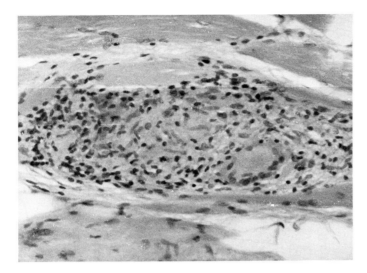

Fig. 16-40. Sarcoid myopathy. (Paraffin section, H&E) A granuloma containing a Langhans-type giant cell separates the muscle fibers. (From Chad.[178])

volvement of muscle is very common, with granulomas (Fig. 16-40) found in 50 to 80 percent of patients with stigmata of sarcoidosis who have been ill for two or more years.[62]

There are three kinds of symptomatic myopathy in sarcoid: a rare, nodular variety presenting with painful areas in parts of certain muscles; an acute form presenting with fever, aches and pains, and proximal muscle weakness; and a chronic, probably most common form seen in perhaps 10 to 15 percent of patients with neurosarcoidosis and presenting with slowly progressive painless proximal weakness, mainly in women over the age of 50.[62] A granulomatous myositis has also been found in Crohn's disease.[63]

Infectious

Pyogenic (bacterial) myositis is uncommon in the developed world except for occasional cases of gas gangrene associated with *Clostridium welchii,* usually the result of complicated mechanical trauma or postoperative wound infection. In the tropics, patients may present with multiple acute muscle abscesses, which are most often due to staphylococci. Pathologically, the affected muscle initially shows acute interstitial edema, followed by a pleomorphic inflammatory infiltrate consisting first of lymphocytes and then of neutrophils. At this stage, the muscle fibers show necrosis, phagocytosis, and regeneration.

Acute viral myositis affects children and adults. Most cases are caused by the influenza virus and the enteroviruses (Coxsackie and Echo groups). The usual clin-

ical syndrome is myalgia occurring in the setting of an acute febrile illness. The patient develops tender and swollen muscles as well as muscle weakness. Serum CK is elevated and there may be myoglobinuria as well as an abnormal EMG. When performed, the muscle biopsy discloses scattered muscle fiber necrosis, regeneration and interstitial inflammatory reaction.[64]

A variety of parasitic infections may involve muscle. The most common is *trichinosis,* which results from ingesting the larvae of the nematode *Trichinella spiralis* in uncooked pork (Fig. 16-41). After maturation of the ingested larvae in the human bowel, fertilized females penetrate the mucosa and deposit large numbers of embryos, which enter venules and lymphatics. These larvae then widely disseminate throughout the body, including the skeletal muscles. During the invasive stage, the affected individual will experience systemic symptoms accompanied by eosinophilia and variable muscle pain and weakness. Biopsy of an affected muscle shows the presence of encysted larvae, variable inflammation, degeneration and phagocytosis of muscle fibers, and focal connective tissue proliferation. In time, the larvae will die and frequently become calcified. Other parasitic infections that may occasionally involve skeletal muscle include cysticercosis (*Taenia solium*), hydatid disease (*Echinococcus*), and toxoplasmosis.

Ischemia

Skeletal muscle is relatively resistant to ischemic injury, because of its rich blood supply with many collat-

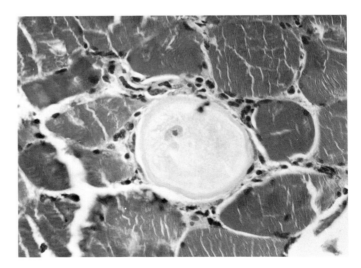

Fig. 16-41. Trichinosis. (Paraffin section, H&E) A degenerating organism is present in the center of the field. A scanty endomysial inflammatory infiltrate is present. The presence of eosinophils or granulomata in the infiltrate should prompt a search for such organisms. (Courtesy of AFIP.)

eral branches. Varying degrees of ischemic damage, however, may occur in the following conditions: (1) occlusion of a major artery to a limb by a thromboembolus; (2) severe arteriosclerosis with occlusion of multiple small peripheral arteries and veins (e.g., diabetes); (3) thrombosis of multiple intramuscular vessels, as in polyarteritis nodosa; (4) Volkmann's ischemic contracture (a rare complication of fractures attributed to arterial spasm); (5) swelling and hemorrhage of certain muscles enclosed in rigid compartments, with secondary compromise of their vascular supply (e.g., anterior tibial syndrome); and (6) trauma.[3]

The histologic changes seen in skeletal muscle subjected to ischemia are similar to those observed in infarction of other tissues of the body. The earliest findings consist of fragmentation of muscle fibers with focal loss of cross-striations. The fibers then become eosinophilic, acquiring a hyaline or waxy appearance. The nuclei become pyknotic and eventually disappear. The interstitium becomes edematous, separating individual fibers, and shows infiltration by polymorphonuclear leukocytes. After about 48 to 72 hours, there is invasion of macrophages, which phagocytize the dead muscle fibers. About this time, there is also beginning proliferation of fibroblasts in the endomysium. Many of the surviving fibers show marked swelling and vacuolization. At the edge of the infarct there is evidence of vigorous regenerative activity. The above changes characterize muscle that has been subjected to a fairly massive ischemic insult, such as a major arterial occlusion leading to gangrene. Lesser degrees of ischemia result in scattered foci of muscle fiber necrosis and regeneration, sometimes accompanied by variable interstitial fibrosis. Relatively little is known about the effects of more chronic ischemia on the skeletal muscle in humans (e.g., chronic arteriosclerotic vascular insufficiency).

Several accounts of the light and ultrastructural features of ischemic injury in experimental animals are available.[3] From these studies, several generalizations can be briefly stated: (1) the average duration of ischemia (usually tourniquet) needed to produce inevitable injury is about 8 hours; (2) the first changes that can be confidently related to the ischemic result are found in the contractile system and in the intracellular organelles: increased intracellular fluid, hypercontraction bands, and swelling of organelles; and (3) later, the cell membranes rupture and cell disintegration follows.

Trauma

Skeletal muscle may be traumatized through application of an external force, in which case the amount of damage is related to the degree of the force, fracture of adjacent bones, and damage to blood vessels.[3] Muscle may also be damaged secondary to violent exertion. This may be the result of herniation of the muscle through a tear in the covering fascia, or through actual rupture of the muscle itself. Histologic examination of the injured muscle shows rupture of many muscle fibers, with tearing of their sarcolemmal sheaths. Adjacent fibers may show granular, vacuolar, or waxy degeneration. These changes are often accompanied by interstitial edema and hemorrhage. The cellular reaction ranges from predominantly neutrophilic in the early stages to mononuclear later on, with phagocytosis of dead fibers and evidence of regenerative activity. Associated ischemic changes secondary to vascular damage are common. If the parallel arrangement of the endomysial tubes is disrupted, this may lead to marked fibrous tissue proliferation, which prevents effective regeneration. The gap is then replaced by a mass of scar tissue.

Primary hemorrhage into skeletal muscle may be secondary to trauma, thrombosis of intramuscular veins (due to severe infection), or hemorrhagic diathesis (anticoagulants, thrombotic thrombocytopenic purpura).[3] Histologically, there is dissociation of muscle fibers by variable amounts of blood. The intervening muscle fibers are normal or may show hyaline degeneration. At the margins of the clot, the red blood cells will eventually undergo phagocytosis, with the formation of hemosiderin pigment as early as the sixth or seventh day. There is also proliferation of fibrous connective tissue around the clot, which, if complete, will lead to formation of a white scar containing scattered hemosiderin-laden macrophages. If organization is incomplete, the connective tissue will form a capsule surrounding a cyst filled with degenerating red blood cells and blood pigment.

Occasionally following an unusually severe traumatic blow or tear, or sometimes following repeated episodes of minor trauma to a muscle, formation of bone may occur within the injured muscle—this is known as traumatic *myositis ossificans*.[3] The muscles most typically affected are the anterior thigh muscles (quadriceps femoris) and brachialis anticus. About 1 to 4 weeks after the initial traumatic event, a painful mass may develop in the affected muscle. This mass is usually readily palpable and may limit motion. Ossification after episodes of lesser trauma may be asymptomatic or may cause slowly progressive limitation of motion, as well as discomfort.

The initial injury affects the muscle and adjacent soft tissues and is almost always associated with a variable amount of hemorrhage. There may also be injury to the adjacent bone and periosteum. Following the initial injury, there is proliferation of intramuscular connective tissue, in which islands of cartilage and bone subsequently develop. The bone may form directly from the fibrous tissue or may arise in the islands of cartilage. The bone is cancellous and resembles the bone of callus formation in healing fractures. The muscle fibers themselves are not involved in the process of ossification but may be incorporated in or compressed by the calcifying tissue. The pathogenesis of myositis ossificans is thought to be related to (1) trauma of the adjacent periosteum with displacement of osteoblasts into the adjacent muscle and subsequent bone formation; (2) activation by trauma or hemorrhage of periosteal implants already present in the muscle; (3) metaplasia of pluripotential intramuscular connective tissue, with formation of cartilage and bone; and (4) metaplasia of fibrocartilage, a normal constituent of many muscle tendons.[3] (See Chapter 14 for a further discussion of the histologic appearance.)

Congenital Myopathies

The congenital myopathies constitute a group of disorders defined largely on the basis of the morphologic appearance of the muscle. Most of these conditions share common (although not invariable) clinical features, including onset in early life, nonprogressive or slowly progressive course, proximal or generalized muscle weakness, and hypotonia.[2,65] Individuals affected at birth or in early infancy may present as floppy babies. A genetic predisposition is usually apparent, although the mode of inheritance can be quite variable. Some patients may have associated dysmorphic skeletal abnormalities. Serum muscle enzymes are usually normal or only slightly elevated, and the EMG shows myopathic features. Because of the similarities in the clinical presentation of these disorders, accurate diagnosis depends on study of the muscle biopsy. This must always include the use of histochemical and electron microscopic techniques, since many of the characteristic morphologic features cannot be reliably identified on conventional paraffin-embedded material. Undue emphasis should not be placed on the histopathology alone, since none of the morphologic alterations seen in these disorders is entirely specific. It is generally the predominance of the morphologic change in a given biopsy in conjunction with the clinical features of the case which allow the diagnosis of a congenital myopathy to be made.

The major congenital myopathies discussed in this section include (1) central core disease, (2) nemaline myopathy, (3) centronuclear (myotubular) myopathy, and (4) congenital fiber type disproportion. In addition to these disorders, there is a smaller, more heterogeneous group of congenital myopathies, characterized chiefly by the presence of abnormal subcellular organelles, such as fingerprint body myopathy,[66] sarcotubular myopathy,[67] zebra body myopathy,[68] cytoplasmic body myopathy,[69] and reducing-body myopathy.[70] The reader is referred to the appropriate literature for discussion of these very rare conditions.

Central Core Disease

Central core disease was the first of the morphologically distinct congenital myopathies to be described.[71] The disorder may be inherited as an autosomal-dominant trait or may occur sporadically. The disease usually presents at birth or shortly thereafter, although some cases may have their onset later in life. Typically, it is characterized by hypotonia and nonprogressive weakness involving proximal more than distal musculature. Skeletal deformities, most commonly congenital dislocation of the hip and kyphoscoliosis, may be present. On occasion, the histologic features of central core disease have been seen in adult patients who are nearly asymptomatic. An association between central core disease and the malignant hyperthermia syndrome has been noted.[72]

Histologic examination of the muscle reveals a virtually pathognomonic picture. Many fibers show a central (or sometimes eccentric) area of pallor best recognized in frozen sections stained with an oxidative enzyme reaction such as NADH-TR (Fig. 16-42). On H&E- and trichrome-stained sections, the cores appear slightly pale, having the same color as but appearing more "homogeneous" than the surrounding sarcoplasm. The cores also show decreased glycolytic enzyme activity, as evidenced by reduced staining on the PAS and myophosphorylase reactions. On longitudinal sections, the cores extend the entire length of the fibers. Cores are only found in type 1 fibers, and most cases show a striking type 1 fiber predominance. On electron microscopy, the cores usually show some disruption of the sarcomeric pattern with degeneration of myofilaments and Z bands and diminution or loss of mitochondria, sarcoplasmic reticulum, and glycogen (Fig. 16-43). Cores have been further subdivided into structured and unstructured types.[73] In the former, the normal myofibrillar banding pattern and ATPase activity are retained, whereas in the "unstructured" core, ATPase staining and myofibrillar banding are lost. Both types of cores can occur in the same muscle, although in most cases the "unstructured" type of core tends to predominate.[74] Cases have also been described in which central cores and nemaline bodies have been found in the same muscle.[75,76]

The histogenesis of the cores is unknown. Because of the similarity of the cores to target and targetoid fibers, at both the light and electron microscopic level, the most frequently proposed explanation is that they result from an abnormality in innervation of the muscle, although there is little evidence to support this.[77] Structural changes somewhat resembling cores have been produced experimentally by tenotomy.[78]

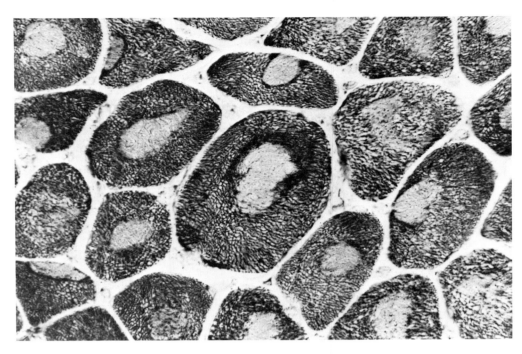

Fig. 16-42. Central core disease. (Frozen section, NADH-TR) Most of the fibers have a central (or sometimes eccentric) area of pallor. The cores occur only in type 1 fibers, and the ATPase stain usually shows a marked type 1 predominance.

Another congenital myopathy morphologically similar to but distinct from central core disease has been described as minicore or multicore disease.[79] This rather uncommon myopathy is characterized by the presence of multiple small foci of myofibrillar degeneration and loss of mitochondrial enzyme activity; these ultrastructurally resemble unstructured cores.

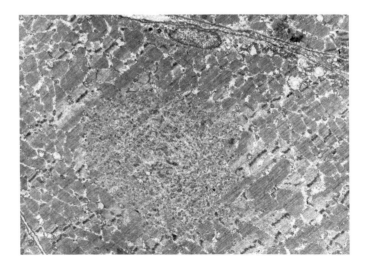

Fig. 16-43. Central core disease. (×1,900) The core consists of degenerated myofibrils and loss of formed membranous organelles. (Courtesy of AFIP.)

Nemaline Myopathy

This congenital myopathy was first described in 1963 by two independent groups of investigators.[80,81] The disorder can present in early childhood as well as in later life. Usually the clinical course in infancy is nonprogressive despite the presence of weakness, hypotonia, and delayed motor development. However, sometimes the course can be rapidly progressive and fatal. The weakness tends to involve the proximal limb muscles most severely and can also affect the facial and bulbar musculature. Skeletal abnormalities such as narrow face, high-arched palate, kyphoscoliosis, and clubbed feet may be present. The mode of inheritance is variable.

The pathologic hallmark of this disorder is the nemaline or rod body. Rod bodies are best visualized in frozen sections stained by the modified trichrome method, appearing as aggregates of red-purple granular or bacilliform structures, 2 to 7 μm in length, which tend to accumulate in the subsarcolemmal regions of the muscle (Fig. 16-44). They are difficult to detect in paraffin-embedded sections stained with H&E but can be seen with phosphotungstic acid hematoxylin (PTAH) stain. Nemaline rods are not stained by the oxidative enzyme or ATPase reactions. They occur predominantly in type 1 fibers. A variable degree of type 1 fiber predominance may be present. The number of fibers containing rod bodies, as well as the number of rods present in a given muscle fiber, can vary

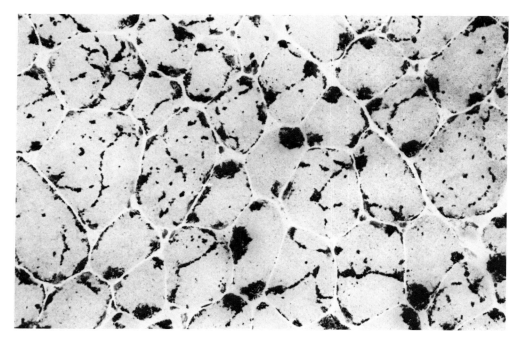

Fig. 16-44. Nemaline myopathy. (Frozen section, MGT) The nemaline (rod) bodies are visualized as aggregates of red-purple granular or bacilliform structures located predominantly in the subsarcolemmal regions of the fibers. The rod bodies are found mainly in type 1 fibers, and there is often a type 1 predominance. (From Chad et al.[176])

considerably from case to case.[82] On electron microscopy, nemaline rods appear as moderately electron-dense, lattice-like structures with periodic lines oriented parallel and perpendicular to the long axis (Fig. 16-45). They closely resemble normal Z bands and can often be observed in continuity with them.[83] The "free" ends of the rod bodies appear to be continuous with the thin myofilaments. Biochemical studies have shown that the major component of the nemaline bodies is α-actinin, which is also the major protein component of Z bands.[84,85] Present evidence thus suggests that nemaline rods are most likely derived from Z-band material. Although rod bodies are by no means specific for nemaline myopathy, in the appropriate clinical setting they are highly characteristic of the disorder. The precise relation of the nemaline bodies to the clinical muscle weakness is poorly understood.[82]

Centronuclear (Myotubular) Myopathy

This condition was first described by Spiro et al.[86] in 1966 and given the name myotubular myopathy because of the resemblance of the affected muscle fibers to fetal myotubes. Shortly thereafter, another group of investigators,[87] not convinced that the muscle fibers actually represented arrested myofiber maturation at the myotube stage, coined the term centronuclear myopathy for this

group of disorders. Both terms remain in current usage. Several clinical variants with different modes of inheritance are recognized.[47] The most common form, inherited as an autosomal-recessive trait, presents in infancy or early childhood and clinically shows prominent in-

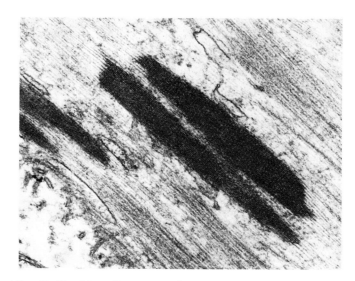

Fig. 16-45. Nemaline myopathy. ($\times 18,000$) The red granular structures seen by light microscopy correspond to these electron-dense rod-shaped masses that seem to arise from the Z disc. (Courtesy of AFIP.)

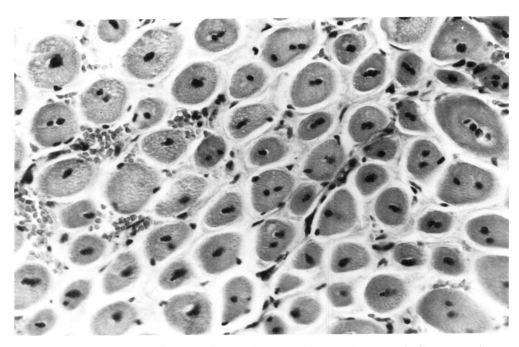

Fig. 16-46. Centronuclear myopathy. (Paraffin section, H&E) Most of the muscle fibers contain a centrally located nucleus. (From Chad et al.[176])

volvement of extraocular and facial muscles in addition to hypotonia and slowly progressive limb muscle weakness. Other less common variants include a severe X-linked recessive form characterized by marked hypotonia and respiratory distress[88-90] and milder, often later-onset autosomal-dominant[91,92] and sporadic[93,94] forms.

The characteristic pathologic feature of this group of disorders is the presence of a centrally located nucleus in the majority of the muscle fibers (Fig. 16-46). The central nuclei are often surrounded by a clear perinuclear halo that histochemically lacks ATPase activity and ultrastructurally is devoid of myofibrils and may show increased numbers of mitochondria and glycogen. The central nuclei are usually confined to type 1 fibers but can occur in both types. Usually there is a predominance of type 1 fibers, and these fibers are often smaller than usual. The term type 1 hypotrophy has been used for the latter situation, in keeping with the suggestion that the fibers have failed to attain normal size.[95]

The pathogenesis of the disorder remains unclear.[47] The original hypothesis of myofiber maturation arrest at the myotube stage has not been clearly proved or disproved. The disease appears to be a primary disorder of muscle; there is as yet no firm evidence implicating an abnormality of innervation.

Congenital Fiber Type Disproportion

Congenital fiber type disproportion was first described as a distinct clinicopathologic entity by Brooke in 1973.[96]

The disease presents in early infancy with hypotonia, proximal muscle weakness, and delayed motor development. Approximately one half of affected persons have skeletal abnormalities, including congenital hip dislocation, joint contractures, foot deformities, high-arched palate, and kyphoscoliosis. Respiratory difficulties may be present. The mode of inheritance is unclear.

The muscle biopsy characteristically shows type 1 fibers which are uniformly smaller than type II fibers by 12 percent or more[2] (Figs. 16-47 and 16-48). This size dispar-

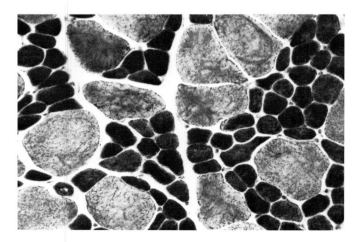

Fig. 16-47. Congenital fiber type disporportion. (Frozen section, NADH-TR) Note the two populations of fibers. The small (dark) fibers are exclusively type 1. (From DeGirolami and Smith.[175])

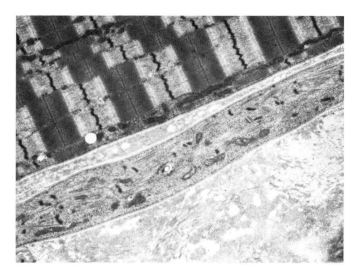

Fig. 16-48. Congenital fiber type disproportion. (×6,500) A small fiber is present next to a normal fiber. The ultrastructural appearance of the small fiber is similar to that in neurogenic atrophy. (From DeGirolami and Smith.[175])

ity is dramatically illustrated in histograms showing two distinct peaks. The type II fibers are of normal size or slightly hypertrophied. Type 1 fiber predominance is often present. With conventional H&E stain, the histologic appearance of the muscle could be easily confused with neurogenic atrophy (e.g., Werdnig-Hoffman disease) or a dystrophic myopathy, hence the need for histochemistry.

The status of congenital fiber type disproportion as a distinct clinicopathologic disorder was recently challenged.[47] It is known that the pattern of fiber size disproportion described above can also be seen in other neuromuscular disorders occurring in childhood, such as infantile facioscapulohumeral dystrophy,[97] Pompe's disease,[98] fetal alcohol syndrome,[98] Krabbe's disease,[99] etc. Furthermore, such well defined conditions as congenital myotonic dystrophy, myotubular myopathy, and nemaline myopathy may have associated hypotrophy of type 1 fibers.

Metabolic Myopathy

The term metabolic myopathy, as used in the present context, implies that there is some abnormality in the metabolism of the muscle that results in abnormal function. This may be caused by a generalized abnormal state of metabolism due to problems in other organs (hepatic failure, endocrinopathy, or renal failure) or to a primary metabolic lesion of the skeletal muscle itself, such as myophosphorylase deficiency in McArdle's disease. In some situations, we suspect that there is a metabolic lesion of some sort that is yet to be identified or defined. Sometimes, storage of abnormal amounts of materials

such as glycogen or lipid is associated with the myopathy, but at other times the metabolic lesion results in weakness with little or no morphologic change or in lysis of the muscle (rhabdomyolysis), especially with exercise. In some cases, no structural abnormality is recognized, but histochemical studies can demonstrate the absence of a given enzyme activity. The list of diseases that may affect skeletal muscle function and structure is long. The following discussion will be limited to the most important entities.

Glycogen Storage Diseases

In the course of intracellular digestion, glycogen is hydrolyzed within lysosomes by acid maltase. When this process fails to take place, glycogen, accumulating within lysosomal vacuoles, leads to muscle fiber damage, the clinical consequence of which is painless, progressive muscle weakness. Glycogen in the cytosol is a major fuel for glycolytic, fast twitch, type IIA and IIB fibers. As it is metabolized anaerobically to pyruvate and lactate, ATP is generated. Abnormalities in glycolytic enzymes lead to glycogen accumulation in the sarcoplasm, reduced lactate production, reduced formation of ATP, and impairment in muscle fiber metabolism, leading to rhabdomyolysis. Thus, clinical manifestations include myalgia (aches, cramps, and pains), fatigue, and myoglobinuria.

Acid Maltase Deficiency (Pompe's Disease, Type II Glycogenosis)

In 1963, Hers[100] discovered that a deficiency of acid maltase (α-1,4-glucosidase) caused a rapidly fatal disorder of infancy characterized by accumulation of glycogen in skeletal muscle, heart, and nervous system (Figs. 16-49 and 16-50). Elucidation of the enzyme defect led to the recognition of milder, later-onset forms.[101] Both the severe and more benign forms are inherited as autosomal-recessive traits. The gene that codes for acid maltase has been mapped to region 2 of the long arm of chromosome 17 and cloning of complementary DNA (cDNA) containing acid maltase sequences has been reported.[102] The various phenotypes are thought to stem from genetic differences but specific mutations have not been fully elucidated.

The infantile form (Pompe's disease) is first noted at about 1 month of age, with severe hypotonia, weakness and heart failure. There is enlargement of the heart, liver, and tongue. Death occurs by 2 years of age from cardiac and respiratory failure. The childhood form has a later onset. There is a delay in reaching motor milestones, followed by progressive weakness of proximal limb and trunk muscles. The liver and tongue may be enlarged but cardiomegaly is rare. Death occurs before the end of the second decade from respiratory insufficiency. In the

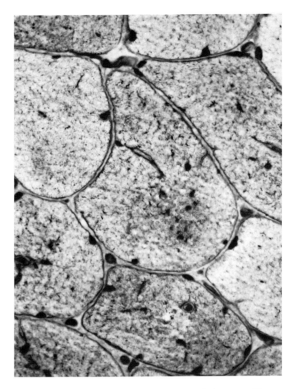

Fig. 16-49. Adult-onset acid maltase deficiency. (Frozen section, PAS) The muscle fibers contain scattered coarse granules of PAS-positive (and diastase-sensitive) material. (Courtesy of AFIP.)

adult form[103] symptoms begin in the third or fourth decade, with slowly progressive weakness and wasting of proximal limb and trunk muscles, with sparing of bulbar musculature. Respiratory muscle weakness may occur and rarely results in death from ventilatory failure. The heart and liver are not affected. The adult variant can present as a limb girdle dystrophy, polymyositis, or spinal muscular atrophy.

CK is elevated in most patients. The EMG discloses myopathic motor unit potentials, fibrillations, positive sharp waves, bizarre high frequency discharges, and true myotonic bursts.[101] Occasionally, reduced recruitment with long duration, high amplitude motor unit potential suggests a neurogenic component.[103]

Of all the glycogenoses, AMD has the most distinct morphologic pattern.[104] Since acid maltase is a lysosomal enzyme, a deficiency or absence of this enzyme leads to the accumulation of glycogen within lysosomes. It is therefore the only glycogenosis that presents as packets of membrane-bound glycogen. There is a massive accumulation of granules and vacuoles of varying size filled with diastase-sensitive, PAS-positive material[105] (Fig. 16-51). Strangely, in spite of the marked devastation of the muscle fiber and the replacement of its contents with membrane-bound glycogen, there is little in the way of regenerative activity. Many fibers show almost complete dissolution of the myofibrillar content, but without apparent activation of the satellite cells or evidence of a reparative process. Indeed, the satellite cells themselves can be shown to contain membrane-bound glycogen. Electron microscopy shows clusters of glycogen granules free in the cytoplasm, in membranous sacs and in autophagic vacuoles with other cytoplasmic products[101] (Fig. 16-52).

In adult cases, the glycogen-containing vacuoles may be few and small, making identification of the disease

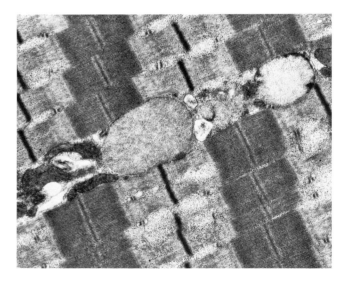

Fig. 16-50. Adult-onset acid maltase deficiency. (×12,000) Same biopsy as Figure 16-49. Distended membrane-bound sacs are filled with glycogen granules. (Courtesy of AFIP.)

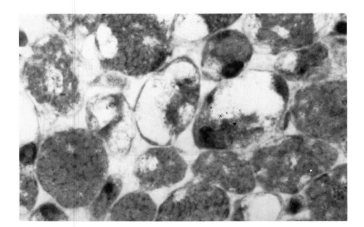

Fig. 16-51. Pompe's disease. (Frozen section, H&E) Most of the muscle fibers have variably sized granules and vacuoles that, with appropriate stains, can be shown to contain glycogen.

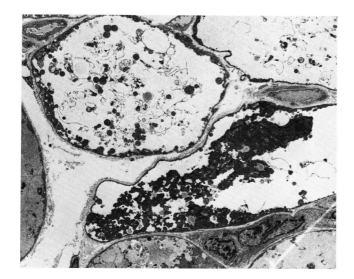

Fig. 16-52. Pompe's disease. (×2,400) Several fibers are almost empty, with remnants of membranes, scattered mitochondria, and a few membrane-bound vesicles that contain glycogen granules (based on higher magnification). Two fibers (bottom) are filled with glycogen, much of which is membrane-bound. Very few myofibrils are visible. (Courtesy of AFIP.)

difficult. The histology of clinically unaffected muscles may be normal, and even in biopsies from weakened muscles abnormalities may be slight.[103] Most vacuoles contain PAS-positive granules which are removed by diastase and show high acid phosphatase activity.[101]

The mechanisms of muscle fiber injury in AMD are thought to involve at least two factors.[102] The first is the excessive storage of undegraded lysosomal material that could displace, compress, and replace vital cellular structures. The second is an abnormal increase in lysosomal autophagic activity which could have deleterious effects on a variety of organelles.

Glycogen of normal structure is greatly increased in amount in the infantile form, somewhat less elevated in the childhood and adult onset forms, and occasionally may be present in normal quantity.[102] The enzyme deficiency can be demonstrated by biochemical assay of muscle tissue or by demonstrating decreased urinary excretion.[106]

At least two hypotheses have been proposed to account for the observed clinical variability in the three forms and the variability in organ involvement in a particular patient. Angelini and Engel[107] found neutral maltase present in the liver and muscle of adults but absent in liver, muscle, and heart of infants. They postulated that neutral maltase was a compensatory factor preventing glycogen accumulation and tissue damage in the more mild adult cases. However, others[108] noted neutral maltase deficiency in the heart of an adult; thus, the age-dependent variability of AMD cannot be explained by different tissue levels of neutral maltase.[102] A second theory attributes mild forms of the disease to residual acid maltase activity, absent from infants but present in most children and adults.[108] However, this theory, too, has been questioned because some cases of infantile AMD do have residual acid maltase and some cases of adult disease do not.[102]

During the past decade, much has been learned about AMD but many problems remain unsolved, including the nature of molecular differences between the different clinical types and how acid maltase regulates glycogen metabolism. Finally, there is no satisfactory treatment for this disease and finding effective therapy remains a major challenge for the future.

Phosphorylase Deficiency (McArdle's disease)

Phosphorylase deficiency was the first hereditary myopathy in which a specific enzyme defect was identified. In 1951, McArdle[109] described a 30-year-old man with a history of cramps and exercise intolerance since childhood. He postulated that the disorder was caused by a defect in glycogen breakdown. Later, it was shown that skeletal muscle phosphorylase was absent and muscle glycogen increased.[110,111]

In most cases, the disease is inherited as an autosomal-recessive trait, although autosomal-dominant transmission has been reported.[112] Males outnumber females by a ratio of 3:1. In childhood, there is easy fatiguability and mild weakness. Later, vigorous activity is accompanied by painful cramps in the exercising muscles. In about one half of patients, muscle necrosis and myoglobinuria occur. Renal failure, a life-threatening complication of myoglobinuria, occurs in 8 percent. Patients learn to avoid sudden bursts of activity and prefer less intense but sustained exercise such as walking. Many patients experience a prominent second wind phenomenon attributable to mobilization of fatty acids and increased muscle blood flow that occurs with exercise.[113] Between attacks, patients are well and can lead reasonably normal lives. Mild, permanent weakness is present in 20 percent.[112] Rarely, the disease presents with weakness and wasting in adult life without exercise intolerance, suggesting an acquired late-onset myopathy.[114,115] Phosphorylase deficiency has also been reported as a cause of the floppy baby syndrome.[116]

In patients suspected of having the disease, ischemic forearm exercise should be performed under standard conditions.[117] The peak level of venous lactate occurs within 3 to 5 minutes after exercise in normal subjects, reaching three to five times the resting pre-exercise level. Because patients with McArdle's disease are unable to break down glycogen, venous lactate fails to rise. Reduced lactate production, however, is not specific for McArdle's disease and is seen with other defects of the glycolytic pathway.

The CK is elevated in most patients at rest and the EMG is abnormal in almost half of patients, showing myopathic potentials especially in patients with permanent weakness.[112]

The biopsy specimen may be structurally normal, except for the complete absence of phosphorylase activity. Often, however, in addition to a negative phosphorylase stain there are subsarcolemmal vacuoles that are filled with glycogen (Fig. 16-53). Biopsies often also show scattered necrotic and regenerating fibers, especially prominent if the patient has had a recent episode of myoglobinuria. Ultrastructural studies demonstrate that the glycogen granules are not membrane bound (Fig. 16-54). The diagnosis of McArdle's disease is specifically dependent on the demonstration of the complete absence of myophosphorylase activity by histochemical or quantitative biochemical techniques[112]; the histochemical reaction for phosphorylase, however, is present in blood vessel walls and regenerating fibers.[118]

Glycogen of normal structure accumulates to a modest degree in skeletal muscle. The defect of phosphorylase activity is restricted to skeletal muscle.[112] Isoenzymes presumably under separate genetic control are present in other tissues. Phosphorylase activity is present in muscle cultures from patients with McArdle's disease[119] and in biopsied specimens that include regenerating fibers.[118] This enzyme activity is possibly due to a fetal iso-enzyme whose genetic control is distinct from that of a mature enzyme.[120] A number of studies demonstrate biochemical heterogeneity in McArdle's disease.[112] In some cases, the enzyme protein is not detectable by a variety of methods whereas in others, enzymatically inactive phosphorylase

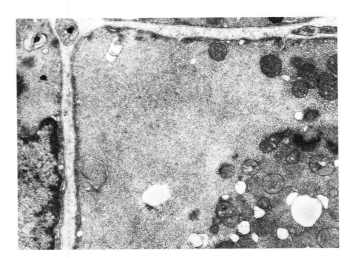

Fig. 16-54. McArdle's disease. (×12,000) The subsarcolemmal vacuoles contain nonmembrane-bound glycogen. This is not specific and can be seen in other glycogenoses or in diseases not related to glycogenosis. (Courtesy of AFIP.)

protein can be demonstrated by a reaction with antibody prepared against normal enzyme.

The best approach to treatment is to avoid bursts of activity that depend on the glycolytic pathway; exercise of moderate intensity that favors aerobic metabolism, intact in patients with McArdle's disease, can be easily achieved.

Phosphofructokinase Deficiency

In 1965, Tarui and colleagues[121] described three siblings with a clinical picture identical to McArdle's disease. Phosphofructokinase (PFK), the glycolytic enzyme that catalyzes the conversion of fructose 6-phosphate to fructose 1,6-diphosphate, was absent in muscle. Tarui et al. also noted that their patients had a mild hemolytic anemia and found that red blood cell PFK activity was reduced by 50 percent. Since these original observations, a number of workers have demonstrated that PFK is a tetramer consisting of combinations of three different subunits—a muscle or M subunit, a liver or L subunit (the subunit present in the red blood cell), and the platelet or P subunit, found in platelets and fibroblasts.[122] Only one isoenzyme is found in adult muscle, and this is a tetramer of four M subunits. By contrast, in erythrocytes, five different isoenzymes are found, made up of combinations of both M and L subunits. This molecular analysis of PFK explains the presence of myopathy and hemolysis in the typical syndrome where there is a defective M subunit. The typical clinical syndrome is very similar to McArdle's disease (exercise intolerance with cramps and sometimes myoglobinuria), but some patients

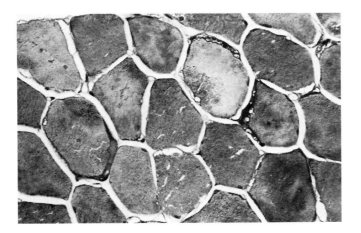

Fig. 16-53. McArdle's disease. (Frozen section, PAS) Note subsarcolemmal collections of PAS-positive (darkly staining) material. (From DeGirolami and Smith.[175])

have been described with onset of weakness in middle life and without cramps or myoglobinuria.[123] An infantile myopathy with delayed motor development has also been described.[124]

Morphologic findings are identical to those of McArdle's disease except that, unlike phosphorylase deficiency, hyaline polysaccharide inclusions have been found in some cases. This polysaccharide stains with PAS but is not digested by salivary diastase. The accumulated material is similar to that found in patients who lack debranching enzyme. These polysaccharide inclusions are perhaps best explained as a secondary disorder of glycogen synthesis caused by greatly increased glucose 6-phosphate (G6P), an activator of glycogen synthetase.[123] In patients with PFK deficiency, there is absence of PFK activity as determined by histochemical or quantitative biochemical techniques.[122] Management is similar to that outlined for patients with McArdle's disease.

Debranching Enzyme Deficiency

Debranching enzyme deficiency is an autosomal-recessive disease that begins in infancy with hepatomegaly, growth retardation, fasting hypoglycemia, and cirrhosis. The enzyme defect has been demonstrated in muscle, liver, leukocytes, and red blood cells.[125] In the absence of debranching enzyme activity, phosphorylase may hydrolyze the 1,4-glycosidic linkages to the point of branching. The resultant glycogen molecule has an excess number of exposed 1,6-glycosidic linkages and is referred to as limit dextrin. Myopathy is sometimes difficult to recognize in very ill infants, but it is not unusual to find hypotonia, lethargy or delayed motor milestones.[125] The disease has also been recognized as a cause of slowly progressive weakness in adult life.[126] Unlike McArdle's disease and PFK deficiency, cramps and myoglobinuria are not seen.

Venous lactate does not rise during ischemic exercise. Serum CK may be markedly elevated. The EMG shows myopathic features or a mixture of myopathic and neurogenic patterns. The muscle biopsy shows subsarcolemmal, coarse, PAS-positive vacuoles. Ultrastructural studies show findings similar to those seen in McArdle's disease.

Other Glycogenoses

Newly recognized defects in distal glycolysis include deficiencies of phosphoglyceratekinase, phosphoglyceratemutase, and lactate dehydrogenase.[127] Defects in all three may produce muscle pain, weakness, and, when exercise persists in the face of myalgia, myoglobinuria. None of these enzyme defects produces a complete block of the glycolytic pathway, and thus severe glycogen accumulation does not occur. The muscle biopsy may show little evidence of glycogen storage.

Myoadenylate Deaminase Deficiency

In 1978, Fishbein et al.[128] described what was at the time a new metabolic myopathy: symptoms of exertional weakness and cramping with morphologically normal muscle biopsies and complete absence of adenosine monophosphate deaminase (AMP-DA) as shown by a histochemical technique. Since that description there have been several reports indicating that AMP-DA deficiency is found in about 1.5 percent of muscle biopsies. It is therefore the most common enzymatic defect of skeletal muscle discovered to date. However, some argue that the true significance of this deficiency is not yet known[129]: It could be a common and clinically inconsequential enzyme defect, or its absence could decrease the muscle's reserve for exercise and only cause symptoms during an excessive workload.

The enzyme plays an important but nonessential role in muscle metabolism, and is normally severalfold higher in type II than in type I fibers. It is activated when the metabolic requirement of the muscle rises and there is a need for increased amounts of ATP. It catalyzes the deamination of AMP, resulting in the formation of IMP and ammonia. Both products, IMP and ammonia, enhance glycolysis and the Krebs cycle, thus promoting efficient metabolism.[130]

Symptoms generally come on in middle age, when patients become aware of postexertional fatigue or weakness along with soreness or cramping of muscle.[130] Unlike the glycolytic enzyme defects, rhabdomyolysis and myoglobinuria do not occur. Unlike acid maltase deficiency and carnitine deficiency, progressive weakness is not a feature of MDD. The disease is essentially benign but diagnosis is important, for the exertional pain may be confused with polymyositis and other metabolic myopathies. Inheritance appears to be autosomal-recessive with a complete block of the gene that codes for a unique skeletal muscle, AMP-DA isozyme. Patients with AMP-DA deficiency have normal levels of the enzyme in other tissues. In about one half of cases the CK is mildly to moderately elevated, and the EMG may show nonspecific abnormalities. The diagnosis is by histoenzymatic examination of muscle with biochemical confirmation. In patients with AMP-DA deficiency alone, the muscle is morphologically normal on biopsy. However, about half the cases of enzyme deficiency are associated with another neuromuscular disorder (e.g., polymyositis, muscular dystrophy, motor neuron disease), and in these cases the biopsy will show the abnormalities expected for that specific disease entity. The patient lacking AMP-DA will fail to generate ammonia during an ischemic exercise test but lactate increases normally.

Mitochondrial Myopathies

For many years a condition was referred to as a mitochondrial myopathy if muscle biopsy disclosed abnormal accumulations of mitochondria in a subsarcolemmal location. Olson et al.[131] noted that mitochondria appeared as purple, subsarcolemmal masses when the Gomori trichrome stain was used and coined the descriptive term ragged-red fiber, which has come to be synonymous with mitochondrial myopathy (Figs. 16-55 and 16-56). However, it has become clear that such abnormal-appearing fibers may be found in a host of diverse conditions including muscular dystrophy and congenital and inflammatory myopathies, and in none of these conditions is an abnormality in mitochondrial function believed to be central to pathogenesis.[132] It is interesting that, even in conditions known to be caused by a mitochondrial abnormality, such as defects in mitochondrial substrate utilization, such as carnitine palmityltransferase (CPT) deficiency and carnitine deficiency, mitochondrial structural abnormalities and ragged red fibers are not seen. Thus, morphologic appearance alone is probably not a good way to determine if a myopathy is due to a primary mitochondrial abnormality. The most appropriate definition of a mitochondrial myopathy would be one in which myopathic symptoms and signs arise as a consequence of a demonstrable abnormality in mitochondrial function.[132] Presuming that such a biochemical abnormality is indeed primary, mitochondrial myopathies can be divided into three groups according to the area of mitochondrial metabolism affected: substrate utilization; oxidation and phosphorylation coupling; or the respiratory chain.[132] The disorders of substrate utilization include CPT and carnitine deficiencies as well as alterations of pyruvate metabolism. Morphologic alterations in mitochondria are lacking in patients with these disturbances; these alterations are considered in the section on lipid myopathy. The second type of disturbance in metabolism affects oxidation and phosphorylation coupling and produces a hypermetabolic state characterized by fever, sweating, heat intolerance, polydypsia and polyphagia.[133,134] Mitochondria are morphologically and functionally abnormal; ragged red fibers are seen and there is loose coupling of oxidative phosphorylation; the precise molecular abnormality is not known. The third category of mitochondrial myopathy occurs as a consequence of a defect somewhere along the respiratory chain. To date, a number of

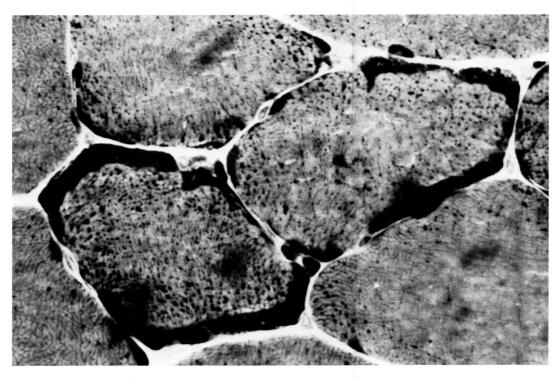

Fig. 16-55. Ragged red fibers. (Frozen section, MGT) The fibers have a red-purple granular-reticular network, often with prominent subsarcolemmal deposits. This material stains positively with the NADH-TR and succinic dehydrogenase reactions, indicating that it represents mitochondria. (From Chad et al.[176])

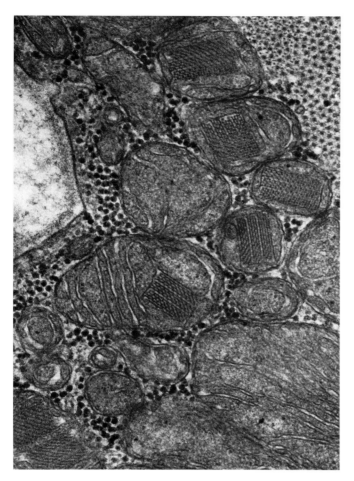

Fig. 16-56. Ragged red fiber. (×57,000) The granular deposits seen by light microscopy consist of pleomorphic abnormal mitochondria, some of which have paracrystalline structures. (Courtesy of AFIP.)

defects have been recognized, including abnormalities in nonheme iron sulfur proteins, and in cytochrome b, cytochrome c1, coenzyme Q, and cytochrome c oxidase. Patients with the last condition appear to have a multisystem disorder marked by progressive weakness, glycosuria, phosphaturia and generalized aminoaciduria; in most of the patients who have been described, the muscle biopsy shows ragged-red fibers.[132]

One distinctive syndrome which is very likely to be caused by a defect in the mitochondrial respiratory chains is the *Kearns-Sayre syndrome,* first described as a clinical entity in 1958.[135] Except for one family, patients have a sporadic disorder that begins by the age of 20 and is distinguished by the clinical triad of chronic progressive external ophthalmoplegia, retinitis pigmentosa, and heart block.[136] Many patients have elevated cerebrospinal fluid (CSF) protein (in excess of 100 mg/dl). Muscle weakness, ataxia, sensorineural hearing loss and lac-

tic acid acidosis are other commonly encountered features. Muscle biopsy discloses ragged-red fibers.

Disorders of Lipid Metabolism

Fatty acids are the major fuel for muscle at rest, in the fasting state and during prolonged, low intensity aerobic exercise. They are mobilized from fat deposits and oxidized in muscle mitochondria. Short chain fatty acids penetrate the mitochondrial membrane with ease, but long chain fatty acids (palmitic and oleic) are impermeable unless combined with *carnitine,* which facilitates their transport to intramitochondrial sites. Inside the muscle fiber, fatty acids are activated to fatty acyl-CoA derivatives. On the outer mitochondrial membrane, these are joined to carnitine by CPT I to form a permeable derivative, fatty acylcarnitine, which moves across the mitochondrial membrane into the mitochondria. There, CPT II catalyzes the reverse reaction, with the formation of fatty acyl-CoA, which can then undergo oxidation.[137]

Two main categories of disordered muscle lipid metabolism have been identified: (1) carnitine deficiency, characterized by progressive weakness and excessive muscle fiber lipid storage; and (2) CPT deficiency, causing recurrent muscle pain and myoglobinuria with little muscle fiber lipid accumulation. Other conditions will be associated with lipid storage myopathy if there is a biochemical defect that interferes with the regulation of lipid metabolism. In mitochondrial myopathies with respiratory chain protein defects, for example, muscle biopsies show lipid droplet accumulation in addition to ragged-red fibers.

Carnitine Deficiency

In 1972, Engel and Siekert[138] described a 19-year-old woman with lifelong mild generalized weakness that rapidly progressed, rendering her bed-fast and in need of respiratory support. Muscle biopsy disclosed excessive lipid accumulation, especially in type I fibers. Subsequently, it was shown that the lipid accumulation was associated with muscle carnitine deficiency.[139] Since that description, some 40 cases have been further described which fall into two seemingly distinct groups. In the first, the *myopathic* form, carnitine deficiency is limited to muscle and the major clinical manifestation is myopathy. In the second, the *systemic* form, carnitine deficiency is widespread and clinical features are dominated by both weakness and hepatic failure.

In the myopathic form there is progressive weakness, most marked in proximal and trunk muscles, generally beginning in childhood. Rarely, there is rapid worsening associated with respiratory failure; heart involvement may give rise to cardiomyopathy. The serum CK is moderately increased in most patients and the EMG shows

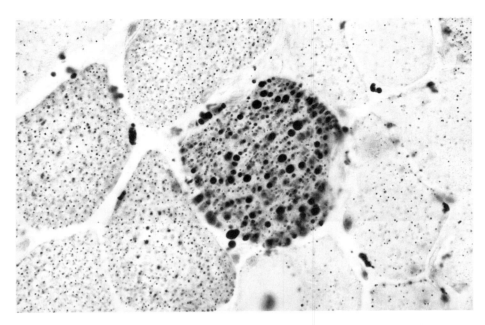

Fig. 16-57. Lipid storage myopathy. (Frozen section, oil-red O). The muscle fiber in the center contains an excessive number of coarse lipid globules.

myopathic changes. The muscle biopsy shows intrafiber lipid droplets, most marked in type I fibers (Fig. 16-57). There is less lipid accumulation in the fibers with reduced oxidative capacity (the type IIA and the type IIB fibers). Ultrastructurally (Fig. 16-58), droplets are not membrane bound and accumulate in parallel rows between myofibrils or beneath the sarcolemma.[139] The condition has responded to corticosteroids and oral administration of carnitine.

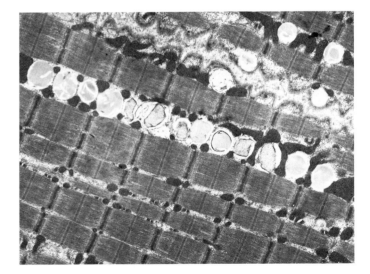

Fig. 16-58. Lipid storage myopathy. (×10,000) Note subsarcolemmal and intermyofibrillar irregular electron-lucent lipid globules. (From DeGirolami and Smith.[175])

The systemic form was first described by Karpati et al.,[140] who described an 11-year-old boy with lifelong clumsiness, thin muscles and a short history of generalized weakness. At ages three and nine he had episodes of unexplained liver failure with hepatic encephalopathy, but recovery was good. The muscle biopsy showed lipid accumulation in most type I fibers, and carnitine was virtually absent from muscle and reduced by 80 to 90 percent in liver and plasma. Since the original report, some 16 cases have been reported. Onset is generally in childhood and the main clinical features are progressive weakness and recurrent hepatic encephalopathy with metabolic acidosis. Death from respiratory failure has occurred before the age of 20 in most cases.[139] Laboratory studies are similar to those found in the myopathic form. Autopsy studies, however, show lipid storage in liver, heart and tubular epithelial cells of the kidney.[139]

Carnitine Palmityltransferase Deficiency

Carnitine palmityltransferase deficiency is the second type of lipid metabolism disorder, first described by Bank et al.[141] in 1975. These workers described two brothers with episodic myoglobinuria. Biochemical studies excluded glycogen storage disease but demonstrated virtual absence of CPT activity in crude muscle extracts and mitochondrial fractions. The disease begins in childhood and shows a striking male predominance.[142] It is probably transmitted as an autosomal-recessive trait, but women may be less susceptible than men to the development of myoglobinuria and may therefore go undetected.[142] The major clinical feature is myoglobinuria associated with muscle pain provoked by prolonged exercise, fasting or a combination of the two. The frequency of myoglobinuria appears to be much higher in CPT deficiency than in McArdle's disease and the other glycolytic defects.[142] Between attacks, patients are well and there is no permanent weakness. Although the pain and myoglobinuria suggest McArdle's disease, there is no intolerance to brief strenuous exercise, no second wind phenomenon, and contracture cannot be induced by exercise under ischemic conditions.[141] The muscle biopsy is usually normal unless there has been a previous episode of myoglobinuria, in which case scattered necrotic and regenerating fibers are found. Lipid accumulation is generally mild or not seen. It is unclear as to why CPT and carnitine deficiency present in different fashions and why the former shows lipid accumulation and the latter does not.

Endocrine Myopathies

Many of the generalized endocrine disorders can be associated with a myopathy. In most cases, evidence of muscle involvement may even be subclinical, revealed only by special studies (e.g., serum enzymes, EMG, muscle biopsy) performed in the course of evaluation of the endocrine disorder. However, in some instances (e.g., thyrotoxicosis), the muscle symptoms may be a prominent, often presenting feature of the endocrine disorder. Most of these myopathies are readily reversed after correction of the underlying endocrine disturbance. As a general rule, the histologic changes present in the muscle tend to be relatively mild and nonspecific, sometimes even in the face of severe muscle weakness and wasting. The endocrinopathies most consistently associated with myopathic features include hyperthyroidism, hypothyroidism, hyperparathyroidism, hyperadrenalism (Cushing's disease), hypoadrenalism (Addison's disease), and acromegaly. These will be briefly discussed below.

Hyperthyroidism

Four different neuromuscular disorders may be seen in hyperthyroidism: thyrotoxic myopathy, myasthenia gravis, thyrotoxic periodic paralysis, and exophthalmic ophthalmoplegia.[2] Only the first condition is discussed in this section.

A chronic myopathy manifested largely by generalized proximal muscle weakness is a commonly observed finding in hyperthyroidism. It may at times precede other signs of thyrotoxicosis. The EMG may show myopathic abnormalities in about 90 percent of cases of hyperthyroidism.[143] Nevertheless, light microscopic examination of the muscle may show essentially no abnormality or

only mild myofiber atrophy.[144-146] Other relatively minor histologic changes reported have included interstitial edema, single fiber necrosis, glycogen depletion, increased subsarcolemmal nuclei, and fatty infiltration. Ultrastructural abnormalities that have been described include papillary projections on the muscle fiber surface, various mitochondrial abnormalities, focal myofibrillar degeneration, tubular aggregates, and subsarcolemmal glycogen deposits.[147,148] Neither the light microscopic nor the ultrastructural changes are specific for thyrotoxicosis.

Hypothyroidism

Patients with hypothyroidism often have a myopathy characterized by proximal weakness, slowed movements and reflexes, stiffness, myalgias, and less commonly cramps and/or muscle enlargement.[143] Serum CK is usually elevated. Muscle biopsy specimens usually show nonspecific myopathic changes such as fiber atrophy (most often involving type 2 fibers), increased internal nuclei, glycogen accumulation, ring fibers, and endomysial fibrosis.[149-152] Ultrastructural changes may include mitochondrial abnormalities, myofibrillar degeneration, glycogen accumulation, dilated sarcoplasmic reticulum, T-tubule proliferation, lipid granules, and autophagic vacuoles.[150,151,153] Basophilic degeneration has been described in long-standing cases of hypothyroidism.[154] None of the light or electron microscopic changes appears sufficient to explain the cause of the weakness in these patients.

Hyperparathyroidism

Both primary and secondary hyperparathyroidism may be associated with a myopathy.[143] Clinically, this affects mainly proximal muscles, often with associated pain and fatiguability, waddling gait, and hyperreflexia. The histologic changes seen in muscle biopsies from these patients are often surprisingly mild and have included nonspecific fiber atrophy, type 2 fiber atrophy, and focal vacuolar and degenerative changes.[155-157]

Hyperadrenalism

Patients with Cushing's disease frequently have a myopathy characterized by proximal muscle weakness and wasting affecting especially the lower extremities. A myopathy can also be seen in association with exogenous corticosteroid therapy. The most consistent and characteristic histologic change observed in muscle biopsies in both conditions is selective atrophy of type II fibers.[158] Sometimes this may involve more specifically the type IIB fibers. Occasionally type I fibers may show excess lipid deposition.[159] Electron microscopy may show an apparent increase in glycogen within type II fibers.[147,160] Other light microscopic and ultrastructural changes have been described but appear to be much less common and not as well documented.

The various theories concerned with the etiology of steroid myopathy have been reviewed in detail by Ruff.[143] Suffice it to say, current evidence indicates that glucocorticosteroids alter muscle carbohydrate and protein metabolism and may interfere with the function of the sarcoplasmic reticulum. However, the precise interaction of these factors in the causation of steroid myopathy remains unknown. There is little evidence to support a viral, electrolyte imbalance, ischemic, or neurogenic etiology.

Hypoadrenalism (Addison's disease)

A myopathy characterized by severe generalized muscle weakness, cramping, and fatigue may occur in 25 to 50 percent of patients with adrenal insufficiency, regardless of its etiology.[143] Serum muscle enzymes and EMG are usually normal. The muscle biopsy usually appears normal, except perhaps for some glycogen depletion.[161]

Acromegaly

Proximal muscle weakness and diminished exercise tolerance may be present in about 50 percent of patients with acromegaly. The muscle weakness may be insidious in onset, slowly progressive, and associated with some diminution in muscle bulk.[143] Serum CK levels may be slightly elevated. EMG may show myopathic changes in about 50 percent of acromegalics. Histologic examination of muscle biopsy specimens has shown the following abnormalities: single fiber necrosis, nuclear enlargement with prominent nucleoli, proliferation and hypertrophy of satellite cells, increased glycogen, lipofuscin accumulation, and, rarely, mononuclear inflammatory infiltrates.[162–166] Hypertrophy of type I and/or type II fibers has also been described. Electron microscopic studies have shown excessive accumulation of glycogen and lipofuscin, myofibrillar degeneration, capillary basement membrane thickening, and increased satellite cells.[162–165] These light and electron microscopic abnormalities have generally not been considered sufficient to explain the muscular weakness in these patients.

Periodic Paralysis

Periodic paralysis constitutes a group of disorders that share in common the clinical feature of attacks of paralysis with associated flaccidity, and a tendency to remit and relapse. Three forms of the disorder are recognized, classified according to the level of serum potassium present during an attack.[167,168] All three variants are usually inherited as autosomal-dominant traits, although they can also occur sporadically. The *hypokalemic* variant is the most common form of periodic paralysis. It is more common in males and usually has its onset between the ages of 20 and 35. The disorder is characterized by the appearance of sudden attacks of generalized muscle paralysis with relative sparing of the external ocular and respiratory muscles. The attacks usually occur at night and are precipitated by prior strenuous exercise, a high carbohydrate meal, or exposure to cold. Serum potassium levels during an attack are low. Between attacks, patients are usually normal, although there may be some residual muscle weakness. The *hyperkalemic* variant usually begins in childhood and tends to affect both sexes equally. Unlike the hypokalemic variant, the attacks often occur during the daytime and are usually briefer but more frequent. There may be considerable variation in the extent and severity of weakness. Some patients may display myotonia, especially of face and hand muscles. Characteristically, there is a rise in serum potassium levels during an attack, although the elevation may at times be quite minimal. The attacks may be precipitated by exercise or exposure to cold, and can also be induced by the administration of potassium chloride. *Normokalemic* periodic paralysis shares many clinical features in common with the hyperkalemic variant. Serum potassium levels typically remain unchanged during an attack.

In addition to the primary periodic paralysis syndromes, secondary forms of both hypo- and hyperkalemic periodic paralysis may occur.[168] Among the more common secondary hypokalemic forms are thyrotoxic periodic paralysis, periodic paralysis secondary to urinary or gastrointestinal potassium loss, and barium-induced periodic paralysis. Periodic paralysis due to hyperkalemia may be seen in patients with renal or adrenal failure.

The pathologic findings in all forms of periodic paralysis are qualitatively similar but tend to be most pronounced in the hypokalemic variant. The principal light microscopic abnormality consists of the presence of variable numbers of vacuoles within myofibers[168,169] (Fig. 16-59). The vacuoles are more often encountered in biopsy specimens taken from individuals during an acute attack; the muscle may, in fact, appear fairly normal between episodes. The most conspicuous vacuolar changes, however, are seen in muscle biopsies obtained from patients who have a permanent myopathy resulting from long-standing disease with recurrent episodes of paralysis. The vacuoles vary in size but can be quite large, and they tend to occupy the interior rather than periphery of the fiber. Multiloculated vacuoles can also be seen. The vacuoles usually appear "empty" but may occasionally contain PAS-positive, diastase-digestible granular material and rarely calcium.[170] In addition to the vacu-

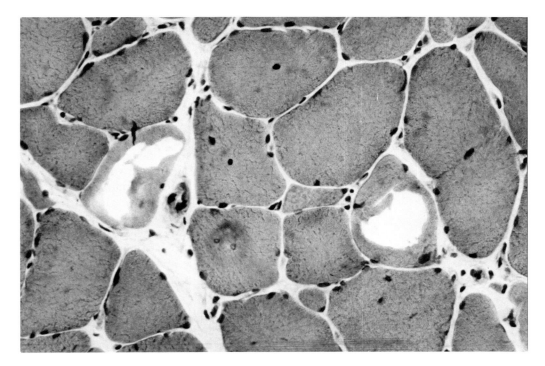

Fig. 16-59. Periodic paralysis. (Frozen section, H&E) Several fibers contain prominent clear vacuoles. The muscle also shows variability in fiber size and internalized nuclei.

oles, biopsies from patients with a permanent myopathy may also show other myopathic features including variation in fiber size, internal nuclei, fiber necrosis, motheaten fibers, and proliferation of connective tissue. Detailed electron microscopic studies by Engel[168,170,171] have shown that the vacuoles arise from the proliferation, degeneration, and autophagic destruction of membranous organelles derived chiefly from the sarcoplasmic reticulum and T-system tubules.

Another morphologic change often encountered in periodic paralysis, especially in the hyperkalemic and normokalemic variants, is the presence of tubular aggregates.[28] In H&E-stained sections, they appear as basophilic deposits found in both the interior and periphery of muscle fibers. They stain intensely red with the modified trichrome method and dark blue with the NADH-TR reaction, but fail to stain with the succinic dehydrogenase (SDH) reaction, thereby distinguishing them from mitochondria (Fig. 16-60). They are found predominantly, but not exclusively, in type 2 fibers. Ultrastructurally, tubular aggregates consist of fascicular arrays of parallel double-walled tubules having a diameter of 60 to 90 nm (Fig. 16-61). On cross-section, they form a hexagonal profile. The tubules can sometimes be observed in continuity with the dilated terminal cisterns of the sarcoplasmic reticulum, from which they are thought to be derived. (See Engel[168] for a comprehensive review

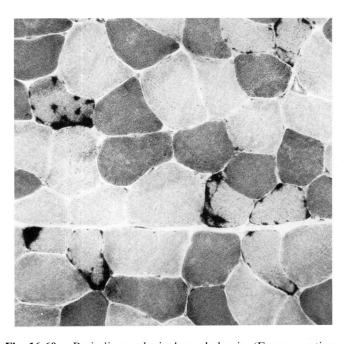

Fig. 16-60. Periodic paralysis, hyperkalemic. (Frozen section, NADH-TR) Scattered fibers contain large deposits of material that stains intensely with NADH-TR. These represent tubular aggregates. (Courtesy of AFIP.)

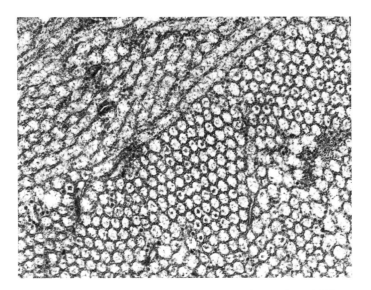

Fig. 16-61. Periodic paralysis, hyperkalemic. (×38,000) Ultrastructure of tubular aggregate consisting of fascicular arrays of parallel double-walled tubules, 60 to 90 nm in diameter. (Courtesy of AFIP.)

of the pathophysiologic mechanisms involved in periodic paralysis.)

Myoglobinuria

Myoglobinuria is a clinical term that refers to the excretion of myoglobin in the urine. It almost always results from a process known as rhabdomyolysis, in which there is extensive destruction or necrosis of skeletal muscle with resultant loss of the integrity of the muscle cell membrane and extrusion of myoglobin into the circulation. As such, myoglobinuria is actually a symptom of massive muscle fiber necrosis rather than a disease process in and of itself. The types of disorders that may be associated with rhabdomyolysis and myoglobinuria are quite varied.[167,172] Many of these conditions occur sporadically and include massive trauma (e.g., crush injury), ischemia, extreme exertion, excessive heat, toxins (especially alcohol), drugs, electrolyte imbalances, certain bacterial and viral infections, and inflammatory myopathies. Other causes of rhabdomyolysis/myoglobinuria that may have a genetic predisposition include the malignant hyperthermia syndrome, certain metabolic myopathies (e.g., McArdle's disease, PFK deficiency, carnitine palmityltransferase deficiency), and occasionally some forms of muscular dystrophy.

During an acute attack of rhabdomyolysis, regardless of the cause, the muscles become tender, swollen, and weak. There may be a history of prior muscle cramps. Serum muscle enzymes are markedly elevated. As a con-

sequence of the severe muscle fiber necrosis, myoglobin is released into the circulation, which in turn is readily cleared by the kidney and excreted into the urine. This can sometimes be severe enough to cause grossly discolored urine and, in some cases, renal shutdown.

Histologic examination of the muscle during the acute phase of an attack may show surprisingly little change: the fibers may appear edematous, with depletion of glycogen as seen on PAS staining, and the nuclei may be slightly vesicular. Over time, however, the muscle fibers will show more obvious histologic evidence of myofiber necrosis, which is accompanied by brisk phagocytosis. After several weeks, the muscle will show considerable regenerative activity. Between attacks, the muscle may appear quite normal (unless the patient also has an underlying myopathy). Sometimes mineralized fibers may be observed as sequelae of previous episodes of necrosis.[28]

Myasthenia Gravis

The neuromuscular junction consists of pre- and postsynaptic components. The former is created by an expansion of the axon terminal. Within the terminal there are abundant vesicles and mitochondria. Vesicles are filled with ACh and congregate at the presynaptic membrane around dense bars, corresponding in their placement to junctional peaks of the postsynaptic membrane, where ACh receptors (AChR) are concentrated. When a nerve impulse arrives at the axon terminal, the ACh-filled vesicles are released and interact with the AChR giving rise to muscle fiber depolarization. The postsynaptic membrane is highly folded, with AChR concentrated at the peaks; acetylcholinesterase (AChE), an enzyme that degrades ACh and thereby terminates its physiologic action, is present in the valleys.

Myasthenia gravis is an autoimmune disease that results from an antibody-mediated attack upon these nicotinic AChR. The main clinical features of the illness are weakness and fatiguability. The weakness has a special predilection for cranial nerve-innervated muscles. It affects all age groups but is especially common in young adult women and older men. Diplopia and ptosis are common presenting manifestations. Other early symptoms include dysphagia, dysarthria, difficulty in chewing, and difficulty in holding up the head. As the disease progresses, involvement of muscles of the shoulder and pelvic girdles as well as trunk muscles develops. In advanced cases and rarely, early in the course of the disease, respiratory muscles are affected.

Laboratory studies disclose antibodies to AChR in 90 percent of patients. Repetitive nerve stimulation at low rates (2 Hz) is abnormal because of a decremental motor response. Ten to 15 percent of patients (especially the

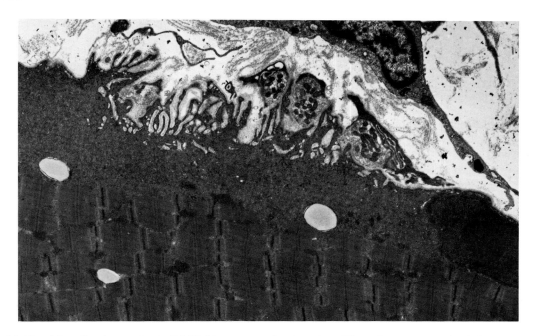

Fig. 16-62. Myasthenia gravis. (×7,000) Neuromuscular junction. The primary synaptic clefts are shallow and the secondary synaptic clefts are widened and shortened. The nerve terminals appear relatively normal.

older men) will be found to have a thymoma, usually well demonstrated by computed tomography (CT) scan of the mediastinum.

Routine muscle biopsy is usually normal. Patients who have been receiving corticosteroids will often have type II fiber atrophy. Rarely, collections of lymphocytes (lymphorrhages) are seen. These could represent macrophages invading neuromuscular junctions.[173] Electron microscopic studies of the muscle end-plate region show a remarkably simplified postsynaptic region with degeneration of junctional folds (Fig. 16-62). When the myasthenic postsynaptic junction is stained for AChR few are found on the terminal expansions of junctional folds, normally sites densely packed with AChR.

Special immunocytochemical studies show IgG, complement components C3 and C9, and the membrane attack complex all localized to the neuromuscular junction. This suggests that complement fixation and activation of the lytic phase of the complement reaction sequence occur in myasthenia gravis.[173]

The etiology of this disease is unknown, but much has been learned of its pathogenesis.[173] First, there is complement-mediated lysis of the postsynaptic membrane, which causes loss of AChR. Second, autoantibodies bind to the AChR and result in accelerated degradation of receptor molecules. The first mechanism reduces membrane surface available for the insertion of new AChR. Third, autoantibodies may directly block the access of ACh to the receptor.

The disease can be successfully treated in most patients. The first line of therapy consists of AChE inhibitors, which increase the physiological effect of ACh. The next line of treatment is corticosteroids, beneficial in 70 to 80 percent of patients, or thymectomy (in the patient below the age of 50), beneficial (sometimes curative) in 40 to 70 percent. Plasmapheresis is reserved for the patient with rapidly progressing fulminant weakness or for the severely weakened myasthenic who has not responded to other treatment modalities.

REFERENCES

1. Engel AG, Banker BQ (eds): Myology. McGraw-Hill, New York, 1986
2. Dubowitz V: Muscle Biopsy. A Practical Approach. Baillière Tindall, London, 1985
3. Kakulas BA, Adams RD: Diseases of Muscle. Pathological Foundations of Clinical Myology. Harper & Row, Philadelphia, 1985
4. Carpenter S, Karpati G: Pathology of Skeletal Muscle. Churchill Livingstone, New York, 1984
5. Burke RE: Motor units: Anatomy, physiology and functional organization. p. 345. In Brooks VB (eds): Handbook of Physiology. Section I: The Nervous System. Vol. 2: Motor Systems. American Physiological Society, Washington DC, 1981
6. Pearson ML, Epstein H (eds): Muscle Development: Mo-

lecular and Cellular Control. Cold Spring Harbor Laboratory, Cold Spring Harbor, NY, 1982

7. Emerson C, Fishman DA, Nadal-Ginard B, Siddiqui MAQ (eds): Molecular Biology of Muscle Development. Alan R Liss, New York, 1985

8. Guth L: Trophic influences of nerve on muscle. Phys Rev 48:645, 1968

9. Gutmann E: Neurotrophic relations. Annu Rev Physiol 38:177, 1975

10. Weiss L: Histology. Elsevier, New York, 1983

11. Boyd IA, Gladden M (eds): The Mammalian Muscle Spindle. Macmillan, London, 1985

12. Engel AG, Stonnington HH: Morphological effects of denervation on muscle. A quantitative study. Ann NY Acad Sci, 228:68, 1974

13. Karpati G, Engel WK: Neuronal trophic function. Arch Neurol 17:542, 1967

14. Mendell JR, Engel WK: The fine structure of type II muscle fiber atrophy. Neurology (NY) 21:358, 1971

15. Pellegrino C, Franzini C: An electron microscope study of denervation atrophy in red and white skeletal muscle fibers. J Cell Biol 17:327, 1963

16. Shafiq SA, Milhorat AT, Gorycki MA: Fine structure of human muscle in neurogenic atrophy. Neurology (NY) 17:934, 1967

17. Engel WK, Brooke MH, Nelson PG: Histochemical studies of denervated or tenotomized cat muscle: Illustrating difficulties in relating experimental animal conditions to human neuromuscular diseases. Ann NY Acad Sci 138:160, 1966

18. Ringel SP, Bender AN, Engel WK: Extrajunctional acetylcholine receptors. Alterations in human and experimental neuromuscular diseases. Arch Neurol 33:751, 1976

19. Morris CJ, Raybould JA: Fibre type grouping and end-plate diameter in human skeletal muscle. J Neurol Sci 13:181, 1971

20. Brooke MH, Engel WK: The histologic diagnosis of neuromuscular diseases: A review of 79 biopsies. Arch Phys Med Rehab 47:99, 1966

21. Karpati G, Engel WK: "Type grouping" in skeletal muscles after experimental reinnervation. Neurology (NY) 18:447, 1968

22. Engel WK: Muscle target fibres, a newly recognized sign of denervation. Nature (Lond) 191:389, 1961

23. Schotland DL: An electron microscopic study of target fibers, target-like fibers, and related abnormalities in human muscle. J Neuropathol Exp Neurol 28:214, 1969

24. Kovarsky J, Schochet SS Jr, McCormick WF: The significance of target fibers: A clinicopathologic review of 100 patients with neurogenic atrophy. Am J Clin Pathol 59:790, 1973

25. DeCoster W, DeReuck J, Vander Eecken H: The target phenomenon in human muscle. A comparative light microscopic histochemical and electron microscopic study. Acta Neuropathol (Berl) 34:329, 1976

26. Mrak RE, Saito A, Evans OB, Fleischer S: Autophagic degradation in human skeletal muscle target fibers. Muscle Nerve 5:745, 1982

27. Dubowitz V: Pathology of experimentally re-innervated skeletal muscle. J Neurol Neurosurg Psychiatry 30:99, 1967

28. Schochet SS Jr: Diagnostic Pathology of Skeletal Muscle and Nerve. Appleton & Lange, East Norwalk, CT, 1986

29. Drachman DB, Murphy SR, Nigam MP, Hills JR: "Myopathic" changes in chronically denervated muscle. Arch Neurol 16:14, 1967

30. Achari AN, Anderson MS: Myopathic changes in amyotrophic lateral sclerosis. Pathologic analysis of muscle biopsy changes in 111 cases. Neurology (NY) 24:477, 1974

31. Schwartz MS, Sargeant M, Swash M: Longitudinal fibre splitting in neurogenic muscular disorders—Its relation to the pathogenesis of "myopathic" change. Brain 99:617, 1976

32. Byers RK, Banker BQ: Infantile muscular atrophy. Arch Neurol 5:140, 1961

33. Gomez MR: Motor neuron diseases in children. p. 1993. In Engel AG, Banker BQ (eds): Myology. McGraw-Hill, New York, 1986

34. Reyes MG, Goldbarg H, Bouffard A: Muscle pathology of congenital Werdnig-Hoffman disease: Is there a prepathologic stage? Neurology (NY) 32:A201, 1982 (abst)

35. Mastaglia FL, Walton JN: Histological and histochemical changes in skeletal muscle from cases of chronic juvenile and early adult spinal muscular atrophy (the Kugelberg-Welander syndrome). J Neurol Sci 12:15, 1971

36. Rowland LP: The membrane theory of Duchenne dystrophy: Where is it? It J Neurol Sci 3(suppl. 1):13, 1984

37. Mokri B, Engel AG: Duchenne dystrophy: Electron microscopic findings pointing to a basic or early abnormality in the plasma membrane of the muscle fiber. Neurology (NY) 25:1111, 1975

38. Carpenter S, Karpati G: Duchenne dystrophy: Plasma membrane loss initiates muscle cell necrosis unless it is repaired. Brain 102:147, 1979

39. Engel AG, Banker BQ (eds): Duchenne dystrophy. p. 1185. In Myology. Vol. 2. McGraw-Hill, New York, 1986

40. Bradley WG, Jones MZ, Mussini JM, et al: Becker-type muscular dystrophy. Muscle Nerve 1:111, 1978

41. Munsat T: Facioscapulohumeral dystrophy and the scapuloperoneal syndrome. p. 1251. In Engel AG, Banker BQ (eds): Myology. Vol. 2. McGraw-Hill, New York, 1986

42. Victor M, Hayes R, Adams RD: Oculopharyngeal muscular dystrophy. A familial disease characterized by dysphagia and progressive ptosis of the eyelids. N Engl J Med 267:1267, 1962

43. Smith TW, Chad D: Intranuclear inclusions in oculopharyngeal dystrophy. Muscle Nerve 7:339, 1984

44. Harper P: Myotonic dystrophy. Major Problems in Neurology. Vol. 9. WB Saunders, Philadelphia, 1979

45. Harper P: Myotonic disorders. p. 1267. In Engel AG, Banker BQ (eds): Myology. McGraw-Hill, New York, 1986

46. Bradley WG: The limb girdle syndromes. p. 443. In Vinken PJ, Bruyn GW (eds): Handbook of Clinical Neurology. Vol. 40. Elsevier, Amsterdam, 1979

47. Banker BQ: Congenital muscular dystrophy. p. 1367. In Engel AG, Banker BQ (eds): Myology. McGraw-Hill, New York, 1986

48. Takada K, Nakamura H, Tanaka J: Cortical dysplasia in congenital muscular dystrophy with central nervous system involvement. J Neuropathol Exp Nerve 43:395, 1984

49. Bohan A, Peter JB, Bowman RL, et al: A computer-assisted analysis of 153 patients with polymyositis and dermatomyositis. Medicine (Baltimore) 56:255, 1977

50. Carpenter S, Karpati G, Heller I, et al: Inclusion body myositis: A distinct variety of idiopathic inflammatory myopathy. Neurology (NY) 28:8, 1978

51. Schwarz MI, Matthay RA, Sahn SA, et al: Interstitial lung disease in polymyositis and dermatomyositis: Analysis of six cases in review of the literature. Medicine (Baltimore) 55:89, 1976

52. Kehoe RF, Bauernfeind R, Tommaso C, et al: Cardiac conduction defects in polymyositis. Electrophysiologic studies in four patients. Ann Intern Med 94:41, 1981

53. Barnes BE: Dermatomyositis and malignancy. A review of the literature. Ann Intern Med 84:68, 1976

54. Lakhanpal, Bunch TW, Ilstrup DM, Melton LJ: Polymyositis-dermatomyositis and malignant lesions: Does an association exist? Mayo Clin Proc 61:645, 1986

55. Banker BQ, Engel AG: The polymyositis and dermatomyositis syndromes. p. 1385. In Engel AG, Banker BQ (eds): Myology. McGraw-Hill, New York, 1986

56. Carpenter S, Karpati, G, Rothman S, Watters G: The childhood type of dermatomyositis. Neurology (NY) 26:952, 1976

57. Mikol J: Inclusion body myositis. p. 1423. In Engel AG, Banker BQ, (eds): Myology. McGraw-Hill, New York, 1986

58. Ringel SP, Carry MR, Aguilera AJ, Starcevich JN: Quantitative histopathology of the inflammatory myopathies. Arch Neurol 43:1004, 1986

59. Whitaker JN, Engel WK: Vascular deposits in immunoglobulin and complement in idiopathic inflammatory myopathy. N Engl J Med 286:333, 1972

60. Kissel JT, Mendell JR, Rammohan KW: Microvascular deposition of complement membrane attack complex in dermatomyositis. N Engl J Med 314:329, 1986

61. Hewlett RH, Brownell B: Granulomatous myopathy: Its relationship to sarcoidosis and polymyositis. J Neurol Neurosurg Psychiatry 38:1090, 1975

62. Delaney P: Neurologic manifestations in sarcoidosis. Review of the literature with a review of 23 cases. Ann Intern Med 87:336, 1977

63. Menard DB, Haddad H, Blaine JG, et al: Granulomatous myositis and myopathy associated with Crohn's colitis. N Engl J Med 295:818, 1976

64. Hays AP, Gamboa ET: Acute viral myositis. p. 1439. In Engel AG, Banker BQ, (eds): Myology. McGraw-Hill, New York, 1986

65. Banker BQ: The congenital myopathies. p. 1527. In Engel AG, Banker BQ (eds): Myology. McGraw-Hill, New York, 1986

66. Engel AG, Angelini C, Gomez MR: Fingerprint body myopathy. A newly recognized congenital muscle disease. Mayo Clin Proc 47:377, 1972

67. Jerusalem F, Engel AG, Gomez MR: Sarcotubular myopathy. A newly recognized, benign, congenital, familial muscle disease. Neurology (NY) 23:897, 1973

68. Lake BD, Wilson J: Zebra body myopathy. Clinical, histochemical and ultrastructural studies. J Neurol Sci 24:437, 1975

69. Jerusalem F, Ludin H, Bischoff A, Hartmann G: Cytoplasmic body neuromyopathy presenting as respiratory failure and weight loss. J Neurol Sci 41:1, 1979

70. Brooke MH, Neville HE: Reducing body myopathy. Neurology (NY) 22:829, 1972

71. Shy GM, Magee KR: A new congenital non-progressive myopathy. Brain 79:610, 1956

72. Frank JP, Harati Y, Butler IJ, et al: Central core disease and malignant hyperthermia syndrome. Ann Neurol 7:11, 1980

73. Neville HE, Brooke MH: Central core fibers: Structured and unstructured. p. 497. In Kakulas BA (ed): Basic Research in Myology. Excerpta Medica, Amsterdam, 1973

74. Isaacs H, Heffron JJA, Badenhorst M: Central core disease. A correlated genetic, histochemical, ultramicroscopic, and biochemical study. J Neurol Neurosurg Psychiatry 38:1177, 1975

75. Afifi AK, Smith JW, Zellweger H: Congenital nonprogressive myopathy. Central core disease and nemaline myopathy in one family. Neurology (NY) 15:371, 1965

76. Fardeau M, Godet-Guillain J, Tomé FMS, et al: Congenital neuromuscular disorders: A critical review. p. 164. In Aguayo AJ, Karpati G (eds): Current Topics in Nerve and Muscle Research. Excerpta Medica, Amsterdam, 1979

77. Ringel SP, Bender AN, Engel WK: Extrajunctional acetylcholine receptors. Alterations in human and experimental neuromuscular diseases. Arch Neurol 33:751, 1976

78. Karpati G, Carpenter S, Eisen AA: Experimental core-like lesions and nemaline rods. A correlative morphological and physiological study. Arch Neurol 27:237, 1972

79. Engel AG, Gomez MR, Groover RV: Multicore disease. A recently recognized congenital myopathy associated with multifocal degeneration of muscle fibers. Mayo Clin Proc 46:666, 1971

80. Conen PE, Murphy EG, Donohue WL: Light and electron microscopic studies of "myogranules" in a child with hypotonia and muscle weakness. Can Med Assoc J 89:983, 1963

81. Shy GM, Engel WK, Somers JE, Wanko T: Nemaline myopathy. A new congenital myopathy. Brain 86:793, 1963

82. Nienhuis AW, Coleman RF, Brown WJ, et al: Nemaline myopathy. A histopathologic and histochemical study. Am J Clin Pathol 48:1, 1967

83. Engel AG, Gomez MR: Nemaline (Z disk) myopathy: Observations on the origin, structure, and solubility properties of the nemaline structures. J Neuropathol Exp Neurol 26:601, 1967

84. Jennekens FGI, Roord JJ, Veldman H, et al: Congenital nemaline myopathy. I. Defective organization of alpha-actinin is restricted to muscle. Muscle Nerve 6:61, 1983

85. Stuhlfauth I, Jennekens FGI, Willemse J, Jockusch BM: Congenital nemaline myopathy. II. Quantitative changes

in alpha-actinin and myosin in skeletal muscle. Muscle Nerve 6:69, 1983

86. Spiro AJ, Shy GM, Gonatas NK: Myotubular myopathy. Persistence of fetal muscle in an adolescent boy. Arch Neurol 14:1, 1966

87. Sher JH, Rimalovski AB, Athanassiades TJ, Aronson SM: Familial centronuclear myopathy: A clinical and pathological study. Neurology (NY) 17:727, 1967

88. van Wijngaarden GK, Fleury P, Bethlem J, Meijer AEFH: Familial ''myotubular'' myopathy. Neurology (NY) 19:901, 1969

89. Barth PG, van Wijngaarden GK, Bethlem J: X-linked myotubular myopathy with fatal neonatal asphyxia. Neurology (NY) 25:531, 1975

90. Ambler MW, Neave C, Tutschka BG, et al: X-linked recessive myotubular myopathy. 1. Clinical and pathologic findings in a family. Hum Pathol 15:566, 1984

91. Bergen BJ, Carry MP, Wilson WB, et al: Centronuclear myopathy: Extraocular- and limb-muscle findings in an adult. Muscle Nerve 3:165, 1980

92. Edstrom L, Wroblewski R, Mair WGP: Genuine myotubular myopathy. Muscle Nerve 5:604, 1982

93. Harriman DGF, Haleem MA: Centronuclear myopathy in old age. J Pathol 108:237, 1972

94. Goulon M, Fardeau M, Got C, et al: Myopathie centronucléaire d'expression clinique tardive. Étude clinique, histologique et ultrastructurale d'une nouvelle observation. Rev Neurol 132:275, 1976

95. Engel WK, Gold GN, Karpati G: Type I fiber hypotrophy and central nuclei. A rare congenital muscle abnormality with a possible experimental model. Arch Neurol 18:435, 1968

96. Brooke MH: Congenital fiber type dysproportion. p. 147. In Kakulas, BA (ed): Clinical Studies in Myology. Part 2. Excerpta Medica, Amsterdam, 1973

97. Brooke MH, Carroll JE, Ringel SP: Congenital hypotonia revisited. Muscle Nerve 2:84, 1979

98. Martin JJ, Clara R, Ceuterick C, Joris C: Is congenital fibre type disproportion a true myopathy? Acta Neurol Belg 76:335, 1976

99. Dehkharghani F, Sarnat HB, Brewster MA, Roth SI: Congenital muscle fiber-type disporportion in Krabbe's leukodystrophy. Arch Neurol 38:585, 1981

100. Hers HG: Alpha-glucosidase deficiency in generalized glycogen storage disease (Pompe's disease). Biochem J 86:11, 1963

101. Engel AG, Gomez MR, Seybold ME, et al: The spectrum and diagnosis of acid maltase deficiency. Neurology (NY) 23:95, 1973

102. Engel AG: Acid maltase deficiency. p. 1629. In Engel AG, Banker BQ, (eds): Myology. McGraw-Hill, New York, 1986

103. Karpati G, Carpenter S, Eisen A, et al: The adult form of acid maltase (alpha-1, 4-glucosidase) deficiency. Ann Neurol 1:276, 1977

104. Hudgson P, Fulthorpe JJ: The pathology of type II skeletal muscle glycoginosis. A light and electron-microscopic study. J Pathol 16:139, 1974

105. Cardiff RD: Histochemical and electron microscopic

study of skeletal muscle in a case of Pompe's disease (glycoginosis II). Pediatr 37:249, 1966

106. Mehler M, DiMauro S: Late-onset acid maltase deficiency. Detection of patients and heterozygotes by urinary enzyme assay. Arch Neurol 33:692, 1976

107. Angelini C, Engel AG: Comparative study of acid maltase deficiency; biochemical differences between infantile, childhood and adult types. Arch Neurol 26:344, 1972

108. DiMauro S, Stern LZ, Mahler M, et al: Adult-onset acid maltese deficiency: A postmortem study. Muscle Nerve 1:27, 1978

109. McArdle B: Myopathy due to a defect in muscle glycogen breakdown. Clin Sci 24:13, 1951

110. Pearson CM, Rimer DG, Mommaerts WFHM: A metabolic myopathy due to absence of muscle phosphorylase. Am J Med 30:502, 1961

111. Schmid R, Mahler R: Chronic progressive myopathy with myoglobinurias: Demonstration of a glycogenolytic defect in the muscle. J Clin Invest 38:2044, 1959

112. DiMauro S, Bresolin N: Phosphorylase deficiency. p. 1585. In Engel AG, Banker AQ, (eds): Myology. McGraw-Hill, New York, 1986

113. Pernow BB, Havel RJ, Jennings DB: The second wind phenomenon in McArdle's syndrome. Acta Med Scand 472:294, 1967

114. Engel WK, Eyerman EL, Williams, HE: Late-onset type of skeletal muscle phosphorylase deficiency. A new familial variety with completely and partially affected subjects. N Engl J Med 268:135, 1963

115. Mastaglia CG, McCollum JPK, Larson PF, et al: Steroid myopathy complicating McArdle's disease. J Neurol Neurosurg Psychiatry 33:111, 1970

116. DiMauro S, Hartlage PL: Fatal infantile form of muscle phosphorylase deficiency. Neurology 28:1124, 1978

117. Munsat TL: A standardized forum ischemic exercise test. Neurology (NY) 20:1171, 1970

118. Roelofs RI, Engel WK, Chauvin PB: Histochemical phosphorylase activity in regenerating muscle fibers from myophosphorylase-deficient patients. Science 177:795, 1972

119. Meienhofer MC, Askansas V, Proux-Daegelen J, et al: Muscle-type phosphorylase activity present in muscle cells cultured from three patients with myophosphorylase deficiency. Arch Neurol 34:779, 1977

120. DiMauro S, Arnold S, Miranda A, et al: McArdle's disease: The mystery of reappearing phosphorylase activity in muscle culture: A fetal isoenzyme. Ann Neurol 3:60, 1978

121. Tarui S, Okuno G, Ikua Y, et al: Phosphofructokinase deficiency in skeletal muscle. A new type of glycogenosis. Biochem Biophys Res Commun 19:517, 1965

122. Rowland LP, DeMauro S, Layzer RB: Phosphofructokinase deficiency. p. 1603. In Engel AG, Banker AQ (eds): Myology. McGraw-Hill, New York, 1986

123. Hays AP, Hallet M, Delfs J, et al: Muscle phosphofructokinase deficiency: Abnormal polysaccharide in a case of late-onset myopathy. Neurology (NY) 31:1077, 1981

124. Danon MJ, Carpenter S, Manaligod JR, Schlisefeld LH: Fatal infantile glycogen storage disease; deficiency of

phosphofructokinase and phosphorylase B kinase. Neurology 31:1303, 1981

125. Brown BI: Debranching and branching enzyme deficiencies. p. 1653. In Engel AG, Banker AQ (eds): Myology. McGraw-Hill, New York, 1986

126. DiMauro S, Hartwig GB, Hays A, et al: Debrancher deficiency: Neuromuscular disorder in five adults. Ann Neurol 5:422, 1979

127. DiMauro S, Bresloin N: Newly recognized defects in distal glycolysis. p. 1619. In Engel AG, Banker AQ (eds): Myology. McGraw-Hill, New York, 1986

128. Fishbein WN, Armbrustmacher VW, Griffin JL: Myoadenylate deaminase deficiency: A new disease of muscle. Science 299:545, 1978

129. Brooke MH: A Clinician's View of Neuromuscular Diseases. 2nd Ed. Williams & Wilkins, Baltimore, 1986

130. Fishbein WN: Myoadenylate deaminase deficiency. p. 1745. In Engel AG, Banker AQ (eds): Myology. McGraw-Hill, New York, 1986

131. Olson W, Engel WK, Walsh GO, et al: Oculocraniosomatic neuromuscular disease with (ragged-red) fibers. Arch Neurol 26:193, 1972

132. DiMauro S, Bonilla E, Zeviani M, et al: Mitochondrial myopathies. Ann Neurol 17:521, 1985

133. Luft R, Ikkos D, Palmieri G, et al: A case of severe hypermetabolism of non-thyroid origin with a defect in the maintenance of mitochondrial respiratory control: A correlated clinical, biochemical and morphological study. J Clin Invest 41:1776, 1962

134. Haydar NA, Kahn HL, Afifi A, et al: Severe hypermetabolism with primary abnormality of skeletal muscle mitochondria. Ann Intern Med 74:548, 1971

135. Kearns TP, Sayre GP: Retinitis pigmentosa, external ophthalmoplegia and complete heart block. AMA Arch Ophthalmol 60:280, 1958

136. Berenberg RA, Pellock JM, DiMauro S, et al: Lumping or splitting? "Orhthalmoplegia-plus" or Kearns-Sayer syndrome. Ann Neurol 1:37, 1977

137. Bressler RR: Carnitine and the twins. N Engl J Med 282:745, 1970

138. Engel AG, Siekert RG: Lipid storage myopathy responsive to prednisone. Arch Neurol 27:174, 1972

139. Engel AG: Carnitine deficiency syndromes and lipid storage myopathies. p. 1663. In Engel AG, Banker BQ (eds): Myology. McGraw-Hill, New York, 1986

140. Karpati G, Carpenter S, Eisen A, et al: The syndrome of systemic carnitine deficiency. Neurology (NY) 25:16, 1975

141. Bank WJ, DiMauro S, Bonilla E, et al: A disorder of muscle lipid metabolism and myoglobinuria. N Engl J Med 292:443, 1975

142. DiMauro S, Papadimitriou A: Carnitine palmitoyltransferase deficiency. p. 1697. In Engel AG, Banker AQ (eds): Myology. McGraw-Hill, New York, 1986

143. Ruff RL: Endocrine myopathies (hyper- and hypofunction of adrenal, thyroid, pituitary, and parathyroid glands and iatrogenic steroid myopathy). p. 1871. In Engel AG, Banker BQ (eds): Myology. McGraw-Hill, New York, 1986

144. Harvard CWH, Campbell EDR, Ross HB, Spence AW: Electromyographic and histological findings in the muscles of patients with thyrotoxicosis. Q J Med 32:145, 1963

145. Satoyoshi E, Murakami K, Kowa H, et al: Myopathy in thyrotoxicosis. With special emphasis on an effect of potassium ingestion on serum and urinary creatine. Neurology (NY) 13:645, 1963

146. Ramsay ID: Electromyography in thyrotoxicosis. Q J Med 34:255, 1965

147. Engel AG: Electron microscopic observations in thyrotoxic and corticosteroid-induced myopathies. Mayo Clin Proc 41:785, 1966

148. Engel AG: Neuromuscular manifestations of Graves' disease. Mayo Clin Proc 47:919, 1972

149. Åström K-E, Kugelberg E, Muller R: Hypothyroid myopathy. Arch Neurol 5:472, 1961

150. Norris FH, Panner BJ: Hypothyroid myopathy. Clinical, electromyographical, and ultrastructural observations. Arch Neurol 14:574, 1966

151. Afifi AK, Najjar SS, Mire-Salman J, Bergman RA: The myopathology of the Kocher-Debre-Semelaigne syndrome. Electromyography, light- and electron-microscopic study. J Neurol Sci 22:445, 1974

152. Khaleeli AA, Gohil K, McPhail G, Round JM, Edwards RHT: Muscle morphology and metabolism in hypothyroid myopathy: Effects of treatment. J Clin Pathol 36:519, 1983

153. Godet-Guillain J, Fardeau M: Hypothyroid myopathy. Histological and ultrastructural study of an atrophic form. p. 512. In Walton JN, Canal N, Scarlato G (eds): Muscle Diseases. Excerpta Medica, Amsterdam, 1970

154. Ho K-L: Basophilic degeneration of skeletal muscle in hypothyroid myopathy. Arch Pathol Lab Med 108:239, 1984

155. Frame B, Heinze EG, Block MA, Manson GA: Myopathy in primary hyperparathyroidism. Ann Intern Med 68:1022, 1968

156. Cholod EJ, Haust MD, Hudson AJ, Lewis FN: Myopathy in primary familial hyperparathyroidism. Clinical and morphologic studies. Am J Med 48:700, 1970

157. Patten BM, Bilezikian JP, Mallette LE, et al: Neuromuscular disease in primary hyperparathyroidism. Ann Intern Med 80:182, 1974

158. Pleasure DE, Walsh GO, Engel WK: Atrophy of skeletal muscle in patients with Cushing's syndrome. Arch Neurol 22:118, 1970

159. Harriman DGF, Reed R: The incidence of lipid droplets in human skeletal muscle in neuromuscular disorders: A histochemical, electron-microscopic and freeze-etch study. J Pathol 106:1, 1972

160. Afifi AK, Bergman RA, Harvey JC: Steroid myopathy. Clinical, histologic and cytologic observations. Johns Hopkins Med J 123:158, 1968

161. Vilchez JJ, Cabello A, Benedito J, Villarroya T: Hyperkalaemic paralysis, neuropathy and persistent motor neuron discharges at rest in Addison's disease. J Neurol Neurosurg Psychiatry 43:818, 1980

162. Mastaglia FL, Barwick DD, Hall R: Myopathy in acromegaly. Lancet 2:907, 1970

163. Mastaglia FL: Pathological changes in skeletal muscle in acromegaly. Acta Neuropathol (Berl) 24:273, 1973

164. Stern LZ, Payne CM, Hannapel LK: Acromegaly: Histochemical and electron microscopic changes in deltoid and intercostal muscle. Neurology (NY) 24:589, 1974

165. Pickett JBE, Layzer RB, Levin SR, et al: Neuromuscular complications of acromegaly. Neurology (NY) 25:638, 1975

166. Nagulesparen M, Trickey R, Davies MJ, Jenkins JS: Muscle changes in acromegaly. Br Med J 2:914, 1976

167. Dubowitz V: Muscle Biopsy. A Practical Approach. 2nd Ed. London, Bailliere Tindall, 1985, pp. 560–564

168. Engel AG: Periodic paralysis. p. 1843. In Engel AG, Banker BQ (eds): Myology. McGraw-Hill, New York, 1986

169. Pearson CM: The periodic paralyses: Differential features and pathological observations in permanent myopathic weakness. Brain 87:341, 1964

170. Engel AG: Evolution and content of vacuoles in primary hypokalemic periodic paralysis. Mayo Clin Proc 45:774, 1970

171. Engel AG: Electron microscopic observations in primary hypokalemic and thyrotoxic periodic paralysis. Mayo Clin Proc 41:797, 1966

172. Penn AS: Myoglobinuria. p. 1785. In Engel AG, Banker BQ (eds): Myology. McGraw-Hill, New York, 1986

173. Engel AG: Acquired autoimmune myasthenia gravis. p. 192. In Engel AG, Banker BQ (eds): Myology. McGraw-Hill, New York, 1986

174. Armbrustmacher VW: Skeletal muscle in denervation. Pathol Annu 13 (Pt 2):1, 1983

175. DeGirolami U, Smith TW: Pathology of skeletal muscle diseases. Teaching monograph. Am J Pathol 107:235, 1982

176. Chad D, Munsat TL, Adelman LS: Diseases of muscle. p. 569. In Rosenberg RN (ed): The Clinical Neurosciences. Vol. 1. Churchill Livingstone, New York, 1983

177. Chad D, Good P, Adelman L, et al: Inclusion body myositis associated with Sjögren's syndrome. Arch Neurol 39:186, 1982

178. Chad DA: Involvement of skeletal muscle in general medical diseases. p. 2. In Neurology and Neurosurgery Update Series. Vol. 3, No. 28. Continuing Professional Education Center, 1982

17

The Nasal Cavity, Paranasal Sinuses, and Nasopharynx

Yao Shi Fu
Karl H. Perzin

Specimens are removed from the nasal cavity, paranasal sinuses, and nasopharynx for two main reasons: diagnosis and treatment. The clinician, while examining a patient, may discover a lesion, which is biopsied for diagnosis. The majority of specimens are sent to the surgical pathologist for both reasons. For example, the surgeon may have removed multiple polyps from the nasal cavity, or because of clinical sinusitis, a sinus may have been curetted. These specimens are sent to the pathologist basically to confirm the clinical diagnosis, but the tissue should be carefully studied because completely unsuspected findings may be identified on histologic examination.

TYPES OF SURGICAL SPECIMENS

The majority of specimens received by the surgical pathologist consist of one or more pieces of tissue resected by polypectomy or by curettage. We believe that all specimens should be fixed and then submitted in toto, even if multiple cassettes are required. When the sections are studied, a clinically unsuspected lesion, such as carcinoma, may be discovered, sometimes in only one of the multiple pieces of tissue submitted.

Small biopsy specimens should, of course, be submitted in toto. In addition, we request that the block(s) be cut at three levels; deeper levels through the block may be required because of suspicious findings seen on the first set of slides.

Small biopsy specimens from this area may show considerable crush artifact. If the tissue is so distorted that a diagnosis cannot be made with absolute certainty, the pathologist should ask the clinician to repeat the biopsy. Other reasons for problems in interpretation of small biopsy specimens include tangential cutting and the small amount of tissue available.

The pathologist will also receive large resection specimens from this area. For example, a radical maxillectomy may have been performed for a biopsy-proven carcinoma. All these specimens should be adequately fixed before sections are taken. The gross appearance of the tumor, its dimensions, the patterns of growth, and involvement of adjacent structures should be documented. The slides should show the relationship between tumor and the surgical lines of resection. This can be done by marking the surgical margins with India ink.

When the pathologist receives a large en bloc resection specimen, the anatomy and orientation of the specimen in many cases can be readily determined because of the presence of structures such as the orbital contents, orbital floor, or lateral wall of the nasal cavity. In other cases, such as a partial maxillectomy, the pathologist may not be able to orient the specimen. In these cases, the clinician and the pathologist should study the specimen together before sections are taken to ensure proper orientation.

In some cases, as when tumor involves the frontal, ethmoid, or sphenoid sinuses, a neoplasm may have been removed piecemeal by curettage, and the pathologist will receive multiple small pieces of tissue that cannot be oriented. As mentioned previously, such specimens should be submitted in toto. When the sections are studied, even though the surgical margin cannot be determined, the pathologist should at least examine for the presence of tumor invasion into bone or other structures.

In examining frozen sections of tissue taken from surgical lines of excision in this area, it is essential not to misinterpret pseudoepitheliomatous hyperplasia and squamous metaplasia involving the lining mucosa and secretory glands as carcinoma. Especially adjacent to areas of necrosis, exuberant granulation tissue may appear sarcomatous. The atypical stromal cells may have enlarged, hyperchromatic, and occasionally pleomorphic nuclei. Some of the cells may be multinucleated. These changes are most commonly seen in patients subjected to recent trauma, surgical intervention, or radiotherapy. However, some patients lack such a history. In contrast to sarcomas, numerous small blood vessels lined by reactive-appearing endothelial cells usually are found in the atypical granulation tissue. These problems will be discussed later in this chapter.

We do not believe that a diagnosis of a lesion in this area should be made on the basis of a frozen section examination. Permanent tissue sections of any lesion on which a biopsy can be done should be studied before a diagnosis is rendered. A large resection, performed in the head and neck area, should not be based on a frozen section diagnosis when a biopsy specimen and permanent sections could have been obtained. Too many pitfalls exist in frozen section diagnosis in this area to justify radical surgery.

Needle biopsies, fine needle aspirations, and cytologic studies are not usually performed in this area, so we have insufficient material to make a statement about these modes of diagnosis.

NORMAL HISTOLOGY

Histologically, the anterior nasal vestibule is covered by a thin layer of keratinizing squamous epithelium extending in from the anterior nares. The posterior nasal vestibule and cartilaginous septum are lined by nonkeratinizing squamous epithelium, beneath which are found secretory glands (minor salivary glands).

The nasal cavity and paranasal sinuses have a mucosal lining consisting of ciliated respiratory-type columnar epithelium. The underlying lamina propria contains many secretory glands and has numerous blood vessels of varying sizes. The mucosa and lamina propria in most areas are found close to bone, including the turbinates and the sinus walls. The olfactory areas consist of a specialized ciliated epithelium and olfactory sensory cells.

The nasopharynx in the newborn is lined entirely by ciliated respiratory epithelium. With increasing age, this lining is replaced by nonkeratinizing squamous cells. Af-

ter age 10, most of the posterior wall is covered by a squamous mucosa, whereas the surface of the anterior and lateral walls appears to be covered with equal amounts of squamous and columnar epithelium. Numerous lymphoid aggregates with germinal centers are found beneath the surface. This tissue may undergo hyperplasia (adenoids).

For the purpose of this chapter, we will use the term *upper respiratory tract* to refer only to the nasal cavity, paranasal sinuses, and nasopharynx.

DISEASES INVOLVING THE UPPER RESPIRATORY TRACT
Nasal Polyps

The nasal polyp is the most common upper respiratory tract lesion to be seen by the surgical pathologist. Nasal polyps may be solitary, but they usually are multiple and often involve both nasal cavities as well as the paranasal sinuses. These lesions are usually associated with allergic and/or infectious disorders. Allergic polyps most frequently occur in the turbinate and ethmoid regions. Choanal polyps, found in the posterior nasal cavity, are thought to be mainly of infectious origin.

On gross examination, nasal polyps consist of soft, edematous, semitranslucent masses of tissue of variable size and configuration. On histologic examination, these lesions are composed of edematous connective tissue in which the collagenous fibers of the lamina propria are pushed apart by homogeneous acidophilic proteinaceous fluid. A variable infiltrate of inflammatory cells, including neutrophils, eosinophils, lymphocytes, and plasma cells, is seen. The presence of numerous eosinophils indicates that the lesion probably has an allergic etiology. The surface ciliated respiratory epithelium may show several abnormalities, including basal cell hyperplasia, squamous metaplasia, atrophy, and ulceration. Occasionally, epithelial atypia may be noted. Edematous changes usually occur in the lamina propria above the level of the secretory glands, which are only sporadically seen in these specimens. The ducts leading to the glands are often observed and may be cystically dilated, producing retention cysts. The glands themselves may show atrophic changes, but occasionally they appear hyperplastic. The stroma may have areas of fibrosis, especially when ulceration or infection has occurred. Rarely, large, bizarre, pleomorphic spindle-shaped cells having hyperchromatic nuclei and prominent nucleoli may be observed in the stroma[1,2] (Fig. 17-1). These atypical stromal cells may lead the pathologist to suspect the presence of a malignant tumor such as an embryonal rhabdomyosarcoma. However, these atypical cells are usually seen in the con-

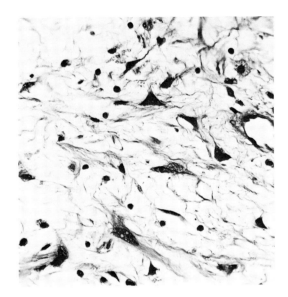

Fig. 17-1. Nasal polyp with stromal cell atypia. Ordinary nasal polyps are composed of an edematous stroma with bland-appearing stromal cells. An occasional totally benign nasal polyp will demonstrate scattered atypical stromal cells with large, pleomorphic, hyperchromatic nuclei.

text of inflamed granulation tissue, have mitoses, and are thought to represent bizarre reactive fibroblasts or histiocytes. The presence of these cells does not indicate that the lesion will recur or behave in a malignant manner.[2]

Approximately 5 to 10 percent of the patients with mucoviscidosis (cystic fibrosis) develop polyps in the nasal cavity and paranasal sinuses.[3] The pathologist should suggest the possibility of this disease when cystically dilated ducts are observed containing inspissated mucoid material in their lumina.

Rarely, children or young adults with storage diseases may present with nasal polyps and airway obstruction. In the case of mucopolysaccharidosis, numerous foamy histiocytes may accumulate in the stroma. Endothelial cells and the surrounding cells also contain vacuolated material, which reacts weakly with periodic acid-Schiff (PAS) and alcian blue stains. Determination of the specific metabolic disorder requires bichemical assay of the serum or urine.

Certain neoplasms involving the upper respiratory passages may produce a polypoid mass (or masses) that project(s) into the involved cavity. These lesions may have the clinical appearance of ordinary nasal polyps and may be resected by polypectomy. The specimen may be sent to the pathologist with the clinical diagnosis of "nasal polyp." For this reason, we believe all specimens that are resected from the nasal cavity, paranasal sinuses, and nasopharynx with the clinical diagnosis of "polyp" should be sectioned in toto and studied histologically. We

have seen a broad spectrum of tumors discovered in this manner, including papillomatosis (papillomas), carcinomas, and nonepithelial tumors (including vascular, smooth muscle, skeletal muscle, and fibrous tissue neoplasms, as well as plasmacytomas and malignant lymphomas).

Nonspecific Infectious Lesions

The surgical pathologist will frequently receive pieces of tissue that have been curetted from one or more paranasal sinuses with the clinical diagnosis of "sinusitis." Pieces of nasal mucosa may also accompany these specimens. We believe all these resected pieces should be studied histologically because unsuspected conditions may be discovered, such as papillomatosis, carcinoma, vasculitis (Wegener's granulomatosis), and so forth.

In cases of sinusitis and rhinitis, the lamina propria is infiltrated by variable numbers of neutrophils, eosinophils, lymphocytes, histiocytes, and plasma cells. Numerous eosinophils indicate an allergic component. The surface mucosa may show a spectrum of changes, including basal cell hyperplasia, squamous metaplasia, atypia, ulceration, and regeneration. The secretory glands may demonstrate variable inflammatory changes.

In some cases a heavy infiltration of mature plasma cells may be seen, a condition that has been called *plasma cell granuloma*. The pathologist should not confuse this entity with a plasmacytoma. Most chronic inflammatory lesions of this area exhibit a mixed polymorphic cell population, including different types of inflammatory cells. In plasma cell granuloma, plasma cells predominate, and very few other inflammatory cells are identified. The plasma cells, however, have the characteristics of mature cells. The presence of Russell bodies would favor a benign diagnosis. In contrast, plasmacytomas are composed of immature cells that have large, atypical, pleomorphic nuclei and demonstrate numerous mitoses. Russell bodies are rarely seen.

A *mucocele* represents one of the complications of sinusitis. The sinus opening into the nasal cavity may be obstructed by inflamed mucosa and its stroma. As a result, the sinus lumen becomes filled with mucus and debris sometimes leading to thinning or even destruction of the bony wall. When the orifice of a secretory gland is obstructed by inflamed tissue or by hyperplastic epithelium, a retention cyst may be formed that may clinically mimic a mucocele. Other causes of mucoceles include osteoma, trauma, and prior surgery to the sinus.

In all these specimens, the pathologist should examine any pieces of bone that may be included with the curetted tissue. If the inflammatory changes involve bone, this fact should be mentioned in the pathology report. The clinician may wish to correlate the changes seen on radiologic studies with the pathologic findings. If the infection has spread into bone, the possibility exists that it may have extended through the bone into adjacent structures such as the cranial or orbital cavities.

Specific Infectious Lesions

Tuberculosis

Tuberculosis may involve the skin of the nose, the mucocutaneous junction, or the nasal cavity itself. When caseating granulomas are found, the pathologist should suspect the presence of tuberculosis and order acid-fast stains.

Leprosy

Leprosy (usually the lepromatous form) may involve the mucous membranes of the nasal cavity and nasopharynx, producing nodular and destructive lesions similar to those seen in the skin. Histologically, the tissues are infiltrated by chronic inflammatory cells, including variable numbers of large, somewhat foamy histiocytes (lepra cells). With the acid-fast stain, *Mycobacterium leprae* can usually be demonstrated in the lepra cell cytoplasm.

Rhinoscleroma

Rhinoscleroma is rarely seen in the United States but may be identified in individuals who have come from areas of the world where this disease is found endemically (parts of Eastern Europe, the Mediterranean area, the Middle East, Central Africa, Pakistan, Indonesia, and parts of Central and South America). This condition affects the mucous membranes of the nasal cavity and the nasopharynx, which gradually become firm, indurated, and somewhat nodular. As a result, the lumen of the passage becomes slowly and progressively narrower. The oropharynx, larynx, and trachea may also be involved.

When the clinician submits a biopsy specimen from one of these lesions, the pathologist should be alerted to the possibility of rhinoscleroma; otherwise the correct diagnosis may be easily missed. Histologically, the lamina propria shows a diffuse, chronic nonspecific inflammatory cell infiltrate, consisting of variable numbers of lymphocytes, plasma cells, and histiocytes (Fig. 17-2). Occasionally, plasma cells predominate, and an incorrect diagnosis of plasmacytoma may be made. Histiocytes with abundant, somewhat foamy cytoplasm, called Mikulicz cells, are found in variable numbers.[4] PAS and Gram stains should demonstrate bacteria in their cytoplasm.

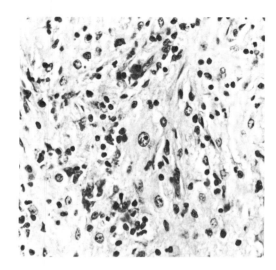

Fig. 17-2.   Rhinoscleroma. The stroma is infiltrated by chronic inflammatory cells. Large histiocytic cells have indistinct borders and abundant finely granular cytoplasm.

The organisms (gram-negative bacilli, *Klebsiella rhinoscleromatis*), are thought to initiate the inflammatory reaction but may only be secondary invaders. An immunoperoxidase technique using rabbit anti-*Klebsiella* capsular antigen III has been found to improve the specificity of histochemical stains and to detect lesions that are otherwise negative by cultures or other special stains.[5] Because of the numerous histiocytes with abundant cytoplasm, leprosy should be considered in the differential diagnosis. The lamina propria may show a variable proliferation of granulation and fibrous tissue. The overlying epithelium is usually found to be intact, but squamous metaplasia and pseudoepitheliomatous hyperplasia may be seen. The inflammatory process usually does not involve the underlying cartilage and bone.

Phycomycosis (Mucormycosis)

Phycomycosis is an infection caused by the class Phycomycetes, which include the orders Mucorales (genera *Rhizopus*, *Mucor*, and *Absidia*) and Entomophthorales. The latter may, rarely, cause indolent chronic granulomatous infection of the sinuses or skin. Most phycomycotic infections are produced by members of the Mucorales group. They normally are identified as saprophytic organisms on the mucosal surfaces of the nasal cavity and paranasal sinuses. Under certain circumstances, these fungi may invade the underlying tissues, causing a serious and often rapidly fatal rhinocerebral form of mucormycosis. Conditions that predispose to invasive mucormycosis include (1) poorly controlled diabetes mellitus (most common); (2) lymphomas, leukemias, and other malignant neoplasms; and (3) immunosuppressed states with suppression of inflammatory cells and/or antibodies by chemotherapeutic agents.[6]

In invasive mucormycosis, the fungi extend directly into the underlying tissues and have a marked tendency to invade blood vessels (Fig. 17-3), especially arteries, leading to thrombosis of vessels and necrosis of the involved tissue. As a result, the nasal and/or ethmoid mucosa appears pale or necrotic (black). From the site of invasion, the organisms may extend into the orbital cavity, producing the clinical picture of a rapidly spreading orbital cellulitis, or into the cranial cavity, causing meningoencephalitis. Progressive tissue necrosis may involve the skin of the eye, the nose, and the maxillary areas.

When invasive mucormycosis is suspected, the clinician will biopsy the nasal or ethmoid mucosa and should alert the pathologist about the suspected diagnosis. Special stains for fungi (PAS, silver-methenamine, or others) should be ordered. These organisms usually can be seen in routine sections but may be identified only with the special stains, especially if only a few fungi are present. Since Mucorales organisms have a special affinity for blood vessels, the pathologist should concentrate on examining blood vessel walls and their lumina, especially in areas where inflammation and necrosis are observed. Mucorales has a typical morphology, consisting of broad, branching, nonseptate hyphae, varying in width from 6 to 50 μm and in length from 100 to 200 μm. Curettings from inflamed and necrotic nasal or sinus tissue may be submitted without an adequate history. The pathologist

should suspect mucormycosis in any case in which blood vessel thrombosis and extensive tissue necrosis are observed. Special stains for fungi should be ordered under these circumstances. Improvement in survival is attributed to early diagnosis followed by aggressive radical resection of affected tissues and systemic amphotericin B therapy.[7] The extent of disease has been shown to be related to the host immune response, especially the serum fungistatic activity.[8]

Phycomycetes organisms should be distinguished from septate hyphae of the Dermatiaceae family, which cause phaeohyphomycosis of the sinuses. These organisms affect mostly immunocompetent children or young adults, who present with nasal obstruction, facial pain, or eye infection. The mucosa of the nasal cavity and sinuses is thickened and polypoid. Histologically, the resected tissue demonstrates marked stromal edema and a nonspecific acute and chronic inflammatory reaction. The hyphae, which are septate and larger than those of Phycomycetes, are found in the impacted mucus of the sinus without invasion of the tissue.[9,10]

Aspergillosis

Aspergillus, a fungus that grows in decaying vegetable matter, is normally found in the air and may be inhaled. As a result, these organisms may be normally present on the mucosal surfaces of the nasal cavity and paranasal sinuses but only rarely produce disease. *Aspergillus* (*fumigatus* and *flavus*) consists of uniform septate hyphae that branch at wide angles and measure 3 to 6 μm in diameter. Sporulating structures (conidial heads or conidiospores) ranging up to 30 μm in diameter may be seen in nature, on culture media, or within air spaces of the body such as paranasal sinuses and bronchi.

In a patient who has a persistent disorder of a paranasal sinus with chronic infection and poor drainage (such as persistent chronic sinusitis), aspergilli may proliferate in the sinus lumen and produce a fungus ball, called an *aspergilloma,* which may be identified in curettings from the involved sinus. The ball is usually composed of hyphae, but conidiospores may also be seen.

In immunosuppressed or otherwise immunocompromised patients, aspergilli may invade the nasal or sinus tissues in a manner similar to that described previously for Mucorales organisms.[11] Less commonly, aspergilli may invade the nasal and sinus tissues in an immunocompetent person. In this case the disease tends to be more localized. The histologic findings vary considerably. In some cases an acute inflammatory reaction with numerous neutrophils and even abscess formation is produced. In other cases fibrosis and chronic inflammation are seen, sometimes associated with caseating and noncaseating granulomas. Giant cells of various types

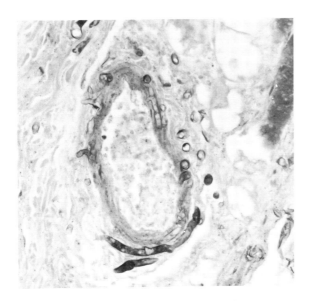

Fig. 17-3. Mucormycosis. The fungal organisms are seen in the wall of a small blood vessel and in adjacent necrotic tissue.

may be observed. Special stains for acid-fast bacteria and fungi should always be ordered when histologic study of any lesion of the nasal cavity and paranasal sinuses demonstrates granuloma formation.

Rarely, aspergillosis presents an allergic sinusitis. The sinuses are filled with dense, mucoid material, which contains numerous eosinophils, desquamated respiratory mucosal cells, cell debris, Charcot-Leyden crystals, and fungal hyphae. The sinus wall shows mild inflammation. Nasal polyps are usually present. Most patients are young and asthmatic and respond to steroid rather than antibiotic therapy.[12]

Rhinosporidiosis

Rhinosporidiosis is a chronic infection caused by the fungus *Rhinosporidium seeberi*. These organisms resemble *Coccidioides immitis*, but the sporocysts attain a larger size, ranging from 100 to 400 μm in diameter. The sporocysts have a thick, double-contoured wall and contain numerous endospores, about the size of red blood cells.

Rhinosporidiosis is rarely seen in the United States but may be identified in persons who come from endemic areas, such as India. Clinically, patients with this disease have multiple broad-based or polypoid lesions involving the nasal cavity and, less commonly, the nasopharynx. The polyps, which bleed easily, may obstruct the nasal passages.

Histologically, these lesions contain variable numbers of sporocysts. A chronic inflammatory reaction, consisting mainly of lymphocytes and plasma cells, is seen, although histiocytes and foreign body giant cells may be associated with collapsed sporocysts. Liberated endospores may induce an acute inflammatory reaction, with neutrophils and microabscesses. These organisms are well demonstrated by special fungal stains.

Myospherulosis

In 1977, Kyriakas[13] described 16 cases of myospherulosis-like organisms involving the nasal cavity, paranasal sinuses, and middle ear. These structures were characterized by "parent bodies" ranging in size from 20 to 120 μm. Spherules, measuring 5 to 7 μm, were found within the parent bodies and also scattered within the tissues. All the patients had been treated with hemostatic packing that contained petrolatum-based ointments and gauze, which suggests that the organisms were introduced via this route.[13] Rosai[14] has reproduced these structures in the test tube by incubating red blood cells and tetracycline ointment at 37°C. Thus, myospherulosis appears to represent altered red blood cells.[14]

Other Granulomatous Lesions

Sarcoidosis

From 3 to 20 percent of patients with systemic sarcoidosis have nasal involvement.[15] People with nasal sarcoidosis usually demonstrate clinical evidence of systemic disease, but occasionally nasal involvement may be the first and only manifestation of this disorder.[16] Sarcoidosis tends to affect mainly the nasal septum and inferior turbinates, but the disease may also be seen in adjacent structures such as the orbital cavity, olfactory tract, and meninges.

In some cases sarcoid granulomas may be found in blind biopsy specimens taken from the nasal cavity (even when the mucosa clinically appears normal).[17] The surgical pathologist may see more of these biopsy specimens in the future as clinicians have become aware that granulomas may be found in the nasal mucosa, where a biopsy can be readily performed.

The histologic features of sarcoidosis involving the mucous membranes of the nasal cavity and paranasal sinuses are similar to those seen in other organs and tissues.

Wegener's Granulomatosis

Wegener's granulomatosis is a rare disease that usually involves the upper respiratory tract (nasal cavity and paranasal sinuses), the lungs, and the kidneys. Less commonly, other organs and tissues may be affected, including skin, eyes, ears, joints, nervous system, and heart.[18] The upper respiratory tract is reported to be involved in 60 to 95 percent of the cases.[18] When diagnosis is made, the disease may be localized in only one site.

When Wegener's granulomatosis involves the nasal cavity early in the course of the disease, the patient may complain only of nasal obstruction. Diffuse nasal mucosal swelling without tissue necrosis may be observed. Most patients are seen later in the course of the disease and have a nasal discharge. Examination usually shows diffuse mucosal destruction with foul-smelling crusts and underlying friable tissue. Perforation of the nasal septum is commonly seen. In descending order of frequency, the maxillary, ethmoid, frontal, and sphenoid sinuses are involved, although pansinusitis is quite frequently identified.[18]

Histologically, the tissues in Wegener's granulomatosis show two major findings: necrotizing granulomatous inflammation and/or vasculitis. The inflammatory cell population includes neutrophils, eosinophils, lymphocytes, plasma cells, and histiocytes, including multinucleated giant cells. Various types of granulomatous inflammation may be seen, including epithelioid

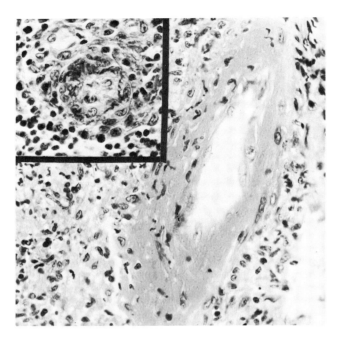

Fig. 17-4. Wegener's granulomatosis. A small artery shows marked "fibrinoid" necrosis, and its wall is infiltrated by neutrophils. In the inset another small artery demonstrates fragmented elastic fibers.

granulomas without necrosis, granulomas with "fibrinoid" necrosis, and granulomas with microabscesses. The vasculitis, which may affect small arteries and/or veins, shows a variable transmural infiltration by inflammatory cells. Fibrinoid necrosis may be found in the vessel wall (Fig. 17-4). Vascular lesions may be difficult to identify because of extensive inflammation and necrosis, but they may be recognized when elastic tissue stains are performed.

The surgical pathologist will encounter nasal and sinus tissues in Wegener's granulomatosis under two different circumstances. In some cases the diagnosis is suspected and a nasal biopsy is performed. In other cases, tissue is curetted from the nasal and/or sinus cavities of patients who have inflammatory lesions in these locations. Wegener's granulomatosis may or may not be suspected. When multiple pieces of tissue have been removed by curettage, the surgical pathologist must study all the resected tissue histologically because diagnostic areas showing granulomas and/or vasculitis may be found only in focal areas. In any case in which extensive tissue necrosis is seen, the pathologist should order elastic tissue stains because the vasculitis in routine sections may be obscured by the inflammation. True vasculitis should be differentiated from the perivascular inflammatory response that is commonly seen in most inflammatory lesions. In vasculitis, the full thickness of the vascular wall

is infiltrated by inflammatory cells. The elastic tissue stains should demonstrate elastic fiber destruction, which may be found only focally in the vessel wall. As described previously, special stains for acid-fast bacteria and fungi should be ordered when granulomas are identified in nasal or sinus tissues.

Allergic Granulomatosis and Angiitis

Churg and Strauss[19] described a syndrome of asthma, fever, eosinophilia, and vasculitis in various organs. In a review of 32 patients with this syndrome, 22 (69 percent) presented with nasal obstruction, nasal polyps, or nasal crusting. The nasal tissue demonstrated eosinophilic infiltrates and extravascular necrotizing, palisading granulomas. Biopsy of subcutaneous nodules of the head and neck region showed granulomas and angiitis. Most patients respond to corticosteroid therapy.[20] The diagnosis of this entity is made by correlation of the clinical and pathologic findings.

Granulomas Secondary to Steroid Injection

A distinctive type of granulomatous lesion involving the nasal mucous membranes may be found after injection of prednisolone acetate (Hydeltra TBA), which is sometimes used to relieve nasal obstruction due to "vasomotor rhinitis," nasal edema, or nasal polyps. This steroid preparation is only slightly soluble and is long-acting. The granulomas are found when the patients are subsequently treated by polypectomy or curettage. These granulomas may be solitary or confluent, have a central zone of amorphous and/or birefringent crystalline material, and are surrounded by a layer of palisading histiocytes with foreign body type giant cells (Fig. 17-5). Wolff[21] first described this entity and postulated that the granulomas were of the foreign body type, induced by the injected material that is not absorbed. The pathologist should be familiar with this type of granuloma, which should be differentiated from other granulomatous lesions.

Lethal Midline Granuloma

The term *lethal midline granuloma* has been used clinically to describe certain necrotizing destructive lesions involving the nose, nasal cavity, and adjacent structures. Nasal collapse, septal perforation, and necrotizing lesions of the sinuses may be seen. This clinical entity may be produced by a spectrum of different diseases, including most commonly Wegener's granulomatosis, malignant lymphoma, and midline malignant reticulosis (a variant of lymphoma), as well as squamous cell carcinoma,

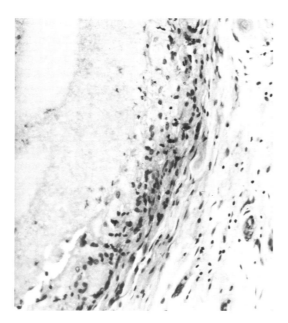

Fig. 17-5. Steroid granuloma. Amorphous, slightly granular material is surrounded by a rim of histiocytic and lymphoid cells.

tuberculosis, leprosy, syphilis, osteomyelitis, various bacterial and fungal infections, giant cell reparative granuloma, eosinophilic granuloma, diabetes, and pemphigus.[22] Thus, we believe the surgical pathologist should never use this term as a pathologic diagnosis since the clinical entity may be produced by many different diseases, each of which has a markedly different treatment and prognosis.

Nasal septal perforation may be associated with "snorting" cocaine. The pathogenesis is not clear, but this drug may produce vasoconstriction, leading to ischemic changes. Increasing numbers of patients with this complication have been seen in recent years as this drug has become more commonly used.

Atrophic Changes of the Mucosa

Atrophic changes may be seen in the surface epithelium and in the secretory glands associated with severe chronic infections. In Sjögren's syndrome, variable atrophic changes occur in major and minor salivary glands, as well as in the lacrimal gland. When this disease involves the nasal cavity, the patient may complain of a dry nose (due to decreased secretions). Histologically, a variable infiltrate of lymphocytes and plasma cells may be found within the secretory glands, associated with varying degrees of acinar atrophy. Hyperplastic changes may be seen within small ducts, leading to almost solid

plugging of these ducts with epithelial and possibly myoepithelial cells ("epimyoepithelial islands").

Hyperplastic Lesions of the Epithelium

Hyperplasia

Hyperplasia of the epithelium lining the nasal cavity and paranasal sinuses is commonly seen in association with inflammatory lesions. Variable degrees of basal cell hyperplasia may lead to thickening of the epithelium. The cells should retain their normal polarity, and maturation should be seen on the surface. Nuclei may be enlarged but should not demonstrate pleomorphism or hyperchromasia. As will be discussed later, these hyperplastic changes should be differentiated from papillomatosis.

Pseudoepitheliomatous Hyperplasia

Pseudoepitheliomatous hyperplasia of the lining epithelium may be seen after various types of injury. This change may be found in the squamous epithelium of the nasal vestibule, where elongated and thickened rete pegs extend into the underlying connective tissue. Pseudoepitheliomatous hyperplasia must be differentiated from invasive squamous cell carcinoma. In the former, rete pegs have a round configuration with smooth borders, and mature squamous cells without hyperchromasia or pleomorphism are identified. In carcinoma, invasive nests have an irregular configuration and vary considerably in size. The cells show varying degrees of anaplasia.

The cells lining the ducts leading to the secretory glands may show varying degrees of hyperplasia, occasionally filling the lumen. These structures usually have a smooth configuration with round borders, and the cells appear benign. These ducts may be mistaken for invasive carcinoma.

Squamous Metaplasia

Squamous metaplasia of the surface columnar respiratory epithelium is frequently seen in nasal polyps and with other chronic inflammatory lesions. Less commonly, squamous metaplasia may be found in the ducts and acini of the underlying secretory glands, especially after mucosal ulceration or necrosis (due to inflammation, trauma, ischemia, or radiation). This change, known as *necrotizing sialometaplasia*, represents a reparative phenomenon but may be confused histologically with carcinoma. This lesion was initially described in the palate[23] but can be seen in the nasal cavity and paranasal sinuses.[24] Histologically, the normal lobular architecture

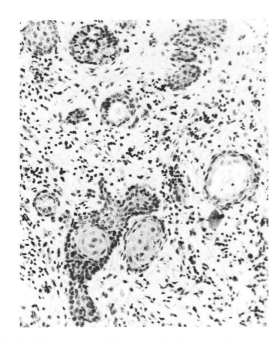

Fig. 17-6. Necrotizing sialometaplasia. An inflammatory reaction has involved this secretory gland. Some duct lumina are still maintained, but most of the lumina have been obliterated by the proliferating reparative cells, which are cytologically benign. Squamous metaplasia can be seen. This process may be misdiagnosed as a carcinoma.

of the secretory glands is preserved (Fig. 17-6). The hyperplastic and metaplastic squamous epithelium partially or completely fills the acini and ducts of the secretory glands, producing a picture of small nests and branching cords lying in an inflamed stroma. The epithelial cells may show reactive changes: nuclei may demonstrate the features of anaplasia or repair (relatively large but uniform nuclei with prominent nucleoli and smooth regular nuclear borders but without pleomorphism or hyperchromatism). In contrast, in invasive carcinoma a lobular configuration should not be maintained, the nests of cells vary more in size and shape, and the cells should show hyperchromatic and pleomorphic nuclei.

Epithelial Atypia (Dysplasia)

Epithelial atypia of the nasal and sinus mucosa may be found incidentally in tissues resected for inflammatory conditions, especially when the epithelium has undergone hyperplasia or squamous metaplasia. More significant dysplasia and carcinoma in situ (CIS) are sometimes identified in nasal papillomatosis or adjacent to invasive carcinoma. The development of abnormal squamous epithelium in the nasal respiratory mucosa has been demonstrated in nickel workers.[25] The affected epithelium begins with the loss of ciliated cells, develops into a metaplastic squamous epithelium, and proliferates in the deep layers with budding rete pegs. Further progression results in mild and moderate dysplasia, with increased mitotic activity and nuclear enlargement, hyperchromasia, and irregularity, especially in the deep layers. In severe dysplasia and CIS, abnormal cells occupy most of the epithelium.[25] These sequential and progressive changes correlate with the amount and duration of nickel exposure.

Benign Epithelial Neoplasms

Squamous Papillomas

Squamous papillomas may arise in the squamous epithelium of the nasal vestibule. These lesions show a marked proliferation of the squamous epithelium, producing an exophytic verrucous growth, with varying degrees of hyperkeratosis. The cells have a benign appearance, without hyperchromatism or pleomorphism. Squamous papillomas may represent hyperplastic rather than neoplastic lesions.

Papillomatosis

Papillomatosis is an uncommon lesion that arises in the respiratory-type epithelium lining the nasal cavity and paranasal sinuses. Many diagnostic terms have been used for this entity, including papilloma, epithelial papilloma, inverted papilloma, squamous papilloma, Schneiderian papilloma, transitional cell papilloma, cylindrical cell papilloma, papillary hypertrophy, and hypertrophic papillary sinusitis. Most investigators now agree that this lesion is a true benign neoplasm, although some authors have suggested that it is a hyperplastic process secondary to inflammation.

Syrjanen et al.[26] recently detected human papillomavirus (HPV) capsid antigen in 50 percent (7 of 14) of these papillomas. By an autoradiographic in situ hybridization method, HPV DNA was demonstrated in the nuclei of 70 percent of papillomas, including two with squamous carcinoma. The specific types of HPV DNA included: type 11 in five papillomas, type 16 in two, and mixed types (11 and 16) in three. Further study will be needed to elucidate the mechanism of transmission and the role of HPV in the development of papillomatosis.

Inflammatory nasal polyps occur 25 to 50 times more frequently than papillomatosis.[27] This lesion comprises 0.5 to 5 percent of all nasal tumors.[27] Papillomatosis is associated with a variety of nonspecific symptoms including nasal stuffiness and fullness, difficulty in breathing through the affected side, rhinorrhea, and epistaxis.[28]

On physical examination, one or more polypoid masses, often having the appearance of ordinary nasal polyps, can be seen projecting into the involved cavity. Occasionally the mucosa shows a diffuse thickening. Some lesions may have an exophytic appearance, with a granular or papillary surface.

Papillomatosis may produce one or more polypoid masses, which are found most often on the lateral nasal walls and less commonly on the septum.[27] In about half the cases, the disease is confined to one nasal cavity; in the other half, a nasal cavity and one or more paranasal sinuses are involved (most commonly the maxillary sinus). In about 10 percent of cases, both nasal cavities are affected.[28]

Histologically, papillomatosis shows a variable proliferation of basal cells, leading to a thickened epithelium. In some areas, ciliated cells may still be seen on the surface; in other foci, they are replaced by the proliferating cells, producing a picture resembling transitional epithelium (urothelium). Variable degrees of squamous metaplasia may be found, but little or no surface keratinization usually is seen. In areas where squamous maturation is present, koilocytosis may be noted in the superficial layers. These cells are characterized by having abundant clear cytoplasm, distinct cell borders, and wrinkled, sometimes binucleated, nuclei. In about 5 percent of papillomas, mucin droplets or microcysts may be identified within the proliferating epithelium. In the cylindrical cell or oncocytic variant of papilloma, the epithelium is thickened and composed of cuboidal to columnar cells

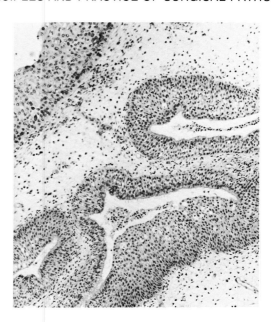

Fig. 17-8. Papillomatosis. An inverted pattern is seen on the right. The cells have uniform, bland-appearing nuclei. On the surface (upper left) a zone of slight epithelial atypia is found.

with abundant eosinophilic cytoplasm. Goblet cells are increased. Numerous microcysts and mucin droplets usually are present.[29] The microcystic pattern may be confused with rhinosporidiosis or adenocarcinoma. The mitotic activity in papillomas is generally low, with 60 percent of cases having fewer than 2 mitoses per 10 highpower fields and only 15 percent having more than 10 per 10 high-power fields.[30]

The proliferating epithelium may produce a papillary or exophytic growth pattern (Fig. 17-7), or an "inverted" pattern may be seen, with large well-formed masses of papillomatous epithelium apparently embedded in the underlying stroma (Fig. 17-8). In some cases the inverted pattern is produced because the tissue has been tangentially cut. In other cases abnormal cells apparently have extended into the ducts leading to the underlying secretory glands. This is proved by the occasional finding of abrupt transition points between the papillomatous epithelium and normal ductal cells deep in the tissue. As a result, the abnormal epithelium may be found close to bone. This finding should not be confused with invasive carcinoma. When papillomatosis involves secretory ducts, the duct usually maintains a smooth outer surface and a round configuration even though its entire lumen has been filled by the proliferating cells.

Papillomas involving the nasal septum, although having a tendency to be exophytic and occurring in younger patients than inverted papillomas, are similar to inverted papillomas in their histologic features and clinical behavior.[31]

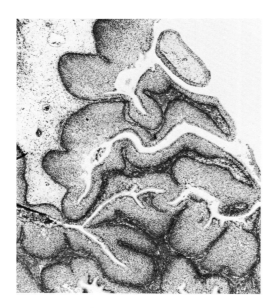

Fig. 17-7. Papillomatosis. The mucosal lining cells have proliferated, leading to marked thickening of the mucosa. Papillary projections and an inverted pattern are seen.

The abnormal epithelium of papillomatosis not only extends into secretory ducts but also probably has the ability to spread laterally into adjacent nasal mucosa and into the paranasal sinuses, gradually replacing the normal respiratory epithelium. The mechanism is probably similar to the manner in which adenomatous epithelium in the colon gradually extends into and replaces adjacent normal mucosal epithelium, producing a lesion that not only projects into the lumen but also grows laterally. In nasal papillomatosis, this lateral extension probably explains the high rate of local recurrence after curettage of the clinically evident lesion. In these cases, the abnormal epithelium has spread microscopically beyond where it can be recognized grossly. We have seen several cases in which recurrences were identified in the nasopharynx, the eustachian tube, or the middle ear, supporting the concept of lateral spread. An alternative explanation would be that papillomatosis can develop in a multicentric manner. This would appear less likely since most recurrences are found near the original lesion and numerous separate primary foci would be required in some cases.

Papillomatosis recurs clinically in about 50 percent of patients.[27,28,32,33] The recurrence rate increases with the duration of follow-up. Most recurrences are seen within the first 5 years after diagnosis, but some lesions recur 10 or more years later.[28,32] Mitotic activity in the original papilloma does not appear to correlate with recurrence, although it often increases in recurrent lesions.[30] In one study, features that were associated with an increased recurrence rate included nuclear atypia, epithelial mucus droplets, and sinus involvement.[28] The mode of therapy also influences the recurrence rate. Limited excisions, such as polypectomy, partial turbinectomy, and Caldwell-Luc curettage, have recurrence rates of 70 to 80 percent, as compared with 6 percent following lateral rhinotomy with maxillectomy and/or ethmoidectomy.[33] In a review of the literature,[34] 64 percent of papillomas recurred following limited excisions and only 11 percent following more complete resections.

In the majority of cases, the cells in papillomatosis show little or no dysplasia. However, changes ranging from atypia to frankly invasive carcinoma may be seen. In one series, 6 percent (4 of 61) of papillomas demonstrated dysplasia, and 3 percent (2/61) demonstrated CIS.[29] The reported frequency of coexisting invasive carcinoma varies from 3 percent,[32,34] to 5 percent,[35] 10 percent,[33] and 15 percent.[30] Invasive carcinoma reportedly develops following excision of papillomas in 3 to 6 percent of patients.[30,34,35] In a review of the literature, the frequency of concurrent and subsequent invasive carcinoma was 8 and 4 percent, respectively.[35] Thus, approximately 10 to 15 percent of papillomas are associated with malignant transformation. The majority of invasive carci-

nomas, concurrent or subsequent, are unilateral and poorly differentiated, usually squamous cell carcinomas. A few are mucoepidermoid carcinomas or resemble undifferentiated nasopharyngeal carcinomas.[29,30] Rarely, squamous cell carcinoma is bilateral and multifocal.[36]

Curettage specimens from the nasal cavity and paranasal sinuses should be submitted in toto for histologic examination, even though the clinical diagnosis is nasal polyps or sinusitis. In some of these cases, completely unsuspected findings such as papillomatosis may be identified. If papillomatosis is discovered histologically and only representative sections have been taken, the remaining tissue certainly should be studied. We have seen cases in which the original sections showed only papillomatosis, but when all the tissue was submitted, invasive carcinoma was also identified (Fig. 17-9).

One of the most difficult problems confronting the pathologist when evaluating specimens from this area is the histologic differentiation between hyperplastic mucosa and papillomatosis. Many nasal polyps and other inflammatory lesions will show focal areas of epithelial hyperplasia. One cannot always precisely draw the line between papillomatosis and hyperplasia. In some cases the proliferative changes can only be described and the possibility of papillomatosis suggested. In general, to diagnose papillomatosis, the lining epithelium should have a thickness of more than 8 to 10 nuclei, and the changes should be seen over a broad surface. The character of the stroma

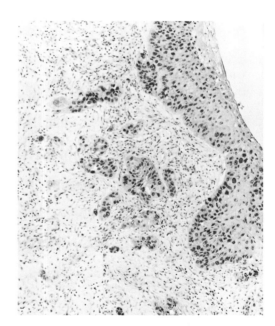

Fig. 17-9. Papillomatosis with invasive carcinoma. Same case as Fig. 17-8. A focus of invasive carcinoma, composed of irregular nests of pleomorphic cells, is seen. The surface epithelium shows moderate to marked atypia.

does not help, because in papillomatosis the supporting connective tissue may show edema and inflammatory changes similar to those found in inflammatory polyps.

The pathologist must differentiate between papillomatosis with atypia and CIS. We usually diagnose carcinoma in situ only when dysplastic cells have involved the full thickness of the epithelium. The pathologist must also differentiate tangentially cut papillomatosis from invasive carcinoma. In general, tangentially cut papillomatosis that is confined to surface or ductal epithelium forms large cellular nests with round, smooth borders. In contrast, invasive carcinoma usually consists of smaller nests and cords with irregular borders. The degree of cellular anaplasia may be misleading because some tangentially cut areas of papillomatosis may have epithelium with severe dysplasia or CIS. Thus, the configuration of the nests of cells more than cellular details helps in differentiating papillomatosis from invasive carcinoma.

Salivary Gland Tumors

Benign salivary gland tumors are seen infrequently in the nasal cavity and only rarely in the paranasal sinuses. These neoplasms may be divided into benign mixed tumors (pleomorphic adenomas) and myoepitheliomas. Oncocytomas are rarely found.

Benign Mixed Tumors

When occurring in the nasal cavity, most benign mixed tumors (pleomorphic adenomas) originate in the bony or cartilaginous nasal septum, but they may arise from the lateral nasal wall, usually involving a turbinate.[37] These neoplasms grow by expansion and may extend into an adjacent paranasal sinus. Physical examination usually shows a polypoid, exophytic, dome-shaped mass, usually covered by an intact mucosa. Histologically, these neoplasms exhibit all the features seen in mixed tumors of the major salivary glands. However, in the nasal cavity these lesions tend to be highly cellular, with the closely packed oval epithelial cells arranged in nests and sheets. Ductal structures are observed infrequently. Epithelial elements usually predominate over the stromal component, which may be inconspicuous. In one study of 40 cases of intranasal mixed tumors,[37] local recurrence was found in three patients (7.5 percent).

Myoepithelioma

A rare variant of benign mixed tumor, myoepithelioma, is composed of uniform, spindle-shaped cells that do not show pleomorphism or mitotic activity. Because of their histologic features, myoepitheliomas are often diagnosed as some type of benign nonepithelial tumor, such as neurilemoma, leiomyoma, fibroma, or myxoma.

On ultrastructural study, myoepitheliomas have cells that are filled with microfilaments (6 to 8 μm thick), are joined by desmosomes, and are surrounded focally by a basal lamina.[38] In cellular benign mixed tumors and in myoepitheliomas, the reticulin stain should show nests of cells devoid of reticulin fibers. In contrast, nonepithelial tumors should have a heavy reticulin fiber pattern throughout the entire lesion. Myoepithelial cells usually are shown to contain S-100 protein in immunoperoxidase studies.

Malignant Tumors

Malignant tumors arising in the nasal cavity, paranasal sinuses, and nasopharynx are uncommon lesions. Their exact incidence is difficult to determine. Lewis and Castro[39] have stated that "cancer of the nasal cavity and paranasal sinuses comprises about 2 percent of cancer in the human body." According to American Cancer Society statistics, 985,000 new cases of cancer were projected in the United States for 1988. Of these, 168,300 tumors would arise in the respiratory tract, including 152,000 in the lung, 12,200 in the larynx, and 4,100 in "other sites" (mainly the nasal cavity, paranasal sinuses, and nasopharynx).[40] Therefore, malignant tumors arising in the upper respiratory tract would at most comprise 2.4 percent of all respiratory tract cancers and 0.41 percent of all malignant neoplasms.

The incidence of malignant neoplasms arising in the upper respiratory passages in relation to other head and neck malignancies is difficult to determine because most studies in the literature investigate tumors of a particular site. However, we have found one study[41] that reported 792 malignant tumors of the head and neck (exclusive of skin) with the following sites of origin: larynx 281; pharynx 229; major salivary glands 81; tongue 58; paranasal sinuses 44; palate 28; nasopharynx 28; buccal mucosa 16; nasal cavity 10; ear 8; and unknown 9. Thus, within the upper respiratory passages malignant neoplasms in this study occurred most frequently in the paranasal sinuses, followed by the nasopharynx and the nasal cavity.

Several studies[39,42,43] have reported on the distribution of malignant neoplasms involving the nasal cavity and paranasal sinuses. These indicate that the maxillary sinuses are affected most frequently. In Table 17-1 the sites involved by malignant tumors, as found in these studies, are listed.

These reports also indicate the squamous cell (epidermoid) carcinoma is the most common malignant tumor found in the nasal cavity and paranasal sinuses. The types of malignant neoplasms reported in these studies are listed in Table 17-2. To investigate the relationship between different histologic types of carcinoma and site

TABLE 17-1. Sites Involved by Malignant Tumors of the Nasal Cavity and Paranasal Sinuses

	Jackson et al.[42]	Lewis and Castro[39]	Hopkin et al.[43]
Maxillary sinus	77 (67%)	451 (58%)	295 (53%)[b]
Nasal cavity	19 (16%)	237 (31%)	147 (26%)
Ethmoid sinus	15 (13%)	75 (10%)	107 (19%)
Frontal sinus	3 (3%)	6 (0.6%)	7 (1.2%)
Sphenoid sinus	1 (1%)	3 (0.4%)	5 (0.9%)
Total	115	772[a]	561

[a] Includes 538 primary tumors (69%) and 234 secondary neoplasms (31%).

[b] Includes 77 patients (14%) who also had involvement of ethmoid sinus.

TABLE 17-2. Types of Malignant Tumors Reported in the Nasal Cavity and Paranasal Sinuses

	Jackson et al.[42]	Lewis and Castro[39]	Hopkin et al.[43]
Squamous cell (epidermoid) carcinoma	61 (53%)	496 (64%)	201 (36%)
Undifferentiated carcinoma	11 (10%)		92 (17%)
Adenoid cystic carcinoma	8 (7%)		30 (5%)
Adenocarcinoma	7 (6%)	129 (17%)	40 (7%)
Papillary adenocarcinoma	2 (2%)		
Transitional cell carcinoma	2 (2%)		60 (11%)
Malignant melanoma	7 (6%)	34 (4%)	39 (7%)
Olfactory neuroblastoma	5 (4%)		3 (1%)
Neuroblastoma	1 (1%)		
Fibrosarcoma	3 (3%)		11 (2%)
Rhabdomyosarcoma			
Angiosarcoma	1 (1%)		
Chondrosarcoma	1 (1%)		
Malignant lymphoma	3 (3%)	40 (5%)	35 (6%)
Plasmacytoma	2 (2%)	13 (2%)	8 (1%)
Carcinosarcoma	1 (1%)		
Other sarcomas		23 (3%)	16 (3%)
Unclassified tumors			
Other		37 (5%)	25 (5%)
Total	115	772	561

of origin within the upper respiratory passages, we examined the files of the Laboratory of Surgical Pathology of the Columbia Presbyterian Medical Center. During the 20 years between 1959 and 1978 a total of 230,000 cases were seen in this laboratory (not including obstetric, gynecologic, pediatric, and neuropathologic specimens, which are studied in other laboratories). As can be seen in Table 17-3, 350 cases of carcinoma involving the upper respiratory tract were studied during this period. Carcinomas arose most frequently in the nasopharynx, followed by the maxillary sinus. Squamous cell carcinoma was the most frequent diagnosis, followed by undifferentiated carcinoma. We should note that this table does not indicate the number of new cases, but only how often a diagnosis was made in a particular site. Some of these lesions represented recurrences of tumor in a patient who had a previously diagnosed carcinoma.

Clinically, malignant tumors involving the upper respiratory tract produce nonspecific symptoms similar to those caused by benign neoplasms and by inflammatory lesions. Symptoms include nasal obstruction, epistaxis, nasal discharge, and pain. Tumors of the maxillary sinus may produce a mass or swelling that projects into the cheek, palate, or orbital cavity. The patient may be first seen by a dentist because of loosening of teeth. Nasopharyngeal neoplasms may also cause middle ear symptoms secondary to eustachian tube obstruction, or they may produce cranial nerve paralysis or enlarged cervical lymph nodes when the tumor has spread beyond the primary site.

On physical examination, a mass may be seen projecting into the involved cavity. These tumors have a variable appearance including polypoid, fungating, or ulcerating. Radiologic studies may show sinus opacification, a mass, and/or bone destruction. In some cases a neoplasm is not suspected and is only discovered when curettage specimens are studied histologically.

Malignant neoplasms arising in the upper respiratory tract may readily spread by direct extension into adjacent

TABLE 17-3. Diagnoses of Carcinoma of the Upper Respiratory Tract, 1959–1978

Diagnosis	Total	Site					
		Nasal Cavity	Maxillary Sinus	Ethmoid Sinus	Sphenoid Sinus	Frontal Sinus	Nasopharynx
Squamous cell carcinoma	219	33[a]	50	8	8	6	114
Undifferentiated carcinoma	51	10	8	1	2	2	28
Adenoid cystic carcinoma	33	6	13	2	3		9
Mucoepidermoid carcinoma	17	3	11				3
Malignant mixed tumor	3	1	1				1
Papillary adenocarcinoma	6	2	2		1		1
Carcinoma, other or unspecified	21	6	9	3	1	–	2
Total	350	61	94	14	15	8	158

[a] Including six in the nasal vestibule.

606

structures since the bony wall in many areas is relatively thin. Malignant tumors of the nasal cavity may extend into adjacent sinuses. Lesions arising in the frontal, ethmoid, and sphenoid sinuses may grow inferiorly into the nasal cavity, superiorly into the adjacent cranial cavity, and, if sufficiently anterior, into the orbital cavity. Neoplasms of the maxillary sinus may extend medially into the nasal cavity, laterally into the soft tissues of the cheek, inferiorly into the palate and oral cavity, posteriorly into the nasopharynx, or superiorly into the orbital cavity or ethmoid region. Tumors of the nasopharynx may grow into the retropharyngeal space and spread from there.

Carcinoma of the Nasal Cavity and Paranasal Sinuses

As described in the preceding section, carcinomas involving the nasal cavity and paranasal sinuses most commonly arise in the maxillary sinus, followed by the nasal cavity. The ethmoid, frontal, and sphenoid sinuses are less frequently affected.

Little is known about the pathogenesis of carcinomas of the nasal cavity and paranasal sinuses. Lewis and Castro[39] reported that 23 percent of their patients had previous sinus surgery and another 24 percent had prior nasal polypectomy. These findings suggest the possibility that previous inflammatory lesions may predispose to the development of carcinoma. The number of patients in this series with previous nasal and sinus surgery certainly exceeds the number of individuals in the general population who have had similar operations. Long-term smoking has been implicated in one study.[44] An increased incidence of adenocarcinoma of the nasal cavity and paranasal sinus has been found in wood and furniture workers.[45,46] Nickel workers appear to have an increased incidence of nasal carcinoma, as do leather workers.[45,46] Maxillary sinus carcinomas, both squamous and glandular types, have been observed many years after Thorotrast instillation.[47]

Squamous Cell Carcinoma

As indicated previously, squamous cell carcinoma is by far the most common malignant tumor to be found in this area. Histologically, these tumors may be divided into keratinizing and nonkeratinizing variants.[48] These lesions show a broad range of differentiation.

In the *invasive keratinizing squamous cell carcinomas,* the tumor cells exhibit keratinization, intercellular bridges, and "pearls." Irregular nests and cords of cells are seen. Tumor cells have enlarged, hyperchromatic, pleomorphic nuclei. As described previously, invasive squamous cell carcinomas may be confused histologi-

cally with such benign lesions as pseudoepitheliomatous hyperplasia, necrotizing sialometaplasia, and papillomatosis. The configuration of the nests and the character of the cells should aid in differentiating squamous cell carcinoma from these other lesions.

A *"nonkeratinizing" type of squamous cell carcinoma* occurs in the upper respiratory passages. These tumors tend to form solid nests of variable size (Fig. 17-10). These masses may have relatively smooth borders. Individual tumor cells usually exhibit uniform, large, round or oval nuclei with prominent nucleoli. The cytoplasm varies from pale acidophilic to amphophilic to vacuolated. The cells may have distinct borders. Occasionally, individual cell keratinization may be identified, supporting the concept that these tumors actually are variants of squamous cell carcinoma. The terminology used for these tumors may produce confusion. These lesions have been classified as undifferentiated carcinoma, "transitional cell" carcinoma, or "Schneiderian" carcinoma. The transitional cell variant is characterized by peripheral nuclear palisading and a smooth configuration of the invasive nests, with surrounding basement membrane-like material. Focal squamous differentiation is sometimes present.[49] Patients with this type of tumor appear to have a slightly better prognosis than those with the squamous type. A highly anaplastic and aggressive carcinoma involving the nasal and sinus cavity has been re-

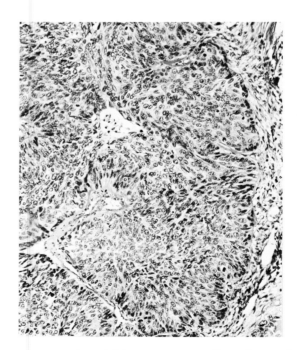

Fig. 17-10. Nonkeratinizing squamous cell carcinoma. Large nests of tumor are composed of spindle-shaped cells. As compared with papillomatosis (inverted papilloma), these nests have an irregular and confluent pattern.

ported.[50,51] At diagnosis, the majority of patients have bony, cranial, or orbital involvement. The tumor cells appear undifferentiated and without keratinization. Medium-sized polygonal cells form irregular nests and sheets and reveal prominent nucleoli and high mitotic activity (higher than 10 per 10 high-power fields). Scattered isolated cell necrosis is a prominent feature. One third of patients developed metastases in cervical lymph nodes. The survival rate at 3 years is about 30 percent.[50] Rarely, poorly differentiated carcinomas may have the appearance of spindle cell sarcoma[52] or endodermal sinus tumor.[53]

The differential diagnosis includes malignant melanoma, olfactory neuroblastoma, and certain adenocarcinomas, all of which may grow in solid nests of cells. Special stains for melanin granules should help in identifying a melanoma. Mucin stains may show secretions, indicative of an adenocarcinoma. Rosettes may be seen, helping to identify a neuroblastoma. Furthermore, this type of carcinoma may be confused with papillomatosis (Figs. 17-7 and 17-8), especially when papillomatosis lesions have been tangentially cut, show an inverted pattern, involve a secretory duct, or demonstrate foci of atypia. As compared with carcinoma, the nests of cells in papillomatosis are larger and more uniform, have smoother borders, and demonstrate a blander cell population. The differential diagnosis, however, may produce considerable difficulty in a small biopsy specimen. Occasionally, a malignant lymphoma may be part of the differential diagnosis. With the reticulin stain, carcinomas should show solid nests of cells devoid of reticulin fibers, whereas lymphomas have a meshwork of fine and coarse fibers. Immunohistochemical studies for leukocyte common antigen, epithelial membrane antigen, and keratin should differentiate between a lymphoma and a carcinoma.

Verrucous squamous cell carcinoma, which is more commonly seen in the oral cavity, is occasionally found in the nasal cavity and paranasal sinuses.[48]

Salivary-Gland-Type Carcinomas

Adenoid Cystic (Cylindromatous) Carcinoma. Adenoid cystic carcinoma (ACC) is the most common type of adenocarcinoma found in the upper respiratory passages[42,54] (Table 17-3). Furthermore, in one study,[55] the nasal and paranasal sinus area was the most common site among many different sites to be involved by this tumor. When arising in the upper respiratory tract, ACC occurs most frequently in the maxillary sinus.[54]

Histologically, these tumors are similar to ACC that arises in the major salivary glands. Small hyperchromatic cells are arranged in tubular, cribriform, or solid patterns.[55] The latter two patterns predominate in ACC aris-

ing in the upper respiratory tract.[55] In most cases the diagnosis can be made without difficulty, based on the distinctive cribriform pattern exhibited by this tumor. However, the correct diagnosis may be difficult to establish in a small biopsy specimen. Some ACCs, especially in this area, consist mainly of solid nests of cells and may be misinterpreted as undifferentiated carcinomas on biopsy. Other ACCs are composed predominantly of small tubular structures and may be confused with a benign mixed tumor. Only when the larger resection specimen is studied may ACC be recognized.

ACC widely infiltrates bone and involves nerves, so that the lesion has usually spread much beyond what is suspected clinically and radiologically. When studying a maxillectomy or other large resection specimen, the pathologist should examine histologically the lines of resection. ACC may be cured if no tumor is found on the surgical margins.[55] However, these neoplasms are almost always identified on the lines of resection in specimens resected from this area.

Mucoepidermoid Carcinoma. Overall, mucoepidermoid carcinoma (MECa) is the most common malignant tumor to develop in the major and minor salivary glands. MECa is found most often in the parotid but may arise in minor salivary glands. In a series of 60 MECas,[56] 8 (13 percent) involved the upper respiratory passages (7 maxilla, 1 nasal cavity).

Histologically, these neoplasms have a distinctive pattern.[56] In better differentiated tumors, mucous, epidermoid, and intermediate cells are found in cystic or glandular structures. Less well differentiated lesions grow in solid nests with a predominance of epidermoid cells. The histologic features usually are sufficiently distinctive to allow the correct diagnosis to be made. However, in some cases small biopsy specimens may only show solid nests of cells, and the lesion may be diagnosed as epidermoid or undifferentiated carcinoma. Only when the larger resection specimen is studied may glandular areas diagnostic of MECa be seen. In our experience some neoplasms of the paranasal sinuses, especially the maxillary sinus, that have been diagnosed as squamous cell or epidermoid carcinomas actually are poorly differentiated mucoepidermoid carcinomas. A tumor that has been interpreted as an "epidermoid" carcinoma arising in the nasal cavity or paranasal sinuses probably should be studied with mucin stains, because some of these neoplasms will show mucin production. However, the overall prognosis does not differ greatly between poorly differentiated epidermoid carcinoma, poorly differentiated mucoepidermoid carcinoma, and undifferentiated carcinoma. Some authors[57] have described tumors designated as "adenosquamous" carcinoma involving the nasal, oral, and laryngeal cavities. These neoplasms probably are variants of mucoepidermoid carcinoma and appear to have the same prognosis as poorly differentiated MECa.

Malignant Mixed Tumors. Malignant mixed tumors (MMT) rarely are found in the upper respiratory passages. In a series of 47 MMTs, 1 involved this area. These lesions have been extensively discussed by LiVolsi and Perzin.[58]

Acinic Cell Carcinoma. Rarely, acinic cell carcinomas have been reported in the nasal cavity and paranasal sinuses.[59,60] Tumor cell cytoplasm may appear eosinophilic, granular, or clear. While nuclei are uniform, nucleoli may be conspicuous. In the case reported by Ordonez and Batsakis,[60] the authors considered the differential diagnosis of rhabdomyoma, chordoma, paraganglioma, melanoma with balloon cells, alveolar soft part sarcoma and ganglioneuroma, before the diagnosis of acinic cell carcinoma was confirmed by immunoperoxidase stain (positive for amylase) and electron microscopy (presence of zymogen granules).

Other Adenocarcinomas

When salivary gland type tumors have been separated, a small group of other adenocarcinomas remain. Rafla,[54] in reporting on 37 mucous gland neoplasms arising in the upper respiratory passages, found the following distribution: adenoid cystic carcinoma, 16; adenocarcinoma 14; mucoepidermoid carcinoma 2; malignant mixed tumor, 2; anaplastic adenocarcinoma 2; and pleomorphic adenoma 1.

Batsakis et al.[61] have divided the other adenocarcinomas into three groups: papillary, sessile, and alveolar-mucoid. The *papillary adenocarcinoma* produces multiple complex papillary fronds lined by cells showing pleomorphism and frequent mitoses. Areas of microinvasion may be identified at the base of the papillae. This tumor must be differentiated from papillomatosis and the surface papillary hyperplasia that may be associated with inflammatory lesions. In general, the papillary fronds seen in papillary adenocarcinoma are much thinner than those found in these other conditions. In addition, the cells show much greater pleomorphism and mitotic activity. This type of adenocarcinoma appears to have a better prognosis than the other variants and has an indolent clinical course with multiple local recurrences. The second type of adenocarcinoma, termed *sessile,* grows over a broad surface and produces glandular structures that are histologically similar to those seen in colonic carcinomas (Fig. 17-11). The columnar cells have no cilia and show variable stratification. Mucin and goblet cells usually can be identified. The *alveolar-mucoid* variant resembles the "colloid" or mucinous adenocarcinomas that may be seen in the breast and in the gastrointestinal

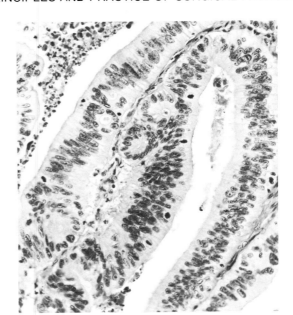

Fig. 17-11. Adenocarcinoma. This nasal cavity tumor is composed of glandular structures lined by cells with spindle-shaped "picket fence" nuclei, mimicking a colonic carcinoma.

tract. Goblet cells, signet-ring cells, and pools of extracellular mucin may be found.[62]

Heffner et al.[63] have divided the other adenocarcinomas into low- and high-grade tumors based on growth patterns, nuclear features, and mitotic activity. This clas-

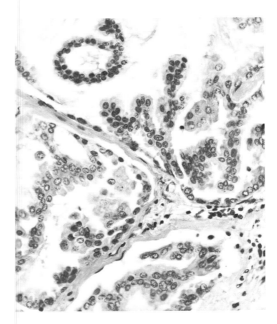

Fig. 17-12. Low-grade adenocarcinoma. This nasal cavity tumor produces glandular and papillary structures lined by cells with uniform nuclei.

sification correlates with prognosis. The following outcomes were observed in their series: in the low-grade group (Fig. 17-12), 78 percent had no evidence of disease, 13 percent were alive with disease, and 9 percent died of disease. In the high-grade group 7 percent had no evidence of disease, 15 percent were alive with disease, and 78 percent had died of disease, including 29 percent with distant metastases. The intestinal variant was classified as high-grade, because most patients with this type died of disease within 3 years of diagnosis. This experience is also shared by other observers.[64] However, in more recent studies the behavior of this type of tumor was found to be most closely related to the extent of disease.[65,66] Based on the 213 cases reported in the literature, 60 percent of patients died of disease (80 percent of these died in 3 years), 53 percent had local recurrences, 8 percent had cervical lymph node metastases, and 13 percent had distant metastases.[66] The intestinal or colonic variant of adenocarcinoma may have the appearance of a colonic adenoma with minimal nuclear atypia, and Paneth cells and enterochromaffin cells may be present. In small biopsies evidence of stromal invasion may be absent. The presence of mucus pools in the stroma should lead to a careful survey of the entire specimen to exclude the possibility of malignancy. In all cases, the patient should be examined for evidence of tumor in these other sites before the neoplasm is accepted as a primary lesion of the upper respiratory passages.

Prognosis of Carcinoma of Nasal Cavity and Paranasal Sinuses

Most carcinomas arising in the nasal cavity and paranasal sinus grow by direct extension into adjacent structures. At the time of diagnosis, most of these tumors have shown extensive local infiltration. Less than 15 to 20 percent of these neoplasms, however, metastasize to cervical lymph nodes.[39] Lymphatics draining the anterior nasal cavity lead to submandibular nodes. From the entire nasal cavity, lymphatics drain to retropharyngeal and anterior jugular nodes. Metastases from the maxillary antrum may be seen in submandibular and other anterior cervical nodes. After surgery, radiotherapy, or both, the 5-year survival rate for nasal carcinoma ranges from 38 to 63 percent and for maxillary carcinoma from 13 to 35 percent.[43,44]

Carcinoma of the Nasopharynx

Nasopharyngeal carcinoma (NPC) differs from carcinomas arising in the nasal cavity and paranasal sinuses in several important respects: clinical, etiologic, and histologic. Since a carcinoma originating in the nasopharynx may remain silent in its primary site, many patients seek medical aid when the disease has spread beyond the nasopharynx. The single most common complaint (32 to 44 percent of cases) is a mass in the neck, which is caused by metastatic disease in a lymph node.[67,68] Nasal symptoms (obstruction, discharge, congestion, epistaxis) are found in 20 to 30 percent of the patients. Middle ear complaints, produced by eustachian tube obstruction, are seen in an equal percentage of patients. Cranial nerve involvement is initially identified in 10 to 15 percent of patients but increases in incidence as the disease progresses. The most frequently affected cranial nerves are III, V, VI, IX, and X.[67,68]

NPC arises most frequently in the superior wall or vault, followed by the pharyngeal recess in the lateral wall. When the nasopharyngoscope is used to visualize this area, tumors may have the following appearance: (1) bulging (elevated, full), (2) infiltrative, (3) exophytic and lobulated, and (4) ulcerative. In some cases, no lesion is seen with certainty, and the carcinoma is only identified when random blind biopsy specimens taken in the nasopharynx are studied histologically.

From its primary site, the tumor may spread directly to the base of the skull, the pterygoid fossa, the paranasal sinuses, or oropharynx. Metastatic disease may be found in cervical lymph nodes, lungs, skeleton, and viscera.

The incidence of NPC varies greatly in differents parts of the world. The highest rates (18 per 100,000 population) are found among southern Chinese and Southeast Asians. For those Chinese who have emigrated to Hawaii and California, the rates (7.8 per 100,000 population) have remained higher than for whites (1 to 2 per 100,000 males and 0.4 per 100,000 females).[69,70] Various risk factors associated with NPC have been reviewed by Henderson et al.[71] and by Lin et al.[72] These include HLA-A_2 with less than two antigens at the B locus, and elevated titers against Epstein-Barr virus (EBV) antigens, including anti-viral capsid antigen (IgA) and anti-early antigen (IgG). Other evidence has implicated environmental factors, especially exposure to wood smoke, fumes, and chemicals, smoking more than 30 cigarettes per day, use of herb drugs, and poor ventilation at the work place.[71,72]

Histologically, the great majority of malignant tumors that arise in the nasopharynx are poorly differentiated squamous cell carcinomas or undifferentiated carcinomas; 10 percent are unclassified, 2 percent adenocarcinoma, and 1 percent sarcoma.[73] According to the World Health Organization (WHO) histologic typing system,[74] NPCs are classified into: type 1, keratinizing squamous cell carcinoma; type 2, nonkeratinizing carcinoma (Fig. 17-13); and type 3, undifferentiated carcinoma (Fig. 17-14), including the lymphoepithelioma, anaplastic, clear cell, and spindle cell variants.[74] Acantholysis may occur rarely in squamous cell carcinomas, producing a pseudoglandular pattern.[75]

PRINCIPLES AND PRACTICE OF SURGICAL PATHOLOGY

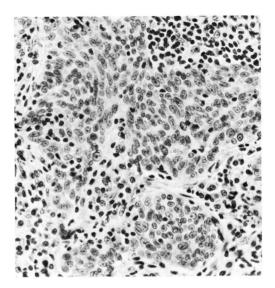

Fig. 17-13. Nasopharyngeal carcinoma (nonkeratinizing type). Here tumor cells focally assume a spindle-shaped configuration.

Based on the WHO classification of NPC, a correlation exists between the histologic type and the presence of antibodies against Epstein-Barr viral capsid antigens and early antigens. These antibodies are detected in 85 percent of North American patients with nonkeratinizing or undifferentiated carcinoma. In contrast, anti-viral capsid antigen is found in 16 percent and anti-early antigen in 35 percent of those having the keratinizing type of tumor.[68]

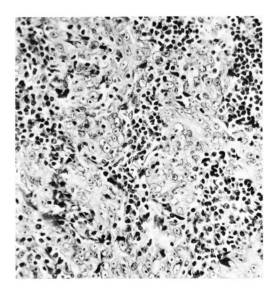

Fig. 17-14. Nasopharyngeal carcinoma (undifferentiated type). Nests of tumor cells merge with the normally present lymphoid tissue. Tumor cells have large clear nuclei with prominent nucleoli.

The WHO classification also correlates well with survival. Among patients with keratinizing carcinomas, the survival rates are 30 percent at 3 years and less than 20 percent at 5 years. Of those having nonkeratinizing or undifferentiated carcinomas, 70 percent survived 3 years and 59 percent 5 years.[68] These survival rates may be related to radiotherapy response; the keratinizing carcinomas respond less well to radiation.

Electron microscopic studies of NPC have shown a varying number of tonofibrils, keratin-like structures, and desmosomal junctions, suggestive of squamous differentiation.[76,77] Some anaplastic carcinomas are composed of highly undifferentiated primitive cells or have cells with a well developed vacuolar system resembling columnar cells.[76] In a study of 10 undifferentiated carcinomas, tonofilaments could not be identified in two neoplasms; the only evidence of epithelial differentiation was the presence of cell junctions.[77] Therefore some poorly differentiated NPC may arise from squamous epithelium and others from respiratory mucosa.[76] Since the nasopharynx is originally lined by ciliated columnar epithelium that later may normally undergo squamous metaplasia, perhaps most poorly differentiated or undifferentiated NPCs might be considered as tumors that arise in the lining epithelium and show either no differentiation, varying degrees of epidermoid differentiation, or less commonly, differentiation toward a mucin-producing cell.[76]

The pathologist will usually receive small biopsy specimens from the nasopharynx. All the tissue must be submitted for histologic examination. We prefer to study three levels of all such specimens. Occasionally, the tumor may be discovered in only one piece on one level. In most cases, nasopharyngeal carcinomas can be readily identified once the pathologist becomes familiar with the various patterns NPC may produce. However, a small focus of tumor, surrounded by a sea of lymphocytes, may be easily missed. A nest of tumor cells may be misinterpreted as a reactive germinal center (and vice versa). In some cases, a malignant lymphoma may be confused with NPC. As mentioned previously, in some carcinomas individual tumor cells are scattered among the lymphoid cells of the nasopharynx, producing a picture that may resemble a malignant lymphoma. In NPC the lymphoid cells appear mature, whereas in lymphomas these cells usually show varying stages of immaturity.

Electron microscopy for cell junctions and tonofilaments and immunoperoxidase studies for cytokeratin and common leukocyte antigen are helpful in differentiating between NPC and lymphoma. In one study using commercially available antibody against broad-spectrum keratin, positive staining was found in all carcinomas of the keratinizing type, 88 percent of those of the nonkeratinizing type, 90 percent of undifferentiated carcinomas, and

50 percent of adenocarcinomas.[78] Common leukocyte antigen was absent in the malignant cells. In patients whose metastatic carcinoma in a cervical lymph node suggests NPC but in whom triple biopsy fails to detect the primary tumor, elevated serum titers for anti-EBV capsid antigen and anti-early antigen provide strong support for the diagnosis of primary NPC.

Most reports have shown that the stage of tumor is the most important factor that determines the prognosis.[67,79] Survival figures vary considerably depending on the method of staging used in the study. When the carcinoma is confined to the nasopharynx, the prognosis is relatively good. When the tumor has metastasized to cervical lymph nodes, the chance of cure is somewhat diminished. Involvement of bone and/or cranial nerves is associated with a poor prognosis. The overall 5-year survival rates vary considerably, ranging from 39 to 62 percent.[67,79]

Metastatic Tumors to Upper Respiratory Tract

Metastatic tumors involving the nasal cavity, paranasal sinuses, and nasopharynx usually are seen as part of widespread metastatic disease. Occasionally, a metastasis to the upper respiratory tract may be the first sign of disease or the first known site of metastatic tumor. Under these circumstances the kidney (renal cell carcinoma) is the most common primary site, followed by lung, breast and colon.[80] Malignant lymphomas and leukemias may also involve this area as part of generalized disease.

Neural and Neuroectodermal Lesions

A small number of neural and neuroectodermal lesions occur in the nasal cavity, paranasal sinuses, and nasopharynx.

Nasal Glioma

Nasal glioma probably results from a congenital malformation and is generally considered to be a form of encephalocele in which the meningeal continuity to the brain has closed during embryonic development. These rare lesions usually are found in infants but occasionally may be identified in older children and adults. The majority of these lesions (approximately 60 percent) present as small, firm subcutaneous nodules at or near the bridge of the nose. Approximately 30 percent produce intranasal masses that are usually attached to the upper part of the nasal cavity and often have a polypoid appearance.[81] A few have been described in the paranasal sinuses (frontal, maxillary) and nasopharynx. Approximately 10 percent are found within both the nasal cavity and the subcutaneous tissue. The intranasal masses may produce symptoms of nasal obstruction. Lesions thought to be nasal gliomas may be resected by local surgical excision. This should not be done, however, if an encephalocele, with connection to the cranial cavity, is suspected clinically. Whether nasal gliomas represent true neoplasms or merely heterotopic glial tissue can be debated. These lesions grow slowly, apparently at the same rate as normal brain tissue. Histologically, nasal gliomas are composed of nests and masses of fibrillary neuroglial tissue with a prominent network of glial fibers. Astrocytic cells may show gemistocytic changes. Neuronal cells are rarely identified. Large astrocytic cells may be misinterpreted as histiocytes. Choroid plexus, ependymal cells, and pigmented cells with retinal differentiation have also been reported.[82] Recurrence after excision is found in 4 to 10 percent of nasal gliomas.[82] Rare cases of heterotopic brain tissue have been reported to occur in the nasopharynx, including one giving rise to an oligodendroglioma.[83,84]

Encephalocele results from herniation of brain tissue and leptomeninges through a bony defect of the skull. The excised tissue has the appearance of normal brain; however, degeneration may result in loss of neurons. In such cases distinction from nasal glioma will require other clinical findings.[82]

Meningiomas

Meningiomas are derived from meningeal arachnoid cells, which are generally considered to be neuroectodermal in origin. Rarely, meningiomas may arise outside the cranial cavity in such sites as the nasal cavity, paranasal sinuses, middle ear, temporal bone, and orbital cavity.[85,86] These ectopic tumors are thought to originate in arachnoid cells that are trapped within or outside bone when the various cranial bones develop and fuse. In a series of 12 nasal and sinus meningiomas, about half had evidence of cranial involvement.[85] In these patients the meningiomas probably originated intracranially, infiltrated locally, and first manifested clinically outside the cranial cavity. Other patients have no demonstrable intracranial lesion, and the tumor can be accepted as an ectopic meningioma. Within the nasal cavity and paranasal sinuses, meningiomas may grow as polyps or space-occupying masses. In these cases the pathologist usually receives curetted pieces of firm, gray tissue. Histologically these lesions have the appearance of intracranial meningiomas. In our experience the meningotheliomatous form is most commonly found in meningiomas of the nasal cavity and paranasal sinuses. Psammoma bodies may or may not be identified. Unless the pathologist remembers that meningiomas may be seen in this area, these lesions may be misdiagnosed as some type of epithelial or soft tissue neoplasm. They particularly may be confused with the psammomatous type of ossifying fibroma, especially in frozen sections.

Pituitary Tumors

Pituitary tumors may occasionally infiltrate locally through the sellar bone and extend into the sphenoid sinus, posterior nasal cavity, and/or superior nasopharynx, there producing polypoid[87] lesions or space-occupying masses leading to nasal obstruction. Some of these tumors may arise in ectopic pituitary tissue, misplaced during the migration of anterior pituitary cells from Rathke's pouch, an evagination from the nasopharyngeal roof. Histologically, these neoplasms are composed of nests and cords of cells, producing an epithelial pattern. Tumor cells may show a moderate degree of nuclear pleomorphism and mitotic activity, leading to an incorrect diagnosis of carcinoma or even plasmacytoma. In many cases the tumor cells have abundant cytoplasm in which fine or coarse granules can be identified, helping to make the correct diagnosis. A few tumors have produced prolactin, TSH, or ACTH with Cushing's syndrome.[87]

Paragangliomas

Paragangliomas rarely occur in the nasal cavity and paranasal sinuses. In a series of 73 paragangliomas of the head and neck region, 3 were reported in the nasal cavity.[88] Symptoms include epistaxis and/or nasal obstruction. These lesions may produce polypoid or space-occupying masses and may locally infiltrate into adjacent bone. They usually are not functional[88,89]; a rare case of ACTH production with Cushing's syndrome has been reported.[90] Histologically these neoplasms have the typical appearance of paragangliomas: small nests of uniform cells lying in a richly vascular stroma. Unless the pathologist remembers this possibility, the lesion may be misinterpreted as some type of epithelial or vascular tumor, perhaps even as an olfactory neuroblastoma or a meningioma.

Schwann Cell Tumors

Schwann cell tumors (neurofibromas, neurilemomas, and malignant schwannomas) only rarely involve the nasal cavity and paranasal sinuses.[91] Robitaille et al.[92] recently reviewed the literature and found only 15 acceptable cases with sinus involvement (including 12 schwannomas, 2 plexiform neurofibromas, 2 neurofibromas, and 1 probable malignant schwannoma). The Schwann cell tumors arising in this area exhibit the same histologic features as those seen elsewhere. Neurilemo-

mas (schwannomas) are encapsulated nodules and are composed of typical Schwann cells arranged in cellular and myxoid patterns. Neurofibromas may produce large bulky masses and may be confused with the myxoma that is seen in this area. Indeed, some lesions diagnosed as myxomas may represent neurofibromas with extensive myxoid change. Neurofibromas should exhibit typical comma-shaped or "teardrop" nuclei with a fine chromatin pattern. In contrast, myxomas are composed of stellate cells with elongated cytoplasmic tails. The nuclei tend to be more hyperchromatic than those found in neurofibromas. The histologic features of malignant schwannoma and the criteria for diagnosis are discussed elsewhere in this book.

Olfactory Neuroblastoma

Olfactory neuroblastomas are thought to arise from the specialized sensory neuroepithelial (neuroectodermal) cells that are normally found in the upper part of the nasal cavity (superior nasal concha, upper part of septum, roof of nose, and cribriform plate of ethmoid).[93,94] This specialized epithelium, in addition to giving rise to neuroblastomas, is probably the progenitor of the "neuroendocrine" tumors that occur in the nasal cavity.[95] Rarely, neuroblastomas are reported to contain carcinomatous elements.[96,97] Since the distinction between olfactory neuroblastoma and neuroendocrine carcinoma is a relatively recent developement, some of the earlier reports of olfactory neuroblastoma probably included an unknown number of neuroendocrine carcinomas.

Clinically, olfactory neuroblastomas may occur in any age group but most often after the age of 40. These tumors most commonly produce nasal obstruction and, less frequently, epistaxis, rhinorrhea, sinus pain, orbital symptoms, and middle ear complaints.[93] On physical examination, a mass, or less often a polyp, is identified in the superior portion of the nasal cavity. Less commonly, facial swelling, orbital enlargement, and cranial nerve paralysis may be found. Radiologic findings include a soft tissue mass involving the intranasal and paranasal areas, sinus opacification, and/or bone destruction. Rare examples of functional olfactory neuroblastomas with secretion of vasopressin causing hypertension and severe hyponatremia have been reported.[98]

Histologically olfactory neuroblastomas are usually composed of cellular nests or masses that are separated into clusters by fine fibrovascular septa. The relatively uniform cells, which are slightly larger than lymphocytes, lie in a finely fibrillar stroma, which may be focally obscured by the cellular proliferation. The cells have round to oval nuclei with a uniformly distributed fine or coarse chromatin pattern (Fig. 17-15). Only occasional prominent nucleoli may be seen. Nuclear pleomorphism is min-

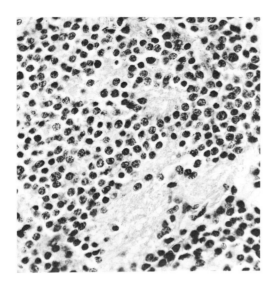

Fig. 7-15. Olfactory neuroblastoma. Tumor cells have round nuclei and indistinct cell borders. Minimal pleomorphism and hyperchromatism are seen. A finely fibrillar stroma is identified focally.

imal and few mitoses are identified. In many of these tumors, pseudorosettes are formed in which rings of neoplastic cells surround finely fibrillar or granular material. True rosettes, defined as ductlike spaces lined by nonciliated column-like cells with basally placed nuclei, are only rarely identified. In a small number of cases, a few mature and immature ganglion cells may be seen.

In a small biopsy specimen of an olfactory neuroblastoma in which considerable crush artifact has occurred, the pathologist may see nests of somewhat dark-staining cells. The neurofibrillar stroma may not be easily recognized. As a result the olfactory neuroblastoma may be misinterpreted as some type of poorly differentiated or undifferentiated carcinoma. As olfactory neuroblastomas become less mature, with fewer pseudorosettes and a less evident fibrillar stroma, the diagnostic areas may be overlooked.

Conversely, other types of nasal tumors may be misinterpreted as olfactory neuroblastoma, including undifferentiated carcinomas, various poorly differentiated adenocarcinomas, malignant lymphomas, and even embryonal rhabdomyosarcomas. Oberman and Rice[99] have described the pitfalls in diagnosis and have illustrated several nasal lesions that were misdiagnosed as olfactory neuroblastoma. We agree with Oberman and Rice that the pathologist, using the light microscope, probably should not diagnose a tumor as an olfactory neuroblastoma in the absence of an intercellular neurofibrillary matrix. The presence of pseudorosettes aids in making the diagnosis. When neurofibrils cannot be identified and when prominent nucleoli, considerable nuclear pleomor-

phism, and many mitoses are found, the diagnosis of olfactory neuroblastoma is difficult to support.

Since olfactory neuroblastomas have some histologic resemblance to ordinary neuroblastomas arising in the adrenal medulla or in sympathetic tissue, a biopsy specimen of a nasal tumor that shows this pattern should lead to the appropriate studies to rule out metastatic disease.

Differentiation between olfactory neuroblastomas and neuroendocrine carcinomas requires special studies. In one report neuroendocrine carcinomas exhibited an organoid, endocrine pattern, lacked a neurofibrillar matrix, and had argyrophilic or argentaffin granules or neurosecretory granules by electron microscopy.[95] However, in a group of 21 olfactory neuroblastomas, most of which contained a neurofibrillar matrix, 80 percent had weakly to moderately positive argyrophilic cells.[94]

By using an immunoperoxidase technique, neuron-specific enolase can be detected in both olfactory neuroblastomas and neuroendocrine carcinomas. In the former, a small number of cells in the periphery of the tumor nests react with the antibodies against S-100 protein and glial filament acidic protein (GFAP).[100] This finding, which is interpreted as evidence of Schwann cell differentiation, is absent in the neuroendocrine carcinomas.[100]

On ultrastructural study, olfactory neuroblastomas contain multiple cytoplasmic processes with neurofilaments and microtubules (Fig. 17-16). Neurosecretory granules about 90 to 240 μm in diameter are found in the cytoplasm and in neural processes. The fibrillary stroma seen with the light microscope corresponds to immature nerve processes.[96] Specific cytoplasmic specialization of normal olfactory neurons, that is, olfactory vesicles or bundles of slender neural fibers resembling proximal processes, have been identified in these tumors.[95] Neuroendocrine carcinomas contain similar neurosecretory granules, but they differ from olfactory neuroblastoma by having desmosomal junctions and tonofilaments and lacking neurofilaments and neuritic processes.[95,103] Additional immunohistochemical and ultrastructural studies will be needed to clearly distinguish olfactory neuroblastomas from neuroendocrine carcinomas.

Olfactory neuroblastomas tend to be slowly growing lesions that infiltrate into adjacent structures. These tumors frequently recur locally after surgical excision. The prognosis appears to be mainly related to extent of disease. Lesions localized to the nasal cavity have a better prognosis than those that involve an adjacent sinus. These neoplasms may infiltrate into the cranial and/or orbital cavities. Cervical lymph node metastases are seen in about 20 percent of cases.[94] If distant metastases are included, the overall rates of metastasis in different series increase to 38 percent[94] and 62 percent.[101] Local recurrences, affecting 30 percent of patients, are most often associated with incomplete excision of the tumor (94).

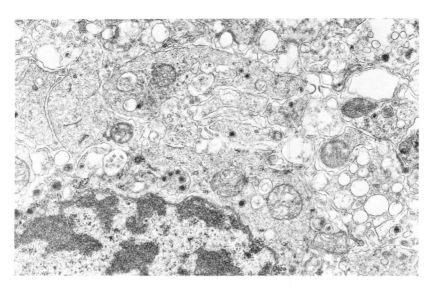

Fig. 17-16. Olfactory neuroblastoma. Membrane-bound neurosecretory granules are present in the cytoplasm and neural processes. Some of the neural processes contain abundant microfilaments and microtubules; others contain dense core and empty vesicles. (×22,500)

The 5-year survival rates are in the range of 58 percent,[101] but the actual cure rate is lower since these tumors may recur many years after initial treatment. Recent reports recommend that these neoplasms be treated with a combination of surgical resection and radiotherapy.[93,101]

Neuroendocrine Carcinoma

Included in the category of neuroendocrine carcinoma are nasal tumors that on light microscopic examination have a histologic appearance ranging from carcinoid tumors to small cell anaplastic carcinomas. Some tumor cells may have an oncocytic appearance with abundant eosinophilic granular cytoplasm,[102] while other have scanty cytoplasm and a high nucleocytoplasmic ratio. Although degree of nuclear atypia and mitotic activity vary from tumor to tumor, the tumors share some of the following features: punctate chromatin pattern, inconspicuous nucleoli, and a distinct organoid arrangement surrounded by a rich vascular network. Some reported neuroendocrine carcinomas have been functional, with secretion of corticotropin, calcitonin, or β-melanocyte-stimulating hormone.[103] By special studies neuroendocrine differentiation can be demonstrated, as described in connection with olfactory neuroblastomatoma. Prognosis has not been clearly defined because of the small number of cases reported; in general, it correlates with degree of differentiation, nuclear anaplasia, and mitotic activity.

Mixed Neuroblastoma and Carcinoma

Olfactory neuroblastomas may, rarely, coexist with adenocarcinomas, squamous carcinomas, or undifferentiated carcinomas.[97] It has been suggested that these mixed neoplasms arise from the basal cells of the olfactory epithelium.[97]

Melanosis and Nevi

Melanosis and nevi are rarely found in this area. When present, the nasal vestibule is most commonly affected, followed by the nasal mucosa. However, when malignant melanomas involving the nasal cavity and paranasal sinuses are studied with special stains for melanin, benign-appearing cells containing melanin granules in their cytoplasm may occasionally be seen in the normal mucosal cell population that lines these structures.[104] Thus, neuroectodermal melanocytic cells probably occur in the nasal and sinus mucosa more frequently than is generally appreciated.

Malignant Melanomas

Malignant melanomas may arise in the nasal cavity and paranasal sinuses. In two large series, 0.6 and 0.7 percent of all malignant melanomas occurred in this area.[105,106] In a series[106] of 660 melanomas originating in the head and neck area (excluding eye), 9 percent were listed as mucosal lesions. A group of 52 melanomas apparently arising in the mucous membranes of the head and neck[105] had the following distribution: oral cavity 26 (50 percent); nasal cavity and sinuses 18 (35 percent)—including nasal cavity 8, maxillary antrum 4, floor of nose 2, ethmoid sinus 2, vestibule 1, and turbinate 1—and pharyngolarynx 8 (15 percent), including nasopharynx and eustachian tube 3. Within the nasal cavity malignant melanomas most commonly involve the nasal septum, followed by the inferior and middle turbinates. In many cases the site of origin cannot be determined with certainty at the time of diagnosis because the lesions are large and involve several structures including the nasal cavity and one or more sinuses.

Clinically, the majority of patients have symptoms of nasal obstruction and/or epistaxis. On physical examination nasal melanomas tend to be large, bulky, friable masses, which bleed with manipulation. The lesions project into the involved cavity and may have a somewhat polypoid configuration.

On gross examination tumor tissue varies in color from white to gray, brown, or black. The consistency has been described as firm, friable, or gelatinous. On histologic examination malignant melanomas arising in this area show the spectrum of changes seen in other melanomas. Most of these tumors grow in sheets or nests of variable size. Polygonal cells of variable size may have vesicular nuclei and prominent nucleoli. In a small number of cases, spindle cells predominate. The amount of melanin pigment varies considerably. With immunohistochemical methods, the diagnosis of malignant melanoma can be readily established by a negative reaction with antikeratin and a positive stain with antibody against S-100 protein.

The prognosis of malignant melanomas arising in the nasal cavity and paranasal sinuses is generally poor because of advanced local disease. In one study only those patients whose melanomas measured less than 8 mm in thickness survived. The reported 5 year survival rates are in the range of 25 percent[107] to 30 percent.[108]

Dermoid Cysts, Teratoid Cysts, Teratomas, and Malignant Teratoid Tumors

Dermoid cysts (dermoid tumors, teratoid tumors, hairy polyps) occurring in the nasopharynx are not true neoplasms but represent development malformations of the first branchial arch resulting in the presence of two germinal layers, ectoderm and mesoderm. These lesions are usually recognized at birth but may be found somewhat later. Clinical problems include difficulty in breathing, sucking, or swallowing. These lesions may produce pe-

dunculated masses attached to the lateral nasopharyngeal wall or to the nasopharyngeal portion of the soft palate. Sessile masses or those with short stalks may lead to complete obstruction of the nasopharynx. Histologically, various tissues have been described including skin, accessory skin structures, fibrous and adipose tissue, smooth and skeletal muscle, and cartilage and bone. Minor salivary glands may be seen, but they may merely be glands secondarily incorporated into the lesion. Treatment consists of surgical excision.

True teratomas, consisting of trigerminal elements, may, rarely, be found. In the head and neck region germ cell tumors occur mainly in newborns and young infants. The most common sites of involvement include the neck, nasopharynx, oropharynx, face, and orbit. The majority are mature teratomas. However, a few immature teratomas or endodermal sinus tumors have been reported. *Epignathi* are teratomas that have differentiated into a parasitic fetus and are usually attached to the sphenoid bone. This entire subject has been reviewed.[109,110]

Malignant teratoid tumors consisting of carcinomatous and sarcomatous tissues have been described in this area.[111,112] The epithelial elements usually consist of mature squamous and immature intestinal or respiratory epithelia. Foci of transitional cell carcinoma and primitive neuroepithelial tumor with rosettes, pseudorosettes, or neurofibrillary matrix are less common. The stromal tissues consist predominantly of fibroblasts and embryonal, immature spindle cells in a myxoid matrix. In addition, islands of cartilage, smooth muscle, and skeletal muscle cells in varying degrees of maturation may be present. These carcinosarcomas histologically resemble immature teratomas; however, none contain seminoma, embryonal carcinoma, or choriocarcinoma. About 35 percent of patients developed cervical lymph node metastases and 60 percent died of tumor in 3 years.[111]

Nonepithelial Tumors

The benign and malignant nonepithelial tumors arising in this area usually produce the same clinical problems caused by epithelial neoplasms (nasal obstruction, epistaxis, etc). Except in a few instances, no specific findings are identified on physical or radiologic examination. In most cases the correct diagnosis is only made when the lesion is examined histologically. The nonepithelial neoplasms that we have studied in our laboratory are listed in Tables 17-4 and 17-5.[113] These tumors are seen much less frequently as compared with epithelial neoplasms and constitute only about 10 to 20 percent of all tumors found in the nasal cavity, paranasal sinuses, and nasopharynx.

TABLE 17.4. Benign Nonepithelial Tumors Involving the Nasal Cavity, Paranasal Sinuses, and Nasopharynx

Vascular tumors	
Angiofibroma	38
Capillary hemangioma	30
Cavernous hemangioma	5
Venous hemangioma	3
Benign hemangioendothelioma	3
Angiomatosis	1
Glomus tumor	1
Subtotal	81
Osseous and fibro-osseous lesions	
Osteoma	31
Fibrous dysplasia	9
Ossifying fibroma	7
Osteoblastoma	1
Giant cell tumor	4
Subtotal	52
Others	
Chondroma	7
Myxoma	6
Fibroma	4
Rhabdomyoma	3
Leiomyoma	2
Lipoma	1
Subtotal	23
Total	156

Vascular Tumors

Hemangiomas

Hemangiomas are found most often in the anterior nasal septum, followed by the turbinates and the vestibule. Capillary hemangiomas are seen most frequently; cavernous hemangiomas, venous hemangiomas, benign hemangioendotheliomas, and angiomatoses are identified

TABLE 17.5. Malignant or Potentially Malignant Nonepithelial Tumors Involving the Nasal Cavity, Paranasal Sinuses, and Nasopharynx

Malignant lymphoma	21
Fibromatosis and fibrosarcoma	19
Rhabdomyosarcoma	16
Osteosarcoma	11
Chondrosarcoma	10
Plasmacytoma	10
Fibrous histiocytoma	9
Leiomyosarcoma	6
Malignant hemangioendothelioma	2
Malignant hemangiopericytoma	2
Malignant giant cell tumor	1
Liposarcoma	1
Total	108

less often. Histologically these lesions have the same appearance as hemangiomas seen elsewhere.[113] *Vascular malformations* may be easily overlooked in multiple pieces of curetted tissue. In contrast to normal vascular channels and to the vessels in hemangiomas, vascular malformations contain numerous closely packed tortuous blood vessels of variable size and configuration.

Angiofibroma

Angiofibroma is the most common nonepithelial neoplasm found in the upper respiratory tract. These lesions most often develop in the nasopharynx of teenage boys. Clinically, angiofibromas produce nasal obstruction, epistaxis, and sometimes massive hemorrhage. Physical examination usually shows a firm, rubbery, bulging nasopharyngeal mass, which may have extended into the posterior nasal cavity. These tumors may infiltrate locally to involve adjacent structures, including the pterygoid region, sphenoid sinus, base of the skull in the ethmoid and sphenoid areas, and pterygomaxillary sulcus to the apex of the orbit and into the orbital cavity, hard and soft palate, and cheek and temple.[114] Grossly, angiofibromas consist of firm, rubbery, gray-white tissue. Microscopically these tumors are composed of a characteristic fibrous stroma in which are found numerous blood vessels of various sizes and shapes (Fig. 17-17). Smaller vascular channels are surrounded only by the fibrous stroma of the tumor. Larger vessels may have an irregular or incomplete smooth muscle coat. Elastic fibers usually

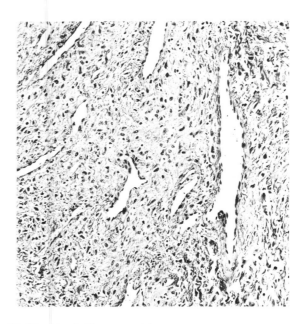

Fig. 17-17. Angiofibroma. This nasopharyngeal tumor is composed of a fibrous stroma in which scattered vascular channels are observed.

THE NASAL CAVITY, PARANASAL SINUSES, AND NASOPHARYNX

cannot be found in the vessel walls, either with elastic tissue stains or with the electron microscope.[113] Stromal cells vary from mature fibrocytes, with small, dense nuclei, to fibroblasts, which have large but regular nuclei with a fine chromatin pattern. On ultrastructural study most of the stromal cells appear to be fibrocytes or fibroblasts, but smooth muscle cells and myofibroblasts have been identified.[113]

In most cases, angiofibromas can be easily diagnosed histologically. Occasionally, the stroma may show focal areas of moderate to marked hypercellularity, suggestive of fibromatosis or fibrosarcoma. The stromal cells in angiofibromas, however, usually still have regular nuclei without pleomorphism or hyperchromatism. Only a few mitoses may be identified. A tumor that demonstrates marked stromal cellularity with numerous mitoses more likely is a sarcoma. Malignant soft tissue tumors arising in this area tend to have a more vascular stroma than similar neoplasms growing elsewhere. However, the blood vessels found in these sarcomas are relatively small compared with the larger vessels seen in angiofibromas. The smaller vascular channels of angiofibromas may become compressed by the stroma, producing a picture reminiscent of hemangiopericytoma, but the vessels rarely exhibit the slitlike pattern that may be found in pericytic tumors.

Because massive bleeding may occur, biopsy or excision of a suspected angiofibroma should be done only in the operating room, where hemorrhage can be controlled. Recurrence after surgical resection varies from 35 to 57 percent.[114,115] In some cases, the lesion appears to regress after puberty. Sarcomatous transformation of angiofibroma has been associated with prior radiotherapy to the area.[116]

Glomus Tumors, Hemangiopericytomas, and Malignant Hemangioendotheliomas (Angiosarcomas)

These vascular tumors may rarely occur in the nasal cavity and paranasal sinuses.[113,117] Hemangiopericytoma-like intranasal tumors have been described.[118] In most of these cases a polypoid mass, which bled easily on manipulation, was identified high in the nasal cavity. Histologically, these neoplasms were composed of uniform, round to spindle-shaped cells without pleomorphism or mitotic activity. Blood vessels of varying sizes and shapes were seen. In contrast to more typical hemangiopericytomas, vascular channels were not dispersed uniformly throughout these tumors and did not show the typical compressed irregular and even slitlike appearance of vessels found in pericytic tumors, having more the appearance of the normal pre-existing vascular channels seen in this area. The spindle-shaped cells were arranged in a more uniform pattern as compared with what is usually found in pericytic tumors. Study of these neoplasms in the future, perhaps with the electron microscope, will demonstrate whether they are hemangiopericytomas, spindle cell epithelial or myoepithelial tumors, leiomyomas, Schwann cell neoplasms, or some other type of lesion. Rare cases of *proliferating systemic angioendotheliomatosis* of the nasal cavity have been reported.[119]

Osseous and Fibro-osseous Lesions

As can be seen in Tables 17-4 and 17-5, osseous and fibro-osseous lesions comprised the second largest group of nonepithelial tumors.

Osteomas

Osteomas most often involve the maxillary and frontal sinuses and may be divided into ivory, mature, and fibrous types. These lesions are composed of varying amounts of mature lamellar bone and mature fibrous tissue.[120]

Fibrous Dysplasia

A fibro-osseous lesion, fibrous dysplasia represents a benign neoplasm or a hamartomatous process in which osseous maturation is arrested at the woven bone stage.[120] The craniofacial bones are normally formed via intramembranous ossification. Osteoid is first deposited in the stroma, developing into a woven fibrous bone. Later, osteoblasts line the surfaces of the woven bone, forming a bony matrix and lamellar bone with regular cement lines. In fibrous dysplasia lamellar bone is usually not seen, the maturation process presumably having stopped at the woven bone stage.

Histologically these lesions are composed of fibrous and osseous tissue in varying proportions. The moderately to highly cellular fibrous stroma consists of relatively mature spindle-shaped fibroblastic cells, which usually do not show hyperchromatism, pleomorphism, or mitotic activity. The osseous component contains irregular trabeculae of woven bone without osteoblasts or regular cement lines. With polarized light, woven bone with irregular birefringent fibers may be identified. In most cases the diagnosis poses no difficulty. However, foci of reactive new bone formation with trabeculae of lamellar bone lined by osteoblasts may be seen at the edges of the lesion where it extends into adjacent normal bone. Similar areas may be found within recurrent lesions of fibrous dysplasia, sometimes obscuring the diagnostic foci of woven bone.

Since these lesions grow slowly, they can usually be treated with conservative local resections. Several surgical excisions may be required for cosmetic reasons. Radical surgical resections should not be performed, and radiotherapy is contraindicated because of the possibility of inducing a sarcoma in the irradiated bone.[120]

Ossifying Fibroma

Ossifying fibroma behaves clinically as a locally aggressive neoplasm, invading locally and destroying adjacent bone. After local excisions, recurrences are frequently seen, and more extensive resection may be required.[120]

Histologically, ossifying fibromas are composed of fibrous and osseous tissue, the former usually predominating. The fibrous stroma varies from moderately to highly cellular. The spindle-shaped fibroblastic cells usually show only minimal pleomorphism and mitotic activity. A wide spectrum of osseous tissue may be seen, including focal deposits of osteoid, "psammoma-like" islands of bone consisting of central bony tissue rimmed by osteoid and occasionally by osteoblasts and of lamellar bone lined by osteoblasts. Transitional stages between osteoid, psammoma-like bone and more fully developed lamellar bone may be found.[120] The psammomatoid variant of ossifying fibroma typically involves the ethmoid region of young children, usually under 10 years of age, with local bone destruction.[120–122]

Ossifying fibromas, especially those with a highly cellular stroma, may be misinterpreted as fibromatosis or well differentiated fibrosarcoma, especially in biopsy material. Fibromatosis and fibrosarcoma may show areas of reactive or metaplastic bone formation, usually where tumor invades pre-existing periosteum or bone. Ossifying fibromas, in contrast, usually have areas of osteoid and bone formation scattered throughout the lesion.

The pathologist may have difficulty in differentiating between an ossifying fibroma and an osteosarcoma, especially in biopsy material. Ossifying fibromas should contain osseous tissue that is relatively uniform and regularly arranged. The fibrous stromal cells should show no more than slight atypia and minimal mitotic activity. In contrast, osteosarcomas contain irregular trabeculae of immature osteoid or bone arranged in a haphazard manner. The stromal cells usually demonstrate greater hyperchromatism, pleomorphism, and mitotic activity as compared with ossifying fibroma. Islands of psammoma-like bone are usually not seen.

In most cases ossifying fibroma and fibrous dysplasia may be differentiated from each other, mainly on the basis of the type of bone formed. However, a small number of lesions demonstrate overlapping features. These mainly have the appearance of fibrous dysplasia, with focal areas of more mature bone formation that appear reparative rather than neoplastic. A lesion that shows areas of woven bone formation should be treated conservatively and will usually exhibit the clinical behavior of fibrous dysplasia.

Giant Cell Tumors

Both benign and malignant giant cell tumors may arise in this area.[120] These neoplasms should be differentiated from other lesions that contain giant cells, including giant cell reparative granulomas, "brown tumors" of hyperparathyroidism, and fibrous histiocytomas. The differential diagnosis has been discussed elsewhere.[120,123]

Osteosarcomas

Osteosarcomas (osteogenic sarcomas) arising in this area[120] are composed histologically of overtly malignant spindle-shaped mesenchymal cells associated with immature malignant-appearing osteoid or bone. Several tumors should be considered in the differential diagnosis, including ossifying fibromas (see the section on ossifying fibroma). Fibrosarcomas growing in the upper respiratory tract may invade pre-existing bone. In these foci, malignant-appearing spindle-shaped cells may be surrounded by irregular and disrupted bone, simulating malignant osteoid and bone formation.[120] In a biopsy specimen this tissue may be incorrectly interpreted as malignant osteoid, and a diagnosis of osteogenic sarcoma may be made. Conversely, a small specimen may show a tumor diagnosed as a fibrosarcoma, but the larger resection specimen may demonstrate unquestionable areas of malignant osteoid or bone. Some neoplasms arising in this area contain both chondrosarcomatous and osteosarcomatous elements. How to classify these tumors remains controversial. Most reports indicate that neoplasms diagnosed as osteosarcoma but in which chondrosarcomatous elements predominate have a better prognosis than ordinary osteogenic sarcomas.[120]

Chordoma

Chordomas occur mainly in the sacrococcygeal and spheno-occipital regions.[124] In the latter site these tumors involve the posterior nasal cavity, sphenoid sinus, sphenoid bone, nasopharynx, and base of the skull. Histologically, tumor cells grow in sheets, nests, and cords, often with a lobulated pattern. The characteristic cell, the physaliferous cell, contains a vacuolated cytoplasm, producing a bubble-like appearance (Fig. 17-18). Some of these cells have multiple fine vacuoles in their cytoplasm, others exhibit a "signet ring" appearance, and some have a clear cytoplasm. With PAS and mucicarmine stains these spaces usually are empty, but a rim of mucin-positive material may be found at the borders of vacuoles. In addition, other cells have a more dense eosinophilic cytoplasm. Many tumor cells of both types contain

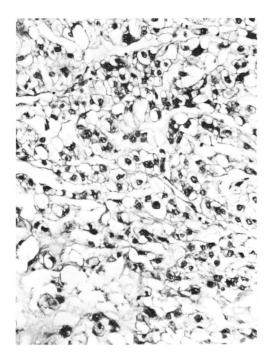

Fig. 17-18. Chordoma. Vacuolated, physaliferous cells are arranged in cords.

finely granular, PAS-positive cytoplasmic material, which is digested by diastase, indicative of glycogen. Because of the presence of vacuolated cells, a carcinoma is frequently considered in the differential diagnosis, especially in small biopsy specimens in this area. In contrast to the findings in chordomas, most mucin-producing epithelial tumors have intracytoplasmic vacuoles filled by mucinous material that is stained either by PAS or by mucicarmine.[125]

In most chordomas the cells show little pleomorphism, hyperchromatism, or mitotic activity. However, in a few cases tumor cells become less differentiated and assume a sarcomatous appearance. These lesions can only be classified as chordoma when more typical areas are recognized. Some chordomas growing in this area contain cartilaginous tissue having the features of chondroma or well differentiated chondrosarcoma. These tumors have been diagnosed as "chondroid chordoma."[124] If physaliferous cells are found in a lesion, a diagnosis of chordoma should be made even though cartilaginous or sarcomatous features are identified.

Chordomas of this region grow slowly, infiltrate locally, and do not metastasize. Following surgery and radiotherapy, long-term survival is possible in spite of multiple recurrences.[125]

Chordomas traditionally have been classified as mesenchymal tumors; however, substantial evidence indicates that they should be interpreted as epithelial tumors.

On ultrastructural study chordoma cells are seen to have desmosomal attachments, and on immunohistochemical examination they are shown to contain keratin in their cytoplasm. Chordomas probably arise from notochord remnants. The notochord probably is an ectodermal structure, which explains the epithelial features manifested by chordomas.[125]

Fibrous Tissue Tumors (Fibroma, Fibromatosis, Fibrosarcoma)

The clinical and pathologic features of fibroma, fibromatosis, and fibrosarcoma have been discussed elsewhere.[126] Several neoplasms should be considered in the differential diagnosis of fibromatosis and fibrosarcomas arising in this area. Various osseous and fibro-osseous lesions, including fibrous dysplasia, ossifying fibroma, and osteosarcoma, have areas of fibroblastic proliferation, but fibromatosis and fibrosarcomas should not demonstrate osteoid or bone formation in the substance of the lesion. Fibrosarcomatous areas may be recognized in many soft tissue tumors, including osteosarcoma, chondrosarcoma, leiomyosarcoma, synovial sarcoma, malignant schwannoma, and fibrous histiocytoma. In general, differentiation toward another type of tissue should lead to a diagnosis other than fibrous tissue neoplasm. Fibromatosis and fibrosarcomas should not contain multinucleate giant cells or cells with large, bizarre, or highly pleomorphic nuclei. If such cells are found, the tumor can usually be identified as some other type of neoplasm.

These fibrous tumors should be distinguished from the *inflammatory pseudotumors* that may infiltrate the surrounding tissues. The lesion consists of hyalinized fibrous tissue mixed with varying numbers of lymphocytes and neutrophils, resembling Riedel's thyroiditis, sclerosing mediastinitis, and retroperitoneal fibrosis. In the head and neck region this lesion has been reported to occur in the parotid gland, maxillary sinus, nose, orbit, and parapharyngeal space and is usually controlled by surgical excision.[127]

Fibrous Histiocytoma

Fibrous histiocytomas involving the upper respiratory passages produce the same clinical features that are associated with other mesenchymal tumors. These neoplasms are histologically similar to fibrous histiocytomas found elsewhere. The degree of differentiation of the cell population appears to correlate with prognosis.[123]

Myxomas

Myxomas growing in this area appear to arise in bone. On gross examination these tumors usually consist of a gray to white multinodular tissue with a firm to gelatinous consistency. Microscopically, myxomas are composed of a relatively avascular myxoid ground substance in which lie scattered spindle-shaped and stellate cells.[128] The cells contain small, dark, elongated or ovoid nuclei and usually demonstrate elongated cytoplasmic tails. In focal areas a more fibrous stroma may be seen in which the cells exhibit the appearance of fibrocytes. Electron microscopic studies have shown that the cells of myxomas arising in this area have the features of fibroblasts.[129]

Various tumors growing in the upper respiratory tract may contain myxoid areas and should be considered in the differential diagnosis. Schwann cell neoplasms should have typical comma-shaped or "teardrop" nuclei, usually demonstrate wavy fibers in their stroma, and may show foci of nuclear palisading. In contrast, myxomas contain cells with elongated cytoplasmic tails and smaller, denser nuclei. Myxoid liposarcomas exhibit a plexiform vascular network and "signet ring" lipoblasts. Embryonal rhabdomyosarcomas demonstrate focal areas of high cellularity and malignant-appearing nuclei. Myxoid change may be seen focally in fibromatosis, fibrosarcoma, fibrous histiocytoma, fibrous dysplasia, ossifying fibroma, and cartilaginous tumors, but thorough examination will usually demonstrate the diagnostic areas in these lesions.

Skeletal Muscle Tumors

Rhabdomyomas may rarely occur in this area.[130–132] *Rhabdomyosarcomas* that arise in the upper respiratory tract usually occur in the first decade; only a few are seen in patients more than 12 years old.[130] When involving the nasal cavity, paranasal sinuses, and/or nasopharynx, these tumors produce large, bulky masses that project into the involved cavity. Some of these lesions have the clinical appearance of multiple nasal polyps.[130,133]

Histologically, rhabdomyosarcomas arising in this area most often have the appearance of embryonal rhabdomyosarcoma or sarcoma botryoides. The alveolar and pheomorphic types are rarely seen. *Embryonal rhabdomyosarcomas* are composed of round to spindle-shaped mesenchymal cells that contain hyperchromatic nuclei and variable numbers of mitoses. Elongated strap-shaped cells and/or small rounded "tadpole" cells, both having acidophilic (eosinophilic) cytoplasm, are usually recognized. Cross striations may be identified. A myxoid stroma may be seen in focal areas. In *sarcoma botryoides* a highly cellular zone of spindle-shaped cells is usually found immediately below the mucosal surface. Cross striations can usually be demonstrated in this area. Deeper in the lesion, these tumors usually become myxomatous and may have an appearance similar to that of embryonal rhabdomyosarcoma. Grossly, sarcoma botryoides usually forms multiple polypoid nodules projecting into the

lumen. The tumor cells in *alveolar rhabdomyosarcomas* are arranged in nests, cords, and bands, producing a pattern suggestive of an epithelial tumor. An alveolar architecture may be seen focally in embryonal rhabdomyosarcomas. In the *pleomorphic* variant, tumor cells exhibit large, bizarre nuclei (sometimes multinucleate) and abundant eosinophilic cytoplasm.

The pathologist may encounter difficulty in establishing the diagnosis of rhabdomyosarcoma, especially in small pieces of biopsy material in which characteristic rhabdomyoblasts cannot be identified. When the specimen consists mainly of myxoid tissue, rhabdomyosarcomas must be differentiated from nasal polyps with stromal atypia, myxomas, and Schwann cell tumors. In highly cellular specimens composed of primitive mesenchymal cells, the differential diagnosis includes malignant lymphoma, histiocytosis, malignant histiocytoma, Ewing's sarcoma, and malignant epithelial neoplasms, especially olfactory neuroblastoma. By immunohistochemistry the majority of rhabdomyosarcomas are shown to have myoglobin, desmin, or both. Electron microscopy may reveal typical or abortive Z, A, and I bands.

Plasmacytomas

Plasmacytomas most often occur within bone. Occasionally these tumors may arise in extraosseous sites, most commonly in the upper respiratory tract.[134] In this area plasmacytomas usually produce raised, smooth-surfaced lesions, which bulge into the lumen of the involved structure. Histologically these neoplasms are composed of a pure population of plasma cells, usually growing in solid sheets. Most of the cells show atypical features including large, pleomorphic nuclei, reversal of the nuclear/cytoplasmic ratio, large, coarse chromatin clumps, and mitotic activity.[134]

In the upper respiratory tract, some inflammatory lesions may contain numerous plasma cells, sometimes almost a pure culture of these cells ("plasma cell granulomas"). The presence of the following features would support the diagnosis of a reactive lesion: (1) numerous small blood vessels lined by large but uniform endothelial cells, (2) mature plasma cells, (3) other types of inflammatory cells, (4) Russell bodies, and (5) polyclonality by immunohistochemistry. Occasionally, a plasmacytoma in which the cells contain relatively little cytoplasm may be misinterpreted as a malignant lymphoma. Some plasmacytomas grow in clusters of cells and may be misdiagnosed as a pituitary tumor or some other epithelial neoplasm.

When the diagnosis of extramedullary plasmacytoma is made, the patient should be examined for evidence of plasma cell disease elsewhere. If none is found, the tumor should be treated as a primary extraosseous lesion.[134] Plasmacytomas may metastasize to cervical lymph nodes.[134]

Malignant Lymphomas

Malignant lymphoma is the most common malignant nonepithelial neoplasm found in the upper respiratory tract,[113] most commonly involving the nasal cavity, the maxillary sinus, and the nasopharynx. Histologically the tumor cells demonstrate a broad spectrum of cellular differentiated lymphoid cells. Diffuse lymphomas are usually found; nodular lymphomas are only rarely seen.[135]

Prognosis appears to be related to the extent of local disease. Overall 5 year survival rates range from 45 to 56 percent.[136,137] The majority of patients who die have systemic lymphoma.[138] Several studies have found a correlation between cell type and prognosis. Patients with T-cell lymphomas of the nasal and Waldeyer's ring areas have lower survival rates than those with B-cell lymphomas.[139] Large cell immunoblastic lymphomas appear to be highly malignant.[136]

A special variety of malignant lymphoma occurring in this area has been called *midline malignant reticulosis*.[140] Both clinically and histologically, these tumors differ from ordinary lymphomas. Midline malignant reticulosis usually shows more extensive swelling of nasal, facial, and periorbital tissues; mucosal ulceration; tissue necrosis; bone destruction; and fistula formation, producing the clinical picture of "lethal midline granuloma."[140] Nasal septal perforation and collapse of the nasal bridge may be seen. Histologically, these tumors are composed of a mixed cell population, including mature lymphocytes, lymphoblasts, and large, immature, pleomorphic, malignant-appearing lymphoid cells (Fig. 17-19). Large atypical cells with bilobed nuclei and prominent nucleoli may be identified, but classical Reed-Sternberg cells are not seen. In addition, a polymorphic inflammatory cell population, consisting of neutrophils, plasma cells, eosinophils, and epithelioid histiocytes, usually is found.[135] Necrosis and abscesses are frequently observed. Tumor cells may infiltrate into blood vessel walls. Necrosis of vessel walls and intravascular tumor thrombi may be found, but true inflammatory vasculitis is not identified. Some authors have suggested that this lesion represents lymphomatoid granulomatosis involving the upper respiratory tract.[141,142] Recent studies have indicated that these lesions are T-cell lymphomas. In addition, lesions that have been designated as lymphomatoid granulomatosis probably also are T-cell lymphomas.[142,143]

Malignant lymphoma and midline malignant reticulosis should be distinguished from an *idiopathic destructive disease* of the midline facial structure.[144] In this disease the cellular infiltrate consists of nonspecific acute and

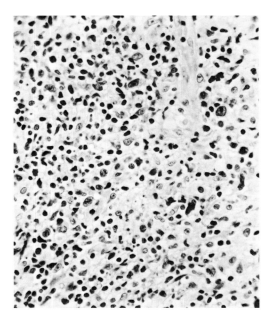

Fig. 17-19. Midline malignant reticulosis. A polymorphic infiltrate consists of mature and immature lymphocytes, histiocytes, and large atypical cells with prominent nucleoli.

chronic inflammation without malignant or atypical lymphoid cells. Inflammatory cells often surround the perivascular area, but vasculitis is absent. Granulomas may be found in a small number of cases. Special stains fail to identify pathogenic organisms. Most patients with this disease have responded to local radiotherapy.[144] It is possible that this disease is equivalent to benign lymphocytic angiitis of the lung.[142,144,145]

In most cases of malignant lymphoma, the diagnosis can be made histologically without difficulty. However, the lymphoma cells may be obscured in heavily inflamed tumors. Occasionally, a malignant epithelial neoplasm may be considered in the differential diagnosis but can be ruled out by appropriate immunohistochemical studies.

Other Nonepithelial Tumors

Other nonepithelial tumors, including *malignant histiocytosis, Ewing's sarcoma, chondromas, chondrosarcomas, leiomyomas, leiomyosarcomas, lipomas,* and *liposarcomas* may arise in the upper respiratory tract; they have been reviewed elsewhere.[146–150]

REFERENCES

1. Smith CJ, Echevarria R, McLelland CA: Pseudosarcomatous changes in antrochoanal polyps. Arch Otolaryngol 99:228, 1974

2. Compagno J, Hyams VJ, Lepore ML: Nasal polyposis with stromal atypia. Review of follow-up study of 14 cases. Arch Pathol Lab Med 100:224, 1976

3. Berman JM, Colman BH: Nasal aspects of cystic fibrosis in children. J Laryngol Otol 91:133, 1977

4. Hoffman EO, Loose ED, Harkin JC: The Mikulicz cell in rhinoscleroma. Am J Pathol 73:47, 1973

5. Meyer PR, Shum TK, Becker TS, et al: Scleroma (rhinoscleroma). Arch Pathol Lab Med 107:377, 1983

6. Yanagisawa E, Friedman S, Kundargi RS, et al: Rhinocerebral phycomycosis. Laryngoscope 87:1319, 1977

7. Parfrey NA: Improved diagnosis and prognosis of mucormycosis. Clinicopathologic study of 33 cases. Medicine (Baltimore) 65:113, 1986

8. Marchevsky AM, Bottone EJ, Geller SA, et al: The changing spectrum of disease, etiology, and diagnosis of mucormycosis. Hum Pathol 11:457, 1980

9. Sobol SM, Love RG, Stutman HR, et al: Phaeohyphomycosis of the maxilloethmoid sinus caused by *Drechslera spicifera:* A new fungal pathogen. Laryngoscope 94:620, 1984

10. Padhye AA, Ajello L, Wieden MA, et al: Phaeohyphomycosis of the nasal sinuses caused by a new species of *Exserohilum.* J Clin Microbiol 24:245, 1986

11. McGill TJ, Simpson G, Healy GB: Fulminant aspergillosis of the nose and paranasal sinuses: A new clinical entity. Laryngoscope 90:748, 1980

12. Katzenstein AA, Sale SR, Greenberger PA: Pathologic findings in allergic aspergillus sinusitis. Am J Surg Pathol 7:439, 1983

13. Kyriakos M: Myospherulosis of the paranasal sinuses, nose and middle ear. Am J Clin Pathol 67:118, 1977

14. Rosai J: The nature of myospherulosis of the upper respiratory tract. Am J Clin Pathol 69:475, 1978

15. Gordon WW, Cohn AM, Greenberg SD, et al: Nasal sarcoidosis. Arch Otolaryngol 102:11, 1976

16. Maillard AAJ, Geopfert H: Nasal and paranasal sarcoidosis. Arch Otolaryngol 104:197, 1978

17. Miglets AW, Viall JH, Kataria YP: Sarcoidosis of the head and neck. Laryngoscope 87:2038, 1977

18. Kornblut AD, Wolff SM, DeFries HO, et al: Wegener's granulomatosis. Laryngoscope 90:1453, 1980

19. Churg J, Strauss L: Allergic granulomatosis, allergic angiitis, and periarteritis nodosa. Am J Pathol 27:277, 1951

20. Olsen KD, Neel HB III, Deremee RA, et al: Nasal manifestations of allergic granulomatosis and angiitis (Churg-Strauss syndrome). Otolaryngol Head Neck Surg 88:85, 1980

21. Wolff M: Granulomas in nasal mucous membrane following local steroid injections. Am J Clin Pathol 62:775, 1974

22. Burston HH: Lethal midline granuloma, is it a pathologic entity? Laryngoscope 69:1, 1959

23. Abrams AM, Melrose RJ, Howell FV: Necrotizing sialometaplasia. Cancer 32:130, 1973

24. Maisel RH, Johnston WH, Anderson HA, et al: Necrotizing sialometaplasia involving the nasal cavity. Laryngoscope 87:429, 1977

25. Trojussen W, Solberg LA, Hogetveit AC: Histopathologic changes of nasal mucosa in nickel workers. A pilot study. Cancer 44:963, 1979

26. Syrjanen S, Happonen R-P, Virolainen E, et al: Detection of human papillomavirus (HPV) structural antigens and DNA types in inverted papillomas and squamous cell carcinomas of the nasal cavities and paranasal sinuses. Acta Otolaryngol (Stockh) 104:334, 1987

27. Ridolfi RL, Leiberman PH, Erlandson RA, et al: Schneiderian papillomas: A clinicopathologic study of 30 cases. Am J Surg Pathol 1:43, 1977

28. Synder RN, Perzin KH: Papillomatosis of nasal cavity and paranasal sinuses (inverted papilloma, squamous papilloma). Cancer 30:668, 1972

29. Barnes L, Bedetti C: Oncocytic Schneiderian papilloma: A reappraisal of cylindrical cell papilloma of the sinonasal tract. Hum Pathol 15:344, 1984

30. Christensen WN, Smith RR: Schneiderian papillomas: A clinicopathologic study of 67 cases. Hum Pathol 17:393, 1986

31. Kelly JH, Joseph M, Carroll E, et al: Inverted papilloma of the nasal septum. Arch Otolaryngol 106:767, 1980

32. Weissler MC, Montgomery WW, Turner PA, et al: Inverted papilloma. Ann Otol Rhinol Laryngol 95:215, 1986

33. Segal K, Atar E, Mor C, et al: Inverting papilloma of the nose and paranasal sinuses. Laryngoscope 96:394, 1986

34. Calcaterra TC, Thompson JW, Paglia DE: Inverting papillomas of the nose and paranasal sinuses. Laryngoscope 90:53, 1980

35. Kristensen S, Vorre P, Elbrond O, et al: Nasal Schneiderian papillomas: A study of 83 cases. Clin Otolaryngol 10:125, 1985

36. Perzin KH, Lefkowitch JH, Hui RM: Bilateral nasal squamous carcinoma arising in papillomatosis: Report of a case developing after chemotherapy for leukemia. Cancer 48:2375, 1981

37. Compagno J, Wong RT: Intranasal mixed tumors (pleomorphic adenomas): A clinicopathologic study of 40 cases. Am J Clin Pathol 68:213, 1977

38. Luna MA, Mackay B, Gamez-Aranjo J: Myoepithelioma of the palate: Report of a case with histochemical and electron microscopic observations. Cancer 32:1429, 1973

39. Lewis JS, Castro EB: Cancer of the nasal cavity and paranasal sinuses. J Laryngol Otol 86:255, 1972

40. Silverberg E, Lubera JA: Cancer statistics, 1988. CA 38:5, 1988

41. Adams GL, Duval AJ: Adenocarcinoma of the head and neck. Arch Otolaryngol 93:261, 1971

42. Jackson RT, Fitz-Hugh GS, Constable WC: Malignant neoplasms of the nasal cavities and paranasal sinuses. Laryngoscope 87:726, 1977

43. Hopkin N, McNicoll W, Dalley VM, et al: Cancer of the paranasal sinuses and nasal cavities. Part I. Clinical features. J Laryngol Otol 98:585, 1984

44. Bosch A, Vallecillo L, Frias Z: Cancer of the nasal cavity. Cancer 37:1458, 1976

45. Roush GC: Epidemiology of cancer of the nose and paranasal sinuses: current concepts. Head Neck Surg 2:3, 1979

46. Brinton LA, Biot WJ, Becker JA, et al: A case-control study of cancers of the nasal cavity and paranasal sinuses. Am J Epidemiol 119:896, 1984

47. Kligerman M, Lattes R, Rankow R: Carcinoma of the maxillary sinus following thorotrast instillation. Cancer 13:967, 1960

48. Bauer WC: Varieties of squamous carcinoma—biologic behavior. Front Radiat Ther Oncol 9:164, 1974

49. Osborn DA: Nature and behavior of transitional tumors in the upper respiratory tract. Cancer 25:50, 1970

50. Helliwell TR, Yeoch LH, Stell PM: Anaplastic carcinoma of the nose and paranasal sinuses. Light microscopy, immunohistochemistry and clinical correlation. Cancer 58:2038, 1986

51. Frierson HF Jr, Mills SE, Fechner RE, et al: Sinonasal undifferentiated carcinoma. An aggressive neoplasm derived from Schneiderian epithelium and distinct from olfactory neuroblastoma. Am J Surg Pathol 10:771, 1986

52. Piscioli F, Aldovini D, Bondi A, et al: Squamous cell carcinoma with sarcoma-like stroma of the nose and paranasal sinuses: Report of two cases. Histopathology 8:633, 1984

53. Manivel C, Wick MR, Dehner LP: Transitional (cylindric) cell carcinoma with endodermal sinus tumor-like features of the nasopharynx and paranasal sinuses. Clinicopathologic and immunohistochemical study of two cases. Arch Pathol Lab Med 110:198, 1986

54. Rafla S: Mucous gland tumors of paranasal sinuses. Cancer 24:683, 1970

55. Perzin KH, Gullane P, Clairmont AC: Adenoid cystic carcinomas arising in salivary glands: A correlation of histologic features and clinical course. Cancer 42:265, 1978

56. Healey WV, Perzin KH, Smith L: Mucoepidermoid carcinoma of salivary gland origin: Classification, clinical-pathologic correlation, and results of treatment. Cancer 26:368, 1970

57. Gerughty Hennigar GR, Brown FM: Adenosquamous carcinoma of the nasal, oral and laryngeal cavities. Cancer 22:1140, 1968

58. LiVolsi VA, Perzin KH: Malignant mixed tumors arising in salivary glands. Cancer 39:2209, 1977

59. Perzin KH, Cantor JO, Johannessen JV: Acinic cell carcinoma arising in nasal cavity: Report of a case with ultrastructural observations. Cancer 47:1818, 1981

60. Ordonez NG, Batsakis JG: Acinic cell carcinoma of the nasal cavity: electron-optic and immunohistochemical observations. J Laryngol Otol 100:345, 1986

61. Batsakis JG, Holtz F, Sueper RH: Adenocarcinoma of nasal and paranasal cavities. Arch Otolaryngol 77:625, 1963

62. Sanchez CG, Devine KD, Weiland LH: Nasal adenocarcinomas that closely simulate colonic carcinomas. Cancer 28:714, 1971

63. Heffner DK, Hyams VJ, Hauck KW, et al: Low-grade adenocarcinoma of the nasal cavity and paranasal sinuses. Cancer 50:312, 1982

64. Mills SE, Fechner RE, Cantrell RW: Aggressive sinonasal lesion resembling normal intestinal mucosa. Am J Surg Pathol 6:803, 1982

65. Klintenberg C, Ologsson J, Hellquist H, et al: Adenocarcinoma of the ethmoid sinuses. A review of 28 cases with special reference to wood dust exposure. Cancer 54:482, 1984

66. Barnes L: Intestinal-type adenocarcinoma of the nasal cavity and paranasal sinuses. Am J Surg Pathol 10:192, 1986

67. Hoppe RT, Goffinet DR, Bagshaw MA: Carcinoma of the nasopharynx. Cancer 37:2605, 1976

68. Neel HB III: Nasopharyngeal carcinoma. Clinical presentation, diagnosis, treatment, and prognosis. Otolaryngol Clin North Am 18:479, 1985

69. Fedder M, Gonzalez MF: Nasopharyngeal carcinoma. A brief review. Am J Med 79:365, 1985

70. Muir CS: Nasopharyngeal carcinoma in non-Chinese populations with special reference to South-East Asia and Africa. Int J Cancer 8:351, 1971

71. Henderson BE, Louie E, Jing JS, et al: Risk factors associated with nasopharyngeal carcinoma. N Engl J Med 295:1101, 1976

72. Lin TM, Chang HJ, Chen CJ et al: Risk factors for nasopharyngeal carcinoma. Int Cancer Res 6:791, 1986

73. Yeh S: A histological classification of carcinomas of the nasopharynx with a critical review as to the existence of lymphoepitheliomas. Cancer 15:895, 1962

74. Shamugaratnam K, Sobin LH: Histological Typing of Upper Respiratory Tract Tumor. International Histological Classification of Tumors, No 19. World Health Organization, Geneva, 1978

75. Zaatari GS, Santoianni RA: Adenoid squamous cell carcinoma of nasopharynx and neck region. Arch Pathol Lab Med 110:542, 1986

76. Lin HS, Lin CS, Yeh S, et al: Fine structure of nasopharyngeal carcinoma with special reference to the anaplastic type. Cancer 23:390, 1969

77. Taxy JB, Hidvegi EF, Battifora H: Nasopharyngeal carcinoma: Antikeratin immunohistochemistry and electron microscopy. Am J Clin Pathol 83:320, 1985

78. Kamino H, Huang SJ, Fu YS: Keratin and involucrin immunohistochemistry of nasopharyngeal carcinoma. Cancer 61:1142, 1988

79. Baker SR, Wolfe RA: Prognostic factors in nasopharyngeal malignancy. Cancer 49:163, 1982

80. Bernstein JM, Montgomery WW, Balogh K: Metastatic tumors to the maxilla, nose and paranasal sinuses. Laryngoscope 76:621, 1966

81. Karma P, Rasanen O, Karja J: Nasal gliomas. A review and report of two cases. Laryngoscope 87:1169, 1977

82. Patterson K, Kapur S, Chandra RS: "Nasal gliomas" and related brain heterotopias: A pathologist's perspective. Pediatr Pathol 5:353, 1986

83. Seibert RW, Seibert JJ, Jimenez JF, et al: Nasopharyngeal brain heterotopia—a cause of upper airway obstruction in infancy. Laryngoscope 94:818, 1984

84. Bossen EH: Oligodendroglioma arising in heterotopic brain tissue of the soft palate and nasopharynx. Am J Surg Pathol 11:571, 1987

85. Perzin KH, Pushparaj N: Nonepithelial tumors of the nasal cavity, paranasal sinuses, and nasopharynx: A clinico-

pathologic study. XIII. Meningiomas. Cancer 54:1860, 1984

86. Ho KL: Primary meningioma of the nasal cavity and paranasal sinuses. Cancer 46:1442, 1980

87. Lloyd RV, Chandler WF, Kovacs K, et al: Ectopic pituitary adenomas with normal anterior pituitary glands. Am J Surg Pathol 10:546, 1986

88. Lack EL, Cubilla AL, Woodruff JM, et al: Paragangliomas of the head and neck region. Cancer 39:397, 1977

89. Schuller DE, Lucas JG: Nasopharyngeal paraganglioma. Report of a case and review of literature. Arch Otolaryngol 108:667, 1982

90. Apple D, Dreines K: Cushing's syndrome due to ectopic ACTH production by a nasal paraganglioma. Am J Med Sci 283:32, 1982

91. Perzin KH, Panyu H, Wechter S: Nonepithelial tumors of the nasal cavity, paranasal sinuses and nasopharynx: A clinicopathologic study. XII. Schwann cell tumors (neurilemoma, neurofibroma, malignant schwannoma). Cancer 50:2193, 1982

92. Rabitaille Y, Seemayer TA, ElDeiry A: Peripheral nerve tumors involving paranasal sinuses. A case report and review of literature. Cancer 35:1254, 1975

93. Djalilian M, Zujko RD, Weiland LH, et al: Olfactory neuroblastoma. Surg Clin North Am 57:751, 1977

94. Mills SE, Frierson HF Jr: Olfactory neuroblastoma. A clinicopathologic study of 21 cases. Am J Surg Pathol 9:317, 1985

95. Silva EG, Butler JJ, Mackay B, et al: Neuroblastomas and neuroendocrine carcinoma of the nasal cavity: A proposed new classification. Cancer 50:2388, 1982

96. Taxy JB, Hidvegi DF: Olfactory neuroblastoma: An ultrastructural study. Cancer 39:131, 1977

97. Miller DC, Goodman ML, Pilch BZ, et al: Mixed olfactory neuroblastoma and carcinoma. A report of two cases. Cancer 54:2019, 1984

98. Singh W, Ranage C, Best P, et al: Nasal neuroblastoma secreting vasopressin. A case report. Cancer 45:961, 1980

99. Oberman HA, Rice DH: Olfactory neuroblastomas: A clinicopathologic study. Cancer 38:2494, 1976

100. Choi HS, Anderson PJ: Immunohistochemical diagnosis of olfactory neuroblastoma. J Neuropathol Exp Neurol 44:18, 1985

101. Olsen KD, DeSanto LW: Olfactory neuroblastoma. Biologic and clinical behavior. Arch Otolaryngol 109:797, 1983

102. Siwersson U, Kindblom LG: Oncocytic carcinoid of the nasal cavity and carcinoid of the lung in a child. Pathol Res Pract 178:562, 1984

103. Kameya T, Shimosato Y, Adachi I et al: Neuroendocrine carcinoma of the paranasal sinus. Cancer 45:330, 1980

104. Cove H: Melanosis, melanocytic hyperplasia and primary malignant melanoma of the nasal cavity. Cancer 44:1424, 1979

105. Conley J, Pack GT: Melanoma of the mucous membrane of the head and neck. Arch Otolaryngol 99:315, 1974

106. Conley J, Hamaker RC: Melanoma of the head and neck. Laryngoscope 87:760, 1977

107. Trapp TK, Fu YS, Calcaterra TC: Melanoma of the nasal and paranasal sinus mucosa. Arch Otolaryngol 113:1086, 1987

108. Lund V: Malignant melanoma of the nasal cavity and paranasal sinuses. J Laryngol Otol 96:347, 1982

109. Chaudhry AP, Lore JM, Fisher JE, et al: So-called hairy polyps or teratoid tumors of the nasopharynx. Arch Otolaryngol 104:517, 1978

110. Lack EE: Extragonadal germ cell tumors of the head and neck region: review of 16 cases. Hum Pathol 16:56, 1985

111. Heffner DK, Hyams VJ: Teratocarcinosarcoma (malignant teratoma?) of the nasal cavity and paranasal sinuses. A clinicopathologic study of 20 cases. Cancer 53:2140, 1984

112. Shanmugaratnam K, Kunaratnam N, Chia KB, et al: Teratoid carcinosarcoma of the paranasal sinuses. Pathology 15:413, 1983

113. Fu YS, Perzin KH: Non-epithelial tumors of the nasal cavity, paranasal sinuses and nasopharynx: A clinicopathologic study. I. General features and vascular tumors. Cancer 33:1275, 1974

114. Conley J, Healey WV, Blaugrund SM, et al: Nasopharyngeal angiofibroma in the juvenile. Surg Gynecol Obstet 126:825, 1968

115. Bremer JW, Neel HB, DeSanto LW, et al: Angiofibroma: Treatment trends in 150 patients during 40 years. Laryngoscope 96:1321, 1986

116. Chen KT, Bauer FW: Sarcomatous transformation for nasopharyngeal angiofibroma. Cancer 49:369, 1982

117. Sarma DP: Angiosarcoma of the nose. Arch Dermatol 116:226, 1980

118. Compagno J, Hyams VJ: Hemangiopericytoma-like intranasal tumors. A clinicopathologic study of 23 cases. Am J Clin Pathol 66:672, 1976

119. Wick MR, Banks PM, McDonald TJ: Angioendotheliomatosis of the nose with fatal systemic dissemination. Cancer 48:2510, 1981

120. Fu YS, Perzin KH: Non-epithelial tumors of the nasal cavity, paranasal sinuses and nasopharynx: A clinicopathologic study. II. Osseous and fibro-osseous lesions, including osteoma, fibrous dysplasia, ossifying fibroma, osteoblastoma, giant cell tumor and osteosarcoma. Cancer 33:1289, 1974

121. DeMello DE, Archer CR, Blair JD: Ethmoidal fibro-osseous lesion in a child. Diagnostic and therapeutic problems. Am J Surg Pathol 4:595, 1980

122. Margo CE, Weiss A, Habal MB: Psammomatoid ossifying fibroma. Arch Ophthalmol 104:1347, 1986

123. Perzin KH, Fu YS: Non-epithelial tumors of the nasal cavity, paranasal sinuses and nasopharynx: A clinicopathologic study. XI. Fibrous histiocytoma. Cancer 45:616, 1980

124. Heffelfinger MJ, Dahlin DC, MacCarty CS, et al: Chordomas and cartilaginous tumors at the skull base. Cancer 32:410, 1973

125. Perzin KH, Pushparaj N: Nonepithelial tumors of the nasal cavity, paranasal sinuses, and nasopharynx: A clinicopathologic study. XIV Chordomas. Cancer 57:784, 1986

126. Fu YS, Perzin KH: Non-epithelial tumors of the nasal cavity, paranasal sinuses and nasopharynx: A clinicopathologic study. VI. Fibrous tissue tumors. Cancer 37:2912, 1976

127. Wold LE, Weiland LH: Tumefactive fibro-inflammatory lesions of the head and neck. Am J Surg Pathol 7:477, 1983

128. Fu YS, Perzin KH: Non-epithelial tumors of the nasal cavity, paranasal sinuses and nasopharynx: A clinicopathologic study. VII. Myxomas. Cancer 39:195, 1977

129. White DK, Chin SY, Mohnac AM, et al: Odontogenic myxoma. A clinical and ultrastructural study. Oral Surg 39:901, 1975

130. Fu YS, Perzin KH: Non-epithelial tumors of the nasal cavity, paranasal sinuses and nasopharynx: A clinicopathologic study. V. Skeletal muscle tumors (rhabdomyoma and rhabdomyosarcoma). Cancer 37:364, 1976

131. Schlosnagle DC, Kratochvil FJ, Weathers DR, et al: Intraoral multifocal adult rhabdomyoma. Report of a case and review of the literature. Arch Pathol Lab Med 107:638, 1983

132. Gale N, Rott T, Kambic V: Nasopharyngeal rhabdomyoma. Report of case (light and electron microscopic studies) and review of the literature. Pathol Res Pract 178:454, 1984

133. Feldman BA: Rhabdomyosarcoma of the head and neck. Laryngoscope 92:424, 1982

134. Fu YS, Perzin KH: Non-epithelial tumors of the nasal cavity, paranasal sinuses and nasopharynx: A clinicopathologic study. IX. Plasmacytoma. Cancer 42:2399, 1978

135. Fu YS, Perzin KH: Non-epithelial tumors of the nasal cavity, paranasal sinuses and nasopharynx: A clinicopathologic study. X. Malignant lymphomas and midline malignant reticulosis. Cancer 43:611, 1979

136. Frierson HF Jr, Mills SE, Innes DJ Jr: Non-Hodgkin's lymphomas of the sinonasal region: Histologic subtypes and their clinicopathologic features. Am J Clin Pathol 81:721, 1984

137. Robbins KT, Fuller LM, Vlasak M, et al: Primary lymphomas of the nasal cavity and paranasal sinuses. Cancer 56:814, 1985

138. Kapadia SB, Barnes L, Deutsch M: Non-Hodgkin's lymphoma of the nose and paranasal sinuses: A study of 17 cases. Head Neck Surg 3:490, 1981

139. Yamanaka N, Harabuchi Y, Sambe S, et al: Non-Hodgkin's lymphoma of Waldeyer's ring and nasal cavity. Clinical and immunologic aspects. Cancer 56:768, 1985

140. Kassel SH, Echevarria RA, Guzzo FP: Midline malignant reticulosis (so-called lethal midline granuloma). Cancer 23:920, 1969

141. Eichel BS, Harrison EG, Devine KD, et al: Primary lymphoma of the nose including a relationship to lethal midline granuloma. Am J Surg 112:597, 1966

142. Crissman JD, Weiss MA, Gluckman J: Midline granuloma syndrome: A clinicopathologic study of 13 patients. Am J Surg Pathol 65:335, 1982

143. Ishii Y, Yamanaka N, Ogawa K, et al: Nasal T-cell lymphoma as a type of so-called "lethal midline granuloma." Cancer 50:2336, 1982

144. Tsokos M, Fauci AS, Costa J: Idiopathic midline destructive disease (IMDD): A subgroup of patients with the "midline granuloma" syndrome. Am J Clin Pathol 77:162, 1982

145. Saldana MJ, Patchefsky AS, Israel HI, Atkinson GW: Pulmonary angiitis and granulomatosis. The relationship between histologic features, organ involvement, and response to treatment. Hum Pathol 4:391, 1977

146. Fu YS, Perzin KH: Non-epithelial tumors of the nasal cavity, paranasal sinuses and nasopharynx: A clinicopathologic study. III. Cartilaginous tumors (chondroma and chondrosarcoma). Cancer 34:453, 1974

147. Fu YS, Perzin KH: Non-epithelial tumors of the nasal cavity, paranasal sinuses and nasopharynx: A clinicopathologic study. IV. Smooth muscle tumors (leiomyoma and leiomyosarcoma). Cancer 35:1300, 1975

148. Fu YS, Perzin KH: Non-epithelial tumors of the nasal cavity, paranasal sinuses and nasopharynx. A clinicopathologic study. VIII. Lipoma and liposarcoma. Cancer 40:1314, 1977

149. Aozasa K: Biopsy findings in malignant histiocytosis presenting as lethal midline granuloma. J Clin Pathol 35:599, 1982

150. Pontius KI, Sebek BA: Extraskeletal Ewing's sarcoma arising in the nasal fossa. Light- and electron-microscopic observations. Am J Clin Pathol 75:410, 1981

18

The Larynx and Trachea

William J. Frable
Mary Ann S. Frable

SPECIMEN HANDLING

Endoscopy is invariably required in establishing a diagnosis of laryngeal and tracheal disease in the presence of any mass lesion. Appropriate biopsy specimens must be taken within a confined space. They are often small and need both precise clinical information, particularly location, and orientation, so that they may be cut perpendicular to the mucosal surface. Affixing small biopsy specimens from these sites on suitable material or using a hand lens at the time of embedding should result in the correct orientation. Biopsy specimens should be appropriately fixed in buffered formalin (usually suitable for most immunohistochemistry) and cut at multiple levels, a minimum of three initially.

Total laryngectomy with or without radical neck dissection provides the most common major specimen received. Specimens for frozen section examination are submitted from these cases for determination of tumor-free margins (the trachea and in the case of supraglottic neoplasms, extension to the base of the tongue, tonsil, pyriform sinus, and wall of the pharynx). Surgeons should avoid submitting margins for frozen section examination separately. It is preferable to complete the resection and then allow the surgical pathologist to view the entire gross specimen for proper orientation and selection of critical margins. Sections should be perpendicular to the nearest point of gross tumor involvement, including the deepest penetration. The free margin should be marked with India ink before freezing to afford the proper orientation in reviewing the subsequently prepared slides. A fast hematoxylin and eosin (H&E) stain is required for a detailed assessment of the margins in terms of diagnosing dysplasia or carcinoma in situ (CIS). A gross margin of less than 5 mm is probably inadequate. There is, however, no evidence in the literature documenting the efficacy of frozen section review of margins in the subsequent management or outcome of the patients with carcinoma of the larynx. A well planned surgical attack with a grossly adequate margin is a more practical approach.

A radical neck dissection specimen is best examined in the fresh state while the larynx is best processed after fixation. Lymph nodes are easier to discriminate from fat and connective tissue within fresh tissue. Nodes are dissected free, and the capsule is sectioned to allow proper penetration of fixative. Consistency is the most important part of labeling lymph nodes from radical neck dissections. We prefer a numerical system referring to levels. Submaxillary salivary gland and nodes are labeled level I. Nodes from the jugular chain are divided into three equal portions from the superior to the inferior: nodes from the upper portion are labeled level II, those from the middle part level III, and those from the lower segment level IV. (The tip of the parotid salivary gland may be included in level II.) Nodes from the posterior cervical chain are labeled level V. Juxathyroid nodes, if they are part of the neck dissection, are labeled level VI, while paratracheal, paraesophageal, and superior mediastinal nodes are labeled level VII (Fig. 18-1). If grossly positive nodes are found, only two from that level need to be submitted, but all questionable and grossly negative nodes should be submitted from other levels.[1]

An alternative method for labeling lymph nodes from radical neck dissections is to identify them strictly by anatomic location. A neck chart should be submitted with

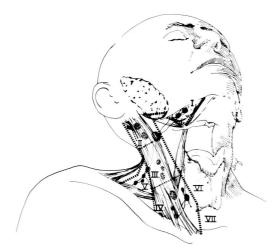

Fig. 18-1. Diagram of lymph node levels from a radical neck dissection.

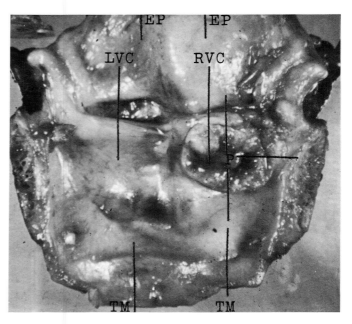

Fig. 18-2. Standard sections that should be submitted from a typical laryngectomy specimen for squamous cell carcinoma of the right true vocal cord with subglottic extension. (Abbreviations: P, primary tumor; RVC, right vocal cord; LVC, left vocal cord; EP, epiglottis; TM, tracheal margin.) Sections from the thyroid and parathyroids, if present, should also be submitted.

the final pathology report, and the positive nodes should be indicated on the chart. Appropriate anatomic terms are: submental, submaxillary, facial (lower border of the jaw), preauricular, parotid, jugular supraomohyoid, jugular infraomohyoid (referring to the muscle), spinal accessory, supraclavicular, pretracheal, and mastoid (behind the ear). The standard radical neck specimen typically includes only the submaxillary, jugular supra- and infraomohyoid, and spinal accessory nodes.

A laryngectomy specimen received for a diagnosis of tumor is opened posteriorly, spread with wooden applicator sticks, and then fixed in formalin. It is usually necessary to crack the thyroid cartilage to open the specimen adequately for fixation. A Polaroid photograph of the fixed larynx taken before section selection is valuable; the sections taken with their orientation may be diagrammed directly on the photograph (Fig. 18-2). Standard sections for a carcinoma of the larynx would include: (1) two to four sections of the primary tumor, demonstrating its depth as well as its superior and inferior margins and including a portion of normal mucosa; (2) one section each of the right and left vocal cords (a portion that is not involved by tumor); (3) a section of the epiglottis; (4) one section of each lobe of the thyroid; (5) one section of any parathyroids discovered; and (6) sections of the tracheal margins and superior margins, particularly the areas at the base of the tongue or wherever gross tumor approximates the line of excision. With a deeply invasive lesion it may be necessary to decalcify the bony and cartilaginous portions of the larynx to document invasion or penetration.

Vertical hemilaryngectomy specimens may be submitted in some glottic carcinomas. The total specimen should be assessed grossly before any attempt at frozen section control of the margins. The relationship between the tumor and its margins is easily destroyed with this type of specimen and compromises the final interpretation with respect to the completeness of the resection. Only the nearest gross margin to the tumor should be taken and then only if a definite therapeutic decision for more surgery is immediately required. This margin should be carefully marked with India ink before sectioning so that it may subsequently be reoriented to the total specimen. If there is a gross tumor-free margin, we believe strongly that the whole specimen should be fixed and that sections should be taken stepwise and perpendicular to the vocal cord to examine the entire mucosa.

EMBRYOLOGY, ANATOMY, AND HISTOLOGY

The beginnings of the respiratory tract, the laryngotracheal groove, are found in the 20 somite (3 mm) embryo. This structure runs lengthwise in the floor of the gut just distal to the pharyngeal pouches. Its epithelium is therefore endodermal in origin, and its supporting connective tissue, striated muscle, and cartilage are derived from mesoderm. All the cartilage and both the intrinsic and extrinsic muscles of the larynx arise from the mesenchyme of the fourth and fifth branchial arches. Because of this origin, the innervation of the muscles of the larynx is primarily through branches of the vagus nerve.[2]

The trachea elongates rapidly during early fetal development, descending nearly eight body segments. The endodermally derived columnar epithelium differentiates into a pseudostratified and a ciliated columnar epithelium throughout the trachea and larynx, excluding the aryepiglottic folds laterally and ventrally, the lingual side of the epiglottis and the upper half of its laryngeal aspect, the vocal folds (true vocal cords), and the upper points of the arytenoid cartilages. These mucosal surfaces are covered by a stratified squamous epithelium. There is a transitional zone of stratified columnar epithelium between adjacent areas of pseudostratified columnar and stratified squamous mucosa.[2,3]

The seromucous glands found throughout the larynx and trachea are derived by invagination of the covering columnar epithelium. They are prominently displayed along the aryepiglottic and ventricular folds and within the lamina propria of the ventricle. A few may be found within the base of the vocal folds. These glands are usually confined to the submucosa, superficial to the lamina propria, but may penetrate the cartilaginous tissue of the epiglottis.[3] Like their counterparts found throughout the oral cavity, they are referred to as aberrant salivary glands. They may give rise to salivary gland–type tumors, hence their importance to the surgical pathologist.

in time after admission to respiratory intensive care, ventilatory assistance, and endotracheal intubation suggests a possible patient to patient transmission through the use of such equipment. An acute bacterial tracheitis may occur in children. The disease can be a medical emergency requiring intubation.[18]

Chronic laryngitis, whose etiology in the past has been attributed to overuse of the voice, today is more commonly associated with continuous exposure to irritating fumes and dust, alcohol abuse, and cigarette smoking. Histologically, a chronic inflammatory exudate is seen. Of more importance are the epithelial alterations (hypertrophy, hyperkeratosis, and regeneration and repair atypia) that must be differentiated from carcinoma (Fig. 18-3). The symptom of hoarseness and the clinical appearance of the vocal cords, with thickening and opacity of the epithelium, strongly suggest preneoplasia or early carcinoma. Biopsy specimens fail to show truly dysplastic cells.

Chronic laryngitis and tracheitis may also be granulomatous, indicating tuberculosis, leprosy, but more commonly a mycotic etiology.[10,19–21] Caseating granulomas strongly suggest tuberculosis, since tuberculoid leprosy is quite rare in the larynx. That structure is involved by the nodular form, with abundant acid-fast organisms demonstrated by special stains (Fite-Faraco).[10,22] Cases of both sarcoidosis and tuberculosis of the trachea are most often extensions from involved mediastinal lymph nodes.[19,23] Blastomycosis of the larynx produces a

NON-NEOPLASTIC CONDITIONS

Inflammatory and Degenerative Disease

The surgical pathologist is seldom involved in the diagnosis of acute laryngitis and epiglottitis.[4–12] Tracheostomy and intubation are sometimes required to treat these conditions. Biopsy specimens of resulting granulation tissue forming either at the site of the tracheostomy or in the subglottic area after intubation may be submitted to the surgical pathologist. Typically featured is a polypoid mass of capillary blood vessels, fibrin, and acute inflammatory cells. Abundant granulation tissue in this situation can lead to laryngeal and tracheal stenosis.[13–15]

Physical agents, particularly thermal burns, produce acute inflammation of the larynx and trachea as part of a generalized effect on the respiratory tract. Secretions submitted for cytologic study from these cases can show severe atypia of regeneration and repair.[16]

Cytologic evidence of herpesvirus may also be found.[17] The infection in the larynx and trachea seems to be incidental in the debilitated immunosuppressed patient who develops acute tracheobronchitis. The clustering of cases

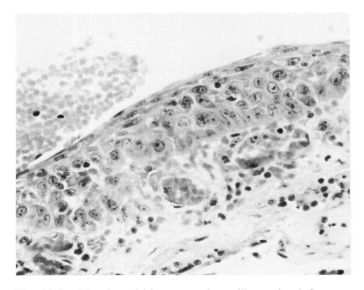

Fig. 18-3. Vocal cord biopsy specimen illustrating inflammatory atypia with active but uniform nuclei. The most prominent feature of these cells is the large nucleoli. The chromatin is bland. Polarity of the cells is only minimally altered. Compare with Fig. 18-6.

marked pseudoepitheliomatous hyperplasia with both acute and chronic inflammation and intraepithelial abscesses. Histoplasmosis evolves as a granulomatous reaction similar to tuberculosis.[20] Of the saprophytic fungi, *Candida albicans* (*Monilia albicans*) is the most likely organism to involve mucosal surfaces of the larynx and trachea as well as the oral cavity. Persistence of candidal infection may be a manifestation of immunosuppression. If oral infection by *Candida* extends to the pharynx, trachea, and/or esophagus, investigation for acquired immune deficiency syndrome (AIDS) should be pursued.[24,25] One case of a fungus ball attributed to candidiasis has been reported in the trachea.[26]

In addition to specific granulomatous disease, other inflammatory and degenerative lesions in the larynx or trachea may form tumorous masses.[27] Rheumatoid arthritis may involve formation at the cricoarytenoid joint of a typical rheumatoid nodule with palisaded epithelioid cells and fibrinoid necrosis.[28] We have seen two cases of gouty tophi of the vocal cord producing a mass and hoarseness.[29] The larynx may also be involved in Wegener's granulomatosis. In two cases, biopsy of a subglottic mass revealed necrotizing granulomas with vasculitis.[30]

So-called amyloid tumors that result in a vocal cord nodule are not composed of true amyloid; however, the larynx and the trachea may be involved by the deposition of true amyloid.[19,31–33] In one unrecognized case of amyloidosis of the trachea, removal of the polypoid masses of amyloid led to fatal tracheal hemorrhage.[34]

Cysts

Cystic masses in the trachea and larynx may be divided into those that are true epithelium-lined structures and those that are herniations of the laryngeal ventricle, termed *laryngoceles*. The latter are both internal (intrinsic to the larynx and presenting with dyspnea and hoarseness) and external (manifesting as a soft tissue mass in the neck). There are also combined forms. True cysts may be lined by either glandular or squamous epithelium, whereas the laryngocele is usually lined by glandular epithelium unless squamous metaplasia occurs. Those cysts arising in the adult result from duct obstruction and retention or from traumatic inclusion of epithelium. Similar cysts may arise in the newborn (congenital cysts) and cause acute airway obstruction.[35,36] Some cysts are also

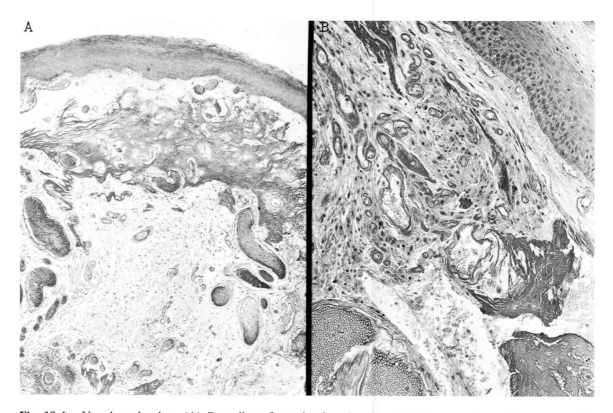

Fig. 18-4. Vocal cord polyp. **(A)** Overall configuration is polypoid, with fibrous and myxoid stroma at the base and varicose and fibrinoid areas beneath the squamous epithelium. **(B)** Details of the fibrinoid and varicose foci.

lined by oncocytic epithelium, but these are not considered to be true neoplasms.[37,38]

Pseudotumors

The *laryngeal nodule*, or *singer's node*, is one of the most common lesions seen by the surgical pathologist. It is attributed to constant irritation of the vocal cord, usually by chronic misuse of the voice. Traditionally four stages—fibrous, polypoid, varicose, and fibrinoid or amyloid—are described, which intermingle and overlap. Initially, a fibrous thickening of the true vocal cord involving Reinke's layer occurs. Thin-walled vessels exude increased amounts of fluid, producing a polypoid projection of the vocal cord followed by thinning of the overlying squamous mucosa. The vessels dilate and there is focal hemorrhage, which with organization evolves to the amyloid stage. This substance is not true amyloid, as demonstrated by either special stains or electron microscopy.[10,35] Several composite examples are illustrated in Figure 18-4.

Pseudolymphomas, very rare masses composed of lymphoid tissue, may arise in the upper respiratory tract as well as in other sites.[35,39,40] These pseudotumors show lymphoid tissue with well developed germinal centers. The presence of this exuberant lymphoid collection in the adult has been cause for concern, since true malignant lymphomas do occur in the larynx and upper respiratory tract. The pseudolymphoma also contains a mixture of plasma cells and lymphocytes. Reaction of the overlying squamous epithelium also occurs, producing both acanthosis and hyperkeratosis. This extends into the crypts, giving the appearance of misplaced or greatly hypertrophied tonsillar tissue.[35,39]

NEOPLASMS

Benign Epithelial Neoplasms

The *squamous papilloma* is the most common and important entity among the benign neoplasms of the larynx and trachea. Histologically, it is an easily recognized proliferation of squamous epithelium of the malpighian layer overlying a thin, fibrovascular connective tissue stalk. Squamous papillomas comprise approximately one sixth of the tumors of the larynx and about one eighth of the neoplasms of the trachea.[35] There are two clinical forms, juvenile and adult; in children, the tumors are frequently multiple, whereas in adults they usually are single.[41-43] Two major etiologies have been postulated: endocrine factors (because of the disappearance of the childhood form at puberty) and viral infections.[42] There is a distinct

difference between the juvenile and adult forms in that viral particles have been demonstrated by some investigators but not others in the juvenile form.

A recent report takes issue with the existence of two different forms or with any etiology other than viral infection. Abramson et al.[44] tested 26 patients with laryngeal papillomas for human papillomavirus (HPV) DNA by Southern blot hybridization and found it to be present in all 26. In 11 of 14 cases latent HPV DNA was also detected in clinically uninvolved tissue. Type 6 or type 11 HPV accounted for 92 percent of the cases examined. The authors also reported no correlation with histopathology, age of onset or the clinical pattern of recurrence and remission. They did not find any specific histopathology or clinical features with respect to the type of HPV infection.[44] Transmissibility has been proved experimentally with the juvenile form.[44] Despite a history of maternal genital infection documented in Abramson's series, it is curious that HPV type 6 is more common in genital papillomas than HPV 11, which is the reverse of the situation in the larynx.[44] Malignant transformation, except for the juvenile form treated by irradiation, has been extremely rare.[45,46]

Recurrence of papillomas after local treatment is quite frequent and may occur rapidly in children.[47] While malignant transformation in the juvenile form has been documented in nonirradiated cases, the real threat is the spread of the process throughout the larynx and trachea, multiple recurrences, and sudden asphyxiation. A diffuse form involving the larynx, including not only the glottic but also vestibular areas with extension into the subglottic area and trachea, is found predominantly in younger children. It is very severe.[41,42] The localized form, if it involves the anterior segments of the vocal cords or the anterior commissure, tends to have a good prognosis, with fewer recurrences.

Malignant degeneration, the most serious complication of papilloma, is heralded by proliferation of dysplastic and frankly anaplastic cells. There is also hyperkeratosis and individual cell dyskaryosis with the presence of mitotic figures, some of which may be atypical.[35] With prolonged lesions, nearly exclusively in adults, malignant change becomes more common, being reported in up to 20 percent of cases. The histologic features of a typical case with areas of dysplasia are illustrated in Figure 18-5. As in any papillary neoplasm, invasion is difficult to evaluate unless a biopsy is done at the base of the stalk, along with the removal of the tumor itself.

The varieties of therapy, which include laser, electrodesiccation, cryotherapy, and continued re-excisions, confirm the difficulty of treatment. The objective is removal of tumor without destruction of the larynx and trachea. The use of radiation therapy has been condemned because of a documented increase in malignant

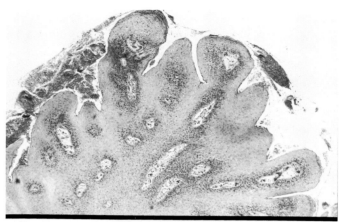

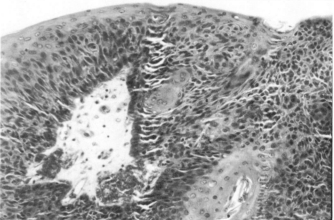

Fig. 18-5. Single squamous cell papilloma of the larynx in an adult. Papillary configuration is obvious in the upper panel. Higher magnification (lower panel) demonstrates areas of mild to moderate dysplasia within the papilloma.

transformation, particularly with juvenile papillomatosis.[46–50]

Hyperplasias, Precancerous Lesions, Carcinoma in Situ

The larynx is unique in that very minimal alterations of the vocal cords will produce symptoms. Therefore the surgical pathologist is likely to see biopsy specimens from a variety of hyperplastic and preneoplastic epithelium unless the patient totally ignores the symptom of hoarseness. A simple classification of epithelial alteration is as follows: (1) keratosis, including hyperkeratosis, hyperplasia, and parakeratosis; (2) keratosis with atypia; and (3) CIS. An alternative term for keratosis with atypia is *dysplasia.* Hyperplasia combined with keratosis shows thickening of the squamous epithelium and surface keratinization, which may be orthokeratotic or parakeratotic.

There is subjectivity in evaluating the degree of cellular atypia in any dysplastic (keratosis with atypia) epithelium, but these biopsies are the most important to access. There is usually thickening of the epithelium, but not invariably. There is cellular alteration, initially confined to the base of the epithelium. Later, with increasing individual cell atypia, more layers of the epithelium are involved. Individual cells and nuclei are irregular in shape and size, and nuclei have a granular irregular chromatin distribution. Accompanying nuclear abnormalities, there is a loss of polarity of the individual cells within the epithelium. In summary, there is a variable irregularity with respect both to individual cells and to cells in relation to each other. A number of comparative examples are found in Figure 18-6; these may be regarded as dysplastic reactions of mild, moderate, and severe degree.[51]

Severe dysplasia overlaps with CIS of the larynx, making that diagnosis also subjective. The full-thickness involvement of intraepithelial neoplasia is seldom seen in laryngeal mucosa, unlike classical carcinoma in situ of the cervix. There is almost always surface keratinization and or parakeratosis. Judgment as to the malignant potential of the epithelium must often be made without a full-thickness epithelial alteration (examples are shown in Figures 18-7 and 18-8). The interpretative problem is further compounded by the projections of neoplastic epithelium, still connected to the surface, into the underlying stroma. Biased cuts will appear to isolate these neoplastic fragments, thereby leading to a false diagnosis of either microscopic or frankly invasive carcinoma. The fact that surface keratinization is present throughout the whole spectrum of dysplasia, CIS, and microinvasive carcinoma makes a confident distinction between a well differentiated, frankly invasive squamous carcinoma and a severe dysplasia sometimes quite difficult. Information about what the otolaryngologist actually saw is extremely important in making a correct diagnosis with any laryngeal biopsy.

In two reports using the terms *hyperkeratosis* and *hyperkeratosis with atypia,* 2 of 65 patients with hyperkeratosis were found to develop carcinoma, versus 13 of 99 with hyperkeratosis plus atypia. The intervals ranged from 6 months to 8 years after the original diagnosis of keratosis.[52,53] Other reports also suggest that there is a considerable difference in what is histologically diagnosed as carcinoma in situ.[54]

A recent study has attempted to reduce the subjectivity of diagnosis of laryngeal squamous cell carcinoma and preneoplasia by using DNA cytophotometry. Results of DNA analysis agreed with histologic interpretation in all cases of definitively benign or malignant lesions. DNA algorithms identified four cases within the group of mild to moderate epithelial dysplasias of the larynx that were proven to be malignant at either follow-up or from an-

Fig. 18-6. Composite photomicrograph of vocal cord biopsy specimens demonstrating dysplasia. **(A)** Mild dysplasia with thin but hyperkeratotic epithelium. Atypical cells occupy the lower one third of the epithelium, are hyperchromatic, vary in size and shape, and have some altered polarity. **(B)** Mild dysplasia with pronounced thickening of the epithelium and parakeratosis. There is minimal nuclear atypia, some individual cell keratinization, and slight alteration of polarity. **(C)** Moderate dysplasia with hyperkeratotic and parakeratotic but thin epithelium. There is altered polarity and nuclei with more distinct chromatin structure demonstrating some variability in size and shape. Downward growth suggests substantial biologic activity. Invasive carcinoma may occur without evolution through full-thickness neoplastic epithelium of classical CIS. **(D)** Moderate dysplasia and marked thickening of the epithelium with hyperkeratosis and parakeratosis. Atypical cells involve about one-half to two-thirds of the epithelium. Biased cuts may isolate portions of the epithelium, suggesting well differentiated invasive squamous cell carcinoma. **(E)** Borderline lesion classified as severe dysplasia. Thin epithelium with marked individual cell atypia and altered polarity essentially reaching to the surface of the biopsy specimen. **(F)** Severe dysplasia with marked thickening of the epithelium and substantial individual nuclear atypia in size, shape, and chromatin structure. This lesion is definitely borderline and could be considered carcinoma in situ.

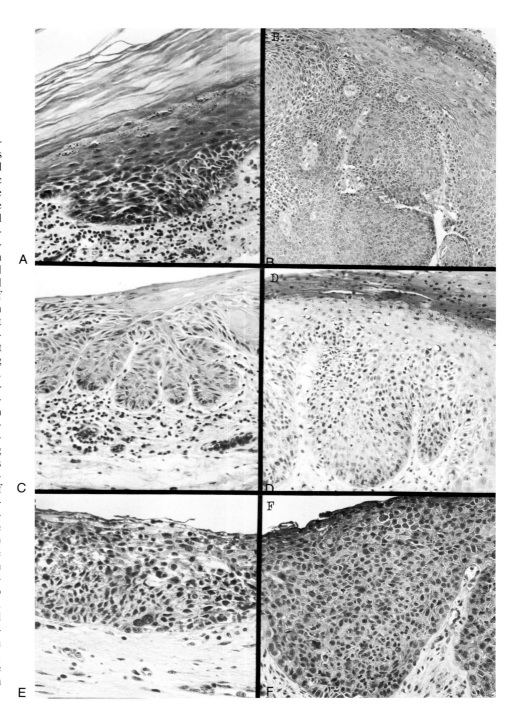

other biopsy site within the larynx. DNA measurements also divided the cases of squamous cell carcinoma into two distinct groups based on their survival.[55]

Regardless of the terminology or subjectivity of the diagnosis, the importance of CIS can be noted from studies in which the mucosa has been examined adjacent to frank invasive carcinoma. Bauer,[56] for example, in 354 cases found that 76 percent had carcinoma in situ spreading widely from adjacent invasive carcinoma of the nonkeratinizing variety, whereas 26 percent had CIS that was not far from the edges of a visible keratinizing carcinoma. Experience with cord stripping as reported by Miller and Fisher[57] also substantiates the importance of carcinoma in situ. They reported 25 patients among

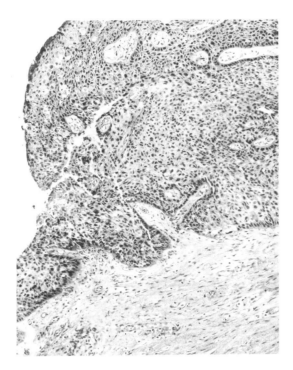

Fig. 18-7. Vocal cord biopsy specimen demonstrating carcinoma in situ without full-thickness epithelial change. Enough individual cells in this epithelium were considered neoplastic to classify the lesion as CIS rather than severe dysplasia. Irregular downgrowth and beginning of exophytic proliferation suggest even an early invasive tumor rather than dysplasia or CIS.

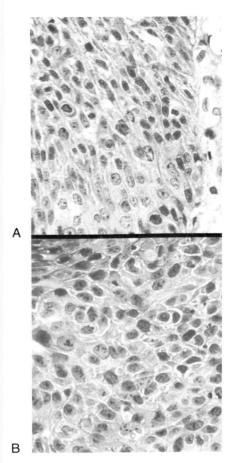

Fig. 18-8. Two vocal cord biopsy specimens illustrating carcinoma in situ with full-thickness neoplasia. In **(A)** the cells are spindle-shaped with poorly defined cell boundaries. The cells in **(B)** have more cytoplasm but greater variation in size and shape and altered polarity.

whom the reappearance of carcinoma was invasive in 13 and in situ in 12. All these studies have implications in the treatment of stage I carcinomas of the larynx in view of the popularity of hemilaryngectomy.

Malignant Epithelial Tumors

Squamous Cell Carcinoma

Squamous cell carcinoma of the larynx is overwhelmingly the most common malignant epithelial neoplasm of the upper respiratory tract. Primary squamous cell carcinoma of the trachea is quite rare.[35] Laryngeal squamous cancer is closely related to cigarette smoking and alcohol consumption.[58] Cigarettes and alcohol together create a powerful carcinogenic effect throughout the respiratory tract, particularly on the larynx.[59] Intrathecally administered polynuclear hydrocarbons in experimental animals will induce laryngeal tumors, including carcinomas. Cigarette smoke inhalation causes preneoplastic and early neoplastic lesions of the larynx, including some invasive carcinomas.[58]

Clinical carcinoma of the larynx is staged by the TNM system of the American Joint Committee for Cancer

Staging and End Results Reporting.[60] The endolarynx is divided into three regions in order to provide for appropriate treatment and prognosis: (1) the *supraglottic* compartment, which includes the laryngeal surface, arytenoids, epiglottis including its tip, aryepiglottic fold, ventricular bands (false vocal cords), and the mucosa of the ventricle; (2) the *glottic* compartment, which includes the true vocal cords and the anterior commissure; and (3) the *subglottic* compartment, which includes the area below the vocal cords to the level of the first tracheal cartilage. Squamous cell carcinomas are classified according to the region in which they arise. Carcinomas are also designated *transglottic* when they extend within all the above areas and below the ventricle.

Studies of whole larynx sections demonstrate that laryngeal carcinomas do not respect arbitrary anatomic boundaries. As pointed out by Olofsson,[61] there are certain weak points through which carcinoma of the larynx will spread, depending on its point of origin. Glottic carcinomas tend to extend vertically but also invade intrinsic laryngeal muscles. The most common site of breakthrough is the thyroid cartilage in the anterior midline. This spread has been frequently found with extension through the cricothyroid membrane anteriorly. Supraglottic carcinomas invade both upward and laterally. Subglottic carcinomas tend to spread up into the thyroarytenoid muscle and also invade the laryngeal cartilages, particularly the cricoid and thyroid. Pre-epiglottic space invasion is quite common among the carcinomas arising on the epiglottis. This is uncommon if the supraglottic tumor arises on the ventricular bands without involvement of the epiglottic cartilage. In summary, clinical methods do not permit accurate assessment of deep invasion of larynx cancer and tend to underestimate it substantially.[61] Carcinoma of the trachea is even more lethal because it is relatively silent until clinically manifest at an advanced stage.[62,63]

Squamous cell carcinoma histologically is either keratinizing or nonkeratinizing. Clinical differences and biologic behavior are summarized in Table 18-1. The non-keratinizing carcinoma has extensive intramusocal neoplasia and pushing margins rather than predominantly infiltrating margins as seen with keratinizing carcinoma. Hence, study of margins is much more likely to be significant in the presence of nonkeratinizing squamous cell carcinoma.[56]

Prognostic Pathology of Squamous Cell Carcinoma of the Larynx

As part of the Centennial Conference on Laryngeal Cancer, an entire workshop was devoted to pathologic features of prognostic importance in determining the outcome of squamous cell carcinoma of the larynx.[64-69,70] Michaels[64] noted that microscopic differentiation of squa-

mous cell cancer of the larynx into well, moderately well, and poorly differentiated types correlates well with clinical prognosis. The quantitative method of Broders' classification did not correlate any better and is more time-consuming. Michaels noted increased differentiation of squamous tumors after radiation therapy and chemotherapy (bleomycin) both in clinical practice and with an experimental system. This was felt to be due to selective destruction of less differentiated tumor cells. Fisher[65] reported on the grading of biopsy specimens with respect to the grade of the entire tumor. He observed that biopsy specimens tended to be undergraded. Jakobson[66] used a more sophisticated grading system, reporting upon eight morphologic criteria, of which four represent the tumor cell population (structure, differentiation, nuclear polymorphism, and mitoses) and four the tumor-host relationship (mode of invasion, stage of invasion, vascular invasion, and host cellular response). A multivariate analysis and prediction of 5-year results showed an excellent correlation. In Jakobsson's series and that of McGavran and Bauer,[67] infiltrative growth (that is, in strands and cords versus pushing-type margins) also correlated with the presence or absence of lymph node metastasis. This has been confirmed by Kashima,[68] who also found that supraglottic location alone portended a very high likelihood of metastatic involvement of cervical lymph nodes. He described a somewhat different morphologic subdivision of peripheral tumor growth patterns, classifying them as pushing, clubbing, shattering, splintering, and infiltrating. Pushing patterns include clubbing, shattering, and true pushing margin, whereas splintering and infiltrating are considered infiltrating patterns.[69]

More recently, DNA ploidy measurements have been correlated with prognosis in laryngeal cancer. Goldsmith et al. found that diploid tumors had a worse prognosis than aneuploid tumors with high levels of DNA after adjustments for tumor status, stage, and node involvement.[70] The finding of diploid tumors having a worse prognosis is at variance with many other studies of malignant tumors in which aneuploidy is more often found to indicate aggressive tumor behavior. This has been documented by Holm, who studied both oral mucosal and laryngeal carcinomas. Diploid squamous cell carcinoma of the oral mucosa had a better prognosis than aneuploid cases. Interestingly, four cases of aneuploid carcinoma of the larynx had the best prognosis.[71] In the series reported by Goldsmith et al. radiation therapy was the predominant treatment. They speculated that aneuploid tumors respond better to this mode of therapy, hence the correlation with a better prognosis for these tumors than for diploid tumors.[71] This study is also in contrast to the DNA measurements of dysplastic laryngeal epithelium.[51]

Batsakis et al.[72] found that stomal recurrence was one of the most serious complications of laryngeal carci-

TABLE 18-1. Comparison of Keratinizing and Nonkeratinizing Carcinoma of the Larynx

	Keratinizing	Nonkeratinizing
Age of patient	Same	Same
Percentage of women	4%	12%
Major site	Glottic-infraglottic	Supraglottic
Gross appearance	Ulcerate, fungating, hyperkeratotic	Tumor mass with fissured mucosa, small ulcer; may be papillary
Mucosal spread	Infrequent	Major mode of spread
Surface tumor margins	Sharply limited	Often poorly defined
Deep growth pattern	Infiltrating	About half with pushing margins
CIS	Less common at edge of tumor	Common and extensive

(From Bauer,[56] with permission.)

636

TABLE 18-2. Pathologic Features and Prognosis of Carcinoma of the Larynx

Site	Glottic, supraglottic, subglottic, or transglottic
Size	Actually measured; use laryngography
Differentiation	Use of multifactorial histologic assessment
Tumor-host interface	Pushing versus infiltrating

(From McGavran,[69] with permission.)

noma. It leads to uncontrolled disease, involving both local spread and a high incidence of distant metastasis. In summary, Table 18-2 indicates the major points of the workshop in terms of pathologic features of prognostic importance. Also of significance in the treated patient is the persistence of laryngeal edema beyond 6 months following irradiation. Edema makes biopsy difficult and tends to obscure persistent carcinoma. Ward et al.[73] have provided an excellent review of this problem. Weymuller[74] found that postirradiation clinical examination was unreliable for detecting recurrence. In preoperatively irradiated patients undergoing laryngectomy, prognosis was best for those patients who were found to be tumor-free in the subsequent pathologic specimen. This was only true, however, in cases in which radical neck dissection showed negative nodes.

It should also be noted that larynx cancer is not infrequently associated with other primary carcinomas of the head and neck. In one series it was the index primary in 12 percent of cases of multiple primary head and neck carcinomas, the highest proportion for any location within that series.[75]

Other Carcinomas of Surface Epithelium

Other varieties of mucosal carcinoma much less frequently seen are verrucous squamous cell carcinoma, lymphoepithelial carcinoma (lymphoepithelioma), undifferentiated carcinoma of large cell type, and oat cell or small cell carcinoma, now referred to as *neuroendocrine* carcinoma. In a large series of cases Ferlito[76] found the following percentages of these other types of carcinoma: verrucose 3.7 percent; lymphoepithelioma 0.5 percent; undifferentiated large cell 7.2 percent; and oat cell (small cell or neuroendocrine) 0.5 percent.

Verrucous Carcinoma

Examples of verrucous carcinoma are illustrated in Figures 18-9 and 18-10. This specific clinical and pathologic entity can be difficult to recognize. It demonstrates an exuberant proliferation of squamous epithelium with hyperkeratosis. It is a pale, wartlike growth clinically. The absence of significant cell anaplasia belies the malignant nature of this lesion, which pushes and penetrates

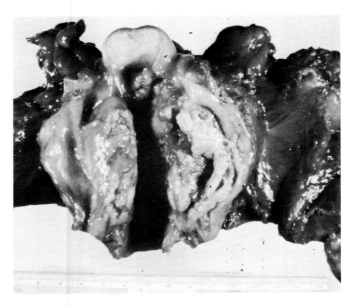

Fig. 18-9. Extensive verrucous carcinoma of the larynx. The tumor had invaded a tracheostomy, the thyroid cartilage, which was partially ossified, the base of the epiglottis, and the pyriform sinus on the right. No clinically positive lymph nodes were present in the cervical area.

into soft tissue. Microabscesses will form in response to keratin debris, and pressure of the neoplasm may actually cause necrosis of cartilage, and the tumor has even invaded the thyroid. While the amount of local neoplasm may be quite extensive, metastases from this tumor are exceedingly rare. The presence or absence of a basement membrane cannot be used as a reliable criterion of invasion.[77] A recent study has detected HPV type 16 in five cases of verrucous carcinoma of the larynx and adjacent normal tissue by DNA hybridization.[78]

Some good results have been achieved with radiotherapy in control of this tumor in the larynx, but undifferentiated neoplastic transformation has occurred when this same lesion in the oral cavity has been treated by radiation.[79] Batsakis et al. do not believe that this should be a factor in selection of the radiation versus surgical therapy for this tumor.[80]

Anaplastic Large Cell Carcinoma

Anaplastic carcinoma with large cells has been described by Ferlito,[76] who collected several cases from the literature. On review, these appear to be undifferentiated forms of squamous cell carcinoma, not necessitating a separate classification. Alternative terminology has been *transitional* and *basaloid* carcinoma, the implication of which in terms of a specific cell of origin is not warranted.[76] These tumors are aggressive, as can be inferred from their histologic characteristics.

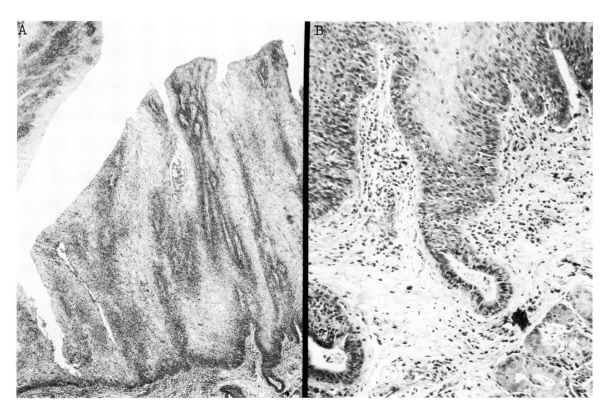

Fig. 18-10. Verrucous carcinoma. **(A)** Column-like exophytic growth of squamous epithelium is seen. **(B)** The base is the only clue to its true malignancy. Differentiating small tumors from squamous papillomas may be very difficult.

Anaplastic Small Cell Carcinoma

Oat cell or small cell carcinoma of the larynx is now a well defined entity. This tumor may be metastatic from the lung, but at least 66 primary cases in the larynx have been reported.[81] In Ferlito's series small cell, oat cell, or neuroendocrine carcinoma (the terms are used interchangeably) accounted for less than 0.5 percent of primary and secondary laryngeal cancers. Electron microscopy detected at least a few neurosecretory granules in all cases.[76,81,82]

Oat cell carcinoma must be differentiated from malignant lymphoma, typical and atypical carcinoid, and small cell squamous carcinoma involving the larynx. Lymphoma is exceedingly rare and does not reveal the conspicuous nuclear molding in the tissue sections or the extensive clumping artifact produced by massive amounts of denatured DNA and the necrosis found in typical oat cell carcinoma. Leukocyte common antigen may be used to separate lymphomas from epithelial malignancies in problem cases. Argyrophil staining methods will be positive with oat cell carcinoma and argentaffine negative. *Carcinoids,* even atypical examples, have an organoid pattern of growth despite features of high mitotic rate in some cases.[83] They have larger and more prominent neurosecretory granules and will usually stain immunohistochemically for a variety of peptide hormones and amine precursors.[81,84,85] Small cell forms of squamous cell carcinoma do not have detectable neurosecretory granules.[81]

The course of oat cell carcinoma of the larynx, as with that of the lung, is often rapidly fatal, but some long-term survivors have been reported.[84] Despite their more organized appearance, most reported carcinoids of the larynx have been aggressive. Unlike oat cell carcinoma they are resistant to radiation and chemotherapy.[85]

The consensus as to histogenesis is that the neuroendocrine carcinomas originate from Kulchitsky cells or a common stem cell, with the ability for divergent differentiation into predominantly or exclusively a neuroendocrine type of tumor, carcinoid, atypical carcinoid, or oat cell (small cell) carcinoma and even paraganglioma. Combination forms with differentiated squamous cell and adenocarcinoma have been reported.[81] Primary oat cell carcinoma has not been described in the trachea.

Spindle Cell Squamous Carcinoma With or Without Pseudosarcomatous Stroma and Carcinosarcoma

Since the report by Lane in 1957 of polypoid sarcoma-like masses in association with a squamous cell carcinoma of the mouth, fauces, and larynx, a controversy has continued over the nature of this lesion. Of the original 10 cases reported by Lane, 4 were in the larynx (base of the epiglottis, pyriform sinus, aryepiglottic fold, and vocal cord). The tumors were polypoid (Fig. 18-11) and made up predominantly of a peculiar spindle cell stroma with giant cells and even atypical mitotic figures. Usually inconspicuously present and frequently seen only on the surface of the lesion was a squamous cell carcinoma. Because of a relatively favorable outcome, with limited therapy in some cases, it was felt that this neoplasm was a pseudosarcomatous stromal reaction in conjunction with or as a response to an intramucosal or superficially infiltrating squamous cell carcinoma.[86] As noted by Lane, this tumor had probably been previously reported under the term *carcinosarcoma* by Saphir and Vass in 1938. That report included 13 cases from the respiratory tract, 6 within the larynx and 7 from the lung, as part of an analysis of 153 cases of carcinosarcoma.[87] Those authors also found that the carcinoma was usually focal in nature but remarked that the metastatic rate of the sarcomatous portion was extraordinarily low.

Subsequent reports, which included histochemical and ultrastructural data, have supported the concept that

some of these cases represent a pseudosarcomatous reaction of the stroma to squamous cell carcinoma.[88,89] However, there have also been conflicting reports, indicating that both the carcinomatous and sarcomatous elements may metastasize, either separately or together, with ultrastrucutral demonstration that the stroma is a transitional form of the carcinoma.[90,91] The review of Hyams[92] indicating a 2-year mortality of 40 percent, refutes the contention that this is a low-grade malignancy. The majority of the lesions in his series were polypoid. He supports the concept that the biphasic pattern represents a squamous cell carcinoma with an anaplastic spindle cell metaplasia. He and other authors restrict the term carcinosarcoma to a dual growth, or collision, tumor of sarcoma and carcinoma, which in metastasis will demonstrate both elements.[92,93] Supporting this concept of different histogenesis for these peculiar polypoid lesions is an electron microscopic study of two clinically similar cases, one demonstrating fusiform cells of mesenchymal type and the other spindle and giant cells of squamous origin.[94]

Recent application of immunohistochemistry to this type of case has not resolved the issue of histogenesis. The case illustrated in Figure 18-12 demonstrates a superficial squamous cell carcinoma, with in situ areas merging with a poorly differentiated small cell carcinoma and surrounded by a spindle cell sarcomatous stroma that in some areas resembles osteoid. This tumor showed cross reactivity for cytokeratin and desmin in the same spindle cells.

Immunohistochemical cross reactivity in similar tumors from the oral cavity has been reported by Ellis and colleagues.[95] Ophir et al. attempted to show that the mesenchymal portion of this tumor type was different from the carcinomatous part on the basis of staining with the intermediate filament vimentin versus cytokeratin.[96] This is not a correct interpretation. Azumi and Battifora have demonstrated coexpression of vimentin and cytokeratin in 10 to 57 percent of carcinomas, depending upon primary site. The only exception to coexpression in their series was neuroblastoma.[97] Also to be considered is the transference of positivity from one cell to another. Examining our case very carefully, one notes that the positive staining for keratin of the spindle cell tumor is seen best where these cells closely approximate definite squamous tumor cells. Where the spindle cell component occurs in wide tumor bands away from differentiated squamous cells, there is no keratin staining. There is also no vimentin staining noted in differentiated epithelial cancer cells in our case. Rosai has had a similar experience, observing that metastatic tumors to the thyroid staining positively for thyroglobulin in areas that are adjacent to recognizable thyroid epithelium with colloid (Rosai J, personal communication).

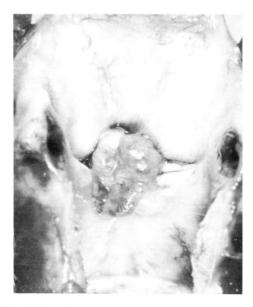

Fig. 18-11. Polypoid squamous cell carcinoma with pseudosarcomatous stroma. Gross polypoid configuration is a rather typical clinical manifestation of this lesion.

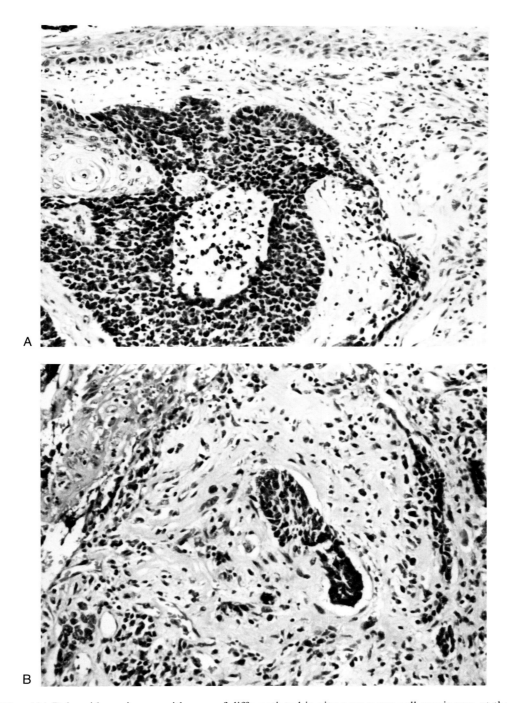

Fig. 18-12. **(A)** Polypoid carcinoma with area of differentiated in situ squamous cell carcinoma at the top, merging at the left with poorly differentiated small cell neuroendocrine-appearing carcinoma. Beneath the base of the in situ carcinoma is a spindle cell sarcomatous pattern, which contained some cells staining positively for cytokeratin. **(B)** Another area of this tumor, showing differentiated squamous cell carcinoma at the top left, small cell pattern of carcinoma in the center, and surrounding sarcoma with the appearance of osteoid.

In summary, this clinical entity perhaps represents three different types of neoplasm:

1. A superficial or intramucosal squamous cell carcinoma, usually well differentiated or moderately well differentiated, with a peculiar sarcomalike stromal reaction. This lesion is often polypoid and potentially carries a good prognosis.
2. Squamous cell carcinoma with spindle cell sarcomatous metaplasia, in which the spindle cells are malignant and of squamous origin. This tumor may be polypoid or infiltrative and carries the prognosis of poorly differentiated squamous cell carcinoma.
3. A true collision tumor of carcinoma and sarcoma in which one or both elements may metastasize. This lesion is apparently quite rare and difficult to document specifically. The sarcoma may be of various histologic types.

Malignant and Benign Glandular Tumors

Adenocarcinoma

Throughout the larynx and trachea there are collections of acini and ducts with morphologic features identical to salivary gland tissue. Tumors arising in these structures are the counterparts of benign and malignant neoplasms of major salivary glands. They are quite rare (less than 1 percent of laryngeal tumors) and are either nonspecific adenocarcinoma or adenoid cystic carcinoma.[98] Over a 30 year period Spiro and associates collected 20 cases arising in the larynx and 11 cases primary in the trachea.[99,100] In a similar 30 year period, Houston et al. reported 21 cases arising in the trachea.[101]

The nonspecific adenocarcinomas, which have variable glandular morphologic features and differing degrees of pleomorphism, are usually found supra- or transglottically.[102] There is a marked male preponderance and patients are often elderly.[99] The location corresponds to the concentration of seromucous glands in the false cords and just inferior to the anterior commissure.[98] Although this neoplasm manifests the typical symptom of hoarseness, in the majority of cases reported the patients had advanced tumors when first seen. The prognosis has been dismal despite radical surgery, not unlike the nonspecific adenocarcinoma counterpart of these tumors in major salivary glands.[99] Their tendency to widespread metastasis is also similar.

Adenoid Cystic Carcinoma

Adenoid cystic carcinoma, with its characteristic pattern of cylinders of mucoid substance surrounded by small, uniform epithelial cells, may be grossly circumscribed but microscopically infiltrative. It grows along tissue planes and is frequently found surrounding

nerves.[98] Olofsson and Van Nostrand[103] collected 60 cases from the literature and reported 4 additional ones. The lesions arose almost exclusively in the subglottic and supraglottic areas. In four cases whole laryngeal sections demonstrated marked local spread of the tumor with multiple skip areas. This tumor has a protracted clinical course with multiple recurrences, usually leading to death.[104] Distant metastases have appeared in at least half of the patients, even in reports with minimal follow-up periods.[98]

Because of the insidious nature of adenoid cystic carcinoma and its infiltrative character, patients do not usually seek medical attention until they experience dyspnea. This is particularly true of this tumor since it occurs throughout the trachea. It is the most common adenocarcinoma of the trachea, and in both the larynx and the trachea there is a female preponderance.[100-106] A more aggressive form has been reported in which the epithelial cells occur in broad sheets, with few of the cylindrical structures and marked areas of necrosis.[104,107]

Other Epithelial Tumors

In a comprehensive review, Ferlito[76] has collected case reports under a variety of terms as follows: giant cell carcinoma, clear cell carcinoma, adenosquamous carcinoma, malignant mixed carcinoma (malignant mixed tumor), mucoepidermoid carcinoma, acinic cell carcinoma, and carcinoid tumors. Most of these appear to be variants of tumors arising from either the surface epithelium, the glandular epithelium of salivary gland type, or both.[98,108,109]

An oncocytic carcinoma has been reported that arose in the arytenoid. While the cells had abundant eosinophilic cytoplasm, there was no indication of hyperplasia of mitochondria.[110] *Benign oncocytic tumors* are quite common in the larynx and pharynx, some of them forming the typical papillary cystic lesions with lymphoid tissue that are analogous to true Warthin's tumor of salivary gland type (Fig. 18-13). The spectrum of oncocytic hyperplasia and metaplasia that may be seen in the larynx casts some doubt on the true neoplastic nature of these tumors.[111]

While several cases have been reported, Fechner is not convinced that a true *malignant mixed tumor* of salivary gland type has been found in the larynx.[76,98] We have not personally seen such a case, either in the larynx or the trachea, and could not find a well documented example reported in the literature. A case reported in 1986 produced ulceration and atypical squamous metaplasia of the vocal cord, resulting in an initial misdiagnosis of squamous cell carcinoma.[112]

Chan et al.[113] collected 13 acceptable and 5 probable

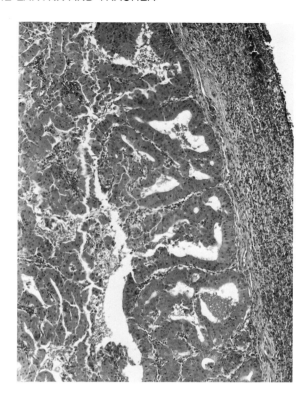

Fig. 18-13. Benign oncocytic tumor found incidently in larynx biopsy specimen. Some of these lesions become papillary with lymphoid stroma, identical to Warthin's tumor of salivary gland type.

cases of *benign mixed tumor* of the trachea and reported 1 additional case. The prognosis and histopathology are those of benign mixed tumors of major salivary glands. They are much less common than the rare squamous cell carcinoma of the trachea and are found predominantly in middle-aged men.

Carcinoid tumors of the larynx[76] and trachea[114] have been reported rarely. Several of these neoplasms were aggressive and metastasized.

Metastatic Tumors

Metastatic tumors to the larynx have been reviewed by Whicker et al.[115] These authors reported one case of carcinoma of the colon metastatic to the larynx among 490 laryngeal carcinomas seen at the Mayo Clinic in a 10-year period. In their literature review melanoma and hypernephroma were the most common metastatic cancers reported. Other, less frequent primary malignant neoplasms metastatic to the larynx were carcinomas of breast and lung. There is no site of predilection within the larynx for metastatic tumors, which may be the initial sign of disseminated cancer, particularly if the bulging

mass causes obstruction or hoarseness. Metastasis to the laryngeal cartilage may expand that structure or may be totally asymptomatic.[98] While not truly metastatic, direct extension by thyroid carcinoma occasionally compromises the larynx. There were 18 cases of laryngeal invasion reported among 2,000 patients treated for thyroid cancer; these 18 included 7 follicular, 6 papillary, 4 anaplastic, and 1 medullary thyroid carcinoma.[116]

Miscellaneous Tumors

Lawson and Zak[117] described glomus body paraganglia of the human larynx between the thyroid and cricoid cartilages. In a prior report paraganglia had been identified just below the epithelium at the anterior end of the vocal cords.[118] *Nonchromaffin paragangliomas* may arise from these structures, and 24 cases have been collected from the literature, only 4 of which were primary in the trachea.[119-121] These tumors are relatively benign but will bleed rather extensively on biopsy. Patients had marked spasmodic pain in the larynx, moving upward towards one ear, on swallowing. Paragangliomas were small lesions and occasionally quite difficult to see. Most of them were in the arytenoid region. The tumor tended to recur, and cervical lymph node metastasis was a frequent feature, although it took many years to develop.[119,120]

Malignant melanoma, while seen more frequently in the upper respiratory tract than benign nevus, is still an exceedingly rare neoplasm of both the larynx and trachea. In a review of 26 cases of malignant melanoma of the upper respiratory tract, Moore and Martin[122] found two cases that occurred in the larynx. We have seen two similar cases primary in the larynx in 23 years of practicing of surgical pathology. It is important to demonstrate junctional activity for a diagnosis of primary malignant melanoma (Fig. 18-14), since the larynx is a potential site of metastatic melanoma. Mori et al.[123] collected five cases of primary malignant melanoma of the trachea and added one of their own. Like other mucous membrane melanomas, those in the upper respiratory tract and trachea are clinically aggressive.

Neurogenic Tumors

Both *neurofibroma* and *neurilemoma* have been reported in the larynx.[35,119,124-127] It is rare, however, for the larynx to be involved in neurofibromatosis (Von Recklinghausen's disease).[126] One reported neurofibroma had an associated squamous cell carcinoma.[127] Most of the tumors occur in the supraglottic area, causing hoarseness. Their histologic appearance is discussed in detail in Chapter 49.

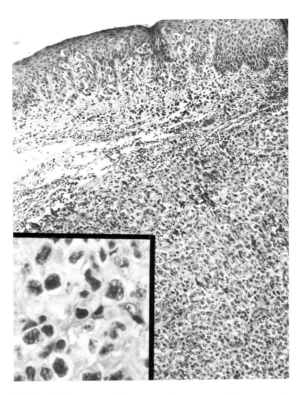

Fig. 18-14. Primary malignant melanoma of the vocal cord. Junctional nesting of the melanoma cells is evident. Details of the underlying invasive melanoma are seen in the inset. Without the presence of pigment in some areas of this tumor and the junctional component, a deep biopsy specimen might have been confused with a malignant lymphoma.

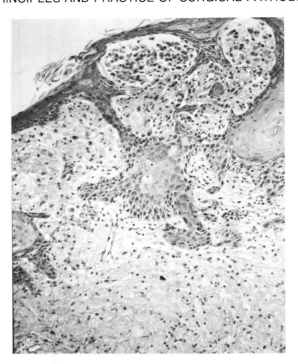

Fig. 18-15. Granular cell tumor of vocal cord. Tumor is composed of cells with small central nucleus and granular cytoplasm. Pseudoepitheliomatous hyperplasia is evident over the surface of this tumor. A superficial biopsy may lead to an erroneous diagnosis of squamous cell carcinoma.

Although controversial, the *granular cell "myoblastoma"* appears to be of neural origin, at least in many of the cases (Fig. 18-15). These neoplasms may be heterogeneous, but a significant number of cases studied ultrastructurally demonstrate origin from Schwann cells with a peculiar granular alteration of the cytoplasm.[128,129] Other origins proposed have been skeletal muscle cells, histiocytes, fibroblasts, and mesenchymal cells. Booth and Osborne[130] reported five cases and collected over 100 from the literature.[119,130,131] Only 10 cases have been reported primary within the trachea.[132] The granules are periodic acid–Schiff (PAS)-positive; some of them will have an angular shape as described by Bangle,[133] but this feature is not uniformly present. The tumor is seen predominantly in the fourth through the fifth decade and is grossly polypoid. Its most important pathologic feature is pseudoepitheliomatous hyperplasia of overlying squamous epithelium. In one review, this occurred in 64 percent of the cases and was severe in 22 percent.[134] It is possible to mistake this hyperplasia for squamous cell carcinoma.[134] It should be remembered that in any pseudoepitheliomatous squamous proliferation it is im-

portant to study the underlying tissue for the presence of granular cells.

A malignant example of granular cell tumor has not been described in the trachea or the larynx, and we have not seen a case, although this tumor recurs in a small number of instances.[35,135,136]

Benign Connective Tissue Tumors

At least one case has been reported in the literature for practically all the connective tissue tumor types. In a large review, Batsakis and Fox[124] collected 10 cases of *lipoma* of the larynx, which usually arises on the arytenoid or in the pyriform fossa. The lipomas all showed a structure typical of adipose tissue.[35,124]

True *fibromas* are exceedingly rare. They are almost invariably found in men over 60 years of age. They should be examined carefully, particularly if there is any pleomorphism, for the possibility of an associated squamous cell carcinoma, the so-called pseudosarcoma tumor described earlier.[35,86] A case has been reported in a 5-day-old boy, possibly attributable to a defect in the development of the sixth branchial arch structure.[137] We were unable to find another case of similar type in a literature search. Pollak et al. reviewed benign tracheal tumors while reporting a fibromyxoma. The majority are soft tissue tumors of mesenchymal origin, and they typically occur in the lower third of the trachea, except for benign mixed tumors and granular cell "myoblastomas."[138]

One case of a *xanthoma* has been reported; it occurred in the aryepiglottic fold in a 37-year-old man.[35] Several cases of *fibrous histiocytomas* primary in the trachea have been reported.[139–147] Fibrous histiocytoma has been found predominantly in children and young adults. Although reportedly benign, in several cases the tumor showed aggressive behavior or infiltration at the time of surgery.[141,142] One lesion recurred in the second year of follow-up after simple excision.[139] A true *myxoma* of the larynx or trachea has not been reported; however, myxoid change is common in laryngeal nodules (polyps). Two *leiomyomas* have been reported in the trachea of adults and one in the larynx of a child.[35,148] Miller[149] also mentions leiomyoma in a large collective review of benign tumors of the lung and tracheobronchial tree.

In 1976 Winther[150] reported two cases of extracardiac *rhabdomyoma* and reviewed 53 cases from the literature. Nine tumors were in the larynx and hypopharynx. The tumors resemble differentiated skeletal muscle, composed of large round to oval cells with a pale, pink-staining, very finely granular cytoplasm. The cells may be vacuolated, and cross striations can usually be found in a few cells.[150] Batsakis and Fox[124] have described a haphazard crystal-like arrangement in some of the cells that corresponds ultrastructurally to the hypertrophied Z band, which is similar in structure to that seen in nemaline myopathy.[124] The age range of reported cases is quite broad, 11 months to 55 years. There is some vague resemblance to granular cell "myoblastomas," but cross striations have never been demonstrated in that tumor, and histochemical and ultrastructural features of granular cell tumor are very different.[124,151,152] Clinical recurrence of the lesion followed if it was incompletely excised, but this does not necessarily indicate a malignant nature.[124]

Hemangiomas usually occur in infants as bulging masses below the cords, whereas in adults they are usually proximal to the vocal cords[153,154]; adults account for 90 percent of the cases.[124,155] The adult form is seen nearly exclusively in men, while there is a preponderance of girls in the infantile form. Airway obstruction is the most common symptom in the infantile form.[153,154] The lesion may be compressible. While relieving the airway obstruction is the most important clinical consideration, biopsy should be avoided because of the marked vascularity. Spontaneous regression has been noted in the infantile form after 6 months of age. This neoplasm is usually of the capillary or cavernous type histologically, often circumscribed but occasionally infiltrating.[35]

Only one case of *lymphangioma* has been reported in a review of 722 benign tumors of the larynx.[156] Holinger et al.[157] found two lymphangiomas among a large series of infants requiring tracheostomy in the first year of life.

Chondromas represent the most common tumor arising in skeletal tissue in the larynx. Tiwari et al. have recently described three new cases and briefly reviewed the literature[158]; 80 percent of the cases were considered benign. They occur predominantly in men (in a ratio of 5:1) and are located principally in the posterior midline involving the cricoid cartilage.[35,158,159] Radiographs reveal irregular calcification in 80 percent of the cases. The tumor projects as a smooth mass, which gradually enlarges and causes obstructive symptoms. This neoplasm can recur if not completely removed. It histologically poses the same problem as cartilaginous tumors in other sites at which minor alterations, such as binucleate cells and atypism, may be considered evidence of low-grade malignancy.

Most reporters of cases seem to favor conservative therapy, that is, an attempt at local excision without laryngectomy, in those chondromas that are clearly benign or at least of no more than borderline malignancy.[160] Biopsy of the lesion is quite difficult, frequently removing only the overlying mucosa without penetration of the actual tumor.[124,159] The problem of predicting behavior on a histologic basis becomes apparent in a review of a report in which 18 cases had microscopic evidence suggesting malignancy. While six tumors recurred, none metastasized.[161] Chondroma of the trachea is rare.[162,163]

Osteoma of the larynx or trachea has not been reported. Two conditions that are pseudotumors, *tracheopathia osteoplastica* and *ossification of the tracheal cartilages,* may have to be differentiated from true chondromas or osteochondromas. The latter condition is simple ossification of the tracheal and laryngeal cartilages and is more common in the larynx. It is essentially an incidental finding. In tracheopathia osteoplastica, however, multiple nodules of cartilage and bone develop and grow between the cartilaginous rings of the trachea and may present within the mucosa. The condition is quite rare but has been reported in conjunction with pulmonary thromboembolic disease.[35,164]

Malignant Tumors of Connective Tissue, Cartilage, and Bone

Among the malignant connective tissue tumors, a rare group, *fibrosarcoma* appears to be the most common, 32 acceptable laryngeal cases having been collected by Batsakis and Fox.[124] Of these patients, 70 percent were over 50 years of age, and there was a male preponderance of 4:1. The tumors manifest as nodular or pedunculated masses, most commonly located on the anterior portion of the vocal cord or at the anterior commissure. As Batsakis and Fox have proposed, this lesion is best divided into two histologic types, well differentiated and poorly differentiated. The prognosis correlates well with the degree of differentiation.[124,165–167] Roncoroni et al. reported a case of primary fibrosarcoma of the trachea, finding only three other acceptable cases in the English literature.[168]

Sixteen cases of *malignant fibrous histiocytoma* of the larynx have been reported.[145,169] One case, following radiation for papillary carcinoma of the thyroid, has been described within the trachea.[170] The differential diagnosis is frequently that of the pseudosarcomatous lesion of Lane versus a true carcinosarcoma or a spindle cell squamous carcinoma with a very pleomorphic pattern. The case reported by Ferlito[169] of simultaneous malignant fibrous histiocytoma and squamous cell carcinoma is probably a carcinosarcoma or spindle cell carcinoma, based on a review of the histopathology presented.

Friedmann[167] found four cases of laryngeal *leiomyosarcoma* in the literature, which in his opinion were well documented. A differential diagnosis from fibrosarcoma requires special stains and/or ultrastructural studies.[167]

Haerr et al.[171] recently reported the eleventh case of *rhabdomyosarcoma* of the larynx and reviewed the literature. This tumor is usually of embryonal type, occurs in children, and, like its counterpart in the orbit, seems to have a good prognosis, perhaps based on early diagnosis. Other authors have reported pleomorphic and alveolar rhabdomyosarcomas in older patients.[172,173] One example of this tumor has recently been reported in a child.[174] Documentation of all the pleomorphic tumors is subject to close scrutiny, since none was confirmed by ultrastructural studies.

An accurate determination of the number of *hemangiosarcomas* has proved quite difficult.[124] Pratt and Goodof[175] collected 15 cases, but in the opinion of Batsakis and Fox[124] only their own case provided convincing photographs of a malignant vascular tumor. Hemangiosarcoma of the larynx or trachea is not specifically listed in the compilation of tumors by the Armed Forces Institute of Pathology.[35] Ferlito et al. have recently reported a case and reviewed the literature. Their case is documented only with conventional light microscopy.[176]

Pesavento and Ferlito found five cases of primary malignant *hemangiopericytoma* of the larynx in a review of the literature and reported one of their own. No special studies were performed to confirm the identity of this tumor beyond conventional light microscopy and a reticulin stain. Data are lacking on biologic behavior. Either there was a short follow-up or none at all or the patients died during or immediately after therapy.[177] Kaposi's sarcoma of the larynx has also been reported.[167]

Synovial sarcomas have been reported in the hypopharynx as a distinct entity, the first reported case in the larynx being that of Miller et al.[178] Harrison et al.[179] reviewed five cases of this lesion reported up until 1961. It was Enzinger who confirmed the histogenesis of these hypopharyngeal tumors as synovial. Fourteen similar cases have been collected by the Armed Forces Institute of Pathology.[35] Synovial elements are not infrequent in the neck as a potential source of the tumor. The tumor in this location has been somewhat better differentiated, demonstrating histochemical features of the mucinous substance that supports the derivation from synovial tissues. The prognosis is also somewhat better than for the same lesion in the extremities. The biphasic pattern is consistently demonstrated.[35]

Allsbrook et al. have reported the eighth case of *liposarcoma* of the larynx as well as reviewing the prior cases.[180]

Ferlito and colleagues indicate that approximately 150 *chondrosarcomas* of the larynx have been reported.[181] The true incidence is quite difficult to determine because the lesion kills by recurrence, with dissemination being exceedingly rare.[124] This is particularly true of the well differentiated tumors with occasional binucleate cartilaginous cells but otherwise essentially no atypia. Even the less differentiated lesions, which are unequivocally malignant, recur and infiltrate rather than disseminating to distant sites.[182] Only two cases of primary chondrosarcoma of the trachea have been reported.[183]

No acceptable cases of *osteosarcoma* of the trachea or larynx are listed either in the Armed Forces Institute of Pathology Registry material or in the review by Batsakis and Fox.[35,124] We believe, however, that at least three such cases have been reported.[184–186]

Malignant Lymphomas and Plasmacytomas

Given the large amount of lymphoid tissue in the nasopharyngeal area, the presence of malignant lymphoma either as a primary lesion or as part of generalized disease is not unexpected. Involvement of the larynx is extremely rare. Swerdlow et al. have recently reported a case of non-Hodgkin's lymphoma and reviewed the English language literature.[187] A bona fide case occurring primarily in the trachea could not be found. Lymphomas of the respiratory tract do not differ histologically from those primary in lymph nodes.

Approximately 10 percent of upper respiratory tract solitary plasmacytomas have occurred in the hypopharynx and larynx,[35] some of which have been of long duration.[188] Plasmacytomas have had a male predominance with a ratio of 3:1, usually occurring in the older age group (50–70 years).[188,189] Pahor[190] reported one case in a 62-year-old man and collected 31 additional cases of solitary plasmacytoma of the larynx. Rawson et al.[191] have listed the important differential features of plasmacytoma versus an inflammatory reaction with a preponderance of plasmacytes. For plasmacytomas, they are as follows: broad masses of plasma cells that lie in a delicate stroma composed of thin capillary blood vessels; adjacent tissue replaced by plasma cell sheets; prominent red nucleoli; increase in nuclear/cytoplasmic ratio; and atypical nuclear characteristics with multinucleate cells.[191] It is said that most of these tumors result in multiple myeloma, but of the 31 cases collected by Pahor,[190] only 6 showed recurrence while 4 eventuated in disseminated myeloma during the follow-up period. While these were all solitary lesions, the larynx can be involved by multiple myeloma as part of a generalized dissemination, although this is rare.[192]

A report by Hood et al.[193] documents a case of primary presentation of mycosis fungoides in the larynx. Cutaneous lesions appeared 2 years after the original biopsy, and death eventually ensued with widespread involvement. The authors did not find any other cases in the English literature. One case has been reported of primary mast cell sarcoma of the larynx.[194]

FUTURE DIRECTIONS

While classifications of some laryngeal tumors remains controversial, the most important aspect of surgical pathology is the correct diagnosis of preneoplasia and intraepithelial neoplasia of the vocal cords. The limits of morphology as a predictor of biologic behavior of these tumors have probably been reached, as they have for other examples of in situ carcinomas. The advent of microlaryngoscopy, precise biopsy, and therapeutic techniques using lasers makes it mandatory that progress be made in a systematic classification of these lesions for better measurement of their ultimate malignant potential. Sophisticated measurements of DNA with a determination of the degree of cell aneuploidy, as undertaken for cervical intraepithelial neoplasia, may hold promise. In terms of function, application of correct and limited therapy in intraepithelial neoplasia of the larynx is of paramount importance.

REFERENCES

1. Fitzgerald PJ: Manual for Pathology Fellows. Revised Ed. Department of Pathology, Memorial Hospital for Cancer and Allied Diseases, New York, 1977
2. Arey LB: Developmental Anatomy. A Textbook and Laboratory Manual for Embryology. 7th Ed. WB Saunders, Philadelphia, 1974
3. Weiss L, Greep RO: Histology. 4th Ed. McGraw-Hill, New York, 1977
4. Johnson GK, Sullivan JL, Bishop JA: Acute epiglottis. Review of 55 cases and suggested protocol. Arch Otolaryngol 100:333, 1974
5. Davidson FW: Acute laryngeal obstruction in children. A fifty-year review. Ann Otol Rhinol Laryngol 87:606, 1978
6. Hannallah R, Rosales JK: Acute epiglottis: Current management and review. Can Anaesth Soc J 25:84, 1978
7. Molteni RA: Epiglottis: Incidence of extraepiglottic infection: Report of 72 cases and review of the literature. Pediatrics 58:526, 1976
8. Scheidemandel HH: Did George Washington die of quinsy? Arch Otolaryngol 102:519, 1976
9. Darnell JD: Acute epiglottis in adults—report of a case and review of the literature. J Indiana State Med Assoc 69:21, 1976
10. Ash JE, Raum M: An Atlas of Otolaryngic Pathology. Armed Forces Institute of Pathology, Washington, 1956
11. Pang LQ: Allergy of the larynx, trachea, and bronchial tree. Otolaryngol Clin North Am 7:719, 1974
12. Hancock BD: Tracheostomy in measles laryngo-tracheo-bronchitis. J Laryngol Otol 86:23, 1972
13. Eschapasse H, Lacomme Y, Hassani M, et al: Laryngeal and tracheal stenoses after intubation and/or tracheotomy. A review of 32 cases including 39 lesions and 33 operations. (Authors' transl.) Acta Chir Belg 76:381, 1977
14. Pahor AL: Tracheal polyp complicating tracheostomy in an infant. Ear Nose Throat J 56:249, 1977
15. Smith RO, Hemenway WG, English GM: Post-intubation subglottic granulation tissue: Review of the problem and evaluation of radiotherapy. Laryngoscope 79:1227, 1969
16. Cooney W, Dzura B, Harper R: The cytology of sputum from thermally injured patients. Acta Cytol 16:433, 1972
17. Frable WJ, Frable MA, Seney FD Jr: Virus infections of the respiratory tract. Cytopathologic and clinical analysis. Acta Cytol (Baltimore) 21:32, 1977
18. Friedman EM, Jorgensen K, Healey GB et al: Bacterial tracheitis—two year experience. Laryngoscope 95:9, 1985
19. Mukherjee DK: Solitary tuberculoma of the larynx: A case report. Tubercle 58:9, 1977
20. Bennett DE: Histoplasmosis of the oral cavity and larynx: A clinicopathologic study. Arch Intern Med 120:417, 1967
21. Batsakis JG: Coccidioidomycosis of the larynx. Ann Otol Rhinol Laryngol 93:528, 1984
22. Luna LG: Manual of Histologic Staining Methods of the Armed Forces Institute of Pathology. 3rd Ed. McGraw-Hill, New York, 1960
23. Ellefsen P: Tracheal dystonia and sarcoidosis. Acta Otolaryngol (Stockh) 70:438, 1970
24. Tashjian LS, Peacock JE: Laryngeal candidiasis. Report of seven cases and review of the literature. Arch Otolaryngol 110:806, 1984
25. Rosenberg RA, Schneider KL, Cohen NL: Update on

AIDS (editorial). Otolaryngol Head Neck Surg 95:127, 1986

26. Spear RK, Walker PD, Lampton LM: Tracheal obstruction associated with a fungus ball. A case of primary tracheal candidiasis. Chest 70:662, 1976

27. Bienstock H, Ehrlich GE, Freyberg RH: Rheumatoid arthritis of the cricoarytenoid joint. A clinicopathologic study. Arthritis Rheum 6:48,1963

28. Moloney JR: Relapsing polychondritis—its otolaryngological manifestations. J Laryngol Otol 92:9, 1978

29. Lefkovits AM: Gouty involvement of the larynx. Report of a case and review of the literature. Arthritis Rheum 8:1019, 1965

30. Waxman J, Bose WJ: Laryngeal manifestations of Wegener's granulomatosis: Case reports and review of the literature. J Rheumatol 13:408, 1986

31. Simon JL: Primary amyloid tumor of the trachea. A case report. Radiology 103:555, 1972

32. Barnes EL, Zafar T: Laryngeal amyloidosis, clinicopathologic study of seven cases. Ann Otol Rhinol Laryngol 86:856, 1977

33. Jones AW, Chaterji AM: Primary tracheobronchial amyloidosis with tracheobronchopathia osteoplastica. Br J Dis Chest 71:268, 1977

34. Shaheen NA, Salman SD, Nassar VH: Fatal bronchopulmonary hemorrhage due to unrecognized amyloidosis. Arch Otolaryngol 101:259, 1975

35. Ash JE, Beck MR, Wilkes JD: Tumors of the Upper Respiratory Tract and Ear. Atlas of Tumor Pathology. Fasc. 12, & 13. Armed Forces Institute of Pathology, Washington, 1964

36. Denson SE, Taussig LM, Pon GD: Intraluminal tracheal cyst producing airway obstruction in the newborn infant. J Pediatr 88:521, 1976

37. Gallagher JC, Puzon BA: Oncocytic lesions of the larynx. Ann Otol Rhinol Larynol 78:307, 1969

38. Oliveria CA, Roth JA, Adams GL: Oncocytic lesions of the larynx. Laryngoscope 87:1718, 1977

39. Saleem TI, Peale AR, Robbins R: Lymphocytic pseudotumor (pseudolymphoma) of the larynx. Report of a rare case and review of the literature. Laryngoscope 80:133, 1970

40. Mabry ML: Lymphoid pseudotumors of the larynx. J Laryngol Otol 81:441, 1967

41. Lynn RB, Takita H: Tracheal papilloma: Case report and review of the literature. Can Med Assoc J 97:1354, 1967

42. Mounier-Kuhn P, Gaillard J, Dumolard P: Papilloma of the larynx and trachea in children. Int Surg 59:483, 1974

43. Aylward TD, Flege JB Jr: Primary papilloma of the trachea. Ann Thorac Surg 16:620, 1973

44. Abramson AL, Steinberg BM, Winkler B: Laryngeal papillomatosis: Clinical, histopathologic and molecular studies. Laryngoscope 97:678, 1987

45. Zur Hausen H: Human papilloma viruses and their possible role in squamous cell carcinomas. Curr Top Microbiol Immunol 78:1, 1977

46. Shapiro RS, Marlowe FI, Butcher J: Malignant degeneration of nonirradiated juvenile laryngeal papillomatosis. Ann Otol Rhinol Laryngol 85:101, 1976

47. Hollinger PH, Schild JA, Maurizi DG: Laryngeal papilloma: Review of etiology and therapy. Laryngoscope 78:1462, 1968

48. Shilovitseva AS: The complex treatment of patients affected with papillomatosis of the larynx and trachea. Arch Otolaryngol 89:552, 1969

49. Gibb AG, Khan JA: Papilloma of the trachea. J Laryngol Otol 85:1205, 1971

50. Strong MA, Vaughan CW, Healy GB, et al: Recurrent respiratory papillomatosis. Ann Otol Rhinol Laryngol 85:508, 1976

51. Friedmann I: Precancerous lesions of the larynx. p. 122. In Alberti PW, Bryce DP (eds): Workshops from the Centennial Conference on Laryngeal Cancer. Appleton & Lange, East Norwalk, CT, 1976

52. Fechner RE: Laryngeal keratosis and atypia. p. 110. In Alberti PW, Bryce DP (eds): Workshops from the Centennial Conference on Laryngeal Cancer. Appleton & Lange, East Norwalk, CT, 1976

53. Rubio CA, Soderberg G: Management of carcinoma in situ. Lancet 1:421, 1969

54. Kleinsasser O, Heck KH: Über das sogenannte Carcinoma in Situ des Larynx. Arch Otolaryngol 174:210, 1959

55. Bocking A, Auffermann W, Vogel H, et al: Diagnosis and grading of malignancy in squamous epithelial lesions of the larynx with DNA cytophotometry. Cancer 56:1600, 1985

56. Bauer WC: Concomitant carcinoma in situ and invasive carcinoma of the larynx. p. 127. In Alberti PW, Bryce DP (eds): Workshop from the Centennial Conference on Laryngeal Cancer. Appleton & Lange, East Norwalk, CT, 1976

57. Miller AH, Fisher JR: Clues to the life history of carcinoma in situ of the larynx. Laryngoscope 81:1475, 1971

58. Saffiotti U, Kaufman DG: Carcinogenesis of laryngeal carcinoma. Laryngoscope 85:454, 1975

59. Wynder EL, Mushinski MH, Spivak JC: Tobacco and alcohol consumption in relation to the development of multiple primary cancers. Cancer 40:1872, 1977

60. Batsakis JG: Tumors of the Head and Neck. Clinical and Pathologic Considerations. Williams & Wilkins, Baltimore, 1974

61. Olofsson J: Growth and spread of laryngeal carcinoma. p. 40. In Alberti PW, Bryce DP (eds): Workshops from the Centennial Conference on Laryngeal Cancer. Appleton & Lange, East Norwalk, CT, 1976

62. Senyszyn JJ, Jacox HW: Primary carcinoma of the trachea followed by primary carcinoma of the esophagus after a six-year interval. A case report. Radiology 92:1346, 1969

63. Martini N, Goodner JT, D'Angio GJ: Tracheoesophageal fistula due to cancer. J Thorac Cardiovasc Surg 59:319, 1970

64. Michaels L: Differentiation of squamous carcinoma of the larynx as a determinant of prognosis. p. 835. In Alberti PW, Bryce DP (eds): Workshops from the Centennial Conference on Laryngeal Cancer. Appleton & Lange, East Norwalk, CT, 1976

65. Fisher HR: Grading of biopsies of laryngeal carcinomas

by multiple criteria. p. 843. In Alberti PW, Bryce DP (eds): Workshops from the Centennial Conference on Laryngeal Cancer. Appleton & Lange, East Norwalk, CT, 1976

66. Jakobsson PA: Histologic grading of malignancy and prognosis in glottic carcinoma of the larynx. p. 847. In Alberti PW, Bryce DP (eds): Workshops from the Centennial Conference on Laryngeal Cancer. Appleton & Lange, East Norwalk, CT, 1976

67. McGavran MH, Bauer WC: Sinus histiocytosis and cervical lymph nodal metastases from transglottic epidermoid carcinoma of the larynx. p. 865. In Alberti PW, Bryce DP (eds): Workshops from the Centennial Conference on Laryngeal Cancer. Appleton & Lange, East Norwalk, CT, 1976

68. Kashima KH: The characteristics of laryngeal cancer correlating with cervical lymph node metastasis. p. 855. In Alberti PW, Bryce DP (eds): Workshops from the Centennial Conference on Laryngeal Cancer. Appleton & Lange, East Norwalk, CT, 1976

69. McGavran MH: Pathologic features of prognostic importance. p. 877. In Alberti PW, Bryce DP (eds): Workshops from the Centennial Conference on Laryngeal Cancer. Appleton & Lange, East Norwalk, CT, 1976

70. Goldsmith MM, Cresson DS, Postma DS, et al: Significance of ploidy in laryngeal cancer. Am J Surg 152:396, 1986

71. Holm LE: Cellular DNA amounts of squamous cell carcinoma of the head and neck region in relation to prognosis. Laryngoscope 92:1064, 1982

72. Batsakis JG, Hybels R, Rice DH: Laryngeal carcinoma: Stromal recurrences and distant metastases. p. 868. In Alberti PW, Bryce DP (eds): Workshops from the Centennial Conference on Laryngeal Cancer. Appleton & Lange, East Norwalk, CT, 1976

73. Ward PH, Calcaterra TC, Kagan AR: The enigma of post-radiation edema and recurrent or residual carcinoma of the larynx. Laryngoscope 85:522, 1975

74. Weymuller EA Jr: Prognostic importance of the tumor-free laryngectomy specimen. Arch Otolaryngol 104:505, 1978

75. Shikhani AH, Matanoski GM, Jones MM, et al: Multiple primary malignancies in head and neck cancer. Arch Otolaryngol 112:1172, 1986

76. Ferlito A: Histological classification of larynx and hypopharynx cancers and their clinical implications. Pathologic aspects of 2052 malignant neoplasms diagnosed at the ORL Department of Padua University from 1966 to 1976. Acta Otolaryngol (Stockh), suppl, 342:1–88, 1976

77. Ferlito A: Diagnosis and treatment of verrucous squamous cell carcinoma of the larynx. A critical review. Ann Otol Rhinol Larygol 94:575, 1985

78. Abramson AL, Brandsma J, Steinberg B et al: Verrucous carcinoma of the larynx. Possible human papillomavirus etiology. Arch Otolaryngol 111:709, 1985

79. Proffitt SD, Spooner TR, Kosek JC: Origin of undifferentiated neoplasm from verrucous epidermal carcinoma of oral cavity following irradiation. Cancer 26:389, 1970

80. Batsakis JG, Hybels R, Crissman JD, et al: The pathology of head and neck tumors: Verrucous carcinoma. Part 15. Head Neck Surg 5:29, 1982

81. Ferlito A: Diagnosis and treatment of small cell carcinoma of the larynx: A critical review. Ann Otol Rhinol Laryngol 95:590, 1986

82. Myerowitz RL, Barne EL, Myers E: Small cell anaplastic (oat cell) carcinoma of the larynx: Report of a case and review of the literature. Laryngoscope 88:1697, 1978

83. Blok PH, Manni JJ, Van Den Broek P, et al: Carcinoid of the larynx: A report of three cases and a review of the literature. Laryngoscope 95:715, 1985

84. Porto DP, Wick MR, Ewing SL, et al: Neuroendocrine carcinoma of the larynx. Am J Otolaryngol 8:97, 1987

85. Patterson SD, Yarington CT Jr: Carcinoid tumor of the larynx: The role of conservative therapy. Ann Otol Rhinol Laryngol 96:12, 1987

86. Lane N: Pseudosarcoma (polypoid sarcoma-like masses) associated with squamous cell carcinoma of the mouth, fauces, and larynx. Cancer 10:19, 1957

87. Saphir O, Vass A: Carcinosarcoma. Am J Cancer 33:331, 1938

88. Friedel W, Chambers RG, Atkins JP Jr: Pseudosarcomas of the pharynx and larynx. Arch Otolaryngol 102:286, 1976

89. Goellner JR, Devine KD, Weiland LH, et al: Pseudosarcoma of larynx. Am J Clin Pathol 59:312, 1973

90. Litchtiger B, MacKay B, Tessmer CF: Spindle cell variant of squamous carcinoma. Cancer 26:1311, 1970

91. Appleman HD, Oberman HA: Squamous cell carcinoma of the larynx with sarcoma like stroma. Am J Clin Pathol 44:135, 1965

92. Hyams VJ: Spindle cell carcinoma of the larynx. p. 489. In Alberti PW, Bryce DP (eds): Workshops from the Centennial Conference on Laryngeal Cancer. Appleton & Lange, East Norwalk, CT, 1976

93. Minckler DS, Meligro CH, Norris HT: Carcinosarcoma of the larynx. Cancer 26:195, 1970

94. Lasser KH, Naeim F, Higgins J, et al: "Pseudosarcoma" of the larynx. Am J Clin Pathol 3:397, 1979

95. Ellis GL, Langloss JM, Enzinger FM: Coexpression of keratin and desmin in a carcinosarcoma involving the maxillary alveolar ridge. Oral Surg 60:410, 1985

96. Ophir D, Marshak G, Czernobilsky B: Distinctive immunohistochemical labeling of epithelial and mesenchymal elements in laryngeal pseudosarcoma. 97:490, 1987

97. Azumi N, Battifora H: The distribution of vimentin and keratin in epithelial and nonepithelial neoplasms. Am J Clin Pathol 88:286, 1987

98. Fechner RE: Adenocarcinoma of the larynx. p. 466. In Alberti PW, Bryce DP (eds): Workshops from the Centennial Conference on Laryngeal Cancer. Appleton & Lange, East Norwalk, CT, 1976

99. Spiro RH, Lewis JS, Hajdu SI, et al: Mucus gland tumors of the larynx and laryngopharynx. Ann Otol Rhinol Laryngol 85:498, 1976

100. Hadju SI, Huvos AG, Goodner JT: Carcinoma of the trachea. Clinicopathologic study of 41 cases. Cancer 25:1448, 1970

101. Houston WE, Payne WS, Harrison EG Jr: Primary cancers of the trachea. Arch Surg 99:132, 1969

102. Cohen J, Guillamondegui OM, Batsakis JG, et al: Cancer of minor salivary glands of the larynx. Am J Surg 150:513, 1985

103. Olofsson J, Van Nostrand AW: Adenoid cystic carcinoma of the larynx: A report of four cases and a review of the literature. Cancer 40:1307, 1977

104. Stillwagon GB, Smith RR, Highstein C, et al: Adenoid cystic carcinoma of the supraglottic larynx: Report of a case and review of the literature. Am J Otolaryngol 6:309, 1985

105. Frable WJ, Wheelock MC: Carcinoma of the trachea. Acta Otolaryngol 76:174, 1962

106. Cleveland RH, Nice CM Jr: Primary adenoid cystic carcinoma (cylindroma) of the trachea. Radiology 122:597, 1977

107. Eby LS, Johnson DS, Baker HW: Adenoid cystic carcinoma of head and neck. Cancer 29:1160, 1972

108. Kaznelson DJ, Schindel J: Mucoepidermoid carcinoma of the air passages: Report of three cases. Laryngoscope 89:115, 1979

109. Frable WJ, Elzay RP: Tumors of minor salivary glands. A report of 73 cases. Cancer 25:932, 1970

110. Johns ME, Batsakis JG, Short CD: Oncocytic and oncocytoid tumors of the salivary glands. Laryngoscope 83:1940, 1973

111. Yamase HT, Putman HC: Oncocytic papillary cystadenomatosis of the larynx. A clinicopathologic entity. Cancer 44:2306, 1979

112. MacMillan RH, Fechner RE: Pleomorphic adenoma of the larynx. Arch Pathol Lab Med 110:245, 1986

113. Chan KM, Fine G, Lewis J, et al: Benign mixed tumors of the trachea. Cancer 44:2260, 1979

114. Briselli M, Mark GJ, Brillo HC: Tracheal carcinoids. Cancer 42:2870, 1978

115. Whicker JH, Carder GA, Devine KD: Metastasis to the larynx. Report of a case and review of the literature. Arch Otolaryngol 96:182, 1972

116. Djalilian M, Beahrs OH, Devine KD: Intraluminal involvement of the larynx and trachea by thyroid cancer. Am J Surg 128:500, 1974

117. Lawson W, Zak FG: The glomus bodies (paraganglion) of the larynx and trachea by thyroid cancer. Laryngoscope 84:98, 1974

118. Kleinsasser O: Das Glomus laryngicum inferius. Ein bisher unbekanntes, nicht chromafinnes Paraganglion vom Bau der sogenannten Carotisdruse im menschlichen Kehlkopf. Arch Otorhinolaryngol 184:214, 1964

119. Michaels L: Neurogenic tumors, granular cell tumor, and paraganglioma. p. 501. In Alberti PW, Bryce DP (eds): Workshops from the Centennial Conference on Laryngeal Cancer. Appleton & Lange, East Norwalk, CT, 1976

120. Tobin HA, Harris HH: Nonchromaffin paraganglioma of the larynx. Case report and review of the literature. Arch Otolaryngol 96:154, 1972

121. Liew SH, Leong AS, Tang HM: Tracheal paraganglioma: A case report with review of the literature. Cancer 47:1387, 1981

122. Moore ES, Martin H: Melanoma of the upper respiratory tract and oral cavity. Cancer 8:1167, 1955

123. Mori K, Cho H, Som M: Primary "flat" melanoma of the trachea. J Pathol 121:101, 1977

124. Batsakis JG, Fox JE: Supporting tissue neoplasms of the larynx. Surg Gynecol Obstet 131:989, 1970

125. Schaeffer BT, Som PM, Biller HF, et al: Schwannomas of the larynx: Review and computed tomographic scan analysis. Head Neck Surg 8:469, 1986

126. Chang-Lo M: Laryngeal involvement in von Recklinghausen's disease: A case report and review of the literature. Laryngoscope 87:435, 1977

127. Gregg JB, Myrabo AK: Combined neurofibroma and carcinoma in the larynx. Arch Otolaryngol 69:307, 1959

128. Fisher ER, Wechsler H: Granular cell myoblastoma, a misnomer. Electron microscopic histochemical evidence concerning its Schwann cell derivation and nature (granular cell Schwannoma). Cancer 15:936, 1962

129. Garancis JC, Komorowski RA, Kuzma JF: Granular cell myoblastoma. Cancer 25:542, 1970

130. Booth JB, Osborn DA: Granular cell myoblastoma of the larynx. Acta Otolaryngol (Stockh) 70:279, 1970

131. Helidonis E, Dokianakis G, Pantazopoulos: Granular cell myoblastoma of the larynx. J Laryngol Otol 92:525, 1978

132. Muthuswamy PP, Alrenga DP, Marks P, et al: Granular cell myoblastoma: Rare localization in the trachea. Report of a case and review of the literature. Am J Med 80:714, 1986

133. Bangle RA: Morphologic and histochemical study of the granular cell myoblastoma. Cancer 5:950, 1952

134. Compagno J, Hyams VJ, Ste-Marie P: Benign granular cell tumors of the larynx: A review of 36 cases with clinicopathologic data. Ann Otol Rhinol Laryngol 84:308, 1975

135. Coates HL, McDonald TJ, Devine KD, et al: Granular cell tumors of the larynx. Ann Otol Rhinol Laryngol 85:504, 1976

136. Frable MA, Fischer R: Granular cell myoblastoma. Laryngoscope 84:2051, 1976

137. Tsui HN, Loré JM Jr: Congenital subglottic fibroma in the newborn. Laryngoscope 86:571, 1976

138. Pollak ER, Naunheim KS, Little AG: Fibromyxoma of the trachea. A review of benign tracheal tumors. Arch Pathol Lab Med 109:926, 1985

139. Kaplan MS, Livingston PA, Baker DC Jr: Diagnosis of tracheal tumors. Ann Otol Rhinol Laryngol 82:790, 1973

140. Siegel MJ, McAlister WH: Tracheal histiocytoma: An inflammatory pseudotumor. J Can Assoc Radiol 29:273, 1978

141. Sandstrom RE, Proppe KH, Trelstad RL: Fibrous histiocytoma of the trachea. Am J Clin Pathol 70:429, 1978

142. Hakimi M, Pai RP, Fine G, et al: Fibrous histiocytoma of the trachea. Chest 68:367, 1975

143. Moersch HJ, Claggett T, Ellis HF: Tumors of the trachea. Med Clin North Am 38:1091, 1954

144. Cohen SR, Landing BH, Isaccs H: Fibrous histiocytoma of the trachea. Ann Otol Rhinol Laryngol 87:2, 1978

145. Ferlito A, Nicolai P, Recher G, et al: Primary laryngeal malignant fibrous histiocytoma: Review of the literature and report of seven cases. Laryngoscope 93:1351, 1983

146. Rolander T, Kim OJ, Shumrik DA: Fibrous xanthoma of the larynx. Arch Otolaryngol 96:168, 1972

147. Wetmore RF: Fibrous histiocytoma of the larynx in a child. Case report and review. Clin Pediatr 26:200, 1987

148. Paludetti G, Rosignobi M: Leiomyoma of the trachea: Report of a case and review of the literature. J Laryngol Otol 98:947, 1984

149. Miller DR: Benign tumors of lung and trachealbronchial tree. Ann Thorac Surg 8:542, 1969

150. Winther LK: Rhabdomyoma of the hypopharynx and larynx. Report of two cases with a review of the literature. J Laryngol Otol 90:1041, 1976

151. Bagby RA, Packer JT, Iglesias RG: Rhabdomyoma of the larynx. Report of a case. Arch Otolaryngol 102:101, 1976

152. Battifora HA, Eisenstein R, Schild JA: Rhabdomyoma of the larynx: Ultrastructural study and comparison with granular cell tumors (myoblastomas). Cancer 23:183, 1969

153. Maier HD: Hemangiomas of the subglottic region, trachea, and mediastinum in infancy and childhood. Ann Thorac Surg 3:514, 1967

154. Flege JB, Valencia G, Zimmerman G: Obstruction of a child's trachea by a polypoid hemangioendothelioma. J Thorac Cardiovasc Surg 56:144, 1968

155. Ferguson GB: Hemangiomas of the adult and of the infant larynx. Arch Otolaryngol 40:189, 1940

156. New GB, Erich JB: Benign tumors of the larynx. A study of seven hundred and twenty-two cases. Arch Otolaryngol 28:841, 1938

157. Holinger PH, Brown WT, Maurizi DG: Tracheostomy in the newborn. Am J Surg 109:771, 1965

158. Tiwari RM, Snow GB, Balm AJ, et al: Cartilagenous tumours of the larynx. J Laryngol Otol 101:266, 1987

159. Barsocchini LM, Moody G: Cartilaginous tumors of the larynx. A review of the literature and a report of four cases. Ann Otol Rhino Laryngol 77:146, 1968

160. Huizenga C, Balogh K: Cartilaginous tumors of the larynx. A clinicopathologic study of 10 new cases and a review of the literature. Cancer 26:201, 1970

161. Goethels PL, Dahlin DC, Devine KD: Cartilaginous tumors of the larynx. Surg Gynecol Obstet 117:77, 1963

162. Brewster DC, MacMillan IK, Edwards FR: Chondroma of the trachea: Report of a case and review of the literature. Ann Thorac Surg 19:576, 1975

163. Foxwell DB: Solitary chondroma of the trachea. J Laryngol Otol 69:419, 1955

164. Smith CC, Dixon MF: Tracheopathia osteoplastica with pulmonary thromboembolic disease. Br J Dis Chest 66:192, 1972

165. Flanagan P, Cross RM, Libcke JH: Fibrosarcoma of the larynx. J Laryngol Otol 79:1049, 1965

166. Prasad JN: Fibrosarcoma of larynx. J Laryngol Otol 86:267, 1972

167. Friedmann I: Sarcomas of the larynx. p. 479. In Alberti PW, Bryce DP (eds): Workshops from the Centennial Conference on Laryngeal Cancer. Appleton & Lange, East Norwalk, CT, 1976

168. Roncoroni AJ, Puy RJ, Goldman E, et al: Malignant fibrous xanthoma of larynx. Arch Otolaryngol 101:135, 1975

169. Ferlito A: Simultaneous malignant pleomorphic fibrous histiocytoma and squamous cell carcinoma in situ of the larynx. Acta Otorhinolaryngol Belg 30:390, 1976

170. Louie S, Cross CE, Amott TR, et al: Postirradiation malignant fibrous histiocytoma of the trachea. Am Rev Respir Dis 135:761, 1987

171. Haerr RW, Turalba CI, El-Mahdi AM, et al: Alveolar rhabdomyosarcoma of the larynx: Case report and literature review. Laryngoscope 97:339, 1987

172. Frugoni P, Ferlito A: Pleomorphic rhabdomyosarcoma of the larynx. A case report and review of the literature. J Laryngol Otol 90:687, 1976

173. Winter LK, Lorentzen M: Rhabdomyosarcoma of the larynx. Report of two cases and a review of the literature. J Laryngol Otol 92:417, 1978

174. Dodd-o JM, Wieneke KF, Rosman PM: Laryngeal rhabdomyosarcoma. Case report and literature review. Cancer 59:1012, 1987

175. Pratt LW, Goodof II: Hemangioendothelial sarcoma of larynx. Arch Otolaryngol 87:484, 1968

176. Ferlito A, Nicolai P, and Caruso G: Angiosarcoma of the larynx. Case report. Ann Otol Rhinol Laryngol 94:93, 1985

177. Pesavento G, Ferlito A: Hemangiopericytoma of the larynx. A clinico-pathological study with review of the literature. J Laryngol Otol 96:1065, 1982

178. Miller LH, Sanatella-Latimer L, Miller T: Synovial sarcoma of larynx. Trans Am Acad Ophthalmol Otolaryngol 80:448, 1975

179. Harrison EG Jr, Black BM, Devine KD: Synovial sarcoma primary in the neck. Arch Pathol 71:137, 1961

180. Allsbrook WC Jr, Harmon JD, Chongchitnant N, et al: Liposarcoma of the larynx. Arch Pathol Lab Med 109:294, 1985

181. Ferlito A, Nicolai P, Montaguti A, et al: Chondrosarcoma of the larynx: Review of the literature and report of three cases. Am J Otolaryngol 5:350, 1984

182. Poole AG, Hall R: Chondrosarcoma of the larynx: A case report and review of the literature. Aust NZ J Surg 56:281, 1986

183. Daniels AC, Conner GH, Straus FH: Primary chondrosarcoma of the tracheobronchial tree. Report of a unique case and brief review. Arch Pathol 84:615, 1967

184. Dahm LJ, Schaefer SO, Cardea HM: Osteosarcoma of the soft tissue of the larynx. Report of a case with light and electron microscopic studies. Cancer 42:2343, 1978

185. Morley AR, Cameron DS, Watson AJ: Osteosarcoma of the larynx. J Laryngol Otol 87:997, 1973

186. Sprinkle PM, Allan MS: Osteosarcoma of the larynx. Laryngoscope 76:325, 1966

187. Swerdlow JB, Merl SA, Davey RF, et al: Non-Hodgkin's lymphoma limited to the larynx. Cancer 53:2546, 1984

188. Cohen SR, Landing BH, Isaacs H, et al: Solitary plasmacytoma of the larynx and upper trachea associated with systemic lupus erythematosus. Ann Otol Rhinol Laryngol 87:11, 1978

189. Gorenstein A, Neal HB III, Devine KD: Solitary extramedullary plasmacytoma of the larynx. Arch Otolaryngol 103:159, 1977

190. Pahor AL: Plasmacytoma of the larynx. J Laryngol Otol 92:223, 1978

191. Rawson AJ, Eyler PW, Horn RC Jr: Plasma cell tumors of the upper respiratory tract. A clinicopathologic study with emphasis on the criteria for histologic diagnosis. Am J Pathol 26:445, 1950

192. East D: Laryngeal involvement in multiple myeloma. J Laryngol Otol 92:61, 1978

193. Hood AF, Mark GJ, Hunt JV: Laryngeal mycosis fungoides. Cancer 43:1527, 1979

194. Horny HP, Parwaresch MR, Kaiserling E, et al: Mast cell sarcoma of the larynx. J Clin Pathol 39:596, 1986

19

Diffuse Diseases of the Lungs

Roberta R. Miller
William M. Thurlbeck

This chapter deals with medical lung disease and the subsequent one with surgical lung disease. The distinction is not always clear. Surgical lung conditions are usually found in patients under the care of surgeons, and the surgical procedures are lung resection, intended to be curative. Patients with medical lung disease are generally treated by internists and undergo surgery for diagnostic purposes. Conditions such as Wegener's granulomatosis, lymphomatoid granulomatosis, bronchocentric granulomatosis, and allergic angiitis and granulomatosis are dealt with in Chapter 20 because of Dr. Saldana's special expertise, although they are more properly thought of as medical conditions.

First we will deal with basic histology, then definitions and concepts, with some emphasis on pathophysiology that all surgical pathologists should know, and finally specific diseases under the broad categories of infiltrative lung disease, obstructive lung disease, and pulmonary vascular disease.

NORMAL HISTOLOGY

This section will describe the normal histology relevant to this chapter, arbitrarily considered to be that of bronchioles, the gas-exchanging units of the lung, and the pulmonary vessels. Of necessity the review must be brief; excellent reviews of lung structure are available.[1-5]

Bronchi are defined as airways that have cartilage in their walls, and the airways distal to them, without alveoli in their walls, are referred to as (membranous) *bron-*

chioles. Bronchioles have an irregular dichotomous branching pattern except for their distal three orders, which show regular dichotomy. An important feature is that while each succeeding generation has a smaller diameter than the preceding one, the total cross-sectional area increases with succeeding generations, since each daughter bronchiole has more than half the diameter of the parent one. It is this increase in total cross-sectional area, which becomes rapid distally, that accounts for the fact that there is little resistance to flow in the peripheral airways (see chronic air flow obstruction, below). Their bronchiolar mucosa lacks the compound mucus-secreting subepithelial glands so characteristic of bronchi. The lining epithelium of even the largest bronchioles when fully distended loses most of the pseudostratified appearance of bronchi. The great majority of the cells lining the bronchioles are ciliated. Their nuclei are basal, rather square in shape, and arranged in a single row in the smaller bronchioles, but the epithelium of larger bronchioles is still pseudostratified. Scattered basal cells with elongated nuclei lie deep to the nuclei of the ciliated cells and provide focal regions where the epithelium is pseudostratified. Mucus-secreting cells are extremely scanty in nonsmokers. When these cells are distended with mucus, they are referred to as *goblet cells.*

Neuroendocrine cells (K cells, Kulchitsky cells) of the lung occur either singly or in clusters, the latter being termed *neuroepithelial bodies.* By hematoxylin and eosin (H&E) staining, these cells have a clear or slightly eosinophilic cytoplasm; with appropriate silver stains, they may be argyrophilic. They are considerably more numerous in fetal than in adult lungs and are distributed mostly in the epithelium of subsegmental bronchi. They are a part of the amine precursor uptake and decarboxylation (APUD) cell system throughout the body and ultrastructurally contain characteristic cytoplasmic dense core granules. Normally they may be shown to contain bombesin, leu-enkaphalin, calcitonin, serotonin, and neuron-specific enolase, although the precise role of these substances in the regulation of growth, development, and gas exchange is unknown. Carcinoid tumors and small cell carcinomas show differentiation toward neuroendocrine cells. In addition to bombesin and other indigenous peptides, these tumors may also produce hormones such as adrenocorticotropin (ACTH) and antidiuretic hormone, which are not demonstrable in normal lung epithelium.[6,7]

The columnar, nonciliated secretory cell (*Clara cell*) is inconspicuous in humans as compared with small laboratory animals. In laboratory animals Clara cells are the progenitor cells of the bronchioles and may differentiate into Clara cells, ciliated cells, or mucus-secreting cells. The epithelial basement membrane is very thin since there is little collagen associated with the true basal lamina, and it is the collagen that makes the basement membrane visible by light microscopy. An elastic tissue net is closely applied to the basal lamina. The muscle of the bronchioles is arranged in a geodesic pattern. A few mononuclear inflammatory cells are present in most bronchioles, but even a modest collection of cells, and any neutrophils, should be regarded as abnormal. In inflated lung specimens the walls of the bronchioles are smooth; however in uninflated specimens the walls often have a crenated appearance. Outside of the muscular layer the arteries and bronchioles may share a common adventitia. Outside of this there is loose connective tissue, forming part of the lung interstitium. Surrounding connective tissue becomes progressively scantier in the smallest bronchioles.

The last purely conducting bronchiole, without alveoli in its walls, is the terminal bronchiole. Distal to it is the gas-exchanging unit of the lung, known as the *acinus*. In order, it comprises respiratory bronchioles, alveolar ducts, and alveolar sacs. Respiratory bronchioles have both alveolated and nonalveolated walls. The latter have epithelium like that of bronchioles except that the cells are flatter. The majority of the cells are still ciliated. There is a relatively abrupt transition between the ciliated cells and flattened epithelium, resembling that of the alveoli. A simplified model of the acinus is shown in Figure 19-1. Respiratory bronchioles have more alveoli in their walls in succeeding generations and are succeeded by alveolar ducts, entirely alveolated conducting structures. The terminal unit of the acinus is the alveolar sac, which is likewise entirely alveolated. The acinus is important as the gas-exchanging unit of the lung, and it is enlargement

COMPONENT PARTS OF ACINUS

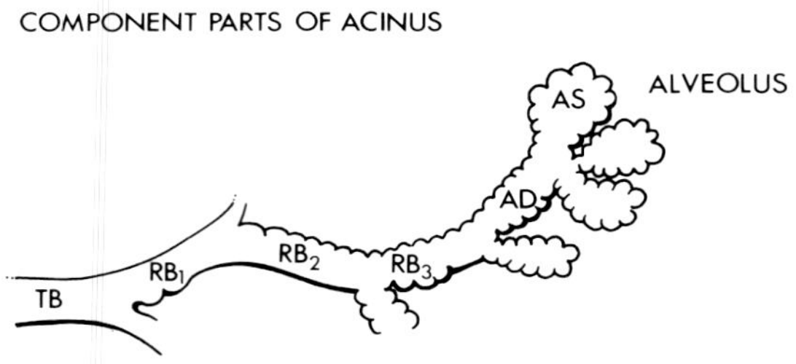

Fig. 19-1. The acinus is the gas-exchanging unit of the lung and consists in series of respiratory bronchioles (RB), alveolar ducts (AD), and alveolar sacs (AS). (From Thurlbeck,[247] with permission.)

and destruction of this structure that results in emphysema.

The surface of human *alveoli* is lined by two types of cells. Most of the surface is covered by the thin, greatly extended cytoplasm of type I epithelial cells, which contain few organelles. There are actually more type II epithelial cells, but because they are columnar, they cover only about 5 percent of the surface of the alveoli. They are characteristically situated in the angles of the alveoli and are thus sometimes called *corner* or *niche* cells. They contain large numbers of organelles and the characteristic osmiophilic lamellar bodies that when secreted into the alveolus constitute the surface-active material essential for alveolar stability. Type II cells have another vital function, that of being the progenitor cells of alveolar epithelium. They have the ability to divide and produce two type II cells, and this happens during lung development and following injury. They can also divide to form one type II cell and one type I cell, and this is a normal process in mature lungs and in the recovery phase of lung injury. Type I and type II cells are joined by tight junctions and thus represent the major barrier to passage of large molecules from the capillary lumen to the air space.

Alveolar macrophages play a major role in the lung's defense mechanism. Their source is controversial. Some consider that they are mainly derived from the bone marrow, undergo a maturation division in the alveolar interstitium, and then pass into the air spaces. Considerable multiplication of macrophages also may occur within air spaces, especially in the neonatal period.[8] Alveolar macrophages differ from peritoneal macrophages in that the former are more dependent on aerobic metabolism.

The interstitium of the alveolar wall contains capillaries (although many would argue these are not part of the interstitium), collagen fibers, elastic fibers, glycosaminoglycans, and interstitial cells. The latter include mast cells, smooth muscle cells, occasional lymphocytes, pericytes, and connective tissue cells. The connective tissue cells are usually referred to as *fibroblasts*, but they appear quiescent and have few organelles. Bundles of filaments identified as actin and myosin have been noted in these cells, and it has been suggested that they may have a contractile role and may control perfusion in the lung. Capillary endothelial cells are joined by tight or "semitight" junctions. The latter are relatively sparse but permit the passage of large molecules. Endothelial cells are metabolically active and metabolize serotonin, norepinephrine, acetylcholine, adenine monophosphate, adenine triphosphate, bradykinin, angiotensin I, very low density lipoproteins, and prostaglandins E_1, E_2, and F_2. A hierarchy of susceptibility to injury exists in the cells of the alveolar wall. The type I cell is the most sensitive, and damage leads to increased permeability and alveolar edema. The capillary endothelium is the next most sensitive, followed by the type II cell. The alveolar wall has a "thin" and a "thick" side. On the thin side the basal lamina of epithelial cells and that of endothelial cells fuse, and gas exchange is most easily accomplished here. On the thick side the basal laminae are separate, and in this space lies another part, the interstitium of the lung, with the components noted above. There is a single capillary layer in the alveolar wall, and capillaries wind from one side of the alveolus to the other.

The *pulmonary vascular tree* is a high capacitance system, and the resistance vessels are the muscular pulmonary arteries. Pulmonary arteries accompany the airways, and it is common to refer to this arrangement together with the common adventitia as the bronchovascular bundle. It is important to recognize that age-dependent structural differences exist in the pulmonary arterial system, and there is increased intimal thickening with age. In the adult, elastic arteries, with more than two elastic laminae, are larger than 1 mm in diameter, and arteries between 100 and 200 μm are muscular, with the muscle enclosed by an internal and an external elastic lamina. Smaller vessels may be muscular (when the muscle is spirally arranged around the vessel so that parts of the wall appear muscular and parts nonmuscular), and nonmuscular. The two elastic laminae fuse where muscle is absent, and a single fragmented elastic lamina separates the intima from the adventitia. The term *pulmonary arteriole* (arterial vessels less than 100 μm in diameter) has become obsolete. The appearance, in terms of vessel size, is surprisingly similar in adults, children, and fetuses,[4] but this is because vessels of similar size represent different generations of artery in infants as compared with adults. When compared by position in the lung, the structure of vessels is very different at different ages. In the fetus and soon after birth, the intra-acinar arteries are all nonmuscular. There is increasing muscularity of the intra-acinar arteries during childhood, but even at age 11 this process is not complete, muscle extending only to the level of the alveolar ducts. In the adult, arterial muscle reaches the alveoli. The ratio of arterial wall thickness

to external arterial diameter is a useful parameter to assess abnormality, but it should be noted that values are low for arteries distended with contrast medium at high pressure. In undistended muscular arteries, the ratio of medial thickness to external arterial diameter (external elastic lamina to external elastic lamina) is about 5 percent (3 to 7 percent).

Pulmonary veins commence at the distal end of alveolar capillaries and proceed in the interstitium of the lung toward the lobular septa. Small pulmonary veins are indistinguishable from nonmuscular pulmonary arteries by histology, but the distinction can be made by the juxta-airway position of pulmonary arteries. The veins drain proximally in the septa, and then form larger structures that lie separate from arteries and airways. The walls of veins are much thinner than those of arteries and in general have a single, poorly formed external elastic lamina and no muscle. Larger veins may contain more than one elastic lamina, also poorly formed. Muscle is scanty. Larger veins are seldom seen in open lung biopsies.

Pulmonary lymphatics are not present between alveolar walls but start where alveoli are juxtaposed to lobular septa and the bronchovascular bundles. Others may commence within the interstitium of the lung. They are very thin-walled vessels with a lining of endothelial cells lying on a basal lamina, embedded in a loose connective tissue matrix. They contain valves that direct the flow of lymph. Lymphatics proceed centrally with the bronchovascular tree, in lobular septa, and with veins, and also to the pleural surface. Pleural lymphatics course on the surface of the lung and send numerous connections into the interior of the lung to anastomose with perivenous lymphatics.

The *interstitium of the lung* is an important concept. It has never been officially defined but our understanding is that it is tissue between structures concerned with gas exchange. Thus it is the loose connective tissue outside of airways and arteries, veins and lymphatics, and is the tissue between the capillary and epithelium on the thick side of the alveolar wall.

TERMINOLOGY AND CONCEPTS

Diffuse Infiltrative Lung Disease and Diffuse Interstitial Lung Disease

A more detailed discussion of the concept of diffuse infiltrative lung disease can be found elsewhere.[9] It implies in large part a diffuse increase in tissue in the interstitium of the lung, the supporting tissue around airways, vessels, lobular septa, and the thick side of the alveolar wall (see the above section on normal histology). However, certain conditions such as bronchiolitis obliterans with organizing pneumonia (BOOP), diffuse pulmonary hemorrhage, and pulmonary alveolar proteinosis are mainly intra-alveolar processes with only slight (or no) interstitial component. Thus, we prefer the term *diffuse infiltrative lung disease,* meaning an increase in tissue within the interstitium and sometimes air spaces. A rigid definition cannot be applied—for example, widespread bronchopneumonia might fall under this definition. The increased amounts of tissue produce radiologically observable opacities, which are generally diffuse and bilateral. However, it is worth noting that 7.7 percent of chest radiographs are normal in patients with chronic infiltrative lung disease on biopsy.[10]

End-Stage or Honeycomb Lung

When alveolar walls are damaged in infiltrative lung disease, fibrosis of the lung may ensue. This has best been described in usual interstitial pneumonia (UIP) (fibrosing alveolitis).[11] It is thought that damage to and disruption of alveolar basal laminae constitute an essential part of this process. Granulation tissue forms within alveolar walls and is then covered by surface epithelium. In other alveoli the granulation tissue protrudes as a polypoid mass into alveolar lumina and then becomes re-epithelialized. Multiplication of fibroblasts and secretion of collagen within the interstitium also occur. The granulation tissue retracts, and the end result is gradual obliteration of alveoli. As this happens, more and more gas-exchanging tissue is lost and becomes incorporated into scars. The airways proximal to the scar (respiratory bronchioles and proximal alveolar ducts) dilate, and alveolar epithelium in them disappears and is replaced by other epithelium. The epithelium lining the spaces is highly variable—it may consist of type I epithelium, type II epithelium, bronchiolar cells, or squamous (epidermoid) cells. Generally a mixture of cell types lines the spaces, which are dilated airways rather than true cysts[12] but are greatly distorted in shape. Consequently, secretions accumulate. The final picture on cut section is of multiple cysts, usually 0.5 to 2 mm in diameter, lined by various types of epithelium and containing secretions. They are separated from each other by connective tissue

of varying thickness and cellularity, and smooth muscle, even fat, may be present.

This appearance is referred to as *end-stage lung* or *honeycomb lung.* The former term is preferable since the resemblance to a honeycomb requires imagination and a penchant for inaccuracy. The concept of end-stage lung is critical. A variety of diseases such as UIP, desquamative interstitial pneumonia (DIP), extrinsic allergic alveolitis, sarcoidosis, and asbestosis may all end up this way. Similarly, focal areas of scarring resembling end-stage lung may occur in otherwise normal lungs. End stage lung is nonspecific and should be thought of in the same way as end-stage renal disease. A common error is to confuse end-stage lung with UIP.

Restrictive Lung Disease

There is no universally accepted definition of *restrictive lung disease.* Most often the term is applied to patients with extensive bilateral pulmonary radiopacities. Under these circumstances a relatively uniform clinical picture emerges in terms of symptoms, signs, radiologic findings, and pulmonary function. These patients correspond closely to patients who have infiltrative lung disease, and on that account the lungs may be stiff. However, the picture is incomplete, and a wider concept is sometimes useful.

In the broadest concept, restrictive lung disease implies impaired maximal filling of the lung with air, that is, diminished total lung capacity. The amount of air that the lung can contain depends on the force applied to the respiratory system, the degree to which the respiratory system can respond to the force applied to it, and whether or not the air spaces in the lung can be filled with air. Thus, in simplistic terms, restrictive lung disease can be classified by both the mechanism and the site of limitation (Table 19-1).

By far the most common cause of restrictive lung disease is diffuse infiltrative lung disease, and this may be the consequence of approximately 100 different conditions. Because they have lung stiffness in common, these conditions show fairly uniform alterations of pulmonary function test data. Compliance—an expression of lung

TABLE 19-1. Pathogenesis of Restrictive Lung Disease

Mechanism of Limitation	Site of Limitation		
	Chest Wall	Pleura	Lungs
Increased stiffness of respiratory system (decreased compliance)	Kyphoscoliosis, chest wall scarring	Pleuritis	Infiltrative lung disease (*e.g.,* fibrosing alveolitis)
Normal compliance of the respiratory system	Paralysis of muscles, obesity	Pleural effusion	Tumor masses, alveolar edema

distensibility in terms of the increase in volume of the lung per increase in transpulmonary pressure (in centimeters of water column), generally expressed in the tidal volume range—is decreased because the lung is stiff. The effects on lung volumes are predictable. Total lung capacity is decreased, because at high lung volumes the respiratory muscles are relatively weak and cannot stretch the stiffened lung to reach maximal volume. Functional residual capacity is the resting volume of the lungs and is determined by the balance between the force of the lungs, which tend to collapse inward, and the force of the chest wall, which tends to spring outward at low lung volumes. In fibrotic lung disease this balance of forces occurs at a lower lung volume because the lung has increased recoil and overcomes the outward recoil force of the chest wall at a lower lung volume. In those other than young subjects, residual volume is mainly determined by airway closure. Because of increased recoil pressure, airways will be kept open at lower lung volumes in patients with infiltrative lung disease, and residual volume will decrease. Total lung capacity is affected to a greater extent than residual volume, and vital capacity is therefore reduced. Thus, characteristically, all the major lung volumes—residual volume, functional residual capacity, total lung capacity, and vital capacity—will be decreased in restrictive lung disease due to infiltrative lung disease.

The results of standard tests of expiratory function may be anomalous. Because vital capacity is decreased, expiratory volumes will be reduced; therefore, tests of expiratory flow, such as the forced expiratory volume in 1 second (FEV_1) and the maximal midexpiratory flow rate, will be reduced when expressed as a percentage of the predicted values. However, because the recoil pressure is increased, the driving force applied to the lungs (recoil pressure) is increased, and the airways are held open more widely at corresponding lung volumes. Thus, the flows may be supernormal when corrected for the compromise in lung volume, and this is best seen in the ratio of FEV_1 to forced vital capacity or to vital capacity, which is characteristically abnormally high in pulmonary fibrosis. Total airway resistance is primarily dependent on large airway size and is unchanged. However, peripheral airway resistance is increased because of distortion and narrowing of the airways (since peripheral resistance contributes little to total airway resistance, the increase in peripheral airway resistance has little effect on total airway resistance).

Most characteristically, the diffusing capacity (transfer factor) for carbon monoxide is reduced in patients with infiltrative lung disease. The main reason for this reduction is an abnormality in ventilation to perfusion matching rather than alteration in diffusion, although the latter abnormality is now regarded as contributing about 20 per-

cent of the abnormality in gas exchange. Ventilation/perfusion abnormalities are brought about by varying degrees of alteration of lung compliance within the lung and by varying degrees of small airway resistance. In addition, increased pulmonary artery pressure shifts blood flow to the upper part of the lung, normally relatively poorly ventilated. Diffusion limitation may be an important factor in the increased hypoxemia that patients with infiltrative lung disease characteristically develop on exercise. Blood gas abnormalities are also characteristic. For an unknown reason, patients with restrictive lung disease due to infiltrative lung disease tend to ventilate much more than patients with equivalent hypoxemia due to other causes. Overventilation does little to increase oxygen content of the blood since patients are generally breathing on the "flat" part of the oxygen dissociation curve. This means that pulmonary venous blood from overventilated parts of the lung does not contain much more oxygen than normal. When mixed with pulmonary venous blood from the underventilated parts of the lung, the oxygen content of the blood is in the low to low-normal range. By contrast, overventilation has a marked effect on the carbon dioxide content of the blood since patients are on the "steep" slope of the carbon dioxide dissociation curve. The carbon dioxide content of blood from overventilated parts of the lung is greatly decreased, and when such blood is mixed with blood from the underventilated areas, the resulting carbon dioxide content of the blood is generally in the low-normal or normal range until advanced states of the disease. Classically, the ratio of the dead space to tidal volume is increased.

As pointed out earlier, not all patients with restrictive lung disease have infiltrative lung disease. Equally, not all patients with infiltrative lung disease have restrictive lung disease; for example, lung volumes are often normal in desquamative interstitial pneumonia and increased in lymphangiomyomatosis. In general terms, however, it is useful to equate restrictive lung disease with infiltrative lung disease. However, one is a functional concept and the other is a morphologic one. Thus, it is not surprising that the intersection space is not complete.

Basic Patient Biopsy Considerations

Many patients with diffuse infiltrative lung disease will ultimately require tissue diagnosis. The type of biopsy, site of biopsy, and laboratory procedures all depend on a few basic clinical and radiologic questions.

1. Is the patient apparently immunocompromised or nonimmunocomprised?
2. Is the process acute or chronic?

3. Is the process central or peripheral?
4. Is the process localized or diffuse?
5. How critically ill is the patient and how quickly is a laboratory diagnosis required?

In this era of high-dose chemotherapy for malignant tumors, aggressive immunosuppression for autoimmune diseases and transplant recipients, and acquired immunosuppression in acquired immunodeficiency syndrome (AIDS), lung disease in the immunocompromised host has become common. These patients ordinarily present acutely (on Friday night), and the differential diagnoses ordinarily are infection, drug reaction, recurrent cancer, and pulmonary hemorrhage. The cited yield of different diagnostic techniques is variable. Bronchoalveolar lavage is highly sensitive in detecting *Pneumocystis carinii* (Pc) pneumonia in AIDS patients[13] and possibly will prove to be effective in the diagnosis of cytomegalovirus (CMV) infection in the future.[14] Transbronchial lung biopsy, usually in conjunction with bronchoalveolar lavage, is a reasonably sensitive method of diagnosing infection in the immunocompromised host.[15] Open lung biopsy is still the major means of diagnosing noninfectious infiltrates in the immunocompromised host.[16] If an open lung biopsy is required, the biopsy site should ordinarily be from the area of worst involvement, since this increases the probability of finding diagnostic abnormalities.[17] Preliminary bacteriologic results, fluorescence studies for viral antigens, and histologic examination for pattern of reaction, viral inclusions, and fungal or *Pneumocystis carinii* organisms should be available within 24 hours. Thus, should the patient undergo biopsy on Friday or Saturday, touch preparations and frozen sections with H&E and silver stains are often required.

Occasionally, an apparently nonimmunocompromised patient will present with acute infiltrative lung disease, the etiology of which eludes diagnostic techniques less invasive than open biopsy. Considerations of site of biopsy and laboratory procedure, in general, are similar to those pertaining to the immunocompromised host. One is likely to find nonspecific diffuse alveolar damage, presumably due to viral infection in most instances, but one may be surprised on occasion to find lymphangitic carcinoma, *Legionella* pneumonia, an unusual infection in an unsuspected AIDS patient, and so forth.

In a nonimmunocompromised patient with chronic infiltrative lung disease, the principles of type and site of biopsy and laboratory procedure are different. Transbronchial lung biopsy is likely to be fruitful in patients with sarcoidosis and lymphangitic carcinoma[18] and nondiagnostic in most other disease processes. Furthermore, should open lung biopsy be required, the object is to sample areas of "average" involvement rather than areas of worst involvement because of the likelihood of

obtaining end-stage lung in the latter sites.[17] Recent advances in computed tomography (CT) of the lungs potentially play a major role in the preoperative evaluation of these patients. CT is useful in distinguishing sarcoidosis and lymphangitic carcinoma from other types of chronic infiltrative lung disease, thus assisting in the decision of whether or not to attempt a transbronchial biopsy.[19] CT is also useful in assessing the distribution of disease, thus directing the surgeon to the area of accessible average involvement.[17] While routine avoidance of the lingula and right middle lobe was once the recommended policy, this no longer seems to be necessary, especially in view of the additional information provided by CT.[17] Frozen section is rarely indicated in chronic infiltrative lung disease, microbiologic studies may be done on a routine rather than urgent basis, and special stains for organisms may also be performed routinely on paraffin sections.

Lung Biopsy

The basic principles for deciding upon the type and site of biopsy have been discussed in the previous section. Transbronchial lung biopsy is reasonably likely to be diagnostic in Pc and CMV pneumonia in the immunocompromised host and sarcoid and lymphangitic carcinomatosis in the nonimmunocompromised patient. Otherwise, a transbronchial lung biopsy is likely to show either normal lung or nonspecific inflammation and/or fibrosis. In the immunocompromised host a nondiagnostic lavage or transbronchial biopsy is ultimately likely to represent either noninfectious disease or sampling error.[15] In the nonimmunocompromised patient little correlation has been found between nonspecific findings on transbronchial biopsy and definitive diagnosis established by subsequent open lung biopsy.[18]

Handling of Biopsied Tissue

Transbronchial Biopsy

In transbronchial biopsy, all the tissue is embedded in paraffin or plastic. Routine blind sampling for electron microscopy is not particularly useful. Serial sections should be obtained for H&E staining, special staining as indicated, and unstained slides, in order to use the limited amount of tissue as efficiently as possible.

Open Lung Biopsy

It is of the upmost importance that open lung biopsy material be fixed in the inflated state for adequate interpretation. There are two methods by which to achieve this objective.

The technique of Carrington and Gaensler[10] is to biopsy the lung while it is inflated with air by the anesthetist, maintain closure of the cut surface by clamps, and immerse the clamped sample into fixative, relying on transpleural diffusion for adequate fixation. This technique necessitates additional sampling for cultures, electron microscopy, mineral analysis, snap freezing, and so forth. We use an alternative and simpler approach whereby the lung sample is divided or wedged out by using a GIA stapler. The staple line of the specimen is excised and used for microbiology examination. The remainder of the wedge can be sampled as desired for frozen sections, electron microscopy, etc. Inflation of the remaining lung sample is achieved by gentle infusion of fixative into the cut surface via a small-bore syringe. Fixation in inflation at least 2 to 3 hours should be allowed before sectioning into blocks, and all the tissue should be processed.

As will be apparent from the following sections of this chapter, different diseases give rise to different architectural patterns. For example, the lesions of sarcoid and lymphangitic carcinomatosis are preferentially distributed along bronchovascular bundles and interlobular septa, eosinophilic granuloma is distributed as randomly dispersed stellate scars, primary pulmonary hypertension is primarily a vascular abnormality, and respiratory syncytial virus infection is primarily a bronchiolar abnormality. A low-power survey is useful to determine the general architectural pattern, and specific attention should be given to conducting airways, vessels, pleura, and alveoli. Polarized light microscopy should always be performed, and various special stains for organisms, elastin, fibrous tissue, and so forth obviously should be performed as indicated.

The Concept of Diffuse Alveolar Damage

The lung can only respond to injury in a limited number of ways, so many agents may produce a similar, if not identical, appearance. The initial lesion after injury may be characteristic for a particular substance. For example, capillary endothelium is primary affected in oxygen toxicity,[20] type I epithelial cells in paraquat poisoning,[21] type II cells in N-nitrosaminethiourea administration,[22] and the vascular endothelium of small vessels in bleomycin toxicity.[23] However, other cells become damaged, the initial specific lesions become obscured in a matter of days, and the appearance becomes nonspecific.

After the initial injury, which in general has been characterized by electron microscopic evidence of damage, more extensive damage occurs to the various cell types.[24] When type I cells are damaged, the integrity of the alveolar wall to fluid is lost, leading to increased permeability and alveolar edema. Passage of proteins, and probably fibrinogen in particular, together with tissue debris, leads to the formation of hyaline membranes in the alveolar spaces (Fig. 19-2). If the basement membrane remains intact and the damage limited, there is proliferation of type II cells to line the alveolar walls. The degree and nature of the cellular infiltration depend on the nature of the insult, but a mononuclear, especially macrophage, accumulation usually occurs and in large part represents

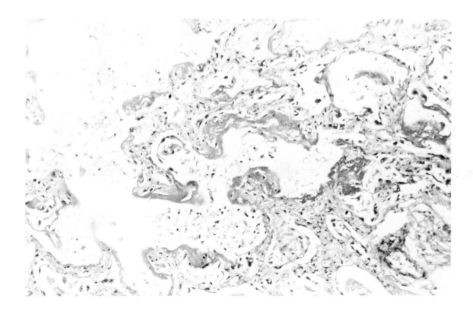

Fig. 19-2. Diffuse alveolar damage in the adult respiratory distress syndrome, showing hyaline membrane formation.

the attempt on the part of the host to clear the space of debris. At the same time there is proliferation of the interstitial cells to form many active fibroblasts, which lay down collagen in the interstitium. Collagen is formed first, and elastic tissue is not synthesized until after several weeks. If the basement membrane remains intact and the insult is limited, the amount of fibrous tissue laid down and the disorganization of lung structure are small. Thus, after a limited insult, such as experimental oxygen poisoning, there is only slight residual tissue alteration consistent with a return to normal, or almost normal, in lung function.[20] Similarly, most patients who recover from the adult respiratory distress syndrome (ARDS) have no or trivial functional effects.[25]

SPECIFIC CAUSES OF INFILTRATIVE LUNG DISEASE

Acute Infiltrative Lung Disease

It is convenient to divide infiltrative lung diseases into acute and chronic. The former have a course that is generally measured in days or weeks, the latter a course measured in months or years.

Adult Respiratory Distress Syndrome

At the time the first edition of this book was written there was considerable doubt as to whether the lesions in ARDS were intrinsic or due to concomitant oxygen therapy. While oxygen is undoubtedly a potent lung toxin (as described below), few doubt the existence of ARDS and that the lesions observed are due in greater or lesser part to the syndrome itself. A role separate from oxygen in the production of ARDS is supported by the obvious observation that lung involvement precedes (and indeed demands) oxygen administration and the facts that lesions have been described in patients who have not had high levels of oxygen[26] and that there is no consistent relationship between the amount of oxygen given and the severity of the lesion. ARDS was first clearly delineated in 1967 by Ashbaugh et al.[27] The usefulness of the term has been disputed,[28] since known conditions such as thromboemboli or specific viruses may cause the syndrome.

Characteristically, a previously well person, or at least one with previously normal lungs, suffers a sudden event such as nonthoracic trauma, generally with shock.[26] After an apparently stable period, dyspnea ensues and the chest radiograph shows rapidly progressive opacification until the lung becomes "whited out." Respiratory failure occurs, requiring ventilatory assistance and varying concentrations of inspired oxygen. About half of the patients recover from this episode with gradual radiologic clear-

ing. The remainder require progressively more aggressive ventilation, with higher ventilator end expiratory pressures and higher concentrations of oxygen. The lung becomes progressively stiffer, chest infiltrates progress, ventilation becomes more difficult, and the patient expires. This is a common condition. Although precise figures are not available, it has been estimated that there are 150,000 cases per year in the United States.

The causes of the syndrome are numerous. Shock of any etiology may result in ARDS. Nonthoracic trauma of any sort is the commonest cause, and excessive bleeding, either spontaneous or related to surgery, may also be complicated by ARDS. Traumatic fat embolism is a well known cause. Another important cause is infection, especially Gram-negative septicemia or viral infections. Aspiration of liquid such as gastric content or that occurring in near drowning is another cause, as is inhalation of a variety of toxic gases and fumes. Drug overdosage, notably heroin but also methadone, propoxyphene, and barbiturates, is another cause. Occasional cases appear to occur spontaneously.[29]

ARDS may be divided into four phases, the first of which is the *preclinical phase*, in which the patient has suffered one of the causes of ARDS but respiratory symptoms and evidence of respiratory failure are not yet apparent. Considerable effort has been made to predict those who will develop ARDS and those who will not, but no clear-cut predictors have yet emerged. Most of the data concerning this stage are naturally derived from experimental animals, but a remarkable study in human trauma[30] has shown that lung weight and hemoglobin content in the lung double in patients dying 0 to 1 hour after trauma, as compared with those dying immediately. Experimental studies have shown that the first lesion is subtle endothelial and alveolar epithelial damage, associated with capillary leak. The damage is thought to be due to aggregation of polymorphonuclear leukocytes (PMNs) after activation of the complement cascade. The PMNs produce damage to the endothelium by release of their lysosomal enzymes or by generation of free radicals. Another remarkable study has shown aggregations of PMNs in capillaries in lung biopsies performed in humans in the acute phase.[31] More florid edema now occurs, and survival after 1 hour is accompanied by further increase in lung weight.

The next phase is the *exudative phase,* which is characterized morphologically by acute diffuse alveolar damage, with less obvious edema, beginning epithelial necrosis, and hyaline membrane formation. Clinically, respiratory failure occurs. This phase merges into the next one, the *proliferative phase,* in which alveolar injury is more prominent and cellular reaction becomes apparent, with type II cell metaplasia of the air spaces, fibroblastic proliferation, and fibrosis. Functionally, the lungs become stiff. The process is apparently reversible for some period and leads presumably to a *healing phase,* which has not been observed in any detail morphologically. Alternatively, at some stage fibrosis becomes progressive and leads to a condition not dissimilar to bronchopulmonary dysplasia of neonates.[32]

As indicated below, ARDS may complicate infections in the immunocompromised host, and most lung biopsies in ARDS are performed under these circumstances. Biopsy may be performed in nonimmunocompromised patients to exclude other conditions or to establish the presence of infection, which complicates and aggravates ARDS.

Oxygen Poisoning

Lung toxicity to increased oxygen levels has been known for many years in animals, and physiologic effects on lung function have been documented in healthy volunteers for some years. That lesions follow prolonged inhalation of high levels of oxygen is not disputed, and they are well documented in retrospective autopsy studies.[33-35] However, prospective studies have suggested that normal lungs are relatively resistant to oxygen and that it is damaged lungs that are particularly susceptible.[35]

Experimental studies have shown that alveolar endothelial cells are first affected by oxygen poisoning. Experimentally and in human cases, the fibrosis is often exquisitely interstitial, with relative preservation of alveolar architecture so that the fibrotic phase may contrast with the lesions of paraquat poisoning and ARDS in some instances. An interesting lesion has been ascribed to oxygen poisoning.[36] This consists of fibroblastic proliferation within alveolar ducts and sacs with relative preservation of alveolar wall architecture (Fig. 19-3). It differs from the lesions of paraquat toxicity in that there are often central spaces of fibrous tissue, sometimes filled with blood and structures that superficially resemble blood vessels. Another difference is that in oxygen toxicity there is not the complete continuity between alveolar wall and exudate that is seen in paraquat poisoning, and there is irregularity of the alveolar wall-exudate contact.

Paraquat (1,1'-Dimethyl-4,4'-dipyridylium Dichloride)

Paraquat is a potent herbicide, which releases hydrogen peroxide and superoxide free radicals during its cyclic oxidation and reduction.[37] In plants it is thought to act on chloroplasts, and in animals by damage to cell membranes. Paraquat in high concentrations is very irri-

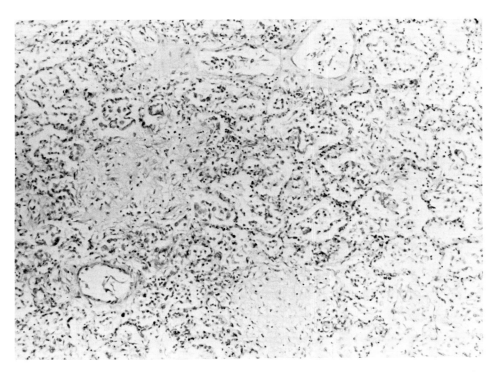

Fig. 19-3. Adult respiratory distress syndrome treated with high concentrations of oxygen. There is mild interstitial thickening with type II cell hyperplasia. In alveolar ducts and sacs, there is fibroblastic proliferation.

tating, and the initial lesion in humans may be an ulcerative oropharyngitis. Transient renal and hepatic dysfunction follows in the next few days, and the patient appears to be recovering when, 5 to 7 days after ingestion, respiratory distress and a radiologic pattern of patchy pulmonary edema develop. Evidence of lung restriction and diminished diffusing capacity may precede the pulmonary symptoms. The delayed effect on the lung is thought to be due to the fact that the concentration of paraquat remains high in the lungs for several days, whereas in other organs there is a rapid fall 24 to 36 hours after ingestion.[38] Once pulmonary symptoms appear, the course is usually rapidly progressive, with increasing dyspnea and increasing radiologic opacities, which may clear slightly to be followed by cysts appearing in the lung fields. Lung involvement was thought to be invariably fatal, but cases have now been reported in which clinical recovery has occurred, and a case has also been described in which a patient was found to have pulmonary fibrosis radiologically after having had a previously normal chest film. On questioning, he admitted to ingestion of paraquat in the intervening period.[39] Paraquat lung lesions are not well documented in sprayers of paraquat.[40] A topic of past interest was whether lesions occurred in smokers of marijuana that had been sprayed with paraquat, since inhaled paraquat in rabbits produces lung disease.[41] No convincing evidence is available linking marijuana smoking with paraquat lung disease.

The lesions vary with the postingestion period. Experimental evidence in animals indicate that the first pulmonary lesions appear in the type I cells of the alveolar epithelium.[21] Nonspecific degenerative changes occur within 12 to 18 hours, and epithelial necrosis occurs by 24 hours. At this stage alveolar edema and congestion are apparent. Type II cell and endothelial damage then occur, and the findings are those of acute diffuse alveolar damage. Fibroblastic proliferation and fibrosis appear next. In the usual patient who dies or on whom a biopsy is performed 1 week to 10 days after ingestion, a striking pattern is seen.[42] There is extensive distortion of the lung architecture, dilatation of bronchioles and alveolar ducts, and alveolar collapse and fibrosis. Cysts may form that are quite large, and which may be lined by alveolar walls and are then emphysematous spaces.[43] A very distinctive form of fibrosis has been described, which may be pathognomonic for paraquat.[44,45] The lung structure remains intact, but all the distal air spaces are filled with loose fibrous tissue. The skeletons of alveolar walls can be made out and are emphasized by the congested alveolar capillaries. The picture is of a completely homogeneous, solid lung. This may represent organization of fibrin-rich "reticulated" edema fluid.[43] Both the acute and subacute phases may be irregularly distributed through the lung.

Drug Reactions

Parenterally or orally introduced substances may produce a variety of lesions within the lung.[46] These include diffuse alveolar damage, pulmonary edema, asthma, eosinophilic pneumonia, and UIP, but only the first of these has major relevance to this section. The features of diffuse alveolar damage induced by antineoplastic therapeutic agents include proliferation of type II cells, which line air spaces, interstitial fibrosis, and relative preservation of lung structure. Advanced honeycombing is not common. A characteristic feature of *all* antineoplastic drug-induced conditions is the presence of large type II cells, which frequently have atypical hyperchromatic nuclei with prominent nucleoli. Electron microscopically, the nuclei often contain tubular structures thought to represent the products of altered nucleic acid metabolism brought about by the anticancer agents.[47]

A myriad of drugs have been associated with pulmonary lesions. Because of a general lack of clinical or pathologic features, the best method of diagnosing drug-induced lesions is by combining a high index of suspicion with a thorough clinical history. The topic of drug-related injury can be approached as a classification of the drugs involved[48]; a classification of reaction involved, such as allergic, overdosage, and so forth; or a classification of target organ effects.[49]

Nitrofurantoin

Nitrofurantoin is a bacteriostatic agent used chiefly to treat urinary tract infection. Both acute and chronic reactions can occur.[50] Acute reactions appear approximately 9 days after administration and consist of fever, dyspnea, bilateral pneumonia on the chest film, and often peripheral eosinophilia. Approximately 20 percent of the patients also have gastrointestinal symptoms, headaches, or myalgia. Histologically, mild interstitial inflammation and vasculitis are present; granulomas may occasionally be identified. Intra-alveolar eosinophils and macrophages are found, and a desquamative interstitial pneumonia pattern may result.[51] The chronic reactions manifest after 1 to 6 months of treatment. Dyspnea in these patients is mild, and systemic reactions are rare. Autoantibodies are occasionally present.[52] Microscopy shows interstitial inflammation and fibrosis accompanied by vascular sclerosis.

Cytotoxic Chemotherapeutic Drugs

The most common drugs that produce diffuse alveolar damage are antitumor agents, which by definition are seen in the immunocompromised host (see above). A reasonably safe working assumption is that any antineoplastic drug may produce diffuse alveolar damage. However, from the clinical point of view there are some drugs (5-Fluorouracil, Vinblastine, cytarabine, Adriamycin, thiotepa, azathioprine) that never or very rarely produce pulmonary lesions. With the increasing number of effective agents coming on the market, the number of toxic agents will increase. A comprehensive list has recently been compiled.[9] It is therefore superfluous to provide a long list of agents, and only two will be mentioned: *bleomycin,* because it is common and a useful prototype of diffuse alveolar damage, and *methotrexate,* because it is unusual in its tissue reactions.

Bleomycin is a glycopeptide that has found use in the treatment of epidermoid carcinoma, lymphoma, and malignant testicular tumors.[53] The drug is concentrated in skin, lungs, and lymph. Pulmonary lesions appear to be dose-related and are not related to pre-existing areas of disease, although prior radiotherapy may predispose to toxicity.[54] Studies have shown toxicity at a mean total dose of 100 to 150 mg/m²,[55] with a significant increase at 450 mg/m².[56] Symptoms consist of a dry cough with progressive dyspnea. Rales, usually in the basal segments, are the earliest physical sign. Radiographs do not exhibit changes until symptoms are present, and then they show a diffuse linear pattern in the lower lung fields. Restrictive lung disease occurs functionally. Histologically, the initial site of injury is at the venous endothelial cell.[23] The cell cytoplasm becomes attenuated and vacuolated. The perivascular tissue is edematous and contains an infiltrate of lymphocytes and plasma cells. Type I pneumocytes then become focally necrotic, allowing fibrin and other proteinaceous material to leak into the alveolus. There is subsequent type II hyperplasia as a regenerative phenomenon, and bizarre-appearing type II cells appear (Fig. 19-4). As the intra-alveolar fibrin becomes organized by fibroblasts, a characteristic intra-alveolar fibrosis occurs.[55] Interstitial fibroblasts are also active, causing septal widening.

Methotrexate exerts its toxicity largely through a hypersensitivity reaction.[57] There is no apparent dose relationship, although intravenous administration is associated with more toxic effects. A cough occurring 12 to 100 days after administration is followed by malaise, increased temperature, and increased dyspnea, and in 50 percent of the patients, peripheral eosinophilia. Microscopically there is an interstitial infiltrate of lymphocytes, plasma cells, and eosinophils. Granulomas with flattened multinucleate giant cells are common. Symptoms last 10 to 40 days, with gradual subsidence after discontinuation of the drug.

Amphophilic Drugs

Amphophilic drugs include the antihistamine chlorcyclizine; haloperidol; chloroquine; the anorectics chlorphentermine and fenfluramine; and the tricyclic antidepressants prinadol, aminotryptyline hydrochloride, imip-

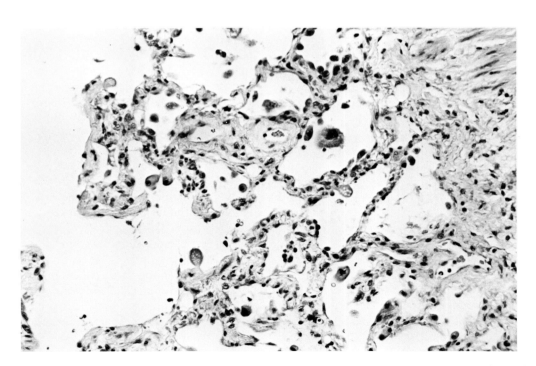

Fig. 19-4. Bleomycin toxicity. Note the hyperchromatic nuclei in enlarged type II cells and intra-alveolar and interstitial fibrosis.

ramine, and clomipramine.[58] Grossly, the lungs are slightly heavy, and lesions appear as white nodules formed of collections of large macrophages that contain numerous lipid vacuoles. The drugs appear to act initially on the capillary endothelial cells, causing degeneration. Interstitial edema follows, and an interstitial infiltrate of macrophages appears. Type II pneumocytes become hyperplastic and contain large secretory vacuoles. Foam cells and amorphous material accumulate in the alveoli, giving a picture similar to that of alveolar proteinosis. Ultrastructurally, numerous lamellar inclusions are identified, both free and within macrophages. The drugs appear to act by alteration of physicochemical properties of phospholipid and to impair metabolism in phagosomes by complexing with phospholipids.

Analgesics

A common serious drug reaction is that produced by heroin.[59] Methadone and propoxyphene cause similar reactions,[60] as does aspirin.[61] Toxicity is due to overdosage, either accidental or intentional. The characteristic lesion is pulmonary edema, which may be complicated by aspiration. The conditions only become a surgical pathology problem when talc is added to or is contained in the narcotic and then acts as an embolus, lodging in the microvasculature and inciting a granulomatous foreign body reaction. The talc is strongly doubly refractile. Some addicts may have diffuse infiltrative lung disease for which a diagnostic biopsy is done.

Vasoactive Agents

Methysergide is used in the treatment of migraine headaches. A fibrotic reaction is incited, resulting in pleural, pulmonary, mediastinal, and retroperitoneal fibrosis. The increased collagen is interstitial and is not accompanied by an inflammatory reaction. The first drug recognized as causing lung lesions was hexamethonium, and other agents such as pentolinium, mecamylamine, and apresoline have been associated with pulmonary lesions. Apresoline is of interest since it has been known to produce lupus erythematosus or a lupus-like syndrome. These drugs are no longer in use and will not be discussed further.

Miscellaneous

Patients receiving *chrysotherapy* for rheumatoid arthritis may develop diffuse reversible pulmonary injury. Histologically, this appears as an interstitial pneumonitis, with a lymphocyte and plasma cell infiltrate accompanied by an increase in interstitial fibrous tissue.[62] Granulomas and vasculitis are not features. Some patients exhibit peripheral eosinophilia with elevated IgE levels, suggesting

hypersensitivity.[63] Such individuals may or may not show cutaneous signs of toxicity. The differential diagnosis of rheumatoid lung is difficult to exclude histologically, but clinically it does not develop with the rapidity of gold toxicity.

Radiation Pneumonitis

Pulmonary damage due to radiation is a common occurrence. Fajardo and Berthrong[64] found that 5 to 20 percent of patients irradiated for thoracic neoplasms developed clinical pneumonitis, which was the cause of death in 8 percent. Effects are proportional to the volume irradiated, total dose, and number of dose fractions delivered, as well as to the total treatment time. Concurrent infection,[65] chemotherapeutic drugs,[66] and steroid withdrawal[67] have all been known to potentiate radiation damage.

Clinical signs and symptoms often are initially absent or very mild. Cough, usually harsh and nonproductive, is a manifestation of bronchial epithelial damage. Progressive dyspnea may be noted 2 to 3 months after irradiation. Pulmonary function tests show a restrictive process. The radiograph in the acute phase shows air space consolidation with loss of lung volume, while in the chronic stage it is distinguished by fibrosis and severe volume loss with obliteration of architecture.

Two main morphologic phases of radiation damage have been described.[68,69] The *initial phase* starts in 1 to 2 hours and lasts for approximately 2 months. The differential diagnosis at this stage in the irradiated patient who develops lung infiltrates includes opportunistic infection and tumor infiltration, as well as irradiation change. The lung at biopsy is likely to be firm and plum-colored. Diffuse alveolar damage is the predominant histologic finding. Vascular changes may be inapparent, and special stains may be needed to identify intravascular fibrin. The interstitial space becomes widened, and the alveoli become filled with exudate, forming prominent hyaline membranes. Macrophages migrate to the alveoli and mononuclear cells are present in the septa, but a neutrophilic response is absent. There is necrosis of type I alveolar epithelial cells and subsequent proliferation of type II cells, which classically appear large and bizarre, with hyperchromatic nuclei, and which must be distinguished from tumor cells. Fibroblast invasion and collagen deposition in the damaged capillaries produce incomplete recanalization. The myointimal cells also undergo proliferation, forming prominent intimal foam cells. Since opportunistic infections, which may coexist with radiation damage, produce diffuse alveolar damage, special stains should be used to exclude their presence.

An *intermediate* or *latent phase* has been suggested by some authors, who believe the immune mechanism is stimulated at this time.[70] The *chronic* or *late* manifestations of radiation damage are characterized by fibroblastic repair. The hyaline membranes become phagocytosed or incorporated into intra-alveolar fibrous tissue. The interstitium becomes thickened and irregular, and there is broadening of the interlobular septa. The microvasculature becomes obliterated. The medium and small arteries now show progressive vascular sclerosis, which is present in an eccentric and discontinuous fashion along the vessels. The resultant ischemia stimulates additional fibrosis, and a vicious circle is established. Bronchioles are not initially affected but become distorted by the fibrosis, with obstruction, stasis, and the onset of chronic bronchiolitis.

Chronic radiation fibrosis may be distinguished from UIP in that it tends to be reasonably confined to the radiation port, while UIP is usually most marked in the lower lobes. The hyaline membranes of the acute stage of radiation damage are not present in UIP, nor do the hyperplastic type II cells and alveolar macrophages show the bizarre cellular features of radiation damage. Although there is vascular sclerosis of the large to medium-sized vessels in UIP, the microvasculature is not involved. Radiation damage to larger vessels, in contrast to the symmetric sclerosis of UIP, is eccentric and discontinuous in nature.

Information on radiation pneumonitis goes back a long time and precedes both modern anticancer therapeutic agents and a considerable improvement in radiotherapeutic techniques. Expert opinion[71] is that the lesions of antitumor drugs and radiation pneumonitis are effectively identical microscopically, except for foam cells within the intima and media. The usual practical problem is whether a pulmonary infiltrate in a previously irradiated patient is due to tumor, infection, or radiation pneumonitis. It is generally possible to diagnose or exclude the first two; the third is diagnosed on the basis of clinical and morphologic information. The lesion is limited to, or near, the radiation port, and the morphologic lesion consists of diffuse alveolar damage with nuclear atypia.

Infections of the Lung

In the immunocompromised host, opportunistic infection is a major differential diagnostic consideration with pulmonary infiltrates. Occasionally, biopsy is necessary to diagnosis infection in a nonimmunocompromised patient. Viral, bacterial, fungal, protozoal, or mixed organisms may be found to be responsible, and many of these infections have relatively specific histologic changes.

Bacterial Infections

Bacterial pathogens in the ICH are often *Gram-negative* and often cause extensive necrotizing pneumonia

with abscesses. *Mycobacterial* infections, either typical or atypical,[72,73] can cause devastating disseminated disease in the ICH and are particularly common in AIDS patients.[74,75] Tuberculosis is discussed more extensively in Chapter 20. The typical reaction pattern of necrotizing granulomas may not be well developed in immunocompromised hosts, and the diagnosis could be overlooked without fluorescent or histochemical demonstration of the organisms.

Legionnaires' disease is an acute respiratory infection caused by *Legionella pneumophila,* so named after this organism was found to be responsible for a 1976 epidemic with several fatalities at an American Legion convention in Philadelphia. In retrospect, the same organism was found to have caused earlier outbreaks of respiratory disease in Pontiac, Michigan, Washington, DC, and Philadelphia.[76] The organism requires complex media for growth in culture, stains best in tissue with a silver-based Dieterle stain rather than a gram stain, and has six antigenically different serogroups, which can be differentiated by direct fluorescence on secretions or tissue. Serotype I is by far the most common. Many of the patients who develop life-threatening *L. pneumophila* pneumonia are immunocompromised. A related organism, *Legionella micdadei,* causes a similar life-threatening pneumonia, apparently exclusively in the immunocompromised host.[76] Grossly, the lungs show lobular or confluent lobular consolidation, with abscesses in approximately 25 percent of cases.[76] Lobar pneumonia is a less frequent gross pattern. Microscopically, the classic finding is alveolar filling by an exudate of fibrin, polymorphonuclear leukocytes, and macrophages (Fig. 19-5). Leukoytoclasis with nuclear dust in the exudate is characteristic. Bronchitis and bronchiolitis are common,[77] but there is some evidence that the changes start in the distal acinus and involve larger airways secondarily.[78] The pattern is nonspecific and the diagnosis must be confirmed by Dieterle stain (Fig. 19-6), direct fluorescence, and/or culture. Diffuse alveolar damage has been described in a few cases, but this reaction pattern may be related more to oxygen therapy than to the primary infection.[77] Extrapulmonary involvement is uncommon.

Viral Infections

The viruses that cause lower respiratory tract infection and are likely to be seen in lung biopsy material, as well as the general patient profile,[79] are listed in Table 19-2.

Influenza. This is the most common cause of viral pneumonia in the nonimmunocompromised adult. Three patterns of reaction may be seen in biopsy or autopsy material: viral pneumonia followed by bacterial superinfection, concurrent influenza and bacterial pneumonia, and "pure" influenza pneumonia. The last is characterized by a combi-

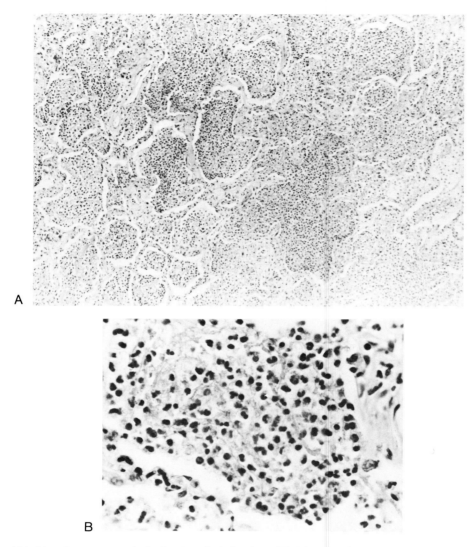

Fig. 19-5. **(A)** Alveolar pneumonia in *Legionella* infection. **(B)** The alveolar exudate consists of polymorphonuclear leukocytes and macrophages.

nation of diffuse alveolar damage and necrotizing bronchitis/bronchiolitis. Concurrent or subsequent bacterial infection is characterized by intra-alveolar collections of PMNs, with or without demonstrable bacteria by tissue Gram stain. There are no specific influenza virus inclusions.

Measles. Asymptomatic radiologic infiltrates and symptomatically mild pneumonia are common in nonimmunocompromised patients with measles (rubeola) infection. Serious measles pneumonia is rare in nonimmunocompromised patients but is well recognized in immunocompromised children. Indicators of a difficult course include absence of rash, persistence of tissue giant cells, persist-

ence of culturable virus, and a poor antibody response. In biopsy or autopsy tissue there is a combination of bronchitis, bronchiolitis, and diffuse alveolar damage. In contrast to influenza, inclusions are found in submucosal glands and alveolar epithelium. Inclusion-bearing cells are characteristically multinucleate (Fig. 19-7). While intranuclear and intracytoplasmic inclusions both occur, the former are more conspicuous and consist of eosinophilic structures surround by a halo, present in each nucleus within the cell.

Respiratory Syncytial Virus. Respiratory syncytial virus (RSV) is the most common cause of serious lower respiratory tract infection in children under 1 year of age.

TABLE 19-2. Viral Pneumonias

Virus	Usual Patient
RNA	
Influenza	NICH[a] (adults)
Measles	ICH[a]
Respiratory syncytial virus	NICH (infants)
DNA	
Adenovirus	NICH (children)
	ICH
Herpes simplex	ICH
Varicella-zoster	NICH (adults)
	ICH
Cytomegalovirus	ICH

Abbreviations: NICH, nonimmunocompromised host; ICH, immunocompromised host.

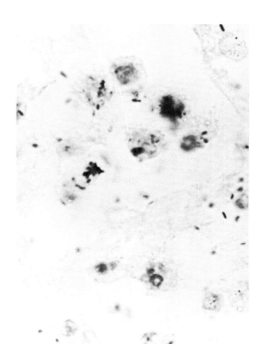

Fig. 19-6. *Legionella* infection. Short, rod-shaped organisms are seen with the Dieterle stain.

Rarely, RSV may cause life-threatening pneumonia in immunologically intact adults. The typical histologic appearance is that of a striking bronchiolitis with epithelial necrosis, acute inflammatory debris in bronchiolar lumina, and a mononuclear cell peribronchiolitis (Fig. 19-8). There is little associated alveolitis, so the bronchiolar lesions are particularly prominent in contrast. Inclusions may be seen in the bronchiolar epithelium early in the course of the disease. They are small intracytoplasmic eosinophilic structures, which are difficult to find but

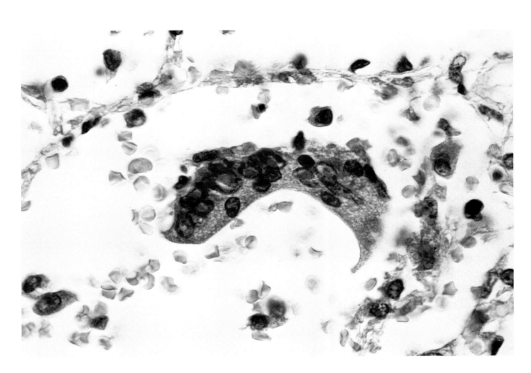

Fig. 19-7. Measles pneumonia with multinucleate epithelial cell containing an inclusion in each nucleus.

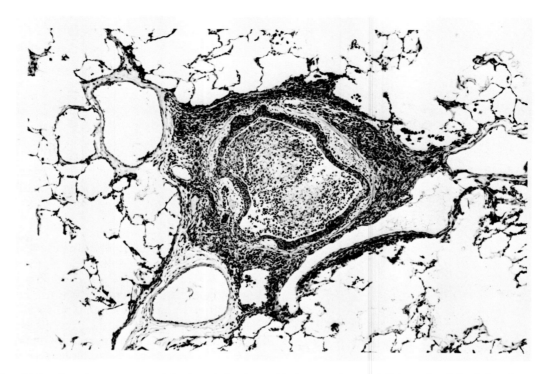

Fig. 19-8. Respiratory syncytial virus infection with intense bronchiolitis and minimal involvement of adjacent alveoli.

which may be highlighted by the Giemsa stain or specific fluorescence.

Adenovirus. *Adenovirus* is an important cause of lower respiratory tract infection in children, particularly since it carries a high risk of long-term sequelae such as bronchiectasis or bronchiolitis. Most adult cases occur in the ICH or, oddly enough, in military recruits. The pattern of reaction of adenovirus pneumonia includes necrotizing bronchitis, necrotizing bronchiolitis, and diffuse alveolar damage. Two types of inclusions are found, primarily in epithelial cells (Fig. 19-9). The smaller, less numerous, and earlier formed inclusion is an intranuclear irregular and granular inclusion surrounded by a halo. This inclusion by itself could be mistaken for herpes simplex virus (see below), but it is accompanied by larger, basophilic, and more numerous "smudge" cell inclusions, in which the nuclear membrane is disrupted and the entire nucleoplasm and cytoplasm are packed with virus particles. Electron microscopy is rewarding in adenovirus infection, since the virions form a characteristic crystalline array.

Herpes Simplex Virus. *Herpes simplex virus* (HSV) pneumonia is seen primarily in immunocompromised hosts. Two patterns of reaction are seen, which probably represent different pathogenetic events. HSV tracheobronchitis begins as ulcerative lesions in the upper airways and extends distally down the airways to reach the bronchioles and parenchyma. This pattern of reaction is seen in a wide variety of seriously ill patients. The other type of HSV pneumonia occurs in profoundly immunosuppressed patients and consists of nonbronchial-related hemorrhagic, variably inflamed miliary nodules. This type is often found in conjunction with multisystem herpetic infection and is thought to represent viremic seeding. Both herpetic ulcers and hemorrhagic nodules contain the characteristic nuclear herpetic inclusions. Nuclear enlargement with a slightly basophilic diffuse ground glass alteration of the nucleoplasm is the first recognizable inclusion. Subsequently, there is coalescence of intranuclear material into a single eosinophilic inclusion surrounded by a halo. Multinucleate inclusion-bearing cells are rare in respiratory tract tissue. The inclusions may be difficult to identify with certainty, and

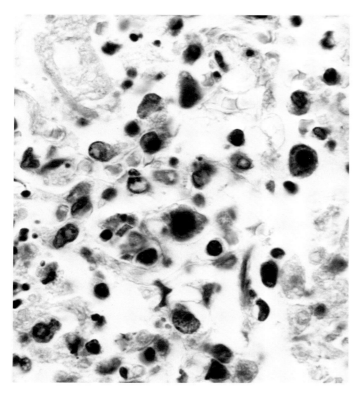

Fig. 19-9. Adenovirus pneumonia with several smudge cell inclusions.

immunoperoxidase, electron microscopy or in situ hybridization may be useful in verifying the diagnosis.

Herpes Varicella-Zoster. Primary varicella infection (chickenpox) ordinarily occurs in childhood, and in immunocompetent children pulmonary complications are found in less than 1 percent of cases. Primary varicella infection in adults is associated with radiologic evidence of pneumonia in approximately 15 percent of cases. Reactivation of varicella infection occurs in the form of zoster, which is a painful cutaneous vesicular rash distributed along dermatomes. In immunologically intact patients, primary varicella and zoster seldom cause life-threatening respiratory illness. In immunocompromised patients both types of infections may cause serious pneumonia in the form of hemorrhagic nodules similar to those described above for HSV. Ulcers of the conducting airways are considerably less common in herpes varicella-zoster (HVZ) than in HSV infection.

Cytomegalovirus. CMV pneumonia is seen almost exclusively in immunocompromised patients. Renal transplant patients, AIDS patients, and bone marrow transplant pa-

tients seem to be particularly prone to this illness, and it is catastrophic in the last population, with a mortality rate of over 80 percent. The classic pattern of reaction in CMV pneumonia is hemorrhagic nodules analogous to those of HSV and HVZ as described above. These hemorrhagic nodules are accompanied by diffuse alveolar damage to a variable degree. Involvement of bronchi and bronchioles is most unusual. The CMV inclusion is characterized by dramatic nuclear and cellular enlargement. The involved nucleus contains one prominent central inclusion surrounded by a halo and marginated chromatin. Cytoplasmic inclusions are also found, characterized by perinuclear basophilic specks (Fig. 19-10). Ultrastructurally, the nucleus contains free uncoated virions, while the cytoplasm contains coated virions in membrane-bound vesicles (Fig. 19-10).

Fungal Infections

A variety of fungal infections give rise to granulomatous pulmonary inflammation, with variable degrees of caseous necrosis, acute inflammation, fibrosis and adenopathy. These organisms all may cause significant disease in nonimmunocompromised patients, and much more serious disease in immunocompromised hosts. The precise diagnosis depends on the morphology and culture of the offending organism, and the differential diagnostic considerations include *Histoplasma capsulatum*,[80] *Cryptococcus neoformans*,[81] coccidioidomycosis,[82,83] *Blastomyces dermatitidis*,[84,85] and *Sporothrix schenckii*.[86] (See Chapters 3 and 4 for further discussion.)

Aspergillus infection may be seen in the form of allergic bronchopulmonary aspergillosis,[87] in which fungal hyphae colonize bronchial mucus plugs, and fungus balls, in which fungi colonize pre-existent pulmonary cavities. However, the most common setting in which aspergillus lung infection is seen in surgical pathology material is in the immunocompromised host.[88] Typically, the organisms invade blood vessels, giving rise to infected infarcts, which often cavitate. *Mucormycosis*[89] is less common than aspergillosis and occurs almost exclusively in either diabetics or immunocompromised patients. It typically gives rise to a similar pattern of lung injury, namely septic thrombi with infarction. *Candidiasis* is a common infection in immunocompromised patients.[90] The usual patterns of reaction are either endobronchial-related fungal colonies or multiple abscesses based around small vessels containing yeasts and pseudohyphae (Fig. 19-11). However, we have seen cases of *Candida* infection causing septic thrombi in large arteries, mimicking *Aspergillus*, and cases of granulomatous infection mimicking tuberculosis. The pseudohyphae can be very difficult to

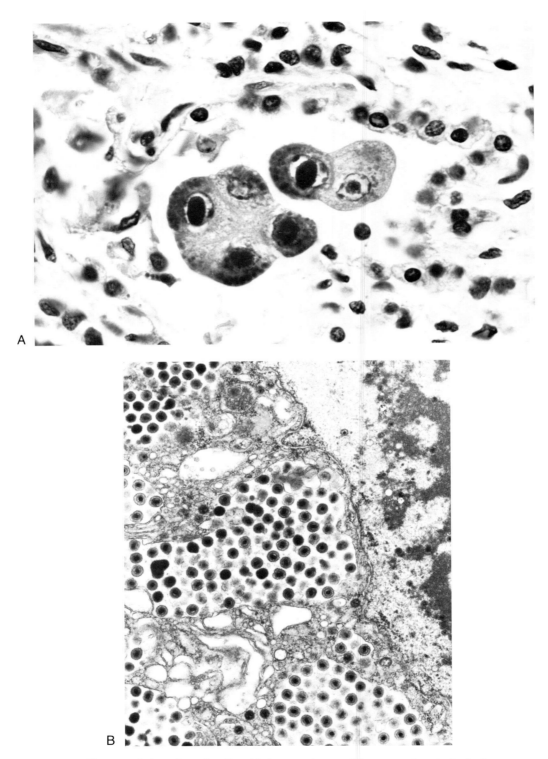

Fig. 19-10. **(A)** Characteristic enlarged cells with intranuclear and intracytoplasmic inclusions are seen in CMV infection. **(B)** Ultrastructural findings in CMV infection consist of uncoated intranuclear virions and coated cytoplasmic virions in membrane-bound vesicles. (×27,360.)

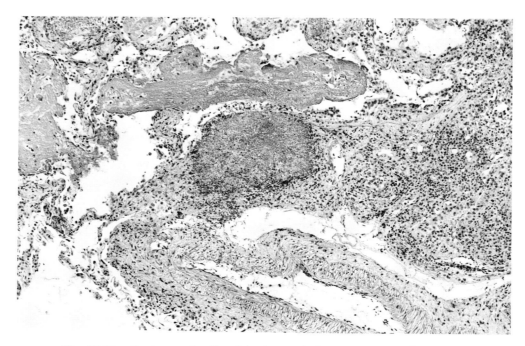

Fig. 19-11. Juxtavascular *Candida* abscess in immunocompromised host.

distinguish from *Aspergillus* by silver stains of tissue sections, and culture is essential for a specific diagnosis.

Pneumocystis

Pneumocystis carinii (Pc) is a protozoan commonly seen as a cause of pulmonary infiltrates in immunocompromised patients in general[91] and in AIDS patients in particular[74] (see also Ch. 4). Extrapulmonary involvement is rare but has been described.[92] Diagnosis depends on the demonstration of the organisms, which may be achieved by open biopsy or bronchoalveolar lavage. Most recently the accuracy of sputum examination has been emphasized.[74] Pc is often seen, but not definitively identified, on H&E stains. Methenamine-silver stains demonstrate the cysts, which are approximately 6 μm in diameter and are folded or cup-shaped (Fig. 19-12). Giemsa stain demonstrates six to eight individual inner bodies within each cyst. The classic H&E appearance of lung tissue infected with Pc is that of a foamy eosinophilic intra-alveolar exudate (which contains the organisms), along with a mild mononuclear interstitial infiltrate. It should be emphasized, however, that many, if not most, cases of Pc pneumonia are not histologically classical. Absence of the foamy exudate, marked interstitial inflammation, marked intra-alveolar histiocytic reaction, and granulomatous inflammation have all been described in Pc pneumonia,[91] so it is imperative that silver stains be performed on all lung biopsies in immunocompromised patients. CMV and various other pathogens

may be found in addition to Pc in any immunocompromised patients, but especially in AIDS patients.

Diffuse Pulmonary Hemorrhage

Diffuse pulmonary hemorrhage (DPH) is a syndrome characterized by hemoptysis, anemia, and radiologic pulmonary infiltrates, which typically are alveolar and show rapid worsening and clearing. The general anatomic correlate is hemorrhage and hemosiderin in alveolar spaces without a grossly visible endobronchial abnormality.[93–95]

There are many etiologies of the DPH syndrome, so it is of considerable importance that one have a classification algorithm for the diagnostic approach to these patients (Fig. 19-13).

Antiglomerular Basement Membrane Disease

Antiglomerular basement membrane (AGBM) disease, also referred to as *Goodpasture's syndrome,* consists of the triad of AGBM antibody, DPH, and glomerulonephritis.[93–95] The disease occurs most commonly in young adult males, and presenting symptoms are usually respiratory rather than renal. The diagnostic abnormality by renal biopsy is linear deposits of IgG along the glomerular basement membrane. The usual pattern of glomerular reaction is a diffuse crescentic glomerulonephritis, although occasionally the glomeruli are normal by ordinary light microscopy. The diagnosis may

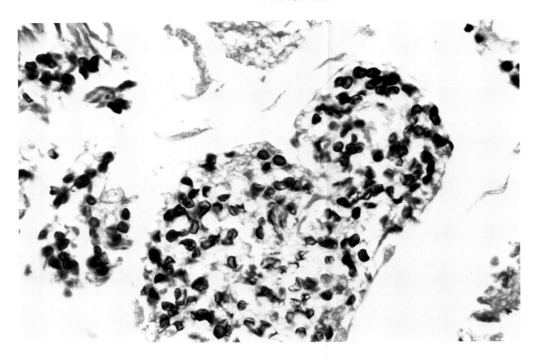

Fig. 19-12. Pneumocystis infection. Numerous organisms staining with methenamine-silver are seen in the alveolar exudate.

also be established by the finding of AGBM antibody in the serum, with radioimmunoassay and enzyme-linked immunosorbent assay (ELISA) having sensitivity and specificity rates in excess of 95 percent.[96] Lung biopsy is a less desirable diagnostic procedure. The findings are nonspecific, consisting of hemorrhage, hemosiderin deposition, and variable interstitial inflammation and fibrosis. The immunofluorescent findings are not as reliable in the lung as they are in the kidney.[96]

Diffuse Pulmonary Hemorrhage Associated with Collagen Vascular Disease

There are a number of immune-complex-related vasculitides and collagen vascular diseases in which DPH may occur, including polyarteritis nodosa, systemic lupus erythematosus, Wegener's granulomatosis, cryoglobulinemia, rheumatoid arthritis, crescentic glomerulonephritis, and scleroderma.[93–96] The common feature is an acute

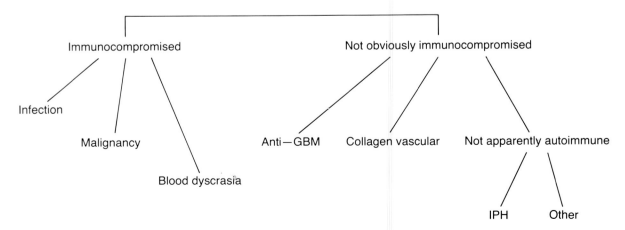

Fig. 19-13. Diagnostic approach to patients with diffuse pulmonary hemorrhage syndrome. (GBM = glomerular basement membrane; IPH = idiopathic pulmonary hemorrhage.)

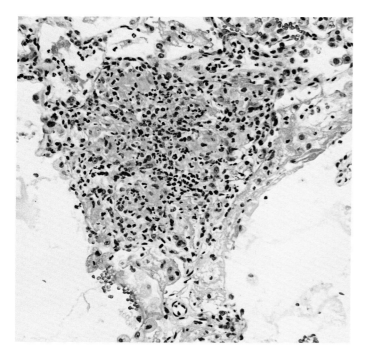

Fig. 19-14. Acute necrotizing capillaritis with fibrin exudate in acute lupus-related pulmonary hemorrhage.

capillaritis with or without larger vessel lesions and with or without renal lesions (Fig. 19-14).

Idiopathic Pulmonary Hemosiderosis

Idiopathic pulmonary hemosiderosis is characterized by diffuse pulmonary hemorrhage with resultant anemia

and radiologic infiltrates in the absence of renal disease or demonstrable immunologic disease. The most common patient populations are children less than 10 years old and young adults in the second to third decades; there is an equal sex ratio in the former group and male predominance in the latter group. The histologic features are similar to those found in AGBM disease, namely hemorrhage, hemosiderin-laden macrophages, and variable degrees of interstitial inflammation and fibrosis (Fig. 19-15). Tissue immunoglobulin studies and electron microscopy show no diagnostic abnormalities.

Miscellaneous Causes of Diffuse Pulmonary Hemorrhage

In the host not apparently immunocompromised there are a myriad of miscellaneous causes of DPH, some of which may be obvious from the clinical setting, and some of which may be extremely elusive. They should always be kept in mind in the differential diagnosis of DPH, particularly in cases that are atypical from a clinical and pathologic standpoint. *Drug reaction* to penicillamine, trimetallic anhydride, and lymphangiography have all been described as causing DPH.[95] Cardiovascular disorders such as mitral stenosis, pulmonary veno-occlusive disease, severe pulmonary edema[94] and amyloidosis may cause DPH. *Blood dyscrasias* such as anticoagulation therapy, disseminated intravascular coagulation, and drug-induced[94] or immune thrombocytopenias[97] may be complicated by DPH. *Lung injury*, either traumatic, in-

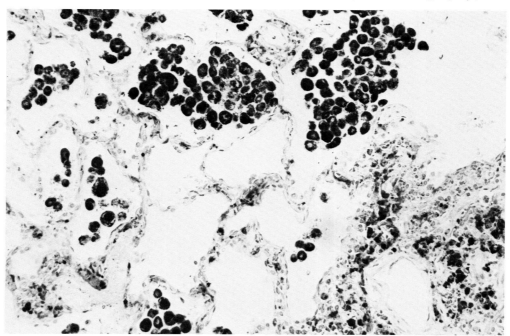

Fig. 19-15. Prussian blue stain of lung biopsy in idiopathic pulmonary hemosiderosis, showing intra-alveolar and interstitial hemosiderin deposits.

halation, or as a manifestation of necrotizing pneumonia and/or diffuse alveolar damage, may result in DPH. Primary and metastatic cancers, particularly angiosarcomas,[95,98] may present as DPH. *Chronic eosinophilic pneumonia* may be complicated by hemoptysis due to DPH.[99]

In immunocompromised patients with progressive pulmonary infiltrates, particularly those with hematologic neoplasia and/or marrow transplantation, some degree of DPH is common although overt hemoptysis is surprisingly unusual.[100,101] In this population the primary differential diagnostic considerations are infection, malignancy, and uncomplicated hemorrhage, presumably related to thrombocytopenia. A variety of *infections* have been associated with DPH, including fungal infections (most commonly *Aspergillus*), viral infections (most commonly CMV), various necrotizing bacterial infections, and Pc.[100,101] *Malignancy* as a cause of DPH in the ICH is considerably less common than is infection,[100] with Kaposi's sarcoma in AIDS being the best documented.[102] The occurrence of DPH presumably due to uncomplicated *thrombocytopenia* is more controversial, since it has been suggested[103] that some degree of diffuse alveolar damage must be present for DPH to occur. Nevertheless, large series[100,101] report approximately 5 percent of immunocompromised patients with pulmonary infiltrates to have apparently uncomplicated pulmonary hemorrhage.

Chronic Infiltrative Lung Disease

Diseases without Distinctive Histologic Features

Lung biopsy is most commonly performed in patients with chronic infiltrative lung disease. Numerous diseases may result in the syndrome; the common causes are listed in Table 19-3. This comes from Carrington and Gaensler's report of the largest series of open lung biopsies that has been analyzed (490 cases).[10] Their report is meant as a guide to the frequency of diagnosis in chronic infiltrative lung disease. One peculiarity of this series is the high percentage of pneumoconiosis, especially asbestosis. This represents Gaensler's interest in occupational lung disease. The other peculiarity is the 4:3 ratio of UIP versus desquamative interstitial pneumonia (DIP); a more realistic figure is 10:1.

The Interstitial Pneumonias

Usual Interstitial Pneumonia (Fibrosing Alveolitis). The large number of terms (Hamman-Rich syndrome, fibrosing alveolitis, cryptogenic fibrosing alveolitis, idiopathic pulmonary fibrosis, widespread pulmonary fibrosis, idio-

TABLE 19-3. Biopsies in Chronic Diffuse Infiltrative Lung Disease[a]

Interstitial pneumonias	24.9%
Usual interstitial pneumonia (12.5%)	
Desquamative interstitial pneumonia (9.2%)	
Lymphoid interstitial pneumonia (0.9%)	
Environmental lung disease	21.6%
Asbestosis (11.8%)	
Silicosis, coal, graphite (4.3%)	
Allergic alveolitis (1.0%)	
Sarcoidosis	13.2%
Nonspecific	13.1%
Unusual specific disorders	9.4%
Eosinophilic granuloma (3.1%)	
Alveolar proteinosis (2.7%)	
Diffuse pulmonary hemorrhage (1.6%)	
"Allergic" reactions	4.5%
Eosinophilic pneumonia (4.3%)	
Infections	3.8%
Pulmonary vascular disease	3.5%
Malignant neoplasm	2.9%
Chronic passive congestion	1.4%
No diagnosis	1.0%

[a] Diagnosis in 490 lung biopsies. The percentage of major categories is shown and, within them, the percentage of subcategories, all expressed as a percentage of the 490 biopsies. (Modified from Carrington and Gaensler,[10] with permission.)

pathic interstitial fibrosis of the lung, usual interstitial pneumonia) used to designate this condition indicates that there is no one term that describes the condition precisely and adequately. Hamman and Rich[104] described a small group of patients who had diffuse, rapidly progressive, fibrosis of the lungs and evidence of subacute inflammation. These patients differed clinically and pathologically from most patients with UIP as it is understood today, and thus many feel that the term Hamman-Rich syndrome or disease is no longer applicable. Most commonly, patients with usual interstitial pneumonia have an insidious onset of breathlessness; 25 to 40 percent date the onset of their symptoms to a flu-like illness. No age is exempt, but most patients are between 40 and 70 years of age, and men are slightly more commonly affected than women. Characteristic clinical findings include clubbing (but not pulmonary osteoarthropathy), late fine inspiratory crackles ("Velcro crackles") at the lung bases, and the final development of pulmonary hypertension and right ventricular hypertrophy and failure. A high erythrocyte sedimentation rate is common, and polycythemia is rare. Most patients die of respiratory failure, often precipitated by pulmonary infection. The average duration of symptoms in one series was 3 years,[105] and the mean survival from time of diagnosis was 4 years, with a range of 0.4 to 20 years, in another series.[106] The radiologic features are variable and include ground-glass, reticular, reticulonodular, linear, nodular, and ill-defined densities. The reticulonodular and ground glass densities are generally equally frequent, and the bases are more severely involved than the apices. Terminal stages show coarse reticulation, often associated with cystic lesions, which are more usually seen in the lower zones of the lung.[107] CT has added another dimension to the diagnosis of UIP. Characteristically the abnormalities are worst in the periphery of the lower half of the lung.[108] The exact precision of diagnosis using CT scanning remains to be determined.

Classification. Identical clinical, radiologic, and morphologic changes may be seen in the lungs of patients with systemic sclerosis (scleroderma), systemic lupus erythematosus, dermatomyositis, and rheumatoid arthritis (see below). In addition, a substantial number of patients have some of the serologic stigmata of the collagen vascular diseases without the complete clinical syndrome. About 60 percent of the patients had non-organ-specific autoantibodies in one series, including 27 percent with rheumatoid factor and 40 percent with antinuclear antibodies.[109] In another series the proportion of these antibodies was lower, but elevated cryoglobulins were found in 41 percent and elevated IgA in 39 percent.[105] It has therefore been suggested that patients with UIP should be classified into three categories:

1. Patients with clinical features of collagen vascular disease
2. Patients without clinical features of collagen vascular disease but with immunologic serum abnormalities
3. Patients with neither clinical features of collagen vascular disease nor immunologic serum abnormalities

The proportion of patients falling into each of the categories is uncertain since no series contains a sufficiently large number of cases to determine the figures precisely. Referral patterns would likely affect certain series, and accumulation of case reports in the literature is unsatisfactory since particular cases are likely to be preferentially reported. UIP has also been reported in association with other diseases such as tubular acidosis[110,111] and celiac disease.[112]

Etiology and Pathogenesis. The association of fibrosing alveolitis with the collagen vascular diseases suggests that immunologic mechanisms may be involved in the production of fibrosing alveolitis. Complement and immunoglobulins have been found in the lung parenchyma in some patients,[109] as have circulating immune complexes together with deposition of immunoglobulins in lung tissue.[113]

Bronchoalveolar lavage studies (at present a controversial topic) have shown an increased number of inflammatory cells, and neutrophils constitute an average of 33 percent of the cells obtained.[114] Eosinophils are invariably present and remain after corticosteroid treatment. In contrast to allergic alveolitis, the number of lymphocytes is not increased. Finally, 95 percent of the patients with UIP have been found to have circulating T-lymphocytes, which produce migration inhibitory factor when exposed to type I collagen.[115] These findings suggest that pulmonary fibrosis results from continued injury to the alveolar interstitium, brought about by mediators from cells that aggregate at the site of collagen-induced, cell-mediated, immunologic phenomena.

Familial fibrosing alveolitis is well documented, and it has been suggested that familial cases may constitute as many as 20 percent of the cases of fibrosing alveolitis in children.[116] While the true figure is likely much lower, even in children, this may indicate that particular HLA antigens may be involved.[117]

Morphologic and Diagnostic Features. At surgery, the lung often has a characteristic hobnailed external surface, and this appearance can also be recognized in lung biopsy tissue. After fixation, the tissue is firm and the cut surface gray-white, often with a fine multicystic appearance with cysts 0.3 to 2 mm in diameter. A characteristic feature of the lung biopsy specimen grossly and microscopically is a heterogeneity (Fig. 19-16) of lesions,[105] and the appearance is characteristically variable even within a given biopsy specimen or slide. The condition is usually more chronic and advanced (honeycombed) in the lower zones of the lung, especially subpleurally. In about 25 percent of the cases fibrosis is focal, and most of the alveolar septa are normal; in another 25 percent there is more fibrous than normal tissue; and in the remainder, most of the lung tissue is very abnormal.[105] The appearance of extensive fibrosis is clearly not compatible with life; it represents the selective nature of a biopsy. Increased collagen, by definition, is always present, although biochemical assays have not shown an increased amount of collagen per unit weight of lung. This anomaly is not completely explained. In part it may be due to the change in the unit weight of lung as well as in the amount of collagen, and in part it may represent a shift from type III collagen (which does not stain histologically) to type I collagen (typical histologic collagen), so the total amount of collagen is assayed biochemically may be little altered.[118]

Foci of end-stage lung are generally present. Interstitial inflammation is always observed, but its severity is variable. In 13 percent of cases it is heavy; in 54 percent it is moderate; and in 33 percent only scattered inflammatory cells are apparent.[105] The bulk of the cells are lymphocytes, macrophages, and plasma cells. Nodular collections of lymphocytes and lymphoid follicles are present in about half the cases. Neutrophils and eosinophils can usually be found, although they are generally not striking and are often found in the cystic spaces of bronchiolectasis. Other evidence of subacute inflammation includes the presence of active granulation tissue in the walls of alveoli and air spaces. This represents a problem with differential diagnosis of BOOP, which is discussed further below. In general, the new granulation tissue is not extensive and is obviously limited to the air space walls. In BOOP, the granulation tissue is within air spaces, often not in continuity with their walls, which are relatively normal. Another feature is the presence of macrophages in the air spaces. These are invariably present, but when present in large numbers, are characteristic of desquamative interstitial pneumonitis (see below). A less well recognized feature is the distortion and narrowing of bronchioles, together with peribronchiolar fibrosis and inflammation. This observation accounts for the functional evidence of small airway obstruction that is found in fibrosing alveolitis.[119] An interesting finding is the presence of cholesterol ester clefts within air spaces.

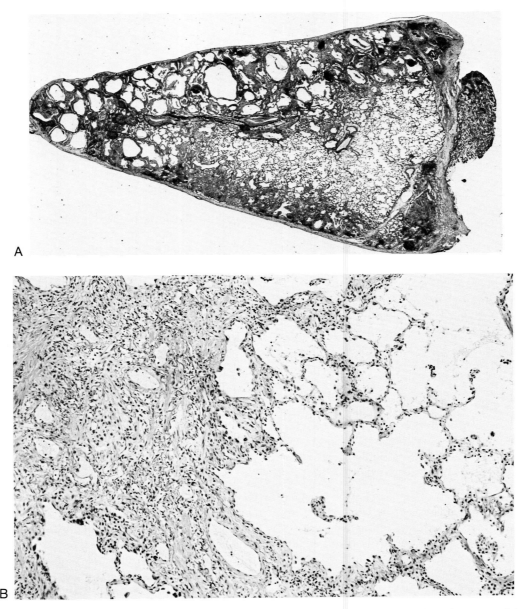

Fig. 19-16. **(A)** Scanning microscopic view of lung biopsy in UIP. Note heterogeneity of abnormalities and subpleural distribution of honeycombing. **(B)** UIP with mildly cellular scarring adjacent to nearly normal alveoli. (*Figure continues.*)

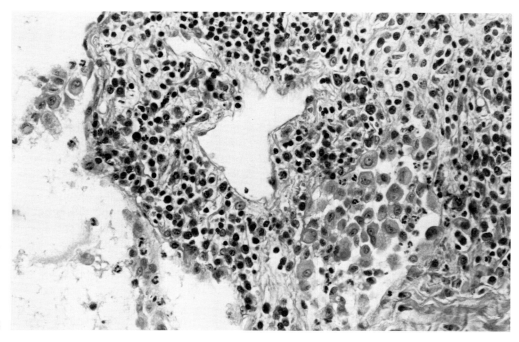

C

Fig. 19-16 (*continued*). (C) More cellular area in UIP with a mononuclear interstitial infiltrate as well as intra-alveolar histiocytes.

These clefts are associated with more severe pulmonary fibrosis and pulmonary hypertension.[105] The pulmonary vessels usually have grossly thickened walls.

It is important to exclude other causes of pulmonary fibrosis, since conditions with a specific microscopic appearance may be nonspecific in their end stage.[107] Thus, it is important to search carefully for any specific lesions and to make quite certain that there are no clues to the etiology from the clinical history or radiographs. In particular, asbestosis may be a problem, but this may reflect the particular experience of one of us while working on a workmen's compensation board. While asbestosis is usually easily recognized by the presence of obvious asbestos bodies and by the pattern of fibrosis, cases are seen in which the lesions appear typical of UIP, yet only an occasional asbestos body is found. Occasionally, no asbestos bodies may be found although the patient has been exposed to asbestos. Under these circumstances the diagnosis of idiopathic fibrosing alveolitis (UIP) seems unreasonable. As indicated, all cases of pulmonary fibrosis should be examined with polarized light, and it may be wise to include a stain for iron, since the occasional asbestos body may be hard to recognize and asbestos bodies are not doubly refractile.

Desquamative Interstitial Pneumonia. In 1965 Liebow et al.[120] described 18 cases that differed in many respects from UIP. The patients were on the average slightly younger, symptoms were usually milder, clubbing was not such a characteristic feature, and radiologically the patients usually had ground-glass opacities, particularly at the bases and at the costophrenic angles. The patients had less evidence of restrictive lung disease, and in many, lung volumes were relatively normal. The striking histologic feature was the presence of numerous cells filling the air spaces (Fig. 19-17). The cells resembled either macrophages or type II cells, and multinucleate cells were present. The original description emphasized the presence in the cytoplasm of cells in the air spaces of green-brown pigment that stained strongly with periodic acid–Schiff (PAS) stain and was diastase-resistant; only occasional iron-staining granules were present. Liebow et al. thought that the cells were chiefly desquamated alveolar lining cells, hence the term *desquamative interstitial pneumonia*. However, it is now known that the cells within the air spaces are macrophages, whereas the cells that line them are mainly type II epithelial cells.[121]

Additional features include the relative preservation of lung architecture, with mild thickening of alveolar walls and absence of severe fibrosis or honeycombing. Interstitial mononuclear inflammation is present, with the formation of lymphoid follicles. Eosinophilic intranuclear inclusions have been described in both the cells lining the air spaces and the cells lying free in air spaces in 5 to 80 percent of cases. They were originally described as "virus-like," but electron microscopically they consist of myelin figures.[122] Liebow and co-workers recognized intracytoplasmic "blue bodies" in the cells in the air spaces

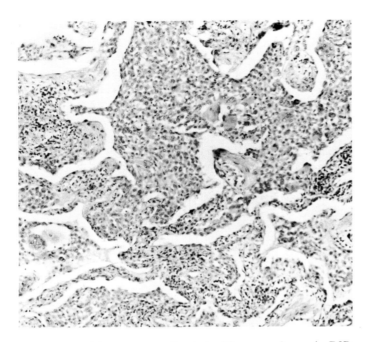

Fig. 19-17. Air spaces are flooded with macrophages in DIP. Occasional giant cells are present. There is mild interstitial pneumonia with type II cell metaplasia.

in about 10 percent of the cases. These bodies are 15 to 25 μm in diameter, stain deeply with hematoxylin and have a central round or oval core surrounded by a clear space, with an outer rim of granular brown material. As seen electron microscopically, the central core consists of radially arranged fibrillar material. It is thought that this material may be connective tissue mucin, and that the outer rim stains for iron.[123] The blue bodies differ considerably in appearance from Michaelis-Guttman bodies, and one case described as malacoplakia of the lung is probably an example of DIP.[124] Large nodular masses were present in both lower lobes, and classical Michaelis-Guttman bodies were seen in the other reported case of malacoplakia of the lung.[125]

Liebow et al. regarded DIP as a separate entity from UIP, but this notion has been challenged. The histologic appearance of DIP is not specific. It is commonly focally present in UIP and has also been reported in asbestosis[126] and other dust-caused diseases[127] and following nitrofurantoin therapy,[51] and is typically found in air spaces adjacent to the nodules of eosinophilic granuloma. It is also true that cases have been reported in which classic DIP "progressed to fibrosing alveolitis."[128,129] It is thus clear that DIP represents a nonspecific reaction to injury and that the differences between DIP and UIP are quantitative rather than qualitative. It is critical to distinguish between DIP and UIP since even if they are related conditions, it has been shown clearly that the clinical fea-

tures are different, the prognosis is much better in DIP, and the response to steroids is greater[130] in DIP (Table 19-4). In classical instances the distinction between DIP and fibrosing alveolitis is easy, but in many cases it is not. The main distinguishing features of DIP are the massive numbers of cells in the air spaces, the general maintenance of alveolar architecture, and a mild degree of fibrosis. The most important feature is the massive intra-alveolar collections of cells, and the diagnosis should thus be made even in the presence of distortion of lung parenchyma and pulmonary fibrosis.

Lymphoid Interstitial Pneumonia. In the interesting but as yet poorly understood condition known as lymphoid interstitial pneumonia (LIP), there is an exquisitely interstitial infiltrate of lymphocytes, plasma cells, and large mononuclear cells. There is a distinct clinical overlap between it, "pseudolymphoma of the lung," Sjögren's syndrome, Waldenström's macroglobulinemia, and involvement of the lung by lymphoma. Spencer[124] has grouped the conditions together as "prelymphomatous states," and Gibbs and Seal[131] have referred to them as "primary lymphoproliferative conditions of the lung."

In 1966 Liebow and Carrington[132] briefly presented a group of cases and used the term lymphoid interstitial pneumonia to describe them, amplifying this description two years later. In 1973 they described 18 cases of LIP with associated dysproteinemia.[133] The proportion of patients with LIP who have dysproteinemia is not completely certain; it is likely to be the majority, since 10 of 13 patients in the only other large series reported had dysproteinemia.[134] LIP is uncommon, and in one series was only one tenth as frequent as DIP.[10] It is commonest between 40 and 70 years of age, but may occur in persons of all ages, including children. Cough and insidious dyspnea are the most common complaints, but pneumonia was the initial symptom in a significant proportion of the cases. Arthralgia, arthritis, and positive rheumatoid factor occurred only rarely. Radiologically, bilateral reticular or reticulonodular infiltrates are most common, but a coarsely nodular pattern has been seen in patients

TABLE 19-4. Clinical Features of DIP and UIP

	DIP	UIP
Average age at diagnosis (years)	42.3	50.9
Duration of symptom (years)	0.9	2.5
Survival (years)	12.2	5.6
Improved	61.5%	11.5%
Worse	27%	69.2%
Mortality	27.5%	66.0%

(From Carrington et al.,[130] with permission.)

with raised IgG levels.[133] Pleural effusion, in each instance on the right side, occurred in 3 of 18 patients.[133] Functionally, a restrictive defect is present.

The characteristic lesion is a diffuse infiltrate limited to the interstitium of the lung, consisting of lymphocytes, plasma cells, and large mononuclear and reticuloendothelial cells. The infiltrates are typically polymorphous, and either lymphocytes or plasma cells are dominant (Fig. 19-18). The general characteristics of the infiltrate are similar to those described by Saltzstein[135] in his description of "pseudolymphoma of the lung," but the two conditions differ in that pseudolymphoma of the lung is generally a localized disease. It is also true that the existence of pseudolymphoma, especially the nodular form, has been questioned.[136] Poorly formed granulomas, consisting of localized accumulations of large reticuloendothelial cells, mononuclear cells, epithelioid cells, and Touton giant cells, were seen in 4 of 18 cases.[133] The granulomas were not as compact as in sarcoidosis, and hyalinization was not seen. Similar granulomas were seen in the lymph nodes in one instance.

LIP can be regarded as the pulmonary analogue of Sjögren's syndrome. In addition, it is very difficult in the lung, just as it is in other organs in Sjögren's syndrome, to distinguish benign from malignant infiltrates, and clearly a spectrum exists.[137] It may also be that LIP may "transform" into lymphoma, and in one instance a pa-tient with LIP and Sjögren's syndrome developed lymphomatoid granulomatosis.[138] LIP has also been described in association with pernicious anemia, the autoerythrocyte sensitization syndrome, and chronic active hepatitis. We have seen a case associated with polymyositis. A more important association is with AIDS. This association was originally reported in children[139,140] but is now well documented in adults.[141,142]

The histologic differential diagnosis is primarily between a benign infiltrate of the lung (LIP) and a malignant infiltrate. The distinction from pseudolymphoma is made by radiologic evidence in LIP of diffuse disease and by histologic demonstration that the lesion is primarily interstitial rather than nodular. Extrinsic allergic alveolitis is usually excluded by the extent of the infiltrate, which is more extensive and severe in LIP. Furthermore, the characteristic bronchiolitis and granulomas with foreign bodies of extrinsic allergic alveolitis are absent in LIP. Lymphomatoid granulomatosis may sometimes also be included in the differential diagnosis, but differs in that the infiltrate is often, indeed characteristically, cytologically atypical, with angioinvasion and angiodestruction. Large areas of necrosis may result from the angioinvasive infiltrate. The exact status of "benign lymphocytic angiitis and granulomatosis"[143] is uncertain. It may be the same condition as LIP.

The distinction between benignity and malignancy is

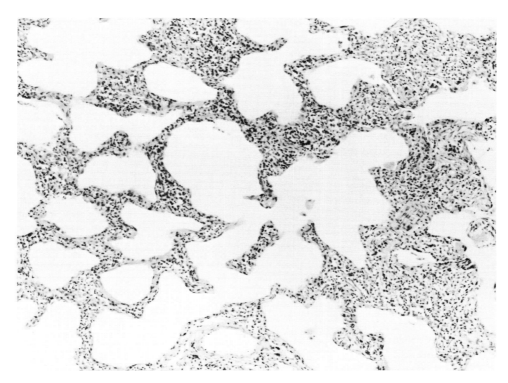

Fig. 19-18. Lymphoid interstitial pneumonia. There is an exquisitely interstitial infiltrate, in this instance consisting of lymphocytes.

made on the characteristics of the infiltrate, the nature of the involvement of the lung, and evidence of extra-pulmonary disease. In LIP the infiltrate is classically polymorphous, and the more purely lymphocyte-dominant the infiltrate, the more likely it is to be malignant. Involvement of the pleura is an important distinguishing feature. While LIP may involve the deep layers of the pleura, extension through all layers of the pleura is more characteristic of lymphoma, and involvement of the parietal pleura and adjacent fat is diagnostic of lymphoma. Extensive involvement of airways, with epithelial ulceration and destruction of cartilage, is also an indication of lymphoma, which is also said to "track" along lymphatic channels.[136] More definitive criteria of malignant lymphoma include involvement of extrapulmonary sites, usually intrathoracic lymph nodes, extrathoracic nodes, or the spleen. Clinical evidence of splenic enlargement is inadequate; histologic confirmation is required.

Giant Cell Interstitial Pneumonia. Giant cell interstitial pneumonia (GIP) is the least well described variant of chronic interstitial pneumonia, with only seven cases reported in detail.[144] The clinical manifestation has been similar to that of UIP or DIP: progressive dyspnea, cough, chest pain, fatigue, and weight loss, with clubbing and fine basal rales on physical examination. The chest radiograph usually shows bilateral patchy, nodular infiltrates involving the midlung fields or upper zones of the lung, with sparing of the apices and costophrenic angles. In other cases flame-shaped opacities have been described, while in still others the radiograph has resembled that seen in DIP. The majority of patients have benefited from steroid treatment, although this has not been uniform. Histologically GIP is characterized by the presence of many large, rather bizarre multinucleate cells in the alveolar spaces. These cells are characteristically cannibalistic, engulfing other cells. Discrete, desquamated macrophages fill the alveolar spaces, and there is an interstitial infiltrate of mononuclear cells, mostly lymphocytes. Since giant cells may be encountered in DIP, the distinction between GIP and DIP is one of degree, and it may be that this rare condition is a variant of DIP.

Cryptogenic Organizing Pneumonitis or Bronchiolitis Obliterans and Organizing Pneumonia. The term *bronchiolitis obliterans* has been used in so many different ways that it has become so ambiguous to be functionally useless. Probably three types of bronchiolar lesions fall under this heading: the presence of loose granulation tissue within the lumina of bronchioles, partially or totally occluding them; occlusion of the lumina of bronchioles by loose fibrous tissue with preservation of the wall, as in rheumatoid bronchiolitis or measles (see below); and total obliteration of bronchioles with disappearance of the airway. The paradox is that once the airway is totally

obliterated, it cannot be seen; perhaps the best example of this sort of bronchiolar obliteration is in bronchiectasis, where loss of airways is well documented.[145] It should also be borne in mind that classical bronchiolitis obliterans (i.e., the presence of loose granulation tissue within bronchioles) may be seen in extrinsic allergic alveolitis, rheumatoid arthritis, and eosinophilic pneumonia.

The issue is further clouded by the description of bronchiolitis obliterans interstitial pneumonia (BIP)[132] in relation to other forms of interstitial pneumonia, namely, UIP, DIP, LIP, and GIP. Precisely what was originally meant by this term is not clear. Our interpretation is that while active young connective tissue is commonly seen in UIP, it is seldom the dominant lesion; when it is dominant, then perhaps this was the condition referred to as BIP. A further complication is that the review of cases of bronchiolitis obliterans from the late Dr. Liebow's file clearly showed a spectrum of various diseases,[146] and nothing but confusion resulted from Liebow and Carrington's paper.[132]

Fortunately one entity, BOOP, has emerged,[147] which is also referred to by the British as cryptogenic organizing pneumonitis.[148] This description actually preceded the North American description, but BOOP has become the term of choice. BOOP fits better into the category of diffuse infiltrative lung disease rather than that of airway diseases associated with chronic air flow obstruction (CAO), since BOOP is not particularly associated with CAO.[149] Although both the radiology and pathology show mainly air space filling, BOOP is an important part of the differential diagnosis of clinical infiltrative lung disease and UIP.

A reasonable consensus has emerged.[147-150] Clinically the average age is about 60 years, the previous history is short (weeks to months) and frequently follows a respiratory infection, sometimes in the immunocompromised host. Dyspnea is present in only half the patients, and fever is present in a small minority. Clubbing is rare. In one study restrictive lung disease was present in 40 percent of cases, but this is less common than in UIP, and the diffusing capacity (D_LCO) was reduced in only half.[150] However, a better documented study showed that evidence of lung restriction was about the same in UIP and BOOP, and D_LCO was not significantly different between the groups.[149] The radiology of the chest is quite often characteristic,[151] with the appearance of bilateral patchy nonsegmental air space consolidation. Small round opacities occur in the lower lobes. In one series[149] 10 of 11 cases were diagnosed correctly by radiology. However, the striking feature is the relatively good prognosis—in about half the patients the condition resolves, mainly as a response to steroids, and 12.5 to 25 percent die, usually in about 3 months. The clinical features of UIP and BOOP are compared in Table 19-5.

TABLE 19-5. Clinical Features of BOOP and UIP

	BOOP	UIP
Average age (years)	57	55
Duration of symptoms	3 months	2 years
Dyspnea	50%	100%
Fever	58%	13%
Respiratory infection	21%	0%
Clubbing	15%	60%
Restrictive lung disease	50%	100%
Decreased diffusing capacity	50%	100%
Chest radiograph		
Air space opacities	70%	0
Interstitial opacities	38%	100%
Outcome		
Resolution	40%	0%
Residual disease	33%	31%
Death from disease	12.5%	62.5%
Mean survival to death	2.7 months	15 months

TABLE 19-6. Distinguishing Morphologic Features of BOOP and UIP

	BOOP	UIP
Distribution of lesions	Patchy, peribronchiolar	Diffuse, random
Location of lesion	Dominantly air space	Predominantly interstitial
Temporal appearance	Uniform, recent	Varying ages
Type of fibrosis	Fibroblastic	Mainly collagen
Honeycombing	Unusual	Common
Foamy macrophages	Common	Unusual

(Modified from Katzenstein et al.,[150] with permission.)

Morphologically, the major feature is organizing pneumonia, mainly in alveoli, alveolar ducts, and respiratory bronchioles (Fig. 19-19), and this is patchy and peribronchiolar. All the lesions appear to be recent and of about the same age. Granulation tissue is often not present in membranous bronchioles and at times may not even be seen in respiratory bronchioles,[148] but this should not be a deterrent to the diagnosis of BOOP. Interstitial pneumonia and type II cell metaplasia are common, but extensive interstitial fibrosis is uncommon, and honeycombing is quite unusual. Obstruction of bronchioles may produce endogenous lipid ("golden") pneumonia. Vascular changes are slight.

Pathologically, the differential diagnosis involves primarily UIP. This is generally easy, but discrepancies may occur even between expert pathologists, as in the National Institutes of Health Interstitial Lung Disease Clinical Trial. The difficulty arises when there is exuberant granulation tissue but it may not be clear whether this is within the air spaces or their walls. As indicated previously, we suspect that such difficult cases were the cases originally described as BIP. Distinguishing morphologic features of UIP and BOOP are listed in Table 19-6.

The etiology is unknown. The morphologic appearance suggests an infective process, but as yet microbiologic investigation has been unproductive despite extensive search in some instances.

Neurofibromatosis (von Recklinghausen's Disease)

Diffuse lung disease is seen in about 10 percent of all patients with neurofibromatosis and in about 20 percent in those who are over the age of 30. At least 31 cases have been reported.[152] Pulmonary involvement appears to be radiologically characteristic, with a mixture of linear or nodular increased markings, particularly in the lower zones of the lung, and large bullae in the upper zones of the lungs. Diffuse interstitial fibrosis was present radiologically in 21 of the 31 reported cases, and bullae were present in 26. Bullae may rupture, with consequent spontaneous pneumothorax. The functional pattern is of either restrictive or obstructive lung disease depending on whether the bullous process or interstitial fibrotic lung disease dominates. The morphologic features of the lung lesions have not been described in detail but appear not to differ from those of classical UIP alveolitis, although hyperplasia of the neurilemmal cells of intrapulmonary nerves and formation of glomus-like structures in small branches of the pulmonary arteries have been described. Patients with bullae but without radiologic evidence of interstitial fibrosis may have histologic evidence of UIP.[153] Adenocarcinoma arising in fibrosing alveolitis has been described in neurofibromatosis,[152] presumably as a reflection of the increased frequency of carcinoma in pulmonary fibrosis.

Collagen Vascular Disease

All the collagen vascular diseases may involve the respiratory system, and each of these diseases may involve it in several different ways. With a few exceptions (e.g., rheumatoid nodules), the morphologic abnormalities are not specific for collagen vascular disease in general or for any one collagen vascular disease in particular. Ultrastructurally, tubular inclusions within endothelial cells have been described[154] in a variety of collagen vascular diseases, but these are not entirely diagnostic. Immune complexes are not reliably demonstrated in lung tissue by either ultrastructural or immunohistochemical techniques.

Rheumatoid Arthritis. At least half of patients with rheumatoid arthritis (RA) have one or more forms of rheumatoid lung disease.[155] In general, patients with more severe

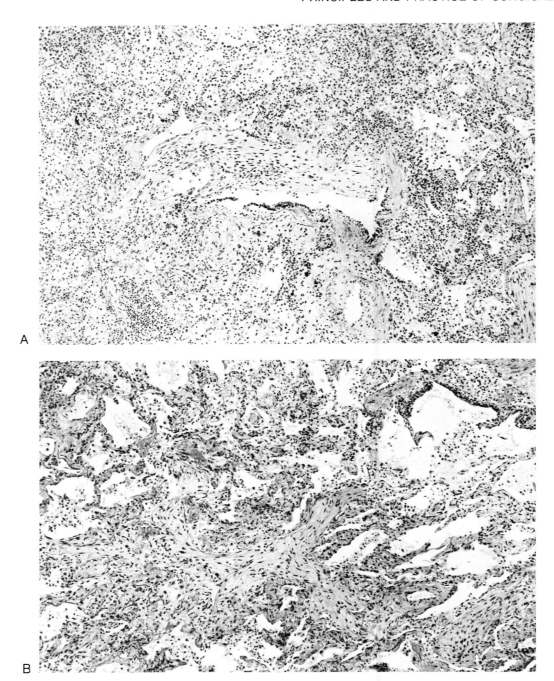

Fig. 19-19. **(A)** Proximal respiratory bronchiole in BOOP, showing granulation tissue plug occupying approximately half of the lumen. **(B)** Granulation tissue branching along the course of alveolar ducts in BOOP. Note scattered intra-alveolar histiocytes.

joint involvement are more likely to develop pleuropulmonary manifestations. The latter usually, but not always, follow the development of clinical arthropathy. At least seven forms of pleuropulmonary disease have been established in association with RA.

Pleural effusion or *pleuritis* is the most common complication of RA and may be found in up to 50 percent of patients at autopsy. Clinically most patients have no symptoms, and radiologically detected pleural effusions occurred in 7.9 percent of men and 1.6 percent of women in one large series.[156] About one third of the patients with pleural effusions have pulmonary manifestations of RA in the form of nodules or interstitial fibrosis.[157]

Rheumatoid lung nodules are the most distinctive histologic lesions in the lung and are relatively common in biopsy material from patients with RA.[158] Radiologically, multiple well defined nodules, ranging from a few millimeters to several centimeters in diameter are seen throughout the lung, and the usual differential diagnosis is metastatic carcinoma. Occasionally, the nodules may be single. Rheumatoid nodules in the lung are more common in patients with subcutaneous nodules, and the lung nodules may wax and wane with the skin nodules.[159] Cavitated solitary nodules may mimic a lung abscess or a cavitated lung cancer. The histologic appearance is similar to that of rheumatoid nodules elsewhere (see Ch. 14). Nodules with or without cavitation may occur in patients treated with steroids, and tuberculosis must then be included in the clinical and pathologic differential diagnosis. Under these circumstances the histologic distinction may not be easy, but the characteristic palisading, the presence of few giant cells, and the absence of organisms are important criteria favoring RA.

In their large series of patients, Walker and Wright[157] found that 1.6 percent had radiologic evidence of *fibrosing alveolitis,* but pulmonary function abnormalities suggesting fibrosing alveolitis have been found in 30 to 40 percent of patients with RA.[160,161] In about half of the patients the chest film was normal, but the majority showed interstitial fibrosis if biopsies were done.[160] The observed difference in frequency may depend on the condition of the patients studied (i.e., the more severe the RA the more frequently will fibrosing alveolitis be found). Radiologically and histologically, the lesions are usually indistinguishable from those of UIP. However, nodules may be seen in the lung parenchyma and occasionally in the walls of airways. In some instances the infiltrate may be quite cellular with little fibrosis (cellular interstitial pneumonia), and in occasional instances, a DIP pattern may be seen.[158] Foci of lymphocytes with germinal centers are often seen in biopsies of RA but are by no means specific for it.

The term *Caplan's syndrome* refers to the occurrence of necrobiotic nodules in the lung in industrially exposed workers. First described in coal miners, the syndrome is characterized by the rapid development of single or multiple nodules 1 to 5 cm in diameter. Similar nodules have been described in workers exposed to silica, aluminum, asbestos, and roof tiles, as well as in boiler scalers.[155] Histologically the lesions consist of a central necrotic area, together with dust and collagenization. The necrotic area is surrounded by palisaded fibroblasts, and very characteristically there is an accumulation of polymorphonuclear leukocytes (PMNs) at the junction of the two zones, often in the region of a cleft-like space. Endarteritis is common and is usually seen in and adjacent to the nodules.

Lymphoid hyperplasia with germinal centers may be found distributed along bronchovascular bundles and interlobular septa[158] (see the section on follicular bronchitis/bronchiolitis on p. 699). If accompanied by a cellular or fibrotic interstitial infiltrate, this merges with cellular interstitial pneumonia or UIP as described above. We have seen a case of rheumatoid-associated lymphoid hyperplasia without diffuse interstitial pneumonitis presenting radiologically as miliary nodules.

Pulmonary hypertension is the rarest[155] pulmonary disorder seen in association with RA. The clinical presentation is that of primary pulmonary hypertension, and the lesions are indistinguishable histologically.

Obliterative bronchiolitis is discussed more fully later.

Systemic Lupus Erythematosus. Systemic lupus erythematosus (SLE) commonly involves the lungs and pleura.[155] Painful pleuritis with or without effusion is the most common abnormality. Acute lupus pneumonitis is a potentially disastrous complication, characterized by acute capillaritis with diffuse alveolar damage. Diffuse pulmonary hemorrhage may occur in SLE with or without demonstrable vasculitis. Fibrosing alveolitis may be seen in SLE, but this complication is relatively uncommon.

Progressive Systemic Sclerosis. Progressive systemic sclerosis (PSS) leads to some degree of fibrosing alveolitis in nearly all cases.[155] In addition, vascular sclerosis, usually without an identifiable actual vasculitis, is typical. Patients with long-standing PSS-related fibrosis are at high risk for the development of bronchioloalveolar carcinoma. Pleural disease is considerably less common in PSS than in RA or SLE.

Ankylosing Spondylitis. Extensive upper zonal pulmonary fibrosis may appear in patients with ankylosing spondylitis, usually 10 years or more after the onset of the disease. The precise frequency of pulmonary involvement is not known, and a range of 0 to 30 percent has been reported. The largest single series indicates a frequency of about 1 percent.[162] Radiologically, the process begins as apical pleural involvement, and then an apical infiltrate develops and progresses to cyst formation. Generally, the disease begins unilaterally and becomes bilateral. The chest film may mimic that of tuberculosis closely. Symptoms are usually absent, but the cavities become secondarily infected, most commonly by *Aspergillus fumigatus,* although a variety of uncommon organisms may also infect the cavities. The histologic lesions consist of nonspecific inflammation and fibrosis. Bronchiolitis obliterans, together with a distal lipid pneumonia, is commonly present.[124]

Mixed Connective Tissue Disease. Mixed connective tissue disease (MCTD) is commonly associated with radiologic and functional evidence of interstitial pulmonary disease and/or pleural effusions.[155] In many cases the abnormalities respond quite well to corticosteroid therapy, but in a few instances severe and progressive pulmonary disease occurs.[163] In these instances the process is described as either fibrosing alveolitis or pulmonary hypertension.

Sjögren's Syndrome. The common pulmonary lesions of Sjögren's syndrome are analogous to the salivary gland lesions, namely a marked lymphoreticular infiltrate in the submucosal glands of the tracheobronchial tree.[155] As described previously, these patients also occasionally develop a lymphoproliferative disorder involving the pulmonary interstitium, ranging from relatively low-grade lymphoid interstitial pneumonia to a high-grade malignant lymphoma. Fibrosing alveolitis and pleural disease are seen in patients with other concurrent autoimmune features such as RA or SLE.

Behçet's Disease. Behçet's disease is an uncommon disease, which uncommonly involves the lung.[164] While the major components of the syndrome include oral and genital ulcers and iridocyclitis, multiorgan involvement on the basis of an immune complex vasculopathy is well recognized, and lung involvement is seen in this context. The characteristic lung abnormalities include a necrotizing mononuclear nongranulomatous vasculitis involving all levels of the arterial, venous, and capillary network. A polymorphonuclear leukocyte infiltrate is believed to follow, rather than precede, the mononuclear cell component. Elastin and muscle destruction occurs, leading to the development of aneurysms, arterial and venous thrombi, and pulmonary infarcts. Erosion of aneurysms into adjacent bronchi leads to hemoptysis, which is a common presentation of pulmonary involvement by Behçet's disease. Fibrosing alveolitis and pleural disease are not features of this disorder.

Polymyositis/Dermatomyositis. Polymyositis and dermatomyositis are uncommonly associated with pulmonary involvement, the reported incidence being only approximately 5 percent.[155] The pattern of involvement is typically fibrosing alveolitis.

Diseases with Distinctive Morphologic Features

While we have divided patients with chronic infiltrative lung disease into two categories—those with distinguishing features and those without—this distinction is to some extent arbitrary. As is apparent from the previous section, there are certain morphologically suggestive features even in the previously listed conditions. It is also true that conditions that may have had a specific morphology at some time may have a nonspecific appearance subsequently. This is especially true of eosinophilic granuloma and extrinsic allergic alveolitis. Thus, it is always

essential to take the clinical history into account when one is diagnosing UIP.

Sarcoidosis

Sarcoidosis is a systemic disorder characterized by both intrathoracic and extrathoracic granulomatous inflammation, which is typically noncaseating. The etiology of the disease is unknown. It is much more common in black persons than in most white populations,[165] and familial cases have been described.[166] Untoward reactions, possibly with immune complexes, to acid-fast organisms, viruses, and various environmental substances have been postulated. A sarcoid-like reaction to malignant tumors is well known, and a few patients with cancer seem to develop sarcoidosis following successful therapy.[167] The considerable amount of work on the immunology of sarcoid has been reviewed,[165,166] and the interrelationships of the participating cells are quite complex. It seems that the tissue reaction begins as a helper T-lymphocyte and monocyte alveolitis, with subsequent accumulation of suppressor T-cells, activated macrophages, and an appreciable number of B-lymphocytes.[168] Since over 90 percent of patients have intrathoracic involvement, the staging of the disease is based on pattern of involvement radiologically. Type I sarcoid is characterized by radiologic hilar adenopathy only, type II by hilar and parenchymal involvement, and type III by parenchymal involvement only. While overall the disease usually either resolves or improves, and only 5 to 10 percent of patients develop life-threatening pulmonary fibrosis, type I patients are most likely to have a favorable outcome, type III patients are most likely to progress, and type II patients are intermediate. Acute onset of disease and associated erythema nodosum seem to be independent favorable prognostic signs.

The hallmark of sarcoidosis in lung tissue is the presence of noncaseating granulomas distributed along the lymphatics of the bronchovascular bundles, interlobular septa, and pleura (Fig. 19-20). The alveolitis that is postulated etiologically is not characteristic histologically; rather, the alveoli not involved by the granulomas are relatively normal. Occasional foci of necrosis within the granulomas are permissible, and asteroid and Schaumann bodies within giant cells are common but not diagnostic. Since the disease process follows bronchovascular bundles and interlobular veins, it is not surprising that some degree of vascular involvement is common (as is discussed later). In spite of the presence of granulomas around pleural lymphatics, radiologically evident pleural effusions or pleural thickening are seen in only 10 percent of cases.[169]

The plain radiograph is characteristic in most cases, and the CT appearance is perhaps even more characteristic in terms of defining the nodular pattern along the distribution of the lymphatics.[19] With a high index of clinical

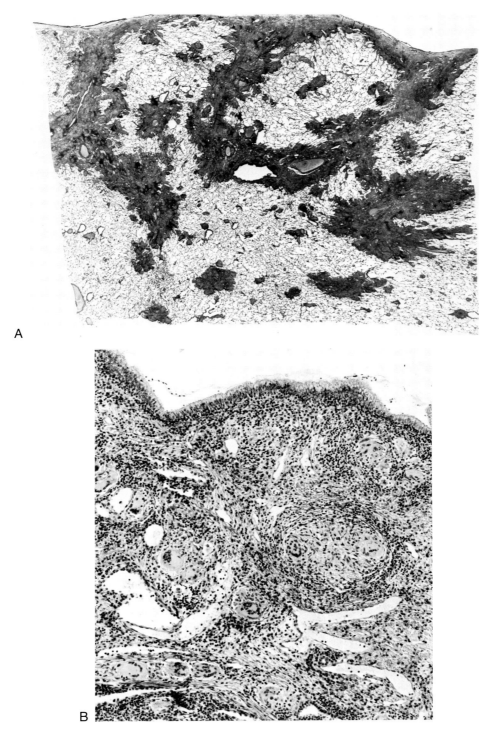

Fig. 19-30. **(A)** Scanning microscopic view of peripheral lung involvement in sarcoidosis. Note distribution of infiltrate along interlobular septa and pleura. **(B)** Noncaseating granulomas in bronchial submucosa in sarcoidosis.

and radiologic suspicion, one is more likely to receive a transbronchial biopsy than an open biopsy in these patients. Sarcoidosis is one of the few types of diffuse infiltrative lung diseases that can be diagnosed by transbronchial biopsy with a high degree of success.[18]

In 1973 Liebow[170] described a disease that he termed *necrotizing sarcoid granulomatosis*. The histologic criteria included granulomatosis or giant cell vasculitis, variable parenchymal necrosis with or without cavitation, and a pneumonitis with sarcoid-like granulomas, which often show central necrosis. He emphasized that various types of angiitis occurred. Extensive granulomatous inflammation occurred with occlusion of vessels. He also observed that granulomas occurred around the external elastic lamellae, resembling the giant cells around the external lamellae in temporal arteritis, as well as a mononuclear infiltrative and occlusive vasculitis. The clinical presentation and radiologic findings are variable; hilar adenopathy and extrathoracic involvement are unusual. In contrast to other pulmonary angiitides, the patients tend to do well with surgical, steroid, or even no therapy.[171-173] While one report suggested that necrotizing sarcoid granulomatosis may be a hypersensitivity reaction to *Aspergillus*,[171] most investigators view it as a variant of sarcoidosis.[172-173]

Extrinsic Allergic Alveolitis and Similar Conditions

Lung disease can result from inhalation of a variety of vegetable and animal dusts, but the lesions and their clinical syndromes may not be identical. In the majority of these, the disease is immunologically mediated, primarily through a type III reaction, although the immunologic mechanisms have not been well documented in all conditions,[174] The prototypical example is *farmer's lung,* which has been the best studied. It is more common in Britain and Europe than in North America and is caused by hypersensitivity to thermophilic actinomycetes (*Micromonospora vulgaris* and *Thermophylliae polyspora*), which grow in moldy hay. In North America *Micropolyspora faeni* is the common cause. Characteristically, the condition occurs when the summers are wet. Since cut hay is not gathered until it is dry, there is abundant multiplication of the organisms in the hay in the intervening period. The farmer is exposed to the moldy hay, usually during winter feeding in an enclosed space. Symptoms appear some hours later, consisting of fever, malaise, cough, and dyspnea. Wheezing is not a usual symptom. The symptoms pass and may reappear when the patient is re-exposed. Radiologic examination shows a diffuse reticulonodular pattern, which is more common in the lung bases. The acute symptoms may not be recognized in some patients, or the initial symptoms may not be remembered, and the patients develop progressive dyspnea. Functionally, restrictive lung disease occurs. Precipitating antibodies to the fungi are found in a high percentage of affected subjects as compared with nonaffected workers in the same environment.[175]

The histologic features depend on the stage at which the disease is seen. Most biopsies are taken in the subacute phase, and characteristically there is extensive chronic interstitial pneumonia, with an infiltrate predominantly of lymphocytes admixed with a minority of plasma cells. Overall lung structure is intact, and alveoli can usually be distinguished. The dominant lesion is interstitial pneumonia, with only few scattered poorly formed granulomas seen in the interstitium. Although it is often said that they are sarcoid-like, the resemblance is seldom more than superficial. The epithelioid cells are loosely arranged and mixed with lymphocytes. Very characteristically, scattered giant cells of the foreign body type are seen and may contain cleft-like spaces or small doubly refractile particles, the exact nature of which is not known (Fig. 19-21). There is involvement of distal bronchioles and respiratory bronchioles. These display chronic inflammation of their walls, often with destruction, distortion, and even obliteration. Lipid-laden macrophages may be found in alveolar spaces, representing the consequences of bronchiolar obstruction, but the macrophages are also seen in alveolar walls. It was once thought that these lesions were features of avian allergic alveolitis (see below), but this is probably not specific for this condition. The largest series reported[176] has been analyzed for the frequency of morphologic lesions, and these are shown in Table 19-7.

The electron microscopic appearance of extrinsic allergic alveolitis has been reported in 18 cases by Kawanami et al.[177] They pointed out that the primary infiltrating cell was the lymphocyte and noted that the deposition of interstitial connective tissue was often associated with masses of loose connective tissue located within air spaces ("alveolar buds"). In the acute phase there may be edema both in air spaces and alveolar walls and a slight infiltrate of plasma cells. In one patient who died 10 to 12 days after the onset of symptoms[178] there was an acute respiratory bronchiolitis with destruction of the bronchiolar walls, fibrin thrombi in adjacent alveolar walls, and an infiltrate of neutrophils, eosinophils, and mononuclear cells. As the condition becomes more chronic, fibrosis occurs with distortion of lung architecture, varying degrees of end-stage lung disease, and occasionally extensive pleural fibrosis. At this stage the lesions may not be distinguishable from fibrosing alveolitis, since the lymphocytic infiltrate diminishes and granulomas may not be apparent.

The clinical syndrome and lesions in *avian allergic alveolitis* are essentially similar. In this instance, the allergens are bird proteins, and precipitating antibodies to extracts of feathers, droppings, serum, and egg white may

TABLE 19-7. Farmer's Lung: Frequency of Histologic Findings, %

Interstitial infiltrate	100	Granulomas	70
Foam cells	65	Interstitial fibrosis	65
Unresolved pneumonia	65	Foreign bodies	60
Bronchiolitis obliterans	50	Pleural fibrosis	48

(From Reyes et al.,[176] with permission.)

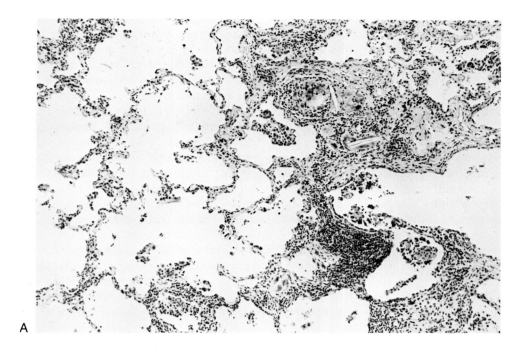

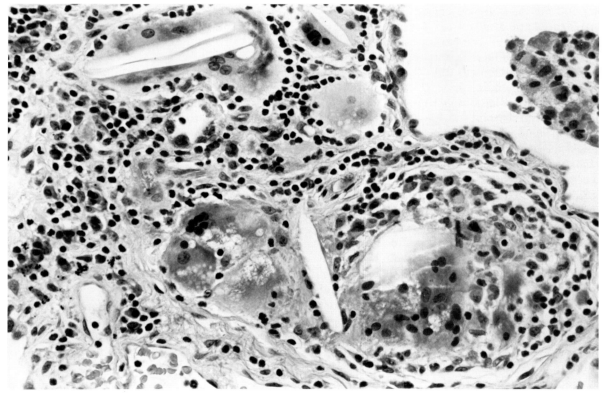

Fig. 19-21. **(A)** Extrinsic allergic alveolitis with mononuclear cell bronchiolitis, interstitial infiltrates with little fibrosis, and granulomas. **(B)** Granulomas in extrinsic allergic alveolitis are relatively ill defined, and the giant cells often show cleft-like spaces.

be present in the blood.[179] The condition has been found in pigeon breeders, pigeon fanciers, poultry farmers, and owners of parakeets. Extrinsic allergic alveolitis has also resulted from infestation of humidifiers and air conditioners by thermophilic actinomycetes.[180] The possibility of extrinsic allergic alveolitis is easily overlooked in this instance since no occupational or leisure activity history is present.

It seems likely that allergic alveolitis is the basic lesion in several other situations, although the lesions and the serum findings have not been completely worked out. These include pituitary snuff takers' lung,[181] furriers' lung, maple bark strippers' lung,[182] suberosis (cork workers' lung),[183] sequoisis (redwood workers' lung),[184] and malt workers' lung.[185] In maple bark strippers' lung, granulomas containing spores of *Cryptostami (Coniosporum) corticale* are seen, although the condition is thought to result from hypersensitivity to the spores rather than from a direct effect. In sequoisis, foreign body giant cells containing doubly refractile material that dissolves during tissue processing are described. Lamellar bodies resembling Schaumann bodies and containing a central particle of redwood dust are also described.

Thesaurosis should be discussed at this point, although there is some question as to whether the condition exists, and if it does, it is not certain that it represents an allergic alveolitis. Thesaurosis is thought to be lung disease consequent to inhalation of hair spray.[186] The original description stressed the finding of macrophages containing PAS-positive material within the air spaces, together with interstitial granulomas resembling sarcoid. Epidemiologic studies showed no increased frequency of lung disease in hairdressers, the population most likely to suffer from excess exposure to hair spray, and thus many do not believe in the existence of the condition.[187] However, we have seen isolated cases in which the lung lesions appeared to be directly related to inhalation of hair spray and disappeared after cessation of exposure. In both its course and the lung lesions the disease resembled sarcoid more closely than allergic alveolitis.

Two important and common conditions have several features in common with extrinsic allergic alveolitis. *Bagassosis* is a lung disease caused by inhalation of sugar cane after the sugar has been expressed from the cane. This residue, bagasse, is compressed for various industrial uses, and the disease may result from hypersensitivity to fungal spores that proliferate during the storage of bagasse. Almost 50 percent of the workers exposed to high levels of bagasse develop symptoms that resemble those of allergic alveolitis, although radiologic changes are more extensive in the upper zones of the lung.[124] Antibodies to thermophilic actinomycetes occur in about two-thirds of the patients with bagassosis.[188] Lung lesions resemble those of extrinsic allergic alveolitis in early

stages, and giant cells containing spindle- and rod-shaped particles are seen. Electron microscopy has shown bacteria and fungi in varying degrees of dissolution and undergoing phagocytosis.[124] In the later stages of the disease, there is extensive pulmonary fibrosis, and emphysema has been described.

Byssinosis results from inhalation of cotton dust, but the relationship to allergic alveolitis is less clear. The clinical features differ in that bronchoconstriction is a prominent feature, occurring characteristically at the beginning of the work week and diminishing over the succeeding days. There is no serologic evidence for sensitivity to cotton dust, but extracts of the cotton bract of pods contain a substance that causes histamine release.[189] The lung lesions are poorly described but appear different from those of allergic alveolitis. Extensive lung pigmentation and peribronchial fibrosis with bronchial distortion, together with fibrous nodules throughout the lung, have been described. "Byssinosis bodies" have been seen in the nodules; these are large, approximately 200 μm $\times$ 50 μm, with a central birefringent hematoxophilic core, which appears to represent a cotton fiber.[190] The fiber is coated with brown iron-containing pigment.

Eosinophilic Granuloma

Eosinophilic granuloma (EG) of the lung has been considered to be one of the manifestations of histiocytosis X, the Hand-Schüller-Christian syndrome and Letterer-Siwe disease being the more aggressive forms of the condition. The common feature in all these disorders is proliferation of a particular type of histiocyte, historically termed the *X cell*.[191] The X cell has been found to have immunologic and ultrastructural characteristics of Langerhans cells of the epidermis,[191,192] and thus EG is more properly viewed as an infiltrative lung disease of Langerhans-type histiocytes. Whether the nature of the disease is inflammatory or neoplastic is unresolved, and its precise relationship to the Hand-Schüller-Christian syndrome and Letterer-Siwe disease is likewise unresolved.

EG is confined to the lung in about 80 percent of cases. Identical histologic lesions may be seen in the bones or elsewhere in the body, which suggests some overlap with Hand-Schüller-Christian syndrome and Letterer-Siwe disease. Isolated involvement of the lung can occur at any age but is most common in young men.[193] Spontaneous pneumothorax is the presenting complaint in about 20 percent of cases; the patients usually have systemic complaints of malaise, dyspnea, and weight loss, and many have fever. Radiologically, the infiltrate is worst in the upper zones of the lung, and often there is a honeycomb pattern. The prognosis is unclear, and there is no series large enough to determine it accurately. It is gener-

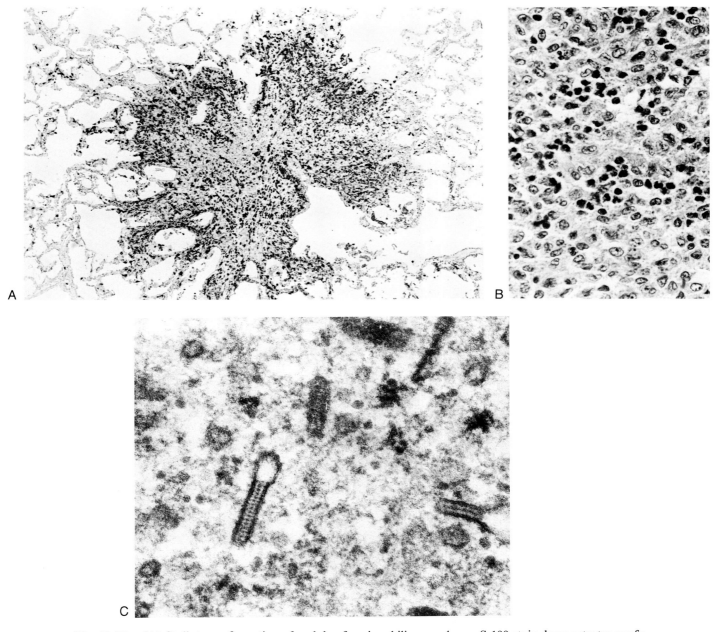

Fig. 19-22. **(A)** Stellate configuration of nodule of eosinophilic granuloma. S-100 stain demonstrates profusion of Langerhans histiocytes. **(B)** Langerhans' histiocytes with indented nuclei and abundant cytoplasm alternate with eosinophils. **(C)** Birbeck granules of Langerhans' histiocyte. (×117,500.)

ally regarded as favorable in perhaps three quarters of patients with lesions limited to the lung,[194] but some authors have suggested that the prognosis is less favorable.[193] Involvement of bones or systemic involvement carries a poorer prognosis. Radiologically, the infiltrates of EG are worst in the upper lung zones, and this distribution of disease is readily demonstrable in long-standing cases. In earlier cases the nodules of EG are irregularly dispersed, affecting the proximal and distal parts of the acinus. Distal acinar subpleural involvement predisposes to spontaneous pneumothorax, which, as mentioned, is well known in this disease. Proximal acinar involvement may compress pulmonary arteries and bronchioles, leading to pulmonary hypertension and obstructive dysfunction, respectively.

The nodules of EG have irregular margins with a stellate configuration (Fig. 19-22A). In early cases there is an admixture of eosinophils and Langerhans-type histiocytes (Fig. 19-22B). The latter cells have an indented nucleus with one or two nucleoli, and an abundant finely vacuolated or faintly eosinophilic cytoplasm.[195] These cells have characteristic ultrastructural cytoplasmic inclusions termed *Birbeck granules,* which consist of linear or racket-shaped bodies derived from and continuous with the external cell membrane (Fig. 19-22C). Immunoperoxidase stains for S100 protein are strongly positive in these cells. In florid EG there are more than 75 staining cells per high-power field.[192] S100-staining cells were also present in this study in other conditions, including less florid EG, but were fewer than 35 per high-power field. In addition to the eosinophils and Langerhans histiocytes, there is an admixture of lymphocytes, macrophages, and fibroblasts within the nodules of EG. With chronicity, the eosinophils and finally the Langerhans histiocytes drop out, and one is left with nonspecific fibrosis and cyst formation,[196] and at this point a definitive diagnosis may be impossible. The usual method of tissue diagnosis is open lung biopsy, since transbronchial biopsies are unlikely to be fruitful. It has been suggested[197] that EG can be diagnosed by the finding of Langerhans histiocytes in sputum. We cannot accept this approach, since these cells may be demonstrated in a variety of interstitial lung diseases,[198] including UIP, DIP, collagen vascular diseases, extrinsic allergic alveolitis, and end-stage fibrosis. Langerhans cells also occur in the stroma of bronchoalveolar carcinoma.[199] Not only is the simple presence of Langerhans histiocytes in the lung not diagnostic of EG, but other cells within the lung stain positively for S100 protein, including myoepithelial cells of the tracheobronchial glands, ''reticulum cells'' of bronchus-associated lymphoid tissue, and cartilage. Thus, as is the case for most of the interstitial lung diseases, the pattern of lung involvement is as important as cytologic details in establishing the diagnosis of EG.

There are two additional potential sources of misdiagnosis in EG. One is an erroneous diagnosis of DIP due to the common phenomenon of a localized, quite striking, DIP-like reaction immediately adjacent to the nodules. The other potential pitfall in the diagnosis of EG is eosinophilic infiltration of the pleura following an episode of spontaneous pneumothorax in young adults.[200] In this condition the eosinophilic infiltrate may extend into the underlying lung, which is usually fibrotic, but the absence of nodules of Langerhans histiocytes and the presence of severe pleural reaction in spontaneous pneumothorax should guide the pathologist to the correct diagnosis.

Tuberous Sclerosis and Lymphangiomyomatosis

The morphologic appearance of the lesions of the lung is identical in tuberous sclerosis and pulmonary lymphangiomyomatosis although the pulmonary lymphangiomyomatosis syndrome is quite distinct from tuberous sclerosis.[201]

Pulmonary lymphangiomyomatosis is confined to women of childbearing age. Dyspnea or pneumothorax is the common presenting complaint, but some patients may have hemoptysis or chylous pleural effusions. Pneumothorax, chylous pleural effusions or ascites, and hemoptysis each occur in about half of the patients during the course of their illness. Initially, the radiologic appearance is that of fine linear and nodular densities, mainly at the lung bases, which progress to bullous and honeycomb changes throughout the lungs. In contrast to fibrosing alveolitis, lung volumes progressively increase radiologically. The pulmonary function pattern is either restrictive, obstructive, or a mixture of the two. Most patients die within 10 years of diagnosis. Because the disease has been almost completely limited to women in the childbearing period, the possibility of hormonal influence has been recognized for a long time. More recently, emphasis has been placed on hormone receptors in the proliferating cells[202,203] and on estrogen suppression, including oophorectomy, in its treatment.[204]

The lung lesions are characterized by an irrational proliferation of smooth muscle within the lung, which involves all peripheral structures—bronchioles, small veins and arteries, and lymphatics (Fig. 19-23A). Smooth muscle also occurs in alveolar walls. Widespread cystic change occurs throughout the lung (Fig. 19-23B), which is thought to be due to smooth muscle proliferation of the bronchioles, with air trapping distal to them. This is the likely mechanism leading spontaneous pneumothorax. Proliferation of venular smooth muscle leads to venous obstruction, intra-alveolar hemorrhage, and hemoptysis. Hemosiderosis is present in about half the cases. Lymphatic smooth muscle proliferation may lead to extrusion of lymph into alveoli, and dilated lymphatic channels may be apparent in the centers of smooth muscle proliferation. Smooth muscle proliferation also occurs in lymph nodes and in the main lymphatic ducts, resulting in chylothorax and chylous ascites.

The differential diagnosis includes UIP, in which extensive smooth muscle proliferation may also occur. However, at this stage there is obvious bronchiolectasis, type II cell proliferation, fibrosis, and interstitial pneumonia, none of which are features of pulmonary lymphangiomyomatosis. It is worth noting that a curious ''adenomatoid'' proliferation of smooth muscle and epithelium occurs in some patients with pulmonary lymphangiomyomatosis, but this is easily distinguishable from UIP.[201] In *benign metastasizing leiomyomas,* the lesions are nodular and discrete, both histologically and radiologically. In *leiomyomatous hamartomas,* the nodules are clearly distinct from the surrounding lung, are formed of fascicles of smooth muscle cells, and may have

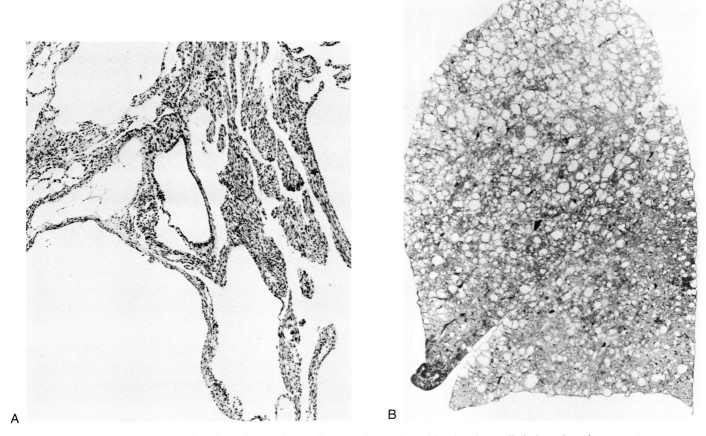

Fig. 19-23. **(A)** Proliferation of smooth muscle around vessels and in alveolar walls in lymphangiomyomatosis. **(B)** Widespread cystic changes in lymphangiomyomatosis (paper-mounted whole lung section).

a glandular component. If single, they are seen predominantly in men, but the multiple form is almost exclusively confined to middle-aged women. The distinction between benign metastasizing leiomyomas and leiomyomatous hamartomas has been questioned. Proliferations of the Kapanci cell,[205] a specialized interstitial cell containing myofilaments, have not been reported, although ultrastructural similarities between the proliferating cells in lymphangiomyomatosis and the pulmonary interstitial cells have been noted.[206]

The relationship between tuberous sclerosis and pulmonary lymphangiomyomatosis is not completely clear. As indicated, the pulmonary lesions are identical. The age of presentation of tuberous sclerosis is different, both sexes are affected, and about 25 percent of patients have a family history. Patients with lymphangiomyomatosis occasionally have renal angiomyolipomas, as do patients with tuberous sclerosis. A family history of lymphangiomyomatosis has not been reported, but in two instances patients with lymphangiomyomatosis have had retarded children.[201] The simplest concept is that tuber-

ous sclerosis and lymphangiomyomatosis represent variations of the same spectrum of the disease process, although it is not precise to regard lymphangiomyomatosis as a forme fruste of tuberous sclerosis.

Eosinophilic Pneumonia

A number of different conditions have been described in which the air spaces of the lungs contain a large number of eosinophils.[207,208] It is easier to regard them all as variants of eosinophilic pneumonia than to regard them as separate disease entities. The term *Loeffler's syndrome* is generally applied to the mildest form of the condition, in which the patients are asymptomatic. The term *pulmonary infiltrates with eosinophilia* syndrome has been used to describe a syndrome of pulmonary infiltrates with blood eosinophilia. The use of the term has little justification, since the same lung lesions and symptoms occur in patients with either transient or no peripheral eosinophilia. The presence of pulmonary infiltrates, often with eosinophilia, has long been recognized in patients with *asthma,* but it is easier to express the same phenomenon by noting that about 20 percent or more of patients with eosinophilic pneumonia have asthma. In all the above-mentioned circumstances the etiology of eosinophilic pneumonia is not known, but there are some well recognized associations of eosinophilic pneumonia. The best examples include sensitivity to nitrofurantoin and other drugs. In some instances these cases are referred to as *hypersensitivity angiitis,* and it is better to regard them as due to a more specific cause of eosinophilic pneumonia (Table 19-8). Pulmonary infiltrates with peripheral eosinophilia are common in tropical countries and likely represent a reaction to migration of parasites through the lung. Eosinophilic pneumonia, usually with asthma, may be a manifestation of *periarteritis nodosa,* and this may or may not be the same as *Churg-Strauss syndrome* or *allergic angiitis and granulomatosis* (see Ch. 20). Finally, eosinophilic pneumonia, together with asthma, may be a manifestation of aspergillosis (*allergic bronchopulmonary aspergillosis*).

Patients with eosinophilic pneumonia often manifest a typial clinical syndrome and radiographic appearance.[209] The condition is almost entirely confined to adults, 80 percent of whom are women, and is most common in middle age, with an average age of onset of 50 years. Severe systemic effects, including fever, sweats, and loss of weight are usual, together with cough and dyspnea. Asthma occurs in about one quarter of the cases, and nasal symptoms occur in about one third. Eosinophilia of the blood is usually found, but it is important to recognize that this may be transient or absent. The chest film shows subpleural parenchymal densities with poorly defined margins, commonly seen at the apices and in the axillary region. In the most extreme example, the infiltrates surround the peripheral portions of the lung and spare the central region, resulting in an appearance described as the "photographic negative of pulmonary edema."[209] The infiltrates may disappear spontaneously and recur in the same position. About three quarters of the cases have a distinctive radiograph. The response to steroids is dramatic and may even be used as a diagnostic test, since the symptoms may disappear within hours and the radiologic abnormalities within days. Lung biopsy can usually be avoided, but there are a sufficient number of atypical cases that biopsy is required from time to time to establish the diagnosis.

The histologic features are flooding of alveolar spaces with eosinophils and macrophages and an associated mild interstitial pneumonia. In some instances the interstitial pneumonia and diffuse alveolar damage may be quite severe, with type II hyperplasia together with large numbers of macrophages in the air spaces, and this may lead to a mistaken diagnosis of DIP. Necrosis of the cellular exudate may occur, resulting in a granulomatous appearance, or actual sarcoid-like granulomas may form. Angiitis of small vessels may be seen. Bronchiolitis obliterans is present in a minority of cases, is usually mild, and is particularly associated with the curious syndrome of rheumatoid arthritis and eosinophilic pneumonia.[210] Occasionally, it may be severe, and it may be difficult to separate eosinophilic pneumonia from bronchiolitis obliterans. Eosinophilic infiltration of any degree of severity is not a feature of bronchiolitis obliterans. The histologic appearance of eosinophilic pneumonia is in general characteristic, but it is important to recognize that the features also include necrosis of the exudate, granulomas, diffuse alveolar damage, and bronchiolitis obliterans.

Alveolar Proteinosis (Lipoproteinosis)

Pulmonary alveolar proteinosis is an infiltrative lung disease characterized by an intra-alveolar accumulation of lipoproteinaceous, surfactant-like material.[211] The disease may be seen in one of four clinical settings: as an idiopathic disease, as an occupational disease, as a drug-induced disease, and as an infiltrate in the immunocompromised host.[211–213] In the idiopathic variety, there is a male predominance, and the usual age range is 30 to 50 years. The usual presenting symptom is dyspnea; cough, while present, is often not as productive as one might imagine from the histology.[214] Pulmonary alveolar proteinosis of demonstrable occupational etiology is most commonly associated with crystalline material and silica, although other substances have also been implicated both experimentally and clinically.[212] Lesions resembling proteinosis have been discussed previously in relation to amphophilic drugs. In the immunocompromised host the underlying disease is overwhelmingly leukemia or lymphoma.[213,215]

TABLE 19-8. Drugs Causing Pulmonary Eosinophilia and/or Polyarteritis

Drug	Pulmonary Eosinophilia	Polyarteritis
Allopurinol		+
Aspirin	+	
Busulfan		+
Hydantoins		+
Hydralazine		+
Imipramine	+	
Iodides		+
Gold salts		+
Nitrofurantoin	+	+
Penicillins	+	+
Sulfonamides	+	+

The histologic appearance is similar in all the clinical settings. The alveolar spaces are filled by granular, relatively hypocellular, intensely eosinophilic material, which is strongly PAS-positive and diastase-resistant (Fig. 19-24). There may be some degree of type II pneumocyte proliferation, but interstitial and intra-alveolar inflammation is characteristically absent. By light microscopy, discrete eosinophilic bodies may be seen within air spaces. By electron microscopy, the granular material consists of free myelin-like figures and laminated bodies, free membrane-bound vacuoles, and electron-dense debris. Immunohistochemistry demonstrates the intra-alveolar material to contain surfactant, although this reaction is said to be more strongly and diffusely positive in the idiopathic and occupational settings than in the immunocompromised host.[211,212] It is of considerable importance to investigate all patients—and particularly immunocompromised patients—with pulmonary alveolar proteinosis for superinfection. The lipoproteinaceous material serves as an excellent culture medium, and a variety of associated fungal, viral, mycobacterial, nocardial, and protozoal superinfections have been described.[213,215]

The pathogenesis of the disease is still a matter of speculation. There is no good evidence of excessive surfactant production. Rather, the defect appears to be a failure of surfactant clearance, which is normally a function of both type II pneumocytes and alveolar macrophages.[212]

The surfactant material itself has been found directly toxic to macrophages. Demonstrable abnormalities of macrophage number, morphology, and phagocytic function have been shown in patients with alveolar proteinosis, as well as abnormalities in function of normal macrophages exposed in vitro to alveolar proteinosis lavage fluid.[216] The current understanding is that nonspecific factors lead to a transient localized surfactant clearance failure, and before this failure is corrected, the material accumulates sufficiently to directly suppress clearance mechanisms.

The usual means of diagnosis is open lung biopsy. Transbronchial lung biopsy and examination of lavage fluid[217] may also be diagnostic, but with these two techniques one is more restricted in examination for superimposed infection and for occupational markers. Treatment with sequential lavage usually induces remission with excellent long-term survival, particularly in nonimmunocompromised patients.

Pulmonary Alveolar Microlithiasis

Alveolar microlithiasis is a rare condition. Fewer than 100 cases have been reported, and about half of these are familial.[218] The Mayo Clinic recorded only eight cases in a 46 year period.[219] Although the condition is frequently described in siblings, there is only one recorded instance of its occurrence in both a parent and a child. Most cases

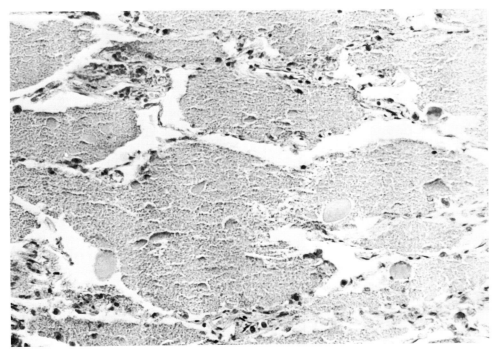

Fig. 19-24. Alveolar proteinosis. Air spaces are filled with eosinophilic, PAS-positive material. Well defined bodies are present.

are diagnosed in adult life, but microlithiasis has been described in a pair of premature stillborn twins,[220] and a number of cases in children have been reported. It is likely that the condition is a congenital metabolic disorder, with slow progression through life. In some instances, however, there may be rapid progression, and the condition may also appear in old age.[221] The chest film may also remain static for many years. The patients may be asymptomatic, or they may have varying degrees of dyspnea, succumbing finally in respiratory failure. The patients exhibit a restrictive pulmonary defect,[222] typically quite mild when compared with the appearance of the chest film, especially in young patients. The chest radiograph is usually immediately diagnostic, with an appearance of sand-like micronodular opacities involving both lungs diffusely, the lower zones being more opaque than the upper. The lung fields may appear almost completely opaque on routine radiographs, but the distinctive discrete opacities can be seen on overpenetrated films.

Grossly, the lung tissue is firm and gritty and maintains its shape. Histologically, the air spaces contain large numbers of concentrically laminated calcified bodies, which also show radial striations. They are termed *calcispherites* and contain calcium and phosphorus, in similar concentrations to those found in bone, and small amounts of magnesium and iron. They are fairly uniform in size and are generally about 0.25 mm in diameter, but some may be as large as 1 mm or more. Ossification may occur. The calcispherites are nearly all in air spaces, but some may occur interstitially. In the stillborn infants referred to, the calcispherites appeared to form in the alveolar wall epithelium and were extruded into the air spaces. The intervening alveolar wall may be relatively normal,[223] but it usually shows interstitial fibrosis with a mild chronic inflammatory cell infiltrate, particularly when there are large aggregates of calcispherites. Calcispherites have to be distinguished from the corpora amylacea that may be found in the air spaces of the lung, especially in patients with chronic heart failure. Corpora amylacea are likewise laminated but are smaller, are not calcified, and often contain a central black core.

Pulmonary Lymphangitic Carcinomatosis

As the name implies, pulmonary lymphangitic carcinomatosis is characterized by metastatic tumor growth, primarily in the pulmonary lymphatics. The cell type is usually adenocarcinoma, and the most common primary sites are lung, breast, and gastrointestinal tract.[224,225] The prognosis in general is grim, with only approximately 15 percent of patients surviving over 6 months, but with occasional long-term survivors.[224]

Pulmonary lymphangitic carcinomatosis has received considerably more attention in the radiologic than in the pathologic literature.[224-227] While the plain chest radiograph appearances are often subtle and nonspecific, CT findings are highly characteristic and accurately reflect the macroscopic abnormalities in this disease. Since the major lymphatic vessels in the lung are located in the pleura, interlobular septa, and bronchovascular bundles, the obvious abnormalities are found primarily in this distribution and consist of thickening and accentuation of these structures. Microscopically, tumor cells are found as plugs within lymphatic vessels, with variable associated amounts of free interstitial tumor, intra-alveolar tumor, hematogenous tumor, edema, inflammation, and interstitial fibrosis.[224-226] The presence of tumor cells in the lymphatics of the bronchovascular bundles is of considerable practical significance, since it explains the fact that lymphangitic carcinoma is one of the few infiltrative lung diseases that can be reliably diagnosed by bronchial or transbronchial lung biopsy.[18]

The pathogenesis of this peculiar pattern of tumor growth is still a matter of speculation. Seeding of the lymphatics from blood vessel emboli is the favored theory, since hematogenous tumor is almost invariably found in the lungs and other organs of patients with lymphangitic carcinoma.[224,226] The notion that lymphangitic carcinomatosis is due to retrograde growth of tumor from an involved thoracic duct or mediastinal/hilar nodes seems less likely since these structures are tumor-free, or nearly tumor-free, in at least half of the cases.[226,227]

Pneumoconioses

The term *pneumoconiosis,* defined literally according to its Greek roots, means "dust in the lung." Organic or nonmineral dusts are implicated in a variety of conditions, which are usually immunologically mediated, and have been discussed earlier. The reaction of the lung to inorganic dust depends on several factors. The composition of the minerals is important because of individual solubilities and toxic reactions. The size of the particles determines the site of deposition within the respiratory tract, while their concentration determines load.[228] Particles greater than 5 μm in aerodynamic diameter tend to impact in the nose and large airways. Because of Brownian movement, particles less than 1 μm in diameter are precipitated in the peripheral airways and air spaces. The ability of the respiratory system to clear or to isolate particles effectively and its competence in repairing damage are factors relating to the type of lesion produced. Finally, individual susceptibility is an enigma preventing one person from acquiring disease, while an identically exposed individual develops marked lesions. In assessing patients with pneumoconiosis, the clinical history, pulmonary function tests, radiologic features, and pathologic material must all be correlated. Such a correlation was performed by Gaensler[229] and his co-workers in 1972 in 52 patients. Histologic lesions were found to predate functional or radiologic changes, which became apparent at various rates depending on the disease. Identification of the injurious dust may be essential; methods of determining dusts within the lung, such as electron probe microanalysis, are discussed in detail in a 1987 monograph, which also provides a comprehensive review of occupational lung disease.[230]

Only those inorganic dusts will be discussed here that are encountered reasonably frequently at biopsy; complete data are available in recent monographs and chapters on occupational lung disease.[230–233]

Asbestosis. Asbestosis is the name given to pneumoconiosis caused by inhalation of a group of fibrous silicates that have varying combinations of magnesium, iron, aluminum, manganese, calcium, sodium, and potassium.[234] There are two main types, serpentine and amphibole.[235] Chrysotile is the only example of the former, but the latter has many subtypes, of which crocidolite (Cape Blue asbestos) and amosite are the best known. The two types differ both in composition and lattice structure, with chrysotile having a central core. Asbestos is found in many industries and in many forms, and occupational and other exposures may be legion.[231]

Clinically, insidiously developing shortness of breath is the first symptom of asbestosis. This is associated with late inspiratory crackles, found initially in the lung bases but becoming widespread as the disease progresses. Finger clubbing is present in about 75 percent of the patients, but its severity is not proportional to the radiologic extent of disease. Pulmonary function tests show a restrictive pattern. Although it has been well documented that early in experimental asbestosis there is fibrosis of respiratory bronchioles and/or alveolar ducts, it is only recently that attention has been drawn to airway lesions in human asbestos disease.[236] Fibrosis of distal (membranous) bronchioles and respiratory bronchioles has been noted, and clinically there is evidence of air flow obstruction in some patients exposed to asbestos (and other) dust.[236] Radiologically, asbestosis is seen predominantly in the lower lung fields, and the earliest changes are seen in the costophrenic angles bilaterally, where there is an increase in vessel markings, with formation of bead-like opacities. Significant morphologic and functional abnormalities may be present even when the chest film is normal.[229] The fine reticulation progresses to irregular opacities and prominent interstitial reticulation.

The pulmonary consequences of asbestos exposure include diffuse interstitial fibrosis (asbestosis), conglomerate massive fibrosis, pleural effusion, pleural plaque, mesothelioma, and lung cancer.[230–233] At 6 months after first exposure, typical asbestos bodies can be seen. These are composed of a central core of asbestos, encrusted with iron. Characteristically, they have knobs at each end, and the body appears beaded (Fig. 19-25). Besides the classical asbestos body, a variety of other iron-encrusted bodies of various shapes and sizes may be seen. Asbestos fibers are found both free and surrounded by macrophages and are not doubly refractile. The iron is most likely derived from phagocytosed red cells and is transferred to the fiber while it is enclosed within a phagolysosome. This coating may represent an attempt by macrophages to neutralize the injurious particle.[237] All hemosiderin-coated bodies are not asbestos bodies, however. A wide variety of substances may produce iron-coated bodies (ferruginous bodies), and these include diatomaceous earth, aluminum silicate, fiberglass, and fragments of lung elastin.[238] However, the classical beaded asbestos body is rarely encountered in routine sections other than after asbestos exposure.

The alteration of lung structure in asbestosis is variable. In some instances there is diffuse, fine fibrosis of the alveolar wall with relative retention of alveolar structure. In other instances, however, there is organization and reorganization of lung tissue, resulting in an appearance resembling that in UIP. Kuhn and Kuo[239] have found cytoplasmic hyaline inclusions, resembling Mallory bodies, in alveolar epithelium, and interpret this as an early reaction to injury. These, however, have also been found in UIP, radiation pneumonitis, and organizing pneumonia.[240] Giant cells containing asteroid bodies are fairly frequently encountered.

Although, in general, a significant dose-related response has been identified in workers exposed to asbestos, the amount of asbestos in the lung and the extent of fibrosis may have little relation. Ashcroft and Heppleston[241] assessed asbestos concentration in lungs with varying degrees of fibrosis and found no correlation between

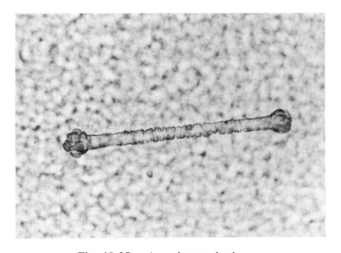

Fig. 19-25. An asbestos body.

the concentration of fibers and the degree of fibrotic reaction. This finding has important implications since, as an extreme example, one may find a histologically atypical example of asbestosis, resembling UIP, with only occasional asbestos bodies. Under these circumstances, the differential diagnosis between UIP and asbestosis may be difficult.

Progressive massive fibrosis (nodular lesions more than 1 cm in diameter) may occur throughout the lung fields.[242] Tuberculosis does not appear to be a factor, and this complication is rare unless the patient has also been exposed to silica. Pleural effusions due to asbestos are usually unilateral and resolve slowly.[243] There is no definite association between pleural plaques and pleural effusion. The development of pleural plaques is unexplained; they tend to be bilateral and involve only the parietal pleura. Common sites are over the ribs, at the lung bases, and in the aponeurotic areas of the diaphragm. Grossly, they are lobulated, white thickenings of the pleura. Microscopically, a plaque is formed of acellular hyaline fibrous tissue with interlacing bands of collagen, producing a basket weave pattern. Asbestos bodies are rarely found.

Malignant mesothelioma of the pleura (see Ch. 25) has a confirmed association with asbestos exposure. The bulky, lobulated neoplasm has a tendency to spread along serosal membranes and to encase the lung. Individuals exposed to asbestos also appear to have a higher risk of developing lung carcinoma than the general population. Smoking has an additive and possibly multiplicative risk effect. Other lesions thought to be related to asbestos exposure include ovarian, gastrointestinal, and hematologic neoplasms.

Silicosis. Silicosis is a chronic fibrosing pulmonary disease caused by prolonged exposure to free silica. Silicon dioxide occurs naturally in three crystalline forms—quartz, cristobalite, and tridymite. Quartz is the most common form and is found in many rocks. Siliceous minerals are ubiquitous and thus can be found in a multitude of industries and occupations. Particles that range from 0.5 to 5 μm in diameter are the ones most likely to cause disease. The concentration and size of the particles determine the likelihood of developing silicosis.[231]

The disease process begins with phagocytosis of the inhaled particles by alveolar macrophages.[244] The silica is initially contained in a phagolysosome. Owing to an unknown toxic effect, possibly to reactive silanol groups, the lysosomal membrane breaks down and releases acid hydrolases into the cell. This results in death of the macrophage and liberation of silica, so the cycle is repeated. The nonlipid material released from the macrophage stimulates fibroblasts, and fibrogenesis is initiated. The fibrosis is not confined to the regions where dust is en-

countered but is also present in the lymph nodes to which the macrophages migrate. An immunologic mechanism has been implicated because of increased serum levels of γ-globulin, the presence of antinuclear antibodies in the serum, and the presence of γ-globulins in the silicotic lesions in many patients. Three morphologic types of silicosis have been described: simple nodular silicosis, conglomerate silicosis (progressive massive fibrosis), and acute silicosis.

Macroscopically, the *nodular form* displays a thickened pleura with many adhesions. Gray-black, well circumscribed nodules 0.5 to 5 mm in diameter are present in the lung parenchyma. If tuberculosis is present, these may be cavitated. The hilar lymph nodes are frequently enlarged and may be calcified, typically at the rim of the node ("eggshell calcification"). Microscopically, the dust particles can be found within macrophages or free in the alveolar septa. Respiratory bronchioles often show aggregates of particles in their walls. The diagnostic lesion is the silicotic nodule, or islet, which contains a central hyalinized whorled mass of acellular collagen (Fig. 19-26). Peripheral to this are layers of macrophages and plasma cells. Small quantities of dust can be identified, but if the dust is high in quartz and small in particle size, very little of it can produce severe fibrosis. It should be noted that silica is poorly refractile; the highly refractile, usually abundant, material often seen is due to associated silicates. Continuing dust exposure increases the number and size of existing nodules. After exposure ceases, the nodules may continue to grow owing to the migration of macrophages peripherally, which leads to continued fibrogenesis, or owing to continued immune perpetuation.

Conglomerate silicosis (progressive massive fibrosis) has the same general features as chronic silicosis, but larger nodules are formed, which often coalesce to form large masses, and the time course is shorter. Cavitation due to superimposed *tuberculosis* is also seen, and tuberculosis has been implicated in the production of conglomerate silicosis even in the absence of cavitation; conventional pulmonary tuberculosis is a major cause of morbidity in silicotic patients, who also have a high incidence of tuberculosis.[245] Tuberculosis is known to increase and perpetuate cellular reactions to dust particles and make them progressive. Silica has an inhibiting effect on the ability of macrophages to contain the growth of mycobacteria. Not only is *Mycobacterium tuberculosis* found, but also the atypical mycobacteria.

Acute silicosis is a rare lesion resulting from an overwhelming exposure to free silica. The particles involved are small, usually between 1 and 2 μm in diameter, and with a high quartz concentration. These conditions are found particularly during sandblasting, which is the usual method of exposure leading to acute silicosis. The sili-

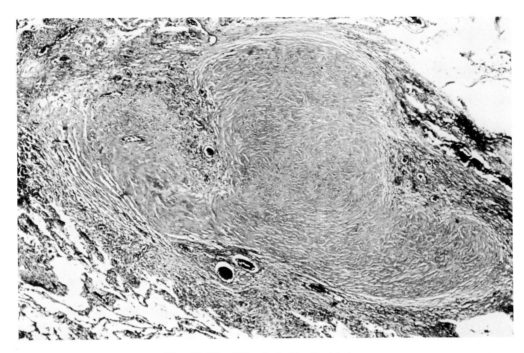

Fig. 19-26. Whorled silicotic islet.

cotic process develops rapidly. Nodules are sparse, and instead the lungs have a gray, consolidated appearance, with diffusely increased interstitial markings. Microscopically, the alveoli are filled by an eosinophilic foamy exudate containing many macrophages. There is prominent type II cell hyperplasia with interstitial fibrosis. The histologic features may resemble those of alveolar proteinosis or desquamative interstitial pneumonia. The exact mechanism of production of the acute lesion is not known.

Clinically, the main symptoms of silicosis develop late. Cough and expectoration are accompanied by progressive shortness of breath. Infections with mycobacteria or fungi give rise to weight loss and other constitutional symptoms and signs. Nodular silicosis runs a protracted course and is usually only associated with minor symptoms and pulmonary function abnormalities. Conglomerate silicosis progresses over a period of years and is associated with major functional abnormalities. Pulmonary function tests are not specific; they may be normal early in the disease or may show an obstructive or a restrictive defect or both. Diffusing capacity is decreased, and exercise-induced hypoxia can occasionally be observed. Patients with acute silicosis may develop symptoms within 6 months after exposure, followed by progressive deterioration and intractable hypoxia, and may have a severe restrictive defect.

Berylliosis. Beryllium aluminum silicate was first recognized as an occupational hazard in fluorescent lamp work-

ers. Use of beryllium in this industry was discontinued, but because of its structural characteristics, it is used in metallic, alloy, and oxide forms in numerous industries. Berylliosis may be either an acute or chronic disease. The acute disease is usually seen in refinery workers and results in the nonspecific pathologic changes of diffuse alveolar damage. Chronic berylliosis is a multiorgan disease in which the lung is most severely involved; it is characterized by a granulomatous inflammatory reaction, which is indistinguishable from sarcoidosis.[246]

Other Dusts. A variety of other dusts may be encountered in the lung, some of which are fibrogenic and others of which are not. These are indicated in Table 19-9.

CHRONIC AIR FLOW OBSTRUCTION

The Concept of Flow Obstruction

Lung biopsy is seldom indicated in patients with chronic air flow obstruction and when done it usually represents clinical misdiagnosis or excessive clinical curiosity. The exception is in cases with unexplained air flow obstruction (i.e., apparently not associated with smoking, chronic bronchitis, or emphysema). Useful clinical and anatomic pathologic criteria exist for the diagnosis of chronic bronchitis, asthma, and emphysema, but the interest in these diseases to the surgical pathologist is small and the volume of information large.[247] Thus,

TABLE 19-9. Less Common Pneumoconioses

Dust	Industry	Presence of Fibrosis	Characteristic Features
Aluminum	Metal refining	Idiosyncratic interstitial fibrosis	Occasional granulomas, black interstitial dust
Antimony	Mining alloy	No	Dust-bearing macrophages
Coal (anthracosis)	Coal workers	No	Black dust in peribronchial aggregates
Barium (baritosis)	Miners, grinders, aspiration	Minimal	Macrophages containing granules of dust
Fiberglass	Manufacturing	No	Particle as negative space
Fuller's earth (aluminum silicate)	Toiletry manufacture	Confluent in upper lobe	No foreign body giant cells; large particles, 15–30 μm
Iron (siderosis)	Welders' oxyacetylene, silver finishers	No	Iron dusts
Magnesium silicate (talcosis)	Talc inhalation, narcotic abuse	Lower lobe fibrosis that cavitates	Doubly refractive particles, often needle-shaped
Tin dioxide (stannosis)	Tin smelting, mining, refining	No	Macrophage aggregates in small nodules
Titanium	Dye	No	Particles within macrophages

the content of this section will be limited to a brief consideration of the concept of chronic air flow obstruction, since this is common knowledge expected of every physician, and to a consideration of those few medical conditions in which biopsies can be expected to be performed.

Chronic obstructive lung disease, better referred to as *chronic air flow obstruction (CAO)* or *chronic air flow limitation,* is a syndrome, and no more specific a condition than anemia or fever. It is recognized clinically by abnormalities of tests of expiratory flow, and disability is determined by the degree to which flow is diminished. Flow is determined by only two factors, the force that is applied to the lungs and the resistance to air flow within the lungs. The former is determined by the elastic recoil of the lung. Emphysema is thought to be associated with loss of elastic recoil, so that flow limitation may occur in emphysematous lungs even if the airways are normal. Resistance to flow may be caused by a number of lesions in the airways, including intraluminal mucus, airway irritability, narrowing of the airway lumina, and inflammation of the airways.

An important concept is that the *peripheral airways,* defined as conducting (i.e., nonalveolated) airways less than 2 mm in internal diameter, contribute only about 20 percent of the total resistance to flow in the respiratory system.[248] Therefore, significant obstruction can occur in the peripheral airways without markedly altering air flow resistance. For example, if every other peripheral airway were destroyed, then peripheral airway resistance would double. However, this would only increase total airway resistance by 20 percent, a change that is barely detectable. Tests of expiratory function thought to reflect total airway resistance, such as the FEV_1, might be normal. The low proportion that peripheral airways contribute to total airway resistance is presently being challenged,[249,250] and it is also true that the FEV_1 has been described as abnormal in the presence of mild bronchiolar abnormalities.[251] It is also important to recognize that lesions in the peripheral airways are the usual cause of obstruction in patients with significant air flow obstruction. As indicated, biopsy specimens in this setting are rarely submitted to the surgical pathologist, but the problem of CAO does arise from time to time. Should it be necessary, for whatever reason, to quantitate peripheral airway lesions, for example in lung resection specimens in this setting, the details of a grading system have been published,[252] and a panel of grading pictures can be obtained from Dr. J.C. Hogg (Pulmonary Research Laboratory, St. Paul's Hospital, Burrard Street, Vancouver, B.C., V6Z 1Y5, Canada).

Bronchiolitis or Small Airway Disease

Biopsies may be performed in patients with air flow obstruction due to peripheral airway disease under a number of circumstances. Sometimes, this may occur because of a mistaken diagnosis of infiltrative lung disease. A broad classification of bronchiolitis is given in Table 19-10.

TABLE 19-10. Bronchiolitis

Lesions in bronchioles in patients with typical chronic air flow
   obstruction
      Mild air flow obstruction ("small airways disease")
      Severe air flow obstruction

Lesions in bronchioles in patients with unusual chronic
   air flow obstruction
      Irritants and viral infections
      Rheumatoid bronchiolitis
      Diffuse panbronchiolitis
      Graft versus host disease
      Heart-lung transplantation
      Follicular bronchiolitis
      Respiratory bronchiolitis
      Cryptogenic bronchiolitis

Bronchiolar Lesions in Patients with Typical Chronic Air Flow Obstruction

Bronchiolitis is an integral part of the lesions found in patients with typical CAO—smokers with chronic bronchitis and varying degrees of pulmonary disability. As indicated, these are of limited concern to surgical pathologists. It is important to recognize that the lesions in patients with mild CAO may be different, not only quantitatively, from those in patients with severe CAO. In mild CAO bronchiolar inflammation plays the most important role; in severe CAO narrowing and tortuosity of the bronchioles are the dominant lesions. In both mild and severe CAO, goblet cell metaplasia is important. These lesions and their functional correlations have been reviewed in detail elsewhere.[253,254]

Bronchiolar Lesions in Patients with Unusual Forms of Chronic Air Flow Obstruction

CAO may occur in settings other than the above, and over the last decade a variety of clinicopathologic syndromes have been defined.

Irritants and Viral Infections

A large number of irritant gases, if respired at the appropriate concentrations, may produce severe bronchiolitis, with acute ulceration and inflammation, followed by occlusion of the airways by loose granulation tissue and finally by complete stenosis and obliteration. The best known of these agents are nitrogen dioxide,[255] sulfur dioxide,[256] and ammonia.[257] Another important set of causes consists of viral infections, perhaps the most important one of which is presently adenovirus.[258] *Mycoplasma pneumonia* should also be recognized as a frequent cause.[259] Measles is now an uncommon cause. The

course of events is similar to that for the toxic gases above. Extensive bronchiectasis may result because of bronchiolar obliteration. Only in rare instances is a lung biopsy performed and then usually because of clinically unusual air flow obstruction, often in a young person. The airway lesions are of course nonspecific, and the diagnosis depends on past history.

Rheumatoid Bronchiolitis

First described in 1977 by Geddes et al.,[260] this is now a well recognized condition. These authors described six patients, five with classical rheumatoid arthritis and the sixth with positive antinuclear antibody, who developed rapidly progressive dyspnea and air flow obstruction. All were nonsmoking females, and death occurred 5 to 18 months after the onset. Radiologically, the lungs were characterized by gross overinflation, but without the peripheral arterial insufficiency of emphysema. The diffusing capacity and volume-pressure curves were normal. Morphologically, scattered occlusion of small bronchi and bronchioles was observed, which was due to loose connective tissue in their lumina (Fig. 19-27). One of us has seen a case in which all gradations from rheumatoid-like granulomas in the walls of airways to fibrous obliteration were present. From the practical point of view, the lesion is spotty within the airways, often in bronchi, and may not be apparent in a biopsy specimen. Because of the widespread recognition of rheumatoid bronchiolitis, biopsy is rarely performed today.

It has now become apparent that CAO is more common in rheumatoid arthritis than previously recognized,[261] and has a frequency that is approximately doubled, whether in smokers or nonsmokers. Even in patients with more severe CAO, the course has not been as malignant as the original cases.

Diffuse Panbronchiolitis

Diffuse panbronchiolitis is a curious condition that appears to be confined to Japanese in Japan. It is quite common, and between 1977 and 1980 there were 1,238 cases recorded in the Japanese panbronchiolitis registry.[262] Men are more commonly affected than women, and the age range is 20 to 60 years. The presenting complaints are chronic productive cough and dyspnea, and three fourths of patients have sinusitis. Radiologically there is variable hyperinflation, and multiple scattered fine opacities less than 2 mm in diameter are seen, which are more profuse in the lower zones. Functionally there is CAO, which is progressive, terminating in respiratory failure. Morphologically the lesion is distinctive. There is severe chronic inflammation of respiratory bronchioles with a mural infiltrate of lymphocytes, plasma cells, and

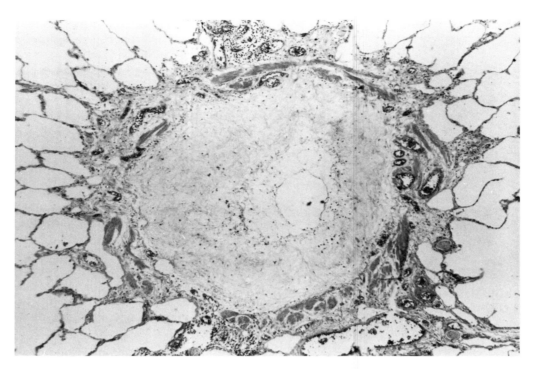

Fig. 19-27. End-stage rheumatoid bronchiolitis showing mucosal erosion and near total luminal obliteration by loose fibrous tissue.

histiocytes. As the lesions progress, there is extension to involve distal bronchioles. The walls of the airways become fibrotic and thickened, and the more proximal bronchioles dilate and become irregular in shape. The lesions are widespread but worse in the lower than in the upper lobes. One of us has seen nine cases in consultation (including that of a Japanese-American born in Hawaii) and is convinced that this is a specific entity. The Japanese have speculated that the condition occurs in the United States and is unrecognized. They have suggested that some of the cases of "obstructive disease of the small airways" reported by Macklem et al.[263] and some cases of "bronchiolitis obliterans" reported by Gosink et al.[146] were examples of diffuse panbronchiolitis. However, a subsequent review of Macklem et al.'s cases has not shown lesions similar to those of diffuse panbronchiolitis. An as yet unemphasized feature of diffuse panbronchiolitis is the accumulation of a large number of macrophages with abundant clear cytoplasm (presumably lipid) in the walls and lumina of bronchioles and in adjacent air spaces.

Many of the clinical features resemble bronchiectasis as seen in North America, but the condition does not date back to childhood respiratory infection. Morphologically, dilatation occurs in more proximal airways (bronchi) in bronchiectasis, and peripheral bronchiolar disease is also more central and more obliterative, involving dis-

tal bronchi and proximal bronchioles. Lymphoid follicles in airway walls are not a feature of diffuse panbronchiolitis.

Graft-Versus-Host Disease

Bronchiolitis has become a well recognized complication of graft-versus-host disease in patients treated with bone marrow transplantation since the first case was reported by Roca et al.[264] in 1982. It has been estimated that it occurs in about 4 to 10 percent of patients[265,266] following bone marrow transplantation. The clinical appearance is of rapidly progressive air flow obstruction, with radiologic evidence of overinflation, starting 3 months to 2 years after transplantation. Other manifestations of graft-versus-host reaction are present, and treatment is of the reaction, which may be effective. A necrotizing bronchiolitis together with bronchiolitis obliterans has been described,[264,267] as well as interstitial fibrosis, mild interstitial inflammation, and peribronchiolar fibrosis.[268]

A lymphocytic bronchitis/bronchiolitis is commonly (87 percent) present at autopsy in patients following bone marrow transplantation, together with bronchial epithelial necrosis and occasional submucosal gland necrosis. The airway lesions are more obvious in patients with severe graft versus host disease.[269]

Heart-Lung Transplantation

Airway disease is now recognized as a serious complication in patients undergoing heart-lung transplantation and was the major cause of death in 5 of 16 patients surviving beyond the postoperative period. The patients had recurrent bronchopulmonary infections and developed dyspnea and air flow obstruction 6 months to 2 years post-transplantation. Radiologically, peribronchial and interstitial infiltrates were seen.[270] Morphologically, there was widespread bronchiolitis obliterans and mucus plugging. Extensive bronchiectasis was present in two of the five cases. Pleural scars, patchy interstitial fibrosis, and accelerated arterial and venous arteriosclerosis also occurred.[271]

The cause is unknown, but there is no shortage of possibilities. These include repeated bronchopulmonary infection, bronchial artery ligation, mucociliary defect, cyclosporine and other drugs, and aspiration due to loss of the cough reflex. This lesion does not seem to occur in unilateral lung transplant recipients.

Follicular Bronchitis/Bronchiolitis

In Yousem et al.'s review of a large series of surgical lung biopsies, 19 biopsies were encountered that showed lymphoid follicles with coalescent germinal centers adjacent to small bronchi and/or bronchioles in the absence of evidence of bronchiectasis or CAO.[272]

These authors classified their patients into three groups: (1) autoimmune (seven patients, of whom six had rheumatoid arthritis and the seventh had unclassifiable collagen-vascular disease); (2) immunodeficient (four patients showing immunodeficiency of varying sorts); (3) hypersensitive (eight patients, with adequate information available to determine that seven of the eight had peripheral eosinophilia). The age range was wide—1.5 to 77 years—and two thirds (13 patients) were female. The commonest symptom was progressive dyspnea or dyspnea on exertion, which occurred in 15 patients. Bilateral interstitial infiltrates, reticular or nodular, were seen radiographically. In general, patients under the age of 30 years had progressive disease.

Respiratory Bronchiolitis

Respiratory bronchiolitis—the presence of green-brown pigmented macrophages in the lumina, walls, and adjacent air spaces of respiratory bronchioles—has been a recognized result of cigarette smoking for a number of years. It has been thought to be the precursor of centrilobular emphysema since it occurs in the same region within the acinus (respiratory bronchioles) and the same region within the lungs (upper zones). It has also been shown to be associated with thickening of the walls of respiratory bronchioles, and it is thought to be a cause of mild CAO in smokers.[273]

In 1987 it was suggested by Myers et al. that respiratory bronchiolitis may be a cause of infiltrative lung disease.[274] These authors reported six heavy-smoking young (mean age 36 years) patients, five of whom presented with cough and dyspnea (one was asyptomatic); four of the six had mild restrictive lung disease and diminished diffusing capacity. All had abnormal chest radiographs, five having diffuse fine reticulonodular densities. Evidence of air flow obstruction was minimal. All had the features of respiratory bronchiolitis, as described above, on lung biopsy. Peribronchiolar inflammation extended into adjacent alveolar septa and was associated with patchy type II cell metaplasia. Aggregates of macrophages were also seen in more peripheral air spaces. Mild localized interstitial fibrosis was observed. The main differential diagnosis was with DIP, but this condition differed in the almost selective aggregation of the macrophages in and around respiratory bronchioles. It can also be distinguished from diffuse pulmonary hemorrhage by the fine granularity of the pigment in the macrophages, which stained for iron. Classical "smokers' inclusions" of kaolinite were seen ultrastructurally.

Cryptogenic Bronchiolitis

Some idea of the frequency of unexplained CAO can be obtained from an interesting study by Turton et al. from the Brompton Hospital, London, England.[275] These authors examined the records of 2,094 patients who had an FEV_1 of less than 60 percent of predicted. They excluded any patients with asthma, chronic bronchitis, or emphysema, current smokers and ex-smokers, and patients with specific lung disease, such as lung cancer. Ten patients remained, nine women and one man, with an age range of 27 to 60 years. Five had RA and presumably rheumatoid bronchiolitis, and the others had air flow obstruction of unknown cause but thought to be due to bronchiolitis. The most likely cause is a viral infection, unrecognized at the time.

Spontaneous Pneumothorax in Young Adults

Pneumothorax is the presence of air in the pleural space. It may be traumatic, iatrogenic, or spontaneous. In the last instance either it may complicate known underlying disease such as extensive emphysema or cavitory lung infections (secondary pneumothorax) or the lungs may be thought to have been hitherto normal (primary pneumothorax). About 70 percent of spontaneous pneumothoraces are primary,[276] and they usually occur in young adults. Spontaneous pneumothorax is a reasonably common condition, affecting about 1 in 400 of the population at some time. Typically, a tall young man, while exercising vigorously, experiences sudden pain in the chest followed by dyspnea. A pneumothorax is discovered clinically and confirmed radiologically. Frequently the condition recurs, and the patient may undergo surgery for wedge bullectomy. Spontaneous pneumothorax is classically thought to be due to rupture of paraseptal emphysema into the pleura to form blebs and rupture through the pleura into the pleural space.[247] *Distal acinar emphysema* is the preferable term since it describes the way in which the acinus is involved: the distal parts of the pulmonary acini (alveolar ducts and sacs) are preferentially enlarged and destroyed. It is not as simple as that, however. *Blebs* have a precise definition as collections of air within the pleura; the term is, however, generally used loosely. The classic study is that of Lichter and Glynne,[277] who noted apical cysts, 0.2 to 1 cm in diameter, surmounting fibrotic lung, approximately 2 × 3 cm in dimension. Most of the cysts were emphysematous ones rather than blebs; similarly, the great bulk of cysts were considered emphysematous bullae in another study.[278] The underlying tissue showed varying degrees of fibrosis and air space enlargement and an infiltrate of chronic inflammatory cells. Small arteries showed marked thickening of their walls. In most instances the emphysema cannot be classified; the lesions are best referred to as *air space enlargement and fibrosis*. If a biopsy is done, the specimen usually shows subacute inflammation, characterized by an infiltrate of lymphocytes and eosinophils and cuboidal metaplasia of the pleural mesothelial cells. The tissue eosinophilia, together with the plump mesothelial cells, may superficially mimic the appearance of eosinophilic granuloma.[200] Since the latter frequently manifests as a spontaneous pneumothorax and also often involves younger male subjects, it is important that pathologists be aware of the appearance of the lung in spontaneous pneumothorax.

The scarring and air space enlargement is presumably a sequel to inflammation. The apex of the lung is subjected to the most negative intrapleural pressure, which is greatest in tall subjects and becomes even more negative with exercise. This force presumably precipitates the episode of spontaneous pneumothorax described above.

Central Airway Lesions

Both chronic bronchitis and asthma are important common conditions that may produce diagnostic lesions on bronchial biopsy. However, the diagnosis of neither condition should be made at biopsy, since they are clinically defined and recognized. It is inappropriate to discuss these lesions here, and the reader is referred elsewhere.[247] One lesion of the central airways may be important at biopsy. It is now apparent that ultrastructural alterations of the cilia may be associated with abnormal ciliary motility and result in chronic airway inflammation or bronchiectasis.[279]

Immotile Cilia Syndrome (Ciliary Dyskinesia Syndrome, Kartagener's Syndrome)

Electron microscopic studies have shown that the fine structure of all cilia, irrespective of species or organ, is the same. The axoneme of the cilia consists of an outer ring of nine paired microtubules (doublets) and two centrally situated single microtubules. This arrangement is often referred to as the *9 + 2 configuration*. The doublets are connected to each other by single strands known as *nexin links*. The central tubules are surrounded by a sheath and connected to each doublet by radial spoke links (Fig. 19-28). The A tubules, or the clockwise positioned tubule of the doublets, have two hooked sidearms of dynein, an ATPase protein. These are referred to as *dynein arms* and are thought to link adjacent doublets and to induce a sliding movement between them, rather like the cross bridges that cause sliding between actin and myosin in muscle.

A number of syndromes now appear to be associated with defects in the detailed structure of the tubules or

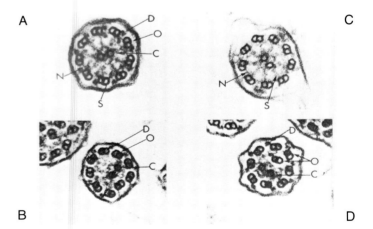

Fig. 19-28. Immotile cilia syndromes. **(A)** Normal cilium. Nine pairs of outer doublets (O) and two single inner tubules are seen (C). Dynein arms (D) are seen on the doublets that are connected to each other by nexin links (N). The central tubules are connected to the doublets by radial spoke links (S). **(B)** In Kartagener's syndrome, dynein arms are absent, but nexin links (N) and radial spokes (S) are seen. **(C)** In radial spoke deficiency, radial spokes are absent, but dynein arms (D) and nexin links can be seen. The central tubules (C) are eccentric. **(D)** A doublet (O) is displaced centrally in a cilium in radial spoke deficiency. (From Sturgess et al.,[283] with permission.)

their interconnections, with consequent ineffective or absent beating of respiratory cilia. The best known is dynein arm deficiency. The abnormalities were first encountered in studies of infertile men who had immotile spermatozoa (which have an identical 9 + 2 structure in their tails). Kartagener's syndrome of bronchiectasis, sinusitis, and situs inversus has been well recognized for years, and affected men are generally sterile.[280] The condition is familial, but the precise genetic abnormality is uncertain. It is now known that absence of the dynein arms of the doublets (Fig. 19-28) is associated with this syndrome.[281] There is loss of mucociliary clearance of the airways, and this predisposes to airway infection and the development of bronchiectasis, which is morphologically identical with the usual "postinfective" bronchiectasis. Why dynein arm deficiency should lead to situs inversus is unclear, but bronchiectasis and sinusitis without situs inversus have been well documented in relatives of patients with Kartagener's syndrome. At this time it is appropriate to refer to patients with the complete triad, together with dynein arm deficiency, as having Kartagener's syndrome, and patients without situs inversus as having dynein arm deficiency. In addition, it has long been known that bronchiectasis is unusually common in Polynesians, specifically Maoris in New Zealand and Samoan Islanders. It was shown in 1978 that dynein arm deficiency is characteristic of these subjects, although situs inversus is very uncommon in them.[282]

Since then many other abnormalities of the axoneme have been shown to be associated with the immotile cilia syndrome. In general, the clinical features are similar to the above because of defective or absent ciliary beat. These include absence of the radial spoke between the central tubules and outer doublets[283] (Fig. 19-28), selective absence of the spoke heads,[284] or selective absence of inner and outer dynein arms.[284] Complex abnormalities have also been reported. These include combined absence of the inner dynein arm and spoke head[285]; absence of the entire axoneme[286,287]; and microtubular transposition, in which the two central microtubules are absent and one of the peripheral doublets crosses to the center of the lower third of the axoneme to take a central position.[288] Secondary ciliary changes may be seen ultrastructurally in affected patients. Normally, the planes of the central singlet tubules are parallel and the basal feet project from the basal bodies in the same direction. In the immotile ciliary syndrome, orderly orientation may be lost.[289] Some patients have cilia with supernumerary microtubules. When the primary defect involves radial spokes, there is loss of the regular spacing of the peripheral doublets from the central pair.[289]

A variety of nonspecific abnormalities may be seen in the cilia of human tracheobronchial epithelium; these are primarily due to cigarette smoking. Mucociliary clear-

ance is often impaired in such subjects, and therefore they may be thought of as having acquired, rather than congenital, airway ciliary dysfunction.

Screening can be carried out by light microscopic examination of the motility of living ciliated cells. Nasal biopsy not infrequently fails to provide ciliated cells, but an adequate sample for light microscopy and electron microscopy can be obtained from the inferior turbinate with a curet or bronchial brush.[290] Adding 0.1 percent tannic acid to the fixative for electron microscopy improves the visualization of the axoneme. A sufficient number of properly oriented cilia should be examined to determine that a consistent abnormality is seen in the great majority, if not all, of the cilia. Some abnormal cilia are found in normals, and more are found in those with bronchial disease. The abnormalities include compound cilia, abnormalities of microtubules, especially the central pair, and minor loss of dynein arms. Only a few cilia are affected as compared with the consistent changes in the immotile cilia syndrome.

PULMONARY VASCULAR SYSTEM
Pulmonary Arterial Hypertension

Cases of pulmonary hypertension can be divided according to cause: precapillary, capillary, and postcapillary. Precapillary hypertension may be caused by increased flow or by increased resistance; usually the alveolar walls are normal or nearly so. Capillary hypertension is associated with destruction of alveoli or distortion of the alveolar capillary bed, such as may occur in emphysema or pulmonary fibrosis. Postcapillary hypertension is associated with passive congestion of alveolar parenchyma.

Precapillary Pulmonary Hypertension

With the advent of cardiovascular surgery, much attention was paid to the morphologic changes in the pulmonary arterial tree in patients with congenital heart disease, and biopsy has been used for prognostic purposes.[4] Heath and Edwards[291] described six grades of structural changes in pulmonary arteries. Grade 1 is seen in patients with congenital heart disease and pulmonary hypertension from birth, and represents retention of the fetal pulmonary vessel morphology. The muscular media of small arteries and arterioles is thickened to up to 25 percent of the vessel diameter, but there is no intimal fibrosis. Grade 2 is seen in vessels less than 300 μm in diameter and is characterized by intimal proliferation. In grade 3 the proliferative intimal changes extend into the medium-sized vessels from 300 to 500 μm in diameter, and in this grade the limit of medial hypertrophy is reached, with medial thickness being up to 30 percent of wall diameter. Although hypertrophy is the rule, it is at this stage that dilatation is first noted, with thinning of the media near an area of occlusion. Dilatation lesions are the hallmark of grades 4 to 6. There are four types of dilatation lesions: plexiform, vein-like branches, angiomatoid lesions, and cavernous lesions. The plexiform lesion is composed of a small muscular artery, which is greatly distended. Leaving this sac-like structure are thin-walled channels, which form alveolar wall capillaries. Thrombotic material is usually present in the sac, with a proximal mass of anastomosing cords of proliferating endothelium, giving the lesion its name. Vein-like branches are large, thin-walled vessels, which arise from a hypertrophied and fibrotic muscular artery. The angiomatoid lesion is composed of thin-walled vessels emanating from a muscular artery. These vessels themselves contain intraluminal vascular formations with walls of elastic tissue. The intraluminal vessels leave their parent vessel and form a mass around it, giving rise to other thin-walled vessels supplying the alveolar capillaries. The cavernous lesion appears to be intermediate between the vein-like branches and the angiomatoid lesion. In addition to dilatation lesions, grade 5 displays hemosiderosis. Grade 6 lesions are uncommon and are characterized by necrotizing arteritis.

Recently, attention has focused on the management of congenital heart disease by lung biopsy. Using a different technique of assessing changes in the pulmonary vasculature, Reid and her colleagues[4] have shown that peripheral extension of muscle, that is, extension of muscle into small arteries previously free of muscle, was characteristic of high flow states. Workers from her laboratory have suggested a different grading system in children less than 2 years of age.[292] Diameter and thickness of arterial walls, peripheral extension of muscle, and the alveolar/arterial ratio are assessed, and three grades of disease—A, B, and C—are proposed. In grade A there is peripheral extension of vascular smooth muscle into the acinus. This is the earliest stage and is associated with increased pulmonary blood flow but not with pulmonary hypertension. Grade B is characterized by increased medial thickness, thus corresponding to Heath and Edwards' grade I. More severe degrees of this grade are usually associated with pulmonary hypertension. There also may be an associated decrease in size of the intra-acinar pulmonary arteries. In grade C, in addition to the changes of grades A and B, there is a reduction in the arterial/alveolar ratio. This grade is associated with marked pulmonary hypertension and is usually accompanied by grade III changes of Heath and Edwards. The changes of the A, B, and C grading system are uniform through the lung, except for the lingula.[293] This system of grading has not been widely accepted, and it also appears that grade C changes have little predictive value and may be reversible.[294] In gen-

eral, the Heath-Edwards system may still be the best estimate of reversibility. Medial hypertrophy regresses readily, as do cellular intimal proliferation and the early stages of concentric laminar intimal fibrosis. However, severe intimal laminar fibrosis does not reverse, and dilatation lesions and fibrinoid necrosis are ominous findings.[295]

Blockage to pulmonary blood flow at the precapillary level can be due to emboli of all kinds, but is most often the result of *multiple recurrent pulmonary emboli*. The clinical signs and symptoms depend on the size, number, and location of the emboli; the time interval between embolic episodes; whether vessel occlusion is complete or partial; and the presence or absence of cardiopulmonary disease. Symptomatology may thus range from complete absence to cardiac arrhythmias, hypotension, and sudden death. Pulmonary hypertension is not sustained until 50 to 70 percent of the pulmonary vascular bed is occluded. The obstruction to flow in thromboembolic disease is found to involve muscular arteries rather than the elastic arteries. Although widespread, the lesions are focal in nature and vary in age.[296] Thus, one may find early thrombi, organized and recanalized vessels, or fibrous bands and intimal plaques marking the site of an embolic episode.

The clinical features of *primary pulmonary hypertension* (*plexogenic pulmonary arteriopathy*) are well documented.[297–299] There is a striking female predominance, except under the age of 12, where sex incidence appears equal. Patients are young, the median age at death being 34 years.[300] Cardiac catheterization reveals pulmonary hypertension in the face of a normal wedge pressure. Dyspnea is characteristic and is associated with anginal pains and signs of congestive heart failure. Hemoptysis, syncope, and palpitations are less frequent. The electrocardiogram shows evidence of right ventricular hypertrophy. Enlargement of the main pulmonary artery branches with ischemia of the peripheral fields is seen radiologically. The latter is confirmed on angiography with demonstration of vascular "pruning."

By definition, primary pulmonary hypertension is of unknown etiology. Many factors may thus play a part in this disease, and many diagnoses must be excluded. Wagenvoort and Wagenvoort[301] studied 156 patients with the diagnosis of primary hypertension and were able to exclude 46 cases on the basis of other histologically recognizable diagnoses. Drugs, including Aminorex[302] and Crotalaria,[303] have been identified either epidemiologically or by experimental evidence as causing pulmonary hypertension. Studies have suggested that an inherited trait plays a major role in primary pulmonary hypertension,[304] while others have implicated the immune system.[300] The possibility of unrecognized pulmonary emboli producing the hypertension has been a vexing problem, particularly since thrombi are often seen in the vessels. Inglesby and co-workers[305] found abnormally elevated antiplasmin levels in 7 of 10 members of a four-generation kindred. They suggested that the pulmonary hypertension was related to inability to lyse undocumented microemboli.

The distinction between multiple recurrent pulmonary emboli and primary pulmonary hypertension may be difficult and only made at autopsy. Recent evidence suggests that the differentiation can be made at lung biopsy. In primary pulmonary hypertension, there is a decrease in the number of arteries less than 40 μm in dimension, whereas this does not occur in multiple recurrent pulmonary emboli. In both conditions there is thickening of the media of the pulmonary arteries, but there is no muscularization of nonmuscular arteries in primary pulmonary hypertension.[4] Other features include the occurrence of concentric laminar intimal fibrosis, which is thought to be specific for primary pulmonary hypertension.[295] Eccentric intimal fibrosis is not specific for multiple recurrent pulmonary emboli, but organizing thromboemboli are highly suggestive, and intravascular fibrous septa (webs) are diagnostic.

Postcapillary Pulmonary Hypertension

Pulmonary venoocclusive disease typically affects individuals between 15 and 20 years of age, and the symptoms often date from an influenza-like illness.[306] The clinical presentation is very similar to that of primary pulmonary hypertension, with progressive dyspnea and development of pulmonary hypertension and cor pulmonale. Radiographically, the lung parenchyma is abnormal, with evidence of chronic passive congestion, notably the presence of edematous interlobular septa (Kerley B lines). Interestingly, the venous pressure, as assessed by the pulmonary wedge pressure, is often normal. Histologically, the parenchymal abnormalities are often more obvious than the venous change. There is hemosiderosis with alveolar wall thickening, and quite considerable interstitial fibrosis may occur. The alveolar capillaries are congested, and the process is often strikingly focal. Curious granulomas may be present, in which fragmented elastic fibers are encrusted with iron and calcium and engulfed by giant cells. Elastic fibers of both alveolar walls and blood vessels are involved. The small pulmonary veins show varying degrees of intimal proliferation. In some instances the occlusion is total; in others there is partial recanalization; and in yet others there is eccentric proliferation of fibrous tissue. The lesions are generally old in appearance. As indicated, venous changes may not be very obvious especially in H&E-stained sections. Similar fibrous occlusions of the pulmonary arteries are seen in about half of the cases.[307] Since

the patients have severe pulmonary arterial hypertension, there are extensive arterial changes of pulmonary hypertension.[308] The condition should always be suspected when a biopsy specimen shows hemosiderosis in addition to pulmonary fibrosis and/or evidence of pulmonary arterial hypertension.

REFERENCES

1. Kuhn C III: Ciliated and Clara cells. p. 91. In Bouhuys A (ed): Lung Cells in Disease. North Holland, Amsterdam, 1976
2. Breeze RG, Wheeldon EB: The cells in the pulmonary airways. p. 111. In Murray JF (ed): Lung Diseases, State of the Art. American Lung Association, New York, 1976–1977
3. Kuhn C III: Ultrastructure and cellular function in the distal lung. p. 1. In Thurlbeck WM, Abel MR (eds): The Lung. Structure, Function and Disease, Williams & Wilkins, Baltimore, 1978
4. Reid LM: The pulmonary circulation: Remodeling in growth and disease. The 1978 J. Burns Amberson lecture. Am Rev Respir Dis 119:531, 1979
5. Kuhn C III: Normal anatomy and histology. Ch. 2. Thurlbeck WM (ed): In Pathology of the Lung. Thieme International, New York, 1988
6. Gail DB, Lenfant CJM: Cells of the Lung: Biology and clinical implications. Am Rev Respir Dis 128:366, 1983
7. Gould VE, Linnoila RI, Memoli VA, Warren WH: Neuroendocrine components of the broncho pulmonary tract; hyperplasias, dysplasias and neoplasms. Lab Invest 49:519, 1983
8. Evans MJ, Sherman MP, Campbell LA, Shami SG: Proliferation of pulmonary alveolar macrophages during postnatal development of rabbit lungs. Am Rev Respir Dis 136:384, 1987
9. Colby TV, Carrington CB: Infiltrative lung disease. In Thurlbeck WM (ed): Pathology of the Lung. Thieme International, New York, 1988
10. Carrington CB, Gaensler EA: Clinical-pathologic approach to diffuse infiltrative lung disease. p. 58. In Thurlbeck WM, Abell MR (eds): The Lung. Structure, Function and Disease. Williams & Wilkins, Baltimore, 1978
11. Basset F, Ferrans V, Soler P et al: Intraluminal fibrosis in interstitial lung disease. Am J Pathol 122:443, 1986
12. Pimentel JC: Tridimensional photographic reconstruction in a study of the pathogenesis of honeycomb lung. Thorax 22:444, 1967
13. Ognibene FP, Shelhamer J, Gill V, et al: The diagnosis of *Pneumocystis carinii* pneumonia in patients with the acquired immunodeficiency syndrome using subsegmental bronchoalveolar lavage. Am Rev Respir Dis 129:929, 1984
14. Clark JG, Crawford SW: Diagnostic approaches to pulmonary complications of marrow transplantation. Chest 91:477, 1987

15. Canham EM, Kennedy TC, Merrick TA: Unexplained pulmonary infiltrates in the compromised patient. Cancer 52:325, 1983
16. Wetstein L: Sensitivity and specificity of lingular segmental biopsies of the lung. Chest 90:383, 1986
17. Miller RR, Nelems B, Muller NL, et al: Lingular and right middle lobe biopsy in the assessment of diffuse lung disease. Ann Thorac Surg 44:269, 1987
18. Wall CP, Gaensler EA, Carrington CB, Hayes JA: Comparison of transbronchial and open biopsies in chronic infiltrative lung diseases. Am Rev Respir Dis 13:280, 1981
19. Bergin CJ, Muller NL: CT in the diagnosis of interstitial lung disease. AJR 145:505, 1985
20. Kapanci Y, Weibel ER, Kaplan HP, et al: Pathogenesis and reversibility of the pulmonary lesions of oxygen toxicity in monkeys. II. Ultrastructural and morphometric studies. Lab Invest 20:101, 1969
21. Smith P, Heath D: The ultrastructure and sequence of the early stages of paraquat lung in rats. J Pathol 114:117, 1974
22. Ryan SF, Loomis-Bell AL Jr, Barrett CR Jr: Experimental acute alveolar injury in the dog. Morphologic-mechanical correlations. Am J Pathol 82:353, 1976
23. Adamson IYR, Bowden DH: The pathogenesis of bleomycin-induced pulmonary fibrosis in mice. Am J Pathol 77:185, 1974
24. Katzenstein AL, Bloor CM, Liebow AA: Diffuse alveolar damage. The role of oxygen, shock and related factors. Am J Pathol 85:209, 1976
25. Lakshminarayan S, Stanford RE, Petty TL: Prognosis after recovery from adult respiratory distress syndrome. Am Rev Respir Dis 113:7, 1976
26. Bachofen A, Weibel ER: Alterations of the gas-exchange apparatus in adult respiratory insufficiency associated with septicemia. Am Rev Respir Dis 116:589, 1977
27. Ashbaugh DG, Bigelow DB, Petty TL, et al: Acute respiratory distress in adults. Lancet 2:319, 1967
28. Murray JF: The adult respiratory distress syndrome (may it rest in peace). Am Rev Respir Dis 111:716, 1975
29. Petty TL, Ashbaugh DG: The adult respiratory distress syndrome: Clinical features, factors influencing prognosis and principles of management. Chest 60:233, 1971
30. Joachim H, Riede UN, Mittenmeyer CH: The weight as a diagnostic criterion (distinction of normal lungs from shock lungs by histologic, morphometric and biochemical investigations). Pathol Res Pract 162:24, 1978
31. Schlag, G, Voight WH, Redl H, Glatzel A: Vergleichende Morphologie des posttraumatischen Lungenversagens. Anaesth Intensivther Notfallmed 15:315, 1980
32. Churg A, Golden J, Fliegel S, Hogg JC: Bronchopulmonary dysplasia in the adult. Am Rev Respir Dis 127:117, 1983
33. Nash G, Blennerhassett JB, Pontoppidan H: Pulmonary lesions associated with oxygen therapy and artificial ventilation. N Engl J Med 276:368, 1967
34. Pratt PC: Pathology of pulmonary oxygen toxicity. Am Rev Respir Dis 110:51, 1974
35. Hogg JC, Katzenstein ALA: Pulmonary edema and diffuse alveolar injury. Ch. 16. In Thurlbeck WM (ed): Pathology of the Lung. Thieme International, New York, 1988
36. Pratt PC: Pathology of adult respiratory distress syndrome. p. 43. In Thurlbeck WM, Abell MR (eds): The Lung, Structure, Function and Disease. Williams & Wilkins, Baltimore, 1978
37. Fletcher K: Paraquat poisoning. p. 86. In Forensic Toxicology. J Wright & Son, Bristol, England, 1974
38. Rose MS, Lock A, Smith IL, et al: Paraquat accumulation: Tissue and species specificity. Biochem Pharmacol 25:419, 1976
39. Anderson CG: Paraquat and the lung. Australas Radiol 14:409, 1970
40. Fairshter RD: Paraquat poisoning: An update. West J Med 128:56, 1978
41. Zavala DC, Rhodes ML: An effect of paraquat on the lungs of rabbits. Its implication in smoking contaminated marihuana. Chest 74:418, 1978
42. Dearden LC, Fairshter RD, McRae DM, et al: Pulmonary ultrastructure of the late aspects of human paraquat poisoning. Am J Pathol 93:667, 1978
43. Rebello G, Mason JK: Pulmonary histological appearances in fatal paraquat poisoning. Histopathology 2:53, 1978
44. Copland GM, Kolin A, Schulman HS: Fatal pulmonary intra-alveolar fibrosis after paraquat ingestion. N Engl J Med 291:290, 1974
45. Thurlbeck WM, Thurlbeck SM: Pulmonary effects of paraquat poisoning. Chest 69(suppl. 2):276, 1976
46. Gillett DG, Ford GT: Drug-induced lung disease. p. 21. In Thurlbeck WM, Abell MR (eds): The Lung. Structure, Function and Disease. Williams & Wilkins, Baltimore, 1978
47. Min KW, Gyorkey F, Gyorkey P: An electron microscopic study of "busulfan lung." Am J Pathol 74:107a, 1974
48. Rosenow EC III: The spectrum of drug-induced pulmonary disease. Ann Intern Med 77:977, 1972
49. Cole P: Drug-induced lung disease. Drugs 13:422, 1977
50. Sovijärv A, Lemola M, Stenius B: Nitrofurantoin-induced acute, subacute and chronic pulmonary reactions. Scand J Respir Dis 58:41, 1977
51. Bone RC, Wolfe J, Sobonya RE, et al: Desquamative interstitial pneumonia following chronic nitrofurantoin therapy. Chest 69(suppl. 2):296, 1976
52. Lundgren R, Bäck O, Wiman LG: Pulmonary lesions and autoimmune reactions after long-term nitrofurantoin treatment. Scand J Respir Dis 56:208, 1975
53. Holoye PY, Luna MA, MacKay B, et al: Bleomycin hypersensitivity pneumonitis. Ann Intern Med 88:47, 1978
54. Samuels ML, Johnson DE, Holoye PY, et al: Large-dose bleomycin therapy and pulmonary toxicity. A possible role of prior radiotherapy. JAMA 235:1117, 1976
55. De Lena M, Guzzon A, Monfardini S, et al: Clinical, radiologic, and histopathologic studies on pulmonary toxicity induced by treatment of bleomycin (NSC-125066). Cancer Chemother Rep 56(pt 1): 343, 1972
56. Blum RH, Carter SK, Agre K: A clinical review of bleomycin—a new antineoplastic agent. Cancer 31:903, 1973

57. Clarysse AM, Cathey WJ, Cartwright GE, et al: Pulmonary disease complicating intermittent therapy with methotrexate. JAMA 209:1861, 1969

58. Kruban Z: Pulmonary changes induced by amphophilic drugs. Environ Health Perspect 16:111, 1976

59. Siegel H: Human pulmonary pathology associated with narcotic and other addictive drugs. Hum Pathol 3:55, 1972

60. Rosenow EC: Drug-induced pulmonary disease. Clin Notes Respir Dis 16:3, 1977

61. Davis PR, Burch RE: Pulmonary edema and salicylate intoxication. Ann Intern Med 80:553, 1974

62. Winterbauer RH, Wilske KR, Wheelis RF: Diffuse pulmonary injury associated with gold treatment. N Engl J Med 294:919, 1976

63. Geddes P, Brostoff J: Letter to editor. N Engl J Med 295:506, 1976

64. Fajardo LF, Berthrong M: Radiation injury in surgical pathology. Pt. 1. Am J Surg Pathol 2:159, 1978

65. Bennett DE, Million PR, Ackerman LV: Bilateral radiation pneumonitis: A complication of the radiotherapy of bronchogenic carcinoma. (A report and analysis of seven cases with autopsy.) Cancer 23:1001, 1969

66. Phillips TL, Wharham MD, Margolis LW: Modification of radiation injury to normal tissues by chemotherapeutic agents. Cancer 35:1678, 1975

67. Castellino RA, Glatstein E, Turbow MM, et al: Latent radiation injury of lungs or heart activated by steroid withdrawal. Ann Intern Med 80:593, 1974

68. White DC: The histopathologic basis for functional decrements in late radiation injury in diverse organs. Cancer 37(suppl. 2):1126, 1976

69. Gross NJ: Pulmonary effects of radiation therapy. Ann Intern Med 86:81, 1977

70. Roswit B, White DC: Severe radiation injuries of the lung. AJR 129:127, 1977

71. Katzenstein ALA, Askin FB: Surgical Pathology of Nonneoplastic Lung Disease. Major Problems in Pathology. Vol. 13. WB Saunders, Philadelphia, 1982, p. 37

72. Kaplan MH, Armstrong, D, Rosen P: Tuberculosis complicating neoplastic disease. A review of 201 cases. Cancer 33:850, 1974

73. Wolinsky E: State of the art: nontuberculous mycobacteria and associated diseases. Am Rev Respir Dis 119:107, 1979

74. Murray JF, Garay SM, Hopewell PC, et al: Pulmonary complications of the acquired immunodeficiency syndrome: An update. Am Rev Respir Dis 135:504, 1987

75. Handwerger S, Mildvan D, Senie R, McKinley FW: Tuberculosis and the acquired immunodeficiency syndrome at a New York City hospital: 1978–1985. Chest 91:176, 1987

76. Winn WC Jr, Myerowitz RL: The pathology of the *Legionella* pneumonias. A review of 74 cases and the literature. Hum Pathol 12:401, 1981

77. Hernandez FJ, Kirby BD, Stanley TM, Edelstein PH: Legionnaires' disease. Postmortem pathologic findings of 20 cases. Am J Clin Pathol 7:488, 1980

78. Hicklin MD, Thomason BM, Chandler FW, Blackman JA: Pathogenesis of acute Legionnaires' disease pneumonia. Immunofluorescent microscopic study. Am J Clin Pathol 73:480, 1980

79. Miller RR: Viral infections of the respiratory tract. In Thurlbeck WM (ed): Pathology of the Lung. Thieme International, New York, 1988

80. Goodwin RA, Des Prez RM: State of the art: Histoplasmosis. Am Rev Respir Dis 117:929, 1978

81. Massachusetts General Hospital, Case Records, 37–1978. N Engl J Med 299:644, 1978

82. Beller TA, Mitchell DM, Sobonya RE, Barbe RA: Large airway obstruction secondary to endobronchial coccidiomycosis. Am Rev Respir Dis 120:939, 1979

83. Massachusetts General Hospital, Case Records, 3–1980. N Engl J Med 302:218, 1980

84. Sarosi GA, Davies SF: Blastomycosis. Am Rev Respir Dis 120:911, 1979

85. Atkinson JB, McCurley TL: Pulmonary blastomycosis: Filamentous forms in an immunocompromised patient with fulminating respiratory failure. Hum Pathol 14:186, 1983

86. England DM, Hochholzer L: Primary pulmonary sporotrichosis. Am J Surg Pathol 9:193, 1985

87. Greenberger PA, Patterson R: Allergic bronchopulmonary aspergillosis. Chest 91:165S, 1987

88. Orr DP, Myerowitz RL, Dubois PJ: Pathoradiologic correlation of invasive pulmonary aspergillosis in the compromised host. Cancer 41:2028, 1978

89. Bigby TD, Serota ML, Tierney LM Jr, Matthay MA: Clinical spectrum of pulmonary mucormycosis. Chest 89:435, 1986

90. Dubois PJ, Myerowitz RL, Allen CM: Pathoradiologic correlation of pulmonary candidiasis in immunosuppressed patients. Cancer 1026, 1977

91. Weber WR, Askin FB, Dehner LP: Lung biopsy in *Pneumocystis carinii* pneumonia: A histopathologic study of typical and atypical features. Am J Clin Pathol 67:11, 1977

92. Grimes MM, LaPook JD, Bar MH et al: Disseminated *Pneumocystis carinii* infection in a patient with acquired immunodeficiency syndrome. Hum Pathol 18:307, 1987

93. Leatherman JW, Davies SF, Hoidal JR: Alveolar hemorrhage syndromes: Diffuse microvascular lung hemorrhage in immune and idiopathic disorders. Medicine (Baltimore) 63:343, 1984

94. Albelda SM, Gefter WB, Epstein DM, Miller WT: Diffuse pulmonary hemorrhage: A review and classification. Radiology 154:289, 1984

95. Miller RR: Diffuse pulmonary hemorrhage. In Thurlbeck WM (ed): Pathology of the Lung. Thieme International, New York, 1988

96. Leatherman JW: Immune alveolar hemorrhage. Chest 91:891, 1987

97. Martinez AJ, Maltby JD, Hurst DJ: Thrombotic thrombocytopenic purpura seen as pulmonary hemorrhage. Arch Intern Med 143:1818, 1983

98. Spragg RG, Wolf PL, Haghighi P, et al: Angiosarcoma of the lung with fatal pulmonary hemorrhage. Am J Med 74:1072, 1983

99. Carrington CB, Addington WW, Goff AM, et al: Chronic eosinophilic pneumonia. N Engl J Med 280:788, 1969

100. Kahn FW, Jones JM, England DM: Diagnosis of pulmonary hemorrhage in the immunocompromised host. Am Rev Respir Dis 136:155, 1987

101. Cordonnier C, Bernaudin JF, Bierling P, et al: Pulmonary complications occurring after allogeneic bone marrow transplantation: A study of 130 consecutive transplanted patients. Cancer 58:1047, 1986

102. Nash G, Fligiel S: Kaposi's sarcoma presenting as pulmonary disease in the acquired immune deficiency syndrome. Hum Pathol 15:999, 1984

103. Smith LJ, Katzenstein ALA: Pathogenesis of massive pulmonary hemorrhage in acute leukemia. Arch Intern Med 142:2149, 1982

104. Hamman L, Rich AR: Acute diffuse interstitial fibrosis of the lungs. Bull Johns Hopkins Hosp 74:177, 1944

105. Crystal R, Fulmer JD, Roberts WC, et al: Idiopathic pulmonary fibrosis. Clinical histologic, radiographic, physiologic, scintigraphic, cytologic and biochemical aspects. Ann Intern Med 85:769, 1976

106. Stack BHR, Choo-Kang YF, Heard BE: The prognosis of cryptogenic fibrosing alveolitis. Thorax 27:535, 1972

107. Genereux GP: The end-stage lung: Pathogenesis, pathology, and radiology. Radiology 116:279, 1975

108. Muller N, Miller RR, Webb WR, et al: Fibrosing alveolitis: CT–pathologic correlation. Radiology 160:585, 1986

109. Turner-Warwick M, Haslam P, Weeks J: Antibodies in some chronic fibrosing lung diseases: II. Immunofluorescent studies. Clin Allergy 1:209, 1971

110. Mason AMS, McIllmurray MB, Golding PL, et al: Fibrosing alveolitis associated with renal tubular acidosis. Br Med J 4:596, 1970

111. Zalin AM, Weeple J, Gumpel M: Fibrosing alveolitis and renal tubular acidosis. Br Med J 4:804, 1970

112. Smith MJL, Benson MK, Strickland ID: Coeliac disease and diffuse interstitial lung disease. Lancet 1:473, 1971

113. Dreisin RB, Schwarz MI, Theophilopoulos AN, et al: Circulating immune complexes in the idiopathic interstitial pneumonia. N Engl J Med 298:353, 1978

114. Reynolds HY, Di Sant'Agnese PA, Zierdt CH: Analysis of cellular and protein content of broncho-alveolar lavage fluid from patients with idiopathic pulmonary fibrosis and chronic hypersensitivity pneumonitis. J Clin Invest 59:165, 1977

115. Kravis TC, Ahmed A, Brown TE, et al: Pathogenic mechanisms in pulmonary fibrosis: Collagen-induced migration inhibition factor production and cytotoxicity mediated by lymphocytes. J Clin Invest 58:1223, 1976

116. Donohue WL, Laski B, Uchida I, et al: Familial fibrocystic pulmonary dysplasia and its relation to the Hamman-Rich syndrome. Pediatrics 24:786, 1959

117. Solliday NH, Williams JA, Gaensler EA, et al: Familial chronic interstitial pneumonia. Am Rev Respir Dis 108:193, 1973

118. Fulmer JD, Crystal RG: The biochemical basis of pulmonary function. p. 419. In Crystal RG (ed): The Biochemical Basis of Pulmonary Function. Marcel Dekker, New York, 1976

119. Ostrow D, Cherniack RM: Resistance to airflow in patients with diffuse interstitial lung disease. Am Rev Respir Dis 108:205, 1973

120. Liebow AA, Steer A, Billingsley JG: Desquamative interstitial pneumonia. Am J Med 39:369, 1965

121. Farr GH, Harley RA, Hennigar GR: Desquamative interstitial pneumonia. An electron microscopic study. Am J Pathol 60:347, 1970

122. Tubbs RR, Benjamin SP, Osborne DG, et al: Surface and transmission ultrastructural characteristics of desquamative interstitial pneumonia. Hum Pathol 9:693, 1978

123. Gardiner IT, Uff JS: "Blue bodies" in a case of cryptogenic fibrosing alveolitis (desquamative type)—an ultrastructural study. Thorax 33:806, 1978

124. Spencer H: Pathology of the Lung. Vols. 1, 2. Text Ed. WB Saunders, Philadelphia, 1977

125. Gupta RK, Schuster RA, Christian WD: Autopsy findings in a unique case of malacoplakia. A cytoimmunohistochemical study of Michaelis-Guttman bodies. Arch Pathol 93:42, 1972

126. Corrin B, Price AB: Electron microscopic studies in desquamative interstitial pneumonia associated with asbestos. Thorax 27:324, 1972

127. Coates EO, Watson JHL: Diffuse interstitial lung disease in tungsten carbide workers. Ann Intern Med 75:709, 1971

128. McCann BG, Brewer DB: A case of desquamative interstitial pneumonia progressing to "honeycomb lung." J Pathol 112:119, 1974

129. Patchefsky AS, Israel HL, Hoch G, et al: Desquamative interstitial pneumonia: Relationship to interstitial fibrosis. Thorax 28:680, 1973

130. Carrington C, Gaensler EA, Coutu RE, et al: Natural history and treated course of usual and desquamative interstitial pneumonia. N Engl J Med 298:801, 1978

131. Gibbs AR, Seal RME: Primary lymphoproliferative conditions of the lung. Thorax 33:140, 1978

132. Liebow AA, Carrington CB: The interstitial pneumonias. p. 109. In Simon M, Potchen EJ, LeMay M (eds): Frontiers of Pulmonary Radiology. Pathophysiologic, Roentgenographic and Radioisotopic Considerations. Grune & Stratton, Orlando, FL, 1969

133. Liebow AA, Carrington CB: Diffuse pulmonary lymphoreticular infiltrations associated with dysproteinaemia. Med Clin North Am 57:809, 1973

134. Strimlan CV, Rosenow EC III, Weiland LH, et al: Lymphocytic interstitial pneumonitis. Review of 13 cases. Ann Intern Med 88:616, 1978

135. Saltzstein SL: Pulmonary malignant lymphomas and pseudolymphomas. Classification, therapy, and prognosis. Cancer 16:928, 1963

136. Colby TV, Carrington CB: Lymphoreticular tumors and infiltrates of the lung. In Sommers S (ed): Pathology Annual 1983. (Part I). Appleton & Lange, East Norwalk, CT, 1983

137. Anderson LG, Talal N: The spectrum of benign and malignant lymphoproliferation in Sjögren's syndrome. Clin Exp Immunol 9:199, 1972

138. Weisbrodt IM: Lymphomatoid granulomatosis of the lung, associated with a long history of benign lymphoepithelial lesions of the salivary glands and lymphoid

interstitial pneumonitis. Report of a case. Am J Clin Pathol 66:792, 1976

139. Joshi VV, Oleske JM, Minnefor AB, et al: Pathologic pulmonary findings in children with the acquired immunodeficiency syndrome. Hum Pathol 16:241, 1985

140. Joshi VV, Oleske JM: Pulmonary lesions in children with the acquired immunodeficiency syndrome: A reappraisal based on data in additional cases and follow-up study of previously reported cases. Hum Pathol 17:641, 1986

141. Solal-Celigny P, Coudere LJ, Herman D, et al: Lymphoid interstitial pneumonitis in acquired immunodeficiency syndrome-related complex. Am Rev Respir Dis 131:956, 1985

142. Grieco MH, Chinoy-Acharya P: Lymphoid interstitial pneumonia associated with the acquired immune deficiency syndrome. Am Rev Respir Dis 131:952, 1985

143. Israel HL, Pachefsky AS, Saldana MJ: Wegener's granulomatosis, lymphomatoid granulomatosis and benign lymphocytic angiitis and granulomatosis. Ann Intern Med 87:691, 1977

144. Sokolowski JW, Cordray DR, Cantow EF, et al: Giant cell interstitial pneumonia. A report of a case. Am Rev Respir Dis 105:417, 1972

145. Reid LM: Reduction in bronchial subdivisions in bronchiectasis. Thorax 5:233, 1950

146. Gosink BB, Friedman PJ, Liebow AA: Bronchiolitis obliterans. Roentgenologic-pathologic correlation. AJR 117:816, 1973

147. Epler GR, Colby TV, McLoud TC, et al: Bronchiolitis obliterans organizing pneumonia. N Engl J Med 312:152, 1985

148. Davidson AG, Heard BE, McAllister WC, Turner-Warwick MEH: Cryptogenic organizing pneumonitis. Q J Med 52 (new series): 382, 1983

149. Guerry-Force ML, Muller NL, Wright JL, et al: A comparison of bronchiolitis obliterans with organizing pneumonia, usual interstitial pneumonia and small airways disease. Am Rev Respir Dis 135:705, 1987

150. Katzenstein ALA, Myers JL, Prophet WD, et al: Bronchiolitis obliterans and usual interstitial pneumonia. A comparative clinicopathologic study. Am J Surg Pathol 10:373, 1986

151. Muller NL, Guerry-Force ML, Staples CA, et al: Differential diagnosis of bronchiolitis obliterans with organizing pneumonia. Clinical, functional and radiologic findings. Radiology 162:151, 1987

152. Webb WR, Goodman PC: Fibrosing alveolitis in patients with neurofibromatosis. Radiology 122:189, 1977

153. Massaro D, Katz S, Matthews MJ, et al: Von Recklinghausen's neurofibromatosis associated with cystic lung disease. Am J Med 38:233, 1965

154. Hammar SP, Winterbauer RH, Bockus D, et al: Endothelial cell damage and tubuloreticular structures in interstitial lung disease associated with collagen vascular disease and viral pneumonia. Am Rev Respir Dis 127:77, 1983

155. Hunninghake GW, Fauci AS: Pulmonary involvement in the collagen vascular diseases. Am Rev Respir Dis 119:471, 1979

156. Walker WC, Wright V: Pulmonary lesions and rheumatoid arthritis. Medicine (Baltimore) 47:501, 1968

157. Walker WG, Wright V: Rheumatoid pleuritis. Ann Rheum Dis 26:467, 1967

158. Yousem SA, Colby TV, Carrington CB: Lung biopsy in rheumatoid arthritis. Am Rev Respir Dis 131:770, 1985

159. Portner MM, Gracie WA: Rheumatoid lung disease with cavitary nodules, pneumothorax, and eosinophilia. N Engl J Med 275:697, 1966

160. Frank ST, Weg JG, Harkleroad LE, et al: Pulmonary dysfunction in rheumatoid disease. Chest 63:27, 1973

161. Laitinen O, Nissilä M, Salorinne Y, et al: Pulmonary involvement in patients with rheumatoid arthritis. Scand J Respir Dis 56:297, 1975

162. Rosenow EC, Strimlan CV, Muhm JR, et al: Pleuropulmonary manifestations of ankylosing spondylitis. Mayo Clinic Proc 52:641, 1977

163. Wiener-Kronish JP, Solinger AM, Warnock ML, et al: Severe pulmonary involvement in mixed connective tissue disease. Am Rev Respir Dis 124:499, 1981

164. Slavin RE, deGroot WJ: Pathology of the lung in Bechet's disease. Am J Surg Pathol 5:779, 1981

165. Hunninghake GW: Staging of pulmonary sarcoidosis. Chest 89:178S, 1986

166. Thomas PD, Hunninghake GW: Current concepts of the pathogenesis of sarcoidosis. Am Rev Respir Dis 135:747, 1987

167. Abdi EA, Nguyen GK, Ludwig RN, Dickout WJ: Pulmonary sarcoidosis following interferon therapy for advanced renal cell carcinoma. Cancer 59:896, 1987

168. Daniele RP, Rossman MD, Kern JA, Elias JA: Pathogenesis of sarcoidosis. Chest 89:174S, 1986

169. Wilen SB, Rabinowitz JG, Ulreich S, Lyons HA: Pleural involvement in sarcoidosis. Am J Med 57:200, 1974

170. Liebow AA: Pulmonary angiitis and granulomatosis. The J. Burns Amberson Lecture. Am Rev Respir Dis 108: 1, 1973

171. Koss MN, Hochholzer L, Feigin DS, et al: Necrotizing sarcoid-like granulomatosis: Clinical, pathologic and immunopathologic findings. Hum Pathol 11(S):510, 1980

172. Singh N, Cole S, Krause PJ, et al: Necrotizing sarcoid granulomatosis with extrapulmonary involvement. Am Rev Respir Dis 124:189, 1981

173. Leavitt RY, Fauci AS: Pulmonary vasculitis. Am Rev Respir Dis 134:149, 1986

174. Salvaggio JE, Karr RM: Hypersensitivity pneumonitis: State of the art. Chest 75:(suppl 2):270, 1979

175. Pepys J, Jenkins PA: Precipitin (FLH) test in farmer's lung. Thorax 20:21, 1965

176. Reyes CN, Wenzel FJ, Lawton BR, Emanuel DA: Pulmonary pathology in farmers' lung. Chest 81:142, 1982

177. Kawanami O, Basset F, Barrios R, et al: Hypersensitivity pneumonitis in man: Light and electron microscopic studies of 18 lung biopsies. Am J Pathol 110:275, 1983

178. Barrowcliff DF, Arblaster PG: Farmer's lung. A study of an early acute fatal case. Thorax 23:490, 1968

179. Moore VL, Fink JN, Barboriak JJ, et al: Immunologic events in pigeon breeders' disease. J Allergy Clin Immuol 53:319, 1974

180. Fink JN, Banaszak EF, Thiede WH, et al: Interstitial pneumonitis due to hypersensitivity to an organism contaminating a heating system. Ann Intern Med 74:80, 1971

181. Mahon WE, Scott DJ, Ansell G, et al: Hypersensitivity to pituitary snuff with miliary shadowing in the lungs. Thorax 22:13, 1967

182. Emanuel DA, Lawton BR, Wenzel FJ: Maple-bark disease. Pneumonitis due to *Coniosporium corticale*. N Engl J Med 26:333, 1962

183. Pimentel JC, Avila R: Respiratory disease in cork workers ("suberosis"). Thorax 28:409, 1973

184. Cohen HL, Merigan TC, Kosek JC, et al: A granulomatous pneumonitis associated with redwood sawdust inhalation. Am J Med 43:785, 1967

185. Grant IW, Blackadder ES, Greenberg M, et al: Extrinsic allergic alveolitis in Scottish maltworkers. Br Med J 1:490, 1976

186. Bergmann M, Flance IJ, Kurz PT, et al: Thesaurosis due to inhalation of hair spray. Report of twelve new cases, including three autopsies. N Engl J Med 266:750, 1962

187. Gowdy JM, Wagstaff MJ: Pulmonary infiltration due to aerosol thesaurosis. A survey of hairdressers. Arch Environ Health 25:101, 1972

188. Salvaggio J, Arquembourg GP, Seabury J, et al: Bagassosis. IV. Precipitins against extracts of thermophilic actinomycetes in patients with bagassosis. JAMA 46:538, 1969

189. Nicholls PJ, Nicholls GR, Bouhuys A: p. 93. In Davies CN (ed): Inhaled Particles and Vapors. 2nd Ed. Pergamon Press, Oxford, 1964

190. Ruttner JR, Spycher MA, Engeler MR: Pulmonary fibrosis induced by cotton fibre inhalation. Pathol Microbiol 32:1, 1968

191. Basset F, Soler P, Wyllie L, et al: Langerhans' cells and lung interstitium. Ann NY Acad Sci 278:499, 1976

192. Webber D, et al: S-100 staining in the diagnosis of eosinophilic granuloma of the lung. Am J Clin Pathol 84:447, 1985

193. Lewis JG: Eosinophilic granuloma and its variants with special reference to lung involvement. A report of twelve patients. Quart J Med 33:337, 1964

194. Colby TV, Lombard C: Histiocytosis X presenting in the lung. Hum Pathol 14:847, 1983

195. Basset F, Corrin B, Spencer H, et al: Pulmonary histiocytosis "X". Am Rev Respir Dis 188:811, 1978

196. Brody AR, Kanich RE, Graham WG, et al: Cyst wall formation in pulmonary eosinophilic granuloma. Chest 66:576, 1974

197. Hammar SP, Winterbauer R, Bockus D: Diagnosis of pulmonary eosinophilic granuloma by ultrastructural examination of sputum (letter). Arch Pathol Lab Med 102:606, 1978

198. Kawanami O, et al: Pulmonary Langerhans' cells in patients with fibrotic lung disorders. Lab Invest 44:227, 1981

199. Hammar S, Bockus D, Remington F: Metastatic tumor of unknown origin. Ultrastruct Pathol 10:281, 1986

200. Askin FB, McCann BG, Kuhn C: Reactive eosinophilic pleuritis: A lesion to be distinguished from pulmonary eosinophilic granuloma. Arch Pathol Lab Med 101:187, 1977

201. Corrin B, Liebow AA, Friedman PJ: Pulmonary lymphangiomyomatosis. Am J Pathol 79:348, 1975

202. Brentani MM, Carvalho RR, Saldiva PH, et al: Steroid receptors in pulmonary lymphangiomyomatosis. Chest 85:96, 1984

203. Graham ML, Spelsberg TC, Dines DE, et al: Pulmonary lymphangiomyomatosis; with particular reference to steroid-receptor assay studies and pathologic correlation. Mayo Clin Proc 59:3, 1984

204. Svendsen TL, Viskym K, Hansborg N, et al: Pulmonary lymphangiomyomatosis: A case of progesterone receptor positive lymphangiomyomatosis treated with medroxyprogesterone, oophorectomy and tamoxifen. Br J Dis Chest 78:264, 1984

205. Kapanci Y, Costabella PM, Gabbiani G: Location and function of contractile interstitial cells of the lungs. p. 69. In Bouhuys A (ed): Lung Cells in Disease. North Holland, Amsterdam, 1976

206. Kane PB, Lane BP, Cordice JWV, et al: Ultrastructure of the proliferating cells in pulmonary lymphangiomyomatosis. Arch Pathol Lab Med 102:618, 1978

207. Carrington CB, Addington WW, Goff AM, et al: Chronic eosinophilic pneumonia. N Engl J Med 289:787, 1969

208. Liebow AA, Carrington CH: The eosinophilic pneumonias. Medicine (Baltimore) 48:251, 1969

209. Gaensler EA, Carrington CB: Peripheral opacities in chronic eosinophilic pneumonia. The photographic negative of pulmonary edema. AJR 128:1, 1977

210. Cooney TP: Inter-relationship of chronic eosinophilic pneumonia, bronchiolitis obliterans and rheumatoid disease: A hypothesis. J Clin Pathol 34:129, 1981

211. Singh G, Katyal SL, Bedrossian CWM, Rogers RM: Pulmonary alveolar proteinosis; staining for surfactant apoprotein in alveolar proteinosis and in conditions simulating it. Chest 83:82, 1983

212. Miller RR, Churg AM, Hutcheon M, Lam S: Pulmonary alveolar proteinosis and aluminum dust exposure. Am Rev Respir Dis 130:312, 1984

213. Bedrossian CWM, Luna MA, Conklin RH, Hiller WC: Alveolar proteinosis as a consequence of immuno suppression. Hum Pathol 11(S):527, 1980

214. Davidson JM, MacLeod WM: Pulmonary alveolar proteinosis. Br J Dis Chest 63:13, 1969

215. Green D, Dighe P, Ali NO, Katele GV: Pulmonary alveolar proteinosis complicating chronic myelogenous leukemia. Cancer 46:1763, 1980

216. Gonzales-Roth RJ, Harris JO: Pulmonary alveolar proteinosis. Further evaluation of abnormal alveolar macrophages. Chest 90:656, 1986

217. Martin RJ, Coalson JJ, Rogers RM, et al: Pulmonary alveolar proteinosis: The diagnosis by segmental lavage. Am Rev Respir Dis 121:819, 1980

218. Ravines HT: Pulmonary alveolar microlithiasis: Report of nine cases with a familial incidence in seven of the nine cases among three families. Am J Clin Pathol 52:767a, 1969

219. Prakash UBS, Barham SS, Rosenow EC, et al: Pulmonary alveolar microlithiasis. Mayo Clin Proc 58:290, 1983

220. Caffrey PR, Altman RS: Pulmonary alveolar microlithiasis occurring in premature twins. J Pediatr 66:758, 1965

221. Sears MR, Change AR, Taylor AJ: Pulmonary alveolar microlithiasis. Thorax 26:704, 1971

222. Fuleihan FJD, Abboud RT, Balikian JP, et al: Pulmonary alveolar microlithiasis: Lung function in five cases. Thorax 24:84, 1969

223. Sosman MC, Dodd GD, Jones WD, et al: The familial occurrence of pulmonary alveolar microlithiasis. AJR 77:947, 1957

224. Heitzman ER: The Lung: Radiologic-Pathologic Correlations. 2nd Ed. CV Mosby, St. Louis, 1984, pp. 413–421

225. Munk PL, Muller NL, Miller RR, Ostrow DN: Pulmonary lymphangitic carcinomatosis: CT and pathologic findings. Radiology 166:705, 1988

226. Janower ML, Blennerhassett JB: Lymphangitic spread of metastatic cancer to the lung. A radiologic-pathologic classification. Radiology 101:267, 1971

227. Stein MG, Mayo J, Muller NL, et al: Pulmonary lymphangitic spread of carcinoma: Appearance on CT scans. Radiology 162:371, 1987

228. Becklake M: Asbestos-related diseases of the lung and other organs: Their epidemiology and implications for clinical practice. Am Rev Respir Dis 114:187, 1976

229. Gaensler EA: Pathological, physiological and radiological correlations in the pneumoconioses. Ann NY Acad Sci 200:574, 1972

230. Churg A, Green FHY (eds): Pathology of Occupational Lung Disease. Igaku-Shoin, New York, 1987

231. Parkes WR: Occupational Lung Disorders. London, Butterworth, 1974

232. Morgan WKC, Seaton A: Occupational Lung Diseases, 2nd Ed. WB Saunders, Philadelphia, 1984

233. Heppleston AG: Environmental lung disease. In Thurlbeck WM (ed): Pathology of the Lung. Thieme International, New York, 1988

234. Hendry NW: The geology, occurrences and major uses of asbestos. Ann NY Acad Sci 132:12, 1965

235. Gaze R: The physical and molecular structure of asbestos. Ann NY Acad Sci 132:23, 1965

236. Churg A, Wright JL: Small airways disease and mineral dust exposure. p. 233. In Sommers S (ed): Pathology Annual. Part II. Vol. 18. Appleton & Lange, East Norwalk, CT, 1983

237. Suzuki Y, Churg J: Structure and development of the asbestos body. Am J Pathol 55:79, 1969

238. Gaensler EA, Addington WW: Asbestos or ferruginous bodies. N Engl J Med 280:488, 1969

239. Kuhn C III, Kuo TT: Cytoplasmic hyaline in asbestosis. A reaction of injured alveolar epithelium. Arch Pathol Lab Med 95:190, 1973

240. Warnock WL, Press M, Churg A: Further observations on cytoplasmic hyaline in the lung. Hum Pathol 11:59, 1980

241. Ashcroft T, Heppleston AG: The optical and electron microscopic determination of pulmonary asbestos fibre concentration and its relations to the human pathological reaction. J Clin Pathol 26:224, 1973

242. Gough J: Differential diagnosis in the pathology of asbestosis. Ann NY Acad Sci 132:368, 1965

243. Gaensler EA, Kaplin AI: Asbestos pleural effusion. Ann Intern Med 74:178, 1971

244. Ziskind M, Jones RN, Weill H: Silicosis. Am Rev Respir Dis 113:643, 1976

245. Snider DE: The relationship between tuberculosis and silicosis. Am Rev Respir Dis 118:455, 1978

246. Matilla A, Galera H, Pascual E, et al: Chronic berylliosis. Br J Dis Chest 67:308, 1973

247. Thurlbeck WM: Chronic Airflow Obstruction in Lung Disease. WB Saunders, Philadelphia, 1976

248. Hogg JC, Macklem PT, Thurlbeck WM: Site and nature of airway obstruction in chronic obstructive lung disease. N Engl J Med 278:1355, 1968

249. Kappos AD, Rodarte JR, Lai-Fook SJ: Frequency dependence and partitioning of respiratory impedance in dogs. J Appl Physiol 61:621, 1983

250. Van Brabandt H, Caubergs M, Verbeken E, et al: Partitioning of pulmonary impedance in excised human lungs. Functional-structural relationships. J Appl Physiol 55:1733, 1983

251. Berend N, Woolcock AJ, Marlin GE: Correlation between the function and structure of the lung in smokers. Am Rev Respir Dis 119:695, 1979

252. Wright JL, Cosio M, Wiggs B, Hogg JC: A morphologic grading system for membranous and respiratory bronchioles. Arch Pathol Lab Med 109:163, 1985

253. Thurlbeck WM: Chronic airflow obstruction. p. 129. In Petty TL (ed): Correlation of Structure and Function in Chronic Obstructive Pulmonary Disease. 2nd Ed. (revised and expanded). Marcel Dekker, New York, Basel, 1985

254. Thurlbeck WM: Chronic airflow obstruction. In Thurlbeck WM (ed): Pathology of the Lung. Thieme International, New York, 1988

255. Horvath EP, DoPico GA, Barbee RA, Dickie HA: Nitrogen dioxide–induced pulmonary disease. J Occup Med 20:103, 1978

256. Woodford DM, Coutu RE, Gaensler EA: Obstructive lung disease from acute sulphur-dioxide exposure. Respiration 38:238, 1979

257. Close LG, Catlin FI, Gohn AM: Acute and chronic effects of ammonia burns of the respiratory tract. Arch Otolaryngol 106:151, 1980

258. Becroft DMO: Bronchiolitis obliterans, bronchiectasis and other sequelae of adenovirus type 21 infection in young children. J Clin Pathol 24:72, 1971

259. Edwards C, Penny M, Newman J: *Mycoplasma* pneumonia, Stevens-Johnson syndrome and chronic obliterative bronchiolitis. Thorax 38:867, 1983

260. Geddes DM, Corrin B, Brewerton DA, et al: Progressive airway obliteration in adults and its association with rheumatoid disease. Q J Med 46:427, 1977

261. Geddes DM, Webley M, Emerson PA: Airways obstruction in rheumatoid arthritis. Ann Rheum Dis 38:222, 1979

262. Homma H, et al: Diffuse panbronchiolitis. A disease of the transitional zone of the lung. Chest 83:63, 1983

263. Macklem PT, Thurlbeck WM, Frazer RG: Chronic ob-

structive lung disease of the small airways. Ann Intern Med 74:167, 1971

264. Roca J, Granana A, Rodriguez-Roisom R, et al: Fatal airway disease in an adult with chronic graft-versus-host disease. Thorax 37:77, 1982

265. Krowka MJ, Rosenow EC III, Hoagland HC: Pulmonary complications of bone marrow transplantation. Chest 87:237, 1986

266. Ralph D, Springmeyer SC, Sullivan SC, et al: Rapidly progressive air-flow obstruction in marrow transplant recipients. Possible association between obliterative bronchiolitis and chronic graft vs. host disease. Am Rev Respir Dis 129:641, 1984

267. Kurzrock R, Zanda A, Kanojia M, et al: Obstructive lung disease after allogenic bone marrow transplantation. Transplantation 37:156, 1984

268. Johnson FL, Stokes DC, Ruggiero M, et al: Chronic obstructive airway disease after bone marrow transplantation. J Pediatr 105:370, 1984

269. Beschorner WE, Saral R, Hutchins GM, et al: Lymphocytic bronchitis associated with graft-versus-host disease in recipients of bone marrow transplants. N Engl J Med 299:1030, 1978

270. Burke CM, et al: Post-transplant obliterative bronchiolitis and other late sequelae in human heart-lung transplantation. Chest 86:824, 1984

271. Yousem SA, Burke CM, Billingham ME: Pathologic pulmonary alterations in long-term heart-lung transplantation. Hum Pathol 16:911, 1985

272. Yousem SA, Colby TV, Carrington CB: Follicular bronchitis/bronchiolitis. Hum Pathol 16:700, 1985

273. Wright JL, Hobson J, Wiggs BR et al: Effect of cigarette smoking on structure of the small airways. Lung 165:91, 1987

274. Myers JL, Veal CF, Shin MS, Katzenstein ALA: Respiratory bronchiolitis causing interstitial lung disease. A clinicopathologic study of six cases. Am Rev Respir Dis 135:880, 1987

275. Turton CW, Williams G, Green M: Cryptogenic obliterative bronchiolitis in adults. Thorax 36:805, 1981

276. Killem DA, Gobbel WG: Spontaneous Pneumothorax. Little, Brown, Boston, 1968

277. Lichter I, Glynne JF: Spontaneous pneumothorax in young subjects. A clinical and pathological study. Thorax 26:409, 1971

278. Ohata M, Suzuki H: Pathogenesis of spontaneous pneumothorax with special reference to the ultrastructure of emphysematous bullae. Chest 77:771, 1980

279. McDowell EM, Barrett LA, Harris CC, et al: Abnormal cilia in human bronchial epithelium. Arch Pathol Lab Med 100:429, 1976

280. Kartagener M, Stucki P: Bronchiectasis with sinus inversus. Arch Pediatr 79:193, 1962

281. Eliasson R: The immotile cilia syndrome. A congenital ciliary abnormality as an etiologic factor in chronic airway infections and male sterility. N Engl J Med 297:1, 1977

282. Waite D, Steele R, Ross I: Cilia and sperm tail abnormalities in Polynesian bronchiectasis. Lancet 2:132, 1978

283. Sturgess JM, Chao J, Wong J, et al: Cilia with defective radial spokes: A cause of human respiratory disease. N Engl J Med 300:53, 1979

284. Afzelius BA, Eliasson R: Flagellar mutants in man on the heterogeneity of the immotile cilia syndrome. J Ultrastruct Res 69:43, 1979

285. Schneeberger EE, McCormack J, Issenberg HJ, et al: Heterogeneity of ciliary morphology in the immotile-cilia syndrome in man. J Ultrastruct Res 73:34, 1980

286. Buccetti B, Burini AG, Pellini V: Spermatozoa and cilia lacking axoneme in an infertile male. Andrologia 12:525, 1980

287. Fonzi L, Lungarella G, Palatresi R: Lack of kinocilia in the nasal mucosa in the immotile cilia syndrome. Eur J Respir Dis 63:158, 1982

288. Sturgess JM, Chao J, Turner JAP: Transposition of ciliary microtubules. Another cause of impaired ciliary motility. N Engl J Med 303:318, 1980

289. Veerman AJP, Van Delden L, Feenstra L, Leene W: The immotile cilia syndrome, phase contrast microscopy, scanning and transmission microscopy. Pediatrics 65:698, 1980

290. Rutland J, Cole PJ: Non-invasive sampling of nasal cilia for measurement of beat frequency and study of ultrastructure. Lancet 2:564, 1980

291. Heath D, Edwards JE: The pathology of hyperactive pulmonary vascular disease. A description of six grades of structural changes in the pulmonary arteries with special reference to congenital cardiac septal defects. Circulation 18:533, 1958

292. Rabinovitch M, Haworth SG, Vance Z, et al: Early pulmonary vascular change in congenital heart disease studied in biopsy tissue. Hum Pathol 11:499, 1980

293. Haworth SG, Reid L: A morphometric study of regional variation of lung structure in infants with pulmonary hypertension and congenital cardiac defect: A justification of lung biopsy. Br Heart J 40:825, 1978

294. Langston C, Holder P: Pulmonary vascular changes in infants and children. p. 57. In Will JA, Dawson CA, Weir EK, Buckner CK (eds): The Pulmonary Circulation in Health and Disease. Academic Press, Orlando, FL, 1987

295. Wagenvoort CA: The pathology of human pulmonary hypertension pattern recognition and specificity. p. 15. In Will JA, Dawson CA, Weir EK, Buckner CK (eds): The Pulmonary Circulation in Health and Disease. Academic Press, Orlando, FL, 1987

296. Edwards WD, Edwards JE: Recent advances in the pathology of the pulmonary vasculature. In Thurlbeck WM, Abell MR (eds): The Lung, Structure, Function and Disease. Williams & Wilkins, Baltimore, 1978

297. Shepherd JT, Edwards JE, Burchell HB, et al: Clinical, physiologic and pathologic considerations in patients with idiopathic pulmonary hypertension. Br Heart J 19:70, 1957

298. Heath D, Edwards JE: Configuration of elastic tissue of pulmonary trunk in idiopathic pulmonary hypertension. Circulation 21:59, 1960

299. Scully RE, Goldabini JJ, McNeely BU (eds): Case records

of the Massachusetts General Hospital. N Engl J Med 294:433, 1976

300. Walcott G, Burchell HB, Brown AL: Primary pulmonary hypertension. Am J Med 49:70, 1970

301. Wagenvoort CA, Wagenvoort N: Primary pulmonary hypertension. A pathologic study of the lung vessels in 156 clinically diagnosed cases. Circulation 42:1163, 1970

302. Kay JM, Smith P, Heath D: Aminorex and the pulmonary circulation. Thorax 26:262, 1971

303. Kay JM, Heath D, Smith P, et al: Fulvine and the pulmonary circulation. Thorax 26:249, 1971

304. Thompson P, McRae C: Familial pulmonary hyperten-

sion. Evidence of autosomal dominant inheritance. Br Heart J 32:758, 1970

305. Inglesby TV, Singer JW, Gordon DS: Abnormal fibrinolysis in familial pulmonary hypertension. Am J Med 55:5, 1973

306. Carrington CB, Liebow AA: Pulmonary veno-occlusive disease. Hum Pathol 1:322, 1970

307. Wagenvoort CA, Wagenvoort N, Takahashi T: Pulmonary veno-occlusive disease: Involvement of pulmonary arteries and review of the literature. Hum Pathol 16:1033, 1985

308. Heath D, Scott O, Lynch J: Pulmonary veno-occlusive disease. Thorax 26:663, 1971

20

Localized Diseases of the Bronchi and Lungs

Mario J. Saldana

Pathologic processes affecting the tracheobronchial tree and lung parenchyma can be classified as diffuse and localized. The didactic value of this simple approach to the pathologic diagnosis of pulmonary lesions is enhanced by practicality: most diffuse processes are medical conditions, whereas localized processes are frequently amenable to surgical treatment.

Diffuse processes are almost always bilateral, involve the lung in a widespread manner, and result in a degree of respiratory insufficiency. In contradistinction, localized processes have a discrete character and need not affect the overall function of the lung. Examples of localized processes include roughly spherical lesions up to 3 cm in diameter (nodules) or greater than 3 cm (masses). Localized lesion of irregular shape are simply designated as infiltrates and can be subsegmental, segmental, or lobar in extent. Nodules, masses, and infiltrates can be solid or undergo cavitation with or without formation of an air-liquid interface. Cystic lesions do quality as localized processes, and they are also discussed.

Localized processes can be single (isolated) or multiple. In the latter case, our approach requires that the intervening lung parenchyma be disease-free, except perhaps for some degree of emphysema, a common condition in persons past middle age. One must realize that localized lesions can and do occur on a background of diffuse disease; for example, carcinoma (localized) can arise in a lung with advanced emphysema (diffuse); progressive massive fibrosis (localized) is seen in pneumoconiosis characterized by extensive interstitial fibrosis (diffuse).

Localized processes have been grouped into five main categories according to their impact on the practicing pathologist: tumors, inflammatory lesions, infiltrative vasculopathies, maldevelopmental processes, and miscellaneous. For additional information on individual subjects, the reader is referred to Spencer's classic textbook of lung pathology.[1] Also recommended are two recent textbooks, one edited by Dail and Hammar[2] and another by Thurlbeck.[3]

TUMORS OF THE LUNG

Cancer of the lung is the most important human cancer in the United States. An estimated 35 percent of all deaths in males and 20 percent in females will be due to lung cancer in 1988.[4] In its rich histologic variety, cancer of the lung certainly mirrors the complex organization of this organ; yet, it should be noted that about 90 percent of all tumors arise from the epithelial lining of bronchi and submucosal glands. It is also true in the lung that malignant tumors vastly outnumber benign tumors.[5]

At the beginning of the twentieth century, lung cancer was a rarity in the United States, as noted by Adler.[6] He could not have guessed that in the 50 year span from the 1930s to the 1980s, cancer of the lung would show a 15-fold increase in males and ninefold increase in females.[4] It is estimated that 100,000 new cases of lung cancer in men and 52,000 in women occurred in 1988 alone.[4] If current trends continue unabated, it is projected that close to 300,000 new cases of lung cancer will occur by 2,000.[7]

It is almost universally accepted that inhaled tobacco smoke is the single main etiologic agent in lung cancer, but other environmental carcinogens acting alone or synergistically also increase the risk of this disease.[7,8] Such agents include inorganic ducts such as asbestos, arsenic, beryllium, chromate, coal tar products, iron oxide, mustard gas, petroleum, and nickel; organic chemicals such as benzopyrene, vinyl chloride, and bischloromethyl ether; and radioactive materials such as uranium, radon, and thorium.

Retrospective as well as prospective studies[8] have shown that the risk of developing lung cancer increases in direct proportion to the number of cigarettes smoked per day, and to the years of smoking. In people who stop smoking, the risk of cancer diminishes steadily and by 15 years of abstention returns to that of nonsmokers. Most cigar and pipe smokers do not have a greatly increased risk of developing lung cancer because they do not inhale; those who inhale have the same risk as cigarette smokers.

Several epidemiologic studies[8] have suggested that smoking low-tar cigarettes diminishes the risk of lung cancer, but this important question needs further investigation. Likewise, there is some evidence[9–11] indicating that passive inhalation of cigarette smoke increases the likelihood of lung cancer, but the matter remains controversial.

Some technical developments of importance in the diagnosis of lung cancer have recently taken place. The major development, perhaps, was the introduction of the flexible fiberoptic bronchoscope with the possibility of obtaining small diagnostic samples of tissue and cells from lesions previously unapproachable with the rigid bronchoscope.[12] Fine needle aspiration (FNA) is now routine in the diagnosis of peripheral lesions and complements the value of fiberoptic bronchoscopy. It has also become clear that cytologic examination of bronchial secretions, effusions, and aspirates of cancer cells is a highly reliable technique in the hands of experienced observers. Indeed, cytologic examination surpasses tissue analysis in providing cell detail, a matter of crucial importance in typing tumors or when dealing with artifactually altered biopsy specimens. The electron microscope remains an indispensable research tool in lung carcinogenesis and also provides useful diagnostic information even when applied to minute bronchial biopsies.[13] The application of the immunoperoxidase technique has added considerably to our understanding of the histogenesis of lung tumors and their pathologic diagnosis.

The pathology of lung tumors has been the subject of important publications such as Liebow's[14] original fascicle of 1952, a cornerstone in the study of these conditions. An updated second edition was completed by Carter and Eggleston in 1979.[15] The first World Health Organization (WHO) classification of lung tumors, edited by Kreyberg et al.,[16] appeared in 1957. A second updated version, edited by Yesner and Sobin,[17] was published in 1977 and is presented in Table 20-1. More recent reviews by Hammar,[18] Dail,[19] and Churg[20] contain a wealth of information.

TABLE 20-1. World Health Organization Histologic Classification of Lung Tumors, 1977

Epithelial tumors
  Benign
    Papillomas
      Squamous cell papilloma
      Transitional papilloma
    Adenomas
      Pleomorphic adenoma (mixed tumor)
      Monomorphic adenomas
    Others
  Dysplasia and CIS
  Malignant
    Squamous cell carcinoma (epidermoid carcinoma)
      Variant
        Spindle cell (squamous) carcinoma
    Small cell carcinoma
      Oat cell carcinoma
      Intermediate cell type
      Combined oat cell carcinoma
    Adenocarcinoma
      Acinar adenocarcinoma
      Papillary adenocarcinoma
      Bronchiolo-alveolar
      Solid carcinoma with mucus formation
    Large cell carcinoma
      Variants
        Giant cell carcinoma
        Clear cell carcinoma
    Adenosquamous carcinoma
    Carcinoid tumor
    Bronchial gland carcinomas
      Adenoid cystic carcinoma
      Mucoepidermoid carcinoma
      Others
    Others

Soft tissue tumors

Mesothelial tumors
  Benign mesothelioma
  Malignant mesothelioma
    Epithelial
    Fibrous (spindle cell)
    Biphasic

Miscellaneous tumors
  Benign
  Malignant
    Carcinosarcoma
    Pulmonary blastoma
    Malignant melanoma
    Malignant lymphomas
    Others

Secondary tumors

Unclassified tumors

Tumor-like lesions
  Hamartoma
  Lymphoproliferative lesions
  Tumorlet
  Eosinophilic granuloma
  Sclerosing hemangioma
  Inflammatory pseudotumor
  Others

LOCALIZED DISEASES OF THE BRONCHI AND LUNGS

For the purpose of the present discussion, we follow a classification of lung tumors that, although simplified, adheres closely to the terminology and histologic criteria set forth by the WHO (Table 20-2). Mesothelioma, a tumor of increasing frequency and importance, is discussed in Chapter 25.

In order to determine the operability of lung cancer, to establish prognosis, and to compare the efficacy of several regimens of treatment, in a meaningful manner, familiarity with staging procedures is required. According to the TNM system (T, tumor; N, lymph node metastasis; M, distant metastasis),[21,22] the following situations exist:

Occult carcinoma: Malignant cells present in bronchopulmonary secretions, but no lesion demonstrable radiographically or bronchoscopically

Stage 0: Carcinoma in situ (CIS)

Stage I: Tumors up to 3 cm in diameter, completely surrounded by lung tissue and visceral pleura (T1) with or without metastasis to ipsilateral peribronchial and hilar nodes (N1); tumors greater than 3 cm in diameter without metastasis, and tumors of any size invading visceral pleura or a lobar bronchus more than 2.0 cm distal to the carina (T2) also rated stage I

Stage II: Tumor classified as T2 with metastasis to ipsilateral peribronchial and hilar lymph nodes (N1)

Stage III: Tumors with metastasis to mediastinal lymph nodes (N2) or distant metastasis (M1); tumors that invade chest wall, diaphragm, or mediastinal contents (T3) also determine that the case in stage III

TABLE 20-2. Classification and Prevalence of Primary Lung Tumors by Histologic Type

Tumor	No. of Cases	%
Usual epithelial tumors		
Adenocarcinoma	435	30
Squamous cell carcinoma	360	25
Small cell carcinoma	270	18
Large cell carcinoma	225	15
Carcinoid tumors	45	3
Rare epithelial tumors		
Submucosal bronchial gland tumors	8	0.5
Bronchial papillary tumors	6	0.4
Mixed epithelial-mesenchymal tumors (carcinosarcoma, blastoma, teratoma)	12	0.8
Nonepithelial tumors		
Lymphoproliferative lesions	21	1.4
Mesenchymal (soft tissue) tumors	18	1.2
Pleural tumors (mesothelioma)	60	4
Miscellaneous tumors	10	0.7
Total	1,470	100

Table based on 1,470 cases studied by biopsy and fine needle aspiration at Jackson Memorial Hospital of Miami, Florida (1977–1987).

A new international staging system for lung cancer[23] was recently introduced and will certainly replace the previous TNM system. In the international system, stage I is defined by the absence of lymph node metastasis. Stage II patients have peribronchial, hilar, or mediastinal lymph node metastasis on the ipsilateral side alone. In what is called stage IIIA disease, the tumor may invade the chest wall (Pancoast tumors included) and there may be hilar or mediastinal lymph node metastasis on the ipsilateral side only. Patients with stage I, II, and IIIA tumors are candidates for surgical therapy.

Stage IIIB is defined by the presence of contralateral hilar, mediastinal, scalene, and supraclavicular lymph node metastasis; or tumors directly invading mediastinal structures (heart, great vessels, vertebrae, esophagus, trachea, carina); or tumors with associated malignant pleural effusion. Stage IV is characterized by distant metastasis (e.g., brain, liver, bone, adrenals). Patients with stage IIIB and IV disease fall within the realm of radiotherapy and chemotherapy.

Usual Epithelial Tumors

Adenocarcinoma

Adenocarcinoma has long been known to be the most common histologic type of lung cancer in Japan and China.[24,25] Only during the past decade has it surpassed squamous cell carcinoma as the most common lung cancer type in the United States[26,27] (Table 20-2). Although epidemiologic data supporting a relationship with cigarette smoking are not as strong as for squamous cell and small cell carcinomas, most patients with adenocarcinoma do have a history of smoking.[18,28] It is also known that when nonsmoking individuals develop lung cancer, it is adenocarcinoma.[29] Whether the predominance of adenocarcinoma reflects the switch from nonfilter to filter cigarettes in smokers' habits over the past three decades or the long-term effects of passive smoking is a fundamental question that remains to be answered. We currently include three anatomic-clinical variants under the designation adenocarcinoma (Table 20-3). Approximately 80 per-

TABLE 20-3. Classification of Pulmonary Adenocarcinoma

Peripheral bronchogenic adenocarcinoma (80%)
  Usual subtypes: acinar, papillary, combined acinar-papillary, adenosquamous carcinoma
  Unusual subtypes: solid carcinoma with mucin production, colloid carcinoma, signet-ring cell carcinoma, intestinal-like, prostatic-like, endodermal tumor resembling fetal lung
Bronchiolo-alveolar carcinoma (15%)
  Histologic subtypes: nonpapillary, papillary, solid
Adenocarcinoma in diffuse interstitial fibrosis (1%)
Central bronchogenic adenocarcinoma (4%)

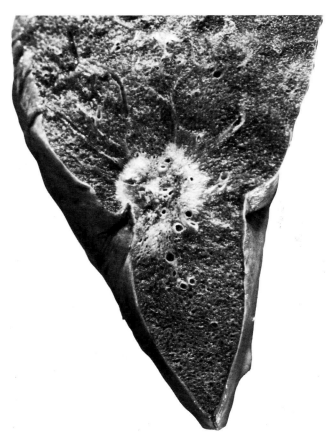

Fig. 20-1. Gross appearance of adenocarcinoma of lung presenting as a peripheral nodule. The tumor grows around a pigmented central scar that contains small bronchi and vessels and produces pleural retraction.

cent of all adenocarcinomas arise in distal bronchi much smaller than those in which squamous cell and small cell carcinomas arise. In our experience such bronchi measure 3 mm or less in diameter. Grossly, adenocarcinomas are firm or hard masses of white to gray tissue characteristically located at the periphery of the lung and covered by a fibrotic puckered pleura (Fig. 20-1). On cut section, they have a solid or a mucoid appearance. Necrosis may be evident, but frank cavitation is rare.

A sprinkling of anthracotic pigment is apparent in the substance of the tumor, and in a large proportion of cases adenocarcinomas are centered around a pigmented scar that produces the pleural retraction. The size of these tumors varies from a few millimeters to several centimeters, depending on the stage of development. Rarely, adenocarcinomas arise in a more proximal position in relation to larger bronchi. A rare form of adenocarcinoma produces a diffuse thickening of the pleura, and the gross appearance simulates mesothelioma.[30]

Histologically, most pulmonary adenocarcinomas are acinar or gland-forming tumors and they occur in well,

moderately, and poorly differentiated forms in approximately equal proportions. Adenocarcinoma cells have abundant clear or basophilic cytoplasm. Their nuclei are vesicular, with a thin, well defined membrane and prominent nucleoli. Most tumors show a papillary component (Fig. 20-2); less frequently, they have a fundamentally papillary structure, but this feature implies no difference in biologic behavior. Mucin secretion is noted in about 80 percent of cases and should be routinely investigated by periodic acid-Schiff (PAS)-diastase or mucicarmine stains. Immunohistochemically, adenocarcinomas are positive for CEA and negative for keratin in formalin-fixed, paraffin-embedded tissue. Both low- and high-molecular-weight keratins are expressed if frozen tissue is used or when paraffin-embedded material undergoes prior trypsinization.

Adenocarcinomas that invade lung tissue elicit a desmoplastic response, so a clear relationship to a parent bronchus within or near the scar is effaced. In other

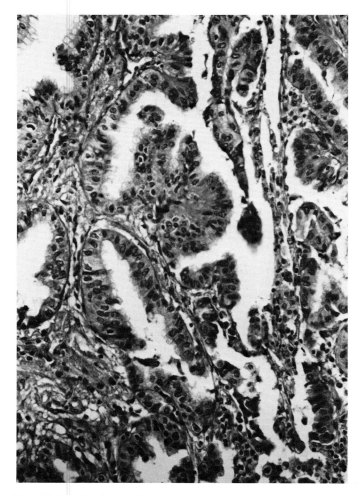

Fig. 20-2. Mucin-producing adenocarcinoma of the lung combining acinar and papillary features.

cases, chance sections reveal small bronchi with in situ changes indicating the origin of the tumor. At the periphery, the tumor cells extend on the framework of alveolar septa, simulating bronchiolo-alveolar carcinoma.

Adenosquamous Carcinoma

Tumors combining adenocarcinoma and squamous cell carcinoma features account for about 2 percent of all lung cancers.[31,32] We interpret adenosquamous carcinoma, fundamentally, as adenocarcinoma with squamous differentiation, a view supported by the histologic findings (Fig. 20-3), their occurrence in the periphery of the lung, and a poor clinical behavior identical to that of adenocarcinomas. Histologically, they are usually poorly differentiated variants; moderately differentiated versions are less frequent and well differentiated adenosquamous carcinomas are exceedingly rare.

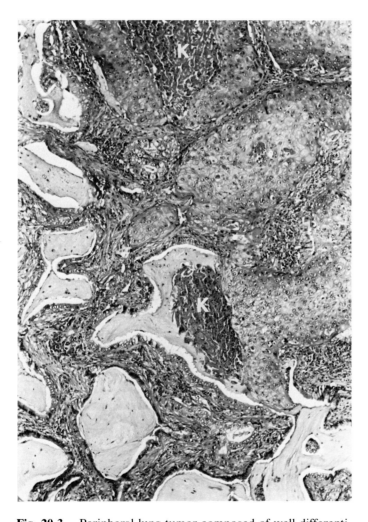

Fig. 20-3. Peripheral lung tumor composed of well differentiated, mucin-producing adenocarcinoma and squamous cell carcinoma (adenosquamous carcinoma). The squamous component of the lesion arises within the confines of the glandular elements, progresses to obliterate them and matures into solid masses of squamous cell carcinoma with production of keratin (K).

Other Adenocarcinomas

Tumors previously designated as large cell carcinomas with intracellular mucin are now considered to be poorly differentiated (solid) variants of adenocarcinoma with no recognizable acinar features. It is also clear that the full range of morphologic expression of adenocarcinomas has not received proper attention in the past; we now recognize tumors that resemble gastric adenocarcinomas of the colloid and signet-ring variants (Fig. 20-4A) and intestinal-type carcinomas indistinguishable from colonic cancer. We have seen a rare example composed of small glands and cells resembling prostatic adenocarcinoma, and the clinical course was highly aggressive (Fig. 20-4B). Another unusual variant, designated endodermal tumor resembling fetal lung,[33–36] is composed of clear glands identical to those of blastoma, but the stroma of this tumor is lacking. The presence of epithelial morules and neuroendocrine features characterize this peculiar form of adenocarcinoma.

Scar Carcinoma

In my experience, most peripheral adenocarcinomas are associated with a central scar. Less frequently squamous cell carcinomas, large cell carcinomas and even rare examples of small cell carcinomas may have an associated central scar. Traditionally the latter has been interpreted as preceding the development of the tumor.[37] Indeed, such an impression is gained from the tumor, best seen at the periphery of the scar, and the heavy anthracotic pigment deposition of the latter suggesting chronicity (see Fig. 20-1). However, following the careful morphologic analysis by Shimosato et al.[24] and biochemical and histochemical analysis of the scar by Madri and Carter[38] and by Barsky et al.,[39] scars are interpreted as a desmoplastic response to the tumor rather than its cause. It is also possible, as proposed by Kung et al.,[25] that so-called scars represent collapse of lung tissue following obstruction of airways by tumor. It is clear, however, that fibrosis and hyalinization develop once the tumor becomes infiltrating. For Shimosato et al.,[24] scars with extensive hyalinization are frequently associated with metastasis. We have also noted that poorly differentiated scar cancers with vascular invasion (best seen by elastic tissue stains) and with necrosis have an unfavorable prognosis.

The only curative therapy for adenocarcinoma is surgery. In stage I disease—the small peripheral nodule detected by chest radiography—the 5 year survival rate is 51 percent. Most cases, when discovered, are in stage III, with distant metastasis notably to the brain, and the 5 year survival rate is 11 percent. Few cases are discovered

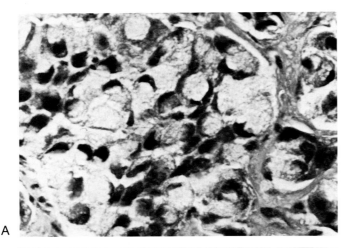

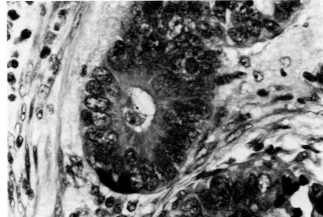

Fig. 20-4. **(A)** Pulmonary adenocarcinoma composed entirely of mucinous signet-ring cells. A gastrointestinal source was ruled out at postmortem examination. **(B)** Another rare histologic pattern of adenocarcinoma of the lung resembling prostatic carcinoma. The latter was ruled out clinically and by negative prostatic acid phosphatase and prostate-specific antigen by the immunoperoxidase technique.

in stage II, and those that are have a survival rate of 21 percent.[15,21,22] Recently, combined chemotherapy has been effective in inducing remission in about one half of patients, and survival of over 1 year has been noted.

Bronchiolo-alveolar Carcinoma

Bronchioloalveolar carcinoma is a distinctive histologic subtype seen in 15 percent of all pulmonary adenocarcinomas (see Table 20-3). These tumors arise in the periphery of the lung beyond a grossly recognizable bronchus and spread on the walls of air spaces, which serve as the stroma for the neoplastic growth.[40] Classically, bronchiolo-alveolar carcinomas are well differentiated tumors, and the alveolar walls on which the tumor spreads may be of normal thickness or discretely thickened by fibrosis and chronic inflammation.

Grossly, bronchiolo-alveolar cancers appear as parenchymal nodular or patchy bland infiltrates. Less often the appearance is that of a multicentric, unilateral or bilateral, nodular process. Still another pattern is that of a confluent or lobar type of pneumonia with a mucoid appearance traditionally compared with *Klebsiella* pneumonia.

Histologically, the cells are columnar in type, and contain mucin and basally located, benign-appearing nuclei (Fig. 20-5A). Mitoses may be difficult to detect. Nonmucin-producing forms do occur, and they exhibit a picket-fence type of cellular growth (Fig. 20-5B). Other variations include multinucleated and giant cells with acidophilic nuclear inclusions, a fact that should suggest type II pneumocyte differentiation.[41] Bronchiolo-alveolar car-

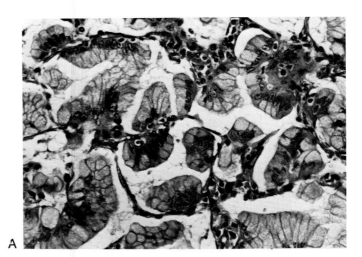

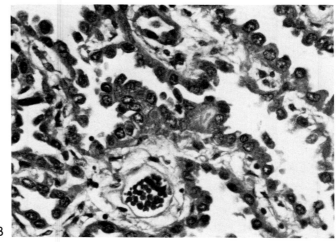

Fig. 20-5. Two different patterns of bronchiolo-alveolar carcinoma. **(A)** Tumor is composed of tall columnar, mucin-producing cells. **(B)** Neoplastic cells are peg-shaped and produce no mucin. The alveolar walls they grow on are slightly thickened by fibrosis. (Fig. A Courtesy of Dr. Carlos Bedrossian, St. Louis, MO.)

cinoma presenting as an isolated nodule or infiltrate has a high resectability rate (87 percent), and the 5 year survival rate is 70 percent. Multinodular and pneumonic forms have a poor prognosis. It should also be noted that metastatic adenocarcinoma from sites such as breast, the colorectal region, and pancreas may simulate bronchiolo-alveolar carcinomas, and this possibility must always be ruled out. Immunohistochemical investigations are of little help in this regard, and one must rely heavily on clinical data.

The histogenesis of bronchiolo-alveolar carcinoma remains a matter of considerable controversy.[42–44] About one third to one half of cases—those exhibiting abundant mucin production—arise from bronchiolar epithelium that has undergone mucoid metaplasia. A large proportion of mucin-negative forms probably arise in nonciliated Clara cells of the bronchiolar epithelium. The possibility that some tumors differentiate as type II pneumocytes is accepted. The evidence for such derivation is the demonstration of cells with features of type II pneumocytes—cytoplasmic lamellar structures—in metastases to the CNS[45] and lymph nodes.[46] The same cells have been shown in tissue cultures from one tumor.[47] Furthermore, Jaagziekte, a viral disease of sheep morphologically indistinguishable from bronchiolo-alveolar carcinoma, represents a proliferation of type II pneumocytes, an additional confirmation of the neoplastic potential of such cells.[48] Finally, Singh et al.[41] showed that type II pneumocyte differentiation of some bronchiolo-alveolar carcinomas is characterized by intranuclear tubular inclusions that stain immunohistochemically for the apoprotein portion of surfactant.

It is not generally recognized that there exist histologic variants of bronchioloalveolar carcinoma exhibiting an exuberant papillary growth; in fact, this feature can be so striking as to suggest a metastasis from sites such as the thyroid or the ovary (Fig. 20-6). Most of these cancers, when examined with the electron microscope, exhibit features of Clara cell (Fig. 20-7) or type II pneumocyte differentiation. The observation can be extended to solid types of bronchiolo-alveolar adenocarcinoma interpreted by light microscopy as large cell undifferentiated carcinoma of bronchus but showing ultrastructural features of Clara cell[49] or type II pneumocyte differentiation[50] (Figs. 20-8 and 20-9). Both papillary and solid tumors do represent histologic variants of bronchiolo-alveolar carcinoma, but their clinical behavior in comparison with the usual, nonpillary tumors remains to be ascertained.

So-called papillary adenomas with features of Clara cell or type II pneumocyte differentiation by electron microscopy are not uncommon in rodents and can be induced experimentally.[51] The designation *adenoma* apparently alludes to their benign histologic features and to their ability to remain confined to the lung in spite of their

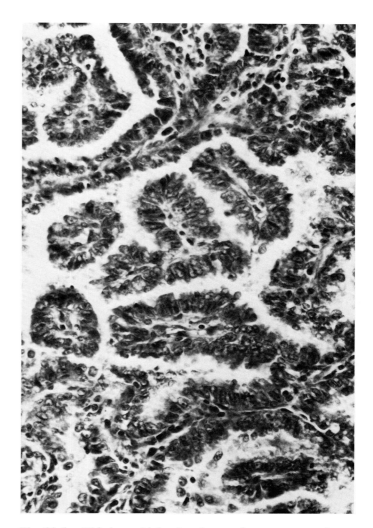

Fig. 20-6. This bronchiolo-alveolar carcinoma presented as a peripheral nodule in a nonsmoking 68-year-old woman. The tumor had striking papillary features throughout. Possible thyroid or ovarian primaries were ruled out clinically and by immunohistologic techniques.

large numbers. However, as noted by Kimura,[52] a malignant potential, including the ability to metastasize, can be noted in some of these tumors after serial transplantation.

In humans, the designation *papillary adenoma* has been seldom used,[53,54] and it is not yet clear whether the two examples on record represent benign tumors or very low-grade bronchiolo-alveolar carcinomas. Against the latter, one of the tumors[53] was present, unchanged, for 10 years prior to surgery. As their animal counterparts, both tumors exhibited features of Clara cell and type II differentiation, suggesting an origin from a common stem cell. Their larger size should help differentiate these putative adenomas from acinar atypical proliferations of the lung, which are microscopic.[55]

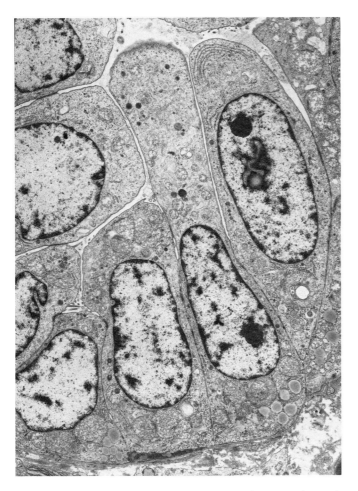

Fig. 20-7. Electron microscopic features of tumor shown in Figure 20-6. It is composed of tall columnar cells with junctional complexes and electron-dense apical granules consistent with Clara cell differentiation.

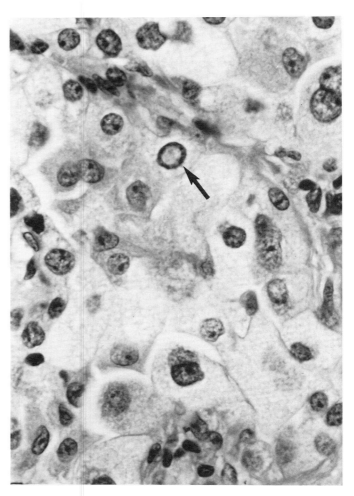

Fig. 20-8. Solid variant of bronchiolo-alveolar adenocarcinoma presenting as a peripheral pulmonary nodule. It was originally interpreted as large cell undifferentiated carcinoma of bronchus. Note nuclear pseudoinclusion indicative of type II pneumocyte differentiation (arrow).

In our experience, bronchiolo-alveolar carcinoma is almost never associated with pigmented scars. Usual bronchogenic adenocarcinomas grow at the periphery of scars in a *lepidic* fashion and can be misinterpreted as bronchiolo-alveolar carcinoma. Careful histologic examination of the scar in such cases will demonstrate a bronchogenic source. Yet, there is a type of pulmonary scarring that is related to the development of bronchioloalveolar carcinoma, i.e., interstitial fibrosis and honeycombing.

Adenocarcinoma in Interstitial Fibrosis. Meyer and Liebow[55] noted the presence of atypical bronchiolar and alveolar cell proliferations in association with interstitial fibrosis and honeycombing. Considerable experience is needed not to overdiagnose such changes as malignant. These workers also showed that adenocarcinomas, frequently of the bronchioloalveolar type, may develop in such lungs, a fact already known in idiopathic interstitial

fibrosis and in scleroderma.[56] However, in a review by Turner-Warwick et al.,[57] no increased incidence of bronchiolo-alveolar carcinoma was noted in a large group of patients with cryptogenic fibrosing alveolitis, as idiopathic interstitial fibrosis is termed in England. These investigators did find an excess relative risk of lung cancer of 14.1 in these patients as compared with the general population. The distribution of lung cancer by histologic type was, however, not different from that found in lung cancer without pulmonary fibrosis. A similar situation exists in patients with lung cancer and asbestosis, which is also a form of pulmonary fibrosis.[58,59]

With increasing frequency, pathologists are asked to render opinions, or to testify in a court of law, on whether lung cancer is causally related to prior *asbestos exposure*. Although this relation is complex and funda-

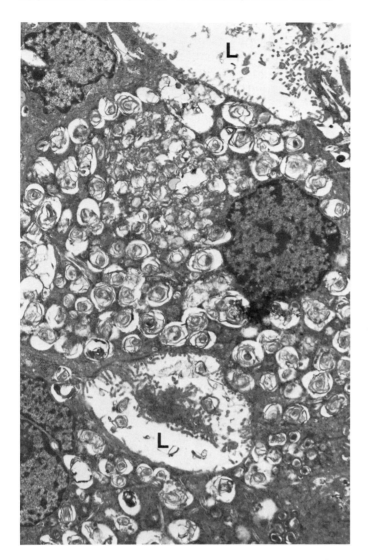

Fig. 20-9. Electron microscopic features of tumor cells illustrated in Figure 20-8. The cytoplasm of the cells is packed with lamellar structures, a feature of type II pneumocytes. The tumor cells frequently form luminal spaces (L).

whether there is asbestosis as well. The latter has been proven histologically present in 18 percent of patients with normal chest radiographs.[59] Fibrosis of the lung as a desmoplastic response to carcinoma should not be misinterpreted as asbestosis. The latter should be searched for away from the areas of carcinoma, both in alveolar tissue and/or around small airways. Since the combination of asbestos exposure and cigarette smoking sharply raises the risk of lung cancer, it is fair to assume, even in the absence of asbestosis, that both asbestos and cigarette smoke played a role in the genesis of lung cancer. The relative contribution of each agent is still impossible to ascertain by scientific means. Many of these cases probably should be compensated, but the measure of the award usually hinges on how the case is argued and the reaction of the jury to the presented facts.

Much simpler and much rarer is the case of cancer of the lung in association with asbestosis, that is, interstitial fibrosis of the lung associated with asbestos bodies (see Ch. 19). It may be correctly stated that asbestos was probably a major agent in the genesis of the lung cancer, and significant compensation is to be expected. In the absence of asbestosis, the presence of asbestos material in lung tissue (asbestos bodies and fibers), or pleural plaques, merely indicates prior exposure but establishes no direct causal relation.

It is also true that cancer developing within 10 years from first exposure to asbestos is probably unrelated, the peak occurrence of these cases being 30 years. In assessing the relative importance of cigarette smoking, it is safe to assume that if the patient stopped smoking 15 years or more before the development of lung cancer, the two are probably unrelated.

Only 4 percent of all adenocarcinomas arise in *large or medium-size bronchi* (see Table 20-3), a location favored by squamous and small cell cancers, and the possibility of a metastatic lesion must be considered. Such tumors originate in the surface epithelium or in submucosal bronchial glands. They are frequently bulky masses histologically composed of lobules rich in mucin and having a complex cribriform appearance.

Squamous Cell Carcinoma

Squamous cell carcinoma is the second most common type of bronchogenic carcinoma (see Table 20-2). As for adenocarcinomas, the full histologic expression of this tumor has not been fully explored, and Table 20-4 summarizes our approach to this problem. Approximately 90 percent of squamous cell carcinomas arise in subsegmental or larger bronchi (Fig. 20-10). They are usually fungating intrabronchial masses composed of gray, white, or yellow tissue. The tumor has a tendency to grow centrally toward the main stem bronchus and to infiltrate

mental points have yet to be worked out, it is helpful to keep in mind certain basic facts when rendering opinions. Against earlier views, it is safe to assume that, in locations within the lung, the gross appearance and cell type of asbestos-related lung cancers are not different from those in the general population.[59] Thus, there are no specific pathologic markers that allow one to state with certainty that a given case of lung cancer is asbestos-related.

The most common and difficult situation deals with patients with a valid and significant history of asbestos exposure but without clinical asbestosis, who have developed lung cancer and who also smoke. The pathologist's task in such cases is not only to confirm the presence of lung cancer in biopsy or autopsy material but to ascertain

TABLE 20-4. Classification of Squamous Cell Carcinoma

Keratinizing subtypes (97%)
  Well differentiated
  Moderately differentiated
  Poorly differentiated
Special subtypes (3%)
  Small cell squamous cell carcinoma
  Spindle cell squamous cell carcinoma (pseudosarcomatous or sarcomatoid squamous cell carcinoma)
  Lymphoepithelioma-like carcinoma

underlying bronchial cartilage, lymph nodes, and adjacent lung parenchyma. Obstructive (lipid) as well as organizing penumonia are seen around the main tumor mass. About 10 percent of squamous cell carcinomas arise peripherally in association with small bronchi, a situation more frequently seen with adenocarcinomas. A large proportion of these tumors are well differentiated and have a great tendency to cavitate, probably as the result of excessive keratin production and poor blood supply. Close to one half of superior sulcus or Pancoast tumors are also of this type. About 15 percent of scar cancers of the lung are squamous cell carcinomas.[37]

Histologically, keratinizing squamous cell carcinomas are classified as well, moderately, and poorly differentiated (Fig. 20-11). Well differentiated squamous cell carcinomas exhibit distinct stratification and extensive keratin production in layers of parallel array and/or forming kera-

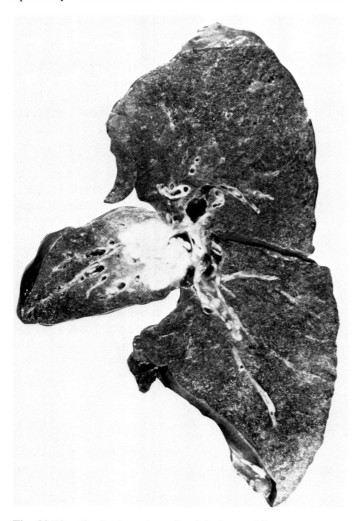

Fig. 20-10. Sagittal section of a right lung with squamous cell carcinoma. The tumor arose in the main bronchus to the right middle lobe. Note the presence of bronchiectasis and obstructive pneumonia distal to the tumor. Hilar node metastases were present.

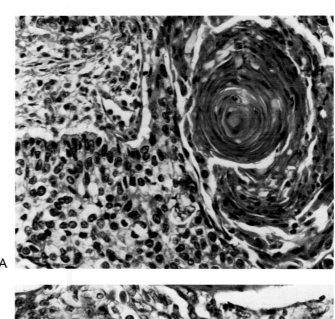

A

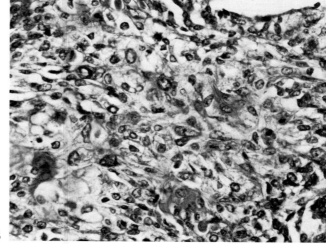

B

Fig. 20-11. (A) Moderately differentiated squamous cell carcinoma. Keratin pearl formation is noted in area of squamous differentiation. (B) Poorly differentiated squamous cell carcinoma for comparison. The darker areas in this largely undifferentiated tumor represent foci of acidophilic keratinous differentiation. Intracellular bridges could be easily detected at a higher magnification.

tin pearls. In moderately differentiated squamous cell carcinomas, there is much less evidence of keratinization. For a tumor to be classified as such, about 20 percent of the tumor area under scrutiny must show evidence of keratinization, the remaining 80 percent being composed of undifferentiated cells. Poorly differentiated forms are composed fundamentally of large undifferentiated cells, and the reason they are considered squamous is the presence of distinct intercellular bridges and/or foci of individual cell keratinization.[15] Most squamous cell carcinomas of the lung are either moderately or poorly differentiated. Well differentiated squamous cell carcinomas are relatively rare in the lung; the finding of a well differentiated epidermoid carcinoma in a cervical lymph node or in soft tissues should suggest a metastasis from a primary tumor in the oropharynx, larynx, or esophagus, rather than lung.[60,61]

Squamous cell carcinoma is the one type of bronchogenic carcinoma in which premalignant and in situ stages have been documented.[15] Grossly, the in situ lesion appears as red granular plaques or gray leukoplakic patches spreading from subsegmental or segmental bronchi to larger bronchi for distances up to several centimeters. Changes of this type can be seen alone or in association with invasive carcinoma. Occasionally, these tumors reach the margin of resection of a lobectomy or pneumonectomy specimen.

Three unusual variants of squamous cell carcinoma are also noted. In *small cell squamous carcinoma*,[62] the tumor is composed of relatively small cells with a tight epithelial arrangement and sharp cytoplasmic borders (Fig. 20-12). Distinct stratification and a basaloid disposition of the cells at the tumor edges are noted; larger squamoid cells at the superficial strata also help in their recognition. Coagulative eosinophilic necrosis within the tumor masses closely resembles small cell carcinoma. By immunohistochemistry and electron microscopy markers of squamous differentiation are demonstrated and neuroendocrine features are absent or seen exceptionally. These tumors behave more like squamous cell carcinomas and the patients should not be given chemotherapy as for small cell carcinoma.

Another variant is *spindle cell squamous carcinoma* resembling a sarcoma; for such tumors the designation pseudosarcomatous or sarcomatoid squamous carcinoma would be appropriate.[63] These tumors tend to be bulky with extensive necrosis and inflammatory changes. The spindle cells of the tumor mimic malignant fibrous histiocytoma, but the recognition of foci of squamoid differentiation aids in the diagnosis. The separation of these tumors from carcinosarcomas is difficult—spindle cell squamous carcinomas usually lack metaplastic heterologous components, a feature more in keeping with carcinosarcoma. Positivity for keratin by the immunoperox-

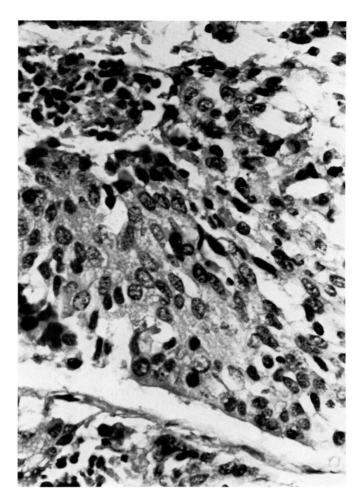

Fig. 20-12. Squamous cell carcinoma formed by relatively small spindle cells, originally interpreted as small cell carcinoma of bronchus. To the upper left portion of the picture the pyknotic and necrotic cells do resemble small cell carcinoma. Immunohistochemical markers for neuroendocrine differentiation were negative and low-molecular-weight keratin was present. At necropsy, the tumor was largely confined to the chest.

idase technique and demonstration of desmosomes and tonofilaments by electron microscopy in the spindle cell component of the lesion argues for spindle cell squamous carcinoma.[64,65] These tumors are aggressive and the prognosis is frequently poor.

Lymphoepithelial carcinoma, a tumor common in the upper respiratory passages, has been described in the lung in association with Epstein-Barr virus (EBV) infection.[66] We have seen an example presenting as a lung mass with extensive spread to hilar and mediastinal lymph nodes (Fig. 20-13). The lesion was highly responsive to radiotherapy.

Squamous cell carcinoma is the most common type of lung cancer associated with cigarette smoking; the risk of

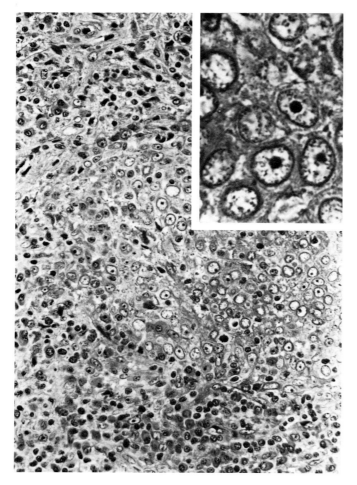

Fig. 20-13. Lymphoepithelial carcinoma of the lung in an Oriental man. The tumor is composed of large polygonal cells in tight epithelial arrangement, with vesicular nuclei and prominent nucleoli. The inset shows the detail of the tumor cells, which were positive for low-molecular-weight keratin and negative for leukocyte common antigen.

developing this cancer increases proportionally to the number of cigarettes smoked. They are in general fast-growing lung masses, with less propensity to distal metastasis than adenocarcinoma.[60,61] The treatment of choice is surgery. The prognosis is dependent on the clinical stage and degree of histologic differentiation of the tumor. In the preclinical stage, there is a high resectability rate (81 percent), and the 5 year survival rate is in the order of 75 percent. A disturbing feature is the development of a second primary tumor in up to 25 percent of patients. Patients with stage I disease had a 54 percent 5 year survival rate; stage II, 36 percent; and stage III, 22 percent. The overall 5 year survival rate for squamous cell carcinoma is 37 percent, the highest among lung cancer types.[15]

In Katlic and Carter's study,[15] the overall 5 year survival rate for poorly differentiated squamous cell carcinoma was 7 percent, 20 percent for moderately differentiated, and 39 percent for well differentiated. The difference between the poorly differentiated group and the combined moderately and well differentiated groups was statistically significant.

Small Cell Carcinoma

Small cell carcinoma is a histologically distinct type of cancer[67–71] that accounts for 18 percent of all lung tumors (see Table 20-2). It is highly malignant and arises from small basal cells or reserve cells of the bronchial epithelium. In about one third to one half of cases, neurosecretory granules can be seen with the electron microscope, but only in some of the cells and in small numbers.[72] The tumor is characterized by its ability to metastasize early and widely, so that clinical manifestations are frequently those due to metastases rather than the primary lesion. One common presentation is as a mediastinal mass without a recognizable lung lesion, and the differential diagnosis includes lymphoma or thymoma.

An in situ stage is usually not recognizable in this tumor. Even in the presence of extensive invasion, endobronchial changes may be entirely missing or consist of slightly raised, velvety gray plaques obliterating the normal mucosal markings. Kato et al.[69] noted that the bronchial mucosa appeared to be normal in 22 of 41 tumors proved to be small cell carcinoma by biopsy. Late in the course of the disease, the bronchi may appear infiltrated and stenosed, but intrabronchial masses of tumor are distinctly rare.

The tumor starts in the bronchial mucosa and extends in a centrifugal fashion to involve the walls of bronchi, peribronchial spaces, and lung parenchyma. The lymph nodes of hilar and mediastinal regions appear full and totally replaced by soft, white tissue. Invasion and obstruction of the superior vena cava is frequently observed (Fig. 20-14). Rarely, small cell carcinoma occurs in the periphery of the lung as an isolated nodule, and the designation *atypical carcinoid* might be applied to such lesions.[73,74]

Microscopically, small cell carcinomas show three different variants: oat cell or lymphocyte-like, intermediate or polygonal-fusiform, and combined patterns (Table 20-5). The so-called *oat cell* variant is rare and represents only 15 percent of all small cell cancers. The cells are twice the size of a lymphocyte or about 20 μm in diameter. They have scant or indistinct cytoplasm, and the nuclei are round to oval to spindled in shape. They are vesicular in character and contain finely dispersed chromatin and indistinct nucleoli. Mitoses are difficult to identify.

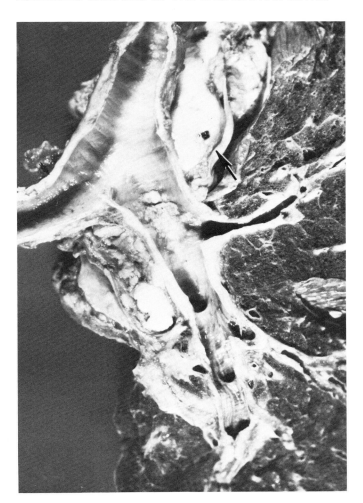

Fig. 20-14. Gross appearance of small cell carcinoma. This rear view of the tracheobronchial tree and lung shows large masses of tumor in the subcarinal and right paratracheal regions. The superior vena cava is filled with tumor (arrow). Flat and granular patches of tumor are also noted in the mucosa of the right mainstem bronchus.

The cells of oat cell carcinoma are arranged in irregular sheets and with no desmoplastic response or secondary inflammatory changes. In other cases, the tumor shows nests, ribbons, or trabeculae supported by a delicate fibrovascular stroma (Fig. 20-15A,B). Near areas of necrosis there may be a peculiar staining of the walls of vessels by an intensely basophilic material shown to be nuclear DNA material from necrotic cells (Fig. 20-16). Another lead to the diagnosis is the presence of the ''crushing'' artifact of tumoral cells. Because the latter can also be seen with lymphocytes, malignant cells should be clearly identified before making a diagnosis of small cell cancer (Fig. 20-16).

Argyrophilic stains containing external reducing agents (Grimelius, Sevier-Munger) and argentaffine stains (Fon-

TABLE 20-5. Small Cell Carcinoma: Histologic Subtypes

Intermediate cell variant (polygonal-fusiform) (70%)
Oat cell (lymphocyte-like) (15%)
Combined (15%)
   Small cell carcinoma: squamous cell carcinoma
   Small cell carcinoma: adenocarcinoma
   Small cell carcinoma: adenocarcinoma: squamous carcinoma
   Small cell carcinoma: large cell carcinoma
   Small cell carcinoma: giant cell carcinoma
   Small cell carcinoma in atypical carcinoid
   Small cell carcinoma in blastoma

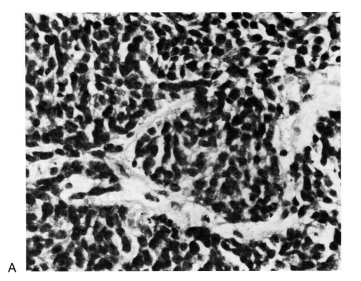
A
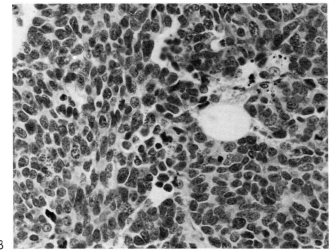
B

Fig. 20-15. **(A)** Microscopic view of the lymphocytelike pattern of small cell carcinoma. Tumor composed of rounded cells with hyperchromatic nuclei. The fibrovascular stroma aids in the recognition of the tumor. **(B)** Oat cell carcinoma composed of rounded and ovoid cells containing nuclei with finely granular chromatin and inconspicuous nucleoli.

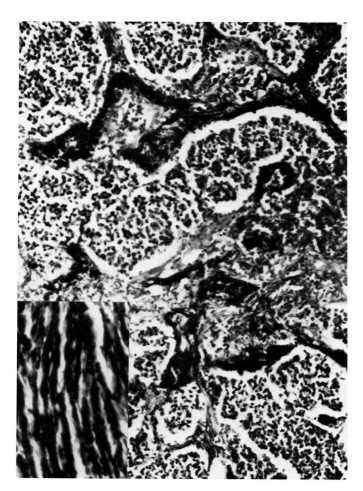

Fig. 20-16. Small cell carcinoma of oat cell type with extensive basophilic staining of vascular structures (Azzopardi's change). The inset shows extensive crushing artifact with no recognizable tumor cells.

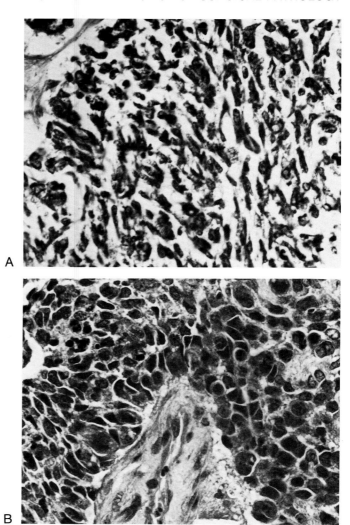

Fig. 20-17. **(A)** Microscopic view of small cell carcinoma, fusiform type. The cells are larger than those in Figure 20-15 and have a well defined spindle shape. **(B)** Cells have a polygonal outline.

tana-Masson) are uniformly negative in these tumors. Immunohistochemically they may express low molecular weight cytokeratins, carcinoembryonic antigen in some cases, neuron-specific enolase and epithelial membrane antigen. Chromogranin is usually negative, reflecting the absence or small numbers of neurosecretory granules.[18]

The greatest proportion of small cell carcinomas (70 percent) belong to the *intermediate cell* variant. The cells are larger than those of the oat cell type and measure, on the average, 30 μm or three times the diameter of a lymphocyte. In some cases, the cells are polygonal in shape, in others fusiform, or a combination (Fig. 20-17A,B). A faintly eosinophilic cytoplasm can be seen in these cells, and mitoses are more readily identified than in oat cell tumors. Occasional giant cells for formed by fusion of tumor cells (Fig. 20-18). Both the basophilic staining of vessels and the crushing artifact can be present.

The remaining 15 percent of small cell carcinomas rep-

resent *combined types*. One such type is characterized by an abrupt transition of small cell carcinoma to squamous cell carcinoma (Fig. 20-19A); transition into adenocarcinoma and to large cell carcinoma has also been noted (Fig. 20-19B). Maturation of part or all of small cell carcinoma into squamous cell carcinoma has been noted spontaneously or following radiotherapy. Striking morphologic changes with appearance of bizarre giant cells can occur spontaneously or following chemotherapy. Foci of transformation into adenocarcinoma are frequently noted in metastases, particularly those in the brain. The combination small cell carcinoma/large cell carcinoma[75] is less responsive to chemotherapy than is pure small cell carcinoma. So-called *atypical carcinoids* are frequently associated with foci of small cell carcinoma.[70] Cases of *blas-

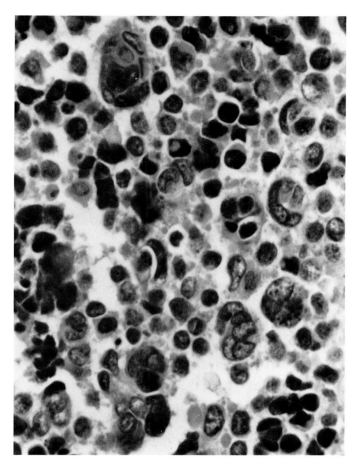

Fig. 20-18. Small cell carcinoma with numerous giant cells. The patient had not received treatment at the time of this biopsy.

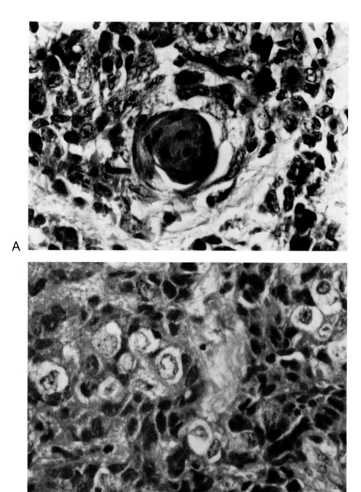

Fig. 20-19. Two examples of small cell carcinoma exhibiting (**A**) squamous differentiation and (**B**) large cell differentiation.

toma of the lung in which the epithelial component was fundamentally small cell carcinoma have been described[76] (Fig. 20-20).

Small cell carcinoma occurs in middle-aged and elderly people, with a mean age at the time of diagnosis of 60 years. It is more common in men than in women, and it has been associated with cigarette smoking, radiation, and exposure to chloromethyl ether. Rarely, patients may develop Cushing's syndrome, ADH syndrome, and Eaton-Lambert syndrome.[15]

The histogenesis of this tumor has been the subject of much controversy and speculation. Some of these tumors, when examined by electron microscopy, exhibit cells with granules of neurosecretory type, but a neural crest origin has been ruled out, and all available evidence points toward endodermal derivation. Other tumors show, in addition to neurosecretory granules, tonofilaments and desmosomes indicating a dual neurosecretory and squamous differentiation. In the case described by McDowell and Trump,[77] individual cells showed tripar-

tite differentiation: neurosecretory granules, tonofilaments and junctional complexes, and mucous granules.

The treatment of choice of small cell carcinoma, regardless of subtype, is combined chemotherapy with or without radiotherapy. With chemotherapy alone, patients with limited disease achieve a complete remission in 90 percent of cases and their average survival is 18 months. Patients with disseminated disease achieve complete remission only in one third of cases, and the average survival is less than 1 year. Occasionally a patient may survive for 3 years or even longer.

Large Cell Carcinoma

Large cell carcinoma is composed of three subtypes: large cell undifferentiated carcinoma, giant cell carcinoma, and clear cell carcinoma.[15,17]

PRINCIPLES AND PRACTICE OF SURGICAL PATHOLOGY

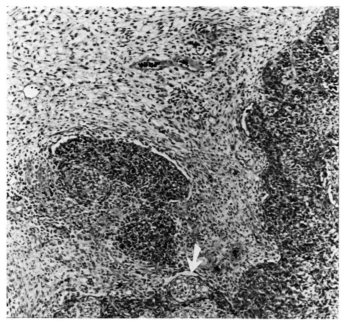

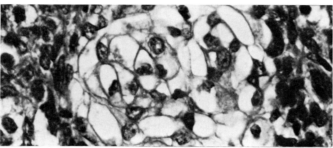

Fig. 20-20. Blastoma of lung composed of a mesenchymal spindle cell proliferation (light areas) and darker epithelial masses of small cell carcinoma. Within the epithelial component, there is a squamous morule (arrow and inset).

Large Cell Undifferentiated Carcinomas

Large cell undifferentiated carcinomas are bulky, soft masses of gray, tan, or pink color, with extensive necrosis. Approximately one half of these tumors involve bronchi of subsegmental size or larger, a figure lower than for squamous cell carcinomas and higher than for adenocarcinomas. The remaining one half are peripheral and subpleural in location, indistinguishable from adenocarcinomas.

The cells in this tumor type are comparatively larger than in the other types of lung cancer, and round to ovoid, polygonal, or spindled in shape. The nuclei are vesicular, occasionally with pink nuclear inclusions. Individual cells may have giant nuclei, and giant multinucleated cells are frequently observed. The cells grow in sheets without organization or pattern. Although a strong des-

moplastic reaction is uncommon, lymphocytes and plasma cells are seen infiltrating a scant fibrovascular stroma.

The most important feature of this tumor is the absence of maturation toward squamous cell or adenocarcinoma.[78] Electron microscopic and immunohistochemical observations[79–82] have shown, however, differentiation along adenocarcinomatous, squamous, adenosquamous, and neuroendocrine lines, and only rarely is the tumor truly undifferentiated. Immunoperoxidase stains may be positive for low molecular weight keratin and for CEA. Nonspecific staining for vimentin is also common. Treatment for large cell undifferentiated carcinoma of the lung is fundamentally surgical, and the prognosis is comparable to that of adenocarcinoma.

Giant Cell Carcinoma

A variant of undifferentiated carcinoma, giant cell carcinoma has bulky necrotic masses with no distinguishing features and is usually found in the periphery of the lung.[83,84] Histologically, the main element is a polygonal, spindle or strap giant cell with one or several nuclei and prominent nucleoli. The cytoplasm can be uniformly eosinophilic or finely vacuolated, and prominent acidophilic nuclear inclusions are frequently noted. A complement of smaller undifferentiated cells is present and little desmoplastic response is noted. In fact, the tumor cells frequently grow in a characteristic noncohesive manner. A characteristic finding is the presence of collections of polymorphonuclear leukocytes within giant cells, apparently phagocytosing cytoplasmic contents, a phenomenon designated as *emperipolesis*. (Fig. 20-21A).

Giant cell carcinomas follow a highly malignant course that parallels that of small cell carcinoma, with development of widespread lymphangitic and hematogenous metastases. These tumors are usually inoperable when discovered and the survival is less than 1 year in spite of any form of therapy. Longer survivals have been reported, but these probably represent less aggressive forms of giant cell carcinoma combined with adenocarcinoma.[15] The differential diagnosis of giant cell carcinoma of the lung includes pleomorphic rhabdomyosarcoma, malignant fibrous histiocytoma, and metastatic adrenocortical carcinoma. Simple stains for mucins (mucicarmine, PAS-diastase) will solve many diagnostic problems. Electron microscopy and immunostaining for epithelial markers (keratin, carcinoembryonic antigen), mesenchymal markers (desmin, actin) and histiocytic markers (alpha-1-antichymotrypsin) are also valuable diagnostic tools.

Clear Cell Carcinoma

Many squamous cell carcinomas, adenocarcinomas, and large cell undifferentiated carcinomas exhibit a com-

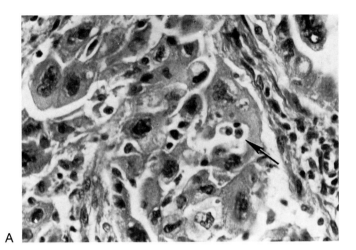

A

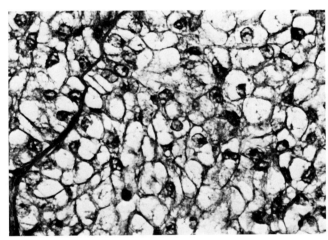

B

Fig. 20-21. **(A)** Microscopic appearance of giant cell carcinoma. Some of the giant cells are intimately associated with clusters of polymorphonuclear leukocytes (emperipolesis) as shown by arrow. **(B)** Clear cell carcinoma. The tumor was a large mass composed entirely of clear cells containing abundant glycogen.

plement of clear cells rich in glycogen. Such a change represents degeneration and has no bearing on biologic behavior and prognosis of the tumor[85,86]. By contrast, primary lung cancers composed entirely of clear cells are extraordinarily rare (Fig. 20-21B) and should prompt a search for a primary tumor in sites such as the kidney. Primary clear cell carcinomas of the lung should also be distinguished from benign clear cell ("sugar") tumors, an entity to be discussed later.

Carcinoids and Other Neuroendocrine Proliferations

The spectrum of neuroendocrine cell proliferations of the human lung is presented in Table 20-6. Normally the

TABLE 20-6. Carcinoid and Other Cellular Proliferations with Neuroendocrine Differentiation

Neuroepithelial bodies
Tumorlets
Typical carcinoids
  Central
  Peripheral (spindle cell)
Atypical carcinoids (well differentiated neuroendocrine carcinoma)
Small cell carcinoma (oat cell and intermediate variants) with neuroendocrine differentiation (poorly differentiated neuroendocrine carcinoma)
Large cell tumors (large cell carcinoma, adenocarcinoma, squamous cell carcinoma, adenosquamous carcinoma) with neuroendocrine differentiation (atypical endocrine tumors)

respiratory epithelium is endowed with a sparse population of neuroendocrine cells analogous to the Kultchitsky cell of the gastrointestional mucosa (K-cell).[87,88] Such a phenomenon is not surprising since embryologically the lung originates as an outpouching of the foregut. K-cells are more frequent in the lungs of fetuses, infants, and children; they proliferative in the event of pathologic conditions such as fibrosis. They occur in focal aggregates designated *neuroepithelial bodies*.[89] Because of their close association with nerves and blood vessels, and degranulation noted following hypoxia or hypercapnia, neuroepithelial bodies are recognized as chemoreceptors.

The designation *tumorlet* was applied by Whitwell[90] to foci of neuroendocrine cells resembling minute carcinoids. As opposed to neuroepithelial bodies, which are normal microscopic structures, tumorlets are usually multiple and measure up to 3 to 4 mm in diameter each. Although they have been observed in normal lungs, they are distinctly more frequent in cases of bronchiectasis and extensively scarred lungs. Their association with solitary or multiple peripheral carcinoids has also been noted.[15]

Histologically, tumorlets consist of small nests of neuroendocrine cells within bronchioles and fibrotic parencymal foci (Fig. 20-22). A relation to small bronchioles or air sacs may not be evident, and their appearance is that of an infiltrative process. However, the cells are histologically benign and no significant pleomorphism, mitosis, or necrosis is observed. Their relation to carcinoids has been further strengthened by the demonstration of argyrophilia and of neurosecretory granules with the electron microscope.

Tumorlets are almost always benign, and their demonstration is a resected specimen does not warrant further evaluation or treatment. However, a few cases with hilar node metastases are on record.[91–93] The patient reported by Rodgers-Sullivan et al.[92] development widespread disseminated carcinoid following the demonstration of tumorlets.

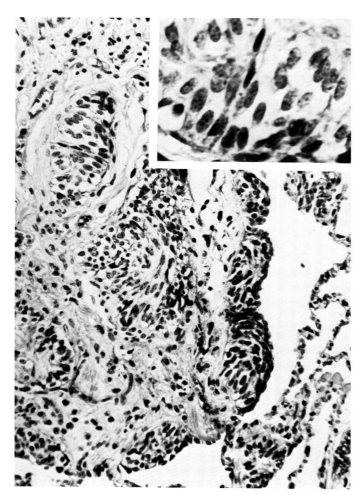

Fig. 20-22. Pulmonary tumorlet. A fibrotic pulmonary nodule contains clusters of oval to spindled carcinoid cells. Cellular detail in inset shows the finely granular nuclear chromatin and the absence of malignant features.

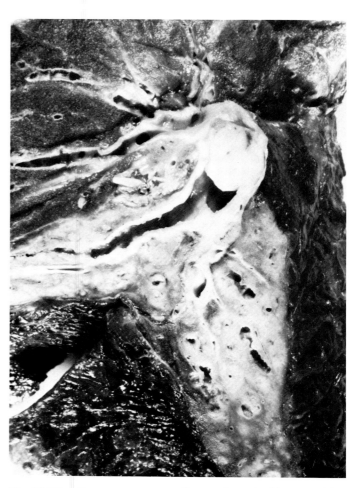

Fig. 20-23. Gross appearance of central carcinoid tumor. The tumor was a round, white-tan mass arising in the bronchus intermedius and had led to obstructive and suppurative pneumonia of the right middle and right lower lobes.

Carcinoid Tumors

Bronchial carcinoids represent 3 percent of all lung tumors (see Table 20-2). They occur in both sexes with equal frequency, but whites appear to be affected more frequently than blacks. The mean age of presentation of the tumor is 40 years, considerably earlier than in the other forms of lung cancer. No association has been noted with cigarette smoking or other carcinogens. A discussion of carcinoid tumors should include the following anatomic-clinical variants: central carcinoid tumors, peripheral carcinoids, and atypical carcinoids.[15,18,20]

Central Carcinoid Tumors. Approximately 90 percent of all carcinoid tumors arise in main, lobar, or segmental bronchi. Characteristically, they grow in a polypoid, exophytic manner within the bronchial lumen (Fig. 20-23). The tumor is a smooth, bosselated, fleshy mass covered by intact bronchial mucosa. On cut section, the color varies from gray to tan to dark red, largely depending on the degree of vascularization.

Only rarely is the tumor entirely exophytic. More frequently it infiltrates the bronchial wall and surrounding lung parenchyma in a dumbbell or iceberg fashion. Most carcinoids measure 2 to 4 cm in mean diameter. However, they vary from 2 mm nodules found incidentally at autopsy at bronchial bifurcations to masses as large as 10 cm in diameter.

Carcinoids are composed of uniform cells with abundant eosinophilic cytoplasm and centrally placed round to ovoid nuclei. The latter are vesicular, with well defined membranes and finely dispersed chromatin (Fig. 20-24). Mitoses are absent or very difficult to find. The tumor commonly grows in a mosaic pattern composed of nests of cells with an intervening delicate fibrovascular stroma. Another pattern, also common in carcinoids elsewhere,

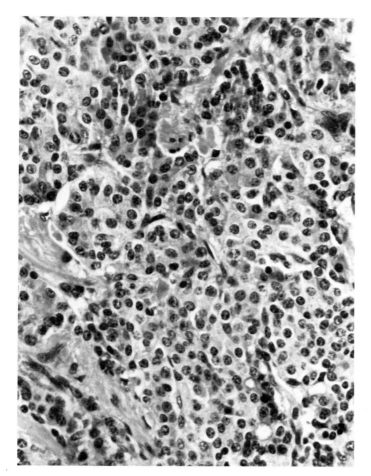

Fig. 20-24. Microscopic features of central carcinoid. This so-called mosaic or solid pattern is frequently seen in these tumors. Note the characteristic interlacing fibrovascular stroma.

neurosecretory granules measuring 50 to 500 nm in many of the cells (Fig. 20-25).

Central carcinoid tumors probably arise from K-cells located at the basal layer of the respiratory epithelium. These cells tend to be concentrated at the neck of bronchial mucous glands.[87] K-cells are also located peripherally in respiratory bronchioles, where they probably are the precursor of peripheral carcinoids. Central carcinoids give rise to metastases in only 5 percent of cases. The metastases are usually to regional lymph nodes. Distant metastases can also occur, and those in bone are characteristically osteoblastic. Liver involvement by metastases is associated with the carcinoid syndrome. The same slow-growing ability of the main tumor is shared by the metastases, and patients with such metastases may survive for many years.[15] Treatment of central carcinoids is surgical and usually involves lobectomy or pneumonectomy. Endobronchial resection is not practiced anymore because of the danger of hemorrhage and the inabil-

consists of cords, ribbons, and trabeculae; a combination of these two patterns is not rare. Prominent oncocytic features are seen rarely in some of these tumors. Another unusual histologic feature of carcinoid is a papillary configuration with carcinoid cells covered by Clara cells.[94]

The delicate fibrovascular stroma of carcinoids may undergo extensive hyalinization and, occasionally, osseous metaplasia.[95] Carcinoids with amyloid stroma are also on record.[96] The overlying bronchial mucosa is frequently intact or may show squamous metaplasia. Not surprisingly, cytologic examination of sputum is frequently negative in these patients, and only brushings of the tumor may succeed in harvesting characteristic carcinoid cells. Argyrophilic stains (Grimelius, Sevier-Munger) usually demonstrate numerous positive cells but argentaffin stains (Fontana-Masson) are infrequently and only focally positive. Mucin production can be seen in significant amounts in those cases with distinct acinar features. Ultrastructural studies demonstrate abundant

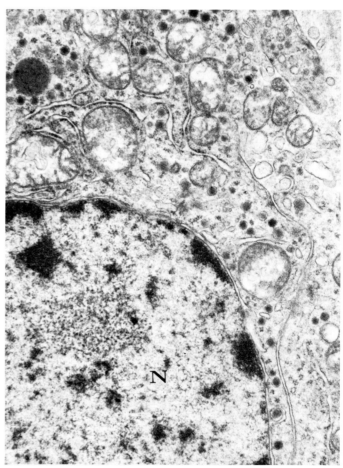

Fig. 20-25. Electron microscopic view of a central carcinoid cell. The cytoplasm contains abundant dense core granules of neurosecretory type. N, nucleus. (×10,000)

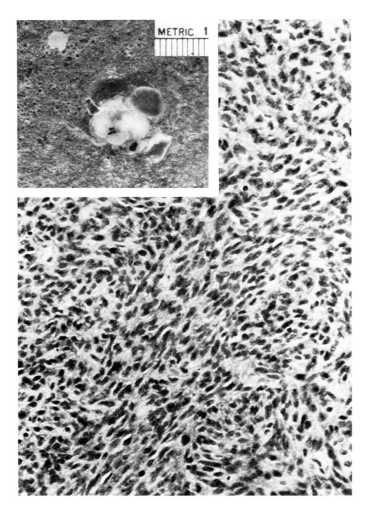

Fig. 20-26. Peripheral carcinoid with spindle cell features. Grossly, there were two independent lesions as shown in inset. Mitoses are more easily identifiable than in central carcinoids.

ity to remove the portion of tumor embedded in the bronchial wall.

Peripheral Carcinoid Tumors. Approximately 10 percent of pulmonary carcinoid tumors are peripheral nodules with no apparent connection to bronchi.[97–101] These fleshy, nonencapsulated nodules or masses have a pale tan to brown parenchyma. Such tumors can also be multiple (Fig. 20-26).

Histologically, peripheral carcinoid tumors may display the patterns noted in central carcinoids. Frequently, however, they have a more disorderly histology with a predominance of spindle cells. Thus, they resemble neurilemoma, smooth muscle neoplasms, and paragangliomas. Pigmented carcinoids due to the presence of melanin have also been described.[100,101] The clue to the diagnosis of peripheral carcinoids rests on the recognition of foci with the ''endocrine'' pattern of central carcinoids.

There is a greater variability in the appearance of nuclei, and mitoses are more easily found than in the central carcinoids. The tinctorial qualities with silver stains are comparable to those of central carcinoids, as is the presence of neurosecretory granules by electron microscopy. Peripheral carcinoids are treatable by surgical excision.

Atypical Carcinoid Tumors. Approximately 10 percent of carcinoids, whether central or peripheral, may exhibit disturbing gross and microscopic features that correlate with a more aggressive biologic behavior.[102–104] These atypical carcinoids are frequently larger than typical carcinoids and may show gross areas of necrosis and hemorrhage. Histologically, they are more pleomorphic and show large, hyperchromatic nuclei, frequent mitoses, and multiple foci of necrosis (Fig. 20-27). The designation

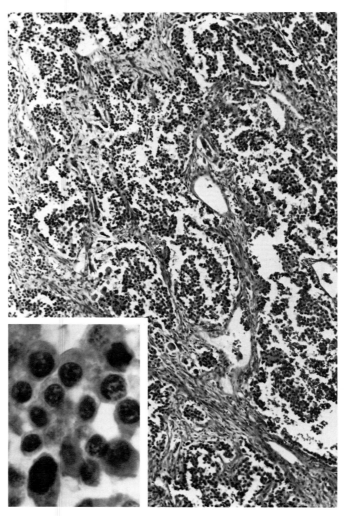

Fig. 20-27. Atypical carcinoid of bronchus showing considerable epithelial disarray and focal necrosis. The organoid structure of carcinoid is still recognizable. (Inset) The cells show marked pleomorphism and frequent mitoses.

well differentiated neuroendocrine carcinoma has been applied to this tumor by Gould et al.[88] While true atypical carcinoids exist, not infrequently examples of small cell carcinoma presenting as a peripheral nodule have been misinterpreted as atypical carcinoids.[73,74] Not surprisingly, such patients are in their 60s and have a significant history of smoking, and their tumors follow a highly malignant course. In a study by Arrigoni et al.[102] of 216 bronchial carcinoids, 23 (11 percent) were atypical carcinoids. Seventy percent of these patients developed metastases, and 30 percent died as the result of tumor. These investigators noted that 5.6 percent of typical carcinoids developed metastases as well. Therapy for atypical carcinoids is complete surgical removal if feasible, followed by radiation therapy to local areas containing metastasis. Those examples of peripheral small cell carcinomas mislabeled peripheral carcinoid should receive chemotherapy as for central lesions.

Other Neuroendocrine Proliferations

A proportion of small cell carcinomas of the oat cell and intermediate variants may express neuroendocrine differentiation by immunohistologic and ultrastructural criteria. To such tumors Gould et al.[88] have applied the designation *poorly differentiated neuroendocrine carcinoma* (Table 20-6). It is not possible by routine histologic stains to separate these small cell carcinomas from those lacking neuroendocrine differentiation. In the opinion of the majority of authors, the presence of neuroendocrine features does not seem to impart a particular biologic behavior.

Finally, a small proportion of squamous cell carcinomas, adenocarcinomas, adenosquamous carcinomas and large cell carcinomas, when studied by electron microscopy, have shown neurosecretory granules. Such tumors are designated *large cell neuroendocrine carcinoma or atypical endocrine tumor of the lung.*[105] Again, there is no practical gain in classifying these tumors by criteria other than their light microscopic appearance.

Rare Epithelial Tumors

Submucosal Bronchial Gland Tumors

Tumors of submucosal gland origin are listed in Table 20-7. The most important member of this group, the central carcinoid tumor, differs in several important aspects from the other tumors. (See the discussion under Usual Epithelial Tumors.)

Benign Mucous Gland Adenoma

This benign tumor,[106] also called papillary cystadenoma of the bronchus, bronchial cystadenoma and ade-

TABLE 20-7. Submucosal Gland Tumors

Benign
  Mucous gland adenomas
  Monomorphic adenoma (oncocytoma)
  Pleomorphic adenoma (mixed tumor of salivary gland type)
Malignant
  Central carcinoid
  Adenoid cystic carcinoma
  Mucoepidermoid carcinoma
  Acinic cell tumor
  Adenocarcinoma

nomatous polyp of the bronchus, represents a true adenoma arising from bronchial mucous glands. Grossly, it projects into the lumen of a major bronchus as a polypoid structure. Histologically, it is composed of dilated glandular spaces filled with mucin (Fig. 20-28).

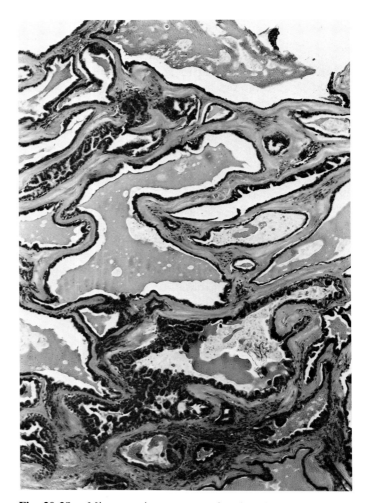

Fig. 20-28. Microscopic structure of an intrabronchial nodule composed of large, mucin-containing cystic spaces lined by flattened and low cuboidal epithelial cells. Because of the bland histologic features and lack of invasion of the bronchial wall, the lesion was interpreted as mucous gland adenoma or cystadenoma of bronchus.

Oncocytoma

A distinction should be made between carcinoid tumors with oncocytoid features and monomorphic adenomas composed of true oncocytes. The latter are large acidophilic cells with granular cytoplasm representing packed mitochondria when examined by electron microscopy. Examples of the former have been reported by Black[107] and Ghadially and Block[108]; of the latter by Fechner and Bentnick[109] and Santos-Briz et al.[110]

Pleomorphic Adenomas and Adenoid Cystic Carcinoma

Also called benign mixed tumors of salivary gland type, pleomorphic adenomas have been described in the tracheobronchial tree.[111] As their salivary gland counterparts, they may recur following inadequate local excision. Among the malignant tumors of bronchial gland origin, *adenoid cystic carcinomas*[112-115] represent the most frequent tumor after central carcinoid. They occur in the trachea and larger bronchi, particularly in the former, where they represent 20 to 35 percent of all cancers. Grossly, these tumors appear as polypoid masses or annular excrescences of firm, white tissue extending for several centimeters over the mucosa. They are notorious for their propensity to infiltrate the cartilaginous rings of the airways and invade surrounding tissues.

Microscopically, the complex glandular structures contain in their lumina both mucin and basement membrane material (Fig. 20-29A). The tumor frequently invades perineural spaces and can metastasize to distant sites. Its biologic behavior is peculiar and well known, with a tendency to recur locally in spite of treatment. Fifteen percent of patients die within 5 years, 45 percent at 10 years, and 80 percent at 20 years. In one patient, death from recurrent disease occurred 30 years after the initial treatment.[15]

Mucoepidermoid Carcinomas

Mucoepidermoid carcinomas[116-121] arise in bronchial submucosal glands of large bronchi and less frequently in the trachea. Their gross appearance is that of an exophytic polypoid mass up to 5 cm in diameter producing bronchial obstruction and atelectasis. Histologically, a distinction should be made between low-grade forms and the much rarer high-grade tumors.

Low-grade mucoepidermoid carcinomas show an admixture of large epidermoid cells and mucous cells. The former grow in sheets and show little keratin and few intercellular bridges. Interspaced among these cells are mucin-producing clear cells, arranged as single cells or in small clusters (Fig. 20-29B). There may be also a component of well defined, mucin-producing glands. Both epidermoid and mucin-producing cells are cytologically benign. Mitoses are absent or very difficult to detect.

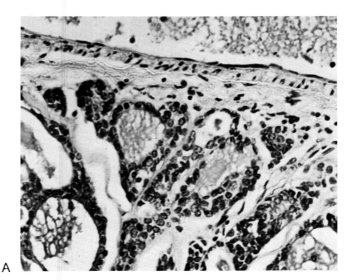

A

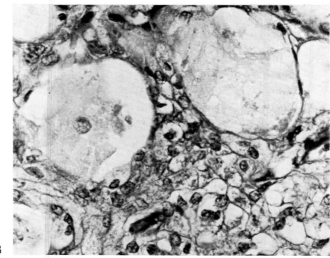

B

Fig. 20-29. **(A)** Adenoid cystic carcinoma (cylindroma) of bronchus extending to the adventitia of an artery. The glandular spaces of the tumor are filled with mucin and basement membranelike material. **(B)** Mucoepidermoid carcinoma of well differentiated type. The solid areas consist of polygonal cells in pavement-like arrangement and with minimal squamous differentiation. Mucin-filled spaces are interspaced among these cells. Note the absence of atypical features in either solid or glandular components.

In high-grade mucoepidermoid carcinomas, the epidermoid component shows distinct atypical nuclear features, focal necrosis, and frequent mitoses. A predominance of glands can be noted in other tumors. They produce mucicarmine-positive material and are composed of atypical cells. Some cases may resemble follicular carcinomas of the thyroid. Low-grade mucoepidermoid carcinomas are locally aggressive but lack a potential for metastases. In high-grade forms, the prognosis is always guarded and many of these patients develop metastases.[119,120] Rarely, a low-grade tumor may have a high-grade biologic potential, as in the case described by Barsky et al.[121]

Acinic Cell Tumor

This type of cancer is well recognized in major salivary glands. Two cases have been described in the lung.[122,123] We have seen another example of this tumor with extensive metastatic spread within and outside the lung (Fig. 20-30). Histologically, the tumor consists of sheets of lightly basophilic cells with finely granular cytoplasm and small, eccentric nuclei. There is extensive and uniform glandular differentiation. The cytoplasmic granules are positive with the PAS stain and negative with mucicarmine, Alcian blue, and argentaffin stains. Ultrastructural observations[122] support an origin of the tumor from ser-

ous cells of the submucosal glands. Salivary gland acinic cell tumors have been associated with metastases more than 10 years after removal of the primary. The follow-up period of the two pulmonary patients has been too short to rule out this eventuality. The case seen by us followed a highly malignant course.

Adenocarcinoma

Mention has already been made of adenocarcinomas arising in bronchial submucosal glands of larger bronchi and their tendency to form lobules and produce large quantities of mucin; they are probably not different in their clinical behavior from other adenocarcinomas of bronchial origin.

Bronchial Papillary Tumors

Also designated papillary tumors of surface epithelium, bronchial papillary tumors are exophytic masses with a distinctive papillary or verrucuous appearance. They occur in the trachea and bronchi and can be benign or malignant.[124-133] Different types are listed in Table 20-8.

Benign (Solitary) Papilloma

Patients with benign papillomas are usually adults.[124,125] The tumors arise in lobar or segmental bronchi and are visible by bronchoscopy. They are sometimes associated with bronchiectatic bronchi. Histologically, the great majority are squamous cell papillomas identical to those in the skin. In older patients, small foci of carcinoma in situ (CIS) may develop in the tumor itself or in the adjacent bronchial epithelium.[124]

Other papillomas may show transitional cell features and resemble tumors of the nasopharynx and paranasal sinus.[125] Still others may exhibit a combination of several types including columnar, cuboidal, undifferentiated multilayered, ciliated, and well differentiated squamous

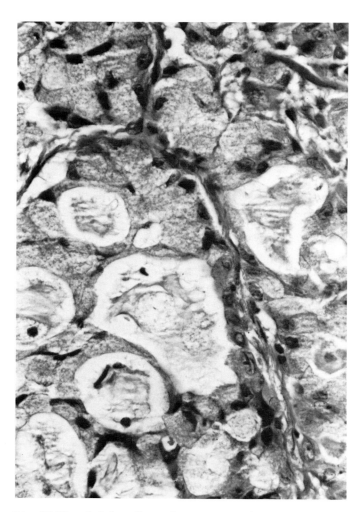

Fig. 20-30. Acinic cell carcinoma presenting as a bronchial mass with extensive lymphangitic spread within the lungs and at distant sites. The basophilic finely granular cytoplasm of the tumor cells is characteristic. (Courtesy of Dr. Margarita Salazar, Mexico City.)

TABLE 20-8. Bronchial Papillary Tumors

Benign (solitary papilloma)
  Squamous type
  Transitional type
  Mixed type
  Mixed type associated with underlying bronchial mucous gland
    adenoma
Potentially malignant
  Juvenile tracheobronchial papillomatosis
Malignant
  Squamous carcinoma
  Mucoepidermoid carcinoma
  Adenocarcinoma
  Transitional cell carcinoma
  (Metastatic thyroid carcinoma)

epithelium. The underlying stroma frequently shows granulation tissue with microscopic foci of hyalinization. Spencer et al.[124] described two papillomas of this type in association with underlying mucous adenoma of bronchus and made reference to a third case in the literature.

Papillomatosis of the Lower Respiratory Tract

Papillomatosis of the lower respiratory tract has also been referred to as juvenile laryngotracheal papillomatosis.[126-130] It is characterized by the presence of innumerable squamous papillomas of varying size studding the mucosa of trachea, bronchi, bronchioles, and even alveoli. The disease is seen in the first, second, and third decades

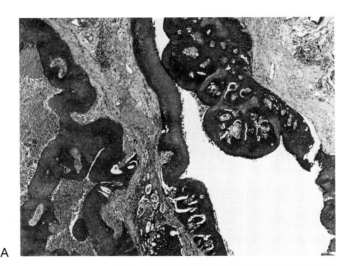

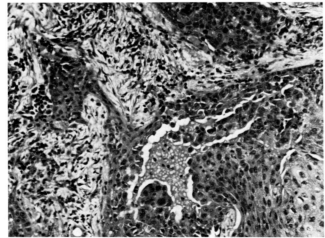

Fig. 20-31. Tracheobronchial papillomatosis evolving into squamous cell carcinoma. **(A)** Extension of papillomata into bronchi and distal air spaces. **(B)** Mediastinal node totally replaced by squamous cell carcinoma. The patient was a 31-year-old man who had a history of laryngeal papillomatosis since childhood.

of life and it is almost invariably associated with laryngeal papillomatosis.

An estimated 2 to 3 percent of patients with laryngeal papillomatosis will develop papillomatosis of the lower respiratory tract.[126] Those affected are younger than 5 years of age, have had numerous recurrent papillomas of the larynx and had been treated by tracheostomy rather than endoscopic removal of the lesions. The disease is suspected of being viral in origin but virus-like particles have been demonstrated only in the laryngeal lesion.[127]

Transformation of papillomatosis into squamous cell carcinoma has occurred in a handful of cases (Fig. 20-31A,B). One such case reported by Moore and Lattes[128] terminated in invasive squamous cell carcinoma after a 34 year course. Malignant transformation is likely to occur in patients who have received radiation therapy[129] and less likely in nonirradiated patients.[130]

Small series of papillary carcinomas forming exophytic intraluminal bronchial masses have been described by Smith and Dexter[131] and Sherwin et al.[132] (Fig. 20-32). The tumors were composed of fibrous fronds lined by neoplastic squamous epithelium resting on a basement membrane. There was only focal and limited superficial infiltration of the bronchial submucosa by tumor. Recognition of such cases is important because the prognosis is better than in the usual infiltrative squamous cell carcinoma.

Mucoepidermoid carcinomas can also arise in the surface epithelium of bronchi and grow in a papillary fashion. All five such cases described by Sniffen et al.[133] were low-grade malignant tumors comparable to their bronchial gland counterparts. *Adenocarcinomas* and *transitional cell carcinomas* can grow in bronchi and have papillary features; little is known of the biology of these tumors. As noted by Spencer et al.[124] and included in Table 20-8 for the sake of completeness, metastatic papillary thyroid carcinomas can infiltrate the trachea and bronchi and simulate a primary papillary tumor of the airways.

Mixed Epithelial-Mesenchymal Tumors

Two main tumors are included in this group: blastoma and carcinosarcoma. Other complex mixed malignant tumors and teratomas are conveniently included in this section. Both blastomas and carcinosarcomas are composed of an admixture of epithelial and mesenchymal elements. They are generally regarded as separate entities based on important differences such as the age distribution of patients, gross features, microscopic appearance, presumed histogenesis, and prognosis. Others believe that blastoma is a variant of carcinosarcoma, a concept supported by the observation of transitional forms showing a combination of both tumors.[134,135]

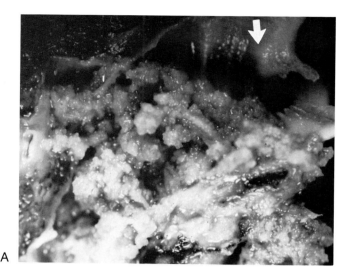

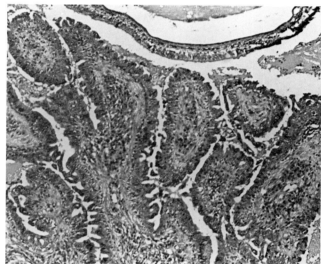

Fig. 20-32. **(A)** This malignant papillary tumor grew within large bronchi (arrow). **(B)** Histologically, it was composed of fibrovascular fronds and papillae lined by malignant transitional and squamous epithelium. No hilar node metastases were present in the resected specimen.

Pulmonary Blastoma

The average age of patients with blastoma of the lung is 40 years, and there is a distinct predilection for men in a ratio of 3 : 1 over women.[134–142] The lesions vary in size from 2 cm in diameter to massive. Most tumors are located in the periphery of the lung, and only rarely an intrabronchial pattern of growth has been documented. On cut section, they are soft and partly necrotic and their color is yellow, white, tan, or gray. The histologic appearance of the tumor is described as biphasic, that is, composed of a primitive, highly cellular, spindle cell stroma containing epithelial elements arranged in solid branching cords and glandular structures. The stroma that surrounds solid cords tends to be poorly differentiated and myxomatous. It is highly cellular and spindly when associated with developed glandular elements.

The glandular component of blastoma is formed by single or multilayered, nonciliated cuboidal or columnar epithelium. Vacuolization, particularly of the subnuclear region of the cells, is noted, and variable amounts of glycogen can be demonstrated in such cells. Mitoses are easily found in both the glandular and stromal components. The latter may also show foci of immature cartilage, bone, and striated muscle (Fig. 20-33).

Pulmonary blastomas have a striking histologic resemblance to the fetal lung. Originally, this led Barnard[136] to use the term "embryoma" for these lesions. Spencer,[137] who studied three such tumors in 1965, proposed the term *blastoma* analogous to neophroblastoma (Wilms' tumor). Based on Waddell's studies on organoid differentiation of the lung, Spencer conceptualized that the tumor arose in a pulmonary primitive mesenchyme or blastema

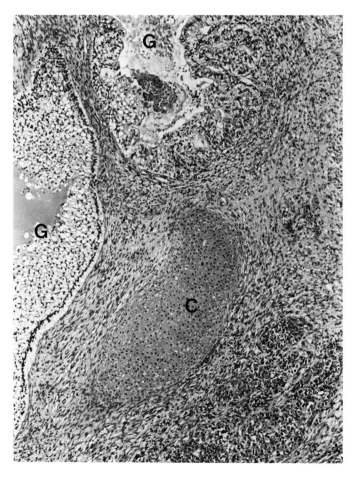

Fig. 20-33. Histologic features of blastoma. Same case depicted in Figure 20-20. A spindle cell mesenchyme with cartilagenous differentiation (C) contains many glandular structures composed of clear cells (G).

with the ability to differentiate toward epithelial and mesenchymal components. The current understanding of lung embryogenesis is inconsistent with this hypothesis. Blastomas are probably endodermally derived carcinomas with the ability to undergo metaplasia into mesenchymal elements such as cartilage, bone, and muscle. This concept is consistent with the observation of pulmonary adenocarcinomas purely composed of the epithelial portion of blastomas.[33–36] At least some examples of blastoma are truly congenital neoplasms.[141]

The biologic behavior of pulmonary blastomas is unpredictable. After adequate resection, the prognosis appears better than in usual bronchogenic carcinoma. As noted by Karcioglu and Someren,[138] the tumor recurred in one half of patients undergoing local resections, and distant metastases were noted.

Carcinosarcoma

Carcinosarcomas are bulky masses measuring 1 to 14 cm in greatest dimensions.[64,65,143–146] Two thirds of lesions are predominantly intrabronchial or combined endobronchial and parenchymal (Fig. 20-34). Such patterns of growth are common to carcinosarcomas in other hollow viscera. In the remaining one third of cases, the tumors occur in the periphery of the lung. The mean age of patients with carcinosarcoma is 64 years, 24 years older than for blastomas.

Histologically, the epithelial component is squamous cell carcinoma and the stroma represents fibrosarcoma in 75 percent of cases (Fig. 20-35). In the remaining 25 percent, the epithelial component is adenocarcinoma or undifferentiated carcinoma. The stromal spindle cells are larger than those in blastomas, and there is distinct collagen production. Foci of cartilage, osteoid, and other mesenchymal tissues have been described.

The prognosis of carcinosarcoma is less favorable than that of blastoma, although patients with the endobronchial pattern of growth do better than those with the peripheral form. There have been patients surviving for more than 3 years, and one for 6 years, following resection of the tumor.[15] The large majority of patients, however, develop disseminated metastases. As for blastomas, carcinosarcomas probably represent carcinomas with metaplastic transformation into mesenchymal elements. As such, they would represent one extreme of a morphologic continuum represented by carcinoma at the other extreme and by sarcomatoid squamous cell carcinoma in the middle.[64,65]

Teratomas

Teratomas of the lung can occur in children and adults.[151–153] They are usually intraparenchymal masses, although in the case reported by Bateson et al.,[153] the

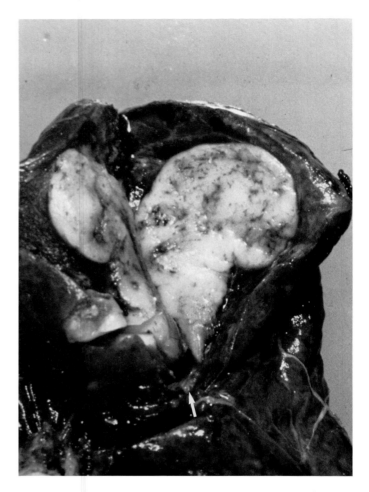

Fig. 20-34. Gross appearance of carcinosarcoma growing as a pale fleshy mass within the substance of the lung but arising in a bronchus (arrow).

teratoma grew endobronchially and was associated with bronchiectasis and bronchiolectasis. We have seen a case of the same description (Fig. 20-36).

Histologically, lung teratomas have a composition similar to that of mediastinal teratomas and include ectodermal, mesodermal, and endodermal derivatives. The tumors may be solid or cystic and may include a variety of tissues such as skin with adnexa, brain, GI epithelium, and pancreas. Benign teratomas are more frequent than malignant forms. They must be removed to alleviate the obstruction or pressure phenomena exerted on the lung.

Other Complex Mixed Tumors

There have been reports of pulmonary tumors composed of complex combinations of epithelial and mesenchymal tissues, such as the malignant mixed tumor reported by Vadillo-Briceno et al.[147] The tumor arose in the right middle lobe of a 67-year-old man and terminated in

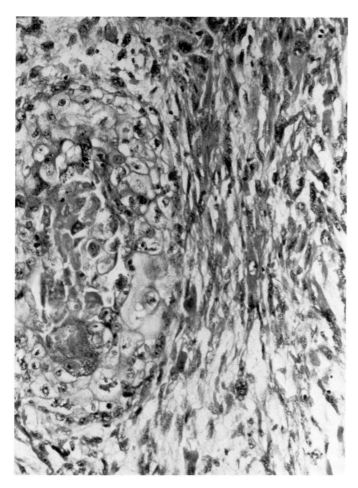

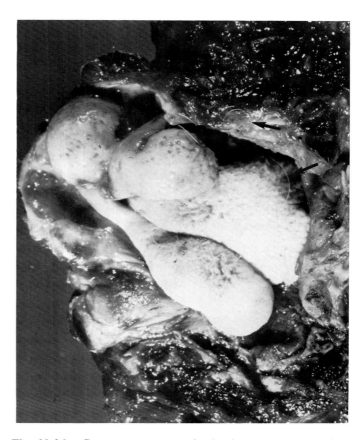

Fig. 20-36. Gross appearance of a benign teratoma growing entirely within a large bronchus that has become bronchiectatic. Histologically, the tumor was composed of mature endodermal, mesodermal, and ectodermal derivatives, including hairs (arrows).

Fig. 20-35. Histologic picture of tumor shown in Figure 20-34. Toward the left side of the picture there is a mass of squamous cell carcinoma. The mesenchymal element, to the right side of the picture, is made of a fibroblastic proliferation and few darker cells representing rhabdomyoblasts. The latter stained positively for desmin and myoglobin by the immunoperoxidase technique.

disseminated metastatic disease. Microscopically, the main tumor mass was composed of a mixture of three different carcinomatous components (small cell carcinoma, epidermoid, and adenocarcinoma) and several mesenchymal tissues (cartilage, adipose, and myxoid). The latter were mature and benign.

In the case reported by Edwards et al.,[148] the epithelial component consisted of squamous cell carcinoma, undifferentiated carcinoma, and clefts lined by bland epithelial cells. The supporting stroma was composed of pleomorphic sarcoma, fibrosarcoma, chondrosarcoma, osteosarcoma, and indeterminate mesenchymal tissue. Subcutaneous metastases showed poorly differentiated pleomorphic sarcoma.

Flanagan et al.[149] described the case of a 46-year-old man with a lung tumor designated squamous cell carci-

noma of the lung with osteocartilaginous stroma. Flanagan and co-workers ruled out the possibility of carcinosarcoma because of the absence of malignant features in the stromal components. Oyasu et al.[150] described the histologic features of a polypoid mass arising from the left lower lobe bronchus in a 57-year-old man. Microscopically, the tumor was characterized by mononuclear cells admixed with multinucleated giant cells similar to those seen in giant cell tumors at bone. Also found were typical squamous cell and spindle cell carcinoma. On the basis of their light microscopic and ultrastructural findings, Oyasu's group suggested that the tumor represented a metaplastic squamous cell carcinoma showing mesenchymal cell differentiation.

Nonepithelial Tumors

Lymphoproliferative and Myeloproliferative Lesions

Malignant lymphomas and other lymphoproliferative and myeloproliferative lesions represent, in our experience, 1.4 percent of all lung tumors (see Table 20-2). As a group, they are slightly more prevalent than all mesenchymal (soft tissue) tumors combined.

Freeman et al.[154] in 1972 noted that 24 percent of all lymphomas in the United States were extranodal in origin. Most commonly they arose in the stomach (24 percent), skin and small intestine (8 percent each), soft tissues (6 percent), bone and salivary glands (5 percent each), and colon and lung (4 percent each). For a long time our understanding of lung lymphomas was based on Saltzstein's classic paper[155] of 1963, but some of the major conclusions of this study are no longer tenable.

There is no doubt that our better understanding of lymphoid disorders of the lung is a reflection of the great advances in the field of lymphomas in general and of outstanding contributions[156–163] over the past decade. It seems no longer justifiable to fix in formalin whole open lung biopsies or autopsy tissues from patients suspected of having a lymphoid pulmonary lesion. A portion of the specimen should be snap-frozen for phenotyping of lymphocytes by monoclonal antibodies and for studies of clonality by DNA hybridization techniques. For better histologic detail a portion of the biopsy should also be fixed in mercuric chloride solutions (B-5 or Zenker's fixative). Attention to cell detail, including observation with the oil immersion lens, is crucial in typing lymphomas.

Secondary pulmonary involvement by systemic lymphoma is far more frequent than primary lung lymphoma and should be suspected from the clinical history and/or physical findings. As in lymph nodes, relapse of a primary or secondary lymphoma may show features different from the original tumor, such as large cell lymphoma in patients with lymphocytic lymphoma or Hodgkin's disease. Above all, infection should always be suspected in patients with known lymphoma and pulmonary infiltrates. Another important cause of pulmonary lesions in this situation is drug-induced disease, which is characterized, among other findings, by striking cytologic abnormalities of alveolar lining cells (see Ch. 19).

Whereas small lymphocytic lymphomas are frequently asymptomatic, mixed and large cell lymphomas usually present with fever, cough, sputum production, and chest pain, and the picture may progress to respiratory failure.[164] The radiographic picture is of little help in establishing the type of lymphoma, although mixed and large cell lymphomas tend to appear as bulky, frequently cavitated masses. For diagnostic purposes, it is probably correct to assume that the entire spectrum of lymphoma affecting lymph nodes also occurs in the lung. Thus, the principles of the working formulation[165] for the classification of nodal lymphomas should be extrapolated to lung lymphomas whenever feasible (see Ch. 12).

Both 'nodular' and 'diffuse' lymphomas occur in the lung, the latter being more frequent. The site of origin is most probably the bronchial-associated lymphoid tissue (BALT). However, in addition to the peribronchial and peribronchiolar location, they follow the lymphatic routes along the interlobular septa and pleura. This phenomenon of "tracking" along lymphatic routes is best appreciated on low power examination and should be interpreted in the context of the cellular composition of the infiltrate. By itself "tracking" is not diagnostic of lymphomas since it can be noted at the periphery of lesions with a clear inflammatory character.[163]

It has also become clear that the traditional requirement of monomorphism of the cellular population is too restrictive and that lymphomas can be mixed in composition (i.e., include small and large cells). They should, however, be uniform in composition from field to field, while reactive inflammatory lesions have a high topographic variability.[163] Moreover, T-cell lymphomas, of relatively late recognition, add peculiar features of 'polymorphism" including large numbers of plasma cells, eosinophils, granuloma formation and vascular invasion. Bronchiolitis obliterans with resulting endogenous lipid pneumonia is a frequent accompanying feature and adds to the cellularity and deceptively benign appearance of these lymphomas.

The most common form of primary lymphoma of the lung is *small lymphocytic lymphoma*. The gross appearance is that of single or multiple nodules or masses involving the parenchyma and pleura. On cut section they have a uniform, white, pink, or yellow appearance (Fig. 20-37). Necrosis, cavitation, and calcification are not features of these lesions. Invasion of the bronchi and vessels occur, and the cartilage of the former may be destroyed. The pleura is frequently infiltrated by the tumor with resulting effusion. Histologically, there is a dense accumulation of lymphocytes with obliteration of the alveolar architecture (Fig. 20-37). The lesions may be either diffuse or nodular, and in the latter case the nodules should not be interpreted as germinal centers. At the periphery of the mass, the infiltrate extends in an interstitial fashion. The regional lymph nodes may be secondarily involved.

The term *pseudolymphoma*[155] has been used in the past for lymphoid nodules or masses that were indistinguishable from well differentiated lymphocytic lymphoma. Histologically the infiltrate was described as mixed and composed of lymphocytes, plasma cells and histiocytes. Another well recognized feature of pseudolymphoma was the presence of germinal centers. The regional lymph nodes were characteristically uninvolved, and the prognosis following surgical excision was excellent. It is now clear that most if not all pseudolymphomas represent lymphocytic lymphomas with a very indolent course. The presence of germinal centers, which are probably residual in character, is no indication that the lesion is benign.[163]

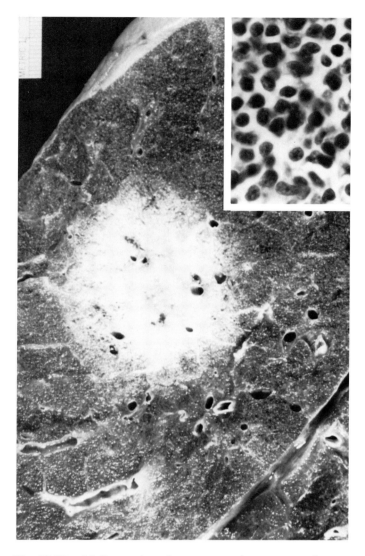

Fig. 20-37. Malignant lymphoma presenting as a round mass in the lung. There is central consolidation but at the periphery the tumor extends in an interstitial manner. (Inset) Histologically, the lesion is composed of a dense proliferation of small lymphocytes.

It has also become clear that many examples of well differentiated lymphocytic lymphomas have a predominant pulmonary presentation[160] and that the radiologic and pathologic features of such cases resemble lymphoid interstitial pneumonia (see Ch. 19). In common with differentiated lymphocytic lesions elsewhere, the rate of progression of these lymphomas is extremely slow and explains why some of these lesions were interpreted as inflammatory in the past.

A variant of well differentiated lymphocytic lymphoma is characterized by the presence of plasmacytoid lymphocytes. Identical lesions are seen in *Waldenström's macroglobulinemia*,[166,167] a systemic disorder characterized by an insidious clinical picture, monoclonal IgM eleva-

tions, and infiltrates of several organs. Radiologically, the process is characterized by diffuse reticular infiltrates, asymmetric reticulonodular lesions, and pleural involvement with effusion.

Well differentiated lymphocytic lymphomas, particularly those with plasmacytoid features, have an excellent prognosis. When localized they are amenable to surgical resection, and cures can be seen in about 80 percent of cases. In the remainder, local recurrence and dissemination occur.

Large cell lymphomas affect mainly adults. They present as large isolated or multiple masses which are sharply separated from the surrounding lung parenchyma. They cavitate in about 50 percent of cases. Noncavitary lesions can be firm or even hard and sclerotic on sectioning. Histologically, they are easy to recognize because of the presence of sheets of uniform large cells. Cytologically they can be composed of cleaved or noncleaved cells. The differential diagnosis include large cell undifferentiated carcinoma, metastatic renal cell carcinoma, melanoma, and seminoma.

Both large cell lymphomas and mixed small cell/large cell lymphomas have a worse prognosis than small lymphocytic lymphomas. When they present as isolated masses, however, they are amenable to surgical resection and cures have been noted. Pertinent to this discussion is the striking bilateral and extensive interstitial involvement of the lung in malignant histiocytosis[168] that can progress to respiratory failure.[169] Undifferentiated lymphomas of Burkitt's and non-Burkitt's type seldom affect the lung as part of a systemic disorder.

Secondary involvement of the lung is common in *Hodgkin's disease*. In the study conducted by Whitcomb et al.,[170] 26 of their 29 patients had the nodular sclerosing variant. In contradistinction, primary Hodgkin's disease of the lung is rare. Kern and colleagues,[171] in 1961, reported 4 patients and found 14 additional case reports in the literature. More recently, Yousem et al.[172] presented clinicopathologic observations in 15 such patients. About one half had clinical manifestations (B symptoms). The pulmonary lesions were single nodules in one third of the patients and multiple nodules in one half. The remainder had bilateral reticulonodular infiltrates or pneumonic consolidation. Patients with primary Hodgkin's disease of the lung should be staged and treated like other patients with the disease. Chemotherapy-induced remissions can be expected in about one half of these patients. Hodgkin's disease presenting as an intrabronchial mass has also been noted.[173]

Plasmacytoma

Rarely, tumor-like masses may develop in the lungs of patients with multiple myelomas. However, none of the 21 patients with myeloma and intrathoracic plasmacytoma studied by Herskovic et al.[174] had tumors of the lung. In a few documented cases, a true neoplastic pulmonary proliferation of abnormal plasma cells has been associated with abnormal serum globulins of the type seen in plasma cell dyscrasias. In the case reported by Kernen and Meyer,[175] the pulmonary lesion preceded the development of multiple myeloma. Extramedullary plasmacytomas in general, even when disseminated, have a better prognosis and respond better to therapy than multiple myeloma.[174–178]

Tumoral infiltrates can develop in the course of chronic myelogenous leukemia and they are designated as *granulocytic sarcoma* or *chloroma*. Bones and soft tissues are more commonly affected, but in the study by Liu et al.,[179] they were also present in the lungs in 5 percent of patients. Occasionally large tumor-like masses composed of fibrous tissue, myeloid tissue, and large numbers of megakaryocytes occur in *agnogenic myeloid metaplasia*.[180,181]

Other lymphoproliferative lesions of a localized character include *intraparenchymal lymph nodes,* usually appearing as coin lesions.[182–184] *Angiofollicular hyperplasia (Castleman's disease)* has been described in the lung.[185,186] *Intrapulmonary thymomas* have also been noted, and one must be certain that the pulmonary lesion is not a metastasis from a mediastinal thymoma. The cases described by McBurney et al.[187] and Yeoh et al.[188] were both on the right side, and there was no evidence of thymoma elsewhere. Secondary involvement of the lung by *angioimmunoblastic lymphadenopathy* can occur and is sometimes massive.[189,190]

Mesenchymal Tumors

Mesenchymal tumors are extremely rare in the lung. They can be benign or malignant and can present either as intrabronchial masses producing obstruction of the airways or parenchymal nodules or masses. Their gross and microscopic features are the same as those of similar tumors in other organs. Surgical removal of these lesions is almost always indicated for diagnostic and therapeutic purposes.

An important subset of mesenchymal lung tumors arises in the main pulmonary artery and its branches and it is generically designated as *pulmonary artery sarcoma*.[191–193] These tumors grow preferentially within the lumina of the major pulmonary arteries to produce obstruction of variable severity. They may grow through the walls of the vessels and invade surrounding structures, or they may extend proximally toward the pulmonary valve and outflow tract of the right ventricle. A centrifugal type of spread is sometimes noted with extension down to the level of small pulmonary arteries, capillaries, and interstitium, and with progressive entrapment of alveoli by the tumor.

One characteristic feature of pulmonary artery sarcomas is their rich symptomatology. Thus, they have been described in association with hemorrhagic tendency, pheochromocytoma-like manifestations, syncope, intractable heart failure, polycythemia, thrombocytopenia, and pericardial effusion. Most of these tumors eventually result in thromboembolic phenomena to the lungs, metastases, progressive obstruction of the pulmonary vascular bed, cor pulmonale, and death.

Pathologically, pulmonary artery sarcoma does not appear to represent a single specific entity, and it has been described under a variety of names, partly reflecting the pathologist's interpretation of such lesions. The terms include solid sarcomatous pulmonary artery, sarcoma, primary sarcoma, fibrosarcoma, leiomyosarcoma, mesenchymoma, osteosarcoma, intimal sarcoma, and spindle cell sarcoma.

Fibrous Tissue Tumors

Fibrosarcomas, together with leiomyosarcomas, represent, by far, the most common primary pulmonary sarcomas.[194,195] Fibromas also occur,[196] but they are much rarer than their malignant counterparts. In the case reported by Turner and Horne,[197] a clinical picture of diabetes mellitus was corrected on removal of a fibrosarcoma. Tumors designated fibromyxoma or myxoma are also on record.[19]

Smooth Muscle Tumors

Leiomyosarcomas are distinctly more common than leiomyomas.[194,195,198–201] In the case described by Wang et al.,[198] a pulmonary leiomyosarcoma arose in an arteriovenous fistula. As in fibrosarcomas, the prognosis of leiomyosarcomas depends on the size, location, and histologic features of the tumor. Bulky, necrotic masses invading surrounding tissues and exhibiting numerous mitoses have bad prognoses. Small intrabronchial lesions are frequently resectable and have a better outlook.

Skeletal Muscle Tumors

No convincing reports of rhabdomyomas arising in the lung exist to our knowledge. The case reported by Zipkin[202] in 1907 as "adenorhabdomyoma" probably represents a blastoma. On the other hand, 13 cases of rhabdomyosarcoma have been described up to 1981.[203] Rhabdomyosarcomas grow locally and are usually limited to the lung. However, extrathoracic metastases have been noted in three of 13 reported cases.

Adipose Tissue Tumors

Lipomas[204] and more rarely liposarcomas[205] occur in the lung. In their review, Bellin et al.[204] found 31 reported lipomas in the English literature and added two cases of their own. They noted that both of these tumors showed areas of cartilaginous metaplasia, but their features were different from those of fibrochondrolipomas (cartilaginous hamartomas). Wu et al.[205] described the case of a pulmonary liposarcoma in a child with adrenogenital syndrome, most likely a chance association.

Nerve Sheath Tumors

Intrapulmonary tumors of nerve sheath origin have been described in the lung and can be benign or malignant.[206,207] So-called granular cell myoblastoma arises in nerve sheath cells. It is usually benign, but occasionally malignant forms have been recognized. In the lung, such lesions occur in the airways as single or multicentric growths or in the lung parenchyma as coin lesions. In the remarkable case described by Majmudar et al.,[208] multiple granular cell tumors of the tracheobronchial tree were associated with respiratory insufficiency. The association of granular cell tumor of bronchus and hypercalcemia has been recently noted.[209]

Cartilaginous Tumors

Chondromas ,[210,211] chondroblastomas,[15] and chondrosarcomas[212,213] usually arise from tracheobronchial cartilage. It should be pointed out that these tumors originate in areas of pre-existing cartilage and should be sharply separated from cartilaginous hamartomas or fibrochondrolipomas.

Osteogenic Tumors

Liebow,[14] in the first AFIP lung fascicle, illustrated a benign osteochondroma of bronchus. Osteosarcomas are relatively more common and have been described by Nosanchuk and Weatherbee[214] and by Reingold and Amronin.[215] The latter authors described two cases and reviewed three other cases in the literature. All tumors were large, fleshy masses occupying the hilar and central regions of the lung. Histologically they were highly cellular and composed of fibrosarcoma, poorly differentiated mesenchymal tissue, osteoid, and immature cartilage. In four of the cases, there were metastases to lymph nodes and viscera.

Histiocytic Tumors

Katzenstein and Maurer[216] described a benign pulmonary neoplasm composed entirely of histiocytes and made reference to two identical cases in the literature. Malignant fibrous histiocytomas have been described by Viguera et al.,[217] Bedrossian et al.,[218] Kern et al.,[219] Silverman and Coalson,[220] and Lee et al.[221] At least three examples of *mast cell tumor* of the lung have been reported in the literature,[222] all of which were probably benign.

Vascular and Pericytic Tumors

Most benign hemangiomas of the lung actually represent arteriovenous fistulas and are discussed in the section on maldevelopmental lesions. However, a diffuse proliferation of capillaries, or *capillary angiomatosis,*[223] occluding pulmonary veins and leading to veno-occlusive pulmonary hypertension, has been described in the lung. One example of what was designated as *lymphangioma* was reported by Wada and colleagues.[224] Tank et al.[225] described one rare case of *glomangioma* of the lung and noted that by electron microscopy the cells of the tumor showed features of differentiation toward smooth muscle. Fabich and Hafez[226] recently described an identical tumor in the trachea.

Epithelioid Hemangioendothelioma

Epithelioid hemangioendothelioma designates a peculiar neoplasm originally reported by Dail and Liebow in 1975[227] and later by Dail et al.[228] in 1983. Originally, the tumor was thought to represent an intravascular bronchiolo-alveolar tumor (IVBAT).

Grossly, most of these nodules are 0.5 to 2.0 cm in diameter and are located beneath the pleura or in the lung parenchyma. On cut section, they are firm, smooth, and tan. Although unencapsulated they are well demarcated from the surrounding lung parenchyma. Microscopically, there is a distinctive zonal architecture. The center of the nodule is composed of hypocellular, hyaline connective tissue resulting in obliteration of the alveolar architecture. However, remnants of the pre-existing alveolar framework can be seen with reticulin and elastic stains. Peripherally, there are round to spindle cells in an eosinophilic matrix (Fig. 20-38). Another important feature of the lesion is the presence of vascular and/or gland-like structures composed of malignant cells. The latter can also be seen in the lumina of small pulmonary arteries and arterioles that have undergone thrombosis. As shown in subsequent studies,[229–232] the main tumor cell is endothelial in origin. As suggested by Weldon-Linne et al.,[231] an appropriate name for the lesion would be sclerosing angiogenic tumor.

The most important vascular neoplasm of the lung is currently *Kaposi's sarcoma*,[223–235] as it is diagnosed in about 5 percent of living patients with AIDS and in up to

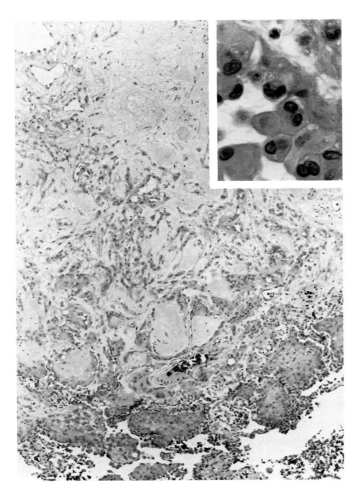

Fig. 20-38. Epithelioid hemangioendothelioma of the lung. Note the contrast between the hyaline core of the lesion (top) and the cellularity at the periphery (bottom). (Inset) In between there are confluent strands and vascular channels lined by large polygonal cells. Immunostaining for factor VIII was positive in these cells, indicating their endothelial identity. (Courtesy of Dr. Samuel Yousem, Pittsburgh.)

25 to 30 percent at necropsy. The tumors occur in the mucoid lining of the tracheobronchial tree, usually in patients with disseminated disease (skin, lymph nodes, GI tract) or in the lung parenchyma as hemorhagic patches that can replace part or all of a lung (Fig. 20.39). Involvement of the pleura can produce a bloody effusion.

Although questioned in the past, the occurrence of *primary angiosarcoma* of the lung has been recently supported by a few reports,[236,237] and we have recently seen one such case. Before this diagnosis can be rendered, however, metastatic angiosarcoma from the right side of the heart must be ruled out. Dense spindle cell proliferations with slit-like vascular spaces and tufting of endothelial cells within vascular structures characterize this tumor in the lung and elsewhere. Away from the main

masses of tumor the lumina of the vessels are filled by the same malignant cells. Immunoperoxidase stain in our case was focally positive for factor VIII.

A relatively large series of 24 patients with primary *hemangiopericytoma* of the lung was collected from the literature by Meade et al.[238] The tumors affected preferentially women of an older age group than men with the same lesion. Recurrence after surgery was noted in about one half of cases. A more recent study on the same tumor has been published by Yousem and Hochholzer.[239]

Combined Mesenchymal Tumors

Two tumors are considered in this category: so-called *cartilaginous hamartoma* or *fibrochondrolipoma* and *mesenchymoma*. Cartilaginous hamartoma or fibrochondro-

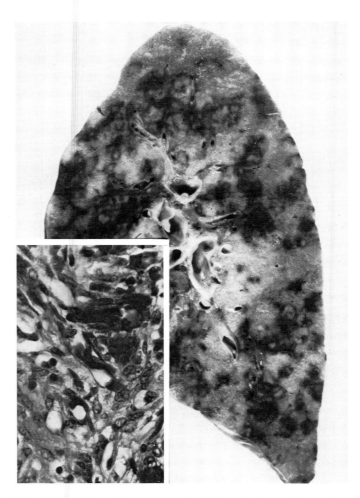

Fig. 20-39. Kaposi's sarcoma involving the lung of a patient with the acquired immunodeficiency syndrome (AIDS). Hemorrhagic, patchy infiltrates replace much of the lung parenchyma. (Inset) Characteristic spindle cell proliferation, vascular spaces, and red cell extravasation of this tumor. (Courtesy of Dr. Joan Mones, Miami.)

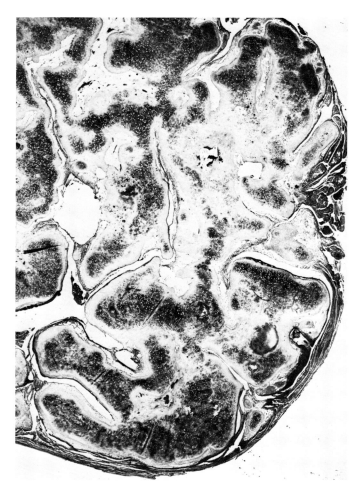

Fig. 20-40. Cartilaginous hamartoma or fibrochondrolipoma. The lesion arose in the periphery of the lung and consisted mainly of calcified cartilage transversed by cleft-like spaces. The latter were lined by benign bronchial epithelium.

lipoma was originally considered to represent a hamartoma or abnormal mixing of normal tissues but is currently considered a neoplasm.[240–244] Its basic component is a loose fibrous or myxoid mesenchyme that undergoes maturation toward cartilage, mature fibrous tissue, and fat in varying combinations (Figs. 20-40 and 20-41). A characteristic feature of the cartilaginous component is the presence of chondrocytes with large and irregular nuclei, but this should not be interpreted as indicative of malignancy. During its growth, the tumor entraps bronchial, bronchiolar, and alveolar epithelium, but this is not an intrinsic component of the lesion. By electron microscopy, the cells nearest the epithelium include mature fibroblasts and a population of glycogen-containing, primitive mesenchymal elements.[242]

Most fibrochondrolipomas occur in the periphery of the lung, unrelated to bronchi, and measure from a few

millimeters to 4 cm in diameter. Calcification and ossification frequently occur. Fifteen percent of the lesions grow endobronchially. Rarely, the lesions are multiple and cystic and may lack altogether the prominent cartilaginous component that characterizes the solitary lesion.

A triad composed of gastric epithelioid leiomyosarcoma, functioning extra-adrenal paraganglioma, and pulmonary chondroma has been described by Carney[243] in two young women. He also referred to a total number of 15 such patients in the literature. It should be noted that the chondroma in the triad represents the lesion currently under discussion.

A case of malignant mesenchymoma arising in the lung has been described by Kalus et al.[245] The tumor was composed of a mixture of undifferentiated malignant mesenchyme, osteosarcoma, chondrosarcoma, and rhabdomyosarcoma. The behavior of this tumor was quite aggressive and resembled that of carcinosarcoma.

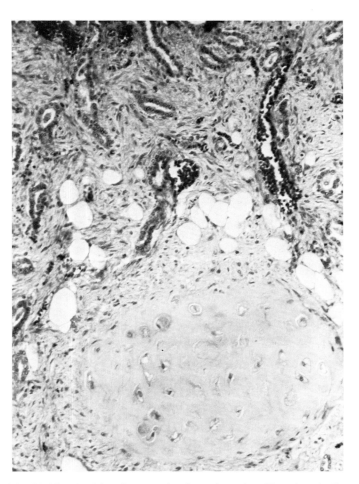

Fig. 20-41. In this microscopic view of another fibrochondrolipoma, the tumor is composed of cartilage, adipose and myxoid tissues, and contains trapped epithelium-lined tubules.

Miscellaneous Group

Miscellaneous tumors are composed of rare tumors of unknown or poorly understood histogenesis (Table 20-9).

Sclerosing Hemangioma

This lesion was originally delineated by Liebow and Hubbell[246] in 1956 on the basis of seven patients. Sporadic publications on the subject have appeared in the literature in the ensuing 26 years. A comprehensive analysis of 51 cases was published in 1980 by Katzenstein et al.[247] The question as to whether the entity represents an inflammatory lesion (postinflammatory pseudotumor) or a neoplasm seems to have been settled, in favor of the latter.

Eighty percent of these patients are adult women (mean age 40 years), and the lesion show a preference for the lower lobes. The patients are usually asymptomatic, and the tumor is discovered incidentally in routine chest radiographs. Grossly, the masses vary from 0.4 to 8.0 cm in diameter. On cut section they are meaty, rubbery, or finely granular. Shades of color vary from gray to tan, yellow, and hemorrhagic. In about 4 percent of the patients the lesions are multiple.

Histologically, Katzenstein et al.[247] described four patterns, usually occurring in combination: solid, hemorrhagic, papillary, and sclerotic (Fig. 20-42). In the solid pattern, sheets of round cells predominate. There is also entrapment of alveolar spaces as the tumor extends, and minute pools of red cells are found interspersed among the round cells. The hemorrhagic pattern is characterized by large, dilated blood-filled spaces resembling a vascular tumor. The papillary pattern is the best recognized and lends the tumor a distinct epithelial character. The sclerotic pattern is seen adjacent to the solid and blood-filled lesions and may contain entrapped alveoli simulating glands. There are also secondary inflammatory changes consisting of foreign body granulomas, cholesterol clefts, hemosiderin deposits, and foci of calcification and necrosis.

The structural complexity of these lesions explains the differences in opinion as to histogenesis when examined

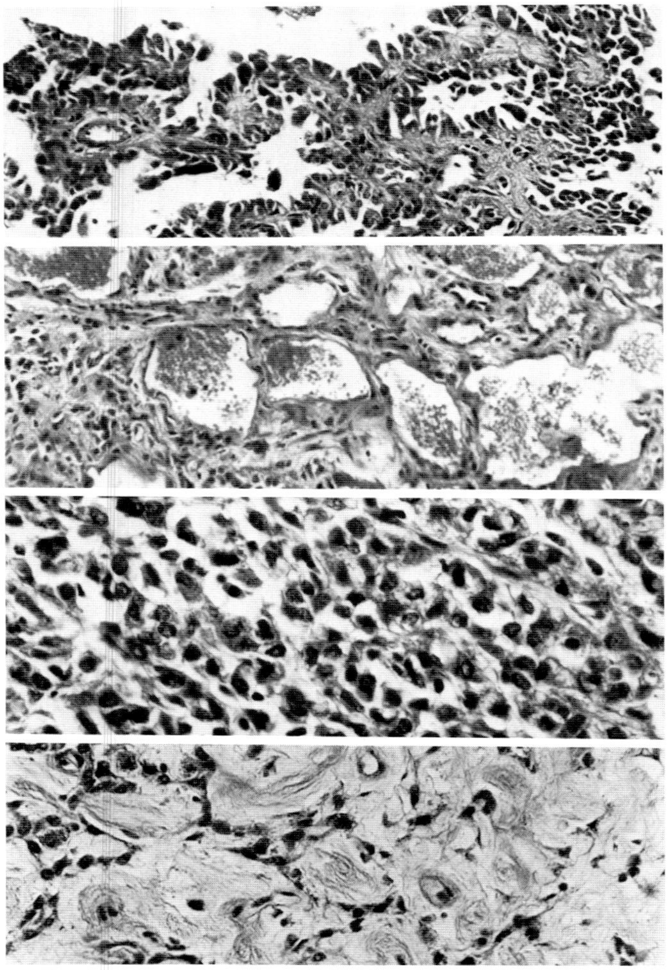

Fig. 20-42. The four characteristic histologic patterns observable in sclerosing hemangioma. (Top to bottom) Papillary, hemorrhagic (cavernous), solid (cellular), and sclerotic.

by electron microscopy. Thus, Hill and Eggleston[248] and Kennedy[249] believe the lesion is epithelial in origin, whereas Haas et al.[250] and Kay et al.[251] favor an endothelial nature. Katzenstein et al.[247] believe that the round cell is epithelial and probably arises in small bronchi, but they do not discount the possibility of a mesothelial source. Dail[19] recently reviewed extensively the results of immunohistologic studies to conclude that the cell of origin of this tumor remains unknown. However, Yousem et al.[252] are of the opinion that the tumor is epithelial in nature and expresses simultaneously bronchiolar epithelial and alveolar pneumocyte differentiation.

Benign Clear Cell Tumor ("Sugar" Tumor)

These tumors may occur in any lobe and appear radiographically as circumscribed peripheral masses ranging in

TABLE 20-9. Lung Tumors: Miscellaneous Group

Sclerosing hemangioma
Benign clear cell tumor ("sugar" tumor)
Melanoma
Paraganglioma
Minute meningothelium-like bodies (chemodectomas)
Intrapulmonary meningioma
Choriocarcinoma
Alveolar adenoma

size from 1 to 6 cm in diameter.[253–257] Grossly, the tumor can vary in color from tan to red, but the yellow color sometimes seen in renal cell carcinoma is absent. It never cavitates or calcifies, and necrosis is absent, except in the case of Sale and Kulander (254). Histologically, the tumor is composed of benign polygonal cells with clear cytoplasm and central, mature nuclei. The most distinctive feature of the lesion is the large content of glycogen demonstrable by PAS stain. Ultrastructurally, the glycogen occurs as monogranular, rosette-forming, and membrane-bound. Fat stains are negative. Another important feature is the sinusoidal blood supply (Fig. 20-43). The histogenesis of this peculiar neoplasm remains to be elucidated. A smooth muscle origin was considered unlikely by Liebow and Castleman.[253] Becker and Soifer[255] proposed a relationship to Kulchitsky cells and carcinoid tumors. Hoch and colleagues[256] thought the tumor represented a variant of leiomyoma or pericytoma, the latter

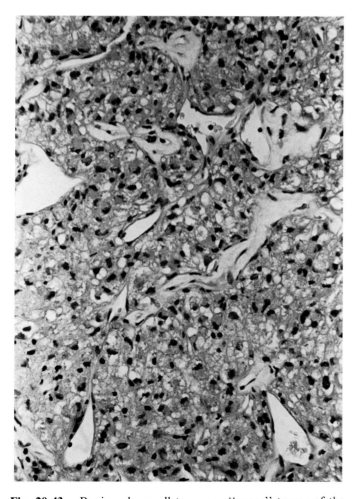

Fig. 20-43. Benign clear cell tumor or ''sugar'' tumor of the lung composed of clear and pink cells with characteristic sinusoidal vascular stroma.

interpretation supported by reticulin stains of the tumor. Benign clear cell tumors must be differentiated from metastatic renal cell carcinoma. The latter frequently contains areas of hemorrhage, necrosis, and thick-walled arterial vessels, and fat stains are positive. The lesion under consideration is invariably benign and surgical resection is curative.

Malignant Melanoma of Bronchus[258–261]

The discovery of a malignant melanoma in a bronchus raises the question of a primary lesion versus a metastasis.[258–261] Generally accepted criteria for primary pulmonary malignant melanoma are (1) the absence of current or past history of melanoma or any resected or cauterized skin lesion of unknown type; (2) a melanin-containing tumor with a pattern indicative of bronchial origin; (3) a long survival period without evidence of melanoma following resection of the pulmonary tumor; and (4) the absence of a primary site elsewhere at necropsy. Cases fulfilling the above criteria have been described. Surgery with or without adjuvant therapy constitutes the treatment of this lesion.

Paraganglioma and Minute Meningothelium-like Bodies

Peripheral nodules interpreted as paragangliomas have been the subject of a 1977 review by Singh et al.[262] They are difficult to distinguish reliably from peripheral carcinoids with spindle cell features. As noted by Singh et al.[262] the intimate association with an arterial wall would favor a paraganglioma. For Dail,[20] there is not yet convincing evidence for the existence of primary lung paragangliomas and the present author concurs with this opinion.

Minute multiple nodules in interstitial location, histologically resembling the carotid body, were described by Korn et al.[263] in 1960. Characteristically, the lesions are centered around venules and measure no more than 1 to 2 mm in diameter (Fig. 20-44). They are fairly common in autopsy material, and their association with thromboembolic disease and other chronic processes has been noted.[264] Costero et al.[265] thought these lesions were mesothelial in origin. Kuhn and Askin[266] and Churg and Warnock[267] noted that the cells lacked the characteristic neurosecretory granules of paraganglioma and that their ultrastructural features resembled those of meningioma.

Intrapulmonary Meningioma

A few examples of primary meningioma of lung have been described.[268,269] As for other forms of extracranial meningiomas, the origin of such tumors is controversial.

748

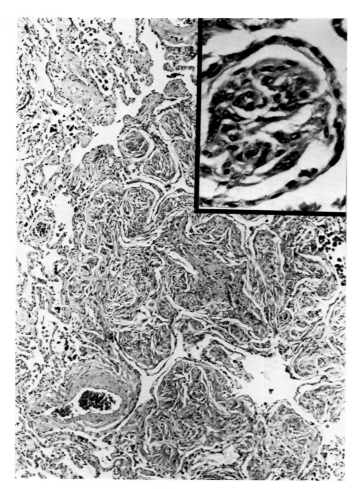

Fig. 20-44. In this rare example there were more than 500 meningothelium-like bodies in the lungs (chemodectomiasis). (Inset) Note the relation of the proliferating cell nests to vessels and their exquisite interstitial location.

Conceivably, a source of origin could be the minute meningothelium-like proliferation already alluded to.

Choriocarcinoma

Primary extragenital choriocarcinoma often develops in midline structures like the retroperitoneum, mediastinum, and pineal region, and in viscera such as the stomach or gallbladder. A primary lung origin is exceptionally rare and undifferentiated carcinoma with giant cell features must be excluded. Increased serum human chorionic gonadotropin (HCG) is of little diagnostic help, since it can also be elevated in cases of undifferentiated large cell carcinoma.

Two instances of primary pulmonary choriocarcinoma have been described by Hayakawa et al.[270] In one patient, a 45-year-old man, the tumor measured 7 × 6 × 5 cm and arose in the left upper lobe. The second patient, a 57-

year-old man, had a 10 × 7 × 6.5 cm tumor located in the right lower lobe. Both patients had gynecomastia, increased HCG levels, and disseminated metastases at necropsy. We have seen another patient with a huge choriocarcinoma of the right upper lobe which was extensively necrotic and hemorrhagic. Metastases to the brain were soon noted.

Alveolar Adenoma

The designation *alveolar adenoma* was recently applied by Yousem and Hochholzer[271] to a group of six isolated pulmonary nodules of a benign character. The lesions could be shelled out with ease and measured 1.8 cm in average diameter. Microscopically they were composed of multiple cystic spaces filled with pink serous or floccular material or by blood (Fig. 20-45). The intervening septa were composed of loose connective tissue con-

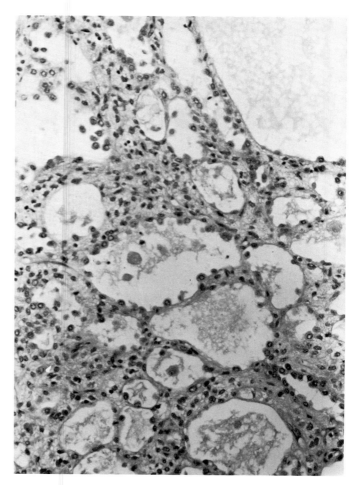

Fig. 20-45. Alveolar adenoma composed of numerous cystic spaces containing floccular fluid. The intervening stroma contains lymphocytes and plasma cells. (Courtesy of Dr. Samuel Yousem, Pittsburgh.)

taining lymphocytes, plasma cells, and macrophages. The lining of the cysts was largely inapparent or consisted of flattened cells. Although the same lesion has been previously interpreted as lymphangioma,[224] much remains to be learned of its histogenesis.

Secondary (Metastatic) Tumors

Rarely, nonpulmonary tumors invade the lung by contiguity, simulating a primary pulmonary cancer.[272] More frequently, however, the tumor reaches the lung via the bloodstream or the lymphatic circulation. It should be pointed out that, in addition to its dual blood supply, the lung is the only organ that receives the entire cardiac output. It is also the final destination of the lymphatic circulation. Thus, ample opportunity exists for tumors arising almost anywhere in the body to metastasize to the lung. This occurred in 30 percent of cadavers with extrapulmonary cancers studied at necropsy by Willis,[273] in 50 percent of patients in the series of Rosenblatt et al.,[274] and in 53 percent in Braman and Whitcomb's study.[275] Cavitation is a common occurrence in metastatic lung tumors.[276]

Discrete metastatic lesions are usually bilateral and multiple and range in size from barely visible to large masses replacing an entire lobe or more. They can occur anywhere in the lung but a predilection for the bases exists. Often, it is impossible to guess correctly the primary source of a metastasis, perhaps with the exception of the brown-black nodules of malignant melanoma, the hemorrhagic and necrotic masses of choriocarcinoma, and the moist, soft, and fleshy masses of sarcomas. The latter characteristically invade the pleura as fungating masses.

Metastases can be single and confined to a lobe, in which case they are amenable to surgical resection. In the study by Habein et al.,[277] 17 percent of 96 patients were alive and free of disease 3 or more years after surgical resection of metastases. These were carcinomas in 73 patients, the most common primary sites being large intestine and breast. Twenty patients had sarcomas, commonly osteosarcomas and fibrosarcomas.

Although the propensity of sarcomas to metastasize early in the course of the disease is well recognized, most favorable surgical results are seen with these lesions, particularly when well differentiated.[277–280] Thus, in the study by Martini et al.,[280] resection of metastatic sarcoma, even when multiple and bilateral, resulted in prolonged survivals in 25 percent of patients.

The value of surgical treatment in metastatic renal cell carcinoma to the lung has been analyzed by Katzenstein et al.[281] Best results were noted with isolated or unilateral metastases and the 5 year survival rate was in the 30 to 40

percent range. Adverse prognostic factors included multiple lesions and involvement of tracheobronchial lymph nodes. This was also Ramming's[282] conclusion in another review. This author also noted the poor survival of patients with metastatic malignant melanoma. Microscopic involvement of bronchi of any size is a common finding in cases of metastatic lung disease. Grossly recognizable metastases to major bronchi, resembling primary bronchogenic carcinoma, are seen, however, in only 2 to 5 percent of patients.[283] The most frequent tumors responsible for this type of lesion are renal cell carcinoma (40 percent) and colorectal cancer (18 percent).

One of the most dramatic forms of metastatic involvement of the lung is *lymphangitic carcinomatosis*.[284] Cancer of the breast accounts for one fourth of these cases, but other sources include stomach, pancreas, prostate, ovary, colon, and uterus. About one half of these patients are dead within 3 months of diagnosis and almost 90 percent within 6 months. With chemotherapy this bleak picture has been altered and patients surviving up to 2 years are on record.

Before leaving the subject of metastatic lung disease, reference should be made to the controversial entity recognized as *benign metastasizing leiomyomas* or *fibroleiomatomatous hamartomas*.[285] The process is characterized by multiple pulmonary nodules, histologically composed of interstitial infiltrates of well differentiated smooth muscle, that in their growth incorporate slit-like spaces lined by benign respiratory epithelium. The great majority of patients with this disease are adult women with a history of previously resected uterine leiomyomas. On review, some of the latter proved to be low-grade leiomyosarcomas. In other patients, inadequate sampling of the uterine tumors was probably responsible for the absence of malignant features.

Wolff et al.[285] reported three male patients and six women with this condition. In the men, the primary source of tumor was respectively the saphenous vein, diaphragm, and soft tissues. The uterus was the common source of tumor in the women. According to these investigators, the term fibroleiomyomatous hamartoma should be discarded.

Benign metastasizing leiomyoma behaves in a benign fashion but, in cases, the nodules encroaching on the functional lung parenchyma lead to respiratory insufficiency and death of the patient. One other interesting aspect of the lesion is its hormonal dependency. In the case described by Horstmann et al.,[286] the lesions were noted to grow in a pregnant patient and to regress spontaneously after delivery. This observation led in another study[287] to the treatment by oophorectomy of one patient with benign metastasizing leiomyoma and another patient with lymphangioleiomyomatosis, and the results were encouraging.

Pseudotumors (Plasma Cell Granuloma)

Plasma cell granuloma[288–295] has also been referred to as postinflammatory pseudotumor, xanthoma, fibroxanthoma, xanthomatous pseudotumor of lung, and histiocytoma. Plasma cell granulomas are usually asymptomatic masses discovered in routine chest roentgenograms. In addition to their pulmonary location they have also been described in the pleura, mediastinum, and many other extrapulmonary locations. They grow intrabronchially as sessile or polypoid masses. More frequently they are found in close juxtaposition with large bronchi, which they compress and distort but do not penetrate. Rarely, the lesion can present as multiple masses.

More than two thirds of the patients with plasma cell granuloma are under 30 years of age. In children under the age of 10 years this represents the most common localized pulmonary process. Radiographically, the masses may be static or increase slowly in size. Cultures of the lesions for bacteria and fungi are consistently negative, as are skin tests.

Microscopically, the lesions are well circumscribed but lack a fibrous capsule. They are composed of mature plasma cells and lymphocytes in a stroma rich in granulation tissue, fibroblasts, foamy histiocytes, and prominent reticuloendothelial cells. Extensive hyalinization of the stroma and entrapment of plasma cells in groups and rows are characteristic features of this lesion (Fig. 20-46). Large numbers of foamy histiocytes characterize certain lesions to which the term *xanthoma* or *fibroxanthoma* has been applied. Invasion of pulmonary vessels by the inflammatory cells and intimal occlusion by fibrosis may mimic a primary lung vasculitis.[292]

Occasionally, the lesions may display a prominent vascular component consisting of numerous hyalinized blood vessels in a loose mesenchymal component.[293] The richness in plasma cells has been considered by some as indicative of plasmacytoma, a term best reserved for the malignant lesion. The prognosis in plasma cell granuloma is excellent, and the treatment is surgical resection.

Spencer[294] introduced the term *plasma cell–histiocytoma complex* to encompass many examples of plasma cell granuloma having a spindle cell component of significance. In some cases the density of the latter component and the presence of a distinct storiform pattern do impart a histiocytic appearance. Spencer believes that at one end of this spectrum plasma cell granuloma blends with malignant fibrous histiocytoma, and two cases in his series behaved in a malignant fashion. However, the possibility exists that some or most of these florid spindle cell proliferations actually represent a reactive process composed mainly of myofibroblasts.

In a recent study of 32 examples of inflammatory pseudotumors of the lung, Matsubara et al.[295] noted that

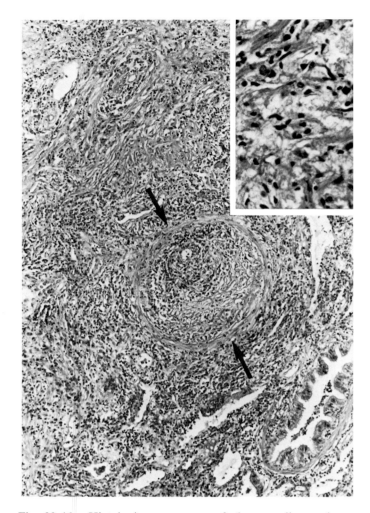

Fig. 20-46. Histologic appearance of plasma cell granuloma with prominent fibrous stroma and blood vessel invasion by plasma cells (arrows). (Inset) Focally, there were collections of foamy histiocytes, a finding that explains the designation fibroxantoma sometimes applied to this lesion.

only 12 percent of the cases had the classic lymphoplasmacytic configuration. Forty four percent were composed of organizing pneumonia and intersitial fibrosis, and a similar proportion were of the fibrous histiocytoma type described by Spencer.[294] They clearly distinguished the latter type from malignant fibrous histiocytoma.

INFLAMMATORY PROCESSES

The discovery of an isolated nodule, mass, or parenchymal infiltrate on a chest radiograph raises the common diagnostic dilemma of malignant versus benign process. Much has been written on this subject, particularly on the decision to operate or not.[296–298] Many of these

TABLE 20-10. Inflammatory Processes of a Preferentially Localized Character

Granulomatous and histiocytic processes
  Tuberculosis (tuberculomas, cavities)
  Atypical mycobacterial infections, malakoplakia, Whipple's disease
    Major fungal infections (histoplasmosis, coccidioidomycosis, cryptococcosis)
  Other processes produced by yeasts
  Lesions due to filamentous or hyphae-forming fungi
  Mycetomas (fungus balls)
  Parasites
  Noninfectious granulomas
Infectious pneumonia
  Mycoplasma pneumonia
  Viral
  Bronchiolitis obliterans
  Bacterial
Suppurative processes
  Actinomycosis
  Nocardiosis
  Bronchiectasis
  Lung abscesses

lesions are inflammatory in nature, particularly granulomatous, and it is the pathologist's task to establish their etiology. Inflammatory processes pertinent to the present discussion are listed in Table 20-10.

Granulomatous and Histiocytic Processes

The proportion of solitary lung lesions found to be granulomas varies considerably in the literature and can be as high as 63 percent[297] or even 75 percent[298] in places where certain fungal diseases are endemic. In general, carcinoma of the lung as a solitary nodule is rare in patients less than 35 years of age, but its frequency increases progressively to 70 percent in patients in the eighth decade and close to 100 percent in the ninth decade.

Ulbright and Katzenstein investigated the morphologic features and etiology of 86 necrotizing granulomas appearing as solitary pulmonary masses. Thirty of their 86 patients (35 percent) showed acid-fast organisms, and fungi accounted for another 35 percent of the cases. Histoplasmosis was by far the most common, and it was found in 24 of the 30 fungal lesions. Five other lesions were due to coccidioidomycosis and one to cryptococcosis. There were 22 necrotizing lesions considered to be granulomatous in which no etiologic agent could be demonstrated. The authors warned of the possibility of erroneously interpreting some of these as examples of pulmonary angiitis and granulomatosis, a group of disorders to be discussed later. They did find a case of Wegener's granulomatosis, two examples of hyalinizing granulomas, and one lesion with fragments of a helminth.[299]

As has been the experience of others, Ulbright and Katzenstein[299] noted that cultures of the granulomas for *Mycobacterium tuberculosis* and fungi were distinctly less helpful in the identification of the agent than direct tissue examination with the Ziehl-Neelsen and Grocott-Gomori methenamine silver stains. The study of two tissue blocks that included the necrotic center of the lesion was sufficient to find the etiologic agent in most cases. In negative cases with histologic features suggestive of infection, the study of additional material is warranted.

Overall, mycobacterial infections are responsible for a majority of solitary necrotizing granulomas of the lung. They are tuberculous in origin in a great proportion of patients, but atypical mycobacterial processes have increased because of the acquired immunodeficiency syndrome (AIDS). Two localized manifestations of tuberculosis are pertinent to this discussion—tuberculomas and cavities.

Tuberculomas

Tuberculomas are round or irregular masses, usually subpleural in location and more frequent in the upper lobes.[300,301] Their size varies considerably and some attain a diameter of 6 cm. On cut section, most tuberculomas exhibit extensive caseous necrosis, calcification, and encapsulation. Some lesions exhibit concentric rings of fibrotic and calcified tissue, a feature also found in some fungal lesions.

Acid-fast organisms are best demonstrated in the necrotic core of the granulomas. At the periphery, chronic inflammatory and granulomatous features are best seen. Both caseating and epithelioid granulomas occur and there is frequently a vasculitis involving arteries and veins. Bronchi and bronchioles may also show necrotic and granulomatous changes.

Tuberculomas represent primary or secondary infection, and it is sometimes impossible to pinpoint the difference. Tuberculomas of primary infection are the result of a well resisted primary infection during which the proliferation of bacilli becomes arrested due to the development of immunity, and the lesion becomes encapsulated. The caseous material gradually becomes inspissated, calcified, ossified, or even resorbed, leaving no trace. During the primary infection the draining lymph nodes of such lesions are also involved, and their size is larger than the pulmonary focus.

Tuberculomas resulting from reinfection are more irregular in outline than primary nodules. They can be observed in the lungs of adults bearing a calcified primary complex. Calcification is less marked and ossification less frequent than in the primary lesion. The term *Simon foci* is applied to caseous nodules with a marked tendency to calcification that develop in the apical portions of the lungs of children as the results of hematogenous dissemination of bacilli after the primary infection has been established.

Tuberculous Cavities

Areas of extensive caseation in secondary tuberculosis may communicate with a bronchus, empty their contents, and give rise to a cavity.[302,303] Early cavities have thick, ragged walls filled with caseous material and abundant bacilli. Later, they become more discrete and develop a fibrous wall. They may close, eventually, either spontaneously or as the result of treatment. Closed healing is most likely to occur in small cavities up to 1 to 2 cm in diameter and follows closure of the communicating

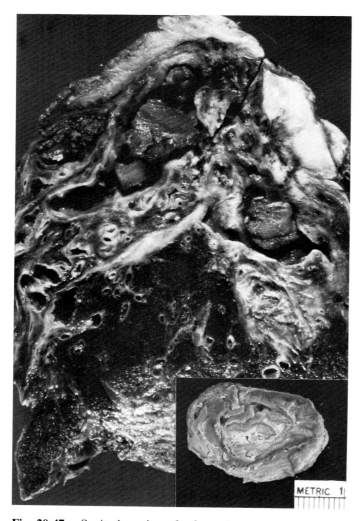

Fig. 20-47. Sagittal section of a formalin-fixed right lung in a case of healed secondary tuberculosis. The interconnecting cavitary lesions contain several fungal balls and masses composed of aspergilli. The inset shows one fungus ball with characteristic concentric layering.

bronchus by inflammation and fibrosis. Air and fluid contents are resorbed and the cavity is sealed off by apposition of its inner lining, composed of granulation tissue; the end result of the process is a star-shaped scar.

Larger cavities can heal while retaining abundant caseous material within them. Grossly, they can be misinterpreted as granulomas. They may eventually establish connection with a bronchus and release their contents, with reactivation of the process. Open healing of cavities occurs frequently following specific chemotherapy. The cavity becomes a spherical cyst filled by air under tension, and a bronchus will nearly always be found entering into it.

Cavities that have healed in the open state are lined by granulation tissue and focally by squamous epithelium extending from the communicating bronchus. They may be secondarily complicated by infection or by colonization by saprophytic fungi (fungus ball) (Fig. 20-47).

According to most authors,[304,305] there are no characteristic gross or microscopic features that permit differentiation of tuberculous lesions from those produced by atypical mycobacteria. In our experience the severity and extent of vascular involvement can be so striking in some atypical mycobacterial lesions as to resemble a vasculitis (Wegener's granulomatosis). Another feature suggestive of atypical mycobateria in Ziehl-Neelsen preparations is the presence of longer, thicker, more bent and coarsely beaded organisms than typical *M. tuberculosis*. Ultimately, the difference must be established by cultures.

Atypical Mycobacterial Infections, Malakoplakia, and Whipple's Disease

Atypical Mycobacterial Infections

Since the advent of the acquired immunodeficiency syndrome (AIDS), atypical mycobacterial infections of the lung and other organs have become more prevalent than before and several reviews on the subject are available in the literature.[306-310] The most important atypical mycobacteria in humans are *M. avium intracellulare* and *M. kansasi*.

Atypical mycobacteria processes in AIDS patients, whether pulmonary or extrapulmonary, appear as bland yellow to gray infiltrates composed of histiocytes containing myriads of organisms, resembling the histiocytes of lepromatous leprosy. Necrosis and granuloma formation are not main features of these lesions.

Malakoplakia

Classically, malakoplakia designates soft yellow tumor-like plaques in the bladder and other organs.[311-314] Five cases of malakoplakia involving the lung have been described. Grossly the lesion appears as single or multiple gray-tan or yellow nodules that may extend through fissures. Histologically the lesions are composed of sheets of vacuolated histiocytes containing PAS-diastase-positive granules in their cytoplasm (Von Hansenman's histiocytes). The presence of round intracytoplasmic blue-gray target-like or owl-eye Michaelis-Guttmann bodies that stain positively for iron and calcium is characteristic of this process.

Whipple's Disease

Classically, the lesions of Whipple's disease affect the submucosa of the small intestine (jejunum) and mesenteric lymph nodes. Rarely the lung may be involved in Whipple's disease, even preceding the characteristic intestinal symptoms of this disorder.[315,316] In the case described by Winberg et al.,[316] peribronchial and parenchymal nodules were composed of typical strongly PAS-positive, enlarged histiocytes containing bacilliform structures by electron microscopy. The differential diagnosis includes atypical mycobacterial infection and malakoplakia.

Major Fungal Infections

Histoplasmosis

Histoplasmosis is worldwide in distribution but more heavily endemic in the central United States.[317] The manifestations of the disease pertinent to this discussion are the cavities and the fibrotic and granulomatous masses usually referred to as *histoplasmomas*. Most of these lesions arise around a primary focus containing necrotic tissue and yeast forms, and surrounded by a fibrotic capsule. Calcification of the pulmonary lesion and hilar-mediastinal lymph nodes is usually more marked than in tuberculosis. Some cases show the distinctive elaboration of collagen in concentric rings.

Cavities are described in chronic pulmonary histoplasmosis, usually in association with emphysematous bullae. These cavities occur in the apex of the lung, and their inner linings contain significant numbers of organisms. *Histoplasma capsulatum* is best demonstrated in tissues by the Grocott-Gomori methenamine silver stain. The organism appears as an oval budding yeast with delicate capsule, measuring 1 to 5 μm in diameter.

Coccidiodomycosis

The coccidiodal granuloma, coccidioidoma or coccidioma, follows the evolution of primary coccidioidal pneumonia to a spherical, dense nodule that tends to occur in the mid-lung fields within 5 cm of the hilum.[318,319] Most frequently, the lesion consists of a single nodule 1 to 4 cm in diameter. Multiple nodules may also co-exist.

Grossly, coccidiomas have a soft, gelatinous center in which *C. immitis* is usually present. Organisms are identifiable in 70 percent of the granulomas and cultured in only 30 percent of cases. Viable organisms have been recovered 15 years after the original infection. The characteristic endosporulating spherules of the organism can be demonstrated with the Grocott-Gomori methanamine silver stain. The PAS stain gives less optimal results, and fluorescent antibody techniques are also available.

Cavitation can occur in the center of a pneumonic infiltrate or within a coccidioma. Initially the cavities have a thick, shaggy wall, but a shelling-out of their contents results in a thin-walled structure that can be confused with a lung cyst. Secondary pyogenic bacterial infections can occur, and fungal contamination may result in a mycetoma or fungus ball.

Coccidiodomycosis is restricted to the Western Hemisphere. In the United States the most endemic regions are the southwestern United States and the bordering regions of northern Mexico. Endemic areas include parts of Arizona, California, Texas, Nevada, New Mexico, and Utah. Great care in the handling of lesions and cultures is required because of the danger of self-contamination.

Cryptococcosis

Cryptococcosis may occur in previously healthy individuals, but it appears more frequently in the immunodepressed and particularly in patients having some form of lymphoma or leukemia.[320,321] The disease is produced by *Cryptococcus neoformans* (*Torula histolytica*), a budding yeast measuring 5 to 10 μm in diameter. It has a thick capsule that creates the impression of a halo around the organism in tissue sections and that can be best demonstrated by Grocott-Gomori methenamine silver and mucicarmine stains. The port of entry of the organism is the lung; other major sites of involvement include the brain, lymph nodes, and bones.

Grossly, the lesions may appear as granuloma-like masses occupying part of the lobe, a bilateral miliary form usually associated with disseminated infection, or a subpleural patchy infiltrate, common in diabetics. However, cryptococcosis as a cause of solitary pulmonary granuloma is much rarer than histoplasmosis or coccidiodomycosis. Of 30 fungal lesions in the study of Ulbright and Katzenstein,[299] only one was due to cryptococcosis.

The microscopic picture of pulmonary cryptococcosis is related to the severity of the infection and to the duration of the process. Early lesions are composed of large numbers of yeasts supported by a fibrinous or light fibrous tissue stroma. These lesions have a characteristic gelatinous appearance due to the abundance of fungal capsular material. They may be single or multiple and can also cavitate.

In more protracted forms of the disease, there is a tissue response composed of large numbers of giant cells of foreign body type containing numerous organisms within cytoplasmic vacuoles. Large numbers of macrophages and lymphocytes are seen, and necrosis may be extensive. With the advent of fibrosis and calcification, the lesion resembles the other fungal granulomas.

Other Granulomatous Infections Produced by Yeast Fungi

Blastomycosis

Blastomycosis is a rare cause of isolated necrotizing granuloma of the lung, and the gross features of the lesion resemble those of histoplasmosis and coccidiodomycosis.[322] The large yeast Blastomyces dermatitidis is occasionally visible on standard hematoxylin and eosin (H&E) preparations and can also be demonstrated by Grocott-Gomori methenamine silver. However, clear separation from other fungi may not be possible due to poor detail. Confusion may arise between the small form of B. dermatitidis and H. capsulatum. Even the presence of a single bud with a broad base of attachment may not be enough to establish the diagnosis of blastomycosis, since occasionally C. neoformans may have a similar appearance. The PAS technique stains B. dermatitidis pink-red and will preserve detail, so that the multiple nuclei of these organisms are clearly seen. All other common fungi have only one nucleus.

Paracoccidioidomycosis

Another name for paracoccidioidomycosis is South American blastomycosis.[323] It occurs mainly in Brazil, Colombia, and Central America. Every patient reported in the United States was originally from these countries or had traveled to South America. The process represents a primary infection of the lung with subsequent dissemination to the skin and mucous membranes. Less frequently, involvement of the reticuloendothelial system (liver, lymph nodes, bone marrow, and spleen) and adrenals occurs. The pulmonary lesions consist of nodules or infiltrates that cavitate in about one third of patients. Histologically, the lesions are similar to those of North American blastomycosis, but the causative organism in the tissues is characterized by the presence of multiple buds.

Sporotrichosis

Sporotrichum schenckii, a fungus of worldwide distribution, usually affects humans in the form of cutaneous or lymph node disease following traumatic introduction of the organism.[324,325] It is thus not surprising that the disease usually occurs in gardeners and florists. Involvement of the lungs in this disease is rare, and even rarer is the presence of isolated pulmonary involvement. The latter has isolated or multiple infiltrates and nodules, occasionally with cavitation.

Pathologically, the lesions of sporotrichosis consist of necrotic foci surrounded by granulomatous inflammation. The organism is difficult to demonstrate in material from the lesions or in tissue sections; however, it can be readily grown in cultures. When visualized, the fungus has a characteristic, polymorphic morphology composed of oval or cigar-shaped budding yeasts that stain positively with Grocott-Gomori methenamine silver; the fungus can form "asteroid" structures. In addition to the primary pulmonary disease, disseminated cutaneous, systemic visceral, arthritic, and osseous forms of sporotrichosis have been described.

Adiospiromycosis

Granulomatous pulmonary adiospiromycosis or hyphomycosis is a disease of rodents and other small mammals produced by the fungi Emmonsia crescens and Emmonsia parva. Rarely, human pulmonary infection occurs in one of two forms: solitary adiospiromycotic granuloma, and disseminated granulomatous pulmonary adiospiromycosis.[326,327]

The inhaled spores of E. crescens measure 2 to 4 μm in diameter. After reaching the alveoli they progressively swell to a diameter of 200 to 700 μm, which represents a volume increase by a factor of one million. Since the fungus does not propagate or disseminate in animal tissues, the resulting pulmonary disability is attributed to encroachment on alveoli and airways by the expanding granulomas. Several examples of this disease have been reported from France, Czechoslovakia, Venezuela, and Honduras.

The capsule of the fungus in the well-developed state measures 24 μm in thickness and stains sharply with the Grocott-Gomori methenamine silver stain. The interior of the spore is usually empty except for numerous small eosinophilic granules. External to the capsule there is a well circumscribed granulomatous response that progresses to hyalinization.

Filamentous (Hyphae-Forming) Fungi

Filamentous fungi are organisms that are a very common cause of morbidity and mortality, particularly in the immunosupressed patient, and pulmonary involvement is frequently a major feature of these infections.

LOCALIZED DISEASES OF THE BRONCHI AND LUNGS

Aspergillosis

In patients with the invasive form of aspergillosis, the lungs are the seat of a pneumonic infiltrate that varies in severity from barely detectable to massive consolidation of several lobes. In other instances the disease is blood borne and characterized by multiple round abscesses with a tendency to cavitate.[328]

Pathologically, the latter lesion consists of necrotic and hemorrhagic nodules. Histologically, tightly packed bundles of aspergilli spread out from the lumina of thrombosed and necrotic vessels into the surrounding lung tissue. Although aspergilli can be seen in standard H&E, they are best demonstrated by Grocott-Gomori methenamine silver and Gridley stains. They appear as dense clusters of septated hyphae, 3 to 4 μm in diameter, characteristically exhibiting a Y-shaped pattern of branching.

Phycomycoses

Phycomycetes or mucorales consist of three genera, *Mucor, Rhizopus,* and *Absedia,* all of which may be responsible for human disease. They produce lesions identical to those produced by aspergilli. On histologic sections the hyphae are broad, nonseptate, and more irregular than those of *Aspergillus* species. They often branch at right angles and do not grow in the characteristic fan-like manner of *Aspergillus.* Mixed infections of *Aspergillus* and phycomycetes are not uncommon. Rarely, phycomycosis may have an isolated pulmonary nodule, as in the case reported by Gale and Kleitsch.[329]

Candidiasis

Although nodules or masses in the lung are uncommon in *Candida albicans* infections, the bronchopulmonary tract may be a primary site of infection in infants, in patients with chronic respiratory infections requiring long-term antibiotic therapy, and in asthmatic patients on chronic corticosteroid therapy. Microscopic involvement of the lung is not rare late in the course of generalized disease. In drug addicts, involvement of the brain and meninges, esophagus, and heart valves is, however, more impressive than lung involvement.

C. albicans appears as oval budding yeasts and as pseudohyphae best demonstrated by the PAS and Grocott-Gomori stains. Routine H&E stains do not as readily reveal the yeasts and pseudohyphae.

Allescheriosis

Monosporium apiospermum (Allescheria boydii) is the case of maduromycosis or mycetoma, a disease occurring in regions in which some inhabitants go barefoot. The disease is more prevalent in the southwestern parts of the United States. The organisms are present in the soil and enter through the skin. In histopathologic sections the disease is identified by the presence of *grains,* the central portion of which are formed by hyphae and the peripheral portion by spores.

Pulmonary infections produced by *Allescheria boydii* have been recorded,[330] and the disease may appear as patchy infiltrates, with or without cavitation, and as fungus balls. In lung tissue the broad septate hyphae must be distinguished from aspergilli. *Allescheria* generally causes more severe injury to the tissues and penetrates deeper in the bronchi than *Aspergillus.* Since both *Allescheria* and *Aspergillus* produce septate hyphae and share some morphologic features, it is conceivable that some errors in histologic diagnosis may occur in the absence of cultural identification.

Mycetomas (Fungus Balls)

The cavities of healed tuberculosis may be the seat of a massive proliferation of saprophytic fungi-forming masses or balls (Fig. 20-47). Cavities due to histoplasmosis, coccidioidomycosis, blastomycosis, sarcoidosis, and lesions such as bronchiectasis, abscesses, or cysts can also be colonized in a similar manner. Rarely, mycetomas can be observed in the course of acute invasive aspergillosis with extensive necrosis of tissue and rapid proliferation of the organism.

The mycetomas can be single or multiple and can reach several centimeters in diameter. They are freely movable within the cavity and are composed or large numbers of hyphae in a complex multilayered arrangement and admixed with blood products, mucus, and cell debris. Fungi most likely to produce mycetomas include members of the genus *Aspergillus (A. fumigatus, A. niger), Allescheria boydii, Cladosporium cladosporoides, Coccidiodes immitis,* and *Phycomycetes.*[328–330] Rarely, the intracavitary masses represent a solid collection of pyogenic bacteria, a condition known as *botryomycosis.*[331]

The clinical importance of fungus balls resides in their association with hemoptysis, sometimes of massive severity, requiring surgical intervention. Fungus balls have been noted to disappear spontaneously or with treatment.

Parasites

Diffuse pulmonary reactions can be the result of parasitic infestation, and they have been associated with two well known syndromes: *Loeffler's syndrome* and *tropical eosinophilia.*[332] Parasites that can be associated with the former include: *Trichuris trichiura, Enterobius vermicularis, Ascaris lumbricoides* and *Ascaris suum, Ancylostoma duodenale, Necator americanus, Trichinella spiralis, Ascaris brazilensis, Toxocara canis* and *Toxocara cati,* the tapeworm *Taenia saginata,* and the liver fluke *Fasciola hepatica.* The syndrome of tropical eosinophilia is produced by some microfilarial forms. *Schistosoma mansoni, Plasmodium falciparum,* and *Pneumocystis carinii* are also causes of diffuse parasitic lung disease. Localized pulmonary reactions pertinent to the present discussion can be seen in the following parasitic infections: *Pneumocystis carinii* infection, amebiasis, opisthorchiasis, schistosomiasis, dirofilariasis, hydatid cyst disease, *Enterobius vermicularis* infestation, and paragonimiasis.

Pneumocystis carinii Pneumonia

We have already discussed the pathology of *Pneumocystis carinii* infection in Chapters 3, 4, and 19. Typically, the disease consists of symptomatic interstitial infiltrates spreading out symmetrically from the hilar regions. Rarely, the process may appear as localized nodular densities as described in patients with AIDS.[333]

Amebiasis

Involvement of the lung in amebiasis follows that of the liver.[334] The usual route of spread is by direct extension from an abscess near the dome of the liver through the diaphragm and into the pleura and right lower lobe. Rarely, the route to the lung is hematogenous, when the organism bypasses the portal circulation and produces single or multiple pulmonary abscesses.

Opisthorchiasis

Opisthorchis viverrini, a liver fluke found in Thailand, can spread to the lung through a hepatopulmonary fistula much in the same way as amebiasis.[335]

Schistosomiasis

Pulmonary involvement by *Schistosoma mansoni* occurs in up to 64 percent of patients with this infection. The lesions are usually diffuse, bilateral, and granulomatous. They form around embolic ova and, more rarely, adult worms. A localized form of the disease forming a tumor-like mass has been described by Thompson et al.[336]

Dirofilariasis

Dirofilaria immitis (dog heartworm) is transmitted to humans via a mosquito that has fed on an infected animal. The larvae migrate throughout the subcutaneous tissue and fascia until they penetrate veins en route to the heart. From there they pass into the pulmonary circulation to produce infarcts with a surrounding zone of fibrosis and granulomatous inflammation. The nodule is characteristically described as a coin lesion in chest radiographs. It can vary in size from 1 to 5 cm in diameter, and it is usually round, with no tendency to calcify or cavitate.[337,338]

Pulmonary nodules produced by other filarial worms resembling *Dirofilaria immitis* are rare since most of these organisms remain on subcutaneous tissues. However, in the case described by Beaver et al.,[339] a living *Brugia malayi*-like filaria produced a pulmonary nodule in a 54-year-old Scotsman living in India for 34 years.

Hydatid Disease

The larvae of *Echinococcus granulosa,* or rarely *Echinococcus multilocularis,* may pass through the portal bed and lodge in the lung to form single or multiple cysts[340] (Fig. 20-48). The latter can also arise in the pleura and mediastinum. If communication with a bronchus occurs, the fluid content of the cyst is expelled, and the patient may experience an anaphylactic reaction to the parasite.

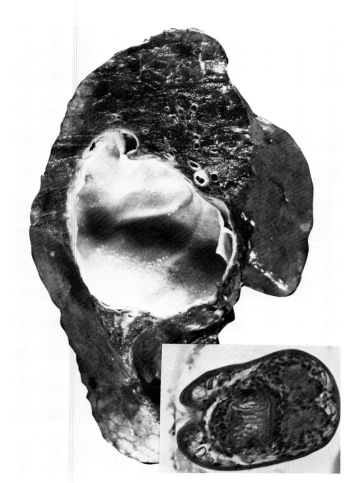

Fig. 20-48. Hydatid cyst in the left upper lobe. Scolices attached to the germinal membrane of the cyst can be discerned in the gross specimen. (Inset) Scolix with hooklet.

An air-fluid level can develop, and secondary infection may take place. Calcification of the cysts occurs in time.

Enterobiasis

The pinworm *Enterobius vermicularis,* or the eggs remaining after disintegration and resorption of other parts of the worm, have been identified in cysts, nodules, or granulomatous lesions in a number of extraintestinal locations, most commonly in the pelvic peritoneum and female genital tract. In the case reported by Beaver and colleagues, a pulmonary nodule was caused by this parasite.[341] The authors quoted a similar case in the literature.

Paragonimiasis

Paragonimiasis is produced by the trematode fluke *Paragonimus westermani.* It is endemic in Japan, China, Korea, the Philippines, Thailand, and some parts of Africa—the Cameroons, Zaire, and Nigeria. It has also been described in South America. The definitive host of *P. westermani* is the human being and other carnivorous mammals such as dogs, cats, and tigers. The adult fluke is small, rounded, and slightly flattened ventrally. It lives in the lungs of the definitive host.[342]

Humans acquire the disease by ingesting raw freshwater crustaceans (crayfish and crab) infested with the parasitic larvae (cercariae). Inside the human body, the larvae migrate to the lung through the gastrointestinal tract, the peritoneum, the diaphram, and the pleural space. In the lungs, the parasite develops into a mature fluke. It deposits a large number of ova in the lung parenchyma, which are eliminated in the sputum, swallowed into the GI tract, and eliminated in the stools. The lesion in the lung varies from early destructive foci that end in abscess formation to late fibrotic cysts that contain necrotic dead adult flukes and eggs and eosinophilic cell debris. Some endarteritis is noted in areas surrounding the cysts.

Noninfectious Granulomas

Sarcoidosis usually is a diffuse, interstitial, and finely nodular pulmonary process accompanied by hilar node enlargement. Rarely, however, striking nodules or masses can be noted in the lung parenchyma, a situation usually referred to as *nodular sarcoidosis.* The nodules may be multiple and cavitary, as described by Tellis and Putnam.[343]

A comparable situation exists for extrinsic allergic alveolitis or *hypersensitivity pneumonitis,* a syndrome characterized by diffuse and bilateral infiltrates. In the patient discussed by Hales,[344] a 34-year-old man with hypersensitivity pneumonitis due to thermophilic actinomy-

cetes, the pulmonary picture was characterized by multiple, bilateral, and almost perfectly rounded nodular masses.

Infectious Pneumonia

Mycoplasma Pneumonia

A most common radiologic picture in *Mycoplasma* pneumonia is that of a unilateral, segmental bronchopneumonia.[345,346] Clinically, the process is less severe than viral pneumonias; however, life-threatening infections and even fatal cases have been observed. Histologically, there is a peculiar combination of suppurative bronchiolitis and interstitial pneumonia rich in lymphocytes, plasma cells, and lymphoreticular elements. Frequently the lesions are hemorrhagic following fibrinous thrombosis of small vessels, possibly associated with the presence of cryoglobulins in the sera of these patients. The organism, as shown by electron microscopy, grows extracellularly in close apposition to the cells lining the airways.

Viral Pneumonia

A fine, focally nodular infiltrate is not an infrequent finding in the chest radiograph of patients with certain viral processes. This is a well recognized occurrence in cytomegalovirus pneumonia[347,348] and can also be noted in herpes virus,[349] varicella,[350] and type 7 adenovirus infection.[351] Many of these lesions are associated with a necrotizing vasculitis, which is frequently overlooked because of the small size of the compromised vessels and the extensive necrosis of the lung tissue. In chickenpox pneumonia, the vascular involvement can be so severe as to produce actual lung infarcts.[350] Healed chickenpox infection in other patients may be associated with striking miliary calcifications.

Bronchiolitis in children is associated with injury to respiratory bronchioles and air passages distal to them. Viruses are the main etiologic agent—respiratory syncytial viruses, adenovirus 3, 7, and 21, rhinoviruses, and parainfluenza viruses (particularly type 3). Less frequently bronchiolitis is secondary to infection by mumps virus, influenza, and mycoplasma (see Ch. 19).

Bronchiolitis Obliterans

Bronchiolitis obliterans[352] of the adult is characterized by the presence of masses of edematous or myxoid exudate (micropolyps) attached to the lumina of respiratory bronchioles, alveolar ducts, and, less frequently, terminal bronchioles. Classically the process has been associated with the inhalation of toxic fumes and gases such as nitrogen dioxide (silo-filler's lung), chlorine, and smoke. Infectious agents include viruses and mycoplasma. In bronchiolitis obliterans organizing pneumonia (BOOP),[353] there is, in addition to the bronchiolar plugs, a significant lymphoplasmacytic lymphoid infiltrate and obstructive pneumonia (golden, lipid or cholesterol pneumonia). Patients with BOOP are highly responsive to corticosteroid therapy and the process should not be confused with interstitial fibrosis of the lung.

Bacterial Pneumonias

Many bacterial pneumonias sometime in their clinical course may present as localized lesions. Vasculitis with focal necrosis of the lung parenchyma is a main pathologic finding in some Gram-negative pneumonias, particularly in *Pseudomonas* infection.[354] *Yersinia enterocolitica* infection may also have a prominent localized component; in the case of Taylor et al.,[355] the multiple pulmonary nodules suggested septic embolization. Melioidosis,[356] produced by the bacterium *Pseudomonas pseudomallei,* is a pneumonic process characterized by multiple, localized infiltrates, indistinguishable from those in granulomatous diseases, including the presence of cavitation.

Suppurative Processes

Actinomycosis

Actinomycosis is produced by *Actinomyces israeli,* a filamentous bacterium that grows in anaerobic cultures.[357] The hallmark of the thoracic involvement in this disease is the presence of lung abscesses and sinus tracts. There is striking involvement of the visceral and parietal pleura, cartilage, fibrous tissue, muscle, subcutaneous tissue, and skin. Involvement of the pericardium with purulent pericarditis and subsequent constrictive pericarditis has been noted. The pulmonary lesions in actinomycosis consists of irregular loculations of pus and extensive fibrosis. "Sulfur granules" composed of *A. israeli* can be grossly discernible or seen only under the microscope. They consist of tangles of branching Gram-positive organisms covered at the periphery of the granule by a radiating fringe of eosinophilic material or clubs. *A. israeli* is acid-fast negative with the classic Ziehl-Neelsen stain but positive with Putt's modification of this stain.

Nocardiosis

Nocardiosis, an infectious process involving the lungs, is produced by *Nocardia asteroides* and *Nocardia brasiliensis,* Gram-positive, filamentous bacteria that frag-

ment into bacillary organisms.[358] *Nocardia asteroides* is responsible for most of these infections in the United States. *Nocardia brasiliensis* primarily involves skin and subcutaneous lymph nodes, but it can penetrate the chest wall and the lung.

The lung lesions in nocardiosis have the gross features of multiple, confluent abscesses with an associated histiocytic or granulomatous response. The absence of extensive scarring, burrowing, or sinus formation differentiates this disease from actinomycosis. Nocardia granules in draining sinuses are less dense, clubs are not formed, and the organisms are weakly acid-fast. Nocardiosis is in our experience an important form of pulmonary infection in patients with AIDS.

Bronchiectasis

The abnormal and permanent dilatation that characterizes bronchiectasis can vary from an isolated, clinically silent lesion to gross distortion of the entire bronchial tree, accompanied by chronic suppuration, debility, and cardiorespiratory insufficiency.[359] A main variant of this disease is so-called postinfective or surgical bronchiectasis. There is very little evidence, however, of an infectious etiology in many of these patients. The designation *surgical* is, likewise, unfortunate, since most of these patients are not operated on nowadays. As Thurlbeck[359] suggested, the term *idiopathic* is perhaps more appropriate. The recent recognition of the immotile cilia syndrome (discussed in Ch. 19) has thrown some light on the pathogenesis of some of these lesions.

Idiopathic bronchiectasis more commonly affects the lower lobes. The left lobe is about twice as often affected as the right lobe. The disease is bilateral in almost half of the patients. In the left lower lobe the posterior basal segment is almost always involved, and the apical segment is frequently spared.

Surgical resection for bronchiectasis is sometimes performed because of hemoptysis. The latter is the result of a remarkable enlargement of the bronchial arteries with development of extensive anastomoses with the pulmonary arteries. Another complication of bronchiectasis is the development of a saprophytic mass of fungi, or fungus ball, with subsequent bleeding. The association of bronchiectasis with peripheral carcinoids of the tumorlet type has already been mentioned.

Lung Abscesses

It is the general consensus that lung abscesses are becoming less common.[360,361] Improvements in anesthesia and operative techniques in oropharyngeal surgery, and particularly the widespread use of antibiotics for pulmonary infections, have played a major role in the declining incidence of lung abscesses. The characteristic distribution of abscesses within the lung has lent strong support to the importance of aspiration. Gravitational forces and the spatial orientation of major bronchi determine that aspiration is more common on the right side than on the left. The posterior segments of both upper lobes and superior segments of the lower lobes are favored sites for aspiration pneumonia. Infected emboli originating in the abdomen or pelvis may produce abscesses anywhere in the lung, usually in a subpleural location.

INFILTRATIVE VASCULOPATHIES

Single or multiple localized lesions can occur in the lung as the result of (1) involvement of pulmonary arteries and veins by a cellular infiltrate of varied composition and significance, progressing to thrombosis, vascular obliteration, and vascular destruction; (2) parenchymal infiltrates centered around the vascular lesions, exhibiting features of granuloma formation and necrosis with or without cavitation; and (3) a nonspecific response of the adjacent lung tissue that includes bronchiolitis obliterans, endogenous (lipid) and organizing pneumonia, and fibrosis.

A characteristic feature of these disorders is their changing and migratory character in the chest radiograph. The presence and type of extrapulmonary involvement also provide important leads toward the correct diagnosis. The latter, however, must be established eventually by open lung biopsy. It is very difficult or even impossible to diagnose such lesions by fiberoptic bronchoscopy due to the small size of the specimen in comparison with the large size and complexity of the lesions. Special stains and cultures for pyogenic bacterial, mycobacteria, and fungi are mandatory—discovery of an infectious agent can result in cure and failure to rule out such agents can lead to unnecessary chemotherapy, complications or even death.

Liebow, in 1973,[362] grouped these disorders under the designation pulmonary angiitis and granulomatosis and classified them on the basis of their histologic features, since little was known in relation to etiology or pathogenesis. Over the past decade, however, it has become clear that the concept of angiitis and granulomatosis embraces both processes of unquestionable inflammatory nature and lymphoproliferative lesions, most of them T-cell lymphomas with a tendency to involve vascular structures. For that reason we presently use the purely descriptive noncommittal term infiltrative vasculopathies of the lung, as listed in Table 20-11.

Group I in this table consists of those true vasculitides having a granulomatous and necrotizing component as a main feature of the lesions. A fourth entity, bronchocen-

TABLE 20-11. Infiltrative Vasculopathies of the Lung

Necrotizing granulomatous vasculitides
  Wegener's granulomatosis (classic and limited variants)
  Allergic granulomatosis and angiitis (Churg-Strauss syndrome)
  Necrotizing sarcoid granulomatosis
  Bronchocentric granulomatosis
Angiocentric lymphoproliferative processes
  Benign lymphocytic angiitis and granulomatosis
  Lymphomatoid granulomatosis
  Angiocentric large cell lymphoma
Miscellaneous
  Classic polyarteritis nodosa of Kussmaul and Maier
  Hypersensitivity vasculitis
  Infectious vasculitis
  Pulmonary vasculitis in IV drug users
  Behçet's disease and the Hughes-Stovin syndrome
  Pulmonary hypertension

tric granulomatosis, although not a true vasculitis, is included nonetheless because the lesions can be easily confused with the other disorders. Group II is composed of three angiocentric lymphoproliferative processes. A third miscellaneous group comprises several entities of interest in the differential diagnosis of primary vascular diseases of the lung. A more detailed treatment of these disorders can be found in a recent review.[363]

Necrotizing Granulomatous Vasculitides

Wegener's Granulomatosis

The classic form of Wegener's granulomatosis (WG) was described by Wegener[364] in 1936 and by Klinger before him.[365] It is characterized by a triad of necrotizing angiitis and aseptic necrosis involving the upper airways (nasal septum and paranasal sinuses) and lung and a focal glomerulitis. A disseminated form of angiitis may sometimes be observed.

The pulmonary lesions of WG usually consist of multiple, bilateral white nodules measuring from a few millimeters to several centimeters. They are sharply circumscribed and frequently cavitated (50 percent). Histologically, there is extensive liquefactive necrosis at the center of the lesions blending with an organizing pneumonia rich in fibroblasts, histiocytes, and giant cells of Langhans, Touton, and foreign body types (Figs. 20-49 and 20-50). Palisading of histiocytes and giant cells is frequently noted around and along the walls of necrotic vessels and at the periphery of the necrotic foci. Rare discrete, sarcoidlike granulomas may be seen in some of these lesions. Eosinophils around the necrotic vessels can be abundant. Lymphocytes and plasma cells are seen in much smaller numbers, particularly toward the periphery of the lesions.

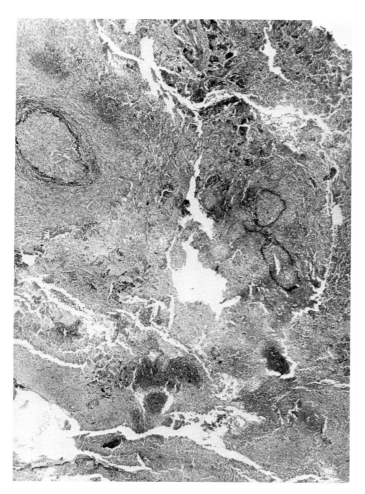

Fig. 20-49. Wegener's granulomatosis. Microscopic view of a lesion showing extensive necrosis of lung tissue. Three pulmonary vessels show inflammation and thrombosis. Weigert's elastic tissue stain with van Gieson counterstain.

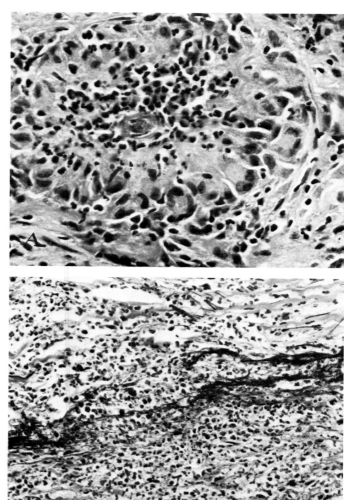

Fig. 20-50. Wegener's granulomatosis. **(A)** Small vessel is surrounded by numerous polymorphonuclear leukocytes and eosinophils. External to that microabscess, there is palisading of histiocytes and giant cells forming a granuloma. There is extensive fibrosis in the surrounding tissue, but lymphocytes are not abundant. (H&E) **(B)** Characteristic liquefactive vasculitis of this disease. (Weigert's elastic tissue stain with van Gieson counterstain.)

A major feature of the lesions is a destructive angiitis involving large muscular arteries and veins within the necrotic core. This change is frequently overlooked in H&E-stained sections but can be detected by elastic tissue stains. Milder degrees of angiitis can be noted away from the necrotic foci. Only in a minority of patients (20 percent), there is hilar adenopathy with involvement similar to that in the lung.

The renal lesion of classic WG is a nonspecific, focal, and segmental glomerulitis with a tendency for rapid progression, crescent formation, and fibrosis. The hypothesis that immunocomplex deposition underlies this disorder has been abandoned; a more recent view implicates the presence of antineutrophilic autoantibodies in the genesis of the lesions and provides a reliable laboratory test for the diagnosis of Wegener's granulomatosis. The upper airway involvement of WG falls within the clinical syndrome of midline granuloma of the face. Frequently,

it is impossible to detect the presence of angiitis or granulomas because of superimposed infection and marked crusting of these lesions.

A rare manifestation of WG is pulmonary hemorrhage associated with neutrophilic capillaritis. The hemorrhage can be massive and dominate the clinical picture. Since such phenomenon can occur in the absence of the characteristic discrete lesions of this disease the differential diagnosis includes Goodpasture's syndrome (immunocomplex-mediated glomerulonephritis with lung hemorrhages). The eventual recognition or development of diagnostic lesions establishes the diagnosis of WG in such cases.

In the limited variant of WG described by Carrington and Liebow in 1970,[366] the process is restricted to the lung or may have very little extrapulmonary extension. These patients are known to have a better response to corticosteroids and a more benign course than those with the classic form of the disease.

It is possible that the limited variant represents a slowly progressive form or a lesser tempo of the disease[367] that may or may not eventuate in glomerular involvement. Regardless of the clinical type, a remarkable therapeutic response to cyclophosphamide has been observed in patients with WG.

Allergic Granulomatosis and Angiitis (Churg-Strauss Syndrome)

Originally described by Churg and Strauss[368] in 1951 on the basis of 14 patients, this process consists of a disseminated necrotizing vasculitis occurring exclusively in asthmatics. Rose and Spencer[369] in 1957 reported 111 autopsy cases of polyarteritis nodosa, 32 of which had identical features to those described by Churg and Strauss. An analysis of 30 patients with this disease was published by Chumbley et al.[370] in 1977. The pulmonary and renal histopathology were studied in four patients by Koss et al.[371] in 1981.

Approximately one fourth of patients with allergic granulomatosis and angiitis have pulmonary involvement. This ranges from transient patchy pneumonic infiltrates to massive bilateral nodular disease or diffuse interstitial disease. Affected vessels are arteries and veins of small caliber that may show a giant cell infiltrate. There is intense eosinophilia within the affected vessels and perivascular tissues, with accompanying lymphocytes, plasma cells, and histiocytes. A characteristic finding is the presence of necrotizing extravascular granulomas composed of histiocytes and giant cells (Fig. 20-51). In rare cases, granulomas are absent altogether in the pulmonary lesion and the diagnosis rests in the demonstration of an eosinophilic vasculitis with thrombotic changes.

In some patients, the vascular lesions blend with extensive areas of eosinophilic pneumonia characterized by numerous histiocytes diffusely intermingled with eosinophils and foci of fibrinoid necrosis. In idiopathic eosinophilic pneumonia, however, vasculitis is not a main feature of the lesions, and the process is more diffuse and affects the peripheral zones of both lungs, giving a picture compared with a negative of the radiograph of pulmonary edema. Bronchial asthma and peripheral blood eosinophilia, previously considered essential for the diagnosis of AGA, can be absent in some patients. The treat-

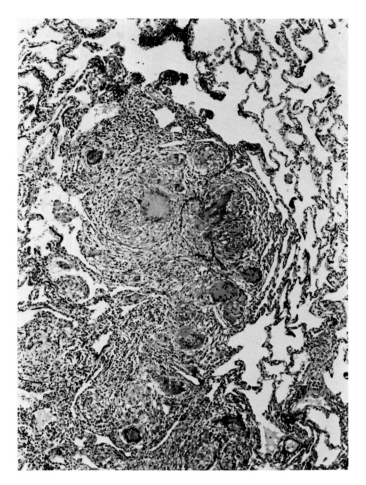

Fig. 20-51. Lesion of allergic granulomatosis and angiitis (Churg-Strauss syndrome) in which multiple granulomas are noted in the wall of an occluded vein and in the adjacent alveolar tissue. There was also dense infiltration by eosinophils. (Courtesy of Dr. Thomas Colby, Rochester, MN.)

ment of choice is corticosteroid therapy, and cytotoxic drugs are seldom needed.

Necrotizing Sarcoid Granulomatosis

Necrotizing sarcoid granulomatosis (NSG) was originally described by Liebow[362] in 1973, on the basis of 11 cases, and reports of close to 100 such cases have accrued in the literature.[363] The pulmonary lesions consist of unilateral or bilateral nodules or infiltrates radiologically indistinguishable from other forms of angiitis and granulomatosis. Pathologically, they consist of massive aggregates of sarcoid-like granulomas surrounding areas of coagulative necrosis (Fig. 20-52). Rarely, the necrosis has suppurative features resembling WG. Bronchial and bronchiolar infiltration by granulomas is frequent. Older lesions exhibit fibrosis and hyalinization.

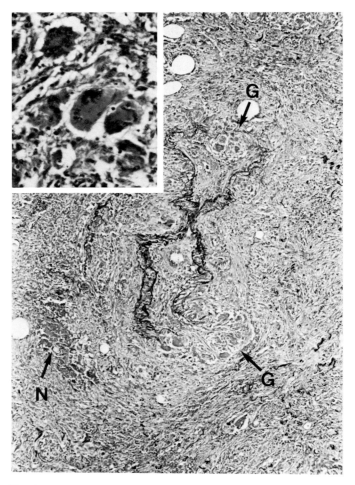

Fig. 20-52. Necrotizing sarcoid granulomatosis showing intrusive granulomas (G) in the wall of a large muscular artery. Necrosis (N) was also a feature of the lesion. (Inset) The alveolar tissue was diffusely infiltrated by confluent granulomas.

The vascular changes are distinctive and striking and both arteries and veins are involved. Large muscular arteries display an alignment of giant cells along the external lamina, for which the designation *giant cell arteritis* seems appropriate. Smaller vessels can be involved in different degrees by intrusive granulomas, to the point of obliteration. Still other vessels may show an intimal lymphoplasmacytic cellular infiltrate associated with fibrosis.

Extrapulmonary involvement does occur in NSG but it is rare. Neurologic involvement has been described in a child by Beach et al.[372] and in another patient by Singh et al.[373] In another patient known to us, the pulmonary lesions responded well to corticosteroid therapy only to be followed by a process of polyarteritis nodosa. Associated disorders in patients with NSG are interesting and include chronic active hepatitis (two patients), granulomatous colitis (one patient), uveitis (two patients), and hypothalamic insufficiency (one patient).

In his review of 32 patients with NSG, Churg[374] concluded that NSG represents so-called nodular sarcoid, but most investigators disagree with this proposition. Against sarcoidosis of any type are the following facts: (1) the radiologic appearance of NSG is most unusual for sarcoidosis and hilar adenopathy is rare in the former disease; (2) although vascular involvement is not unusual in sarcoidosis, it is not so strikingly severe as in NSG; (3) the extent of the necrosis in NSG would be most unusual for sarcoidosis; (4) normal angiotensin-converting enzyme levels in both serum and tissue have been noted in one patient with NSG and three other patients had a negative Kveim test; and (5) systemic vasculitis has been noted in NSG, a feature not seen in sarcoidosis. It is also possible that some examples of *nodular sarcoid* have no relationship to sarcoidosis and represent, in fact, Liebow's NSG. Regardless of its nature, NSG is a benign process and most patients do well with corticosteroids or with no treatment at all.

Bronchocentric Granulomatosis

Bronchocentric granulomatosis (BCG) was originally described by Liebow[362] in 1973 on the basis of nine patients. An enlarged version of this study, based on 23 patients, was published by Katzenstein, et al.[375] in 1975. Katzenstein et al. chose to disregard this disorder as a type of pulmonary angiitis and granulomatosis after noting that the vasculitis could be best interpreted as incidental to the airway involvement. We have decided to include BCG in the present discussion because the lesions not only share some common features with, but are also frequently misdiagnosed as, one or more of the three previously discussed entities. From a practical standpoint, it is important to distinguish BCG because of its much better prognosis.

Bronchocentric granulomatosis is seen on the chest radiograph as unilateral or bilateral infiltrates that can simulate the angiocentric processes already discussed. Katzenstein et al.[375] distinguished a group with a history of asthma and another group, with an older age distribution, that did not have asthma. Histologically, the process is characterized by extensive inflammatory and destructive lesions of small bronchi and bronchioles. The walls of these structures may show extensive caseous-like necrosis, eosinophilia, and granulomas. In other lesions, polymorphonuclear leukocytes rather than eosinophils accumulate in the involved bronchioles. There is also a dense lymphocytic and plasmacytic infiltrate of the airways and distal lung parenchyma and nonspecific changes of broncholitis obliterans and obstructive pneumonia. The inflammatory infiltrate may extend to involve the adjacent pulmonary arteries, which show variable degrees of intimal fibrosis (Fig. 20-53).

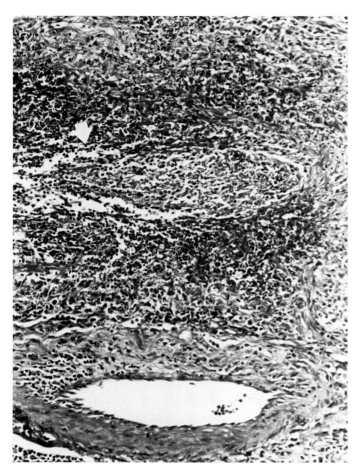

Fig. 20-53. Bronchocentric granulomatosis. A small airway is totally necrotic and shows suppurative as well as granulomatous cellular response (arrow). Eosinophils are numerous in the lesion. (Bottom) Pulmonary artery with mild vasculitis.

Of great interest is the presence in some of these lesions of noninvasive fungi (*Aspergillus, Mucor*), the significance of which is not clear. The association with other processes such as mucoid impaction, allergic bronchopulmonary aspergillosis, and eosinophilic pneumonia has been noted. Patients with rheumatoid arthritis may also exhibit lesions on BCG.

As noted by Liebow,[362] BCG is a lesion rather than a disease, and the lesion may be infectious or due to hypersensitivity phenomena. From a practical standpoint, once this diagnosis is suggested by open lung biopsy, the possibility of ulcerocaseous tuberculosis of bronchi must be ruled out by special stains and cultures. The same applies for other organisms, such as *Aspergillus, Mucor,* or *Sporotrichum*. If an organism is identified, treatment should be directed against the specific cause. In those patients in whom infection has been ruled out, corticosteroids should be used; the effect of the latter is usually curative. Because BCG can be confused with Wegener's

granulomatosis, patients with the former disease may be subjected to unnecessary and dangerous chemotherapy. We know of one such patient in whom cyclophosphamide therapy resulted in sepsis and death.

Angiocentric Lymphoproliferative Processes

The distinctive feature of these disorders is the presence of a lymphoproliferative infiltrate with a propensity to involve vascular structures in the lung and elsewhere in a manner that simulates a vasculitis. The prototype is lymphomatoid granulomatosis (LYG). Angiocentric large cell lymphoma (ALCL) and a less well recognized entity, benign lymphocytic angiitis and granulomatosis (BLAG), will be also discussed.

The description of LYG by Liebow et al.[376] in 1972 represents a turning point in our understanding of these disorders. They noted that in this disease the lesions display an intense lymphoreticular proliferation that is missing in WG, a disease LYG resembles both pathologically and clinically. Presently LYG is interpreted as a T-cell malignant lymphoma with characteristic features of pleomorphism, granuloma formation, and angiocentricity. Features in common with other T-cell proliferations include a tendency to involve extranodal sites (skin, CNS) and to run an unpredictable clinical course.

There appears to be a spectrum of lesions ranging from BLAG to LYG to ALCL. The works of Jaffe[377] and Costa and Martin[378] have supported this concept and have provided interesting data indicating that most of these processes probably represent post-thymic T-cell proliferations.

Benign Lymphocytic Angiitis and Granulomatosis

Patients with BLAG may be erroneously diagnosed as having either Wegener's granulomatosis or lymphomatoid granulomatosis. Although the pulmonary radiologic findings in these three disorders are identical, patients with BLAG are frequently asymptomatic, and extrapulmonary involvement is very rare.[363,379–381]

The most characteristic feature of the pulmonary lesions is the presence of a diffuse, highly cellular but histologically benign infiltrate composed primarily of small lymphocytes, occasional large stimulated lymphocytes, plasmacytoid lymphocytes, and plasma cells. Mitoses are rare, and foci of coagulative necrosis in the centers of the lesions are seen only occasionally. The walls of small arteries and veins show moderate to severe infiltration by the lymphoid cells, but actual occlusion of the lumen is rare (Fig. 20-54). Infiltration of respiratory bronchioles

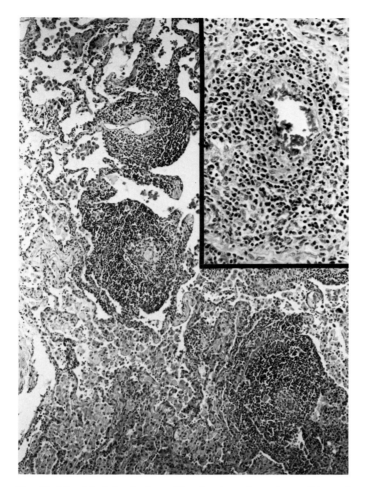

Fig. 20-54. Nodular lesion of benign lymphocytic angiitis and granulomatosis shows a dense perivascular and intravascular infiltrate by lymphocytes. The alveoli are filled by foamy histiocytes (endogenous lipid pneumonia), secondary to bronchiolitis obliterans (not shown in this field). (Inset) Detail of a pulmonary vessel infiltrated by small lymphocytes lacking cytologic atypia and admixed with plasma cells.

giving a picture of bronchiolitis obliterans is also a feature of these lesions. The resulting endogenous lipid pneumonia adds to the cellularity and variegated histologic composition. Sarcoid-like granulomas are another prominent feature of some of these lesions. Of great interest in the observation that chlorambucil therapy results in prompt remissions and dramatic cures in BLAG. Comparable results are not seen in Wegener's granulomatosis and even less so in lymphomatoid granulomatosis; thus, aggressive combined chemotherapy is probably overtreatment in this disease.

Lymphomatoid Granulomatosis

Grossly, the lesions of LYG appear as well localized nodules or pneumonic infiltrates with extensive necrosis (Fig. 20-55). Histologically the centers of the lesions show extensive coagulative necrosis. There is invasion and destruction of pulmonary arteries and veins by a pleomorphic cellular infiltrate composed of small lymphocytes, plasma cells, histiocytes, and large atypical lymphoreticular cells, some of which may resemble Reed-Sternberg cells (Fig. 20-56). Sarcoid-like granulomas and tissue eosinophilia are seen only rarely.

Lesions rich in mature lymphocytes and plasma cells and poor in atypical lymphoreticular elements have a better prognosis than do those in which the latter are numerous and prominent and the lymphocytes and plasma cells comparatively sparse. Involvement of the CNS and nerves is seen in about one third of the patients and constitutes a poor prognostic sign. The characteristic lymphoreticular infiltrates can affect the brain, cranial nerves, and peripheral nerves. The skin is involved in about 40 percent of patients. Typically, the lesions consist of firm, raised nodules up to 3 cm in diameter, with

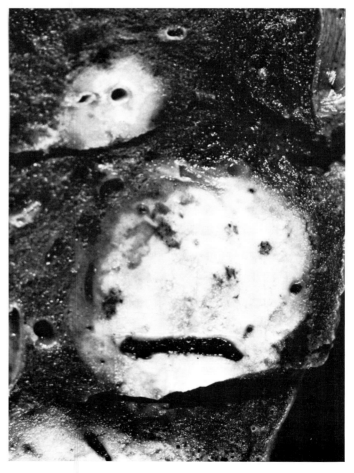

Fig. 20-55. Lymphomatoid granulomatosis. Two highly necrotic, angiocentric nodules in the lung of a patient who died with massive hemoptysis.

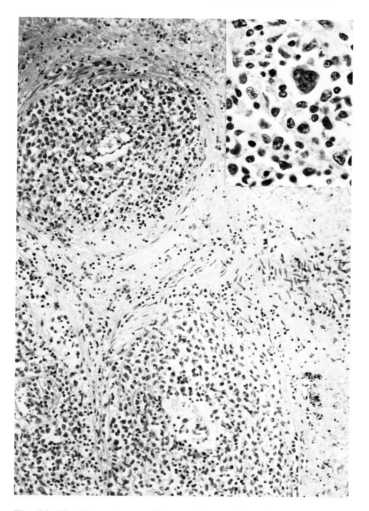

Fig. 20-56. Lymphomatoid granulomatosis. Microscopic view showing extensive necrosis and the atypical lymphoreticular infiltrate characteristic of this disease infiltrating and destroying two pulmonary vessels. (Inset) Detail of the infiltrate, including the presence of large atypical cellular elements resembling Reed-Sternberg cells.

purple discoloration and a tendency to ulcerate. The lower extremities, abdomen, and gluteal regions are preferential sites of occurrence. Sometimes, massive infiltrates have occurred in the trunk, neck and feet. Some of the skin lesions are preceded by a psoriasiform rash.

Sinus and upper airway involvement has been considered unusual in LYG. However, recent reports would indicate that so-called polymorphic reticulosis or midline malignant reticulosis[382] is a nasal lesion histologically identical to LYG and can be followed by systemic manifestations characteristic of the latter disease. Renal involvement is seen in one third of patients with lymphomatoid granulomatosis and consists of nodular or diffuse infiltrates of the kidney parenchyma, but no glomerulitis is observed. Although LYG has been shown to be a pleo-

morphic T-cell malignant lymphoma, progression to a monomorphic large cell lymphoma can develop in 12 percent of patients and indicates a very poor prognosis. Corticosteroid therapy in a few patients with LYG has been associated with significant although transient remissions. A good response to cyclophosphamide, as noted in WG, is, however, lacking and the mortality rate is very high. Appropriate therapy is aggressive combined chemotherapy.

Angiocentric Large Cell Lymphoma

Cases of malignant large cell lymphoma of the lung with angioinvasion and extensive coagulative necrosis can be confused with lymphomatoid granulomatosis. The key to the diagnosis of lymphoma in these cases is the identification of foci, sheets, or uniform infiltrates of large mononuclear atypical lymphoid cells, a feature that is absent in LYG unless it is undergoing conversion to a more easily identified lymphoma. Jaffe et al. (quoted by Saldana)[363] classified seven patients with angiocentric lymphoma according to the New International Working Formulation as diffuse mixed small and large cell (five cases); diffuse large cell (one case); and diffuse large cell immunoblastic (one case). All but one patient achieved complete remission with aggressive combination therapy.

Miscellaneous Vasculitides

Classic Polyarteritis Nodosa of Kussmaul and Maier

Classic polyarteritis nodosa of Kussmaul and Maier[363] is a multisystemic process characterized by necrosis, inflammation, and thrombosis of medium-sized and smaller arteries of many organs. There may be fibrinoid necrosis of the vascular wall, and the inflammatory infiltrate is composed initially of granulocytes with some eosinophils, lymphocytes, and plasma cells. In older lesions, lymphocytes and plasma cells predominate. Eventually, the arterial well is scarred, and the lumen is occluded. Granuloma formation is not a feature of these lesions.

The clinical manifestations of polyarteritis nodosa are the result of ischemic changes and infarcts of the involved organs. Characteristically, acute and healed lesions coexist in the same patient. Focal medial injury leads to aneurysm formation, another feature of diagnostic importance, as such aneurysms can be diagnosed angiographically. Almost any organ can be involved in polyarteritis nodosa, but characteristically the lung and the spleen are almost always spared. At times, microscopic involvement of the bronchial arteries may be detected by histologic examination.

Polyarteritis nodosa is a recognized complication of viral hepatitis. Hepatitis B antigenemia (HBsAg) and circulating HBsAg-anti-HBs immune complexes frequently occur in these patients. Moreover, HBs antigen, immunoglobulins, and complement are noted in the vascular lesions. The occurrence of polyarteritis nodosa in drug addicts may result from the high incidence of hepatitis B antigenemia in such individuals.

Earlier data indicated that approximately two thirds of patients with untreated polyarteritis nodosa died within the first year of the disease, usually of renal failure, or massive hemorrhage in the brain or gastrointestinal tract. With corticosteroid therapy, the 5 year survival rate is approximately 60 percent. More recently cyclophosphamide and plasmapheresis have proven even more beneficial.

Hypersensitivity Vasculitis

Also designated as *microscopic polyarteritis*,[363] hypersensitivity vasculitis encompasses a large and heterogeneous group of clinical syndromes that have in common the predominant involvement of arterioles, venules, and capillaries, in contradistinction to the involvement of medium-sized and small muscular arteries of classic polyarteritis nodosa. Tissue eosinophilia may be seen, but granuloma formation is not a feature of the lesions. Characteristically, the lesions of hypersensitivity vasculitis tend to be of the same age. Skin involvement is frequently observed, and the lung is seldom affected.

Hypersensitivity vasculitis associated with rheumatoid arthritis is frequently a typical leukocytoclastic vasculitis of small venules involving the skin and synovium. Patients with severe erosive and nodular disease and positive rheumatoid factor can develop a fulminant disseminated vasculitis involving pulmonary arterioles and medium-sized muscular arteries and veins. Approximately one fifth of patients with systemic lupus erythematosus (SLE) develop hypersensitivity vasculitis of the skin. Less frequently, a generalized systemic vasculitis, including pulmonary involvement, may develop.

Infections

Mention has already been made of the fact that vasculitis is a common finding in infectious granulomas; these lesions can be easily confused with necrotizing granulomatous vasculitides.[363] Also, bacterial pneumonias of the Gram-negative type, such as *Pseudomonas* pneumonia, show characteristic vascular involvement. Viral and rickettsial infections frequently and characteristically involve the endothelium of capillaries, arterioles, and venules, producing a small vessel vasculitis.

Intravenous Drug Abuse

In drug addicts, self-administration of narcotics and other particulate material can produce striking lesions, including thrombosis, necrotizing arteritis, and plexiform-like lesions, in pulmonary arteries.[363,383]

Behçet's Disease and Hughes-Stoven Syndrome

Behçet's disease is a multisystemic disorder of unknown origin characterized by oral aphthous ulcers, genital ulcers, and relapsing iritis. Associated findings include thrombophlebitis migrans, arthritis, erythema nodosum, and neurologic signs. The age of onset is usually the third decade of life, and men are more frequently affected than women.

The pulmonary vascular pathology in a patient with Behçet's disease has been described by Slavin and de Groat.[384] The basic lesion consists of a lymphocytic and necrotizing vasculitis involving pulmonary arteries, veins, and capillaries. The changes can evolve to aneurysms of elastic pulmonary arteries, some of which may erode into bronchi. Arterial and venous thrombi, pulmonary infarcts, and striking perivascular fibrosis also occur.

The combination of pulmonary artery aneurysms, recurrent thrombophlebitis, and increased intracranial pressure is referred to as the Hughes-Stovin syndrome.[385] Slavin and de Groat[384] reviewed the clinical and pathologic findings in cases of Hughes-Stovin syndrome reported in the literature and found them remarkably similar to those observed in Behçet's disease. The authors believe that the Hughes-Stovin syndrome represents unrecognized or incomplete expressions of Behçet's disease.

Pulmonary Hypertension

Increments in pulmonary arterial blood flow or pressure can lead to damage of pulmonary arteries and arterioles.[363] If the level of pulmonary arterial pressure approaches that of the systemic circulation, a necrotizing arteritis occurs. This has been noted repeatedly in congenital malformations of the heart and idiopathic pulmonary hypertension. It has also been reproduced experimentally. The "angiomatoid" or "plexiform" lesions noted in some of these conditions are apparently the result of a focal vasculitis followed by repair and proliferation of bronchial collateral vessels.

MALDEVELOPMENTAL ANOMALIES

Localized lesions of maldevelopmental character are relatively rare but frequently pose diagnostic difficulties. They have been arranged into three main groups: cystic lesions, vascular anomalies, and ectopic tissues in the lung and pleura. A more detailed list of such conditions is presented in Table 20-12.

Cystic Lesions

Intralobal Sequestration, Extralobar Sequestration, and Bronchopulmonary Foregut Malformation

Pulmonary sequestration is a mass of abnormal pulmonary tissue that does not communicate with the tracheobronchial tree through a normally located bronchus and that receives its arterial blood supply via an anomalous systemic artery. When the pulmonary sequestration is enveloped by visceral pleura, the term *intralobar* is used; in *extralobar* sequestration, the abnormal lung tissue is located outside the confines of the lobe, usually within the left pleural space (Rokitansky's lobe).[386-390] Occasionally, the extrapulmonary sequestration may occur below the diaphragm, as a paragastric mass.

Bronchopulmonary foregut malformation is no more than a pulmonary sequestration, either intralobar or extralobar, that communicates with the alimentary tract, usually the esophagus, by means of a tubular structure resembling a bronchus.[386-389]

Ninety percent of extralobar sequestrations and 60 percent of intralobar sequestrations occur on the left side. Characteristically, their blood supply is by means of an arterial vessel arising from the thoracic or abdominal aorta. The venous drainage of intralobar sequestration is to the pulmonary venous system, that of the extralobar variety to the azygos or portal systems.

TABLE 20-12. Maldevelopmental Lesions

Cystic lesions
    Intralobar sequestration, extralobar sequestration, and bronchopulmonary foregut malformation
    Congenital cystic adenomatoid malformation
    Congenital (infantile) lobar emphysema
    Congenital pulmonary lymphangiectasia
    Other cystic lesions
Vascular anomalies
    Arteriovenous fistulas and hemangiomas
    Systemic-pulmonary arteriovenous fistulas
    Pulmonary varicosities
    Aneurysms of pulmonary arteries
Ectopic tissues in the lung (brain, liver, kidney, adrenal, thyroid, skeletal muscle, GI epithelium, pancreas, endometrium, decidua, bone)

Variations in blood supply do occur and include a double systemic and pulmonary blood supply to an intralobar sequestration, azygos vein drainage in intralobar sequestration, and pulmonary arterial blood supply to extralobar sequestration.[388] A well recognized event is that of a fatal hemorrhage if the artery to a sequestration is inadvertently severed during surgery, particularly when the artery arises in the abdominal aorta.

The most favored location for intralobar sequestration is the posterobasal segment of a lower lobe. Upper lobe location is rare but does occur, particularly on the right side. The sequestration frequently appears as an encapsulated, multiloculated cystic structure filled with mucus and partly surrounded by normal lung tissue. Histologically, the fibrous septa contain thickened vessels and are lined by hyperplastic respiratory epithelium. Suppurative changes may be a prominent feature when infection has supervened.

Since sequestration represents a space-occupying lesion, atelectasis and infection of the surrounding lung tissue are likely to occur. The infection can spread to the sequestration, giving rise to an abscess. The latter eventually erodes the capsule, establishes a connection with a normal bronchus, and drains its contents. Complete resolution of an infected sequestration is, however, difficult to achieve because of inadequate drainage.

In extralobar sequestration, often called *accessory lung,* the mass of abnormal lung tissue is lined by smooth or wrinkled pleura. On cut section, there is spongy tissue with numerous large and small cysts containing clear mucoid fluid (Fig. 20-57). Rudimentary bronchi can be found; bronchioles are intricately branched and lined by tall columnar cells that may show papillary projections.

The gross and microscopic appearance of bronchopulmonary foregut malformation is that of either intralobar or extralobar sequestration. The communication with the foregut is a tubular structure, usually containing creamy mucoid material. Histologically, the fistula shows transition of esophageal to bronchial mucosa and, rarely, gastric mucosa. There is a layer of cartilaginous ring near the entrance of the fistula in the lung.

The most accepted theory on the origin of these malformations was proposed by Eppinger and Schawerstein in 1902 and subsequently supported by others.[390] According to this view, an aberrant lung bud develops in the embryonic foregut distal to the normal tracheobronchial bud. That pluripotential mass of tissue acquires its own blood supply and migrates distally, giving rise to the sequestration. Whether the latter will be intralobar or extralobar is probably determined by the time at which the aberrant bud develops. An early origin of the abnormal bud in the short, primitive foregut will be carried distally by the normal lung and incorporated as an intralobar sequestration. A late origin from the elongated foregut will

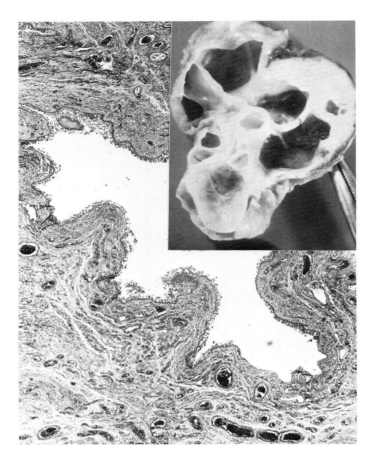

Fig. 20-57. Microscopic view of extralobar sequestration or accessory pulmonary lobe shows large cystic cavities lined by respiratory epithelium. There is extensive fibrosis and the artery supplying the sequestration arises from the aorta. (Inset) Gross features of the lesion, which is multicystic and filled with clear mucoid fluid.

remain outside the lung (extralobar). It is speculated that in sequestration the communication between the aberrant bud and foregut overgrows its vascular supply and undergoes involution; it remains patent in bronchopulmonary foregut malformation.

Of 233 cases of pulmonary sequestration reported before 1962, 199 cases were of the intralobar variety, 30 were extralobar (7 : 1 ratio), and 4 had coexisting intralobar and extralobar sequestration.[387] Intralobar sequestration rarely manifests itself in children and virtually never in neonates. Extralobar sequestration and bronchopulmonary foregut malformation, while occasionally described in adults, are most often seen within the first few months of life, frequently in neonates.

There are reports describing the development of carcinoma,[391] tuberculosis, aspergillosis, and botryomycosis within sequestrations.[392] The severe sclerotic vascular changes presumably due to a systemic to pulmonary fis-

tula are well known, including the development of necrotizing arteritis.[393]

Congenital Cystic Adenomatoid Malformation

Congenital cystic adenomatoid malformation is usually limited to a lobe, but rare instances of involvement of more than one lobe and bilaterality are known to occur. Stocker et al.[394] in 1977 published the results of a comprehensive analysis of this condition. They classify congenital cystic adenomatoid malformation into three main pathologic types.

Type I includes multiple large cysts or a combination of large and smaller cysts with a predominance of the former. This is the most common form of the disease and

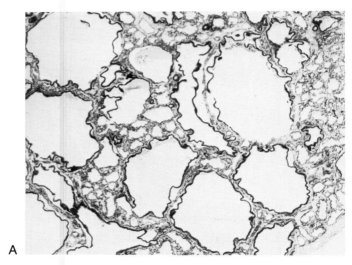

A

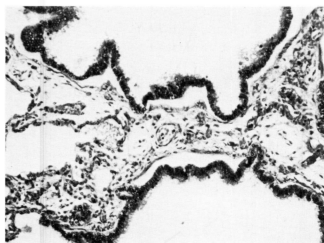

B

Fig. 20-58. Cystic adenomatoid malformation. **(A)** Lesion composed of evenly spaced, relatively uniform cystic spaces lined by respiratory epithelium. **(B)** Between the cystic spaces there are smaller air sacs lined by cuboidal or flattened epithelium.

accounts for approximately 50 percent of the cases. The affected lobe is bulky and causes mediastinal shift and respiratory distress in the newborn period. Type II is characterized by multiple, evenly spaced cysts, none more than 1.2 cm in diameter. It is seen in approximately 40 percent of patients and is the form with which other congenital anomalies are more frequently associated. Type III appears as a bulky, firm mass of uniform, small and evenly spaced cysts (Fig. 20-58).

Approximately 50 percent of patients with congenital cystic adenomatoid malformation of the lung are born prematurely and another 25 percent are stillborn. Congenital hydrops, polyhydramnios, and postnatal anasarca have been described, probably as the result of vena caval compression.

Pathologic features aiding in the diagnosis of congenital cystic adenomatoid malformation include the massive enlargement of the lobe, particularly in type I, and the presence of anastomosing passages resembling terminal bronchioles. The latter are lined by tall columnar epithelium that may be mucus secreting. Poorly developed bronchial cartilage and bronchial mucoserous glands can be seen. Alveolar differentiation is deficient, and the overdistention of the lobe is apparently due to air trapping. Congenital cystic adenomatoid malformation can be complicated by pneumothorax. Surgical intervention is necessary, but the uninvolved lung is often hypoplastic and mortality is high (80 percent).

Congenital (Infantile) Lobar Emphysema

Congenital lobar emphysema is characterized by marked overdistention of a lobe resulting in compression of the ipsilateral normal lung, mediastinal shift, herniation of the emphysematous lung through the anterior mediastinum, and atelectasis of the contralateral lung.[395–402] The onset of symptoms of respiratory distress often occurs in the neonatal period, in at least 50 percent of patients within the first month and in only 5 percent after 6 months of age.[395]

A single lobe involvement is usual, most frequently the left upper lobe (50 percent), the right middle lobe (24 percent), or right upper lobe (18 percent). Lower lobe involvement and multiple lobe involvement are uncommon. Characteristically the affected lobe is overinflated and fails to deflate after excision. Microscopically, the alveoli appear distended and alveolar wall fibrosis can sometimes be observed.[396]

Bronchial obstruction is the accepted explanation for most cases of congenital (infantile) lobar emphysema, and abnormalities of bronchial cartilage in the affected lobe can be demonstrated in about one half of these patients.[397] Other causes include compression of bronchi by bronchogenic cysts or abnormal vessels, bronchial mu-

cus plug, "volvulus" of a lobe, and a proposed ball-valve obstruction of the orifices of segmental bronchi.[387]

Other mechanisms have been proposed for this condition. Using quantitative criteria, Hislop and Reid[399,400] found that alveoli can be normal in size but increased in number, a condition they term *polyalveolar lobe*. They have proposed that a polyalveolar lobe with or without emphysema is responsible for some cases of infantile lobar emphysema.

Congenital Pulmonary Lymphangiectasia

Congenital pulmonary lymphangiectasia consists of a prominent network of cystically dilated lymphatics in the interlobular septa and around the bronchovascular bundles.[403,404] The dilated lymphatics contain lymph and interfere with the normal distention of alveolar tissue. Congenital pulmonary lymphangiectasia occurs under three different circumstances.[403] In group I, representing about 10 percent of cases, the pulmonary process is part of a generalized form of lymphangiectasia that includes intestinal lymphangiectasia. In group II, representing about 20 percent of cases, it is the result of obstruction to pulmonary venous flow, usually associated with congenital heart disease. The latter is, most commonly, total anomalous venous return, but other causes include atresia of pulmonary veins and various forms of hypoplastic left heart syndrome.

Group III is the largest and accounts for about two thirds of all cases. It is composed of patients with a primary developmental defect of the lung lymphatics, and the prognosis is particularly poor in this group. An embryologic explanation has been proposed for this anomaly. Normally, the pulmonary lymphatics appear at the ninth week of fetal life, and by the fourteenth week they form a prominent network in the connective tissue between pulmonary lobules. By the twentieth week, the amount of connective tissue and the caliber of the lymphatics diminish considerably while the lobulation of the lung becomes less distinct. According to Laurence,[404] group III congenital pulmonary lymphangiectasia represents a developmental error in which the normal regression of connective tissue and lymphatics fails to occur after the sixteenth week of intrauterine life. The cause for this failure of the lymphatics to regress is not known. It should be noted that a similar explanation is proposed for congenital lymphangiectasia involving a limb.

Other Cysts

Bronchogenic cysts are congenital anomalies arising from an abnormal budding or diverticulum of the tracheobronchial tree. They can be conveniently divided into central and peripheral (intrapulmonary) cysts. The most common variant of central bronchogenic cyst occurs in the mediastinum, at the level of the carina or lower trachea, and can produce obstruction of major airways.[405] Often no communication exists between the cyst and parent bronchus. The cyst is filled with mucoid secretion, and its internal lining consists of respiratory epithelium. Other components of the wall are cartilage, muscle, and seromucous glands. More aberrant locations for these cysts are the neck, the presternal area, and even the shoulder.[406]

Peripheral (intraparenchymal) congenital cysts probably represent a disorder of bronchial growth at a later stage in fetal life than the more central bronchogenic cysts. Some are filled with serous fluid, and those communicating with the bronchial tree are air filled. Head distinguishes this simple type of bronchogenic cyst from the *batrachian* cyst.[407] The latter probably represents congenital cystic adenomatoid malformation of the lung.

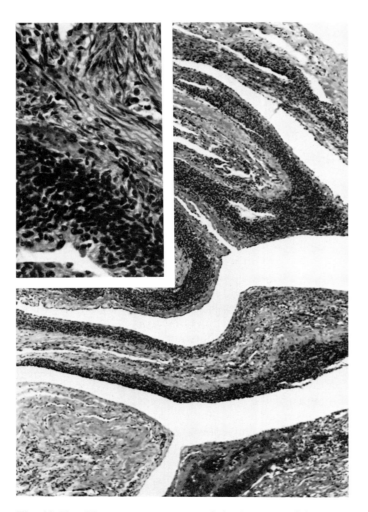

Fig. 20-59. Hamartomatous cyst of the lung containing cambium layer and mesenchymal stroma. (Inset) Detail of the cyst wall. (Courtesy of Dr. Eugene Mark, Boston.)

Multiple and bilateral hamartomatous nodules and cysts containing a cambium layer and primitive mesenchyme have been described by Mark[408] (Fig. 20-59). These curious cystic lesions evolve over many years. Sarcomatous transformation occurred in one of the five lesions described by Mark.

Vascular Anomalies

Pulmonary Arteriovenous Fistula

About 60 percent of patients with pulmonary arteriovenous fistula[409–413] have Rendu-Osler-Weber disease or hereditary telengiectasia, an autosomal-dominant disease. No pulmonary symptoms are noted in the majority of patients, but when present they usually begin in the second or third decade. Commonly observed symptoms are exertional dyspnea, cyanosis, clubbing of fingers, and polycythemia; hemoptysis is rare. A cerebrovascular accident (CVA) or brain abscess may also occur.

The radiographic picture is that of one or more shadows, usually rounded or coinlike, most often in the periphery of the lower lobes. A cardiac murmur is not usually present, but a continuous bruit may be audible over the lesions and become more accentuated by deep inspiration.

Grossly, the lesions vary in size from minute telangiectasia to well circumscribed masses up to 8 cm in greatest dimension. In about one third of patients, the lesions are bilateral and multiple, usually adjacent to the pleura. Histologically, the lesions consist of dilated, tortuous, and confluent blood spaces, representing the confluence of a pulmonary artery, proximally, and a pulmonary vein, distally, with no intervening capillary bed. Rarely, a bronchial artery contribution to the lesion exists. Thrombotic masses have been noted within the aneurysmal sac, the wall of which contains variable amounts of muscle, fibroelastic tissue, and calcium. The treatment of choice is surgery. Angiography is important, especially if an operation is to be performed, because the lesion may be multiple.

A variant of arteriovenous fistula is characterized by multiple small lesions of a saccular type. It may be difficult to recognize these lesions in the chest radiograph, in the angiogram, at gross dissection of the lung, and even under the microscope. They have been shown by injection-corrosion cast techniques at postmortem[412] and by magnification pulmonary angiography in a living patient.[413]

Systemic Artery to Pulmonary Vessel Fistula

Lesions of this type are rare and may be congenital or acquired.[414–418] The patients are usually asymptomatic, and the lesion is discovered because of a continuous murmur or an abnormal chest radiograph. The systemic arterial component is usually supplied by an internal mammary or intercostal artery, or an anomalous branch of the aorta. Bronchial, epicardial, pericardiophrenic, lateral thoracic, and esophageal arteries can also be afferent components. The fistulas empty into a pulmonary artery or into a vein with approximately equal frequency.[417]

In some patients, the lesion is clearly congenital, but other cases are the result of trauma or extensive pleural fibrosis (apical tuberculosis, bronchiectasis) allowing systemic collaterals to enter the lung and establish multiple connections with pulmonary vessels.

The correct diagnosis is established by selective arterial angiography. If surgery is to be performed, the preferred treatment is interruption of the vascular channels and resection of the involved lung. Grossly, the lesions represent a complex, racemose mass of vascular channels that can best be demonstrated by injection-corrosion techniques.

Pulmonary Varicosities

Radiologically, pulmonary varices can simulate coin lesions, pulmonary tuberculosis, bronchogenic carcinoma, mediastinal tumor, lymphadenopathy, and arteriovenous fistulas.[419,420] They are most commonly seen in the right lung, especially in the upper lobe. Pulmonary varicosities are presumed to be of congenital nature because of their occurrence in young people, sometimes coexisting with other congenital abnormalities. However, their reported association with valvular heart disease and pulmonary venous hypertension has led to the speculation that the latter factor may be causally related to dilation and varix formation. Indeed, in one patient, the varix was observed to shrink in size after prosthetic valve replacement.[420]

Aneurysms of Pulmonary Arteries

Aneurysms of pulmonary arteries are rare, usually involving either the main pulmonary artery or its main branches. Charlton and du Plessis[421] reviewed the literature up to 1961 and collected reports of 30 cases of aneurysms of secondary and tertiary branches. In most cases, the aneurysms were of mycotic type, resulting from an episode of bacterial endocarditis in patients with congenital heart defects.

The possibility that some of these aneurysms could be congenital was raised by Plokker et al,[422] who described the case of a 26-year-old patient with an aneurysm of a tertiary branch of the pulmonary artery presenting as a coin lesion and referred to another case with a similar presentation. In view of abnormalities in the elastic con-figuration of the pulmonary artery, these authors proposed a congenital weakness as a main cause of some of these aneurysms.

Ectopic Tissue in the Lung

Glial nodules[423] in the lungs are known to occur in anencephaly; it is assumed that they arise by implantation of glial cells sloughed from the exposed neural plate into the amniotic fluid followed by aspiration by the fetus. Brain tissue may also gain entry into the lung via embolic circulatory pathways due to obstetric trauma or in later life.[424,425]

Gonzalez-Crussi et al.[423] described the case of a newborn with respiratory distress and extensive brain heterotopia resembling cystic adenomatoid malformation. It is possible that, as in those instances of brain heterotopia in the nasal and oral cavities, maldevelopment of the basicranial structures may have allowed brain tissue to be extruded into the nasopharynx and aspirated during intrauterine life.

Migration of *liver* parenchyma through a diaphragmatic defect, thought to represent a persistence of the primitive pleuroperitoneal canal, can result in the presence of a mass of liver tissue in close association with the pulmonary right lower lobe. The ectopic liver tissue may be unconnected with the liver or connected through a pedicle containing vessels and bile ducts.[426,427]

In one report, an intrathoracic liver mass, not connected to the liver, followed trauma to the right upper abdominal quadrant, and was noted to increase in size since the time of detection.[427] Microscopically, the mass was encapsulated and consisted of hyperplastic nodules separated by thin strands of dense fibroconnective tissue. Surgical removal of ectopic liver tissue was curative.

A thoracic *kidney* is a very rare developmental anomaly that radiologically appears as a well demarcated mass with a subphrenic component at the base of a lung and posteriorly.[428,429] The left side is more commonly affected than the right, and one bilateral case has been reported. The excretory urogram is diagnostic in this condition.

Deposits of *adrenal tissue* in the lung are known to occur.[430] Thyroid tissue[431] can occur inside the trachea. The anomaly is three times more frequent in women than in men and may cause tracheal obstruction. Bundles of *striated muscle* fibers can be observed, rarely, in intralobar sequestration and in pulmonary blastomas.

Gastrointestinal epithelium lining mucus-filled cysts has been reported in newborn infants and occasionally in adults. One such lesion measuring 25 cm in diameter and located in the left lower lobe was described by Killett et al.[432] The same report described the presence of masses of *pancreatic tissue* in a cystic intralobar sequestration of the right upper lobe in a 2-month-old child.

The presence of *endometrial* tissue in the lung and pleura is well recognized; there have been 17 reported cases of histologically proven thoracic endometriosis and 27 cases of probably thoracic endometriosis up to 1981.[433] The lesion may be asymptomatic or can be associated with a clinical picture of catamenial pneumothorax, catamenial hemoptysis, or recurrent hemothorax. *Decidua*,[19] usually pleural in location, is an abnormality noted in these patients under hormonal stimulation (pregnancy, progestational therapy).

Nodular deposits of *metaplastic bone* are not infrequent in patients with mitral stenosis and in chronic inflammatory conditions. Ossification with bone marrow metaplasia is seen in tracheobronchial cartilages of elderly people. Idiopathic heterotopic ossification unrelated to any obvious pathological condition may affect all lobes or be restricted to both bases or one lobe. Occasionally, it may be so severe as to transform a whole lobe into a solid mass of bone.[434]

MISCELLANEOUS LESIONS

Miscellaneous localized pulmonary lesions are listed in Table 20-13 and are discussed in the following sections.

Rheumatoid Nodules

Nodules in the chest radiographs of patients with rheumatoid arthritis can be found any time in the course of the disease.[435] They are frequently associated with manifestations such as diffuse interstitial fibrosis and pleural effusion, and the rheumatoid factor is invariably elevated. Most of the nodules are between 1 and 2 cm in diameter and show a preference for the subpleural regions.

Histologically, the rheumatoid nodule has a three-layered structure. The central portion shows features of fibrinoid necrosis with disintegration of the alveolar architecture, focal collections of foamy histiocytes, and dust-laden macrophages. Peripheral to it is a dense prolif-

TABLE 20-13. Localized Pulmonary Lesions: Miscellaneous Group

Rheumatoid nodules
Caplan's nodule
Amyloidoma
Hyalinizing granuloma
Lipoid granuloma
Localized radiation fibrosis
Apical caps
Infarcts and contusions
Rounded atelectasis

eration of histiocytes in palisade arrangement. The third and outermost layer is composed of organizing pneumonia or granulation-like tissue rich in lymphocytes, plasma cells, and fibroblasts. The inflammation extends to neighboring vessels, which also show variable degrees of intimal fibrosis.

Pulmonary nodules in patients with rheumatoid arthritis often coexist with subcutaneous nodules. They may disappear spontaneously, recur, persist indefinitely, or cavitate. Because neoplasms or infections can radiologically resemble these innocuous lesions, surgical resection is frequently performed.

Caplan's Syndrome

The term *Caplan's syndrome*[436,437] was originally applied to the combination of coal worker's pneumonoconiosis, rheumatoid arthritis, and pulmonary nodules. The latter can measure 0.5 to 5.0 cm in diameter and usually occur in a background of category 0 to 1 coal worker's pneumoconiosis. They can develop concomitantly with the arthritic symptoms, precede them by as many as 5 to 10 years, or occur afterward. Calcification is very common and the nodules may also be associated with pleural effusion.

To the naked eye, the Caplan nodule has less dust deposition than the surrounding lung, and it may show a system of concentric layers. Histologically, the center of the nodule is composed of necrotic tissue, dust, and collagen. Outside the necrotic area, there is a cellular zone with dense infiltration of lymphocytes, plasma cells, and histiocytes. Endarteritis with occlusion of vessels is frequently found. A peripheral zone shows acute and chronic inflammation and fibrosis. Since the original description, the concept of Caplan's nodule has been expanded to include similar lesions in other pneumoconioses, such as silicosis and asbestosis.

Pneumoconiosis

Localized masses or infiltrates of various kinds can occur in the lungs of patients with several pneumoconiosis.[437–439] For the purpose of this discussion, some lesions such as progressive massive fibrosis (PMF) and silicosis are briefly discussed. PMF is classically described in complicated coal worker's pneumoconiosis (CWP). PMF consists of massive lesions usually found in the posterior segments of the upper lobes or superior segments of the lower lobes. The pleura underlying the lesions is frequently adherent to the inner chest wall. On cut section, the lesions are composed or solid, amorphous black tissue, and there is frequently cavitation. The cavities may be filled with jet black fluid. Cavitation of PMF lesions is virtually always the result of ischemic necrosis or secondary tuberculosis. In the United States and Britain, the former is true, but tuberculosis is common in those areas of the world where this infection is endemic.

Microscopically, there are many deposits of coal dust and fibrosis, with resulting obliteration of the lung architecture, accompanied by a cellular infiltrate composed of lymphocytes and plasma cells. The fibrous masses encroach upon vessels and bronchi and obliterate them. Vascular involvement is a main feature of PMF lesions; traces of obliterated arteries and veins at the periphery of the lesions can be recognized with elastic tissue stains. The adventitia and media of medium-sized and large pulmonary arteries are often infiltrated by dust-laden cells.

Characteristic lesions in silicosis consist of gray, fibrotic nodules, more profuse in the apical and posterior zones of upper and lower lobes. They vary in size from a few millimeters to large conglomerate masses that may occupy much of a lobe. When cut, the nodules are hard and gritty in consistency. They have a characteristic whorled appearance, also seen in involved lymph nodes. The areas of massive fibrosis may show cavitation due to either ischemic necrosis or tuberculosis. In the latter instance, caseation may be seen in the center of the lesion. Microscopically, silica microcrystals can be easily identified by polarized light at the periphery of the lesions.

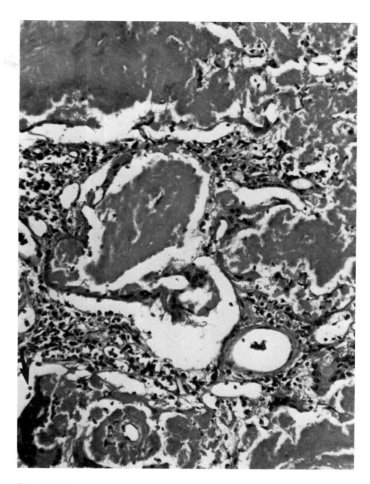

Fig. 20-60. Amyloidoma. The patient had numerous pulmonary nodules composed of amyloid deposits within alveolar spaces and in the walls of vessels. A foreign body giant cell response is noted (arrow). There is also a diffuse cellular infiltrate composed of lymphocytes and plasma cells. (Courtesy of Dr. Morton Robinson, Miami Beach.)

Amyloidoma

Amyloidosis can occur as a disease largely confined to the respiratory tract.[440,441] There are two anatomic-clinical forms: nodular and diffuse tracheobronchial amyloidosis. Patients with the nodular form of the disease are usually older than 60 years. Multiple nodules are more frequent than solitary lesions and the disease is bilateral in 50 percent of patients. The etiology of the condition is unknown, and patients may have other associated processes.

Radiologically, the condition resembles a neoplasm. Grossly, amyloidomas are parenchymal in location, with a preference for the subpleural region. Most of the masses measure between 3 and 6 cm but can be as large as 16 cm in diameter. Smaller lesions have a tan-gray, almost cartilaginous appearance. Large lesions are variegated in appearance, with foci of hemorrhage, necrosis, and calcification. Microscopically, there are extensive amorphous deposits of amyloid in the centers of the lesions with obliteration of the lung architecture (Fig. 20-60). Amyloid deposits are also prominent in the walls of bronchi and bronchioles, and particularly in the walls of vessels. A giant cell granulomatous response is seen around these vessels, and there are large numbers of lym-

phocytes and plasma cells, particularly toward the periphery of the lesions.

Amyloid is recognized in these lesions by crystal violet and Congo red stains. The prognosis of this disease is excellent, and the nodules change little in size over the years. On the contrary, diffuse tracheobronchial amyloidosis is frequently associated with airway obstruction and the prognosis is poor.

Pulmonary Hyalinizing Granuloma

Pulmonary hyalinizing granuloma was described by Engleman et al.[442] in 1977 on the basis of 20 patients. In most of these cases, the lesions were multiple, bilateral, and mildly symptomatic nodules. Four patients had associated fibrosing mediastinitis, and one other patient had

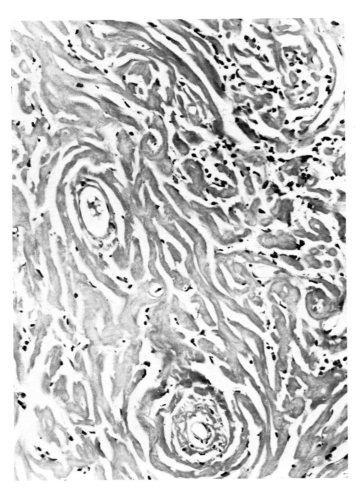

Fig. 20-61. Hyalinizing granuloma. Characteristic perivascular hyaline lamellae and scant lymphoplasmacytic cellular infiltrate. (Courtesy of Dr. Jorge Restrepo, Bogota, Colombia.)

retroperitoneal fibrosis and amyloidosis. The patient described by Drasin et al.[443] had malignant lymphoma and eventually developed multiple myeloma and systemic amyloidosis.

Microscopically, the nodules are composed of homogeneous, pink, hyaline lamellae surrounded by collections of plasma cells, lymphocytes, and histiocytes (Fig. 20-61). Mild perivascular inflammation is frequently seen. Positive staining for amyloid may be seen in only a minority of cases, and the lesions do not calcify or ossify as nodular amyloidosis does. Other differences include the younger age of the patients with hyalinizing granuloma and the association with sclerosing mediastinitis and retroperitoneal fibrosis.

The prognosis of this disease is favorable.[444] The nodules remain stable or enlarge slightly over many years. The differential diagnosis includes amyloidosis, rheuma-

toid nodules, plasma cell granuloma, nodular sarcoidosis, and infectious granulomas (tuberculosis, histoplasmosis).

Lipoid Granuloma

Inhalation of lipid materials can produce single or multiple, sharply circumscribed masses with a marked resemblance to lung tumors, both radiologically and by palpation at the time of thoracotomy.[445,446] Moreover, atypical histiocytes may be found in the sputum or bronchial washings of these patients; they can be erroneously interpreted as malignant cells.

Aspiration of lipid material can occur in two different clinical settings: infants and adults. The infantile type most frequently represents a bilateral, diffuse process following milk aspiration and is very often complicated by bacterial infection. The adult type is usually observed in patients with a history of habitual self-administration of oily substances in the form of nasal drops or sprays or the ingestion of mineral oil.

Grossly, the masses are approximately rounded, frequently multiple, and very hard in consistency. Histologically, the lipid dissolved during histologic preparation appears as rounded, empty vacuoles surrounded by giant cells of foreign body type. There is extensive fibrosis and hyalinization. Lymphocytes and plasma cells are also present. The lumina of the airways contain clusters of lipid-laden histiocytes and giant cells. Stains for lipids (oil-red O) in formalin-fixed or fresh material will be positive in the bubbly spaces of the lesion.

Localized Radiation Fibrosis

Diffuse interstitial pneumonitis and interstitial fibrosis are well recognized complications of radiation to the lung. Less well known is the occurrence of fibrotic masses or infiltrates following radiation to a localized portion of the lung.[447-449] Most common in our experience are unilateral apical lesions in women who had received axillary radiation to breast cancer nodal metastases. Bilateral apical fibrosis has been noted following radiation to the neck for lymphoma or carcinoma. The hilar regions can be similarly involved after radiation to the mediastinum. When a prior history of radiation is not elicited or ignored, patients with such lesions are put through unnecessary diagnostic tests, including biopsy. The latter shows characteristic features of interstitial fibrosis, striking alveolar cell atypia and obliterative vascular changes.

Apical Caps

In about 20 to 25 percent of the general autopsy population, particularly in the older age groups, the pulmonary apices are covered by broad, flattened, fibrotic caps.[450,451] They are usually bilateral and can be calcified. The pathogenesis of this lesion is obscure, but the possibility of tuberculosis has been discarded. Another view is that it represents a nonspecific response of the apex to a situation of relative ischemia. Sometimes an apical cap can be so prominent as to prompt a biopsy. The latter would show nonspecific changes in fibrosis with marked hyalinization and elastosis, chronic inflammation, intra-alveolar pigmented macrophages, and foci of calcification. The possibility that some apical cancers (Pancoast tumor) arise in relation to apical caps has been raised[452] but remains unproven.

Pulmonary Infarcts and Contusions

Radiographic signs of congestive atelectasis and infarction develop in about 10 percent of patients with pulmonary thromboembolism. The picture is that of parenchymal densities ranging from a patchy pneumonic infiltrate to a round nodular lesion. The only distinguishing feature of these lesions is their abutment against the pleura.[453] In civilian life, *pulmonary contusion*[454] is almost frequently seen in automobile accident victims whose chests violently strike steering wheels and dashboards. In military practice, pulmonary contusion is caused by nonpenetrating wounds from high velocity missiles, blows from blunt objects, and the blasts of high velocity missiles. Regardless of etiology, the picture of the lung contusion is one of rupture of blood vessels and alveoli with interstitial and alveolar hemorrhage. The lesions may range from clinically undetectable areas of hemorrhage to the fatal, massive, bloody consolidation of one or both lungs.

Rounded Atelectasis

A little known form of collapse, rounded atelectasis, is occasionally seen on chest radiographs.[455,456] It appears as a rounded or oval mass measuring 2.5 to 5 cm in greatest diameter, pleural-based, and usually lying along the posterior surface of a lower lobe. The lesion appears to be centered on chronically inflamed and fibrotic pleura, and the blood vessels near it gather in a sheaf-like fashion as they converge toward the mass, much like the tail of a comet. Lack of familiarity with this clinically innocuous entity usually leads to a mistaken diagnosis of neoplasm

followed by unneeded thoracotomy. The unaware pathologist may mistakenly interpret such a lesion as a healed infarct. Recently, the relation between asbestos-induced pleural fibrosis and rounded atelectasis has been noted.[456]

REFERENCES

1. Spencer H: Pathology of the Lung. 4th Ed. Pergamon, Oxford, 1985
2. Dail DH, Hammar SP (eds): Pulmonary Pathology, Springer-Verlag, New York, 1988
3. Thurlbeck WM (ed): Pathology of the Lung. Thieme, New York, 1988
4. Silverberg E, Lubera JA: Cancer Statistics 1988. CA 38:5, 1988
5. Arrigoni MG, Woolner LB, Bernat PE, et al: Benign tumors of the lung. A ten-year surgical experience. J Thorac Cardiovasc Surg 60:589, 1970
6. Adler I: Primary Malignant Growths of the Lungs and Bronchi: A Pathological and Clinical Study. Longmans, Green, New York, 1912
7. Gori GB, Peters JA: Etiology and prevention of lung cancer. Prev Med 4:235, 1975
8. Wynder EL: The etiology, epidemiology and prevention of lung cancer. Semin Respir Med 3:135, 1982
9. Hirayama T: Non-smoking wives of heavy smokers have a higher risk of lung cancer: A study from Japan. Br Med J 282:183, 1981
10. Trichopoulos D, Delandidi A, Spanos L, MacMahon B: Lung cancer and passive smoking. Int J Cancer 27:1, 1981
11. Garfinkel L: Time trends in lung cancer mortality among nonsmokers and a note on passive smoking. J Natl Cancer Inst 66:1061, 1981
12. Mark EJ: Lung Biopsy Interpretation. Williams & Wilkins, Baltimore, 1984
13. Elema JD, Keuning HM: The use of electron microscopy for the diagnosis of cancer in bronchial biopsies. Hum Pathol 19:304, 1988
14. Liebow AA: Tumors of the Lower Respiratory Tract. Atlas of Tumor Pathology. section 5. Pt. 17. Armed Forces Institute of Pathology, Washington, DC, 1952
15. Carter D, Eggleston JC: Tumors of the Lower Respiratory Tract. Atlas of Tumor Pathology. second series. Pt. 17. Armed Forces Institute of Pathology, Washington, DC, 1980
16. Kreyberg L, Liebow AA, Uehlinger EA: Histological typing of lung tumors. World Health Organization, Geneva, 1957
17. World Health Organization: The World Health Organization Histological Typing of Lung Tumors. 2nd Ed. Am J Clin Pathol 77:123, 1982
18. Hammar SP: Common neoplasms. p. 727. In Pulmonary Pathology. Dail DH, Hammer SP (eds): Springer-Verlag, New York, 1988
19. Dail DH: Uncommon Tumors. p. 847. In Pulmonary Pa-

thology. Dail DH, Hammar SP (eds): Springer-Verlag, New York, 1988

20. Churg A: Tumors of the Lung. p. 311. In Pathology of the Lung. Thurlbeck WM (ed): Thieme, New York, 1988
21. Carr DT, Mountain CF: Staging of Lung Cancer. Semin Respir Med 3:154, 1982
22. Mountain CF, Lukeman JM, Hammar SP, et al: Lung Cancer Classification: The relationship of disease extent and cell type to survival in a clinical trial population. J Surg Oncol 35:147, 1987
23. Mountain CF: A new international staging system for lung cancer. Chest 89(suppl):2255, 1986
24. Shimosato Y, Hashimoto T, Kodama T, et al: Prognostic implications of fibrotic focus (scar) in small peripheral lung cancers. Am J Surg Pathol 4:365, 1980
25. Kung ITM, Lui IOL, Loke SL, et al: Pulmonary scar cancer: A pathologic reappraisal. Am J Surg Pathol 9:391, 1985
26. Vincent RG, Pickren JW, Lane WW, et al: The changing histopathology of lung cancer. A review of 1682 cases. Cancer 39:1647, 1977
27. Valaitis J, Warren S, Gamble, D: Increasing incidence of adenocarcinoma of the lung. Cancer 47:1042, 1981
28. Taylor AB, Shinton NH, Waterhouse JAH: Histology of bronchial carcinoma in relation to prognosis. Thorax 18:178, 1963
29. Weiss W, Boucot KR, Cooper DA: The histopathology of bronchogenic carcinoma and its relation to growth rate, metastasis, and prognosis. Cancer 26:965, 1970
30. Harwood TR, Gracey DR, Yookoo H: Pseudomesotheliomatous carcinoma of the lung. Am J Clin Pathol 65:159, 1976
31. Ashley DJB, Davies HD: Mixed glandular and squamous-cell carcinoma of the bronchus. Thorax 22:431, 1967
32. Fitzgibbons PL, Kern WH: Adenosquamous carcinoma of the lung: A clinical and pathology study of seven cases. Hum Pathol 16:463, 1985
33. Kradin RL, Young RH, Dickersin R et al. Pulmonary blastoma with argyrophil cells lacking sarcomatous features (pulmonary endodermal tumor resembling fetal lung). Am J Surg Pathol 6:165, 1982
34. Kodama T, Shimosato Y, Watarabe S, et al: Six cases of well-differentiated adenocarcinoma simulating fetal lung tubules in pseudoglandular stage: Comparison with pulmonary blastoma. Am J Surg Pathol 8:735, 1984
35. Manning JT Jr, Ordonez NG, Rosenberg HS, Walker WE: Pulmonary endodermal tumor resembling fetal lung. Arch Pathol Lab Med 109:48, 1985
36. Muller-Hermelink HK, Kaiserling E: Pulmonary adenocarcinoma of fetal type: alternating differentiation argues in favor of a common endodermal stem cell. Virchows Arch [A] 409:195, 1986
37. Auerbach O, Garfinkel L, Parks VR: Scar cancer of the lung. Increase over a 21-year period. Cancer 43:636, 1979
38. Madri JA, Carter D: Scar cancers of the lung: origin and significance. Hum Pathol 15:625, 1984
39. Barsky SH, Huang SJ, Bhuta S: The extracellular matrix of pulmonary scar carcinomas is suggestive of a desmoplastic origin. Am J Pathol 124:412, 1986
40. Liebow AA: Bronchiolo-alveolar carcinoma. Adv Intern Med 10:329, 1960
41. Singh G, Scheithauer BW, Katyal S: The pathobiologic features of carcinomas of type II pneumocytes. Cancer 57:994, 1986
42. Kuhn C: Fine structure of bronchioloalveolar cell carcinoma. Cancer 30:1107, 1972
43. Bedrossian CWM, Weilbaecher DG, Beninck DC, et al: Ultrastructure of human bronchioloalveolar cell carcinoma. Cancer 36:1399, 1975
44. Montes M, Binette JP, Chaudhry AP, et al: Clara cell adenocarcinoma—Light and electron microscopic studies. Am J Surg Pathol 1:245, 1977
45. Johnston WW, Ginn FL, Amatulli JM: Light and electron microscopic observations on malignant cells in cerebrospinal fluid from metastatic alveolar cell carcinoma. Acta Cytol 15:365, 1971
46. Morningstar WA, Hassan MO: Bronchiolo-alveolar carcinoma with nodal metastases. An ultrastructural study. Am J Surg Pathol 3:273, 1979
47. Bonikos DS, Hendrickson M, Bensch KG: Pulmonary alveolar cell carcinoma. Fine structural and in vitro study of a case and critical review of this entity. Am J Surg Pathol 1:93, 1977
48. Nisbet DL, Mackay JMK, Smith W, et al Ultrastructure of sheep pulmonary adenomatosis (Jaagziekte). J Pathol 103:157, 1971
49. Ogata T, Endo K: Clara cell granules of peripheral lung cancers. Cancer 54:1635, 1984
50. Feldman PS, Innes DJ: Pulmonary alveolar cell carcinoma: A new variant. Lab Invest 42:20, 1980 (abst)
51. Kauffman SL, Alexander L, Sass L: Histologic and ultrastructural features of the Clara cell adenoma of the mouse lung. Lab Invest 40:708, 1979
52. Kimura I: Progression of pulmonary tumor in mice. 1. Histological studies of primary and transplanted pulmonary tumors. Acta Pathol Jpn 21:13, 1971
53. Fantone JC, Geisinger KR, Appelman HD: Papillary adenoma of the lung with lamellar and electron dense granules. An ultrastructural study. Cancer 50:2839, 1982
54. Noguchi M, Kodama T, Shimosato Y, et al: Papillary adenoma of type 2 pneumocytes. Am J Surg Pathol 10:134, 1980
55. Meyer EC, Liebow AA: Relationship of interstitial pneumonia, honeycombing and atypical epithelial proliferation to cancer of the lung. Cancer 218:322, 1965
56. Montgomery RD, Stirling GA, Hamer NAJ: Bronchiolar carcinoma in progressive systemic sclerosis. Lancet 2:693, 1962
57. Turner-Warwick M, Lebowitz M, Burrows B, et al: Cryptogenic fibrosing alveolitis and lung cancer. Thorax 35:496, 1980
58. McDonald JC, McDonald AD: Epidemiology of asbestos-related lung cancer. p. 57. In Antman K, Aisner J, eds: Asbestos Related Malignancy. Grune & Stratton, Orlando, FL, 1987
59. Churg A: Neoplastic asbestos-induced diseases. p. 279. In Churg A, Green FHY, eds: Pathology of Occupational Lung Disease. Igaku-Shoin, New York, 1988

60. Matthews MJ: Problems in morphology and behavior of bronchopulmonary malignant disease. p. 23. In Israel L, Chahinian AP (eds): Lung Cancer: Natural History, Prognosis and Therapy. Academic, Orlando, FL, 1976

61. Matthews MJ, Gordon PR: Morphology of pulmonary and pleural malignancies. p. 49. In Straus MJ (ed): Lung Cancer: Clinical Diagnosis and Treatment. Grune & Stratton, Orlando, FL, 1977

62. Churg A, Johnston WH, Stalbarg M: Small cell squamous and mixed small cell squamous-small cell anaplastic carcinomas of the lung. Am J Surg Pathol 4:255, 1980

63. Love GL, Baroca PJ: Bronchogenic sarcomatoid squamous cell carcinoma with osteoclast-like giant cells. Hum Pathol 14:1004, 1983

64. Addis BJ, Corrin B: Pulmonary blastoma, carcinosarcoma and spindle cell carcinoma: An immunohistochemical study of keratin intermediate filaments. J Pathol 147:291, 1985

65. Humphrey PA, Scroggs MW, Rogli VL, Shelburne JD: Pulmonary carcinomas with a sarcomatoid element: An immunocytochemical and ultrastructural analysis. Hum Pathol 19:155, 1988

66. Begin LR, Eskandari J, Joncas J, Panasci, L: Epstein-Barr Virus related lymphoepithelioma-like carcinoma of lung. J Surg Oncol 30:280, 1987

67. Barnard WG: The nature of the "oat-celled sarcoma" of the mediastinum. J Pathol 29:241, 1926

68. Azzopardi JG: Oat-cell carcinoma of the bronchus. J Pathol 78:513, 1960

69. Kato Y, Ferguson TB, Bennett DE, et al: Oat cell carcinoma of the lung. A review of 138 cases. Cancer 23:517, 1964

70. Carter D: Small-cell carcinoma of the lung. Am J Surg Pathol 7:787, 1983

71. Yesner R: Small cell tumors of the lung. Am J Surg Pathol 7:7, 1983

72. Sidhu GS: The ultrastructure of malignant neoplasms of the lung. Pathol Annu 17:229, 1982

73. Mark EJ, Ramirez JF: Peripheral small cell carcinoma of the lung resembling carcinoid tumor. Arch Pathol Lab Med 109:263, 1985

74. Gephardt GN, Grady KJ, Ahmad M, et al: Peripheral small cell undifferentiated carcinoma of the lung. Clinicopathologic features of 17 cases. Cancer 61:1002, 1988

75. Radice PA, Matthews MJ, Ihde DK et al: The clinical behavior of "mixed" small/large cell bronchogenic carcinoma compared to "pure" small cell subtypes. Cancer 50:2894, 1982

76. Case Records of the Massachusetts General Hospital (case 3-1984). N Engl J Med 310:178, 1984

77. McDowell EM, Trump BF: Pulmonary small cell carcinoma showing tripartite differentiation in individual cells. Hum Pathol 12:286, 1981

78. Delmonte VC, Alberti O, Saldiva PHN: Large cell carcinoma of the lung: Ultrastructural and immunohistochemical features. Chest 90:524, 1986

79. Churg A: The fine structure of large cell undifferentiated carcinoma of the lung: Evidence for its relation to squamous cell carcinomas and adenocarcinomas. Hum Pathol 9:143, 1978

80. Horie A, Ohta M: Ultrastructural features of large cell carcinoma of the lung with reference to the prognosis of patients. Hum Pathol 12:423, 1981

81. Albain KS, True LD, Golomb HM, et al: Large cell carcinoma of the lung: Ultrastructural differentiation and clinicopathologic correlations. Cancer 56:1618, 1985

82. Piehl MR, Lee I, Ma Y, et al: Subsets of pulmonary large cell undifferentiated carcinomas defined immunohistochemically (abstract). Lab Invest 56:60A, 1987

83. Nash G, Stout AP: Giant cell carcinoma of the lung: Report of 5 cases. Cancer 2:369, 1958

84. Wang NS, Seemayer TA, Ahmed MN, Knaack J: Giant cell carcinoma of the lung: A light and electron microscopic study. Hum Pathol 7:3, 1976

85. Katzenstein A-LA, Prioleau PG, Askin FB: Histologic spectrum and significance of clear-cell change in lung carcinoma. Cancer 45:943, 1980

86. Edward C, Carlile A: Clear cell carcinoma of the lung. J Clin Pathol 38:880, 1985

87. Bensch KG, Gordon GB, Miller LR: Studied on the bronchial counterpart of the Kultschitzky (argentaffin) cell and innervation of bronchial glands. J Ultrastruct Res 12:668, 1965

88. Gould VE, Linnolla RI, Memoli VA, Warren WH: Neuroendocrine components of the bronchopulmonary tract: Hyperplasias, dysplasia, and neoplasms. Lab Invest 59:519, 1983

89. Lauweryns JM, Godderis P: Neuroepithelial bodies in the human child and adult lung. Am Rev Respir Dis 111:496, 1975

90. Whitwell F: Tumorlets of the lung. J Pathol 70:529, 1955

91. Hausman DH, Weimann RB: Pulmonary tumorlet and hilar node metastasis: Report of a case. Cancer 20:1515, 1967

92. Rodgers-Sullivan RF, Weisland RH, Palumbo PJ, et al: Pulmonary tumorlets associated with Cushing's syndrome. Am Rev Respir Dis 117:799, 1978

93. D'Aggti VD, Perzin KH: Carcinoid tumorlets of the lung with metastasis to a peribronchial lymph node: Report of a case and review of the literature. Cancer 55:2472, 1985

94. Mark EJ, Quay SC, Dickersin R: Papillary carcinoid tumor of the lung. Cancer 48:316, 1981

95. Kinney FJ, Kovarick JL: Bone formation in bronchial adenoma. Am J Clin Pathol 44:52, 1965

96. Al-Kaisi N, Abdul-Karim FW, Mendelsohn G, Jacobs G: Bronchial carcinoid tumor with amyloid stroma. Arch Pathol Lab Med 112:211, 1988

97. Felton WL II, Liebow AA, Lindskog GE: Peripheral and multiple bronchial adenomas. Cancer 6:555, 1953

98. Bonikos DS, Bensch KG, Jamplis RW: Peripheral pulmonary carcinoid tumors. Cancer 37:1977, 1976

99. Ranchod M, Levine GD: Spindle-cell carcinoid tumors of the lung. Am J Surg Pathol 4:315, 1980

100. Cebelin MS: Melanocytic bronchial carcinoid tumor. Cancer 46:1843, 1980

101. Grazer R, Cohen SM, Jacobs JB, Lucas P: Melanin-containing peripheral carcinoid of the lung. Am J Surg Pathol 6:73, 1982

102. Arrigoni MG, Woolner LB, Bernatz PE: Atypical carci-

noid tumors of the lung. J Thorac Cardiovasc Surg 64:413, 1972

103. Mills SE, Walker AN, Cooper PH, Kron IL: Atypical Carcinoid tumor of the lung. Am J Surg Pathol 6:643, 1982

104. Grote TH, Macon WR, Tavis B, et al: Atypical carcinoid of the lung. A distinct clinicopathologic entity. Chest 93:370, 1980

105. Neal MH, Kosinki R, Cohen P, Orenstein JM: Atypical endocrine tumors of the lung: a histologic, ultrastructural and clinical study of 19 cases. Hum Pathol 17:1264, 1986

106. Emory WB, Mitchell WT Jr, Hatch HB Jr: Mucous gland adenoma of the bronchus. Am Rev Respir Dis 108:1407, 1973

107. Black WC III: Pulmonary oncocytoma. Cancer 23:1347, 1969

108. Ghadialy FN, Block HJ: Oncocytic carcinoid of the lung. J Submicrosc Cytol 17:435, 1985

109. Fechner RE, Bentinck DC: Ultrastructure of bronchial oncocytoma. Cancer 31:1451, 1973

110. Santos-Briz A, Terron J, Sastre R, et al: Oncocytoma of the lung. Cancer 40:1330, 1977

111. Payne WS, Schier J, Woolner LB: Mixed tumors of the bronchus (salivary gland type). J Thorac Cardiovasc Surg 49:663, 1965

112. Heilbrunn A, Crosby IK: Adenocystic carcinoma and mucoepidermoid carcinoma of the tracheobronchial tree. Chest 61:145, 1972

113. Payne WS, Fontana RS, Woolner LB: Bronchial Tumors originating from mucous glands: Current classification and unusual manifestations. Med Clin North Am 48:945, 1968

114. Weber AL, Grillo HG: Tracheal tumors: A radiological, clinical and pathological evaluation of 84 cases. Radiol Clin North Am 16:227, 1978

115. Spencer H: Bronchial mucous gland tumors. Virchows Arch [A] 383:101, 1979

116. Turnbull AD, Huvos AG, Goodner JT, et al: Mucoepidermoid tumors of bronchial glands. Cancer 28:539, 1971

117. Leonardi HK, Jung-Lee Y, Legg MA, et al: Tracheobronchial mucoepidermoid carcinoma. Clinicopathological features and results of treatment. J Thorac Cardiovasc Surg 76:431, 1978

118. Klacsmann PG, Olson JL, Eggleton JC: Mucoepidermoid carcinoma of the bronchus. An electron microscopic study of the low grade and the high grade variants. Cancer 43:1720, 1979

119. Seo IS, Warren J, Mirkin D, et al: Mucoepidermoid carcinoma of the bronchus in a 4-year-old child: A high-grade variant with lymph node metastases. Cancer 53:1600, 1984

120. Metcalf JS, Maize JC, Shaw EB: Bronchial mucoepidermoid carcinoma metastatic to skin: Report of a case and review of the literature. Cancer 58:2556, 1986

121. Barsky SH, Martin SE, Mathews M, et al: "Low grade" mucoepidermoid carcinoma of the bronchus with "high grade" biological behavior. Cancer 51:1505, 1983

122. Fechner RE, Bentinck BR, Askew JB Jr: Acinic cell tumor of the lung. A histologic and ultrastructural study. Cancer 29:501, 1972

123. Katz DR, Dubis JJ: Acinic cell tumor of the bronchus. Cancer 38:830, 1976

124. Spencer H, Dail DH, Arneaud J: Non-invasive bronchial epithelial papillary tumors. Cancer 45:1486, 1980

125. Assor D: A papillary transitional cell tumor of the bronchus. Am J Clin Pathol 55:761, 1971

126. Al-Saleem T, Peale AR, Norris CM: Multiple papillomatosis of the respiratory tract: Clinical and pathologic study of 11 cases. Cancer 22:1173, 1968

127. Boyle WF, McCoy EG, Fogarty WA: Electron microscopic identification of virus-like particles in laryngeal papilloma. Ann Otol Rhinol Laryngol 80:693, 1971

128. Moore RL, Lattes R: Papillomatosis of larynx and bronchi. Cancer 12:117, 1959

129. Mayors M, Devine KD, Parkhill EM: Malignant transformation of benign laryngeal papillomas after radiation therapy. Surg Clin North Am 43:1049, 1963

130. Runckel D, Kessler S: Bronchogenic squamous carcinoma in non-irradiated juvenile laryngotracheal papillomatosis. Am J Surg Pathol 4:293, 1980

131. Smith JF, Dexter D: Papillary neoplasms of the bronchus of low grade malignancy. Thorax 18:340, 1963

132. Sherwin RT, La Foret EG, Strieder JW: Exophytic endobronchial carcinoma. J Thorac Cardiovasc Surg 43:716, 1962

133. Sniffen RC, Soutter L, Robbins LL: Muco-epidermoid tumors of the bronchus arising from surface epithelium. Am J Pathol 34:671, 1958

134. Bauermeister DE, Jennings ER, Beland AH, et al: Pulmonary blastoma, a form of carcinosarcoma. Am J Clin Pathol 46:322, 1966

135. Roth JA, Elguezabal A: Pulmonary blastoma evolving into carcinosarcoma. A case study. Am J Surg Pathol 2:407, 1978

136. Barnard WG: Embryoma of lung. Thorax 7:299, 1952

137. Spencer H: Pulmonary blastomas. J Pathol 82:161, 1965

138. Karcioglu ZA, Someren AO: Pulmonary blastoma. A case report and review of the literature. Am J Clin Pathol 61:287, 1974

139. McCann MP, Fu Y, Kay S: Pulmonary blastoma. A light and electron microscopic study. Cancer 38:789, 1976

140. Fung CH, Lo JW, Yonan TN, et al: Pulmonary blastoma. An ultrastructural study with a brief review of literature and a discussion of pathogenesis. Cancer 39:153, 1977

141. Ashworth TG: Pulmonary blastomas: A true congenital neoplasm. Histopathology 7:585, 1983

142. Francis D, Jacobson M: Pulmonary blastoma. Curr Top Pathol 73:265, 1983

143. Cabarcos A, Gomez Dorronsoro M, Lobo Beristain JL: Pulmonary carcinosarcoma: A case study and review of the literature. Br J Dis Chest 79:83, 1985

144. Moore TC: Carcinosarcoma of the lung. Surgery 50:886, 1962

145. Kakos GS, Williams TE Jr, Assor D, et al: Pulmonary carcinosarcoma. Etiologic, therapeutic, and prognostic considerations. J Thorac Cardiovasc Surg 61:777, 1971

146. Diaconita G: Bronchopulmonary carcinosarcoma. Thorax 30:682, 1975

147. Vadillo-Briceno F, Feder W, Albores-Saavedra J: Malignant mixed tumor of the lung. Chest 58:84, 1970
148. Edwards CW, Saunders AM, Collins F: Mixed malignant tumor of the lung. Thorax 34:629, 1979
149. Flanagan P, McCracken AW, Cross RM: Squamous carcinoma of the lung with osteocartilagenous stroma. J Clin Pathol 18:403, 1965
150. Oyasu R, Battifora HA, Buckingham WB, et al: Metaplastic squamous cell carcinoma of bronchus simulating giant cell tumor of bone. Cancer 39:1119, 1977
151. Gautam HP: Intrapulmonary malignant teratoma. Am Rev Respir Dis 200:863, 1969
152. Holt S, Deverall PB, Boddy JE: A teratoma of the lung containing thymic tissue. J Pathol 126:85, 1978
153. Bateson EM, Hayes JA, Woo-Ming M: Endobronchial teratoma associated with bronchiectasis and bronchiolectasis. Thorax 23:69, 1968
154. Freeman C, Berg JW, Cutler SJ: Occurrence and prognosis of extranodal lymphomas. Cancer 29:252, 1972
155. Saltzstein SL: Pulmonary malignant lymphomas and pseudolymphomas: Classification, therapy and prognosis. Cancer 16:928, 1963
156. Mann RB, Jaffe ES, Berard CW: Malignant lymphomas: A conceptual understanding of morphologic diversity. Am J Pathol 94:105, 1979
157. Koss MN, Hochholzer L, Nichols PW, et al: Primary non-Hodgkin's lymphoma and pseudolymphoma of the lung: A study of 161 patients. Hum Pathol 14:1024, 1983
158. Marchevsky A, Padilla M, Kaneko M, et al: Localized lymphoid nodules of lung: A reappraisal of the lymphoma vs pseudolymphoma dilemma. Cancer 51:2070, 1983
159. L'Hoste RJ, Filippa DA, Lieberman PH, et al: Primary pulmonary lymphomas. Cancer 54:1397, 1984
160. Turner RR, Colby TV, Doggett RS: Well-differentiated lymphocytic lymphoma: a study of 47 patients with primary manifestation in lung. Cancer 54:2088, 1984
161. Herbert A, Wright DH, Isaacson PG, et al: Primary malignant lymphoma of the lung: Histopathologic and immunologic evaluation of nine cases. Hum Pathol 15:415, 1984
162. Jaffe ES: Pathologic and clinical spectrum of post-thymic T-cell malignancies. Cancer Invest 2:413, 1984
163. Colby TV, Yousem SA: Pulmonary lymphoid neoplasms. Semin Diagn Pathol 2:183, 1985
164. Cathcart-Rake W, Bone RC, Sobonya RE, et al: Rapid development of diffuse pulmonary infiltrates in histiocytes lymphoma. Am Rev Respir Dis 117:587, 1978
165. National Cancer Institute: Sponsored study of classifications of non-Hodgkin's lymphomas. Summary and description of a working formulation for clinical usage. The non-Hodgkin's lymphoma pathologic classification project. Cancer 49:2112, 1982
166. Ferguson WB Jr, Bachman LB, O'Toole WF: Waldenstrom's macroglobulinemia with diffuse pulmonary infiltration: lung biopsy and response to chlorambucil therapy. Am Rev Respir Dis 88:689, 1963
167. Winterbauer RH, Riggins RCK, Bauermeister DE: Pleuropulmonary manifestations of Waldenstrom's macroglobulinemia. Chest 66:368, 1974
168. Colby TV, Carrington CB, Mark GJ: Pulmonary involvement in malignant histiocytosis: A clinicopathologic spectrum. Am J Surg Pathol 5:61–73, 1981
169. Wongchaowart B, Kennealy JA, Crissman J, et al: Respiratory failure in malignant histiocytosis. Am Rev Respir Dis 12:640, 1981
170. Whitcomb ME, Schwarz MI, Keller AR, et al: Hodgkin's disease of the lung. Am Rev Respir Dis 106:79, 1972
171. Kern WH, Crepeau AG, Jone JC: Primary Hodgkin's disease of the lung. Cancer 14:1151, 1961
172. Yousem SA, Weiss LM, Colby TV: Primary pulmonary Hodgkin's disease: A clinicopathologic study of 15 cases. Cancer 57:1217, 1986
173. Seward CW, Badfar SH: Endobronchial Hodgkin's disease presenting as a primary pulmonary lesion. Chest 62:649, 1972
174. Herskovic T, Andersen HA, Baayrd ED: Intrathoracic plasmacytomas. Presentation of 21 cases and review of the literature. Chest 47:1, 1965
175. Kernen JA, Meyer BW: Malignant plasmacytoma of the lung with metastases. J Thorac Cardiovasc Surg 51:739, 1966
176. Robson AO, Knudsen A: Plasmacytoma of lung and stomach. Br J Dis Chest 53:62, 1959
177. Baroni CD, Mineo TC, Ricci C, et al: Solitary secretory plasmacytoma of the lung in a 14-year-old boy. Cancer 40:2329, 1977
178. Gerewal H, Curie BGM: Aggressive phase of multiple myeloma with pulmonary plasma cell infiltrates. JAMA 248:1875, 1982
179. Liu PI, Ishimaru T, McGregor DH: Autopsy study of granulocytic sarcoma (chloroma) in patients with myelogenous leukemia, Hiroshima-Nagasaki, 1949–1969. Cancer 31:948, 1973
180. Pitcok JA, Reinhzod EH, Justus BW, Mendelsohn RS: A clinical and pathologic study of seventy cases of myelofibrosis. Ann Intern Med 57:73, 1962
181. Ward HP, Block MH: The natural history of agnogenic myeloid metaplasia (AMM) and a critical evaluation of its relationship with the myeloproliferative syndrome. Medicine (Baltimore) 50:357, 1971
182. Trapnell DH: Recognition and incidence of intrapulmonary lymph nodes. Thorax 19:44, 1964
183. Benisch B: An intrapulmonary lymph node presenting as a coin lesion of the lung. Chest 76:336, 1979
184. Kradin RL, Spirn PW, Mark EJ: Intrapulmonary lymph nodes: clinical, radiologic and pathologic features. Chest 87:662, 1985
185. Tung KSK, McCormack LJ: Angiomatous lymphoid hamartoma. Cancer 20:525, 1967
186. Harigaya K, Mikata A, Kageyama K, et al: Histopathological study of six cases of Castleman's tumor. Acta Pathol Jpn 25:355, 1975
187. McBurney RP, Claggett OT, McDonald JR: Primary intrapulmonary neoplasm (thymoma?) associated with myasthenia gravis: Report of a case. Mayo Clin Proc 26:345, 1951

188. Yeoh CB, Ford JM, Lattes R, Wyle RH: Intrapulmonary thymoma. J Thorac Cardiovasc Surg 51:131, 1966

189. Iseman MD, Schwarz MI, Stanford RE: Interstitial pneumonia in angioimmunoblastic lymphadenopathy with dysproteinemia. A case report with special histopathologic studies. Ann Intern Med 85:752, 1976

190. Zylak CJ, Banerjee R, Gailbraith PA, et al: Lung involvement in angioimmunoblastic lymphadenopathy (AIL). Radiology 121:513, 1976

191. Jacques JE, Barclay R: The solid sarcomatous pulmonary artery. Br J Dis Chest 54:217, 1960

192. Hopwood D, McNeill G: Spindle cell sarcoma of the pulmonary trunk: A case report with histochemistry and electron microscopy. J Pathol 128:71, 1978

193. Baker PB, Goodwin RA: Pulmonary artery sarcomas: A review and report of a case. Arch Pathol Lab Med 109:35, 1985

194. Martini N, Hajdu SI, Beattie EJ Jr: Primary sarcoma of the lung. J Thorac Cardiovasc Surg 61:33, 1971

195. Guccion JG, Rosen SH: Bronchopulmonary leiomyosarcoma and fibrosarcoma. a study of 32 cases and review of the literature. Cancer 30:836, 1972

196. Corona FE, Okeson GC: Endobronchial fibroma. An unusual case of segmental atelectasis. Am Rev Respir Dis 110:350, 1974

197. Turner MA, Horne CHW: Primary fibrosarcoma of the lung and diabetes mellitus. Br J Surg 57:713, 1970

198. Wang NS, Seemayer TA, Ahmed MN, et al: Pulmonary leiomyosarcoma associated with an arteriovenous fistula. Arch Pathol 98:100, 1974

199. Vera-Roman JM, Sobonya RE, Gomez-Garcia JL, et al: Leiomyoma of the lung: literature review and case report. Cancer 52:936, 1983

200. Yellin A, Rosenman Y, Lieberman Y: Review of smooth muscle tumours of the lower respiratory tract. Br J Dis Chest 78:337, 1984

201. White SH, Ibraham NBN, Forrester-Wood CP, Jeyasingham K: Leiomyomas of the lower respiratory tract. Thorax 40:306, 1985

202. Zipkin R: Uber ein Adeno-Rhabdomyom der linken Lunge und Hypoplasia der rechten bei einer totgeborenen Frucht. Virchows Arch [A] 187:244, 1907

203. Lee SH, Rengachary SS, Paramesh J: Primary pulmonary rhabdomyosarcoma: A case report and review of the literature. Hum Pathol 12:92, 1981

204. Bellin HJ, Libshitz HL, Patchefsky AS: Bronchial lipoma. Report of two cases showing chondrotic metaplasia. Arch Pathol 92:20, 1971

205. Wu JP, Gilbert EF, Pellet JR: Pulmonary liposarcoma in a child with adrenogenital syndrome. Am J Clin Pathol 62:791, 1974

206. Silverman JF, Leffer BR, Kay S: Primary pulmonary neurilemoma. Arch Pathol Lab Med 100:644, 1976

207. Neilson DB: Primary intrapulmonary neurogenic sarcoma. J Pathol 76:419, 1958

208. Majmudar BM, Thomas J, Gorelkin L, et al: Respiratory obstruction caused by a multicentric granular cell tumor of the laryngotracheobronchial tree. Hum Pathol 12:283, 1981

209. Grabriel JR Jr, Thomas L, Kondlapoodi P, et al: Granular cell tumor of the bronchus: a previously unreported cause of hypercalcemia. J Surg Oncol 24:338, 1983

210. Davidson MA: A case of primary chondroma of the bronchus. Br J Surg 28:571, 1940

211. Shermeta DW, Carter D, Haller JS Jr: Chondroma of the bronchus in childhood. A case report illustrating problems in diagnosis and management. J Pediatr Surg 10:545, 1975

212. Smith EAC, Cohen RV, Peale AR: Primary chondrosarcoma of the lung. Am Intern Med 53:838, 1960

213. Daniels AC, Conner GH, Straus FH: Primary chondrosarcoma of the tracheobronchial tree. Report of a unique case and brief review. Arch Pathol Lab Med 84:615, 1967

214. Nosanchuk JS, Weatherbee L: Primary osteogenic sarcoma in lung. Report of a case. J Thorac Cardiovasc Surg 58:242, 1969

215. Reingold IM, Amronin GD: Extraosseous osteosarcoma of the lung. Cancer 28:491, 1971

216. Katzenstein A, Maurer JJ: Benign histiocytic tumor of lung: Am J Surg Pathol 3:61, 1979

217. Viguera JL, Pujol JL, Reboires SD, et al: Fibrous histiocytoma of the lung. Thorax 31:475, 1976

218. Bedrossian CWM, Verani R, Unger KM, et al: Pulmonary malignant fibrous histiocytoma. Light and electron microscopic studies of one case. Chest 75:186, 1979

219. Kern WH, Hughes RK, Meyer BW, et al: Malignant fibrous histiocytoma of the lung. Cancer 44:1783, 1979

220. Silverman JF, Coalson JJ: Primary malignant myxoid fibrous histiocytoma of the lung: Light and ultrastructural examination with review of the literature. Arch Pathol Lab Med 108:49, 1984

221. Lee JT, Shelbourne JD, Linder J: Primary Malignant fibrous histiocytoma of the lung: A clinicopathologic and ultrastructural study of five cases. Cancer 53:1124, 1984

222. Kudo H, Morinaga S, Shimosato Y. Solitary mast cell tumor of the lung. Cancer 61:2089, 1988

223. Magee F, Wright JL, Kay M, et al: Pulmonary capillary hemangiomatosis. Am Rev Respir Dis 132:922, 1985

224. Wada A, Tateishi R, Terazawa T, et al: Lymphangioma of the lung. Arch Pathol 98:211, 1974

225. Tank CK, Toker C, Foris NP, et al: Glomangioma of the lung. Am J Surg Pathol 2:103, 1978

226. Fabich DR, Hafez G-R: Glomangioma of the trachea. Cancer 45:2337, 1980

227. Dail D, Liebow A: Intravascular bronchioloalveolar tumor. Am J Pathol 78:6a, 1975 (abst)

228. Dail DH, Liebow AA, Gmelich JT, et al: Intravascular, bronchiolar, and alveolar tumor of the lung (IVBAT): An analysis of twenty cases of a peculiar sclerosing endothelial tumor. Cancer 51:452, 1983

229. Corrin B, Manners B, Millard M, et al: Histogenesis of the so-called Intravascular Bronchioloalveolar Tumor. J Pathol 128:163, 1979

230. Ferrer-Roca O: Intravascular and sclerosing bronchio-alveolar tumor. Am J Surg Pathol 4:375, 1980

231. Weldon-Linne CM, Victor TA, Christ ML, et al: Angiogenic nature of the "intravascular bronchioloalveolar tumor" of the lung. Arch Pathol Lab Med 105:174, 1981

232. Sherman JL, Rykwalder PJ, Tashkin DP: Intravascular

bronchiolo-alveolar tumor. Am Rev Respir Dis 123:468, 1981

233. Nash G, Fligiel S: Kaposi's sarcoma presenting as pulmonary disease in the acquired immunodeficiency syndrome: diagnosis by lung biopsy. Hum Pathol 15:999, 1984

234. Pitchenick AE, Fischl MA, Saldana MJ: Kaposi's sarcoma of the trachiobronchial tree. Chest 87:122, 1985

235. Meduri GV, Stover DE, Lee M, et al: Pulmonary Kaposi's sarcoma in the acquired immune deficiency syndrome: Clinical, radiographic and pathologic manifestations. Am J Med 81:11, 1986

236. Spragg RG, Wolf PL, Haghighi P, et al: Angiosarcoma of the lung with fatal pulmonary hemorrhage. Am J Med 74:1072, 1983

237. Yousem S: Angiosarcoma presenting in the lung. Arch Pathol Lab Med 110:112, 1986

238. Meade JB, Whitwell F, Bickford BJ, et al: Primary haemangiopericytoma of lung. Thorax 29:1, 1974

239. Yousem SA, Hochholzer L: Primary pulmonary hemangiopericytoma. Cancer 59:549, 1987

240. Bateson EM: So-called hamartoma of the lung—A true neoplasm of fibrous connective-tissue of the bronchi. Cancer 31:1458, 1973

241. Ramchand S, Baskerville L: Multiple hamartomas of the lung. Am Rev Respir Dis 99:932, 1969

242. Stone FJ, Churg AM: The ultrastructure of pulmonary hamartoma. Cancer 39:932, 1969

243. Carney JA: The triad of gastric epithelioid leiomyosarcoma, functioning extra-adrenal paraganglioma, and pulmonary chondroma. Cancer 43:374, 1979

244. Tomashefski JF Jr: Benign endobronchial mesenchymal tumors: their relationship to parenchymal pulmonary hamartomas. Am J Surg Pathol 6:531, 1982

245. Kalus M, Rahman F, Jenkins DE, et al: Malignant mesenchymoma of the lung. Arch Pathol 95:199, 1973

246. Liebow AA, Hubbell DS: Sclerosing hemangioma (histiocytoma, xanthoma) of the lung. Cancer 9:53, 1956

247. Katzenstein A, Gmelich JT, Carrington CB: Sclerosing hemangioma of the lung. A clinicopathologic study of 51 cases. Am J Surg Pathol 4:343, 1980

248. Hill GS, Eggleston JC: Electron microscopic study of so-called "pulmonary sclerosing hemangioma." Report of a case suggesting epithelial origin. Cancer 30:1092, 1972

249. Kennedy A: "Sclerosing hemangioma of the lung": An alternative view of its development. J Clin Pathol 26:792, 1973

250. Haas JE, Yunis EJ, Totten RS: Ultrastructure of a sclerosing hemangioma of the lung. Cancer 30:512, 1972

251. Kay S, Still WJS, Borochovitz D: Sclerosing hemangioma of the lung: An endothelial or epithelial neoplasm? Hum Pathol 8:468, 1977

252. Yousem SA, Wick MR, Singh G, et al: So-called sclerosing hemangiomas of lung. Am J Surg Pathol 12:582, 1988

253. Liebow AA, Castleman B: Benign clear cell ("sugar") tumors of the lung. Yale J Biol Med 43:213, 1971

254. Sale GE, Kulander BG: Benign clear cell tumor of lung with necrosis. Cancer 37:2355, 1976

255. Becker NH, Soifer I: Benign clear cell tumor ("sugar tumor") of the lung. Cancer 27:712, 1971

256. Hoch WS, Patchefsky AS, Takeda M, et al: Benign clear cell tumor of the lung. An ultrastructural study. Cancer 33:1328, 1974

257. Fukuda T, Machinami R, Toshita T, Nagashuma K: Benign clear cell tumor of the lung in an 8-year-old girl. Arch Pathol Lab Med 110:664, 1986

258. Gephardt GN: Malignant melanoma of the bronchus. Hum Pathol 12:671, 1981

259. Cartens PHB, Kuhns JG, Ghazi C: Primary malignant melanomas of the lung and adrenal. Hum Pathol 15:910, 1984

260. Angel R, Prades M: Primary bronchial melanoma. J Louisiana State Med Soc 136:13, 1984

261. Smith S, Opipari MI: Primary pleural melanoma: A first reported case and literature review. J Thorac Cardiovasc Surg 75:827, 1978

262. Singh G, Lee RE, Brooks DH: Primary pulmonary paraganglioma. Report of a case and review of the literature. Cancer 40:2286, 1977

263. Korn D, Bensch K, Liebow AA, et al: Multiple minute pulmonary tumors resembling chemodectomas. Am J Pathol 37:641, 1960

264. Ichinose H, Hewitt RL, Drapanas T: Minute pulmonary chemodectoma. Cancer 28:692, 1971

265. Costero I, Barroso-Nogel R, Martinez-Palomo A: Pleural origin of some of the supposed chemodectoid structures of the lung. Beitr Pathol 146:351, 1972

266. Kuhn C III, Askin FB: The fine structure of so-called minute pulmonary chemodectomas. Hum Pathol 6:681, 1975

267. Churg AM, Warnock ML: So-called "minute pulmonary chemodectoma." A tumor not related to paragangliomas. Cancer 37:1759, 1976

268. Kemnitz P, Sportmann H, Heinrich P: Meningioma of the lung: first report with light and electron microscopic findings. Ultrastruct Pathol 3:359, 1982

269. Chumas JC, Larelle CA: Pulmonary meningioma: A light and electron microscopic study. Am J Surg Pathol 6:795, 1982

270. Hayakawa K, Takahashi M, Sasaki K, et al: Primary choriocarcinoma of the lung: Case report of two male subjects. Acta Pathol Jpn 27:123, 1977

271. Yousem SA, Hochholzer L: Alveolar adenoma. Hum Pathol 17:1066, 1986

272. Shamsuddin AM, Edelman B, Nguyen T-H, et al: Multifocal malignant pheochromocytoma presenting as a lung tumor. Hum Pathol 12:475, 1981

273. Willis RA: The spread of tumors in the human body. Butterworth, London, 1952, p. 172

274. Rosenblatt MB, Lisa JR, Trinidad S: Pitfalls in the clinical and histologic diagnosis of bronchogenic carcinoma. Dis Chest 49:396, 1966

275. Braman SS, Whitcomb ME: Endobronchial metastases. Arch Intern Med 135:543, 1975

276. LeMay M, Piro AJ: Cavitary pulmonary metastases. Ann Intern Med 62:59, 1961

277. Habein HC Jr, Claggett OT, McDonald JR: Pulmonary resection for metastatic tumors. Arch Surg 78:716, 1959

278. Edlich RF, Shea MA, Foker JE, et al: A review of 26

years' experience with pulmonary resection of metastatic cancer. Dis Chest 49:587, 1966

279. Feldman PS, Kyriakos M: Pulmonary resection for metastatic sarcoma. J Thorac Cardiovasc Surg 64:784, 1972

280. Martini N, Bains MS, Huvos AG, et al: Surgical treatment of metastatic sarcoma to the lung. Surg Clin North Am 54:841, 1974

281. Katzenstein AL, Purvis R Jr, Gmelich J, et al: Pulmonary resection of metastatic renal adenocarcinoma. Pathologic findings and therapeutic value. Cancer 41:712, 1978

282. Ramming KP: Surgery for pulmonary metastases. Surg Clin North Am 60:815, 1980

283. King DS, Castleman B: Bronchial involvement in metastatic pulmonary malignancy. J Thorac Surg 12:305, 1943

284. Janover MD, Blennershassett JB: Lymphangitic spread of metastatic cancer to the lung. A radiologic-pathologic classification. Radiology 101:267, 1971

285. Wolff M, Kaye G, Silva F: Pulmonary metastases (with admixed epithelial elements) from smooth muscle neoplasms. Am J Surg Pathol 3:325, 1979

286. Horstmann JP, Pietra GC, Harman JA, et al: Spontaneous regression of pulmonary leiomyomas during pregnancy. Cancer 39:314, 1977

287. Banner AS, Carrington CB, Emory WB, et al: Efficacy of oophorectomy in lymphangioleiomyomatoses and benign metastasizing leiomyoma. N Engl J Med 305:204, 1981

288. Bahadori M, Liebow AA: Plasma cell granulomas of the lung. Cancer 31:191, 1973

289. Brown WJ, Johnson LC: Post-inflammatory "tumors" of the pleura. Milit Surg 109:415, 1951

290. Spyker MA, Kay S: Plasma cell granuloma of a mediastinal lymph node with extension to right lung. J Thorac Cardiovasc Surg 31:211, 1956

291. Tchertkoff V, Lee BY, Wagner BM: Plasma cell granuloma of the lung. Case report and review of literature. Chest 44:440, 1963

292. Warter A, Satge D, Roeslin N: Angioinvasive plasma cell granuloma of the lung. Cancer 59:435, 1987

293. Tomita T, Dixon A, Watanabe I, et al: Sclerosing vascular variant of plasma cell granuloma. Hum Pathol 11:197, 1980

294. Spencer H: The pulmonary plasma cell/histiocytoma complex. Histopathology 8:903, 1984

295. Matsubara O, Tan-Liu NS, Kenney RM, Mark EJ: Inflammatory pseudotumors of the Lung: progression from organizing pneumonia to fibrous histiocytoma or to plasma cell granuloma in 32 cases. Hum Pathol 19:807, 1988

296. Higgins GA, Shields TW, Keehn RJ: The solitary pulmonary nodule. Arch Surg 110:570, 1975

297. Ray JF III, Lawton BR, Magnin GE, et al: The coin lesion story: Update 1976. Twenty years experience with early thoracotomy for 179 suspected malignant coin lesions. Chest 70:332, 1976

298. Trunk G, Gracey DR, Byrd RB: The management and evaluation of the solitary pulmonary nodule. Chest 66:236, 1974

299. Ulbright TM, Katzenstein A: Solitary necrotizing granulomas of the lung: Differentiating features and etiology. Am J Surg Pathol 4:13, 1980

300. Steer A: Histogenesis of tuberculous pulmonary lesions. Am Rev Respir Dis 95:200, 1967

301. Rich AR: The pathogenesis of tuberculosis. 2nd Ed. Charles C Thomas, Springfield, IL, 1951, pp. 824–880

302. Auerbach O, Green H: The pathology of clinically healed tuberculous cavities. Am Rev Tuberc 42:707, 1940

303. Thompson JR: "Open healing" of tuberculous cavities. Am Rev Tuberc 72:601, 1955

304. Snijder J: Histopathology of pulmonary lesions caused by atypical mycobacteria. J Pathol 90:65, 1965

305. Wolinsky E: Nontuberculous mycobacteria and associated diseases. Am Rev Respir Dis 119:107, 1979

306. Reichart CM, O'Leary TJ, Levens DL, et al: Autopsy pathology in the acquired immune deficiency syndrome. Am J Pathol 112:357, 1983

307. Guarda LLA, Luna MA, Smith JL Jr. et al: Acquired immunodeficiency syndrome: Post-mortem findings. Am J Clin Pathol 81:549, 1984

308. Moskowitz L, Hensley GT, Chan JC, Adams K: Immediate causes of death in acquired immunodeficiency syndrome. Arch Pathol Lab Med 109:735, 1985

309. Sohn C, Schroff RW, Kliewer KE: Disseminated *Mycobacterium avium*-intracellular infection in homosexual men with acquired cell-mediated immunodeficiency: A histologic and immunologic study of two cases. Am J Clin Pathol 79:247, 1983

310. Auerback O, Dail DH: Mycobacterial Infections. p. 173. In Dail DH, Hammar SP (eds): Pulmonary Pathology. Springer-Verlag, New York, 1988

311. Gupta RK, Schuster RA, Christian WD: Autopsy findings in a unique case of malakoplaquia. Arch Pathol Lab Med 93:42, 1972

312. Colby TV, Hunt S, Pelzmann K, et al: Malakoplakia of the lung: A report of two cases. Respiration 39:295, 1980

313. Damjanov I, Katz SM: Malakoplakia. Pathol Annu 16:103, 1981

314. Crouch E, Wright J, White V, Churg A: Malakoplakia mimicking carcinoma metastatic to lung. Am J Surg Pathol 8:151, 1984

315. Dail DH: Metabolic and other diseases. p. 535. In Dail DH, Hammar SP (eds): Pulmonary Pathology. Springer-Verlag, New York, 1988

316. Winberg CD, Rose ME, Rappaport H: Whipple's disease of the lung. Am J Med 65:873, 1978

317. Goodwin RA Jr, Des Prez RM: Histoplasmosis. Am Rev Respir Dis 117:929, 1978

318. Drutz DJ, Catanzaro A: Coccidioidomycosis. Am Rev Respir Dis 117:559, 727, 1978

319. Deppisch LM, Donowho EM: Pulmonary coccidioidomycosis. Am J Clin Pathol 58:489, 1972

320. Campbell GD: Primary pulmonary cryptococcosis. Am Rev Respir Dis 94:236, 1966

321. Hammerman KJ, Powell KE, Christianson CS, et al: Pulmonary cryptococcosis: Clinical forms and treatment. Am Rev Respir Dis 108:1116, 1973

322. Sarosi GA, Davies SF: Blastomycosis. Am Rev Respir Dis 120:911, 1979

323. Giraldo R, Restrepo A, Gutierrez F, et al: Pathogenesis of paracoccidioidomycosis: A model based on the study of 46 patients. Mycopathol Mycol Appl 58:63, 1976

324. Jay SJ, Platt MR, Reynolds RC: Primary pulmonary sporotrichosis. Am Rev Respir Dis 115:1051, 1977

325. Brook CJ, Ravikrishnan KP, Weg JG: Pulmonary and articular sporotrichosis. Am Rev Respir Dis 116:141, 1977

326. Kodousek R, Vortel V, Fingerland A, et al: Pulmonary adiaspiromycosis in man caused by Emmonsia crescens: Report of a unique case. J Clin Pathol 56:394, 1971

327. Watts JC, Callaway CS, Chandler FW, et al: Human pulmonary adiospiromycosis. Arch Pathol 99:11, 1975

328. Pechan WB, Novick AC, Lalli A, et al: Pulmonary nodules in a renal transplant recipient. J Urol 124:111, 1980

329. Gale AM, Kleitsch WP: Solitary pulmonary nodule due to phycomycosis (mucormycosis). Chest 62:752, 1972

330. Arnett JC Jr, Hatch HB: Pulmonary allescheriasis. Report of a case and review of the literature. Arch Intern Med 135:1250, 1975

331. Speir WA, Mitchener JW, Galloway RF: Primary pulmonary botryomycosis. Chest 60:92, 1971

332. Case Records of the Massachusetts General Hospital (case 26-1974). N Engl J Med 291:35, 1974

333. Barrio JL, Suarez M, Rodriguez JL, et al: *Pneumocystis carinii* pneumonia presenting as cavitating and noncavitating solitary pulmonary nodules in patients with the Acquired Immunodeficiency Syndrome. Am Rev Respir Dis 134:1094, 1986

334. Thiruvengadam KV, Madanagopalan N, Solomon V, et al: Pleuropulmonary amebiasis: Report of a case with pleural biopsy findings. Dis Chest 42:111, 1962

335. Priyananda B, Tandhanand S: Opisthorchiasis with pulmonary involvement. Ann Intern Med 54:795, 1961

336. Thompson HG, Pettigrew R, Johnson EA: Solitary pulmonary bilharzioma. Thorax 34:401, 1979

337. Robinson MJ, Viamonte M, Viamonte M Jr: Dirofilariasis: Diagnostic consideration for pulmonary "coin lesions." South Med J 67:461, 1974

338. Awe RJ, Mattox KL, Alvarez BA, et al: Solitary and bilateral pulmonary nodules due to *Dirofilaria immitis*. Am Rev Respir Dis 112:445, 1975

339. Beaver PC, Fallon M, Smith GH: Pulmonary nodule caused by a living Brugia malayi-like filaria in an artery. Am J Trop Med Hyg 20:661, 1971

340. Wolcott MW, Harris SH, Brigg JN, et al: Hydatid disease of the lung. J Thorac Cardiovasc Surg 62:465, 1971

341. Beaver PC, Kriz JJ, Lau TJ: Pulmonary nodule caused by Enterobius vermicularis. Am J Trop Med Hyg 22:711, 1973

342. Mayer GJ: Pulmonary paragonimiasis. J Pediatr 95:75, 1979

343. Tellis CJ, Putnan JS: Cavitation in large multinodular pulmonary disease: A rare manifestation of sarcoidosis. Chest 71:792, 1977

344. Case Records of the Massachusetts General Hospital (case 47-1979). N Engl J Med 301:1168, 1979

345. Murray HW, Masur H, Senterfit LB, et al: The protean manifestation of *Mycoplasma pneumoniae* in adults. Am J Med 58:229, 1975

346. Koletsky RJ, Weinstein AJ: Fulminant *Mycoplasma pneumoniae* infection. Report of a fatal case, and review of the literature. Am Rev Respir Dis 122:491, 1980

347. Goodman N, Daves ML, Rifkind D: Pulmonary roentgen findings following renal transplantation. Radiology 89:621, 1967

348. Beschorner WE, Hutchins GM, Burns WH, et al: Cytomegalovirus pneumonia in bone marrow transplant recipients: Miliary and diffuse patterns. Am Rev Respir Dis 122:107, 1980

349. Nash G, Foley FD: Herpetic infection of the middle and lower respiratory tract. Am J Clin Pathol 54:857, 1970

350. Glick N, Levin S, Nelson K: Recurrent pulmonary infarction in adult chickenpox pneumonia. JAMA 222:173, 1972

351. Simila S, Ylikorkala O, Wasz-Hockert O: Type 7 adenovirus pneumonia. J Pediatr 79:605, 1971

352. Gosink BB, Friedman PJ, Liebow AA: Bronchiolitis obliterans. Roentgenologic-pathologic correlation. AJR 117:816, 1973

353. Epler GR, Colby TV, McLoud TC, et al: Bronchiolitis obliterans organizing pneumonia. N Engl J Med 312:152, 1985

354. Fetzer AE, Werner AS, Hagstrom JWC: Pathologic features of pseudomonal pneumonia. Am Rev Respir Dis 96:1121, 1967

355. Taylor BG, Zafarzai MZ, Humphreys DW, et al: Nodular pulmonary infiltrates and septic arthirtis associated with *Yersinia enterocolitica* bacteremia. Am Rev Respir Dis 116:525, 1977

356. Everett ED, Nelson RA: Pulmonary melioidosis. Am Rev Respir Dis 112:331, 1975

357. Brown RJ: Human actinomycosis: A study of 181 subjects. Hum Pathol 4:319, 1973

358. Frazier AR, Rosenow EC III, Roberts GD: Nocardiosis. Mayo Clin Proc 50:657, 1975

359. Thurlbeck WM: Chronic Airflow Obstruction in Lung Disease. WB Saunders, Philadelphia, 1976

360. Schweppe HL, Knowles JH, Kane L: Lung abscess: An analysis of the Massachusetts General Hospital cases from 1943 through 1956. N Engl J Med 265:1039, 1961

361. Alexander JC, Wolfe, WG: Lung abscess and emphysema of the thorax. Surg Clin North Am 60:835, 1980

362. Liebow AA: Pulmonary angiitis and granulomatosis. The J. Burns Amberson Lecture. Am Rev Respir Dis 108:1, 1973

363. Saldana MJ: Vasculitides and angiocentric lymphoproliferative processes. p. 447. In Dail DH, Hammar SP (eds): Pulmonary Pathology. Springer-Verlag, New York, 1988

364. Wegener F: Über eine eigenartige rhinogene Granulomatose mit besonderer Beteiligung des Arteriensystems und der Nieren. Beitr Pathol Anat 102:36, 1939

365. Klinger H: Grenzformen der Periarteritis nodosa. Frankfurt Pathol 42:455, 1931

366. Carrington CB, Liebow AA: Limited forms of angiitis and granulomatosis of Wegener's type. Am J Med 49:366, 1970

367. De Remee RA, McDonald TJ, Harrison EG, Coles DT: Wegener's granulomatosis. Anatomical correlates, a proposed classification. Mayo Clin Proc 51:777, 1976

368. Churg J, Strauss L: Allergic granulomatosis, allergic angiitis and periarteritis nodosa. Am J Pathol 27:277, 1951

369. Rose GA, Spencer H: Polyarteritis nodosa. Q J Med 26:43, 1957

370. Chumbley LC, Harrison EG, De Remee RA: Allergic granulomatosis and angiitis (Churg-Strauss syndrome). Report and analysis of 30 cases. Mayo Clin Proc 52:477, 1977

371. Koss MN, Antonovych T, Hochholzer L: Allergic granulomatosis (Churg-Strauss syndrome). Pulmonary and renal morphologic findings. Am J Surg Pathol 5:21, 1981

372. Beach RC, Corrin B, Scopes TW, et al: Necrotizing sarcoid granulomatosis with neurologic lesions in a child. J Pediatr 97:950, 1980

373. Singh N, Cole S, Krause PJ, et al: Necrotizing sarcoid granulomatosis with extrapulmonary involvement. Clinical, pathologic, ultrastructural, and immunologic features. Am Rev Respir Dis 124:189, 1981

374. Churg A: Pulmonary angiitis and granulomatosis revisited. Hum Pathol 14:868, 1983

375. Katzenstein A, Liebow AA, Friedman PJ: Bronchocentric granulomatosis, mucoid impaction, and hypersensitivity reactions to fungi. Am Rev Respir Dis 111:497, 1975

376. Liebow AA, Carrington CRB, Friedman PJ: Lymphomatoid granulomatosis. Hum Pathol 3:457, 1972

377. Jaffe ES: Pulmonary lymphocytic angiitis: A nosologic quandary (editorial). Mayo Clin Proc 63:411, 1988

378. Costa J, Martin SE: Pulmonary lymphoreticular disorders. p. 282. In Jaffe ES (ed): Surgical Pathology of the Lymph Nodes and Related Organs. WB Saunders, Philadelphia, 1985

379. Saldana MJ, Patchefsky AS, Israel HI, Atkinson GW: Pulmonary angiitis and granulomatosis: The relationship between histological features, organ involvement, and response to treatment. Hum Pathol 8:391, 1977

380. Israel HL, Patchefsky AS, Saldana MJ: Wegener's granulomatosis, lymphomatoid granulomatosis, and benign lymphocytic angiitis and granulomatosis of lung: Recognition and treatment. Ann Intern Med 87:691, 1977

381. Gracey DR, DeRemee RA, Colby TV, et al: Benign lymphocytic Angiitis and granulomatosis: Experience with three cases. Mayo Clin Proc 63:323, 1988

382. De Remee RA, Weiland LH, McDonald TJ: Polymorphic reticulosis, lymphomatoid granulomatosis: Two diseases or one? Mayo Clin Proc 53:634, 1978

383. Tomashiefski JF, Hirsch CS: The pulmonary vascular lesions of intravenous drug abuse. Hum Pathol 11:133, 1980

384. Slavin RE, de Groat WJ: Pathology of the lung in Behçet's disease. Am J Surg Pathol 5:779, 1981

385. Hughes JP, Stovin PGI: Segmental pulmonary artery aneurysms with peripheral venous thrombosis. Br J Dis Chest 53:19, 1959

386. Gerle RD, Jaretzki A, Ashley CA, et al: Congenital bronchopulmonary foregut malformation: Pulmonary sequestration communicating with the gastrointestinal tract. N Engl J Med 278:1413, 1968

387. Landing BH: Congenital malformations and genetic disorders of the respiratory tract. Am Rev Respir Dis 120:151, 1979

388. Blesovsky A: Pulmonary sequestration: A report of an unusual case and a review of the literature. Thorax 22:351, 1967

389. Heithoff KB, Sane SM, Williams HJ, et al: Broncho-pulmonary foregut malformation: A unifying etiological concept. AJR 126:46, 1976

390. Kyllonen KEJ: Intralobar pulmonary sequestration and a theory as to its etiology. Acta Chir Scand 127:307, 1964

391. Bell-Thomson J, Missier P, Sommers SC: Lung carcinoma arising in bronchopulmonary sequestration. Cancer 44:334, 1979

392. Mattila SP, Kekonen PES, Kyllonen KEJ, et al: Pulmonary sequestration associated with tuberculosis, aspergillosis and pseudomycosis. Ann Chir Gynaecol 64:30, 1975

393. Johnston DG: Inflammatory and vascular lesions in bronchopulmonary sequestration. Am J Clin Pathol 26:636, 1956

394. Stocker JT, Madewell JE, Drake RM: Congenital cystic adenomatoid malformation of the lung. Hum Pathol 8:155, 1977

395. Taber P, Benveniste H, Gans SL: Delayed infantile lobar emphysema. J Pediatr Surg 9:245, 1974

396. Zatzkin HR, Cole PM, Bronsther B: Congenital hypertrophic lobar emphysema. Surgery 52:502, 1962

397. Binet JP, Nezelof C, Fredet J: Five cases of lobar tension emphysema in infancy: Importance of bronchial malformation and value of postoperative steroid therapy. Dis Chest 41:126, 1962

398. Murray FG, Talbert JL, Haller JA: Obstructive lobar emphysema of the newborn infant: Documentation of the "mucus plug syndrome" with successful treatment by bronchotomy. J Thorac Cardiovasc Surg 53:886, 1967

399. Hislop A, Reid L: New pathological findings in emphysema of childhood. 2. Overinflation of a normal lobe. Thorax 26:190, 1970

400. Hislop A, Reid L: New pathological findings in emphysema of childhood. 1. Polyalveolar lobe with emphysema. Thorax 25:682, 1970

401. Henderson R, Hislop A, Reid L: New pathological findings in emphysema of childhood. 3. Unilateral congenital emphysema with hypoplasia and compensatory emphysema of contralateral lung. Thorax 26:195, 1971

402. Shafir R, Jaffe R, Kalter Y: Bronchiectasis: A cause of infantile lobar emphysema. J Pediatr Surg 11:107, 1976

403. Noonan JA, Walters LR, Reeves JT: Congenital pulmonary lymphagiectasis. Am J Dis Child 120:314, 1970

404. Laurence KM: Congenital pulmonary lymphangiectasis. J Clin Pathol 12:62, 1959

405. Eraklis AJ, Griscom NT, McGovern JD: Bronchogenic cysts of the mediastinum in infancy. N Engl J Med 281:1150, 1969

406. Constant E, Davis DG, Edminster R: Bronchogenic cyst of the suprasternal area. Plast Reconstr Surg 52:88, 1973

407. Head JR: Cystic disease of the lung. With emphasis on emphysematous blebs and bullae. Am J Surg 89:1019, 1955

408. Mark EJ: Mesenchymal cystic hamartoma of the lung. N Engl J Med 315:1255, 1986

409. Gomes MR, Bernatz PE, Dines DE: Pulmonary arteriovenous fistulas. Ann Thorac Surg 7:582, 1969

410. Standefer JE, Tabakin BS, Hanson JS: Pulmonary arteriovenous fistulas: Case report with cine-angiographic studies. Am Rev Respir Dis. 89:95, 1964

411. Dines OE, Arms RA, Bernatz PE, et al: Pulmonary arteriovenous fistulas. Mayo Clin Proc 49:460, 1974

412. Hales MR: Multiple small arteriovenous fistulae of the lungs. Am J Pathol 32:927, 1956

413. Sagel SS, Greenspan RH: Minute pulmonary arteriovenous fistula demonstrated by magnification pulmonary angiography. Radiology 97:529, 1970

414. Kuphart RJ, Mackenzie JN, Templeton AW, et al: Systemic-pulmonary arteriovenous fistula of the chest wall and lung. A report of a case and review of the literature. J Thorac Cardiovasc Surg 54:113, 1967

415. Cox PA, Keshishian JM, Blades BB: Traumatic arteriovenous fistula of the chest wall and lung. J Thorac Cardiovasc Surg 54:109, 1967

416. Varma KK, Clarke CP: Congenital systemic-to-pulmonary arteriovenous fistula: Report of a case. Aust NZ J Surg 40:360, 1971

417. Brundage BH, Gomez AC, Cheihin MD, et al: Systemic artery to pulmonary vessel fistulas. Report of two cases and review of the literature. Chest 62:19, 1972

418. Saito T, Matsuda M, Yamaguchi T, et al: A case of traumatic systemic-pulmonary arteriovenous fistula. Jpn Heart J 16:196, 1975

419. Davia JE, Golden MS, Price HL, et al: Pulmonary varix. A diagnostic pitfall. Circulation 49:1011, 1974

420. Hipona FA, Jamseridi A: Observations on Natural history of varicosity of pulmonary veins. Circulation 35:471, 1967

421. Charlton RW, du Plessis LA: Multiple pulmonary artery aneurysms. Thorax 16:364, 1961

422. Plokker HWM, Wagenaar S, Bruschke AVG, et al: Aneurysm of a pulmonary artery branch: An uncommon cause of a coin lesion. Chest 68:258, 1975

423. Gonzalez-Crussi F, Boggs JD, Raffensperger JG: Brain heterotopia in the lungs. A rare cause of respiratory distress in the newborn. Am J Clin Pathol 73:281, 1980

424. Valdes-Dapena M, Arey JG: Pulmonary emboli of cerebral origin in the newborn. Arch Pathol Lab Med 84:643, 1967

425. Levine SB: Embolism of cerebral tissue to lungs. Arch Pathol 96:183, 1973

426. Le Roux BT: Heterotopic intrathoracic liver. Thorax 16:68, 1961

427. Lasser A, Wilson GL: Ectopic liver tissue mass in the thoracid cavity. Cancer 36:1823, 1975

428. Nakata H: Thoracic kidney presentings as a mass in the base of the lung. Chest 71:123, 1977

429. Lundius B: Intrathoracic kidney. AJR 125:678, 1975

430. Bozie C: Ectopic fetal adrenal cortex in the lung of a newborn. Virchows Arch [A] 363:371, 1974

431. Dowling EA, Johnson IM, Collier FCD, et al: Intratracheal goiter: A clinicopathologic review. Ann Surg 156:258, 1962

432. Killett HS, Lepphard O, Willis RA: Two unusual examples of heteroplasia in the lung. J Pathol Bacteriol 84:421, 1962

433. Hibbard LT, Schumann WR, Goldstein GE: Thoracic endometriosis: A review and report of two cases. Am J Obstet Gynecol 140:227, 1981

434. Popelka Ch G, Kleinermann L: Diffuse pulmonary ossification. Arch Intern Med 137:523, 1977

435. Noonan CD, Taylor FB Jr, Engelman EP: Nodular rheumatoid disease of the lung with cavitation. Arthritis Rheum 6:232, 1963

436. Caplan A, Payne RB, Withey JLA: A broader concept of Caplan's syndrome related to rheumatoid factors. Thorax 17:205, 1962

437. Morgan WKA, Seaton A: Occupational Lung Disease. WB Saunders, Philadelphia, 1975

438. Abraham JL: Recent advances in pneumoconiosis: The pathologist's role in etiologic diagnosis. p. 96. In Thurlbeck WM, Abell MR (eds): The Lung. Structure, Function and Disease. Williams & Wilkins, Baltimore, 1978

439. Mark ET: The second diagnosis: The role of the pathologist in identifying pneumoconiosis in lungs excised for tumor. Hum Pathol 12:585, 1981

440. Lee S-C, Johnson HA: Multiple nodular pulmonary amyloidosis. Thorax 30:178, 1975

441. Rubinow A, Celli BR, Cohen AS, et al: Localized amyloidosis of the lower respiratory tract. Am Rev Respir Dis 118:603, 1978

442. Engleman P, Liewbow AA, Gmelich J, et al: Pulmonary hyalinizing granuloma. Am Rev Respir Dis 115:997, 1977

443. Drasin H, Blume MR, Rosenbaum EH, et al: Pulmonary hyalinizing granulomas in a patient with malignant lymphoma with development nine years later of multiple myeloma and systemic amyloidosis. Cancer 44:215, 1979

444. Yousem SA, Hochholzer L: Pulmonary hyalinizing granuloma. Am J Clin Pathol 87:1, 1987

445. Tunell WP, Blades BB: Asynchronous bilateral lipoid pneumonia presenting as solitary nodules in the lung. J Thorac Cardiovasc Surg 63:334, 1972

446. Didolkar MS, Gamarra MC, Hartmann RA, et al: Lipoid granuloma of the lung. J Thorac Cardiovasc Surg 66:122, 1973

447. Ackerman LV: The pathology of radiation effect of normal and neoplastic tissue. AJR 114:447, 1972

448. Gross NJ: Pulmonary effects of radiation therapy. Review. Ann Intern Med 86:81, 1977

449. Fajardo, LF, Berthrong M: Radiation injury in surgical pathology. I. Am J Surg Pathol 2:159, 1978

450. Renner RR, Markarian B, Pernice NJ, Heitzman ER: The apical cap. Radiology 110:569, 1974

451. Butler CI, Kleinerman J: The pulmonary apical cap. Am J Pathol 60:205, 1970

452. Solovay J, Solovay HV: Apical pulmonary tumors—Relation to apical scarring. Dis Chest 48:20, 1965

453. Mosser KM: Pulmonary Embolism. State of the Art (1976–1977). American Lung Association, New York, 1978

454. Shepard GH, Ferguson JL, Foster JH: Pulmonary contusion. Ann Thorac Surg 7:110, 1969

455. Schneider HJ, Felson B, Gonzalez LL: Rounded atelectasis. AJR 134:225, 1980

456. Mintzer RA, Cugell DW: The association of asbestos-induced pleural disease and rounded atelectasis. Chest 81:457, 1982

21

The Cardiovascular System

Hugh A. McAllister, Jr.
Victor J. Ferrans

MYOCARDIUM AND ENDOCARDIUM

Myocardial Biopsies

Procedures used to obtain myocardial tissue include operative resection (infundibular tissue in patients with muscular obstruction to right ventricular outflow, ventricular septal muscle in patients with hypertrophic obstructive cardiomyopathy, left atrial appendage in patients with mitral valvular disease); operative biopsies; and removal by various types of bioptome catheters, which can be used to obtain samples of ventricular endocardium and adjacent myocardium. In the right ventricle, catheter biopsies usually are taken from the septal wall; in the left ventricle, from the free wall. Multiple samples can be obtained, each measuring about $3 \times 2 \times 2$ mm. Because of the risk of perforation of a thin chamber wall, catheter biopsies usually are not taken from the atrial walls or the right ventricular free wall. Transmural samples of ventricular wall also have been obtained (percutaneously or at open thoracotomy) with biopsy needles.

Regardless of the method used to obtain tissue, myocardial biopsies show artifacts (Fig. 21-1) related to the unopposed contraction that the free edges of the tissue undergo as a response to cutting. These artifacts are manifested as hypercontraction bands and are most pronounced in a peripheral zone that extends for 100 to 200 μm into the depth of the tissue. Thus, they constitute a significant drawback to the use of needle biopsies, particularly those taken with needles of small internal diameters. Operative biopsies also may show artifacts (espe-

cially in mitochondria) related to elective cardiac arrest and cardiopulmonary bypass.

Endomyocardial biopsy specimens are to be evaluated systematically to include: (1) endocardium (thickness, cell types and number, stroma, contiguity, and thrombus); (2) cardiac myocytes (size, arrangement, degeneration, storage deposits, sarcoplasmic membrane changes, nuclear changes, organisms such as *Toxoplasma* or trypanosomes, or cytomegalovirus inclusions); (3) myocardial interstitium (cell types and number, stromal composition, storage deposits such as amyloid, organisms such as fungi); and (4) blood vessels (endothelium, basement membrane, wall thickness and composition, thrombus or embolic materials, and organisms such as rickettsiae). Myocardial biopsy specimens need to be properly oriented to include endocardium in the plane of sectioning. For electron microscopic processing this should be done before tissues are darkened by postfixation with osmium tetroxide.

Light microscopic stains routinely used to study formalin-fixed myocardial biopsies are hematoxylin and eosin (H&E) and Masson's trichrome. Movat pentachrome, periodic acid–Schiff (PAS), Congo red, Perls' stain for iron, and stains for organisms are used as needed. For immunohistochemical or biochemical studies, unfixed tissue must be frozen rapidly and kept under appropriate conditions of storage; however, monoclonal antibodies have recently become available that are most useful for the immunohistochemical identification of inflammatory cells and subtypes of lymphocytes (common leucocyte antigen—L26 for B cells and UCHL1 and T12 for T cells), and that can be used with paraffin sections of

788

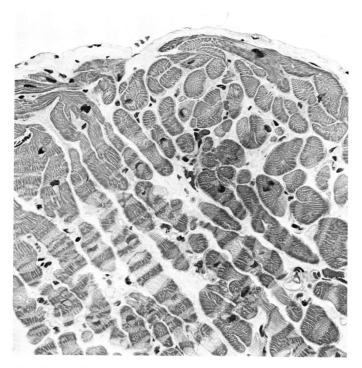

Fig. 21-1. Histologic section of myocardial biopsy specimen obtained from right side of ventricular septum with bioptome catheter. The biopsy, taken from a patient with suspected endomyocardial fibrosis, revealed no abnormalities. Note the thin layer of endocardial connective tissue (top) and the artifactual contraction bands in the muscle cells (lower center).

formalin-fixed tissue. Tissue should not be rinsed with saline before fixation, because this results in severe artifacts. If electron microscopic study is to be performed, the tissue can be fixed either with 2.5 to 3 percent glutaraldehyde or with a mixture of 1 percent glutaraldehyde and 4 percent formaldehyde in 0.1 M phosphate buffer, pH 7.4 (McDowell's fixative). Fixation with this solution allows satisfactory preparations to be made for both light and electron microscopic study. Staining en bloc with uranyl acetate is not necessary for ultrastructural study and may interfere with the staining of glycogen particles.

Cardiac Hypertrophy and Fibrosis

Hypertrophy is evaluated by light microscopy on the basis of the transverse diameters of the muscle cells (normally less than 15μm) and nuclear morphology. If necessary, additional evaluation is made by electron microscopy, which is useful in determining the presence and severity of degenerative changes that occur in the late stages of hypertrophy.[1] Structural alterations resulting from hypertrophy alone are: increased size of nuclei, Golgi complexes, and T-tubules; increased degrees of convolution of intercalated discs; increased numbers of ribosomes; focal accumulations of Z-band material; variability in mitochondrial size; and large accumulations of glycogen granules and mitochondria in perinuclear areas.

Degenerative changes in hypertrophied myocardium (Fig. 21-2) may involve practically every type of subcellular organelle and can occur in hypertrophy of any cause. The enlarged, dilated atria of patients with mitral valvular disease and atrial fibrillation show the most severe cellular degeneration. Perhaps the most important degenerative change is myofibrillar lysis, which results in loss of myofibrils and usually involves the thick (myosin) filaments to a greater extent than the thin (actin) filaments. Because of this, myofibrillar lysis often leaves in the muscle cells numerous actin filaments that are no longer associated with myosin filaments. Z-band material may increase in amount so that Z bands are much wider than normal and actually may become confluent. Some of these Z bands have a highly organized substructure similar to that seen in skeletal muscle in nemaline myopathy. In cells undergoing myofibrillar loss, the sarcoplasmic reticulum (SR) can undergo proliferation and formation of various types of aggregates of SR tubules and cisterns.

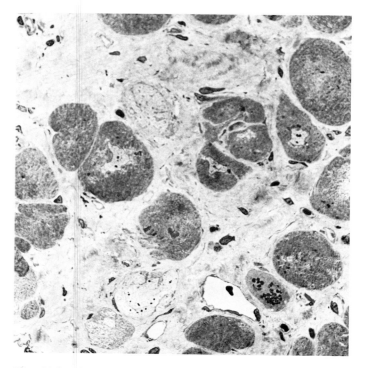

Fig. 21-2. Hypertrophy, interstitial fibrosis, and marked degenerative changes in some of the muscle cells are seen in left ventricular biopsy specimen obtained at the time of valvular replacement in a patient with aortic valvular disease. Several myocytes have pale cytoplasm and are almost completely devoid of myofibrils. (Plastic-embedded tissue, alkaline toluidine blue ×1000.)

Other changes indicative of degeneration of cardiac muscle cells include: intranuclear tubules; intramitochondrial and intranuclear deposits of glycogen (these also can occur in nondegenerated cells); accumulation of tangled masses of intermediate or cytoskeletal (100 Å in diameter) cytoplasmic filaments; dilatation and disorganization of T-tubules; formation of electron-dense concentric lamellae (myelin figures); dissociation of intercellular junctions, and development of unusual (intracytoplasmic) junctions formed by two parts of the plasma membrane of the same cell (rather than by the plasma membranes of two different cells); thickening of the basal laminae of the muscle cells; and formation of spherical microparticles derived from the plasma membrane, particularly in junctional areas. These spherical microparticles should not be confused with viral particles.

Two types of *myocardial fibrosis* are recognizable. The first of these, interstitial fibrosis (Fig. 21-2), is associated relatively frequently with myocardial hypertrophy and is characterized by bands of fibrous connective tissue that encircle the cardiac muscle cells and separate them from adjacent cells. The second type, replacement fibrosis, is associated with the healing of muscle cell necrosis and is characterized by patches of fibrous connective tissue in which cardiac muscle cells are either very scarce or absent. Ultrastructurally, both types are composed of collagen fibrils, spicules and star-shaped granules of proteoglycan material, small elastic fibers, and connective tissue microfibrils. The relative amounts of these components are variable.

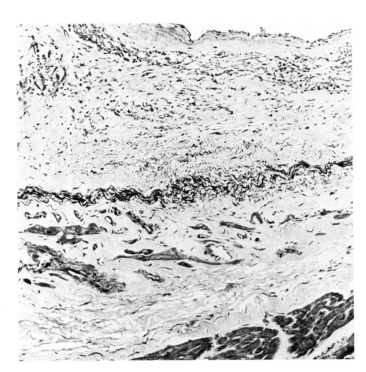

Fig. 21-3. Histologic section of endocardial fibrous plaque in left ventricular outflow tract of a patient with hypertrophic obstructive cardiomyopathy. This plaque has a layered appearance and contains smooth muscle cells, collagenous and elastic fibers, and acid mucopolysaccharide (the last not demonstrated in this illustration). Ventricular septal muscle underlying the plaque is shown at lower right. (Movat pentachrome stain.)

Hypertrophic Cardiomyopathy

Several forms of hypertrophic cardiomyopathy are recognized clinically according to whether or not obstruction to left ventricular outflow and asymmetric hypertrophy of the ventricular septum are present. Cardiomegaly, generalized hypertrophy, thick ventricular walls, a small, slit-shaped left ventricular cavity, and asymmetric hypertrophy of the ventricular septum are present in the majority of patients.[2] In a minority of patients the mass of asymmetrically hypertrophied ventricular septal tissue is localized to the apical region of the left ventricle (apical hypertrophic cardiomyopathy); however, in most patients the asymmetric thickening is maximal in the middle third of the ventricular septum. In patients with the obstructive form of hypertrophic cardiomyopathy, the mitral valve, particularly the ventricular surface of the anterior leaflet, usually is thickened by fibrous and elastic tissue; a plaque of similar fibroelastotic thickening is present on the endocardium of the septal wall of the left ventricular outflow tract (Fig. 21-3). This plaque, thought to result from contact between the septal surface and the anterior mitral leaflet, is removed during left ventricular myotomy-myectomy.

The cardiac muscle shows severe hypertrophy and foci of disarray in which cells are arranged in whorls instead of in parallel, and their myofibrils are oriented in various directions (Fig. 21-4). This disarray is present in the ventricular septum and in the anterior and posterior free walls of the left ventricle. The disarray has been quantified in large histologic sections and found to involve more than 5 percent of the total area of the ventricular septum and the left ventricular free walls. However, it is most pronounced in the central third of the septum, an area that cannot be sampled by using an endomyocardial bioptome. Myocardial fiber disarray is very frequently observed in myocardial biopsies from patients with hypertrophic cardiomyopathy; however, it is not specific for this disorder in a qualitative sense, as it occurs, with involvement of less than 5 percent of myocytes in the ventricular septum, in patients with various other disorders.[3] Therefore, the diagnosis of hypertrophic cardiomyopathy should not be either made or ruled out only on the basis of the findings in the small areas of tissue included in myocardial biopsies.

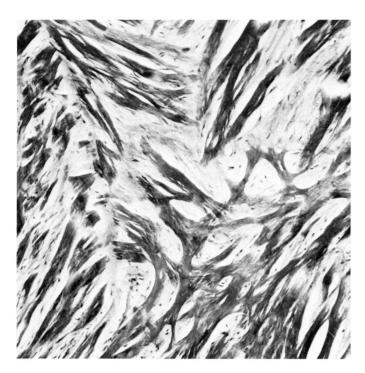

Fig. 21-4. Marked disarray of myocytes is evident in operatively resected ventricular septal muscle of patient with hypertrophic obstructive cardiomyopathy. Delicate interstitial fibrosis is also present. (Masson trichrome stain.)

Dilated Cardiomyopathy

The term dilated cardiomyopathy designates a heterogeneous group of syndromes that are characterized anatomically by: marked cardiac dilatation; mild or no thickening of the ventricular walls; mural thrombosis; atrioventricular valvular regurgitation because of displacement of the papillary muscles toward the apex; and variable degrees of fibrosis and myocardial cellular degeneration. Foci of myocytolysis also may be present. The nonspecific nature of the histologic and ultrastructural changes precludes making the diagnosis of dilated cardiomyopathy on the basis of biopsy findings alone.[1] However, the histologic, immunohistochemical, and ultrastructural findings in dilated cardiomyopathy may be of clinical predictive value. Much attention is being given at the present time to the possibility that in many cases dilated cardiomyopathy develops as a consequence of myocarditis in which most of the inflammatory reaction has subsided, leaving myocyte damage and interstitial fibrosis. Dilated cardiomyopathy of unknown cause, with or without lymphocytic infiltrates, has been reported in some patients with the acquired immune deficiency syndrome (AIDS).

Peripartal cardiomyopathy and *alcoholic* cardiomyopathy are two syndromes of dilated cardiomyopathy that do not have specific microscopic features,[2,4] although they are clinically distinctive. Alcoholic cardiomyopathy may be complicated by thiamine deficiency (which can be determined only by biochemical studies). A significant number of patients with "peripartal" cardiomyopathy actually have lymphocytic myocarditis. Therefore, endomyocardial biopsy is necessary to establish the proper diagnosis. *Anthracycline* cardiomyopathy is a heart muscle disorder induced by the administration of daunorubicin or doxorubicin, two antibiotics currently used in cancer therapy. It is characterized microscopically (Fig. 21-5) by myofibrillar loss and by striking dilatation of the sarcoplasmic reticulum, which imparts a characteristic vacuolated appearance to the affected cells.[5] The severity of these changes can be assessed in a semiquantitative manner in myocardial biopsies.[6,7] This assessment is of value in deciding whether or not to continue administration of these agents to patients suspected of developing anthracycline-induced cardiomyopathy.[7]

Infantile cardiomyopathy with histiocytoid change is another type of cardiomyopathy with distinctive morphologic features.[8] These consist of yellow nodules composed of large, round or elongated cardiac muscle cells that have lost practically all their contractile elements, are filled with mitochondria, lipid droplets, and glycogen, and show various degrees of dissociation of their intercellular junctions (Fig. 21-6). Thus far, these features have

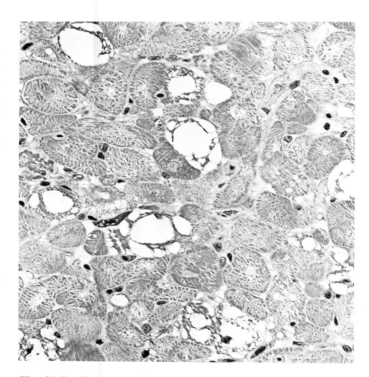

Fig. 21-5. Pronounced vacuolization of myocytes is the characteristic feature of doxorubicin-induced cardiomyopathy. (Plastic-embedded tissue, H&E ×500.)

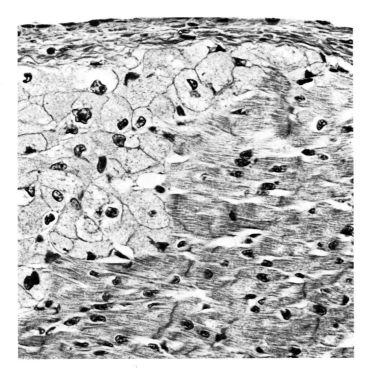

Fig. 21-6. Myocardium of patient with histiocytoid cardiomyopathy, showing part of a nodule of abnormal myocytes (upper left), which are located immediately beneath the endocardium and are adjacent to normal myocytes (lower right).

been reported only in small children presenting with the sudden onset of recurrent tachyarrhythmias, which have been eventually fatal in most cases. The etiology of this disorder remains unknown.

Myocardial Ischemia

Anatomic changes involving the myocardium in ischemic heart disease are: (1) cardiac muscle cell damage, necrosis, and associated inflammatory reaction; (2) myocardial fibrosis; and (3) complications such as perforation of the ventricular septum or a ventricular free wall, various forms of papillary muscle dysfunction (which show variable degrees of necrosis, fibrosis, atrophy, and calcification), ventricular aneurysms, and embolic phenomena related to mural thrombi.[9,10] Necrosis (Fig. 21-7) occurs in two main forms: (1) coagulation necrosis, which is basically limited to central regions of infarcts and is characterized by a relaxed appearance of the sarcomeres and by intramitochondrial flocculent deposits, and (2) necrosis with contraction bands, which is found in peripheral regions of infarcts and is characterized by deeply eosinophilic hypercontraction bands, intramitochondrial calcific deposits, and progression to myocytolysis.[11] Necrosis with contraction bands is thought to

result from reperfusion of the ischemic area surrounding the central zone of coagulation necrosis. This type of necrosis is also observed in patients dying soon after cardiac operations (circumferential hemorrhagic necrosis), and it is characteristically severe in the stone heart syndrome.[10] However, it is a nonspecific lesion, which also can be seen in other conditions, including prolonged hypotension, toxicity of endogenous or exogenous catecholamines, accidental and iatrogenic electrical injury, and myocarditis. The association of contraction band necrosis with coagulation necrosis in a myocardial biopsy specimen should suggest the possibility of acute myocardial infarction, particularly when lymphocytes are not a significant feature of the inflammatory infiltrate. Fibrosis associated with the healing of myocardial infarcts may lead to formation of ventricular aneurysms. These and resected left ventricular papillary muscles (from patients undergoing mitral valve replacement for papillary muscle dysfunction) are the most common surgical pathology specimens related to ischemic heart disease.

Cardiac Aneurysms

The term *cardiac aneurysm* designates a spectrum of gross and microscopic changes associated with aneurys-

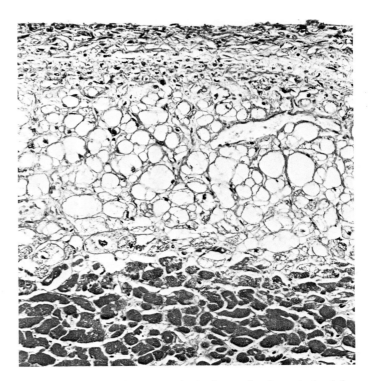

Fig. 21-7. Area of myocytolysis (center), characterized by empty sarcolemmal sheaths, separates endocardium (top) from area of coagulation necrosis (dark zone at bottom) in 3-day-old myocardial infarct.

mal bulging of a segment of the ventricular wall.[9,10] These changes consist of overall thinning of the ventricular wall; endocardial thickening by fibrous and elastic tissue; decrease in the amount of cardiac muscle; and corresponding increase in the amount of fibrous connective tissue in the wall. In their most severe form, these changes lead to the formation of large aneurysmal sacs, which are thin-walled, contain very little cardiac muscle in their walls, may be partially filled by laminated thrombi, and communicate by a large orifice with the main portion of the left ventricular cavity. Calcific deposits may be present in the aneurysmal wall. In less severe forms, the affected areas of the wall show lesser degrees of thinning, fibrosis, and endocardial thickening and contain more numerous cardiac muscle cells. The latter often show degenerative changes. The transition between fibrous aneurysmal wall and uninvolved myocardial wall may be gradual, and the borders of the ventricular aneurysm may be poorly demarcated.

The most common cause of true cardiac aneurysms is infarction of the anterior wall of the left ventricle. However, apical aneurysms, formed by progressively severe thinning of the ventricular wall so that the aneurysmal wall contains practically only endocardium and visceral pericardium, are characteristically found in Chagas' disease[12]; such aneurysms also occur in idiopathic dilated cardiomyopathy[13] and, rarely, in hypertrophic cardiomyopathy.[14]

Pseudoaneurysm of the Heart

A pseudoaneurysm results when the myocardial wall ruptures, but the rupture is contained by adherent thrombus or by pericardial adhesions. The diagnosis is based on the following findings: (1) the orifice by which the pseudoaneurysm communicates with the cardiac chamber is small compared with the size of the pseudoaneurysmal cavity; and (2) myocardial fibers are not present in the wall, which is a fibrous sac derived from parietal pericardium, organizing thrombus, or both. The latter distinction is best made by examining the borders of the resected specimen. The most common causes of cardiac pseudoaneurysm are: (1) transmural myocardial infarction with cardiac rupture; (2) cardiac operations in which incisions are made in the left ventricular wall (or even in the ventricular septum, as in the myotomy-myectomy procedure for hypertrophic obstructive cardiomyopathy); and (3) various forms of trauma. Pseudoaneurysms are much more likely to rupture than are true cardiac aneurysms.[10]

Annular Subvalvular Left Ventricular Aneurysms

Annular subvalvular aneurysms arise from the left ventricular cavity in the area of junction between the fibrous rings of the heart (most commonly the mitral, less frequently the aortic) and the left ventricular myocardium. These aneurysms are outpockets that extend through the tissue just below the ring toward the ventricular septum, the left atrium, or the epicardium.[15] They may contain laminated thrombus. They have a small circular opening with a rim of fibrous tissue, and their walls usually are formed by collagenous tissue and may be partially calcified. They are not related to ischemic heart disease, and their etiology is unknown.[10]

Myocarditis

Inflammatory cell infiltrates (Fig. 21-8) and myocyte damage or degeneration serve as the basis for the diagnosis of myocarditis,[9,10,16] which can be acute (infiltrates composed of polymorphonuclear leukocytes, lymphocytes, or both) or chronic (also including plasma cells, macrophages, and usually some degree of fibrosis). The timing of the endomyocardial biopsy with respect to the onset of the myocarditis is crucial to diagnosis and perhaps to therapeutic outcome. The interstitial cell population changes with time, as demonstrated by studies of

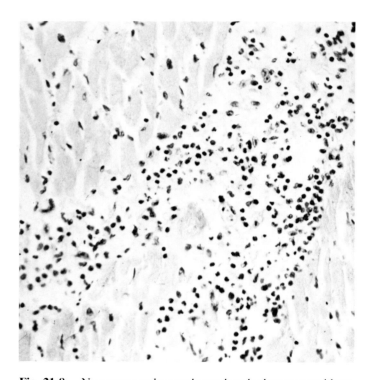

Fig. 21-8. Numerous polymorphonuclear leukocytes and lymphocytes infiltrate heart of a patient with myocarditis due to epidemic hemorrhagic fever.

animal models of viral myocarditis. In patients with progressive disease, decreasing numbers of lymphocytes and increasing numbers of fibroblasts have been observed by electron microscopy in serial endomyocardial biopsies.[16]

Myocarditis can be caused by any one of a heterogeneous group of disorders, which usually present in predictable morphologic patterns, including inflammatory cell infiltrates characterized predominantly by granulomas, eosinophils, neutrophils, or lymphocytes. The morphologic types of myocarditis and their causes are summarized in Tables 21-1 to 21-4.

The most common type of myocarditis recognized by endomyocardial biopsy is lymphocytic myocarditis, which is presumed in most cases to be postviral and to be mediated by an aberrant immune response. However, the histologic criteria for diagnosis of lymphocytic myocarditis are the most controversial, largely because numerous types of mononuclear cells (which are connective tissue cells) in the myocardial interstitium resemble lymphocytes by conventional light microscopy (Table 21-5).

The identification of lymphocytes alone is not enough to establish the diagnosis of myocarditis. The presence of lymphocytes in close approximation to the sarcolemmal membranes of degenerating cardiac myocytes is required to establish the diagnosis of lymphocytic myocarditis.[16] Myocardial lymphocytes may be found in the myocardium of apparently normal individuals[17] and may also be present in such conditions as drug-associated myocardial damage (the consequences of drug hypersensitivity or toxicity)[18,19] or at the periphery of another lesion such as a granuloma[20,21] or in ischemic lesions in the process of healing. Some disorders (lymphomas, leukemia, etc.) are associated with increased numbers of lymphocytes in many tissues of the body, including the myocardium, without evidence of myocyte damage. Large numbers of myocardial lymphocytes may be present in these disorders but usually indicate a noninflammatory or neoplastic condition.

An intensive search using cultures, serologic studies, and appropriate tissue stains must be made for specific etiologic agents such as viruses, rickettsiae, bacteria, fungi, or parasites when indicated. Viruses are considered the most frequent cause of myocarditis but seldom are specifically identified. The value of viral cultures of myocardial biopsy specimens has not been established yet.

Rheumatic Myocarditis and Aschoff Nodules

Aschoff nodules, located in endocardium or in perivascular areas, provide the basis for the diagnosis of the rheumatic process (Fig. 21-9). They undergo a process of evolution, during only part of which they show specific

TABLE 21-1. Causes of Lymphocytic Myocarditis

Infection (viral, fungal, protozoal, rickettsial, bacterial, chlamydial, mycoplasmal)
Infectious mononucleosis
Aberrant immune response (postviral; Kawasaki disease; polymyositis; systemic lupus erythematosus, mixed connective tissue disease, other collagen-vascular diseases)
Drug reaction (hypersensitivity, drug-induced lupus, other)
Sarcoidosis (and other causes of granulomatous myocarditis)
Cardiac allograft rejection
Idiopathic process

TABLE 21-2. Causes of Granulomatous Myocarditis

Collagen-vascular disease (rheumatic fever, rheumatoid arthritis, ankylosing spondylitis, Wegener's granulomatosis)
Metabolic disorder (Farber's disease, gout, oxalosis, granulomatous disease of childhood)
Proliferative disorders of the mononuclear-phagocyte system (juvenile xanthogranuloma, Chester-Erdheim disease, malignant histiocytosis)
Infection (bacterial, mycobacterial, fungal, parasitic, rickettsial, or Whipple's disease)
Sarcoidosis
Hypersensitivity
Foreign body granulomas
Idiopathic

TABLE 21-3. Causes of Eosinophilic Myocarditis

Drug hypersensitivity
Disseminated eosinophilic collagen-vascular disease (Loeffler's syndrome)
Parasitic infestation
Wegener's granulomatosis
Cardiac allograft rejection
Idiopathic process

TABLE 21-4. Causes of Neutrophilic Myocarditis

Infarction
Infection
  Direct (bacterial)
  Indirect (toxic, as in diphtheria, or septic)
Leukoclastic vasculitis (collagen-vascular disease)

TABLE 21-5. Types of Mononuclear Cells in the Myocardial Interstitium

Lymphocytes
Plasma cells
Mast cells
Schwann cells
Smooth muscle cells
Endothelial cells
Perithelial cells
Cardiac histiocytes
Macrophages
Fibroblasts
Undifferentiated mesenchymal cells

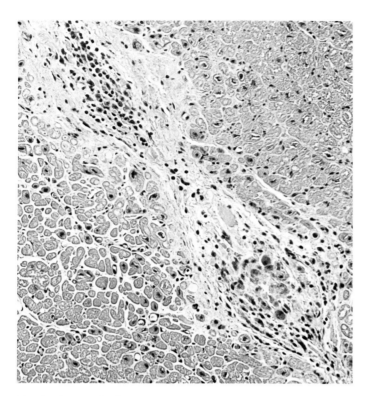

Fig. 21-9. Aschoff nodule in left ventricular papillary muscle excised with mitral valve in a 23-year-old woman with mitral stenosis and regurgitation and recurrent migratory polyarthritis. Ovoid masses of inflammatory cells, including multinucleated Aschoff cells, monocytes, and lymphocytes, are surrounded by fibrous connective tissue.

diagnostic features (Aschoff cells and fibrinoid necrosis). Aschoff cells are large, mono- or polynucleated cells, contain chromatin bars located in the central third of the nucleus, possess amphophilic cytoplasm, and have indistinct cytoplasmic borders. These cells differ from Anitschkow cells (Fig. 21-10), which also have nuclear chromatin bars but are small and elongated, have a scanty cytoplasm lacking basophilia, and constitute a totally nonspecific finding.[1] A nonspecific lymphocytic myocarditis is frequently found in patients with rheumatic fever, and in the absence of Aschoff nodules in a biopsy specimen this rheumatic myocarditis cannot be accurately distinguished from other causes of lymphocytic myocarditis.

Myocardial inflammatory reactions also occur in collagen-vascular diseases and in sarcoidosis. Lesions in collagen-vascular diseases include: nonspecific myocarditis, which occurs in dermatomyositis (with lymphocytic infiltrates) and systemic lupus erythematosus (often in association with fibrinoid necrosis, vasculitis, and pericardial and endocardial lesions); fibrosis, which occurs in scleroderma without being associated with a significant inflammatory reaction; rheumatoid nodules and less distinctive

granulomatous lesions, which are found in rheumatoid arthritis; and myocardial necroses associated with vascular lesions, which occur in periarteritis nodosa, Wegener's granulomatosis, and thrombotic thrombocytopenic purpura.[22] The lesions in myocardial sarcoidosis consist of noncaseating granulomas with epithelioid cells and multinucleated giant cells. Such lesions must be distinguished from other types of myocardial granulomatous processes and from giant cell myocarditis (Table 21-2).[16]

Cardiac Transplantation—Monitoring Rejection

Percutaneous transvenous endomyocardial biopsy remains the most reliable means of detecting acute cardiac rejection and has contributed greatly to the increased survival of cardiac transplant patients. Several systems have been used to grade the degree of cardiac allograft rejection.[23,24] The Stanford system describes rejection as mild, moderate, or severe. At the Texas Heart Institute cardiac allograft rejection is evaluated on a numerical scale ranging from 0 to 10 (Figs. 21-11 to 21-14 and Table 21-6). This scale was developed to give a numerical objectivity to the degree of cardiac allograft rejection and to enhance com-

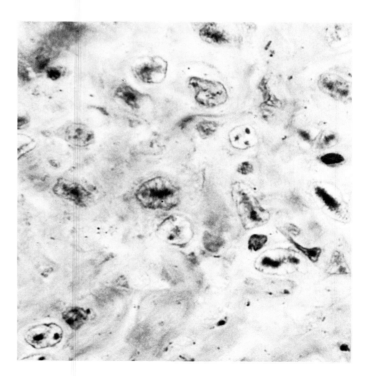

Fig. 21-10. High-magnification view of part of an Aschoff nodule, showing Anitschkow cells with typical nuclei, which contain a serrated, centrally located chromatin bar. Fine strands extend from the chromatin bar toward the nuclear periphery. (Plastic-embedded tissue, alkaline toluidine blue, ×1,200.)

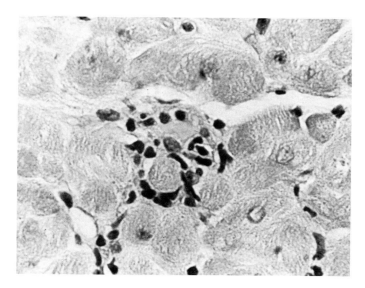

Fig. 21-11. Rejection of transplanted human heart, grade 3, Texas Heart Institute scoring system. Perivascular mononuclear cell infiltrate with focal extension into interstitium but no myocyte degeneration. (H&E.)

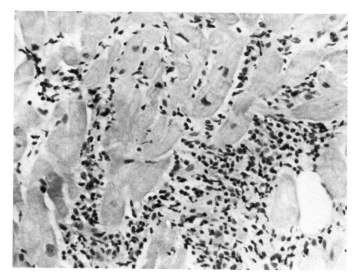

Fig. 21-13. Rejection of transplanted human heart, grade 5, Texas Heart Institute scoring system. More extensive interstitial infiltrate and myocyte degeneration than seen in Fig. 21-12. (H&E.)

munication between the pathologist, surgeon, and cardiologist. A comparison of the Texas Heart Institute and Stanford grading systems of cardiac allograft rejection is illustrated in Fig. 21-15. The prime determinant of higher grades of allograft rejection is the extent of cardiac myocyte degeneration. By plotting the numerical value and the date of the patient's previous endomyocardial

biopsies on the 0 to 10 scale, one can accurately determine the degree of cardiac allograft rejection, the direction of change, and the speed of change. These parameters are important in determining the patient's immunosuppressive regimen and the cardiac allograft biopsy interval.[24]

It is also important to consider the *differential diagnosis* of acute rejection in interpreting endomyocardial biopsies from these patients. During the first two weeks following transplantation, *ischemic injury* secondary to reperfusion is commonly encountered, and is characterized by focal myocytolysis, with an infiltrate of macrophages and neutrophils rather than the predominantly lymphocytic infiltrate of acute rejection. Repeat biopsies frequently demonstrate phenomena of healing at a previous biopsy site, including separation and disorganization of the myocytes by fibrin, granulation tissue, and eventually fibrosis. *Infection* (myocarditis) may also be

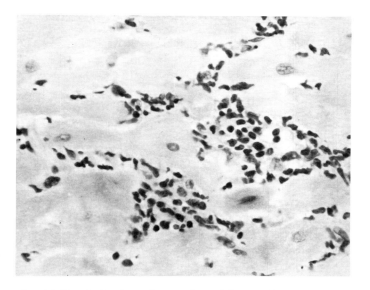

Fig. 21-12. Rejection of transplanted human heart, grade 4, Texas Heart Institute, scoring system. Interstitial mononuclear cell infiltrate with very focal myocyte degeneration (note cell to right of and below center). (H&E.)

TABLE 21-6. Texas Heart Institute's Evaluation of Cardiac Allograft Rejection by Endomyocardial Biopsy

0	No evidence of rejection
1–2	Perivascular aggregates of mononuclear cells
3	Perivascular aggregates of mononuclear cells with extension into the interstitium
4–8	Interstitial mononuclear cells with cardiac myocyte degeneration of increasing severity
9–10	Extensive cardiac myocyte degeneration, interstitial mononuclear cells and polymorphonuclear leukocytes

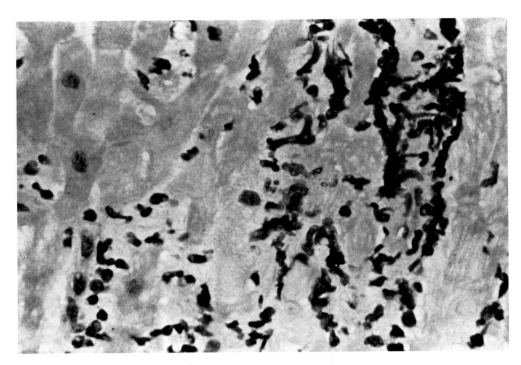

Fig. 21-14. Rejection of transplanted human heart, grade 6, Texas Heart Institute scoring system, H&E. Scattered myocyte degeneration associated with perivascular and interstitial mononuclear cell infiltrate.

seen in these immunocompromised patients, and usually will produce a mixed inflammatory infiltrate rather than a purely mononuclear one; the organism responsible (cytomegalovirus, Toxoplasma, various fungi) may or may not be identified in the biopsy specimen. Eosinophils may be a marker of infection, but are also seen after cyclosporine treatment in the absence of infection. *Resolving rejection* after treatment of an acute rejection episode is characterized by resorption of necrotic myocytes and their replacement by hemosiderin-laden macrophages and fibroblasts. *Chronic rejection* is rarely encountered in endomyocardial biopsy material, and is essentially a vascular phenomenon, with intimal proliferation and adventitial inflammatory infiltration in small and large coronary arteries.

Metabolic and Storage Diseases

The diagnosis of glycogen storage disease should be based not only on the morphologic demonstration of increased amounts of glycogen but also on biochemical analysis of the glycogen structure and on identification of the enzymatic defect (in leukocytes, liver biopsy, and/or tissue culture of skin fibroblasts). Myocardial involvement is most severe in the infantile form or type II (Pompe's disease) but also occurs in types III and IV. In type II the glycogen is morphologically and biochemically normal. In heart muscle it is stored both within lysosomes and in the main cytoplasmic compartment. These deposits are associated with massive cardiomegaly and with a typical lacework appearance of the muscle cells.

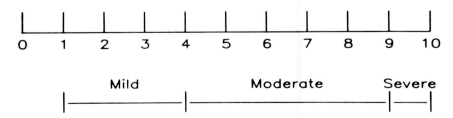

Fig. 21-15. Comparison of the Stanford and Texas Heart Institute scoring systems for grading of transplant rejection. (From McAllister et al.,[24] with permission.)

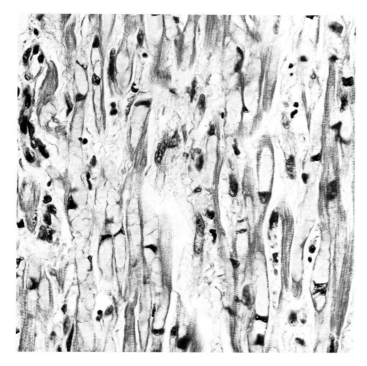

Fig. 21-16. Myocytes in left ventricle of a patient with type IV glycogen storage disease contain basophilic masses of abnormal glycogen.

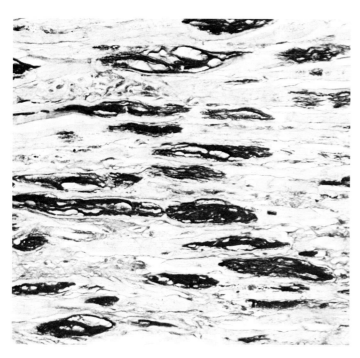

Fig. 21-17. PAS-positive material, considered to be an abnormal polymer of glucose, occupies central regions of cardiac myocytes of patient with the Lafora type of myoclonic epilepsy.

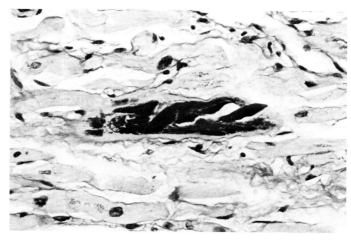

Fig. 21-18. Basophilic degenerative material occupies most of cytoplasm of muscle cell of an elderly patient who died of neoplastic disease.

In type III the glycogen is morphologically normal but biochemically abnormal, and it is free in the cytoplasm. In type IV the glycogen is both biochemically and morphologically abnormal; it is basophilic, is free in the cytoplasm, is very slowly degraded by amylase, and forms fibrils that measure about 40 to 50 Å in diameter and are ultrastructurally similar to those that occur in cardiac muscle cells in *basophilic degeneration* (a frequent, nonspecific incidental finding in the hearts of elderly individuals) and in the Lafora type of myoclonic epilepsy[1,25] (Figs. 21-16 to 21-19). One patient with phosphofructokinase deficiency, glycogen storage disease, and cardiac involvement has been reported,[26] and one patient with glycogen storage disease limited to the heart and associ-

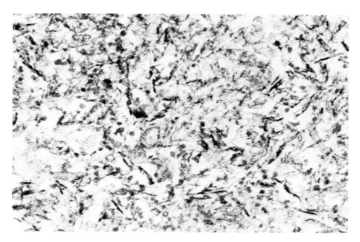

Fig. 21-19. Electron micrograph of basophilic degenerative material similar to that shown in Fig. 21-18. This material is composed of fine fibrils associated with particles resembling glycogen granules. (×65,000.)

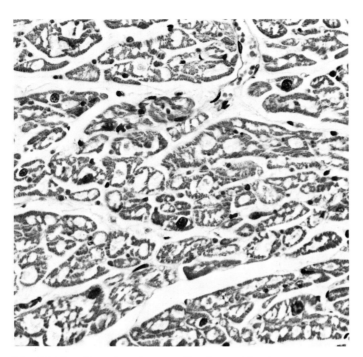

Fig. 21-20. Cytoplasmic vacuolization, which imparts a lace-like appearance to the tissue, is present in myocardium of a patient with Fabry's disease.

ated with deficient activity of cardiac phosphorylase kinase also has been described.[27] Two necessary notes of caution are that myocardial biopsy specimens often contain strikingly prominent pools of glycogen in perinuclear regions of the cells (especially when compared with necropsy specimens), and that glutaraldehyde fixation produces a marked artifactual increase in the intensity of the PAS reaction.

Cardiovascular lesions in the *mucopolysaccharidoses* consist of deposits of acid mucopolysaccharides, and often also of glycolipids (which have not been fully characterized), in pleomorphic (usually vacuolated) inclusions in cardiac muscle cells and in connective tissue cells and smooth muscle cells in endocardium, valves, and vessels. The large, extramural coronary arteries may display severe intimal thickening. Distinction between the cardiovascular morphologic findings in the various types of mucopolysaccharidoses and mucolipidoses is extremely difficult, and these findings should be closely correlated with extracardiac anatomic, clinical, and biochemical observations. The lesions in these disorders also must be distinguished[25] from those in generalized GM$_1$ gangliosidosis, Sandhoff's disease (a type of generalized GM gangliosidosis), and Farber's disease (lipogranulomatosis).

Other disorders associated with lipid storage phenomena within cardiac muscle cells and/or cardiac connective tissue cells include: *Fabry's disease* (Fig. 21-20), in which the deposits contain glycolipids that show strong

birefringence, are soluble in lipid solvents, and form parallel or concentric electron-dense lamellae with a regular periodicity (these deposits also involve coronary endothelium and smooth muscle); *type I* and *type III hyperlipoproteinemia*, in which foam cells (containing neutral lipids) can form yellow patches in endocardium; homozygous *type II hyperlipoproteinemia*, in which cholesterol-rich foam cells can infiltrate the endocardium and coronary arteries; and *Gaucher's disease* and *Niemann-Pick disease*, in which foam cells (containing glucocerebroside and sphingomyelin, respectively) occasionally can infiltrate the myocardial interstitium.[25] The lamellar deposits that occur in the cytoplasm of cardiac myocytes in Fabry's disease and other metabolic disorders must be distinguished from those that occur in *chloroquine toxicity*. In the latter disorder, such deposits are associated with curvilinear bodies.[26,28] *Triglyceride deposits* within cardiac muscle cells are found in numerous disorders, including carnitine deficiency, hypoxia and ischemia, alcoholic cardiomyopathy, Reye's syndrome, thyrotoxicosis, diabetes mellitus, prolonged hypotension, and conditions due to administration of a variety of toxic agents.

Other disease entities that must be considered in the differential diagnosis of myocardial storage disorders are hemochromatosis, hemosiderosis, oxalosis, and amyloidosis.[25] In *hemochromatosis* and *hemosiderosis* the deposits show positive histochemical reactions for iron

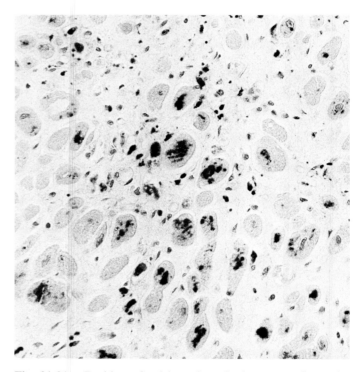

Fig. 21-21. Darkly stained iron deposits in myocardium of a patient with cardiac hemosiderosis due to multiple transfusions of blood. (Perl's stain.)

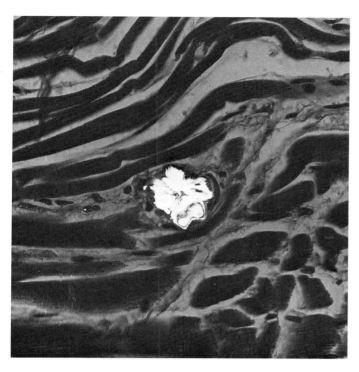

Fig. 21-22. Oxalate crystal in myocardium of a patient with oxalosis. (Polarized light micrograph of section stained with H&E.)

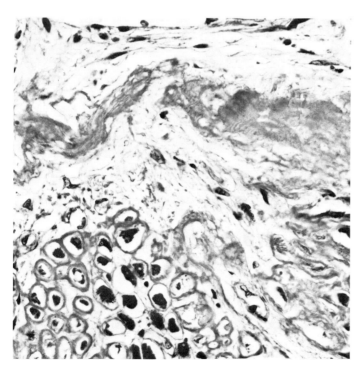

Fig. 21-23. Amyloid deposits are present just beneath the endocardium (top) and surround muscle cells of a patient with cardiac amyloidosis.

(Fig. 21-21). In the various syndromes of primary and secondary oxalosis, the oxalate crystals can be identified in myocardium by polarization microscopy of routine paraffin sections and by specific histochemical staining (Fig. 21-22). The green birefringence of Congo red–stained amyloid deposits and the identification of amyloid fibrils by electron microscopy establish the diagnosis of cardiac involvement in *amyloidosis* (Fig. 21-23). Myocardium, endocardium, valves, and vessels (mainly intramural coronary arteries and arterioles) are involved to some extent in the majority of the syndromes of amyloidosis. Amyloid fibrils in myocardium must be distinguished from connective tissue microfibrils, which are larger in diameter (120 to 150 Å) than amyloid fibrils (100 Å), have a beaded appearance, and can be very numerous in fibrotic hearts. Amorphous deposits of electron-dense material have been observed ultrastructurally in endocardium, myocardium, and blood vessels in light chain disease associated with restrictive cardiomyopathy. Such deposits can be recognized only by ultrastructural study or by immunohistochemical demonstration of the presence of immunoglobulin light chains.[30]

The cardiomyopathy in the *Duchenne* type of progressive *muscular dystrophy* is characterized by myocardial fibrosis that is preferentially distributed in subepicardial areas. Cardiac involvement without distinctive anatomic changes occurs in numerous other heredofamilial neuromuscular disorders.[25]

Myocardial fiber atrophy, interstitial edema, and, rarely, inflammatory cell infiltrates have been described in obese patients having severe, often fatal ventricular arrhythmias while taking a modified *liquid protein diet* as part of a weight reduction program.[25]

Cardiac morphologic lesions reported in *endocrine disorders*[31] include: myocardial hypertrophy and fibrosis in acromegaly; basophilic degeneration of the muscle cells in myxedema; focal myocarditis and myocytolysis in pheochromocytoma; fiber calcification in hypercalcemia; focal vacuolization and hyalinization of the muscle cells in Cushing's syndrome (and also in hypokalemia of other causes); and hypertrophy in hyperthyroidism. Dilated cardiomyopathy has been reported in association with diabetes mellitus, but morphologic findings have been variable and nonspecific.[31] The basement membranes of myocardial capillaries have been reported to be thicker in diabetic and myxedematous patients than in control patients.[32]

Mural Endocardium

Mural endocardium in biopsy or surgical material should be evaluated with respect to: (1) overall thickness; (2) layered arrangement; (3) type and number of cells present; (4) presence of overlying thrombus, and (5) relative amounts of extracellular components of connective tissue (i.e., collagen, elastic fibers, and proteoglycans). The pathologic reactions of mural endocardium to injury generally lead to endocardial thickening, of which several types are recognized on the basis of the predominant changes in the cellular and extracellular components of the endocardium.[1] Regional differences in normal endocardial thickness and layered structure must be taken into account: endocardium is much thicker and contains a much better developed layer of smooth muscle cells in the left atrium than elsewhere.

In *congenital endocardial fibroelastosis* the thickness of ventricular and atrial endocardium is markedly increased, and the elastic fibers are very numerous and larger than normal (Fig. 21-24). *Acquired endocardial fibroelastosis* can be diffuse (a nonspecific finding in many conditions associated with ventricular dilatation) or focal (friction lesions, contact lesions, jet lesions); elastic fibers in these lesions are small and the relative amounts of elastic fibers and collagen are variable.[1] The mural and valvular endocardial lesions in *endomyocardial fibrosis* and *carcinoid heart disease* are described in the section on valves. Selective calcification of elastic fibers, which often assume a characteristic curled appearance (Fig. 21-25), occurs in mural endocardium and systemic vessels of patients with *pseudoxanthoma elasticum*.[25] Small, flat plaques containing amyloid deposits have been described in mural endocardium in amyloidosis.

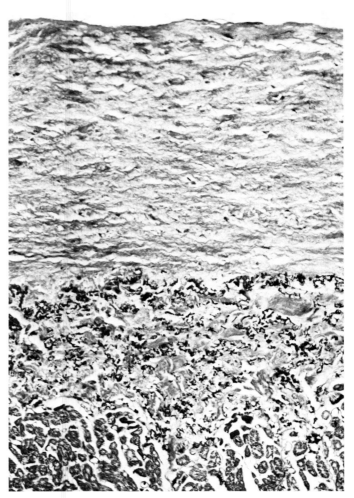

Fig. 21-25. Calcified elastic fibers (lower center) are present in the inner layer of left ventricular endocardium of a patient with pseudoxanthoma elasticum.

Fibrous rings present in the left ventricular outflow tract of patients with *fixed outlet subaortic stenosis* have the usual layered structure of endocardium.[33] *Pacing catheters* inserted into the right ventricle become attached to mural endocardium by a small thrombus, which also forms a thin layer over the catheter surface. Organization of this thrombus leads to the formation of a tightly adherent white fibrous sheath composed of collagen, microfibrils, fibrin, and connective tissue cells.[10]

CARDIAC VALVES

The Collagen Vascular Diseases

Rheumatic Valvulitis

In the *acute phase* of rheumatic valvulitis, the most conspicuous lesions are minute, translucent nodules (verrucae) along the lines of closure (Fig. 21-26). These are

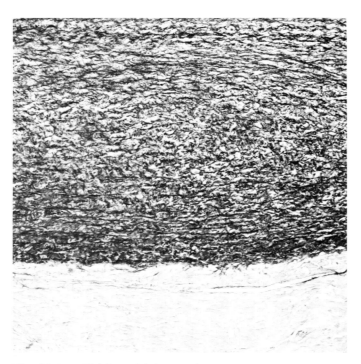

Fig. 21-24. Thickened left ventricular endocardium of a patient with congenital endocardial fibroelastosis. (Elastica-van Gieson.)

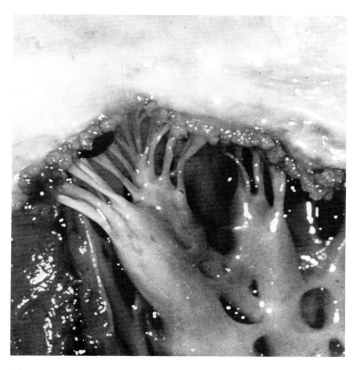

Fig. 21-26. Mitral valve of a child who died with acute rheumatic fever. The verrucae along the line of closure and chordae tendineae represent foci of fibrinoid necrosis.

most frequently observed in the mitral and aortic valves, less often in the tricuspid, and rarely in the pulmonary valve. They vary in diameter from less than 1 mm to 3 mm and are located on the atrial surface of the atrioventricular valves and on the ventricular surface of the semilunar valves.[34] Occasionally, a few verrucae may be distributed elsewhere over the cusps. They are also characteristically present on the chordae tendineae, especially those of the mitral valve, and not infrequently, they extend over the posterior leaflet of the mitral valve onto the endocardium of the left atrium. The verrucae tend to conglomerate on the corpora arantii of the aortic valve and extend in a row along the semilunar cusps. Diffuse thickening of the valves, except the pulmonary, is a less conspicuous but frequent gross alteration.

The inflammatory process is observed most frequently in the auricularis layer of the atrioventricular valves and the ventricularis layer of the semilunar valves. A nonspecific inflammatory process, which may involve the entire valve and ring, consists of edema, increased numbers of capillaries, and a variety of inflammatory cells (mainly lymphocytes, but occasionally polymorphonuclear leukocytes predominate). Plasma cells, fibroblasts, and other mononuclear cells are often present in variable numbers. Usually the valve also contains Anitschkow and Aschoff cells (previously described in the section on myocardium) which may be arranged in nodules or in rows and often surround foci of eosinophilic fragmented

collagen or fibrinoid or both. Aschoff cells may be multinucleated.[1,34] Microscopically, the verrucae may have the appearance of either thrombi, formed by the deposition of platelets and fibrin on the surface of the valve, or extruded collagen that has undergone fibrinoid degeneration. The region immediately adjacent to the vegetation, shows marked proliferation of fibroblasts, as well as edema and numerous lymphocytes (Fig. 21-27).

Gross alterations of the cardiac valves become more pronounced as a result of *recurrent* rheumatic valvulitis. Thickening, irregularity of the surfaces, and gross vascularization are usually present. This thickening is usually most pronounced in the distal third of the valve leaflets.[34] The chordae tendineae become thicker and shorter, with especially prominent thickening at their insertions into the valve leaflets. Verrucae in various stages of activity and healing may be observed. In addition to being thickened, the aortic cusps may be considerably shortened, with their free margins rolled and inverted toward the sinus pocket. Fibrous adhesions are commonly present at the commissures, and verrucae in various stages of activity may extend across the commissures of aortic cusps. In recurrent valvulitis there is a higher incidence of verrucae on the valves of the right side of the heart, and microscopically considerable fibrosis, an apparent increase in elastic tissue, and inflammatory changes in vari-

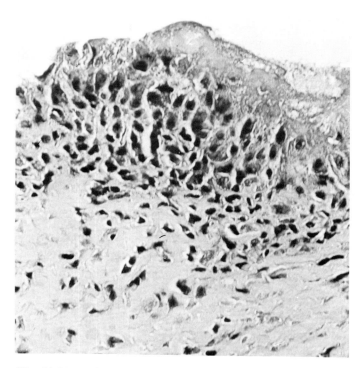

Fig. 21-27. Histologic section of a verruca in the mitral valve of a patient with acute rheumatic carditis. Note inflammatory cells, fibrinoid necrosis, and fibrin superimposed on valvular connective tissue.

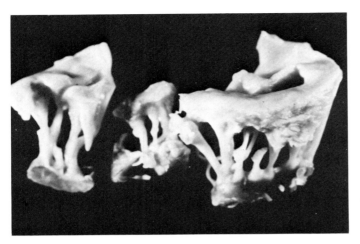

Fig. 21-28. Fibrotic, thickened mitral valve leaflets and chordae resected at operation from a patient with severe mitral stenosis of rheumatic origin.

ous stages of activity are observed.[34] The fibrosis and inflammation involve the rings as well as the leaflets. This histologic pattern differs from that of acute valvulitis, in which the thickening of the valves is the result only of edema and inflammation. Also in contrast to the appearance of acute valvulitis is the presence of numerous arteries with thick muscular walls in the ring and proximal portion of the valve.

In *chronic* rheumatic valvulitis the alterations already described in recurrent valvulitis are more advanced. Usually the diffuse thickening and fibrosis of the valves have resulted in loss of elasticity and in narrowing of the orifice. Thickening, fusion, and shortening of the chordae tendineae of the mitral valve are usually pronounced (Fig. 21-28). In addition, focal deposits of calcium salts may be present. These deposits may be extensive and may project to the atrial and ventricular surfaces, causing further distortion. Ossification complete with hematopoiesis may occur, causing further distortion. Verrucae are less frequent in chronic valvulitis than in recurrent valvulitis and are broad and flat. Active inflammation is less pronounced than in recurrent valvulitis and usually consists of scattered foci of perivascular cuffing with lymphocytes. The grossly apparent thickening is due to an increase in fibrous and elastic tissue throughout the entire leaflet, including the rings and the tips of the valves. The fibrous connective tissue is usually homogeneous and hyaline. These valves are vascularized by capillaries and thick-walled vessels, which are most numerous in the superficial layers. The verrucae no longer consist of material showing fibrinoid necrosis but are organized by fibroblasts and collagen fibers. As chronicity progresses, the number of fibroblasts decreases, and the verrucae become dense, hyalinized scars.

Rheumatoid Valvulitis

Rheumatoid granulomas may occur in any of the cardiac valves but are most common in the mitral and aortic valves.[35] Involvement may be focal or diffuse and is usually most prominent in the midportion or base of the valve. The chordae tendineae are usually uninvolved, but occasionally they may be fibrotic and shortened. Commissural fusion is rare. Rheumatoid nodules are most commonly located within the valve leaflets and are enclosed by fibrous tissue; rarely, a rheumatoid nodule may erode the surface of the valve so that the necrotic center of the nodule communicates with a cardiac cavity. In these unusual occurrences there may be superimposed thrombus or infective endocarditis. Verrucae of fibrinoid necrosis, common in rheumatic valvulitis and systemic lupus erythematosus, are not a feature of pure rheumatoid valvulitis.

Lupus Erythematosus Valvulitis

Lupus erythematosus valvulitis (atypical verrucous endocarditis of Libman and Sacks) is recognized as a specific valvular abnormality occurring in systemic lupus erythematosus (Fig. 21-29). Any valve may be involved, but the mitral and tricuspid valves are most often af-

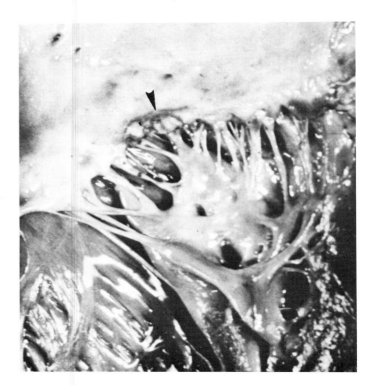

Fig. 21-29. Mitral valve of a 21-year-old woman, illustrating atypical verrucous endocarditis of Libman and Sacks. These foci of fibrinoid necrosis (arrowhead) have no special tendency to occur along the lines of closure of the valves and may be present on the chordae tendineae and mural endocardium.

fected. The verrucae may be located on either side of a valve cusp but most frequently are present on the ventricular surface of the posterior mitral leaflet or in the valve ring; involvement of the anterior mitral leaflet is infrequent. They have no special tendency to occur along the lines of closure of the valves and may be scattered on the chordae tendineae and atrial or ventricular mural endocardium. The lesions are small, usually ranging in size from 1 to 4 mm in diameter, but, rarely, may reach a diameter of 8 to 10 mm. They are sterile, dry, granular pink vegetations that may be single or multiple in conglomerates.[34] Histologically, the verrucae consist of a finely granular, eosinophilic, fibrinoid material, which may contain hematoxylin bodies. In a general sense these hematoxylin bodies are the tissue equivalent of the L.E. cell of the blood and bone marrow.[34] The verrucous endocardial lesions result from degenerative and inflammatory processes of the endocardium and deeper layers of the valves. An intense valvulitis is present, which is characterized by fibrinoid necrosis of the valve substance and which often is contiguous with the vegetations. Exudative and proliferative cellular reactions are present in the deeper layers of the valve. Healing of these lesions may produce foci of granulation tissue, which develop into focal fibrous thickenings in the valves or the mural endocardium. Rarely, bacterial endocarditis may be superimposed on the Libman-Sacks lesions.[35]

Lesions Resembling Collagen Vascular Disease Valvulitis

Although not collagen vascular diseases, three entities that may result in fibrous thickening of the cardiac valves and thickening and fusion of chordae tendineae are Whipple's disease, endomyocardial fibrosis with eosinophilia, and radiation. In *Whipple's disease* the valve most commonly involved is the mitral, followed by the tricuspid and aortic. The gross deformity (Fig. 21-30) closely resembles that seen in chronic rheumatic heart disease, with diffuse thickening and fibrosis of the valve leaflets and chordae tendineae and rolling of the free edges of the leaflets. Microscopically, large macrophages filled with PAS-positive granules identical to those found in the small intestine in patients with this disease are present in the valve substance (Fig. 21-31). Proliferating fibrous tissue and chronic inflammatory cells are commonly associated with the PAS-positive macrophages. Scattered rod-shaped bodies, measuring 1.5 to 2.0 μm in length and 0.2 to 0.4 μm in diameter, are present intracellularly and extracellularly. These bodies, as well as membrane-bound masses of fibrillar material within the macrophages, are identical to those described in jejunal biopsies of patients with Whipple's disease.[36]

In *endomyocardial fibrosis with eosinophilia* (Figs. 21-32 and 21-33), the valves most commonly involved are

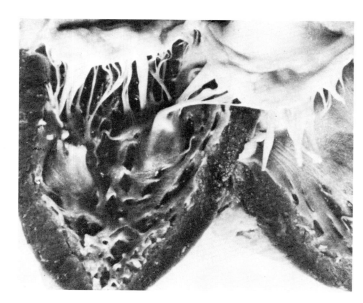

Fig. 21-30. Mitral valve of a 52-year-old man with intestinal lipodystrophy (Whipple's disease), illustrating diffuse thickening and fibrosis of the valve leaflets and chordae tendineae, resembling the gross deformity of chronic rheumatic valve disease.

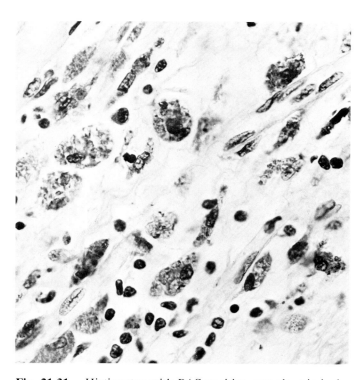

Fig. 21-31. Histiocytes with PAS-positive cytoplasmic inclusions infiltrate the myocardium of a patient with Whipple's disease. (PAS-hematoxylin.)

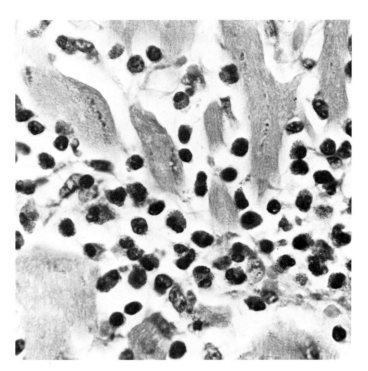

Fig. 21-32. Numerous eosinophils are present between cardiac muscle cells of a patient with hypereosinophilia and endomyocardial fibrosis.

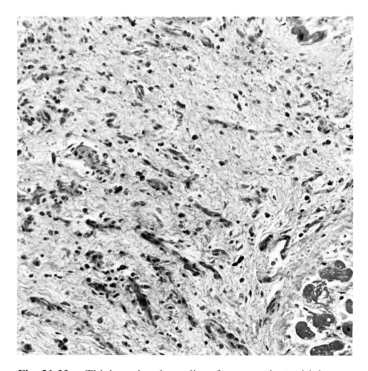

Fig. 21-33. Thickened endocardium from a patient with hypereosinophilia and endomyocardial fibrosis contains dense fibrous tissue, granulation tissue, and scattered eosinophils.

the mitral and tricuspid, with a lesser incidence of aortic valve involvement. There is fibrous thickening of endocardium, with superimposed fibrin thrombus beneath either the posterior mitral leaflet or the posterior or septal tricuspid leaflet. These leaflets become adherent to the underlying mural endocardium, with resulting regurgitation.[37] The aortic valve cusps are occasionally thickened by vascularized fibrous tissue, which is superimposed on the ventricular aspects of the cusps. The commissures of the aortic valve may become fused by fibrous tissue with superimposed fibrin thrombus. Eosinophilic leukocytes in varying numbers are usually present at the periphery of the fibrous lesions.

Rarely, patients receiving *mediastinal irradiation* may develop lesions of the cardiac valves.[38] The valves most commonly involved are the tricuspid and mitral, followed by the aortic and pulmonary. The fibrous valvular thickenings are focal, and the anterior tricuspid leaflet and the anterior mitral leaflet are usually more markedly involved than the posterior leaflets. The chordae tendineae also may be focally thickened with fibrous tissue.

Other Collagen Vascular and Related Diseases

Valvular lesions in *scleroderma* are distinctly rare; the most common lesion is nonbacterial thrombotic endocarditis. In patients with *thrombotic thrombocytopenic purpura*, nonbacterial thrombotic endocarditis frequently is present. In both these diseases, the cardiac valves most commonly involved are the mitral and aortic.[35] Valvulitis is most unusual in *Wegener's granulomatosis*; the mitral valve is most commonly involved by the inflammatory process, which may result in subsequent fibrosis with commissural fusion resembling rheumatic mitral stenosis.[39] Primary valvulitis is not a feature of *dermatomyositis*. Diseases that may result in valvulitis but are manifested most commonly by aortitis (syphilis, ankylosing spondylitis, psoriatic arthritis, Reiter's syndrome, and granulomatous aortitis) are discussed in the section on the aorta.

Endocrine and Metabolic Diseases

In *carcinoid heart disease* there is either focal or diffuse plaque-like thickening of valvular and mural endocardium and occasionally of the intima of the great veins, coronary sinus, pulmonary trunk, and main pulmonary arteries (Fig. 21-34). The fibrous tissue is atypical and limited in the majority of instances to the right side of the heart. When the pulmonary valve is involved, deposition is almost exclusively on the arterial aspect of the valve cusps. When the tricuspid valve is involved, however, the fibrous tissue is located predominantly on the ventricular aspect, often causing the leaflets to adhere to the

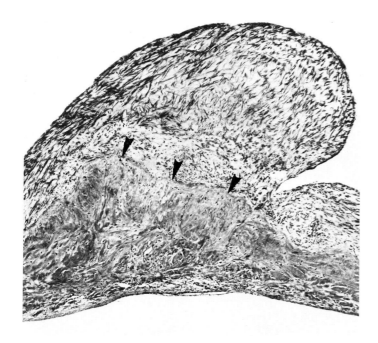

Fig. 21-34. Fibrous plaque containing elongated smooth muscle cells is superimposed on the fibrosa (arrowheads) of tricuspid valve of patient with carcinoid heart disease. (Masson trichrome.)

adjacent ventricular wall.[34] Similar lesions may be observed in the mitral and aortic valves in patients with a patent foramen ovale or with a functioning bronchial carcinoid tumor.[31] In some patients with predominant right-sided carcinoid heart disease, the mitral and aortic valves also may be involved to a lesser degree. Microscopically, these lesions contain fibroblasts, myofibroblasts, and smooth muscle cells embedded in a distinctive stroma, which is rich in collagen and proteoglycans but lacking in elastic fibers. Blood vessels, often thick-walled, may be immediately adjacent to the valve leaflets. Lymphocytes and plasma cells are frequently located adjacent to these blood vessels.

The heart valves are involved in 50 percent of patients with cardiac amyloidosis. Valvular involvement is usually minimal, but discrete nodules measuring from 1 to 4 mm in diameter are occasionally present on the valves, either in the cusps or the annulus.[25] Rarely, valvular involvement is diffuse, resulting in thick rigid cusps and stenotic or regurgitant orifices. The four cardiac valves are affected with almost equal frequency.

All heart valves and valvular annuli, especially the mitral and aortic valves, are sites of heavy pigment deposition in patients with *ochronosis*. Although the pigment deposition is most prominent at the bases of the mitral and aortic valves and annulus fibrosus, the edges of the cusps may be roughened and fused for 1 to 2 mm at their bases; the cusps may be focally calcified. The ochronotic pigment appears blue-black on gross examination and yellow-tan in histologic sections. Infective endocarditis occasionally may be superimposed, especially when the valves are heavily calcified.

The cardiac valves may be involved in any of the *mucopolysaccharidoses*, most frequently in Hurler's disease (mucopolysaccharidosis I).[25] The valves are considerably thickened, particularly the mitral valve; right-sided cardiac valves are less severely affected than those in the left side of the heart. The valvular thickening is most pronounced at the free margins, which have an irregular, nodular appearance. The commissures are not fused. The chordae tendineae of the atrioventricular valves are moderately shortened and thickened. Calcific deposits occur in the angle just beneath the basal attachment of the posterior mitral leaflet (mitral annular calcification), in the mitral leaflets, and in the aortic aspect of the aortic valve cusps. The valves contain large, oval, or rounded connective tissue cells (Hurler cells) filled with numerous clear vacuoles, which are the sites of deposition of acid mucopolysaccharide.[25] This material is extremely soluble and difficult to preserve. In addition, small granular cells are present, which contain membrane-limited electron-dense material associated with fragments of collagen fibrils. The valve thickening is due to the presence of these cells and to an increase in the amount of fibrous connective tissue.

In *Fabry's disease* the glycosphingolipid is deposited within the cardiac valves, and occasionally valvular dysfunction results.[25] The mitral and aortic valves are the two that most commonly present clinical problems. There may be thickening of the valves with interchordal hooding, or there may be attenuation of the chordae with thickening and ballooning of the mitral valve. Commissural fusion is not a feature of Fabry's disease.

Type II hyperlipoproteinemia exists in homozygous and heterozygous forms, which differ in the severity and age of onset of clinical symptoms. Aortic valvular disease is frequent in homozygous patients but usually does not occur in heterozygous patients. The aortic valve may be markedly stenosed by fibrous tissue, deposits of foam cells, and cholesterol clefts in the cusps. Thickening of the mitral valve, resulting in both stenosis and regurgitation, as well as thickening of the pulmonary valve and endocardium by foam cells also occurs.[25]

Patients with *gout* most commonly develop dysfunction due to hypertension secondary to renal damage; however, tophi occasionally may be present in the heart, most commonly in the mitral valve and the endocardium of the left ventricle and less frequently in the mitral annulus and aortic and tricuspid valve leaflets.[25] In order to establish the diagnosis histologically, appreciable amounts of uric acid must be identified in the tophi to distinguish them from small amounts of uric acid that may be deposited upon previously existing fibrocalcific lesions. Urate deposits are histochemically identifiable by fixation in absolute ethanol, followed by staining by the de Galantha method.

Floppy Valve (Myxomatous Degeneration) and Connective Tissue Dyscrasias

Although myxomatous degeneration has been described in tricuspid aortic and pulmonary valves, the mitral valve is most commonly involved, and the posterior leaflet is affected more often and more severely than the anterior leaflet. Grossly, the most outstanding feature is a marked increase in surface area of the affected leaflet. The affected leaflets are voluminous, hooded, and white (Fig. 21-35); however, they transilluminate with ease, especially before fixation. Upon sectioning, the myxomatous consistency of the center of the cusp is often apparent grossly. Small foci of ulceration with occasional superimposed thrombi may be noted on the atrial surface of the affected mitral leaflet.[10] The chordae tendineae often are elongated and thin; however, some localized thickening may be present at their insertions into the valve leaflets. Rupture of the chordae tendineae is common in myxomatous degeneration of the mitral valve; less frequently, myxomatous degeneration may result in

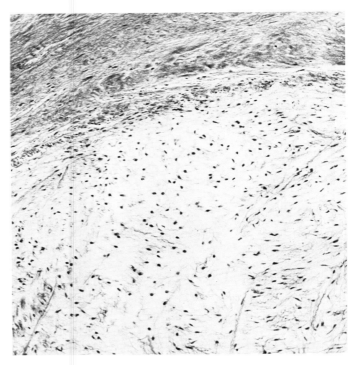

Fig. 21-36. Part of spongiosa (center and bottom) and fibrosa (top) of mitral valve excised from a patient with mitral valvular prolapse. The spongiosa is widened and contains abundant myxoid material. (Plastic-embedded tissue, alkaline toluidine blue.)

aneurysmal dilatation and rupture of a mitral leaflet. Commissural fusion is not a feature of the floppy valve. Since these valves are predisposed to infective endocarditis, gross evidence of this complication must be sought by the surgical pathologist so that appropriate sections can be obtained for culture prior to fixation of the valve.

Microscopically, the spongiosa contains stellate cells embedded in a matrix rich in acid mucopolysaccharides (Fig. 21-36). Characteristically there is focal to extensive replacement of the normal dense, homogeneous collagen of the fibrosa by this myxomatous tissue. This histologic pattern is in contrast to that seen in most valvular heart diseases, in which the spongiosa of the leaflets is either partially or completely replaced by dense fibrous tissue. The collagen in the chordae tendineae may show changes similar to those in the fibrosa. The atrialis leaflet generally contains a variable degree of fibroelastic proliferation, and superficial ulceration with microscopic fibrin deposition is not uncommon. Unless there is superimposed infective endocarditis, there is no evidence of inflammation or vascularization. Ultrastructurally, there is focal loss of the normal orderly cross-banding of collagen fibers. It should be noted that microscopically small areas of myxomatous degeneration are not uncommonly found near the free edges of normal or diseased valves and

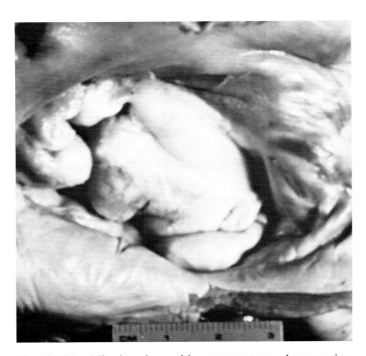

Fig. 21-35. Mitral valve with myxomatous degeneration (floppy mitral valve) viewed from the left atrial aspect. The affected leaflets are voluminous and hooded.

should not be confused with the diffuse microscopic findings in floppy valves.

Myxomatous degeneration of the cardiac valves, with resulting insufficiency, often occurs in connective tissue dyscrasias such as Marfan's syndrome, osteogenesis imperfecta, cutis laxa, and relapsing polychondritis. This group of diseases also may be associated with cystic medial degeneration of the aorta. Adults with *Marfan's syndrome* most commonly have myxomatous degeneration of the aortic valve; however, the mitral valve is more commonly involved in children.[25] The affected mitral and aortic leaflets contain an accumulation of myxoid material, mainly in the spongiosa. The *Ehlers-Danlos syndrome* is a heterogeneous group of several genetically distinct disorders of connective tissue synthesis, which differ in major clinical features, inheritance patterns, and biochemical defects. Cardiovascular lesions have been described in types I to IV; however, myxomatous degeneration and prolapse of the mitral valve appear to be more common in type III, the benign hypermobile form.[25] The most common valvular lesion in *osteogenesis imperfecta* is aortic regurgitation; mitral regurgitation and combined aortic and mitral regurgitation are less common. The aortic regurgitation results from dilatation of the aortic root and deformity of the valvular leaflets, which become abnormally translucent, weak, and elongated. Aneurysms of the sinuses of Valsalva also occur. The mitral annulus is dilated; the mitral leaflets are attenuated, redundant, and tend to prolapse; and the chordae tendineae may rupture.[25] In *cutis laxa* the most common cardiac lesions involve the aorta, pulmonary artery, and pulmonary veins; less commonly, there may be myxomatous degeneration of the aortic or mitral valves.[25] The cardiac valves most commonly involved in *relapsing polychondritis* are the aortic and mitral. Microscopically, lesions identical to those in the other connective tissue dyscrasias may be present.[10]

Congenital Malformations of the Cardiac Valves

The most common congenital malformation of heart valves is the *bicuspid aortic valve*. Unless it is the site of associated dysplasia, this valve is not inherently stenotic, although it frequently becomes stenotic in later life. Stenosis is secondary to fibrosis and calcification of the cusps and not to fusion of the commissures, as is seen in rheumatic aortic stenosis.[40] Classically, the calcific deposits form nodules at the base of the cusps in the sinus of Valsalva and extend to, but frequently do not involve, the free edge of the valve cusps (Fig. 21-37). In addition, there are foci of calcification and extensive fibrosis within the substance of the cusp. Commissural fusion usually is

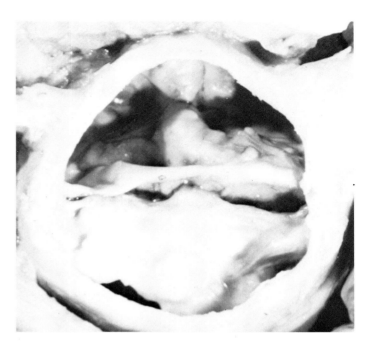

Fig. 21-37. Stenotic bicuspid aortic valve, viewed from the aortic aspect, illustrating fibrocalcific thickening of the base and substance of the cusps; the commissures are not fused.

minimal, involves only one commissure, and only rarely is extensive.[41] Another common reason for surgical excision of a bicuspid aortic valve is infective endocarditis. The extremely high incidence of infective endocarditis in patients with bicuspid aortic valves is well known. Therefore, each of these valves must be examined closely by the surgical pathologist for superimposed infective endocarditis and sections must be taken for microbiologic culture prior to fixation.

The *quadricuspid aortic valve* is far less common than the bicuspid valve. The most frequent indication for surgical excision of these valves is aortic insufficiency. Most commonly, one of the cusps is rudimentary; however, the gross and microscopic appearance of the valves is usually otherwise normal. *Quadricuspid pulmonary valves* rarely cause cardiac dysfunction unless there is associated dysplasia of the valve or a coexisting congenital cardiac defect. As in quadricuspid aortic valves, the fourth cusp is usually small and rudimentary, with the remaining cusps appearing morphologically normal.[42]

Valve dysplasia may affect any of the cardiac valves, most frequently the aortic valve; 25 percent of patients have multiple valve involvement.[43] The dysplastic changes may be severe and extensive, so that the entire valve is distorted, or mild and focal, without evidence of impairment of valve function. A dysplastic stenotic pulmonary valve is frequently present in patients with Noonan's syndrome. The dysplastic semilunar valve may

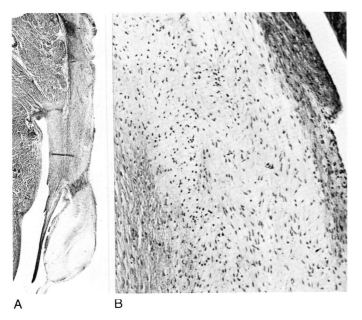

Fig. 21-38. Two views of a histologic section of a dysplastic mitral valve. **(A)** Low-power view on left shows marked thickening of the spongiosa of the valve leaflet. **(B)** Higher magnification view on right illustrates increased cellularity of the spongiosa with small spindle cells that resemble fibroblasts and are surrounded by acid mucopolysaccharide and haphazardly arranged bundles of collagen.

be unicuspid, bicuspid, or tricuspid; failure of development of the commissures also may occur, resulting in a dome-shaped valve. Stenosis is secondary to the marked thickening of the individual valve cusps (Fig. 21-38A). The spongiosa of the dysplastic valve is quite cellular and is composed primarily of small spindle cells resembling fibroblasts, set in an acid mucopolysaccharide matrix and haphazardly arranged bundles of collagen[10] (Fig. 21-38B). This loose connective tissue encroaches upon and often replaces the ventricularis and fibrosa of the valve cusps. The majority of involved cusps consist entirely of this loose connective tissue; however, remnants of the ventricularis and fibrosa, interrupted by accumulations of abnormal loose connective tissue, are often found at the base of the cusps. Inflammation and calcification are not features of the dysplastic valve. The abnormal valve tissue of the dysplastic or incompletely differentiated valve resembles the embryonic connective tissue of the cardiac valves in 8- to 12-week-old fetuses.[43]

Prosthetic Heart Valves

Types

Prosthetic heart valves in current use can be classified into two major groups, rigid-framed (mechanical) valves and tissue valves (bioprostheses). Rigid-framed valves are of three types: (1) valves with a centrally placed occluder (ball or disc), which moves up and down in a metal cage and allows only lateral blood flow; (2) valves with a tilting disc, which permits semicentral flow; and (3) valves with two hinged semicircular plates (Saint Jude type), which allow central flow. Tissue valves include: (1) fresh and variously treated homografts; (2) human dura mater or fascia lata valves; (3) bovine pericardial valves; and (4) porcine aortic valves. The metal and plastic mounting frames and the preimplantation chemical treatments vary from one type of tissue valve to another. Knowledge of this is necessary to interpret morphologic findings in these valves. Also essential for the evaluation of any prosthetic valve is knowledge of the length of time for which the valve was in place and the specific reason for its removal.

Complications

Certain complications are common to all types of prosthetic heart valves. Among these are thrombosis, embolization, infection (Fig. 21-39), dehiscence of the valvular ring, paravalvular leak, disproportion, turbulent flow, and hemolysis. Complications limited to rigid-framed prostheses[44] are related to wear and fracture of mechanical components, resulting in interference with proper motion of the occluder (and sometimes also in embolic phenomena), whereas complications peculiar to tissue

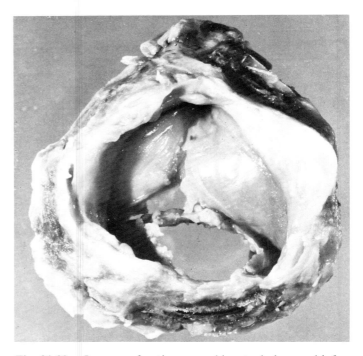

Fig. 21-39. Large perforation caused by staphylococcal infection in a cusp of a porcine aortic valvular bioprosthesis. Note vegetations at edges of perforation.

valves[45] are related to calcification or breakdown of the prosthetic tissue leaflets.

Complications Common to All Types of Prosthetic Valves

Thrombus formation in mechanical prostheses is most common at the base of the struts forming the cage. From this area thrombi can spread and interfere with motion of the occluder, with seating of the occluder on the orifice, or with blood flow. These thrombi can undergo organization, can become infected, or can be sources of emboli. Ball valves with cloth-covered cage struts are less likely to form thrombi than are those with uncovered struts. Tissue valves are least likely to form large thrombi, although aggregates of platelets do develop on their surfaces. Thrombi can splint the cusps of bioprostheses and render them stenotic. Thrombi removed from prosthetic heart valves must be examined (by histology and by culture) for evidence of infection. *Dehiscence of a valvular ring* must be regarded as being due to infection until proved otherwise. *Paravalvular leaks* most frequently result from a prosthesis having been sutured to a ring that is heavily calcified or weakened (as in patients with Marfan's syndrome or other connective tissue disorders). Anemia and renal hemosiderosis are typical findings in *hemolysis* produced by prosthetic heart valves.

Disproportion is caused by prosthetic heart valves that are too large for the chamber in which they are placed. This can result in interference with movement of the poppet, as in the case of large ball valves placed in a small ascending aorta (particularly in patients with combined mitral and aortic valve disease, in whom the aortic root usually is not dilated) or in a small left ventricle (as in patients with combined mitral and aortic stenosis in whom the left ventricle is hypertrophied but not dilated). If a porcine bioprosthesis is improperly placed in the mitral orifice, one of its struts may obstruct the left ventricular outflow tract. In the case of double valve replacement, the prosthetic mitral valve may be inadvertently placed in such a way as to interfere with proper seating of the poppet of the prosthetic aortic valve. Disproportion also may result from normal growth of the heart of a child in whom a small prosthetic valve was implanted at an early age.

Complications Limited to Rigid-Framed (Mechanical) Prosthetic Valves

Turbulent blood flow produced by caged ball prostheses may lead to *diffuse endocardial fibroelastotic thickening* and to intimal proliferation in the ascending aorta, sometimes with extension of the thickening into the coronary arterial ostia. Degeneration (variance) of the silicone rubber poppet was common in the caged ball prostheses implanted before 1967. This complication,

which resulted from surface abrasion and lipid infiltration, has not been reported in the metallic hollow poppet first used at that time. Wear of a caged disc, causing "grooving" and disc cocking, has been described in most caged disc prostheses. Disc cocking remains a potential problem with all caged disc valves, and it may be totally unrecognized as a cause of fatalities. Wear of the cloth covering on the struts and the orifice occurred in some of the older models of completely cloth-covered caged ball prostheses, but strut cloth wear has not been reported in the new Starr-Edwards models with metal tracks. Dislodgement of caged discs and poppets has been reported in association with wear of these components or with fracture of struts.

Complications Limited to Bioprosthetic (Tissue) Valves

The various types of bioprosthetic heart valves developed since the late 1970s have in common the following characteristics: collagen is their major structural component; they are mounted (except for some of the homografts) on metal and plastic stents; the incidence of clinical episodes of thromboembolism is lower with these valves than with rigid-framed valves; and they have problems of long-term durability because they can develop stenosis as a result of calcification and regurgitation related to alterations in collagen.[45]

Porcine Aortic Valves. Porcine aortic valves treated with a low (less than 1 percent) concentration of glutaraldehyde (to cross-link tissue proteins, to sterilize the tissue, and to eliminate problems of antigenicity) and mounted on flexible stents have become the most widely used type of valvular bioprosthesis. During the first 5 years after implantation these valves usually have excellent function, although they can develop extensive anatomic changes (Figs. 21-40 and 21-41). After these first 5 years appreciable incidences of calcification and cuspal damage become evident. Calcific deposits develop more frequently and earlier in children and young adults than in older individuals and also are more frequent in patients with chronic renal disease. Cuspal perforations have no relation to patient age.

A bioprosthetic heart valve removed because of dysfunction should be first examined for evidence of infection, perforation, or calcification, and cultures should be taken as indicated by clinical or anatomic findings; then it should be radiographed and photographed before the cusps are detached from the frame for histologic sectioning. These valves are fragile and should be handled only by the mounting frame in order to avoid producing artifactual damage to the cusps. Connective tissue stains and stains for calcium are useful in evaluating these valves. Transmission electron microscopy provides the best method for studying the collagen, and scanning electron

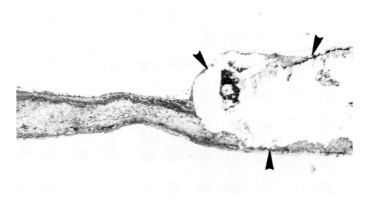

Fig. 21-40. Large calcific deposit (arrowheads) has caused considerable thickening of cusp of porcine aortic valvular bioprosthesis that had been implanted in a young child for 50 months in the mitral position. (Plastic-embedded tissue, alkaline toluidine blue.)

microscopy is the method of choice for examining the surfaces.

Histologically, porcine aortic valves are composed of the following three layers, which also are recognizable in the bioprostheses even after having been in place for long periods of time: (1) the ventricularis, which faces the ventricular cavity when the valve is in its anatomic position and which contains collagen and abundant elastic fibers; (2) the spongiosa, which is the proteoglycan-rich middle layer; and (3) the fibrosa, which contains densely packed collagen but only small, scanty elastic fibers and which faces the aortic wall. Proteoglycans are lost from the spongiosa during commercial processing and soon

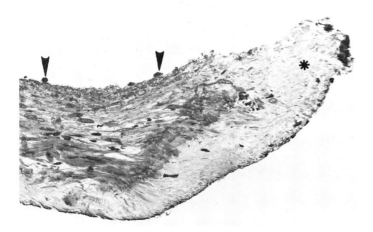

Fig. 21-41. Area of severe degeneration of collagen (asterisk) is adjacent to edge of cuspal tear (far right) in porcine aortic valvular bioprosthesis that had been implanted for 15 months in the aortic position. Aggregates of platelets (arrowheads) are attached to the cuspal surfaces. (Alkaline toluidine blue.)

after implantation of the bioprosthesis, leaving empty spaces that gradually are filled with deposits of plasma proteins. The surfaces of porcine valvular bioprostheses usually do not become endothelialized, although they may be covered by macrophages, multinucleated giant cells, platelet aggregates, and small fibrin deposits. Polymorphonuclear leukocytes are very scanty or absent unless infection is present. Macrophages show little tendency to invade the bioprosthetic tissue, and there is no evidence that immunologic rejection plays a role in its deterioration.

When calcific deposits develop (Fig. 21-40), it is usually in association with collagen in these spaces and with surface thrombi, especially in regions near the commissures; they form yellow, plaque-like or raised lesions. Calcific deposits also develop in the aortic wall just adjacent to the cusps and in cardiac muscle cells in a muscular shelf extending from the ventricular septum into the base of the right coronary cusp of the porcine aortic valve. This cusp is larger than the others, and its base is less translucent. Calcific deposits also can be associated with perforations, perhaps because collagen adjacent to these deposits undergoes severe mechanical stresses. The collagen in bioprostheses undergoes a time-dependent process of degeneration, which may be related to material fatigue and may result in perforation of the cusps. Perforations in porcine valves occur most frequently near the basal attachment of the cusps, where the tissue is thinnest. In pericardial valves, particularly those implanted in the mitral position, cuspal tears are likely to involve the free edge near the attachment to the post. It has been suggested that such tears begin at the attachment suture. Infection of porcine valvular bioprostheses differs from that of rigid-framed valves in that it is likely to involve the cusps (rather than the sewing ring), is less likely to result in formation of a ring abscess, and usually extends into the collagen in the cusps.[45] The incidence of infection in the two types of valves appears to be similar.

Other Bioprosthetic Valves. Aortic valve homografts (either fresh, sterilized with antibiotics, or freeze-dried and chemically treated) have been used only to a limited extent in the United States. In contrast to glutaraldehyde-treated bioprostheses, they become covered with a fibrous sheath of host origin. Their complications include calcification, cuspal rupture, and fibrous retraction of the edges of the cusps. *Autologous fascia lata valves* implanted without any chemical treatment have had a very poor record of durability and a high incidence of degeneration, thrombosis, calcification, and fibrous contraction of the cusps. Their use has been completely discontinued. *Human dura mater valves* preserved by glycerol treatment have been used extensively in Latin America.

Bioprostheses made of *glutaraldehyde-treated bovine pericardium* also have been used as substitute cardiac valves. Both dura mater and pericardium consist of dense collagenous sheets with sparse elastic fibers. Their layered structure is easily distinguishable histologically from that of porcine aortic valves. Complications of pericardial and dura mater valves are similar to those of porcine valves and consist mainly of calcification and cuspal dehiscence.[44]

Conduits. Conduits composed of various synthetic materials have been used to correct hypoplasia or atresia of the pulmonary artery. Valveless conduits were first used; subsequently, conduits containing mechanical (Bjork-Shiley) valves were employed but were found to be prone to valvular thrombosis. More recently, extensive use has been made of pulmonic conduits with bioprosthetic (porcine or pericardial) valves; in addition, left ventricular apical-aortic conduits have had limited use for correction of tunnel aortic stenosis.[44] The most frequent complication of conduits is obstruction, which can result from one or more of the following causes: (1) muscular compression of the proximal end of the conduit during ventricular systole; (2) accumulation of thrombotic or fibrous material (fibrous peel) in the wall of the conduit; (3) compression of the conduit by the sternum; (4) calcific or thrombotic stenosis of the bioprosthesis; and (5) stenosis at the distal end (the most common cause of obstruction) because of small size of the artery at the anastomotic site.

Infective Endocarditis

The relative frequency of involvement of the cardiac valves by infective endocarditis is the same as that of involvement by rheumatic heart disease: mitral, aortic, aortic and mitral combined, tricuspid, and pulmonary valves, in that order, but the last two valves are uncommonly involved. In many cases of combined aortic and mitral involvement, the anterior leaflet of the mitral valve appears to be infected by regurgitant deposition of organisms from the aortic vegetation. Lesions usually originate on the atrial surface of the atrioventricular valves and the ventricular surface of the semilunar valves and vary from tiny granular or flat vegetations to large polypoid masses (Fig. 21-42). They may be single or multiple and may be firm or soft but are usually friable. Grossly, they may appear yellow-white to red or brown.[46] The affected valve exhibits destruction that varies with the extent of tissue loss. Ulceration or perforation may occur, or an aneurysm of the valve may form. Rupture of chordae tendineae is common. Infection may spread into the contiguous structures, resulting in annular or myocardial abscesses or aneurysms of the sinuses of Valsalva. Micro-

scopically, the vegetations are composed of masses of necrotic tissue, fibrin, platelets, erythrocytes, leukocytes, and organisms (Fig. 21-42). Classically, there is a superficial zone of fibrin, organisms, and leukocytes; an intermediate zone of amorphous necrotic material; and a basal zone of granulation tissue extending from the substance of the valve. Small foci of calcification are common.

Bicuspid aortic valves or valves with acquired deformities are most frequently involved; however, infective endocarditis may develop in apparently normal valves, including the pulmonary and tricuspid valves, especially in patients over 60 years of age. In apparently normal valves the lesions tend to be larger, and tissue destruction is more extensive. Staphylococci and Gram-negative organisms are more likely to be the etiologic agents than in the case of infection of deformed valves, where *Streptococcus viridans* is the most common organism encountered. Infected but previously normal valves often show marked necrosis and inflammation, which are less common findings in infected, previously scarred valves.

Although streptococci and staphylococci are the most common microorganisms responsible for infection, a wide variety of bacteria and fungi have been recovered from patients with infective endocarditis. *Candida* spp. in particular are recovered from addicts and patients with

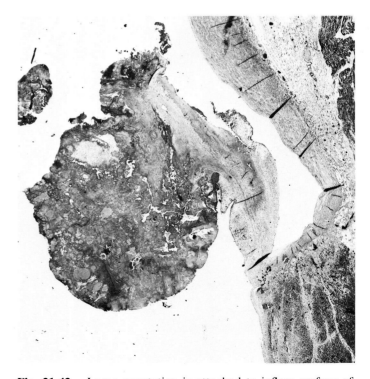

Fig. 21-42. Large vegetation is attached to inflow surface of aortic valve cusp of a young woman with gonococcal endocarditis.

prosthetic heart valves. Gram-negative bacilli account for only a small percentage of infections, despite the relative frequency of Gram-negative bacteremia, and are more likely to be encountered in addicts or in patients with prosthetic heart valves. Rarely, infections are due to other organisms, such as meningococci, pneumococci, gonococci, *Brucella, Hemophilus, Corynebacteria*, mycobacteria, rickettsiae, and *Aspergillus* and other fungal species.[47] Fungal vegetations, in particular, tend to be large and friable, with a tendency to embolization. Because fungal endocarditis is frequently indolent clinically, it is important for the surgical pathologist to obtain appropriate special stains on any thromboembolus removed from a systemic artery. Any valve removed surgically that has gross lesions suggestive of infective endocarditis should have sections taken for microbiologic culture prior to fixation. Merely taking a swab of the surface of the valve for culture is not adequate; indeed, sections of the valve should be taken for culture, even if the valve appears grossly normal, in patients in whom the clinical history or physical findings suggest the possibility of infective endocarditis.

Healing of vegetations may occur as a result of therapy, and perhaps sometimes spontaneously, without antimicrobial therapy.[46] These healed vegetations often result in multiple calcified polypoid lesions on the surface of the valve. Contracture of scar tissue may further reduce the surface area of the valve. The healed vegetations in the heart valves or chordae tendineae are similar

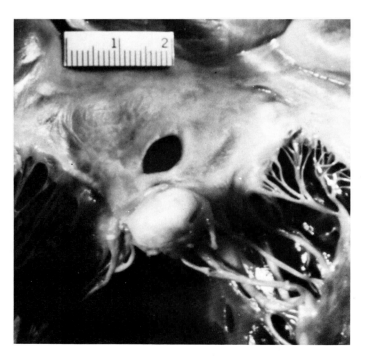

Fig. 21-43. Circumscribed perforation, secondary to healed infective endocarditis, in anterior leaflet of mitral valve.

in gross appearance to those with active infection.[46] Occasionally, well circumscribed defects with smooth edges remain in the heart valve after the healing of perforations due to infective endocarditis (Fig. 21-43). Usually the etiology of these morphologic abnormalities cannot be identified, especially if there is no known antecedent infection. Histologic study rarely helps to resolve such cases because the alterations resulting from the healing of the inflammatory process tend to be similar in their end-stage appearance.[46]

THE AORTA

Aortic Atherosclerosis

The surgical pathology of aortic atherosclerosis is the direct result of advanced lesions and their complications of progressive luminal compromise, aneurysm, and distal embolization. *Saccular aneurysms* of the abdominal aorta are the most common type of aortic aneurysm, and their usual cause is atherosclerosis. Although this process of atherosclerosis occurs primarily in the intima, there is secondary atrophy of the media beneath the atheroma, with resulting weakness of the media being responsible for aneurysm formation. Most commonly these aneurysms begin inferior to the origins of the renal arteries and terminate at the iliac bifurcation of the aorta. Usually, the anterior wall of the aorta is markedly involved while the posterior wall is not. Therefore, erosion of the spine is not commonly observed in these cases. Coincidental occurrence of atherosclerotic aneurysms of the iliac arteries is not unusual. Although thrombus may be present within the aneurysm, the lumen of the aorta usually remains patent. Therefore such aneurysms are not attended by signs of aortic occlusion, which is usually caused by occlusive thrombosis in an atherosclerotic aorta that is not aneurysmal. The major complication of abdominal aortic aneurysm is rupture, which most commonly occurs with large aneurysms measuring 7 cm or more in diameter.[34] However, rupture occasionally may be due to superimposed infection and may occur in lesions of small size. All resected abdominal aortic aneurysms should therefore be cultured and stained for bacteria, especially if they are under 7 cm in diameter. *Embolization* is a common complication of aortic atherosclerosis and may result from atherosclerotic lesions in the tributaries of the aorta, such as the carotid, renal, and iliac arteries. Thromboemboli in the lower extremities predominantly involve the femoral and popliteal arteries. Cholesterol emboli usually are present in small arteries (100 to 200 μm in diameter). Cholesterol emboli have been implicated in the development of gangrene, and it has been suggested that they cause focal ischemic changes of the toes, especially in patients with adequate peripheral pulses.[34,48]

Aortitis

Granulomatous/Sclerosing Aortitis

The most common location of granulomatous aortitis (Takayasu's disease) is the aortic arch; however, any segment or segments of the aorta and its major branches may be involved down to, and including, the femoral artery (Fig. 21-44). The lesions in the aorta range from a florid inflammatory process, consisting mainly of lymphocytes and plasma cells, to a healed fibrotic lesion. Both types of lesions may be seen in the same patient, suggesting a chronic recurrent process.[49]

In the granulomatous phase there is dilatation and medial hypertrophy of the vasa vasorum with marked mononuclear cell infiltration, predominantly in the adventitia and outer two thirds of the media; lymphoid follicles may be abundant in the adventitia (Fig. 21-45). Patchy areas of necrosis develop in the outer two thirds of the media, and the elastic lamellae are fragmented. The breakdown of elastin initiates a foreign body response, and giant cells appear in the wall in proximity to clumps of fragmented elastic tissue (Fig. 21-46). There is marked irregular

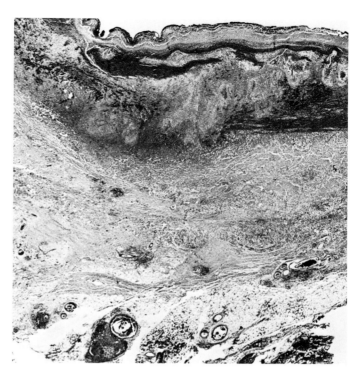

Fig. 21-45. Section of aorta with granulomatous aortitis. The intima (top) is thickened with edema and fibrous tissue, and there is irregular necrosis of the outer portion of the media, with dense adventitial fibrosis. There is marked dilatation and hypertrophy of the vasa vasorum. (Movat stain.)

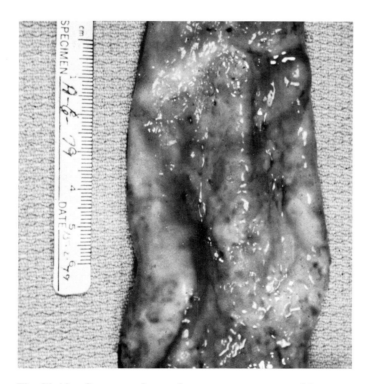

Fig. 21-44. Segment of aorta from a young woman with granulomatous aortitis. Note the sharp demarcation between diseased and normal aorta. Serologic tests for syphilis were negative.

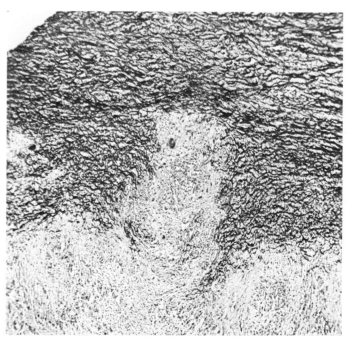

Fig. 21-46. Section of aorta with granulomatous sclerosing aortitis. Adventitial fibrosis (bottom) and fragmentation of elastic fibers in the media are accompanied by a multinucleated giant cell reaction. (Movat stain.)

thickening of the intima with dense fibrous tissue. Grossly, this intimal fibrosis produces the wrinkled "tree bark" appearance formerly thought to be pathognomonic of luetic aortitis. As the inflammatory cells disappear from the outer two thirds of the media and the adventitia, the necrotic areas are replaced by dense fibrous tissue, resulting in thickening of the wall of the aorta and narrowing of the lumen. Final obliteration of the lumen may occur by thrombosis. In some cases fragmentation of the elastic lamellae and necrosis of the media lead to aortic dilatation and aneurysm formation rather than stenosis.[50] The fibrotic intima frequently becomes focally calcified, often with areas that closely resemble atherosclerotic lesions. In those cases in which fibrosis is predominant and inflammation is minimal, the diagnosis of sclerosing aortitis replaces that of granulomatous aortitis (Fig. 21-47). It is important, however, to remember that these are not two separate diseases but indeed represent different phases of the same disease spectrum.

Although considered a disease of arteries, granulomatous aortitis may cause valvular dysfunction by involving the cardiac valves. The cardiac valves most commonly involved are the aortic, mitral, and tricuspid, in that order.

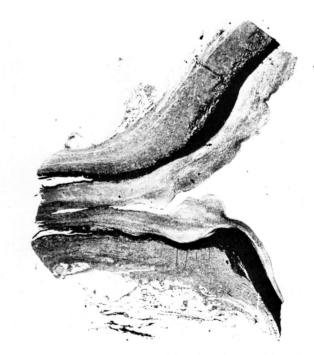

Fig. 21-47. Section of aorta with sclerosing aortitis. There is intimal and adventitial fibrosis, with fibrous replacement of the outer portion of the media. Arteries arising from the aorta (in this case a coronary artery) may also be involved. (Movat stain.)

Syphilitic Aortitis

Syphilitic aortitis is a focal disease of the ascending aorta and aortic arch, with skip areas that are grossly and histologically normal. Microscopically, the pathology of syphilitic aortitis is identical to that of granulomatous aortitis. In syphilitic aortitis, however, progressive sclerosis with luminal compromise is rare, whereas aortic dilatation with aneurysm formation is common.[34,50] Syphilitic aortitis is distinguished from idiopathic granulomatous aortitis serologically or, in rare cases, by demonstration of a microgumma or spirochetes in the aortic lesion. The aortic annulus is frequently dilated, with resulting aortic regurgitation. The aortic valves in these patients usually only display fibrosis on the rolled free margins of the aortic valve cusp. This is probably the result of the hemodynamic effects of aortic regurgitation.

Other Aortitides

A spectrum of gross and microscopic changes identical to those in idiopathic granulomatous/sclerosing aortitis may be seen in patients with *ankylosing spondylitis, psoriatic arthritis, or Reiter's syndrome*. In these disorders the disease process is usually limited to the proximal 3 or 4 cm of the ascending aorta but may directly involve the aortic and mitral valves as well. Patients with *rheumatoid arthritis* may develop rheumatoid granulomas in the aorta.[35] Usually the aorta is affected only in the first 2 or 3 cm, but occasionally its entire length is involved, either continuously or with clearly demarcated skip areas. Patients with rheumatic fever also may develop *rheumatic aortitis,* characterized by elongated foci of fibrinoid degeneration surrounded by infiltrates of lymphocytes and large, frequently multinucleated histiocytes. Healing by fibrosis leads to nonspecific intimal scars. Frequently, rheumatic aortitis is limited to the intima, but the process may extend deeper to involve both the media and adventitia. The initial few centimeters of the ascending aorta are commonly involved in rheumatic aortitis.[34,35] *Tuberculous aortitis* almost exclusively occurs by contiguous spread of the tuberculous process from a tuberculoma in the lungs or a periaortic lymph node.[50] If the aortic wall is sufficiently weakened, an aneurysm may result.

Dissecting Aneurysms of the Aorta

Some form of medial degeneration is an essential prerequisite for aortic dissection. Rare medial lesions associated with dissecting aneurysm include granulomatous aortitis and bacterial aortitis. However, by far the most common medial lesion preceding dissection is *cystic me-*

dial degeneration. In cystic medial degeneration, two basic defects are commonly observed in varying proportions: (1) focal loss and disruption of elastic lamellae of the media; and (2) loss of medial smooth muscle cells. The defects in the aortic media are created by loss and disruption of elastic lamellae and loss of smooth muscle cells and are filled by increased amounts of acid mucopolysaccharide (Fig. 21-48). However, these changes occur to some degree as a consequence of the aging process, and they must be evaluated with account taken of the age of the patient. In contrast to the findings in granulomatous aortitis, the aortic wall affected by cystic medial degeneration is thinned rather than thickened, unless there has been a dissection. Neither the adventitia nor the intima is thickened, and the vasa vasorum are not hypertrophied. In the most common form of cystic medial degeneration, which usually occurs after the age of 40 years, the predominant defect is one of focal smooth muscle cell loss. The less common form, which occurs in younger age groups and is frequently associated with familial diseases such as Marfan's syndrome, Ehlers-Danlos syndrome, osteogenesis imperfecta, or cutis laxa, is characterized predominantly by defects in elastic tissue.[25] In many patients intermediate forms occur in which both types of degeneration coexist. When dissection of the aorta has occurred, the presence of cystic medial degeneration may be missed unless the surgical pathologist examines the thin rim of normal aorta at the proximal and distal ends of the specimen.

Intimal tears in the ascending portion of the thoracic arch are present in approximately 90 percent of dissecting aneurysms. Tears distal to the arch are found in a smaller number of these patients. Approximately 5 percent of dissecting aneurysms do not have an intimal tear, however.[34] The proximal intimal tears are usually found within 5 to 10 cm of the aortic valve. These tears are usually transverse or oblique and are 4 to 5 cm in length, with sharp, clean, but jagged margins. Most commonly, the intimal tear is oriented in the long axis of the aorta. The dissecting aneurysm is characterized anatomically by hemorrhagic dissection within the media of the aorta. This hemorrhage characteristically occurs between the middle and outer thirds of the media.

External blunt trauma is a relatively infrequent cause of aortic dissection, although it is not uncommonly a factor contributing to dissections in peripheral arteries.[50] Most traumatic ruptures of the aorta result in external hemorrhage and not in intramural dissection. The most common site of rupture secondary to blunt trauma is usually the aortic isthmus just distal to the subclavian artery. Less commonly, blunt trauma may result in formation of a post-traumatic, usually false aneurysm. In the presence of pre-existing medial disease, however, comparatively minor trauma may initiate a dissecting aneurysm.

Congenital Defects of the Aorta

Congenital Aneurysms of the Aortic Sinuses

Congenital aneurysms of the aortic sinuses may develop from the right and posterior (noncoronary) sinuses but rarely from the left. There is either a lack of fusion or a separation of the aortic media and the valvular annulus. Owing to the effects of aortic blood pressure, a finger-like endothelial sac extends through the defect, protruding from the base of the affected sinus into the right atrium or right ventricle. The condition is asymptomatic until the aneurysm ruptures, producing an aortocardiac fistula.[34]

Coarctation of the Aorta

Coarctation of the aorta usually occurs opposite or just distal to the aortic insertion of the ligamentum arteriosum. At times, however, it is somewhat proximal to that site. Corresponding to the zone of luminal narrowing there is a concavity of the adventitia of the aorta involving the cephalic, ventral, and dorsal aspects. Although the zone of greatest constriction is frequently short and

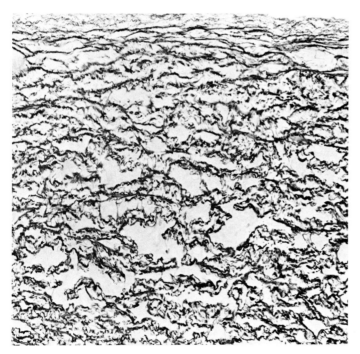

Fig. 21-48. Aorta from a patient with Marfan's syndrome shows areas of disruption of elastic fibers and accumulation of acid mucopolysaccharide material. (Elastica-van Gieson.)

clearly defined, the diameter of the aorta in the portion leading to it tapers gradually. Beyond the constriction, there is commonly a segment exhibiting poststenotic dilatation. Examination of the aortic lumen reveals it to be considerably more restricted at the zone of coarctation than is suggested by the external diameter. Microscopically, the lumen of the aorta is narrowed by deformity and thickening of the aortic media. Specimens from adolescents and adults often display, in addition to the medial deformity, thickening of the intima in the area of aortic narrowing. This intimal thickening in the zone of luminal narrowing is scant or absent in infants. The aortic wall distal to the coarctation is usually thin. Both proximal and distal segments of the aorta may develop cystic medial degeneration. The portion of the aorta distal to the coarctation may exhibit a localized, corrugated patch, which extends above the intimal surface and microscopically consists of fibrous intimal thickening, representing a jet lesion.[34]

Supravalvular Aortic Stenosis

In supravalvular aortic stenosis the site of obstruction is the ascending aorta, most frequently at a level corresponding to the most cephalad extension of the aortic valve cusps.[34] The narrowing results both from thickening of the aortic media and from superimposed fibrous intimal proliferation. Less frequently, the supravalvular obstruction results from diffuse hypoplasia of the entire ascending aorta or from a fibrous membrane just above the aortic sinuses, with a central orifice and an aorta of more normal size.

Aortic Narrowing

Narrowing of the lower thoracic portion of the aorta or of the abdominal aorta is a rarity. This narrowing differs from that of true aortic coarctation in that it usually is of moderate extent, with uniform tapering of the aorta toward the narrowest point.

CORONARY ARTERIES

Large, Extramural Coronary Arteries

Relatively few anatomic abnormalities in large, extramural coronary arteries are likely to come to the attention of the surgical pathologist. *Atherosclerotic lesions* of large, extramural coronary arteries usually are submitted as endarterectomy specimens, which consist of material (cholesterol, fibrous tissue, intimal smooth muscle cells, and calcific and pultaceous debris) from the usual type of complicated atherosclerotic plaque. Other operable coronary lesions include ostial lesions related to *granuloma-*

tous and *luetic aortitis,* and coronary arterial *aneurysms.* The latter may be congenital (due to a medial defect) or acquired (due to atherosclerosis, infection, or inflammatory arteritis) and should be distinguished from dilated arteries supplying coronary arteriovenous shunts. *Emboli* to coronary arteries may result from intracardiac thrombi or tumors, vegetations in infective and noninfective endocarditis, calcific debris from valves or atherosclerotic plaques, and platelet aggregates in cardiopulmonary bypass machines. The coronary arterial aneurysms caused by the coronary arteritis that occurs in Kawasaki's disease have been successfully bypassed, as these lesions tend to involve the most proximal portions of the extramural coronary arteries.[51] Inflammatory coronary arteritides are described in the section on vasculitis. The Gruntzig balloon catheter dilatation procedure has been shown to cause intimal and medial tears (which seem to heal uneventfully) in coronary arteries.[52] *Dissection* of the wall of a coronary artery may occur spontaneously (Fig. 21-49) or, more frequently, as a complication of coronary bypass, coronary angiography, or aortic valve replacement.

Small, Intramural Coronary Arteries

Various abnormalities of small intramural coronary arteries can be recognized on examination of myocardial biopsy material; however, small blood vessels in biopsy

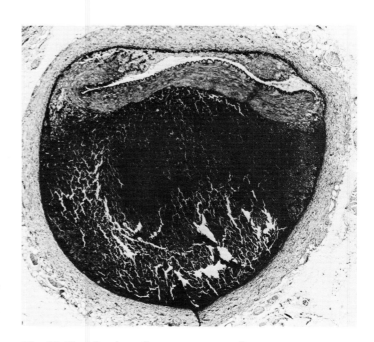

Fig. 21-49. Section of coronary artery from a young woman, illustrating a spontaneous dissecting aneurysm between the outer media and adventitia, resulting in marked luminal compromise. (Movat stain.)

material often are severely contracted or collapsed (marked undulation of the internal elastic lamina is indicative of artifactual contraction), and their walls appear much thicker than they actually are. Therefore, considerable caution is necessary in interpreting pathologic changes in these vessels. Small coronary arteries normally are much thicker-walled in left ventricular papillary muscles than elsewhere in the heart.

Abnormalities of small coronary vessels occur in a number of conditions[53] but usually are not diagnostic of a specific disease. Such changes often are focal, and their extent and clinical significance are difficult to evaluate, particularly in catheter biopsies from the right ventricle. Among these changes are: (1) fibromuscular dysplasia, which occurs in a variety of disorders and also can involve arteries other than coronaries; (2) intimal proliferation, which is found in hypertrophic cardiomyopathy, fixed outlet subaortic stenosis, and Fredreich's ataxia; (3) fibrinoid necrosis, which may be present in periarteritis nodosa, other types of generalized arteritis, and malignant arterial hypertension; (4) medial necrosis, which can be seen in several diseases having in common cardiomyopathy, electrical instability of the heart, syncope, and sudden death; (5) nonspecific inflammatory changes that occur in vasculitides of various causes; and (6) changes due to atherosclerosis (a relatively infrequent finding) and embolic or thrombotic diseases.[53] Several of these types of change may coexist in a given vessel. Subintimal deposits of PAS-positive material have been described in small coronary vessels in diabetes mellitus, in Fredreich's ataxia, and in a few cases of alcoholic cardiomyopathy. Their significance remains uncertain. The bacilli of Whipple's disease have been found in the walls of small coronary arteries.[53]

PERIPHERAL ARTERIES

Atherosclerosis

Among the diseases of the peripheral arteries that result in circulatory insufficiency of the extremities, atherosclerosis is by far the most frequent. The iliac, femoral, popliteal, and tibial arteries are most often affected. Intimal disease is most severe in the proximal arterial tree, and smaller unnamed distal ramifications are relatively spared. Diseased arteries are thickened and tortuous, and their lumina are irregularly narrowed and frequently contain both mural and occlusive thrombi of various ages. Histologically, the intimal thickening represents the advanced, complicated atherosclerotic plaque. The media of sclerotic peripheral arteries is often calcified, and many of these calcified arteries also contain osseous foci.[48]

Medial Sclerosis

Medial sclerosis is characterized by ring-like calcification within the media of medium to small muscular arteries. Although Mönckeberg's medial sclerosis may occur together with atherosclerosis, the two disorders are totally distinct.[34] The blood vessels most severely affected by Mönckeberg's sclerosis are the femoral, tibial, radial, and ulnar arteries and the arterial supply of the genital tract in both sexes. The calcification is not associated with any inflammatory reaction, and the intima and adventitia are largely unaffected. In the pure, uncomplicated form of Mönckeberg's sclerosis, these medial lesions do not encroach on the vessel lumen. However, calcification of the internal elastic lamina and the adjacent media may occur in hyperparathyroidism, vitamin D intoxication or hypersensitivity, pseudoxanthoma elasticum, and juvenile intimal sclerosis (idiopathic arterial calcification of infancy), with associated fibromuscular hyperplasia of the intima resulting in significant luminal compromise. These changes also may involve the coronary arteries. Intimal proliferation associated with medial calcification is particularly prominent in juvenile intimal sclerosis (Fig. 21-50).

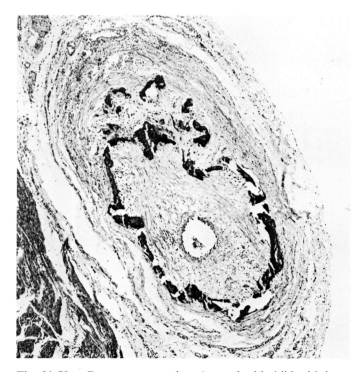

Fig. 21-50. Coronary artery in a 6-month-old child with juvenile intimal sclerosis. There is extensive calcification of the internal elastic membrane, with marked intimal fibrosis.

Fibromuscular Dysplasia

Fibromuscular dysplasia occurs most commonly in the renal arteries; however, any of the muscular arteries and the branches of the aorta may be affected. Those arteries most commonly affected include the cervical portion of the internal carotid artery and the celiac, superior mesenteric, inferior mesenteric, and iliac arteries. Less commonly, the vertebral artery and the branches of the external carotid artery also may be affected.[50]

There are four morphologic types of fibromuscular dysplasia.[54] The first type, medial fibroplasia, is the type generally referred to as *fibromuscular hyperplasia,* although true muscular hyperplasia is not present. In this variant the internal elastic membrane is thinned and replicated, and destruction and thickening of the media are focally present (Fig. 21-51). In the foci of medial thickening much of the muscle is replaced by collagen. However, microaneurysms and small saccular aneurysms may appear in areas of muscular thinning. This is the most common type of fibromuscular dysplasia encountered, and usually it is not complicated by dissection or rupture. A second type of fibromuscular dysplasia consists of *intimal fibroplasia,* characterized by a circumferential accumulation of collagen and intimal smooth muscle cells inside the internal elastic lamina (Fig. 21-52). This type of dysplasia is particularly associated with dis-

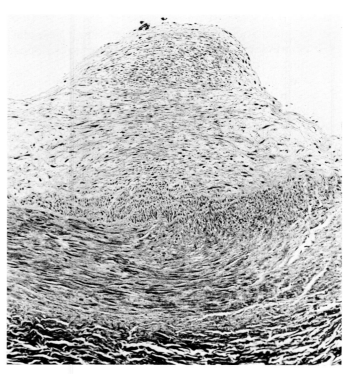

Fig. 21-52. Intimal fibroplasia of a renal artery in a young woman. There is focal fibromuscular hyperplasia of the intima with haphazard nuclear polarity.

secting aneurysms in the arterial wall, and it occurs most commonly in children and young adults. In the third type *true hyperplasia* of smooth muscle and fibrous tissue occurs in the media. This type is not uncommonly associated with rupture of the external elastic lamina and with medial dissection. The fourth type of fibromuscular dysplasia, *adventitial fibrosis,* is characterized by a dense collagenous collar, which produces an external stenosis of the artery. It may involve varying lengths of the artery and often replaces a considerable amount of media. It may be focal but can extend into the segmental renal arteries. It is usually found in young women, most often in the arteries to the right kidney.[54]

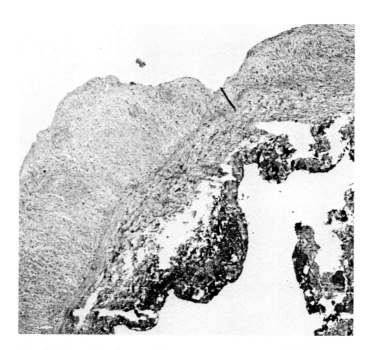

Fig. 21-51. Renal artery from a young woman with fibromuscular dysplasia. Foci of fibrous medial thickening are adjacent to areas of marked medial thinning. Varying degrees of fibromuscular intimal proliferation are present in this vessel.

Thromboangiitis Obliterans (Buerger's Disease)

The arterial occlusive lesions known as thromboangiitis obliterans initially occur in distal medium-sized and small arteries such as the anterior tibial, posterior tibial, radial, ulnar, plantar, palmar, and digital arteries, rather than in the brachial or femoropopliteal arteries. At a later stage the involvement may extend proximally to major arteries.[50,55]

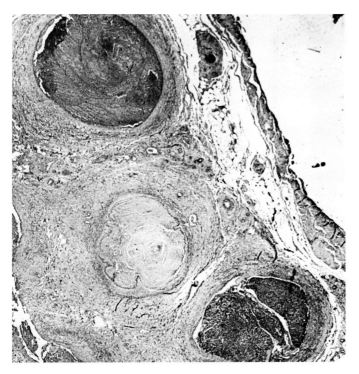

Fig. 21-53. Section of artery, nerve, and vein from the calf of a young man with thromboangiitis obliterans, illustrating arterial and venous thrombosis with dense adventitial fibrosis involving the contiguous connective tissue and enveloping the nerve.

Microscopically, highly cellular organizing and recanalizing thrombi fill the lumina of the diseased arteries. However, the cellularity diminishes with the age of the lesion. Characteristically, there is no evidence of prior intimal or medial disease, and the internal elastic lamina is intact. The intima, media, and adventitia are diffusely infiltrated with lymphocytes, but there is no evidence of necrosis of the vessel wall. As the lesion progresses in age, there is increasing intimal and adventitial fibrosis. Occasionally, a cellular organizing thrombus may contain granulomatous foci and scattered giant cells of the Langhans type. Fresh thrombi, which may contain small suppurative or granulomatous foci, are also observed. The lymphocytic infiltrate of the acute lesion and the dense adventitial fibrosis of the older lesion commonly involve the contiguous connective tissue and adjacent veins (Fig. 21-53). Additionally, nerves in the neurovascular bundle frequently became enveloped in the dense fibrous tissue formed about the vessels. Because this is a remitting and relapsing disease, it is possible to find lesions within the same artery or different arteries at different stages of activity. Superficial migratory thrombophlebitis is present at the early stage of the disease in many patients and may reappear during exacerbations of thromboangiitis obliterans.

Granulomatous Arteritis (Temporal Arteritis, Giant Cell Arteritis, Cranial Arteritis)

Granulomatous arteritis is a focal, granulomatous inflammation of arteries of medium and small size, affecting principally the cranial vessels, especially the temporal arteries in older individuals. In the more severe expressions of this disease, lesions have been found in arteries throughout the body, and in some cases the aortic arch has been involved. The disease is frequently associated with the syndrome of polymyalgia rheumatica. Affected arteries develop nodular enlargements, which may be palpated when arteries are superficial, as in the temporal area. Of importance to the surgical pathologist is the extremely focal nature of the disease in most cases. A biopsy specimen removed from a segment of artery adjacent to a sharply demarcated area of arterial inflammation may be entirely negative. These lesions vary in intensity within a short segment of the artery, and their morphologic appearance depends on the activity of the process. The intima is grossly thickened by a mixed inflammatory cell infiltrate and by edema early in the disease process and by dense fibrous tissue in the more chronic lesions (Fig. 21-54). The internal elastic lamina is

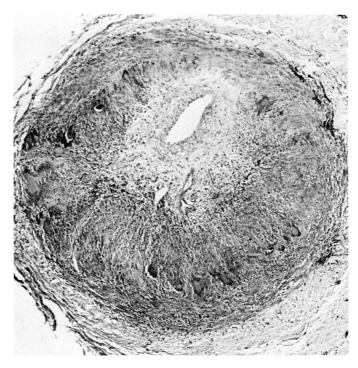

Fig. 21-54. Temporal artery from an elderly patient with polymyalgia rheumatica. The intima is markedly thickened by edema, inflammatory cells, and fibrous tissue. Variable numbers of inflammatory cells are present in the media and adventitia; however, the contiguous connective tissue is not involved.

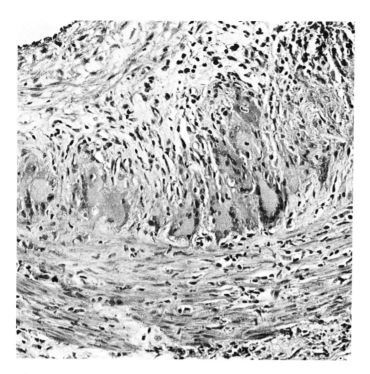

Fig. 21-55. Higher magnification view of the temporal artery illustrated in Fig. 41-54. Multinucleated giant cells are present along the fragmented internal elastic membrane.

fragmented early in the disease process. Later, giant cells of the Langhans type accumulate around the fragmented ends of elastic fibers (Fig. 21-55). The media is infiltrated early by mixed inflammatory cells and later by lymphocytes. The media is usually preserved, but occasionally there can be focal necrosis of medial smooth muscle cells. Involvement of the adventitia is variable, but a cellular infiltrate is frequently found early in the disease process, and delicate adventitial fibrosis predominates in the more chronic lesion. Strikingly, the contiguous connective tissue is usually not involved, either with inflammatory cells or with subsequent fibrosis. In the healed lesion intimal fibrosis predominates, with little cellular reaction remaining; however, elastic tissue stains demonstrate extensive disruption of the internal elastic lamina.

Arteritis Associated with the Collagen Vascular Diseases

Panarteritis Nodosa

Panarteritis nodosa is a form of necrotizing arteritis that chiefly affects medium-sized muscular arteries, especially at their points of bifurcation. Grossly, these lesions appear as nodules measuring 2 to 4 cm in diameter. Microscopically, the active lesion of panarteritis nodosa

consists of segmental necrosis and inflammation of all layers of the arterial wall and contiguous connective tissue (Fig. 21-56). The inflammatory cell population is mixed, but in the active lesion polymorphonuclear leukocytes are the most common cell type. Fibrinoid necrosis is usually present in the intima and inner third of the media, and a superimposed thrombus is frequently encountered. An aneurysm may form in the weakened arterial wall. These lesions are usually present in varying stages of evolution, and the arterial lumen may be occluded by varying combinations of fresh thrombus, granulation tissue, and fibrous tissue. Recanalization also may be observed.

Lesions that are microscopically identical to those of panarteritis nodosa occasionally may be found in an artery adjacent to the cystic duct in patients operated on for acute cholecystitis, in an artery in the periappendiceal adipose tissue in patients operated on for acute appendicitis, and in other localized sites as incidental findings. More often than not, these patients do not have systemic panarteritis nodosa, and caution must be exercised in making this diagnosis in the absence of systemic disease. Necrotizing arteritis, morphologically similar to panarteritis nodosa, may occur in medium-sized muscular ar-

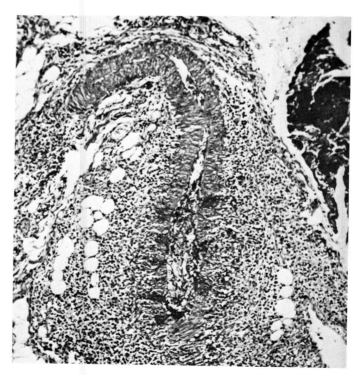

Fig. 21-56. Biopsy specimen of deltoid muscle, illustrating a medium-size muscular artery with panarteritis nodosa. There is segmental necrosis and inflammation of all layers of the arterial wall and contiguous connective tissue, with a predominance of polymorphonuclear leukocytes.

teries distal to the site of surgical repair of aortic coarctation.

Wegener's Granulomatosis

In contrast to panarteritis nodosa, Wegener's granulomatosis predominantly involves small arteries, arterioles, and venules. In this form of necrotizing vasculitis, the blood vessel lesions form the nucleus of a granuloma that consists of acute and chronic inflammatory cells and giant cells in connective tissue. Pulmonary arteries are not usually involved in classic panarteritis nodosa, whereas pulmonary disease is common in Wegener's granulomatosis. Necrotizing granulomas and upper airway disease are characteristic of Wegener's granulomatosis but are not features of panarteritis nodosa.[39]

Other Collagen Vascular Diseases

Disseminated vascular lesions occur with varying frequency in rheumatoid arthritis, rheumatic fever, systemic lupus erythematosus, scleroderma, and dermatomyositis. Except for the occasional occurrence of a classic rheumatoid granuloma in the arterial wall, the morphologic changes in the blood vessels in these disorders are nonspecific.[34] Occasional patients with rheumatoid arthritis may have a fulminant, widespread necrotizing arteritis affecting medium-sized vessels. This arteritis is indistinguishable morphologically from panarteritis nodosa. More commonly, however, in this group of collagen vascular diseases the inflammatory cell infiltrate in the arterial wall is much less extensive than in panarteritis nodosa. Although there may be focal areas of medial necrosis, these are rarely extensive, and aneurysm formation is distinctly uncommon. The internal elastic lamina may be focally disrupted but rarely is extensively destroyed. Although fibrinoid necrosis is not uncommon in blood vessels affected by this group of collagen vascular diseases, superimposed thrombus is unusual.

Infective Arteritis

The inflammatory reaction to infection of an artery depends on the nature of the infecting organisms (bacteria, fungi, viruses, rickettsiae or protozoa) and on the ability of the arterial wall to react to injury. Some organisms elicit little or no inflammatory response, whereas others completely destroy the arterial wall. A great variation is found in the inflammatory response, depending on the type of artery involved, the mode of involvement, and the stage of the reaction. The end results of an infectious process in the arterial wall can be: (1) damage that may be so minimal as to be barely noticeable; (2) thickening and

scarring of the wall, with possible impairment of function; (3) eventual calcification or degeneration of fibrous scars in the wall; (4) thrombosis and subsequent recanalization of the artery; (5) rupture of the artery, with resulting hemorrhage; (6) weakening and dilatation of the arterial wall; and (7) formation of a mycotic aneurysm. Infective arteritis may result from dissemination of organisms from distant intra- or extravascular foci or from direct extension in contiguous tissues.[50] These lesions may be relatively diffuse or localized. In addition to routine histologic examination, cultures for bacteria, mycobacteria, and fungi, as well as serologic studies for viruses, frequently are necessary in order to identify the infective agent. The use of special histochemical stains for organisms and immunohistochemical techniques usually are helpful diagnostic aids.

Drug-Induced Arteriopathy

Vasculitis related to hypersensitivity to therapeutic agents most commonly involves arterioles, capillaries, and venules. Although an inflammatory cell infiltrate is present in all three layers of the involved vessel walls, there is no evidence of necrotizing vascular lesions or of fibrinoid necrosis. Therefore, the media is not weakened and, in contrast to panarteritis nodosa, aneurysm formation is not a feature. The inflammatory cell infiltrate consists primarily of mononuclear cells, mainly lymphocytes, and prominent numbers of eosinophils. Usually there is an extensive perivascular infiltrate consisting of the same population of inflammatory cells. In many organs the inflammatory process appears to spread from the affected blood vessels to adjacent structures. This perivascular infiltrate alone is not sufficient evidence on which to base a diagnosis of hypersensitivity vasculitis. The endothelial lining of the involved vessels appears intact, and thrombosis is not a feature of this disease process.[56]

Intimal proliferation, with or without associated thrombosis, has been found in women taking *oral contraceptives*, in *pregnant* and *postpartum* women, and in a few men with *severe liver disease*.[57] The lesion may occur in any of the branches of the pulmonic, portal, or systemic arteries.[58] Microscopically, the focal areas of intimal thickening are usually eccentric and consist mainly of smooth muscle cells and collagen, with variable amounts of acid mucopolysaccharide (Fig. 21-57). The internal elastic lamina is intact, but in areas of intimal thickening it is usually thickened and replicated into the intima. The arterial media is usually of normal thickness; however, there may be focal areas of apparent decrease in the expected number of smooth muscle cells and of increased amounts of stainable acid mucopolysac-

822

PRINCIPLES AND PRACTICE OF SURGICAL PATHOLOGY

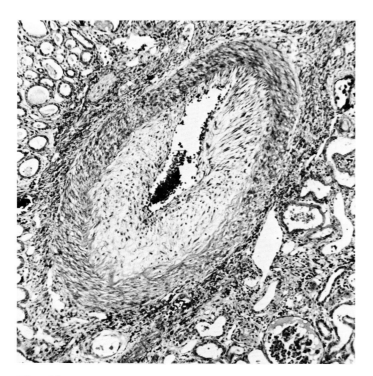

Fig. 21-57. Intraparenchymal renal artery from a young woman who had been taking oral contraceptives. There is intimal thickening consisting of smooth muscle cells, collagen, and acid mucopolyaccharide. (Movat stain.)

charide. The adventitia appears normal. Frequently, there is an occlusive thrombus, which appears loosely attached to the intimal proliferative lesion without intimal ulceration or inflammation. Indeed, inflammatory cells are rare in these lesions, and there is no evidence of a necrotizing arteritis or of fibrinoid necrosis.

The arterial lesions induced by *ergotamine* are those of intimal proliferation and hyalinization and medial hypertrophy, resulting in compromise of the arterial lumen. Superimposed thrombosis completes the occlusion, and gangrene results. The vessels most commonly involved are the tibial, radial, and ulnar arteries or small tributaries down to arterioles.

Methysergide maleate (Sansert)[59,60] and *cocaine*[61] also may produce spasm and occlusive lesions in arteries. Such lesions have been reported in association with chronic abuse of cocaine.[61] Rarely, the intimal proliferation produced by methysergide maleate may be so extensive that distal ischemia persists after withdrawal of the drug.[59,60]

Patients who abuse drugs intravenously may also develop arterial lesions. Disseminated lesions, identical morphologically to those of panarteritis nodosa, are not uncommonly seen in patients taking amphetamines intravenously. The pulmonary arterioles may be occluded by

intimal deposits containing talc or magnesium silicate in those patients who take certain drugs (most commonly Ritalin, Darvon, and the mixture of paregoric and Pyribenzamine known as "blue velvet") intravenously.[59]

Primary Dissecting Aneurysms of Peripheral Arteries

Although extension of hemorrhage from a dissecting aneurysm of the aorta into major arterial branches occurs frequently, primary dissecting aneurysms of the peripheral arteries without involvement of the aorta are rare. The renal artery is most commonly affected, followed by the coronary and intracranial arteries.[34] The length of the dissection in peripheral arteries is variable, but usually in the renal arteries a long segment of artery is dissected with frequent extension into branches, sometimes into intraparenchymal renal arteries. Dissection of the renal artery is commonly associated with fibromuscular dysplasia but occasionally may occur distal to marked stenosis by atherosclerosis at the orifice of the renal artery. However, significant changes of atherosclerosis in the involved portion of the artery are infrequent. The coronary artery most commonly involved is the left anterior descending artery. In contrast to the frequent occurrence of rupture, with resulting hemorrhage, in dissecting aneurysms of the aorta, narrowing of the true lumen, with infarction of the organ supplied by the artery, is the rule in dissecting aneurysms of peripheral arteries. In muscular arteries such as coronary, mesenteric, and hepatic arteries, the dissection most commonly occurs in the outer media immediately adjacent to the external elastic lamina (Fig. 21-49). In those arteries with a more prominent elastic component, such as the carotid, iliac, and brachial arteries, the dissection may occur in any portion of the media but is most common in the outer third. In this latter group of arteries, cystic medial degeneration may be evident microscopically. In the purely muscular arteries, however, microscopic alterations in either smooth muscle or elastic tissue are seldom encountered. In contrast to dissecting aneurysms of the aorta, intimal tears in this group of arteries are not frequent.

Multiloculated cysts that contain abundant acid mucopolysaccharide and are located between the media and adventitia of muscular arteries constitute a lesion quite distinct from focal cystic medial degeneration of the arterial media (Figs. 21-58 and 21-59). These cysts are identical in microscopic appearance to the myxoid cysts of tendon sheaths ("ganglion"). Although these cysts have been described in the external iliac, ulnar, and radial arteries, they are much more common in the popliteal artery. Rarely, a connection between the arterial lumen and the cyst has been present but has not resulted in intramu-

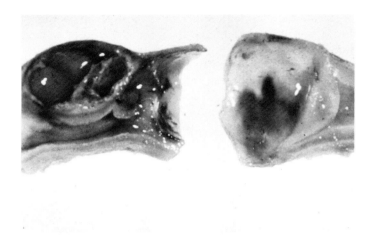

Fig. 21-58. Popliteal artery resected from a young man contains a multiloculated cyst between the media and adventitia (top). The cyst encroaches on the arterial lumen (bottom).

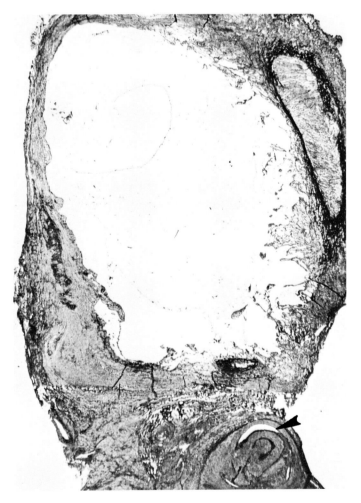

Fig. 21-59. Microscopic section of the popliteal artery cyst illustrated in Fig. 21-58. These cysts are multiloculated and contain acid mucopolysaccharide. There is marked encroachment on the arterial lumen (arrowhead). (Movat stain.)

ral dissection. Progressive enlargement of the multiloculated cysts encroaches upon the arterial lumen, eventually producing thrombosis. The length of the involved arterial segment varies from 2 to 8 cm.[50]

Congenital Lesions of the Peripheral Arteries

The most common congenital lesions of the peripheral arteries of importance to the surgical pathologist are hypoplasia and aplasia of arteries and congenital arteriovenous fistulae. Total failure of canalization of individual arteries (aplasia) is not unusual, nor is the finding of accessory or aberrant arteries of normal morphology. However, congenital hypoplasia of arteries is rare and eventually produces symptoms of arterial insufficiency. Although any artery may be involved, hypoplasia of the iliac arteries is the most common.[52]

Arteriovenous Fistulae

Arteriovenous anastomoses develop normally in certain regions of the body, particularly the palms of the hands, soles of the feet, terminal phalanges of the fingers and toes, nose, ears, eyelids, and tip of the tongue, and persist as normal adult structures. The formation of congenital arteriovenous communications to an abnormal degree, such as to produce a gross vascular lesion, is the result of a failure of differentiation of the involved vessels. These malformations take two forms, diffuse and localized. The lower extremities are most frequently involved, followed by the upper extremities, neck, face, and brain. In any extremity there is a predilection for the distal portion. In more than half of the cases of congenital arteriovenous fistulae, hemangiomas of the skin or subcutaneous tissues are associated. The apparent invasiveness of arteriovenous fistulae, their poorly defined limits, and the ability of pre-existing arteriovenous channels to dilate more widely, causing local or distant recurrences, have led to confusion regarding malignancy. These are not malignant lesions, nor do they have premalignant potential. These veins and arteries often develop intimal thickening and sclerosis, and the smooth muscle in the media may be in disarray, suggesting a hamartoma. In many cases the growth of these lesions is apparently initiated or accelerated by trauma. The history of trauma, however, may mask the diagnosis of congenital arteriovenous fistula, as the two most common complications of arterial trauma are arteriovenous fistula and false aneurysm. A *traumatic arteriovenous fistula* is produced by a penetrating wound that lacerates the artery and adjacent vein, allowing a communication to develop between the openings of these vessels, either directly or by way of false aneurysm sacs. *Traumatic* or *false aneurysms* are formed by the disruption of the wall of an artery, followed by confinement of hemorrhage and hematoma formation by the surrounding fascia and other supporting tissues to define the limits of the aneurysm. These injuries are usually caused by penetrating trauma but also may occur with blunt trauma.[50]

VASCULAR GRAFTS

Aortocoronary Bypass Grafts

Most surgical specimens from components of the coronary circulation consist of grafts that have been implanted as aortocoronary bypasses and have been subsequently removed because of malfunction. The segments of native coronary arteries proximal to the sites of functionally successful bypass grafts may experience a pronounced decrease in blood flow and luminal size.

Aortocoronary Saphenous Vein Bypass Grafts

Aortocoronary saphenous vein bypass grafts should be examined first by radiography to detect calcification and then by multiple transverse sections. Stains for fibrin and connective tissue are useful in their microscopic evaluation. It is indispensable to know how long the graft had been in place before removal and whether or not preoperative angiographic studies indicated the need for special attention to a particular region of the graft. The reason for failure of a graft system may not be evident on study of the graft itself.[62] Vein grafts that appear normal upon removal may have malfunctioned in vivo because they were: (1) either too short (excessive tension and compression) or too long (kinking or torsion predisposing to thrombosis); (2) improperly anastomosed to the coronary artery (anastomosed into or just upstream to an area of marked arterial luminal narrowing or anastomosed by sutures that constrict the arterial lumen). The possibility of dissection of the wall of the coronary artery also must be considered: dissection occurs with surprising frequency when the graft is anastomosed in the area of a plaque.

Changes that represent responses of the venous graft to the implantation procedure and to subsequent hemodynamic alterations can be classified as early or late.[62,63] Early changes (less than 1 week after implantation) consist of endothelial damage, nonocclusive platelet-fibrin aggregates, occlusive and nonocclusive thrombi, smooth muscle cell necrosis, and mild leukocytic infiltration. Intimal thickening and medial and adventitial fibrosis begin to develop during the second week, together with endothelial regeneration (which may be incomplete). Occlusive thrombi may recanalize with formation of multiple small luminal channels. Fibromuscular intimal proliferation occurs to some degree in most aortocoronary vein grafts; however, it is not necessarily a progressive phenomenon leading to graft occlusion, and after the first year it usually stabilizes (Fig. 21-60). Graft occlusion because of thrombosis or severe fibromuscular intimal thickening is most likely to occur within the first 3 months. In some patients late occlusion is related to lipid deposition complicating fibromuscular intimal thickenings. The lesions resulting from the combination of these processes contain foam cells, fibrous tissue, and calcific deposits. They resemble atherosclerotic plaques and tend to be most frequent in patients with hyperlipidemia. Aneurysmal dilatation in aortocoronary bypass grafts is extremely rare. Localized segmental stenoses also can cause late occlusion. Their morphology has not been studied in detail, but it has been suggested that they are related to venous valves.

Other Types of Aortocoronary Bypass Grafts

Systemic arteries have been used as free grafts in the aortocoronary position (radical and internal mammary arteries); they also have been dissected free and anasto-

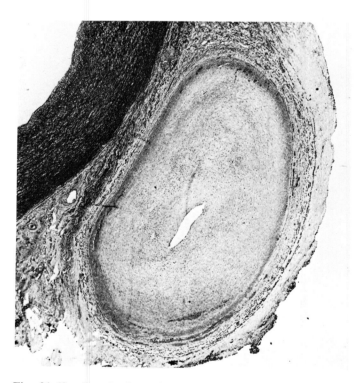

Fig. 21-60. Proximal portion of saphenous vein graft in the aortocoronary position (note aorta at upper left) shows severe luminal narrowing due to fibromuscular intimal proliferation. (Movat stain.)

mosed as pedicled grafts into a coronary artery (internal mammary and splenic arteries). In both instances the implanted vessels undergo variable degrees of fibromuscular intimal hyperplasia, which in the case of radial arteries often is the cause of occlusion. Synthetic grafts made of Dacron or polytetrafluoroethylene have had limited use as aortocoronary bypass grafts and as arteriovenous shunts in chronic hemodialysis; some of these coronary grafts have been reported to thrombose, and the arteriovenous shunts often become infected. Occlusive thrombosis also has been frequently encountered in aortocoronary bypass grafts made of biologic materials, including ficin-treated, dialdehyde-starch tanned, and glutaraldehyde-treated veins.[64]

Other Vascular Prostheses

The problems encountered in the various forms of vascular grafts have been reviewed in detail.[64] Regardless of the type of material of which grafts are composed, they should be evaluated for thickness, cellularity, hyalinization, hemorrhage, layering of the pseudointima, connective tissue ingrowth, and appearance of new blood vessels in the adventitia and between the components (fabric material). Portions of the graft should be submitted for microbiologic culture prior to fixation if infection is suspected.

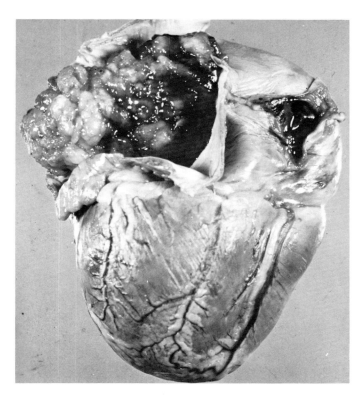

Fig. 21-61. The majority of cardiac myxomas consist of multiple, friable, polypoid fronds and have a distinctive mucoid or gelatinous appearance. Approximately 75 percent of cardiac myxomas arise in the left atrium, as illustrated here.

TUMORS

Primary Tumors of the Heart

Benign Tumors

Cardiac Myxoma

The most common primary tumor of the heart is the cardiac myxoma. Cardiac myxomas vary in clinical presentation, depending on the chamber in which they are located; however, they are similar in gross and microscopic appearance, irrespective of their location.[65,66] Grossly, most myxomas have a short, broad-based attachment and are pedunculated, soft, gelatinous, and polypoid (Fig. 21-61); however, some of these tumors have a rounded, smooth surface. True sessile myxomas are distinctly rare, and most of the so-called sessile myxomas have previously embolized, leaving only the broad base of the polypoid tumor attached to the endocardium. Myxomas frequently contain areas of hemorrhage. They vary from 1 cm to 15 cm in diameter (average 5 to 6 cm).

Microscopically, myxomas consist of a myxoid matrix composed of acid mucopolysaccharide, within which are polygonal cells with scant eosinophilic cytoplasm. These cells are arranged singly, often assume a stellate shape,

and are disposed in small nests; occasionally they are multinucleated. The myxoma surface is covered by these polygonal cells, usually in a monolayer with focal clustering at crevices (Fig. 21-62). These cells also form vessel-like channels, which simulate primitive capillaries, throughout the myxoid stroma. Ultrastructurally the polygonal cells closely resemble multipotential mesenchymal cells. The stroma contains variable amounts of reticular fibers, collagen, elastic fibers, and smooth muscle cells.[67] Large arteries and veins are commonly present at the base of the tumor and communicate with the subendocardium. Lymphocytes and plasma cells are not infrequent, especially at the site of attachment to the subendocardium, and foci of extramedullary hematopoiesis are commonly found throughout the tumor. Foci of microscopic calcification are presently in approximately 10 percent of myxomas, and areas of metaplastic bone occasionally occur. Embolization from cardiac myxomas is a common event and may occur with tumors arising in either the left or the right side of the heart. After a portion of the myxoma has embolized, a thrombus may form over the denuded surface of the tumor; this thrombus also may subsequently embolize. Therefore, the possibility of cardiac myxoma must be considered even if histologic ex-

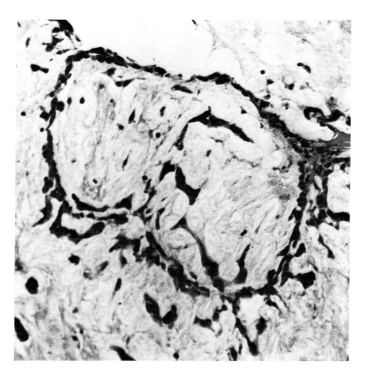

Fig. 21-62. The surface cells of the myxoma usually are arranged in a monolayer; however, foci of multilayered, hyperplastic cells, as illustrated here, are frequent.

amination reveals the pattern of a thromboembolus rather than the classic microscopic appearance of embolic cardiac myxoma.

Complete surgical excision of the myxoma and its base, along with a small rim of grossly unaffected endocardium and myocardium, is the preferred treatment. If not completely excised, the cardiac myxoma can recur. Because of the possibility of recurrence, the pathologist should examine the margins of the grossly unaffected myocardium and endocardium microscopically to be certain that no portion of the myxoma remains.

Papillary Fibroelastomas

Papillary fibroelastomas are usually incidental findings at autopsy or on surgically excised valves and are not associated with cardiac dysfunction in the vast majority of patients. Although they most frequently arise from the valvular endocardium, papillary fibroelastomas may arise anywhere in the heart; occasionally they are multiple. When these tumors occur on the atrioventricular valves, they usually project into the atria, and although they may arise from the free edge of the valve, more commonly they originate from its midportion. On the semilunar valves these tumors arise with nearly equal frequency on the ventricular and arterial side and may be situated anywhere on the valve.[65]

Grossly, a papillary fibroelastoma resembles a sea anemone, with multiple papillary fronds attached to the endocardium by a short pedicle. The fronds consist of a central core of dense connective tissue surrounded by a layer of loose connective tissue and covered by endothelial cells that are frequently hyperplastic. The mantle of loose connective tissue consists of an acid mucopolysaccharide-rich matrix, within which are embedded collagen fibrils, elastic fibers, scattered smooth muscle cells, and occasionally, mononuclear cells. Usually, a fine meshwork of elastic fibers surrounds a central collagen core, but occasionally the entire central core appears to consist of elastic fibers. This core is continous with the connective tissue of the endocardium and merges imperceptibly with it. Similarly, the endothelial cells that cover the papillary fronds are in contiguity with the normal endothelial cells on the surface of the endocardium or the cardiac valve.

Rhabdomyoma

The most common primary, cardiac tumor in infancy and childhood is the rhabdomyoma.[65] In 90 percent of affected patients, cardiac rhabdomyomas are multiple. They occur with nearly equal frequency in the right and left ventricles, including the ventricular septum. In 30 percent of these patients, the atria are also involved. There is no documented rhabdomyoma (or cardiac myxoma) originating in a cardiac valve.

Grossly, rhabdomyomas are white to yellow-tan and vary in size from millimeters to a few centimeters (Fig. 21-63). Microscopically, the tumors are circumscribed but not encapsulated and are easily distinguished from the surrounding myocardium. The rhabdomyoma cells are large (up to 80 μm in diameter) and contain abundant glycogen. The histologic demonstration of glycogen depends on the speed and type of fixation and is best achieved with the PAS reaction on frozen sections from unfixed tissue or after methanol or nonaqueous fixation.[68] Classic "spider cells," with centrally placed cytoplasmic masses containing the nucleus and elongated projections of slender myofibrils extending to the cell periphery, are present in each tumor (Figs. 21-64 and 21-65). Frequently, however, the cytoplasmic mass is eccentrically placed, and the cytoplasmic projections traverse the vacuolated cells. Microscopic calcification within rhabdomyoma cells is rare. In newborns many of the rhabdomyomas contain collections of nucleated red blood cells, myelocytic precursor cells, and occasional megakaryocytes, consistent with extramedullary hematopoiesis.

Ultrastructurally, intercellular junctions resembling intercalated discs are located around the entire periphery of the rhabdomyoma cells. This ultrastructural feature is not found in normal adult cardiac muscle cells, in which

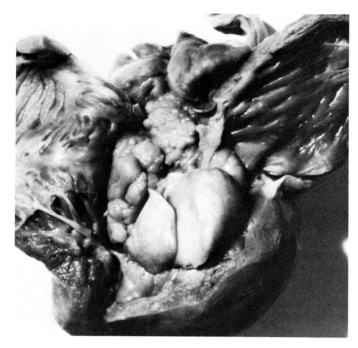

Fig. 21-63. Rhabdomyoma fills the right ventricle and obstructs the tricuspid valve of a newborn infant.

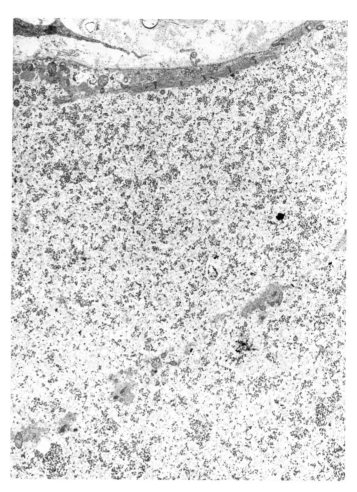

Fig. 21-65. Electron micrograph of peripheral portion of rhabdomyoma cells. A myofibril is subjacent to the plasma membrane, and most of the cytoplasm shown is occupied by glycogen particles. (Uranyl acetate and lead citrate ×11,000.)

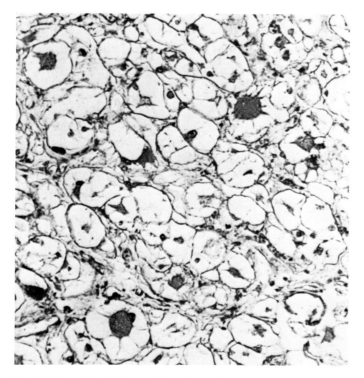

Fig. 21-64. Histologic section of cardiac rhabdomyoma showing typical spider cells with a centrally located cytoplasmic mass and clear peripheral cytoplasm.

most of the junctions are located at the two ends of the cell, but is suggestive of embryonic cardiac muscle cells.[69]

Although the cardiac rhabdomyoma has been repeatedly described in the literature as an inoperable lesion because of its tendency to multiplicity, cardiac rhabdomyomas have been successfully excised in at least five patients. In all five, the rhabdomyomas were at least partially intracavitary and produced symptoms related to obstruction of intracardiac blood flow. These symptoms were relieved by operative resection. Since there is no evidence to suggest that rhabdomyoma cells are capable of mitotic division after birth and tuberous sclerosis appears to be rare in patients with intracavitary rhabdomyomas and cardiac symptoms, patients with cardiac rhabdomyomas will continue to be considered as surgical candidates.[65,68,69]

Fibroma

In contrast to rhabdomyomas, cardiac fibromas are almost always solitary and located in the ventricular myocardium, frequently in the ventricular septum (Fig. 21-66). These firm, gray-white tumors are often large, sometimes exceeding 10 cm in diameter. Although they grossly appear sharply demarcated, microscopically they interdigitate with the adjacent myocardium. Satellite nodules may appear to be present, but when traced these nodules connect to the main tumor mass in a different plane. The central portion of the tumor is composed of hyalinized fibrous tissue, often with multiple foci of calcification (which may be seen on chest radiographs) and cystic degeneration, probably secondary to poor blood supply. Elastic tissue also may be prominent, as it is in many of the fibromatoses of the superficial soft tissues. Indeed, fibromas of the heart are connective tissue tumors derived from fibroblasts and have the same spectrum of appearance and behavior as soft tissue fibromatoses in other areas of the body. These intramyocardial masses of proliferating connective tissue should not be confused with reactive fibrous tissue proliferation in the endocardial or epicardial layers of the heart. Areas of cellular fibrous tissue are present in each tumor, usually at the periphery (Fig. 21-67). Mitotic figures are rare in these areas of fibrous tissue and, as in the extracardiac fibromatoses, cellularity is not an indication of malig-

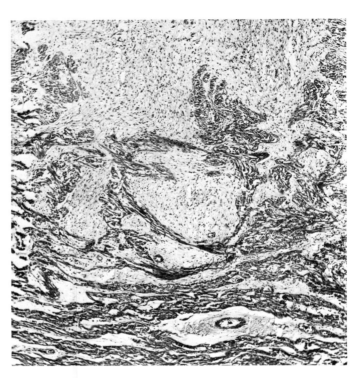

Fig. 21-67. Although grossly fibromas appear encapsulated, microscopically they merge and interdigitate with the surrounding myocardium. Bundles of individual myofibers are entrapped in the expanding fibrous tissue and are often present deep within the fibroma.

nancy. Because of the invasive growth of these tumors, normal cardiac muscle cells are frequently entrapped in the growing fibrous tissue and are left intact deep within the tumor, occasionally in central locations. These myocardial cells eventually degenerate and become vacuolated as they are separated from the remainder of the myocardium. True spider cells, diagnostic of the rhabdomyoma, are not found in the cardiac fibroma.[65]

Lipomatous Hypertrophy

In lipomatous hypertrophy of the atrial septum (interatrial lipoma), the mass of accumulated fat frequently bulges from beneath the atrial septal endocardium, most commonly into the right atrium. Rarely, an interatrial lipoma may protrude far into the atrium. This entity must be considered in the angiographic diagnosis of intracavitary masses. Although the interatrial lipoma cannot be completely resected because of its proximity to the atrioventricular node, a portion of the tumor may be submitted to the surgical pathologist for microscopic examination.

Microscopically, there is a variable mixture of mature adipose tissue cells and granular or vacuolated cells (Fig.

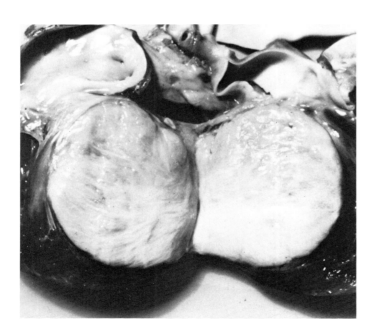

Fig. 21-66. Fibromas are located most frequently in the ventricular septum, are single, and often reach massive proportions. On cross section the tumors are firm and appear trabeculated. Foci of calcification and areas of cystic degeneration are frequently apparent grossly.

21-68). Fat droplets are usually demonstrable with oil red O stain both in the mature fat cells and in the granular cells. With light and electron microscopic examination, the granular cells appear identical to fetal fat cells. The presence of fetal fat is a hallmark of lipomatous hypertrophy of the atrial septum, and occasionally these interatrial masses consist entirely of fetal fat. Myocardial cells are invariably entrapped in the mass, especially at the periphery, and may demonstrate bizarre hypertrophic, atrophic, or degenerative changes. Often the muscle nuclei are large, hyperchromatic, and pleomorphic. Neither classic spider cells nor neoplastic muscle cells are found in the interatrial lipoma, but varying amounts of fibrous tissue and foci of chronic inflammatory cells, predominantly lymphocytes and plasma cells, are frequently present.[65]

Teratoma

The majority of true teratomas of the heart and pericardium are extracardiac but intrapericardial, arise from the base of the heart, are usually attached to the root of the pulmonary artery and aorta, and generally receive their blood supply from the vasa vasorum of these vessels (Fig. 21-69). Although intracardiac teratomas have been

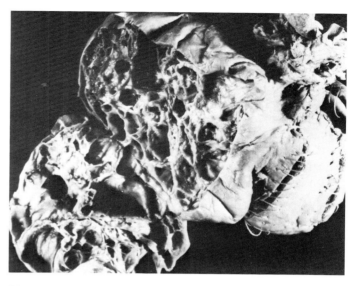

Fig. 21-69. Cardiac teratomas are usually intrapericardial tumors attached to the root of the aorta and pulmonary artery. The tumor may reach massive proportions, and the transected surface is always multicystic.

reported, most reports describe cysts that do not include all three germ layers. Although teratomas may occur in adults, the majority are present in the pediatric age group, and girls are affected much more commonly than boys.[65]

Intrapericardial teratomas may assume massive proportions, measuring up to 15 cm in diameter. They are pear-shaped, usually smooth-surfaced, and lobulated. On sectioning, the teratoma contains numerous multiloculated cysts and intervening solid areas. Microscopically, intrapericardial teratomas resemble teratomas elsewhere in the body, and derivatives of all three germ layers are present. Since teratomas have a malignant potential, all of them should be adequately sampled to avoid overlooking the rare malignant example.

Other Primary Cardiac Tumors

Intracardiac bronchogenic cysts are, with rare exception, incidental findings of no clinical significance. In the unusual exception, surgical excision is indicated for relief of symptoms. Bronchogenic cysts are usually contained within the myocardium, especially the ventricular myocardium, although they may project into a cardiac chamber or into the pericardial space. Rarely exceeding 1 to 2 cm in diameter, bronchogenic cysts are misplaced elements of the respiratory tract, and, unlike teratomas, contain only elements derived from mesoderm and endoderm arranged in an orderly manner resembling a bronchus.

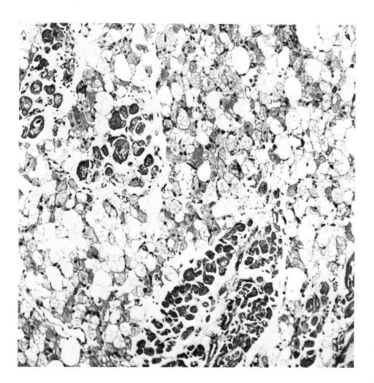

Fig. 21-68. In lipomatous hypertrophy of the atrial septum, there is an accumulation of adipose tissue, and the myofibers are compressed against the endocardium. Islands of atrial myofibers are trapped in the adipose tissue, which is composed of mature fat cells and varying amounts of fetal fat.

Hemangioma

Hemangiomas may occur at any site in the heart or pericardium and may be mainly intramural or mainly intracavitary. Grossly, hemangiomas are red and hemorrhagic. Microscopically they are classified according to the morphologic pattern and interrelationship of the vascular channels, endothelial cells, and supporting stroma. This classification (capillary, cavernous, intramuscular, hemangioendothelioma) is descriptive of varying growth patterns and does not necessarily imply differences of prognosis.[65]

Other Benign Tumors

Lymphangiomas are uncommon in the heart, but, as elsewhere in the body, frequently are diffuse proliferations rather than distinct tumors. Hamartomas composed of more than one type of mesenchymal tissue are rarely present in the heart and most commonly represent arteriovenous malformations (vascular hamartomas).

Paragangliomas usually involve the base of the heart, especially the posterior wall of the left atrium. They are usually invasive and are extremely vascular, making surgical resection difficult. A case has been reported in which one of these tumors was resected by a procedure involving removal and reimplantation of the entire heart.[70]

Rare benign tumors of the heart or pericardium include granular cell tumor, neurofibroma, leiomyoma, heterotopic thymoma, and ectopic thyroid tissue. Microscopically these tumors resemble those of the same type occurring elsewhere in the body.[65]

Malignant Tumors

Angiosarcoma

Angiosarcoma is the most frequently occurring primary cardiac sarcoma and is found two to three times more often in men than in women. The site of origin most frequently is the right side of the heart, especially in the right atrium.[65]

Microscopically, angiosarcomas are composed of malignant cells that form vascular channels; however, there is usually considerable variation in histology even within the same tumor. Most angiosarcomas contain foci of solid areas of spindle cells, and occasionally they are composed almost entirely of sheets of rounded anaplastic cells or spindle cells. Even in these cellular, solid-appearing angiosarcomas, a reticulum stain will usually demonstrate a vascular pattern in at least part of the tumor. The vascular channels vary markedly in size and configuration, but they are usually multiple, anastomosing, and lined by rounded or elongated, often multilayered, endothelial cells. Occasionally these proliferating endothelial cells fill the vascular channels, thus giving the tumor a solid appearance. Pleomorphism and anaplasia may be marked, and mitoses are usually frequent, as are intraluminal tufting projections of multilayered endothelial cells without an intervening stroma. Spindle cell areas usually merge imperceptibly with vascular and solid areas. Anastomosing vascular channels, foci of endothelial tufting, and spindle cell areas are the most reliable indicators of angiosarcoma. In combination with these features, pleomorphism, anaplasia, and mitoses are adjunctive diagnostic aids; alone, however, they are not reliable indicators of malignancy in an endothelial tumor.

Kaposi's Sarcoma

Kaposi's sarcoma involving the heart has recently been described in patients with AIDS and is morphologically identical to Kaposi's sarcoma occurring in other organs.

Rhabdomyosarcoma

Rhabdomyosarcoma, the second most common primary sarcoma of the heart, is a neoplasm composed of malignant cells with features of striated muscle. Unlike angiosarcomas, rhabdomyosarcomas have no propensity to arise in a particular cardiac chamber. Indeed, they originate with equal frequency in the left and right sides of the heart. Microscopically, both juvenile (embryonal or alveolar) and adult forms occur; however, the adult form is much more common.[65] The diagnosis of rhabdomyosarcoma is made by definite identification of rhabdomyoblasts, which often is extremely difficult because these tumors exhibit marked pleomorphism and anaplasia. The nuclei vary widely in size, shape, and chromaticity. Pyknotic nuclei are rare, but giant forms and abnormal mitoses are frequent; these nuclei are often large and vesicular. Spindle cell foci, as well as solid cellular and loose myxoid areas, are frequently present within the same tumor. Microscopic foci of necrosis and hemorrhage are common. This marked variation in microscopic appearance suggests the diagnosis of rhabdomyosarcoma and should initiate a search for rhabdomyoblasts. Cross-striations may be identified by light microscopy in approximately 20 to 30 percent of these tumors. To facilitate ultrastructural studies, suggestive rhabdomyoblasts are initially identified by light microscopy using the phosphotungstic acid-hematoxylin stain; then the appropriate area of the paraffin block is excised and processed for electron microscopic study. Ultrastructurally, both thick and thin filaments (actin and myosin) as well as Z-band material must be identified. Only rarely will these elements be organized into the characteristic sarcomeres of striated muscle; more commonly they are arranged haphazardly throughout the cytoplasm.

Fibrosarcoma and Malignant Fibrous Histiocytoma

Fibrosarcoma and malignant fibrous histiocytoma are malignant mesenchymal tumors that are primarily fibroblastic in their differentiation. These tumors arise with equal frequency on the left and right side of the heart, with no predilection for any single site. They may be nodular or infiltrative and are firm and gray-white.[65]

Microscopically, fibrosarcomas consist of spindle-shaped cells with elongated, blunt-ended nuclei and tapering cytoplasm. Although mitoses are usually frequent, pleomorphism and anaplasia are generally minimal. Nucleoli are not prominent. The spindle cells are arranged haphazardly, occasionally in broad bundles or fascicles that may course at acute angles to one another; however, palisading nuclei and interlacing cords of cells are not features of fibrosarcoma. Tumor necrosis is rare, but foci of myxoid change are common. Metaplastic cartilage and bone are often present and do not provide sufficient reason to classify these tumors as malignant mesenchymomas. A malignant fibrous histiocytoma has fibrosarcomatous areas, but it is differentiated from a fibrosarcoma by a storiform pattern of the spindle cells and the presence of giant cells, often with multiple nuclei. These tumors are discussed in greater detail in Chapter 10.

Malignant Teratoma

Unlike most primary cardiac sarcomas, malignant teratomas occur most commonly in children. Like their benign counterparts, they are primarily intrapericardial, attached to the base of the heart, and more common in females. Elements of the three germ layers are identified in the primary tumor; however, one of these elements has become malignant, either metastasizing or invading adjacent structures. The most common malignant pattern is embryonal carcinoma, but examples of choriocarcinoma and squamous cell carcinoma have been recognized.[65]

Osteosarcoma

When extraskeletal osteosarcoma is primary in the heart, it most commonly arises in the left atrium, usually from the posterior wall near the entrance of the pulmonary veins. Less frequently it may originate in the right atrium or right ventricle. These tumors have fibrosarcomatous areas in close association with areas of osteoid and malignant osteoblasts. Foci of apparent chondrosarcoma are not uncommon; however, pure extraskeletal chondrosarcomas primary in the heart are rarely encountered.[65]

Other Malignant Tumors

The heart is occasionally the primary site of *extranodal lymphoma, thymoma, liposarcoma,* or *leiomyosarcoma.* By both light and electron microscopy these tumors are identical to their counterparts occurring elsewhere in the body.

Metastatic Tumors of the Heart

Metastatic tumors are the most frequently encountered cardiac tumors. The incidence of secondary tumors of the heart is 20 to 40 times as great as that of primary benign and malignant cardiac tumors combined. Nearly every type of malignant tumor from every organ and tissue has been reported to metastasize to the heart. Perhaps the sole exception would be tumors primary to the central nervous system.

Besides direct extension from contiguous structures and lymphatic spread, carcinoma may occasionally reach the heart via direct venous extension, especially in the case of renal cell carcinoma and hepatoma, which may extend up the inferior vena cava into the right atrium. Hematogenous spread, on the other hand, is the main route of metastasis for sarcoma, lymphoma, and leukemia, as well as for melanoma involving the heart.

Metastatic tumor growth in the heart is generally solid, small, and multiple; large tumor masses or confluent tumor nodules are rare, and tumor necrosis is extremely unusual.

Primary Tumors of Major Blood Vessels

Tumors arising in major blood vessels are distinctly uncommon. The majority of tumors of the major blood vessels are of smooth muscle origin; *leiomyomas* and *leiomyosarcomas* account for 70 percent of all reported cases and over 90 percent of tumors arising in large veins.[65]

Approximately 65 percent of all primary tumors of major blood vessels arise in large veins. The majority of smooth muscle tumors of large veins are malignant; indeed, slightly more than 75 percent of all benign and malignant tumors arising in large veins are leiomyosarcomas. Approximately one half of the leiomyosarcomas of the large veins arise in the inferior vena cava; they are eight times as common in women as in men. Veins of the lower extremity are the next most frequently involved (30 percent), followed by veins of the torso (12 percent) and the upper extremities and head and neck (8 percent). Approximately 15 percent of smooth muscle tumors of the veins are benign. They have the microscopic appearance of leiomyomas elsewhere in the body.

Primary neoplasms of large arteries are extremely unusual, and with few exceptions, all of those reported have been malignant. Histologically, approximately one fourth of the sarcomas of the pulmonary artery are leiomyosarcomas. These tumors appear to arise in the main pulmonary artery and may grow in a retrograde fashion involving the pulmonary valve or extend along branches of the pulmonary artery into the lung. Less commonly, fibrosarcoma, angiosarcoma, rhabdomyosarcoma, osteosarcoma, chondrosarcoma, and malignant mesenchymoma primary in the pulmonary artery have been reported.

In the aorta, sarcomas are equally divided between the thoracic and abdominal regions. The sarcomas of the aorta and its major tributaries appear to arise in the wall of the affected vessel. They rarely occlude the vessel lumen but rather grow along the intimal surface. Many of these tumors are confined to the intimal layer of the artery, without evidence of invasion of the muscular wall. The two most common types of sarcoma involving major arteries are leiomyosarcoma and fibrosarcoma. Intimal fibroplasia involving the large arteries must not be confused with sarcoma.[65]

REFERENCES

1. Ferrans VJ, Butany JW: Ultrastructural pathology of the heart. p. 319. In Trump BF, Jones RT (eds): Diagnostic Electron Microscopy. Vol 4. Churchill Livingstone, New York, 1983
2. Ferrans VJ, Rodriguez ER: The pathology of the cardiomyopathies. p. 15. In Giles TD, Sander GE (eds): Cardiomyopathy. PSG Publishing Co., Littleton, MA, 1988
3. Maron BJ, Roberts WC: Quantitative analysis of cardiac muscle cell disorganization in the ventricular septum of patients with hypertrophic cardiomyopathy. Circulation 59:689, 1979
4. Ferrans VJ, Buja LM, Roberts WC: Cardiac morphologic changes produced by ethanol. p. 139. In Rothschild MA, Oratz M, Schreiber S (eds): Alcohol and Abnormal Protein Biosynthesis. Pergamon Press, New York, 1974
5. Ferrans VJ: Overview of cardiac pathology in relation to anthracycline cardiotoxicity. Cancer Treat Rep 62:955, 1978
6. Legha SS, Benjamin RS, Mackey B, et al: Reduction of doxorubicin cardiotoxicity by prolonged continuous intravenous infusion. Ann Intern Med 96:133, 1982
7. Billingham ME, Mason JW, Bristow MR, Daniels JR: Anthracycline cardiomyopathy monitored by morphologic changes. Cancer Treat Rep 62:865, 1978
8. Ferrans VJ, McAllister HA Jr, Haese WH: Infantile cardiomyopathy with histiocytoid change in cardiac muscle cells. Report of six patients. Circulation 53:708, 1976
9. Hudson REB: Cardiovascular Pathology. Williams & Wilkins, Baltimore, 1965
10. Pomerance A, Davies MJ: The Pathology of the Heart. Blackwell, Oxford, 1975
11. Jennings RB, Ganote CE: Ultrastructural changes in myocardium during acute ischemia. Circ Res 35: suppl. 3, 156, 1974
12. Santos-Buch CA: American trypanosomiasis: Chagas' disease. Int Rev Exp Pathol 19:63, 1979
13. Alday LE, Moreyra E, Quiroga C, et al: Cardiomyopathy complicated by left ventricular aneurysms in children. Br Heart J 38:162, 1976
14. Macina G, Singh A, Drew TM, et al: Asymmetric myocardial hypertrophy, left ventricular aneurysm, mural thrombus, and sudden death. Am Heart J 111:175, 1986
15. Barbaresi F, Longhini C, Brunazzi C, et al: Idiopathic apical left ventricular aneurysm in hypertrophic cardiomyopathy. Report of 3 cases, and review of the literature. Jpn Heart J 26:481, 1985
16. McAllister HA Jr: Myocarditis: Some current perspectives and future directions. Tex Heart Inst J 14:331, 1987
17. Billingham M: The diagnostic criteria of myocarditis by endomyocardial biopsy. Heart Vessels (suppl.) 1:133, 1985
18. McAllister HA Jr, Hall RJ: Iatrogenic heart disease. p. 871. In Cheng TO (ed): The International Textbook of Cardiology, Pergamon Press, New York, 1986
19. McAllister HA Jr, Ferrans VJ: Granulomas of the heart and major blood vessels. p. 75. In Ioachim HL (ed): Differential Diagnosis of Granulomas. Raven Press, New York, 1982
20. McAllister HA Jr, Ferrans VJ: Eosinophilic and granulomatous inflammation of the heart. p. 246. In Kapoor AS (ed): Cancer and the Heart: A Textbook of Cardiac Oncology. Springer-Verlag, New York, 1986
21. Edwards WD, Holmes DR Jr, Reeder GS: Diagnosis of active lymphocytic myocarditis by endomyocardial biopsy: Quantitative criteria for light microscopy. Mayo Clin Proc 57:419, 1982
22. McAllister HA Jr: Pathology of the cardiovascular system in chronic renal failure. p. 1. In Lowenthal DT, Pennock RL, Likoff W, et al. (eds): Management of Cardiovascular Disease in Renal Failure. FA Davis, Philadelphia, 1981
23. Billingham ME: Diagnosis of cardiac rejection by endomyocardial biopsy. Heart Transplant 1:25, 1982
24. McAllister HA Jr, Schnee JM, Radovancevic B, Frazier OH: A system for grading cardiac allograft rejection. Tex Heart Inst J 13:1, 1986
25. Ferrans VJ, Boyce SW: Metabolic and familial diseases. In Silver MD (ed): Cardiovascular Pathology. Churchill Livingstone, New York, 1982
26. Hays AP, Hallett M, Delfs J, et al: Muscle phosphofructokinase deficiency: Abnormal polysaccharide in a case of late-onset myopathy. Neurology 31:1077, 1981
27. Eishi Y, Takemura T, Sone R, et al: Glycogen storage disease confined to the heart with deficient activity of cardiac phosphorylase kinase: A new type of glycogen storage disease. Hum Pathol 16:193, 1985
28. McAllister HA Jr, Ferrans VJ, Hall RJ, et al: Chloroquine-induced cardiomyopathy. Arch Pathol Lab Med 111:953, 1987
29. Ratliff NB, Estes ML, Myles JL, et al: The diagnosis of chloroquine cardiomyopathy by endomyocardial biopsy. N Engl J Med 316:191, 1987
30. McAllister HA Jr, Bossart M, Ferrans VJ, et al: Restrictive

cardiomyopathy with kappa light chain deposits in myocardium as a complication of multiple myeloma; histochemical and electron microscopic observations. Arch Pathol Lab Med 112:1151, 1988

31. McAllister HA Jr: Pathology of the heart in endocrine disorders. In Silver MD (ed): Cardiovascular Pathology. Churchill Livingstone, New York, 1982

32. Silver MD, Huckell VF, Lorber M: Basement membranes of small cardiac vessels in patients with diabetes and myxedema: Preliminary observations. Pathology 7:213, 1977

33. Ferrans VJ, Muna WFT, Jones M, et al: Ultrastructure of the fibrous ring in patients with discrete subaortic stenosis. Lab Invest 39:30, 1978

34. Gould SE: Pathology of the Heart and Blood Vessels. 3rd Ed. Charles C Thomas, Springfield, IL, 1968

35. McAllister HA Jr: Collagen diseases and the cardiovascular system. In Silver MD (ed): Cardiovascular Pathology. Churchill Livingstone, New York, 1982

36. McAllister HA Jr, Fenoglio JJ: Cardiac involvement in Whipple's disease. Circulation 52:152, 1975

37. Olsen EGJ, Spry CJF: The pathogenesis of Löffler's endomyocardial disease, and its relationship to endomyocardial fibrosis. Prog Cardiol 8:281, 1979

38. Roberts WC, Dangel JC, Bulkley BH: Nonrheumatic valvular cardiac disease: A clinicopathologic survey of 27 different conditions causing valvular dysfunction. Cardiovasc Clin 5(2):333, 1973

39. Fauci AS, Wolff SM: Wegener's granulomatosis and related diseases. DM 23(7):1, 1977

40. Cheitlin MD, Fenoglio JJ, McAllister HA Jr, et al: Congenital aortic stenosis secondary to dysplasia of congenital bicuspid aortic valves without commissural fusion. Am J Cardiol 42:102, 1978

41. Fenoglio JJ, McAllister HA Jr, DeCastro CM, et al: Congenital bicuspid aortic valve after age 20. Am J Cardiol 39:164, 1977

42. Davia JE, Fenoglio JJ, DeCastro CM, et al: Quadricuspid semilunar valves. Chest 72:186, 1977

43. Hyams VJ, Manion WC: Incomplete differentiation of the cardiac valves. A report of 197 cases. Am Heart J 76:173, 1968

44. Lefrak EA, Starr A: Cardiac Valve Prostheses. Appleton & Lange, East Norwalk, CT, 1979

45. Ferrans VJ, Tomita Y, Hilbert SL, et al: Evaluation of operatively excised prosthetic tissue valves. p. 311. In Waller BF (Ed): Pathology of the Heart and Great Vessels, Churchill Livingstone, New York, 1988

46. Titus JL: Infective endocarditis, active and healed. p. 176. In Edwards JE, Lev M, Abell MR (eds): The Heart. Williams & Wilkins, Baltimore, 1974

47. Freedman LR: Endocarditis updated. DM 26(3):1, 1979

48. Schenk EA: Pathology of occlusive disease of the lower extremities. Cardiovasc Clin 5(1):288, 1973

49. Virmani R, Lande A, McAllister HA, Jr: Pathologic aspects of Takayasu's arteritis. p. 55. In Lande A, Berkmen Y, McAllister HA Jr (eds): Aortitis: Clinical Pathologic and Radiographic Aspects. Raven Press, New York, 1986

50. Whelan TJ Jr, Baugh JH: Non-atherosclerotic arterial lesions, and their management. Parts I–IV. Curr Probl Surg. 4 Feb. 1967; and 3, Mar. 1967

51. Fujiwara H, Hamashima Y: Pathology of the heart in Kawasaki disease. Pediatrics 61:100, 1978

52. Pasternak RC, Baughman KL, Fallon JT, et al: Scanning electron microscopy after coronary transluminal angioplasty of normal canine coronary arteries. Am J Cardiol 45:591, 1980

53. James TN: Small arteries of the heart. Circulation 56:2, 1977

54. Perry MO: Fibromuscular dysplasia. Surg Gynecol Obstet 139:97, 1974

55. Virmani R, McAllister HA Jr: The pathology of the aorta and major arteries. p. 7. In Lande A, Berkmen Y, McAllister HA Jr (eds): Aortitis: Clinical, Pathologic and Radiographic Aspects. Raven Press, New York, 1986

56. Mullick FG, McAllister HA Jr, Wagner BM, et al: Drug related vasculitis, clinicopathologic correlations in 30 patients. Hum Pathol 10:313, 1979

57. Irey NS, Norris HJ: Intimal vascular lesions associated with female reproductive steroids. Arch Pathol 96:227, 1973

58. Irey NS, McAllister HA Jr, Henry JM: Oral contraceptives and stroke in young women. A clinicopathologic correlation. Neurology 28:1216, 1978

59. McAllister HA Jr, Mullick FG: The cardiovascular system. p. 201. In Riddel R (ed): Pathology of Drug-Induced and Toxic Diseases. Churchill Livingstone, New York, 1982

60. Ferrans VJ: Effects of toxic substances on the heart. p. 691. In Sperelakis N (ed): Physiology and Pathophysiology of the Heart, Kluwer Academic Publishers, 1989

61. Simpson RW, Edwards WD: Pathogenesis of cocaine-induced ischemic heart disease. Arch Pathol Lab Med 110:479, 1986

62. Spray TL, Roberts WC: Changes in saphenous veins used as aortocoronary bypass grafts. Am Heart J 94:500, 1977

63. Bulkley BH, Hutchins GM: Pathology of coronary artery bypass graft surgery. Arch Pathol Lab Med 102:273, 1978

64. Sawyer PN, Kaplitt MJ: Vascular Grafts. Appleton & Lange, East Norwalk, CT, 1978

65. McAllister HA Jr, Fenoglio JJ: Tumors of the cardiovascular system. In Atlas of Tumor Pathology. 2nd Ed. Armed Forces Institute of Pathology, Washington, 1978

66. McAllister HA, Jr, Hall RJ, Cooley DA: Surgical pathology of tumors and cysts of the heart and pericardium. p. 343. In Waller BF (ed): Pathology of the Heart and Great Vessels. Churchill Livingstone, New York, 1988

67. Ferrans VJ, Roberts WC: Structural features of cardiac myxomas. Hum Pathol 4:111, 1973

68. Fenoglio JJ, Diana DJ, Bowen TE, et al: Ultrastructure of a cardiac rhabdomyoma. Hum Pathol 8:700, 1977

69. Fenoglio JJ, McAllister HA Jr, Ferrans VJ: Cardiac rhabdomyoma: A clinicopathologic and electron microscopic study. Am J Cardiol 38:241, 1976

70. Hui G, McAllister HA Jr, Angelini P: Left atrial paraganglioma: Report of a case and review of the literature. Am Heart J 113:1230, 1987

22

The Oral Cavity

Robert O. Greer, Jr.

THE NATURE AND HANDLING OF SURGICAL SPECIMENS FROM THE ORAL CAVITY

The vast majority of tissue samples received from the oral cavity will represent one of the following: (1) excisional biopsy, (2) incisional biopsy, (3) bone biopsy, (4) aspiration biopsy, (5) punch biopsy, (6) exfoliative cytology, and (7) curettage biopsy.

The punch biopsy specimen is rarely encountered because of the nearly unlimited access that the clinician has to oral sites using a scalpel. The aspiration or needle biopsy is typically used in the oral cavity to obtain fluid from a cavity of soft tissue or bone for chemical analysis.

Bone biopsy specimens are commonly encountered material from the oral cavity. The hard tissue, of course, requires decalcification before processing. The tissue sample sizes that the surgical pathologist must deal with are frequently rather small (less than 1 cm in diameter). Commercial rapid decalcification solutions can be used; however, they tend to compromise cellular detail. Five percent nitric acid in neutral buffered formalin can be a reasonable alternative; decalcification of course takes longer, but cytologic detail is maintained. The tissue is considered properly decalcified when the decalcification solution that has been in contact with the hard tissue is mixed with 5 ml of ammonium hydroxide and 5 percent ammonium oxalate and a clear solution results. A cloudy or milky solution indicates that further decalcification is necessary. Tissue submitted as curettings from a tooth socket often contain bone fragments. It is wise to decalcify this material to avoid sectioning difficulty.

Most soft tissue biopsy specimens from the oral cavity are small elliptical or wedge-shaped samples. If the tissue is received unfixed, it may be necessary to place thin, flat biopsy specimens (e.g., floor of the mouth lesions) on a thin sheet of cardboard to prevent folding.

In suspected vesiculobullous lesions, overaggressive handling of the delicate tissue can cause separation of epithelium from the underlying connective tissue, which of course impairs histopathologic interpretation.

Teeth are frequently only examined grossly. Often when teeth are submitted, the surgeon is interested in the microscopic findings in soft tissue attachments to the root or crown of the tooth (e.g., dentigerous cyst, periapical cyst, odontogenic keratocyst). It is of paramount importance to submit the attached soft tissue when such differential diagnoses are entertained by the submitting doctor.

Frozen section specimens are handled in much the same manner as tissue from elsewhere throughout the body. Anatomically, considerable fatty tissue can be encountered in oral soft tissue specimens. These can be difficult samples on which to prepare frozen sections. The smaller the quantity of adipose tissue included, the simpler the sectioning process.

Very often artifact occurs as a result of the handling of oral tissues. Several types of artifact can be encountered, including crush artifact, which occurs most commonly in the manipulation of the tissue when it is removed by using forceps or dull scalpel blades. This type of artifact is very dangerous in that it alters tissue morphology and squeezes the chromatin out of the cell nuclei.[1] Inflammatory and tumor cells are the most susceptible to crush damage, and therefore this artifact can render an otherwise adequate specimen nondiagnostic. To prevent crush artifact, tissue has to be handled very delicately, both at removal and at the surgical bench.

A second very common artifact seen in oral tissue specimens is electrosurgery artifact. Electrosurgery of course provides adequate and prompt tissue hemostasis when a tissue sample is removed; however, the effect of electrosurgery on the tissue cytologically is to cauterize it, thereby precipitating protein and causing the resultant cauterization artifact, which microscopically appears as coagulated or shredded tissue. A third type of artifact seen in oral tissue samples is the artifact produced by the application of dyes or colored medicaments to the tissues at the time of surgery. Such medicaments can be introduced by the injection of a local anesthetic in or around the biopsy site. A fourth kind of artifact is dehydration artifact caused by improper fixatives or air drying of the specimen. Ten percent neutral buffered formalin remains the fixative of choice for routine biopsy specimens. The last type of artifact that can inadvertently occur in oral tissue samples is freezing artifact. This frequently occurs in the winter when outpatient biopsy specimens are sent in for evaluation by mail. Ten percent formalin will freeze at $-11°C$, producing a clefting artifact that appears in the epithelium. Freezing artifact can be avoided by using Lillie's AAF (acetic alcohol formalin); this fixative contains 10 parts 40 percent formaldehyde, 5 parts glacial acetic acid, and 5 parts absolute ethyl alcohol. The solution will not freeze until it reaches $-30°C$.[1]

Many of the vesiculobullous diseases of skin and mucous membranes are mediated by immunologic injury. *Immunofluorescence* has thus become increasingly valuable in the study of the mucous membrane diseases. Immunomicroscopic techniques that are commonly used for detecting tissue-bound immunoreactants include: (1) direct immunofluorescence; (2) direct immunoperoxidase; and (3) the peroxidase/antiperoxidase (PAP) technique.[2]

Direct immunofluorescence is the most commonly accepted technique for evaluating mucous membrane tissue samples for vesiculobullous disease. Specimens must be received in a fresh state, unfixed. Tissue may be submitted in Michel's solution or snap-frozen in liquid nitrogen as soon as possible after excision. The preferred biopsy technique involves submission of perilesional tissue. Direct lesional biopsies are not recommended for immunofluorescence evaluation, except for disseminated lupus erythematosus and vasculitis. Lesions from blistering diseases usually contain so much cellular damage that it is frequently impossible to determine if there is a deposit of immunoreactants. A lesional biopsy extending into perilesional mucosa can be bisected to provide satisfactory biopsies for routine hematoxylin and eosin (H&E) evaluation and immunofluorescent evaluation.

Immunohistochemical evaluation of suspected viral oral diseases (papilloma, condyloma, and some epithelial dysplasias) is becoming increasingly important.[3] The PAP technique is extremely sensitive and is suitable for light and electron microscopic examination. Formalin-fixed tissue can be used for in situ DNA hybridization for viral protein, while examination by Southern blot methods requires fresh tissue.

HISTOLOGIC AND TAXONOMIC CONSIDERATIONS

The mucous membrane that lines the oral cavity and contiguous structures is composed of a layer of stratified squamous epithelium, which overlies a fibrous connective tissue lamina propria and fibrofatty submucosa. Nerves, capillaries, and minor salivary glands are abundant throughout the supporting connective tissue. Subjacent to the mucous membrane, one may encounter muscle, as in the tongue or buccal mucosa, or bone or cartilage, as in the mandibular or maxillary alveolar processes that support the teeth.

The Tooth Germ Apparatus

To understand the pathology of tumors arising from the tooth germ apparatus, it is necessary to understand the development of the tooth. The developing tooth germ originates as an invagination of a tubular epithelial extension of basal cells from the stomadeal ectoderm overlying the developing alveolar ridges. This tubular extension is composed of cuboidal epithelial cells enveloped by a basal lamina.

The dynamic relationships observed between tissues of the developing odontogenic apparatus are markedly influenced by epitheliomesenchymal interactions. As the dental lamina progressively invades the underlying connective tissue, differentiation at the terminal end ensues. The lamina degenerates to form the inner enamel epithelium, outer enamel epithelium, and a central zone encased by these two epithelial layers. The central region is composed of an aggregate of stellate cells termed the *stellate reticulum*. The inner enamel epithelium differentiates further to become a layer of tall columnar cells with oval nuclei polarized away from the basal lamina. This characteristic cell, an ameloblast, is a hallmark of enamel epithelium. In juxtaposition to this ameloblastic layer and interposed between the ameloblasts and stellate reticulum is an intermediate layer of cuboidal cells termed the *stratum intermedium*.

As the epithelial element differentiates in this fashion, the underlying connective tissue assumes a unique quality. Subjacent to the epithelial cap of the tooth germ is a condensation of mesenchyme, which will become the vital tooth pulp. The cells are spindle-shaped, and the fibrous element is delicate. At this stage a layer of connective tissue cells begins to differentiate in juxtaposition to the ameloblastic layer. These cells are derivatives of the neural crest and are referred to as *ectomesoderm*. At the interface the ectomesodermal cells (odontoblasts) become elongated and begin to elaborate an eosinophilic matrix, which will become dentin, the principal calcified substance of the tooth. Subsequent to the elaboration of a predentin layer by odontoblasts, the ameloblasts begin to synthesize a keratin matrix, which will eventually calcify as enamel, the surface structure of the tooth. The integrated efforts of the odontoblastic and ameloblastic layers eventually generate the crown of the tooth.

The radicular (root) region is formed in a similar fashion, whereby tubular extensions from the enamel epithelium progressively grow deeper into the developing alveolar bone accompanied by continued differentiation of odontoblasts. After dentin is synthesized along this lattice, the epithelial component degenerates. The connective tissue adjacent to the developing root region buttresses the dentin layer, which was previously shielded by an epithelial layer; these mesenchymal cells differenti-

ate into cementoblasts and generate a layer of cementum, which coats the radicular dentin. Sharpey's fibers become inserted into the cemental tissues and pass through the adjacent fibrous tissue, interlacing with fibers inserted into the developing alveolar osseous tissue to create the periodontal ligament of the tooth. As root development proceeds, an eruptive force is created, pushing the tooth toward the surface epithelium until it erupts into the oral cavity.

As tooth development proceeds, remnants of progenitor cells remain entrapped within the jaws. Three primary sources for oncogenic change remain:

1. Remnants of the dental lamina residing in the mature adult gingiva (rests of Serres)
2. Remnants of the radicular epithelial projections of the tooth germ residing throughout the periodontal ligament (rests of Malassez)
3. Remnants of the ameloblastic layer overlying the crown of a tooth that failed to erupt (reduced enamel epithelium surrounding the crown of impacted teeth)

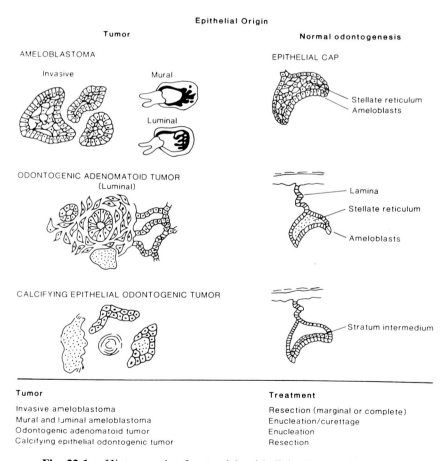

Fig. 22-1. Histogenesis of potential epithelial odontogenic tumors.

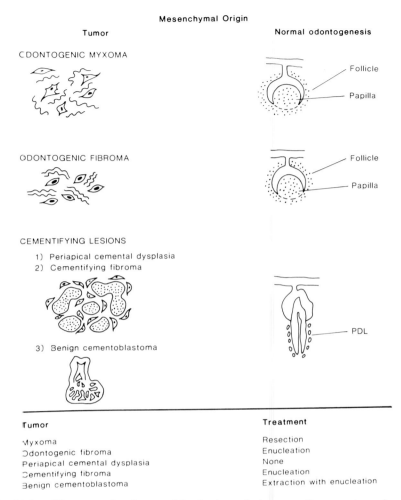

Fig. 22-2. Histogenesis of potential odontogenic tumors of mesenchymal origin.

All these odontogenic epithelial rests can undergo neoplastic transformation. It is theorized that during odontogenic oncogenesis, the epithelial component alone may proliferate; the epithelial component may influence surrounding connective tissue to differentiate and to proliferate in the absence of the epithelium itself; or the neoplasm may recapitulate tooth formation by neoplastic proliferation of both epithelial and mesenchymal tissues. These three possibilities account for classifying tumors as epithelial, mesenchymal, or mixed neoplasms, respectively. Figures 22-1 to 22-3 delineate the proposed histogenesis and treatment of odontogenic neoplasms.

CYSTS OF ODONTOGENIC ORIGIN

The bulk of the cysts that arise from odontogenic epithelium are classified as developmental cysts. In the broadest sense, a cyst that occurs at the root apex in association with a nonvital tooth is also odontogenic in origin, but custom continues to dictate that such cysts are classified as inflammatory cysts. Odontogenic cysts can develop during any stage of odontogenesis, including development within the enamel organ, in reduced enamel epithelium, or in epithelial odontogenic remnants. The etiology of cyst formation is unknown. Figure 22-4 is a schema of the various odontogenic cysts.

Primordial Cyst

The primordial cyst is thought to represent about 5 percent of all follicular cysts and between 1.75 and 6 percent of all odontogenic cysts.[4] The primordial cyst is thought to arise via cystic degeneration of the central stellate reticulum of the developing tooth germ before ameloblastic differentiation and the induction of a calcified product. After this cystic change has occurred, the development of a tooth is nullified, and the cyst thus

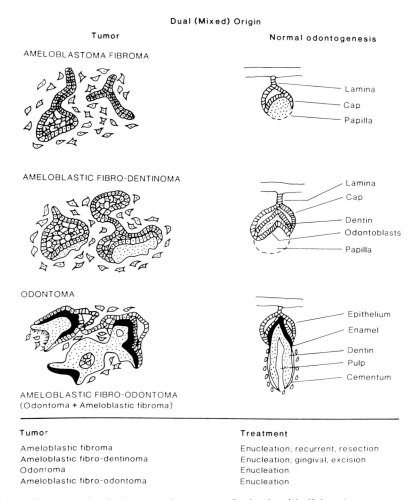

Fig. 22-3. Histogenesis of odontogenic tumors of mixed epithelial and mesenchymal origin.

takes the place of the tooth that would eventually develop. It must be remembered that the primordial cyst may develop from any one of the deciduous or permanent tooth germs, or it may in fact arise from a supernumary tooth germ. Gardner and Sapp[5] and Soskalne and Shear[6] have documented that primordial cysts can also develop from remnants of the dental lamina. Most authorities now believe that this derivation from the dental lamina is probably the most frequent mode of primordial cyst initiation.

Clinical and Radiologic Features

The primordial cyst is typically a lesion of the child or young adult.[7] It is encountered less frequently in adults, but because the lesion grows slowly and usually asymptomatically, it may not be identified until late adulthood. Primordial cysts are most commonly encountered in the mandible, with well over two thirds of the lesions located in the third molar area.[8] There is no apparent sex predilection for the primordial cyst, although a few reports in the world literature document a male predominance.[9,10] These reports presuppose that all primordial cysts are odontogenic keratocysts, an assumption that is not always valid.

The radiologic manifestations of the primordial cyst range from a solitary well circumscribed radiolucency to a large expansile multilocular lesion involving a large segment of the mandible or maxilla[11] (Fig. 22-5). Since other cysts and tumors can have similar appearances, a clinical differential diagnosis of ameloblastoma, odontogenic myxoma, aneurysmal bone cyst, and hemangioma must be entertained.

Pathologic Features

The primordial cyst is typically a sac-like structure lined by a layer of stratified squamous epithelium and

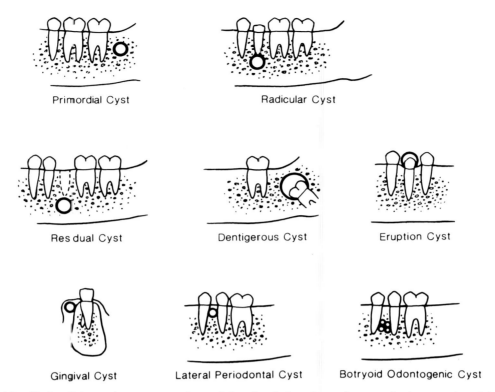

Fig. 22-4. Schematic representatives of the classic locations of cysts of odontogenic origin.

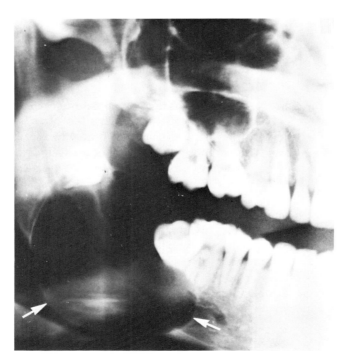

Fig. 22-5. Odontogenic keratocyst (dentigerous type) of the mandible.

supported by a dense relatively avascular connective tissue wall. When the lesion becomes secondarily infected, generally, owing to perforation of the cortical plates of bone, the epithelium may show rete ridge elongation. In such instances the supporting connective tissue will show a generalized inflammatory cell infiltrate.

Frequently, the primordial cyst will display the histologic hallmarks of an odontogenic keratocyst (see the following section). When such features are identified, it is paramount that the clinician and the pathologist understand the biologic behavior differences between the two lesions.

Management of the primordial cyst is discussed in the section on odontogenic keratocyst.

Odontogenic Keratocyst

There has been considerable controversy in the world literature about this cystic lesion since it became a popular term for the primordial cyst. So pervasive has the term *odontogenic keratocyst* become as a synonym for *primordial cyst* that the World Health Organization (WHO) uses the terms interchangeably.[12]

The etiology and pathogenesis of the odontogenic keratocyst remain undetermined although most investigators

THE ORAL CAVITY

suggest that the lesion arises from remnants of the dental lamina. Eversole and associates[13] have suggested that the odontogenic keratocyst and other odontogenic cysts can arise from reduced enamel epithelium as well as from other follicular odontogenic remnants derived from lining epithelial cells. Stoelinga[14] concludes, however, that some of these cysts arise from other sources, perhaps oral epithelium, especially in areas of the mandible such as the ascending ramus, where it is difficult to identify residual dental laminal tissues.

This terminology presupposes that only a cyst arising without association to a tooth can be a keratocyst. Although this may in fact be the general rule, exceptions certainly do occur, and there are numerous well documented reports in the literature that support the fact that dentigerous cysts (those cysts associated with the crown of a tooth)[15] and even residual cysts (those remaining after previous extraction of a tooth or enucleation of a cyst)[16] may have the identical histologic features and a behavioral pattern consistent with that of the insidious odontogenic keratocyst.

A critical fact for the surgical pathologist to remember is that the odontogenic keratocyst may be in direct association with a tooth, or it may occur after tooth extraction. It need not always occur when there is a history of failure of a tooth to develop, as with the primordial variety.

Gardner and Sapp[5] suggest that use of the term *primordial cyst* be discontinued, and that this entity should be viewed purely as a developmental concept. They further suggest that the term *odontogenic keratocyst* be maintained to designate a specific entity with a characteristic microscopic appearance. The latter proposal appears to be a sound one; the former proposal is less acceptable, since although primordial cysts are rare, they nonetheless do occur. To further clarify this confusing issue, a simple and easily understandable sign-out diagnosis that the clinician can appreciate would be "odontogenic keratocyst; primordial, residual, dentigerous, or lateral periodontal type."

Clinical and Radiologic Features

The term *odontogenic keratocyst* was first used by Philipsen[17] in 1956 to describe any odontogenic cyst displaying microscopic keratinization of the epithelial lining. The lesion has since been reported to account for anywhere from 8 to 10 percent of all jaw cysts.[18,19] These cystic lesions show a marked predilection for the posterior body of the mandible and occur most frequently in the second and third decades of life. The lesion shows a variable radiologic pattern (Fig. 22-5). Browne[18] described three distinct radiologic appearances in a series of 83 cases. He documented 56 percent as having a uni-

locular pattern, 20 percent as a solitary cavity with a locular periphery, and 23 percent as multilocular.

The odontogenic keratocyst can have a peripheral radiographic border that is smooth or scalloped. Aggressive lesions may result in displacement of impacted teeth or resorption of the roots of teeth. Extrusion of erupted teeth has also been reported.

The odontogenic keratocyst tends to grow slowly. The patient is frequently symptomless; when a complaint is encountered, it is usually the notation of jaw expansion by the patient, not pain.

Pathologic Features

The salient histologic features of odontogenic keratocyst have been discussed by many authorities but probably were most succinctly described by Gardner and Sapp,[5] who indicate that the following microscopic features are necessary to arrive at a diagnosis: (1) a thin stratified squamous epithelial lining six to eight cells thick, without rete ridge formation; (2) prominent columnar or cuboidal basal cells with dense nuclear staining; (3) a corrugated surface layer of parakeratin, and (4) a thin connective tissue wall (Fig. 22-6).

Not all cysts displaying keratinization are odontogenic keratocysts. One cannot therefore render a diagnosis of odontogenic keratocyst simply because the cyst lumen is filled with keratin. If the salient features described above are not present, the lesion should not be designated an odontogenic keratocyst; it is probably some other form of odontogenic, fissural, or inflammatory jaw cyst.

Two specific histologic variants of the odontogenic keratocyst have been recognized, the parakeratotic and the orthokeratotic subtypes. The predominant form is the parakeratotic.[20] Wright[21] reviewed a series of odontogenic keratocysts and demonstrated a peak incidence in the third decade of life, with a male predominance. The vast majority of the lesions he identified (72 percent) were unilocular. The keratotic variant was found to be somewhat less aggressive than the parakeratotic type and recurred in only 1 of 24 patients, who were followed for periods ranging from 6 months to 8 years.

The high rate of recurrence of this lesion may be related to the frequency of proliferation of daughter cysts in the wall, the penetration or budding of exceedingly thin epithelium into the connective tissue (often resulting in incomplete removal), or the reinitiated proliferation of cyst lining from remnants of the dental lamina.

A frequently noted histologic feature associated with the odontogenic keratocyst has been the separation of the epithelial cyst lining from the supporting connective tissue capsule.[19] Wilson and Ross[22] examined this feature ultrastructurally since it had been hypothesized that the separation very likely accounted for the difficulty in sur-

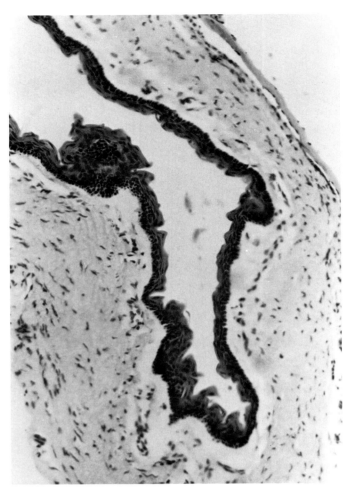

Fig. 22-6. Characteristic parakeratinized corrugated epithelial lining of the odontogenic keratocyst.

gical removal and resultant elevated recurrence rate. These investigators found the basal lamina complex in odontogenic keratocyst to be ultrastructurally normal and could not fully explain the separation phenomenon except to hypothesize that there is somehow increased enzymatic collagen degradation.

Behavior and Management

The most striking clinical feature of the odontogenic keratocyst is its propensity for recurrence. The consistent recurrence rate documented in large reported series is about 25 percent,[18] although reports in the literature range from 6 to 60 percent.[8]

Treatment has ranged from enucleation of unilocular lesions to resection of a considerable portion of the af-

fected jaw in large multilocular, expanding, or erosive lesions.[23]

It has been well documented that odontogenic keratocysts can be a component of the *basal cell nevus syndrome,* with its concomitant multiple cutaneous nevoid basal cell carcinomas and skeletal abnormalities. It is exceedingly important that the clinician and pathologist consider the possibility of this syndrome in any patient with an established diagnosis of odontogenic keratocyst. It is essential to have a high index of syndrome suspicion in patients with multiple odontogenic keratocysts or with a family history of multiple cysts of the jaws.

Botryoid Odontogenic Cyst

The botryoid odontogenic cyst was first described by Weathers and Waldron in 1973.[24] They defined this cyst as an unusual multilocular cyst of the anterior jaw. Since that time very few cases have been reported in the literature, although many authorities consider the lesion to be simply a variant of a lateral periodontal cyst. Kaugars[25] reviewed the limited number of botryoid odontogenic cysts that were available in the literature and found a marked predilection for occurrence in the mandibular canine-premolar region in patients over 50 years of age. The most common symptoms were clinical expansion and tenderness, but occasionally the lesions were asymptomatic.

The botryoid odontogenic cyst is thought to arise from proliferating rests of the dental lamina or displaced rests of Malassez. Kaugers maintains that in order to render a diagnosis of botryoid odontogenic cyst the following criteria are necessary: (1) histologic features similar to those of the lateral periodontal cyst; (2) a multilocular radiographic pattern, which is most often noted but need not absolutely be present; and, (3) there must be no evidence of inflammatory origin from either pulpal or periodontal elements.

The histologic appearance of the botryoid odontogenic cyst is characterized by multiple cystic areas within a lesion showing no evidence of atypia and overlying epithelial keratinization. The polycystic areas are lined by cells with abundant cytoplasm and a lack of keratinization. The cells often pile up in a somewhat lobular pattern extending into the lumen of the cyst and showing linkage and positivity with periodic acid–Schiff (PAS) staining.

The treatment of choice is surgical excision. Because the lesions are often radiographically multilocular, there may be a somewhat increased risk of recurrence or of persistence, and it is recommended that patients who have this diagnosis be given periodic clinical and radiographic examinations.

Calcifying Odontogenic Cyst

Clinical and Radiologic Features

Calcifying odontogenic cyst is a curious lesion first thoroughly described by Gorlin and associates in 1962, although they document that it was reported by Rywland much earlier.[26,27] The calcifying odontogenic cyst typically presents as a slow-growing, asymptomatic central osseous jaw lesion. Extraosseous examples have been documented in the literature, but they represent less than 25 percent of reported lesions.[28,29] The lesion has a marked predilection of the mandible, and although both sexes appear to be equally affected, the lesion appears to occur more frequently in women before the fourth decade and more commonly in men after the fourth decade. Regardless of a maxillary or mandibular occurrence, over 75 percent of the lesions reported in the series of Freedman and associates[28] occurred anterior to the first molar.

Radiologically the intraosseous lesion appears as a unilocular or multilocular cystic radiolucent area. The margins may be well defined or poorly demarcated, and small irregular calcified bodies of varying sizes have been reported in 29 to 37 percent of all reported cases.[30,31]

These calcifications may fill the cyst cavity entirely or may be totally absent; therefore, the presence or absence of such calcifications is of questionable value in unequivocally establishing a radiologic diagnosis. Numerous odontogenic tumors can have radiologic features that are quite similar to the calcifying and keratinizing odontogenic cyst. Such lesions should be included in the radiologic differential diagnosis. They include the calcifying epithelial odontogenic tumor, adenomatoid odontogenic tumor, ameloblastic odontoma, and the so-called cystic odontoma.

Keszler and Gugliemotti[32] reported two calcifying odontogenic cysts associated with odontomas. The WHO International Classification of Odontogenic Tumors and Allied Lesions defies the calcifying odontogenic cyst as a "non-neoplastic lesion that can occur in association with other odontogenic lesions including odontomas."

There has been extended debate in the literature as to whether the calcifying odontogenic cyst represents a cyst or a tumor, since the lesion can present grossly as a cyst or a solid mass. The calcified structures identified radiologically can have the gross appearance of irregular hard tissue fragments or even small teeth or denticle-like structures.

Pindborg and Kramer[12] hold the view that the calcifying odontogenic cyst is non-neoplastic. Gorlin and colleagues[26] have actually demonstrated the lesion originating from the dental epithelium of a developing unerupted tooth. Lesions that develop in an extraosseous site likely develop from remnants of odontogenic epithelium in the gingiva or alveolar mucosa.

Pathologic Features

The calcifying odontogenic cyst can present grossly as a sac-like soft tissue structure or as a solid mass with calcified foci. Histologically, tissue sections reveal a cavity or potential cavity lined by a prominent and well defined basal layer of cuboidal or columnar cells that have some resemblance to ameloblasts. These cells stain deeply basophilic. Overlying the basal epithelial layer, loosely arranged epithelial cells that resemble the central stellate reticulum of the tooth germ can be identified. Interspersed among these cells are large eosinophilic cells, which have been termed *ghost cells* (Fig. 22-7). These cells are thought to have undergone aberrant keratinization, and occasionally they flatten out in a manner similar to normal keratin.[6] The entire lumen of the cyst may be filled with aberrant keratin, and on occasion foreign body giant cell activity is prominent in the cyst lumen and in the supporting capsular connective tissue wall.

Sauk[27] and Freedman and Lumerman[28] have documented that the basal epithelial layer can show prominent budding, and that odontogenic epithelium frequently penetrates deeply into the supporting collagenous wall. Dentin, enamel, and even melanin have been reported proliferating within the wall of calcifying odontogenic cysts.[18]

Behavior and Management

Recurrence of the calcifying odontogenic cyst is exceedingly rare. Even the most conservative form of enucleation appears to be curative. There appears to be little potential for the lesion to develop into an odontogenic tumor, and although there is a single report in the literature of the cyst occurring in association with an ameloblastic fibro-odontoma, there is doubt that the reported case represented a true calcifying odontogenic cyst.[33] The more likely sequence is that the lesion represented cystic change in a true odontogenic tumor.

Dentigerous Cyst

The dentigerous cyst (follicular cyst) is a relatively common odontogenic cyst that occurs in association with the crown of an unerupted tooth. This cyst develops when the enamel-forming apparatus (enamel organ) has been reduced to a few layers of epithelial cells surrounding the tooth crown. Fluid accumulates within the potential follicular space of the organ and a cyst eventuates.

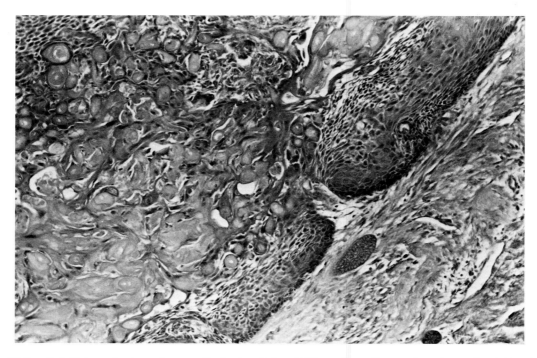

Fig. 22-7. Calcifying odontogenic cyst displaying "ghost"-like cells, adherent keratin, and calcifications. Note prominence of basal epithelial layer.

Typically, the crown of the tooth protrudes into the cystic cavity.

Clinical and Radiologic Features

The dentigerous cyst is most commonly found in association with impacted or partially impacted mandibular third molars, maxillary canine teeth (cuspid teeth), and maxillary third molars. Radiologically, the dentigerous cyst will present as a well defined radiolucent area surrounding the crown of a tooth. The lesion may be displaced to one side of the tooth crown and need not always arise superficial to it.

The radiolucency may be unilocular or multilocular. The lesion has the potential to expand bone, and the cyst may cause extensive destruction of bone, with almost complete replacement of the medullary portion of the ramus and body of the mandible by the cyst.[5] It is not always possible to definitively diagnose a dentigerous cyst radiologically, since odontogenic keratocysts and certain odontogenic tumors such as ameloblastoma and odontogenic myxoma may have similar appearances.

Stanley reviewed a 20 year series of 11,598 radiographs from patients with dentigerous cysts and found little evidence of internal resorption, bone loss adjacent to the distal surface of the approximating second molar teeth, or resorption of adjacent second molars.[34] These data seem to dispute the current practice of early extraction of totally embedded third molars when adverse signs and symptoms are absent. Nonetheless, from a diagnostic point of view a unicystic lesion with clinical and radiologic characteristics of a dentigerous cyst may in fact prove to be an ominous lesion. Ameloblastoma has been shown to be a real consequence of dentigerous cyst formation in South African blacks.

Pathologic Features

Grossly, the lesion will appear as a sac enveloping the tooth. The distinction between a dentigerous cyst and a hyperplastic dental follicle with cystic degeneration is often an arbitrary one because of the histologic similarity between the two. The diagnosis of dentigerous cyst is often based on the size of the gross specimen and the degree of radiologic involvement.

It is extremely important to examine the cyst wall for thickenings and outgrowths since there are well documented instances of ameloblastoma and even squamous cell carcinoma arising in the walls of dentigerous cysts.

Histologically, the dentigerous cyst consists of lining epithelium supported by a fibrous connective tissue wall. The epithelium is generally of the stratified squamous variety and only a few cell layers thick. Occasionally, the cyst may be lined by columnar or mucus-secreting cells.

The cyst wall may be diffusely inflamed or totally free of an inflammatory infiltrate. Frequently, the cyst wall contains extensive cholesterol clefting so as to resemble a radicular or periapical cyst; when this is noted microscopically, only the anatomic location allows one to differentiate between a dentigerous and a periapical cyst.

It is quite common to observe odontogenic epithelial rests in the walls of dentigerous cysts. There is considerable debate as to whether these rests have the potential to develop along neoplastic lines; nonetheless, it is very important to relay to the clinician the presence of rest activity in the walls of all odontogenic cysts. All dentigerous cysts should be examined with multiple histologic sections for ameloblastoma.

Behavior and Management

The dentigerous cyst is most often quite adequately treated by complete surgical excision and curettage. Occasionally, lesions that show extensive bony involvement are managed by multiple surgical enucleation procedures. Recurrence is a possibility in all cysts that have odontogenic epithelial remnants within bone at surgery.

Gingival Cyst

Gingival cysts occur as two distinct entities, those of the new-born and those of the adult.[35] Gingival cysts of the newborn present as single or multiple small white nodules along the crest of the alveolar ridge. These excrescences have been variously reported in the literature as microcysts of the gingiva,[30] Bohn's nodules, and Epstein's pearls.[36] These outgrowths in fact represent cystic degeneration of remnants of the dental lamina. They are usually asymptomatic and exfoliated without consequence. Histologically, they appear as keratin-filled cysts lined by stratified squamous epithelium.

Gingival cysts of the adult are quite common. They also are thought to originate from dental lamina remnants. Gardner and Sapp[5] point out that these lesions may also arise from traumatic implantation of surface epithelium from the oral cavity into the underlying connective tissue. The most frequent site for the gingival cyst of the adult is in the mandibular cuspid and premolar area; interestingly, this is a frequent site for supernumerary teeth as well. Gingival cysts usually present clinically as painless swellings. Histologically, the gingival cyst of the adult mimics that of the newborn. Gingival cysts have little, if any, potential for recurrence, and simple excision is curative.

INFLAMMATORY, FISSURAL, AND NONODONTOGENIC CYSTS

Radicular Cysts

Radicular cysts account for approximately 10 percent of all inflammatory cysts.[37] The radicular cyst is far and away the most common cyst of the jaws. It is also known as periapical cyst, apical periodontal cyst, and dental cyst. Classically, the lesion is the end result of extensive dental caries and pulpal death.

When a carious lesion extends uncontrolled beyond the hard tissue of the tooth, the pulp subsequently becomes inflamed. Ultimately, the process can extend along the root canal of the tooth, beyond the apical foramen, and into the periapical ligamental tissues and bone. The localized inflammatory process that results from the extension of noxious stimuli beyond the apex of the tooth is typically called an *apical granuloma*. It is, of course, not a true granuloma, but an accumulation of chronic inflammatory granulation tissue. Epithelial rests (rests of Malassez) are commonly found around the root apices, and as the inflammatory process continues, these rests frequently proliferate as strands of epithelium into the granulation tissue, with subsequent central degeneration and ultimate cyst formation.

Clinical and Radiologic Features

By the time a periapical cyst has formed, the patient is usually symptom-free. Typically, the pulp is dead and the tooth is nonvital. Radicular cysts expand slowly, and there is usually little if any expansion of the jaw associated with them.

Radiologically, the lesion will present as a fairly well circumscribed area of radiolucency at the root apex. It is impossible to determine from radiologic findings alone whether the lesion represents a periapical cyst, periapical granuloma, or some other form of pathologic alteration.

Pathologic Features

The surgical specimen usually consists of fragments of glistening or granular soft tissue. Rarely is the tooth removed with the cyst intact. If surgical root canal therapy has been performed, the periapical remnants may be submitted as fragments from the surgical site. The cyst lining is only rarely appreciated as a shiny surface, and a lumen containing fluid or cheesy material is seen only when the specimen is submitted intact.

Microscopically, one usually finds fragments of lining and penetrating squamous epithelium supported by a diffusely and chronically inflamed connective tissue wall.

Cholesterol clefts are frequently present in the cyst lumen or wall. Foam cells, plasma cells, lymphocytes, and foreign body type giant cells are also commonly identified. Hyalinized Rushton bodies, thought to be unique to odontogenic cysts, can be identified in about 10 percent of the lesions.[38] This unique finding is often helpful in attempting to separate odontogenic from fissural cysts.

The *residual cyst* is thought to represent a cystic remnant that remains in the jaw after the associated tooth or teeth have been extracted. Most often this term is used to indicate that the lesion is a residual radicular cyst; however, a residual cyst could certainly occur after incomplete removal of any cystic lesion. Most residual radicular cysts remain asymptomatic within the jaws and are only identified via a routine radiologic examination of the area.

Radicular cysts are not considered to have the potential to differentiate along odontogenic tumor lines as do the odontogenic keratocyst and dentigerous cyst. Exceedingly rare cases of squamous cell carcinoma have been reported, apparently arising in association with the wall of radicular cysts.[39]

Fissural Cysts

For decades it has been postulated that fissural cysts are those cysts that arise from remnants of epithelium that were trapped within fusion lines during formation of the face or from remnants of embryologic ductal elements. A schematic representation of the anatomic sites of each of these cysts is presented in Figure 22-8.

Today, there is debate as to whether fissural cysts do in fact develop from epithelial entrapment.[40-42] It has been documented that epithelial entrapment along suture lines occurs only along the medial palatal raphe, leading to the conclusion that the classification of fissural cysts is more a deference to convenience than to developmental biology.[5]

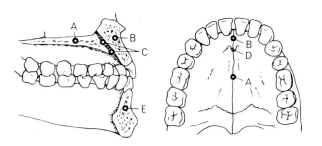

Fig. 22-8. Diagram illustrating the location of the various fissural cysts of the jaws. (A and B) Median palatine cyst; (C) nasopalatine duct cyst (incisive canal cyst); (D) cyst of the palatine papilla; (E) median mandibular cyst.

Nasopalatine Duct Cyst

The nasopalatine duct cyst, also known as the *incisive canal cyst,* is the most commonly encountered of the fissural cysts. It is thought to be derived from residua of the nasopalatine duct, an embryonic structure that actually is housed within the incisive canal of the maxilla.

Clinical and Radiological Features

Linear radiologic surveys of large groups of patients indicate that the nasopalatine duct cyst occurs in approximately 1 percent of those persons examined.[43] The lesions commonly present as well circumscribed, oval, heart-shaped, or occasionally elliptical radiolucencies behind the central incisors in the midmaxilla.

Clinically, an obvious intraoral swelling can be identified, but rarely is the lesion symptomatic unless it is secondarily infected.

At times it is rather difficult to separate a true nasopalatine duct cyst from the normal radiologic shadow of the incisive canal. Gardner and Sapp[5] suggest that any lesion with a diameter greater than 6 mm should certainly be suggestive of a cyst. Cysts occurring in this same area that are wholly within soft tissue and present no radiologic picture are known as *cysts of palatine papilla.* Exceedingly large nasopalatine duct cysts with extensive posterior limits have been variously referred to as *median palatal cysts* or *midpalatine cysts.*

Pathologic Features

Microscopically, the cyst is seen as an epithelially lined cavity rimmed by stratified squamous or respiratory epithelium. Occasionally, mucous glands, cartilage, bone, and nerve bundles are identified within or adjacent to the supporting connective tissue wall.

Nasopalatine duct cysts are treated by surgical enucleation and seldom recur.

Globulomaxillary Cyst

Clinical and Radiologic Features

The globulomaxillary cyst is a relatively uncommon fissural cyst, which develops between the lateral incisor and cuspid teeth in the anterior maxilla. The cyst, which is usually symptomless, is most often identified during a routine dental radiologic survey as a well delineated pear- or heart-shaped radiolucency, which frequently causes the roots of the cuspid and lateral incisor teeth to diverge.

Historically, the globulomaxillary cyst has been considered to be a lesion that arises from entrapped epithelial remnants between the globular portion of the medial nasal process and the maxillary process during the development of the face.[5,43] Christ,[41] however, believes that these cystic lesions develop from odontogenic (tooth germ) epithelium and further postulates that the origin could very reasonably be the epithelium from a supernumerary tooth germ. Cherrick[43] indicates that the globulomaxillary cyst accounts for 3 percent of all the cysts found within the jaws and is typically seen before the age of 30.

A host of lesions should be included in the differential diagnosis of the globulomaxillary cyst. Lesions such as the adenomatoid odontogenic tumor, odontogenic keratocyst, and central giant cell granuloma can all present as asymptomatic radiolucent swellings in this area, and thus all should be considered on clinical grounds.

It is exceedingly important for the surgical pathologist to ascertain whether teeth adjacent to the lesion are vital; if they are not, then the likelihood of the lesion being a routine radicular cyst greatly outweighs the chances of the lesion representing a globulomaxillary cyst.

Pathologic Features

The globulomaxillary cyst most often appears histologically as a cystic cavity lined by stratified squamous, cuboidal, or pseudostratified ciliated columnar epithelium. The supporting connective tissue may show varying degrees of chronic inflammation.

The globulomaxillary cyst is managed by surgical enucleation and rarely recurs.

Nasolabial Cyst

The nasolabial cyst (*nasoalveolar cyst*) is a lesion of soft tissue rather than bone. It is thought to arise from fissural epithelium or residual epithelium derived from the nasolacrimal or nasopalatine duct.

Clinical and Radiological Features

The cyst will usually present as a swelling in the nasolabial fold or as a swelling within the nostril itself. The patient may complain of fullness in the area of the upper lip; pain is seldom a presenting symptom. The lesion may become so large that it totally fills the intraoral labial sulcus. Radiologically, there are usually no findings, unless the lesion has become so large that pressure resorption of the underlying alveolar bone has occurred. Although the majority of nasolabial cysts are unilateral, bilateral occurrences have been documented.

Nearly three quarters of all documented cases of nasolabial cyst have occurred in females.

Pathologic Features

The nasolabial cyst may be lined by stratified squamous, cuboidal, or respiratory-type epithelium. Goblet secretory cells are also frequently encountered within the more prominent squamous epithelial lining. The supporting wall is generally one of avascular, often hyaline-appearing collagen.

For nasolabial cysts, the management modality of choice is surgical enucleation; recurrence is uncommon.

Lymphoepithelial Cyst

The lymphoepithelial cyst (*branchial cleft cyst*) is thought to arise as a result of a developmental entrapment phenomenon. A popular developmental theory is that the cyst arises from crypts of lymphoid tissue that become occluded, resulting in ultimate cystic proliferation of the epithelium.[44] A second theory is that during embryogenesis, epithelium of glandular or ductal origin becomes included with lymphoid tissue, and subsequently this glandular epithelium undergoes cystic proliferation.[45,46]

Clinical Features

The cyst is most often encountered in the floor of the mouth; in addition it has been reported in nearly all other oral sites and in the parotid gland. Lymphoepithelial cysts are usually described clinically as freely movable nodular masses that are totally asymptomatic.

Pathologic Features

Most lymphoepithelial cysts are relatively small. Guinta and Cataldo[46] reviewed a series of 21 lesions and found the average lesion to measure only 6 mm in diameter. The mucosal surface usually appears normal. On sectioning, one may encounter yellow "cheesy material."

The histopathologic findings are rather consistent. Underlying normal oral epithelium is a cyst that is usually lined by a thin, flattened layer of stratified squamous epithelium. The lumen is usually filled with amorphous eosinophilic coagulum, proteinaceous debris, and varying degrees of inflammatory cells. Subjacent to the epithelium one finds well-organized lymphoid tissue, usually encircling the entire cyst. The lymphoid tissue, which often has a typical follicular pattern, is distributed throughout a supporting wall of loose areolar connective tissue.

Total surgical excision is the treatment of choice. In most large reported series, long-term follow-up has documented little tendency for recurrence.[46]

The lymphoepithelial cyst may also occur in the preauricular region in the parotid gland.[47] Very rarely, branchial carcinomas have been reported in lymphoepithelial cysts.[48,49]

Thyroglossal Duct Cyst

The thyroglossal duct cyst is a rather uncommon cyst that is thought to arise from residual epithelium after formation of the thyroid gland Entrapment of this epithelium occurs during a period when the thyroglossal duct extends as a hollow tract from the foramen cecum at the base of the tongue to the thyroid gland. The cyst is commonly identified in close approximation and subjacent to the hyoid bone.

Thyroglossal duct cysts tend to be midline structures, typically arising as subcutaneous soft tissue swellings.

Pathologic Features

The typical thyroglossal duct cyst is lined by ciliated respiratory epithelium, pseudostratified columnar epithelium, or squamous epithelium. The supporting wall of the cyst will frequently contain accumulations of chronic inflammatory cells, and occasionally thyroid acini can be found in the cyst wall. Occasionally mucous glands can be found in the wall. A few instances of carcinoma arising in thyroglossal remnants have been documented. The most common malignancies have been papillary adenocarcinomas.[8] As a differential diagnosis, the rare *thymic cyst* also has to be considered in the face of a midline neck swelling and a biopsy specimen that shows a cystic cavity. Usually, recognizable thymic tissue allows the separation of these two entities.

Surgical excision is the treatment of choice for thyroglossal duct cysts.

Mucocele

Clinical and Radiologic Features

The mucocele (*mucus extravasation phenomenon, mucous retention cyst*) is a common lesion that typically presents as an asymptomatic swelling with a central collection of mucus. Frequently, mucoceles have a so-called blue dome appearance. The etiology of the mucocele has been the subject of considerable scrutiny. One theory postulates that the mucocele occurs as a result of a salivary ductal stenosis or obstruction, which ultimately results in the accumulation of mucin and ductal dilatation that presents clinically as a swelling. This theory assumes that all mucoceles would therefore be epithelially lined; in fact when they are examined closely, most are not. A second theory suggests that some mucoceles result as a consequence of true rupture of the salivary gland duct system, allowing extravasation or precipitation of mucus into the surrounding connective tissue and submucosa. This theory suggests that most mucoceles are not therefore true mucous cysts because they have no epithelial lining.

The most frequent site for the mucocele is the labial mucosa of the lower lip. The upper lip is seldom, if ever, affected, probably because it is not subjected to the amount or degree of trauma that the lower lip and its minor salivary glands receive.

Cysts similar to mucoceles have been reported in the maxillary sinus, including the *mucous retention cyst* of the maxillary sinus and the *surgical ciliated cyst* of the maxilla. The former lesion is best visualized on panoramic radiographs as a smooth, uniform, ovoid dome-shaped radiopacity of the sinus. The surgical ciliated cyst generally occurs as a unilocular or multilocular cystic lesion arising after surgical entry into the maxillary sinus. The maxillary sinus mucous retention cyst fails to have an epithelial lining and is instead lined by flattened fibroblasts and occasionally histiocytes. The surgical ciliated cyst is typically lined by respiratory-type epithelium.

Pathologic Features

Histologically, the typical microscopic picture is that of benign squamous epithelium overlying a connective tissue lamina propria that contains either a dilated duct-like structure that is rimmed by flattened fibroblasts or, very rarely, epithelium. The channel-like structure will contain extravasated mucin, proteinaceous debris, and acute and chronic inflammatory cells. Mucoceles may present in a manner such that all that is identified histologically is extravasated mucin and inflammatory cells in a connective tissue stroma. Minor salivary gland acinar and ductal structures may be identified deep or lateral to the extravasated mucin.

Another common histologic feature is granulation tissue; in fact, it frequently fills central areas of mucoceles, so that 80 to 90 percent of the tissue sample may represent granulation tissue with very little evidence of extravasated mucin. A differential diagnosis that must be entertained in such instances is pyogenic granuloma, and frequently it is difficult to differentiate pyogenic granuloma from mucocele on the basis of histologic characteristics alone.

At times it is difficult to distinguish a mucocele from a low-grade mucoepidermoid tumor histologically. In such instances it is important to remember that grossly the mucoepidermoid tumor will nearly always have the appearance of a solid mass even when a large portion of the tumor is quite mucinous. The mucocele almost always manifests as a cyst.

Behavior and Management

Treatment is often a problem with mucoceles because treatment necessitates total removal of the damaged gland in addition to the associated cystic lining. If the gland is not removed as well as the cyst, mucus may continue to be extravasated into the tissues, and the mucocele will frequently recur. Two management modalities have been used. Most often, total surgical excision of the mucocele and the gland will remove the cause and the pathologic condition. A second surgical procedure that is often used is a marsupialization procedure whereby the cyst is collapsed and its contents aspirated. Alginate is injected into the lesion so it becomes firm and the anatomic outline can be adequately visualized. Finally, excision at the borders of the alginate is used. The technique of marsupialization is one that is reserved for large lesions, typically in the floor of the mouth. The *ranula* is a type of mucocele that is found in the floor of the mouth. The ranula typically develops in either of the two manners that a mucocele does, and surgical excision or marsupialization are the treatment modalities of choice.

BENIGN AND MALIGNANT ODONTOGENIC TUMORS

Benign Epithelial Odontogenic Tumors

Ameloblastoma

Ameloblastoma (adamantinoma) is an odontogenic neoplasm, the etiology of which is unknown. Some authorities believe that the lesion arises in association with the difficult eruption of a third molar or in association with a previous infection or cyst. Hertz[50] and Forsberg[51] suggest that trauma or inflammation are common etiologic agents. Tumors that appear to be histologically compatible with ameloblastoma in humans have been produced in mice by the injection of polyoma virus extracts.[52-54]

Although the root *amelo* is derived from the old French word for enamel, there is little consensus about the histogenesis of the ameloblastoma. Most investigators agree that the tumor is derived from odontogenic epithelium or certain derivatives or residua thereof. The histomorphologic structure is reminiscent of the dental lamina as it penetrates the ectomesenchyme of the forming fetal jaw and differentiates into the epithelial enamel organ.[55] The dental lamina thus remains the most likely parent tissue.[56] The most convincing support for a dental lamina origin centers around the fact that the biologic and physiologic characteristics of the tumor remarkably parallel

those of the dental lamina, a structure that continued to grow from surface oral epithelium, pushing out columns of epithelial cells in an orderly fashion into the supporting connective tissue until the site of ultimate tooth germ formation is reached within bone.

Other sources have been suggested as potential tissues of origin for the ameloblastoma. They include surface oral epithelium, odontogenic cyst epithelium, epithelial rests of Malassez, and the enamel organ.[56] All these, except the enamel organ origin, remain reasonable and likely tissues of origin.[56] Perhaps the most convincing factor against direct enamel organ origin is the fact that enamel deposition is conspicuously absent from the histopathologic features of the ameloblastoma.

Less than 2 percent of all odontogenic tumors and cysts are estimated to be ameloblastoma, yet the lesion continues to fascinate pathologists because of its diversity of microscopic features and surgeons because of its defiance of complete eradication.

Clinical and Radiologic Features

Sehdev and associates[57] have compiled the most complete single review of the clinicopathologic statistics on ameloblastoma. They reviewed 92 lesions, the vast majority of which occurred in the mandible. Maxillary ameloblastomas accounted for slightly less than 20 percent of their reported cases, consistent with other large reported series in the literature.[58] Men and women appear to be affected in nearly equal numbers, and the vast majority of all tumors show a peak incidence in the third and fourth decades.

Painless swelling is the most common early symptom of ameloblastoma in either jaw. Sehdev et al.[57] found that in 14 of 20 patients with maxillary ameloblastoma, the duration of symptoms was less than one year. Nasal obstruction and epistaxis occurred late in the course of the disease. In mandibular ameloblastomas, the typical lesion presents as a slowly expanding swelling that usually causes thin-walled, bulging cortical plates. The lesion appears to be a locally invasive tumor that has a tendency to recur if surgical removal is inadequate. It is estimated that 30 to 35 percent of all ameloblastomas arise within the wall of or in association with a follicular cyst.[59] There appears to be no racial predilection for ameloblastoma.

Radiologically, the majority of ameloblastomas present as intraosseous multilocular or soap-bubble-type radiolucencies, which may communicate with the oral cavity via destruction of the cortical plates (Fig. 22-9). Occasionally, the lesions can have a unilocular cystic presentation, or the crown of a tooth may be found in association with the tumor. In the latter instance the lesion may appear to have a radiopaque quality, but if calcifications are found radiologically, the lesion is probably not an amelo-

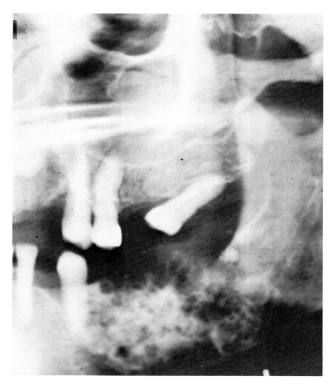

Fig. 22-9. Note the multilocular radiologic appearance of ameloblastoma. (Courtesy of Richard Nelson, D.D.S.)

blastoma. When establishing a differential diagnosis for ameloblastoma on the basis of radiologic information, it is important to remember that lesions such as central giant cell granuloma, aneurysmal bone cyst, odontogenic myxoma, and odontogenic keratocyst may all have similar radiologic appearances.

Pathologic Features

Typically, the tissue sample that is received consists of a solid gray-white tumor mass and a margin of peripheral bone. Resection may include the teeth at the periphery of the resected specimen. The lesion usually appears as an expansile lesion within bone; it may have perforated the cortical plate. When this has occurred, there may be extraosseous tumor beyond the bony margins proliferating into soft tissue structures. On sectioning, the tumor tissue is usually gray-white to gray-brown, depending on the amount of central hemorrhage within the tumor itself. It cuts readily, although there may be a gritty consistency to the tissue. Ameloblastomas do not contain a calcified product, and therefore hard tissue structures of the tooth will not be identified histologically. Occasionally, the tissue sample submitted is a cyst. In such instances one frequently finds a sac-like lining with elevated white nodular areas within; the white nodular areas often represent

mural ameloblastoma proliferation. It is important for the pathologist to examine all of the tissue sample in order not to miss any neoplastic proliferation in the wall of a cyst.

Classically, five histologic patterns have been described for ameloblastoma. The "follicular" variant is composed of tumor epithelium arranged in islands or sheets with a central area of polyhedral cells that resemble primitive stellate reticulum (Fig. 22-10). The plexiform or reticular pattern consists of irregular strands of epithelium bordered by columnar cells that surround an admixture of cells resembling stellate reticulum. The basal cell, granular cell, and acanthomatous variants contain central cells that have a basaloid, granular, or squamous or keratinaceous character, respectively.

Waldron and El Mofty[60] recently reviewed a series of 116 ameloblastomas and identified 14 examples of a new *desmoplastic* variant. The histologic features described for this lesion were unique, characterized by a rather extensive collagenized stroma containing small islands of true epithelium with a rare tendency to form cystic structures. The lesion was most often identified in the anterior portions of the jaws and (rather uncharacteristically for ameloblastoma), half of the examples occurred in the maxilla.

Cystic degeneration is not uncommon within the central portion of the epithelial component of ameloblastomas. Of the five major histologic types of ameloblastoma, the follicular and plexiform patterns appears to be the most frequently encountered on microscopic inspection. Quite frequently, a tumor shows one or more patterns throughout multiple sections of the tumor mass as it proliferates as either sheets, nests, cords, or anastomosing strands of neoplastic epithelium into a well vascularized

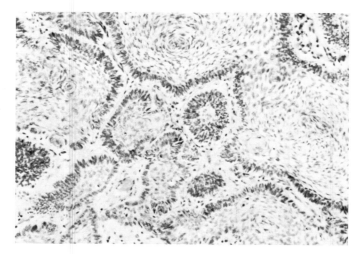

Fig. 22-10. Follicular ameloblastoma. Note discrete islands and nests of tumor cells set in loose collagenous stroma.

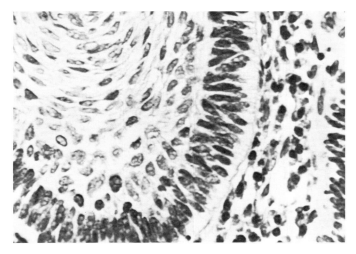

Fig. 22-11. Ameloblastoma. Neoplastic islands showing peripheral columnar cells with apically polarized nuclei and central reticular areas. Note distinct resemblance to immature enamel organ.

connective tissue stroma. Cells that rim individual tumor islands are usually columnar or cuboidal cells resembling preameloblasts (Fig. 22-11). Individual tumor cells usually have oval to vesicular nuclei that are polarized toward the central portion of the follicular tumor nests. The cytoplasm ranges from granular to homogeneous; it is usually eosinophilic. Mitotic activity is minimal in most tissue sections.

Plexiform Unicystic Ameloblastoma

Gardner and Corio[61] coined the term *plexiform unicystic ameloblastoma* in 1984 to describe a variant of ameloblastoma with a low recurrence rate that usually arose in the posterior mandible. Clinically, most of these lesions had previously been thought to be dentigerous cysts. Eversole and Leider[62] further characterized the lesion as *cystogenic ameloblastoma,* with findings similar to those of Gardner and Corio except that their cases demonstrated that the lesion did not have to be radiographically unilocular and could, in fact, be multilocular. Although the plexiform unicystic ameloblastoma is most often associated with unerupted teeth, it can arise in relationship to an erupted tooth.

Histologically, it is a neoplasm composed of an anastomosing network of stratified squamous epithelium within a delicate connective tissue stroma. The basal cells of this epithelium do not exhibit the changes of early ameloblastoma. Instead, a network is recognized of elongated interlacing epithelial strands that often show basal layer budding. Epithelial odontogenic rests are commonly present in the wall of the cystic lesion. This variant of ameloblastoma has been given separate consideration because it manifests a less aggressive behavior and more favorable prognosis than the classic intraosseous ameloblastoma.

Gardner and colleagues recommend that the surgical site of a plexiform unicystic ameloblastoma be radiographed annually for 10 years following surgery. Should the lesion recur, the appropriate treatment should involve an *en bloc* resection with a 1 to 1.5 cm margin of normal bone.

Only within recent years has a malignant potential for ameloblastoma been described.[63] The so-called malignant ameloblastoma is discussed in detail later in this chapter.

Differential Diagnosis

Ameloblastoma is frequently confused histologically with ameloblastic fibroma. Considerable care should be taken to separate the two entities because the ameloblastic fibroma behaves in a much less aggressive manner than ameloblastoma, and management is correspondingly more conservative. The ameloblastic fibroma is composed of both epithelial and mesenchymal tooth germ components. Like the ameloblastoma, it produces no calcified dental structure. Histologically, ameloblastic fibroma consists of islands and cords of odontogenic epithelium that resemble the dental lamina of early tooth development. The stroma is generally composed of fibromyxoid embryonic connective tissue, which closely resembles the dental papilla of a developing tooth germ. Both the epithelial and mesenchymal components of the lesion are considered neoplastic. A useful histologic feature that separates ameloblastic fibroma from ameloblastoma is the fact that the supporting stroma of the former remains primitive and quite cellular, whereas the connective tissue stroma of the ameloblastoma more closely resembles mature collagen. Ameloblastic fibroma also occurs in a much younger age group than ameloblastoma, with an average age of 15.5 years.[64] The mean age of patients with ameloblastoma is about two decades older. Conservative surgical excision remains the treatment of choice, although Trodahl[64] has emphasized that the tumor may have a higher recurrence potential than was previously appreciated.

Although the vast majority of ameloblastomas arise centrally within bone, 22 documented cases of *peripheral (soft tissue) ameloblastoma* had been reported in the literature by 1983. Since that time numerous additional cases have been reported.[65–67] Perhaps the most interesting recent reports involve documentation of a peripheral ameloblastoma of the buccal mucosa, bringing the total number of such cases reported in the world's literature to three.[65] The distinction between basal cell carcinoma and peripheral ameloblastoma in this site is often difficult.

Woo et al.[65] conclude that the histology of the peripheral ameloblastoma is so similar to that of basal cell carcinoma that the distinction ' peripheral ameloblastoma'' may simply represent a semantic preference. The origin of both lesions in the oral cavity is either from pluripotential cells of the basal cell layer or from native or ectopic epithelial rests.

The extraosseous ameloblastoma shows a distinct mandibular predilection. Of the first 22 documented cases, 10 occurred between the ages of 30 and 50. The recommended treatment is excision with a small margin of normal tissue and re-examination of the surgical site periodically.

The *craniopharyngioma* is a rare lesion found in the bone beneath the sella turcica. It is histologically similar to ameloblastoma and is often referred to as a pituitary ameloblastoma. The origins of the two tumors are somewhat similar since Rathke's pouch does originate embryologically by invagination of oral epithelium. One microscopic feature of the craniopharyngioma not generally found in ameloblastoma is the almost universal occurrence of irregular calcified masses of bone and/or cartilage in the former.[68] The craniopharyngioma also tends to occur before the age of 25, much earlier than ameloblastoma.

Ultrastructural studies (Fig. 22-12) of ameloblastoma are sparse.[67,69] Electron microscopic findings generally reveal a biphasic neoplasm; individual tumor islands are composed of peripheral columnar cells surrounding a central area of stellate cells. A continuous basement membrane surrounds the cell islands. Peripheral columnar cells have parallel cellular membranes with little interdigitation of cell processes. Cell membranes are usually in close apposition, but occasionally separate focally, forming intercellular lacunae. Plasma membranes of adjacent tumor cells are intimately connected by desmosomes. Cell nuclei remain oval or elliptical and apically situated in the cells. One to two nucleoli are generally present. The cytoplasm of peripheral cells often contains abundant glycogen granules, frequent mitochondria, and, rarely, lysosomes and rough endoplasmic reticulum. Clear cytoplasmic vesicles slightly larger than mitocohondria and bounded by a single membrane may be prominent. Poorly developed Golgi complexes can occasionally be seen adjacent to the nucleus at the pole pointing to the center of the lesion. Tonofilaments tend to be widely distributed in long, curved, and arching bundles around nuclei and adjacent to the plasma membranes.

The so-called adamantinoma of long bones bears a superficial microscopic resemblance to ameloblastoma. It is doubtful whether any valid relationship between the two can be established.

Surgical excision with adequate margins is generally the treatment of choice for the central osseous ameloblastoma.

Calcifying Epithelial Odontogenic Tumor

The calcifying epithelial odontogenic tumor was first described in 1958 by Pindborg[70] and is now recognized as a distinct entity by WHO. The growth potential and biologic behavior have been authoritatively stated to be similar to those of ameloblastoma,[71] indicating the probability of invasiveness and a prediction of local recurrence if conservatively removed in an advanced developmental stage. Histogenesis of the calcifying epithelial odontogenic tumor is open to debate. The tumor shows a propensity for development in association with a tooth. Pindborg[70] suggests that the lesion develops from reduced enamel epithelium or from stratum intermedium.

Clinical and Radiologic Features

Clinically, the lesion typically appears as a locally invasive central osseous neoplasm and has an aggressive behavior potential similar to that of ameloblastoma. Extraosseous lesions have been reported,[72] and like their extraosseous ameloblastoma counterpart, they have a very low biologic aggressiveness.

The mandible appears to be affected more often than the maxilla, and the most frequent site of occurrence is the premolar/molar region. Typically, the lesion appears

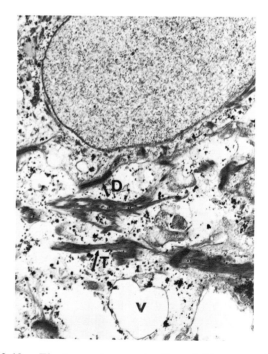

Fig. 22-12. Electron micrograph of ameloblastoma. Cells in central stellate areas have prominent desmosomes (D) and tonofilaments (T). Cytoplasmic vesicles (V) are prominent.

as a radiolucent expansile lesion that is fairly well delineated peripherally. A calcified central area is frequently identified. Half of the lesions that have been reported in the world literature have been in association with an unerupted tooth.[73] Typically, a differential diagnosis of ameloblastoma, calcifying odontogenic cyst, odontoma with cystic change, and ameloblastic fibroma is entertained.

Most lesions are identified in patients in the fourth and fifth decades, although an age range of 3 to 92 years has been reported.

Pathologic Features

The tumor usually consists of a white homogeneous specimen, which may contain calcified material. A tumor capsule is not always appreciated, and frequently the invasive properties of the tumor beyond the periphery into bone are not identified on gross inspection.

The basic histologic pattern of the calcifying epithelial odontogenic tumor has been described as characteristic and unique by recent reviewers.[71,73] These reports maintain a histologic consistency with the original published observation, which is one of sheets and masses of polyhedral epithelial cells with deeply eosinophilic cytoplasm supported by a well vascularized connective tissue stroma. Intracellular bridging is an often noted characteristic, and there may be a moderate degree of cellular pleomorphism, as well as considerable variance in chromaticity of individual cell nuclei (Fig. 22-13). Foci of amorphous, faintly eosinophilic cell product and small round or irregular calcified aggregates, which may be massively coalescent with a concentric ring phenomenon, are an invariable feature of the classic tumor histology (Figs. 22-13 and 22-14).

The eosinopyilic homogeneous material has been variously described as amyloid, keratin, basal lamina, and enamel matrix. The substance stains positively with amyloid stains (thioflavin T and Congo red) and most investigators consider it an amyloid-like product.[74,75]

A survey of 23 cases from the files of the Armed Forces

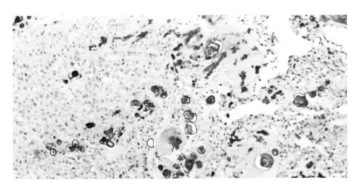

Fig. 22-13. Calcifying epithelial odontogenic tumor. Note sheets of cells with variable density of calcification.

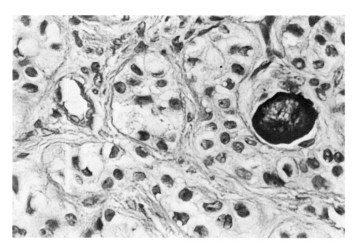

Fig. 22-14. Calcifying epithelial odontogenic tumor composed of epithelial cell clusters with nuclear pleomorphism and variable amounts of cytoplasm. Scattered calcifications are seen.

Institute of Pathology with a discussion of histologic variation was reported by Krolls and Pindborg.[73] They commented on the diagnostic challenge of a "clear cell" variant and found two such tumors in their series. It is significant to note that in both cases there were transition areas to an unequivocal classic tumor histology. Abrams and Howell[76] reported a single instance of clear cell calcifying epithelial odontogenic tumor in a 1967 review of four tumors. In their case, a bimorphic cytoplasmic appearance was observed. The pathologist confronted with a clear cell calcifying odontogenic tumor must consider clear cell types of salivary gland neoplasms, metastatic hypernephroma, and glycogen-rich adenocarcinoma in a differential microscopic diagnosis.[77]

Krolls and Pindborg[73] maintain that the treatment of choice for the calcifying epithelial odontogenic tumor is conservative surgical excision, but one must remember that calcifying epithelial odontogenic tumors with a classic histology have a potential for an aggressive infiltrative course.

The ultrastructure of this lesion has been reviewed by Anderson et al.[78] They were able to demonstrate intracellular bridging and desmosomal attachments, as well as intracytoplasmic tonofilaments and hemidesmosomes in their ultrastructural evaluation of the lesion. Their study supports an epithelial origin for the tumor.

Adenomatoid Odontogenic Tumor

Clinical and Radiologic Features

The adenomatoid odontogenic tumor, also known by the misleading term *adenoameloblastoma,* is a neoplasm of young people, with a propensity to occur in the second or third decade of life. Occasionally, cases have been reported in older people, but this represents the exception rather than the rule. Women appear to be affected much more commonly than men.[79] A common clinical finding is that of a painless, slowly expansile lesion of bone, and although pain may be a factor, it is exceedingly rare. The tumor is usually identified in the maxillary canine, premolar, or incisor area, although a few cases have been reported along the angle of the mandible. Seventy-five percent of the reported cases have been associated with an unerupted or impacted tooth, the most common tooth being the maxillary cuspid. Instances of an extraosseous variant have been documented.[80]

Radiologically the lesion usually presents as a solitary cyst-like lesion. As a differential diagnosis one should include dentigerous cyst, odontogenic keratocyst, and inflammatory cyst of dental origin (radicular cyst). Frequently, calcifications are seen in association with the tumor, producing a faintly detectable radiopacity. The lesion rarely grows to a size that results in penetration of the cortical plates, and if such is the appearance, then the differential diagnosis should include a more aggressive odontogenic neoplasm.

The origin of the lesion has not been identified, although there are theories that indicate that the adenomatoid odontogenic tumor is derived from the enamel organ or its remnants or possibly from remnants of dentigerous cysts. There also seems to be a very distinct morphologic correspondence between the cells that line the duct-like structures of the tumor and the cells of the interenamel epithelium in the tooth germ. The duct-like structures in the tumor may in fact represent nothing more than an abortive attempt at the formation of the enamel organ.

Pathologic Features

Lucas[8] points out that most adenomatoid odontogenic tumors are small, measuring 1 to 3 cm in diameter. The tumor may or may not be encapsulated by a peripheral rim of mature collagen. On cut section one usually identifies a white to yellow firm surface, which may have cystic areas that contain central gelatinous material. The calcified material that is often identified on radiographs may represent poorly formed tooth structure or an aberrant dystrophic type of calcification grossly. The cut section may be quite gritty or granular, resembling the cut surface of a mature central giant cell granuloma.

The dominant histologic feature of the tumor is proliferation of sheets, nests, and cords of neoplastic epithelial cells that differentiate along columnar lines in numerous places to resemble ameloblasts. Frequently, these columnar cells form ducts or tubules, with the central lumen ultimately encased by columnar cells (Fig. 22-15). The peripheral cells stain deeply, and their nuclei are polar-

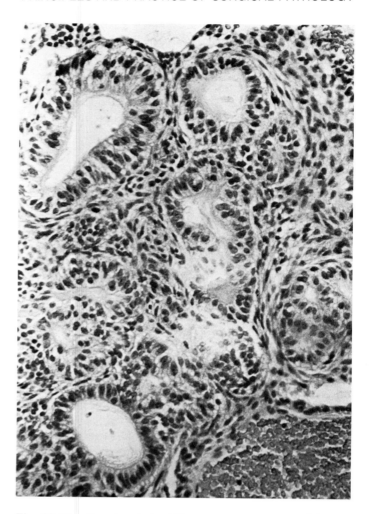

Fig. 22-15. Prominent duct-like structures are noted in this adenomatoid odontogenic tumor. Spindle cells surround the duct-like areas.

ized away from the central portion of the neoplasm in a manner similar to that found in ameloblastoma. In addition to the tubular and ductal structures, bands, sheets, and clusters of cells arranged in a spindlelike pattern may be identified (Fig. 22-15). Occasionally, these areas can take on a cartwheel or cribriform pattern reminiscent of salivary gland tumors, especially the mixed tumor. Tumor nests are supported by a scant connective tissue stroma. On occasion, tumor cells are arranged in a rosette pattern lined by cuboidal or columnar epithelium. Calcified material is common throughout the tumor. These calcifications develop primarily at junctions between aggregates of epithelial cells that form the tumor and the adjacent vascularized stromal tissues. The calcific foci have been shown to resemble enamel, preenamel, or dentin morphologically and have similar staining and tinctorial qualities.

Poulson and Greer[81] reviewed the electron microscopic findings of two adenomatoid odontogenic tumors and identified two distinctly different cell types. One cell was polygonal to columnar and tended to surround the tumor's duct-like structures to form small nodules. These cells seemed to share common features with preameloblasts in that ultrastructurally an abundance of free ribosomes and a paucity of endoplasmic reticulum were identified. A second cell type was identified that appeared similar to cells of the stratum intermedium and stellate reticulum of the tooth germ. These cells were spindle-shaped with ovoid nuclei and appeared to be perpendicular to luminal cells. Their ultrastructure showed dense cytoplasm and numerous filaments and ribosomes.

Histochemical attempts to identify the nature and source of the eosinophilic material that is often observed in the adenomatoid odontogenic tumor suggest that the material is amyloid-like.[81]

Behavior and Management

The tumor appears to grow very slowly and is a relatively benign lesion. It shows no tendency toward recurrence, and conservative surgical excision remains the treatment of choice. It must be pointed out that some authorities feel that this lesion represents a hamartoma and not a true odontogenic tumor. It is exceedingly important to separate this lesion from the ameloblastoma since the behavior patterns are diametrically opposed. Although there is a close morphologic correlation between the cells of the adenomatoid odontogenic tumor and the ameloblastoma, the lesions are quite distinct entities.

Benign Mesodermal Tumors

Myxoma

Myxomas (*odontogenic myxoma, myxofibroma*) of bone are fairly uncommon neoplasms. Regardless of their sparsity, the controversy as to whether or not myxomas of the jaws are odontogenic in origin or of central osseous mesenchymal origin continues. The distinction appears to be primarily of academic interest since the behavior pattern of myxoma of bone tends to remain the same whether or not an odontogenic origin can be demonstrated and whether or not odontogenic epithelial rests are present within the tumor. If one considers that true myxomas do occur, one would conversely have to consider that a distinctive cell, perhaps a "myxoblast," gives rise to the tumor. In fact, most authorities who have evaluated the ultrastructure of myxomas support the theory that the lesion arises from fibroblasts and that

the myxomatous appearance occurs because of the abundant amount of intercellular mucin.[8,82]

Clinical and Radiologic Features

Myxomas of the jaw occur most frequently in the posterior mandible. Maxillary myxomas are rather rare. The tumors present as slow-growing, expansile, nonpainful lesions, most often in the second or third decades of life.[43] Most myxomas appear as sessile swelling of the jaws, with a thin eggshell covering of the cortical bone. Women appear to be affected slightly more often than men.[83] Clinically, the most common finding is that of a multilocular radiolucency or a compartmentalized soap bubble radiolucency; however, there are reported cases in which myxomas have presented as solitary unilocular cyst-like lesions (Fig. 22-16). The tumor borders may be well defined or poorly delineated radiologically. It is not uncommon for the lesion to show scalloping and interdigitation between the teeth. Myxomas have been reported in association with unerupted teeth and congenitally missing teeth; however, the lesion may very well arise in association with developed dental structures.

As noted, the histogenesis of the lesion is open to debate. The probability of the lesion developing from either dental mesenchymal tissue or nondental mesenchymal tissue must be considered, although the vast majority of the reports are of cases that appear to be of dental origin.

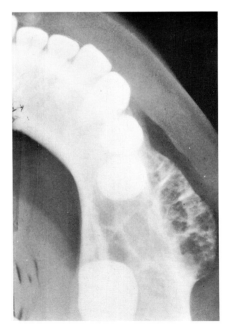

Fig. 22-16. Multilocular lesion of mandible expanding the labial cortex representing the (odontogenic) myxoma. (Courtesy of Richard Glass, D.D.S., Stephen Young, D.D.S., and Michael Rohrer, D.D.S.)

Pathologic Features

The lesion may appear grossly as a gray-white to yellow fibrous mass without a peripheral capsule. The cut surface in such instances will be firm and glistening and will fail to bulge beyond surrounding tissues on sectioning. Myxomas may also present grossly as rather mucoid, slimy specimens with a gelatinous appearance when fixed. In such instances a capsule is not identified, and areas of bone are often present within the cut surface.

Microscopically, myxomas consist primarily of accumulations of triangular to stellate fibroblasts with rather lengthy anastomosing processes and loose mucoid intracellular material (Fig. 22-17). The cytoplasm ranges from slightly basophilic to deeply eosinophilic depending on the degree of collagenization that has taken place. The supporting stroma is typically that of a mucopolysaccharide complex that may contain odontogenic epithelium. Hasleton and colleagues[83] reported islands of odontogenic epithelium at all intervals throughout cases they reported. Odontogenic epithelium can be found in a high percentage of cases of central myxoma of bone involving the jaws, but it may represent nothing more than a fetal remnant and is not necessarily important in the genesis of the tumor. It is nearly impossible to distinguish between jaw myxomas that will behave aggressively and those that will have a totally benign biologic behavior. Farman et al.[84] reviewed 213 cases of jaw myxofibromas and found no mortality related to the tumor. I am aware of three cases resulting in eventual orbital exenteration and maxillectomy. It appears that lesions of the maxilla spread rapidly throughout the surrounding cancellous bone and tend to have a more aggressive behavior than their mandibular counterparts.

The ultrastructural features of the odontogenic myxoma have shed some light on the cell of origin. The theory that is most commonly accepted today is that the tumor cell of origin closely resembles a fibroblast, a cell known to have an active secretory function. Goldblatt[85] has described two types of cells in odontogenic myxomas: a nonsecretory (type I) and a secretory (type II) cell. Both these cells appear to be of connective tissue origin. Redman et al.[86] have ultrastructurally identified cells resembling myofibroblasts in odontogenic myxomas. This finding supports the theory that the cell of origin for the tumor may be periodontal ligament fibroblasts, which have also been shown to have such microfilament systems. The exact function of the myofibroblasts in the tumor is not known, although it has been postulated that their contractile mechanism may be the device for allowing cell motility in the granulation tissue that is often associated with this tumor. Zimmerman and Dahlin[87] have attempted to define benign and malignant varieties of central jaw myxomas on the basis of the cytologic appearance of nuclei and anisocytosis. They have met with only limited success and have been unable to distinguish benign and malignant variants. There is some suggestion that the greater the fibrous component of the tumor, the less aggressive the biologic behavior.

A few examples of myxomas as tumors of the oral soft tissue have been reported.[88] Elzay and Duntz[88] believe that soft tissue myxomas are derived from early embryonic mesenchymal tissues. These investigators maintain that the neoplasms remain quiescent for long periods of time and have the ability to suddenly enlarge. The recommended therapy is surgical excision with adequate margins. The lesion is thought not to have the aggressive potential of its central osseous counterpart.

The complex of soft tissue myomas, spotty skin pigmentation, and endocrine overactivity has recently been recognized as a syndrome, transmitted as an autosomal dominant trait.[89] A serious component of this syndrome is the so-called cardiac myxoma. Many of the patients with this myxoma syndrome complex have clearly visible markers, including mucocutaneous pigmentation.

Odontogenic Fibroma

Clinical and Radiologic Features

There appear to be two distinct histologic variants of the odontogenic fibroma: (1) simple central odontogenic fibroma, and (2) the World Health Organization central odontogenic fibroma (WHO type). The simple type, as described by Gardner,[90] is a very rare neoplasm composed of an uniform proliferation of mature, relatively dense connective tissue, which may or may not have an admixture of small entrapped epithelial odontogenic

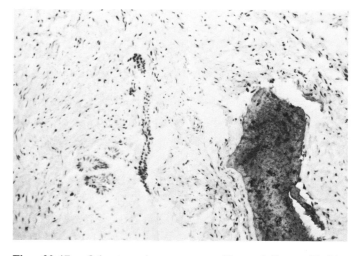

Fig. 22-17. Odontogenic myxoma. Note delicate fibrillar stroma, odontogenic rests, and bone trabeculae.

rests. The WHO variant consists of mature collagenous fibrous connective tissue with prominent islands, strands, and nests of odontogenic epithelium and occasional aggregates of dysplastic dentin, cementum, and calcifications.

Dahl and associates[91] reviewed a series of 11 odontogenic fibromas and found the age distribution to range from 11 to 80 years. The mean age of their patients was 34 years. Five cases were identified in females and six in males. Wesley et al.[92] have documented an age range of 11 to 67 years in their clinical and morphologic studies. The lesion shows no sexual predilection, and the mean age of all patients was 22 years. The lesion remains perhaps the most ill defined and least understood of all odontogenic neoplasms. Wesley and colleagues gleaned only seven cases from the world literature; all tumors were found in close association with the crown of an impacted tooth and presented clinically as slowly enlarging swellings. They usually presented as multiocular radiolucencies, although unilocular lesions were identified.

There are reports in the literature indicating that the tumor can contain calcified material that is visible radiologically.[93] All reported cases have occurred in the mandible.

Pathologic Features

The odontogenic fibroma presents as an encapsulated neoplastic mass with a homogeneous white cut surface that usually glistens. Typically, it is identified in association with an impacted tooth. Microscopically, one usually finds a moderately dense and relatively cellular proliferation of collagen with a uniform distribution of bland fibroblasts. Occasionally amorphous calcifications can be identified in the tissue sample, but only in the supporting collagen. In some of the cases that have been reported, odontogenic epithelium has been identified. The presence of odontogenic epithelium should not negate a diagnosis of odontogenic fibroma. The greatest difference between the odontogenic fibroma and the lesion that closely resembles it microscopically, odontogenic myxoma, is that in the latter the stroma exhibits only scant amounts of collagen and abundant ground substance, whereas in the odontogenic fibroma the stroma is highly collagenous and much more cellular.

Vincent and associates[94] have recently described a variant of odontogenic fibroma using the term "central granular cell odontogenic fibroma." All of their eight reported cases occurred in women as well circumscribed radiolucencies. The age range was 53 to 65 years. Seven tumors occurred in the posterior body of the mandible and one in the premolar region of the maxilla. The lesions were treated by surgical excision, and no recurrences were identified during a follow-up period ranging from 6 to 144

months. Microscopically, the lesions consisted of an abundance of polygonal cells with eosinophilic granular cytoplasm and eccentric ovoid nuclei, and an occasional entrapped epithelial odontogenic rest. Rarely, ovoid calcifications could be identified.

Ultrastructurally, the morphologic characteristics of odontogenic fibroma are quite similar to those of odontogenic myxoma in that cells in both neoplasms exhibit large amounts of endoplasmic reticulum. Two cell types have not been identified in odontogenic fibroma, in contrast to odontogenic myxoma. The lesion is benign and responds well to surgical enucleation, with no tendency to recur or undergo malignant transformation.

Periapical Cemental Dysplasia

Periapical cemental dysplasia (cementoma) is a distinct pathologic entity that most commonly involves multiple periapical regions of mandibular incisor teeth, although it may in fact involve other areas as well. Radiologically, the process is characterized in its initial stages by well defined nonexpansile radiolucencies, which become transformed into radiopaque calcified lesions at a later stage of development. Periapical cemental dysplasia is seen in 2 or 3 of every 1,000 patients screened with routine dental radiographs.[95,96] The average age is usually the late third or early fourth decade, and lesions appear to be more common in blacks than in whites.

There are three apparent radiologic stages of progression: an osteolytic phase, a mixed phase, and a totally osteoblastic phase. The most classic finding is that of a radiopaque mass rimmed by a thin radiolucent line. Rarely do the lesions grow with any rapidity, and typically they do not attain a diameter of greater than 5 to 6 mm. The etiology is unknown. One theory that has been expressed is that the lesions are a result of trauma. A second hypothesis is that the lesions represent a very special form of fibrous dysplasia. The current thinking is that the lesions are of periodontal ligament origin and perhaps represent a proliferation of principal fibers of the periodontal ligament membrane with osseous differentiation.[97]

It is important that the clinician distinguish periapical cemental dysplasia from a radiolucent cyst of dental inflammatory origin. It is important to realize that the tooth is always vital in cases of peripheral cemental dysplasia. Typically, the surgical pathologist should not receive a specimen of this nature since it can be diagnosed on clinical grounds.

Histologically, one generally identifies numerous round, globular, or trabecular deposits of basophilic cementum or cementoid material deposited in a loose fibrous connective tissue stroma. No treatment is warranted.

Cementifying Fibroma

Clinical and Radiologic Features

Cementifying fibroma is a member of the *cementoma* group of lesions. The distinction between these lesions is largely one of location, lesional number, and sex. Additional lesions in the cementoma group include: cementoblastoma, gigantiform cementoma, periapical cemental dysplasia, and florid osseous dysplasia. The cementifying fibroma (*cemento-ossifying fibroma*) is considered to be a lesion of periodontal ligament origin,[97] arising from undifferentiated mesenchymal cells in the periodontal ligament or residuum thereof. Like periapical cemental dysplasia, it occurs chiefly in the mandible, and most of the patients are in the third or fourth decade of life. There is no sex predilection. One feature that distinguishes it from periapical cemental dysplasia is that it presents as a solitary expansile lesion, most frequently in the molar or premolar area, as opposed to the anterior region for periapical cemental dysplasia. Cementifying fibroma can undergo three phases of radiologic development, namely, lytic, blastic, and mixed phases.[98]

The cementifying fibroma has to be considered a true reactive fibro-osseous growth, if not a true neoplasm. It has to be managed surgically, unlike periapical cemental dysplasia.

Pathologic Features

The tumor may consist of a totally calcified mass, but most frequently it is composed of a bosselated mass of soft tissue and interspersed calcified foci. The cut surface may be quite gritty. Although radiologically one may identify what appears to be a distinct capsule, a true fibrous capsule is usually not identified grossly, perhaps because the lesion is usually removed in multiple fragments.

Histologically, the lesion is composed of globular or trabecular calcified masses of cementum. These masses are often basophilic and range in size from quite large to a little more than droplets. A common histologic finding is that as the lesion progressively increases in size, the calcified portions tend to coalesce at the expense of the supporting connective tissue stroma. In the early stages of development, it may be made up almost totally of fibroblastic collagen with a few blood vessels and very little calcified product. The supporting stroma is composed of a proliferation of plump to stellate fibroblasts resembling the periodontal ligament from which the lesion is thought to arise.

The cementifying fibroma is a benign lesion and the treatment of choice is generally surgical enucleation or curettage. There is no great tendency for the lesion to recur. There is little reason to separate this lesion from ossifying fibroma, discussed under fibro-osseous lesions

later in this chapter; however, it is accepted as a distinct odontogenic tumor by WHO, a matter of some confusion to the surgical pathologist.

Benign Cementoblastoma

Clinical and Radiologic Features

The benign cementoblastoma (true cementoma) was initially described in 1930 by Norberg.[99] The lesion was defined as a true neoplasm of cementum or cementum-like tissue formed on the tooth root by accompanying cementoblasts. It typically presents as a slow-growing mass tenaciously attached to the cementum of molar or premolar teeth. Corio et al.[100] recently reviewed a series of 24 cases of cementoblastoma presented in the world literature and added a case of their own. They found that the lesion was not as uncommon as might be thought by its infrequent documentation in the world literature. Their investigations found an age range of 10 to 63 years, the mean age being 23 years.

In most instances, pain is a significant feature of cementoblastoma; well over half of the documented case reports indicate that pain was a primary presenting symptom.[101,102] The cementoblastoma has quite a distinctive radiologic appearance, that of a large radiopaque mass attached to the root of a molar or premolar tooth. The opaque mass is usually surrounded by a thin radiopaque line.

Pathologic Features

Grossly, one can identify a sectioned tooth with an attached globular mass resembling hypercementosis if the specimen is submitted at least partially intact.

The microscopic appearance of cementoblastoma is fairly consistent. Histologically, there is a peripheral rim of radiating columns of cementum lined by large pleomorphic (cemento)blastic cells. In addition, at the peripheral border islands of cementum and cementum-like substance can be seen set in a fibrous stroma. Frequently, the peripheral cementoblasts have quite hyperchromatic nuclei and marked pleomorphism and appear to be stacked in a layer or lattice-like pattern. A portion of the tumor may show reactive cementum with tremendous reversal line activity. Giansanti[103] has demonstrated a fine birefringence compatible with that of cementum in his case studies.

Differential Diagnostic Guidelines

In establishing a differential diagnosis for a cementoid lesion, it is important to evaluate clinical, radiologic, and histologic parameters. Periapical cemental dysplasia is a lesion that is most commonly encountered in the anterior mandible and is frequently identified in the middle-aged woman; there appears to be a black racial predilection, and this should be a prime consideration in trying to establish a differential diagnosis for multiple blastic, lytic, or mixed radiologic lesions in the anterior mandible. Cementifying fibroma, on the other hand, typically presents as a solitary lesion, which may have a peripheral radiopaque border; the lesion is usually identified in the posterior mandibular region, and there is no sex predilection.

Another entity that should be considered in the differential diagnosis of cemental lesions is *gigantiform cementoma*. It is a lesion about which there is considerable confusion in the world literature. It is thought to be a lesion that is predominantly seen in the middle-aged black women. Radiologically it presents as large, dense, sclerotic multifocal masses, typically in the mandible. Some authorities feel that there is a distinct histologic appearance to the lesion, while others, including myself, feel that the lesion represents a variant of ossifying fibroma, probably identical to the multiple endostoses that have been described by Bhaskar and Cutwright.[98]

Benign cementoblastoma is a lesion that is typically seen in the mandibular premolar-molar region. It is found in individuals younger than those with periapical cemental dysplasia, cementifying fibroma, or gigantiform cementoma. Although the histologic features of all these can be strikingly similar, clinical and radiologic diagnostic parameters should help the surgical pathologist differentiate the lesions from one another.

Behavior and Management

Cementoblastoma is thought to have a fairly unlimited growth potential, with a tendency for expansion of the jaw, root resorption, and bone erosion. Even though this potential has been demonstrated, a conservative surgical approach is the treatment of choice. Extraction of the associated tooth is indicated regardless of whether one encounters a vital or nonvital pulp. The tumor can easily be enucleated from adjacent bone, which reinforces the fact that a conservative surgical approach is the treatment of choice. A malignant potential has not been documented for this lesion; therefore, Abrams et al.[102] indicate that the term benign cementoblastoma is redundant.

Dual (Mixed) Benign Epithelial and Mesodermal Tumors

Ameloblastic Fibroma

Clinical and Radiologic Features

The ameloblastic fibroma is an odontogenic neoplasm derived from both ectodermal (ameloblastic) and connective tissue (fibroma) elements of the odontogenic apparatus. Most authorities consider that as the two cell types proliferate, they tend to undergo patterns of normal odontogenesis. The largest series reported in the literature are by Chaudry and associates[104] and Trodahl.[105] Both groups of authors found that the lesions occurred primarily in patients under the age of 20 and that the average age was 15. There is no apparent sex or race predilection.

The classic manifestation is that of a painless swelling in the posterior mandible, although the maxilla may occasionally be involved. Typically, the lesions are identified on routine radiologic screening. The tumor usually manifests radiologically as either a unilocular or multilocular radiolucency. There may be cortical expansion in the case of larger lesions. Trodahl[105] found that 75 percent of the lesions that he identified were associated with the crown of an impacted tooth, and that most of them displayed a multilocular radiologic pattern.

Pathologic Features

Grossly, the ameloblastic fibroma has the consistency of a fibrous tumor, and it may or may not be rimmed by a definitive collagenous capsule. Microscopically, one is able to identify sheets, nests, strands, and cords of epithelial cells set in an embryonal-appearing connective tissue stroma (Fig. 22-18). The epithelial cells often are surrounded by a prominent basement membrane and are composed predominantly of cuboidal or low columnar cells arranged back to back. The epithelial cells are quite similar to the peripheral layer of cells seen around the follicles in the developing tooth germ. Frequently, the epithelial cells are arranged in a branching or linking chain-like pattern. At times, the epithelial cells are composed only of double rows of cells without a central stellate layer, although it is possible for the epithelial component to proliferate to such an extent that a central stellate reticulum akin to that seen in ameloblastoma can be found. Stellate cells, however, are never so prominent as in ameloblastoma. On occasion, the central stellate areas may undergo cystic degeneration.[106]

Van Wyk and associates[107] reported finding an amorphous, eosinophilic, hyaline-like material in ameloblastic fibroma. The material typically surround epithelial islands. Edwards and Coubran[108] reported a cystic ameloblastic fibroma with melanin pigment entrapment. The pigment appeared similar to what Richardson et al.[109] have described in the pigmented calcifying epithelial odontogenic tumor.

Differential Diagnosis

One of the most important distinguishing histologic features that separates ameloblastic fibroma from ameloblastoma is that in ameloblastic fibroma the supporting connective tissue stroma is composed of a loose stellate proliferation of connective tissue cells that resembles

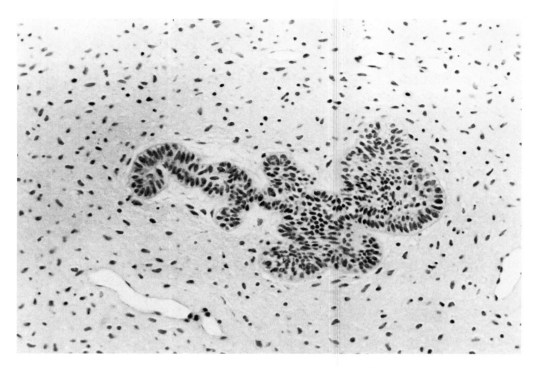

Fig. 22-18. Ameloblastic fibroma. Cell-rich embryonal stroma and odontogenic epithelial island.

that of the normal dental papilla; there is rarely any evidence of the dense collagen formation seen in the supporting stroma of the ameloblastoma.

Ameloblastic fibroma can also be confused histologically with calcifying epithelial odontogenic tumor, adenomatoid odontogenic tumor, and odontoma. The calcifying epithelial odontogenic tumor is also composed of sheets and cords of neoplastic epithelial cells; however, they can be differentiated from the epithelial cells in ameloblastoma because of their strikingly eosinophilic cytoplasm. Columnar ameloblasts with nuclear polarization are also absent. The calcifying epithelial odontogenic tumor also has a mature collagenous stroma, not the immature mesenchymal stroma of ameloblastic fibroma.

Adenomatoid odontogenic tumor occurs in the same age groups as the ameloblastic fibroma. It may also contain elongated and anastomosing cords of epithelium similar to that found in ameloblastic fibroma. A principal distinguishing feature between the two is the fact that adenomatoid odontogenic tumor usually has a thick, fibrous capsule; such a capsule is usually not encountered in ameloblastic fibroma. The adenomatoid odontogenic tumor also often resembles a cyst with luminal epithelial proliferations, a feature that is not seen in ameloblastic fibroma. The stroma of the adenomatoid odontogenic tumor is extremely sparse and does not constitute a major portion of the neoplasm, whereas in ameloblastic fibroma the loose, stellate connective tissue stroma is exceed-

ingly prominent. Finally, in the ameloblastic fibroma there are no organoid rosettes or ductal structures, prominent features of the adenomatoid odontogenic tumor.[106]

Behavior and Management

Until recently, the ameloblastic fibroma was considered to represent a fairly nonaggressive benign odontogenic tumor, which could easily be enucleated and did not show a high recurrence rate, but Trodahl[105] has recently reported a recurrence rate of 43.5 percent. Carr et al.[110] and Tanaka et al.[111] have also documented high recurrence rates for this tumor. It appears that the lesion may be somewhat more aggressive than was originally thought, and therefore many authorities recommend that therapy include excision with adequate margins and not simply surgical curettage.

Ameloblastic Fibro-odontoma

Clinical and Radiologic Features

The ameloblastic fibro-odontoma is an exceedingly rare neoplasm, which manifests radiologically as a unilocular or multilocular cystic lesion with radiopaque central areas. WHO recognizes this tumor as a distinct odontogenic tumor, which affects both sexes equally and occurs at an early age, usually within the second decade of life.[112] There remains, nontheless, considerable debate as to whether or not the lesion should be classified as a separate odontogenic tumor.

Ameloblastic fibro-odontoma was first described in 1967 by Hooker,[113] who differentiated it from ameloblastic odontoma. Histologically, the ameloblastic fibro-odontoma is composed of three principal components: (1) a stroma rich in an immature cellular connective tissue resembling developing dental pulp; (2) an ectodermal component characterized by islands of epithelium composed of palisading columnar or cuboidal cells at the periphery and loosely arranged cells in the central stroma; and (3) a mineralized component made of dental structures composed of either dentin, enamel, or cementum. Gardner[114] has suggested that some reported instances of ameloblastic fibro-odontoma are, in fact, simply developing odontomas.

Because of the histologic resemblance between ameloblastic fibroma and a developing odontoma, consideration of clinical behavior is paramount if a proper diagnosis is to be rendered. A small lesion located on the occlusal surface of an erupting tooth is probably a developing odontoma and not an ameloblastic fibroma or ameloblastic fibro-odontoma. Tsataras[115] reviewed a host of ameloblastic fibro-odontomas and found the median age to be 13 years, with 73.3 percent of the cases occuring in individuals younger than 20 years.

The tumor is a benign neoplasm that should be treated surgically. Curettage with eburnation of surrounding bone seems to be sufficient to resolve most lesions, and recurrence is uncommon.

Pathologic Features

The lesion is composed histologically of an epithelial and connective tissue component resembling ameloblastic fibroma. In addition, a calcified product that resembles enamel or dentin is usually identified in the tissue sample. Many authorities believe that the lesion is nothing more than a variant of, and a slightly more aggressive, ameloblastic fibroma.[116] Richardson and associates[109] maintain that structural variations occurring in more or less familiar lesions such as ameloblastic fibroma do not constitute grounds for creation of a new class of lesion, unless accompanied by distinctively different clinical or behavioral characteristics. They tend to favor the categorization of this lesion as an ameloblastic fibroma with calcification—a unique histologic feature, but one that does not alter the behavior pattern, and therefore a lesion that does not warrant subclassification. Only time and a large series of cases with strict clinical and histologic evaluation will allow us to determine whether or not the ameloblastic fibro-odontoma necessitates a separate subclassification.

Odontoma

Clinical and Radiologic Features

The odontoma is the most common of all odontogenic neoplasms. Odontomas are typically subclassified into compound and complex types. Clinically, the majority of odontomas are identified in adolescents. Budnick[117] reviewed a series of 149 odontomas and found that 76 were of the complex type: a lesion composed of a mass of irregularly arranged dentin, enamel, cementum, and connective tissue arranged in a disorganized pattern not resembling normal tooth morphology. He further documented that 73 were of the compound variety, composed of tooth-like structures arranged in an organized pattern.

Regezi and associates[118] found that 30 percent of 706 odontogenic tumors they reviewed were odontomas. Complex odontomas are more common in the mandible, usually the posterior regions, whereas compound odontomas show a marked predilection for the anterior regions. The most prevalent age for diagnosis and treatment is the second decade of life. Budnick[117] points out that 67 percent of the tumors he reviewed occurred in the maxilla. There was a marked predilection for the anterior maxilla, and a slight male predominance was also documented.

Clinically, the lesions are usually asymptomatic, and the most common complaint, is there is one, is intraoral swelling. Most lesions are identified on the basis of routine radiographs and appear as radiopaque masses, sometimes surrounded by lytic areas. Small denticles or tooth-like structures may also be surrounded by a radiolucent area.

Pathologic Features

Odontomas are composed of enamel, enamel matrix, dentin, cementum, and pulpal tissue arranged in a uniform pattern or in a haphazard pattern, resulting in the subclasses, compound and complex odontomas, respectively.

Grossly, one usually receives a hard tissue structure, often with attached firm soft tissue or, on occasion, granulation tissue. The presence of a calcified dental product in the tissue samples negates a diagnosis of ameloblastoma. It is often exceedingly difficult to distinguish between ameloblastic fibro-odontoma and an early developing complex odontoma, and the distinction may be of academic interest only. Epithelial odontogenic remnants may be prominent throughout odontoma and ameloblastic fibro-odontoma. The important distinguishing feature is the fact that ameloblastic fibro-odontoma has a primitive mesenchymal connective tissue stroma and histologically resembles a composite of ameloblastic fibroma and odontoma.

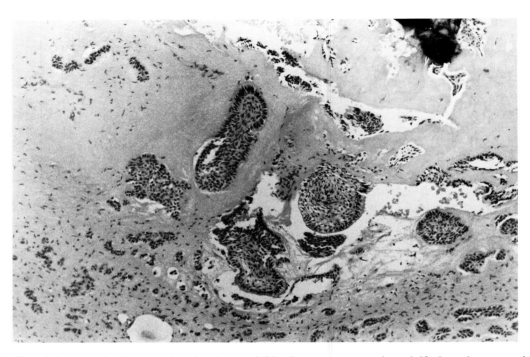

Fig. 22-19. Odontoameloblastoma showing the ameloblastic component and a calcified product resembling osteodentin.

WHO also describes a lesion known as *odontoameloblastoma (ameloblastic odontoma)*. This lesion has the histologic characteristics of an odontoma and a true ameloblastoma (Fig. 22-19). Tooth-like structures surround epithelial ameloblastic islands. The connective tissue stroma is mature. The lesion has the biologic behavior pattern of an ameloblastoma. It seems likely, however, that the lesion is nothing more than an immature complex odontoma with entrapment of epithelial elements and an aggressive natural history.

The credit for separating ameloblastic fibro-odontoma and ameloblastic odontoma is given to Hooker.[118] The ameloblastic odontoma is, in contrast to the ameloblastic fibro-odontoma, a relatively locally aggressive tumor. Its rate of recurrence is thought to be similar to that of the conventional ameloblastoma. The neoplasm is composed of enamel and dentin set within a mature fibrous connective tissue stroma, with an epithelial component that is identical to that of an ameloblastoma. Ameloblastic odontoma and ameloblastic fibro-odontoma have similar radiographic appearances, with well defined radiolucencies and variable irregular radiopacities. Multilocularity appears to be a more common finding in ameloblastic odontoma.

Both the complex and compound odontomas have an exceedingly limited growth potential and even though they may enlarge dramatically, for the most part they behave in a quiescent and totally benign biologic fashion. Local surgical excision is the treatment of choice.

Malignant Odontogenic Tumors

Odontogenic Carcinomas

Few malignant tumors are thought to arise from the odontogenic apparatus. The lesions primarily considered are ameloblastic carcinoma, primary intra-osseous carcinoma, and malignant ameloblastic sarcoma or ameloblastic fibrosarcoma.

Ameloblastic Carcinoma

Perhaps the best classification scheme has been suggested by Elzay.[119] He recognizes three different variants of odontogenic carcinoma: ameloblastic carcinoma, type I, arising from an odontogenic cyst; type II, arising from an ameloblastoma as either a well or a poorly differentiated ameloblastic carcinoma; and Type III, arising as either a keratinizing or a nonkeratinizing neoplasm. Slootweg and Muller[120] reviewed a series of 26 cases of ''malignant ameloblastoma'' and found that the patients had metastatic involvement in 20 instances. The vast majority of the metastases were to the lungs. The second most common site involved was lymph nodes. Patients had a mean age of 31.3 years, and follow-up showed that 11 of 16 patients died during a period of up to 9 years. *Ameloblastic carcinoma,* as defined by Elzay (Types I and II), showed a slightly older mean age of 33.2 years; 80 percent of the tumors were located in the mandible; the most common site of metastasis was to the lungs, just as in malignant ameloblastoma as defined by Slootweg and Muller; and patients died between 1 and 45 years after initial diagnosis of the tumor.

Ikemura et al.[63] have also described a malignant potential for ameloblastoma. They reviewed 14 cases of metastatic ameloblastoma and reported a case of their own in a 54-year-old woman with lung and lymph node metastases. When ameloblastomas do metastasize, they most frequently appear in the lungs, cervical lymph nodes, or vertebrae.

Histologically, ameloblastomas that may metastasize cannot always be differentiated from the more classic benign ameloblastoma. It appears that inadequate surgical resection and a long duration of the tumor have a significant relationship to ultimate metastatic disease occurrence.

Sound judgment is needed to distinguish between malignant ameloblastoma and central osseous jaw tumors of salivary gland origin. Occasionally, squamous cell carcinoma can occur in association with ameloblastoma. When this occurs, it may be extremely difficult to determine if the carcinoma arose within the ameloblastoma or whether, in fact, two tumors exist. Gorlin[121] indicates that malignant ameloblastoma have the cytologic atypia seen in most malignant tumors. Lucas[4] maintains that distant spread of the ameloblastoma is rather like that of basal cell carcinoma; he indicates that metastatic dissemination is quite unlikely although local spread to cervical lymph nodes is possible.

Primary Intraosseous Carcinoma (Type III of Elzay)

Elzay[119] found 12 instances of primary interosseous carcinoma in his review of malignant odontogenic tumors. Two thirds of the lesions were in males, and the vast majority were located in the mandible. The patients seemed to be somewhat older than the patients with a malignant ameloblastoma or a ameloblastic carcinoma, with a mean age of 45.2 years. Of these cases 67 percent showed a plexiform or alveolar pattern of growth, and nearly 60 percent were nonkeratinizing. Elzay reported that the 2-year survival rate in these patients was only 40 percent.

Ameloblastic Sarcoma

Leider and colleagues[122] have reported 17 cases of ameloblastic fibrosarcoma. They regard the lesion as the malignant counterpart of the ameloblastic fibroma. They found that the lesion occurs most frequently in young individuals, with an average age of 30 years, shows no sex predilection, and occurs more often in the mandible than in the maxilla.

Pindborg and Kramer associates[12] define the ameloblastic fibrosarcoma as a neoplasm that appears similar to ameloblastic fibroma, with the distinction that the mesodermal component shows sarcomatous features. Some investigators[123,124] note that a calcified component may be present.

Most patients with an ameloblastic sarcoma present with a chief complaint of pain or swelling. Occasionally paresthesia may also be reported. The lesions have been described as multilocular, resembling ameloblastic fibroma, and occasionally they show a common feature of root resorption. The tumor is composed histologically of an odontogenic epithelial component that may show atypical features and a cellular stroma composed of malignant palisading spindle cells. Dysplastic dentin may occasionally be observed. Ameloblastic sarcoma is a tumor of low-grade malignancy, and there are few reports of tumors that have metastasized. Ameloblastic sarcomas have been reported to develop in pre-existing benign counterparts such as ameloblastic fibroma and ameloblastic fibro-odontoma. Occasionally the tumor will appear to represent a simple fibrosarcoma, with little histologic evidence of an odontogenic epithelial component.

TUMORS OF UNCERTAIN HISTOGENESIS

Melanotic Neuroectodermal Tumor of Infancy

Melanotic neuroectodermal tumor of infancy was first described by Krompecher in 1891.[125] Since that time more than 70 cases have been documented in the world literature. There has been considerable confusion as to the origin of the tumor. The most common of the proposed origins have been the odontogenic tissues and the neural crest. It is generally considered by most authorities today that the lesion is a tumor of neural crest origin. The neoplasm has also been referred to as *melanotic ameloblastoma, retinal anlage tumor,* and *melanotic progonoma.*

The neoplasm is benign, with recurrence rates in the range of approximately 15 percent. Dehner[126] reported a malignant melanotic neuroectodermal tumor in a 4-month-old boy. The tumor eventually metastasized, and the patient died 3 months later. There is some debate concerning whether or not the tumor was originally a neuroblastoma. Nagase and his associates[127] reviewed a series of 17 recurrent melanotic neuroectodermal tumors,

12 of which they interpreted as being rapidly growing tumors but none of which metastasized.

Clinical and Radiologic Features

Clinically, the lesion usually presents as a tumor mass with a subjacent radiographic lucency in the premaxilla (Fig. 22-20). Over 80 percent of all tumors have been identified in this area, although reports in the literature indicate that the lesion can be found in long bones or the bones of the skull.[125] Often the teeth in association with the tumor appear to be floating in space, and a differential diagnosis of histiocytosis X is therefore entertained. The majority of the tumors occur in the first decade of life. They may be locally destructive of bone, but are benign and do not metastasize.

Pathologic Features

The tumor generally separates quite easily from the bone and is usually only partially encapsulated. On cut section, one will usually find a firm, glistening cut surface that is gray-white with numerous speckles or streaks of black and brown material distributed throughout. Occasionally, there may be multiple tumor nodules instead of a single tumor mass.

Microscopically, the tumor is composed of two cell types, pigmented and nonpigmented (Fig. 22-21), both of which are set in a loose connective tissue stroma. The pigmented cells tend to be cuboidal or flattened and are much larger than the smaller nonpigmented cells. The larger cells often contain melanotic granules, while the nonpigmented cells tend to be arranged in solid groups

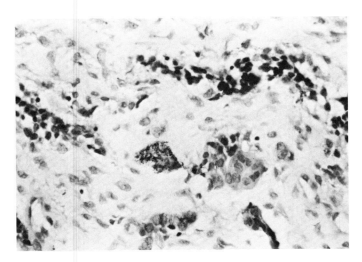

Fig. 22-21. Melanotic neuroectodermal tumor showing large epithelial tumor cells with scattered melanin and smaller lymphocyte-like cells without melanin.

and often form the lining of cleft-like spaces. The nonpigmented cells are typically round and contain a nucleus that stains deeply basophilic and usually fills up the majority of the cell. Pigmented spindle-shaped cells may also be identified within the tumor mass. Misugi et al.[128] have documented ultrastructurally that the pigment-containing cells are quite consistent with melanocytes, and that the nonpigmented cells resemble neuroblasts.

The tumor is usually treated by conservative surgical excision.

NONODONTOGENIC TUMORS AND LESIONS OF ORAL SOFT TISSUES
Developmental Conditions

Median Rhomboid Glossitis

Clinical Features

Median rhomboid glossitis is a relatively common disorder, which appears clinically as a red, angular, diamond-shaped or ovoid area on the dorsal surface of the tongue. It is usually identified at the junction of the anterior two thirds and posterior one third of the tongue. The etiology of the condition is unknown, although most authorities postulate that it arises from a failure of the tuberculum impar to retract at the time of formation of the two lateral halves of the tongue, resulting in a central depapillated overgrowth. It has been proposed that the lesion arises from salivary gland inclusions, odontogenic epithelial rests, and even candidal infection.[129]

The condition is usually symptomless, unless the patient eats hot, spicy foods or drinks exceedingly hot flu-

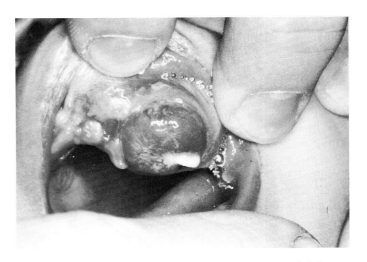

Fig. 22-20. Melanotic neuroectodermal tumor of infancy. (Courtesy of Richard Glass, D.D.S., Stephen Young, D.D.S., and Michael Rohrer, D.D.S.)

ids, and it is brought to the patient's attention by the clinician. A differential diagnosis often includes squamous cell carcinoma; however, squamous cell carcinoma is exceedingly rare on the central portion of the dorsal surface of the tongue.

Pathologic Features

Histologically, findings include acanthotic epithelium devoid of papillae. There may be marked branching and elongation of rete ridges as they penetrate into the supporting connective tissue. The connective tissue is usually mildly inflamed, with increased vascularity.

Treatment usually involves management of symptoms when they occur.

Lingual Thyroid Nodule

Clinical Features

Functioning ectopic lingual thyroid tissue can be found in the oral cavity in the form of a tumor-like mass. This frequently presents a differential diagnostic challenge. Such nodules have been reported on the posterolateral and dorsal surfaces of the tongue and on the floor of the mouth.[130] Lingual thyroid nodules may remain dormant until puberty and then begin to proliferate as nodular masses that can be quite alarming. It is important that the clinician evaluate these nodules thoroughly because on occasion they have been described as the only functioning thyroid tissue in the body.

Pathologic Features

Lingual nodules resemble normal thyroid tissue, but when enlargement occurs, there may be changes that resemble those seen in a colloid goiter. Sauk[131] implemented a study to determine the frequency of ectopic oral thyroid tissue. In a series of 200 consecutively accessioned autopsies, Sauk was able to identify thyroid tissue in 10 percent of the cases, a rather high frequency.

Lesions of Epithelial Origin

Squamous Papilloma

Papillomatous proliferation of squamous epithelium is a common morphologic feature of verruca vulgaris, condyloma acuminatum, inflammatory papillary hyperplasia, and verrucous carcinoma. It is well documented that one or more of 56 types of human papillomavirus serve as the causative infectious agent in verruca vulgaris of the skin and in anogenital condylomata acuminata.[132] Eversole and associates[133] have been able to show human papillo-

mavirus type 2 DNA in oral and labial verruca vulgaris. Detection of human papillomavirus antigen in oral papillary lesions has also been reported by Jin and Toto.[134]

The oral papilloma is a surface epithelial neoplasm and represents one of the most frequently encountered lesions in the oral cavity. Despite its frequency, there are few comprehensive reports on the subject. Bhaskar[135] and Jones[136] report that papillomas represent 80 percent of all the tumors of the oral cavity in children, and Kahn and associates[137] indicate that they are the most frequent benign neoplasm of the soft palate and uvula. Waldron, in an unpublished review of 125 papillomas, noted that over 50 percent occurred in the second to fifth decades of life, with the lip being the most common site. They can present clinically as broad-based, raised, oval swellings, or they may be pedunculated. The surface is typically corrugated or villous. Most tumors in the oral cavity take on a marked degree of keratinization and appear as white lesions, although red lesions may occur in nonkeratinized regions, especially in the posterior pharynx.

Occasionally, multiple oral papillomas can occur in association with verruca vulgaris or condyloma acuminatum of the skin.[138,139] The *focal dermal hyperplasia syndrome* may have multiple oral papillomatosis associated with it. Eversole and Sorenson[140] have reported *florid oral papillomatosis* with Down's syndrome. In an evaluation of 110 lesions, Greer and Goldman[141] found that the age range was 6 to 85, with 38 being the median age. They documented one exceedingly rare inverted oral papilloma, histologically similar to the type of lesion seen in the paranasal sinuses and the bladder.

The most frequent location documented by Greer and Goldman[141] was the tongue. Together the palate and buccal mucosa accounted for nearly as many lesions. The three sites combined accounted for two thirds of the lesions.

Pathologic Features

The papilloma is classically an exophytic lesion demonstrating a complex pattern of multiple finger-like projections of stratified squamous epithelium surrounding a central vascular connective tissue core. The epithelium may be hyperkeratotic or acanthotic, and the supporting collagen may contain chronic inflammatory cells, especially if there has been superficial ulceration of the lesion due to trauma. Occasionally, lesions that are much more aggressive than papillomas may take on a papillomatous appearance clinically. Wertheimer and Stroud[142] have reported a case of peripheral ameloblastoma occurring in a papilloma, but the relationship of this lesion to the more benign papilloma is purely morphologic.

Excision of the papilloma at its base is mandatory to prevent recurrence; although this is the most prevalent form of treatment, cryosurgery has been used as well.

Papillary Hyperplasia

Clinical Features

Inflammatory papillary hyperplasia most often occurs in the oral cavity in association with an ill-fitting maxillary denture or in association with poor oral hygiene. The typical site is the palate, although cases have been reported in the cheeks.[143] It is rather uncommon to find inflammatory papillary hyperplasia in patients who do not wear dentures, but it does occur, with the same clinical appearance as the lesion in a denture-bearing area.

Greer and associates attempted to identify human papillomavirus DNA in smokeless tobacco-associated keratoses from juveniles, adults, and older patients, using papillary hyperplasia cases as control tissue samples.[144] In none of our 35 instances of papillary hyperplasia were we able to identify human papillomavirus DNA.

Typically, the lesions appear as diffuse papillary or warty exophytic lesions affecting denture-bearing areas. They may be so extensive as to take on the appearance of verrucous carcinoma, and verrucous carcinoma has to be included in a differential diagnosis of such lesions. Frequently the epithelium is ulcerated owing to the trauma from ill-fitting dentures. The chief complaint is pain when ulceration occurs.

There has been considerable debate in the literature as to whether or not papillary hyperplasia is a premalignant lesion. Although there are reported cases of the development of squamous cell carcinoma in lesions that were thought to be papillary hyperplasia, there is little evidence to support the theory that this lesion actually leads to the development of squamous cell carcinoma. Differential diagnoses that should be considered on the basis of clinical grounds include florid oral papillomatosis, multifocal condyloma acuminatum, and verrucous carcinoma.

Pathologic Features

Papillary hyperplasia presents as a proliferation of multiple exophytic papillary projections, supported by a connective tissue core that is nearly always chronically inflamed. Very often the chronic inflammatory infiltrate is limited to the superficial connective tissue layer and is composed predominantly of plasma cells and lymphocytes. The epithelium may show marked hyperkeratosis, parakeratosis, or acanthosis. Atypical epithelial changes are rarely, if ever, identified.

The treatment of choice is surgical excision unless the lesion is very small, in which case it may respond to denture relief, relining of the denture, or reconstruction of the denture.

Keratoacanthoma

Clinical Features

Keratoacanthoma is a lesion that typically occurs on sun-exposed skin surfaces. The most common perioral site is the lip. It can occur in the oral cavity, but it is an exceedingly rare intraoral neoplasm. Svirsky et al.[145] have reported a solitary keratoacanthoma on the maxillary gingiva in a 12-year-old boy. Only three additional cases of solitary intraoral keratoacanthoma have been reported in the English literature. Periorally, keratoacanthoma chiefly occurs along the vermilion border of the lip, where it presents as a painless, usually rapidly growing, 1 to 2 cm, firm, raised nodule with a central depressed keratin-filled crater. It tends to occur most frequently in middle-aged and older patients, but there are reports in infants and children.[146] Males appear to be affected twice as frequently as females.

Two variants of keratoacanthoma are now recognized, solitary and multiple.[147,148] In the multiple keratoacanthomatous state the oral mucous membranes are rarely involved; when they are, the histologic appearance of the multifocal keratoacanthoma is similar to that of solitary cutaneous or mucosal keratoacanthoma.[149]

Most investigators concur that keratoacanthomas of the skin arise from a portion of the adnexal hair follicle. There is some debate as to origin of the lesion when it presents entirely on the mucosal surface of the oral cavity. Svirsky and coworkers[145] postulate that an adnexal structure other than a hair follicle may be responsible for the development of intraoral keratoacanthoma, and it is their contention that perhaps sebaceous glands, which are common to the mucous membranes as well as to the skin, may be responsible for the development of keratoacanthoma. In the small number of well documented intraoral cases, it has been rather difficult to demonstrate sebaceous glands in tissue sections; therefore, the hypothesis that the lesion arises from sebaceous adnexal structures remains unsupported histologically. The distinctive microscopic features of keratoacanthoma are detailed in Chapter 9.

Lichen Planus

Clinical Features

Lichen planus is a mucocutaneous disease, most often characterized by the development of white or lacy striae in the oral cavity. Lesions may also present as bullae or ulcers. Lichen planus can mimic traumatic hyperkeratosis, leukoedema, geographic tongue of the ectopic variety, or white sponge nevus. Lesions may also occur on the skin as plaque-like abrasions. Skin lesions may or may not precede oral lesions.

The pathologic process in lichen planus is most likely a cell-mediated response localized to the basement membrane zone and characterized by degeneration of the epithelial cells in the basal layer and disruption of the basement membrane.

An atypical, possibly premalignant form of lichen planus termed *lichenoid dysplasia* has been investigated by Eisenberg and colleagues.[150] These investigators suggest that although superficial similarities exist at the clinical and microscopic levels between lichen planus and lichenoid dysplasia, involucrin immunostaining may allow distinction between the two. Recent research suggests that erosive lichen planus can be treated with systemic isotretinoin and topical retinolic acid.[151]

There is some suggestion that the lesion is aggravated by psychosomatic features, and that patients with the disease frequently are under constant stress or tension. Occasionally, patients with this lesion will subsequently develop oral carcinoma.[152] The pathologic features of lichen planus are discussed at length in Chapter 8.

Nicotine Stomatitis

Clinical Features

Smoking, particularly cigar and pipe smoking, is the etiologic agent responsible for nicotine stomatitis. Nicotine stomatitis is characterized by white palatal proliferations with central red areas representing inflamed or obstructed minor salivary gland ducts. The surrounding and intervening mucosa is frequently white and may show desquamation.

Pathologic Features

Histologically, the pathologist can appreciate hyperkeratinized epithelium and marked squamous metaplasia with deep rete ridge penetration into the connective tissue lamina propria, with diffuse inflammation that frequently surrounds small ducts and associated minor salivary glands. It is often difficult to identify a fortuitous section showing salivary gland to surface epithelial communication, the classic histologic marker of the disorder.

The lesion is benign and shows no progression toward dysplasia. It is important, nonetheless, to at least recall the field cancerization effect that is associated with continued tobacco use, and although nicotine stomatitis is thought to be a reversible benign transformation, the continued use of the tobacco irritant may in fact potentiate a de novo palatal carcinoma, unassociated with the previous nicotine stomatitis.

The treatment of choice is to reduce or refrain from tobacco use.

Leukoplakia and Erythroplakia

The term *leukoplakia* is used to classify a white patch or plaque on the oral mucous membrane that cannot be removed by scraping and cannot be classified clinically or microscopically as another disease entity.[152]

This definition was proposed by the World Health Organization Collaborating Center for Precancerous Lesions at its 1978 conference.[153] Leukoplakia has further been defined to have multiple subtypes by Pindborg and associates[154] and Sugar and Banocyz[155] (Table 22-1). Table 22-1 depicts the various types of leukoplakia described by these investigators. Leukoplakia appears to occur most often before age 40 and shows a predilection for males. In Sugar and Banocyz's study of 670 leukoplakic patients who were followed for over 3 years, 31 percent of the lesions disappeared, 30 percent improved, and 25 percent remained unchanged.[155] Their study and those of Pindborg and others revealed that approximately 6 percent of oral leukoplakias became malignant. Leukoplakia has been reported in all oral sites but appears to be most common in the tongue, lips, and floor of the mouth.

Burkhardt[156] has separated leukoplakia into three microscopic forms corresponding to the verrucous and erosive clinical forms that have been described. These microscopic forms have been described as (1) plain, (2) papillary endophytic, and (3) papillomatous exophytic. However, most authorities consider *leukoplakia* to be exclusively a clinical term, and there is no histologic picture that is characteristic of this process.

Erythroplakia is defined as a red patch that is characteristically velvety and cannot be clinically or pathologically ascribed to any other disease entity. It is considered by many investigators to be the earliest sign of asymptomatic oral cancer.[157] It is important to consider both leukoplakia and erythroplakia together, since in the past both have been considered premalignant lesions.

**TABLE 22-1. Leukoplakia of the Oral Cavity—
Clinical Types**

Authors	Leukoplakia Subtype
Pindborg et al.[154]	Homogeneous: white patch with a variable appearance, smooth or wrinkled; smooth areas may have small cracks or fissures Speckled or nodular: erythematous base with white patches or nodular excrescences
Sugar and Banocyz[155]	Leukoplakia simplex: white, homogeneous keratinized lesion, slightly elevated Leukoplakia verrucosa: white, verrucous lesion, with wrinkled surface Leukoplakia erosiva: white lesion with erythematous areas, erosions, fissures

Although various systemic diseases may appear as white plaques (lichen planus, syphilitic mucous patches, moniliasis, lupus erythematosus), such entities do not in fact represent leukoplakia as defined by WHO, since they have a distinctive histologic appearance.[152]

The prevalence of oral leukoplakia in the general population is unknown, although there are studies that indicate it affects anywhere from 0.2 to 0.5 percent of the population.[152] Typically, patients with leukoplakia are totally asymptomatic, and the lesions are most commonly discovered on routine examination of the oral cavity or because the patient may be aware of a roughness or color change within the mouth. It is mandatory to do a biopsy of such white lesions to determine their exact nature in nearly all instances. The etiologic agents that are most commonly implicated as causal are cigarette smoking, tobacco chewing, snuff dipping, and the concomitant use of alcohol in excess.

Greer and associates[3,144] have identified a special form of leukoplakia (smokeless tobacco leukoplakia) associated with the use of smokeless tobacco products. These investigators have recently identified human papillomavirus capsid antigens and viral protein in such lesions using immunocytochemical and recombinant DNA techniques. They have proposed that the human papillomavirus may have a synergistic role with tobacco to produce the clinically discernible leukoplakic lesions. Dysplasia was not identified in any of these cases.

The possible premalignant nature of leukoplakia has been debated for many years. Silverman and Galante[152] contend that between 2.5 and 6 percent of lesions properly ascribed the name leukoplakia transform into carcinoma. Mashberg and Meyers[157] suggest that erythroplakia is even more likely to develop into cancer. Intermediate forms (speckled leukoplakia or erythroplakia) have also been reported.[158]

The vast majority of white oral plaques, however, are benign, not premalignant hyperkeratoses, and are typically present because of some chronic form of irritation to the oral mucosa. The irritation may be from a prosthetic appliance or from tobacco (nicotine stomatitis). The changes appear to be reversible if the irritant is removed. Histologically, hyperkeratosis, parakeratosis, and acanthosis may be seen, but dyspolarity and atypia are lacking. The most common sites are the tongue, palate, and gingiva.

In summary, leukoplakia is a clinical term designating a lesion that may have a variety of histologic appearances. The pathologist should not use this term but should report biopsies of these lesions in terms of the specific histologic features seen (hyperkeratosis, acanthosis, dysplasia, etc.) The lesions showing *dysplasia* (see below) are those in which progression to carcinoma should be more feared.

Epithelial Dysplasia

Clinical and Pathologic Features

The etiology of oral epithelial dysplasia is thought to be related for the most part to extensive alcohol and tobacco use. Features characteristic of epithelial dysplasia are the classic cytologic abnormalities associated with most epithelial atypias. They include basal layer hyperchromatism, atypical mitoses, altered nuclear/cytoplasmic ratios, loss of cellular polarity, nuclear pleomorphism, prominent nucleoli, and basal layer hyperplasia (Fig. 22-22). Individual cell keratinization in the spinous layer (dyskeratosis) is another hallmark of dysplasia.

Epithelial dysplasia of the oral cavity has not undergone the close scrutiny and extensive categorization that dysplasia of the uterine cervix has. Oral epithelial dysplasia is usually classified as mild, moderate, or severe. In mild dysplasia the severity of the atypical changes is minimal; the most prominent features include basal layer hyperplasia, loss of cellular polarity, and atypical mitoses. The surface layer may be hyperkeratinized, so the lesion appears white clinically. As the atypical cytologic changes increase to include a greater frequency of altered nuclear/cytoplasmic ratios, dyskeratoses, basal layer hyperchromatism, and mitoses, the degree of severity of the dysplasia increases proportionately. There is often considerable debate as to whether lesions that affect the mucosa in continuity with the skin surface should be categorized as actinic keratosis or as a mild, moderate, or severe dysplastic change. It is my feeling that lesions involving the mucosal surface, regardless of contiguous skin surface findings, must be classified according to dysplastic criteria and not simply as an actinic change. The biologic behavior of a dysplastic lesion of the oral mucosa appears to be much more aggressive than corresponding atypical changes of the skin.

Carcinoma in Situ (Intraepithelial Carcinoma)

Clinical and Pathologic Features

The diagnosis of carcinoma in situ should be based on rigid histologic criteria; however, the distinction between carcinoma in situ and severe epithelial dysplasia is often arbitrary. Classically, a carcinoma in situ tissue sample should show all the atypical cytologic criteria necessary for a malignant diagnosis, but these atypical changes must be confined to the epithelial layer. With carcinoma in situ, one must identify an intact basement membrane and top to bottom or through and through epithelial dysplasia. Lesions that are diagnosed as carcinoma in situ may appear red, white, blue, or black clinically, and on occasion they may present as a tumor mass. Mashberg and Meyers[157] indicate that a large percentage of early

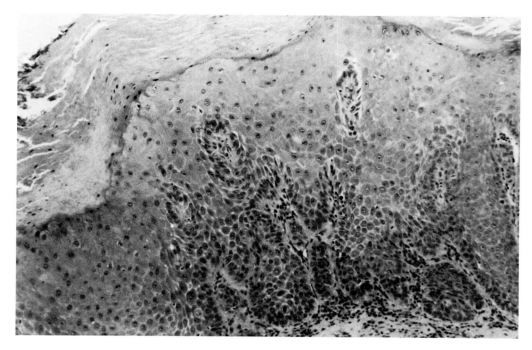

Fig. 22-22. Moderate epithelial dysplasia showing a loss of cellular polarity, nuclear hyperchromatism, dyskeratosis, and basal cell layer hyperplasia.

epithelial changes that present as red lesions clinically show at least some degree of dysplasia, and a large percentage of the lesions represent carcinoma in situ.

Squamous Cell Carcinoma (Epidermoid Carcinoma)

Cancer statistics compiled by the National Cancer Institute predict that over 24,000 new cases of oral cancer will occur in the United States annually. These statistics are based on annual surveys of oral cancer that include cancer of the lips, tongue, floor of the mouth, salivary glands, pharynx, and other unspecified sites within the mouth. Oral cancer continues to account annually for nearly 7 percent of all new cancer cases among both men and women in the United States.[159] Less than 35 percent of the documented oral cancers are cured by present treatment modalities.[159] A marked improvement in this cure rate can be documented if oral cancer is detected at an early stage. Early, well localized cancer of the oral cavity can have a cure rate as high as 90 percent.[160]

Nearly 90 percent of all oral cancers represent squamous cell carcinoma. The vast majority of all remaining malignancies are malignant salivary gland tumors, lymphomas, and assorted malignant neoplasms of mesenchymal origin, including bone. Oral cancers are estimated to account for 6.2 percent of all carcinomas in men and 1.9 percent of all carcinomas in women in the United

States.[161,162] There are very much higher percentages of cancer in other parts of the world, especially some Asiatic countries, where there are reports that oral cancer represents 50 percent of all recorded malignancies.[163,164] Oral cancer tends to be a disease of older age and affects men much more frequently than women. Most patients with oral cancer are over 45 years of age.

Etiology

The cause of squamous cell carcinoma of the oral cavity remains unknown, although the most frequently implicated etiologic agents are tobacco and alcohol or combinations of the two. Heredity undoubtedly plays a role in the development of squamous cell carcinoma, but just how important it is is unknown. There are reports in the Scandinavian literature documenting that patients with the iron-deficient *Plummer-Vinson syndrome* show changes in the mucous membrane that predispose to malignancy.[165] Andreasen[166] indicates that patients with discoid lupus erythematosus have a higher probability of developing squamous cell carcinoma of the lip than patients without lupus. Pindborg et al.[167] indicate that the condition known as *oral submucous fibrosis* is a precancerous lesion. The disorder occurs most frequently in India, although there are reports from Great Britain among Indians and Pakistanis living in that country.

There are many reports in the literature that document

the relationship between excessive alcohol use and oral squamous cell carcinoma and between cirrhosis of the liver and cancer of the tongue and oral mucosa.[152,158] In heavy drinkers who are also heavy smokers, it appears that the neoplastic predisposing factors of alcohol and tobacco work in combination to induce changes in the oral epithelium that eventually lead to malignancy. Recent studies indicate an independent and synergistic relationship between oral cancer and the consumption of tobacco and alcohol.[152] The risk of developing oral and head and neck cancer appears to be six times greater for alcoholics than for nonalcoholics, which is quite similar to the situation with smokers versus nonsmokers.[152]

Risk factors other than alcohol and tobacco have now been reported for oral squamous cell carcinoma, including herpes simplex, lichen planus, and candidiosis.[168–170]

There is strong evidence that the *hairy leukoplakia* identified in patients with acquired immunodeficiency syndrome (AIDS) is *Candida*-associated, but there is no genuine proof that hairy leukoplakia develops into squamous cell carcinoma.[170]

Squamous cell carcinoma may develop as a long-term complication (9 to 25 year latent period) of radiotherapy.[171] Actinic radiation is often responsible for carcinoma of the lip, but it does not seem to be responsible for squamous cell carcinoma arising within the oral cavity. Lip carcinoma is twice as frequent in England and the Scandinavian countries as it is in the United States. Blacks seem to suffer a much lower frequency of squamous cell carcinoma of the lip and the skin surfaces than whites, probably as a result of protective melanin pigmentation.

The tongue is the most common site for squamous cell carcinoma within the oral cavity, although squamous cell carcinoma of the lip is the most common site of cancer if perioral sites are included. The next most common intraoral site after the tongue is the floor of the mouth. Numerous surveys[152,159] indicate varying degrees of frequency in the buccal mucosa and other sites of the oropharynx. Interestingly, Silverman and Galante[152] note that there was a 31 percent decrease in the number of cases of lip cancer reported in California from 1960 to 1973; they relate this to the fact that there appears to be increasing use of protective agents by patients to screen out actinic radiation.

The increased incidence of multiple cancers in association with continued smoking is quite interesting. Fu et al.[172] reviewed 153 carcinomas of the floor of the mouth treated at the University of California, San Francisco, between 1957 and 1973. They found that 15 percent of the patients had at least one subsequent primary oral cancer during the 16 year period. Wynder et al. in a similar study documented an 8.3 percent incidence of second primaries.

There has been lengthy debate as to whether patients with a history of syphilis develop oral squamous cell carcinoma with greater frequency than patients with no such history. Present data indicate that a relationship between a past history of syphilis and oral carcinoma is debatable, but it is a risk factor that must be considered to be of some significance in the development of carcinoma of the tongue.[152,173]

Pathologic Features

Grossly, squamous cell carcinoma of the oral cavity can present as an ulcer, an alteration of mucosal color, or a tumor mass. Ulcerative lesions usually have a crateriform appearance with rolled, elevated borders that are firm because of the infiltration of tumor along the margins. The cut section usually has a gray-white, glistening appearance with little tendency for the lesions to bulge beyond the cut margins. Lesions that appear clinically red often have a granular or gritty appearance, and the cut section frequently has the consistency of granulation tissue as opposed to the firm cut section of ulcers.

Squamous cell carcinoma is characterized by a proliferation of sheets, nests, cords, and neoplastic islands of epithelium that penetrate into the supporting connective tissue lamina propria and submucosa. The neoplasm is usually identified histologically as being well differentiated, moderately differentiated, poorly differentiated, or undifferentiated (nonkeratinizing). In the past, tumors were graded as grades I to IV.[174] This numerical system is much less used by pathologists today.

A uniform method of clinical staging for squamous cell carcinomas in the oral cavity has been recommended by the American Joint Committee for Cancer Staging. The staging process groups squamous cell carcinoma of the oral cavity into four stages.

Stage I: Primary tumors that are limited to an oral site with no evidence of cervical lymph node metastases

Stage II: Tumors that have extended beyond their original site to contiguous oral sites but remain limited to the oral cavity with no discernible cervical lymph node metastasis

Stage III: Tumors limited to a single site or contiguous oral structures, also showing cervical lymph node metastases without fixation of the nodes

Stage IV: Primary tumors that have extended beyond their site within the oral cavity clinically, in concert with palpable fixed cervical lymph node metastases or distant lymph node metastases

Staging, more than any other parameter, allows the clinician and the pathologist to predict the behavior of the tumor.[159] Platz et al.[175] and Lederer et al.[176] have recently

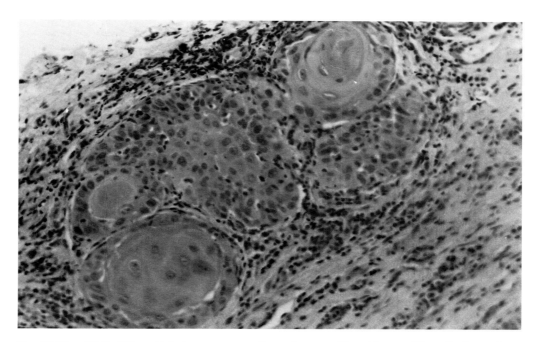

Fig. 22-23. Well differentiated squamous cell carcinoma with evidence of keratin formation.

defined a specific form of microinvasive squamous cell carcinoma, which they have separated from the traditional TNM staging of squamous cell carcinomas. These *microcarcinomas* have a better prognosis than T1 lesions. The findings of these authors suggest that clinical stage and histologic grade do occasionally show a correlation, and that microcarcinomas have more favorable prognoses based on a specific histology.

The neoplastic cells of well differentiated squamous carcinomas bear a striking similarity to the cells of normal squamous epithelium. The cells are generally large, with vesicular to oval nuclei and eosinophilic cytoplasm, intracellular bridging is usually easily discernible, and the degree of nuclear hyperchromatism and bizarre mitotic activity is minimal. Keratin pearl formation is usually quite prominent in well differentiated squamous cell carcinoma, and individual cell keratinization tends to be a hallmark of this form of the disease (Fig. 22-23). The connective tissue lamina propria and supporting fibromuscular submucosa into which neoplastic islands penetrate often show a marked degree of chronic inflammation, predominantly plasma cells and lymphocytes. Squamous cell carcinomas that show a moderate degree of differentiation display a much more varied histologic pattern, and although the tumor cells resemble normal squamous epithelial cells, hyperchromatism, pleomorphism, anisocytosis, and loss of attachment of cells are more prominent. As a rule, the frequency of atypical mitoses is increased, and the frequency of individual cell keratinization and keratin pearl formation is decreased.

In poorly differentiated squamous cell carcinomas, there is very little evidence that the tumor is of squamous origin. Individual cell keratinization is lacking; nuclear-to-cytoplasmic ratios are markedly altered; and there is a tremendous amount of pleomorphism and atypical mitoses (Fig. 22-24). Tumor giant cells may also be prominent in poorly differentiated tumors. Undifferentiated squamous cell carcinomas have also been referred to as nonkeratinizing squamous cell carcinoma. They have little if any resemblance to a neoplasm of squamous epithelial origin, and frequently tumor cells resemble histiocytes, atypical lymphocytes, or spindled fibroblasts. The char-

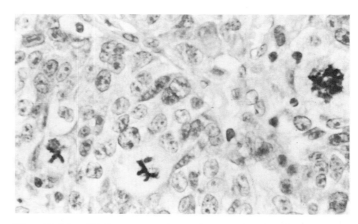

Fig. 22-24. High-power photomicrograph showing cellular atypia in poorly differentiated squamous cell carcinoma.

acteristic histologic features that identify the tumor cells as epithelial may be totally lacking. Electron microscopic evaluation may be the only method of documenting that the tumor is of squamous epithelial origin.

Anatomic Sites

Squamous Cell Carcinoma of the Tongue. Epidermoid carcinoma of the tongue usually manifests as an ulcerative or papillary-type lesion in the middle third of the tongue. There are reported cases of multiple tumors that have coalesced into a single tumor mass at the tip and along the central surface of the tongue. Lymph node metastasis in carcinoma of the tongue is frequent; the average 5 year survival rate is reportedly in the range of 20 to 25 percent. If lymph node metastases are identified at initial surgery, the recurrence rate ranges as high as 40 to 50 percent. Lesions along the anterior portion of the tongue have a much better prognosis than those along the lateral two thirds of the tongue. In 1962 Frazell and Lucas[173] indicated that lesions that are well differentiated have a much better prognosis than those that are poorly differentiated.

Squamous Cell Carcinoma of the Lips. Squamous cell carcinoma affects the lower lip much more commonly than the upper lip. It typically presents as an ulcer or warty growth along the vermilion border. The first lymph nodes involved are the submandibular and submental nodes, with extension into the deeper cervical lymph nodes if the lesion is not managed early. Histologically, the vast majority of squamous cell carcinomas of the lip are well differentiated. Poorly differentiated and highly anaplastic lesions are rare. This form of cancer carries with it a very high 5 year survival rate. Cross and colleagues[177] reported an 80 to 85 percent 5 year survival rate when such lesions were identified without nodal involvement. When squamous cell carcinomas of the lip are identified in concert with lymph node metastases, the survival rate drops to less than 40 percent.

Knapel et al.[178] have reported that carcinomas of the upper lip and commissures are usually less differentiated than those of the lower lip and are thought to grow more insidiously and rapidly. Lymph node metastases of upper lip carcinomas are also thought to be more diffuse.

Squamous Cell Carcinoma of the Buccal Mucosa. The most common buccal mucosal site is the retromolar area posterior or adjacent to the third molar teeth. Very frequently, these lesions present as long-standing white or red lesions, which eventually develop into warty, papillary, or ulcerative growths. Long-standing lesions may invade alveolar mucosa and bone, so it is often difficult to determine where the lesion first began. Microscopically, buccal mucosal lesions usually present as well differenti-

ated tumors, with early spread to the submandibular and upper cervical nodes.

Vanderwall[179] has reported that squamous cell carcinomas of the buccal mucosa, left untreated, are extensively destructive lesions and can show rapid invasion into the pterygomaxillary fossa. Metastasis to regional lymph nodes will occur in about 50 percent of such cases. Five-year survival rates for these lesions are generally in the range of 20 to 30 percent.

Squamous Cell Carcinoma of the Gingiva. Squamous cell carcinoma of the gingiva is rare; when it does occur, it usually presents in the molar and premolar areas. Ulcerations and papillary growths are the most common findings. This lesion can be exceedingly vexing because of its close proximity to bone and its ability to rapidly spread into bone. Although such lesions are frequently well differentiated, 5 year survival rates are only in the range of 20 to 40 percent. Cady and Catlin[180] reviewed 600 patients with carcinoma of the gingiva and found an unusual 50 percent survival rate over a 20 year period. It has been my experience that squamous cell carcinoma of the gingiva is indeed a very rapidly growing and aggressive neoplasm, and that a 50 percent survival rate after 20 years is exceedingly high.

Squamous Cell Carcinoma of the Floor of the Mouth. Carcinoma of the floor of the mouth is usually identified in the anterior portion of the mouth beneath the ventral surface of the tongue. It may present as a red velvety, wart-like, or ulcerative lesion. Histologically, most of the tumors tend to be well differentiated. Lymph node metastases are usually to the submandibular lymph nodes or the anterior jugular nodes. Greer and Wilson[159] found the floor of the mouth to be the most common oral site for squamous cell carcinoma in a review of over 100 cases in a 5 year retrospective study.

Squamous Cell Carcinoma of the Palate. Squamous cell carcinoma is more frequently identified in the soft palate than in the hard palate. It generally presents as an ulcer or papillary growth. The tumors are generally well differentiated, and the prognosis is poor, with 5 year survival rates between 5 and 10 percent. Greer and Wilson[159] found the palate to be the least common site for all squamous cell carcinomas in their 5 year survey.

Variants of Squamous Cell Carcinoma

Adenoid Squamous Cell Carcinoma. Adenoid squamous cell carcinoma has been documented by Jacoway et al. and Tomich and Hutton.[181,182] The lesions that have been reported were identified on the lip as tumor masses in solar-damaged skin. The lower lip is much more commonly affected than the upper lip, and the lesion appears always to be situated along the vermilion border. Most lesions present as ulcerations or elevated slightly crusted nodules. Most cases have been reported in men over the age of 50 years.

Microscopically, the lesions are characterized by a proliferation of squamous cell carcinoma with central acantholysis and the development of cystic spaces filled with desquamated cells. Many cystic spaces have a pseudoglandular arrangement and are rimmed by cuboidal epithelium, hence the name adenoid squamous carcinoma. Typically, the stroma shows a chronic inflammatory infiltrate and degeneration of the collagen typical of the basaloid solar degeneration found in actinic keratosis. The lesions are exceedingly slow growing, and metastases have not been documented.

Spindle Cell Carcinoma. Spindle cell carcinomas have also been referred to as *pleomorphic carcinoma, metaplastic carcinoma,* and *sarcomatoid carcinoma.*

The vast majority of patients with spindle cell carcinoma are men in the sixth or seventh decade of life. Batsakis[183] reports that there are no special studies that are absolutely diagnostic of spindle cell carcinoma so as to enable the pathologist to separate it from other sarcomatoid lesions. Batsakis has further suggested that these tumors are not a homogeneous class of neoplasms.[183,184]

This form of squamous cell carcinoma has been documented consistently in the world literature only in the past 15 years, although similar lesions have long been identified in the breast and skin. Spindle cell carcinomas are most frequently identified on the lips; the lower lip is the most commonly involved oral site. Clinically, they present as polypoid nodular or fleshy lesions.

Grossly, the lesions have a smooth, glistening, often whorled pattern on cut surface. Leifer and colleagues[185] have reviewed a series of spindle cell carcinomas of the oral mucosa with light and electron microscopy. They conclude that the lesions are of squamous epithelial derivation. Histologically, the lesion presents as an undifferentiated or anaplastic proliferation of spindle and stellate cells often arranged in interlacing fascicles, thus resembling a tumor of connective tissue origin. Many authorities indicate that this spindle cell proliferation can always be traced to a continuity with surface epithelium with multiple sections.[186] Often the pathologist must consider differential diagnoses of fibrosarcoma, rhabdomyosarcoma, and liposarcoma. It may be difficult to render a diagnosis of squamous cell carcinoma unless one is able to identify a continuity between the proliferating spindle cell elements and the surface. Electron microscopy with identification of desmosomal attachments and immunohistochemical study of intermediate filaments are useful adjuncts.

When one encounters a tumor composed of interlacing fascicles of cells that are spindle-shaped and highly undifferentiated, serial sectioning of the tumor is mandatory.

Postradiation squamous cell carcinomas can often take on a spindled appearance, and it may be difficult to tell a recurrent neoplasm from a proliferation of mature fibrogranulation tissue, spindle cell carcinoma, or "pseudosarcoma." The fact that in the pseudosarcoma tumor giant cells seem to be found with a greater degree of frequency than in recurrent squamous cell carcinoma is most helpful in the differential diagnosis. Another lesion that can be confused with spindle cell carcinoma is nodular fasciitis. A striking histologic feature of nodular fasciitis that differentiates it from spindle cell carcinoma is the random arrangement of bundles of fibroblasts in a mucoid matrix; such a mucoid matrix is not a feature of spindle cell carcinoma. Another important feature that separates the two is stromal vascularity. The marked vascularity of nodular fasciitis with its fine capillary network is rarely seen in spindle cell carcinoma.

Spindle cell carcinomas can prove exceedingly aggressive. Ellis and Corio[187] found mean survival rates of patients with this disease to be under 2 years. Batsakis found that 27 percent of 166 sarcomatoid carcinomas that he studied metastasized.[183,184]

Verrucous Carcinoma
Clinical Features

Verrucous carcinoma was first reported by Friedell and Rosenthal[188] and popularized by Ackerman[189] as a variant of squamous cell carcinoma. It is chiefly identified after the sixth decade of life and is most common in the mandibular buccal sulcus and along the alveolar mucosa of the mandibular ridge. A few cases of verrucous carcinoma of the maxillary alveolar mucosa have been documented.[190] Our material indicates a male predominance; Shafer et al.[68] document a female predominance.

Verrucous carcinoma is best defined as a clinicopathologic entity. Frequently it goes unrecognized in its earliest stages because of its simple localized papillary or verruciform appearance, often thought to be consistent with a papilloma or verruca vulgaris. Verrucous carcinoma is most likely part of a histologic spectrum in which the definitive lesion arises from a papillary verrucoid leukoplakia over a course of some years.[191] Shear and Pindborg[192] have suggested that the term *verrucous hyperplasia* be considered part of this continuum and propose verrucous hyperplasia as a separate and distinct clinicopathologic entity. Batsakis has suggested, however, that verrucous hyperplasia is simply an early form of verrucous carcinoma. I have had the opportunity to see at least two cases of verrucous hyperplasia developing over a 6-year period into classic verrucous carcinoma, in a 53-year-old woman and a 71-year-old man.

Verrucous carcinoma can undergo multiple phases of clinical development, so that it can appear either as a soft circumscribed lesion, as a fibrotic, rather red granular lesion, as a rough stippled lesion, or as a papillomatous corrugated growth.

Frank invasive squamous cell carcinoma can be identified in verrucous carcinoma in approximately 38 percent of cases. It is exceedingly important, therefore, that verrucous carcinomas be multiply sectioned in order to ensure diagnostic certainty.

Much information in the literature suggests that smokeless tobacco use predisposes to the development of verrucous carcinoma of the oral cavity. Greer and colleagues[144] reviewed a series of 30 smokeless tobacco leukoplakias and were unable to demonstrate even mild dysplasia. Smokeless tobacco use alone did not appear to initiate verrucous carcinoma development; however, human papillomavirus capsid antigens were present in many of the specimens tested and in situ DNA hybridization showed human papilloma viruses type 2 and 6 in 5 of the 30 cases. We postulate that human papillomavirus may often be overlooked as a co-factor in the verrucous carcinoma scenario.

Pathologic Features

Grossly, verrucous carcinoma presents as a papillary or corrugated mass composed of folds of tissue with finger-like clefts between tissue extensions. These papillary folds on cut section are usually gray-white and homogeneous. Microscopically, verrucous carcinoma is characterized by a proliferation of elevated layers of squamous epithelium, which typically penetrate superficially and broadly into the supporting collagen as elongated rete

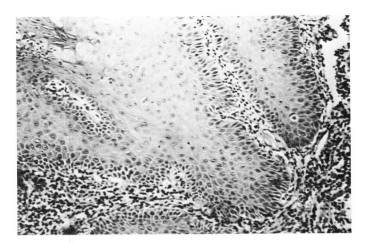

Fig. 22-26. Verrucous carcinoma. Higher power showing neoplastic epithelium with minimal atypia, rimmed by intact basement membrane.

pegs (Figs. 22-25 and 22-26). It is important to note that the cytologic characteristics of the penetrating epithelium are often far from malignant-appearing. More often than not, the pathologist is not able to appreciate the classic cytologic hallmarks of malignancy in the tissue sample. The basement membrane is usually intact, which makes a diagnosis of infiltrating carcinoma difficult, and the epithelium will often extend as a blunt proliferation into the supporting connective tissue along a characteristic broad pushing front as described by Ackerman.[193] Jacobson and Shear[193] indicate that a second characteristic feature of verrucous carcinoma is the manner in which the normal epithelium at the edge of the lesion is bent upon itself by the continued proliferation of the neoplastic epithelium. The supporting collagen typically shows a dense chronic inflammatory infiltrate. Shafer[194] points out that another characteristic feature of verrucous carcinoma is the distinct wedge-like parakeratin plugging between individual finger-like processes of the neoplasm.

Differential Diagnosis

When a diagnosis of verrucous carcinoma is entertained, the most common differential diagnoses considered are pseudoepitheliomatous hyperplasia, oral florid papillomatosis as described by Eversole and Sorenson,[195] papillary hyperplasia, and keratoacanthoma. Keratoacanthoma is an exceedingly rare entity within the oral cavity. The characteristic lipping at the periphery of keratoacanthoma and the glassy hyalinized appearance of keratoacanthoma nearly always serve to separate it from verrucous carcinoma. The distinct parakeratin plugging that is commonly seen in verrucous carcinoma is not identified in keratoacanthoma. A feature characteristic of both lesions is the broad pushing front at the connective

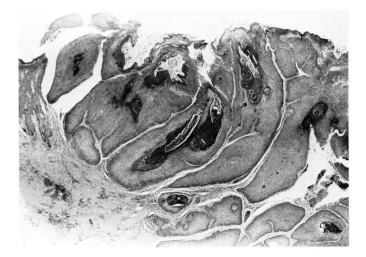

Fig. 22-25. Verrucous carcinoma. Note abundant keratin-plugging of bulbous epithelial masses and invasion on a broad "pushing" front.

tissue margin of growth. Oral florid papillomatosis is characterized histologically by multiple papillary growths supported by a richly vascularized supporting connective tissue stroma. Such vascularity is an unusual finding in verrucous carcinoma. In differentiating pseudoepitheliomatous hyperplasia from verrucous carcinoma, Kraus and Perez-Mesa[196] point out that the bulbous rete ridge pattern of verrucous carcinoma serves to differentiate it from pseudoepitheliomatous hyperplasia, a proliferation in which the rete ridges tend to proliferate as sharp, pointed, elongated, or knife-like structures as they infiltrate the supporting connective tissue. Papillary hyperplasia is usually associated with an ill-fitting denture, is usually palatal, and shows no epithelial atypia.

Verrucous carcinoma must be distinguished from well differentiated squamous cell carcinoma. A lesion that shows cytologic atypia, penetration of the growth beyond the basement membrane, lack of a broad pushing front of neoplastic growth, and no evidence of parakeratin plugging is a well differentiated squamous cell carcinoma. Development of a second oral cancer is not uncommon in patients with a diagnosis of verrucous carcinoma.

There has been considerable debate in the literature as to whether verrucous carcinoma should be treated by surgery or radiation therapy. Most data indicate that the treatment of choice is wide surgical excision. This management modality is supported by Fontz et al.[197] Greer[198] has reported management of a case of long-standing multifocal verrucous carcinoma in a 75-year-old woman using a chemotherapeutic regimen that included methotrexate therapy with citrovorum rescue. Although not the primary management modality of choice, this protocol may prove beneficial in problematic late-stage cases, usually where there may be involvement of bone.

Squamous Cell Carcinoma Arising in Odontogenic Cysts

Malignant transformation of the lining of odontogenic cysts is rare, although there are reports in the literature that document such occurrences.[199] It may be difficult to differentiate squamous cell carcinoma in the wall of the cyst from exuberant odontogenic epithelial rest activity. Characteristically, classic odontogenic epithelial rest activity tends to proliferate as a thin ribbon or small nest-like cluster of cells without the multiphasic finger-like expansions of squamous cell carcinoma.

Toller[200] postulates that the cystic lesion that is most likely to undergo malignant transformation is the odontogenic keratocyst or primordial cyst.

Oral Melanocytic and Other Pigmented Lesions

A host of pigmented lesions affect the oral mucosa. The *amalgam tattoo* is by far the most commonly en-

countered exogenous form of oral pigmentation. It is associated with the entrapment of dental amalgam granules in the oral mucosa and presents as a flat pigmented spot.

Malignant melanoma of the oral cavity is rare, accounting for about 1 to 8 percent of all melanomas. Rapini et al.[201] reviewed a series of 171 cases reported in the oral literature and reported six new cases in 1985. Three of their six patients showed a well developed radial growth phase. The prognosis for oral melanoma is quite poor, with the average survival after diagnosis often no longer than 2 years. Melanoma and other melanocytic tumors and dysplasias are discussed in further detail in Chapter 9.

Benign Epithelial Lesions Resembling Malignant Tumors

Pseudoepitheliomatous Hyperplasia

Clinical Features. Occasionally *hyperplastic odontogenic epithelial cells* may resemble squamous cell carcinoma, as can the *organ of Chievitz,* typically seen in the buccal-temporal space.[202] More common, however, is pseudoepitheliomatous hyperplasia, which may accompany oral mucosal ulceration or be seen alone. It also occurs frequently in association with *granular cell tumor* as a reactive proliferation. Elzay and O'Keefe[203] have reported an instance of primary pseudoepitheliomatous hyperplasia involving the gingiva. Preliminary pathologic diagnoses of inverted papilloma, verrucous carcinoma, squamous odontogenic tumor, verruca vulgaris, and keratoacanthoma need to be entertained when confronted with a possible pseudoepitheliomatous hyperplasia.

Histologic features that separate this entity from verrucous carcinoma and keratoacanthoma have been discussed previously. Rete ridge penetration into the connective tissue is typically in the form of a knife-like or sharp edge in pseudoepitheliomatous hyperplasia (Fig. 22-27); this is an unusual feature in verrucous carcinoma or keratoacanthoma.

Inverted oral papilloma may be a reasonable differential diagnosis, although only three cases have been reported in the world literature.[204] Inverted papilloma in the oral cavity typically shows proliferation of acantholytic squamous epithelium without cystic activity, whereas with oral pseudoepitheliomatous hyperplasia, especially the type identified in young individuals, there are often cystic areas filled with keratin.

Usually when pseudoepitheliomatous hyperplasia is removed, there is no recurrence. Nonetheless, my colleagues and I have had the opportunity to review a case, similar to that reported by Elzay and O'Keefe,[203] that has required three surgical procedures.

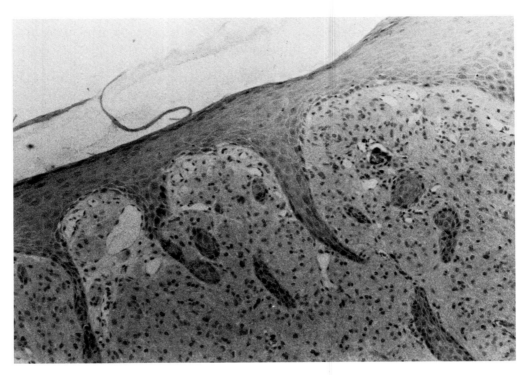

Fig. 22-27. Pseudoepitheliomatous hyperplasia overlying granular cell tumor.

Necrotizing Sialometaplasia

Clinical Features. Necrotizing sialometaplasia is a benign inflammatory process of the minor salivary glands, which typically presents as a deeply excavated, sharply demarcated ulcer. The disorder was first described in 1973 by Abrams and colleague.[205] Most reported cases have been in the hard palate, but cases have been documented involving the mucosa of the mandible.[206]

Necrotizing sialometaplasia usually is identified in adults and often is bilateral. Most patients indicate that the lesion is painful, but there are reported cases in which the lesions were seen without pain as a chief complaint. Occasionally, cases are reported in which there is little or no evidence of ulceration.[207] The cause of necrotizing sialometaplasia is unknown, but trauma has been implicated as an initiating factor. It is postulated that trauma causes intermittent ischemia, followed by infarction and a subsequent mucosal ulcer. Philipsen et al.[208] consider necrotizing sialometaplasia to be the ulcerative or terminal stage of leukokeratosis nicotini palati. Occasionally, patients have prodromal symptoms that include fever, malaise, and swelling. The disease is a benign one, which heals spontaneously in 6 to 10 weeks, usually without treatment.

Recently Poulson and I[209] reported a case of necrotizing sialometaplasia obscuring an underlying embryonal rhabdomyosarcoma. We postulated that the extremely rapid growth of the malignant tumor in the parapha-

ryngeal space probably resulted in physical obstruction or impingement of blood vessels supplying tissues of the oral pharynx, with consequent tissue infarction and a superimposed necrotizing sialometaplasia.

Pathologic Features. Microscopically, necrotizing sialometaplasia is characterized by a central ulcer with a proliferation of reactive epithelial hyperplasia at the edge. The supporting lamina propria may be filled with acute and chronic inflammatory cells. Neutrophils and foamy histiocytes are usually prominent.[205] Within the connective tissue stroma, salivary acinar and ductal elements show marked lobular squamous metaplasia. Lobular ischemic necrosis may be identified and is thought to be a histologic hallmark of the disease. Salivary gland mucin is frequently distributed in microcysts throughout the supporting lamina propria.

Necrotizing sialometaplasia must be differentiated from squamous cell carcinoma and mucoepidermoid carcinoma since mixtures of islands of squamous epithelium with residual mucous cells may lead to a mistaken diagnosis of mucoepidermoid carcinoma. One of the main histologic differences between necrotizing sialometaplasia and both mucoepidermoid carcinoma and squamous cell carcinoma is the regular nuclear morphology of squamous cells in necrotizing sialometaplasia, without cytologic atypia.

Abrams et al.[205] document the following chief histologic features that help differentiate necrotizing sialometaplasia from squamous and mucoepidermoid carcinoma: (1) lobular infarction and necrosis, (2) benign appearing squamous cells, (3) metaplasia of ducts and mucinous acini, (4) a prominent granulation tissue reaction with extensive inflammatory components, and (5) maintenance of lobular architecture. Although necrotizing sialometaplasia is thought to involute on its own, in the vast majority of cases it is surgically excised because of the difficulty in differentiating it from squamous cell carcinoma or a carcinoma of salivary gland origin on clinical grounds.

See Chapter 23 for further discussion of this entity.

Metastatic Tumors Affecting the Oral Tissues

Cancer metastatic to the oral tissues is an infrequent finding. Such metastases account for no more than 1 percent of the neoplasms found in the oral cavity. Meyer and Shklar[210] in a review of the literature found only 25 instances out of a series of over 2,400 malignant oral tumors. Castigliano and Rominger[211] reviewed the literature from 1902 through 1953 and found only 175 reported examples of metastases to the jaws from other primary sites.

Mayer and Shklar found the most common site of the primary lesion to be breast, followed by lung, kidney, thyroid, colon and rectum, prostate, and stomach. Few metastases from primary sites in the liver, testis, bladder, or female urogenital organs were encountered. McDaniel et al.[212] found lung carcinoma to be the most common metastatic tumor to the jaws, followed by carcinoma of the thyroid and prostate, malignant melanoma, and osteogenic sarcoma.

Oral soft tissue metastases are even rarer than central osseous metastases. Hatziotis and colleagues[213] in a 1973 review of the literature found only 48 cases of soft tissue metastases between the years 1945 and 1970. Metastatic tumors to the oral cavity occur late in the course of malignant disease and, except for those that are known to grow slowly, generally receive only palliative treatment. Radiation therapy is often used to decrease the size of the bony expansion if the deformity is interfering with vital function.

Lesions of Mesenchymal Origin

Irritation Fibroma

Clinical Features

Fibromas of the oral soft tissues are not true neoplasms; they are more appropriately classified as inflammatory hyperplasias, generally due to trauma or irritation from cheek biting or ill-fitting dentures. When a fibrous overgrowth occurs clinically as a solitary nodular lesion, it is generally termed an irritation fibroma. The irritation fibroma usually presents as a solitary nodular lesion that is typically pink and takes on the color of the associated mucosa. On occasion, the lesion may be traumatized and thus become markedly hyperparakeratotic and white. Fibromas can occur at any site within the oral cavity, and there seems to be no age or sex predilection. The irritation fibroma probably represents the most common benign fibrous overgrowth that is identified in the oral cavity. The lesions are typically asymptomatic. Occasionally, multiple lesions can be identified. Fibromas have often been called *fibroid epulis* in the literature. Unfortunately, this nonspecific term has also been used for such lesions as peripheral giant cell granuloma and the congenital fibroid epulis of the newborn.

Pathologic Features

The gross surgical specimen is usually that of a soft tissue nodule with a firm, glistening, white cut surface. Histologically, it is composed of benign keratinizing squamous epithelium overlying a lamina propria composed of interlacing fascicles of collagen often having a capsule or pseudocapsule at the periphery. Although these histologic characteristics mimic those of a true neoplasm, the proliferation represents nothing more than a form of hyperplasia. On occasion, the hyperplastic connective tissue is exceedingly well vascularized, and it is difficult to separate the fibroma from a pyogenic granuloma. Some authors[68] indicate that lesions of this type tend to become more fibrous as they mature, and in fact the irritation fibroma in many instances represents only the terminal stage of a pyogenic granuloma. The accepted treatment is simple surgical excision.

Inflammatory Fibrous Hyperplasia

Clinical Features

Inflammatory fibrous hyperplasia is a very common reactive lesion of the oral mucosa. It is most often caused by overextension of dentures into the supporting oral structures such that the surrounding connective tissue becomes hyperplastic. The most common sites are the maxillary and mandibular buccal vestibular mucosa adjacent to the overextended denture border. Usually, the lesions appear clinically as polypoid exophytic redundant masses of tissue. They can become so prominent that the lateral border of the denture may be totally covered; quite frequently the lesions become ulcerated.

The vast majority of the lesions are asymptomatic, and the patient may be unaware of their presence. Classically, the lesions appear as pink polypoid soft tissue extensions; they do not have the firm consistency of a neoplasm. Inflammatory fibrous hyperplasia may affect the gingiva as a development enlargement known as *fibromatosis gingivae* or as a drug-induced enlargement, *Dilantin hyperplasia.*

Pathologic Features

The gross appearance is usually that of a polypoid piece of soft tissue, which may or may not be ulcerated. The cut section is glistening white, and occasionally calcified.

The lesion consists of a polypoid mucosal ellipse covered by keratinizing squamous epithelium and supported by a connective tissue lamina propria composed of interlacing fascicles of collagen. Osseous metaplasia may be seen, and a chronic inflammatory infiltrate is usually identified throughout the connective tissue stroma. Very rarely, a giant cell component may be described.

On occasion, inflammatory fibrous hyperplasia may regress on its own if it is a very small lesion. The vast majority of lesions, however, are greater than 2 cm in length and will not resolve without surgical excision. The lesions do not have a malignant potential; however, there are reports of carcinoma arising in adjacent tissue unrelated to the fibrous hyperplasia.

Pyogenic Granuloma

Clinical Features

The pyogenic granuloma is a very common intraoral reactive proliferation, which classically arises from long-standing chronic irritation. It can be found on any surface of the oral cavity. Chronic irritants may include calculus along the gingival tissues surrounding teeth, ill-fitting prosthetic appliances, fractured teeth with jagged surfaces due to long-standing caries, or a chronic habit such as cheek biting.

The vast majority of the lesions appear as polypoid, nodular, hemorrhagic growths. The most frequent site is the gingiva; frequently interdental papillae are affected, and the patient may complain of spontaneous bleeding from that area or of blood in the mouth on awakening in the morning. Palpation or probing of the lesion will usually elicit the bleeding quite readily. On occasion, the lesions can undergo a rapid growth rate that is alarming, mimicking the growth characteristics of a true neoplasm.

Pathologic Features

Typically, the specimen consists of a nodular, granular, or gritty lesion, which may show surface erosion. The supporting connective tissue usually contains a very marked proliferation of exuberant granulation tissue composed predominantly of vascular channels, proliferating fibroblasts, acute and chronic inflammatory cells,

and hemorrhage. The periphery of the specimen may show maturing collagen and osseous metaplasia.

On occasion, a few giant cell aggregates can be found, but the dominant giant cell proliferation characteristic of giant cell granuloma is not identified. In addition, the supporting stroma does not have the fibroblastic background that is typical of a giant cell granuloma. Frequently the endothelial cell proliferation may be so prominent as to mimic a hemangioma. Pyogenic granuloma can undergo partial fibrosis or sclerosis. Such lesions have been termed *sclerosing pyogenic granulomas* for the sake of convenience.

Occasionally, oral pyogenic granulomas are identified in association with pregnancy; the common terminology for such lesions is pregnancy tumor. The distinction is of academic interest only. Pyogenic granulomas are best treated by simple surgical excision. Pregnancy tumors usually regress postpartum, but on occasion they have to be surgically excised.

Differential Diagnosis

The increased incidence of AIDS makes it mandatory for pathologists reviewing a suspected pyogenic granuloma of the oral cavity to obtain a thorough patient history. *Kaposi's sarcoma,* a component of AIDS, can present as a solitary soft tissue nodule in the oral cavity, mimicking pyogenic granuloma. Histologically, Kaposi's sarcoma demonstrates vascular channels lined by endothelial cells and spindle cells, but unlike pyogenic granuloma, the spindle cell element typically has an anaplastic sarcomatous appearance. A chronic inflammatory infiltrate may make it more difficult to distinguish Kaposi's sarcoma from a nonspecific reactive inflammatory granulomatous inflammation such as pyogenic granuloma.

Papillary endothelial hyperplasia may also be mistaken for a pyogenic granuloma or angiosarcoma.[214] This condition, also referred to as *intravascular angiomatosis,* has been reported in the head and neck with some frequency.[215]

Peripheral Fibroma With Calcification (Peripheral Odontogenic Fibroma)

Clinical Features

The peripheral odontogenic fibroma with ossification is a soft tissue tumor that characteristically presents as a focal gingival overgrowth. Cundiff[216] in a review of 365 lesions noted that 8 percent occurred anterior to the molar area. Cundiff further documented a 16 percent recurrence rate in his series. Bernier defined the peripheral fibroma with calcification simply as an irritation fibroma arising from connective tissues of the periodontium with the added odontogenic potential of that tissue.[217] This pluripotential feature is seen in the formation of bone, cementum, and other calcified tissues.

A clinicopathologic review of 22 cases of peripheral fibroma with ossification has been reported by Greer and Zarlengo[217] who identified the lesions most often in young adults. Women were affected slightly more often then men. A median age of 27 and an age range of 11 to 28 were documented. Twenty lesions occurred in whites, while only two lesions were reported in blacks. The lesions appeared as exophytic, sessile, or pedunculated soft tissue growths of the gingiva, occurring most often anterior to the molars with no predilection for either arch. A 27 percent recurrence rate was documented.

Pathologic Features

In the series of Greer and Zarlengo,[217] 18 of the 22 lesions contained calcified material. These polypoid lesions usually are covered by benign keratinizing squamous epithelium and are supported by an active fibrous proliferation with focal calcified areas (Fig. 22-28). Stellate fibroblasts as well as plump endothelial cells often dominate the stromal histology. Epithelial odontogenic rests (Fig. 22-29) were observed in 9 of the 22 lesions reviewed.

There is considerable debate in the literature as to whether the lesion is a true neoplasm of periodontal ligament origin or a reactive lesion due to injury. Most authorities favor the second theory and maintain that the odontogenic rests identified histologically are only fortuitous findings.

Adequate surgical excision to the base of the lesion is the treatment of choice if recurrence is to be avoided.

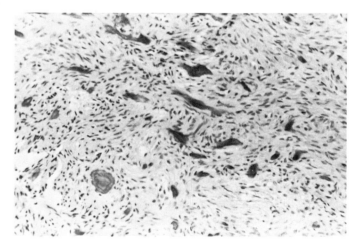

Fig. 22-28. Reactive fibrous proliferation with focal calcified areas in peripheral odontogenic fibroma.

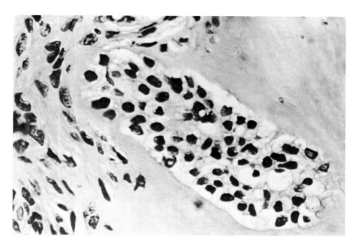

Fig. 22-29. Peripheral odontogenic fibroma. Epithelial rests are occasionally a part of the tumor histology.

Giant Cell Granuloma

Two forms of giant cell granuloma can occur, a soft tissue form and a central osseous variety. The soft tissue form has often been referred to in the past as a giant cell epulis, a nonspecific term, which should be avoided.

Peripheral Giant Cell Granuloma (Giant Cell Reparative Granuloma)

Clinical and Radiologic Features. Peripheral giant cell granuloma most often occurs as a soft tissue overgrowth in the tooth-bearing areas of the jaws. The lesions classically have a hemorrhagic, polypoid appearance and bleed readily on probing. Frequently, the surface is ulcerated.

The lesion may cause a radiologically evident cup or saucerization defect in the underlying bone. Because of this finding, a periapical radiograph may aid in establishing a clinical diagnosis.

Peripheral giant cell granulomas are more common in women than in men, and they tend to involve the anterior portion of the jaws, frequently presenting in the mandibular symphyseal region. Giansanti and Waldron[218] reviewed 720 cases of peripheral giant cell granuloma and found the average age to be 30.

Pathologic Findings. The gross appearance of peripheral giant cell granuloma is typically that of a polypoid mass, which on cut section has a firm or gritty and often hemorrhagic appearance. The texture of the cut surface, although firm, is not solid, and pressure can frequently elicit hemorrhage. Microscopically, the lesion consists of a nonencapsulated proliferation of stellate and reticular fibrous connective tissue with a dominance of ovoid or spindle cells and plump endothelial cells. The stroma contains an abundant proliferation of multinucleate giant cells. The supporting stromal cells may show considerable mitotic activity, and capillary proliferation throughout the mass is usually quite prominent. Hemorrhage, chronic inflammatory cells, and hemosiderin are dominant features, and quite frequently metaplastic bone and calcified structures arranged in globular and trabecular patterns can be identified.

There has been considerable debate in the literature as to the origin of the giant cells in this lesion. Some authors feel that the giant cells arise from endothelial cells, while others debate an osteoclastic origin. Sapp[219] has shown ultrastructurally that the giant cells have features resembling those of osteoclasts.

The histologic differential diagnoses that most often have to be entertained when reviewing a giant cell granuloma microscopically are pyogenic granuloma and hemangioma. These lesions, however, do not contain the characteristic giant cell proliferation seen in giant cell granuloma.

The treatment of peripheral giant cell granuloma is surgical excision to subjacent bone. Recurrences have been reported, and there is often debate as to whether or not teeth adjacent to the lesion should be removed in association with the soft tissue mass. Most authorities consider this contraindicated. A decrease in the reported recurrence rate has been documented since practitioners managing this lesion have gained better understanding of its biologic behavior.

Central Giant Cell Granuloma

Clinical and Radiologic Features. Central giant cell granuloma is an aggressive bony lesion that occurs in young adults, principally in the second or third decades, although Waldron and Shafer[220] have documented age extremes of 7 and 67.

Austin[221] reviewed a series of 968 benign tumors of the jaws and found that central giant cell granulomas accounted for only 3.5 percent of the lesions. Greer and others[222] documented a 3.6 percent incidence in a review of 109 tumors of the oral mucosa and jaws in children.

The granuloma usually presents as a swelling or expansile lesion within bone and is commonly associated with a sensation of increased pressure or pain. The classic radiologic appearance is that of a soap bubble, honeycomb, or locular central osseous radiolucency (Fig. 22-30). The cortical bone may be eggshell thin, and the lesion appears to affect the jaw anterior to the molars much more frequently than the posterior jaw. The mandible is much more frequently affected than the maxilla. On occasion, the lesion can perforate the cortical plates, mimicking an aggressive malignant neoplasm. The soap bubble or honeycomb appearance of the lesion is not pathognomonic, since a host of lesions, including ameloblastoma, odonto-

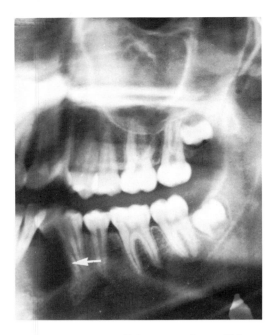

Fig. 22-30. Pear-shaped radiolucency of mandible, spreading cuspid and incisor teeth apart, represents a central giant cell granuloma.

genic myxoma, aneurysmal bone cyst, and hemangioma, can have the same radiologic features.

Perhaps the most heated of the long-standing debates about central giant cell granuloma of bone is whether or not a percentage of these tumors represent true giant cell tumors similar to those described by Austin et al.[221] Shafer[68] points out that even after classifying all giant cell lesions of bone, including the brown tumor of hyperparathyroidism, variants of fibrous dysplasia, aneurysmal bone cyst, cherubism, and central giant cell granuloma, there remains a small group of neoplasms that are exceedingly aggressive and, in fact, have shown metastasis. Dahlin[223] refers to these as true giant cell tumors of bone. Shafer speculates that perhaps a few "true" giant cell tumors represent exceedingly reactive osteogenic sarcomas with nearly undetectable malignant osteoid.

Batsakis[224] concludes that the following features separate the two entities: (1) osteoid formation or the presence of osteogenic activity is not a characteristic of the true giant cell tumor except where a peripheral fracture has occurred; (2) true giant cell tumors are typically devoid of hemosiderin, histiocytes that are laden with lipid, or an inflammatory cellular component; (3) giant cell granulomas are predominantly lesions of the first two decades of life, whereas the true giant cell tumor of bone occurs most often in the third or fourth decade.

Giant cell granulomas of the jaws have to be considered reactive lesions and not true neoplasms with malignant potential. The true giant cell tumor of bone is more often a lesion of long bones, usually identified at the

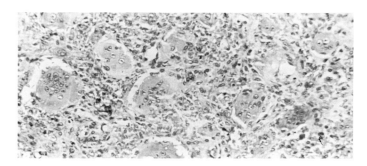

Fig. 22-31. Central giant cell granuloma displaying abundance of multinucleate giant cells, capillaries, and a background stroma of loose fibrillar connective tissue.

lower end of the femur, upper end of the tibia, and lower end of the radius. Giant cell granulomas of the jaws may on occasion behave aggressively, but unequivocal metastases from such lesions have not been documented.

Pathologic Features. Grossly, the central giant cell granuloma is identified as loose, gritty, hemorrhagic tissue, which may contain spicules of bone. Histologically, it is composed of a loose fibrillar connective tissue stroma with a prominent proliferation of endothelial cells and vascular channels. The collagen fibers are loosely arranged and only occasionally are they collected in bundles. Distributed throughout this fibrillar network are nu-

merous giant cells, which contain nuclei abundantly distributed around the periphery of the cell (Figs. 22-31 and 22-32). The cytoplasm of the giant cell is usually granular, and vacuoles can sometimes be identified. Bone and osteoid are frequently identified distributed randomly throughout the tumor. Hemosiderin pigment and extravasated blood are prominent findings in the lesion, particularly at the periphery. Lesions that have perforated the bone may show necrosis or extensive hemorrhage and fibrosis at their periphery.

From a differential diagnostic standpoint, several lesions have to be considered when entertaining a diagnosis of giant cell granuloma. Aneurysmal bone cyst tends to occur in the same age group as giant cell granuloma. It also shows a slight female predilection; however, large cavernous sinusoidal blood spaces and thrombosis are much more prominent in the aneurysmal bone cyst. A diagnosis of cherubism should be entertained whenever evaluating a central giant cell lesion of the jaws; however, the classic multifocal radiologic presentation of cherubism in the jaws allows distinction between the two, although histologic findings very often are identical. The brown tumor of hyperparathyroidism should also be entertained as a diagnosis; its radiologic and microscopic characteristics and those of giant cell granuloma are nearly identical. The brown tumor of hyperparathyroidism tends to occur a decade or two later than the central

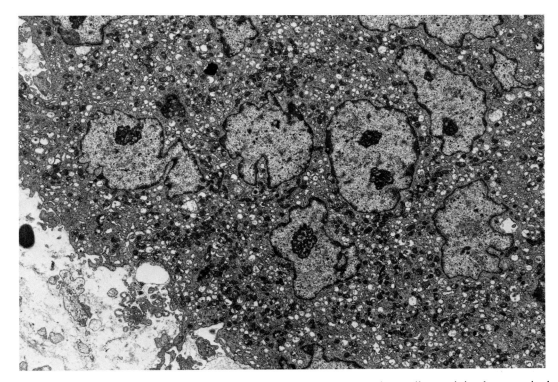

Fig. 22-32. Giant cell granuloma. Electron micrograph of multinucleate giant cell containing large vesicular nuclei and dense nucleoli with irregular configurations.

giant cell granuloma of the jaws. The establishment of a definitive diagnosis of brown tumor is dependent on demonstrating parathyroid disease, kidney abnormalities, or associated systemic disease. Serum calcium level determinations are mandatory when such a diagnosis is entertained. The giant cell granuloma rarely, if ever, results in elevated serum calcium levels.

Behavior and Management. The management of the central giant cell granuloma is generally considered to be thorough curettage and surgical excision to the margins of the lesion. Typically, the lesions fill in with new bone and do not recur. There is a group of these lesions that have been reported to have a somewhat more aggressive behavior than the majority. Andersen and coworkers[225] document a recurrence rate as high as 13 percent in these cases, but recurrences can be managed by similar curettage and wider surgical excision. Radiation therapy is contraindicated in the management of central giant cell granuloma.

Nodular Fasciitis

Nodular fasciitis, also known as pseudosarcomatous fasciitis, is a rather uncommon fibroblastic proliferation, which histologically resembles a well differentiated fibrosarcoma.[226] The lesion was first described by Konwaler et al.[227]; since their original description, it has been documented that approximately 10 percent of all cases of nodular fasciitis occur in the head and neck area.[228]

Werning[229] reported a series of 41 cases from the Armed Forces Institute of Pathology and stated that most occurred in the subcutaneous tissues overlying the zygoma and mandible. A few were reported in the parotid sheath. The lesions are characterized microscopically by an abundant proliferation of fibroblasts set in a richly vascular myxoid matrix containing an abundance of mucopolysaccharide ground substance. The proliferation of fibroblasts is relatively haphazard, with a considerable variation in size and shape. Multinucleated giant cell forms are frequently present. The lesion may be confused with fibrosarcoma or angiosarcoma. The distinction from fibrosarcoma is probably most important. Nodular fasciitis displays a typical haphazard, rather random arrangement of the fibroblasts; with fibrosarcoma a more classic herringbone pattern predominates.

The prominent clinical presentation in nodular fasciitis in the oral cavity is that of a rather discrete nodule.[230] The lesions range from slightly tender to asymptomatic, and range in size from less than 1 cm to more than 10.5 cm.[231] There appears to be no sex predilection, and the lesion can occur at any age. The salient pathologic features are discussed in Chapter 10.

Desmoplastic, Juvenile, or Congenital Fibromatosis

Juvenile or congenital fibromatosis (desmoplastic fibroma) is considered a variant of nodular fasciitis, which, in the head and neck region, is most often identified in the jaws, although lesions of the floor of the mouth have been reported by Takagi and Ishikawa.[232] Freedman and associates[233] reviewed 25 reported cases of desmoplastic fibroma reported in the world literature and documented an additional case of their own. The lesion is predominantly seen in young persons, with a peak incidence in the second decade; there is no apparent sex predilection. Over 75 percent of the desmoplastic fibromas reviewed by Freedman et al. had eroded the buccal or lingual cortical plates, and approximately one third of the cases recurred.

The etiology of this lesion is unknown, although abdominal desmoid-type fibromatosis is undoubtedly related to trauma and to pregnancy. Of the lesions reviewed by Freedman and associates, 34 percent showed some evidence of root resorption, and the radiographic findings were most often a unilocular, well-defined radiolucency of bone.[233] The lesion is characteristically composed of whorls of fibroblasts with oval or fusiform nuclei distributed between collagen bundles. Scattered multinucleated giant cells may be present. The characteristic histologic features are discussed in greater detail in Chapter 10.

Lipoma

Clinical Features

In a 10 year study of benign tumors of the oral cavity, Dockerty and coworkers[234] found that lipomas[235–237] constituted 4.4 percent of the total. The literature was reviewed in 1966 by MacGregor and Dyson,[238] and to their compilation of 45 well documented cases they added 12 of their own. In 1973 Greer and Richardson reviewed 16 additional cases.[237]

Lipomas are generally described as soft, freely movable, or spongy asymptomatic masses. The most frequent location of the tumor appears to be the buccal mucosa. There is no age or sex predilection. The histologic features of lipoma are delineated in Chapter 10.

Granular Cell Tumor

Clinical Features

Granular cell "myoblastoma" (granular cell tumor) is most often a lesion of the tongue, although it has been described in the lip, palate, gingiva, and in extraoral locations including the breast, skin, and gastrointestinal tract.

The lesion is found in all ages, and usually presents as a solitary nodule, which is not painful and grows very slowly. Over one third of all cases documented in the world literature have been reported in the tongue.[239]

Pathologic Features

Histologically, the granular cell tumor presents as a soft tissue nodule, which is usually covered by benign keratinizing squamous epithelium. The epithelium may be quite hyperplastic and may show a marked degree of pseudoepitheliomatous hyperplasia, rendering a differentiation from squamous cell carcinoma a problem (Fig. 22-27). The supporting connective tissue contains a distinct proliferation of large granular cells, which may be arranged in sheets, cords, strands, or nests. The cytoplasm is typically filled with eosinophilic granules, and the nucleus is usually small, round to oval, and vesicular. Mitotic activity is infrequently seen.

Histochemically the granules in the granular tumor myoblastoma are nonlipid and appear to be composed of a glycoprotein substance.[240,241]

There is some controversy about the histogenesis of the granular cell tumor. Some theories suggest a muscle origin for the lesion[242]; others suggest that the condition is a degenerative process affecting muscle fibers. Histologically, cross striations have not been conclusively demonstrated in any of the papers indicating a muscle origin. Azzopardi[243] favors a histiocytic origin. Histochemical studies have not supported this theory. The most prevalent theory in the literature suggests that the granular cell tumor is of Schwann cell origin[244]; however, even electron microscopic evaluation has not absolutely confirmed the origin of this tumor.[245]

The most important point for the surgical pathologist to keep in mind is not to characterize the associated pseudoepitheliomatous hyperplasia as a squamous epithelial neoplasm. A second important point to remember is that a superficial biopsy of the lesion is totally unacceptable. When the lesion is described clinically as a nodule and only a superficial fragment is submitted, a second biopsy is mandatory.

Congenital Epulis of the Newborn

Clinical Features

The congenital epulis of the newborn is a lesion typically found in the anterior maxilla as a pedunculated or sessile soft tissue swelling. Rarely, the lesion may occur on the mandibular mucosal surface. There is a marked female predominance. The etiology is unknown.

Pathologic Features

The pathologic features of the congenital epulis of the newborn are quite similar to those of the granular cell tumor, but the typical pseudoepitheliomatous hyperplasia that is seen with granular cell tumor is not identified. On occasion, odontogenic epithelium has been identified interspersed among the granular cells, as have been focal areas of osseous metaplasia.

The congenital epulis of the newborn must be distinguished from the rare well differentiated rhabdomyoma.[246] Histochemically, the lesions can be differentiated in that the intracellular granules seen in congenital epulis of the newborn are not composed of glycogen and glycoproteins as they are in rhabdomyoma. Cherrick[42] points out that the intracellular granules of granular cell tumor appear to be glycolipid and stain PAS-positive. Campbell[247] suggests that there might be a relationship between ameloblastoma and congenital epulis of the newborn in that the granular cells that are present in the granular cell type of ameloblastoma have identical histochemical reactions to those of congenital epulis. This hypothesis has not been proved and certainly there is no parallel in terms of biologic behavior. Schwann cells and axon fibers have not been identified in cases of congenital epulis that have undergone ultrastructural scrutiny, which negates a neurogenic origin.[248] Two recent immunohistochemical studies show that granular cells of the granular cell tumor of the newborn, unlike those of the granular cell "myoblastoma," do not react with antisera against S-100 protein.[249,250]

The congenital epulis of the newborn is a benign lesion, which is amenable to conservative surgical excision. It does not appear to recur with any frequency.

Nerve Sheath Neoplasms

Tumors arising from neural tissue, specifically tumors of nerve sheath origin, are quite common in the head and neck region, which is their most common location.[251]

These tumors can occur as both soft tissue and bony lesions. Typically, they remain asymptomatic unless they attain appreciable size. When they arise as bony lesions, they generally cause a sensation of pressure, often the patient's chief complaint. Soft tissue tumors typically begin as nodular convex swellings, the tongue being the most common site of involvement.[252]

The two types of tumors documented most frequently are neurilemoma and neurofibroma. The neurilemoma can occur at any age, typically as a solitary tumor. Generally, the lesion presents in subcutaneous tissues, and it may on occasion be multifocal. Rarely is neurilemoma associated with von Recklinghausen's neurofibromatosis, although cases have been reported.

The neurofibroma occurs only rarely as a solitary tumor. It presents principally as a multifocal tumor, usually in association with multiple neurofibromatosis of the skin and internal organs. Both tumors are neoplastic proliferations of neuroectodermal Schwann cells with a collagenous fibrillar matrix. Detailed histology and natural history of these tumors can be found in Chapter 49.

The *traumatic neuroma* is a rarely encountered oral lesion, which does not represent a true neoplasm but rather an exuberant overgrowth of nerve fibers occurring after nerve severance. Considering the amount of trauma that the oral cavity is exposed to through extractions of teeth, prosthetic appliances, and extensive manipulative dental procedures, it is surprising that the lesions are not more common than the literature documents.

The chief symptom of traumatic neuroma is usually isolated pain associated with a pre-existing surgical procedure. The most common sites tend to be the posterior mandibular areas adjacent to the mandibular canal and the tongue.

Harkin and Reed[253] have described a neoplasm termed *myxoma of nerve sheath* (neurothecoma). These tumors are most often lobulated tumors of the skin composed of spindled cells and an abundant mucoid matrix.[254] The nerve sheath myxoma is only rarely identified in the oral cavity. In this location it is usually described clinically as a gradually enlarging painless growth arising on the lower lip. To date, seven cases have been reported involving the oral cavity.[255]

Vascular Lesions

Benign tumor-like proliferations of vascular tissues are exceedingly common in the oral cavity. These tumors probably do not represent true neoplasms but more properly represent developmental anomalies or hamartomas. The hemangioma is the most common of all of these lesions.

An important fact that must be remembered by the surgical pathologist is that many oral angiomatous proliferations are found in association with syndromes that have a systemic vascular counterpart. These syndromes include hereditary hemorrhagic telangiectasia, Sturge-Weber syndrome, and Maffucci's syndrome.

It is also important for the surgical pathologist to recognize that AIDS may be associated with atypical vascular proliferations in the oral cavity. Close scrutiny of such lesions for atypical cytologic features suggestive of Kaposi's sarcoma, including back to back proliferation of vascular channels and proliferation of apparent sarcomatous cells along the walls of thin slit-like spaces, is important.

Other malignant vascular tumors, including malignant hemangiopericytoma and angiosarcoma, have been reported rarely in the oral cavity.[256]

TUMORS OF SALIVARY GLANDS

Salivary gland tumors account for approximately 1 to 4 percent of all tumors in the head and neck region.[43] Frazell[257] has further documented that salivary gland tumors account for 5 percent of all the benign and malignant tumors in the human body, excluding those of the skin. Minor salivary gland tumors are much less common than major salivary gland tumors, accounting for approximately 20 percent of all salivary gland tumors. Documentation of the behavior and pathology of the various histologic types of salivary gland neoplasms can be found in Chapter 23; however, it is important to note certain characteristics of minor salivary gland tumors unique to an intraoral presentation.

When salivary gland tumors are identified intraorally, the most common site will be the palate, followed by the lip. Pleomorphic adenomas account for over 60 percent of all salivary gland tumors in major or minor salivary glands. Adenoid cystic carcinoma and mucoepidermoid tumor (carcinoma) account for a much larger percentage of minor than of major salivary gland tumors.

This difference in the incidence of mucoepidermoid tumors and adenoid cystic carcinoma within the oral cavity is an exceedingly important feature for the surgical pathologist to remember when reviewing minor salivary gland specimens. A second axiom to remember is that salivary gland tumors do occur centrally within the mandible, a feature of note when confronted with a clear cell or apparent mucus-producing intraosseous tumor.

DYSPLASIAS OF BONE

Fibro-osseous lesions are reactive bony lesions that show replacement of normal bone architecture with benign cellular fibrous tissue containing varying amounts of mineralized material. There is considerable variation among pathologists in the terminology and classification of these lesions. At present, the concepts about the lesions are not totally uniform. Three specific lesions will be considered here because of their frequent appearance in the jaws: fibrous dysplasia, ossifying fibroma, and cherubism.

Fibrous Dysplasia
Clinical and Radiologic Features

Fibrous dysplasia was first described by von Recklinghausen in 1891 by the term *osteitis fibrosa disseminata*.[258] The disease generally affects the jaws as a monostotic lesion, although polyostotic forms have been reported. In Waldron and Giansanti's review of 22 lesions,[260] the most classic findings were painless enlargement of involved bones. Ages ranged from 5 to 65, with a mean of 27 years.

The characteristic maxillary appearance is that of a ground-glass or "orange peel" radiopacity. The borders of lesions are often difficult to define, and frequently there appears to be a transitional zone between normal and abnormal bone. Multilocular radiolucencies are occasionally seen.

There has been considerable recent emphasis on trying to separate head and neck fibrous dysplasia from other fibro-osseous lesions; consequently a common term that has been popularized is *craniofacial fibrous dysplasia*. Craniofacial fibrous dysplasia represents fibrous dysplasia of the maxilla, mandible, and bones of the skull. Eversole et al.,[259] in a review of 512 fibro-osseous lesions, found a predilection of craniofacial fibrous dysplasia for the mandible; however, the cases that were adequately documented as polyostotic fibrous dysplasia showed a predilection for the maxilla. Eversole and colleagues point out that the criteria that distinguish between monostotic fibrous dysplasia and ossifying fibroma of the jaws are varied. Their review of the literature indicates that, based on radiologic findings alone, it is often impossible to separate monostotic fibrous dysplasia radiologically from the supposedly better delineated ossifying fibroma.

The diagnosis of fibrous dysplasia is a clinicopathologic one. It is often less than productive for the surgical pathologist to attempt to diagnose fibrous dysplasia (or most fibro-osseous lesions, for that matter) by simple histologic examination of tissue samples. Accurate diagnosis is based on a very thorough evaluation of clinical, radiographic, and histologic parameters. There are no clinical laboratory tests that are absolute in diagnosing fibrous dysplasia, and bone chemistries, including calcium, phosphorus, and alkaline phosphatase, may be normal or increased.

Pathologic Findings

Grossly, the tissue received for pathologic evaluation usually is yellow, gray, or brown, with a gritty cut surface. Normal bone may be replaced by yellow to white homogeneous areas, and occasionally there may be central areas that appear cystic.

Classically, fibrous dysplasia is composed of a stroma that is fibrous in nature. The stroma may be highly cellular or have the appearance of maturing collagen. Distributed randomly throughout the supporting collagenous stroma are bone trabeculae, which usually have large osteocytes within lacunae. The margins of the bone trabeculae often show a streaming of collagen bundles and fibers from the trabeculae into the surrounding stroma (Fig. 22-33). The vast majority of the lesions examined

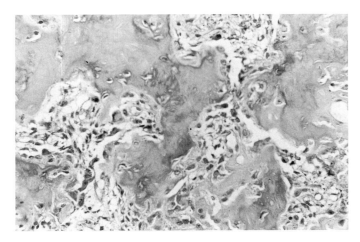

Fig. 22-33. Fibrous dysplasia with proliferating fibrous stromal tissue and irregular osseous trabeculae often rimmed by plump osteoblasts and occasional osteoclasts.

will show areas of woven bone. Many authorities consider the presence of woven bone mandatory for a diagnosis of fibrous dysplasia.[260] However, most reports on craniofacial fibrous dysplasia document that it is not necessary to identify woven bone to render this diagnosis.[258,259] In a series of 150 cases of craniofacial dysplasia, Eversole et al.[258] were able to identify 19 cases in which there were multiple spheroid calcifications in a connective tissue setting; 85 had woven osteoid, 27 had lamellar bone, and 19 showed osteoblastic rimming. These authors also reviewed 75 cases of monostotic fibrous dysplasia and found that once again there was a variance of pattern of bone in the lesions, ranging from spheroid calcifications to woven osteoid to lamellar bone, with areas of osteoblastic rimming. Thus, the old adage that osteoblastic rimming often negates a diagnosis of fibrous dysplasia is best discarded.

Waldron and Giansanti[259] paid particular attention to the relative amounts of woven and lamellar bone in each section of the 65 lesions that they reviewed. They also paid considerable attention to the evidence of osteoblastic rimming in bone. Although they found that the majority of the bone they identified was of the woven type, lamellar bone was constantly seen among the tissue samples. It is important to realize that fibrous dysplasia represents a dynamic series of events in the maturation of bone, as opposed to permanent maturation arrest in the woven bone stage. Spjut et al.[261] have noted that occasional lamellar transformation can be identified in fibrous dysplasia and that this finding should not detract from a diagnosis of fibrous dysplasia if other criteria, especially radiologic and clinical criteria, are fulfilled.

Most lesions diagnosed as fibrous dysplasia tend to stabilize after the completion of normal skeletal development, although continuous growth has been documented in some cases. Conservative and/or cosmetic surgical management is the treatment of choice. The lesions are not radiosensitive, and radiation therapy has been shown in fact to predispose to postradiation sarcoma.

Pathogenesis

A host of theories exist concerning the etiology of fibrous dysplasia, including trauma, atypical mesenchymal bone-forming activity, and a complex of endocrine disturbances with local bone susceptibility.[262] Abnormal activity of mesenchymal cells is the theory that is most often accepted.

Treatment and Prognosis

A few cases of aggressive fibrous dysplasia have been reported in the literature, but there appears to be no distinctive histologic appearance for these particular lesions.[263] Malignant transformation does occur in fibrous dysplasia, most often subsequent to radiation exposure although it can occur without prior radiation damage. In their review of 29 cases of malignant degeneration of fibrous dysplasia, Gross and Montgomery found that 13 of the patients had received previous radiation therapy.[264]

Ossifying Fibroma

Clinical and Radiologic Features

Ossifying fibroma is a distinct pathologic entity, which can be separated quite easily from fibrous dysplasia in cases in which Albright's syndrome or polyostotic disease is identified. However, the distinction is much more difficult when these two features are not appreciated. Waldron and Giansanti[257] document that the lesions are most often distributed equally between the maxilla and the mandible although there seems to be a distinct paucity of lesions reported in the anterior maxilla. A large proportion of ossifying fibromas are found in intimate relationship to the roots of teeth or in the periapical regions of the jaws. There can be quite a variation in the radiologic features of ossifying fibroma, ranging from totally lytic lesions with varying amounts of radiopaque calcific foci to lesions that are totally radiopaque (Fig. 22-34). Most often, ossifying fibroma is well circumscribed radiologically, but occasionally the lesion can have a "punched out" appearance. On rare occasions the lesions tend to blend into normal bone, causing some difficulty in distinguishing them from fibrous dysplasia. Waldron and Giansanti[257] and Hammer and co-workers[265] consider ossifying fibroma to be a lesion of periodontal ligament origin.

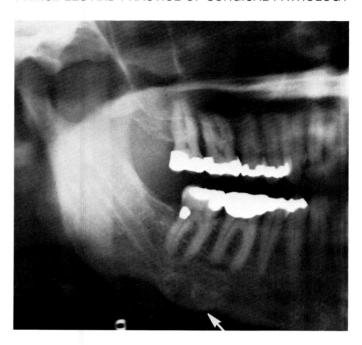

Fig. 22-34. Well-circumscribed ossifying fibroma expanding inferior border of mandible. (Courtesy of Al Oesterle, D.D.S.)

Pathologic Features

Ossifying fibroma usually shells out as multiple gritty or partially calcified gray-white pieces of tissue. Histologically, one is usually able to identify a component of fibrous and osseous tissue. The supporting stroma may be composed of interlacing fascicles of collagen or loose proliferating fibroblasts, which can have a stellate character. A varying amount of vascularity can be appreciated, ranging from areas in which there is total lack of endothelial-lined channels to areas of multiple capillary proliferation.

Lamellar trabeculae may be appreciated either as a distinct osseous component separate from the fibrocellular stroma or as an anastomosing retiform osseous component, which tends to blend into the surrounding stroma. Woven bone may also be identified. Globular calcifications frequently described as cementoid may be seen in the tissue sample. When such globules are seen, the term *cemento-ossifying fibroma* or *cementifying fibroma* (see odontogenic tumors) has been employed (Fig. 22-35). In fact, this terminology probably serves only to further confuse the spectrum of fibro-osseous lesions. The differentiation between cementoid and osteoid material is only of academic interest and does not alter the biologic behavior of the tumor. Surgical excision and occasionally en bloc resection in instances of a recurrent lesion are the accepted therapy.

A lesion referred to as *juvenile active ossifying fibroma*

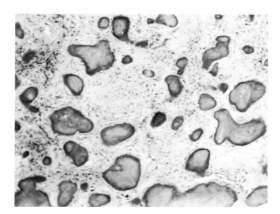

Fig. 22-35. Ossifying fibroma showing spherical masses of tissue that resemble globular ossicles set in a fibrillar stroma.

has been reported in the literature.[259] The lesion is considered to be an aggressive one, which has the potential to be lethal. Many pathologists, however, consider the lesion to be a low-grade osteosarcoma.

The vast majority of pathologists involved in subclassifying fibro-osseous lesions indicate that the distinction between fibrous dysplasia and ossifying fibroma is essentially a clinical and not a histopathologic one. It is important to evaluate the symptomatology and behavior of the lesion and to evaluate thoroughly the radiologic findings. Lesions that are classically identified as ossifying fibroma usually have a thin bony peripheral shell and a distinct boundary on the radiograph, whereas fibrous dysplasia tends to be much more diffuse.

Differential Diagnosis

The most significant feature separating ossifying fibroma from fibrous dysplasia is the classic circumscribed nature of the former. However, clinical and radiographic appearances of the two conditions can occasionally be identical. Waldron and Giansanti[259] report that the stroma of fibrous dysplasia is somewhat more fibrous than that of ossifying fibroma. Cementoblastoma can also mimic ossifying fibroma, from which it is best differentiated by the observations that cementoblastoma is attached to root surfaces and that globules of cementum and layered zones of cementogenesis are typical histologically.

Cherubism

Clinical and Radiologic Features

Cherubism is probably best considered a genetic disorder. It is typically inherited as an autosomal dominant trait with variable expressivity. The vast majority of the lesions are identified in early childhood, and boys appear to be affected more often than girls. When the lesion was first described, it was documented as a solitary lesion in one quadrant of the jaw. Since that time it has been found that lesions frequently progress to involve all four quadrants of the jaws, additional portions of the craniofacial complex, and the long bones. Radiologically the lesions have a typical soap bubble, multilocular, or compartmentalized appearance. The mandible or the maxillary alveolar processes may be expanded, causing occasional perforation of the cortex. Teeth may be irregularly spaced, totally absent, or unerupted. The fact that the lesions are expansile is of special importance in the maxilla since the orbit may be impinged on, causing upward displacement of the eyeball. This classic clinical appearance, with the eyes of the child turned toward the sky and expanded cheeks, is often likened to an angelic or cherubic appearance.

Pathologic Features

Typically, the specimen consists of friable, mottled red-brown, sometimes gritty tissue. The cut surface may show a whorled or lobulated pattern. Microscopically, the typical appearance is that of an admixture of loosely arranged fibrous connective tissue, multinucleate giant cells, and occasional fragments of poorly mineralized bone. Giant cells, although they tend to be the predominant feature, are sometimes present in only small numbers. Thin-walled vessels are often prominent throughout the supporting stroma, and in many cases giant cells tend to aggregate around small vascular spaces. Hemosiderin may also be prominent. When the lesions are mature, the histologic features are often those of mature interlacing collagen fascicles, with only a few scattered giant cells.

Several lesions can appear histologically identical to cherubism, including central giant cell granuloma, aneurysmal bone cyst, and the brown tumor of hyperparathyroidism. Thorough histories and adequate clinical workup are absolutely mandatory in differentiating these lesions. When a familial history is demonstrable along with the classic histologic picture, a diagnosis of cherubism can usually be established.

The lesions of cherubism tend to show marked activity immediately after their appearance, especially in the first decade of life. After puberty, growth tends to slow down, but total regression is not always appreciated. Treatment is not standardized, and in general, no treatment is indicated except for biopsy to arrive at a diagnosis. Cosmetic osseous recontouring may be instituted when the active growth phase has terminated.[266]

TUMORS OF BONE AND CARTILAGE

The principal neoplasms of bone that affect the jaws have essentially the same clinical and microscopic features that are discussed in Chapter 15 of this text. Salient clinical and histologic features exclusive to the jaws are discussed below.

Osteosarcoma tends to occur in the jaws a decade later than in the long bones. An additional exclusive early clinical feature that has been reported by Garrington et al.[267] is a symmetric widening of the periodontal ligament around one or more teeth. Garrington and colleagues contend that this radiologic feature of osteosarcoma appears before any other radiologic change.

Osteosarcoma in the maxilla or the mandible has a mean age of presentation of 34.1 years, with 44 percent of the tumors affecting the maxilla and 55 percent the mandible according to Forteza and associates.[268] Most lesions grow exceedingly rapidly and are painless or minimally painful. Histologically the fibroblastic type is most frequent. Overall survival rates for all therapeutic categories is 75 percent, with a mean disease-free interval of 8 years, according to these investigators. The rare *parosteal osteosarcoma* of the jaws behaves in a less aggressive fashion than the central osseous variety.

Osteoid osteoma and *osteoblastoma* can be identified in the jaws. They have essentially the same histopathologic and clinical features as those found in long bones and other parts of the skeleton. Pain is a characteristic feature of both osteoid osteoma and osteoblastoma. Greer and Berman[269] reviewed all the existing literature on osteoblastoma of the jaws in 1975; information on age and sex was available in 10 of 12 published cases. Ages ranged from 6 to 22, with a mean of 14.7 years. An interesting finding in their review of jaw lesions was that pain was a characteristic feature in 75 percent of the cases. There is a growing body of evidence that suggests that there is no definitive histologic difference between osteoid osteoma and osteoblastoma except for size. This appears to be an even more acceptable proposition in view of the fact that in our review, pain, a feature that is always associated with osteoid osteoma, was a significant finding in 9 of 13 cases of osteoblastoma. Farman and co-workers[270] also deemed the distinction between osteoblastoma and osteoid osteoma so difficult that they consider the two lesions a single entity.

Chondrosarcoma and *mesenchymal chondrosarcoma* are occasionally found in the jaws; they are also discussed in Chapter 15.

REFERENCES

1. Bernstein ML: Biopsy technique: The pathological considerations. J Am Dent Assoc 96:438, 1978
2. Valenzuela R, Bergfeld WF, Deodhar SD: Interpretation of Immunofluorescent Patterns in Skin Diseases. American Society of Clinical Pathology Press, Chicago, 1984, p. 11
3. Greer RO, Poulson TC, Boone ME, et al: Smokeless tobacco associated oral changes in juvenile, adult and geriatric patients: Clinical and histomorphologic features. Gerodontics 2:87, 1986
4. Barnes L (ed): Surgical Pathology of the Head and Neck. Marcel Dekker, New York, 1985, p. 1241
5. Gardner DG, Sapp JP: Odontogenic and fissural cysts of the jaws. Pathol Ann 13 (pt 1): 177, 1978
6. Soskalne WA, Shear M: Observations on the pathogenesis of primordial cysts. Br Dent J 123:321, 1967
7. Shear M, Rachanis CC: Age standardized incidence rates of primordial cyst (keratocyst) on the Witwatersand. Community Dent Oral Epidemiol 6:296, 1978
8. Lucas RB: Pathology of Tumors of the Oral Tissues. 3rd Ed. Churchill Livingstone, London, 1976
9. Panders AK, Hadders HN: Solitary keratocysts of the jaws. J Oral Surg 27:931, 1969
10. Radden BG, Reade PC: Odontogenic keratocysts. Pathology 5:325, 1973
11. Shear M: Radiological features of mandibular primordial cysts (keratocysts). J Maxillofac Surg 6:147, 1978
12. Pindborg JJ, Kramer IRH: Histological Typing of Odontogenic Tumors, Jaw Cysts and Allied Lesions. International Histological Classification of Tumors. World Health Organization, Geneva, 1971
13. Eversole LR, Saves WR, Rovin S: Aggressive growth and neoplastic potential of odontogenic cysts with special reference to central epidermoid and mucoepidermoid carcinomas. Cancer 35:270, 1975
14. Stoelinga PJW, Peters JH: A note on the origin of keratocysts of the jaws. Int J Oral Surg 2:37, 1973
15. Pindborg JJ, Hansen J: Studies on odontogenic cyst epithelium. 2. Clinical and roentgenological aspects of odontogenic keratocysts. Acta Pathol Microbiol Scand 58:283, 1963
16. Mosby EL, Sugg WE Jr: Residual odontogenic keratinizing cyst: Report of a case. US Navy Med 67:222, 1976
17. Philipsen HP: Om keratocyster (kolesteatomer) i kaeberne. Tandlaegebladet 60:963, 1956
18. Browne RM: The odontogenic keratocyst: Clinical aspects. Br Dent J 128:225, 1970
19. Browne RM: The odontogenic keratocyst: Histologic features and correlation with clinical behavior. Br Dent J 131:249, 1971
20. Brannon RB: The odontogenic keratocyst: A clinicopathologic study of 312 cases. Part 1. Clinical features. Oral Surg 42:54, 1976
21. Wright JM: The odontogenic keratocyst: Orthokeratinized variant. Oral Surg 51:609, 1981
22. Wilson DF, Ross AS: Ultrastructure of Odontogenic keratocysts. Oral Surg 45:887, 1978

23. Bramley PA: Treatment of cysts of the jaws. Proc R Soc Med 64:547, 1971

24. Weathers DR, Waldron CA: Unusual multilocular cysts of the jaws (botryoid odontogenic cysts). Oral Surg 36:235, 1973

25. Kaugars SGE: Botryoid odontogenic cyst. Oral Surg 62:555, 1986

26. Gorlin RJ, Pindborg JJ, Clausen FP, et al: Calcifying odontogenic cyst—a possible analogue of the cutaneous calcifying epithelioma of Malherbe (an analysis of fifteen cases). Oral Surg 15:1235, 1962

27. Sauk JJ: Calcifying and keratinizing odontogenic cyst. J Oral Surg 30:893, 1972

28. Freedman PD, Lumerman H, Gee JK: Calcifying odontogenic cyst. A review and analysis of seventy cases. Oral Surg 40:93, 1975

29. Herd JR: The calcifying odontogenic cyst. Aust Dent J 17:421, 1972

30. Fejerskov O, Krogh J: The calcifying ghost cell odontogenic tumor—or the calcifying odontogenic cyst. J Oral Pathol 1:273, 1972

31. Altini M, Farmon AG: The calcifying odontogenic cyst. Eight new cases and a review of the literature. Oral Surg 40:751, 1975

32. Keszler A, Gugliemotti NB: Calcifying odontogenic cyst associated with odontoma: Report of two cases. J Oral Surg 45:457, 1987

33. Farmon AG, Smith SN, Nortje CJ, et al: Calcifying odontogenic cyst with ameloblastic fibro-odontoma: One lesion or two. J Oral Pathol 7:19, 1978

34. Stanley HR: Consequence of neglected "impacted third molars" (abstract 25). American Academy of Oral Pathology 41st Annual Meeting, Scottsdale, AZ, 1987

35. Ritchey B, Orban B: Cysts of the gingiva. Oral Surg 6:765, 1953

36. Fromm A: Epstein's pearls, Bohn's nodules and inclusion-cysts of the oral cavity. J Dent Child 34:275, 1967

37. High AS, Hirschman PN: Age changes in residual radicular cysts. J Oral Pathol 15:524, 1986

38. Rushton MA: Hyalin bodies in the epithelium of dental cysts. Proc R Soc Med 48:407, 1955

39. Eversole LR, Sabes WR, Rovin S: Aggressive growth and neoplastic potential of odontogenic cysts: With special reference to central epidermoid and mucoepidermoid carcinomas. Cancer 35:270, 1957

40. Little JW, Jakoben J: Origin of the globulomaxillary cyst. J Oral Surg 31:188, 1973

41. Christ TF: The globulomaxillary cyst: An embryologic misconception. Oral Surg 30:515, 1970

42. Stafne EC, Austin LT, Gardner BS: Median anterior maxillary cysts. J Am Dent Assoc 23:801, 1936

43. Cherrick HM: The jaws and teeth. p. 95. In Coulson WF: Surgical Pathology. JB Lippincott, Philadelphia, 1978

44. Knappe MJ: Pathology of oral tonsils. Oral Surg 29:295, 1970

45. Bhaskar SN: Lymphoepithelial cysts of the oral cavity: Report of 24 cases. Oral Surg 21:120, 1966

46. Guinta J, Cataldo E: Lymphoepithelial cysts of the oral mucosa. Oral Surg 35:77, 1973

47. Weitzner S: Lymphoepithelial (branchial) cyst of parotid gland. Oral Surg 35:85, 1973

48. Stewart S, Levy R, Karpel J, Stoopack J: Lymphoepithelial (branchial) cyst of the parotid gland. J Oral Surg 32:100, 1974

49. Burnstein A, Scardinio PT, Tomaszewski MM, Cohen MH: Carcinoma arising in a branchial cleft cyst. Cancer 37:2417, 1976

50. Hertz J: Adamantioma. Histopathologic and prognostic studies. Acta Chir Scand 102:405, 1951

51. Forsberg A: A contribution to the knowledge of the histology, histogenesis and etiology of adamantiomas. Acta Odontol Scand 12:39, 1954

52. Stanley HR, Bear PN, Kilham L: Oral tissue alterations in mice inoculated with the Rose stain of polyoma virus. Periodontics 3:178, 1965

53. Main JHP, Dawe CJ: Tumor induction in transplanted tooth buds infected with polyoma virus. JNCI 36:1121, 1966

54. Lucas RB: Odontogenic tumors in polyoma virus-infected mice. Fourth Annual Proceedings of the International Academy Oral Pathology, New York, 1969

55. Greer RO, Richardson JF: Ameloblastoma of mucosal origin. A pathobiologic re-evaluation. Arch Otolaryngol 100:174, 1974

56. Spouge JD: Oral Pathology. CV Mosby, St Louis, 1973, pp 324–350

57. Sehdev MK, Huvos AG, Strong EW, et al: Ameloblastoma of maxilla and mandible. Cancer 33:324, 1974

58. Rockoff WM: A statistical analysis of ameloblastoma. Oral Surg 16:1100, 1963

59. Kane JP: Odontogenic Tumors. A Statistical and Morphological Study of 88 Cases. Thesis. Georgetown University, Washington, 1951

60. Waldron CA, El Mofty SK: A histopathologic study of 116 ameloblastomas with special reference to the desmoplastic variant. Oral Surg 63:441, 1987

61. Gardner DG, Corio RL: Plexiform unicystic ameloblastoma: A variant of ameloblastoma with a low recurrence rate after enucleation. Cancer 53:1730, 1984

62. Eversole LR, Leider AS, Straub D: Radiographic characteristics of cystogenic ameloblastoma. Oral Surg 57:772, 1984

63. Ikemura K, Tashiro H, Fugino H, et al: Ameloblastoma of the mandible with metastasis to the lungs and lymph nodes. Cancer 29:930, 1972

64. Trodahl JN: Ameloblastic fibroma. A survey of cases from the Armed Forces Institute of Pathology. Oral Surg 33:547, 1972

65. Woo S-B, Smith-Williams JE, Schiubba JJ, Lipper S: Peripheral ameloblastoma of the buccal mucosa: The report and review of the English literature. Oral Surg 63:78, 1987

66. Gardner DG: Peripheral ameloblastoma. A study of 21 cases including 5 reported as basal cell carcinoma of gingiva. Cancer 39:1625, 1972

67. Greer RO, Hammond WS: Extraosseous ameloblastoma: Light microscopic and ultrastructural observations. J Oral Surg 36:553, 1978

68. Shafer WG, Hine MK, Levy BM: A Textbook of Oral Pathology. 3rd Ed. WB Saunders, Philadelphia, 1974
69. Mincer HH, McGinnis JP Ultrastructure of three histologic variants of ameloblastoma. Cancer 30:1036, 1972
70. Pindborg JJ: A calcifying epithelial odontogenic tumor. Cancer 2:838, 1958
71. Greer RO, Richardson JF: Clear-cell calcifying odontogenic tumor viewed relative to the Pindborg tumor. Oral Surg 42:775, 1976
72. Patterson JT, Martin TH, DeJean EK, et al: Extraosseous calcifying epithelial odontogenic tumor. Report of a case. Oral Surg 27:363, 1969
73. Krolls JO, Pindborg JJ: Calcifying epithelial odontogenic tumor. A survey of 23 cases and discussions of histomorphologic variations. Arch Pathol 98:206, 1974
74. Liu AR, Liu Z, Shao J: Calcifying epithelial odontogenic tumors: A clinico-pathologic study of nine cases. J Oral Pathol 11:399, 1982
75. El-Labban NG, Lee KW, Kramer IRH, Harris M: The nature of the amyloid-like material in a calcifying epithelial odontogenic tumor: An ultrastructural study. J Oral Pathol 12:366, 1983
76. Abrams AM, Howell FV: Calcifying epithelial odontogenic tumor: Report of four cases. J Am Dent Assoc 74:1231, 1967
77. Mohamed AH, Cherrick HM: Glycogen-rich adenocarcinoma of minor salivary glands: A light and electron microscopic study. Cancer 36:1057, 1975
78. Anderson HC, Kim B, Minkowitz S: Calcifying epithelial odontogenic tumor of Pindborg: An electron microscopic study. Cancer 24:585, 1969
79. Courtney RM, Kerr DA: The odontogenic adenomatoid tumor. A comprehensive study of twenty new cases. Oral Surg 39:424, 1975
80. Giansanti JS, Someren A, Waldron CA: Odontogenic adenomatoid tumor (adenoameloblastoma). Survey of 111 cases. Oral Surg 30:69, 1970
81. Poulson TC, Greer RO: Adenomatoid odontogenic tumor: Clinicopathologic and ultrastructural concepts. J Oral Surg 41:818, 1983
82. White DK, Chess SY, Mohnac AM, et al: Odontogenic myxoma. A clinical and ultrastructural study. Oral Surg 39:901, 1975
83. Hasleton PS, Simpson W. Craig RDP: Myxoma of the mandible—a fibroblastic tumor. Oral Surg 46:396, 1978
84. Farman AG, Nortje CJ, Groteposs FW, et al: Myxofibroma of the jaws. Br J Oral Surg 15:3, 1977
85. Goldblatt LI: Ultrastructural study of an odontogenic myxoma. Oral Surg 42:206, 1976
86. Redman RS, Greer RO, Rutherford RB: Myofibroblasts in odontogenic myxoma (abstract 12). Scientific Session, American Academy of Oral Pathology Annual Meeting, Fort Lauderdale, 1978
87. Zimmerman DC, Dahlin DC: Myxomatous tumors of the jaws. Oral Surg 11:1069, 1958
88. Elzay RP, Dutz W: Myxomas of the perioral soft tissues. Oral Surg 45:246, 1978
89. Cook CA, Lund BA, Carney JA: Mucocutaneous pigmented spots and oral myxomas: The oral manifestations of the complex myxomas, spotty pigmentation, and endocrine over-activity. Oral Surg 63:175, 1987
90. Gardner DG: The central odontogenic fibroma, an attempt at clarification. Oral Surg 50:425, 1980
91. Dunlap CL, Barker BF: Central odontogenic fibroma of the WHO-type. Oral Surg 57:390, 1984
92. Wesley RD, Wysachi GP, Mintz SM: The central odontogenic fibroma. Clinical and morphologic studies. Oral Surg 40:235, 1975
93. Mallow RD, Spatz JJ, Zubrow HJ, et al: Odontogenic fibroma with calcification. Oral Surg 22:564, 1964
94. Vincent SD, Hammond HL, Ellis GL, Juhlin JP: Central granular cell odontogenic fibroma. Oral Surg: 63:715, 1987
95. Chaudry AP, Spink JH, Gorlin RJ: Periapical fibrous dysplasia (cementoma). J Oral Surg 16:483, 1958
96. Stafne EC: Cementoma: Study of 35 cases. Dent Survey 9:27, 1933
97. Waldron C, Giansanti JJ: Benign fibro-osseous lesions of the jaws. A clinical-radiologic-histologic review of 65 cases. Oral Surg 35:340, 1973
98. Bhaskar SN, Cutwright DE: Multiple enostosis: Report of 16 cases. J Oral Surg 26:321, 1968
99. Norberg O: Zur Kenntis der dysontogenetischen Geschwülste der Zieferknochen. Vierteljahrsschrift fur Zahnh. 46:321, 1930
100. Corio RL, Crawford BE, Schaberg SJ: Benign cementoblastoma. Oral Surg 41:524, 1976
101. Cherrick HM, King OH Jr, Lucatorto FM, et al: Benign cementoblastoma. Oral Surg 37:54, 1974
102. Abrams AM, Kirby JW, Melrose RJ: Cementoblastoma. Oral Surg 38:394, 1974
103. Giantsanti JS: The pattern and width of collagen bundles in bone and cementum. Oral Surg 30:508, 1970
104. Chaudry AP, Stickel FR, Gorlin RJ, et al: An unusual odontogenic tumor. Report of a case. Oral Surg 15:86, 1962
105. Trodahl JN: Ameloblastic fibroma. A survey of cases from the Armed Forces Institute of Pathology. Oral Surg 33:547, 1972
106. Shafer WG: Ameloblastic fibroma. J Oral Surg 13:317, 1955
107. Van Wyk CW, Uyver PC: Ameloblastic fibroma with dentinoid formation/immature dentinoma: A microscopic and ultrastructural study of the epithelial connective tissue interface. J Oral Pathol 12:37, 1983
108. Edwards MB, Coubran CF: Cystic, melanotic ameloblastic fibroma with granulomatous inflammation. Oral Surg 49:333, 336, 1980
109. Richardson JF, Balogh K, Merk F, et al: Pigmented odontogenic tumors of jawbone. A previously undescribed expression of neoplastic potential. Cancer 34:1244, 1974
110. Carr RF, Halperin V, Wood C, et al: Recurrent ameloblastic fibroma. Oral Surg 29:85, 1970
111. Tanaka S, Mitsui Y, Mizuno Y, et al: Recurrent ameloblastic fibroma. Report of a case. Oral Surg 30:944, 1972
112. Pindborg JJ, Kramer IRH: Histologic Typing of Odontogenic Tumors, Jaw Cysts and Allied Lesions. p. 27. World Health Organization, Geneva, 1971
113. Hooker SP: Ameloblastic odontoma: An analysis of 26 cases (abstract). Oral Surg 24:375, 1967

114. Gardner DG: The mixed odontogenic tumors. Oral Surg 58:166, 168, 1984

115. Tsataras GT: A review of ameloblastic fibro-odontoma. Thesis. George Washington University, Washington, 1972

116. Cherrick HM: The jaws and teeth. p. 82. In Coulson WF (ed): Surgical Pathology. JB Lippincott, Philadelphia, 1978

117. Budnick SD: Compound and complex odontomas. Oral Surg 42:501, 1976

118. Regezi JA, Kerr DA, Courtney RM: Odontogenic tumor: Analysis of 706 cases. J Oral Surg 36:771, 1978

119. Elzay RP: Primary interosseous carcinoma of the jaws: Review and update of odontogenic carcinomas. Oral Surg 54:299, 1982

120. Slootweg PJ, Muller H: Malignant ameloblastoma or ameloblastic carcinoma. Oral Surg. 57:168, 1984

121. Gorlin RJ, Goldman HM: Thoma's Oral Pathology. Vol 1. 6th Ed. CV Mosby, St. Louis, 1970

122. Leider AS, Nelson JF, Trodahl JN: Ameloblastic fibrosarcoma of the jaws. Oral Surg 33:559, 1972

123. Adekey EO, Edwards NB, Goubran GF: Ameloblastic fibrosarcoma. Oral Surg 46:254, 1978

124. Chomette G, Auriol M, Guilbert F: Ameloblastic fibrosarcoma: A clinical and anatomopathological study of three cases. Histoenzymological and ultrastructural data. Arch Anat Cytol Pathol 30:172, 1982

125. Hoggins GW, Grundy MC: Melanotic neuroectodermal tumors of infancy. Report of a case. Oral Surg 40:34, 1975

126. Dehner LP, Sibley RK, Sauk JJ Jr, et al: Melanotic neuroectodermal tumor of infancy: A clinicopathologic ultrastructural and tissue culture study. Cancer 43:1389, 1979

127. Nagase M, Ueda K, Fukushima M, Nakajima T: Recurrent melanotic neuroectodermal tumor of infancy: Case reported survey of 16 cases. J Maxillofac Surg 11:131, 1983

128. Misugi K, Okajima H, Newton WA, et al: Mediastinal origin of a melanotic progonoma or retinal anlage tumor. Ultrastructural evidence for neural crest origin. Cancer 18:477, 1965

129. Cooke BED: Median rhomboid glossitis—candidiasis and not a developmental anomaly. Br J Dermatol 93:399, 1975

130. Knoblich R: Accessory thyroid in the lateral floor of the mouth. Report of a case with embryologic considerations. Oral Surg 19:234, 1965

131. Sauk JJ Jr: Ectopic lingual thyroid. J Pathol 102:239, 1970

132. Melnick JL, Bunting H, Banfield WS, et al: Electron microscopy of viruses of human papilloma, molluscum contagiosum, and vaccinia, including observations on the formation of virus within cell. Ann NY Acad Sci 54:1214, 1952

133. Eversole LR, Laipis PJ, Green TJ: Human papillomavirus, type II DNA in oral and labial verruca vulgaris. J Cutan Pathol 14:319, 1987

134. Jin, YT, Toto PD: Detection of human papovavirus antigen in papillary lesions. Oral Surg 58:702, 1984

135. Bhaskar SN: Oral tumors of infancy and childhood. J Pediatr 64:195, 1963

136. Jones JH: Non-odontogenic tumors in children. Br Dent J 119:439, 1965

137. Kohn EM, Dahlin DC, Erich JB: Primary neoplasms of the hard and soft palates and uvula. Mayo Clin Proc 38:233, 1963

138. Orlean SL, DaDow CS: Superficial keratoses: Verruca vulgaris and pachyderma oris. J Dent Med 15:108, 1960

139. Orfuss AJ: Profuse warts of the skin and mucous membranes. Arch Dermatol 93:776, 1966

140. Eversole LR, Sorenson HW: Oral florid papillomatosis in Down's syndrome. Oral Surg 37:202, 1974

141. Greer RO, Goldman HM: Oral papillomas: Clinicopathologic evaluation and retrospective examination for dyskeratosis in 110 lesions. Oral Surg 38:435, 1974

142. Wertheimer FW, Stroud DE: Peripheral ameloblastoma in a papilloma with recurrence. Report of a case. J Oral Surg 30:47, 1972

143. Waite DE: Inflammatory papillary hyperplasia. J Oral Surg 19:210, 1961

144. Greer RO, Eversole LR, Poulson TC, et al: Identification of human papillomavirus DNA in smokeless tobacco-associated keratoses from juveniles, adults, and other adults using immunocytochemical and in situ DNA hybridization techniques. Gerodontics 3:87, 1987

145. Svirsky JA, Freedman PD, Lumerman H: Solitary intraoral keratoacanthoma. Oral Surg 43:116, 1977

146. Scofield HH, Werning JT, Shukes RC: Solitary intraoral keratoacanthoma. Oral Surg 37:889, 1974

147. Smith JF: A case of multiple primary squamous cell carcinomata in the skin in a young man with spontaneous healing. Br J Dermatol 46:267, 1934

148. Grzybowski M: A case of peculiar generalized epithelial tumors of the skin. Br J Dermatol 62:310, 1950

149. Young SK, Larsen PE, Markowitz NR: Generalized eruptive keratoacanthoma. Oral Surg 62:422, 1986

150. Eisenberg E, Murphy GF, Krutchkoff DJ: Involucrin as a diagnostic marker on oral lichenoid lesions (abstract 13). American Academy of Oral Pathology, 41st Annual Meeting, Registry Resort, Scottsdale, AZ, 1987

151. Camisa C, Allen CN: Treatment of oral erosive lichen planus with systemic isotretinoin. Oral Surg 62:393, 1986

152. Silverman S Jr, Galante M: Oral Cancer. 6th Ed. University of California at San Francisco Press, 1977

153. Pindborg JJ: World Health Organization Collaborating Center for Oral Precancerous Lesions: Definition of leukoplakia and related lesions: An aid to studies on oral precancer. Oral Surg 46:518, 1978

154. Pindborg JJ, Renstrup G, Poulsen HE, Silverman S Jr: Studies in oral leukoplakias: Five clinical and histologic signs of malignancy. Acta Odontol Scand 21:407, 1963

155. Sugar L, Banocyz J: Untersuchungen bei Präkanzerose der Mundschleimhaut. Dtsch Zahn Mund Kieferheilk 30:132, 137, 1959

156. Burkhardt A: Der Mundhöhlenkrebs und seine Vorstadien. G. Fisher, New York, 1980

157. Mashberg A, Meyers H: Anatomical site and size of 222 early asymptomatic oral squamous cell carcinomas: A continuing prospective study of oral cancer. II. Cancer 37:2149, 1976

158. Greer RO: Lesions of the oral cavity. p. 127. In Wood RP, Northern JL (eds): Manual of Otolaryngology. A Symptom Oriented Text. Williams & Wilkins, Baltimore, 1979

159. Greer RO, Wilson G: Oral cancer: A five year retrospective regional study. Colo Oral Cancer Bull 2:2, 1979

160. Greer RO: Oral cancer: An Overview. Colo Oral Cancer Bull 1:5, 1978

161. Cherrick HM: The mouth and oropharynx. p. 27. In Coulson WF (ed): Surgical Pathology. Philadelphia, JB Lippincott, 1978

162. Dorn HR, Cutler JJ: Morbidity from Cancer in the United States. p. 186. Public Health Monograph No 50. U.S. Government Printing Office, Washington, 1959

163. Malaowalla AM, Silverman S, Mani NJ, et al: Oral cancer in 57,518 industrial workers in Gujarat India. A prevalence and follow-up study. Cancer 37:1882, 1976

164. Pindborg JJ: Oral cancer from an international point of view. Can Dent Assoc J 31:219, 1965

165. Ahlbom HE: Simple achlorhydric anemia, Plummer-Vinson syndrome, and carcinoma of the mouth, pharynx and esophagus in women. Br Med J 2:331, 1936

166. Andreasen JO: Oral manifestations in discoid and systemic lupus erythematosus. I. Clinical investigation. Acta Odontol Scand 22:295, 1964

167. Pindborg JJ, Mehta IS, Gupta DC, Daftary DK: Prevalence of oral submucous fibrosis among 50,915 Indian villagers. Br J Cancer 22:646, 1968

168. Silverman S, Griffith M: Studies on oral lichen planus: #2. Follow-up on 200 patients: Clinical characteristics and associated malignancy. Oral Surg 37:705, 1974

169. Cawson, RA: Chronic oral candidiasis and leukoplakia. Oral Surg 22:582, 1966

170. Belton CM, Eversole LR: Oral hairy leukoplakia: ultrastructural features. J Oral Pathol 15:493, 1986

171. Slaughter DP, Southwick HW: Mucosal carcinomas as a result of irradiation. Arch Surg 74:420, 1957

172. Fu KK, Lichter A, Galante M: Carcinoma of the floor of the mouth: An analysis of treatment results and the sites and courses of failures. Int J Radiat Oncol Biol Phys 1:829, 1976

173. Frazell EL, Lucas JC: Cancer of the tongue. Report of management of 1,554 patients. Cancer 15:1085, 1962

174. Broders AC: Carcinomas of the mouth: Type and degrees of malignancy. AJR 17:90, 1927

175. Platz H, Fries R, Hudec M, et al: Prognostic relevance of minimal invasion of the oral cavity: A retrospective DOSAK study. Clin Onco 1:467, 1982

176. Lederer B, Managetta JB: Morphological analysis of minimal invasion carcinoma (microcarcinoma) of the oral mucosa. Clin Oncol 1:475, 1982

177. Cross JE, Guralnick E, Daland EM: Carcinoma of the lip. A review of 563 case records of carcinoma of the lip at the Pondville Hospital. Surg Gynecol Obstet 87:153, 1948

178. Knapel MR, Koranda FC, Panje WR, Grand DJ: Squamous cell carcinoma of the upper lip. J Dermatol Surg Oncol 8:487, 1982

179. Vanderwall I: Squamous cell carcinoma: Clinical and histopathological aspects. p. 33. In Vanderwall I, Snow GB (eds): Oral Oncology, Martinus Nijhoff, Boston, 1984

180. Cady B, Catlin D: Epidermoid carcinoma of the gum. A 20-year survey. Cancer 23:551, 1969

181. Jacoway JR, Nelson JF, Boyers RC: Adenoid squamous cell carcinoma (adenoacanthoma) of the oral labial mucosa. A clinicopathologic study of fifteen cases. Oral Surg 32:444, 1971

182. Tomich CE, Hutton CE: Adenoid squamous cell carcinoma of the lip. Report of cases. J Oral Surg 30:592, 1972

183. Batsakis JG: Pathology of tumors of the oral cavity. p. 48. In Thawley SE, Panje WR (eds): Comprehensive Management of Head and Neck Tumors. WB Saunders, Philadelphia, 1987

184. Batsakis JG, Rice DH, Howard DR: The pathology of head and neck tumors: Spindle cell lesions (sarcomatoid carcinomas, nodular fasciitis, and fibrosarcoma) of the aerodigestive tracts. Part 14. Head Neck Surg 4:499, 1982

185. Leifer C, Miller AS: Spindle cell carcinomas of the oral mucosa. A light and electron microscopic study of apparent sarcomatous metastasis to cervical lymph nodes. Cancer 34:597, 1974

186. Greene GW, Bernier JL: Spindle cell squamous carcinoma of the lip. Report of four cases. Oral Surg 12:1008, 1959

187. Ellis GL, Corio RL: Spindle cell carcinoma of the oral cavity: A clinicopathologic assessment of 59 cases. Oral Surg 50, 523, 1980

188. Friedell HL, Rosenthal LM: The etiologic role of chewing tobacco in cancer of the mouth. Report of eight cases treated with radiation. JAMA 116:2130, 1941

189. Ackerman LV: Verrucous carcinoma of the oral cavity. Surgery 23:670, 1948

190. Biller HF, Ogura JH, Bauer WC: Verrucous carcinoma of the larynx. Laryngoscope 81:1323, 1971

192. Shear M, Pindborg JJ: Verrucous hyperplasia of the oral mucosa. Cancer, 46:1855, 1980

193. Jacobson S, Shear M: Verrucous carcinoma of the mouth. J Oral Pathol 1:66, 1972

194. Shafer WG: Verrucous carcinoma. Int Dent J 22:451, 1972

195. Eversole LR, Sorenson JW: Oral florid papillomatosis in Down's syndrome. Oral Surg 37:202, 1974

196. Kraus FT, Perez-Mesa C: Verrucous carcinoma. Clinical and pathologic study of 105 cases involving oral cavity, larynx, and genitalia. Cancer 19:26, 1966

197. Fonts EA, Greenlaw RH, Rush BF, et al: Verrucous squamous cell carcinoma of the oral cavity. Cancer 23:152, 1969

198. Greer RO: Oral cancer: An overview. Colo Oral Cancer Bull 1:5, 1978

199. Baker R, D'Onofrio ED, Cario B, et al: Squamous cell carcinoma arising in a lateral periodontal cyst. Oral Surg 47:495, 1979

200. Toller PA: Origin and growth of cysts of the jaws. Ann R Coll Surg Engl 40:306, 1967

201. Rapini RP, Golitz LE, Greer RO Jr, et al: Primary malignant melanoma of the oral cavity. A review of 177 cases. Cancer 55:1543, 1985

202. Tschen JA, Fechner RE: The juxtaoral organ of Chievitz. Am J Surg Pathol 3:147, 1979

203. Elzay RP, O'Keefe EM: Unusual gingival proliferation:

Primary pseudoepitheliomatous hyperplasia. Oral Surg 47:436, 1979

204. Greer RO: Inverted oral papilloma. Oral Surg 36:400, 1973

205. Abrams AM, Melrose RJ, Howell FV: Necrotizing sialometaplasia. A disease stimulating malignancy. Cancer 32:130,1973

206. Forney SK, Foley JM, Sugg WE, et al: Necrotizing sialometaplasia of the mandible. Oral Surg 43:720, 1977

207. Bronstein SL, Greer RO, Steffen K: Necrotizing sialometaplasia. A benign disease simulating malignancy. Colo Oral Cancer Bull 1:12, 1978

208. Philipsen HP, Peterson JK, Simonsen BH: Necrotizing sialometaplasia of the palate. Int J Oral Surg 5:292, 1976

209. Poulson TC, Greer RO, Ryser RW: Necrotizing sialometaplasia obscuring an underlying malignancy: Report of a case. J Oral Maxillofac Surg 44:570, 1984

210. Meyer I, Shklar G: Malignant tumors metastatic to the mouth and jaws. Oral Surg 20:350, 1969

211. Castigliano SG, Rominger CJ: Metastatic malignancy of the jaws. Am J Surg 87:496, 1954

212. McDaniel RK, Luna MA, Stimson PG: Metastatic tumors of the jaws. Oral Surg 31:380, 1971

213. Hatziotis J, Constantinidou H, Papanayotou PH: Metastatic tumors of the oral soft tissue. Review of the literature and report of a case. Oral Surg 36:544, 1973

214. McClatchey KD, Batsakis JG, Young SK: Intravascular angiomatosis. Oral Surg 46:70, 1978

215. Heyden G, Dahl I, Angervall L: Intravascular papillary endothelial hyperplasia in the oral mucosa. Oral Surg 45:83, 1978

216. Cundiff EJ: Peripheral Ossifying Fibroma. A Review of 365 Cases. Thesis, Indiana University, Bloomington, 1972

217. Greer RO, Zarlengo WD: Peripheral odontogenic fibroma. A reappraisal of biologic behavior. J Colo Dent Assoc 57:11, 1979

218. Giansanti JS, Waldron CA: Peripheral giant cell granuloma: Review of 720 cases. J Oral Surg 27:787, 1969

219. Sapp JP: Ultrastructure and histogenesis of peripheral giant cell reparative granuloma of the jaws. Cancer 30:1119, 1972

220. Waldron CA, Shafer WG: The central giant cell reparative granuloma of the jaws. An analysis of 38 cases. Am J Clin Pathol 45:437, 1966

221. Austin LT, Dahlin DC, Royer RQ: Giant cell reparative granuloma and related conditions affecting the jawbones. Oral Surg 12:1285, 1959

222. Greer RO, Mierau GW, Favara B: Tumors of the Head and Neck in Children. Praeger, New York, 1983, p. 240

223. Dahlin DC: Bone Tumors. 2nd Ed. Charles C Thomas, Springfield, IL, 1967

224. Batsakis JG: Tumors of the Head and Neck. Clinical and Pathologic Considerations. 2nd Ed. Williams & Wilkins, Baltimore, 1979, p. 395–400

225. Andersen L, Fejerskov O, Philipsen HP: Oral giant cell granulomas. A clinical and histologic study of 129 new cases. Acta Pathol Microbiol Scand 81A:606, 1973

226. Vickers RA: Mesenchymal (soft) tissue tumors of the oral region. In Gorlin RJ, Goldman HM: Thoma's Oral Pathology. Vol 1. 6th Ed. CV Mosby, St. Louis, 1970

227. Konwaler WE, Keasler L, Kaplan L: Subcutaneous pseudosarcomatous fibromatosis (fasciitis). Am J Pathol 24:241, 1955

228. Stout AP, Lattes R: Tumors of the Soft Tissue. Atlas of Tumor Pathology, Ser. 2, Fasc. 1. Armed Forces Institute of Pathology, Washington, 1967

229. Werning JT: Nodular fasciitis of the orofacial region. Oral Surg 48:441, 1979

230. Miller R, Cheris L, Stratigos GT: Nodular fasciitis. Oral Surg 40:399, 1975

231. Shuman R: Mesenchymal tumors of soft tissue. p. 565. In Anderson WAD (ed): Pathology. 6th Ed. CV Mosby, St Louis, 1971

232. Takagi M, Ishikawa G: Fibrous tumor of infancy—report of a case originating in the oral cavity. J Oral Pathol 2:293, 1973

233. Freedman PD, Cardo V, Kerpel SM, et al: Desmoplastic fibroma (fibromatosis) of the jawbones. Oral Surg 46:386, 1978

234. Dockerty MB, Parkhill EM, Dahlin DC, et al: Tumors of the Oral Cavity and Pharynx. p. 155. In Atlas of Tumor Pathology. Fasc. 106. Armed Forces Institute of Pathology, Washington, 1968

235. Osment LS: Cutaneous lipomas and lipomatosis. Surg Gynecol Obstet 127:129, 1962

236. Gellhorn A, Marks PA: The composition and biosynthesis of lipids in human adipose tissue. J Clin Invest 40:925, 1961

237. Greer RO, Richardson JF: The nature of lipomas and their significance in the oral cavity. Oral Surg 36:551, 1973

238. MacGregor AJ, Dyson DP: Oral lipomas. A review of the literature and a report of twelve new cases. Oral Surg 21:770, 1966

239. Herschfus L, Wolter JG: Granular cell myoblastoma of the oral cavity. Oral Surg 29:341, 1970

240. Matthews JB, Mason GI: Oral granular cell myoblastoma: An immunohistochemical study. J Oral Pathol 11:343, 1982

241. Stefansson K, Wollman RL: S-100 protein in granular cell tumors (granular cell myoblastomas). Cancer 49:1634, 1982

242. Willis RA: Pathology of Tumors. 4th Ed. Butterworth, London, 1967

243. Azzopardi JG: Histogenesis of the granular cell myoblastoma. J Pathol Bacteriol 71:85, 1956

244. Fisher ER, Wechsler H: Granular cell myoblastoma—a misnomer. Electron microscopic and histochemical evidence concerning its Schwann cell derivation and nature. Cancer 15:936, 1962

245. Garancis JC, Komorowski RA, Kuzma JF: Granular cell myoblastoma. Cancer 25:542, 1970

246. Misch KA: Rhabdomyoma purum: A benign rhabdomyoma of tongue. J Pathol Bacteriol 75:105, 1958

247. Campbell JAH: Congenital epulis. J Pathol Bacteriol 70:233, 1955

248. Kay S, Elzay RP, Willson MA: Ultrastructural observations on a gingival granular cell tumor (congenital epulis). Cancer 27:674, 1971

249. Armin A, Connelly E, Rowden G: An immunoperoxidase

investigation of S-100 protein in granular cell myoblastomas: Evidence for Schwann cell derivation. Am J Clin Pathol 79:37, 1983

250. Monteil RA, Loubiere R, Charbit Y, Gillette JY: Gingival granular cell tumor of the newborn: Immunoperoxidase investigation with anti-S-100 antiserum. Oral Surg 64:78, 1987

251. Ellis GL, Abrams AM, Melrose RJ: Intraosseous benign neural sheath neoplasms. Report of seven cases and review of the literature. Oral Surg 44:731, 1977

252. Cherrick HM, Eversole LM: Benign neurosheath neoplasms of the oral cavity: Report of 37 cases. Oral Surg 32:900, 1971

253. Harkin JC, Reed JJ: Tumors of the Peripheral Nervous System. Atlas of Tumor Pathology. Ser. 2. Fasc. 3. Armed Forces Institute of Pathology, Washington, 1969

254. Gallager RL, Helwig EB: Neurothekoma—a benign cutaneous tumor of nerve origin. Am J Clin Pathol 74:759, 1980

255. Mason MR, Knepp DR, Herbold DR: Nerve sheath myxoma (neurothekoma): a case involving the lip. Oral Surg 62:185, 1986

256. Wesley RK, Mintz SM, Wertheimer FW: Primary malignant hemangioendothelioma of the gingiva. Oral Surg 39:103, 1975

257. Frazell E: Clinical aspects of tumors of the major salivary glands. Cancer 7:637, 1954

258. Eversole LR, Sabes WR, Rovin S: Fibrous dysplasia: A nosologic problem in the diagnosis of fibro-osseous lesions of the jaws. J Oral Pathol 1:189, 1972

259. Waldron CA, Giansanti JS: Benign fibro-osseous lesions of the jaws. A clinical and radiologic-histologic review of sixty-five cases. Part I. Oral Surg 35:190, 1973

260. Reed RJ: Fibrous dysplasias of bone. Arch Pathol 75:480, 1963

261. Spjut JJ, Dorfman HD, Fechner RE, et al: Tumors of Bone and Cartilage. Atlas of Tumor Pathology, Ser. 2. Fasc. 5. Armed Forces Institute of Pathology, Washington, 1970

262. Marlow CD, Waite DE: Fibro-osseous dysplasia of the jaws: Report of a case. J Oral Surg 23:632, 1965

263. Schonfield IDF: An aggressive fibrous dysplasia. Oral Surg 38:29, 1974

264. Gross CW, Montgomery WW: Fibrous dysplasia and malignant degeneration. Arch Otolaryngol 85:653, 1967

265. Hammer JE, Scofield HH, Cornyn J: Benign fibro-osseous jaw lesions of periodontal membrane origin. Cancer 22:861, 1968

266. Eversole LR: Clinical Outline of Oral Pathology: Diagnosis and Treatment. Lea & Febiger, Philadelphia, 1978, p. 206

267. Garrington GE, Scofield HH, Cornyn J, et al: Osteosarcoma of the jaws. Analysis of 56 cases. Cancer 20:377, 1967

268. Forteza G, Colmenero B, Lopez-Barea F: Osteosarcoma of the maxilla and mandible. Oral Surg 62:179, 1987

269. Greer RO, Berman DN: Osteoblastoma of the jaws: Current concepts and differential diagnosis. J Oral Surg 36:304, 1978

270. Farman AG, Nortje CJ, Grotepass F: Periosteal benign osteoblastoma of the mandible: Report of a case and review of the literature pertaining to benign osteoblastic neoplasms of the jaws. Br J Oral Surg 14:12, 1976

23

The Major Salivary Glands

James J. Sciubba
John G. Batsakis

Tumors of the major salivary glands, and especially malignant ones, do not represent a major diagnostic load in nonspecialized hospitals. As an example, cancers of the parotid gland represent approximately 1 percent of all human neoplasms and are said to account for only 650 deaths per year in the United States.[1] In addition to this low frequency, other aspects of salivary gland tumors can serve as pitfalls in the diagnosis and management of the lesions. Despite numerous functional, embryologic, and morphologic similarities between the exocrine pancreas and the major salivary glands, the neoplastic expressions of the latter are far more diverse and almost unique in their variation. The biologic behavior of the tumors as a group is also peculiar. Salivary gland carcinomas do not follow the pattern of other more well known cancers. Three and 5 year follow-up periods are inadequate for delineating prognosis. In many instances, the tumors may be so slow growing that a 20 year survival with active disease is possible.

Histopathologic diagnosis is the cornerstone for therapeutic planning. For salivary gland tumors, two other factors modify this cornerstone: histologic grade and clinical stage. Of the two, stage is the most important, and the size of the mass is a prominent factor in staging parotid cancer. Table 23-1 presents the 1988 American Joint Committee on Cancer's (AJC) staging system[2] Other versions have preceded the AJC system. Spiro et al.[3] have done a considerable amount of work correlating stage of disease with prognosis, incidence of lymph node metastasis, and distant metastasis. They have reported 5 year survival rates of 85 percent for T1 parotid cancers, 67 percent for T2 cancers, and 14 percent for T3 cancers.

Using the same staging system as Spiro, Fu and co-workers[4] found a 5 year survival rate of 88 percent and a 10 year determinate survival rate of 83 percent for stage I cancers, a 5 year survival rate of 76 percent, and a 10 year survival rate of 76 percent for stage II cancers, and a 5 year survival rate of 49 percent and a 10 year survival of 32 percent for stage III cancers.

Correlation of stage with distant metastases is notable in the study by Spiro et al.[3] These workers found that stage I lesions had a 2 percent incidence of distant spread, whereas stage III cancers had a 39 percent incidence. Furthermore, they were able to correlate recurrence rates with stage of disease. T1 lesions recurred in only 7 percent of cases, whereas T3 lesions had a 58 percent recurrence rate. In their study of mucoepidermoid carcinomas, they found that lymph node metastases, distant metastases, recurrence, and overall survival correlated well with stage of the neoplasm.

Attempts at correlating biologic course and prognosis with histologic grade have not been as successful. High-grade carcinomas such as poorly differentiated, high-grade mucoepidermoid carcinoma and high-grade adenocarcinomas are also those presenting with high-stage lesions. The histologic grading of adenoid cystic carcinomas into high and low grades has produced inconsistent correlation, and here again grade yields to stage as the superior prognosticator. Grading of acinic cell carcinoma has not been shown to afford reasonable expectations as to biologic aggressiveness.[5] The most successful application of grading has been the division of mucoepidermoid carcinomas into low-grade, intermediate-grade, and high-grade lesions.[6] Even here, however, size and anatomic

TABLE 23-1. American Joint Committee on Cancer T-N-M Staging Classification for Major Salivary Glands

T (Primary Neoplasm)[a]	
TX	Cannot be assessed
T0	No evidence of primary neoplasm
T1	Neoplasm 2 cm or less in greatest dimension
T2	Neoplasm more than 2 cm but less than 4 cm in greatest dimension
T3	Neoplasm more than 4 cm but less than 6 cm in greatest dimension
T4	Neoplasm more than 6 cm in greatest dimension
N (Lymph node)	
NX	Regional lymph nodes cannot be assessed
N0	No regional lymph node metastasis
N1	Metastasis in a single ipsilateral lymph node, 3 cm or less in greatest dimension
N2	Same as N1, but more than 3 cm and less than 6 cm in greatest dimension, or in multiple ipsilateral lymph nodes, none larger than 6 cm, or in bilateral or contralateral lymph nodes, none more than 6 cm in greatest dimension
N2a	Metastasis in a single ipsilateral lymph node, more than 3 cm but not more than 6 cm in greatest dimension
N2b	Metastasis in multiple ipsilateral lymph nodes, none larger than 6 cm
N2c	Metastasis in bilateral or contralateral lymph nodes not larger than 6 cm in greatest dimension
N3	Metastasis in a lymph node more than 6 cm in greatest dimension
M (Distant metastasis)	
MX	Cannot be assessed
M0	No distant metastasis
M1	Distant metastasis
G (Histopathologic grade)	
GX	Cannot be assessed
G1	Well differentiated
G2	Moderately well differentiated
G3	Poorly differentiated
G4	Undifferentiated
Histopathologic type	

[a] T categories are further subdivided into: (a) no local extension, (b) local extension. Local extension is clinical or grossly visible evidence of invasion of skin, soft tissues, bone, or nerve. Microscopic evidence only is not defined as local extension in the T classification.

site of the carcinoma play a more important modifying role.

Salivary gland tumors afford the surgical pathologist the opportunity to bring into play nearly all his armamentarium—cytology, frozen sections, histochemistry, and electron microscopy. Routine hematoxylin and eosin (H&E)-stained sections, however, are the most important, and accurate diagnoses can be made from them in the great majority of cases. Recalling that electron microscopic detail does not define malignancy, fine structural analysis of salivary gland tumors is used to identify cell types by their cytoplasmic organelles, for example, mitochondria in oncocytes and synthetic products in glycogen-containing, mucinous or serous cells. In nearly all these examples, appropriate histochemical procedures will obviate the need for electron microscopy. Preopera-

tive needle aspirate cytology for diagnosis of salivary gland tumors has been used for more than two decades.[7] The success of the procedure varies directly with the experience of the cytopathologist *and* of the procurer of the specimen. The major failing in the past has been an unacceptable false negative rate. Even with reduction of that rate, however, the clinical value of the procedure remains to be substantiated.[7] For tumors of the salivary glands, preoperative cytologic diagnoses *may* provide the surgeon with a more precise operative plan but, as we have indicated earlier, size of the tumor and extrasalivary extension are equally important, and these variables cannot be accurately assessed until the tumor is surgically exposed.

Intraoperative histologic diagnosis is provided by frozen section studies, but this is but one purpose of the frozen section examination. In our opinion, just as valuable a contribution is the assessment of adequacy of excision. This assessment is on tissue selected by the surgeon and not from sections cut from the specimen by the surgical pathologist.

The fine needle aspirate and the frozen section sample are just two of the types of specimens the surgical pathologist should be prepared to deal with in his evaluation of lesions of the major salivary glands. Incisional biopsy, except perhaps for sublingual gland tumors, should not be encouraged, for the contemporary surgical principles of major salivary gland surgery are such that the usual minimal specimen from the parotid gland is the lateral or superficial lobe, and the entire gland if the lesion is in the submandibular gland. In both instances, the specimen is an excisional biopsy. Exceptions to this are deep-lobe parotid tumors where a near total parotidectomy is performed and when the conservation-minded surgeon removes a superficial lobe lesion with a cuff of normal salivary tissue.

Because of the importance of stage, two maneuvers are mandatory in the gross examination of the intact salivary gland lesion: (1) measurement of the tumor and (2) delineation of margins. India ink marking is recommended for the latter evaluation. Description of the gross characteristics is axiomatic, but it is also clear that few salivary gland tumors have diagnostic gross features. The benign mixed tumor and Warthin's tumor are exceptions. Circumscription, encapsulation, multilobulation, and apparent satellite nodules should be noted. Areas of necrosis or softening in an otherwise benign mixed tumor are often ancillary findings of malignant transformation and must be sectioned for microscopic examination.

There is no routine number of sections to be taken from a tumor of a major salivary gland. Deep and other margins are required for all tumors, benign or malignant. Since intraparotid extension by infiltrative growth is also important, such gross areas are also required to be sampled. It is in these foci that perineural invasion, intravascular extension and other indications of biologic aggressiveness are best evaluated.

In both parotid and submandibular gland specimens, lymph nodes are included because of the intimacy of the nodes to the glands, especially the relatively rich system in and about the parotid gland. In the latter, these lymph nodes are within the parotid gland fascia and sections will usually demonstrate them. Except for high-grade carcinomas, true lymphatic metastases are not common and even in the high-grade lesions are not usually manifest at the time of primary surgery.

In the salivary glands, mucoprotein histochemistry and enzyme histochemistry have been extensively studied but have not been of any particular diagnostic usefulness. There are variable quantities of both sialo- and sulphomucins in salivary glands, and there is a rather pronounced degree of mucin heterogeneity in humans, not merely from gland to gland but even from cell to cell. Enzyme histochemistry (e.g., phosphatases, peroxidase, ATPase) of salivary tissues is very dependent on the integrity of the cell and its functional state.[7] These account for the variable data produced by such studies.

Given the variability of reactive products and also variation in stain techniques, histochemical analysis of a salivary gland tumor provides only little diagnostic aid. The demonstration of mucous cells will distinguish a high-grade mucoepidermoid carcinoma from a squamous cell carcinoma but does little else. Periodic acid-Schiff (PAS) techniques provide pretty color contrasts but lack specificity (mucins, collagen, basement membranes, secretory granules). PAS after diastase digestion will permit the characterization of intracellular glycogen, but this too is dependent on the functional status and fixation of the cell.

In short, there is no specific histochemical battery unique to salivary gland pathology. A high-quality mucin stain (alcian blue, ph 2.5) is necessary, but all others are ancillary rather than diagnostic.[7]

Immunocytochemical studies of the carbohydrate and proteins of the neoplasm, including lectins, epithelial membrane antigens, high- and low-molecular-weight keratins, S-100 protein antigen, and muscle-specific actin, have contributed to our understanding of the complicated constituency of salivary gland tumors and of their histogenesis.[8–15] These studies have made for greater recognition and appreciation for the contributions made to the neoplasms by myoepithelium. It is now evident that myoepithelial cells are major players, not just passive participants, in nearly all salivary gland tumors taking origin from the intercalated duct portion of the salivary duct unit. These neoplasms include pleomorphic adenomas, adenoid cystic carcinomas, epimyoepithelial carcinomas, terminal duct adenocarcinomas, many monomorphic adenomas, and myoepithelioma and myoepithelial carcinoma. In general, salivary gland neoplasms with a

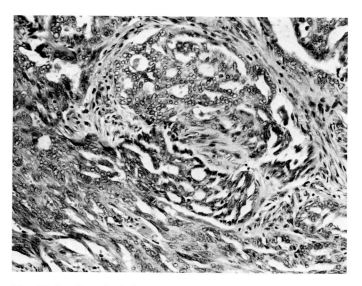

Fig. 23-1. Terminal duct adenocarcinoma of the soft palate. Note the dual cell population of small epithelial ducts and spindled myoepithelial cells.

prominent myoepithelial component are those with a low to intermediate grade of biologic behavior (Fig. 23-1). High-grade carcinomas, such as ductal carcinoma and primary squamous cell carcinoma, lack a myoepithelial element.[16]

EMBRYOGENESIS AND HISTOGENESIS OF SALIVARY GLANDS

The major salivary glands (parotid, submandibular, and sublingual) and salivary tissue from the lips to the anterior faucial pillars are ectodermally derived.[17] They originate from the stomodeal lining (oral mucosa) as simple epithelial proliferations or invaginations into the underlying mesenchyme. All salivary glands undergo similar patterns of development with a solid cord or primordium connecting the surface invagination to the advancing or "invading" ectodermal element. A basal lamina or basement membrane similar to that seen in developing teeth, hair follicles, and cutaneous adnexa separates ectodermal and mesodermal tissues.

Progression of ectodermal penetration deeper into the mesenchymal elements allows generalized tissue-to-tissue interaction to occur: cytodifferentiation and morphodifferentiation[17,18] As penetration into deeper mesenchyme occurs, there is a concomitant elongation of the main duct primordium. This elongation is probably related to cell proliferation along its length, as well as to an increase in cell number at the proximal and distal ends of the primordium.

Progressive branching characterizes further development and morphogenesis. Branching morphogenesis is a result of tissue-to-tissue interaction with the extracellular materials, notably collagen and epithelial (ectodermal) basement membrane playing the critical role in establishing this pattern.

As branching proceeds as solid ductal structures, acinar or end-piece differentiation begins. Each branch or strand with terminal clusters is surrounded by highly cellular, richly vascular mesenchyme. By 5 months gestation, a lumen becomes recognizable within the strands that become future ductal components. A tubuloalveolar pattern is formed when terminal cell clusters differentiate into round or oblate alveoli. As the tubuloalveolar pattern is established, further cytodifferentiation of ductal and secretory end-piece (acinous) elements occurs. The secretory end piece is connected to the developing ductal system by the terminal tubule complex.[17,18]

Donath et al.[18] defined three stages in parotid gland development: (1) anlage stage from 0 to 12 weeks of development, (2) differentiation of lobular and ductal elements, which occurs from 12 to 36 weeks of development, and (3) structural and functional refinement, including myoepithelial cell maturation, from the thirty-sixth to fortieth week.

At 6 and 8 weeks of gestation, respectively, the submandibular and sublingual glands appear as an ectodermal invagination just lateral to the base of the tongue in the floor of the mouth. From this point, the primordium migrates distally and inferiorly with subsequent branching into two distinct glandular aggregates. A similar early pattern of development is noted for intraoral minor salivary tissue. Budding invaginations from oral ectoderm invade the mesenchyme at 10 weeks gestation. Branching morphogenesis begins after a relatively short cord (duct) is formed.

The most active part of the embryonic salivary duct unit is at the junction of the intercalated ducts and secretory end pieces or acini. Reserve cells in the intercalated ducts persist throughout adult life and are the putative source for replenishment of acinous cells, intercalated duct cells, and proximally related striated duct cells. It is also from this cellular zone of the salivary duct unit that most salivary gland tumors arise.[17]

CLASSIFICATION OF SALIVARY TUMORS

Several approaches to the classification of salivary neoplasms have been published. Some of these have had morphologic features as their basis, while histogenesis has served to support a taxonomic scheme in another study.[20] The latter approach emphasizes the importance of the reserve cell population within the intercalated and excretory components of the duct system. If one considers a postembryonic dedifferentiation of a cell within the reserve cell population as the primary biologic event, neoplasia will result. Whether the result of this epigenetic neoplastic event is benign or malignant will depend on the overall extent of genome dedifferentiation within the reserve cell component.

Despite attempts at histogenetic classification of salivary neoplasms, most current and workable systems rely on morphologic and biologic features. When the array and complexity of salivary neoplasia is considered, it becomes clear that a flexible and pragmatic system is difficult to formulate. In a practical context, the scheme used by Foote and Frazell[21] with some modification is one that offers flexibility and usefulness. One of our modifications of that system relates to the expected behavioral pattern of mucoepidermoid and acinic cell carcinomas (Table 23-2). We strongly believe that they should be classified as cancers but with variable histologic grades and corresponding behavior patterns. Personal experiences have shown that so-called low-grade lesions have metastasized and in some cases have killed.

Finally, the classification in Table 23-2 is as comprehensive a listing as we have been able to define. Some of the lesions are rarely encountered in practice, but their inclusion permits placement of the lesions into a clinicopathologic category to assist in consideration of therapy.

We believe that the monomorphic adenoma group of tumors should be provided with more than simple listing. Since the identification and separation of this group by Kleinsasser and Klein,[22] numerous studies and single case reports have served to broaden and/or confuse their status. The basic difference between pleomorphic and monomorphic adenoma for our purposes relates to the presence or absence of histologically definable alterations of stroma such as those with myxoid or chondroid features.

The biologic potential of the monomorphic adenoma group remains as yet unclear due to the short follow-up periods of the published studies. One particular feature of the monomorphic group worthy of thought is the potential relationship between it and the mixed tumor or pleomorphic adenoma, as well as the adenoid cystic carcinoma. Our contention is that the basal cell type of monomorphic adenoma and the membranous variant be considered as benign homologues of adenoid cystic carcinoma.

Within this system, we have included tumors of clear cell morphology with both benign and malignant forms. This done despite our belief that clear cell tumors are best regarded as at least low-grade carcinomas.[23]

Some taxonomic confusion has arisen about malignancy and the mixed tumor. Most commonly, carcinoma

TABLE 23-2. Classification of Salivary Gland Tumors

Benign epithelial
   Pleomorphic adenoma (mixed tumor)
   Warthin's tumor (papillary cystadenoma lymphomatosum)
   Monomorphic adenoma
      Basaloid
      Dermal analogue (membranous)
      Ductal
      Sebaceous
      Oncocytoma
      Myoepithelioma
      Clear cell
   Ductal papilloma
      Inverted
      Intraductal
      Sialadenoma papilliferum

Malignant primary epithelial
   Mucoepidermoid carcinoma
   Adenoid cystic carcinoma
   Acinic (acinous) cell carcinoma
   Epimyoepithelial duct carcinoma (clear cell carcinoma)
   Myoepithelial carcinoma
   Ductal carcinoma
   Papillary and nonpapillary adenocarcinoma
   Mucinous adenocarcinoma
   Oncocytic carcinoma
   Carcinoma ex pleomorphic adenoma
   Squamous cell carcinoma
   Carcinoma ex monomorphic adenoma
   Basaloid carcinoma
   Carcinosarcoma (true malignant mixed tumor)
   Undifferentiated carcinoma with lymphoid stroma (lymphoepithelial
     carcinoma)
   Undifferentiated carcinoma
   Neuroendocrine carcinoma
   Carcinoma ex Warthin's tumor

Malignant primary nonepithelial
   Osteosarcoma
   Malignant peripheral nerve sheath tumors
   Lymphomas
   Other sarcomas

Metastatic neoplasms

Benign nonepithelial
   Hemangioma
   Lipoma
   Neural tumors

Tumorlike conditions
   Oncocytosis
   Sialadenosis
   Necrotizing sialometaplasia
   Lymphoepithelial lesion
   Sialocysts
   Mucocele and ranula

Unclassified or indeterminate
   Embryoma (sialoblastoma)
   Osteoclast-like giant cell tumor

arises *within* a pre-existing benign mixed tumor—a carcinoma *ex* mixed tumor. Here, the carcinoma usually develops after many years or may develop after several recurrences of inadequately treated benign mixed tumor. In such instances, only the carcinomatous component will metastasize. Most commonly, the cancer is a poorly defined type of ductal adenocarcinoma. This particular form of cancer must be separated from the true malignant mixed tumor, which is truly a biphasic malignancy or carcinosarcoma. The true malignant mixed tumor is an extremely rare neoplasm with dim prognostic features.

MAJOR SALIVARY GLAND NEOPLASIA

Incidence

Among the various sites of salivary gland tumors, the parotid gland is by far the most common. In a large study of more than 2,500 tumors in the parotid, submandibular, and palatal glands, Eneroth[24] found that 85.8 percent were located in the parotid gland, while 6 percent and 7 percent were in the submandibular gland and palatal glands, respectively. These figures are similar to those of smaller series.[22,25,26]

In the parotid gland, as in all other major salivary glands, the benign mixed tumor predominates.[21,27–29] In the parotid, it is diagnosed in 25 to 27 percent of cases, whereas in the submandibular gland, it is diagnosed in 37 to 60 percent. In the parotid, the superficial lobe is the site most often involved, especially the tail or the infra-auricular region, while parapharyngeal or deep lobe extension accounts for approximately 10 percent of parotid tumors. Deep presentations of surface tumors may be related to herniation of the tumor laterally through the stylomandibular tunnel with the tumor assuming a dumbbell shape. In a large series of deep lobe parotid tumors, the mixed tumor accounted for 74 percent of all diagnoses, while mucoepidermoid carcinoma, acinic cell carcinoma, and adenoid cystic carcinoma accounted for 8 percent, 4 percent, and 1 percent, respectively.

Of interest when comparing malignant epithelial tumors in parotid and submandibular glands is the much higher incidence of adenoid cystic carcinoma in the submandibular gland; in the intraoral minor salivary glands this relationship is magnified still further. Eneroth[24] noted twice the incidence of malignant tumors in the submandibular gland when compared with the parotid gland, although the relative incidence of malignancy was even higher in minor glands of the palate.

As noted previously, the parotid gland is the principal major salivary gland involved by neoplasia. Much of the data presented in subsequent pages relate to tumors of the parotid gland, since experience and the literature have been concentrated on parotid tumors as being prototypes. There are, however, apparently significant biologic differences between similar tumors in the submandibular and sublingual glands and the parotid. The following section addresses these differences.

TUMORS OF THE SUBMANDIBULAR AND SUBLINGUAL GLANDS

A mass in the region of the submandibular gland is most often a result of a benign inflammatory disorder and most likely is related to obstruction of the duct system of the gland. The typical history of intermittent swelling and pain after eating can usually be elicited.

Of all salivary gland neoplasms, those of the submandibular gland account for about 10 percent, whereas 80 percent involve the parotid gland. There is, however, a higher incidence of malignancy in the former. In the event of a submandibular gland neoplasm, the chances are nearly 50 percent that the lesion will be malignant. Table 23-3 amplifies this predilection in 778 epithelial neoplasms of the submandibular gland, where 46.5 percent are histologically malignant.[30–38]

Neoplasms of the submandibular gland are usually painless masses. Advent of pain follows local extension and is most often a late symptom. Preoperative motor nerve paralysis is highly indicative of submandibular malignancy but it is uncommon. This is attributable to the lack of a direct relationship between the gland and adjacent motor nerves. The inferior surface of the superficial part of the gland is related to the cervical branch of the facial nerve and the medial surface to the glossopharyngeal nerve, the lingual nerve, the hypoglossal nerve, and the submandibular ganglion. The deep portion of the gland is related to the lingual nerve above and the hypoglossal nerve below.

Benign neoplasms occur more often in women and malignant tumors in men. The peak age incidence also differs by a decade; the fifth decade for benign tumors, sixth for malignant.

TABLE 23-3. Primary Epithelial Neoplasms of the Submandibular Gland

Classification	No. of Cases	Percentage of Total
Mixed tumor	416	53.5
Adenoid cystic carcinoma	142	18.3
Mucoepidermoid carcinoma	61	7.8
Carcinoma ex pleomorphic adenoma	42	5.4
Squamous cell carcinoma	38	4.9
Adenocarcinoma	36	4.6
Poorly or undifferentiated carcinoma	33	4.2
Warthin's tumor	4	0.5
Acinous cell carcinoma	3	0.4
Oncocytoma	3	0.4
	778	100

Morbidity, except for recurrence, with benign mixed tumors is unusual. A definitive incidence of recurrence is elusive. Spiro et al.[30] record a 2.2 percent rate after surgical treatment that ranged from enucleation to complete removal of the gland. As judged by an absence of recurrence in 37 patients treated by total excision of the gland by Trail and Lubritz[38] that is the treatment of choice.

For malignant tumors, recurrences are almost axiomatic and for adenoid cystic carcinomas have ranged from 35 to 85 percent.[30] Other malignant variants follow essentially the same pattern. Taking stage only as a consideration, Stage I and II carcinomas of the submandibular gland have a recurrence rate of 4:1 over carcinomas of similar stage in the parotid gland. Furthermore, stage-by-stage comparison of histologic types of carcinomas of both major salivary glands clearly points to a more accelerated biological aggressiveness and lethality of those of the submandibular gland. Only low-grade carcinoma—acinous cell, low-grade adenocarcinoma and mucoepidermoid carcinomas—do not share this ominous behavior. Unfortunately, all three types represent a distinct minority of the carcinomas in the submandibular gland.

Therapeutic failures are attributable to uncontrolled local disease, involvement of regional lymph nodes, and distant metastases. Extension of the primary tumor may be in any direction. The platysma, skin, and mandible are invaded by anterior or superficial growth. The anterior belly of the digastric muscle and the mylohyoid muscle are involved by posterior or deep infiltration. From these points, the neoplasm gains access to the floor of the mouth. Inferior extension leads to invasion of the wall of the pharynx. Invasion of adjacent nerves may be found with any of the high-grade carcinomas but is most prevalent in adenoid cystic carcinomas.

The submandibular gland is supplied with a fairly rich lymphatic capillary network, which lies in the interstitial spaces. Lymph flow is toward the capsule, and four collecting pathways are usually present. From the lateral and superior portions of the gland, flow is to the prevascular or preglandular submandibular nodes. The posterior part of the gland's lymphatic drainage is directly to the anterior subdigastric nodes of the internal jugular chain.

Lymphatic spread to regional lymph nodes from a salivary gland carcinoma of the submandibular gland is quite high, even for adenoid cystic carcinoma, a neoplasm not particularly noted for such an occurrence. Bardwil et al.[27] record an overall incidence of 46 percent and point out that the rate is *three times* that for tumors of the same histologic type in the parotid gland. Thirty-seven of 121 (30 percent patients studied by Spiro et al.[30]) manifested histologically proven metastases to regional lymph nodes. Squamous cell and high-grade glandular carcinomas (adenocarcinoma, mucoepidermoid and anaplastic) manifest the highest individual rates. While there is not a direct correlation, carcinomas with histologic evidence of nerve invasion are more likely to have nodal metastases.

The incidence of distant metastases from carcinoma of the submandibular gland also exceeds that for the parotid gland.[39] Spiro et al.[30] record an overall incidence of 39 percent and indicate their belief that this is an underestimate. Table 23-4 presents their data according to histologic type. On a subjective basis, it would appear that neoplasms with a prolonged course and persistent local disease exhibit the highest incidence of distant spread. Conversely, carcinomas such as squamous cell carcinomas declare their lethality earlier, and lymph node metastasis rather than distant dissemination is the usual event.

The factors leading to a more malignant behavior for carcinomas of the submandibular gland are translated into low cure rates and low survivals. Hanna and Clairmont[35] claim a 28 percent 5 year survival rate for patients with submandibular gland carcinoma, whereas those with carcinoma of the parotid had a 72 percent 5 year survival rate. Spiro et al.[30] offer comparable data; 5 and 10 year cure rates of 32 percent and 24 percent for submandibular primaries and 62 percent and 54 percent for parotid carcinomas.

Neoplasms of the smallest of the major salivary glands—the sublingual—comprise only 0.5 to 1 percent of all epithelial tumors arising in these glands. The observed inverse relationship between size of gland and malignancy is dramatically emphasized for neoplasms of sublingual gland origin. A fairly accurate assessment of the relative incidence of malignancy is: parotid gland, 20 percent, submandibular gland, 50 percent; and sublingual gland, 80 percent. Most of the carcinomas are mucoepidermoid. Adenoid cystic carcinomas follow closely.[39]

TABLE 23-4. Submandibular Gland Carcinoma: Distant Metastases

Histologic Type	Percentage with Distant Metastases
Adenoid cystic	57
Adenocarcinoma	50
Carcinoma ex pleomorphic adenoma	48
Undifferentiated	33
High-grade and intermediate-grade mucoepidermoid	21
Squamous cell carcinoma	0
All other forms	0

MONOMORPHIC ADENOMA

Separation of the monomorphic adenoma group from the benign mixed tumor was done by Kleinsasser and Klein[22] in 1967. Several reports since this original description have established the histologic heterogeneity within this group of neoplasms with the elaboration of classification schemes based on this histologic variation (Table 23-5).[40–42] We must consider that the term *monomorphic* does not necessarily equate with unicellularity. Indeed, even at the light microscopic level, a degree of cellular heterogeneity may be evident. This is supported by our own unpublished ultrastructural observations as well as those of others.[41] The multiplicity of cell types is further emphasized by demonstration of histochemically dissimilar mucosubstances comparable with those of myoepithelial and ductal cell origin.[41] A more detailed explanation of the cells of origin in monomorphic adenomas and histogenetic concepts as well as their possible role in hamartomatous relationships has been offered by Batsakis and Brannon.[41]

The basaloid type of monomorphic adenomas comprises the most common type within this group, accounting for approximately 54 percent of all monomorphic adenomas in our series.[42] Except in rare instances, the parotid gland is the most common site of involvement, with slow growth rate and evolution over several years.[43] While of a low order, multifocality is more common in this group of neoplasms than in mixed tumors, which exhibit multifocal origin in less than 0.5 percent.[42]

Of the basaloid adenomas, the trabecular-tubular form (Fig. 23-2) is the most common; the solid type is of intermediate occurrence; and the canalicular form is the least

TABLE 23-5. Histogenic Classification of Monomorphic Adenomas

Terminal duct origin
  Basal cell or basaloid adenoma
    Solid
    Trabecular-tubular
    Canalicular
  Membranous adenoma
    Dermal analogue tumors
  Clear cell (nonmucinous) adenoma
  Salivary duct adenoma

Terminal or striated duct origin
  Apocrine
    Sebaceous lymphadenoma
    Sebaceous adenoma

Striated duct origin
  Cystadenolymphoma
  Oncocytoma

Proximal duct origin
  Mucinous adenoma
  Epidermoid papillary adenoma

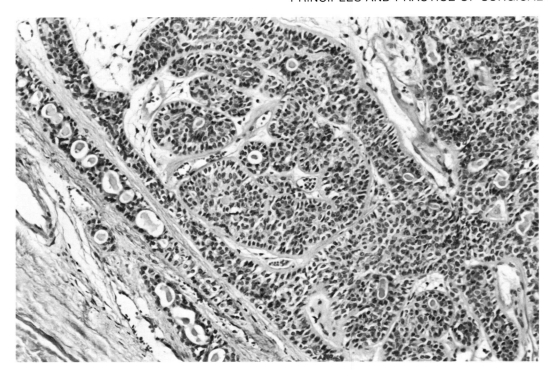

Fig. 23-2. Monomorphic adenoma of tubular-trabecular type.

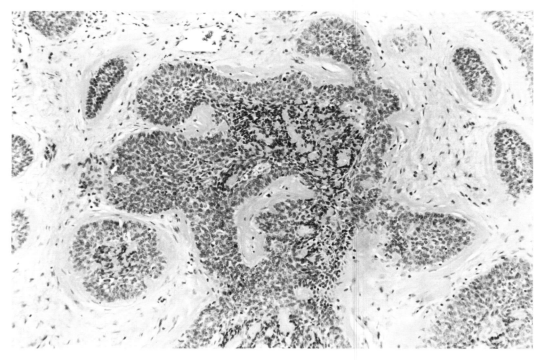

Fig. 23-3. Monomorphic adenoma, dermal analogue type. The abundant interepithelial basement membrane material, growth pattern, and cells are reminiscent of the dermal cylindroma.

common in the major salivary glands. Adenomas with an excessive amount of hyaline, eosinophilic, basal lamina material may be classified as membranous adenomas.[41–44] These variants have a relatively high incidence of multifocality and the least orderly appearance. Distribution of the hyaline material is around vascular channels within the tumor, at the tumor-stromal interface among epithelial cells as droplets and as large coalescent masses that displace the epithelial cells. The membranous adenoma (Fig. 23-3) bears a strong resemblance to the dermal eccrine cylindroma, leading to the consideration of this form as a dermal analogue tumor.[41–44] There appears to be a conceptual, clinical and pathologic link between the dermal cylindroma and the membranous form of basaloid adenoma vis-à-vis the cutaneous basal or germinative layer and the terminal duct or intercalated duct reserve cell system.[41–44] Indeed, it is proposed that in cases of salivary gland-skin tumor diathesis, a single pleiotropic gene may be acting on stem cells that are of similar ontogenic origin.[44]

Further insight into the overall character of the entire group of monomorphic adenomas may be gained by considering the trabecular-tubular form. While exhibiting the greatest degree of structural orderliness within the overall group of basaloid adenomas, they also demonstrate the most interepithelial stroma. This stroma does not manifest those featues or characteristics of the mixed tumor. This observation may serve as the initial thought in considering potential relationship between monomorphic and pleomorphic adenomas. Other considerations involve the so-called hybrid form of basal cell adenoma, which implies coexistence and blending of monomorphic

adenoma with another benign (usually mixed tumor) or more rarely malignant lesion (adenoid cystic carcinoma).[45] The premise to be tested is that certain monomorphic adenomas may merely represent transitions or stages in development of a mixed tumor or pleomorphic adenoma. To our mind, most monomorphic adenomas possess sufficient structural singularity that such transitions would be difficult to reconcile. Only duct adenomas and certain basaloid adenomas seem to provide the basis for formulating such hypothesis. In time, clarification of the myoepithelial cell's participatory role in both monomorphic and pleomorphic adenomas may help answer the question.

Clean, extirpative surgical excision is usually curative for monomorphic adenomas. Recurrence, or more aptly persistence, is the result of multifocal origin in some of the monomorphic adenomas and absence of a capsule.

Earlier we alluded to the salivary-cutaneous syndrome, in which patients have synchronous or metachronous cutaneous adnexal tumors and seemingly analogous major salivary gland tumors, particularly in the parotid gland. The dermal analogue salivary tumors[41] not only have a considerably higher recurrence rate than that of other monomorphic adenomas, they are also more often progenitors of carcinomas—carcinomas *ex* monomorphic adenomas. Table 23-6, prepared from a review of the literature and the addition of cases from the University of Texas M. D. Anderson Cancer Center, is illustrative of these events. Nine of the 11 carcinomas *ex* monomorphic adenomas arose in dermal analogue parotid adenomas. Their clinical behavior is primarily one of local aggressiveness. Regional and distant metastases are rare.

TABLE 23-6. Monomorphic Adenomas and Carcinomas ex Monomorphic Adenomas

Clinicopathologic Features	Monomorphic Adenomas (Exclusive of Dermal Analogue Adenomas)	Dermal Analogue Monomorphic Adenomas	Carcinomas ex Monomorphic Adenomas
Number of patients	222	24	11
Sex of patients (Male/Female ratio)	1.2 : 1	5 : 1	1.5 : 1
Age of patients at diagnosis (years)	0–83 ($\bar{m}$ 58.2)	34–81 ($\bar{m}$ 58.6)	55–79 ($\bar{m}$ 68.3)
Number of patients with dermal appendage tumors	0	9 (37.5%)	2 (18.1%)
Salivary gland site			
Parotid	123	24	9
Minor salivary glands	102	2	1
Submandibular	6	2	1
Not designated	3	0	0
Multicentric primary neoplasms	6 (2.8%)	12 (50.0%)	7 (63.3%)
Size of primary neoplasm (cm)	1.2–8 ($\bar{m}$ 2.4)	1.5–5 ($\bar{m}$ 3.5)	3–14 ($\bar{m}$ 5)
Number of patients with recurrences	2 (0.8%)	6 (27.8%)	6 (54.5%)

Abbreviation: $\bar{m}$, mean.

BENIGN MIXED TUMOR (PLEOMORPHIC ADENOMA)

The most common of all salivary gland tumors of minor or major gland origin is the benign mixed tumor or pleomorphic adenoma. Rauch[46] found that among 4,245 cases of mixed tumor 85 percent were located within the parotid gland, while the submandibular gland and minor salivary glands of the oral cavity and sinonasal tract accounted for 8 percent and 6.5 percent respectively. Similarly, Foote and Frazell[21] noted that within the major glands, 90 percent of the mixed tumors were located within the parotid. Mixed tumors arising in the upper lip are more common than those in the lower lip—a trait that holds true for all salivary gland pathologic conditions with the exception of the extravasation type of mucocele.

From a clinical standpoint, the growth of mixed tumors is very slow. If untreated for long periods of time or after periods of relative quiescence, there may be sudden enlargement. In certain cases, an initial early perceptible growth phase may be followed by a rather torpid or even static pattern of development. In the parotid gland, the mixed tumor is usually a nontender and painless mass present below or anterior to the ear in close relation to the angle of the mandible. When found in the cheek, its location may range from the tragus of the ear to nearly the commissure of the mouth, but always below the level of the zygoma. Those lying between the posterior border of the mandible and mastoid tip may be grooved by the ramus. Mixed tumors in the tail of the parotid may be a few centimeters below the mandibular angle and anterior to the sternomastoid muscle.

Deep lobe tumors of the parotid gland are 10 times less common than superficial lobe lesions.[47] Mixed tumors arising within this deep lobe or medial pharyngeal extension of the gland may manifest as a parapharyngeal mass displacing the tonsil and faucial pillars medially. Access to this potential space is by way of the stylomandibular tunnel, which is formed by the base of the skull above, by the posterior border of the mandible and medial pterygoid muscle anteriorly, and by the styloid process and stylomandibular ligament posteriorly. Pressure on the superior pharyngeal constrictor muscle may produce pain, dysphagia, and dysphonia. These symptoms along with a parapharyngeal mass could lead to an erroneous diagnosis of peritonsillar abscess. The overall shape of tumors growing in this manner is that of a dumbbell.

A large variation in size is noted for mixed tumors. While some may be a few millimeters to a few centimeters in diameter, a few attain gigantic proportions and produce a great deal of disfigurement.

The overall surface topography can vary from nodular to lobular, whereas the outline is usually clearcut and distinct (Fig. 23-4). The primary mixed tumor is solitary;

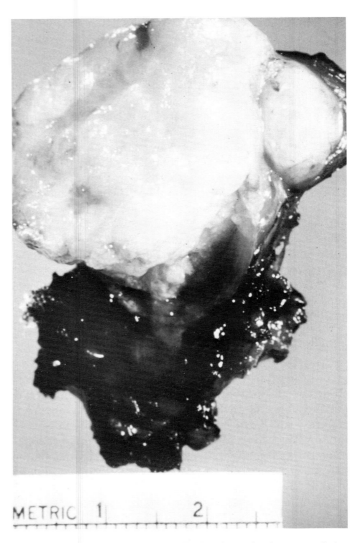

Fig. 23-4. Gross appearance of a benign mixed tumor of the parotid gland.

multinodularity is the gross pathologic hallmark of a recurrent lesion.

While the term *capsule* is used in describing marginal features at the gross level, this so-called capsule is often incomplete and of variable density and thickness. Regardless of the presence or lack of this capsule, the tumor is always clearly demarcated. Actual infiltration of the capsular structure does appear, however, to play a prognostic role.[48] On examination of serial sections of the capsular-tumor interface, it may be noted that apparent satellite nodules at variable distances from the main tumor mass are actually outgrowths or pseudopods of this mass in a tangential plane to the surface.

Mixed tumors are generally firm to hard or cartilaginous. Small tumors (those up to a few centimeters in size) are quite mobile, whereas larger lesions of the parotid are less movable and have a more lobular, bosselated surface. In the case of deep lobe or parapharyngeal tumors, a degree of fixation may be noted, since anatomic confines and overlying structures tend to limit mobility.

Establishing the diagnosis of mixed tumor relies on the demonstration of epithelial and mesenchymal components (Fig. 23-5). In most instances, this is not difficult. On occasion, the differential diagnosis may include a monomorphic adenoma or, even more rarely, an adenoid cystic carcinoma. Mixed tumors may exhibit considerable histologic variation; one third of tumors manifest epithelial and mesenchymal components in equal proportions, whereas 12 percent are extremely cellular and 22 percent are predominantly epithelial.[49] In an attempt to correlate histologic features with behavioral patterns, VandenBerg et al.[26] noted that mixed tumors composed solely or predominantly of epithelial elements actually had a better prognosis than those that were less cellular. This has been confirmed in later studies where higher rates of recurrence in mixed tumors were associated with less cellular lesions containing chondroid, myxoid and chondromyxoid background stromal features (Fig. 23-6).

Related to if not directly responsible for the structural complexity and diversity of the mixed tumor group of neoplasms is the role of the myoepithelial cell.[13,50,51] This cell (Fig. 23-7) assumes a facultative as well as a modulating role in its relation to elements of ductal reserve cell

origin. The myoepithelial cell, in its numerous interactions, is believed responsible for production of mesenchymal mucin, chondroid material, bone, and cartilage. Our own ultrastructural studies indicate that mixed tumors contain cells of ductal and myoepithelial character, with precursor cells and transitional forms also present. Many forms of the myoepithelial cell can be noted to differentiate along stromal or mesenchymal tissue lines to form fibroblasts, osteoblasts, and chondroblasts.[52,53] The ratio and relation between ductal and myoepithelial elements, as well as the degree of stromal metaplasia by the latter, contribute to structural variation and diversity from one lesion to another as well as within individual lesions. Confirmation of the significant role played by the myoepithelial cell in the formation of this tumor has been accomplished by ultrastructural and immunohistochemical methods. It is the myoepithelial cell that appears to modulate the tumor's morphologic appearance, its intermediate filament composition and the capacity to produce large amounts of matrix substances.[13,51]

Studies by Takeguchi et al.[52] defined two types of mixed tumor. In the myoepithelial cell-rich variant there is a great deal of mucin production with chondroitin 6 and 4 sulfates as well as heparin sulfate. A second type of tumor is predominantly epithelial. Tumors with composite features also occur.

Reports of salivary gland tumors composed totally or

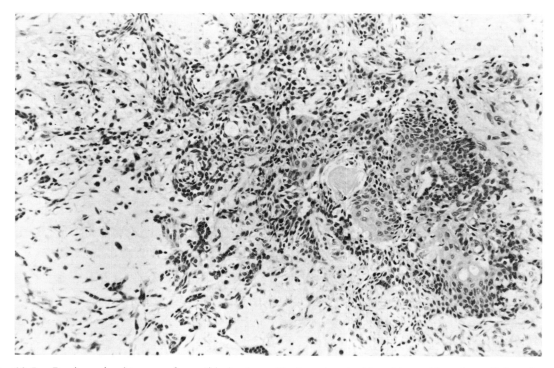

Fig. 23-5. Benign mixed tumor of parotid gland manifesting chondroid, epidermoid, and small ductal components.

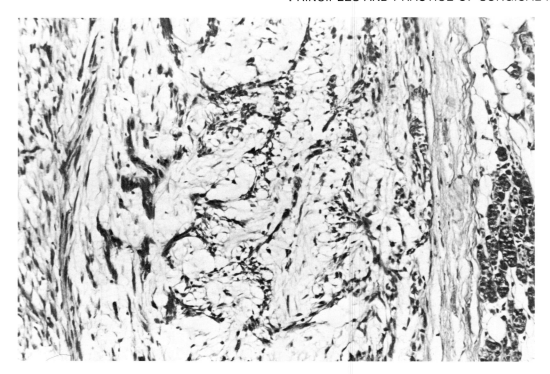

Fig. 23-6. Mixed tumor with thin capsule and a prominent myxoid composition.

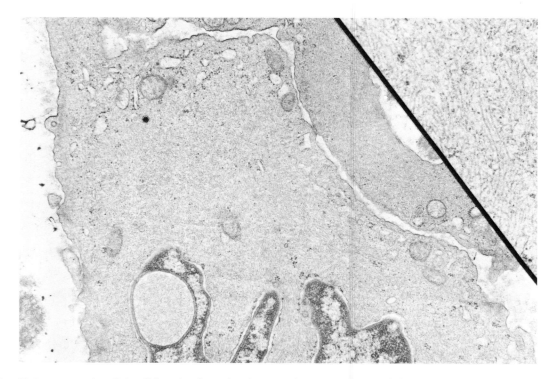

Fig. 23-7. Myoepithelial cell in a benign mixed tumor demonstrating a minimal flocculent basement membrane-like material at the cell border. An occasional pinocytotic vesicle is present. Dense aggregates of myofilaments fill the cytoplasm (inset shows filament detail). (×24,000; inset ×80,000.)

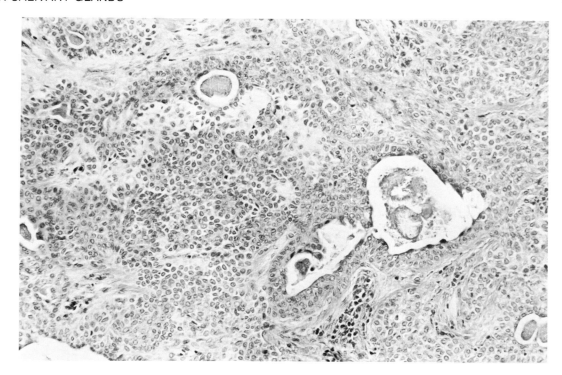

Fig. 23-8. Plasmacytoid (hyaline) cells in a mixed tumor of the parotid gland.

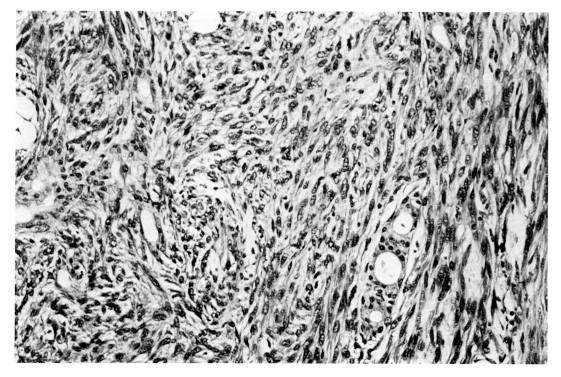

Fig. 23-9. Spindle cells of myoepithelial derivation outnumber ductal epithelial elements in this myoepithe-liomatous mixed tumor.

almost completely of myoepithelial cells have been published.[16] These cells may assume a plasmacytoid appearance (Fig. 23-8) as in these three reports, or as in Luna's case, a spindle cell (Fig. 23-9) outline may be present.[54] Support for the myoepithelial derivation of the plasmacytoid cell derives from a study which termed these cells hyaline cells.[55]

Most recurrent mixed tumors seem to occur within the surgical scar or closely associated with it. They are usually multiple and widely distributed and separate from each other within the area of primary surgery. Nodules will vary in size, some being minute.

Most recurrences grow at the same rate as the primary lesions, with most appearing between two to seven years after initial treatment. Current surgical management of major gland mixed tumors by removal of at least the gland in cases of submandibular gland involvement or lateral lobectomy in instances of parotid gland disease has produced low rates of recurrence. At one institution this approach has led to a decrease in recurrences from 8 to 2 percent,[24] while in another a 0 percent recurrence rate has resulted.[25]

Two distinct mixed tumors—the true malignant mixed tumor and carcinoma arising within a previously benign mixed tumor, the carcinoma *ex* mixed tumor—are discussed later in the section on malignant mixed tumors.

WARTHIN'S TUMOR (PAPILLARY CYSTADENOMA LYMPHOMATOSUM, ADENOLYMPHOMA)

Warthin's tumor is the most common oncocytic tumor in the parotid gland and is the second most common benign salivary gland tumor. It is almost always located in the parotid gland and preferentially in the gland's inferior portion.

In the parotid gland, this lesion appears as a soft, sometimes fluctuant or cystic mass that is painless and smooth with a slow uniform growth rate. It may reach 4 to 5 cm in size before growth ceases. Most cases are found in men, especially in the fifth and sixth decades of life. Of interest is the occurrence of bilateral lesions as well as unilateral multifocal lesions. In the review by Kavka[56] 21 examples of bilaterality and 4 cases of bilateral simultaneous occurrence were noted. As emphasized by Batsakis,[57] the rare reports of Warthin's tumor arising in the submandibular gland can be accounted for by the close proximity of this gland to the tail of the parotid gland. Oncocytic lesions are not restricted to the parotid gland and can occur in any salivary tissue. In these instances, however, the unique bicellular (oncocytes and lymphoid tissue) composition of Warthin's tumor is lacking.[57]

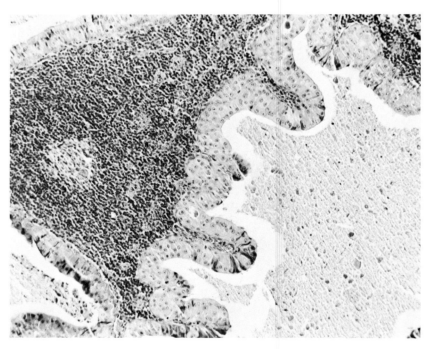

Fig. 23-10. Warthin's tumor. Two tissues comprise this tumor: lymphoid and oncocytic ductal cells.

In the parotid, the most acceptable theory of origin is related to the developmental sequence and interrelationship between parenchymal elements and lymphoid tissue.[58] The lack of a definitive capsule and the overall loose arrangement of glandular tissue and subsequent entrapment of lymph nodes early in development is the initial series of events. This is followed by relatively late encapsulation, which permits ductal and acinar elements to be intermixed within extraoral intraglandular lymph nodes. Within this overall context, a transition from normal ductal epithelium to tumor epithelium has been noted. While the epithelial component is clearly oncocytic, there appears to be variation in the overall state of epithelial differentiation and in the ratio of the oncocytic and lymphoid components. Using the above-mentioned criteria, Seifert et al.[59] have noted four subtypes of such lesions, with 90 percent of cases being composed of tumors that were at least 50 percent epithelial.

Microscopically, the epithelial/oncocytic component forms a double layer—an inner or basal cuboidal one and an outer or peripheral columnar layer (Fig. 23-10). Nuclear features of the former are essentially vesicular, whereas the nuclei of the outer cell layer are luminally oriented and more pyknotic. Other epithelial cell types such as goblet, sebaceous, and squamous cells may also be noted. The associated lymphoid tissue is benign but may manifest varying degrees of reactivity and plasma cell participation.

Surgical excision is the treatment of choice, and it is generally considered that given adequate removal, recurrences are few. Multicentric origin, however, can defeat too conservative an excision. In rare instances, malignancy can arise from either the epithelial or lymphoid components of the tumor.

ONCOCYTOMA AND ONCOCYTIC LESIONS

The oncocytoma accounts for 0.1–1 percent of all salivary gland neoplasms.[60] While almost all oncocytomas are benign lesions with a predictable behavior pattern, on rare occasions malignant forms may be encountered. Oncocytes are characterized by a large size with acidophilic densely packed cytoplasmic granules (Fig. 23-11). Ultrastructural studies have identified dense arrays of abnormally formed mitochondria as being the source of the acidophilic granularity at the light microscopic level.[61,62] This level of examination may be necessary to characterize cytoplasmic granularity in certain instances to rule out the presence of lysosomal granules, excessive proliferation of smooth endoplasmic reticulum, or secretory granules (Fig. 23-12).

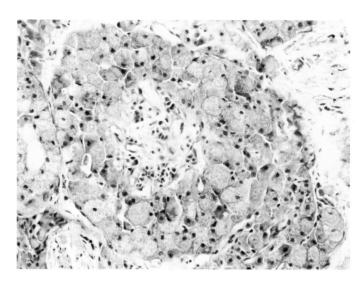

Fig. 23-11. Enlarged, eosinophilic granular cells (oncocytes) in a parotid gland oncocytoma.

The actual origin and behavioral-functional pattern of the oncocyte is somewhat unclear, although most investigators would agree that the cell arises as a somatic mutation. Their presence in salivary gland parenchymal and ductal components is unusual before the fifth or sixth decade of life, whereas they are nearly universal in patients over 70 years of age. In adult or mature salivary tissue, the true oncocyte should possess a high degree of mitochondrial oxidative activity and large numbers of mitochondria that are enlarged, pleomorphic, or structurally abnormal. The functional significance of such oxidative capacity is unknown. When considering the fact that the volume fraction occupied by mitochondria approaches 60 percent of the cytoplasm in conjunction with the intact oxidative metabolic pathways, the question of function becomes intriguing.[63]

In addition to its presentation as non-neoplastic oncocytic foci or multinodular oncocytosis accompanying aging, the oncocyte may be found in association with distinctive salivary tumors such as the mixed tumor, adenoid cystic carcinoma, and mucoepidermoid carcinoma.

We consider solid oncocytic nodules to be neoplastic (oncocytoma). These are treated by parotidectomy. Recurrences after such a procedure are unusual. If recurrence is noted, however, it usually occurs within 5 years after the initial surgical procedure.

Malignant tumors of oncocytic origin (malignant oncocytoma) are rare. Johns et al.[61] accepted only 11 cases reported as of 1977. Attempts at defining cytologic criteria for malignancy within the oncocytic group of neo-

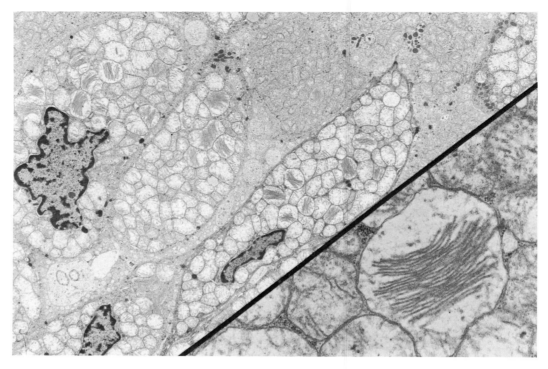

Fig. 23-12. Oncocytes with numerous abnormally shaped mitochondria. Inset presents detail of an abnormal mitochondrion with stacks of centrally placed cristae. (×6,000; inset ×30,000.)

plasms have not been successful.[64] Features such as local extension, local recurrence, and focal cellular pleomorphism, while implying local aggressiveness, do not necessarily imply malignancy.

ADENOID CYSTIC CARCINOMA

In the parotid gland adenoid cystic carcinoma accounts for less than 4 percent of all neoplasms, whereas in the submandibular gland it accounts for 10 percent. Of interest is the much higher incidence within the minor salivary glands, where this lesion is the most commonly diagnosed malignancy. Of adenoid cystic carcinomas of the head and neck region, the minor salivary glands account for 58 to 70 percent of all reported cases.[65–67]

The overall growth rate is rather slow, and the clinical appearance is that of a firm, usually unilobular mass generally measuring 2 to 4 cm in diameter at the time of diagnosis. An indication as to the overall aggressive nature of this neoplasm is the early invasion of the facial nerve, with facial nerve paralysis noted in 4 percent of cases as an initial finding. Furthermore, 18 percent of the patients have been reported to have pain as a symptom when first seen.[66] These clinical findings have been attributed to perineural invasion, a frequent histologic finding.

Intercalated or terminal duct elements are thought to give rise to this tumor. Ultrastructural and immunochemical studies have demonstrated that the state of cellular differentiation parallels that of the developing intercalated duct cell.[14,68]

It has also become clear that the so-called cystic spaces are not glandular lumina but rather pseudocysts (Fig. 23-13) that contain replicated, multilayered basal lamina material.[68] Similar, if not identical, material may be found at the stromal-tumor cell interface of some forms of this tumor, producing a characteristic cribriform or cylindromatous appearance.

Cribriform and so-called cylindromatous growth patterns characterize the standard or well accepted light microscopic patterns of adenoid cystic carcinoma (Fig. 23-14). Tubular forms are less common (Fig. 23-15) whereas the solid-basaloid form represents the least commonly encountered variant. Distinction among these histologic variants is probably of little value in terms of overall behavioral prediction. More important factors include the size of the primary lesion, its anatomic location, the presence or absence of metastasis and facial nerve involvement, and the results of surgical treatment regarding margins. The view of Perzin et al.[61] is in essential agreement with this philosophy, although they state that the solid or basaloid type is associated with the worst overall prognosis. Eby et al.[69] point to the finding of areas

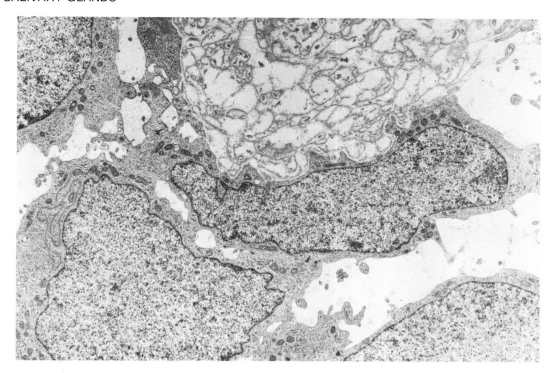

Fig. 23-13. Pseudocystic space (top) in an adenoid cystic carcinoma of the parotid gland. Such spaces may dominate the light microscopic appearance of this carcinoma. At the ultrastructural level, they contain replicated or multilayered basal lamina material. The absence of microvilli serves to distinguish this space from a true lumen. (×8,000.)

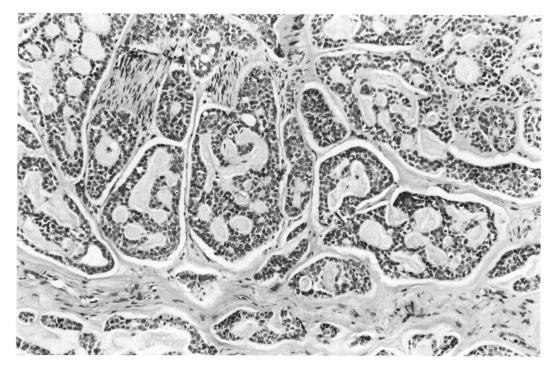

Fig. 23-14. Cribriform and cylindromatous type of adenoid cystic carcinoma of parotid gland. Note the invasion of nerves by this highly neurotropic carcinoma.

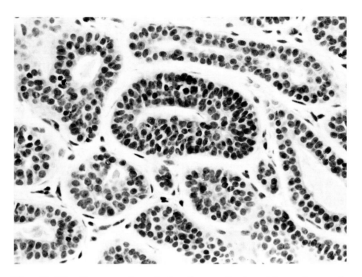

Fig. 23-15. Low-grade tubular form of adenoid cystic carcinoma.

of central necrosis within the solid clusters of cells as indicating a more aggressive, fulminant form of the disease with a correspondingly poor clinical outcome.

Cells comprising the tumor are small and isomorphic with disproportionately large nuclei. Little or no nuclear atypism or mitotic activity is present. Chromatin is arranged as dense aggregates, while the nuclear outline is even. These components are those of a basaloid cell with features of an intercalated duct precursor population.

Pseudocystic spaces, which many consider the morphologic hallmark of this neoplasm, have been found to contain a variety of mucosubstances on histochemical analysis. This material consists chiefly of sulfated mucopolysaccharides. This is in contrast to the mucins contained within tumor ducts or "true lumina," which react histochemically as neutral glycoproteins and sialomucins.[70]

Although details about treatment vary among institutions, the primary modality of therapy remains surgery. When this lesion involves the parotid gland a wide resection involving superficial parotidectomy or superficial and deep lobectomy is the treatment of choice. Some surgeons believe that the facial nerve should not be spared, while others recommend nerve resection only if tumor surrounds or invades the nerve.[1]

The increasing use of postoperative radiotherapy has improved overall survival rates of adenoid cystic carcinoma of the major salivary glands.[1,4]

Long-term survival in cases of adenoid cystic carcinoma must be viewed not at the 5 year mark but at 10 and even 20 years to obtain an accurate assessment of the insidious nature of this neoplasm, as well as of other

salivary cancers. Generally, survival rates are poor, as evidenced by the studies of Spiro et al.,[65] who noted only 10 percent determinate survival at 15 years.

Patterns of recurrence relate to local extension. Lymph node involvement may occur rarely via the embolic pathway and more often by direct extension.[71] Metastatic disease is more likely to occur as the result of a vascular or hematogenous process, most commonly to lung. Lung metastases have been said to outnumber those to the lymph nodes by a 3 : 1 margin. Spiro et al.[65] noted a 43 percent incidence of distant metastases.

A positive correlation has been reported between location of the tumor, clinical stage, duration of symptoms and histologic pattern of growth and overall prognosis.[72,73] A parotid gland location is associated with a better prognosis, as are limited stage (I and II), a less than one-year clinical presence, and a cribriform or tubular architecture (Fig. 23-15), as opposed to a solid pattern of growth.

MUCOEPIDERMOID CARCINOMA

We consider lesions categorized under the histologic designation *mucoepidermoid* to be carcinomas, albeit of varying lethality, and not simply tumors.[6,74] Of all malignant salivary gland tumors, the mucoepidermoid carcinoma is perhaps the most common, accounting for up to 9 percent of these lesions.

Clinical manifestation is related to the degree of infiltration and to the histologic quality or grade of the tumor, as well as to the stage or extent of the disease.[1,74] Low-grade carcinomas may often be indistinguishable from mixed tumors in the major salivary glands. As with the mixed tumor, they tend to be firm and lobulated when palpated and asymptomatic. The average duration of the lesion before diagnosis is just over six years. These tumors vary in size, but low-grade lesions rarely measure more than 3 cm. In contrast to low-grade lesions, in many instances the high-grade form clinically manifests fixation to adjacent tissues, pain, or paralysis of the facial nerve. In the palate, the high-grade forms often are ulcerated and may be associated with loosening of teeth secondary to invasion and destruction of underlying alveolar bone. Loosening of teeth was rarely noted, however, in Spiro's[74] comprehensive study of 367 cases of mucoepidermoid carcinoma. This series demonstrated that nearly all lesions of the maxillary sinus or nasal cavity were large, with marked bony destruction evident. Metastatic spread to lymph nodes occurred in 29 percent of patients, especially in cases involving the submandibular gland and in recurrences of high-grade lesions.

A dual population of cells is generally considered essential to the diagnosis of mucoepidermoid carcinoma,

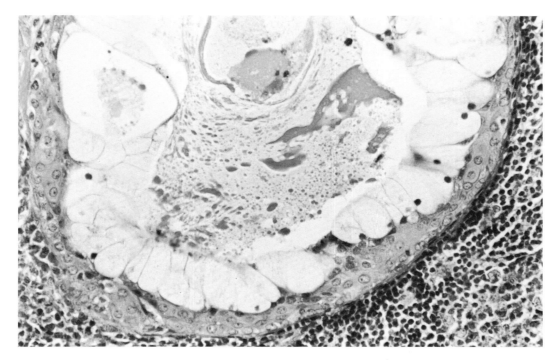

Fig. 23-16. Low-grade mucoepidermoid carcinoma exhibiting mucous cells and epidermoid cells arranged around a mucin-filled lumen.

that is, the mucous cell and the squamous or epidermoid cell.[75,76] In the low-grade lesion, these elements frequently are arranged around cystic spaces, which are often mucin-filled (Fig. 23-16). Lumen diameter of such cysts may be rather large at times, whereas less commonly microcystic features may predominate. Low-grade lesions are characterized by a predominance of well differentiated mucous cells, often with goblet cell features, as well as more cuboidal elements with vacuolated to eosinophilic cytoplasm. In lesions of this grade, the minority of the cell population is composed of squamous cells, while rare clear cells may be scattered within the squamous component. On occasion, clear cells may predominate, forming almost all the tumor and producing an appearance that may resemble a metastatic hypernephroma and must be distinguished from it. Both mucous and squamous elements within the low-grade tumor show little evidence of dysplasia or cellular pleomorphism.

A cell type that has been described as the intermediate cell has been postulated as a transitional form by Foote and Frazell.[21] These cells are free of mucin and lipid vacuoles as well as PAS-positive material within the cytoplasm. The designation of intermediate cell relates not to its morphologic properties but rather to its putative or potential ability to differentiate toward mucous or epidermoid cells and even clear cells.

Sikowara[75] identified several other cell types in the mucoepidermoid carcinoma. Within this system, the progenitor for all other cells is termed the maternal cell.

The histologically intermediate subgroup exhibits fewer cystic or gland-like spaces and greater cellularity when compared with the low-grade tumor. Much of the lesion is composed of squamous or epidermoid cells and intermediate cells; in addition, a proportional decrease in mucus-filled cysts and goblet or secretory cells is evident. A higher degree of cellular atypia and invasiveness is also present (Fig. 23-17).

A predominant squamous or epidermoid element characterizes the high-grade form. A considerable degree of cytologic atypia characterizes the epidermoid population of cells; mitotic activity and invasiveness are quite evident. Tumor cell aggregates form sheets and islands, which may be indistinguishable from squamous cell carcinoma. Easily identifiable mucous cells are rarely noted, although cellular mucin may be prominent (Fig. 23-18).

Treatment must be directed toward complete surgical removal since most authors consider this a lesion of low radiosensitivity.

Recurrence rates for mucoepidermoid carcinoma are rather high in most series.[76] Frazell[77] reported a range of 15 to 60 percent for low- and high-grade lesions. A 75 percent rate of recurrence was reported by Stevenson and Hazard,[78] whereas a 30 percent recurrence rate was

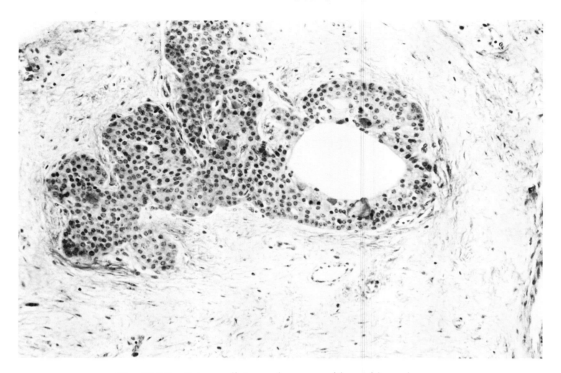

Fig. 23-17.   Intermediate-grade mucoepidermoid carcinoma.

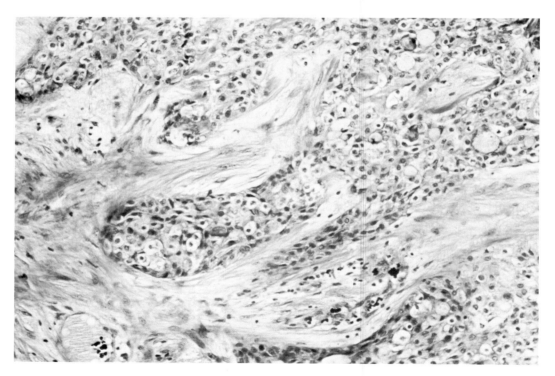

Fig. 23-18.   High-grade mucoepidermoid carcinoma. This is but one appearance of these high-grade forms. Others are more epidermoid or glandular.

noted by Batsakis[79] and Jakobsson.[80] In a study of 60 cases, Healey et al.[81] noted that recurrences were related to the degree of histologic differentiation and the presence or absence of tumor at the line of resection. When no tumor was evident at the surgical margin, the lesion recurred in only 1 of 31 cases, while in the 28 instances where tumor was present at margins, 19 recurrences developed. Recurrent lesions tend to retain their original cellular composition.[82] It should be noted, however, that metastases from mucoepidermoid carcinomas may be clonal, with only components of higher grade carcinoma identified.

ACINIC (ACINOUS) CELL CARCINOMA

Acinic cell carcinoma accounts for between 2.5 and 4 percent of all parotid gland tumors and ranks second only to Warthin's tumor in its frequency of bilateral parotid gland involvement—approximately 3 percent. It is rare in salivary tissues other than the parotid gland.[83,84]

Although characteristically seen in patients who are in the fifth decade of life, the acinic cell carcinoma can occur throughout life, and figures prominently in salivary gland malignant tumors of childhood. In children, only mucoepidermoid carcinomas are more common.

Acinic cell neoplasms are usually derived (by neoplastic differentiation of the cells responsible for normal acinar replenishment) from two cell sources: (1) the reserve cells of the terminal tubule, or (2) intercalated ducts.[85] Less commonly, these neoplasms may arise from more mature acinar cells. In the fullest expression of neoplastic development and differentiation, an acinic cell carcinoma will appear histologically as an enlarged caricature of a normal salivary lobule. In the acinic cell carcinoma manifesting the least differentiation, there is a striking resemblance to the early phases of embryonic development of the functional salivary unit.[5]

Between these two histomorphologic extremes, acinic cell neoplasms present a variety of histologic patterns (Figs. 23-19 and 23-20). Although a single pattern often dominates the microscopic appearance, admixtures occur. The growth patterns are categorized as solid, papillary-cystic, follicular, and microcystic. Of these growth patterns, the solid, lobular form is observed most frequently. The acinic cell carcinoma, perhaps more than any other salivary gland neoplasm except Warthin's tumor, may also be multifocal.[5] On occasion, this multifocal growth originates from entrapped salivary gland tissue in extraparotid or intraparotid lymph nodes; this distinctive histogenesis is also shared with Warthin's tumor. In general, nearly all the acinic cell carcinomas ap-

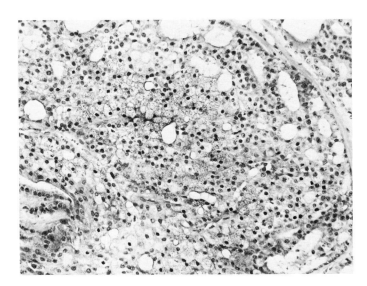

Fig. 23-19. Acinic cell carcinoma of parotid gland manifesting in its most typical form. Note the secretory granules. Microliths may be present.

pear circumscribed either by a condensation of stroma or by an apparent capsule. The latter is unusual in our experience. On the other hand, a solitary, macrocystic presentation of the neoplasm is not unusual.

The cells participating in the aforementioned growth patterns of the acinic cell carcinoma range from granulated serous-type cells to more primitive tubular cells or undifferentiated polymorphic cells. Predominance of one cell type is usual. Histochemical reactions are inconsistent and do not aid in the differential diagnosis.[85] Foci of undifferentiated cells can be found in these carcinomas.[86]

A lack of definable histologic criteria of malignancy in many acinic cell carcinomas is not justification for ignoring the biologic course of the neoplasms.[6] A determinate survival rate of 89 percent at 5 years and 56 percent after a 20 year follow-up period should remove doubt about the malignancy of this tumor.[87] Similar survival figures have been provided by others,[5,21,88] with local recurrence, metastasis, and death due to tumor reported in 30 percent, 14 percent, and 13 percent, respectively, of a total of 278 cases. Metastases occur to regional lymph nodes in approximately 10 percent of cases. Distant metastases (to lungs and bone) occur in approximately 15 percent of cases.

Attempts at predicting biologic course based on histomorphologic findings have not been fruitful.[6] This failure led Eneroth et al.[89] to evaluate the DNA content of the tumor cells. From their investigations, it is suggested that the DNA content of acinic cell carcinomas is equivalent to that of cells from a poorly differentiated adenocarcinoma. Furthermore, they pointed to a strong correlation

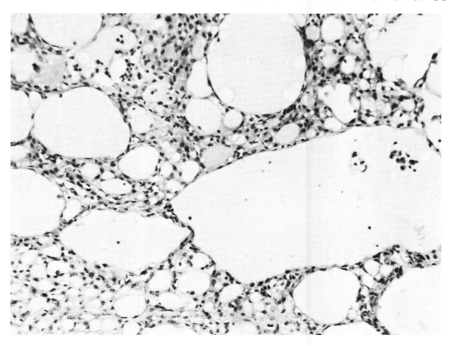

Fig. 23-20. Follicular type of acinic cell carcinoma.

between DNA content and the invasiveness of the carcinoma.

ADENOCARCINOMAS AND UNDIFFERENTIATED CARCINOMAS

Adenocarcinomas and undifferentiated carcinomas of the salivary glands are malignant epithelial neoplasms that do not fulfill histologic criteria allowing them to be placed in other categories of classification. The term adenocarcinoma is used in a specific sense since, generically, all carcinomas of the salivary glands are adenocarcinomas. As such, adenocarcinomas can arise from any portion of the salivary duct system. They may be muciparous or nonmuciparous carcinomas and may be solid or papillary (Fig. 23-21).

The true incidence of adenocarcinoma of the major salivary glands is difficult to define, but they probably do not constitute more than 3 percent of all major salivary gland tumors. Most originate from the larger intralobular ducts or excretory ducts.[90]

A rather distinctive form of adenocarcinoma has strong histologic similarities to ductal carcinomas of the breast, that is, intraductal papillary proliferation, mucoid variants, cribriform pattern, and occasionally areas like sclerosing adenosis (Fig. 23-22). Called *salivary duct carcinoma,* this form of adenocarcinoma is one of the most

lethal carcinomas of the major salivary glands.[91,92] It manifests a male predilection and is characterized by a high incidence of regional and distant metastases. Death occurs in two thirds of patients within 5 years. Table 23-7 compares this high-grade carcinoma with the terminal duct adenocarcinoma of the oral cavity. The contrast between carcinomas arising from the intercalated duct portion of the salivary duct unit (terminal duct adenocarci-

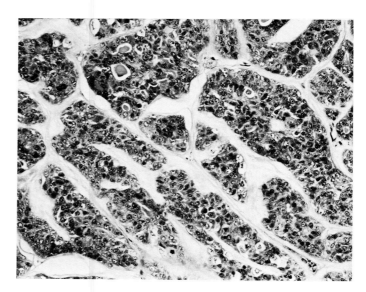

Fig. 23-21. Adenocarcinoma of parotid gland.

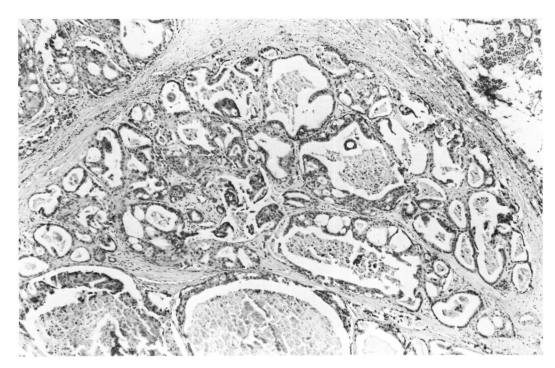

Fig. 23-22. Salivary duct carcinoma of the parotid gland. Note the cytoarchitectural similarity to ductal carcinomas of the breast.

noma) and the larger ducts (salivary duct carcinoma) is evident.[91–94]

An *undifferentiated carcinoma* of the major salivary glands is one whose light microscopic phenotypic expression does not allow it to be placed into other categories of classification.[95–97] The carcinoma is devoid of differentiation features and presents as islands, cords, or sheets of neoplastic epithelial cells, at times deceptively uniform, but with necrosis and a high mitotic index. Those with an associated lymphoid stroma are called lymphoepithelial carcinomas or undifferentiated carcinomas with lymphoid stroma.[98] These are somewhat more distinctive in

that they often manifest a close resemblance to undifferentiated carcinomas of nasopharyngeal type. This resemblance is further accentuated by a pathogenetic relation with Epstein-Barr virus.[99,100] No such relation is evident with other forms of undifferentiated carcinoma.

All of the undifferentiated carcinomas are high-grade malignant tumors. They are predominantly parotid gland in origin and have a clinical course marked by multiple recurrences and regional lymph node metastasis with distant spread. More than two thirds of patients are dead of their disease within 5 years.

A small number of apparently undifferentiated carcino-

TABLE 23-7. Terminal Duct Adenocarcinoma versus Salivary Duct Carcinoma

Clinicopathologic Features	Terminal Duct Adenocarcinoma	Salivary Duct Carcinoma
Number of patients	69	30
Sex	Female, 48; male, 21	Female, 7; male, 23
Mean age at diagnosis (years)	49 (23–79)	64 (27–83)
Salivary gland site	Palate 45, buccal mucosa 10, upper lip 7, retromolar 5, others 2	Parotid gland 25, sub-mandibular gland 5
Patients with recurrences	8 (12%)	20 (55%)
Patients with cervical lymph node metastases	7 (10%)	20 (66%)
Patients with distant metastases	0	20 (66%)
Patient deaths attributed to neoplasm	1 (10 yr)	21 (70%) (7 mo. to 3 yr)

mas exhibit electron microscopic and immunocytochemical evidence of neuroendocrine differentiation.[97] These features have no bearing on biologic course or response to therapy.

MALIGNANT MIXED TUMORS

In an historic sense, the early reports indicating frequent recurrence after inadequate surgical treatment of mixed tumors led to the supposition that all mixed tumors were of at least low-grade malignant potential. After a long period of quiescence, the inadequately treated tumors recurred, often in a multinodular pattern with a somewhat rapid growth rate. Also in an historic sense, we would like to call attention to the interchangeable use of the terms malignant mixed tumor and carcinoma *ex* mixed tumor. In reality, these are separate and distinct entities in terms of cell or tissue of origin, history, and histomorphology.

Of the two, the malignant mixed tumor is far less common,[101,102] to the point of being considered a rarity. The so-called true malignant mixed tumor exists in two forms: the histologically benign but inexplicably metastasizing mixed tumor and the heterologous carcinoma and sarcoma occurring simultaneously—that is, a carcinosarcoma. The former type will demonstrate areas of histologically benign mixed tumor at both the primary and metastatic sites. In all acceptable cases reported, the parotid gland has been the site of the primary tumor, and the age range has been from 16 to 48 years. The metastasis-free interval has ranged from 5 to 22 years. Of great interest is that while some investigators emphasize this particular form of malignant mixed tumor as more akin to a transplantation process than a metastatic one, others have demonstrated increased mitotic activity and infiltrative growth patterns, criteria that we suggest be adopted when the term malignancy is used. These structural criteria will help eliminate instances in which multiple benign recurrences and accidental dissemination or transplantation may have occurred. The second type of malignant mixed tumor, or heterologous malignancy, will demonstrate metastatic features of obvious carcinoma and sarcoma with overall resemblance to the primary tumor.

Carcinoma *ex* mixed tumor, the more common type of malignant mixed tumor, also has two distinct forms, although these distinctions are made more on clinical grounds than on morphologic ones. The more common form is usually found in patients approximately one to

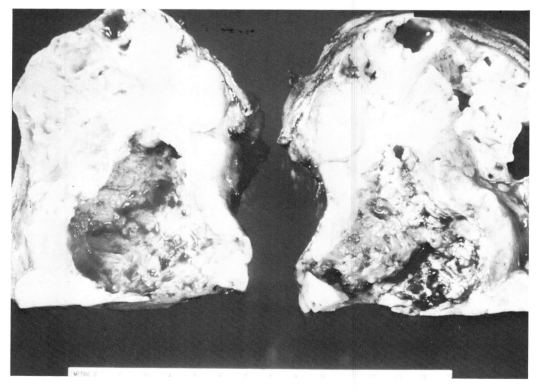

Fig. 23-23. Malignant transformation in a mixed tumor (carcinoma *ex* pleomorphic adenoma). The bosselation, cystic necrosis, and softening are gross indicators of such a malignant change.

two decades older than for benign mixed tumor (Fig. 23-23). In most cases, a previously untreated benign mixed tumor has existed for many years, or multiple recurrences of benign mixed tumor are noted within which malignant transformation has occurred. This biologic event is underscored when noting that benign mixed tumors of long duration (over 15 years) compared with those of short duration show a small proportion of tetraploid cells. The second clinical form of carcinoma *ex* mixed tumor is that which is diagnosed in a patient whose initial course was brief. In this type, the patient population tends to be 10 to 30 years younger than that with the more common form.

The incidence of carcinoma *ex* mixed tumor ranges from 1.5 to 6.5 percent of cases in the mixed tumor category.[103–105] The parotid gland is the most common site of origin, followed by the submandibular gland and minor salivary glands of the palate, lip, and paranasal sinuses.

Histomorphologic indications in an otherwise benign mixed tumor or pleomorphic adenoma that may lead away from a benign diagnosis include zones of necrosis with or without areas of dystrophic mineralization and infiltration of epithelial cords into a background supportive element that is usually well hyalinized. This latter feature has been emphasized by Boles et al.[104] as being an important feature to evaluate in such cases. Epithelial cells in these areas will demonstrate discrete cytologic features of malignancy, while solid lobular areas of epithelial cells and peripheral infiltrative destructive growth further identify the malignant features of this lesion (Figs. 23-24 and 23-25).

The malignant mixed tumor/carcinoma *ex* mixed tumor demonstrates one of the highest rates of distant metas-

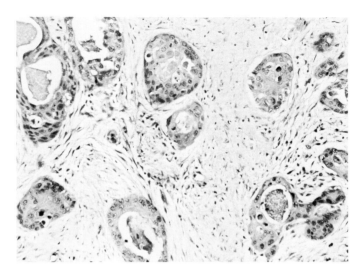

Fig. 23-25. Ductal adenocarcinoma arising in a mixed tumor. This is but one histologic expression of the epithelial malignancies found in carcinoma *ex* pleomorphic adenoma.

tases and recurrences and therefore a dismal prognosis. Local recurrences and distant metastasis are found in 38 to 71 percent of cases. Favored sites of metastasis indicate a preference for hematogenous spread, since distant spread occurs more frequently than local or regional lymph node metastases. Overall survival figures as reported by Spiro et al.[103] have been considered in terms of determinate cure rates. At 5, 10, and 15 year intervals these figures were 40 percent, 24 percent, and 19 percent, respectively.

CLEAR CELL TUMORS

Light microscopic clear cells occur in a variety of salivary gland tumors, but ultrastructural subclassification indicates that there is a variety of cellular forms encompassed by this descriptive term. A clear property of the cytoplasm may be the result of minimal cellular differentiation and lack of organelles or may be caused by storage and/or accumulation of cytoplasmic contents (glycogen, mucus, lipid, clear secretory granules).[106] The cells are most often of the duct system (striated and intercalated), less often myoepithelial cells, and rarely acinous cells. Table 23-8 lists various clear cells and their fine structural characteristics. As can be seen, clear cells are likely to be present in a number of otherwise definable salivary gland tumors: mucous clear cells in mucoepidermoid carcinomas (Fig. 23-26), sebaceous clear cells in sebaceous lymphadenomas, or accompanying other forms of salivary gland tumors such as the organelle-poor cells in

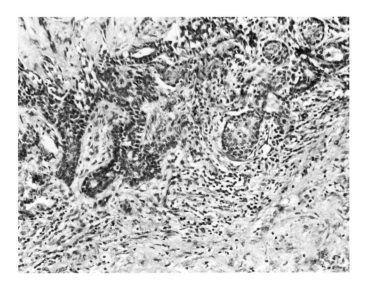

Fig. 23-24. Destructive, infiltrative growth by malignant epithelium in a carcinoma *ex* pleomorphic adenoma.

TABLE 23-8. Clear Cells in Salivary Tissues and Tumors

Type of Cell	Fine Structural Characteristics
Intercalated duct reserve cell	Minimal organelles
Storage cell (striated duct)	Glycogen granules
Myoepithelial cell	Glycogen granules, myofilaments, hemidesmosomes
Clear epidermoid cell	Tonofilaments
Goblet and mucous cells	Mucin granules and vacuoles
Sebaceous cells	Lipid
Clear acinic cell	Clear secretory granules, reduced organelles

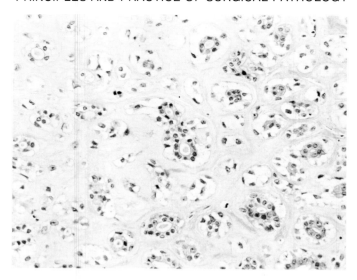

Fig. 23-27. Typical appearance of one form of clear cell carcinoma. This example shows the eosinophilic intercellular stroma and the biphasic glandular component: an outer mantle of clear cells surrounding small ducts.

mixed tumors, acinic cell carcinomas, and monomorphic adenomas.

There is, however, a distinctive group of salivary gland tumors that are composed wholly, or nearly so, of clear cells. These cells are mucin- and lipid-negative and usually contain glycogen. Glycogen positivity varies not only with the manner with which the tissue is processed but also with the differentiation of the cell itself.[92,107]

These clear cell tumors have been reported in the literature under a number of diagnostic terms: glycogen-rich clear cell adenoma or carcinoma, clear cell myoepithelioma and adenomyoepithelioma, among others. Seifert and Donath[106,108] consider the cells to be either organelle-poor and indifferent duct cells or myoepithelial or both. In Figure 23-27, both ductal cells and apposed clear cells are evident, and this form of clear cell lesion has been designated epithelial-myoepithelial carcinoma of interca-

lated ducts. The outer mantle of larger cells usually is glycogen rich. By their location and ultrastructural features, these cells are myoepithelial. A distinctive intercellular hyalinelike ground substance is usually present.

The combination of two cell types, hyaline stroma, and glycogen positivity is not duplicated by any other salivary gland tumor, but the histologic appearance varies from tumor to tumor and even within a given tumor. When myoepithelial clear cells predominate, the lesion appears as sheets of clear cells with rarely encountered duct cells or lumina.

Examination with the electron microscope confirms the biphasic cellular composition of the classic form of clear cell tumor. The inner, epithelial cell layer is similar to the epithelium of the intercalated ducts. The glycogen-containing outer layer of cells manifests many of the fine structural features attributed to myoepithelial cells. Immunohistochemical studies also point to an intercalated duct origin with a differentiation toward both myoepithelial and ductal elements.[107]

The tumors may arise in any salivary tissue, but there is a reported preference for the parotid glands, where they have been estimated to comprise less than 1 percent of that gland's tumor population. Table 23-9 presents the clinicopathologic features of the epimyoepithelial carcinoma.[107]

Before leaving clear cell lesions, a word about the so-called clear cell variant of acinic cell carcinoma is necessary. We doubt whether such a lesion is definable. Clear cell areas in an otherwise typical acinic cell carcinoma occur because (1) the cells contain clear secretory granules as a result of disordered protein synthesis, (2) the

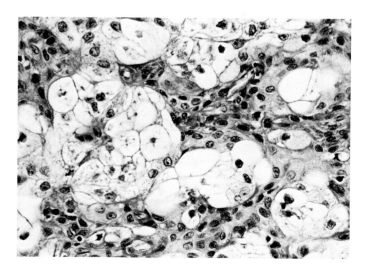

Fig. 23-26. Clear cell area in a mucoepidermoid carcinoma. Mucin content of cells, which may be scant, and the presence of clusters of nonclear intermediate cells serve to distinguish this lesion from other forms of clear cell lesions.

TABLE 23-9. Clinical Characteristics of Epimyoepithelial Carcinomas

Feature	Number
No. patients	35
Sex of patients	Female, 24; male, 11
Mean age at diagnosis (range, years)	62 (31–89)
Salivary gland site	27 parotid 4 submandibular 1 buccal 1 maxillary sinus
Patients with recurrences (%)	13 (37)
Patients with regional node metastases (%)	6 (17)
Patients with distant metastases (%)	3 (8.9)
Patient deaths attributed to carcinoma (%)	3 (8.9)

cells are organelle-deficient intercalated duct cells, or (3) the cells are clear because of processing artifacts.

TUMORS OF SEBACEOUS ORIGIN

Although sebaceous gland elements in the parotid gland may be considered as normal findings, sebaceous neoplasms are the least frequently encountered tumors of salivary tissues.[109] The most frequently reported form is the sebaceous lymphadenoma. Sebaceous adenomas and sebaceous carcinomas are rare.

The sebaceous lymphadenoma very likely shares a histogenetic basis with Warthin's tumor since both have a conspicuous lymphoid component. The lymphoid tissue, often an intraparotid or juxtaparotid lymph node, contains sebaceous glands, ductal elements, and areas of epidermoid differentiation. The often superficial position allows ready excision, and recurrences are unusual.[110]

Before ascribing an intraparotid origin to a sebaceous cell carcinoma, invasion from a contiguous cutaneous sebaceous cell carcinoma or metastasis from an extraparotid primary must be excluded.[109] Indeed, such instances exceed the number of primary carcinomas. Malignant sebaceous cells may also be a part of or dominate the histologic appearance of a carcinoma *ex* pleomorphic adenoma.

SQUAMOUS CELL CARCINOMA

Exclusion of metastases and forms of mucoepidermoid carcinoma has led to a remarkably constant incidence for primary squamous cell carcinoma of 0.3 to 0.5 percent of all parotid gland tumors.[111]

In our experience, primary squamous cell carcinomas of the parotid gland have been well or moderately well differentiated carcinomas. There is no mucus production, and intracellular keratinization, intercellular bridging, and keratin pearl formation are often noted.

Local recurrence and regional lymph node metastases are the usual course of primary squamous cell carcinomas.

The submandibular gland has a higher incidence of primary squamous cell carcinoma—approximately 3.5 percent of all tumors of that gland. The difference in incidence exhibited by the two major salivary glands is attributed to the much higher frequency of obstructive duct disease in the submandibular gland.

METASTASES TO SALIVARY GLANDS

Metastatic involvement (in the broadest context) of the parotid gland may arise from (1) lymphatic spread, (2) hematogenous dissemination, or (3) contiguous extension. The last is common with sarcomas of the parotid region, while the parotid gland as a focus of metastasis from a distant primary is unusual.

Lymphatic metastases to the gland may be direct without involvement of the paraglandular or extraglandular lymph nodes, may be secondary from a metastatic focus in a paraglandular lymph node, or may be from a retrograde extension from massive metastases in the neck.

The parotid gland and the juxtaparotid area are rather abundantly supplied by lymph nodes and lymphatics. The lymph nodes may be divided into intraglandular and extraglandular groups.[112] An average of 20 intraparotid lymph nodes may be identified after serial sectioning of the normal parotid gland.[113,114] These are definable nodes with capsules and sinuses, and their number does not include the normally present aggregates of lymphocytes and lymphoid tissue without nodal characteristics. Intraglandular nodes are located along the posterior facial vein between the superficial and deep parts of the parotid gland and are both superficial and deep parts of the parotid gland and are both superficial and deep to the facial nerve. Extraglandular nodes are usually subdivided into pre-auricular and infra-auricular groups and are predominantly in the preauricular area, along the superficial temporal vessels.

The intraglandular and extraglandular groups, while separable by the topography, are a single functional unit. Afferent lymphatics arise from the lateral and frontal scalp, eyelids, conjunctivae, lacrimal gland, molar area, root of nose, external auditory meatus, auditory tube, and cranial vault. The sinonasal, nasopharyngeal, and oropharyngeal regions also have lymphatic connections.

While carcinomas of these sites are all capable of yielding parotid node metastases, the high risk group of patients are those with deeply invasive melanomas or poorly differentiated squamous cell carcinomas in the skin of the ipsilateral eyelid, frontal, temporal, posterior cheek, and anterior ear regions.[115]

The paraglandular lymph nodes are most often the site of the metastases. These are relatively more abundant in the pre- and supratragal areas. The anterior portion of the parotid gland is rarely involved as a metastatic focus in either intraglandular or paraglandular lymph nodes.

In accordance with the risk potential, the predominant histologic types of metastases are melanomas and squamous cell carcinomas. On occasion, the metastasis may be present as a lesion from an occult primary.

Carcinomas and melanomas of mucosal surfaces involve the parotid group of lymph nodes less frequently, but they too may manifest as the signal metastasis. Distant sites with metastases to the parotid region and parotid gland are unusual and are led by carcinomas of the kidney, lung, and breast. Seifert et al[116] noted that less than 1 percent of tumors involving the parotid and submandibular glands were from distant sites; most of these (60 percent) originated in the head and neck. Metastases to the two parotid groups of lymph nodes not only may pose problems in clinical assessment of the mass but also often perplex the pathologist, particularly those who are unaware of the aggregation of lymph nodes in this region. Unless the lymph node is overrun by the metastasis, the identification of its capsule and circumscription from the parotid parenchyma serves to point to a lymphatic metastasis (Fig. 23-28). The dominance of melanoma and squamous cell carcinoma in the statistics of tumors metastatic to the parotid further serves as a distinction, since both cancers are rare as parotid gland primaries. Hematogenous metastases, besides their histologic differences from primary neoplasms of the parotid gland, usually involve the inter- and intralobular fibrous septa of the gland, only secondarily extending into the parenchyma.

Metastatic cancer in the parotid gland lymph nodes is usually an ominous prognostic sign that is worsened by concomitant cervical lymph node metastases. Some enhancement may be provided by surgical excision coupled with postoperative irradiation. In the series reported by Cassisi et al,[117] the recurrence rate in the parotid gland/ipsilateral neck was reduced from 75 percent to 20 percent by this combination therapy.

EPITHELIAL NEOPLASMS IN CHILDREN

Less than 5 percent of all salivary gland tumors occur in children and, exclusive of hemangiomas, fewer than 0.25 percent are found in children under 10 years of age.[118] Within the first decade of life, the perinatal (congenital or neonatal) epithelial salivary gland tumor is rare. During the perinatal period, the epithelial tumors

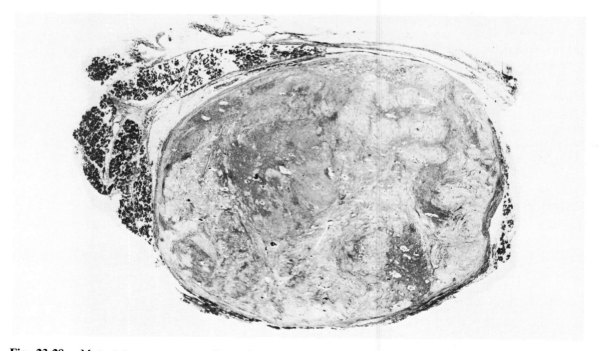

Fig. 23-28. Metastatic squamous cell carcinoma to an intraparotid lymph node. The tumor is entirely confined to the lymph node.

assume either a histologically malignant appearance (25 percent) and behave accordingly, with local and distant metastases, or an appearance evocative of stages during the embryonic development of the salivary glands.[118] Acinar differentiation in the latter is an exception. The tumors recall the preacinar stages of development, with mitotically active and primitive cell masses attempting to form ducts and pseudoductular spaces. A loose, investing mesenchyme, also with an embryonic appearance, further supports the impression of an abortive embryogenesis.

The perinatal tumors are not readily accommodated into contemporary classification schemes. Those fulfilling criteria for classifiable adult tumors, e.g., pleomorphic adenomas, monomorphic adenomas, and carcinomas, should be so designated. Those not so suited should be called *embryomas* or *sialoblastomas* in deference to their organoblastic appearance.[119] The rarity and attendent histopathologic uncertainty of embryomas should serve as constraints against too aggressive management. In the older child and adolescent, the pleomorphic adenoma is the most common benign tumor. Mucoepidermoid and acinic cell carcinomas are the two leaders among the carcinomas.

LYMPHOMA

Primary presentation of a lymphoma in the major salivary glands is much less common than secondary involvement. Although such lymphomas are nominally considered extranodal, the lymphomatous process, in either instance, most often begins within lymph nodes associated with the salivary glands.

The parotid gland is involved far more often than the submandibular, and a primary lymphoma of the sublingual gland is a medical curiosity. The predilection for the parotid gland is related to the normal presence of lymph nodes and lymphoid tissue within the gland proper. Lymph nodes and encapsulated aggregates of lymphoid tissue are absent in embryonic and adult submandibular and sublingual glands.

Salivary gland lymphomas fall into two pathogenic categories: (1) those associated with autoimmune disease, such as *Sjögren's* or *sicca syndrome;* and (2) those without such a probable relationship. In each, histologic evidence of a pre-existing salivary lesion with the characteristics of lymphoepithelial lesion may be present, although these findings are more often seen in patients with systemic immune disease.

With or without an associated immune disorder, salivary gland lymphomas have been classified most often as diffuse large cell in type. Diffuse and nodular poorly differentiated lymphomas follow in order of prevalence.

LYMPHOEPITHELIAL LESION

The lymphoepithelial lesion is a distinctive, yet not pathognomonic, sialadenopathy. Expressed solely in histomorphologic terms, the lymphoepithelial lesion is a progressive disorder that begins with a focal, periductal lymphoreticular reaction and culminates in a total or near total replacement of acinar parenchyma, duct disruption, and duct cell metaplasia. In its end stage, the salivary gland presents a picture of dispersed epimyoepithelial islands set in a matrix of lymphocytes, plasma cells, and other immunocytes[120] (Fig. 23-29).

This rather stereotyped histopathologic description contrasts sharply with the clinical diseases and syndromes with which the lymphoepithelial lesion is associated. Among these, *Sjögren's syndrome* stands foremost.

There is no facile definition of Sjögren's syndrome. It exists as a complex interrelated clinicopathologic spectrum that ranges from a disease limited to exocrine glands to an exocrine gland disease with extraglandular manifestations to disease with other autoimmune connective tissue disorders, especially rheumatoid arthritis and systemic lupus erythematosus.[121]

The presence or absence of a coexisting autoimmune disease has led to separation of the syndrome into primary and secondary forms.[121] The pure primary form is an exocrinopathy resulting from a lymphocyte-mediated destruction of exocrine glands that leads to decreased or absent glandular secretions and consequent mucosal dryness. Principal exocrine targets are the major and minor salivary glands in the head and neck, but exocrine elements in the lungs, gastrointestinal tract, and elsewhere can also be affected. The designation *sicca complex* has

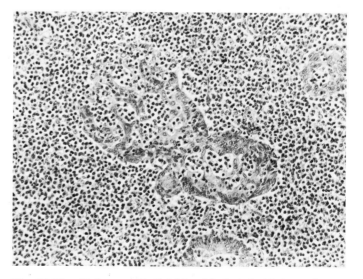

Fig. 23-29. Epimyoepithelial island in lymphoid tissue from a lymphoepithelial lesion.

been used as an alternative to primary Sjögren's syndrome. The secondary form of the syndrome is defined as the exocrinopathy preceded or followed by another autoimmune systemic disease.

The pathogenetic relationship between primary and secondary forms of Sjögren's syndrome is best highlighted by a described variant of the primary type—primary Sjögren's syndrome with extraglandular manifestations. Extraglandular in this context refers primarily to a lymphoproliferative process involving extrasalivary sites such as the reticuloendothelial system, kidneys, skeletal muscle, and lungs. Such lymphoproliferative lesions may be benign, malignant, or histologically indeterminate, the so-called pseudolymphomas.[121] In addition to the lymphoproliferative component of the extraglandular lesions, patients can also have purpura, vasculitis, myositis, and mononeuritis multiplex. An immune complex glomerulonephritis has also been described.

In company with the diverse clinical manifestations of Sjögren's syndrome, there is abundant evidence that the syndrome reflects B-cell hyperactivity with or without abnormalities of immunoregulation.[121] The findings include polyclonal hypergammaglobulinemia and nonorgan-specific autoantibodies such as rheumatoid factor and antibodies to extractable nuclear antigens. Four separate autoantibodies are known to be found in sera from patients with Sjögren's syndrome.[121] One is the organ-specific antisalivary duct antibody; the other three are nonorgan specific. Assay for the latter can provide some assistance in differential diagnosis. Rheumatoid arthritis-associated nuclear antigen (RANA) is not found in the primary form of the syndrome but is present in sera from patients with rheumatoid arthritis (with or without the syndrome). The SS-A antigen is found in primary Sjögren's syndrome, but not in secondary forms. SS-B antigen is present in patients with primary Sjögren's syndrome and in patients with Sjögren's syndrome associated with lupus erythematosus.

Paradoxically, antisalivary duct antibodies are of little help in diagnosis. Their concentration is inversely related to the degree of lymphoreticular infiltrate in salivary tissues, and only 25 percent of patients with primary Sjögren's syndrome manifest increased antibody levels.[121] Patients with rheumatoid arthritis only have an equal degree of reactivity, and patients with secondary Sjögren's syndrome and rheumatoid arthritis have nearly a 70 percent reactivity rate.

From the preceding immunologic data there has evolved the premise that the salivary glands are secondarily involved, albeit with high selectivity, by an autoimmune process. The process is unlike Hashimoto's thyroiditis and is closely related to rheumatoid arthritis and lupus erythematosus. Translation of this premise to the histopathologic changes in salivary glands cannot be done. Once again, the limited repertoire of response by tissue to different stimuli defeats specific etiologic correlations.

The lymphoepithelial lesion *is* the salivary gland's tissue response in patients with primary and secondary forms of Sjögren's syndrome. It is *not*, however, diagnostic of the syndrome and can be found in patients who have localized, limited (unilateral or unifocal) salivary gland disease. Figure 23-30 presents the possible existing relationships of the lymphoepithelial lesion to the four major clinical presentations. Each of the four may be self-contained entities, or they may evolve through the full spectrum to secondary Sjögren's syndrome.

The development of lymphoma in patients with Sjögren's syndrome is significant, so patients should not be lost to followup, especially women.

Data presented by Moutsopoulos[121] indicate a relative risk of lymphoma in women with Sjögren's syndrome

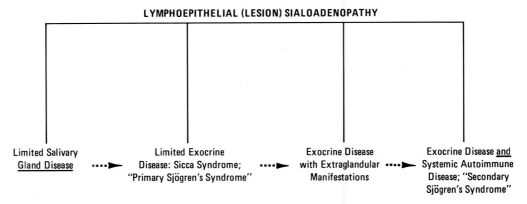

LYMPHOEPITHELIAL (LESION) SIALOADENOPATHY

Limited Salivary Gr Gland Disease ····▶ Limited Exocrine Disease: Sicca Syndrome; "Primary Sjögren's Syndrome" ····▶ Exocrine Disease with Extraglandular Manifestations ····▶ Exocrine Disease <u>and</u> Systemic Autoimmune Disease; "Secondary Sjögren's Syndrome"

Fig. 23-30. Disorders in which the lymphoepithelial lesion may be found in major salivary glands. The horizontal arrows also indicate the possible biologic progression from a limited salivary gland disease to secondary Sjögren's syndrome.

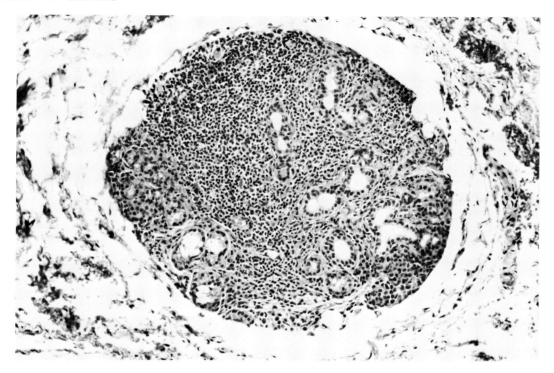

Fig. 23-31. Minor salivary gland lobule in a labial biopsy specimen from a patient with Sjögren's syndrome. This would be regarded as a high-score focus, since the inflammatory infiltrate is intense and many acini have been destroyed.

with or without rheumatoid arthritis of over 40 times that of controls. The lymphomas are almost exclusively non-Hodgkin's in type and are most often extrasalivary.

Clinicopathologic monitoring of patients with the various forms of Sjögren's syndrome has been facilitated by biopsy of minor salivary tissue: lip, palate, and nasal (septum) mucosa.[122] Since the syndrome is an exocrinopathy, biopsy specimens from these sites reflect extent and progress of the disease in the major salivary glands. The degree of correlation is high. Aggregates of lymphocytes within minor salivary tissue acini are scored (Fig. 23-31). Each aggregate of 50 or more cells is considered to represent a *focus*. The number of foci within 4 mm² of salivary tissue is determined and constitutes a *focus score*.[122] A focus score of more than 1 is considered characteristic of Sjögren's syndrome and is found in less than 1 percent of either normal or necropsy controls.

HEMANGIOMA AND OTHER SUPPORTING TISSUE LESIONS

Supporting tissue tumors, except vasoformative lesions, most often *incorporate* the salivary glands in their growth rather than take origin from structures or tissues within the glands themselves. Lipomas, neurilemmomas

of the facial nerve, and hemangiopericytomas, while unusual, are the most commonly reported lesions other than hemangiomas.

Vasoformative tumors (almost exclusively hemangiomas) are the most common lesions of the major salivary glands during infancy and early childhood.[123] Of the salivary gland tumors manifesting during the first year of life, and especially in the first six months, the *hemangioma* of the parotid gland is the predominant tumor. Clinical presentation of a parotid hemangioma in late childhood or in adults is very unusual. More than 90 percent of salivary gland hemangiomas are parotid in origin; the remainder are found in the submandibular gland. Hemangiomas of the parotid gland may be present at birth and are almost always evident within the first few months of life. There is a striking female predilection and an observed left-sided preference.

The tumors are usually asymptomatic masses occurring at the angle of the jaw and often extending over the ramus of the mandible. Large, deforming lesions may result from rapid growth or intralesional hemorrhage. Some tumors are cystic to palpation, others firmer or sponge-like.

Much has been made of associated regional and cutaneous hemangiomas as a preoperative diagnostic aid. Such a relation is quite variable and, in our personal opinion, is more uncommon than usual. More commonly, there is a bluish discoloration of the overlying skin which is accentuated when the patient cries or the head is inverted.

Surgically excised specimens convey the gross impression of a hypertrophied gland, indicating a confinement of the angiomatous proliferation to the gland proper. The size increase may be two to five or more times that of the normal infantile parotid. On cut section, the tumor is congested, deep red, and spongy.

The microscopic appearance is characteristic and variations from a highly cellular endothelial and capillary proliferation are minimal (Fig. 23-32). An increase in size of the vascular spaces may be noted in the older child as compared with the lesion in infancy, but cavernous hemangiomas are almost exclusively found in the adolescent or adult.[124]

The lobular architecture of the salivary gland is preserved and even accentuated. The lesional tissue replaces the acinar parenchyma and isolates the ducts, which remain as islands. Nuclear pleomorphism and atypia are absent, but the mitotic rate may be increased. On occasion, proliferating vasoformative foci are also found in periparotid soft tissues.

Hemangiomas of the salivary glands in adults are histologically unlike those of the infant, the former being characteristically of a cavernous form. Lymphangiomas are rarely localized intrasalivary lesions. The salivary glands are much more often incorporated by lymphangiomas of the adjacent tissues. Angiosarcomas primary in salivary glands are medical curiosities.

Because of the rather unique clinical and demographic features of the infantile hemangiomas of the major salivary glands, diagnosis is often possible without resort to tissue examination. This diagnostic advantage, coupled with the facts that malignant salivary gland tumors occur later in childhood and adolescence and many *cutaneous* hemangiomas undergo spontaneous involution, have led to debate over the management of the tumors.[123,125] Protagonists support either an expectant, nonintervention approach or surgical removal. Spontaneous resolution is clearly possible. In like manner, a noninvolution has been also documented. In those patients manifesting resolution, the return of functional secretory parenchyma is testimony to the replenishment abilities of the terminal duct system. Since a rather rapid growth is usual during the fourth to sixth month, it in itself is not a clear indication for surgical intervention. Sustained growth, exten-

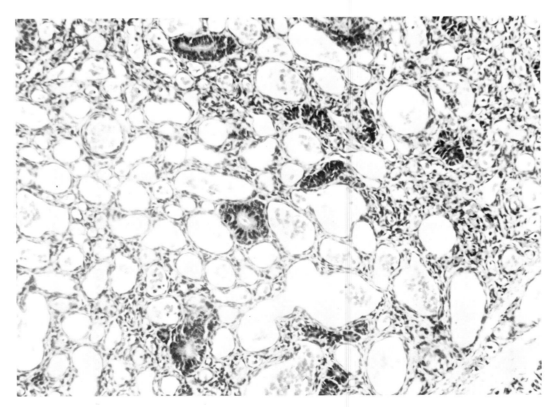

Fig. 23-32. Hemangioma of the parotid gland. The only parenchyma remaining is represented by scattered ducts. The remainder is lesional tissue composed of proliferating capillaries.

sive hemorrhage in the tumor, and unsureness of diagnosis are indications for surgery. Recurrences are of a low order.

INFLAMMATORY LESIONS

The salivary glands, like other tissues, can be the site of a large number of inflammatory and infectious diseases. The lymphoepithelial lesion, discussed in detail earlier because of its propensity to manifest as a space-occupying tumor, is actually the most important of these inflammatory lesions. Others include acute purulent sialadenitis due to bacterial infection and specific infections such as tuberculosis, syphilis, and viral diseases such as that caused by cytomegalovirus; these are usually not encountered in surgical material and are discussed in more detail in Chapter 3.

Lesions seen by the surgical pathologist are predominantly *nonspecific chronic sialadenitis* and *necrotizing sialometaplasia*. The former is often associated with duct ectasia, frequently as a result of intraductal calculi, and is characterized histologically by acinar atrophy, lymphoid infiltration, and fibrosis. Residual ductal elements, some-

times with squamous metaplasia, trapped within dense fibrous tissue must not be confused with carcinoma.

In necrotizing sialometaplasia,[126-128] the simulation of mucoepidermoid or squamous cell carcinoma is even more striking. This condition occurs as solitary or multiple ulcers usually on the hard palate of adults and does not recur after local excision or appropriate oral hygiene. Similar lesions can be seen in the soft palate and in major salivary glands after previous surgical procedures. Histologically, as the nomenclature suggests, the dominant processes are necrosis of acinar cells and the partial or total replacement of acini by foci of squamous metaplasia (Fig. 23-33). Pseudoepitheliomatous hyperplasia at the ulcer margins adds to the confusion with malignancy, but the preservation of lobular architecture within the lesion should enable the correct diagnosis to be made.

In the major salivary glands, necrotizing sialometaplasia is a vascular-based lesion.[128] Nearly all reported examples followed a surgical resection of the parotid gland, and necrotic or occluded medium-sized arteries could be found in sections of the gland with the necrotizing sialometaplasia. These observations, along with the vulnerability of palatine arteries, are strong support for an ischemic basis for the lesion in any salivary tissue site.[128]

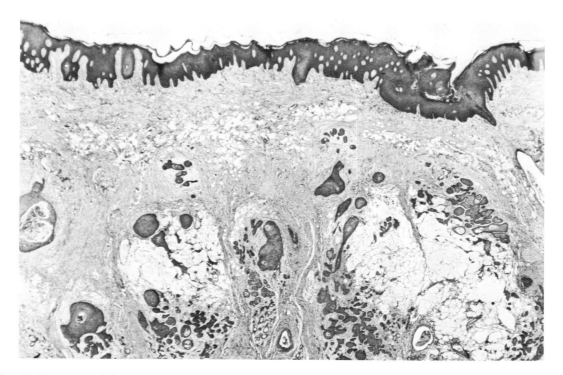

Fig. 23-33. Necrotizing sialometaplasia of the hard palate. Metaplastic (epidermoid) ducts and acini lie within or adjacent to lobules of altered minor salivary glands. This architecture and the nonmalignant appearance of the metaplasia serve to distinguish this lesion from squamous cell carcinoma and mucoepidermoid carcinoma.

OTHER NON-NEOPLASTIC LESIONS

Sialocysts and Mucoceles

Sialocysts of salivary glands are greatly outnumbered by pseudocystic lesions, exemplified by mucoceles. In the major salivary glands, sialocysts are predominantly lesions of the parotid glands, where they are classified as (1) salivary duct cysts, (2) lymphoepithelial cysts, or (3) dysgenetic or congenital cysts.[129] All arise from salivary ducts and have no relation to the branchial apparatus.

Salivary duct cysts are the most common and are no more than unilocular or occasionally multilocular ectatic salivary ducts with or without an oncocytic lining. They occur randomly in the parenchyma from the intralobular or interlobular ducts and are not associated with a lymphoid component.

Lymphoepithelial cysts always have an associated lymphoid tissue, have a variable epithelial lining (often metaplastic squamous in type), arise from enclaved salivary ducts, and in recent years have been found in increasing numbers in patients with acquired immune deficiency syndrome (AIDS) or AIDS-related complex (ARC).[130–132]

Polycystic (dysgenetic) disease of the parotid glands is the most rare of the nonmucocele group of non-neoplastic cystic lesions.[129] The light microscopic appearance of the lesion is distinctive, if not pathognomonic, and the clinical manifestations are such that a presumptive clinical diagnosis can be made: (1) it has been found only in females; (2) overt clinical signs are usually delayed, even into adulthood; (3) the affliction is bilateral; (4) a history of fluctuating, nontender parotid swelling for several years is antecedent to surgical intervention; (5) sialograms show cystic alterations with the main parotid duct uninvolved; and (6) surgical procedures are for diagnosis or cosmesis.

From the perspective of light microscopic appearance, the only variable in an otherwise uniform expression is the amount of residual acinar parenchyma. A lobular configuration is usually persistent, but the lobules are replaced or permeated by dilated cystic ducts. A honeycomb appearance is conveyed, with a few unaffected ducts and acini in stromal interstices. The cystic spaces are lined by an epithelium that varies from attenuated, flattened cells to cuboidal cells. Secretory products within the cysts range from watery fluid to inspissated, often laminated, microliths or spheroliths.

Mucoceles are preponderantly labial and intraoral benign extravasation lesions and are only unusually encountered in the parotid or submandibular glands. Here they are the result of either surgical disruption of ducts or secondary to neoplastic obstruction of ducts. The singular exception is the *ranula,* a benign, space-occupying lesion of sublingual gland origin.[133] An intraoral ranula is usually readily recognized by its characteristic location and appearance. A blue, translucent, and fluctuant swelling in the floor of the mouth, sometimes with a history of spontaneous rupture and expulsion of viscid fluid, is nearly pathognomonic. Considerably less familiar is the presentation of the ranula as a soft tissue neck mass, with or without an oral component. Known as a plunging or burrowing ranula, the cervical ranula should be added to the clinical differential diagnosis of benign cystic neck masses.

A painless, soft, ballotable neck mass is the most common clinical presentation. Parapharyngeal extension may be present. The cervical ranulas are variable in size at the time of treatment. Usually above the hyoid and in the submental or submandibular region, they may extend deeply into the neck, to the supraclavicular region and upper mediastinum, or posteriorly to the skull base.

Establishment of the sublingual gland as the origin of cervical ranulas has replaced theories of an extrasalivary origin and has thereby dictated appropriate management.[133] Surgical excision of the adjacent sublingual gland decreases or eliminates recurrence or persistence of the ranula.

Most ranulas, whether oral or cervical, are pseudocysts without an epithelial lining. Mucus extravasated from the sublingual glands enters the soft tissues and dissects between fascial planes. The histologic appearance of the ranula varies in accordance with time. Those with a short clinical history and without prior surgical intervention manifest a loose, vascularized connective tissue surrounding collections of mucin, microscopically simulating a bursa or even an angioma. Numbers of histiocytes and mucocytes lie in the wall of the pseudocyst and may even dominate areas of histologic sections. With progression, the mucin, histiocytes, and mucocytes became less prominent, and the appearance of the ranula is that of a dense, still well vascularized, fibrous connective tissue pseudocyst.

Heterotopias and Accessory Salivary (Parotid) Glands

Heterotopic salivary tissue is well known and has been described in the parathyroid gland, hypophysis, external ear canal, mastoid, upper and lower neck, and mandible and along the tract of a thyroglossal duct. Neoplasms arising from these heterotopias are rare unless the salivary tissues are those enclaved within parotid or periparotid lymph nodes.[134]

The accessory parotid gland is not rare. Approximately 20 percent of human parotid glands manifest accessory tissue. The accessory parotid tissues are variable in size, position, and shape. The tissue most often lies on or above the parotid duct and between the buccal branch of the facial nerve and the duct. One or several tributaries empty from the accessory tissue into the duct. While the tissue may be found in communication with the oral sub-mucosal part of Stensen's duct, the farthest removed ac-cessory gland from the parotid gland proper is usually on the buccal fat pad at the anterior border of the masseter muscle. An average distance from the anterior edge of the main parotid gland is 6 mm. There is no histologic difference between accessory tissue and the parotid gland proper.

Accessory parotid tissue is heir to all diseases afflicting the parotid gland proper. The spectrum of neoplasms is also similar, with pleomorphic adenomas the most com-mon benign tumor and mucoepidermoid carcinoma the most often encountered carcinoma. Approximately 50 percent of accessory parotid tumors are histologically malignant.[134]

Because of therapeutic considerations, it is important to recognize accessory parotid tissue as the source of a salivary gland tumor. The most important distinction is that dealing with tumors arising in the anteriofacial pro-cess or partially sequestered part of the parotid gland.

Sialadenosis

Sialadenosis or sialosis belongs in the differential diag-nosis of bilateral and, far less often, unilateral swellings of the parotid glands. The disorder is a noninflammatory parenchymatous disease brought about by a secretory and metabolic disturbance of the acinar parenchyma. In most instances, sialadenosis presents as a painless, re-current bilateral swelling of the parotid glands.

Because of the conspicuous (50 percent) association of sialadenosis with disorders of the nervous system, al-tered nutritional states, endocrinopathies, and pharmaco-logic effects of medication, it has been classified into three major groups: neurogenic, dystrophic-metabolic, and hormonal.[135] Experimental evidence points to a dysregulation of the autonomic innervation of the sali-vary acini as the unifying factor in all forms of sialade-nosis.

The heterogeneous and seemingly disparate synchrotic disorders (starvation, malnutrition, forcefeeding, alco-holism, bulimia, anorexia nervosa, diabetes mellitus, ovarian and thyroid disease, hepatic disorders) associ-ated with sialadenosis all produce their salivary effects through an aberrant intracellular secretory cycle within the acinar cell. The abnormality of the cycle is a result of

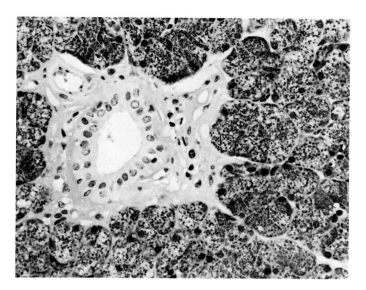

Fig. 23-34. Sialadenosis in a 24-year-old woman. An interlo-bular duct is surrounded by swollen, granule-rich acini.

a neurohormonally elicited interference on the neurore-ceptor of the glandular cell.

Changes in the secretory behavior of an acinus can be caused by either an excessive stimulation or an inhibition of secretion, both initiated through a neuropathic altera-tion in the autonomic innervation of the acini. With this in mind, sialadenosis can then be considered a result of a peripheral autonomic neuropathy.

Biopsy specimens from humans and parotid sections from experimental animals with sialadenosis, either stim-ulatory or inhibitory in type, characteristically manifest an increased acinar diameter. There is uniform hypertro-phy and likely a hyperplasia of the functional acinar parenchyma (Fig. 23-34). The cytoplasm of the swollen acinar cells is either granular or alveolate-translucent, or a mixture of both. Ultrastructurally, the secretory gran-ules of different optical densities correspond to the light microscopic cytoplasmic structure. Donath and col-leagues[136] distinguished three different types of sialad-enosis on the basis of electron microscopic appearance: dark granular, light granular, and mixed granular. The dark granular cells manifest protein-rich granules but are without evidence of an increased synthesis of proteins. Granules of low optical density and increased synthesis of protein characterize the light granular type. It should be noted, however, that there is no correlation between these ultrastructural forms and the clinical presentations of the sialadenosis. It is likely that intrinsic differences in the secretory cycle of the acini and their autonomic con-trol account for the predominance of the parotid glands as affected sites in sialadenosis.[135]

REFERENCES

1. Johns ME: Parotid cancer: A rational basis for treatment. Head Neck Surg 3:132, 1980
2. Beahrs OH, Henson DE, Hutter RVP, Myers MH (eds): American Joint Committee on Cancer: Manual for Staging of Cancer. 3rd Ed. JB Lippincott, Philadelphia, 1988
3. Spiro RH, Huvos AG, Strong EW: Cancer of the parotid gland. Am J Surg 139:452, 1975
4. Fu KK, Leibel SA, Levine ML, et al: Carcinoma of the major and minor salivary glands. Cancer 40:2882, 1977
5. Batsakis JG, Chinn EK, Weimert TA, et al: Acinic cell carcinoma: A clinicopathologic study of thirty-five cases. J Laryngol Otol 93:325, 1979
6. Batsakis JG: Mucoepidermoid and acinous cell carcinomas of salivary tissues. Ann Otol 89:91, 1980
7. Batsakis JG: Histopathological considerations. p. 25. In Suen JY, Myers, EN (eds): Cancer of the Head and Neck. Churchill Livingstone, New York, 1981
8. Gustafsson H, Carlsoo B, Kjorell U, et al: Ultrastructural and immunohistochemical aspects of carcinoma in mixed tumors. Am J Otolaryngol 7:218, 1986
9. Virtanen I, Miettinen M, Lehto V-P: Diagnostic application of monoclonal antibodies to intermediate filaments. Ann NY Acad Sci 455:635, 1986
10. Batsakis JG: Intermediate filaments and salivary gland tumors. Am J Otolaryngol 7:231, 1986
11. Zarbo RJ, Regezi JA, Batsakis JG: S-100 protein in salivary gland tumors: An immunohistochemical study of 129 cases. Head Neck Surg 8:268, 1986
12. Stead RH, Qizilbash AH, Kontozoglou T, et al: An immunohistochemical study of pleomorphic adenomas of the salivary gland: Glial fibrillary acidic protein-like immunoreactivity identifies a major myoepithelial component. Hum Pathol 19:32, 1988
13. Dardick I, van Nostrand AWP, Phillips MJ: Histogenesis of salivary gland pleomorphic adenoma (mixed tumor) with an evaluation of the myoepithelial cell. Hum Pathol 13:62, 1982
14. Caselitz J, Schulze J, Seifert G: Adenoid cystic carcinoma of the salivary glands: An immunohistochemical study. J Oral Pathol 15:308, 1986
15. Azumi N, Battifora H: The cellular composition of adenoid cystic carcinoma. Cancer 60:1589, 1987
16. Batsakis JG, Kraemer B, Sciubba JJ: The pathology of head and neck tumors: The myoepithelial cell and its participation in salivary gland neoplasia. Head Neck Surg 5:222, 1983
17. Batsakis JG: Salivary gland neoplasia: An outcome of modified morphogenesis and cytodifferentiation. Oral Surg 49:229, 1980
18. Donath K, Dietrich H, Seifert G: Entwicklung und ultrastrukturelle Cytodifferenzierung der Parotis des Menshen. Virchows Arch 378:297, 1978
20. Eversole LR: Histogenic classification of salivary tumors. Arch Pathol 92:433, 1971
21. Foote FW, Frazell EL: Tumors of the major salivary glands. Cancer 6:1065, 1953

22. Kleinsasser O, Klein HJ: Basalzellademme der Speicheldrusen. Arch Klin Exp Ohren Nasen Kehlkopfheilkd 189:302, 1967
23. Batsakis JG: Clear cell tumors of salivary glands. Ann Otol 89:196, 1980
24. Eneroth C-M: Salivary gland tumors in the parotid gland, submandibular gland and the palate region. Cancer 27:1415, 1971
25. Skolnik EM, Friedman M, Becker S, et al: Tumors of the major salivary glands. Laryngoscope 87:843, 1977
26. VandenBerg HJ, Kambouris A, Pryzbylski T: Salivary tumors: Clinicopathologic review of 190 patients. Am J Surg 108:480, 1964
27. Bardwil JM: Tumors of the parotid gland. Am J Surg 114:498, 1967
28. Eneroth C-M: Histological and clinical aspects of parotid tumors. Acta Otolaryngol 191(suppl.):1, 1964
29. Woods JE, Weiland LH, Chong GC, et al: Pathology and surgery of primary tumors of the parotid. Surg Clin North Am 57:565, 1977
30. Spiro RH, Hajdu SI, Strong EW: Tumors of the submaxillary gland. Am J Surg 132:463, 1976
31. Rafla S: Submaxillary gland tumors. Cancer 26:821, 1970
32. Eneroth C-M, Hjertman L, Moberger G: Malignant tumors of the submandibular gland. Acta Otolaryngol (Stockh) 64:514, 1967
33. Byers RM, Jesse RH, Guillamondegui OM, et al: Malignant tumors of the submaxillary gland. Am J Surg 126:458, 1973
34. Lower JT, Farmer JC: Submaxillary gland tumors. Laryngoscope 84:542, 1974
35. Hanna DC, Clairmont AC: Submandibular gland tumors. Plast Reconstr Surg 61:198, 1978
36. Simons JN, Beahrs OH, Woolner LB: Tumors of the submaxillary gland. Am J Surg 108:485, 1964
37. Conley J, Myers E, Cole R: Analysis of 115 patients with tumors of the submandibular gland. Ann Otol 81:323, 1972
38. Trail M, Lubritz J: Tumors of the submandibular gland. Laryngoscope 84:1225, 1974
39. Batsakis JG: Carcinomas of the submandibular and sublingual glands. Ann Otol Rhinol Laryngol 95:211, 1986
40. Seifert G, Schulz C-P: Das monomorphe Speichelgangadenom. Klassifikation und Analyse von 79 Fällen. Virchows Arch [A] 383:77, 1979
41. Batsakis JG, Brannon RB: Dermal analogue tumours of major salivary glands. J Laryngol Otol 95:155, 1981
42. Batsakis JG, Brannon RB, Sciubba JJ: Monomorphic adenomas of salivary glands: A histologic study of 96 tumors. Clin Otolaryngol 6:129, 1981
43. Mintz GA, Abrams AM, Melrose RJ: Monomorphic adenomas of the major and minor salivary glands. Oral Surg Oral Med Oral Pathol 53:375, 1982
44. Headington JI, Batsakis JG, Beals TF, et al: Membranous basal cell adenoma of parotid gland, dermal cylindromas and trichoepitheliomas. Cancer 39:2460, 1977
45. Bernacki EG, Batsakis JG, Johns ME: Basal cell adenoma. Distinctive tumor of salivary glands. Arch Otolaryngol 99:84, 1974

46. Rauch S: Die Speicheldrusen des menschen. Thieme, Stuttgart, 1959
47. Chu W, Strawitz JG: Parapharyngeal growth of parotid tumors. Arch Surg 112:709, 1977
48. Eneroth C-M: Mixed tumors of major salivary glands. Prognostic role of capsular structure. Ann Otol 74:944, 1965
49. Naeim F, Forsberg MI, Waisman J: Mixed tumors of the salivary glands: Growth pattern and recurrence. Arch Pathol Lab Med 100:271, 1976
50. Hubner G, Klein HG, Kleinsasser O, et al: Role of myoepithelial cell in the development of salivary gland tumors. Cancer 27:1255, 1971
51. Erlandson RA, Cardon-Cardo C, Higgins PJ: Histogenesis of benign pleomorphic adenoma (mixed tumor) of the major salivary glands. Am J Surg Pathol 8:803, 1984
52. Takeguchi J, Soube M, Yoshida M, et al: Pleomorphic adenoma of the salivary gland. With special reference to histochemical and electron microscopic studies and biochemical analysis of glycosaminoglycans in vivo and vitro. Cancer 36:1771, 1975
53. Hamper H: The myothelia (myoepithelial cells): Normal state: Regressive changes: Hyperplasia: tumors. Curr Top Pathol 53:162, 1970
54. Luna MA, MacKay B, Gomez-Araujo J: Myoepithelioma of the palate. Cancer 32:1429, 1973
55. Lomax-Smith JD, Azzopardi JJ: The hyaline cell: A distinctive feature of mixed salivary tumors. Histopathology 2:77, 1978
56. Kavka SJ: Bilateral simultaneous Warthin's tumors. Arch Otolaryngol 91:302, 1970
57. Batsakis JG: Tumors of the Head and Neck: Clinical and Pathological Considerations, 2nd Ed. Williams & Wilkins, Baltimore, 1979
58. Azzopardi JG, Hou LT: The genesis of adenolymphoma. J Pathol 88:213, 1964
59. Seifert G, Bull HG, Donath K: Histologic subclassification of the cystadenolymphoma of the parotid gland. Virchows Arch [A] 388:13, 1980
60. Ellis GL: "Clear cell" oncocytoma of salivary gland. Hum Pathol 19:862, 1988
61. Johns ME, Regezi JA, Batsakis JG: Oncocytic neoplasms of salivary glands: An ultrastructural study. Laryngoscope 87:862, 1977
62. Tandler B, Hutter RVP, Erlandson RA: Ultrastructure of oncocytoma of the parotid gland. Lab Invest 22:567, 1970
63. Carlsoo B, Domeij S, Helander HF: A quantitative ultrastructural study of a parotid oncocytoma. Arch Pathol Lab Med 103:471, 1979
64. Gray SR, Cornog, JL, Seo IS: Oncocytic neoplasms of salivary glands. A report of fifteen cases including two malignant oncocytomas. Cancer 38:1306, 1976
65. Spiro RH, Huvos AG, Strong EW: Adenoid cystic carcinoma of salivary origin. Am J Surg 128:512, 1974
66. Conley J, Dingman DL: Adenoid cystic carcinoma of the head and neck (cylindroma). Arch Orolaryngol 100:81, 1974
67. Perzin KH, Gullane P, Clairmont AC: Adenoid cystic carcinomas arising in salivary glands. Cancer 42:265, 1978
68. Tandler B: Ultrastructure of adenoid cystic carcinoma of salivary gland origin. Lab Invest 24:504, 1971
69. Eby LS, Johnson DS, Baker HW: Adenoid cystic carcinoma of the head and neck. Cancer 29:1160, 1972
70. Bloom GD, Carlsoo B, Gustaffson H, et al: Distribution of mucosubstances in adenoid cystic carcinoma. Virchows Arch [A] 375:1, 1977
71. Allen MS, Marsh WL: Lymph node involvement by direct extension in adenoid cystic carcinoma. Absence of classic embolic lymph node metastasis. Cancer 38:2017, 1976
72. Matsuba HM, Simpson JR, Mauney M, et al: Adenoid cystic salivary gland carcinoma: A clinicopathologic correlation. Head Neck Surg 8:200, 1986
73. Nascimento AG, Amaral LP, Prado LAF, et al: Adenoid cystic carcinoma of salivary glands. Cancer 57:312, 1986
74. Spiro R, Huvos AG, Berk R, et al: Mucoepidermoid carcinoma of salivary gland origin. A clinicopathologic study of 367 cases. Am J Surg 136:461, 1978
75. Sikowara L: Mucoepidermoid tumors of salivary glands. Polish Med J 3:1345, 1964
76. Laudadio P, Caliceti V, Cerasoli PT, et al: Mucoepidermoid tumour of the parotid gland: A very difficult prognostic evaluation. Clin Otolaryngol 12:177, 1987
77. Frazell EL: Clinical aspects of tumors of the major salivary glands. Cancer 7:637, 1954
78. Stevenson GF, Hazard JB: Mucoepidermoid carcinoma of salivary gland origin. Cleve Clin Q 20:445, 1953
79. Batsakis JG, Chinn E, Regezi JA, et al: The pathology of head and neck tumors: Salivary glands, 2. Head Neck Surg 1:167, 1978
80. Jakobsson PA, Eneroth C-M: Mucoepidermoid carcinoma of the parotid gland. Cancer 22:111, 1968
81. Healey WV, Perzin KW, Smith L: Mucoepidermoid carcinoma of salivary gland origin. Classification, clinical-pathologic correlation, and results of treatment. Cancer 26:368, 1970
82. Hamper K, Schimmelpenning H, Caselitz J, et al: Mucoepidermoid tumors of the salivary glands. Correlation of cytophotometrical data and prognosis. Cancer 63:708, 1989
83. Spiro RH, Huvos AG, Strong EW: Acinic cell carcinoma of salivary origin: A clinicopathologic study of 67 cases. Cancer 41:924, 1978
84. Ellis GL, Corio RL: Acinic cell adenocarcinoma. A clinicopathologic analysis of 294 cases. Cancer 52:542, 1983
85. Batsakis JG, Wozniak KJ, Regezi JA: Acinous cell carcinoma: A histogenetic hypothesis. J Oral Surg 35:904, 1977
86. Regezi JA, Batsakis JG: Histogenesis of salivary gland neoplasms. Otolaryngol Clin North Am 10:297, 1977
87. Chong GC, Beahrs OH, Woolner LB: Surgical management of acinic cell carcinoma of the parotid gland. Surg Gynecol Obstet 138:65, 1974
88. Abrams AM, Coryn J, Scofield HH: Acinic cell adenocarcinoma of the major salivary glands. A clinicopathologic study of 77 cases. Cancer 18:1145, 1965
89. Eneroth C-M, Silfversward C, Zetterberg A: Malignancy

of acinic cell tumours elucidated by microspectrophotometric DNA analysis. Acta Otolaryngol (Stockh) 77:126, 1974

90. Batsakis JG, Regezi JA: The pathology of head and neck tumors: Salivary glands, 4. Head Neck Surg 1:340, 1979

91. Hui KH, Batsakis JG, Luna MA, et al: Salivary duct carcinomas: A high grade malignancy. J Laryngol Otol 100:105, 1986

92. Luna MA, Batsakis JG, Ordonex NG, et al: Salivary gland adenocarcinomas: A clinicopathologic analysis of three distinctive types. Semin Diagn Pathol 4:117, 1987

93. Batsakis JG, Pinkston GR, Luna MA, et al: Adenocarcinomas of the oral cavity: A clinicopathologic study of terminal duct carcinomas. J Laryngol Otol 97:825, 1983

94. Batsakis JG, Luna MA: Low-grade and high-grade adenocarcinomas of the salivary duct system. Ann Otol Rhinol Laryngol 98:162, 1989

95. Nagao K, Matsuzaki O, Saiga H, et al: Histopathologic studies of undifferentiated carcinoma of the parotid gland. Cancer 50:1572, 1982

96. Gnepp DR, Corio RL, Brannon RB: Small cell carcinoma of the major salivary glands. Cancer 58:705, 1986

97. Kraemer BB, Mackay B, Batsakis JG: Small cell carcinoma of the parotid gland. A clinicopathologic study of three cases. Cancer 52:2115, 1983

98. Saw D, Lau WH, Ho JHC, et al: Malignant lymphoepithelial lesion of the salivary gland. Hum Pathol 17:914, 1986

99. Saemundsen AK, Albeck H, Hansen JPH, et al: Epstein-Barr virus in nasopharyngeal and salivary gland carcinomas of Greenland Eskimos. Br J Cancer 46:721, 1982

100. Huang DP, Ng HK, Ho YH, et al: Epstein-Barr virus (EBV)-associated undifferentiated carcinoma of the parotid gland. Histopathology 13:509, 1988

101. Tortoledo ME, Luna MA, Batsakis JG: Carcinomas ex pleomorphic adenoma and malignant mixed tumors. Arch Otolaryngol 110:172, 1984

102. Stephen J, Batsakis JG, Luna MA, et al: True malignant mixed tumors (carcinosarcomas) of salivary glands. Oral Surg 61:597, 1986

103. Spiro RH, Huvos AG, Strong EW: Malignant mixed tumor of salivary origin. A clinicopathologic study of 146 cases. Cancer 39:388, 1977

104. Boles R, Johns ME, Batsakis JG: Carcinoma in pleomorphic adenomas of salivary glands. Ann Otol 82:684, 1973

105. LiVolsi VA, Perzin KH: Malignant mixed tumors arising in salivary glands. I. Carcinomas arising in benign mixed tumors. A clinicopathologic study. Cancer 39:2209, 1977

106. Donath K, Seifert G, Schmitz F: Zur Diagnose und Ultrastruktur des tubularen Speichelgangcarcinoms. Epithelial-myoepitheliales Schaltstuckcarcinoma. Virchows Arch [A] 356:16, 1972

107. Luna MA, Ordonez NG, Mackay B, et al: Salivary epithelial-myoepithelial carcinomas of intercalated ducts: A clinical, electron microscopic and immunocytochemical study. Oral Surg 59:482, 1985

108. Seifert G, Donath K: Uber das Vorkommen Sog. heller Zellen in Speicheldrusentumoren. Ultrastruktur und Differetialdiagnose. Z Krebsforsch 91:165, 1978

109. Batsakis JG, Littler ER, Leahy MS: Sebaceous gland lesions of the head and neck. Arch Otolaryngol 95:151, 1972

110. Gnepp DR, Brannon R: Sebaceous neoplasms of salivary gland origin. Cancer 53:2155, 1984

111. Batsakis JG, McClatchey KD, Johns ME, et al: Primary squamous cell carcinoma of the parotid gland. Arch Otolaryngol 102:355, 1976

112. Conley J, Arena S: Parotid gland as a focus of metastasis. Arch Surg 87:757, 1963

113. Batsakis JG: Parotid gland and its lymph nodes as metastatic sites. Ann Otol Rhinol Laryngol 92:209, 1983

114. McKean ME: The distribution of lymph nodes in and around the parotid gland: An anatomical study. Br J Plast Surg 38:1, 1985

115. Storm FK, Eiber FR, Sparks FC, et al: A prospective study of parotid metastases from head and neck cancer. Ann J Surg 134:115, 1977

116. Seifert G, Hennings K, Caselitz J: Metastatic tumors to the parotid and submandibular glands—Analysis and differential diagnosis of 108 cases. Pathol Res Pract 8:484, 1986

117. Cassisi NJ, Dickerson DR, Million RR: Squamous cell carcinoma of the skin metastatic to parotid nodes. Arch Otolaryngol 104:336, 1978

118. Batsakis JG, Mackay B, Ryka AF, et al: Perinatal salivary gland tumours (embryomas). J Laryngol Otol 102:1007, 1988

119. Taylor GP: Congenital epithelial tumor of the parotid—sialoblastoma. Pediatr Pathol 8:447, 1988

120. Ferlito A, Cattai N: The so-called 'benign lymphoepithelial lesion': 1. Explanation of the term and of its synonomous and related terms. J Laryngol Otol 94:1189, 1980

121. Moutsopoulos HM: Sjögren's syndrome (Sicca syndrome): Current issues. Ann Intern Med 92:212, 1980

122. Daniels TE: Labial salivary gland biopsy in Sjögren's syndrome: Assessment as a diagnostic criterion in 362 suspected cases. Arthritis Rheum 27:147, 1984

123. Schuller DE, McCabe BF: The firm salivary mass in children. Laryngoscope 87:1891, 1977

124. Mussbaum M, Tan S, Som ML: Hemangiomas of the salivary glands. Laryngoscope 86:1015, 1976

125. Koop CE: Surgical pros and cons. Surg Gynecol Obstet 135:274, 1972

126. Abrams AM, Melrose RJ, Howell FV: Necrotizing sialometaplasia. Cancer 32:130, 1973

127. Fechner RE: Necrotizing sialometaplasia. A source of confusion with carcinoma of the palate. Am J Clin Pathol 67:315, 1977

128. Batsakis JG, Manning JT: Necrotizing sialometaplasia of major salivary glands. J Laryngol Otol 101:962, 1987

129. Batsakis JG, Bruner JM, Luna MA: Polycystic (dysgenetic) disease of the parotid glands. Arch Otolaryngol Head Neck Surg 114:1146, 1988

130. Weidner N, Geisinger KR, Sterling RT, et al: Benign lymphoepithelial cysts of the parotid gland. A histologic, cytologic and ultrastructural study. Am J Clin Pathol 85:395, 1988

131. Shugar JMA, Som PM, Jacobson AL, et al: Multicentric

parotid cysts and cervical adenopathy in AIDS patients. A newly recognized entity: CT and MR manifestations. Laryngoscope 98:772, 1988

132. Smith FB, Rajdeo H, Panesar N, et al: Benign lymphoepithelial lesions of the parotid gland in intravenous drug users. Arch Pathol Lab Med 112:742, 1988

133. Batsakis JG, McClatchey KD: Cervical ranulas. Ann Otol Rhinol Laryngol 97:561, 1988

134. Batsakis JG: Accessory parotid gland. Ann Otol Rhinol Laryngol 97:434, 1988

135. Batsakis JG: Sialadenosis. Ann Otol Rhinol Laryngol 97:94, 1988

136. Donath K, Spillner M, Seifert G: The influence of the autonomic nervous system on the ultrastructure of the parotid acinar cells. Experimental contribution to the neurohormonal sialadenosis. Virchows Arch [A] 364:15, 1974

24

The Mediastinum and Thymus

William Ray Salyer
Diane Cereghino Salyer

THE MEDIASTINUM

The mediastinum is the area in the median portion of the thorax separating the pleura of the lungs. It extends from the sternum anteriorly to the vertebral column posteriorly and from the thoracic inlet superiorly to the diaphragm inferiorly.

The age of the patient is a valuable diagnostic aid, since some mediastinal lesions characteristically occur in children, whereas others are rare in pediatric patients.

Anatomic subdivision of the mediastinum into anterior, middle, and posterior serves a purpose because the various lesions have a tendency to occur in predictable compartments (Table 24-1). The specific site of origin is necessary information in the evaluation of a specimen from the mediastinum.

Anterior mediastinum. Germ cell tumors and lymphomas occur in children, but the other anterior mediastinal lesions are uncommon in childhood. In adults all the entities listed in Table 24-1 occur.

Middle mediastinum. Lymph node enlargement, the clinically predominant mediastinal abnormality, is largely a lesion of the middle mediastinum in both children and adults. The most frequent causes of lymph node enlargement are metastatic tumors, infections in association with primary lung involvement, and lymphoma. Bronchogenic cysts usually occur in this location, but they may present in any of the three compartments.

Posterior mediastinum. Neurogenic tumors are the most common primary mediastinal neoplasms and by far the most common primary tumors in the posterior mediastinum in both children and adults. Tumors of sympathetic nervous system origin—neuroblastoma, ganglioneuroblastoma, and ganglioneuroma—occur predominantly in children and young adults. Tumors of neural sheath origin (Schwann cell origin)—neurofibromas, neurilemmomas, and neurofibrosarcomas—are usually seen in adults.

Many mediastinal lesions are asymptomatic and are detected incidentally on chest films. Some patients have pain or symptoms and signs referable to involvement of one of the critical mediastinal structures, such as dyspnea, dysphagia, or superior vena cava syndrome.[1]

The appearance of many mediastinal lesions on routine radiologic examination may be identical. For this reason, surgical exploration is preferred over attempts to establish a diagnosis with limited approaches such as needle biopsy. An exception is the biopsy of lymph nodes via mediastinoscopy in the evaluation of some patients with lung carcinoma. Computerized tomography (CT) seems more sensitive in detecting mediastinal masses, in providing a specific preoperative diagnosis of some lesions (for example, cysts and lipomas), and in defining metastases from the lung.[2] Nuclear magnetic resonance (NMR) imaging can allow distinction of cystic structures and may also differentiate vascular from nonvascular structures without the need for contrast media.[3]

Developmental Abnormalities

Cervical Thymus

Failure of thymic descent is discussed in the section on the thymus.

TABLE 24-1. Mediastinal Lesions by Compartment and Age Group

Compartment	Children	Adults
Anterior	Lymphoma Germ cell neoplasms Developmental cysts	Thymic lesions Lymphoma Germ cell neoplasms Developmental cysts Paraganglioma Thyroid lesions Parathyroid lesions
Middle	Lymph node enlargement Developmental cysts	Lymph node enlargement Developmental cysts
Posterior	Sympathetic nervous system neoplasms	Nerve sheath neoplasms

Mediastinal Parathyroid

The lower parathyroid glands and the thymus are derived from the third and fourth branchial pouches. During development one or both lower parathyroids may descend into the mediastinum. The overall incidence of this occurrence is approximately 20 percent.[4]

Parathyroid adenoma and parathyroid hyperplasia can develop in glands situated in the mediastinum. In one study 84 of 400 patients with hyperparathyroidism had a mediastinal parathyroid adenoma.[5] The glands are most often immediately adjacent to the thymus superiorly in the mediastinum and can be removed through a low collar incision without sternotomy; this was the case in 62 of the 84 patients in the study cited.[5]

Mediastinal Thyroid

Cases in which all thyroid tissue is located in the mediastinum are quite rare.[6] Slightly more common and representing 0.2 to 1 percent of all cases of enlarged glands[7] are mediastinal thyroid goiters, with a blood supply derived from mediastinal vessels and no connection with cervical thyroid tissue.[8,9] Most examples of mediastinal thyroid represent substernal extension of an enlarged thyroid gland.[7,8] The enlargement is usually due to multiple colloid or adenomatoid nodules. Thyroiditis, hyperplasia, and neoplasia also may affect mediastinal thyroid tissue. In one series 3 percent of enlarged glands involved the mediastinum; most of these were continuous with the cervical thyroid and had a cervical blood supply.[7] In these instances mediastinal involvement is due largely to mechanical factors. Caudal extension is the path of least resistance for an enlarging gland. Respiratory motion, negative intrathoracic pressure, and increased gland weight also are contributory. The aortic arch partially obstructs growth to the left, and this is thought to explain the higher incidence of mediastinal goiter on the right than on the left.[7]

The clinical manifestation of mediastinal thyroid enlargement is commonly due to compression of structures in the thoracic inlet. The gland may be asymptomatic and may be an incidental finding on chest films. Radioiodine scans provide a noninvasive technique for diagnosis when mediastinal thyroid tissue is suspected.

Benign Developmental Cysts of the Mediastinum

Benign developmental mediastinal cysts are uncommon. They are often asymptomatic and are discovered incidentally on imaging examinations done for screening or for evaluation of an unrelated problem. Bronchogenic and gastroenteric cysts may be symptomatic because of infection, secretion, or pressure. Cysts that have been infected may have a nonspecific histologic appearance due to destruction of the inner mucosal lining and fibrosis. The surgical accessibility of these lesions, which may be preoperatively diagnosed as neoplasms, necessitates awareness of their anatomic and histologic characteristics.

Pericardial Cysts

Pericardial cysts are considered to be derived from a persistence of the ventral recesses of the primitive pericardial cavity as the two thoracic coeloms join ventrally. The caudal portion of this process of cavitary formation is the septum transverum, which becomes the diaphragm. Pericardial cysts are located therefore in the anterior cardiophrenic angle, and they commonly are associated with the diaphragm. A suprapericardial location of pericardial cysts is infrequent and may, therefore, be overlooked as a diagnostic possibility.[10] This location is explained by an early detachment of the cyst from the septum transversum that descends in development. There is no embryologic explanation for the observation that pericardial cysts occur more frequently on the right side.[10]

Pericardial cysts vary from less than 1 cm to more than 10 cm in diameter. They are almost always unilocular and contain clear thin fluid. Histologically, a single layer of mesothelial cells is seen to overlie a thin strand of smooth muscle and connective tissue (Fig. 24-1A). Mild chronic inflammation is common, but acute inflammation is absent. Calcification may be present.[11]

Bronchogenic and Esophageal Cysts

The distinction between bronchogenic and esophageal cysts may be difficult because of their similar location and occasionally similar histologic features. An under-

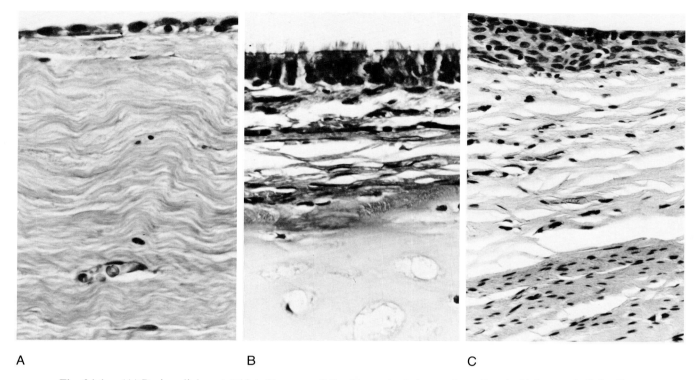

A   B   C

Fig. 24-1. (**A**) Pericardial cyst. Thick fibrous wall lined by a single layer of small, cuboidal mesothelial cells. (**B**) Bronchogenic cyst. Cartilage in cyst wall lined by respiratory-type epithelium. (**C**) Esophageal cyst. Smooth muscle in cyst wall lined by a nonkeratinizing squamous epithelium.

standing of the embryologic development of the tracheo-bronchial tree, as related to the development of the esophagus, clarifies the relationship and similarities of cysts of these organs[12] (Fig. 24-2). The respiratory diverticulum is initially openly connected to the foregut. With the development of an esophagotracheal septum, the respiratory tree is separated from the esophagus except in the region of the laryngeal orifice.[13]

Bronchogenic cysts are thought to arise as supernu-

merary lung buds, a theory supported by the occurrence of small diverticula of the right primary bronchus, a region where many larger bronchogenic cysts are located.[13] Bronchogenic cysts occur anywhere along the tracheo-bronchial tree to the level of the secondary bronchi. They are often found in the subcarinal region, which is also a common site for tracheoesophageal fistula. Cysts in the subcarinal region, hilar region, and along the esophagus may have esophageal attachments. These cysts can be

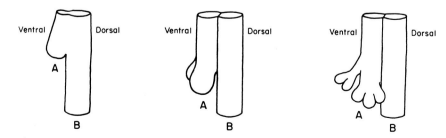

Fig. 24-2. (*Left*) Lateral view of respiratory system at 3 weeks of gestation (A, respiratory diverticulum; B, foregut). (*Center*) Lateral view at 4 weeks of gestation. Esophagotracheal septum is present (A, bronchial buds developing in respiratory diverticulum; B, esophagus). (*Right*) Lateral view at 5 weeks of gestation (A, trachea with lung buds dividing in three right and two left mainstem bronchi; B, esophagus). (From Salyer et al.[12] with permission.)

found, rarely, within the pericardium. Attachments at the point of origin may be tenuous or no longer recognizable at the time of operation.

Bronchogenic cysts range in size from 1 to 6 cm. Cartilage and bronchial glands are often found in the cyst wall, but they are not invariably present. Focal calcification may be present. The cysts are characteristically unilocular, thin-walled, and spherical. The cysts are lined by ciliated columnar epithelium (Fig. 24-1B). In many cases, however, there is focal or extensive squamous metaplasia or extreme attenuation of the mucosa, so that the cysts are partially lined by a simple, flattened, epithelial layer. The underlying stroma is hyaline connective tissue, often with strands of smooth muscle and fibrous tissue. The contents of the cysts may be serous or mucinous.

Esophageal cysts are less common than bronchogenic cysts. Most evidence supports the theory that the esophageal cysts arise as a persistence in the wall of vacuoles that form and coalesce longitudinally in the embryologic process of forming a lumen in a solid tube.

Problems in making the distinction between bronchogenic cysts and esophageal cysts are related to their close relationship embryologically. If continuity with the bronchial tree is not maintained, a bronchial cyst may become intrapulmonary, or it may become attached to the esophageal wall. Cysts located entirely within the wall of the esophagus but containing cartilage and ciliated columnar epithelium have been described. If a cyst closely associated with or within the esophageal wall has only ciliated columnar epithelium but no cartilage formation, then the origin of the cyst cannot be determined, since the esophagus is lined by ciliated columnar epithelium very early in development, and this lining may persist in esophageal cysts. The presence of a definite double layer of smooth muscle surrounding a cyst that does not contain cartilage suggests that the cyst is esophageal in origin[12] (Fig. 24-1C). Neither bronchogenic cysts nor esophageal cysts are associated with other developmental abnormalities.

Gastroenteric Cysts

There are several theories on the derivation of thoracic gastroenteric cysts. The most cogent theory, that of Fallon et al.[14] and Veneklaas,[15] is that the endodermal tube adheres focally to the notochord, to which it is closely approximated. With development and growth of the embryo, a ''traction diverticulum'' forms, which later separates to form a gastroenteric cyst. This theory is attractive because of the constant relationship of these cysts to vertebrae and the high incidence of associated vertebral malformation. Other mechanisms of formation, such as sequestrations of foregut nodules and duplications of the intestinal tract, may be applicable in some cases. There is a low association of thoracic enteric cysts with intra-abdominal enteric cysts.

Gastroenteric cysts are rare. They are often symptomatic since they are lined by any of a variety of types of gastrointestinal mucosa, which may secrete fluid.[16] Acid secretion has been reported, and the cysts have been known to ulcerate and rupture.

Inflammatory Disorders of the Mediastinum

Acute Mediastinitis

Acute infections of the mediastinal soft tissues, most often due to bacteria, may result from trauma, as a complication of thoracic surgery, or by extension from a perforated viscus, such as esophageal perforation. Mediastinitis is a documented complication of odontogenic infections.[17] The infection may remain localized, or it may spread as a diffuse cellulitis, depending on the cause of the infection, type of organism, host factors, and therapy. Acute mediastinitis is a very serious problem clinically. The mortality is high, in part owing to the nature of the underlying processes. The inflammatory response with subsequent repair is not specific histologically.

Granulomatous Mediastinitis

Any of the organisms that ordinarily elicit a granulomatous inflammatory reaction may affect the mediastinum, but histoplasmosis and tuberculosis are most common. The process may be recognized as an asymptomatic radiologic mass, or symptoms and signs referable to involvement of a vital structure may be present.[18] When the inflammatory process does not remain localized but spreads extensively along mediastinal tissue planes, extensive scarring may result. In a series of 47 patients with mediastinal granuloma,[19] the inflammatory process progressed to chronic sclerosing mediastinitis in 12.

Chronic Sclerosing Mediastinitis

In chronic sclerosing mediastinitis there is diffuse replacement of mediastinal connective tissue with densely collagenized, sparsely cellular fibrous tissue (Fig. 24-3). A mild chronic inflammatory component is usually present. The process may infiltrate vital mediastinal structures with resultant functional compromise. In one review, this occurred in 64 of 77 cases (83 percent).[18]

The clinical and radiologic features depend on the structures involved. The most common findings are mediastinal widening and a superior vena cava syndrome.[18,20] Compromise of pulmonary veins or bronchi also may occur.[20]

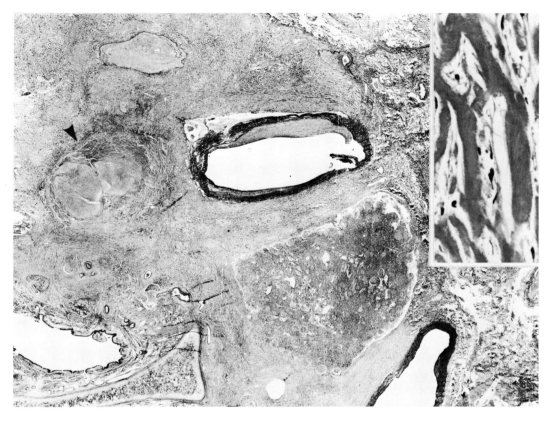

Fig. 24-3. Sclerosing mediastinitis. Dense fibrous connective tissue with scattered chronic inflammatory cells infiltrates bronchus, lung parenchyma, and vessels. Old granuloma is present in the midst of fibrosis (arrowhead). (Inset) Sparsely cellular, densely collagenized connective tissue. Broad bands of collagen are identical to those of a hypertrophic scar (keloid).

In some cases evidence of a coexisting mediastinal granulomatous infection has been apparent (Fig. 24-3). The infection that has been most often documented is histoplasmosis, but other mycoses and tuberculosis can be seen.[19,21,22,23] Some authors have suggested that most, if not all, examples of sclerosing mediastinitis are postinfectious.[20,21]

The pathogenesis of the extensive fibrosis is unclear. Goodwin et al.[22] suggested that the process represents a host response to a continued release of antigens from organisms within a granuloma. Others, noting the morphologic similarity of sclerosing mediastinitis, keloids, retroperitoneal fibrosis, Riedel's thyroiditis, sclerosing cholangitis, sclerosing cervicitis, and orbital pseudotumor,[24] have suggested that all these conditions represent an idiosyncratic abnormality in collagen organization. Descriptions of patients with more than one of these processes provide support for this hypothesis.[24,25] In the case of sclerosing mediastinitis, the stimulus usually is granulomatous inflammation.

Lymph Nodes

Reactive Hyperplasia

Enlargement of mediastinal lymph nodes usually occurs in association with pulmonary infections. The histologic changes are identical to those seen in reactive lymph nodes elsewhere in the body.[26,27] The nodal enlargement is seldom great enough to be of clinical or radiologic significance, and the clinical course is determined by the pulmonary infection.

Giant Lymph Node Hyperplasia

Giant lymph node hyperplasia has been interpreted as a peculiar variety of lymphoid hyperplasia possibly resulting from faulty immune regulation.[28] No specific infectious agents have been identified. Keller et al.[29] found that 129 of 183 cases (71 percent) occurred in the mediastinum. It should be noted, however, that 46 of the 183 cases in this review were from the Pulmonary and Mediastinal Pathology Branch of the Armed Forces Institute of Pathology. Dorfman and Warnke have emphasized the extramediastinal location of identical lesions.[26] In addition to the originally described monocentric form of giant lymph node hyperplasia, a multicentric variant has been described.[28,30,31]

Histologically, the localized form of giant lymph node hyperplasia has been divided into two categories, the hyaline vascular and plasma cell types.[29] In the initial series of monocentric cases, the hyaline vascular type accounted for 74 of 81 cases.[29] The age range was 8 years to 66 years with no sex preference. Eight were extrathoracic. A single mass, 1.5 to 15 cm in greatest dimension, was discovered on routine chest radiographs in 46 patients. In 15 cases there were symptoms due to compression of tracheobronchial structures or chest pain. Systemic manifestations usually were absent. The radiologic appearance of the thoracic lesions was that of a rather well circumscribed, solitary, mediastinal or hilar mass. Clinically, the mass variably simulated a thymoma, a proximal lung tumor, or a neurogenic neoplasm. Complete surgical excision has been curative.

Histologically the hyaline-vascular type of giant lymph node hyperplasia has small lymphoid follicles distributed diffusely throughout the mass (Fig. 24-4). The follicles contain a prominent, central vascular component, often with hyalinization of the vessel walls simulating thymic Hassall's corpuscles. In some cases there is a layering of lymphocytes in a concentric fashion around the small follicles. Usually there is also a striking interfollicular distribution of hyalinized vessels with prominent endothelial cells. A polymorphic cell population of small lymphocytes, plasma cells, immunoblasts, and eosinophils is present between the follicles and the vascular component.

The plasma cell type of giant lymph node hyperplasia, which occurs in a minority of cases, is similar to the hyaline-vascular type in many clinical respects. There were, in some cases, associated systemic manifestations such as anemia, hyperglobulinemia, and fever.[29] Histologically, this type is characterized by sheets of plasma cells distributed between large reactive lymphoid follicles (Fig. 24-5). The follicles may contain proteinaceous material. Although there may be prominent vessels in the interfollicular area, the hyalinized vessels within small follicles generally are absent.

There may be features of both types of giant lymph node hyperplasia in the same mass (Fig. 24-5). All multicentric cases of giant lymph node hyperplasia have been interpreted histologically to be the plasma cell variant. They have been associated with systemic manifestations, as in the monocentric plasma cell type of giant lymph node hyperplasia. The localized and multicentric entities,

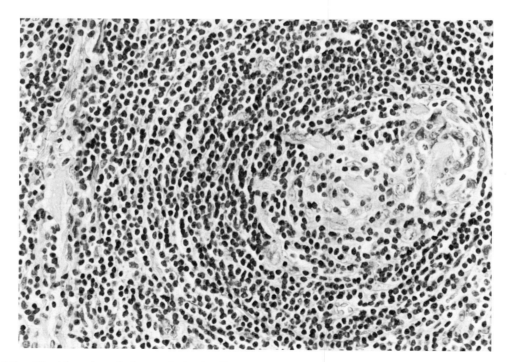

Fig. 24-4. Giant lymph node hyperplasia, hyaline-vascular type. Small reaction centers are surrounded by concentric layers of small lymphocytes. There is marked hyalinization of small vessels, both within the follicle and in the interfollicular region.

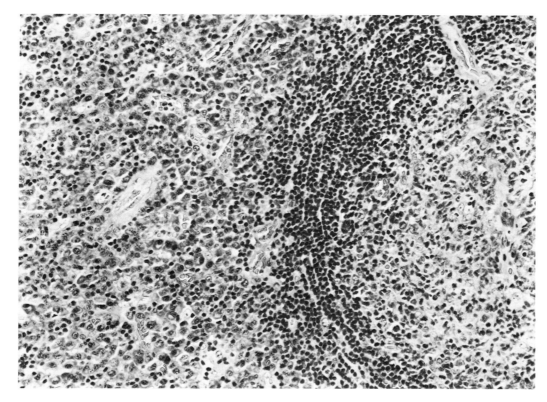

Fig. 24-5. Giant lymph node hyperplasia, plasma cell type. Sheets of plasma cells in interfollicular region. The concentric layering of lymphocytes around the germinal center and hyalinization of vessels are usually absent in this type of giant lymph node hyperplasia.

despite their histologic similarities are, however, different in age distribution, gross appearance, and clinical presentation.[28,30] Importantly, the multicentric type of presentation is frequently associated with an aggressive clinical course and with lymphoid malignancy.[31] It has been suggested that the current concept of giant lymph node hyperplasia is too restrictive, and that a diverse histologic and clinical spectrum exists.[28,32] Most immuno-histochemical studies confirm a reactive nature for both the current subtypes of giant lymph node hyperplasia and even for the aggressive multicentric variants.[31–34] These studies support the concept of an unusual type of immune response.

The hyaline-vascular type, when located in the mediastinum, has been confused with thymoma. There is a superficial resemblance of the hyalinized vessels to Hassall's corpuscles, which are, in fact, uncommon in thymoma.[29] Careful inspection will reveal the absence of keratinizing squamous cells, which constitute Hassall's corpuscles. The polymorphic cell population is not seen in thymoma, and many of the features that characterize thymoma, such as broad connective tissue bands and perivascular spaces,[35] are absent in giant lymph node hyperplasia.

A lymph node partially involved by Hodgkin's disease with residual follicles should be considered in the differential diagnosis. Reed-Sternberg cells are absent in giant lymph node hyperplasia, and the hyalinized vasculature and follicles would be unusual in Hodgkin's disease. The polymorphic cell population and small, hyalinized follicles should allow the exclusion of nodular lymphoma.

The plasma cell type of giant lymph node hyperplasia closely resembles reactive lymph nodes of patients with rheumatoid arthritis, and the clinical features are similar. None of the patients in the series of Keller et al.[29] had evidence of this disease, however. While there is often diffuse adenopathy in rheumatoid arthritis, the formation of a large localized mass is uncommon.

Lymph Node Granulomas

Granulomatous inflammation in mediastinal lymph nodes is often associated with mycobacterial or fungal pulmonary infection, and the clinical course is dominated by the lung involvement. Occasionally the lymph node lesion is predominant. Enlargement of lymph nodes may compromise a bronchus, usually that of the right middle lobe, leading to obstructive pneumonia. Extension of infection from lymph nodes to other mediastinal structures is the usual mode of spread of infection within the thorax, for example, in tuberculous pericarditis. As discussed in the section on inflammatory disorders of the mediastinum, spread of infection from lymph nodes to mediastinal soft tissue is thought to be responsible for at least some cases of chronic sclerosing mediastinitis.

Infectious granulomas in lymph nodes often can be distinguished histologically from those due to sarcoidosis. Unlike granulomas due to identifiable organisms, in sarcoid the granulomas are commonly distributed diffusely through the node, are approximately the same size, are in about the same stage of development, and usually show no necrosis. However, special stains for organisms should be obtained in all cases with granuloma formation. In a patient with strong clinical evidence of sarcoidosis, mediastinal lymph node biopsy by mediastinoscopy usually will contribute to the diagnosis. In one series of 55 patients with sarcoidosis, granulomatous inflammation was documented in 54 by mediastinoscopy.[36]

Metastatic Tumor

The most common of all mediastinal abnormalities is metastatic tumor in mediastinal lymph nodes. The lung is the most common site of primary tumor, but mediastinal lymph nodes may be involved by metastases from any primary site, particularly when the lungs also contain metastatic deposits.

The mediastinal lymph nodes are the most common site of metastases from lung carcinoma. The presence of tumor in lymph nodes is regarded as evidence of nonresectability, since the 4 year survival is less than 10 percent when metastases are present versus 30 to 40 percent when no tumor is found in the mediastinum.[37] At the time of clinical presentation, over 40 percent of the patients with lung carcinoma have demonstrable mediastinal involvement.[37] Scalene lymph node biopsies also are not reliable indicators of resectability.[37]

Mediastinoscopy—direct visual examination and biopsy of mediastinal lymph nodes—has been refined in an attempt to stage patients with lung carcinoma preoperatively. Its use has been proposed in evaluation of all patients with presumed primary tumors of the lung. After a negative examination by mediastinoscopy, only about 3.4 percent of neoplasms are found to be unresectable at subsequent thoracotomy.[38]

In a review of 4,983 cases of lung carcinoma, a positive mediastinoscopic biopsy was obtained in 39 percent.[37] Thus, 61 percent of patients were subjected to two proce-dures—mediastinoscopy and thoracotomy. Attempts to select patients most at risk for mediastinal metastases and to eliminate unnecessary mediastinoscopic proce-dures have established that patients with one or more of the following should undergo mediastinoscopy: central localization of tumors, large lymph nodes radiologically, and laryngeal nerve involvement. The results of mediastinal biopsy were positive in 22 of 27 patients satisfying these criteria. In a group of 27 patients with none of the above findings, 23 of 27 had a negative mediastinoscopic examination.[39]

Mediastinoscopy with biopsy is useful also in establishing a tissue diagnosis before initiation of nonsurgical modes of therapy in patients with both obviously inoperable modes of therapy in patients with both obviously inoperable primary lung carcinoma and metastatic disease from other primary sites. It is also valuable in the case of metastatic breast carcinoma as a means to obtain tissue for receptor assays.[40]

The morphology of metastatic tumor in mediastinal lymph nodes is similar to the appearance of the primary lesion. The presence of anthracosilicotic nodules and scarring or healed granulomatous disease may increase the difficulty in interpretation. The presence of a small number of scattered, usually nonnecrotic granulomas may be a clue to the presence of nearby tumor but, of course, is nonspecific.[41,42]

In general, mediastinoscopic and needle biopsies are not the procedures of choice in the evaluation of mediastinal masses.[43] The small amounts of tissue obtained are often inadequate for accurate diagnosis in these conditions. Furthermore, as will be discussed later, all anterior mediastinal masses, including lymphoma, should be excised as completely as possible. A diagnosis made by biopsy, therefore, does not eliminate the need for thoracotomy. The newer imaging techniques have little impact in assessing these patients, since there is poor correlation between size of lymph nodes and presence of metastases.[43]

THYMUS

Development and Anatomy

Embryologically the thymus is derived from the third and, to a lesser degree, the fourth pairs of pharyngeal pouches. It is primarily an epithelial organ, and the epithelial cords normally descend into the anterior mediastinum and proliferate. The two lobes are joined but not completely fused. By the third month of development the epithelium is infiltrated by lymphocytes and other mesenchymal cells.

The thymus is located both in the thorax and in the neck. Superiorly, each thymic lobe is attached to the thyroid by thyrothymic ligaments. Posteriorly, the thymus is bounded by the trachea superiorly and the pericardium and great vessels within the thorax. The cervical fascia and strap muscles and the sternum are anterior to the thymus in the neck and the thorax, respectively.

Grossly, the thymus is a lobulated pink-tan organ in infancy. With increasing age it acquires a softer consistency and yellow color due to infiltration by adipose tissue. The average weight of the thymus at birth is 15 g. The weight increases with age to an average of 35 g at puberty. After puberty, the quantity of thymic tissue diminishes, but it does not disappear entirely. At age 70 the average weight is 5 g.[44] There is a great deal of variation in weight and shape among individuals, which has led to much confusion about the significance of thymic size in association with other diseases.

During infancy and childhood the thymus is larger relative to the size of the anterior mediastinum than in later life. The thymic shadow is normally seen on chest films. Failure to realize this in the past led to irradiation of the thymus as therapy for respiratory illness in the belief that

thymic enlargement and tracheobronchial compression were responsible. The irradiation has resulted in an increased incidence of thyroid tumors in these patients in later life.[45]

Histologically the normal thymus is divided into small lobules. Each lobule is subdivided into cortex and medulla, and normally this subdivision can be appreciated at low magnification (Fig. 24-6). The main substance of the thymus is composed of epithelial cells and lymphocytes. The epithelial cells are indistinct relative to the lymphoid cells in ordinary hematoxylin and eosin (H&E) sections. This is particularly true in the cortical regions, where there is a higher concentration of lymphoid cells.

The epithelial nature of the background cells of the thymus has been demonstrated by tissue culture,[46] electron microscopy,[47] and immunohistochemistry.[48] Electron microscopic studies of the normal human thymus have shown a bland epithelial-type cell with smooth margins and little interdigitation with adjacent cells. Filopodia are not usually seen. The epithelial cells contain thick cytoplasmic tonofilaments, which extend into desmosomes. A basal lamina is present at all sites of interface of epithelial cells with connective tissue, such as the thymic

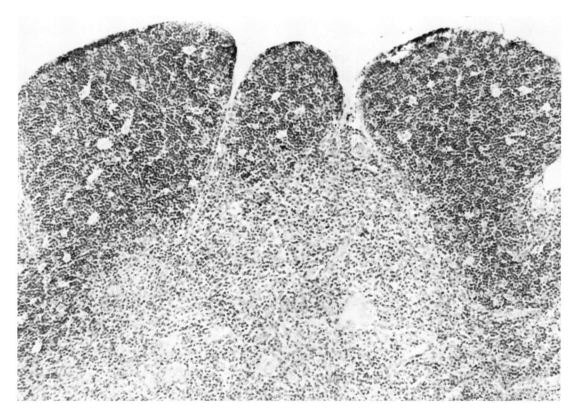

Fig. 24-6. Normal thymus. Lobulation and encapsulation are apparent. The corticomedullary junction is distinct. The cortex contains a greater concentration of lymphocytes, and individually distributed epithelial cells are difficult to discern. The medulla contains fewer lymphocytes, and epithelial cells are present in aggregates and Hassall's corpuscles.

capsule and around blood vessels.[47,48] Differences between cortical and medullary epithelial cells can be seen ultrastructurally.[35] Keratin staining of thymic epithelial cells has been demonstrated by immunohistochemistry.[48–50] In the medulla thymic epithelial cells are more prominent, and they are often arranged in small groups. Squamous differentiation may be obvious, with keratinization in the center of small nests (Hassall's corpuscles).

Normal thymic epithelial cells are in close contact with thymic lymphoid cells and are believed to be responsible for the production of thymic hormones[51,52] and maturation of thymic lymphoid cells.[35,53,54] The immunohistochemical characteristics of normal thymic epithelial cells vary with cortical or medullary location.[51,55,56]

The lymphocytes in the normal thymus are thought to originate from bone marrow precursors. They undergo a maturation process in the thymus from cortex to medulla, presumably influenced by the surrounding cellular environment. The surface markers of all thymic lymphoid cells are distinct from the surface markers of similar T-cells in the peripheral lymphoid tissue.[57] They are designated *thymocytes* or immature T-lymphocytes.[57,58] The surface markers of thymocytes differ according to cortical or medullary location within the normal thymus.[53,56,58] The relatively more mature medullary thymocytes have some surface markers in common with peripheral T-cells.[53] The classification of surface markers on epithelial cells and thymocytes promotes understanding of the role of the thymus in normal and abnormal immune states and in neoplastic conditions.

Developmental Abnormalities

Failure of Descent

Because of failure of descent into the mediastinum, the entire thymus, one lobe, or variable portions of a lobe may remain in a cervical location and may present as a cervical mass.[59,60] Any of the thymic abnormalities to be discussed may occur in the neck. Thymic tissue in the neck is often associated with a parathyroid gland. Hassall's corpuscles within such "ectopic" thymic tissue may be confused with metastatic squamous cell carcinoma on frozen section.

Thymic Cysts

Thymic cysts result from failure of obliteration of the thymopharyngeal duct during development.[61–64] They may occur anywhere along a line from the angle of the jaw to the midline of the neck and in the anterior mediastinum.[61] These lesions usually are not detected until later in life as a result of gradual enlargement. The enlargement occurs because of accumulation of secretions pro-

duced by the lining epithelium or because of secondary changes such as hemorrhage or seepage of plasma into the cyst lumen.

Although cysts are more common in the mediastinum, cysts in the cervical region are more likely to result in a mass lesion or to manifest symptoms of compression.[62] Thymic cysts in the mediastinum are often asymptomatic and are found incidentally on chest films or at autopsy.

Cysts may be unilocular or multilocular and contain serous or hemorrhagic fluid. Small quantities of necrotic debris may be present. The lining epithelium is variable and may be squamous, columnar, or cuboidal. A mixture of cell types is present in some cases. The lining may be partially or entirely absent as a result of hemorrhage, degeneration, and cholesterol granulomas. Thymic tissue is often separated from the cyst by a thick fibrous capsule.[62]

There may be a large cystic component in thymomas and in occasional cases of other tumors involving the thymus. A careful search for solid, nodular areas in the wall of thymic cysts is necessary to exclude this possibility.

Diffusely enlarged and cystic Hassall's corpuscles have been recorded in the past as an indication of congenital syphilis (DuBois' abscesses). They are not specific, however, and are seen also as an incidental finding at autopsy.

Immunodeficiency Diseases

Significant changes are seen in the thymus in numerous conditions involving T-cell immunodeficiencies (Table 24-2). The conditions are heterogeneous and predominantly congenital, and most of them include other disorders. The thymus may be absent (*aplasia*) or markedly reduced in size (*hypoplasia*). In many T-cell immunodeficiencies the thymus is small and composed of spindled

TABLE 24-2. T Cell Immunodeficiency Diseases and the Thymus

Syndrome	Thymus
Severe combined immunodeficiency syndrome	Dysplasia
Nezelof's disease	Dysplasia
Immunodeficiency with nucleoside phosphorylase deficiency	Involution
DiGeorge's syndrome	Aplasia
DiGeorge's syndrome (incomplete form)	Hypoplasia, precocious involution
Ataxia-telangiectasia	Dysplasia or aplasia
Wiskott-Aldrich syndrome	Involution or normal
Chronic mucocutaneous candidiasis	Involution
Acquired immune deficiency syndrome (AIDS)	Dysplasia

epithelial cells and only rare lymphocytes and rare or absent Hassall's corpuscles, with an indistinct cortico-medullary junction (*dysplasia*) (Fig. 24-7). In some conditions the thymus shows histologic evidence of involution.

It is not usual for the morphology or the immunologic function of the thymus to be altered in the many disorders of the B-cell system.[65]

Acquired immune deficiency syndrome (AIDS) has been associated with a dysplastic appearance.[65] There is evidence for a direct viral effect on the thymus in acquired immunodeficiency.[66] The distinction between neonatal acquired immunodeficiency and other congenital immunodeficiency syndromes can be made on the basis of serologic information.

In the DiGeorge syndrome the thymus is absent or extremely small. Numerous sections of mediastinal and cervical connective tissue may be necessary to detect thymic tissue which, if present, is morphologically normal.[35,67]

In the combined immunodeficiency diseases associated with adenosine deaminase deficiency, the thymus is normal but appears to have undergone involution.[68]

Monoclonal antibody studies, which have made it possible to distinguish stages of T-cell maturation, have been used to study some immunodeficiency diseases as diseases of variable differentiation arrest.[65] Bone marrow or thymic transplantation has been used to restore immunologic competence in small numbers of patients with immune deficiency diseases.[69–71]

Involution

Acute Involution

Acute, or stress, involution of the thymus involves a reduction in thymic mass, most commonly associated with severe illness.[72] This results from secretion of adrenal corticosteroids, which have a lymphocytolytic effect. Steroid therapy can produce the same effect, as can irradiation. A "starry-sky" appearance, particularly in the cortex, results from necrosis of lymphocytes and phagocytosis of cell debris (Fig. 24-8). Loss of corticomedullary distinction and fibrosis may result, especially in the irradiated thymus. These changes may be seen at any age

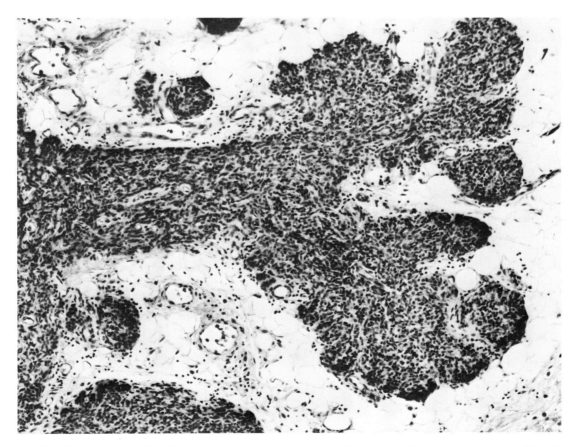

Fig. 24-7. Thymic dysplasia. Absence of corticomedullary zonation, markedly reduced number of lymphocytes, and spindled epithelial cells. Hassall's corpuscles are absent.

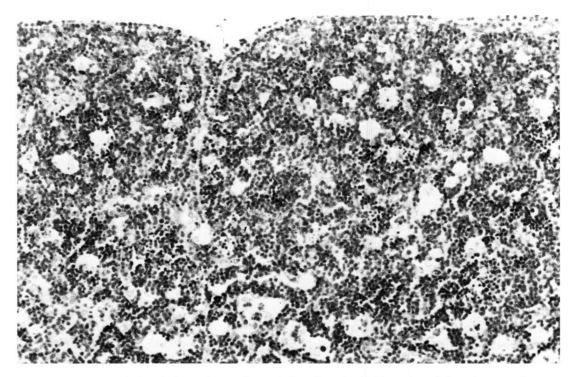

Fig. 24-8. Acute thymic involution. The corticomedullary junction is blurred, and there is extensive necrosis of thymic lymphocytes. "Starry-sky" appearance results from macrophages with phagocytized cell debris.

but are most obvious in young patients, before marked age involution has occurred. Acute involution usually is an incidental autopsy finding, and its significance is uncertain.

Age Involution

The quantity of thymic tissue gradually diminishes with time as a result of loss of lymphocytes. The cortex is thin, epithelial cells may be spindled, and Hassall's corpuscles are cystic or calcified. There is replacement by mature adipose tissue. Only scattered small nests of thymic tissue, difficult to identify, remain. Although the phenotypic involution of lymphocytes has been detailed, its impact on the immune system is not understood.[73]

Thymic Hyperplasia

Follicular Hyperplasia

Hyperplasia, as it refers generally to an increased number of cells in a given organ or portion of the organ, is rare in the thymus. The term *thymic hyperplasia* is used in practice to mean the presence of germinal centers in the medullary area of the thymus. The thymus usually is normal in size and may be small.

The presence of follicular hyperplasia historically has been associated with diseases of presumed autoimmune etiologies. The association is strongest for myasthenia gravis; about 65 percent of patients with this disease have thymic germinal centers.[74–76] Thymic follicles have also been described in patients with systemic lupus erythematosus, scleroderma, rheumatoid arthritis, thyrotoxicosis, and Addison's disease.[35]

The association of follicular hyperplasia with immune disorders must be viewed with caution. It was once assumed that germinal centers normally do not occur in the thymus.[75] It is now clear that the incidence of follicles is dependent on the case population studied. Illness and stress appear to result in disappearance of the follicles.[77] The incidence of follicles is less than 10 percent in routine autopsy studies, but thymic follicles are found in 51 percent of the patients who die suddenly and accidentally.[78] The incidence of germinal centers also was shown to be related to the duration of illness before death.[78] Several authors have noted, however, that the size of the germinal centers is larger in patients with myasthenia gravis than in unaffected persons.[77,78]

In follicular hyperplasia, the germinal centers vary somewhat in number and size. They may be present diffusely, or only occasional follicles may be seen. They involve the thymic medulla exclusively, with expansion of the medulla and compression of the overlying cortex. The germinal centers are morphologically and histochemically identical to the follicles of lymph nodes.[79] Thymic epithelial cells are absent.[79,80]

The germinal centers are composed of cells revealing B cell differentiation.[81] This seems paradoxical in view of the T cell nature of the thymus. However, Tamaoki et al.[79] and Levine and Bearman[80] have shown by electron microscopy that the follicles are located in the perivascular space of the thymus. Thus, they are separated from the true thymic parenchyma by the epithelial basal lamina.

The significance of the association between thymic follicular hyperplasia and myasthenia gravis is discussed subsequently.

True Thymic Hyperplasia

Rare instances of apparent true thymic hyperplasia in children have been reported.[82,83] The thymuses of these patients were markedly enlarged (224 and 420 g), but morphologically they were unremarkable. Peripheral lymphocytosis was present in both cases. The latter resolved, and the patients did well after thymectomy.

True thymic hyperplasia also has been described in association with diffuse thyroid hyperplasia (Graves' disease). Its significance is unknown.

Myasthenia Gravis

Myasthenia gravis is a neuromuscular disease characterized by skeletal muscle weakness that increases in severity with increased activity. The disease process is mediated by autoantibodies to acetylcholine receptors of muscle.[84] The thymus is normal in approximately 25 percent of patients with myasthenia gravis. There is follicular hyperplasia of the thymus in 65 percent and thymoma in 10 percent.[76] Despite the fact that myasthenia gravis is a particularly well characterized disease immunologically, the exact role of the thymus is poorly understood. The relationship of thymic hyperplasia and increased B-cells in germinal centers to the presence of autoantibodies to acetylcholine receptors is obscure.[85] In patients with thymoma and myasthenia gravis there are invariably antibodies to striated muscle.[86,87] These antibodies cross-react with surface receptors on the epithelial cells of thymomas but not with normal thymic epithelial cells. Monoclonal antibody studies are being used to study the role of T-cells and epithelial cells in the development of autoantibodies.[85,86]

Thymectomy retains an important role in the therapy of myasthenia gravis in spite of the wide use of corticosteroids, the increase in use of cytotoxic agents, and the use of plasmapheresis. A decrease in antibodies to acetylcholine receptors occurs in a significant number of patients after thymectomy.[85] The response to surgery in patients without thymoma is particularly good; about 30 percent experience complete remission and another 30 percent are improved.[88]

Thymoma

Although the term thymoma means "tumor of the thymus," these tumors are considered to be neoplasms of the epithelial component. The lymphoid component is regarded as secondary. The neoplastic thymic epithelial cells recapitulate immunohistochemically the nature of normal thymic epithelial cells,[89,95–99] with some minor differences. The epithelial cells may be either of cortical or medullary type or both.[52,89,97,99] Analysis of the cortical or medullary epithelial surface markers has been studied in relation to clinical course.[97,99] Currently, clinical and macroscopic features appear to provide more uniformly accepted indicators of prognosis than do phenotypic classification of epithelial cells.[99] The epithelial cells of thymoma may also stain for the presence of thymosin.[100] Neoplasms that arise in or involve the thymus but are not composed of thymic epithelial cells should be recognized and separated because of their greatly different biologic behavior. Terms such as *granulomatous thymoma* (for Hodgkin's disease involving the thymus) and *seminomatous thymoma* (for anterior mediastinal germinoma) should be abandoned.

The T-cell origin of the lymphocytic component of thymomas has been documented, and these cells are thymocytes cytochemically, as opposed to mature T-cells.[52,89–94] The thymocytes are variably cortical or medullary in type.[92] The cortical or medullary subclassification of thymocytes has not been shown conclusively to relate to prognosis or clinical features of thymomas.

About 2 percent of thymomas arise in a cervical location,[101,102] and thymomas have been described in association with thyroid tissue.[103] A peculiar variant of thymoma with hamartomatous elements has been described in supraclavicular and suprasternal locations.[104,105] This variant exhibits a mixed histologic pattern, which includes spindled epithelial elements, epithelial islands, adipose tissue, and lymphocytes. Immunoperoxidase stains can help distinguish these ectopic thymomas from other lesions that occur in this location,[103,104] and the electron microscopic appearance is consistent with the usual thymoma.[101,104]

Thymoma is the most common primary tumor of the anterior mediastinum. Anecdotal reports of thymoma in siblings exist.[106,107] The median age at the time of detection is 50 years,[108] thymoma is rare in children.[109] The

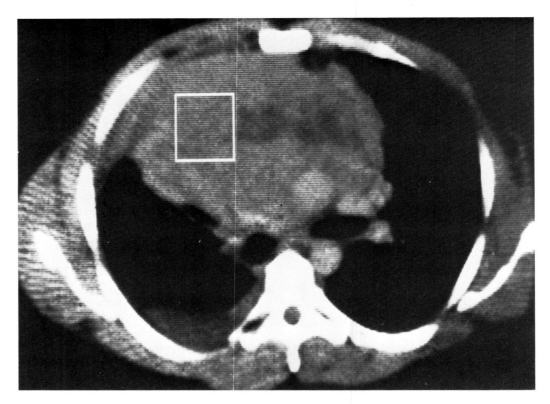

Fig. 24-9. Large anterior mediastinal mass demonstrated by CT scanning. Lesion is a thymoma.

majority of thymomas are asymptomatic and are incidental findings on chest films. About 2 percent arise in a cervical location. They may result in a variety of symptoms due to compression or invasion of adjacent mediastinal structures. Some patients seek medical attention because of symptoms of an associated syndrome such as myasthenia gravis.[35,108,110–112]

Radiologically, the appearance of a thymoma is not distinctive. The tumors tend to be somewhat lobulated and may show calcification, especially peripherally.[35] They may be apparent only on lateral views. Occasionally, small thymomas are inapparent on radiographs and are incidental findings following thymectomy for myasthenia gravis. They usually are obvious when CT techniques are used (Fig. 24-9).

The gross appearance of thymomas may be quite distinctive.[110,111] They are characteristically nodular, with varying sized lobules of gray or tan tissue separated by broad bands of firm connective tissue (Fig. 24-10). Grossly apparent cysts with amber or dark red fluid are present in about 50 percent of cases. There are often small foci of hemorrhage or necrosis. Most thymomas range between 5 and 10 cm in greatest dimension, although much larger lesions have been reported.[35] A small rim of nonneoplastic thymus may be identified at the tu-

mor periphery. This should be examined histologically, especially if an associated syndrome exists, to detect follicular hyperplasia. Most thymomas are surrounded by a dense fibrous capsule.

Architecturally, thymomas almost always are divided into varying sized lobules by fibrous septa that are continuous with the capsule (Fig. 24-11). The lobules are well

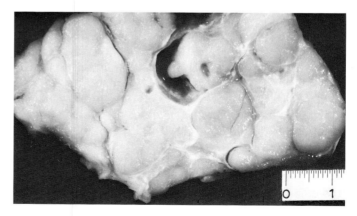

Fig. 24-10. Thymoma, with variable-sized lobules divided by fibrous septa. Cysts are often present.

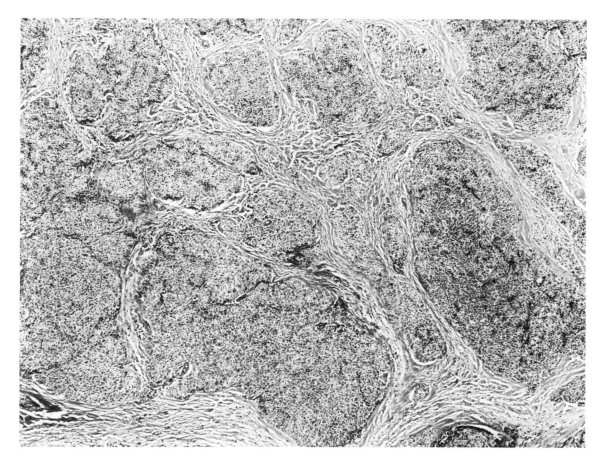

Fig. 24-11. Thymoma, tumor lobules of variable sized divided by prominent fibrous septa.

demarcated and usually angular. The septal connective tissue does not extend into the lobules of tumor. A mottled appearance on low magnification results from variable numbers of lymphocytes in different areas of a thymoma. This appearance has been termed *medullary differentiation,* since areas with fewer lymphocytes and more prominent epithelial cells are reminiscent of the normal thymic medulla[35,113] (Fig. 24-12). A characteristic of about 50 percent of thymomas is the presence of dilated perivascular spaces[35] (Fig. 24-13). These may reach cyst-like proportions. Plasma and lymphocytes often are apparent in the dilated spaces. Organization of the spaces with hyalinization may be prominent.

Cytologically, the identification of thymomas rests on the recognition of the variable appearance of the epithelial cells. In tumors in which lymphocytes predominate, epithelial cells are individually distributed and have a histiocytic appearance, recapitulating the histology of normal thymic cortex (Fig. 24-14). In tumors in which lymphocytes are few, the epithelial cells often are arranged in sheets and nests of cohesive cells with a squamoid appearance, reminiscent of the normal thymic medulla (Fig. 24-15). Formation of Hassall's corpuscles and keratinization, however, are unusual. A morphologic spectrum exists between the extremes of lymphocyte predominance, with few epithelial cells, and epithelial predominance, with few lymphocytes (Fig. 24-16). Different areas of the same thymoma may have markedly different appearances.

The epithelial cells of many thymomas show a variable extent of cytoplasmic elongation, or spindling. However, in only a small number of tumors is epithelial spindling the predominant pattern (Fig. 24-17). The formation of isolated glandular spaces or of pseudorosettes by the epithelium also is seen occasionally (Fig. 24-18).

Nuclear atypia, necrosis, and mitoses in the epithelial cells are uncommon in conventional thymomas.[35,101,104] The lymphocytes may be small and normal in appearance. However, atypical lymphocytes and numerous mitoses are not unusual[35,113] (Fig. 24-14). A "starry-sky"

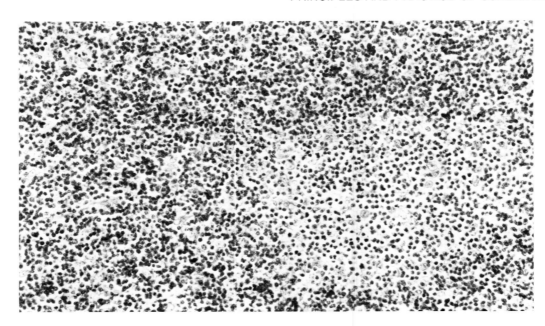

Fig. 24-12. Thymoma, with "medullary differentiation." Lighter-stained zone is similar to normal thymic medulla with few lymphocytes and more prominent aggregates of epithelial cells in these foci.

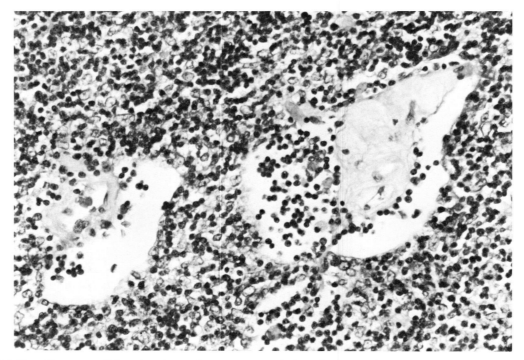

Fig. 24-13. Thymoma. Dilated perivascular spaces contain lymphocytes. The spaces often contain proteinaceous material, which may organize with resulting hyalinization, as in the perivascular space on the right.

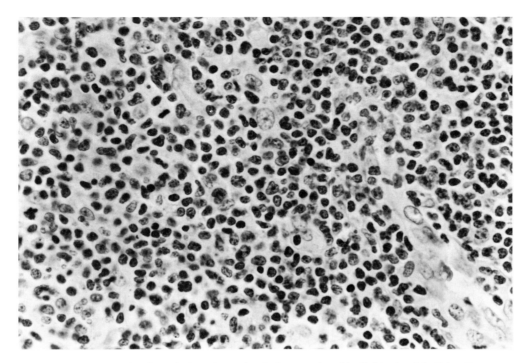

Fig. 24-14. Thymoma, predominantly lymphocytic. Only occasional individual epithelial cells are present in a background of lymphocytes. The lymphocytes may be small and round or appear reactive. There may be lymphocytes in mitosis, and distinction from lymphocytic lymphoma may be difficult.

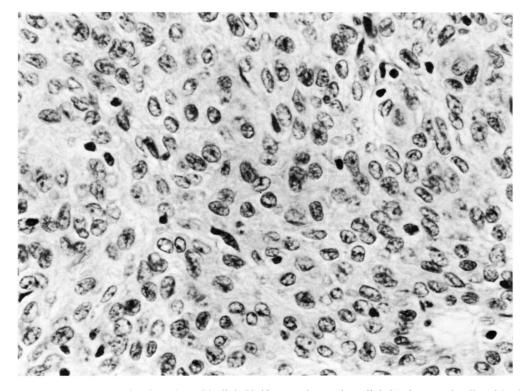

Fig. 24-15. Thymoma, predominantly epithelial. Uniform polygonal to slightly elongated cells with obvious epithelial features and only rare lymphocytes.

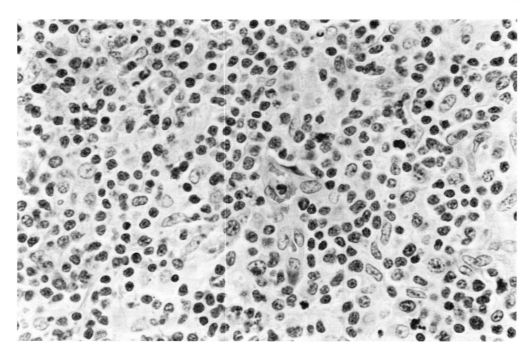

Fig. 24-16. Thymoma with approximately equal mixture of epithelial cells and lymphocytes. The epithelial cells have histiocytoid appearance and are present individually and in small groups.

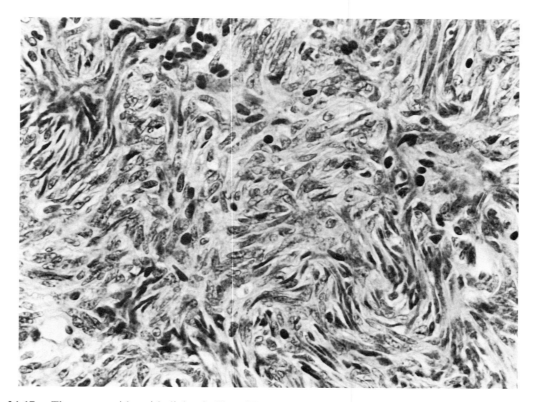

Fig. 24-17. Thymoma with epithelial spindling. Note scattered lymphocytes. Cells have elongated, bland nuclei and indistinct cytoplasmic margins. Small foci of spindled epithelium are quite common; predominantly spindled neoplasms are unusual.

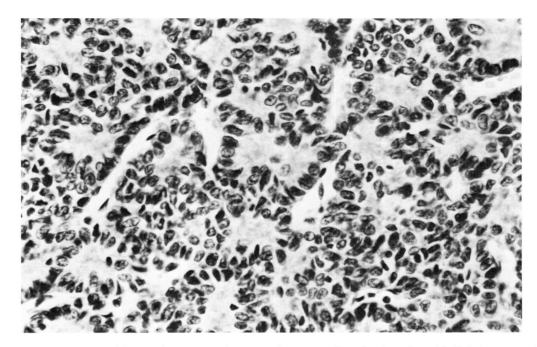

Fig. 24-18. Thymoma with pseudorosettes. An unusual pattern of predominantly epithelial thymoma. Nuclei are at periphery, and cytoplasmic processes occupy the center of the pseudorossettes. In contrast to carcinoid tumors, no lumen is formed. Compare with Fig. 24-21. This pattern usually is admixed with more common architectural varieties of thymoma.

appearance may even result from the phagocytosis by macrophages of cell debris resulting from increased lymphocyte turnover.

The usual classification of thymomas, based on the proportion of lymphocytes and on the arrangement of the epithelial component,[111] emphasizes the wide morphologic spectrum that exists in thymomas, but it correlates poorly with the variable natural history of these lesions. With the exception of the rare thymic carcinoma (see the following section), the local aggressiveness, the ability to metastasize, and the existence of associated syndromes cannot be predicted on histologic grounds.[108]

Invasion beyond the tumor capsule into adjacent mediastinal structures is the most important anatomic prognostic factor. It is present at the time of surgery in 10 to 50 percent of patients with thymoma.[35,106,108,114,115] The presence or absence of invasion is best documented by the surgeon. Metastases of conventional thymomas outside the thorax are rare, but undoubted examples have been reported.[116,117] Immunoperoxidase stains may help distinguish metastatic thymoma from other diagnostic possibilities.[116] Conventional thymomas that are locally invasive or metastatic are histologically indistinguishable from benign ''encapsulated'' thymomas and are classified as malignant because of their behavior.[35,108,116]

The course even of invasive tumors usually is slow, and patients may live with tumor for many years. Mor-

bidity and mortality result from invasion of vital mediastinal structures. Complete surgical excision is the treatment of choice for all thymomas. Recurrence after excision of an encapsulated tumor is rare, and no further therapy is necessary.[115,118–120] Radiotherapy has been successful in the control of invasive tumors in some cases.[121]

A number of diseases are associated with thymoma in a greater than expected incidence[112] (Table 24-3). About 10 percent of patients with myasthenia gravis have a thymoma. These tumors do not differ from those unassociated with myasthenia,[108,110] although their average size is somewhat smaller, and predominantly spindled thymomas are unusual in patients with myasthenia gravis.[35,74]

A thymoma is present in about 50 percent of patients with red cell hypoplasia. Most often the thymoma is of

TABLE 24-3. Syndromes Associated with Thymoma

Myasthenia gravis
Erythroid hypoplasia
Hypogammaglobulinemia
Myocarditis
Polymyositis
Rheumatoid arthritis
Systemic lupus erythematosus
Adrenal atrophy
Pemphigus vulgaris
Chronic mucocutaneous candidiasis

the predominantly spindled type, but there are no other morphologic correlates. Erythroid hypoplasia may be accompanied by reduced platelets and/or granulocytic elements. The red cell hypoplasia is seldom cured by tumor removal.[122]

The other listed diseases are less common, but some of them, especially acquired hypogammaglobulinemia, polymyositis, myocarditis, and systemic lupus erythematosus, have been associated with thymoma often enough to suggest a relationship.[112] The pathogenesis of these disorders and of their association with thymoma is unknown, but abnormal immune mechanisms are regarded as most likely.

The most important prognostic factors for thymoma are the presence or absence of tumor invasion and the presence or absence of associated disease. All patients with a noninvasive thymoma who did not have myasthenia gravis were cured, whereas there are few 10 year survivors in patients with invasive tumors and myasthenia gravis.[123] The 10 year cumulative survival rates for patients with a thymoma with and without myasthenia gravis were 32 and 67 percent, respectively, in the Massachusetts General Hospital series.[123] These data are in close agreement with the survival figures in a series from The Johns Hopkins Hospital, in which all associated diseases were included.[108]

Histologically, thymomas may resemble a number of other neoplasms. Predominantly lymphocytic thymoma can be confused with lymphocytic lymphoma. The lymphocytic component in thymoma does not have the monotonously and uniformly atypical features with nuclear clefts found in poorly differentiated lymphocytic lymphoma. Scattered individual epithelial cells can be found even in predominantly lymphocytic thymomas. They may be recognized most easily at the periphery of lobules adjacent to the fibrous septa. Electron microscopic demonstration of cytoplasmic tonofilaments or desmosomes in the epithelial component may be helpful in occasional cases to exclude lymphoma with certainty, particularly well differentiated lymphocytic lymphoma. Primary mediastinal involvement by the latter is unusual, however.

Predominantly spindled thymomas may be very difficult to distinguish from fibrous mesothelioma. The presence of a lymphocytic component and other features of thymoma may allow distinction, but electron microscopy may be necessary in some cases.

Electron microscopy[48,125] also may be required to distinguish between histiocytic (large cell lymphocytic) lymphoma and undifferentiated carcinoma, a situation that also exists in evaluation of nasopharyngeal tumors. Immunoperoxidase stains for keratin will highlight the epithelial nature of thymomas.[48,123,124]

The criteria for differentiating thymoma from thymic carcinoid tumors are presented later.

The difficulty of histologic differential diagnosis in many cases has important implications. Surgical exploration, rather than needle biopsy or other limited procedure, is preferred to obtain sufficient material for accurate diagnosis. Since surgical excision, as far as is possible, is indicated for all anterior mediastinal tumors, needle biopsy has no advantage in the operable patient in most instances. Anterior mediastinal tumors should be thoroughly sampled, and, in anticipation of diagnostic difficulty, tissue should be frozen and retained for immunoperoxidase studies and fixed for electron microscopy.

Thymic Carcinoma

Rare thymomas are composed partially or entirely of cytologically malignant epithelial cells, and these tumors are separately classified as thymic carcinomas.[35,113,126,127] In these cases there are nuclear pleomorphism, mitotic activity, and nuclear alterations that satisfy classical cytologic criteria for malignant neoplasms. These tumors may show squamous differentiation (Fig. 24-19) and may contain clear cells reminiscent of renal cell carcinoma. The lesions may be undifferentiated or sarcomatoid,[126] or they may resemble nasopharyngeal carcinoma (lymphoepithelioma) (Fig. 24-20) or may be identical to small cell anaplastic carcinoma of the lung. The last is discussed further under thymic carcinoid tumors. Obviously, a diagnosis of primary thymic carcinoma should be made only after exclusion of other primary sites, particularly the lung. Thymic carcinomas are more likely to be invasive than conventional thymomas, but curative resection has been accomplished in some cases.[113] They have a marked propensity for widespread metastasis.[126] The lymphoepithelioma-like thymic carcinoma has been associated with Epstein-Barr virus, a finding that supports the similarity of this lesion to the lesion that occurs in the nasopharynx.[126–128]

Thymic Carcinoid Tumor

Originally regarded as a peculiar type of thymoma, it is now recognized that neoplasms that are morphologically similar to carcinoid tumors elsewhere in the body occur as primary tumors in the thymus.[129–131] Their cellular differentiation is similar to that of Kulchitsky cells, which are present in the normal thymus of animals and humans. Thymic carcinoid tumors should be distinguished from true thymomas because of their morphologic features, functional attributes, and natural history.[35,129–131]

These neoplasms occur almost exclusively in adults, with 43 the median age.[129] The tumor may be detected

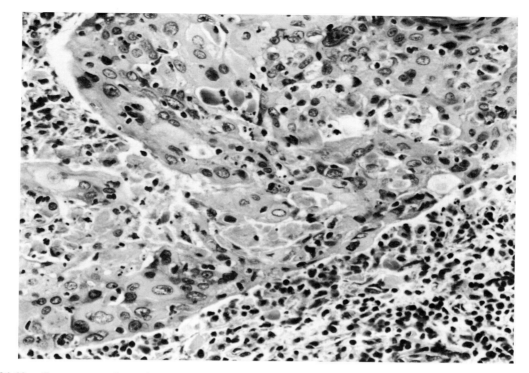

Fig. 24-19. Squamous cell carcinoma of thymus. Rarely, primary thymic neoplasms are cytologically malignant and show squamous differentiation. Squamous cell carcinoma metastatic to the mediastinum is much more common and must be excluded on clinical grounds.

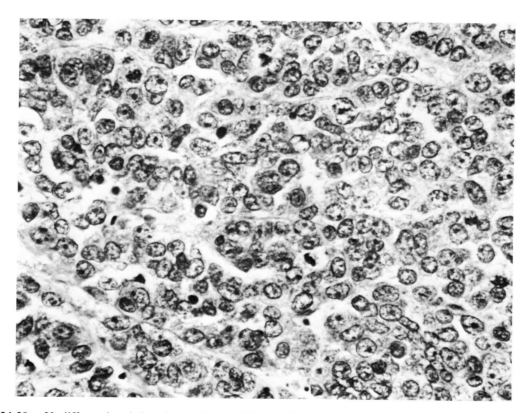

Fig. 24-20. Undifferentiated thymic carcinoma. Sheets of large cells, often with a syncytial appearance, necrosis and numerous mitoses. There may be an admixture of lymphocytes. These neoplasms are identical to undifferentiated nasopharyngeal carcinoma and must be distinguished from "histiocytic" lymphoma. Undifferentiated carcinoma metastic to the mediastinum is much more common than primary thymic carcinoma.

incidentally on a chest film, may result in symptoms due to compression of mediastinal structures, or may lead to abnormal endocrinologic features. Other than evident hormone secretion, there are no specific clinical or radiologic characteristics of thymic carcinoid tumors.

About 34 percent of the patients with thymic carcinoid tumors have had Cushing's syndrome.[130,131] Originally it was thought that this association was present in patients with epithelial thymomas. It is now clear that Cushing's syndrome is present only in patients with thymic carcinoid tumors, not conventional thymomas. Corticotropin has been demonstrated chemically in some cases.[131] In patients with recurrent and/or metastatic tumors associated with Cushing's syndrome, the latter may dominate the clinical course. Approximately 15 percent of the patients have had thymic carcinoid tumors as a part of the type 1 multiple endocrine neoplasia syndrome.[129,131]

Thymic carcinoid tumors manifest as rounded, usually well-circumscribed mass lesions on chest radiographs. Small flecks of calcification are common, but the peripheral rim of mineralization occasionally seen in the capsule of thymomas is not evident. The tumors tend to be large with an average greatest dimension of 11 cm.[132] The tumors are composed of fleshy pink-tan tissue and often have foci of hemorrhage and necrosis. The broad fibrous septa that are typical of thymomas are absent. Rosai et al.[132] have suggested grading these tumors based on their degree of differentiation. Some thymic carcinoid tumors share many similarities with carcinoid tumors of other sites. The tumors are composed of moderately small round cells with clear to granular eosinophilic cytoplasm. The nuclei contain coarsely clumped chromatin. Nucleoli are not prominent, and there is little variation in cell or nuclear size and shape. The cells are set in a vascular stroma with foci of erythrocyte extravasation. Fine fibrovascular septa divide rather large groups of cells into nests, cords, and ribbons. Rosette or gland formation with central lumina is common. Mitotic activity is minimal, and necrosis is absent. Argyrophilia, but not argentaffinity, is present in occasional cells. Such thymic carcinoid tumors are described as grade 1 by Rosai et al.[132] (Fig. 24-21).

Most thymic carcinoid tumors, however, closely resemble the atypical carcinoid tumor of the lung. Mitoses, often exceeding 10 per 10 high-power fields, mild pleomorphism, and necrosis, often in the center of large nests and with dystrophic calcification, are the rule. Cytologically there may be nuclear enlargement and cellular pleomorphism. The majority of thymic carcinoid tumors share these features and are considered grade II by Rosai et al. (Fig. 24-22).

Neoplasms with the unusual features that carcinoid tumors from other sites may exhibit also have been described. Spindled carcinoids[133] and carcinoid tumors with

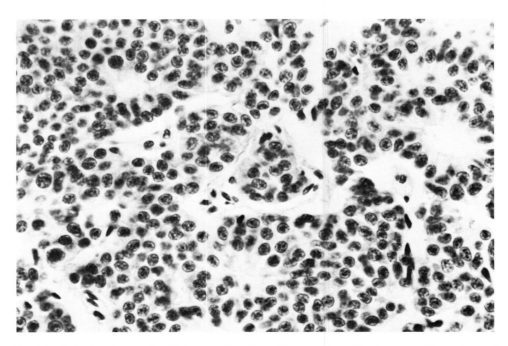

Fig. 24-21. Typical thymic carcinoid tumor. Small, uniform cells with "peppered" nuclear chromatin pattern are arranged in ribbons and rosettes. No true lumina are formed in the rosettes, in contrast to thymoma with pseudorosettes (see Fig. 24-18).

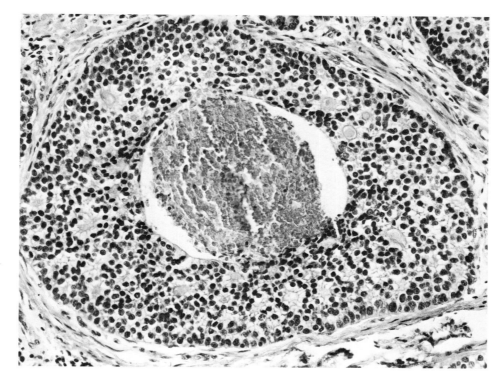

Fig. 24-22. Atypical thymic carcinoid tumor. Necrosis, often in the center of cell nests, is present. The necrosis, scattered mitoses, and a variable degree of pleomorphism characterize atypical carcinoid tumors.

focal squamous metaplasia[132] are examples. It is to be expected that lesions with osteoid formation or glandular differentiation with mucin production also will be described. Thymic spindled tumors with amyloid stroma and calcitonin production[134] reflect capacity for differentiation like that of thyroid medullary carcinoma and the presence in the normal thymus of C cells.[132]

The functional and ultrastructural similarities between bronchial carcinoid tumor and small cell anaplastic carcinoma of the lung are present also in the thymus. Because of the common occurrence of extensive mediastinal metastases of bronchial small cell carcinoma, it is very difficult to prove a thymic origin for such a tumor. However, there appear to be rare examples of primary small cell carcinoma of the thymus in which a bronchial origin has been excluded convincingly.[132] Such neoplasms occupy one end of the morphologic spectrum in the schema of Rosai et al.[132] (grade III carcinoid tumors). They are identical histologically to oat cell carcinoma in the lung (Fig. 24-23). It should be remembered that small cell anaplastic carcinomas may retain the capacity for cellular organization, with formation of ribbons, nests, and rosettes.

Ultrastructurally, thymic carcinoids, regardless of the degree of differentiation, are identical to other foregut

carcinoids. There are intracytoplasmic dense core granules, which are small, round, and uniform in size and shape. Desmosomes are infrequent and tonofilaments are absent. The treatment of thymic carcinoid tumors is primarily surgical. Postoperative irradiation also should be considered, particularly if gross invasion is observed at surgery. Radiotherapy has been successful as a palliative measure in some patients.[124]

Thymic carcinoid tumors are more aggressive than conventional thymomas. In about two thirds of the cases, invasion was present initially or the lesions recurred. Distant metastases developed in approximately 30 percent.[129,131] Although they usually are slow-growing, the invasive neoplasms result in death, often after several years, due to involvement of critical mediastinal structures.

There are a number of clinical and morphologic differences that distinguish conventional thymomas from thymic carcinoid tumors[129] (Table 24-4). Cushing's syndrome occurs only in association with the latter, and immunoperoxidase staining has shown corticotropin to be associated with carcinoid tumor cells.[131] Myasthenia gravis, red cell hypoplasia, and other thymoma-related diseases have not been described in patients with thymic

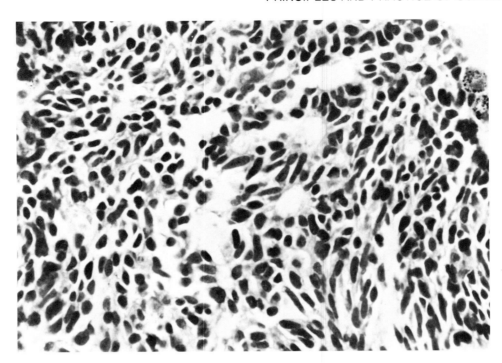

Fig. 24-23. Small cell anaplastic carcinoma of thymus. The tumor is identical in appearance to small cell carcinoma of the lung, which must be distinguished on clinical grounds. An endocrine-like pattern with rosette formation is common in these neoplasms.

carcinoid tumor. Complete resection of carcinoid tumors always is curative of the syndrome; this is not the case with thymoma-related diseases, which may appear even after tumor removal.[108,135,136] It is also apparent that a much more ominous prognosis obtains for patients with thymic carcinoid tumors.

There is usually little difficulty in differentiating thymomas from thymic carcinoid tumors by light microscopy. The thick fibrous septa, cystic perivascular spaces, and biphasic population of epithelial cells and lympho-

cytes are absent in carcinoid tumors. The pseudorosettes in thymomas lack true central spaces, unlike the rosettes of carcinoid tumors (compare Figs. 24-18 and 24-21). Predominantly spindled thymomas may be confused with spindled carcinoids. However, in the former other features of conventional thymomas usually are present, mitoses are rare, nuclear chromatin is finely dispersed, and cytoplasmic boundaries are indistinct.[132] Carcinoid tumors will usually stain positively with neuron-specific enolase.[124] Carcinoid tumors may stain positively with low molecular weight keratin stains, but they are negative for high molecular weight or mixed keratin stains, unlike thymomas.[124] Electron microscopic examination may be necessary for differential diagnosis in rare instances.

Other entities that may be confused with thymic carcinoid are separable easily on clinical or morphologic grounds. Ectopic parathyroid adenoma is almost always responsible for chemically detectable hypercalcemia. The small groups of rather large cells (''Zellballen'') that characterize paraganglioma are absent in carcinoid tumors. Metastatic bronchial carcinoid or islet cell tumor in the anterior mediastinum in the absence of evidence of tumor at the primary site is very unusual. As noted earlier, it is not possible to distinguish small cell anaplastic carcinoma that is primary in the lung from that primary in the thymus.

TABLE 24-4. Differing Features of Thymoma and Thymic Carcinoid

	Thymoma	Thymic Carcinoid
Cushing's syndrome	−	+
Myasthenia gravis, hypoplastic anemia	+	−
More than one syndrome, same patient	+	−
Syndrome development after tumor removal	+	−
Syndrome always cured by tumor removal	−	+
Associated with multiple endocrine neoplasia	−	+
Demonstration of substance that causes syndrome within tumor	−	+
Good prognosis (see text)	+	−

(Modified with permission from Salyer et al,[129] with permission.)

Thymolipoma

Thymolipoma should be distinguished from lipomas arising in the mediastinum outside the thymus. These tumors are unusual; they probably represent involution of a previously truly hyperplastic thymus.[35] They usually are asymptomatic, although instances associated with systemic disease (Graves' disease[137] and aplastic anemia[138]) have been reported. One patient with lipomas of the thymus, thyroid, and pharynx has been described.[139] The average age when first discovered was 22 years in one review.[139] Radiologically, thymolipomas appear as lobulated anterior mediastinal masses of low density, resulting in confusion with cystic lesions. The tumors are often quite large; the average weight is 1,000 g.[140]

Thymolipomas are grossly identical to lipomas elsewhere, with uniformly soft, lobulated yellow tissue, except that small foci of gray-white thymic tissue are scattered within the fat. A thin fibrous capsule surrounds the mass. Microscopically, the adipose tissue is mature, and the thymic tissue is morphologically normal.

GERM CELL TUMORS

Germ cell tumors may arise within or near the thymus in the anterior mediastinum. There is no longer any doubt that most of these lesions are primary in this location. Metastasis to the mediastinum as the sole manifestation of a primary gonadal germ cell tumor is most unusual.[141] Testicular surgery is not warranted if the gonads are normal clinically.[141,142] Ultrasonography is a sensitive technique in investigating for an occult testicular primary.[143] The histogenesis of extragonadal germ cell tumors is uncertain. It is theorized that they originate either from primordial germ cells that have not completed migration from yolk sac endoderm to the urogenital ridge, or from totipotential embryonic cells that have escaped the influence of regulators and organizers during normal embryogenesis.[148]

Germ cell tumors of every type may occur in the mediastinum, and they are identical to the gonadal tumors grossly, histologically, and ultrastructurally[144–147] (Table 24-5). The reader is referred to Chapter 42 for a description of the morphologic features of these neoplasms.

Benign germ cell tumors are mature teratomas. These are equally common in men and women.[148] They are found incidentally on chest radiographs as rounded, well circumscribed masses. Symptoms may result from compression of adjacent structures.

Pure immature teratoma is rare in the mediastinum. Unlike the other malignant germ cell tumors, there is an approximately equal sex incidence.[149] Although the number of cases in the literature is small and the follow-up

TABLE 24-5. Germ Cell Neoplasms of the Mediastinum

Benign
  Mature teratoma
Malignant
  Germinoma
  Embryonal carcinoma
  Endodermal sinus tumor
  Choriocarcinoma
  Immature teratoma
  Mixed

data are incomplete, it appears that the prognosis of infants with immature teratoma is much better than that of children over the age of 2.[150]

The vast majority of malignant germ cell tumors other than immature teratoma occur in men in the third and fourth decades of life.[151] These tumors most often are symptomatic as a result of their rapid growth and invasive qualities. Radiologically they tend to be poorly circumscribed (Fig. 24-24). Pleural effusions may be present.

The most common malignant germ cell tumor is germinoma, the counterpart of testicular seminoma and ovarian dysgerminoma. As noted in Chapter 42, these tumors often contain numerous lymphocytes admixed with the neoplastic cells. This admixture may be confusing and may suggest a diagnosis of thymoma, but the markedly different cytologic appearance of germinoma cells allows separation. A slightly more cohesive growth pattern and the polymorphic cell population distinguish germinoma from histiocytic lymphoma. When only small biopsy specimens are available, ultrastructural examination[144] or immunoperoxidase studies[48,124,154] may be necessary to differentiate the lesion from thymoma, thymic carcinoma, and in particular, large cell lymphoma.

Like those in the gonads, mediastinal germinomas are extremely sensitive to radiotherapy. The survival rate is reported to be 80 to 90 percent,[35,142,151,153] and patients may be cured by irradiation even after the development of metastasis.[153] The overall survival rate, however, has not been as high as that for testicular seminoma,[158] perhaps because of greater tumor size at the time of discovery. The recommended therapy is surgical excision and postoperative radiotherapy.

Pure embryonal carcinoma,[141,152] endodermal sinus tumor,[145,146,156,157] and choriocarcinoma[159,160] primary in the mediastinum are rare. These tumors are highly malignant and are usually extensively invasive at the time of surgery. The diagnosis and subclassification may be facilitated by the use of immunoperoxidase stains.[124,156,160,161] Mixed germ cell tumors are composed of an admixture of two or more different malignant germ cell neoplasms. All recognized components should be reported when dealing with mixed germ cell tumors.

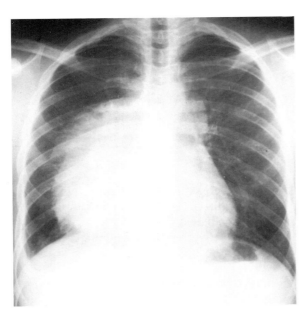

Fig. 24-24. Embryonal carcinoma of anterior mediastinum extending into right lung field.

An association between mediastinal germ cell tumors and hematologic malignant neoplasms has been described.[157,162] An association between mediastinal germ cell tumors and Klinefelter's syndrome has also been reported.[155]

In the past, most patients with embryonal carcinoma, endodermal sinus tumor, choriocarcinoma, immature teratoma, and mixed germ cell tumor of the mediastinum died of locally invasive disease and/or metastases. With the exception of infants with immature teratoma, the prognosis for these patients is poor, but improvements in systemic chemotherapy regimens may improve the outlook.[158]

LYMPHOMAS

In patients with malignant lymphoma, a mediastinal mass may represent involvement of the thymus or mediastinal lymph nodes. The lymph nodes of the anterior, middle, or posterior mediastinal compartments may be affected. Nodular sclerosing Hodgkin's disease and T-lymphoblastic lymphomas are two lymphomas known to originate in the thymus. Mediastinal lymphoma, exclusive of these two entities, often implies widespread nodal disease.

Hodgkin's Disease

Anterior mediastinal involvement by Hodgkin's disease is the most frequent of the primary mediastinal lymphomas. The thymus and/or contiguous lymph nodes may be affected. The lesion is detected on routine chest radiographs in many patients; in others, there are symptoms or signs of mass lesions or systemic abnormalities such as fever or weight loss. Systemic diseases that are associated with conventional thymoma have been described in patients with mediastinal Hodgkin's disease, but such an occurrence is rare.[163,164]

Radiologically, the mass may appear lobulated and well circumscribed if only the thymus is involved or multinodular and poorly circumscribed when extrathymic and/or lymph node spread has occurred.

Almost all examples of Hodgkin's disease of the anterior mediastinum are of the nodular sclerosing type. This often is apparent grossly. Wide, firm fibrous bands separate fleshy gray or tan nodules. In some cases the entire mass is fibrous. Small cysts and foci of necrosis may be apparent.

Histologically, the nodules contain an admixture of lymphocytes, eosinophils, and Reed-Sternberg cell variants. The latter often are set in a clear space (lacunar cells), an artifact of formalin fixation. They may be present in clusters. Classical Reed-Sternberg cells may be difficult to find. The intervening bands consist of sparsely cellular, birefringent collagen. An apparent increase in thymic epithelial cells may be present, and these cells may appear reactive. Hassall's corpuscles within the nodules are not uncommon (Fig. 24-25). It is this mixture of residual thymic epithelium with elements of Hodgkin's disease that led to the concept of "granulomatous thymoma." The lesion was incorrectly regarded as a subtype of thymoma rather than Hodgkin's disease involving the thymus.

A syncytial variant of nodular sclerosing Hodgkin's disease has been described, in which 5 of 18 cases occurred in the mediastinum and 6 of 18 in the cervical area.[165] In these cases sheets of Reed-Sternberg cells may simulate thymoma or metastatic neoplasm on routine light microscopy.

A distinction between thymoma and Hodgkin's disease is not difficult if adequate tissue is available. Fibrous septa are present in both tumors. In thymoma the septa are usually distinct from the tumor nodules and branch irregularly, producing angulated lobules. In Hodgkin's disease the fibrous tissue is admixed with the cellular aggregates, which are usually round or ovoid. The histologic features of thymoma, such as perivascular spaces, are absent in Hodgkin's disease. Lacunar cells and Reed-Sternberg cells are not seen in thymomas. Thymic cysts coexisting with Hodgkin's disease may obscure the true nature of the neoplasm (Fig. 24-25). Absence of keratin positivity by immunoperoxidase staining in large malignant cells excludes thymoma as a diagnostic consideration.[48,124,165] Immunologic marker studies have been

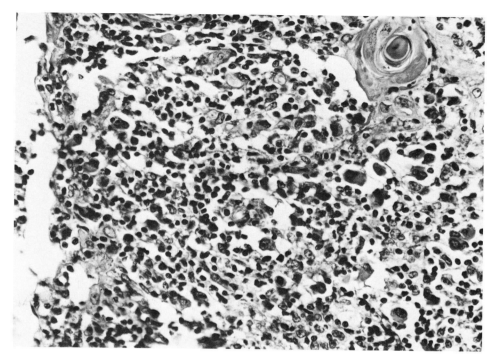

Fig. 24-25. Hodgkin's disease of the thymus. Hassall's corpuscle and reactive epithelial cells are admixed with atypical mononuclear "Hodgkin's" cells and lymphocytes. An associated thymic cyst (left) is common and may obscure the diagnosis.

done in attempts to define antigens that support a diagnosis of Hodgkin's disease.[166]

Hodgkin's disease that is primary in the mediastinum has a good prognosis. In one series of 267 patients, all survived 8 years.[167] In 85 percent of these cases there had been no relapse after initial radiation therapy. A poor prognostic feature of primary mediastinal Hodgkin's disease is the presence of an initially large mediastinal mass, as defined by mediastinal measurements taken on upright posteroanterior radiography.[167–169] Since relapse and recurrence of disease are related to the size of the initial lesion, a more aggressive therapeutic approach has been advocated in these cases.[167,169]

Lymphoblastic Lymphoma

T-cell lymphoblastic lymphoma (Fig. 24-26) is often seen in children and young adults but occurs in all age groups.[170,171] The disease is characteristically associated with an anterior mediastinal thymic mass,[170] and presentation with mediastinal mass is more common in the younger patients.[172] Initially, leukemic cells are not often present, but 30 to 50 percent of patients will develop a leukemic phase with circulating cells that are morphologically indistinguishable from the cells of acute lym-

phoblastic leukemia.[170,171] Pleural effusions are common, and multiple thoracic lymph node groups may be involved. Many patients are symptomatic as a result of compression of vital structures or of respiratory compromise due to infiltration of the trachea and airways.[173] Death due to acute respiratory insufficiency before therapy can be instituted is not uncommon. Radiologically, the neoplasm tends to be large and poorly circumscribed. Grossly the tissue is fleshy and pink-tan with foci of necrosis and hemorrhage. There is often extensive invasion of mediastinal structures and soft tissues.

Surface marker studies show that the majority of lymphoblastic lymphomas are of thymic origin.[172] There is some evidence that the variable phenotypic expression reflects the stages of immature thymocyte maturation.[174] Considerable overlap exists between the phenotypic characterization of T-cell acute lymphoblastic leukemia and T-cell lymphoblastic lymphoma, so that in a majority of cases no clear malignant T-cell surface marker distinctions can be made between the two entities.[171] In some studies a change in surface antigens is observed in patients with lymphoblastic lymphoma in leukemic relapse, with a shift toward "dedifferentiation" and an expression of immature antigens.[175]

Although there often is a rapid objective response of lymphoblastic lymphomas to radiotherapy or chemother-

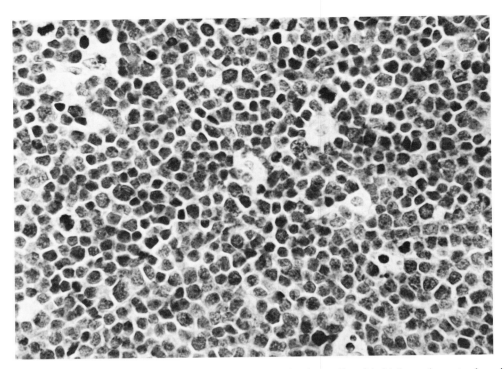

Fig. 24-26. Lymphoblastic lymphoma. Sheets of poorly cohesive cells with high nucleocytoplasmic ratio and numerous mitoses. The chromatin is finely distributed. A "starry-sky" appearance is due to phagocytic macrophages.

apy, remissions usually are of short duration. A median survival time of 8 months from diagnosis was noted in the series of Nathwani et al.[170] Some improvement in survival data has been noted with the use of early systemic chemotherapeutic regimens.[176]

Large Cell Lymphocytic Lymphoma

It is uncommon for non-Hodgkin's lymphoma other than lymphoblastic lymphoma to present in the mediastinum; fewer than 5 percent of non-Hodgkin's lymphoma cases present in this location. These lymphomas are usually large cell lymphocytic lesions with a diffuse pattern and accompanying sclerosis. Surface marker studies have shown that these lesions can be subclassified in the standard manner and that B-cell lymphomas and B- and T-cell immunoblastic lymphomas are represented.[177–179] The prognostic implications of subclassification are not entirely clear, and these lesions have such similar clinicopathologic features that they are often discussed as a single entity.

The non-Hodgkin's lymphomas often present in young adults, and they are usually symptomatic. They have a poor prognosis[177–180] and respond poorly to therapy. They infiltrate the thorax extensively, and they may extend outside the thorax.

Morphologically, the cells in a mediastinal large cell lymphoma usually have vesicular nuclei, with angulated chromatin and prominent nucleoli. Nuclear clefts may or may not be present. The amount of sclerosis is variable (Fig. 24-27) and is occasionally extensive.[178] The differential diagnosis may include thymoma, seminoma, Hodgkin's disease, and carcinoma.

Immunoperoxidase stains are sufficiently useful in making an accurate diagnosis that electron microscopy may be unnecessary. Lymphomas will stain with a variety of leukocyte surface markers. Thymomas and carcinoma are keratin-positive, unlike lymphoma and seminoma. In addition, thymomas typically contain thymocytes with phenotypes resembling those found in normal thymus.[124] Seminomas that appear pure in type morphologically may still stain positively for human chorionic gonadotropin, and seminomas are usually ferritin-positive.[124]

Other Non-Hodgkin's Lymphomas

Any of the other varieties of lymphomas may involve the mediastinum primarily but usually do so as part of

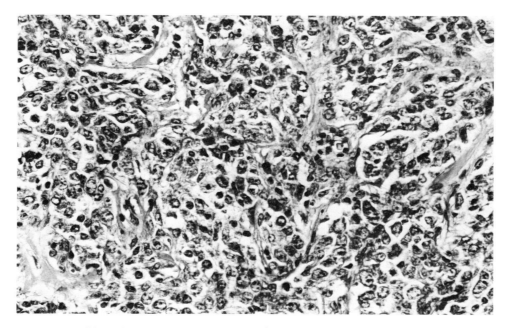

Fig. 24-27. Large cell lymphoma. Large, poorly cohesive cells with vesicular nuclei. In this field, groups of cells are separated into compartments by bands of collagen, imparting an epithelial appearance ("sclerosing histiocytic lymphoma").

systemic disease. The clinical and morphologic features of these neoplasms are described in Chapter 12. The distinction between thymoma and lymphocytic lymphoma is discussed in the section on thymoma. The diagnosis is facilitated by use of immunoperoxidase stains for keratin, which is positive in thymoma, and leukocyte common antigen, which is positive in lymphoma.[124]

NEURAL TUMORS

Neural tumors are the most common primary tumors of the mediastinum, constituting 20 to 40 percent of all primary mediastinal lesions in large series.[1,181] They are divided into three groups based on their presumed histogenesis: (1) tumors of nerve sheath origin, (2) tumors of sympathetic nervous system origin, and (3) tumors of paraganglionic origin (Table 24-6).

Nerve Sheath Tumors

Neurilemmoma (Schwannoma)

About 50 percent of neural tumors of the mediastinum are neurilemomas.[182–184] They occur almost exclusively in adults. Although they may develop in association with any nerve, more than 95 percent arise in the posterior mediastinum.

Neurilemmomas are found incidentally in approximately half the cases. Symptoms due to sensory or motor nerve impairment or to compression of adjacent structures are present in the remaining 50 percent of the cases.[184] Because neurilemmomas may develop within a posterior spinal nerve near the vertebral foramen, spinal cord compression can occur.

Radiologically, mediastinal neurilemmomas are usually large, well circumscribed homogeneous masses. Small calcified foci may be observed. Most tumors are solitary; multiple tumors occur only in patients with neurofibromatosis (von Recklinghausen's disease).

TABLE 24-6. Neural Tumors of the Mediastinum

Children
  Sympathetic nervous system neoplasms
    Neuroblastoma
    Ganglioneuroblastoma
    Ganglioneuroma

Adults
  Sympathetic nervous system neoplasms
    Ganglioneuroma
  Nerve sheath neoplasms
    Neurilemoma
    Neurofibroma
    Malignant peripheral nerve sheath tumor
  Paraganglionic neoplasms
    Branchiomeric paraganglioma
    Aorticosympathetic paraganglioma

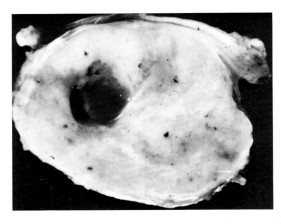

Fig. 24-28. Neurilemmoma. Cyst and myxoid areas (lighter zones) within solid tumor mass. Large nerve trunk is apparent over surface of neoplasm.

Neurilemmomas in the posterior mediastinum may be extremely large. They usually are solid, firm, and tan to white. An associated major nerve may be apparent grossly (Fig. 24-28). Those involving the spinal canal as well as the posterior mediastinum have an hourglass configuration. Small cysts or areas of softening may be present. Histologically, they are identical with their counterparts elsewhere (see Ch. 49), with a variable ad-

mixture of Antoni A and B patterns (Fig. 24-29). Immunohistochemical stains for the acidic protein S-100 are positive in neurilemoma. Some tumors are markedly cellular and contain bizarre and pleomorphic nuclei. These cellular features combined with the large size of the tumor may suggest a diagnosis of sarcoma.[185,186] The development of sarcoma in a neurilemmoma is, however, regarded as a very rare occurrence.[187] Most authors considered the bizarre nuclei as degenerative in origin.

Neurofibroma and Malignant Peripheral Nerve Sheath Tumor

Mediastinal neurofibromas are uncommon and constitute about 14 percent of mediastinal neural tumors.[183] The majority occur in patients with neurofibromatosis. Otherwise the clinical and radiologic features do not differ from those of neurilemoma. They are identical morphologically to neurofibromas elsewhere, although they tend to be larger.

Approximately 10 percent of mediastinal nerve sheath tumors are malignant.[183,184] The term *malignant peripheral nerve sheath tumor (neurofibrosarcoma)* should be reserved for those malignant neoplasms that either obviously arise from a major nerve or show definite schwan-

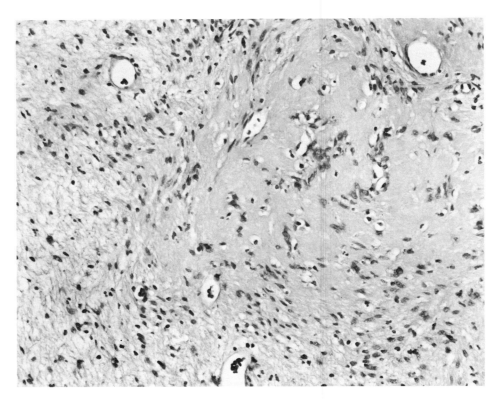

Fig. 24-29. Neurilemmoma. Loose myxoid area (Antoni B) merges with more organized solid zone with palisaded nuclei (Antoni A).

nian differentiation. In the mediastinum most examples of neurofibrosarcoma occur in patients with neurofibromatosis,[183] and many are associated with contiguous plexiform neurofibromas (Fig. 24-30). A diagnosis of sarcoma should not be based solely on cellularity and nuclear pleomorphism. A mitotic activity of greater than 10 mitoses per 10 high-power fields or tumor necrosis are reliable criteria for malignancy. These criteria are easily satisfied in most neurofibrosarcomas.

Sympathetic Nervous System Tumors

Malignant neoplasms presumed to be of sympathetic nervous system origin occur predominantly but not exclusively in children.[188–191] The benign ganglioneuroma is found most commonly in children and young adults. Most sympathetic nerve neoplasms develop in the abdomen, but 20 to 25 percent arise from the sympathetic chain in the posterior mediastinum. Morphologically, these lesions are identical at all sites.

The tumors of the sympathetic nervous system show variable cellular differentiation. There is a spectrum ranging from tumors composed entirely of small neuroblasts with little or no maturation (neuroblastoma) (Fig. 24-31) to neoplasms containing an admixture of neuroblasts and ganglion cells (ganglioneuroblastoma) (Fig. 24-32) to benign lesions containing ganglion cells and nerve sheath elements (ganglioneuroma) (Fig. 24-33). A sharp division into the different types cannot be made because one type may blend into another. The survival rate in patients with neoplasms of the sympathetic nervous system is directly related to the degree of differentiation. All neoplasms with neuroblastic elements should be regarded as potentially malignant. Increased urinary excretion of catecholamines and their metabolites occurs in many neuroblastomas, ganglioneuroblastomas, and ganglioneuromas. Measurement of these substances may be used for screening, detection, and evaluation of therapy.[192,193]

Neuroblastomas usually produce clinical symptoms and signs. In some series survival figures are better for mediastinal than for abdominal neuroblastoma.[191] The prognosis gradually worsens with increasing age of the patient for neuroblastoma in all sites.[189,191]

Ganglioneuromas most often are asymptomatic and incidental radiologic findings. They are assumed to develop from complete maturation of neuroblastic tissue,[187] but

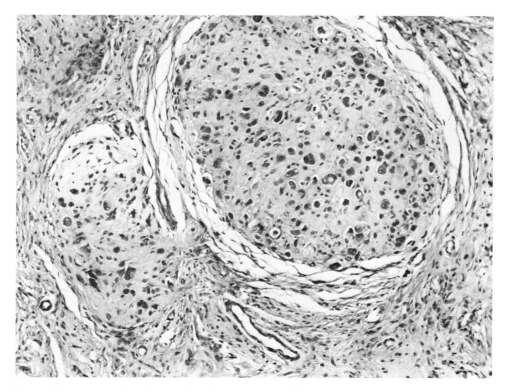

Fig. 24-30. Malignant peripheral nerve sheath tumor (neurofibrosarcoma). Pleomorphism and mitoses support the diagnosis of sarcoma. The arrangement of the cells in nerve-like bundles suggests origin in a preexisting plexiform neurofibroma. Areas of recognizable neurofibroma are present elsewhere, and the patient has neurofibromatosis.

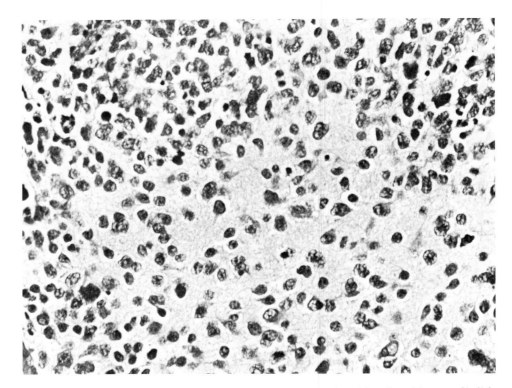

Fig. 24-31. Neuroblastoma. Sheets of small, pleomorphic cells associated focally with neurofibril formation. The latter is evidence of neural differentiation in what is otherwise an undifferentiated small cell tumor by light microscopy.

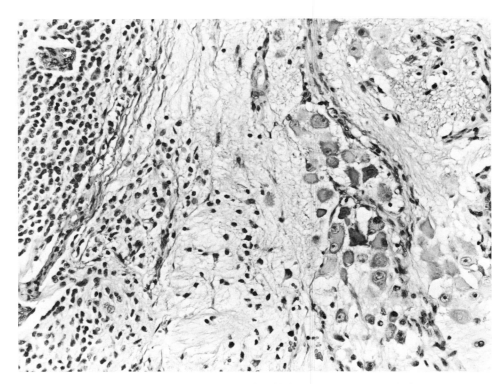

Fig. 24-32. Ganglioneuroblastoma. Immature cells with fibrillar processes are admixed with well developed ganglion cells. The latter lack satellite cells and a few show multinucleation.

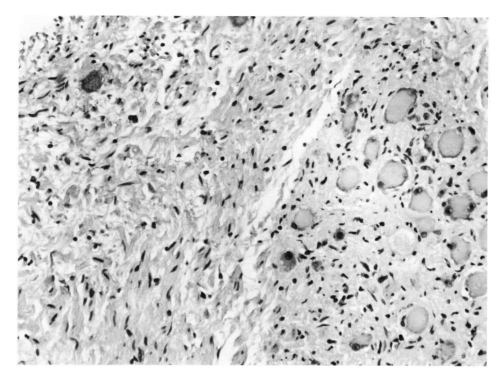

Fig. 24-33. Ganglioneuroma. Mature ganglion cells set within a loose neurofibroblastic stroma. Satellite cells are absent, and the ganglion cells may be multinucleate. No immature neural tissue is present.

they may continue to enlarge as a result of proliferation of the nerve sheath component.

The prognosis for ganglioneuroblastoma of the mediastinum is better than for neuroblastoma or for intra-abdominal ganglioneuroblastoma.[189] Prediction of prognosis based on the pattern of growth of the mature and immature elements has been attempted.[189] Clearly, the clinical stage of the tumor is most significant, with surgery being curative in stage I lesions,[189,190] while stage IV lesions have a poor prognosis despite aggressive therapy.[189,190]

It may be difficult to distinguish a ganglioneuroma from a neurilemoma with entrapped normal ganglion cells. The ganglion cells in the former often are binucleate and lack satellite cells (Fig. 24-33).

Paragangliomas

Although paragangliomas have been classified according to chromaffin or nonchromaffin staining properties, this histochemical reaction can be unreliable. The most useful classification is based on anatomic site of origin, as proposed by Glenner and Grimley.[194] They divided extra-adrenal paragangliomas into four types based on location: branchiomeric, aorticosympathetic, intravagal, and visceral-autonomic. Neoplasms of the first two classes occur in the mediastinum.

Branchiomeric paragangliomas arise in normal paraganglionic tissue that is associated with arteries and cranial nerves of the branchial arches.[194] In the mediastinum, paraganglia occur in subclavian, aortico-pulmonary, coronary, and pulmonary locations. Neoplasms of these paraganglia are uncommon. Fewer than 50 cases have been reported.[195] The age range is 21 to 79 years. Most occur in the anterior mediastinum, and the clinical presentation is indistinguishable from that of thymoma.

Aorticosympathetic paragangliomas of the mediastinum develop in association with the thoracic sympathetic chain. They have been variously referred to as nonchromaffin paraganglioma, chemodectoma, and pheochromocytoma. They almost always occur in the costovertebral sulcus in the posterior mediastinum. Fewer than 32 cases have been described.[196]

Neoplasms arising in the branchiomeric paraganglia usually resemble the normal tissue, with small rounded groups of cells ("Zellballen") separated by fibrovascular septa (Fig. 24-34). This arrangement may be inapparent on frozen section. They usually are extremely vascular. There is abundant amphophilic to eosinophilic, slightly granular cytoplasm. The nuclei may be quite atypical, with marked variability from cell to cell in size and shape, but mitotic activity is unusual.

The microscopic appearance of aorticosympathetic

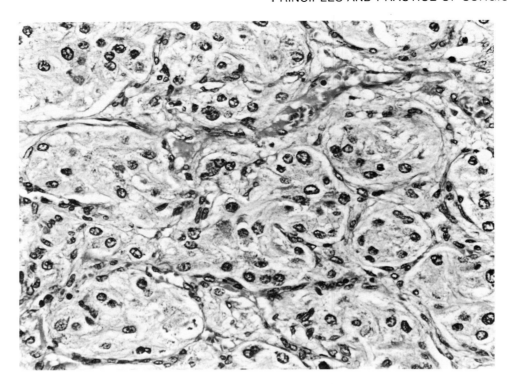

Fig. 24-34. Branchiomeric paraganglioma. Polygonal to spindled cells with granular cytoplasm are divided into rather uniform small nests by fibrovascular septa.

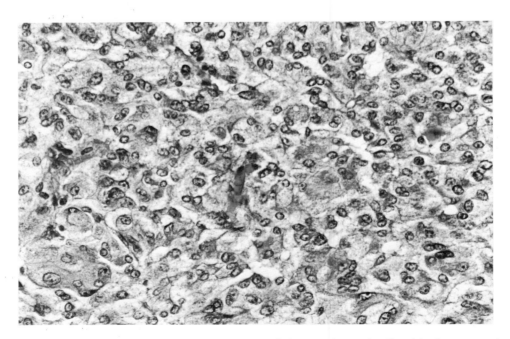

Fig. 24-35. Aorticosympathetic paraganglioma. Sheets of plump polygonal cells with plump granular cytoplasm. Although often quite vascular, this lesion lacks the fibrovascular septa of the usual branchiomeric paraganglioma. It has the morphologic features of the usual adrenal paraganglioma (pheochromocytoma).

paragangliomas is variable. Although those located in the abdomen usually resemble branchiomeric tumors, in the mediastinum they more often simulate adrenal medullary paragangliomas (pheochromocytomas).[194] The Zellballen pattern is less conspicuous or absent. The cells are arranged in sheets or trabeculae (Fig. 24-35). Abundant fine vascular septa coursing irregularly through the neoplasm impart an "endocrine" appearance. In some cases posterior mediastinal paragangliomas are identical to branchiomeric tumors, or a blending of the two patterns is present.

Branchiomeric paragangliomas are rarely functional. Aorticosympathetic tumors of the posterior mediastinum are more likely to be associated with hypertension due to catecholamine secretion.[196,197] Functional neoplasms are classified by some authors as extra-adrenal pheochromocytomas. Ultrastructurally, both types of mediastinal paraganglioma contain similar dense core cytoplasmic granules.[194,196]

Paragangliomas in all anatomic sites may show aggressive, invasive, local growth or distant metastases. The incidence of such behavior varies.[195] Branchiomeric paragangliomas of the mediastinum more often are malignant than those of some sites, such as carotid bodies, probably because of the large size that they may attain before detection in a relatively "silent" location. In one review,[195] of 41 patients 8 died of tumor; another 7 patients had unresectable neoplasms. The most important prognostic factor is the initial resectability.[195] Tumors with aggressive local behavior or metastases cannot be distinguished histologically from those that are not aggressive and do not recur. Posterior mediastinal paragangliomas less often are associated with aggressive behavior. Less than 10 percent are malignant,[196] which is comparable with the incidence of malignant adrenal paragangliomas.

Mediastinal paraganglioma must be distinguished from carcinoid tumor and spindled thymoma. The cells of typical carcinoid tumors are more uniform with less nuclear pleomorphism. The nests of cells are more variable in size and shape than those of paraganglioma. Central necrosis in cell aggregates is common in carcinoid tumors, but it is unusual in paraganglioma, and true rosettes are found in carcinoid tumors. Spindled thymomas usually have a lymphocytic component and lack the Zellballen cellular arrangement.

SOFT TISSUE TUMORS

Benign and malignant mesenchymal neoplasms identical to those elsewhere in the body may occur in the mediastinum.[198–210] They are often larger at the time of initial diagnosis than their counterparts in other soft tissue locations. Histologically, they are identical, and subclassification may be facilitated by immunoperoxidase stains for tumor antigens[206] (also see Ch. 10). The prognosis is related to the grade of the tumor, the clinical stage, and the resectability.

Tumor-like masses composed of *hematopoietic tissue* have been described in patients with severe chronic anemia, usually hereditary spherocytosis or thalassemia.[211–213] The masses occur in the posterior mediastinum, characteristically in a paravertebral location, with an asymmetric bilateral distribution. The radiologic appearance of extramedullary hematopoiesis is often accompanied by the vertical striations of chronic anemia in adjacent vertebrae. In the appropriate clinical setting, the appearance of these masses, without bony erosion, is sufficiently characteristic that tissue studies may not be necessary.[212] Certainly this tissue should not be removed, and needle biopsy risks hemorrhage in this well vascularized tissue.[212,213]

Mesothelioma may rarely present in the mediastinum. Its pathologic features are discussed in detail in Chapter 25.

ABNORMALITIES OF BLOOD VESSELS

Lesions of the major arteries and veins must be considered in the differential diagnosis of mediastinal masses (see Ch. 21). Aortic aneurysms are most common, but aneurysms or congenital anomalies of any vessel may result in a radiologic abnormality.[214] Angiography often is useful in determining the precise nature of these lesions preoperatively.

SUMMARY

The wide variety of benign and malignant neoplasms and of nonneoplastic conditions that occur in the mediastinum must be properly classified if appropriate clinical evaluation and therapy are to proceed. The patient's age, location of the lesion, and radiologic appearance may suggest a diagnosis, but surgical exploration almost always is required for definitive diagnosis. There is much overlap in the clinical and radiologic manifestations of the various lesions.

The differential diagnosis of many of the entities is difficult. An attempt at complete surgical excision is the initial therapy of choice for all mediastinal cysts and neoplasms. Diagnostic procedures such as needle biopsy have a small role in the diagnosis of primary mediastinal lesions.[215] Also, because of the frequent difficulties in light microscopic diagnosis, tissue should be frozen, processed for immunoperoxidase studies, and fixed for electron microscopic study whenever possible.

REFERENCES

1. Wychulis AR, Payne WS, Claggett OT et al: Surgical treatment of mediastinal tumors: A 40 year experience. J Thoracic Cardiovasc Surg 62:379, 1971

2. Graeber GM, Shriver CD, Albus RA, et al: The use of computed tomography in the evaluation of mediastinal masses. J Thoracic Cardiovasc Surg 91:662, 1986

3. Webb WR, Gamsu G, Stark DD, et al: Evaluation of magnetic resonance sequences in imaging mediastinal tumors. AJR 143:723, 1984

4. Kurtay M, Crile G: Aberrant parathyroid glands in relationship to the thymus. Am J Surg 117:705, 1969

5. Nathaniels EK, Nathaniels AM, Wang C: Mediastinal parathyroid tumors: A clinical and pathological study of 84 cases. Ann Surg 171:165, 1970.

6. Mark JBD: Ectopic mediastinal thyroid: Features in diagnosis and factors in treatment. Chest 45:412, 1964

7. Lindskog BI, Malm A: Diagnostic and surgical considerations on mediastinal (intrathoracic) goiter. Chest 47:201, 1965

8. Nwafo DC: Heterotopic mediastinal goitre. Br J Surg 65:505, 1978

9. McCort JJ: Intrathoracic goiter. Its incidence, symptomatology, and roentgen diagnosis. Radiology 53:227, 1949

10. Stoller JK, Shaw C, Matthay RA: Enlarging atypically located pericardial cyst. Recent experience and literature review. Chest 89:402, 1986

11. Zhao F: Calcified pericardial cyst: A case report and the roentgenologic and pathologic differentiation from other calcified mediastinal cysts. J Thorac Cardiovasc Surg 32:193, 1984

12. Salyer DC, Salyer WR, Eggleston JC: Benign developmental cysts of the mediastinum. Arch Pathol Lab Med 101:136, 1977

13. Langman J: Medical Embryology: Human Development—Normal and Abnormal. Williams & Wilkins, Baltimore, 1963, p. 205

14. Fallon M, Gordon ARG, Lendrum AC: Mediastinal cysts of foregut origin associated with vertebral abnormalities. Br J Surg 41:520, 1954

15. Veeneklaas GMH: Pathogenesis of intrathoracic gastroenteric cysts. Am J Dis Child 83:500, 1952.

16. Sirivella S, Ford WB, Zikria EA, Miller WH: Foregut cysts of the mediastinum: Results in 20 consecutive surgically treated cases. J Thorac Cardiovasc Surg 90:776, 1985

17. Wurster CF, Krespi YP: Mediastinitis occurring as a complication of odontogenic infections. Laryngoscope 96:747, 1986

18. Schowengerdt CG, Suyemoto R, Main FB: Granulomatous and fibrous mediastinitis. A review and analysis of 180 cases. J Thorac Cardiovasc Surg 57:365, 1969

19. Strimlan CV, Dines DE, Payne WS: Mediastinal granuloma. Mayo Clin Proc 50:702, 1975

20. Farmer DW, Moore E, Amparo E, et al: Calcific fibrosing mediastinitis: Demonstration of pulmonary vascular obstruction by magnetic resonance imaging. AJR 143:1189, 1984

21. Goodwin RA, Loyd JE, Des Prez RM: Histoplasmosis in normal hosts. Medicine (Baltimore) 60:231, 1981

22. Goodwin RA, Nickell JA, Des Prez RM: Mediastinal fibrosis complicating healed primary histoplasmosis and tuberculosis. Medicine (Baltimore) 51:227, 1972

23. Wieder S, Rabinowitz JG: Fibrous mediastinitis: A late manifestation of mediastinal histoplasmosis. Radiology 125:305, 1977

24. Light AM: Idiopathic fibrosis of mediastinum: A discussion of three cases and review of the literature. J Clin Pathol 32:78, 1978

25. Mitchinson MJ: The pathology of idiopathic retroperitoneal fibrosis. J Clin Pathol 23:681, 1970

26. Dorfman RF, Warnke R: Lymphadenopathy simulating the malignant lymphomas. Hum Pathol 5:519, 1974

27. Burns BF, Wood BS, Dorfman RF: The varied histopathology of lymphadenopathy in the homosexual male. Am J Surg Pathol 9:287, 1985

28. Frizzera G, Peterson BM, Bayrd ED, et al: A systemic lymphoproliferative disorder with morphologic features of Castleman's disease: Clinical findings and clinicopathologic correlations in 15 patients. J Clin Oncol 3:1201, 1985

29. Keller AR, Hochholzer L, Castleman B: Hyaline-vascular and plasma-cell types of giant lymph node hyperplasia of the mediastinum and other locations. Cancer 29:670, 1972.

30. Weisenburger DD, Nathwani BN, Winberg CD, et al: Multicentric angiofollicular lymph node hyperplasia: A clinicopathologic study of 16 cases. Hum Pathol 16:162, 1985

31. Miller RT, Mukai K, Banks PM, et al: Systemic lymphoproliferative disorder with morphologic features of Castleman's disease: Immunoperoxidase study of cytoplasmic immunoglobulins. Arch Pathol Lab Med 108:626, 1984

32. Carbone A, Manconi R, Volpe R, et al: Immunohistochemical, enzyme histochemical, and immunologic features of giant lymph hyperplasia of the hyaline vascular type. Cancer 58:908, 1986

33. De Paoli P, Carbone A, Reitano M, et al: Giant lymph node hyperplasia: A disease of primary follicle/mantle zone lymphocytes. Clin Immunol Immunopathol 40:371, 1987

34. Harris NL, Bhan AK: "Plasmacytoid T cells" in Castleman's disease. Am J Pathol 11:109, 1987

35. Rosai J, Levine GD: Tumors of the Thymus. Atlas of Tumor Pathology, Series 2. Fasc. 13. Armed Forces Institute of Pathology, Washington, 1976

36. Stanford W, Steele S, Armstrong RG, et al: Mediastinoscopy. Its application in central versus peripheral thoracic lesions. Ann Thorac Surg 19:121, 1975.

37. Goldberg EM, Shapiro CM, Glicksman AS: Mediastinoscopy for assessing mediastinal spread in clinical staging of lung carcinoma. Semin Oncol 1:205, 1974

38. Coughlin M, Des Lauriers J, Beaulieu M: Role of medias-

tinoscopy in pretreatment staging of patients with primary lung cancer. Ann Thorac Surg 40:556, 1985

39. Acosta JL, Manfredi F: Selective mediastinoscopy. Chest 71:150, 1977

40. Neifeld JP, Ingle JN, Tormey DC, et al: Mediastinoscopy. A diagnostic aid in metastatic carcinoma of the breast. Cancer 37:1973, 1976

41. Gorton G, Linell F: Malignant tumours and sarcoid reactions in regional lymph nodes. Acta Radiol [Diagn] (Stockh) 47:381, 1957

42. Nadel E, Ackerman LV: Lesions resembling Boeck's sarcoid in lymph nodes draining an area containing a malignant neoplasm. Am J Clin Pathol 20:952, 1950

43. Unruh H, Chiv RC-J: Mediastinal assessment for staging and treatment of carcinoma of the lung. Ann Thorac Surg 41:224, 1986

44. Hammar JA: Die Menschen Thymus in Gesundheit und Krankheit. Z Mikrosk Anat Forsch 16: suppl., 733, 1928

45. Pifer JW, Toyooka ET, Murray RW, et al: Neoplasms in children treated with X-rays for thymic enlargement. I. Neoplasms and mortality. JNCI 31:1333, 1963

46. Weiss L: The Cells and Tissues of the Immune System. Englewood Cliffs, NJ, Prentice-Hall, 1972

47. Bearman RM, Levine GD, Bensch KG: The ultrastructure of the normal human thymus: A study of 36 cases. Anat Rec 190:755, 1978

48. Battifora H, Sun TT, Raja MB, et al: The use of anti-keratin antiserum as a diagnostic tool: Thymoma versus lymphoma. Hum Pathol 11:635, 1980

49. Nagle RB, McDaniel KM, Clark VA, et al: The use of antikeratin antibodies in the diagnosis of human neoplasms. Am J Clin Pathol 79:458, 1983

50. Savino W, Dardenne M, Marche C, et al: Thymic epithelium in AIDS: An immunohistologic study. Am J Pathol 122:302, 1986

51. Goldstein AL, Low TLK, Thurman GB, et al: Current status of thymosin and other hormones of the thymus gland. Recent Prog Horm Res 37:369, 1981

52. Savino W, Dardenne M: Thymic hormone-containing cells. VI. Immunohistologic evidence for the simultaneous presence of thymolin, thymopoietin, and thymosin 1 in normal and pathological human thymuses. Eur J Immunol 14:987, 1984

53. Bahn AK, Reinherz EL, Poppema S, et al: Location of T cell and major histocompatibility complex antigens in the human thymus. J Exp Med 152:771, 1980

54. Savino W, Berrih, Dardenne M: Thymic epithelial antigen, acquired during ontogeny and defined by the anti-pig monoclonal antibody, is lost in thymomas. Lab Invest 51:292, 1984

55. Haynes BF, Robert-Guroff M, Metzger RS, et al: Monoclonal antibody against human T cell leukemia virus p19 defines a human thymic epithelial antigen acquired during ontogeny. J Exp Med 157:907, 1983

56. Janossy G, Thomas JA, Bollum FJ, et al: The human thymic microenvironment: An immunohistochemical study. J Immunol 125:202, 1980

57. McCaffrey R, Harrison TA, Parkman R, et al: Terminal deoxy nucleotidyltransferase in human leukemic cells and in normal human thymocytes. N Engl J Med 292:775, 1975

58. Mokhtar N, Hsu SM, Lad RP, et al: Thymoma: The lymphoid and epithelial components mirror the phenotype of normal thymus. Hum Pathol 15:378, 1984

59. Weller GL: Development of the thyroid, parathyroid, and thymus glands. Man Contrib Embryol Carnegie Inst 24:93, 1933

60. Gilmour JR: Some developmental abnormalities of the thymus and parathyroids. J Pathol Bacteriol 52:213, 1941

61. Indeglia RA, Shea MA, Grage TB: Congenital cysts of the thymus gland. Arch Surg 94:149, 1967

62. Bieger RC, McAdams AJ: Thymic cysts. Arch Pathol 82:535, 1966

63. Mikal S: Cervical thymic cyst. Case report and review of the literature. Arch Surg 109:558, 1974

64. Fahmy S: Cervical thymic cysts: Their pathogenesis and relationship to branchial cysts. J Laryngol Otol 88:47, 1974

65. Nezelof C: The pathology of the thymus in immunodeficiency states. Curr Top Pathol 75:151, 1986

66. Joshi VV, Oleske JM, Saad S, et al: Thymus biopsy in children with acquired immunodeficiency syndrome. Arch Pathol Lab Med 110:837, 1986

67. Dische MR: Lymphoid tissue and associated congenital malformations in thymic agenesis. Findings in one infant and two severely malformed stillborns. Arch Pathol 86:312, 1968

68. Huber J, Kersey J: Pathological findings. p. 289. in Meuwissen HJ, Pickering RJ, Pollara B, et al. (eds): Combined Immunodeficiency Disease and Adenosine Deaminase Deficiency. A Molecular Defect. Academic Press, New York, 1975

69. Bortin MM, Rimm AA: Severe combined immunodeficiency disease. Characterization of the disease and results of transplantation. JAMA 238:591, 1977

70. Shearer WT, Wedner HJ, Strominger DB, et al: Successful transplantation of the thymus in Nezelof's syndrome. Pediatrics 61:619, 1978

71. Thong YH, Robertson EF, Rischbieth HG, et al: Successful restoration of immunity in the DiGeorge syndrome with fetal thymic epithelial transplant. Arch Dis Child 53:580, 1978

72. Dourov N: Thymic atrophy and immune deficiency in malnutrition. Curr Top Pathol 75:127, 1986

73. Steinman GG: Changes in the human thymus during aging. Curr Top Pathol 75:43, 1986

74. Alpert LI, Papatestas A, Kark A, et al: A histologic reappraisal of the thymus in myasthenia gravis. A correlative study of thymic pathology and response to thymectomy. Arch Pathol 91:55, 1971

75. Castleman B, Norris EH: The pathology of the thymus in myasthenia gravis. A study of 35 cases. Medicine (Baltimore) 28:27, 1949

76. Castleman B: The pathology of the thymus gland in myasthenia gravis. Ann NY Acad Sci 135:486, 1966

77. Vetters JM, Barclay RS: The incidence of germinal centres in thymus glands of patients with congenital heart disease. J Clin Pathol 26:583, 1973

78. Middleton G: The incidence of follicular structures in the

human thymus at autopsy. Aust J Exp Biol Med Sci 45:189, 1967

79. Tamaoki N, Habu S, Kameya T: Thymic lymphoid follicles in autoimmune disease. II. Histological, histochemical and electron microscopic studies. Keio J Med 20:57, 1971

80. Levine GD, Bearman R: Electron microscopy of the thymus. In Johannessen JV (ed): Electron Microscopy in Human Medicine. McGraw-Hill, New York, 1978

81. Staber FG, Fink U, Sack W: B lymphocytes in the thymus of patients with myasthenia gravis. N Engl J Med 292:1032, 1975

82. O'Shea PA, Pansatiankul B, Farnes P: Giant thymic hyperplasia in infancy: Immunologic, histologic, and ultrastructural observations, abstracted. Lab Invest 38:391, 1978

83. Katz SM, Chatten J, Bishop HC, et al: Massive thymic enlargement. Report of a case of gross thymic hyperplasia in a child. Am J Clin Pathol 68:786, 1977

84. Drachman DB: Myasthenia gravis. N Engl J Med 198:136, 186, 1978

85. Penn AS, Jaretki A, Wolff M, et al: Thymic abnormalities: Antigen or antibody? Response to thymectomy in myasthenia gravis. Ann NY Acad Sci 377:786, 1981

86. Willcox N, Schluep M, Ritter MA, et al: Myasthenic and non-myasthenic thymoma: An expansion of a minor cortical epithelial subset? Am J Pathol 127:447, 1987

87. Dardenne M, Savino W, Bach JF: Thymomatous epithelial cells and skeletal muscle share a common epitope defined by monoclonal antibody. Am J Pathol 126:194, 1987

88. Buckingham JM, Howard FM, Bernatz PE, et al: The value of thymectomy in myasthenia gravis: A computer-assisted matched study. Ann Surg 184:453, 1976

89. Van der Kwast TH, van Vliet E, Cristen E, et al: An immunohistologic study of the epithelial and lymphoid components of six thymomas. Hum Pathol 16:1001, 1985

90. Sato Y, Shaw W, Mukai K, et al: An immunohistochemical study of thymic epithelial tumors. II. Lymphoid components. Am J Surg Pathol 10:862, 1986

91. Chan WC, Zaatar GS, Tabei S, et al: Thymoma: An immunohistochemical study. Am J Clin Pathol 82:160, 1984

92. Musiani P, Maggiano N, Aiello F, et al: Phenotypical characteristics and proliferative capabilities of thymocyte subsets in thymoma. Clin Immunol Immunopathol 40:385, 1986

93. Reddick RL, Jennette JC: Immunologic and ultrastructural characterization of the small cell population in malignant thymoma. Hum Pathol 14:377, 1983

94. Kornstein MJ, Hoxie JA, Levinson AI, et al: Immunohistology of human thymomas. Arch Pathol Lab Med 109:460, 1985

95. Takacs L, Savino W, Monostori S, et al: Cortical thymocyte differentiation in thymomas: An immunohistologic analysis of pathologic microenvironment. J Immunol 138:687, 1987

96. Chilosi M, Ianucci AM, Pizzolo G, et al: Immunohistochemical analysis of thymoma. Case report. Am J Surg Pathol 8:309, 1984

97. Ring NP, Addis BJ: Thymoma: An integraged clinicopath-

ological and immunohistochemical study. J Pathol 149:327, 1986

98. Kodama T, Watanabe S, Sato Y, et al: An immunohistochemical study of thymic epithelial tumors. I. Epithelial component. Am J Surg Pathol 10:26, 1986

99. Marino M, Muller-Hermelink HK: Thymoma and thymic carcinoma. Relation of thymoma epithelial cells to the cortical and medullary differentiation of thymus. Virchows Arch [A] 407:119, 1985

100. Van den Tweel JG, Taylor CR, McClure J, et al: Deletion of thymosin in thymic epithelial cells by an immunoperoxidase method. Adv Exp Med Biol 114:511, 1979

101. Martin JME, Randhawa G, Temple WJ: Cervical thymoma. Arch Lab Pathol Med 110:354, 1986

102. Neill J: Intrathyroid thymoma. Am J Surg Pathol 10:660, 1986

103. Havzach HR, Day ES, Franssila KO: Thyroid spindle-cell tumor with mucous cysts: An intrathyroid thymoma. Am J Surg Pathol 9:525, 1985

104. Rosai J, Limas C, Husband EM: Ectopic hamartomatous thymoma: A distinctive benign lesion of lower neck. Am J Surg Pathol 8:501, 1984

105. Smith PS, McClure J: Unusual subcutaneous mixed tumor exhibiting adipose, fibroblastic and epithelial components. J Clin Pathol 35:1074, 1982

106. Wick MK, Scheithauer BW, Dines DE: Thymic neoplasia in two male siblings. Mayo Clin Proc 57:653, 1982

107. Pascuzzi RM, Sermas A, Phillips L, et al: Familial autoimmune MG and thymoma: Occurrence in two brothers. Neurology 36:423, 1986

108. Salyer WR, Eggleston JC: Thymoma. A clinical and pathological study of 65 cases. Cancer 37:229, 1976

109. Dehner LP, Martin SA, Sumner HW: Thymus related tumors and tumor-like lesions in childhood with rapid clinical progression and death. Hum Pathol 8:53, 1977

110. Lattes R: Thymoma and other tumors of the thymus. An analysis of 107 cases. Cancer 15:1224, 1962

111. Castleman B: Tumors of the Thymus. Atlas of Tumor Pathology, Series 1. Fasc. 19. Armed Forces Institute of Pathology, Washington, 1955

112. Rosenow EC, Hurley BT: Disorders of the thymus: A review. Arch Intern Med 144:763, 1984

113. Levine GD, Rosai J: Thymic hyperplasia and neoplasia: A review of current concepts. Hum Pathol 9:495, 1978

114. Gray, GF, Gutowski WT: Thymoma: A clinicopathologic study of 54 cases. Am J Surg Pathol 3:235, 1979

115. Maggi G, Giaccone G, Donadio M, et al: Thymoma: A review of 169 cases, with particular reference to results of surgical treatment. Cancer 58:765, 1986

116. Jose B, Yu AT, Morgani TF, et al: Malignant thymoma with extrathoracic metastasis: A case report and review of the literature. J Surg Oncol 15:259, 1980

117. Salter DM, Krajewski AS: Metastatic thymoma: A case report and immunohistological analysis. J Clin Pathol 39:275, 1986

118. Fugimura S, Kondo T, Handa M, et al: Results of surgical treatment for thymoma based on 66 patients. J Thorac Cardiovasc Surg 93:708, 1987

119. Fechner RE: Recurrence of noninvasive thymomas. Re-

port of four cases and review of literature. Cancer 23:1423, 1969

120. Monden Y, Nakahara K, Ioka S, et al: Recurrence of thymoma: Clinicopathologic features, therapy and prognosis. Ann Thorac Surg 39:165, 1985

121. Marks RD, Wallace KM, Pettit HS: Radiation therapy control of nine patients with malignant thymoma. Cancer 41:117, 1978

122. Souadjian JV, Enriquez P, Silverstein MN, et al: The spectrum of diseases associated with thymoma. Arch Intern Med 134:374, 1974

123. Taylor RT: Immunomicroscopy: A diagnostic tool for the surgical pathologist. In Bennington JL (ed): Major Problems in Pathology. WB Saunders, Philadelphia, 1986

124. Spagnolo DV, Michie SA, Crabtree GS, et al: Monoclonal anti-keratin (AEI) reactivity in routinely processed tissue from 166 human neoplasms. Am J Clin Pathol 84:697, 1985

125. Osborne B, Mackay B, Battifora H: Thymoma: A clinicopathologic study of 23 cases. Pathol Annu 20:289, 1985

126. Wick MR, Scheithauer BW, Weiland LH, et al: Primary thymic carcinomas. Am J Surg Pathol 6:613, 1982

127. Rosai J: "Lymphoepithelioma-like" thymic carcinoma: Another tumor related to Epstein-Barr virus? N Engl J Med 312:1320, 1985

128. Leyvraz S, Henle W, Chahinian AP, et al: Association of Epstein-Barr virus with thymic carcinoma. N Engl J Med 312:1296, 1985

129. Salyer WR, Salyer DC, Eggleston JC: Carcinoid tumors of the thymus. Cancer 37:958, 1976

130. Rosai J, Higa E: Mediastinal endocrine neoplasm, of probable thymic origin, related to carcinoid tumor. Clinicopathologic study of 8 cases. Cancer 29:1061, 1972

131. Wick MR, Scott RE, Li CY, et al: Carcinoid tumor of the thymus. A clinicopathologic report of seven cases with a review of the literature. Mayo Clin Proc 55:246, 1980

132. Rosai J, Levine G, Weber WR, et al: Carcinoid tumors and oat cell carcinomas of the thymus. Pathol Annu 11:201, 1976

133. Levine GD, Rosai J: A spindle cell variant of thymic carcinoid tumor. A clinical, histologic, and fine structural study with emphasis on its distinction from spindle cell thymoma. Arch Pathol 100:293, 1976

134. De Lellis RA, Wolfe JH: Calcitonin in spindle cell thymic carcinoid tumors. Arch Pathol 100:340, 1976

135. Namba T, Brunner NG, Brob D: Myasthenia gravis in patients with thymoma with particular reference to onset after thymectomy. Medicine (Baltimore) 57:411, 1978

136. Azer MS, Zikria E, Ford WB: Myasthenia gravis appearing after removal of a thymoma. Report of a case and review of the literature. Am Surg 37:109, 1971

137. Benton C, Gerard P: Thymolipoma in a patient with Graves' disease: Case report and review of the literature. J Thorac Cardiovasc Surg 51:428, 1966

138. Barnes RDS, O'Gorman P: Two cases of aplastic anemia associated with tumours of the thymus. J Clin Pathol 15:264, 1962

139. Trites AEW: Thyrolipoma, thymolipoma, and pharyngeal lipoma: A syndrome. Can Med Assoc J 95:1254, 1966

140. Peake JB, Zeigler MG: Thymolipoma: Report of three cases. Am Surg 43:477, 1977

141. Luna MA, Valenzuela-Tamariz J: Germ-cell tumors of the mediastinum. Postmortem findings. Am J Clin Pathol 65:450, 1976

142. Bagshaw MA, McLaughlin WT, Earle JD: Definitive radiotherapy of primary mediastinal seminoma. AJR 105:86, 1969

143. Kirschling RJ, Kvols LK, Charboneau JW, et al: High-resolution ultrasonographic and pathologic abnormalities of germ-cell tumors in patients with clinically normal testes. Mayo Clin Proc 58:648, 1983

144. Levine GD: Primary thymic seminoma—a neoplasm ultrastructurally similar to testicular seminoma and distinct from epithelial thymoma. Cancer 31:729, 1973

145. Vuletin JC, Rosen Y, Brigati DJ, et al: Endodermal sinus tumor of the mediastinum. Ultrastructural study. Chest 72:112, 1977

146. Mukai K, Adams WR: Yolk sac tumor of the anterior mediastinum. Case report with light- and electron-microscopic examination and immunohistochemical study of alpha-fetoprotein. Am J Surg Pathol 3:77, 1979

147. Harms D, Jänig U: Immature teratomas of childhood. Report of 21 cases. Pathol Res Pract 179:388, 1985

148. Gonzalez-Crussi F: Extragonadal Teratomas. Atlas of Tumor Pathology. Series 2. Fasc 18. Armed Forces Institute of Pathology, Washington, 1982

149. Canty TG, Siemens R: Malignant mediastinal teratoma in a 15-year-old girl. Cancer 41:1623, 1978

150. Lack EE, Weinstein HJ, Welch KJ: Mediastinal germ cell tumors in childhood: A clinical and pathological study of 21 cases. J Thorac Cardiovasc Surg 89:826, 1985

151. Pachter MR, Lattes R: "Germinal" tumors of the mediastinum: A clinicopathologic study of adult teratomas, teratocarcinomas, choriocarcinomas, and seminomas. Chest 45:301, 1964

152. Cox JD: Primary malignant germinal tumors of the mediastinum. A study of 24 cases. Cancer 36:1162, 1975

153. Schantz A, Sewall W, Castleman B: Mediastinal germinoma. A study of 21 cases with an excellent prognosis. Cancer 30:1189, 1972

154. Warnke RA, Coatter KC, Falini B, et al: Diagnosis of human lymphoma with monoclonal antileukocyte antibodies. N Engl J Med 309:1275, 1983

155. McNeil MM, Leong AS, Sage RE: Primary mediastinal embryonal carcinoma in association with Klinefelter's syndrome. Cancer 47:343, 1981

156. Kuzur ME, Gobleigh MA, Greco FA, et al: Endodermal sinus tumor of the mediastinum. Cancer 50:766, 1982

157. Truong LD, Harris L, Mattioli C, et al: Endodermal sinus tumor of the mediastinum. A report of 7 cases and review of the literature. Cancer 58:730, 1986

158. Sterchi M, Cordell AR: Seminoma of the anterior mediastinum. Ann Thorac Surg 19:371, 1975

159. Sandhaus L, Strom RL, Mukai K; Primary embryonal-choriocarcinoma of the mediastinum in a woman. A case report with immunohistochemical study. Am J Clin Pathol 75:573, 1981

160. Kathuria S, Jablokow BR: Primary choriocarcinoma of

the mediastinum with immunohistochemical study and review of the literature. J Surg Oncol 34:39, 1987

161. Mukai K, Adams WR: Yolk sac tumor of the anterior mediastinum: Case report with light and electron microscopic immunohistochemical study of alpha feto-protein. Am J Surg Pathol 1:77, 1979

162. De Ment SH, Eggleston JC, Spivak JL: Association between mediastinal germ cell tumors and hematologic malignancies. Am J Surg Pathol 9:23, 1985

163. Remigo PA: Granulomatous thymoma associated with erythroid hypoplasia. Am J Clin Pathol 55:68, 1971

164. Null JA, LiVolsi VA, Glenn WWL: Hodgkin's disease of the thymus (granulomatous thymoma) and myasthenia gravis. A unique association. Am J Clin Pathol 67:521, 1977

165. Strickler JG, Michie SA, Warnke RA, et al: The "syncytial variant" of nodular sclerosing Hodgkin's disease. Am J Surg Pathol 10:470, 1986

166. Sheibani K, Battifora H, Burke JS, et al: Leu M1 antigen in human neoplasms. An immunohistologic study of 400 cases. Am J Surg Pathol 10:227, 1986

167. Mauch P, Gorshein D, Cunningham J, et al: Influence of mediastinal adenopathy on site and frequency of relapse in patients with Hodgkin's disease. Cancer Treat Rep 66:809, 1982

168. Ryoo MC, Kagan AR, Wollin M, et al: Observations on the treatment of mediastinal masses in Hodgkin's disease. Am J Clin Oncol 10:185, 1987

169. Anderson H, Jenkins J, Brigg DJ, et al: The prognostic signficance of mediastinal bulk in patients with Stage IA–IVB Hodgkin's disease. Clin Radiol 36:449, 1985

170. Nathwani BN, Diamond LW, Winberg CD, et al: Lymphoblastic lymphoma: A clinicopathologic study of 95 patients. Cancer 48:2347, 1981

171. Harden EA, Haynes BF: Phenotypic and fractional characterization of human malignant T cells. Semin Hematol 22:13, 1985

172. Weiss LM, Bindl JM, Picozzi VJ, et al: Lymphoblastic lymphoma: An immunophenotype study of 26 cases with comparison to T cell acute lymphoblastic leukemia. Blood 67:474, 1986

173. Rosen PJ, Feinstein DI, Pattengale PK, et al: Convoluted lymphocytic lymphoma in adults. A clinicopathologic entity. Ann Intern Med 89:319, 1978

174. Feller AC, Parwaresch MR, Stein H, et al: Immunophenotyping of T-lymphoblastic lymphoma/leukemia: Correlation with normal T cell maturation. Leuk Res 10:1025, 1986

175. Donlon JA, Jaffe ES, Braylan RC: Terminal deoxynucleotidyl transferase activity in malignant lymphomas. N Engl J Med 297:461, 1977

176. Coleman CN, Picozzi VJ, Cox RS, et al: Treatment of lymphoblastic lymphoma in adults. J Clin Oncol 4:1628, 1986

177. Addis BJ, Isaacson PG: Large cell lymphoma of the mediastinum: A B-cell tumor of probable thoracic origin. Histopathology 10:379, 1986

178. Perrone T, Frizzera G, Rosai J: Mediastinal diffuse large cell lymphoma with sclerosis. A clinicopathologic study of 60 cases. Am J Surg Pathol 10:176, 1986

179. Yousem SA, Weiss LM, Warnke RA: Primary mediastinal non-Hodgkin's lymphomas: A morphologic and immunologic study of 19 cases. Am J Clin Pathol 83:676, 1985

180. Menestrina F, Chilosi M, Bonetti F, et al: Mediastinal large cell lymphoma of B-type, with sclerosis: Histopathological and immunohistochemical study of eight cases. Histopathology 10:589, 1985

181. Ingels GW, Campbell DC, Giampetro AM, et al: Malignant schwannomas of the mediastinum. Report of 2 cases and review of the literature. Cancer 27:1190, 1971

182. Oberman HA, Abell MR: Neurogenous neoplasm of the mediastinum. Cancer 13:882, 1960

183. Ackerman LV, Taylor FH: Neurogenous tumors within the thorax. A clinicopathological evaluation of forty-eight cases. Cancer 4:669, 1951

184. Gale AW, Jelihovsky T, Grant AF, et al: Neurogenic tumors of the mediastinum. Ann Thorac Surg 17:434, 1974

185. Fletcher CD, Davies SE, McKee PH: Cellular schwannoma: A distinct pseudosarcomatous entity. Histopathology 11:21, 1987

186. Woodruff JM, Godwin TA, Erlandson RA, et al: Cellular schwannoma: A variety of schwannoma sometimes mistaken for malignant tumor. Am J Surg Pathol 5:733, 1981

187. Harkin JC, Reed RJ: Tumors of the Peripheral Nervous System. Atlas of Tumor Pathology. Series 2. Fasc. 3. Armed Forces Institute of Pathology, Washington, 1969

188. Mackay B, Luna MA, Butler JJ: Adult neuroblastoma. Electron microscopic observations in nine cases. Cancer 37, 1334, 1976

189. Adam A, Hochholzer L: Ganglioneuroblastoma of the posterior mediastinum: A clinicopathologic review of 80 cases. Cancer 47:373, 1981

190. Bove KE, McAdams AJ: Composite ganglioneuroblastoma. An assessment of the significance of histological maturation in neuroblastoma diagnosed beyond infancy. Arch Pathol Lab Med 105:325, 1981

191. Hughes M, Marsden HB, Palmer MK: Histologic patterns of neuroblastoma related to prognosis and clinical staging. Cancer 34:1706, 1974

192. Kaser H: Catecholamine-producing neural tumors other than pheochromocytoma. Pharmacol Rev 18:659, 1966

193. Bond JV: Clinical significance of catecholamine excretion levels in diagnosis and treatment of neuroblastoma. Arch Dis Child 50:691, 1975

194. Glenner GG, Grimley PM: Tumors of the Extra-Adrenal Paraganglion System (Including Chemoreceptors). Atlas of Tumor Pathology. Series 2. Fasc. 9. Armed Forces Institute of Pathology, Washington, 1974

195. Olson JL, Salyer WR: Mediastinal paragangliomas (aortic body tumor). A report of four cases and a review of the literature. Cancer 41:2405, 1978

196. Gallivan MV, Byungkyu C, Rowden G, et al: Intrathoracic paravertebral malignant paraganglioma. Arch Pathol Lab Med 104:46, 1980

197. Ogawa J, Inoue H, Koide S, et al: Functioning paragangli-

oma in the posterior mediastinum. Ann Thorac Surg 33:507, 1982

198. Rasaretnam R, Panabokke RG: Leiomyosarcoma of the mediastinum. Br J Dis Chest 69:63, 1975

199. Standerfer RJ, Armistead SH, Paneth M: Liposarcoma of the mediastinum: report of two cases and review of the literature. Thorax 36:693, 1981

200. Ikeda T, Ishihara T, Yoshimatsu H, et al: Primary osteogenic sarcoma of the mediastinum. Thorax 29:582, 1974

201. Pacter MR, Lattes R: Mesenchymal tumors of the mediastinum. I. Tumors of fibrous tissue, adipose tissue, smooth muscle, and striated muscle. Cancer 16:74, 1963

202. Gindhart TD, Tucker WY, Choy SH: Cavernous hemangioma of the superior mediastinum. Report of a case with electron microscopy and computerized tomography. Am J Surg Pathol 3:353, 1979

203. Pacter MR, Lattes R: Mesenchymal tumors of the mediastinum. II. Tumors of blood vascular origin. Cancer 16:95, 1963

204. Pacter MR, Lattes R: Mesenchymal tumors of the mediastinum. III. Tumors of lymph vascular origin. Cancer 16:108, 1963

205. Gibbs AR, Johnson NF, Giddings JC: Primary angiosarcoma of the mediastinum: Light and electron microscopic demonstration of Factor VIII-related antigen in neoplastic cells. Hum Pathol 15:687, 1984

206. Chen W, Chan CW, Mok CK: Malignant fibrous histiocytoma of the mediastinum. Cancer 50:797, 1982

207. Mills SA, Breyer RH, Johnston FR, et al: Malignant fibrous histiocytoma of the mediastinum and lung: A report of three cases. J Thorac Cardiovasc Surg 84:367, 1982

208. Besznyak I, Svastits E, Krasnai G, et al: Malignant fibrous histiocytoma of the lung. J Thorac Cardiovasc Surg 33:106, 1985

209. Natsuaki M, Yoshikawa Y, Itoh T, et al: Xanthogranulomatous malignant fibrous histiocytoma arising from posterior mediastinum. Thorax 41:322, 1986

210. Barva NR, Patel AR, Takita H, et al: Fibrosarcoma of the mediastinum. J Surg Oncol 12:11, 1979

211. Toback A, Hasbrouck DJ, Blaustein J, et al: Granulocytic sarcoma of the anterior mediastinum. Am J Med Sci 290:206, 1985

212. Falappa P, Danza FM, Leone G, et al: Thoracic extramedullary hematopoiesis: Evaluation by conventional radiology. Diagn Imaging 51:19, 1982

213. Catinella FP, Boyd AD, Spencer FC: Intrathoracic extramedullary hematopoiesis simulating anterior mediastinal tumor. J Thorac Cardiovasc Surg 89:580, 1985

214. Kelley MJ, Mannes EJ, Ravin CE: Mediastinal masses of vascular origin. A review. J Thorac Cardiovasc Surg 76:559, 1978

215. Sinner WN: Directed fine needle biopsy of anterior and middle mediastinal masses. Oncology 42:92, 1985

25

The Pleura and Pericardium

W.T. Elliott McCaughey
Virginia M. Walley

THE PLEURA

Normal Structure and Function

The pleura is a continuous membrane that lines the pleural cavities. The visceral pleura invests the lungs; the parietal pleura lines the thoracic cage, the lateral aspect of the mediastinum, the thoracic inlet, and the superior surface of the diaphragm. The membrane consists of a single row of flat mesothelial cells and a thin underlying layer of connective tissue containing elastic laminae. Ultrastructurally, the mesothelial cells have numerous long microvilli on their free surfaces. They also show desmosomes and cytoplasmic tonofilaments. The microvilli facilitate fluid absorption, and by localizing lubricant (hyaluronic acid) at the cell surface, they seem to aid friction-free movement of the lungs against the chest wall. Mesothelial cells express both low and high molecular weight cytokeratins immunocytochemically whereas the subserosal cells express vimentin. However, when subserosal cells are involved in reactive proliferation, they may coexpress vimentin and low molecular weight cytokeratin, a finding that reflects their ability to differentiate into mesothelium.[1]

The visceral pleura is supplied by the pulmonary and bronchial arterial systems and the parietal pleura by the systemic system. The greater hydrostatic pressure in the parietal pleural circulation causes the passage of fluid into the pleural space. Reabsorption occurs mainly at the venous ends of the capillaries of the visceral pleural circulation. Although several liters of fluid enter the pleural space every 24 hours, only a few milliliters are present at any one time. Changes in the permeability of the pleural capillary network as a result of disease processes may cause accumulation of fluid in the pleural cavity. The extensive pleural lymphatic network also participates in fluid transport, and obstruction of the lymphatic channels or lymph nodes may contribute to a pleural effusion. Outward flow of lymph from the lung parenchyma to the visceral pleura occurs, a factor that may facilitate spread of pulmonary cancer to the visceral pleura.

Pleural Effusion

Accumulation of fluid in the pleural cavity is the commonest manifestation of pleural disease. Classically, effusions are categorized as transudates and exudates. Transudates have a low protein content (less than 3 g/dl); in exudates the protein content is higher than 3 g and the specific gravity is greater than 1.015. Transudates are due to systemic factors such as cardiac failure or hypoalbuminemia, which affect capillary hydrostatic or oncotic pressures in the Starling equation. Exudates result from irritative disease processes involving the serous membrane. Common causes include cancer, pneumonia, and pulmonary infarction. Many types of metastatic cancer may cause pleural effusion, but lung and breast carcinomas and lymphomas account for two thirds of cases.[2,3] Chylous effusions are particularly likely to be associated with lymphomas.[4] Pleural effusions due to metastatic cancer are commonly bilateral. Unilateral pleural effusion is the usual finding in patients with diffuse pleural mesothelioma, although bilateral effusion may occur in the later stages.

Diagnostic Specimens

Diagnostic specimens are obtained in order to determine the nature of an effusion or of a pleural thickening or mass. Pleural fluid is usually the first diagnostic specimen to be sent for analysis. Tissue is sometimes necessary for diagnosis and may be obtained by needle biopsy, thoracoscopy, or open biopsy.

Pleural Fluid

Effusion fluids are usually studied microbiologically and cytologically. Cytologic examination is valuable for diagnosing cancer. Fresh fluid for cytology is put into a container to which heparin (3 units per milliliter of fluid anticipated) has been added and is immediately centrifuged. The optimal volume of fluid is 100 ml, but as little as 2 to 3 ml has been used successfully. Preliminary wet mounts stained with toluidine blue can be used to gain information about the cellularity of the fluid and its nature as a guide to further handling. Smears are prepared from the centrifuge cell pellet and fixed in 95 percent alcohol. The remainder of the pellet is used for preparation of a cell block and, where indicated, for electron microscopy. Cell block material should be fixed in acetified methyl alcohol (1 part glacial acetic acid, 9 parts methyl alcohol) or in Bouin's solution and after routine processing is embedded in paraffin. Cell blocks are particularly useful for immunostains as well as ordinary stains such as those for mucin. For electron microscopy, a portion of the cell pellet is fixed in 3 percent glutaraldehyde.

Filter or cytocentrifuge preparations are valuable when little fluid is available or few cells are present. Filter specimens are prepared by gravity or light suction filtration of the fluid through a filter (pore size 8 μm for bloody specimens, 5μm for clear ones).

When fluids for cytology cannot be processed immediately, they may be left overnight when mixed with equal volumes of 50 percent ethanol and 2 volume percent Carbowax 1540.

Needle Biopsy

The value of needle biopsy (with a Cope or an Abrams needle) in the diagnosis of pleural disease is largely limited to cases in which there is widespread involvement of the serous membrane. It is less sensitive than cytology in detecting the presence of cancer. In one large study, pleural malignant disease was established by cytology in 57.6 percent of cases and by needle biopsy in 43 percent. Together the two techniques established the diagnosis in 64.7 percent of cases.[5] It is more difficult to establish the cell type of a cancer in needle than in cytology specimens, although increasing use of immunostaining and electron microscopy has helped greatly with cell characterization in both types of sample. Needle biopsy is of limited value in inflammatory disease other than for the detection of diffuse granulomatous processes such as tuberculosis.

Thoracoscopy (Pleuroscopy)

Thoracoscopy is very helpful in the diagnosis of pleural cancer, permitting direct visualization of the process and the taking of multiple biopsy specimens.[6,7] It has permitted diagnosis in most cases of pleural mesothelioma.[7]

Open Biopsy

Many tissue specimens are still obtained through thoracotomy, especially when mesothelioma enters the differential diagnosis. If the pleural space is obliterated, tissue can be obtained from a minithoracotomy.[6]

Pleuritis

Pleural inflammation is usually secondary to underlying lung disease, especially pneumonia, and is often accompanied by a fibrinous or fibrinopurulent exudate. When due to infection, pleuritis may advance to the accumulation of pus in the pleural cavity and the formation of an empyema. For the most part pleural inflammatory reactions due to various infections have no specific morphologic characteristics, and identification of the infectious agent involved depends on culture. However, in active tuberculous pleurisy granulomas are present. Granulomatous involvement of the pleura is also found occasionally in sarcoidosis.

Reactive eosinophilic pleuritis[8] may occur secondary to rupture of pleural blebs into the pleural cavity. It is characterized by diffuse or nodular collections of histiocytes and eosinophils in the visceral or parietal pleura. Giant cells may also be present. Active pleural inflammation may occur in connective tissue diseases such as rheumatoid arthritis, systemic lupus erythematosus, or progressive systemic sclerosis. In rheumatoid arthritis the inflammatory process occasionally may derive some specificity from the presence of rheumatoid nodules.

Hyperplasia and shedding of mesothelium is a common reaction to serosal irritation in all the serosal cavities. Reactive mesothelial cells are often numerous in effusion fluid. They are frequently rounded and single but may form small sheets or clusters. The cells may show considerable pleomorphism, including the presence of multinucleate forms (Fig. 25-1), and their pleomorphism, cou-

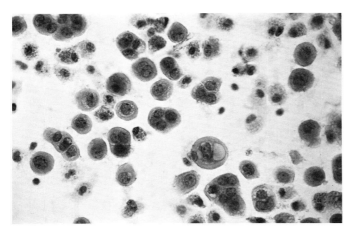

Fig. 25-1. Reactive mesothelial cells in an effusion. There is some cellular pleomorphism with scattered multinucleate cells and occasional cytoplasmic vacuolation.

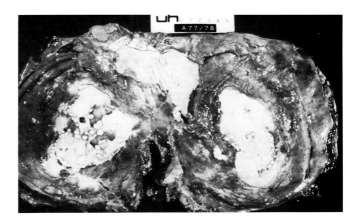

Fig. 25-3. Pleural plaques on the superior surface of the diaphragm. The plaques were hard and partly calcified. The nodularity on the surface of one plaque is a not uncommon finding.

pled with an increased nuclear/cytoplasmic ratio and prominent nucleoli, may create a close resemblance to cancer cells, especially those of malignant mesothelioma. Their cytoplasm is often optically dense, although there may be some peripheral pallor or foaminess. Cytoplasmic vacuolation, mainly due to accumulation of hyaluronic acid, may be present. Intercellular articulations, including embracing and engulfing of cells by other cells, are sometimes seen. These various cellular features are observed in biopsy specimens as well, and here also differentiation from tumor may be very difficult when hyperplasia is marked and there is cytologic atypia[9] (Fig. 25-2).

Pleural fibrosis is often a complication of bacterial pneumonia but is also seen in association with pneumoconioses, connective tissue diseases, and hypersensitiv-

ity pneumonitis, as well as following trauma. In persons exposed to asbestos, diffuse fibrous thickening of the visceral pleura may accompany the characteristic interstitial pulmonary fibrosis of asbestosis. Persons inhaling asbestos may also develop fibrous plaques in the parietal pleura; these often occur in the absence of asbestosis or scarring of the visceral pleura. These plaques occur in the lower half of the pleural cavity and are commonly observed on the superior surface of the diaphragm (Fig. 25-3). They are composed of dense hyaline fibrous tissue, which has a basketweave pattern (Fig. 25-4) and may become partly calcified. The lesions are usually several centimeters in diameter but may be as big as a human palm. Because they may be mistaken for tumor at the time of surgery or may become incorporated in the substance of tumor, they are frequently seen in biopsy tissue.

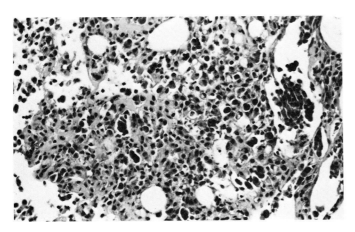

Fig. 25-2. Atypical mesothelial hyperplasia in a pleural biopsy. There is considerable nuclear pleomorphism. Follow-up confirmed that the process was not neoplastic.

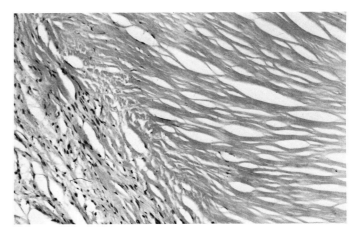

Fig. 25-4. Pleural plaque. The hyaline collagen has a basket weave pattern and is poorly cellular. Adjacent pleural tissue is seen at bottom left.

Primary Pleural Tumors

Primary pleural neoplasms, which are uncommon, may be divided into localized and diffuse forms (Table 25-1). Localized tumors of pleura are mainly fibrous and benign and are usually called localized (or solitary) mesotheliomas or, less frequently, fibromas. Very rarely, localized papillary mesotheliomas are noted on the pleura (Fig. 25-5). The diffuse tumors are invariably malignant, and virtually all are mesotheliomas. Rarely, angiosarcomas may involve the pleura diffusely.[10] Diffuse mesotheliomas are more common than localized pleural tumors, especially in areas where occupational exposure to asbestos has been common.

A few malignant pleural tumors have gross characteristics intermediate between those of the localized and diffuse forms.

Localized Fibrous Mesothelioma

Some 80 percent of localized fibrous mesotheliomas arise from the visceral pleura, from which they frequently project into the pleural cavity as a rounded, pedunculated mass. A few lie largely or entirely within lung parenchyma while maintaining contact with the visceral pleura. The small proportion arising from the parietal pleura usually expand into the pleural cavity. Most localized mesotheliomas are benign, but some 20 percent recur locally or metastasize.[11] Malignant tumors are usually large (more than 10 cm in diameter) at the time of initial surgery; larger neoplasms may also be associated with a pleural effusion. Localized mesotheliomas may be accompanied by extrathoracic joint symptoms[12] and occasionally by hypoglycemia[11] and galactorrhea.[12]

In most localized tumors, fibrous or collagenized areas are prominent microscopically (Fig. 25-6). Cellular fields composed of oval or spindle-shaped cells are also frequently seen (Fig. 25-7). The presence of numerous

TABLE 25-1. Classification of Primary Pleural Tumors

Localized
  Fibrous mesothelioma
    Benign
    Malignant
  Benign papillary mesothelioma (very rare)
  Angioma (very rare)

Diffuse
  Malignant mesothelioma
    Epithelial
      Tubulopapillary or tubular
      Solid (mesothelial)
    Sarcomatous (including desmoplastic)
    Biphasic
    Undifferentiated
  Angiosarcoma (very rare)
  ? Other sarcomas

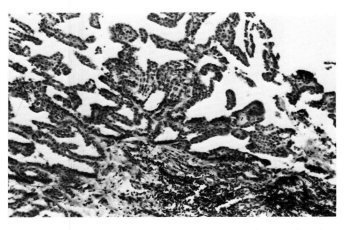

Fig. 25-5. Solitary benign papillary mesothelioma. The slender fronds are covered by a layer of uniform cuboidal cells.

rounded or branching vascular spaces may create a resemblance to hemangiopericytoma (Fig. 25-8). When the tumors project into lung substance, their pulmonary surfaces frequently become covered by a layer of cuboidal or low columnar epithelium. In some cases this non-neoplastic epithelium lines clefts, which dip into the substance of the tumor (Fig. 25-9) and give the impression of a biphasic neoplasm.

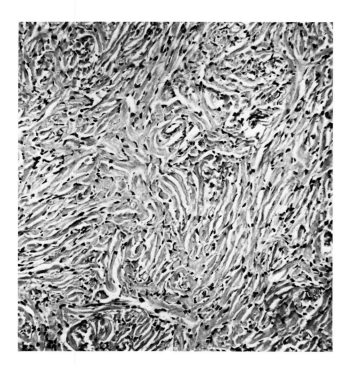

Fig. 25-6. Localized fibrous mesothelioma. The tumor is composed of a meshwork of hyaline collagen strands with moderate numbers of associated spindle cells.

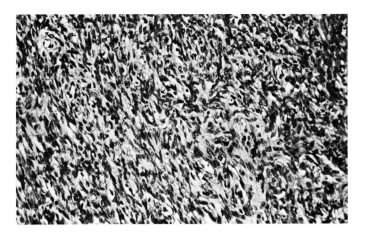

Fig. 25-7. Localized fibrous mesothelioma. The tumor is cellular in this area.

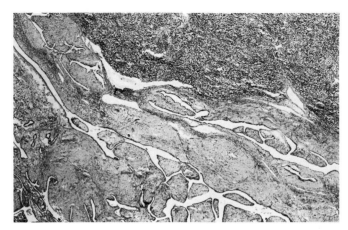

Fig. 25-9. Localized fibrous mesothelioma. Branching spaces lined by non-neoplastic cuboidal epithelium of bronchiolar type dip into the substance of the tumor and create a complex pseudopapillary appearance.

Recent immunocytochemical and ultrastructural studies give support to the view that at least some of these tumors are of mesothelial origin.[13]

Diffuse Pleural Mesothelioma

Etiology

It is widely accepted that some 60 to 80 percent of diffuse pleural mesotheliomas are caused by inhaled asbestos dust, although the percentage of cases with an occupational history of asbestos exposure varies greatly in different series. Usually the asbestos exposure has taken place in an occupational setting, but paraoccupational, neighborhood, domestic, and environmental exposures may also be involved. The main forms of asbestos used commercially (chrysotile, amosite, and crocidolite) have all caused pleural mesothelioma, but there is evidence that chrysotile, which accounts for most of the asbestos used in the Western world in recent decades, may be less potent than the other commercial forms in this regard. Also, it is not clear to what extent the ability of chrysotile to cause mesothelioma is due to the chrysotile fiber itself or to the fibers of the tremolite form of asbestos, which sometimes contaminates the chrysotile ore. The capacity of asbestos to cause mesothelioma is related to the physical characteristics of the fiber, long, thin asbestos fibers being the most carcinogenic.[14,15] Thus, it is not surprising that nonasbestos mineral fibers having the same physical characteristics as asbestos can cause mesothelioma to develop in both humans[16] and experimental animals.[17] It is possible also that factors or agents other than mineral fiber may be involved in the causation of some mesotheliomas.[18]

From the epidemiologic and medicolegal standpoint it is important that the surgical pathologist carefully study any parenchymal lung tissue associated with mesothelioma biopsy material for evidence of asbestos exposure in the form of asbestos bodies or asbestosis. Wet tissue should always be retained in case specialized asbestos fiber analysis is required as part of a more detailed investigation.

The latent interval between the first exposure to asbestos and the initial clinical manifestation of the tumor is usually in the 20 to 50 year range.

Epidemiology

The incidence of diffuse mesothelioma continues to rise,[19] a reflection of widespread industrial use of asbes-

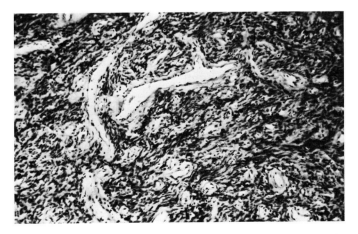

Fig. 25-8. Localized fibrous mesothelioma. The appearance in this vascular area of tumor bears some resemblance to a hemangiopericytoma.

tos in the past and the inadequate safety practices then in effect. It has been estimated that 1,600 cases occurred in 1980 in the United States.[20] Marked geographic variations in frequency are largely explained by the distribution of industries such as shipbuilding that have used asbestos extensively in the past. Those who work alongside asbestos workers or live with them have also been at increased risk.[21,22] Occasionally striking examples of family clustering are seen.[23] The incidence of diffuse mesothelioma rises with increasing age, occasional cases being seen in childhood. Nearly three quarters of these cancers originate in the pleura, most of the remainder being peritoneal.

Clinical Presentation

Pleural effusion is usually the first clinical finding. After drainage, pleural thickening may be apparent radiographically, but frequently is not obvious for at least several months after the effusion is detected. Sometimes, also, the chest radiograph or computed tomography (CT) scan may show a localized mass that is difficult to distinguish from lung cancer; only later does the diffuse nature of the pleural tumor become obvious. The effusion tends to disappear with fusion of the thickened layers of pleura in the later stages. Subcutaneous tumor nodules may appear in the chest wall, especially in relation to aspiration needle tracts and thoracotomy scars.[24] Evidence of extension of the tumor into the mediastinum, the peritoneum, or the opposite pleural cavity is fairly common in the later stages, and involvement of axillary or supraclavicular lymph nodes may be noted at this time. Occasionally there is bilateral pleural or peritoneal involvement at an early stage. However, metastases are seldom obvious during life. Thrombocytosis and thromboembolic episodes are common[25]; hypoglycemia[26] and inappropriate secretion of antidiuretic[27] and gonadotropic hormones[28] are occasionally seen.

Gross Appearance and Behavior

Diffuse pleural mesotheliomas in their early stages usually appear as granulations, multiple nodules, or plaques, which are often most numerous on the parietal pleura.[7] Occasionally at this stage there is a dominant mass of tumor with relatively inconspicuous satellite nodules. With progression the tumor nodules increase in number and size and eventually coalesce to form a continuous layer, which obliterates the pleural cavity and encases the lung (Fig. 25-10). The cancer emphasizes its malignancy particularly by direct infiltration of adjacent tissue such as lung, chest, mediastinum, and diaphragm. At the hilum the tumor may compress a major bronchus and occasionally infiltrates its wall. Lymph node metastases, usually regional, are common, and dissemination to the

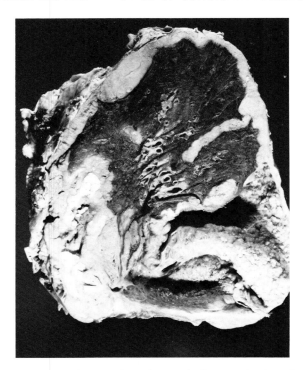

Fig. 25-10. Malignant pleural mesothelioma. The lung is encased by a thick layer of tumor, which also extends along the interlobar fissure. The cancer projects into lung substance at several points.

opposite lung, liver, kidney, adrenal gland, and bone is not infrequent in the late stages.[29]

Cytology

Epithelial mesotheliomas usually exfoliate large numbers of cells, which are generally larger than benign mesothelial cells but may vary considerably in size (Fig. 25-11). Cell clusters or morulae may be prominent. Well differentiated mesothelioma cells, like reactive mesothelial cells, often have dense cytoplasm, and their nuclei may show only subtle malignant changes. Cytoplasmic vacuolation is sometimes prominent. Poorly differentiated mesothelioma cells are often impossible to distinguish from other types of malignant cells.

Histology

Four main histologic groups of diffuse pleural mesothelioma can be recognized: epithelial, sarcomatous, biphasic, and poorly differentiated/undifferentiated.[29] In addition, some tumors, usually of the sarcomatous type, contain large amounts of dense fibrous tissue and are known as *desmoplastic* mesotheliomas.[30]

Tumors of purely epithelial type account for some 50 percent of cases and show much variation in appearance. Often there are epithelial tubulopapillary or tubular for-

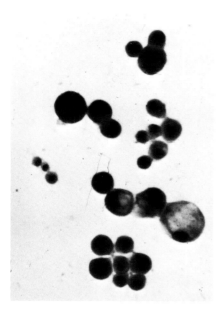

Fig. 25-11. Malignant mesothelioma cells in effusion fluid. The cells show marked variation in size. Cytoplasmic vacuolation is present.

mations (Figs. 25-12 and 25-13); much less frequently there is a predominantly papillary or microcystic pattern. The epithelial cells in the better differentiated glandular areas are often medium-sized and cuboidal or flattened, with marked uniformity of the nuclei, which are sometimes vesicular and have prominent nucleoli. In other glandular areas there may be considerable nuclear pleomorphism, and the tumor cells may assume a columnar form. Some tumors of epithelial form may be composed in part or in whole of sheets or clumps of polygonal cells,

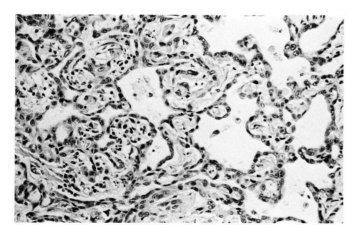

Fig. 25-12. Diffuse malignant mesothelioma. The tumor has a well developed tubulopapillary pattern. The tumor cells are cuboidal or flattened.

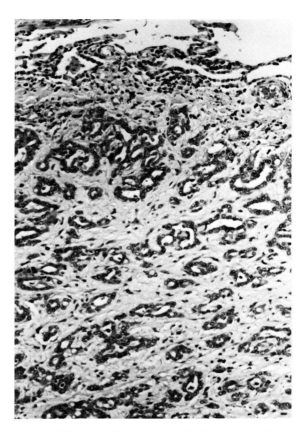

Fig. 25-13. Diffuse malignant mesothelioma. Cuboidal tumor cells form tubules. The tumor cell nuclei are vesicular and uniform.

which when well differentiated may closely resemble hyperplastic mesothelium (Fig. 25-14) but in more poorly differentiated tumors may be difficult to distinguish from other undifferentiated neoplasms. The presence of large cytoplasmic vacuoles that do not stain for mucin may help to exclude adenocarcinoma (Fig. 25-15). Not infrequently the degree of differentiation varies considerably within the same tumor, a fact that emphasizes the importance of adequate histologic sampling. The stroma of epithelial-type mesotheliomas may be composed of dense collagenous tissue or looser collagen fibers. Desmoplasia is sometimes very prominent, but on occasion the stroma takes on a markedly myxoid or edematous appearance (Fig. 25-16).

An entirely sarcomatous structure is seen in 15 to 20 percent of diffuse mesotheliomas. In these tumors spindle-shaped tumor cells may take up storiform, whorled, or even herringbone patterns, the appearances resembling those seen in soft tissue tumors such as malignant fibrous histiocytoma, fibrosarcoma, or malignant schwannoma (Fig. 25-17). Dense fibrous elements are dominant in the desmoplastic variant of sarcomatous mesothe-

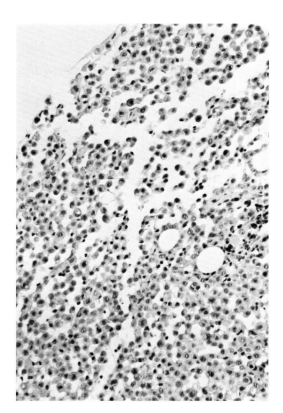

Fig. 25-14. Diffuse malignant mesothelioma. The tumor is composed of sheets of rounded, relatively uniform, polyhedral cells resembling those of hyperplastic mesothelium.

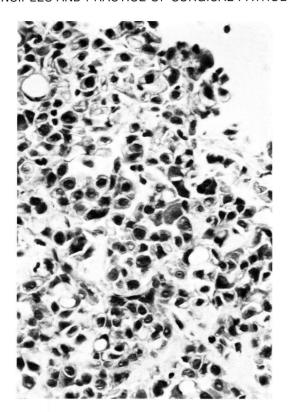

Fig. 25-15. Diffuse malignant mesothelioma. The tumor cells are poorly differentiated and pleomorphic and could be readily confused with those of other poorly differentiated tumors. The presence of prominent cytoplasmic vacuoles that did not stain for mucin supported the diagnosis of mesothelioma.

lioma (Fig. 25-18) and may simulate reactive fibrosis. Even with generous sampling, desmoplastic mesothelioma and fibrous pleurisy may be very difficult to distinguish.[9]

In a further 15 to 20 percent of tumors, epithelioid and sarcomatous areas are both present. In these biphasic tumors the two phenotypes of tumor may occur in different parts of its substance (Fig. 25-19) or may be intimately admixed (Fig. 25-20).

Undifferentiated tumors consist of sheets of poorly differentiated and pleomorphic cells similar to those occurring in many different types of tumor (Fig. 25-21). They are recognized as mesotheliomas only on the basis of their localization, behavior, and immunocytochemical and ultrastructural appearance.[31]

Differential Diagnosis

The range of the histologic differential diagnosis is shown in Table 25-2. Aside from metastatic carcinoma, the distinction of mesothelioma from other entities still depends largely on the application of classical pathologic principles and knowledge. Thus, in the case of well differentiated mesothelioma, separation from mesothelial

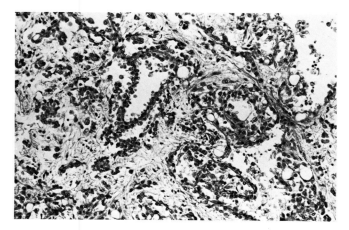

Fig. 25-16. Diffuse malignant mesothelioma of tubulopapillary epithelial type with a prominent myxoid stroma.

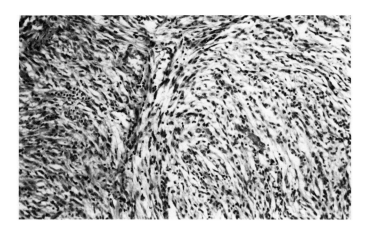

Fig. 25-17. Sarcomatous diffuse malignant mesothelioma. The appearance is indistinguishable from that found in many spindle cell sarcomas.

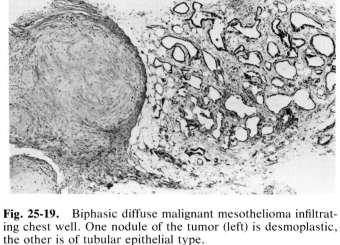

Fig. 25-19. Biphasic diffuse malignant mesothelioma infiltrating chest well. One nodule of the tumor (left) is desmoplastic, the other is of tubular epithelial type.

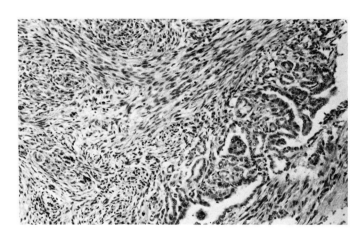

Fig. 25-20. Biphasic diffuse malignant mesothelioma. Sarcomatous and tubulopapillary areas (bottom right) are admixed.

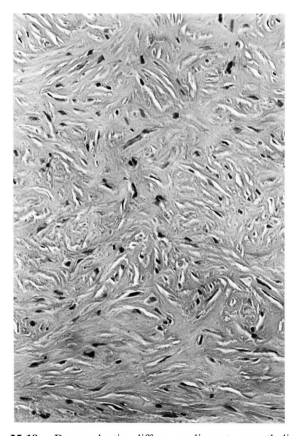

Fig. 25-18. Desmoplastic diffuse malignant mesothelioma. The nuclear atypia distinguishes the tumor from reactive fibrosis.

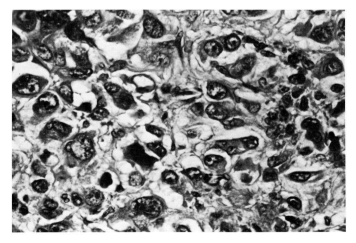

Fig. 25-21. Poorly differentiated diffuse mesothelioma. The tumor is composed of plump polyhedral cells with dense cytoplasm and pleomorphic nuclei with prominent nucleoli.

TABLE 25-2. Differential Diagnosis of Diffuse Malignant Mesothelioma

Epithelial mesothelioma
  Well differentiated papillary or solid
    Mesothelial hyperplasia
  Moderately differentiated tubulopapillary
    Adenocarcinoma
  Poorly differentiated
    Any poorly differentiated carcinoma

Biphasic (mixed) mesothelioma
  Other biphasic tumors (e.g., synovial sarcoma, carcinosarcoma)
  Carcinoma with cellular stroma
  Mesothelial hyperplasia with serosal fibrosis

Sarcomatoid and desmoplastic mesothelioma
  Sarcomas arising in adjacent tissues or metastatic sarcoma
  Fibrosis

hyperplasia rests primarily on the extent of mesothelial proliferation and nuclear atypia, although when other factors such as necrosis and tissue invasion are present in biopsies, they provide valuable support for the diagnosis of mesothelioma.[9] With mesotheliomas in which a biphasic histologic pattern is well developed, the chances of misdiagnosis should be small because of the rarity of this pattern in other tumors that might involve the pleura. Sarcomatous mesotheliomas in most instances cannot be distinguished from other sarcomas microscopically. In this situation knowledge of the gross characteristics of the tumor is very helpful, since sarcomas that arise in the lung or chest wall or that have metastasized to the pleura from remote sites rarely, if ever, involve the pleura diffusely. Separation of desmoplastic mesothelioma from pleural fibrosis may depend largely on the detection of subtle degrees of cytologic atypia and tissue patterns.[9,30]

Special stains and electron microscopy may be very helpful in effecting a distinction between malignant mesothelioma and carcinoma.[31–40]

Special Stains

Many adenocarcinomas contain cytoplasmic mucin vacuoles, whose nature can be confirmed by mucicarmine staining or by a positive periodic acid–Schiff (PAS) reaction that persists after diastase digestion (D-PAS-positive). Granular PAS-positive cytoplasmic staining is seen quite often in mesotheliomas, but the reaction is nearly always effaced by prior diastase digestion. Scanty D-PAS- or mucicarmine-positive cytoplasmic granules or vacuoles are seen in occasional tumors in which all other criteria for the diagnosis of mesothelioma are met, but the presence of more abundant positively staining material effectively excludes the diagnosis.[29] Cytoplasmic vacuoles that do not stain for mucin are found in many mesotheliomas (Fig. 25-15). These sometimes react positively with alcian blue or colloidal iron, the staining being eliminated or reduced by prior hyaluronidase treatment. As hyaluronic acid and other acid mucopolysaccharides are soluble in aqueous fixatives, the absence of a reaction with colloidal iron or alcian blue may simply reflect use of an inappropriate fixative. As acid mucopolysaccharides are a normal component of connective tissue, their presence in the stromal or sarcomatous portion of a tumor is of no diagnostic significance. Tissue extraction studies have shown that hyaluronic acid constitutes an average 45 percent of total glycosaminoglycans in mesotheliomas and 28 percent in lung cancers.[32]

Immunoperoxidase staining techniques for the detection of cell markers are now used extensively to help distinguish mesothelioma from metastatic adenocarcinoma. Carcinoembryonic antigen is a useful marker in this respect since immunostaining for this antigen is often strongly positive in adenocarcinomas and negative or only weakly positive in mesotheliomas.[33,34] Leu M-1 and B72.3 are other markers that are found quite often in adenocarcinomas and rarely, if ever, in mesotheliomas.[33,35]

Cytoplasmic keratins of various molecular weights are usually present in both adenocarcinomas and mesotheliomas. Discriminatory profiles for diagnostic purposes have not yet emerged, but higher molecular weight keratins are found more often in mesotheliomas than in adenocarinomas.[33,36] Moreover, as observed in cell blocks, positive staining for keratin tends to be perinuclear in mesotheliomas whereas it is more likely to be at the periphery of the cell in adenocarcinomas.[34] More specific for mesothelioma is the coexpression of cytokeratins and vimentin in some tumors.[1,37] Sarcomatoid mesotheliomas usually stain positively for keratin, unlike many sarcomas (synovial and epithelioid sarcomas are exceptions). Some benign pleural fibrous lesions stain for keratin and epithelial membrane antigen but benign localized fibrous mesotheliomas are said to be negative.[38]

Electron Microscopy

The hallmark of well differentiated mesothelioma cells is the presence of numerous long slender microvilli on the cell surfaces or within cytoplasmic lumina[39,40] (Fig. 25-22). In less well differentiated mesotheliomas, the microvilli may be shorter and less numerous and thus indistinguishable from those often seen in adenocarcinoma cells.[40] Intercellular junctions and intermediate cytokeratin filaments are often prominent in mesotheliomas. The latter may be organized as tonofilament bundles or as aggregates, and filament distribution is often perinuclear. Some sarcomatous mesotheliomas show evidence of epithelial differentiation in the form of microvilli and desmosome-like intercellular junctions. In poorly differentiated

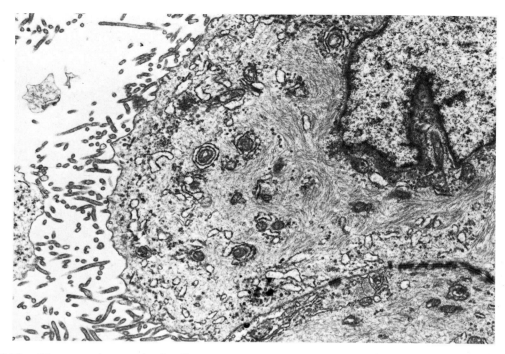

Fig. 25-22. Electron micrograph of malignant mesothelioma. There are numbers of long, slender microvilli projecting from the luminal surface of the tumor cell. Large numbers of intermediate filaments are present in the cytoplasm, and there are multiple desmosomes at the lateral margin.

mesotheliomas the microvilli, intermediate filaments, and cell junctions may be entirely absent. Even in these circumstances the mosaic arrangement of the tumor cells, the presence of long, narrow cytoplasmic processes running parallel to adjacent plasma membranes, the small number of organelles in the abundant cytoplasm, and the disaggregation of nuclear chromatin may help to distinguish the tumor from adenocarcinoma.[31]

Prognosis

In the past the average survival time of patients with diffuse pleural mesothelioma from the onset of symptoms has been in the 12 to 15 month range.[41] However, the limited therapeutic advances of recent years, particularly those associated with the use of chemotherapy, seem to have increased average survival by at least several months. A small number of patients have survived for a number of years following chemotherapy or have had complete remissions.[42,43] Radical surgery has occasionally been associated with extended survival.[44,45]

Patients with epithelial-type diffuse mesotheliomas survive significantly longer than those whose tumors are sarcomatous, with biphasic tumors occupying an intermediate position.[24,46] Tumors with an edematous or mucoid stroma may also have a better prognosis.[44]

Secondary Pleural Tumors

Metastatic tumors in the pleura are far more common than mesotheliomas. Most are adenocarcinomas, with lung in men and breast in women being the most frequent

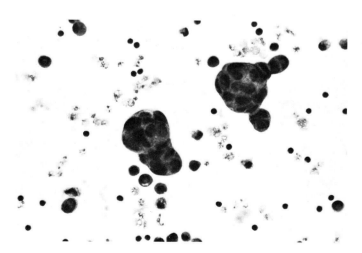

Fig. 25-23. Breast cancer cells in pleural fluid. The cancer cells form clumps as well as being dispersed individually. The nuclear hyperchromatism and pleomorphism and the increased nuclear-to-cytoplasmic ratio indicate that the cells are cancerous.

primary sites. The metastatic tumor frequently takes the form of multiple granules or nodules on the visceral pleura and is often accompanied by an effusion in which cancer cells are found (Fig. 25-23). The bronchioloalveolar form of pulmonary adenocarcinoma may occasionally infiltrate pleura diffusely and mimic diffuse mesothelioma grossly.[47] Rarely, other forms of lung carcinoma and carcinomas arising elsewhere may invade the pleura diffusely.[48] Squamous cell carcinoma occasionally has involved the pleura in patients with persistent pleurocutaneous fistula or extrapleural pneumothorax.[49]

THE PERICARDIUM

Structure and Function

The pericardial cavity is a smooth-surfaced fibrous sac, which is lined by mesothelium and which normally contains up to 50 ml of serous fluid.[50] Its function is still a matter of conjecture, but it probably distributes diastolic pressures over the four heart chambers.[51]

Developmental Defects

The pericardial cavity may be absent, partially or completely.[52] *Diverticula* of the pericardial sac may cause clinical confusion if they produce masses on chest radiography. It is rare for cardiac structures to be torsed in such diverticular defects and surgery to be required. *Cysts* of mesothelial or bronchogenic origin similarly may confuse the differential diagnosis clinically, the mesothelial ones often producing right costophrenic angle masses.[53]

Pericarditis

Purulent pericarditis may be caused by a number of bacterial pathogens, most commonly pneumococci, staphylococci, and streptococci.[51,54] Nowadays it is commonly secondary to penetrating trauma or recent surgery. Tuberculosis is the best known infection causing chronic pericarditis. Sterile acute or chronic pericarditis may be associated with diverse conditions, including renal failure, myocardial infarction, recent radiotherapy, drug therapy, or systemic disorders such as collagen-vascular diseases. The possibility that pericarditis is part of a viral myopericarditis must be kept in mind. Any time the pericardium or myocardium is disturbed by surgery, infarct, or trauma, there is the potential for a delayed autoimmune myocarditis, the so-called postpericardotomy or Dressler's syndrome.

Pericardial Effusion

Any form of pericardial inflammation or neoplasm may be associated with an effusion.[51,54] Hemorrhagic effusions are most often associated with cancer, tuberculosis, blood dyscrasias, recent surgery, or other trauma. Frank hemopericardium is usually related to a ruptured myocardial infarct or to a ruptured vessel as in aortic dissection. Chylous effusion may be idiopathic or may result from abnormalities, especially traumatic, of lymph nodes and thoracic duct drainage in the posterior mediastinal space. Rare cases of cholesterol pericarditis have been reported.[54]

Pericardial Tamponade

Tamponade is a condition in which the heart chambers cannot sufficiently dilate to accommodate venous return in diastole, because of raised intrapericardial pressure.[51,54] It may be caused by as little as 150 ml of fluid accumulating quickly in the pericardial sac, but if fluid accumulates slowly, much larger amounts are required. Although the pericardium is often left open after cardiac surgery, this may not prevent tamponade.[55] Hemopericardium is the commonest cause of tamponade.

Pericardial Constriction

In pericardial constriction the heart cannot dilate during diastole because the pericardial cavity is obliterated and converted to a rigid fibrous hull. This may result from a host of conditions associated with pericarditis and adhesions, and in areas where tuberculosis is endemic this infection is a common cause. Constriction may be associated with neoplastic involvement. Previous hemopericardium and cardiac surgery have also led to constriction.[56] Unusual associations include idiopathic retroperitoneal fibrosis.[57] In many instances the original inciting insult may be obscure, the initiating disease process having resolved years earlier. Occasional cases are difficult to differentiate from restrictive cardiomyopathy and may require endomyocardial biopsy in the workup.[58]

Pericardial Neoplasms

Rare benign neoplasms, hamartomas, and heterotopias include lipomas, teratomas, and ectopic thyroid or thymic tissue.[53] Multiple lipomas may be associated with tuberous sclerosis.[53] Teratomas are most often seen in children and found at the base of the heart or the great vessels.[59] The great majority of malignant neoplasms are metastases.[53,59] As in the case of the pleural cavity, the breast and lung are the most common primary sites. Leukemia, lymphoma, and melanoma also have an unusual propensity to involve the heart and pericardium. Metastatic tumor usually takes the form of discrete nodules but may occasionally assume a diffuse sheet-like form resembling mesothelioma. Metastases may be associated with an effusion and sometimes with tamponade or constriction.

Malignant mesothelioma is the commonest primary pericardial neoplasm.[53] This tumor progresses to encase the heart and attachments of the major vessels. Other primary cardiac malignancies such as angiosarcoma, rhabdomyosarcoma, and fibrosarcoma may involve the pericardium as well. Malignant mesothelioma and angiosarcoma invade the pericardium diffusely, the others more often focally. Occasional mesotheliomas have been associated with asbestos exposure[60] or with direct application of asbestos and fiberglass to the pericardium.[61] Pericardial Kaposi's sarcoma in patients with acquired immunodeficiency syndrome (AIDS) has been reported.[62] Primary pericardial lymphoma has also been described.[63]

Pericardiocentesis and Pericardial Window

Pericardiocentesis or catheter drainage may be used therapeutically to relieve tamponade or diagnostically to provide material for hematocrit determination, culture, biochemistry, or cytology[64]. In pericardial constriction or in recurrent effusion, surgical decortication of the heart and removal of pieces of pericardium of varying size may be required.[65] Creation of a window for drainage into the peritoneal or pleural cavity may be useful.

REFERENCES

1. Bolen JW, Hammar SP, McNutt MA: Reactive and neoplastic serosal tissue. A light microscopic, ultrastructural and immunocytochemical study. Am J Surg Pathol 10:34, 1986
2. Leuallen EC, Carr DT: Pleural effusions. N Engl J Med 252:79, 1955
3. Hausheer FH, Yarbro HW: Diagnosis and treatment of malignant pleural effusions. Semin Oncol 12:54, 1985
4. Roy PH, Carr DT, Payne WS: The problem of chylothorax. Mayo Clin Proc 42:457, 1967
5. Prakash UBS, Reiman HM: Comparison of needle biopsy with cytologic analysis for the evaluation of pleural effusion: Analysis of 414 cases. Mayo Clin Proc 60:158, 1985
6. Lewis RJ, Sisler GE, MacKenzie JW: Diffuse mixed malignant pleural mesothelioma. Ann Thorac Surg 31:53, 1981
7. Boutin C, Viallat JR, Rey F: Thoracoscopy in diagnosis, prognosis and treatment of mesothelioma. p. 301. In

Antman K, Aisner J (eds): Asbestos-Related Malignancy. Grune & Stratton, Orlando, FL, 1987
8. Askin FB, McCann BG, Kuhn C: Reactive eosinophilic pleuritis. A lesion to be distinguished from pulmonary eosinophilic granuloma. Arch Pathol Lab Med 101:187, 1977
9. McCaughey WTE, Al-Jabi M: Differentiation of serosal hyperplasia and neoplasia in biopsies. Pathol Annu 21(Part 1):271, 1986
10. McCaughey WTE, Dardick I, Barr JR: Angiosarcoma of serous membranes. Arch Pathol Lab Med 107:304, 1983
11. Dalton WT, Zolliker AS, McCaughey WTE, et al: Localised primary tumors of the pleura. Cancer 44:1465, 1979
12. Briselli M, Mark EJ, Dickersin GR: Solitary fibrous tumors of the pleura. Cancer 47:2678, 1981
13. Doucet J, Dardick I, Srigley JR, et al: Localised fibrous tumours of serous surfaces. Immunohistochemical and ultrastructural evidence for a type of mesothelioma. Virchows Arch [A] 409:349, 1986
14. Stanton W: Some etiologic considerations of fiber carcinogenesis. p. 289. In, Bogouski P, Gilson JC, Wagner JC (eds): Biological Effects of Asbestos. International Agency for Research on Cancer, Lyons, 1973
15. Timbrell V: Physical factors as etiologic mechanisms. p. 295. In Bogouski P, Gilson JC, Wagner JC (eds): Biological Effects of Asbestos. International Agency for Research on Cancer, Lyons, 1973
16. Baris YI, Artvinli M, Sahin AA: Environmental mesothelioma in Turkey. Ann NY Acad Sci 330:423, 1979
17. Suzuki Y, Bohl AN, Langer AM, Selikoff IJ: Mesothelioma following intraperitoneal administration of zeolite. Fed Proc 39:640, 1980
18. Peterson JT, Greenberg SD, Buffler PA: Non-asbestos related malignant mesothelioma. A review. Cancer 54:951, 1984
19. Spirtas R, Beebe GW, Connelly RR, et al: Recent trends in mesothelioma incidence in the United States. Am J Ind Med 9:397, 1986
20. Asbestiform Fibers. Non-occupational Health Risks. National Academy Press, Washington, 1984
21. Anderson HA, Lilis R, Daum SM, et al: Household-contact asbestos neoplastic risk. Ann NY Acad Sci 271:311, 1976
22. Vianna NJ, Polan AK: Non-occupational exposure to asbestos and malignant mesotheliomas in females. Lancet 1:1061, 1978
23. Risberg B, Nickels J, Wagermark J: Familial clustering of malignant mesothelioma. Cancer 45:2422, 1980
24. Elmes PC, Simpson MJC: The clinical aspects of mesothelioma. J Med (NS) 45:427, 1976
25. Chahinian AP, Paj AK, Holland JF, et al: Diffuse malignant mesothelioma. Prospective evaluation of 69 patients. Ann Intern Med 96:746, 1982
26. Jara F, Takita H, Rao UNM: Malignant mesothelioma of pleura. NY State J Med 77:1885, 1977
27. Perks WH, Crow JC, Green M: Mesothelioma associated with the syndrome of inappropriate secretion of antidiuretic hormone. Am Rev Respir Des 117:789, 1978
28. Rich S, Presant CA, Meyer J, et al: Human chorionic gonadotropin and malignant mesothelioma. Cancer 43:1457, 1979

29. McCaughey WTE, Kannerstein M, Churg J: Tumors and pseudotumors of serous membranes. Atlas of Tumor Pathology, Series 2. Fasc. 20. Armed Forces Institute of Pathology, Washington, 1986

30. Cantin R, Al-Jabi M, McCaughey WTE: Desmoplastic diffuse mesothelioma. Am J Surg Pathol 6:215, 1982

31. Dardick I, Al-Jabi M, McCaughey WTE, et al: Ultrastructure of poorly differentiated diffuse epithelial mesothelioma. Ultrastruct Pathol 7:151, 1984

32. Chiu B, Churg A, Tengblad A, et al: Analysis of hyaluronic acid in the diagnosis of malignant mesothelioma. Cancer 54:2195, 1984

33. Otis CN, Carter D, Cole s, Battifora H: Immunohistochemical evaluation of pleural mesothelioma and pulmonary adenocarcinoma. A bi-institutional study of 47 cases. Am J Surg Pathol 11:445, 1987

34. Cibas ES, Corson JM, Pinkus GS: The distinction of adenocarcinoma from malignant mesothelioma. The role of routine mucin histochemistry and immunohistochemical assessment of carcinoembryonic antigen, keratin proteins, epithelial membrane antigen and milk fat globulin derived antigen. Hum Pathol 18:67, 1987

35. Szpak CA, Johnston WW, Roggli V, et al: The diagnostic distinction between malignant mesothelioma of the pleura and adenocarcinoma of the lung as defined by monoclonal antibody. Am J Pathol 122:252, 1986

36. Blobel GA, Moll R, Franke WW, et al: The intermediate filament cytoskeleton of malignant mesotheliomas and its diagnostic significance. Am J Pathol 121:235, 1985

37. Churg A: Immunohistochemical staining for vimentin and keratin in malignant mesothelioma. Am J Surg Pathol 9:360, 1985

38. Epstein JI, Budin RE: Keratin and epithelial membrane antigen immunoreactivity in nonneoplastic fibrous pleural lesions: Implications for the diagnosis of desmoplastic mesothelioma. Hum Pathol 17:514, 1986

39. Warhol MJ, Corson JM: An ultrastructural comparison of mesotheliomas with adenocarcinomas of the lung and breast. Hum Pathol 16:50, 1985

40. Dardick I, Jabi M, McCaughey WTE, et al: Diffuse epithelial mesothelioma: A review of the ultrastructural spectrum. Ultrastruct Pathol 11:503, 1987

41. Legha SS, Muggia FM: Pleural mesothelioma: Clinical features and therapeutic implications. Ann Intern Med 87:613, 1977

42. Yap B-S, Benjamin RS, Burgess A, Bodey GP: The value of Adriamycin in the treatment of diffuse malignant pleural mesothelioma. Cancer 42:1692, 1978

43. Rossof AH: Treatment 11: Chemotherapy in the management of mesothelioma. p. 73. In Kittle CF (ed): Mesothelioma: Diagnosis and Management. Year Book Medical Publishers, Chicago, 1987

44. Butchart EG, Ashcroft T, Barnsley WC, Holden MP: Pleuropneumonectomy in the management of diffuse malignant mesothelioma of the pleura. Experience with 29 patients. Thorax 31:15, 1976

45. Kittle CF: Treatment 1: The surgical treatment of mesothelioma. p. 61. In Kittle CF (ed): Mesothelioma: Diagnosis and Management. Year Book Medical Publishers, Chicago, 1987

46. Griffiths MH, Riddell RJ, Xipell JM: Malignant mesothelioma. Pathology 12:591, 1980

47. Harwood TR, Gracey DR, Yokoo H: Pseudomesotheliomatous carcinoma of the lung. Am J Clin Pathol 65:159, 1976

48. McCaughey, WTE: Criteria for the diagnosis of diffuse mesothelial tumors. Ann NY Acad Sci 132:608, 1965

49. Rüttner JR, Heinzl S: Squamous cell carcinoma of the pleura. Thorax 32:497, 1977

50. Roberts WC, Spray TL: Pericardial heart disease: A study of its causes, consequences and morphologic features. In Spodick DH (ed): Pericardial Diseases. FA Davis, Philadelphia, 1976

51. Shabetai R: The pericardium. Grune & Stratton, Toronto, 1981

52. Nasser WK: Congenital defects of the pericardium. p. 51. In Fowler NO (ed): The Pericardium in Health and Disease. Futura Publishing, Mt. Kisco, NY, 1985

53. McAllister HA Jr, Fenoglio JJ: Tumors of the cardiovascular system. In Atlas of Tumor Pathology. Series 2. Fas. 15. Armed Forces Institute of Pathology, Washington, 1978

54. Fowler NO: The Pericardium in Health and Disease. Mount Kisco. Futura Publishing, Mt. Kisco, NY, 1985

55. Nelson RM, Jenson CB, Smoot WM III: Pericardial tamponade following open heart surgery. J Thorac Cardiovasc Surg 58:510, 1969

56. Kutcher MA, King SB III, Alimurung BN, et al: Constrictive pericarditis as a complication of cardiac surgery: Recognition of an entity. Am J Cardiol 50:742, 1982

57. Hanley PC, Shub C, Lie JT: Constrictive pericarditis associated with combined idiopathic retroperitoneal and mediastinal fibrosis. Mayo Clin Proc 59:300, 1985

58. Schoenfeld MH, Supple EW, Dec GW, et al: Restrictive cardiomyopathy versus constrictive pericarditis: Role of endomyocardial biopsy in avoiding unnecessary thoracotomy. Circulation 75:1012, 1987

59. Chan HSL, Sonley MJ, et al: Primary and secondary tumors of childhood involving the heart, pericardium and great vessels: A report of 75 cases and review of the literature. Cancer 56:825, 1985

60. Kahn EI, Rohl A, Barrett EW, et al: Primary pericardial mesothelioma following exposure to asbestos. Environ Res 23:270, 1980

61. Churg A, Warnock ML, Bersch KG: Malignant mesothelioma arising after direct application of asbestos and fiberglass to the pericardium. Am Rev Respir Dis 118:419, 1978

62. Cammarasano C, Lewis W: Cardiac lesions in acquired immune deficiency syndrome (AIDS). J Am Coll Cardiol 5:703, 1985

63. Case Records of the Massachusetts General Hospital: Case 22-1987. N Engl J Med 316:1394, 1987

64. Krikorian JG, Hancock EW: Pericardiocentesis. Am J Med 65:808, 1978

65. Robertson JM, Mulder DG: Pericardiectomy: A changing scene. Am J Surg 148:86, 1984

26

Retroperitoneum, Mesentery, Omentum, and Peritoneum

Gerald Fine
Usha B. Raju

A variety of primary neoplastic and non-neoplastic diseases may be encountered in the retroperitoneum, mesentery, omentum, and peritoneum in addition to those that originate from adjacent or distant organs. Some are common to more than one of these sites, while others more frequently or exclusively involve only one. Because of the intimate relation of these structures to one another, it may be difficult or impossible at times to determine the primary site of involvement; this is particularly true of the large neoplasms.

Benign and malignant tumors in these locales, exclusive of those arising in contiguous organs and lymph nodes, are relatively rare, principally mesenchymal in origin, and similar to those occurring elsewhere in the soft tissues. These are discussed more fully in Chapter 10. A survey of the literature indicates involvement by these tumors in order of decreasing frequency in the retroperitoneum, mesentery, and omentum (Tables 26-1 and 26-2). In studies conducted by Russell et al.[1] and Hashimoto et al.[2] of 1966 soft tissue sarcomas, 276 (14.5 percent) were retroperitoneal and 11 (0.55 percent), all leiomyosarcomas, were mesenteric; none was omental. Tumors are more commonly malignant in the retroperitoneum, benign in the mesentery, and essentially equally distributed between benign and malignant in the omentum. In four studies of 611 primary retroperitoneal tumors, excluding lymphomas and cysts, malignant tumors varied from 76 to 96 percent.[3–6]

The prevalence of the various primary neoplasms varies not only as to site but as to patient age as well. Most are encountered in the retroperitoneum of adults. There are several notable exceptions:

1. Mesotheliomas: except for rare retroperitoneal involvement, restricted to the peritoneum in adults
2. Neurogenic tumors: neuroblastomas common in the retroperitoneum of children; ganglioneuromas and schwannian and paraganglionic tumors more common in the retroperitoneum of adults
3. Teratomas and rhabdomyosarcomas: more commonly encountered in the retroperitoneum of children

Clinical signs and symptoms vary and often are manifest only after the tumor has attained huge proportions, becoming obvious as an abdominal mass, ascites, or by pressure on or infiltration of adjacent structures. This is particularly true of the expansile growths, in contrast to the aggressive infiltrating growths, which are more apt to produce early clinical problems and lead to investigation earlier in the course of the tumor.

Surgical management of these tumors is generally difficult, and the prognosis is often poor, since the tumor has frequently attained a large size and/or become adherent to or infiltrated adjacent structures, making removal difficult or impossible. Although the histologic features may be benign, recurrence and impingement on surrounding

TABLE 26-1. Reported Malignant Tumors of the Retroperitoneum, Mesentery, and Omentum

Tumor	Retroperitoneum	Mesentery	Omentum
Liposarcoma	635	19	7
Leiomyosarcoma	341	16	4
Fibrosarcoma	146	18	19
Rhabdomyosarcoma	180	4	1
Sarcoma, unclassified	204	66	40
Malignant fibrous histiocytoma	113[a]	—	—
Xanthogranuloma	18	6	—
Xanthosarcoma	6	—	—
Inflammatory malignant fibrous histocytoma	7	1	—
Mesenchymoma	62	—	—
Hemangiopericytoma	52	3	4
Angiosarcoma	11	—	12
Myxosarcoma	12	1	8
Fibromyxosarcoma	2	—	1
Extraskeletal Ewing's sarcoma	6	—	—
Mesothelioma	2	—	—
Synovial sarcoma	5	—	—
Chondrosarcoma	3	—	—
Clear cell sarcoma	1	—	—
Osteosarcoma	—	1	—
Plasmacytoma	—	—	1
Alveolar soft part sarcoma	2	—	—
Malignant schwannoma	59	1	—
Neuroblastoma	67	—	—
Sympathicoblastoma	32	—	—
Paraganglioma	17	—	—
Teratoma	—	—	1
Sacrococcygeal	176	—	—
Retroperitoneal	16	—	—
Seminoma	13	—	—
Choriocarcinoma	5	—	—
Embryonal carcinoma	35	—	—
Endodermal sinus tumor	12	—	—
Extrarenal Wilms' tumor	16	—	—
Papillary serous carcinoma	1	—	—
Papillary mucinous carcinoma	3	—	—
Mixed müllerian tumor	4	—	—
Adrenal carcinoma	19	—	—
Renal cell carcinoma	6	—	—
Adenocarcioma	8	—	—
Anaplastic carcinoma	15	—	—
Carcinoid	—	1	—
Totals	2,312	137	98

[a] Abdominal histiocytomas reported by Enjoji et al.[86] and by Weiss and Enzinger[94] were not segregated from retroperitoneal tumors.
(Data from references 1–80, 83–131, and 133–173.)

TABLE 26-2. Reported Benign Tumors of the Retroperitoneum, Mesentery, and Omentum

Tumor	Retroperitoneum	Mesentery	Omentum
Lipoma	293	55	14
Lipoblastoma	5	4	—
Hibernoma	2	—	—
Fibromatosis	—	91	5
Fibroma	17	45	3
Lymphangioma	13	114	26
Lymphangiomyoma	14	—	—
Hemangioendothelioma	5	2	—
Hemangioma	5	4	—
Hemangiomatosis	—	1	—
Leiomyoma	18	10	10
Leiomyoblastoma	—	2	6
Mesenchymoma	14	4	—
Myxoma	11	9	1
Myxoid hamartoma	—	—	3[a]
Osseous tumor	—	1	—
Fibrocartilagonous tumor	—	2	—
Elastofibroma	—	—	1
Giant LN hyperplasia	20	10	—
Neurofibroma	23	7	2
Neurilemoma	9	—	—
Ganglioneuroma	167	5	—
Paraganglioma	59	2	—
Gran. cell myoblastoma	11	—	—
Dermoid	18	16	26
Teratoma	—	2	—
Sacrococcygeal	865	—	—
Retroperitoneal	140	—	—
Serous cystadenoma	18	—	—
Mucinous cystadenoma	6	—	—
Mesonephric adenoma	—	1	—
Plasma cell granuloma	—	1	—
Totals	1,733	388	97

[a] Tumors involved omentum and mesentery.
(Data from references 1–80, 83–131, and 133–173.)

vital structures may result in the death of the patient. Information regarding prognosis of tumors in these sites is limited, being most plentiful for retroperitoneal tumors. Histologic tumor grade and completeness of tumor resection are better prognostic indicators than histologic type. Following what was considered to be complete ex-

cision of retroperitoneal tumors, Cody et al.[7] found the 5-year survival rate for low and high grade tumors was, respectively, 80 percent and less than 10 percent. The disease-free 5-year survival, which varied from 2 percent to 10.2 percent during varying time intervals in the period 1926 to 1974, was in marked contrast to the 63 percent obtained following complete excision of sarcomas in the extremities. This, together with a 77 percent recurrence rate among patients in whom complete excision of the tumor was believed to have been accomplished, emphasizes the need for adjuvant therapy for retroperitoneal sarcomas. Death from sarcoma in all three sites is often related to local tumor recurrence(s) and to involvement of neighboring organs as well as distant metastasis. Meager data regarding the incidence and pattern of metastasis indicate involvement of lung, liver, bone, and brain, in order of decreasing frequency, among retroperitoneal sarcomas and the liver, peritoneum, and lung in mesenteric and omental malignant neoplasms.

TUMORS OF THE RETROPERITONEUM, MESENTERY, AND OMENTUM

Primary

Tumors of Adipose Tissue

Tumors of adipose tissue are among the most frequently encountered mesenchymal tumors of the retroperitoneum, far surpassing those in the mesentery and omentum.[8-18] Approximately 20 percent are pelvic, and 80 percent are abdominal, with the perirenal area the most frequent site involved.

Liposarcoma

Liposarcoma in the retroperitoneum is far more common than in the mesentery and omentum, and accounted for 30 percent of 249 retroperitoneal lipomatous tumors in three studies,[8-10] 19 percent of 1808 soft tissue liposarcomas in seven studies,[1,11-16] and 25 percent of 434 primary retroperitoneal sarcomas, excluding lymphomas, in three studies.[1,2,7] They have been more frequent than lipomas in the retroperitoneum but not in the mesentery and omentum. All the tumors have occurred in adults except for five in the retroperitoneum of children, three of which were not accepted by Shmookler and Enzinger[19] as malignant.[11,20] They are generally very large, lobulated, soft, yellow or grey, mucoid masses, infrequently of fibrous consistency. The mean weight of 24 retroperitoneal tumors was 17.5 lbs, but they have been reported to weigh as much as 63 lbs.[18] Their gross circumscription generally is deceiving, since the tumors frequently infiltrate imperceptibly into surrounding organs, necessitating their removal to effect a complete tumor extirpation.

The varied histology found in peripheral soft tissue liposarcomas may be encountered and accounts for the complex terminology employed in early reports: fibroliposarcoma, lipomyxosarcoma, and fibromyxoliposarcoma. Distinction of the well differentiated (lipomalike) sarcoma from lipoma may be very difficult and may require extensive sampling before the nuclear abnormality and/or cellularity of the sarcoma is found. Care must be exercised not to interpret focal firm gross areas with moderate increase in cellularity and atypia resulting from necrosis as representing sarcoma. Other problems in microscopic diagnosis are encountered in the differentiation of the dedifferentiated (fibroblastic) variant of liposarcoma from fibrous histiocytoma and fibrosarcoma (Fig. 26-1). Distinction among these tumors may be impos-

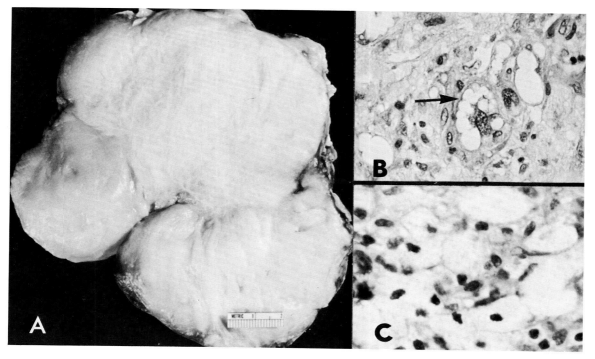

Fig. 26-1. Fibroblastic liposarcoma of the retroperitoneum. **(A)** Gross appearance. **(B)** The spindle cell fibrous appearance of this retroperitoneal tumor was interpreted as a fibrous histiocytoma until lipoblastic cells were identified in some portions of tumor (arrow). These cells are to be distinguished from the xanthomatous (foam) cells **(C)** that may be found in the histiocytic tumors.

sible, particularly when dealing with small tumor samples. Lipid stains demonstrating intracellular lipid may be helpful in identifying an adipose tissue tumor, but it should be borne in mind that occasional lipid droplets can be found in many tumors and that fatty differentiation of the liposarcoma may be focal and require a good deal of sampling to identify lipogenesis. Cellular lipid may be found in the histiocytic tumors, but it occurs in a cell whose bland nucleus and finely vacuolated cytoplasm are unlike that of the uni- or multivacuolated lipoblast. Differentiation of myxoid liposarcoma from myxoma likewise presents a problem; it is resolved by the rich capillary network and evidence of lipogenesis in the myxoid liposarcoma.

Liposarcomas in distant sites occurring simultaneously with, subsequent to, or preceding retroperitoneal or omental liposarcomas have been considered multicentric tumors.[11,14,21,22] Most have involved the lower extremities and preceded a retroperitoneal tumor by less than 1 to 19 years. Spermatic cord neoplasms have preceded or followed retroperitoneal involvement by 1 to 10 years.[11] The single omental tumor was preceded by a forearm liposarcoma 8 years earlier.[21]

The behavior of liposarcoma can be correlated with the degree of tumor differentiation and completeness of its resection. Local recurrence(s), variable but often frequent in the retroperitoneum (28 to 95 percent),[8,9,11] may be delayed for as long as 10 to 12 years[15] and are undoubtedly related to unrecognized tumor infiltration and the limitations placed on the surgical extirpation by the relationship between tumor and vital organs. Kindblom et al.[11] found recurrences to occur in 35 and 71 percent, respectively, in radically and nonradically excised well differentiated and myxoid retroperitoneal liposarcomas. Metastasis—more commonly to the peritoneum, liver, and lungs and infrequently to lymph nodes, mediastinum, and heart—occurred in 27 of 79 retroperitoneal tumors.[11,15] The 5 and 10 year survival rates, respectively 24 to 41 percent and 4 to 15 percent in different studies, are inferior to the 55 to 70% and 42 to 50% obtained in liposarcomas in the extremities, likely related to differences in resectability at these sites.[9,11,15,18] There have been long-term survivors among patients with pleomorphic liposarcomas, but only patients with well differentiated or myxoid neoplasms were free of disease at 6 to 30 years.[15]

The beneficial effect of radiation therapy to the tumor observed by some authorities has not been experienced by others.[11,12,15] Enterline et al.[12] found it beneficial in myxoid but not in nonmyxoid liposarcomas. Kinne et al.[15] observed a prolongation of the disease-free interval from 16 to 32 months, and in one instance radiation provided a 30 year cure following biopsy of the tumor.

Lipoma

Lipoma, also more common in the retroperitoneum than in the mesentery and omentum, may contain other tissues—fibrous, myxomatous, or vascular—which have been incorporated into the name in the early literature, creating the terms *fibrolipoma, myxolipoma,* and *fibromyxolipoma.*[8,23,24] Rarely, hematopoietic foci may be present in retroperitoneal tumors to justify the designation of myelolipoma.[25] Adults are predominately affected; only 21 tumors—14 retroperitoneal, 5 mesenteric, and 2 omental—have been reported in children, the youngest under 1 year of age.[26–29] They have been among the largest tumors, weighing as much as 179 pounds in the adult and 50 pounds in children.[16,27] Encapsulation is the rule, but they may infiltrate or encompass adjacent structures, compromising their function and resulting in the patient's demise. Recurrence(s) following surgical excision have been encountered but with less frequency than in their malignant counterpart. Von Wahlendorf[8] recorded a 14 percent recurrence rate among 132 lipomas and 28 percent among 21 liposarcomas in the retroperitoneum. Among patients with complete tumor excision, DeWeerd and Dockerty[9] recorded recurrence in 3 of 9 lipomas and in 20 of 21 liposarcomas. Microscopic changes of malignancy evident in some recurrences should not be interpreted a priori as a malignant transformation of the lipoma but as a disclosure of a previously undiscovered focus of malignancy in the original large lipomatous tumor.

Lumbosacral lipoma is usually an unencapsulated growth, which affects principally female children from birth to 10 years of age, and only occasionally adults.[30,31] Its connection with the spinal canal by a stalk may result in spinal cord traction and ischemia producing leg paralysis and/or neurogenic bladder. Initially, it may be asymptomatic but clinically evident as a mass in the lumbosacral region, frequently associated with spina bifida or sacral dysgenesis.

Pelvic Lipomatosis

Pelvic lipomatosis in the perirectal, perivesical, or periureteral region chiefly affects black men during the third and fourth decades of life.[32,33] Early in the disease perineal pain and urinary frequency may be the only clinical manifestations but progression to hydronephrosis, uremia, and death may ensue.

Lipoblastoma

Lipoblastoma has been reported infrequently in the retroperitoneum and mesentery and, with the exception of one mesenteric tumor, only in children aged 7 months to

12 years.[34-37] Circumscribed and noncircumscribed forms have been encountered with the lobular histology and benign behavior similar to those occurring in other sites. Lobulation and absence of anaplastic lipoblasts distinguish it from the well differentiated liposarcoma.

Hibernoma

A histologically distinct, uncommon, benign adipose tissue tumor, hibernoma has been reported infrequently in the periadrenal, perirenal, and paraortic areas—sites in which brown fat is to be found.[38,39]

Tumors of Muscle Tissue

Smooth muscle tumors in the retroperitoneum, much more common than in the mesentery and omentum, comprise approximately 50 percent of all soft tissue smooth muscle tumors, are more frequent in women than men, and are rare in children.[1,40-49] Except for the infrequent epithelioid variant, all are the conventional spindle cell variety or a mixture of the two.

Leiomyosarcoma

Leiomyosarcoma, with its propensity toward cystic degeneration, is much more frequent than its benign counterpart in the retroperitoneum but not in the mesentery and omentum. In three studies leiomyosarcomas represented 23.5 percent of 434 primary retroperitoneal sarcomas excluding lymphomas.[1,2,7] Well differentiated tumors present no diagnostic problems, but the less dif-

ferentiated growths possessing a varied histologic pattern may be misdiagnosed as other neoplasms, including hemangiopericytoma, fibrous histiocytoma, fibrosarcoma, and neurofibrosarcoma. Care must be taken not to include large myomatous tumors arising in, and inconspicuously connected to, the gastrointestinal (GI) tract as primary mesenteric or omental tumors (Fig. 26-2). Likewise, the mesenteric epithelioid myomatous tumor must be distinguished from nonchromaffin paraganglioma, for which we believe it has been mistaken and reported.[50,51] Absolute criteria of malignancy cannot be established among smooth muscle tumors. A greater degree of tumor aggressiveness generally is best correlated with increased tumor cell mitotic activity and anaplasia and tumor size and necrosis. However, tumors with as few as one mitosis per 10 high-power fields (hpf) and as little as 7.5 cm in greatest diameter have metastasized to one or more sites: lungs, liver, soft tissue, bone, lymph nodes, and GI tract.[52] Surgical removal has been difficult and often impossible. Even after apparent successful excision, local recurrence, metastasis, or death resulting therefrom frequently ensues in 2 years or less. Five year survival free of tumor is uncommon. Only eight patients among 60 with retroperitoneal tumors survived 6 to 15 years free of tumor.[2,49,52]

Rhabdomyosarcoma

Rhabdomyosarcoma is rare in the mesentery and omentum, but in the retroperitoneum it accounted for 7 percent of 924 soft tissue rhabdomyosarcomas in four studies[1,14,53,54] and 10.6 percent of 434 primary retroperi-

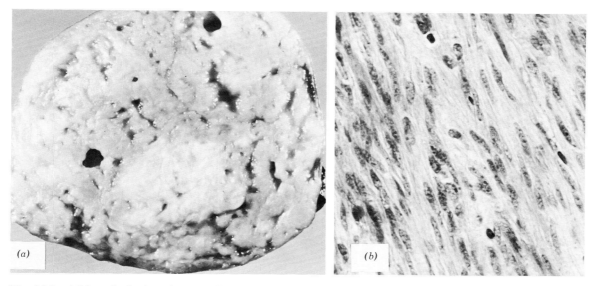

(a)   *(b)*

Fig. 26-2. This soft, fleshy, circumscribed, cellular leiomyosarcoma was attached to the stomach serosa by a thin short fibrous pedicle. **(A, B)**

toneal sarcomas, excluding lymphomas, in three studies.[1,2,7] The embryonal, alveolar, and mixed embryonal-alveolar types occur principally but not exclusively in children and predominate over the pleomorphic type, which chiefly afflicts adults.[6,7,53–57] The embryonal tumors must be distinguished from other small cell tumors (neuroblastoma, lymphoma, and extraskeletal Ewing's tumor), and the pleomorphic rhabdomyosarcoma from other pleomorphic sarcomas, most notably, malignant fibrous histiocytoma. Dependency on cytology and growth pattern in tissue sections for this differentiation is no longer necessary. Electron microscopy and, more recently, immunocytochemistry have provided additional methods for identifying the rhabdomyosarcoma.

When first encountered, they frequently have been unresectable or disseminated. In one instance, hypoglycemia was associated with an embryonal retroperitoneal tumor.[58] The prognosis has been poor, with a varying tumor response to multimodality chemotherapy. A greater than 50 percent tumor response was achieved in 14 of 18 patients, four of whom were alive and free of active tumor 10 to 30 months from diagnosis.[59]

Rhabdomyoma

Rhabdomyoma, adult or fetal, has not been reported in the retroperitoneum, mesentery, or omentum.

Tumors Arising from Fibrous Tissue

Benign fibrous tumors, recorded as fibromas in the older literature and now classified as *fibromatosis*, occur principally in the mesentery and infrequently in the retroperitoneum and omentum of adults and seldom in children.[60–70] Generally they are solitary in one site; rarely, there may be synchronous involvement in the mesentery, retroperitoneum, or abdominal wall scar.[14,69,70] Frequently, the tumor may be associated with familial colonic polyposis, Gardner's syndrome, or a previous abdominal operation, but they may arise unrelated to these conditions.[63,64] Such is the case in *pelvic fibromatosis*, which occurs chiefly in young women and may encroach on and compress pelvic organs and/or blood vessels. Local infiltration makes surgical eradication of fibromatosis difficult and recurrence highly probable. Surgical excision may be curative but recurrence(s) and local infiltration may result in the patient's demise. Absence of an inflammatory cell component and lack of tumor cell anaplasia and mitotic activity serve to distinguish this lesion from idiopathic fibrosis and differentiated fibrosarcoma.

The rarity of *fibrosarcoma* in the retroperitoneum, mesentery, and omentum experienced by ourselves and others is not supported by the frequency with which it has been reported by some investigators.[1–7,71–80] Among 434 primary retroperitoneal sarcomas excluding lymphomas in three studies, fibrosarcoma accounted for 9 percent of tumors, with a 1 to 13 percent frequency range in individual studies.[1,2,7]

Variants of other spindle cell neoplasms, such as malignant schwannoma, leiomyosarcoma, malignant fibrous histiocytoma, and dedifferentiated liposarcoma, must be considered when making a diagnosis of a less differentiated fibrosarcoma. Fibromatosis must be distinguished from the well differentiated fibrosarcoma. The six mesenteric fibrosarcomas reported by Stout[79] were reclassified as fibromatosis in a publication subsequent to his enunciation of the concept of fibromatosis.[40] It is likely that some of the 37 mesenteric and omental fibrosarcomas (see Table 26-1), many of which were reported prior to Stout's[81,82] fibromatosis papers, would also be reclassified. An interesting clinical finding associated with four retroperitoneal fibrosarcomas is hypoglycemia.[14,83]

Tumors of Histiocytes

Histiocytic tumors were not reported as such in the retroperitoneum, mesentery, or omentum until 1964.[84] Before this time, they were recorded as xanthogranuloma in the retroperitoneum or mesentery or classified as other neoplasms.[5,6,40,80] Since 1964, they have been observed with increasing frequency, principally in the retroperitoneum, where they represented 1.8 percent of 1966 soft tissue sarcomas in two studies[1,2]; 9.2 percent of 295 malignant fibrous histiocytomas (MFH) of soft tissues in two studies[1,85]; and 12.7 percent of 276 primary retroperitoneal sarcomas excluding lymphomas in two studies.[1,2] Storiform, pleomorphic, myxoid, xanthogranulomatous, xanthosarcomatous, inflammatory, and malignant fibrous xanthoma subtypes have been reported; giant cell, angiomatoid, and malignant histiocytoma variants have not been reported.[84–94]

The status of xanthogranuloma has been problematic, since it was described in 1935 and considered to be a benign inflammatory process.[88] Reassessment of its histology and behavior has made it apparent that the term xanthogranuloma had embraced two entities—a reactive inflammatory process and a neoplasm. The banal lipid and nonlipid histiocytic-inflammatory cell morphology of the latter, clouding an inconspicuous, sometimes storiform, fibroblastic component, and the similar but atypical anaplastic cellularity of the xanthosarcoma are now recognized as variants of MFH and are classified as the subtype inflammatory malignant fibrous histiocytoma (IMFH).[14,87,89–92] The behavior of these xanthomatous-histiocytic tumors can be deduced to some degree from the anaplasia and mitotic activity of the tumor cells. Among 27 tumors (20 retroperitoneal and 7 mesenteric), there were 16 tumor deaths: 8 of 17 xanthogranulomas, 4 of 4 xanthosarcomas, and 4 of 6 IMFH.[87,89–92] Recurrence(s) following surgical excision occurred in four xanthogranulomas, two xanthosarcomas, and three IMFH. Local recurrence(s) and metastasis have been frequent among other subtypes of retroperitoneal MFH, occurring respectively in 59 percent and 37 percent of 49 patients in three studies.[85,93,94] Among 27 patients with follow-up data, there were 20 tumor deaths (17 from recurrent local tumor and 3 from metastasis) and 7 patients living (4 with metastasis and 2 with and 1 without local tumor).[85,93] There were only two 5-year survivals, both with pulmonary metastasis.

Tumors Arising from Blood and Lymphatic Vessels

Benign vascular tumors are more common than malignant tumors, involving the mesentery, omentum, and retroperitoneum in order of decreasing frequency. Lymphangioma is most common in all three sites, but most frequently the mesentery[14,95–100] (Fig. 26-3). The tumor originally called *lymphangiopericytoma* and subsequently renamed *lymphangiomyoma* has involved only the retroperitoneum of women.[101–104] It has been nonme-tastasizing but has been part of a syndrome consisting of chylous ascites and similar tumors in the lung and/or pleura and, less commonly, tuberous sclerosis. *Hemangiomas* and *hemangioendotheliomas* are rare and were not encountered in the omentum.[66,105–108] Thrombocytopenia and intravascular coagulation have been striking findings in a number of hemangioendotheliomas of the retroperitoneum and mesentery of children.[106–108]

Malignant vascular tumors, not as common as their benign counterpart, have been hemangiopericytoma and angiosarcoma.[2,3,5,14,40,45,109–111] The former, exceeding the latter in incidence, has involved all three sites, predominantly the retroperitoneum, whereas angiosarcoma has been noted only in the omentum and retroperitoneum.

Other Mesenchymal Tissue Tumors

Mesenchymoma

Reported only in the retroperitoneum and mesentery, mesenchyoma has been more frequent in the former site (19:1 among 80 tumors)[3,40,112,113] (see Tables 26-1 and 26-2). Malignant tumors were retroperitoneal and benign tumors were retroperitoneal and mesenteric. The retroperitoneum was the second most common site of involve-

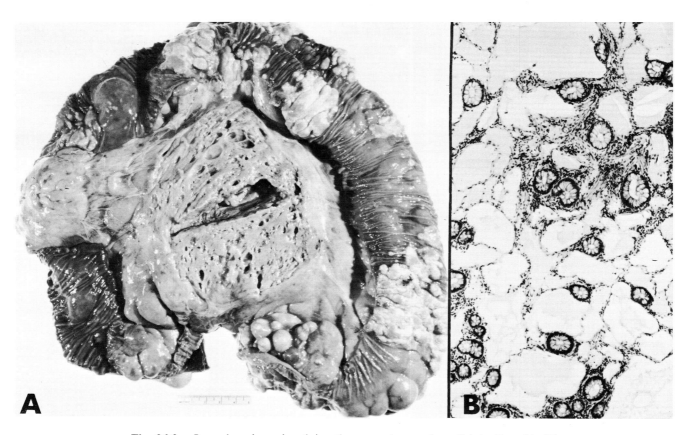

Fig. 26-3. Lymphangioma involving the mesentery and small intestine. **(A, B)**

ment, accounting for 16 percent of 225 malignant mesenchymomas in the surgical pathology laboratory of Columbia University.[112]

Myxomas

Myxomas with abundant myxoid stroma and stellate cells mimicking primitive mesenchyme have been reported 21 times—11 retroperitoneum, 9 mesentery, and 1 omentum.[45,65,77,113,114] Growth to an extremely large size and infiltration of surrounding tissues are not uncommon, but metastasis has not been reported. Their morphology may mimic other myxoid tumors, in particular, myxoid liposarcoma. They lack the florid delicate vascularity of the liposarcoma and they do not possess the cellular elements found in other myxoid tumors (myxoid fibrous histiocytoma, neurofibroma, and botryoid rhabdomyosarcoma).

Myxosarcoma and Fibromyxosarcoma

Considered by some investigators to be malignant counterparts of the myxoma, myxosarcoma and fibromyxosarcoma have been reported with approximately the same frequency as the myxoma but with a different distribution.[4,71,77,115] Fourteen tumors were retroperitoneal, nine were omental, and one was mesenteric. It is not possible to determine their status in the present histogenetic classification of soft tissue tumors because of the lack of descriptive or photographic information. They may represent myxoid variants of a number of tumors—liposarcoma, neurofibrosarcoma, or, as suggested by Enzinger and Weiss[14] for the fibromyxosarcoma, a malignant fibrous histiocytoma.

Myxoid Hamartoma

Simultaneously involving the omentum and mesentery in three infants aged 4 to 6 months, myxoid hamartoma represents another example of classification difficulty among myxoid tumors.[116] Their embryonal cellular makeup suggested a malignant neoplasm, but this has not been borne out by the 1 to 10 year survival in spite of incomplete removal of the tumor.

Tumors Arising from Nerve Tissue

Neuroblastoma

Neuroblastoma is one of the most common malignant neurogenic tumors in the retroperitoneum, occurring almost exclusively in children.[117,118] Extra-adrenal tumors are approximately half as frequent as those of adrenal origin. Generally solitary, they may be multiple with as many as six retroperitoneal tumors having been observed. Rarely, they have been observed in teratomas.

Spontaneous differentiation, purported to be more common in the pelvic retroperitoneal and cervical-thoracic tumors, occurs in primary and metastatic sites. It may vary in different portions of the same tumor and may progress to a point where ganglioneuromatous masses are enveloped by neuroblastic tissue.

Differentiation from other small cell tumors—lymphoma, Ewing's sarcoma, and embryonal rhabdomyosarcoma, also common in children, and anaplastic small cell carcinoma in adults—may be difficult, particularly in the absence of rosettes or neurofibrils. Electron microscopy and, more recently, immunocytochemistry have aided in the recognition and separation of neuroblastomas from these other neoplasms.

The prognosis is generally grave, with metastases occurring frequently to one or more of many sites, with bone, regional nodes, liver, skull, and lungs being most frequent. Patient age, tumor differentiation, extent of involvement, and primary tumor location influence the prognosis. It is better in younger children and in tumors of the pelvis and retroperitoneum than in those of the adrenal.

Ganglioneuroma

Ganglioneuroma, more frequent in the retroperitoneum than in the mesentery (33 : 1 in Table 26-2), affects an older age group than does neuroblastoma.[119–121] Unlike neuroblastoma, extra-adrenal tumors are more common than those arising in the adrenal.

Malignant Peripheral Nerve Sheath Tumor

Except for one mesenteric tumor,[78] malignant schwannoma, or neurofibrosarcoma, has involved the retroperitoneum of adults, representing 7.6 percent of 434 primary retroperitoneal sarcomas excluding lymphomas in three studies.[1,2,7] Spindle cell, spindle-cell epithelioid, or epithelioid morphology occurs in that order of decreasing frequency[1–3,7,122,123] (Fig. 26-4). Glandular inclusions are rarely encountered. Unless grossly identified as arising from a nerve, their histology may be misinterpreted as another variety of neoplasm, particularly fibrosarcoma or leiomyosarcoma. Identification of malignant schwannoma is aided by the demonstration of nerve fibers, more likely to be found at the periphery of the tumor, and/or S-100 protein in the tumor cells, and by electron microscopy.

Neurofibroma and Neurilemoma

Neurofibroma and neurilemoma are also more frequent in the retroperitoneum; only the neurofibroma has been reported in the mesentery and omentum.[40,113,120,124–126] Recurrence has been observed in several of the retroperitoneal neurofibromas.[120]

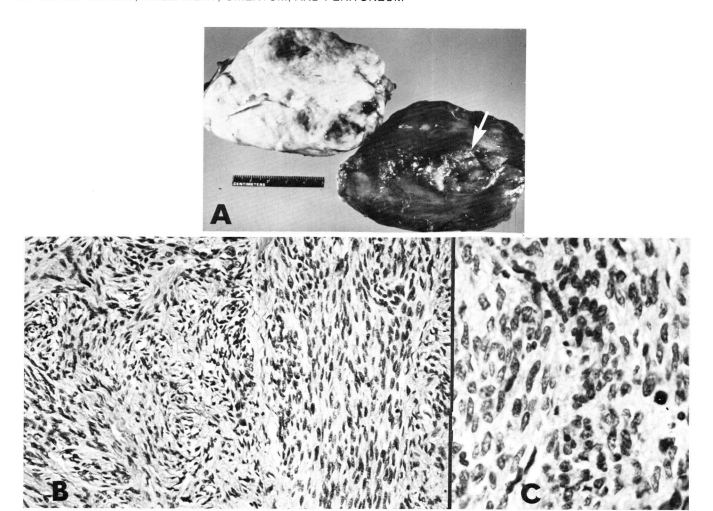

Fig. 26-4. **(A, B, C)** The cell arrangement, cellularity, and pleomorphism in this retroperitoneal tumor are those of a malignant schwannoma. The tumor infiltrated the cortex of a vertebra to which it was attached (arrow indicates site of attachment). Other retroperitoneal tumors removed were neurofibromas.

Paraganglioma

Paragangliomas occur most frequently as functioning tumors of the adrenal gland (pheochromocytoma), but 10 to 20 percent are extra-adrenal, generally benign, non-chromaffin, and nonfunctioning, associated with the autonomic nervous system or Zukerkandl's organ.[127–131] Generally solitary, they may be multiple in the retroperitoneum or associated with neoplasms of similar or dissimilar type (gastric leiomyoblastoma and pulmonary chondroma) in other sites.[129,130] A distinctive organoid and vascular histology, generally but not always present, is usually sufficient for their recognition (Fig. 26-5). In some instances, however, histochemical and/or electron microscopic studies may be necessary to distinguish them from other neoplasms, most notably alveolar soft part sarcoma, regarded as a malignant nonchromaffin

paraganglioma by some authors, and epithelioid smooth muscle tumors.[131] Cytoplasmic granules that are argyrophilic, chromogranin- or chromaffin-positive, and periodic acid-Schiff (PAS)-negative in the paraganglioma are in contrast to the cytoplasmic granular and crystalline PAS-positive diastase-resistent polysaccharide of the alveolar soft part sarcoma. The epithelioid myomatous tumor may possess an organoid cellular arrangement but it lacks the cellular-vascular relationship and the cytoplasmic histochemical positivity of the paraganglioma.

In a study of 12 extra-adrenal paragangliomas, Lack et al.[127] identified argyrophil granules in all the tumors, a positive chromaffin reaction in the four tumors that were properly fixed for this examination, and elevated catecholamines with symptoms in three patients. Symptoms attributable to norepinephrine elaboration by the tumor, more common than in other paragangliomas, have been

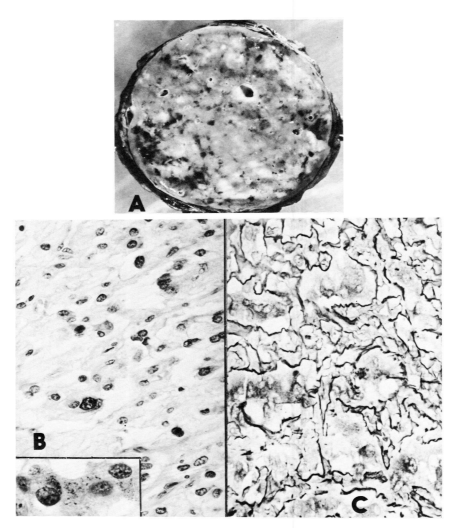

Fig. 26-5. Paraganglioma. The cell aggregates are brought out by the reticulin stain (**C**) in this tumor, which was located at the bifurcation of the aorta. It was found incidentally during arteriography for atherosclerosis of the aorta. Argyrophilic cytoplasmic granules are seen in the Grimelius stain. (Inset)

reported in 25 to 60 percent of tumors.[128] Extra-adrenal paragangliomas are more aggressive than those of adrenal origin, with a 20 to 40 percent metastatic rate compared with a 2 to 10 percent rate for those of adrenal origin.[14,128] Histologic recognition of their malignancy has been problematic. Mitotic activity and/or vascular invasion by the tumor, features supportive of malignancy, were readily identifiable in three of the five malignant tumors but were lacking in the remaining nine tumors studied by Lack et al.[127]

Tumors Arising from Heterotopic Tissue

An array of ectopic tissues (urogenital, neurenteric, spleen, ovary, and adrenal) and primary tumors (germinal, teratoma, dermoid, and carcinoma) have been recorded principally in the retroperitoneum.[132,133]

Teratoma

Teratomas, predominantly retroperitoneal and exceedingly rare in the mesentery and omentum, are more often benign than malignant (5 : 1).[113,134–151] Any level of the retroperitoneum may be involved, but the sacrococcygeal area of infants and children (female to male: 3–4 : 1) and, much less frequently, adults, is the most common site, representing the location of 45 to 60 percent of all childhood teratomas. This sex and age prevalence has not been as striking among teratomas in other areas of the retroperitoneum. Their tissue composition is variable in type and maturity. Neuroepithelial tissue represents the most frequent, and metanephric and mesenchymal tissue the least frequent of the immature components. Histologic grading (based on the quantity of immature and embryonal tissue, tumor necrosis, and cellular atypia and mitotic activity) and the clinical staging of the tumor have been useful prognostic indicators.[138] Local recurrence following surgical extirpation is greatly minimized among tumors of lower grade and stage and when the coccyx is removed with the tumor. Interestingly, glial tissue dissemination as seen in the peritoneum with ovarian teratomas has not been reported in the retroperitoneum despite the neural tissue content of the teratoma. While local recurrence has occurred even with grade 0 tumors, particularly when the coccyx has not been resected, death attributable to tumor has been negligible even in the higher grade neoplasms unless they bear a malignant component. In the presence of the latter, most frequently embryonal carcinoma or endodermal sinus tumor and rarely other neoplasms such as choriocarcinoma, neuroblastoma, and rhabdomyosarcoma, death within 5 years can be expected in 90 percent of patients.[135] Serum α-fetoprotein (AFP) has been an invaluable aid in detecting the presence of endodermal sinus tumor prior to surgical removal. Malignancy among sacrococcygeal teratomas (17 percent of 1041 tumors) is more frequent than at other retroperitoneal levels (10 percent of 156 tumors) and has shown a patient age relationship not noted elsewhere in the retroperitoneum (see Tables 26-1 and 26-2). Malignancy increasing from 5 to 10 percent in the first 2 months of life to 50 to 90 percent thereafter makes paramount the early recognition and complete removal of the tumor.[142–144]

Dermoid Cysts

Dermoid cysts, more frequent than teratomas in the abdomen (14 : 1), have been reported in order of decreasing frequency in the omentum, retroperitoneum, and mesentery, more often in women than men or children.[152–156] Synchronous involvement of the omentum and ovary with a dermoid cyst has suggested to some investigators that abdominal dermoids arise by implantation rather than representing imperfectly developed teratomas from germ cells. Such an origin is refuted by the more frequent occurrence of omental dermoids with normal ovaries. Supernumerary omental ovary which has been the nidus for teratoma development does not appear to account for all omental dermoids.[156] Symptoms from abdominal dermoids, often diverse and perplexing, result from torsion of the omentum, intestinal obstruction, volvulus, or inflammation in the cyst wall and adjacent structures. The latter may prevent the cyst's removal and necessitate marsupialization to relieve the symptoms.

Other Germ Cell Tumors

Germ cell tumors identical to those of the gonads are infrequent in the retroperitoneum unless associated with a teratoma.[3,133,136–141,157,158] Like teratomas, they may occur at any level of the retroperitoneum but are more fre-

quent in the sacrococcygeal area of children, less common in men, and exceedingly rare in women. The frequency with which testicular tumors metastasize to the retroperitoneum makes the acceptance of a primary retroperitoneal germ cell tumor in men problematic. Ultrasound can be helpful to detect nonpalpable testicular neoplasms. Embryonal carcinoma and endodermal sinus tumors are most frequent in the sacrococcygeal area of children. Seminoma and choriocarcinoma are infrequent in the retroperitoneum of men. A sacrococcygeal germinoma in a woman with normal ovaries was cited by Conklin and Abell.[141]

Wilms' Tumor

Extrarenal Wilms' tumors have been reported in different areas of the retroperitoneum with and without teratomatous elements. With the exception of one male patient, all tumors were in children.[159–163]

Serous/Mucinous Cystadenoma, Cystadenocarcinoma, Carcinosarcoma, and Mesonephric Tumors

Serous and mucinous cystadenoma and cystadenocarcinoma and carcinosarcoma, histologically identical to müllerian tumors, and cystic tumors with glomeruli and tubules have been reported in the retroperitoneum, predominantly in women, and rarely in men and children.[133,164–170] Origins considered for these have been heterotopic ovarian tissue, paramesonephric or mesonephric tissue, and müllerian metaplasia and subsequent neoplasia of invaginated peritoneal mesothelium. One adenoma considered mesonephric in origin was reported by Yannopoulos and Stout.[40]

Other Primary Carcinomas

Other primary carcinomas in the retroperitoneum have been recorded as undifferentiated, adenocarcinoma, and adrenal or renal cell (hypernephroid) type not involving adrenal or kidney.[3,5,171] Suggested sources for these tumors have been heterotopic adrenal tissue and metanephric blastema.

Tumors of Lymphoid Tissue

Malignant lymphoma (Hodgkin's and non-Hodgkin's) and plasmacytoma rarely may present in the retroperitoneum or mesentery and remain the only site of involvement. Generally, the tumor is part of a yet undiscovered generalized involvement. Angiofollicular lymph node hyperplasia (angiomatous lymphoid hamartoma or hyperplasia, giant lymph node hyperplasia, lymph nodal hamartoma) of the type more commonly found in the

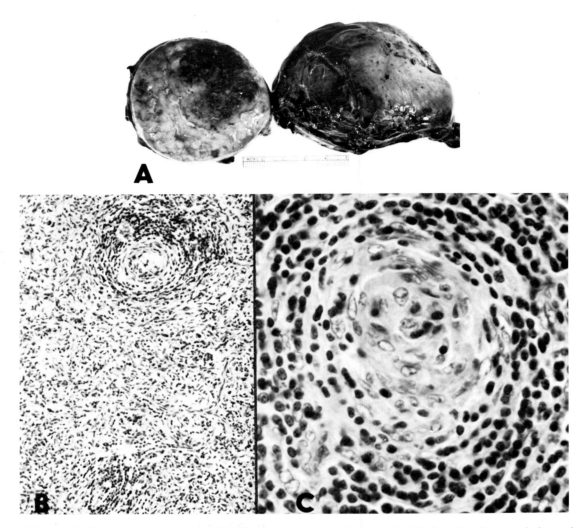

Fig. 26-6. **(A)** This retroperitoneal angiofollicular lymph node hyperplasia **(B)** has the characteristic angiomatous fibrous relacement of lymphoid tissue and **(C)** the fibrotic Hassall's corpuscle-like appearance of the germinal centers.

cervical and mediastinal regions is occasionally encountered in the retroperitoneum or mesentery[172,173] (Fig. 26-6). The angiomatous and fibrous appearance with germinal centers of lymphoid follicles that are fibrotic or resemble Hassall's corpuscles serve to distinguish the process from the various malignant lymphomas.

Tumors Rarely Encountered

These include extraskeletal Ewing's sarcoma,[14] mesothelioma,[5] chondrosarcoma,[2,174,175] clear cell sarcoma,[2] and synovial sarcoma,[1–3,7] in the retroperitoneum; osseous and fibrocartilagenous tumor,[176] plasma cell granuloma,[40] osteogenic sarcoma,[113] and carcinoid[177] in the mesentery; and elastofibroma,[178] and plasmacytoma[179] in the omentum.

Tumors of Uncertain Histogenesis

Tumors of disputed origin, granular cell myoblastoma and alveolar soft part sarcoma, have been reported infrequently in the retroperitoneum.[7,80] Histologic distinction of the latter tumor from paraganglioma is discussed above. The controversial ancestry of both tumors is considered in Chapter 10.

Metastatic Tumors

Secondary neoplasms in the mesentery and omentum are generally derived from carcinomas of the GI tract, ovary, pancreas, and gallbladder. The retroperitoneal space is involved as a result of tumor extension from primary bone neoplasms, notably saccrococcygeal chordoma, and from pancreatic carcinoma or retroperitoneal lymph node metastases principally from the testis, prostate, pancreas, kidney, urinary bladder, uterine cervix, and endometrium.

CYSTS OF THE RETROPERITONEUM, MESENTERY, AND OMENTUM

Cysts are encountered as acute problems or incidental findings in the mesentery, omentum, and retroperitoneum (in that order of decreasing frequency), in children and adults, accounting for 1 in 100,000 to 150,000 hospital admissions. They may be embryonic or developmental (lymphatic, enteric, urogenital, and dermoid); traumatic; postinflammatory; neoplastic; and infective (parasitic, mycotic).[180–186] Their preoperative diagnosis may be facilitated by angiographic and ultrasound studies.

Lymphatic cysts are the most common, presenting as unilocular or multilocular masses containing serous or milky fluid.[180–182] They are lined by flat or cuboidal epithelium and have a thin fibrous wall with a variable smooth muscle component. Lymphoid cell aggregates may be present in the surrounding adventitia. The small bowel mesentery is more frequently involved than the large bowel mesentery, omentum, or retroperitoneum. Histologic distinction of lymphatic and mesothelial cysts may require special techniques. Their removal is generally uncomplicated and recurrences are rare, being more frequent among the retroperitoneal cysts.

Enteric cysts have a mucosal lining and muscular wall and are more common in the small bowel and mesentery. Their surgical extirpation is complicated, due to a blood supply common to the adjacent bowel. They occur rarely in the retroperitoneum as a result of an abnormal splitting of the notochord during embryogenesis.[183,184]

Urogenital cysts, considered to be of mesonephric or paramesonephric origin, are rare and have been described in the retroperitoneum.[185,186]

Parasitic cyst in the retroperitoneum has been reported with *Echinococcus* infestation.[187]

NONNEOPLASTIC CONDITIONS OF THE RETROPERITONEUM, MESENTERY, AND OMENTUM
Retroperitoneum

Retroperitoneal abscess is generally secondary to pyelonephritis, diverticulitis, pancreatitis, appendicitis, or tuberculous spondylitis but may originate from infections in distant sites. *Hemorrhage* in the adult is most often the result of aortic aneurysm, trauma, anticoagulant therapy, or hemorrhagic diathesis, and less commonly is of adrenal origin. It may become encapsulated and mimic a cyst or neoplasm.[188] *Malakoplakia* involving the retroperitoneum may be confused with histiocytoma if the Michaelis-Gutmann bodies are absent or obscured by a florid histiocytic or fibrous histiocytic reaction.[189,190] *Idiopathic fibrosis* (Ormond's disease) more commonly affects adults, but it has been reported in 13 children, the youngest being a stillborn of 7 months gestation.[191–196] It may be focal, but generally it is diffuse above the brim of the pelvis, beginning medially, encircling the aorta and iliac arteries, and extending laterally to involve the ureter and rarely forward into the mesentery and mesocolon. Its association with Reidel's struma, mediastinal and pericardial fibrosis, sclerosing cholangitis, and pseudotumor of the orbit lends credence to its being part of a systemic process.[194–196] The dense, poorly cellular fibrous tissue may simulate fibromatosis, but the presence of lymphocytes and plasma cells and the arrangement of the fibrous tissue serve to distinguish it from the latter entity. Drugs (methysergide, haloperidol, ergotamine, and β-blockers), α_1-antitrypsin deficiency, and autoallergy to ceroid elaborated in atherosclerotic plaques have been considered to play a role in the pathogenesis.[197–201] In rare instances, malignant neoplasms, notably malignant lymphoma and gastric carcinoma associated with chronic inflammation and fibrosis, may clinically and grossly mimic retroperitoneal fibrosis.[202] Tumor cells may be widely scattered and difficult to find and identify in this situation. Immunoperoxidase studies may be helpful in identifying sclerosing lymphoma.[203]

Endometriosis isolated in the retroperitoneum has been responsible for ureteral obstruction.[204,205]

Mesentery

Inflammatory and fibrous lesions involving the mesentery and retroperitoneum have similar histologic features. While they generally occur in one of the two areas, they may be associated with, and have been considered to be part of, a systemic process (see under Retroperitoneum). In some instances, there is a self-limited acute and chronic productive inflammation, usually of the root of the small intestine and less often the mesocolon or omentum, which has variously been termed mesenteric panniculitis, lipogranuloma, and isolated lipodystrophy, and likened to Weber-Christian disease.[206–208] This may result in a significant mass that may or may not be symptomatic. A more severe fibrotic and hyaline scarring process with retraction of the mesentery, which may result in distortion of intestinal loops and varying degrees of

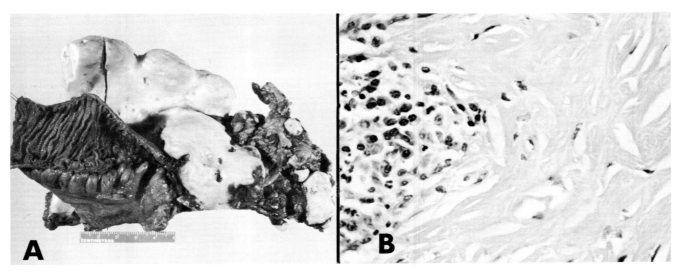

Fig. 26-7. Retractile mesenteritis. **(A)** Firm plaques of **(B)** dense fibrous tissue with foci of plasma cells and lymphocytes. The plaques distort the lumen of the small intestine. **(B)**

intestinal obstruction and pain, has been designated *retractile mesenteritis* (Fig. 26-7).

Omentum

Torsion of the omentum secondary to adhesions or tumor or strangulation in a hernia sac may result in hemorrhagic infarction, producing signs and symptoms misdiagnosed as acute appendicitis or cholecystitis.[209,210] Similarly, *epiploic appendages* may become infarcted, resulting in altered, sometimes calcific adipose tissue that may grossly simulate a neoplastic process (Fig. 26-8). Microscopic examination readily clarifies their nature.

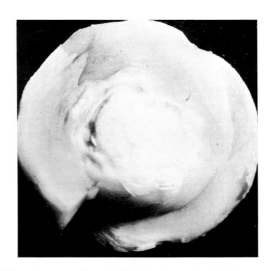

Fig. 26-8. A centrally calcified infarcted epiploic appendage was an incidental finding at laparotomy.

Symptoms may suggest a variety of clinical conditions: pelvic disease, appendicitis, small bowel obstruction, diverticulitis, and colon carcinoma. Death has resulted from peritonitis and intestinal obstruction.

Oxyuriasis producing an omental nodule and acute abdominal pain and distention has been observed as a result of the female worm migrating from the anus into the peritoneum via the vagina, uterus, and fallopian tubes.[211]

Endometriosis, nodular in the omentum and producing a massive bloody ascites, has been observed in young women, predominantly nulliparous and of African descent.[212]

Cryptococcus involvement of the omentum was responsible for an 8 cm mass and epigastric pain in an otherwise healthy young man.[213]

PERITONEUM

Inflammation

Inflammation, diffuse or localized, acute or chronic, is frequently encountered in the peritoneum, resulting from a variety of agents: bacteria, parasites or their ova, fungi, viruses, chemical or foreign material.[214–217] The acute variety is most frequently associated with diseases of abdominal organs with or without perforation: appendicitis, salpingitis, diverticulitis, perforated duodenal ulcer, cholecystitis, intestinal infarction, and hemorrhage related to a variety of conditions, most commonly ruptured ectopic pregnancy. Less frequently encountered is primary peritonitis caused by hemolytic streptococci or pneumococci.[214] Tuberculous peritonitis may be part of disseminated tuberculosis associated with intestinal involvement or secondary to urogenital tuberculosis.[218] Microscopic distinction from neoplasm is not a problem, but the peritoneal granulomas may be misinterpreted grossly as primary or metastatic malignancy. *Malakoplakia* involving the peritoneum as seed-like nodules may also be confused grossly with a neoplastic process.[219]

Irritants

Irritants may be responsible for peritonitis. These include contents of ruptured hollow organs; hemorrhage from ectopic pregnancy, rupture of a corpus luteum or aneurysm; foreign material (*Lycopodium* spores, talc, and starch used as dusting powder in surgical gloves); therapeutic and diagnostic agents (oily materials used in salpingography, barium sulfate administered for diagnostic radiologic study and escaping from the bowel, and sclerosing agents used in the treatment of hernia).[220–222] The inflammatory nature of the response to many of these agents is readily recognized grossly and/or microscopically, but in some situations a granulomatous response may be productive of a mass that may be impossible to distinguish grossly from tumor. In some instances the marked cellular response may even mimic neoplasia microscopically (e.g., the cellular fibrous proliferation occurring after the injection of sclerosing agents for the treatment of inguinal hernia). Some of these iatrogenic reactions are discussed in more detail in Chapter 5.

Adhesions

Intraperitoneal adhesions are secondary to abdominal operations or inflammation of abdominal or pelvic organs. The former are related to drying of the serosa, blood in the peritoneal cavity, and a local depression of peritoneal plasminogen activator.[223,224]

Extensive peritoneal fibrosis (*sclerosing peritonitis*), attributed to asbestos, carcinoid tumor, and β-adrenergic blocking drugs, may simulate tuberculosis grossly and result in bowel obstruction.[225,226]

Periodic Disease

Periodic disease (familial Mediterranean fever, familial recurring polyserositis) is responsible for intermittent bouts of pain, particularly in the abdomen, but also in the chest and joints.[227] Between attacks the patients are in excellent health. In the involved serosal surfaces, one may encounter sterile exudates consisting of focal collections of neutrophils, fibrin strands, and ecchymoses, but only rarely are fibrous adhesions and scars produced despite the many attacks. Amyloid of the perireticular type in the kidneys, spleen, adrenals, pulmonary alveolar capillaries, and hepatic sinusoids, but not in other organs, may result in the patient's death, but generally the course of the disease is protracted. It is a genetic disorder of unknown etiology and pathogenesis affecting patients of Armenian, Arab, or Jewish ethnic origin, the last being predominantly the non-Ashkenazi Jews (the Sephardic and Iraqi ethnic groups).

Ascites

Ascites is commonly encountered associated with liver cirrhosis or other causes of portal hypertension and with primary or metastatic neoplasia in the peritoneum. The properties of the fluid are those of a transudate, in contrast to the fluid associated with inflammation and the chylous fluid related to obstruction of the thoracic duct, usually by neoplasm. Examination of the cells in the fluid by smear, Millipore filter preparations, and/or cell blocks is of help in determining whether the underlying cause of the ascites is neoplastic. The recognition of neoplastic cells generally offers less difficulty than the identification of the primary tumor site. Difficulty is particularly encountered in distinguishing mesothelioma, metastatic carcinoma, and mesothelial cell hyperplasia.[228] False positive diagnoses may occur in cases of tuberculosis, hepatic cirrhosis, and congestive heart failure as a result of mesothelial cell enlargement and aberrations including mitotic figures, pseudoacinar formation, multiple nuclei, and signet ring cell appearance.[229–231] The use of histochemical and immunoperoxidase techniques and the morphologic features of the mesothelial cells in most instances permit the distinction between mesothelioma and metastatic carcinoma, but there still remain cases in which the distinction cannot be made from the cytologic preparations alone.[232]

Cysts

Mesothelial cell-lined cysts, solitary or multiloculated, have been described free in the abdominal cavity or attached to the fallopian tube, the ovary, and occasionally the bowel.[233–235] Although they may be associated with pelvic inflammatory disease (PID) in women, a morphologic separation from benign cystic mesothelioma may not always be feasible. These cysts show an epithelial cell lining with occasional focal squamous metaplasia, a serous fluid content, and a thin fibrous wall, which distinguish them from lymphatic cysts with their flat endothelial cell lining, milky fluid content and thin fibrous wall that may also contain smooth muscle. Where the distinction is not evident, special techniques may be helpful. These include staining for mucosubstances, which may be present in mesothelial cells but are absent in endothelial cells; factor-VIII-related antigen and *Ulex* immunochemical staining, which is positive in endothelial cells and negative in mesothelial cells; and ultrastructural differences between mesothelial and endothelial cells. Cysts resulting from *Echinococcus* and *Blastomyces* have been reported.[216,217]

Splenosis

Implantation of splenic fragments following splenic rupture results in asymptomatic nodules in the peritoneum. There is no sex preference but, when these nodules occur in women, they grossly resemble endometriosis.[236]

Hyperplasia

The response of the serosal lining cells and underlying mesenchymal tissue of the peritoneum to irritants may be profuse, producing papillary, glandular, or solid proliferations. In men and boys, they are most commonly observed in hernial sacs.[237] In women they are often associated with pelvic inflammatory disease and may be accompanied by mesothelium-lined cysts.[233,238] These lesions can be distinguished from primary and metastatic peritoneal neoplasms by virtue of their banal cellular characteristics and lack of invasive qualities.

Metaplasia

Although the peritoneum of both sexes responds similarly to irritants of various type and shares some similar primary neoplasms, the peritoneum in women exhibits an assortment of benign and malignant lesions that are not observed in men. These are attributed to a secondary müllerian system represented by the peritoneal mesothelium and underlying connective tissue, which have the same embryologic ancestry as the müllerian duct.[239] Metaplasia and proliferation of one or both of these cellular layers results in a variety of lesions that are principally epithelial, stromal, or an admixture of these.

Endosalpingiosis, a term originally restricted to lesions featuring tubal epithelium, has come to be identified with a proliferation of one or more types of müllerian epithelium—tubal, endometrial, or endocervical.[240-244] Glands, cysts, papillae, or solid epithelial aggregates, frequently admixed with psammoma bodies, constitute the microscopic or 1 to 2 mm macroscopic nodules (Figs. 26-9 and 26-10). Any area of the peritoneum and even the pelvic, paraortic, and inguinal lymph nodes may be involved, but there is a predilection for the ovarian surfaces, pelvic peritoneum, and omentum. The lesions may be isolated incidental findings, but not infrequently they have occurred with diseases involving the upper female genital tract. The frequency with which they have been found associated with tubal inflammation and tubal pregnancy has suggested to Zinsser and Wheeler[240] that an implantation of regurgitated tubal epithelium was the pathogenesis for their cases with omental involvement. Involvement of the peritoneum or pelvic lymph nodes

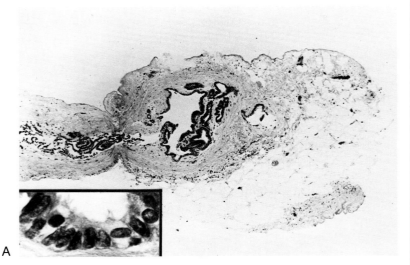

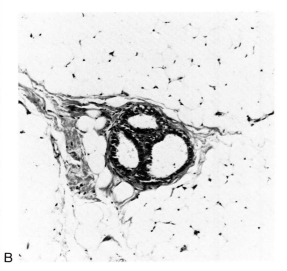

Fig. 26-9. Endosalpingiosis. The lesions were incidental findings in the cul-de-sac **(A)** and omentum **(B)** during abdominal exploration for an ovarian dermoid cyst in a 48-year-old woman. Glands are lined by bland columnar epithelium and include few ciliated cells. (Inset)

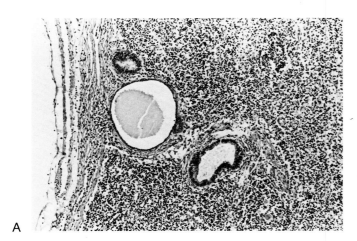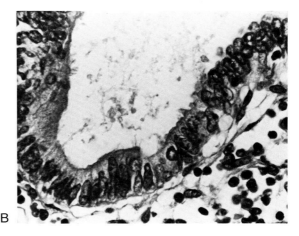

Fig. 26-10. Gland inclusions in retroperitoneal lymph nodes were an incidental finding in a woman at autopsy. They are lined by tubal type epithelium and include few ciliated cells. **(A, B)**

synchronous with, or subsequent to, differentiated serous ovarian or other adenocarcinomas has been observed and must not be regarded as representing metastases.[238,243] The distinction can be made on the basis of the banal and mitotically inactive epithelium that is often tubal and ciliated and lacks the infiltrative and destructive properties of carcinoma.

The course of peritoneal endosalpingiosis thus far appears to be benign, with evidence for spontaneous regression. Whether these lesions may represent the nidus for the development of peritoneal serous carcinomas must remain speculative. However, glandular inclusions in lymph nodes have been the site of development of a malignant or borderline tumor.[243]

Walthard rests represent another form of epithelial metaplasia that is commonly seen on the serosal surface of the fallopian tube and only rarely in other peritoneal sites.[238] The microscopic similarity to urothelial cells and Brenner tumor cells has also been noted ultrastructurally.[245]

Endometriosis of the peritoneum, like other sites of extrauterine involvement, has a disputed pathogenesis. While coelomic metaplasia may not explain all cases of peritoneal involvement, there is evidence to support its role in endometriosis. Unlike endosalpingiosis, there is participation of both mesothelium and underlying mesenchymal tissue. The glands and stroma are identical to those of the endometrium and their response to ovarian hormones may produce symptoms, which are not observed in endosalpingiosis. A variety of changes ranging from benign atypical epithelial proliferation and glandular hyperplasia to malignant transformation may be observed in ectopic endometrium. Malignancy may occur in any or all of the cellular constituents. Carcinoma is the most frequent type of malignant tumor, but sarcomas, carcino-

sarcoma, or malignant mixed mesodermal tumor similar to those observed in the uterus may develop.[238]

Papillary serous peritoneal tumors, histologically identical to the corresponding ovarian tumors, may arise from the peritoneum as solitary, multifocal or diffuse proliferations independent of or synchronous with similar ovarian tumors (Fig. 26-11). A histologic spectrum similar to their ovarian counterpart can be observed.[241,246–250] The well differentiated borderline tumors have well defined connective tissue cores covered by crowded columnar pseudostratified cells and few ciliated cells; they may contain frequent psammoma bodies. Less differentiated tumors display cellular atypia, pleomorphism, mitotic activity, and invasive properties not observed in the borderline tumors. Foci of endosalpingiosis may be present adjacent to the neoplasm. Their behavior is commensurate with the histopathology.

Excision of the borderline tumor is associated with long disease-free survival, but the prognosis of the high grade invasive carcinoma is poor, despite responses to the same chemotherapeutic regimens used for ovarian carcinoma.

Leiomyomatosis peritonealis disseminata is a rare disorder in which the peritoneal surfaces are covered by well demarcated, gray-white firm nodules.[243,251–253] Women of reproductive age, many of whom are pregnant or taking contraceptive steroids, are affected. They are generally asymptomatic and the lesions are discovered at the time of cesarean section or tubal ligation. When symptoms are present, they are usually due to coexistent endometriosis or uterine leiomyomata. The lesions arise in the subcoelomic mesenchymal tissue and consist of uniform bland smooth muscle cells. Decidual cells and rarely endometriosis may be present in the nodules.[253] Despite an ominous gross appearance, the histopathol-

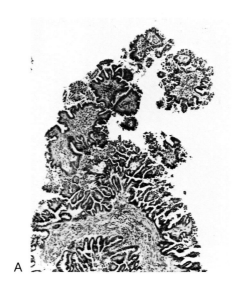
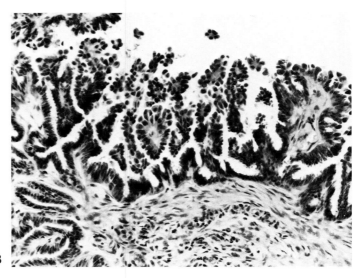

Fig. 26-11. Serous papillary peritoneal tumor of borderline malignancy. This 5 cm cauliflower-like mass involved the peritoneum of the right mesosalpinx, fallopian tube, and appendix of a 19-year-old woman. Crowded columnar cells, vertically oriented, covered the papillary cores or formed solid epithelial tufts **(A, B)**. There was no invasion. Psammoma bodies were numerous.

ogy and clinical course are benign. Ultrastructurally, the smooth muscle composition of the lesions has been identified along with fibroblasts, myofibroblasts, and decidual cells.[252,253]

Hormonal imbalance as a causative factor in the disease is suggested in some cases in which there has been regression of the nodules following termination of a pregnancy and subsequent recurrence when the patient becomes pregnant again.

Endometrial stromal tumor, malignant mixed müllerian tumor, and carcinoma, reported in the peritoneum unrelated to endometriosis, further illustrate the versatility of the subcoelomic mesenchyme and mesothelium in women in the formation of neoplasms.[164,165,167,254,255]

Decidual reaction may occur in the subcoelomic connective tissue in any area of the hormonally sensitive pelvic or abdominal peritoneum of women. As incidental findings,[256] the nodules may be solitary or multiple and occasionally may show cytologic atypia.[238]

Benign Mesothelioma

Four benign patterns of peritoneal mesothelioma have been observed: papillary, cystic, adenomatoid, and the rare solitary fibrous variety common in the pleura.

Papillary mesothelioma in the peritoneum occurs as a solitary or multifocal tumor with a papillary or tubulopapillary architecture (Fig. 26-12). The broad papillae with loose fibrous tissue are covered by a single layer of uniform mesothelial cells. Psammoma bodies may be present but are infrequent. An adenomatoid pattern was observed in one tumor.[257] They occur in both sexes, but the multifocal lesions are more common in women.[247,248,258] Information regarding their behavior is meager, but it indicates an indolent course unlike diffuse malignant mesothelioma.

Cystic mesothelioma is infrequently encountered, occurring predominantly in women and rarely in men and children.[259–261] The cysts contain thin serous fluid and are lined by a single layer of flat to cuboidal cells that are occasionally squamous or arranged in a papillary pattern. The differentiation of this lesion from lymphangioma may require special studies for identification. Cystic mesothelioma may develop numerous local recurrences but does not metastasize.

Adenomatoid tumor, frequent in the fallopian tube and the uterine serosa, is rarely found in other peritoneal sites.[262] The origin from mesothelial cells has been substantiated in ultrastructural studies. They are discussed more fully in Chapter 42.

Malignant Mesothelioma

Malignant mesothelioma in the peritoneum occurs predominantly in men, infrequently in women and rarely in children.[247,250,263,264] Exposure to asbestos has been responsible for an increase in its incidence. It occurs in one of three histologic patterns: epithelium-like (tubular and tubulopapillary), fibrous, or a combination of these. There are two gross patterns: diffuse and solitary. The

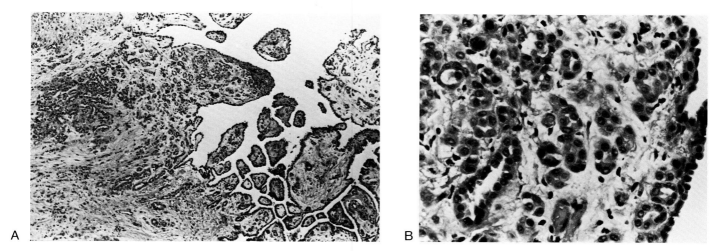

Fig. 26-12. Well differentiated papillary mesothelioma. Small cauliflower-like growths were found on the free edge of the omentum near the right ovary at laparoscopy for infertility in a 29-year-old woman. The right ovarian surface had similar but smaller papillary excresences. Endometriosis was documented clinically in the posterior cul-de-sac. The papillae and tubules are lined by uniform cuboidal mesothelial cells.

solitary fibrous form is rarely seen in the peritoneum.[265,266] The diffuse epithelial variant is the most common form encountered, and its histologic differentiation from metastatic carcinoma (particularly of ovarian origin) and mesothelial cell hyperplasia may be difficult and at times impossible, a definitive diagnosis becoming evident only after thorough necropsy examination has been carried out (Fig. 26-13). Histochemical stains may be helpful in distinguishing mesothelioma from carcinoma. The presence of alcian blue-positive hyaluronidase-labile mucosaccharide and/or periodic acid-Schiff (PAS)-positive diastase-digestible polysaccharide in the mesothelial cells is in contrast to the Alcian blue-positive hyaluronidase-stable mucosaccharide and PAS-positive diastase-resistant polysaccharide of other epithelial neoplasms. Immunocytochemistry has been cited to be an aid in differentiating mesothelioma from pulmonary adenocarcinoma by virtue of the negative and positive carcinoembryonic antigen (CEA) reaction, respectively, in mesothelioma and pulmonary adenocarcinoma.[267,268] This reaction does not have the same significance for peritoneal mesotheliomas in women by virtue of the finding of

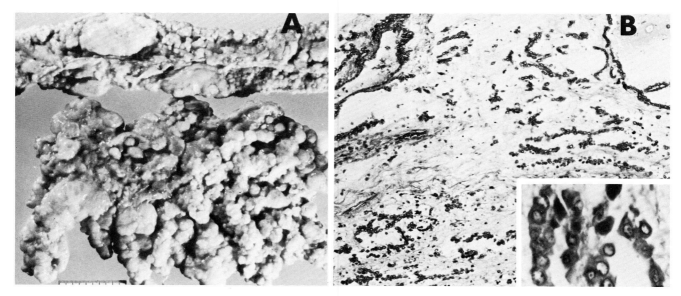

Fig. 26-13. Tubular (epithelial) diffuse mesothelioma. Nodules of tumor were limited to the peritoneum of this man. No other tumor was found at necropsy.

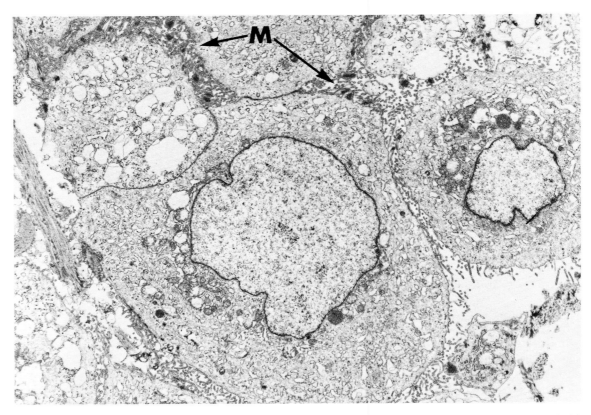

Fig. 26-14. The long numerous microvilli (M) are features of the cells of normal mesothelium and this epithelial-like mesothelioma of the peritoneum. (×5,000)

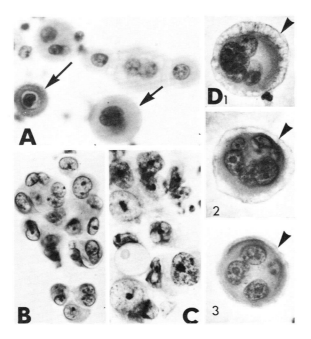

Fig. 26-15. The peripheral lucent zone (arrows) of malignant mesothelial cells (d), corresponding to their microvilli, is helpful in their identification and distinction from other malignant cells such as metastases from prostate (b) or lung (c). Increased cell and nuclear size with increased nuclear: cytoplasmic ratios as well as nuclear atypia serve to distinguish the malignant (d) from the hyperplastic (a) mesothelial cell. (Courtesy of Dr. Sudha Kini, Henry Ford Hospital.)

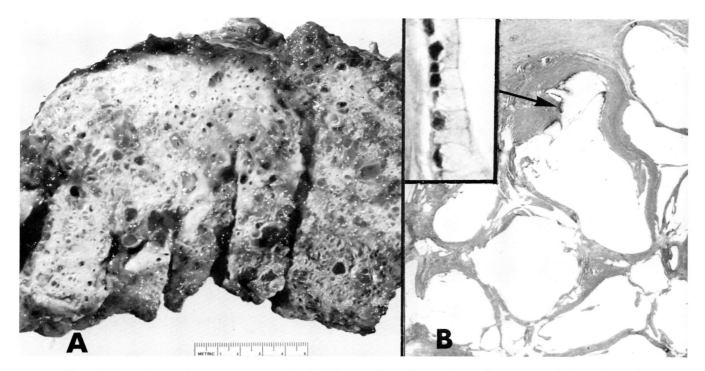

Fig. 26-16. **(A)** Pseudomyxoma peritonei. **(B)** Masses of cystic gelatinous tissue covered the peritoneal surfaces at necropsy. Infrequent cysts were partially lined by a mucus-containing benign-appearing epithelium (arrow and inset). A mucocele of the appendix had been removed 12 years previously.

Bane et al.[269] that more than 50 percent of ovarian carcinomas were CEA-negative. The numerous long slender microvilli of the differentiated mesothelial cell may also aid in differentiation from metastatic carcinoma. These are most easily visualized at the ultrastructural level, but they may be observed in smears of the ascitic fluid (Figs. 26-14 and 26-15). While mesotheliomas may remain confined to the peritoneal cavity, resulting in recurrent ascites, they may also infiltrate locally or metastasize distantly. They may coexist with a pleural mesothelioma and may be associated with hypoglycemia, which may subside after removal of the neoplasm, but unfortunately removal is only rarely possible.[270]

Metastatic Tumors

Metastatic tumors are more common in the peritoneum than are primary neoplasms, representing dissemination principally from epithelial tumors of adjacent or distant organs. The GI tract and its related organs, ovary, endometrium, breast, and lung are common primary sites. Unique presentations of peritoneal metastasis are *pseudomyxoma peritonei* and *gliomatosis peritonei*. The former term refers to a diffuse involvement of the peritoneal surface by mucinous material, often with little par-

ticipation of a histologically bland mucinous or serous-type epithelium[271] (Fig. 26-16). The appendix or ovary or both are generally the primary sites from which the peritoneum is involved. Unlike other instances of peritoneal metastases, there is a protracted course with restriction of the involvement to the peritoneal cavity.

Gliomatosis peritonei is the presence of benign glial implants on peritoneal surfaces secondary to immature ovarian teratoma. The implants may remain without change, undergo malignant change, or regress.[272]

REFERENCES

1. Russell WO, Chohen J, Enzinger FM, et al: A clinical and pathological staging system for soft tissue sarcomas. Cancer 40:1562, 1977
2. Hashimoto H, Tsuneyoshi M, Enjoll M: Malignant smooth muscle tumors of the retroperitoneum and mesentery. A clinicopathologic analysis of 44 cases. J Surg Oncol 28:177, 1985
3. Scanlan DB: Primary retroperitoneal tumors. J Urol 81:740, 1959
4. Duncan RE, Evans AT: Diagnosis of primary retroperitoneal tumors. J Urol 117:19, 1977
5. Melicow MM: Primary tumors of the retroperitoneum; a clinicopathologic analysis of 162 cases: Review of the lit-

erature and tables of classification. J Int Colloq Surg 19:401, 1953

6. Pack GT, Tabah EJ: Primary retroperitoneal tumors. A study of 120 cases. Int Abst Surg 99:209, 1954, 313, 1954

7. Cody HS, Turnbull AD, Fortner JG, et al: The continuing challenge of retroperitoneal sarcomas. Cancer 47:2147, 1981

8. Von Wahlendorf L: Ueber retroperitoneale lipome. Arch Klin Chir 115:751, 1921

9. DeWeerd JH, Dockerty MB: Lipomatous retroperitoneal tumors. Am J Surg 84:397, 1952

10. Farbman AA: Retroperitoneal fatty tumors. Arch Surg 60:343, 1950

11. Kindblom LG, Angervall L, Svendsen P: Liposarcoma. A clinicopathologic, radiographic and prognostic study. Acta Pathol Microbiol Scand 83(suppl):253, 1975

12. Enterline HT, Culberson JD, Rochlin DB: Liposarcoma. A clinical and pathological study of 53 cases. Cancer 13:932, 1960

13. Evans HL: Liposarcoma. A study of 55 cases with a reassessment of its classification. Am J Surg Pathol 3:507, 1979

14. Enzinger FM, Weiss SW: Soft Tissue Tumors. CV Mosby, St Louis, 1983

15. Kinne DW, Chu FCH, Huvos AG et al: Treatment of primary and recurrent retroperitoneal liposarcoma. Twenty-five year experience at Memorial Hospital. Cancer 31:53, 1973

16. Stout AP: The malignant tumor of lipoblasts. Ann Surg 119:86, 1944

17. Menne FR, Burge RF: Primary liposarcoma of the great omentum. Arch Pathol Lab Med 22:823, 1936

18. Enzinger FM, Winslow DJ: Liposarcoma: A study of 103 cases. Virchows Arch [A] 335:367, 1962

19. Shmookler BM, Enzinger FM: Liposarcoma occurring in children. An analysis of 17 cases and review of the literature. Cancer 52:567, 1983

20. Groff DB, Horwitz A: Liposarcoma. Am J Surg 107:725, 1964

21. Hassan MA: Subcutaneous liposarcoma of forearm followed by liposarcoma of omentum. Br J Surg 57:393, 1970

22. Ackerman LV: Multiple liposarcomas. Am J Pathol 20:789, 1944

23. Lin JJ, Lin F: Two entities in angiolipoma. A study of 459 cases of lipoma with review of literature on infiltrating angiolipoma. Cancer 34:720, 1974

24. Cattell RB, Warren KW: Retroperitoneal lipoma. Surg Clin North Am 27:659, 1947

25. Benson PA, Janko AB: Pelvic myelolipoma (rare presacral tumor). Am J Obstet Gynecol 92:884, 1965

26. Harvard BM: Retroperitoneal lipoma in children: Report of a case and review of literature. J Urol 70:159, 1953

27. Pinto VC, Mattos AG, Pimenta E, et al: Retroperitoneal myxolipoma—report of a case in a child 7 years of age. Pediatrics 14:11, 1954

28. Weitzner S, Blumenthal BI, Moynihan PC: Retroperitoneal lipoma in children. J Pediatr Surg 14:88, 1979

29. Ikins RG, Arbogast JL: Lipomata of the omentum. J Indiana Med Assoc 35:354, 1942

30. Jacobi A: Congenital lipoma. Arch Pediatr 1:65, 1984

31. Lassman JP, James CCM: Lumbosacral lipomas: Critical survey of 26 cases submitted to laminectomy. J Neurol Neurosurg Psychol 30:174, 1967

32. Bender L, Koss M: Periureteral lipomatosis: Case report. J Urol 103:293, 1970

33. Engels EP: Sigmoid colon and urinary bladder in high fixation: Roentgen changes simulating pelvic tumor. Radiology 72:419, 1959

34. Jimenez JF: Lipoblastoma in infancy and childhood. J Surg Oncol 32:238, 1986

35. Stringel G, Shandling B, Mancer K, et al: Lipoblastoma in infants and children. J Pediatr Surg 17:277, 1982

36. Chung EB, Enzinger FM: Benign lipoblastomatosis: An analysis of 35 cases. Cancer 32:482, 1973

37. Fisher MF, Fletcher BD, Dahms BB, et al: Abdominal lipoblastomatosis: Radiographic, echographic and computed tomographic findings. Radiology 138:593, 1981

38. Rigor VU, Goldstone SE, Jones J, et al: Hibernoma. A case report and discussion of a rare tumor. Cancer 57:2207, 1986

39. Leiphart CJ, Nudelman EJ: Hibernoma masquerading as a pheochromocytoma. A case report. Radiology 95:659, 1970

40. Yannopoulos K, Stout AP: Primary solid tumors of the mesentery. Cancer 16:914, 1963

41. Stout AP, Hendry J, Purdie FJ: Primary solid tumors of the great omentum. Cancer 16:231, 1963

42. McCullough CD, Cahill K: Primary leiomyoma of the omentum. Am J Surg 104:785, 1962

43. Ranchod M, Kempson RL: Smooth muscle tumors of the gastrointestinal tract and retroperitoneum. A pathologic analysis of 100 cases. Cancer 39:255, 1977

44. Wile AG, Evans HL, Romsdahl MM: Leiomyosarcoma of soft tissue. A clinicopathologic study. Cancer 48:1022, 1981

45. Dixon AY, Reed JS, Dow N, et al: Primary omental leiomyosarcoma masquerading as hemorrhagic ascites. Hum Pathol 15:233, 1984

46. Hartz PH, Van DeStadt FR: Leiomyoma angiomatosum of the mesentery. Am J Clin Pathol 19:639, 1949

47. Golden T, Stout AP: Smooth muscle tumors of the gastrointestinal tract and retroperitoneum. Surg Gynecol Obstet 73:784, 1941

48. Botting AJ, Soule EH, Brown AI Jr: Smooth muscle tumors in children. Cancer 18:711, 1965

49. Kay S, McNeill DD: Leiomyosarcoma of retroperitoneum. Surg Gynecol Obstet 129:285, 1969

50. Areán VM, DeArellano R: Intra-abdominal non-chromaffin paraganglioma. Ann Surg 144:133, 1956

51. Arneill JR, Haigler HS, Gamboa LG: Malignant intra-abdominal nonchromaffin paraganglioma. Report of a case with survival of eleven years. J Int Coll Surg 22(6):656, 1954

52. Shmookler BM, Lauer DH: Retroperitoneal leiomyosarcoma. A clinicopathologic analysis of 36 cases. Am J Surg Pathol 7:269, 1983

53. Sutow WW, Sullivan MP, Ried HL, et al: Prognosis in childhood rhabdomyosarcoma. Cancer 25:1384, 1970

54. Lloyd RV, Hajdu SI, Knapper WH: Embryonal rhabdomyosarcoma in adults. Cancer 51:557, 1983

55. Weichert KA, Bove KC, Aron BS: Rhabdomyosarcoma in children. A clinicopathological study in 35 patients. Am J Clin Pathol 66:692, 1976

56. Lawrence W, Jegge G, Foote FW Jr: Embryonal rhabdomyosarcoma. Cancer 17:361, 1964

57. Horn RC Jr, Enterline HT: Rhabdomyosarcoma: A clinicopathological study and classification of 39 cases. Cancer 11:181, 1958

58. McPeak CJ, Papaioannow AN: Nonpancreatic tumors associated with hypoglycemia. Arch Surg 93:1019, 1966

59. Ransom JL, Pratt CB, Hustu HO, et al: Retroperitoneal rhabdomyosarcoma in children. Cancer 45:845, 1980

60. Bruton OC: Fibroma of mesentery. Report of a case in a six-day-old infant. J Pediatr 8:63, 1936

61. Adams JT, Kutner FR: Pure fibroma of the mesentery. Am J Surg 111:734, 1966

62. Bonello J, Schultz L, Delaney JP: Primary benign solid tumor of the mesentery. Minn Med 60:405, 1977

63. Mathias JR, Smith WG: Mesenteric fibromatosis associated with familial polyposis. Am J Dig Dis 22:741, 1977

64. Richards RC, Rogers SW, Gardner EJ: Spontaneous mesenteric fibromatosis in Gardner's Syndrome. Cancer 47:597, 1981

65. Schmid HH: Über retroperitoneale und mesenteriale tumoren. Arch Gynakol 118:490, 1923

66. Braasch JW, Mon AB: Primary retroperitoneal tumors. Surg Clin North Am 47:663, 1967

67. Norman FW: Fibrous tumors of the omentum. Calif Med 99:407, 1963

68. Suarez V, Hall C: Mesenteric fibromatosis. Br J Surg 72:796, 1985

69. Schweitzer RJ, Robbins GF: A desmoid tumor of multicentric origin. Arch Surg 80:488, 1960

70. Bach C: Desmoid tumors of the abdominal wall in children. Ann Pediatr 11:239, 1964

71. Ransom HK, Samson PC: Malignant tumors of the greater omentum. Ann Surg 100:523, 1934

72. Guernsey CM: Primary tumors and cysts of the omentum. Proc Mayo Clin 14:694, 1939

73. Jacobson S, Juul-Jorgensen S: Primary retroperitoneal tumors. A review of 26 cases. Acta Chir Scand 140:498, 1974

74. Heller EL, Sieber WK: Fibrosarcoma. A clinical and pathological study of sixty cases. Surgery 27:539, 1950

75. Bizer LS: Fibrosarcoma. Report of sixty-four cases. Am J Surg 121:586, 1971

76. Lawler RH, Fox PF: Primary fibrosarcoma of the great omentum. Am J Surg 69:135, 1945

77. Rankin FW, Major SG: Tumors of the mesentery. Surg Gynec Obstet 54:809, 1932

78. Warren S, Sommer GNJ: Fibrosarcoma of the soft parts with special reference to recurrence and metastasis. Arch Surg 33:425, 1936

79. Stout AP: Fibrosarcoma. Cancer 1:30, 1948

80. Ackerman LV: Tumors of the peritoneum and retroperitoneum. Atlas of Tumor Pathology. Fasc. 23, 24. Armed Forces Institute of Pathology, Washington, DC, 1954

81. Stout AP: The fibromatoses. Clin Orthop 19:11, 1961

82. Stout AP: Fibrous tumors of the soft tissues. Minn Med 43:455, 1960

83. Heath AO, Wagner FB: Retroperitoneal fibrosarcoma without hypoglycemia. Arch Surg 92:198, 1966

84. O'Brien JE, Stout AP: Malignant fibrous xanthoma. Cancer 17:1445, 1964

85. Kearney MM, Soule EH, Ivins JC: Malignant fibrous histiocytoma. A retrospective study of 167 cases. Cancer 45:167, 1980

86. Enjoji M, Hashimoto H, Tsuneyoshi M, et al: Malignant fibrous histiocytoma. A clinicopathologic study of 130 cases. Acta Pathol Jpn 30:727, 1980

87. Kyriakos M, Kempson RL: Inflammatory fibrous histiocytoma. An aggressive and lethal lesion. Cancer 37:1584, 1976

88. Oberling C: Retroperitoneal xanthogranuloma. Am J Cancer 23:477, 1935

89. Patel VC, Meyer JE: Retroperitoneal malignant fibrous histiocytoma. Cancer 45:1724, 1980

90. Merino MJ, LiVolsi VA: Inflammatory malignant fibrous histiocytoma. Am J Clin Pathol 73:276, 1980

91. Kahn LB: Retroperitoneal xanthogranuloma and xanthosarcoma (malignant fibrous xanthoma). Cancer 31:411, 1973

92. Kay S: Inflammatory fibrous histiocytoma (? xanthogranuloma). Report of two cases with ultrastructural observations in one. Am J Surg Pathol 2:313, 1978

93. Usher SM, Beckley S, Merrin CE: Malignant fibrous histiocytoma of the retroperitoneum and genitourinary tract: a clinicopathological correlation and review of the literature. J Urol 122:105, 1979

94. Weiss SW, Enzinger FM: Malignant fibrous histiocytoma. Cancer 41:2250, 1978

95. Kalish M, Dorr R, Hoskins P: Retroperitoneal cystic lymphangioma. Urology 6:503, 1975

96. Takiff H, Calabria R, Yin L, et al: Mesenteric cysts and intra-abdominal cystic lymphangiomas. Arch Surg 120:1266, 1985

97. Molander ML, Mortensson W, Udén R: Omental and mesenteric cysts in children. Acta Paediatr Scand 71:227, 1982

98. Savage JL: Omental lymphangioma. Quart Bull Northwestern Univ Med School 33:262, 1959

99. Krahe Von T, Schneider B, Schmidt Ch: Zystisches lymphangiom des omentum majus. ROFO 143:476, 1986

100. Daniel S, Lazarevic B, Attia A: Lymphangioma of the mesentery of the jejunum: Report of a case and brief review of the literature. Am J Gastroenterol 78:726, 1983

101. Wolff, M: Lymphangiomyoma: Clinicopathologic study and ultrastructural confirmation of its histogenesis. Cancer 31:988, 1973

102. Bhattacharyya AK, Balogh K: Retroperitoneal lymphangiomyomatosis. A 36-year benign course in a postmenopausal woman. Cancer 56:1144, 1985

103. Cornog JL, Enterline HT: Lymphangiomyoma, a benign lesion of chyliferous lymphatics synonymous with lymphangio-pericytoma. Cancer 19:1909, 1966

104. Jao J, Gilbert S, Masser R: Lymphangiomyoma and tuberous sclerosis. Cancer 29:1188, 1972

105. Ward GE, Stewart EH Jr: Retroperitoneal cavenous hemangioma. Am J Surg 80:470, 1950

106. Pearl GS, Mathews WH: Congenital retroperitoneal hemangioendothelioma with Kasabach-Merritt Syndrome. South Med J 72:239, 1979

107. Weinblatt ME, Kahn E, Kochen JA: Hemangioendothelioma with intravascular coagulation and ischemic colitis. Cancer 54:2300, 1984

108. Hansen RC, Castellino RC, Lazerson J, et al: Mesenteric hemangioendothelioma with thrombocytopenia. Report with angiographic findings. Cancer 32:136, 1973

109. Stout AP: Hemangioendothelioma: A tumor of blood vessels featuring vascular endothelial cells. Ann Surg 118:445, 1943

110. Herdman JP: Retroperitoneal tumors. Br J Surg 40:331, 1953

111. Kalisher L, Straatsma GW, Rosenberg BF, et al: Primary malignant hemangioendothelioma of the greater omentum. Cancer 22:1126, 1968

112. Lattes R: Tumors of the soft tissues. Atlas of Tumor Pathology. Fasc. 1. Revised Second Series. Armed Forces Institute of Pathology, Washington, DC, 1982

113. Hart JT: Solid tumors of the mesentery. Ann Surg 104:184, 1936

114. Stout AP: Myxoma, the tumor of primitive mesenchyme. Ann Surg 127:706, 1948

115. Judd ES, Larson LM: Retroperitoneal tumors. Surg Clin North Am 13:823, 1933

116. Gonzalez-Crussi F, de Mello DE, Stotelo-Avila C: Omental-mesenteric myxoid hamartomas. Infantile lesions simulating malignant tumors. Am J Surg Pathol 7:567, 1983

117. Bodian M: Neuroblastoma. Pediatr Clin North Am 6:449, 1959

118. Gross RE, Farber S, Martin LW: Neuroblastoma sympathicum; a study and report of 217 cases. Pediatrics 23:1179, 1959

119. Stout AP: Ganglioneuroma of the sympathetic nervous system. Surg Gynecol Obstet 84:101, 1947

120. Carpenter WB, Kernohan JW: Retroperitoneal ganglioneuromas and neurofibroma. A clinicopathological study. Cancer 16:788, 1963

121. Donhauser JL, Bigelow NA: Primary retroperitoneal tumors. Arch Surg 71:234, 1955

122. Armstrong JR, Cohn I Jr: Primary malignant retroperitoneal tumors. Am J Surg 110:937, 1965

123. Gill W, Carter DC, Durie B: Retroperitoneal tumors; a review of 134 cases. J R Coll Surg Edinb 15:213, 1970

124. Castleman B: Multiple neurofibromas of omentum. Case records of the Massachusetts General Hospital. N Engl J Med 265:1064, 1961

125. Harrington JL Jr, Edwards LW: Massive retroperitoneal neurilemoma, with emphasis on technical problems encountered during surgical removal. Surgery 57:366, 1965

126. North JP: Primary tumors of the retroperitoneum. Ann Surg 151:693, 1960

127. Lack EF, Cubilla AL, Woodruff JM, et al: Extra-adrenal paragangliomas of the retroperitoneum. A clinicopathologic study of 12 tumors. Am J Surg Pathol 4:109, 1980

128. Glenner GG, Grimley PM: Tumors of extra-adrenal paraganglion system. Atlas of Tumor Pathology, fasc. 9. Second series. Armed Forces Institute of Pathology. Washington, DC, 1973

129. Olson JR, Abell MR: Nonfunctional nonchromaffin paragangliomas of the retroperitoneum. Cancer 23:1358, 1969

130. Carney JA, Sheps SG, Go VLW, et al: The triad of gastric leiomyosarcoma, functioning extra-adrenal paraganglioma and pulmonary chondroma. N Engl J Med 296:1517, 1977

131. Smetena HF, Scott WJ Jr: Malignant tumors of nonchromaffin paraganglia. Milit Surg 109:330, 1951

132. Finkbeiner AE, DeRidder PA, Ryden SE: Splenic-gonadal fusion and adrenal cortical rest associated with bilateral cryptorchism. Urology 10:337, 1977

133. Hansmann GH, Budd JW: Massive unattached retroperitoneal tumors based on remnants of the embryonic urogenital apparatus. Am J Pathol 7:631, 1931

134. Ordonez NG, Manning JT, Ayala AG: Teratoma of the omentum. Cancer 51:955, 1983

135. Mahour GH, Woolley MM, Trivedi SN, et al: Sacrococcygeal teratoma: A 33 year experience. J Pediatr Surg 10:183, 1975

136. Valdiserri RO, Yunis EJ: Sacrococcygeal tumors. A review of 68 cases. Cancer 48:217, 1981

137. Lack EE, Travis WD, Welch KJ: Retroperitoneal germ cell tumors in childhood. A clinical and pathologic study of 11 cases. Cancer 56:602, 1985

138. Gonzalez-Crussi F, Winkler RF, Mirkin DL: Sacrococcygeal teratomas in infants and children. Relationship of histology and prognosis in 40 cases. Arch Pathol Lab Med 102:420, 1978

139. Noseworthy J, Lack EE, Kozakewich HPW: Sacrococcygeal germ cell tumors in childhood: An updated experience with 118 patients. J Pediatr Surg 16:358, 1981

140. Chreitien PB, Milam JD, Foote FW: Embryonal adenocarcinoma (a type of malignant teratoma) of the sacrococcygeal region. Clinical and pathologic aspects of 21 cases. Cancer 26:522, 1970

141. Conklin J, Abell MR: Germ cell neoplasms of sacrococcygeal region. Cancer 20:2105, 1967

142. Altman RP, Randolph JG, Lilly JR: Sacrococcygeal teratoma: American Academy of Pediatrics Surgical Section Survey—1973. J Pediatr Surg 9:389, 1974

143. Donnellan WA, Swenson O: Benign and malignant sacrococcygeal teratomas. Surgery 64:834, 1968

144. Gonzalez-Crussi F: Extragonadal teratomas. Atlas of Tumor Pathology. Fasc. 18. Second series. Armed Forces Institute of Pathology, Washington, DC, 1982

145. Izant RJ, Filston HC: Sacrococcygeal teratomas. Analysis of forty-three cases. Am J Surg 130:167, 1975

146. Palumbo LT, Cross KR, Smith AN, et al: Primary teratomas of the lateral retroperitoneal spaces. Surg 26:149, 1949

147. Polsky MS, Shackelford GD, Weber CH Jr, et al: Retroperitoneal teratoma. Urology 8:618, 1976

148. Arnheim EE: Retroperitoneal teratomas in infancy and childhood. Pediatrics 8:309, 1951

149. Engel RM, Elkins RC, Fletcher BD: Retroperitoneal teratoma. Review of the literature and presentation of an unusual case. Cancer 22:1068, 1968

150. Berry CL, Keeling J, Hilton C: Teratomata in infancy and childhood. A review of 91 cases. J Pathol 98:241, 1969

151. Shkolnik Z, Deutsch AA, Reiss R: Retroperitoneal choriocarcinoma in the male. Br J Urol 55:335, 1983

152. Meyer K, Shapiro P: Dermoid cyst of the lesser omental bursa. Am J Surg 27:551, 1935

153. Judd ES, Fulcher OH: Dermoid cysts of the abdomen. Surg Clin North Am 13:835, 1933

154. Warfield JO: Omental dermoid cyst. Am Surg 22:652, 1956

155. James CF Jr: Dermoid cysts of the mesentery. Am J Surg 65:116, 1944

156. Printz JL, Choate JW, Townes PL, et al: The embryology of supernumerary ovaries. Obstet Gynecol 41:246, 1973

157. Buskirk SJ, Evans RG, Farrow GM, et al: Primary retroperitoneal seminoma. Cancer 49:1934, 1982

158. Abell MR, Fayos JV, Lampe I: Retroperitoneal germinomas (seminomas) without evidence of testicular involvement. Cancer 18:273, 1965

159. Carney JA: Wilms' tumor and renal cell carcinoma in retroperitoneal teratoma. Cancer 35:1179, 1975

160. Todd DW, Roskos R, Baldwin J: Extrarenal Wilms' tumor. Minn Med 67:635, 1984

161. Adam YG, Rosen A, Oland J, et al: Extrarenal Wilms' tumor. J Surg Oncol 22:56, 1983

162. Akhtar M, Kott E, Brooks B: Extrarenal Wilms' tumor. Report of a case and review of the literature. Cancer 40:3087, 1977

163. Ward SP, Dehner LP: Sacrococcygeal teratoma with nephroblastoma (Wilms' tumor): A variant of extragonadal tumor in childhood. A histologic and ultrastructural study. Cancer 33:1355, 1974

164. Ulbright TM, Kraus FT: Endometrial stromal tumors of extra-uterine tissue. Am J Clin Pathol 76:371, 1981

165. Ferrie RK, Ross RC: Retroperitoneal müllerian carcinosarcoma. Can Med Assoc J 97:1290, 1967

166. Douglas GW, Kastin AJ, Huntington RW: Carcinoma arising in a retroperitoneal müllerian cyst, with widespread metastasis during pregnancy. Am J Obstet Gynecol 91:210, 1965

167. Hasiuk AS, Peterson RO, Hanjani PH, et al: Extragenital malignant mixed müllerian tumor. Case report and review of the literature. Am J Clin Pathol 78:726, 1984

168. Fujii S, Konishi I, Okamura H, et al: Mucinous cystadenocarcinoma of the retroperitoneum: A light and electron microscopic study. Gynecol Oncol 24:103, 1986

169. Ulbright TM, Morley DJ, Roth LM, et al: Papillary serous carcinoma of the retroperitoneum. Am J Clin Pathol 79:633, 1983

170. Roth LM, Ehrlich LE: Mucinous cystadenocarcinoma of the retroperitoneum. Obstet Gynecol 49:486, 1977

171. Smith BA, Webb EA, Price WE: Retroperitoneal hypernephroid mesonephroma. J Urol 94:616, 1965

172. Spencer TD, Maier RV, Olson HH: Retroperitoneal giant lymph node hyperplasia. A case report and review of the literature. Ann Surg 50:509, 1984

173. Bainbridge ET: Angiomatous lymphoid hamartoma of the pelvis. Br J Obstet Gynaecol 83:823, 1976

174. Fukudo T, Ishikawa H, Ohnishi Y, et al: Extraskeletal myxoid chondrosarcoma arising from the retroperitoneum. Am J Clin Pathol 85:514, 1986

175. Dhaliwal US, Singh A, Dhaliwal SS, et al: Retroperitoneal mesenchymal chondrosarcoma. J Indian Med Assoc 83:62, 1985

176. Harris HL, Herzog M: Solid mesenteric tumors with a report of case. Ann Surg 104:66, 1897

177. Barnardo DE, Stavrow M, Bourne R, et al: Primary carcinoid of the mesentery. Hum Pathol 15:796, 1984

178. Sutsumi AT, Kawabata K, Taguchi K, et al: Elastofibroma of the greater omentum. Acta Pathol Jpn 35:233, 1985

179. Peison B, Benisch B, Williams MC, et al: Primary extramedullary plasmacytoma of the omentum associated with adenocarcinoma of the colon. Hum Pathol 11:399, 1980

180. Kyrtz RJ, Heimann TM, Holt J, et al: Mesenteric and retroperitoneal cysts. Ann Surg 203:109, 1986

181. Caropreso PR: Mesenteric cysts. A review. Arch Surg 108:242, 1974

182. Walker AR, Putnam TC: Omental, mesenteric and retroperitoneal cysts. A clinical study of 33 new cases. Ann Surg 178:13, 1973

183. Barr WB, Yamashita T: Mesenteric cysts: Review of the literature and report of a case. Am J Gastroenterol 41:53, 1964

184. Bentley JFR, Smith JR: Developmental posterior enteric remnants and spinal malformations. The split notochord syndrome. Arch Dis Child 35:76, 1960

185. Steinberg L, Rothman D, Drey NW: Müllerian cyst of the retroperitoneum. Am J Obstet Gynecol 107:963, 1970

186. Lloyd FA, Bonnett D: Müllerian duct cysts. J Urol 64:777, 1950

187. Singh RS, Sahay S: Retroperitoneal primary hydatid cyst of pelvis. J Indian Med Assoc 83:64, 1985

188. Leake R, Wayman TB: Retroperitoneal encysted hematomas. J Urol 68:69, 1962

189. Povysil C: Extravesical malakoplakia. Arch Pathol 97:273, 1974

190. Terner JY, Lattes R: Malakoplakia of colon and retroperitoneum. Report of a case with a histochemical study of the Michaelis-Gutmann inclusion bodies. Am J Clin Pathol 44:20, 1965

191. Osborne BM, Butler JJ, Bloustein P, et al: Idiopathic retroperitoneal fibrosis (sclerosing retroperitonitis). Hum Pathol 18:735, 1987

192. Chan SL, Johnson HW, McLoughlin MG: Idiopathic fibrosis in children. J Urol 122:103, 1979

193. Mitchinson MJ: The pathology of idiopathic retroperitoneal fibrosis. J Clin Pathol 23:681, 1970

194. Binder SC, Deterling RA, Mahoney SA, et al: Systemic idiopathic fibrosis. Report of a case of the concomitant occurrence of retractile mesenteritis and retroperitoneal fibrosis. Am J Surg 124:422, 1972

195. Hanley PC, Shub C, Lie JT: Constrictive pericarditis associated with combined idiopathic retroperitoneal and mediastinal fibrosis. Mayo Clin Proc 59:300, 1984

196. Stewart TW Jr, Friberg TR: Idiopathic retroperitoneal fibrosis with diffuse involvement: Further evidence of systemic idiopathic fibrosis. South Med J 77:1185, 1985

197. Mitchinson MJ: Retroperitoneal fibrosis revisited. Arch Pathol Lab Med 110:784, 1986

198. Ahmad S: Methyldopa and retroperitoneal fibrosis. Am Heart J 105:1037, 1983

199. Lege-Savary D, Vallières A: Ergotamine as a possible cause of retroperitoneal fibrosis. Clin Pharm 1:179, 1982

200. Jeffries JJ, Lyall WA, Bezchlibnyk K, et al: Retroperitoneal fibrosis and haloperidol. Am J Psychiatry 139:1524, 1982

201. Palmer PE, Wolfe HJ, Kostas CI: Multisystem fibrosis in alpha-1-antitrypsin deficiency. Lancet 1:221, 1978

202. Jonsson G, Linstedt E, Rubin SO: Two cases of metastasizing scirrhous gastric carcinoma simulating idiopathic retroperitoneal fibrosis. Scand J Urol Nephrol 1:299, 1967

203. Waldron JA, Newcomer LN, Katz ME, et al: Sclerosing variants of follicular center cell lymphomas presenting in the retroperitoneum. Cancer 52:712, 1983

204. Buckspan MB, Cooter NB, Goldfinger M, et al: Endometriosis an unusual cause of ureteral obstruction. Can J Surg 28:447, 1985

205. Lichtenheld FR, McCauley RC, Staples PP: Endometriosis involving the urinary tract. A collective review. Obstet Gynecol 17:762, 1961

206. Thompson GT, Fitzgerald EF, Somers SS: Retractile mesenteritis of the sigmoid colon. Br J Radiol 58:266, 1985

207. Durst AL, Freund H, Rosemann E, et al: Mesenteric panniculitis. Review of the literature and presentation of cases. Int Surg 62:207, 1977

208. Crane JT, Aguilar MJ, Grimes OR: Isolated lipodystrophy, a form of mesenteric tumor. Am J Surg 90:169, 1955

209. Epstein LI, Lempke RE: Primary idiopathic segmental infarction of the greater omentum: Case report and collective review of the literature. Ann Surg 167:437, 1968

210. Carmichael DH, Organ CH: Epiploic disorders. Conditions of the epiploic appendages. Arch Surg 120:1167, 1985

211. Reyes CV, Foy BK, Aranha GV, et al: Omental oxyuriasis: Case report. Milit Med 149:682, 1984

212. Naraynsingh V, Raju GC, Ratan P, et al: Massive ascites due to omental endometriosis. Postgrad Med J 61:539, 1985

213. Chong PY, Panabokke RG, Chew KH: Omental crytococcoma. Arch Pathol Lab Med 110:239, 1986

214. Davis JH: Current concepts of peritonitis. Am Surg 33:673, 1967

215. Chandrasoma PT, Mendis KN: Enterobius vermicularis in ectopic sites. Am J Trop Med Hyg 26:644, 1977

216. Barnett L: Hydatid cysts; their location in various organs and tissues of body. Aust NZ J Surg 12:240, 1943

217. Thieme GA, Bundy AL, Fleischer AC, et al: Blastomycosis presenting as a peritoneal inflammatory cyst. J Clin Urol 13:205, 1985

218. Gonnella JS, Hudson EK: Clinical patterns of tuberculous peritonitis. Arch Intern Med 117:164, 1966

219. Rose G, Morrison EA, Kirkham N, et al: Malakoplakia of the pelvic peritoneum in pregnancy. Br J Obstet Gynaecol 92:170, 1985

220. Cox KR: Starch granuloma (pseudo-malignant seedlings). Br J Surg 57:650, 1970

221. Kay S: Tissue reaction to barium sulfate contrast medium: Histopathologic study. Arch Pathol Lab Med 57:279, 1954

222. Eiseman B, Seeling MG, Womack N: Talcum powder granuloma; frequent and serious postoperative complication. Ann Surg 126:820, 1947

223. Bockman RF, Woods M, Sargent L, et al: A unifying pathogenetic mechanism in the etiology of intraperitoneal adhesions. J Surg Res 20:1, 1976

224. Ryan GB, Grobety J, Majno G: Postoperative peritoneal adhesions. A study of the mechanisms. Am J Pathol 65:117, 1971

225. Baddeley H, Lee REJ, Marshall AJ, et al: Sclerosing peritonitis due to practolol. Br Med J 2:192, 1977

226. Brown P, Read AE, Baddeley H, et al: Sclerosing peritonitis, an unusual reaction to a β-adrenergic blocking drug (Practolol). Lancet 2:1477, 1974

227. Meyerhoff J: Familial mediterranean fever: Report of a large family, review of the literature, and discussion of the frequency of amyloidosis. Medicine (Baltimore) 59:66, 1980

228. Naylor B: The exfoliative cytology of diffuse malignant mesothelioma. J Pathol Bacteriol 86:293, 1963

229. Johnson WD: The cytological diagnosis of cancer in serous effusion. Acta Cytol 10:161, 1966

230. Foot NC: The identification of neoplastic cells in serous effusions. Am J Pathol 32:961, 1956

231. Takagi F: Studies on tumor cells in serous effusion. Am J Clin Pathol 24:663, 1954

232. Walts AE, Said JW, Banks-Schlegel S: Keratin and carcinoembryonic antigen in exfoliated mesothelial and malignant cells: An immunoperoxidase study. Am J Clin Pathol 80:671, 1983

233. McFadden DE, Clement PB: Peritoneal inclusion cysts with mural mesothelial proliferation. Am J Surg Pathol 10:844, 1986

234. Lees RF, Feldman PS, Brenbridge AN, et al: Inflammatory cysts of the pelvic peritoneum. AJR 131:633, 1978

235. Lascano EF, Villamayor RD, Lauró JL: Loose cysts of the peritoneal cavity. Ann Surg 152:836, 1960

236. Watson WJ, Sundwall DA, Bensen WL: Splenosis mimicking endometriosis. Obstet Gynecol 59(suppl.):518, 1982

237. Rosai J, Dehner LP: Nodular mesothelial hyperplasia in hernial sacs. A benign reactive condition simulating a neoplastic process. Cancer 35:165, 1975

238. Gompel C, Silverberg SG: Pathology in Gynecology and Obstetrics. 3rd Ed. JB Lippincott, Philadelphia, 1985

239. Lauchlan SC: The secondary müllerian system. Obstet Gynecol Surv 27:133, 1972

240. Zinsser KR, Wheeler JE: Endosalpingiosis in the omentum. A study of autopsy and surgical material. Am J Surg Pathol 6:109, 1982

241. Raju U, Fine G, Greenawald KA, et al: Primary papillary

serous neoplasia of the peritoneum. A clinicopathological and ultrastructural study of eight cases. Hum Pathol 20:426, 1989

242. Burmeister RE, Fechner RE, Franklin RR: Endosalpingiosis of the peritoneum. Obstet Gynecol 34:310, 1969

243. Farhi DC, Silverberg SG: Pseudometastases in female genital cancer. Pathol Ann 17(pt 1):47, 1982

244. Kheir SM, Mann WJ, Wilkerson JA: Glandular inclusions in lymph nodes. The problem of extensive involvement and relationship to salpingitis. Am J Surg Pathol 5:353, 1981

245. Roth LM: The Brenner tumor and the Walthard cell nest: An electron-microscopic study. Lab Invest 31:15, 1974

246. Bell DA, Scully RE: Serous borderline tumors of the peritoneum. Lab Invest 56:5A, 1987

247. McCaughey WTE: Papillary peritoneal neoplasms in females. Pathol Ann 20(2):387, 1985

248. Foyle A, Al-Jobi M, McCaughey WTE: Papillary peritoneal tumors in women. Am J Surg Pathol 5:241, 1981

249. Genadry R, Poliakoff S, Rotmensch J, et al: Primary, papillary peritoneal neoplasia. Obstet Gynecol 58:730, 1981

250. Kannerstein M, Churg J, McCaughey WTE, et al: Papillary tumors of the peritoneum in women: Mesothelioma or papillary carcinoma. Am J Obstet Gynecol 127:306, 1977

251. Valente PT: Leiomyomatosis peritonealis disseminata. A report of two cases and review of the literature. Arch Pathol Lab Med 108:669, 1984

252. Tavassoli FA, Norris HJ: Peritoneal leiomyomatosis (leiomyomatosis peritonealis disseminata). A clinicopathologic study of 20 cases with ultrastructural observations. Int J Gynecol Pathol 1:59, 1982

253. Kuo T, London SN, Dinh TV: Endometriosis in leiomyomatosis peritonealis disseminata. Ultrastructural study and histogenetic consideration. Am J Surg Pathol 4:197, 1980

254. Ober WB, Black MD: Neoplasms of subcelomic mesenchyme. Arch Pathol 59:698, 1955

255. Czernoblisky B, Lancet M: Broad ligament adenocarcinoma of Müllerian origin. Obstet Gynecol 40:238, 1972

256. Kwan D, Pang LS: Deciduosis peritonei. J Obstet Gynaecol Br Commonw 71:804, 1964

257. Hanrahan JBA: Combined papillary mesothelioma and adenomatoid tumor of the omentum. Cancer 16:1497, 1963

258. Goepel JR: Benign papillary mesothelioma of peritoneum: A histologic, histochemical and ultrastructural study of six cases. Histopathology 5:21, 1981

259. Miles JM, Hart WR, McMahon JT: Cystic mesothelioma of the peritoneum. Report of a case with multiple recurrences and review of the literature. Cleve Clin Q 53:109, 1986

260. Sienkowski IK, Russell AJ, Dilly SA, et al: Peritoneal cystic mesothelioma: an electron microscopic and immunohistochemical study of two male patients. J Clin Pathol 39:440, 1986

261. Silberstein MJ, Lewis JE, Blair JD, et al: Congenital peritoneal mesothelioma. J Pediatr Surg 18:243, 1983

262. Craig JR, Hart WR: Extragenital adenomatoid tumor. Evidence for the mesothelial theory of origin. Cancer 43:1678, 1979

263. Favara BE, Odom LF: Malignant peritoneal mesothelioma in a child. Pediatr Pathol 5:411, 1986

264. Talerman A, Montero JR, Chilcote RR, et al: Diffuse malignant peritoneal mesothelioma in a 13-year-old girl. Report of a case and review of the literature. Am J Surg Pathol 9:73, 1985

265. Stout AP: Solitary fibrous mesothelioma of the peritoneum. Cancer 3:820, 1950

266. Hill RP: Malignant fibrous mesothelioma of the peritoneum. Cancer 6:1182, 1953

267. Corson JM, Pinkus GS: Mesothelioma: Profile of keratin proteins and carcinoembryonic antigen. An immunoperoxidase study of 20 cases and comparison with pulmonary adenocarcinomas. Am J Pathol 108:80, 1982

268. Wang N, Huang S, Gold P: Absence of carcinoembryonic antigen-like material in mesothelioma. An immunohistochemical differentiation from other lung cancers. Cancer 44:937, 1979

269. Bane B, Raju U, Greenawald KA, et al: Mesothelioma: A reappraisal of the diagnostic approach. Lab Invest 54:4A, 1986

270. Saeed SM, Fine G, Horn RC Jr: Hypoglycemia associated with extrapancreatic tumors. An immunofluorescent study. Cancer 24:158, 1969

271. Sandenberg HA, Woodruff JD: Histogenesis of pseudomyxoma peritonei. Review of 9 cases. Obstet Gynecol 49:339, 1977

272. Truong LD, Jurco S, McGavran MH: Gliomatosis peritonei. Am J Surg Pathol 6:443, 1982

27

The Esophagus

Scott H. Saul
Horatio T. Enterline
John Jones Thompson

EMBRYOLOGY

The esophagus is recognizable at about the 2.5 mm stage (third week of gestation). In contrast to some reports based on other species, it maintains a lumen throughout development. The earliest epithelial lining consists of two or three layers of stratified epithelium; this subsequently becomes vacuolated and is then replaced by ciliated epithelium by the 60 mm stage (about 10 weeks). Ciliated epithelium in turn is replaced focally by mucin-secreting cells in the proximal and distal esophagus. At about the 90 mm stage (16 weeks), stratified squamous epithelium appears in the mid-esophagus and proceeds to line virtually the entire organ.[1,2] The presence of occasional goblet cells in the fetal esophagus is controversial.

NORMAL ANATOMY AND HISTOLOGY

The adult esophagus is 24 to 30 cm in length, being slightly shorter in women than in men. Its termination at the esophagogastric junction (EGJ) is located approximately 38 to 40 cm from the dental incisors; however, individual variation exists. Surprisingly, there is still debate about important details of the histology and anatomy of the esophagus. All the usual layers of the gastrointestinal (GI) tract are represented. The mucosa is composed of nonkeratinized stratified squamous epithelium. A basal zone is present and normally is not more than two or three cells thick, or more than 15 percent of the total epithelial thickness. Argyrophil cells may be found in the basal cell layer. Mitoses are infrequent and confined to the basal zone. Papillae of the lamina propria extend through no more than two thirds of the total epithelial thickness.[3,4] Small numbers of intraepithelial lymphocytes (primarily of the cytotoxic/suppressor class) and Langerhans cells can be found.[5] A few lymphocytes and plasma cells as well as occasional lymphoid aggregates are present normally in the lamina propria. The muscularis mucosae is quite thick, particularly distally, and should not be misinterpreted as muscularis propria on suction biopsies.

Small mucus-secreting glands similar to those of the gastric cardia, referred to as cardiac or superficial glands, occur in the lamina propria (Fig. 27-1). They communicate to the surface via a channel lined by a layer of mucus-secreting cells which may replace small areas of squamous mucosa at these foci. These glands are inconstant, being most common in the distal esophagus and less so in the upper esophagus.[6] Ham[7] states that there are only a few scattered glands in the submucosa. However, a study by Umlas and Sakhuja[8] of three normal esophagi sectioned transversely at intervals of 0.5 cm showed an average of four submucosal glands at each level (Fig. 27-2). These glands may demonstrate serous acini as well as the more common mucinous type, thus resembling most minor salivary gland tissue.[6] They empty into ducts lined by cuboidal to columnar epithelium, which becomes stratified squamous as it reaches

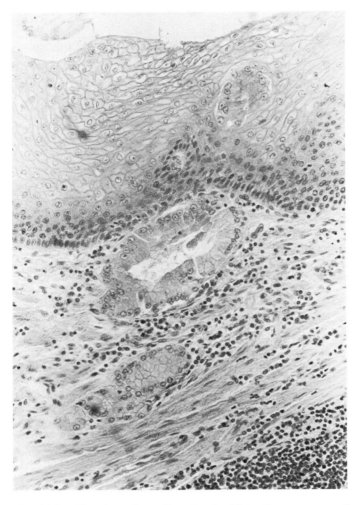

Fig. 27-1. Esophageal cardiac glands. Note the presence of mucus-secreting glands in the lamina propria and their connection to the surface. Small areas of the squamous epithelium on the surface may be replaced by mucous cells from the duct orifice.

the surface. Sometimes metaplastic squamous epithelium lines nearly the entire duct and may replace some of the acini.

The muscularis propria is striated in the upper third, smooth muscle in the lower third, and is mixed in the middle third. Innervation is by parasympathetic fibers from the vagus and from the sympathetic trunks and celiac ganglia. The usual myenteric (Auerbach's) ganglionic plexi are present.[7] The muscularis propria is covered by adventitia rather than a serosa, except for the most distal 1 to 2 cm which is intra-abdominal.

The arterial supply is multiple, consisting of branches of the aorta and inferior thyroid, bronchial, intercostal, inferior phrenic and left gastric arteries. Veins accompany the arteries and form a plexus communicating with the gastric coronary and azygous veins. This creates a connection between the portal and systemic venous sys-

tems—the well known reason for esophageal varices in portal hypertension.[9]

Defining the EGJ has traditionally been a problem, as this does not necessarily coincide with the squamocolumnar junction.[10] The presence of columnar mucosa in the distal 2 to 3 cm of the esophagus has been observed in normal persons.[11] The EGJ often has a irregular zigzag configuration (Z line) of interdigitating gray squamous and pink columnar mucosa. The distal esophagus at the EGJ is best identified microscopically by the presence of submucosal glands, which are not found in the stomach. Other features include a thicker muscularis mucosae and the presence of two rather than three layers of muscularis propria in the esophagus. Clinically, the manometric localization of the lower esophageal sphincter aids in defining the EGJ.

LYMPHATICS

The esophagus contains a rich plexus of mucosal lymphatics connecting with a less rich submucosal plexus that, in turn, communicates with widely spaced longitudinal channels in the muscle coats. Lymph (and tumor) spreads more freely in a longitudinal direction than circumferentially. There is normally little connection between mucosal lymphatics of the esophagus and stomach. In general, lymph from the esophagus below the tracheal bifurcation passes through the para-aortic nodes or the celiac axis region. Lymph from above this point drains upward to paraesophageal nodes, upper paratracheal nodes, and finally to nodes in the region of the inferior thyroid artery.[12] There is individual variation.

PHYSIOLOGY

The esophagus is said to begin with the cricopharyngeus muscle, which connects anteriorly with the cricoid cartilage and spreads in a fan-shaped fashion to surround the upper esophagus. It variably contributes to the outer longitudinal fibers of the esophagus[13] and constitutes the upper esophageal sphincter (UES). The lower esophageal sphincter (LES) represents a specialized segment of circular muscle in the distal 2 to 3 cm of esophagus. Although not identifiable grossly, it functions to separate the positive intra-abdominal pressure from the esophagus, where the pressure is negative compared with the atmosphere. Basal LES pressure is 15 to 30 mmHg in normal persons.[14,15] The complexity of this region is illustrated by a wide variety of excitatory and inhibitory neurotransmitters such as acetylcholine (ACh), norepinephrine, vasoactive intestinal polypeptide (VIP), substance P, neuropeptide Y, and encephalin, all of

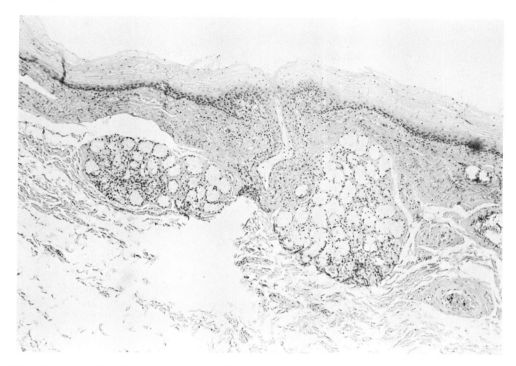

Fig. 27-2. Esophageal submucosal glands. Several glands seen in the submucosa are connected to the surface by a central duct. The gland cells are largely mucinous.

which have been demonstrated by immunohistochemistry.[16] LES pressure is quite sensitive to the effects of many exogenously administered neurotransmitters, hormones, and miscellaneous compounds.[2,14]

The UES and LES are normally closed. Swallowing consists of a coordinated opening of the UES, a rapid distally moving ring of contraction beginning in the upper esophagus, followed by relaxation of the LES.[17]

EMBRYONIC REMNANTS AND HETEROTOPIAS

Foci of columnar mucin-secreting and ciliated cells have been reported in 6.3 percent and 4.2 percent, respectively, of esophagi of infants and children at autopsy.[18] In the same study, foci of gastric body-type epithelium (presence of parietal cells) were about half as common. These were distributed in the upper two thirds of the esophagus and were often accompanied by an inflammatory infiltrate. Recently, Jabbari et al.[19] found patches of gastric body-type mucosa at the time of endoscopy in the region of the upper esophageal sphincter (inlet patch) in 3.8 percent of adults. These foci varied from 3 to 30 mm in greatest diameter. Macroscopically, they were pink and velvety. Parietal and chief cells were virtually always present, as was an associated chronic inflammatory infiltrate. The remainder of the esophagi were

nearly always unremarkable. Acid secretion could be demonstrated in the larger patches, suggesting that peptic-induced disease may be responsible for the occasional symptomatic case. Whether these foci represent true heterotopias or inadequate squamous replacement of columnar mucosa followed by parietal and chief cell differentiation is unclear. The fact that Schridde was able to detect gastric mucosa in the upper esophagus in 70 percent of cases in a meticulous autopsy study emphasizes that this is not an uncommon finding.[20] Less than 10 well documented cases of adenocarcinoma arising in ectopic gastric mucosa of the upper esophagus have been reported.[21] These should be distinguished from those arising in Barrett's esophagus.

Sebaceous glands have been found in 2 percent of carefully examined esophagi at autopsy.[22] These foci are typically 1 to 5 mm in diameter and round and yellow and can be single or multiple. They have been identified endoscopically in both the proximal and distal esophagus.[23,24]

ESOPHAGEAL AND GASTROENTERIC CYSTS

Cysts of the esophagus and paraesophagus are rare lesions. Nonetheless, cysts (type unspecified) are said to be the second most common benign tumor in the Mayo Clinic experience.[25] They may be divided into *retention cysts* and *developmental cysts*. Within the latter group, gastroenteric (gastroenterogenic) cysts are best separated from other cysts more closely akin to bronchogenic cysts. Retention cysts, also sometimes called mucoceles, represent dilations of the ducts of submucosal glands. They are usually small and more common in the distal esophagus.[2,6] Numerous retention cysts have been termed esophageal intramural pseudodiverticulosis (which is discussed later). Developmental cysts are discussed in detail in Chapter 24.[2,26–31]

ATRESIA, STENOSIS, AND TRACHEOESOPHAGEAL FISTULA

Atresia of a portion of the esophagus, with or without a tracheoesophageal fistula, and a related phenomenon, congenital stenosis, are well known pediatric and neonatal problems. Fistula may also occur independently of atresia or stenosis. In the most common situation (90 percent of cases), the proximal esophagus ends in a blind pouch, and a tracheoesophageal fistula connects with the lower segment of the esophagus. Approximately one third of infants with esophageal atresia will have an additional major malformation.[2] In addition to regurgitation and signs of aspiration, children with the most common form of tracheoesophageal fistula show contained air in the stomach and intestine.[2,31,32] Separation of congenital from acquired stenosis may be quite difficult if not impossible. The three main forms are congenital stricture due to tracheobronchial remnants (chondroepithelial choristoma, cartilaginous esophageal ring), congenital esophageal web and congenital idiopathic muscular hypertrophy.[31,33,34] Tracheobronchial remnants result in a fusiform stenotic segment of about 2 cm in length. Incomplete cartilaginous rings, bronchial-type submucosal glands and lymphoid aggregates are found beneath a normal esophageal squamous mucosa.

RINGS AND WEBS

The terms *rings* and *webs* have been used more or less interchangeably for annular membranes typically having eccentric lumina. They are nearly always composed of epithelium and lamina propria with an absent or inconspicuous smooth muscle component. Their pathogenesis is obscure for the most part, although a few are clearly postinflammatory adhesions, such as those reported in benign mucous membrane pemphigus.[35,36] The most common site clinically recognized is the upper esophagus, and nearly one half of these cases occur in women with the Plummer-Vinson (Patterson-Kelley) syndrome. The histology is that of a fold of squamous mucosa with a mild chronic inflammatory infiltrate in the lamina propria. There is an increased risk of developing squamous cell carcinoma of the hypopharynx and oropharynx as well as the upper esophagus (see under Squamous Cell Carcinoma).[35]

Rings and webs may also occur in the mid- and lower esophagus. Those lesions at the squamocolumnar junction are referred to as Schatzki rings. These lower esophageal rings (webs) are surfaced on the proximal side by stratified squamous epithelium and on the distal side by columnar epithelium. Significant inflammatory changes are absent.[36,37] Goyal and co-workers[36,37] report that a lower ring can be demonstrated at autopsy in 10 percent of the population when properly searched for and may be the most common cause of esophageal dysphagia. These investigators also recognize a less common muscular ring, always proximal to the site of the mucosal ring when both are present. Their origin is debatable. Mid-esophageal rings are quite rare. Annular fibrous strictures of the lower esophagus are typically secondary to reflux esophagitis.[36,37]

PATHOLOGY OF ESOPHAGEAL MOTILITY DISORDERS

The smooth coordination of the sphincteric and peristaltic function of the esophagus is important in the swallowing mechanism (see the section Physiology). A number of conditions, defined by manometric methods, are caused or complicated by hyperfunction, hypofunction, and/or incoordination of esophageal motor activity.[2,14,38,39] These include diffuse esophageal spasm, primary and secondary forms of achalasia, the so-called nutcracker esophagus, and others.[14,38,39] It is possible that these disorders represent a spectrum of disease rather than well defined individual entities. The clinical importance of the nutcracker esophagus, characterized manometrically by high-amplitude peristaltic contractions in a patient who often complains of anginal-type chest pain, is controversial.[40] As its pathologic features are unknown, it is not discussed further. Several complications of dysmotility such as diverticula and esophageal ruptures and tears are also discussed in this section. Systemic disorders such as scleroderma may also cause dysmotility, as can myopathies such as myotonic dystrophy. The common entity of reflux esophagitis is discussed in detail later in this chapter.

Diffuse Esophageal Spasm

With increased use of manometric studies, a group of patients has been found who have simultaneous, repetitive, high-amplitude and nonperistaltic contractions aris-

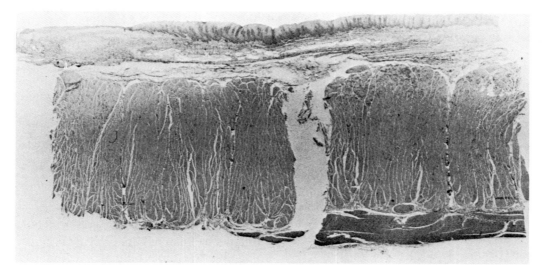

Fig. 27-3. Idiopathic muscular hypertrophy. Low-power photomicrograph shows the regular thickening of the circular layer most commonly seen in idiopathic hypertrophy.

ing from the smooth muscle portion of the esophagus. These occur in the face of some preservation of normal peristaltic function. Although the abnormal contractions may be associated with various forms of organic disease, the term diffuse esophageal spasm has been used when no obvious underlying cause is found. The importance of this disorder, which occurs primarily in males, is its association with dysphagia and angina-type chest pain. The barium esophagram often demonstrates a curled or corkscrew appearance.

The pathologic correlate of diffuse esophageal spasm appears to be what is called *idiopathic* or *diffuse muscular hypertrophy* (IMH) of the esophagus[2,41–45] by pathologists (see also under Nonepithelial Tumors) (Fig. 27-3). The esophagus, particularly distally, demonstrates a uniform thickening of the muscularis propria, especially the inner circular layer which may be five times the thickness of the outer longitudinal layer. The muscular thickening, which may be as great as one centimeter, does not classically involve the EGJ. The lumen may be markedly narrowed in the affected segment. A recent report suggests that the smooth muscle is actually hyperplastic rather than hypertrophic.[44] While the number of ganglion cells in the myenteric (Auerbach's) plexus is invariably within normal limits, a lymphocytic infiltrate in the plexus (ganglionitis) may be present. It is interesting that the muscular thickening noted in this disorder is similar to that seen in the sigmoid colon in patients with diverticular disease, another entity associated with abnormal motor function. The precise pathogenesis of diffuse esophageal spasm-related muscular hypertrophy (hyperplasia) is unclear.

Achalasia

Achalasia may generally be defined as "failure of relaxation of smooth muscle fibers at any junction of one part of the gastrointestinal tract with another." However, unless otherwise stated, achalasia refers to a condition of the esophagus characterized manometrically by (1) complete absence of peristalsis; (2) failure of the LES to relax completely upon swallowing; the resting LES pressure is typically, but not necessarily elevated; (3) low amplitude, nonperistaltic contractions; and (4) increased intraesophageal pressure.[14,38,39] These abnormalities are present in the smooth, but not the skeletal, muscle of the esophagus. Achalasia leads to functional obstruction of the distal esophagus with a dilated fluid- and food-filled proximal portion. At times the dilation is extreme and is termed megaesophagus. Patients are typically 20 to 40 years of age, but a wide range exists.[2] They usually present with progressive dysphagia. Regurgitation, aspiration, and weight loss are also common manifestations. In so-called vigorous achalasia, an added manometric finding is the presence of high-amplitude nonperistaltic contractions similar to those of diffuse esophageal spasm. The caliber of the esophagus in this subgroup of patients is close to normal. Although the precise etiology of achalasia is unknown, it appears that it is a neuronal rather than a myopathic disorder. Most observers agree that the number of ganglion cells in Auerbach's plexus is markedly decreased or commonly absent in the dilated esophageal body.[2,46,47] The same degree of paucity of ganglion cells in the distal nondilated esophagus may not be present, but this is controversial. Similar to diffuse esophageal spasm, a variable lymphocytic infiltrate in the myenteric plexus may be present. Lewy bodies identical to those seen in Parkinson's disease have been described in ganglion cells in the myenteric plexus as well as the dorsal motor nucleus of the vagus.[48] These findings, as well as the presence of wallerian degeneration of vagal fibers and a decreased number of small intrinsic esophageal nerve fibers, emphasize the role of a primary neuropathy.[45,46] Denervation hypersensitivity can be demonstrated pharmacologically.[2]

The esophageal wall is often thickened secondary to smooth muscle hypertrophy, particularly of the inner circular layer of the muscularis propria. This is generally true distally and is more variable in the dilated proximal esophagus, which may actually demonstrate thinning.[43,46] The dilated nature of the esophagus and the paucity of ganglion cells distinguishes achalasia from diffuse esophageal spasm/idiopathic muscular hypertrophy. Esophagitis secondary to stasis may be present.

Secondary forms of achalasia are well described.[2,48] In 100 percent of patients with Chagas' disease of the esophagus, a similar set of pathologic findings is noted, and an associated achalasia is also present clinically. The trypanosome responsible for this disease (*Trypanosoma cruzi*) is known to elaborate a neurotoxin that destroys ganglion cells in the myenteric plexus.[49] Tumors of the lower esophagus and mediastinum may also cause an achalasia-like pattern; therefore, a thorough diagnostic evaluation is required for all patients in whom achalasia is suspected.

The frequency of squamous cell carcinoma is increased in patients with achalasia (see the section on squamous cell carcinoma). Heller myotomy is the standard treatment of choice.[38] By disrupting the LES, this also causes reflux esophagitis. Barrett's esophagus and adenocarcinoma have been reported to occur in this clinical situation.[50]

Rupture and Partial-Thickness Tears

Spontaneous rupture, or Boerhaave's syndrome (BS), and partial-thickness tears, or Mallory-Weiss syndrome (MWS), of the esophagus are well known conditions, associated in 90 percent of cases with an episode of vigorous vomiting. Many cases occur during an alcoholic episode, while others have been described during episodes of coughing, hiccupping, and chest massage.[2,51,52] The ruptures and partial tears are longitudinally oriented, with most ruptures occurring in the left posterior aspect of the distal esophagus, while the tears of MWS are typically found in the gastric cardia. Extension into the esophagus occurs in 9 percent of cases of MWS. The generation of a large pressure gradient between the stomach and esophagus is important in the pathogenesis of these two conditions. In MWS, the LES appears to be inappropriately closed, while in BS it is the UES that has failed to relax.[2,51,52] MWS currently accounts for 5 to 15 percent of all upper GI bleeding episodes, with a mortality rate of less than 5 percent.[52] BS, on the other hand, is rare and is less commonly associated with massive bleeding. However, because of spillage of gastric contents into the mediastinum and pleural cavity there is an associated high (approximately 50 percent) mortality.[53]

Diverticula

Incoordination of the upper sphincter, that is the cricopharyngeus, is now accepted as the basic cause of the relatively common Zenker's (pharyngoesophageal) diverticulum, a posterior outpouching of the uppermost esophagus. Patients are generally middle-aged or elderly. They typically present with regurgitation of food that was swallowed hours earlier.[2] The diverticula gradually enlarge, causing food retention and secondary aspiration. All layers of the posterior pharyngeal wall are generally involved, although the muscle layer is often greatly attenuated.[2] An increased frequency of squamous cell carcinoma is recognized in Zenker's diverticula, ranging from 0.31 percent to 0.7 percent[54,55]; therefore, the excised specimen should be adequately sectioned to detect cancer (Fig. 27-4). Diverticulectomy and/or myotomy are the treatments of choice.[56] Most mid-esophageal diverticula in the region of the tracheal bifurcation have been reported as traction diverticula due to scarring of tuberculous lymph nodes or similar conditions[57] (Fig. 27-5). More recently, however, esophageal dysmotility has been reported as an important cause of pulsion-type diverticula in both the mid-esophagus and more commonly the distal esophagus.[58]

Muscular Dystrophies

A recent study demonstrated abnormal esophageal motor function in patients with myotonic, but not nonmyotonic, forms of muscular dystrophy.[59] The predominant motor dysfunction was in the skeletal muscle in the region of the UES and esophageal body. There was marked skeletal muscle fiber size variation, with many fibers demonstrating internal nuclei and pyknotic clumps. Focal necrosis and fiber regeneration were seen, but inflammation was absent. Although motility was also abnormal in the distal (smooth muscle) esophagus, this was histologically normal, suggesting that this finding was secondary to the proximal skeletal muscle damage. A previous report on progressive muscular dystrophies did describe atrophy of smooth muscle in the esophagus and the remainder of the GI tract.[60]

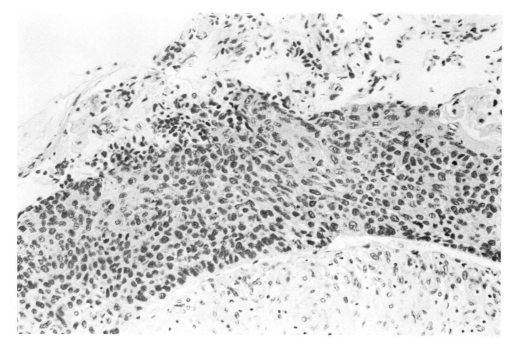

Fig. 27-4. CIS in a Zenker's diverticulum. The entire thickness of the epithelium is replaced by atypical cells showing no evidence of surface maturation. Note the character of the sloughing surface cells that might be seen on cytologic examination. In other areas, invasive carcinoma was present.

Systemic Sclerosis (Scleroderma)

Systemic sclerosis (SSc), nearly always associated with Raynaud's disease, affects the esophagus in 90 percent of cases.[61] By definition, it is considered a component of the CREST (calcinosis cutis, Raynaud's phenomenon, esophageal dysmotility, sclerodactyly, and telangectasia) variant of SSc. It involves the smooth muscle of the distal two thirds of the esophagus and clinically is detectable by diminution and disappearance of peristaltic waves. The lower sphincter becomes incompetent, and reflux esophagitis frequently occurs. The early stages

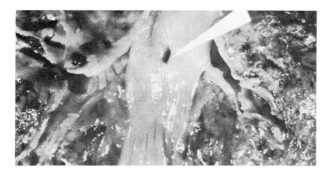

Fig. 27-5. Traction diverticulum of esophagus. Small diverticulum is indicated by the arrow. The lesion is located at the tracheal bifurcation adjacent to the underlying carinal lymph nodes.

are marked by smooth muscle atrophy with little fibrosis and the changes are thought to be related to a neural defect.[62] At autopsy, the upper esophagus is typically dilated, while the distal esophagus is usually thickened and narrowed and demonstrates the later stages of the disease.[2] Extensive erosions related to reflux esophagitis may be seen. The latter may be complicated by Barrett's epithelium and adenocarcinoma.[63] The most striking change is the prominent but patchy atrophy of the smooth muscle of the muscularis propria, particularly of the inner circular layer.[2] The muscularis mucosae has been described as either atrophic or hypertrophic. The degree of fibrosis is variable but can be considerable. The excess collagen is found in areas of myofiber dropout and in the submucosa. Intimal thickening of blood vessels can be marked. Ganglion cells are preserved. Other areas of the GI tract are frequently involved as well.

ESOPHAGITIS

In a recent study by Mitros,[4] 62 percent of 569 consecutive surgical pathology specimens obtained from the esophagus over a period of about 2 years demonstrated esophagitis. While its causes are diverse, esophagitis related to reflux of gastroduodenal contents is by far the most common type. In general, the histopathologic features of esophagitis are nonspecific, although the presence of viral inclusions or fungal elements may indicate a specific etiology. Various drugs, caustic substances, chemotherapeutic agents, instrumentation, irradiation or multisystem disorders such as Crohn's, Behçet's, or graft-versus-host disease may cause esophagitis.

Reflux Esophagitis

Introduction and Pathophysiology

Symptomatic gastroesophageal reflux is a common problem affecting nearly 10 percent of the population.[64] An unknown number of persons also have asymptomatic reflux. This disorder is usually associated solely with varying degrees of discomfort (heartburn), which can be treated medically, although occasionally surgical intervention is required. Development of a columnar-lined (Barrett's) esophagus with its associated risk of adenocarcinoma has caused difficulties in patient management for clinicians and pathologists alike.[11,65]

Although the precise mechanism of reflux esophagitis remains elusive, the degree of damage of the esophageal mucosa appears related to (1) the nature of the refluxing fluid (i.e., the presence of acid-pepsin with a variable contribution by alkaline bile), and (2) the duration of exposure. The gastroduodenal contents reflux into the esophagus through an incompetent LES, which often has an abnormally low resting pressure. Delayed clearance may be related to esophageal dysmotility and delayed gastric emptying. Although a sliding hiatal hernia is frequently present, it is not necessary for the production of reflux esophagitis.[2,66]

Histopathology and Diagnostic Criteria

The diagnosis of reflux esophagitis is one that is in search of a gold standard.[4] The clinical evidence of reflux esophagitis, such as symptomatology, endoscopic appearance, abnormal LES pressure, patient response to acid drip test (Bernstein test) and 24 hour pH monitoring often give contradictory data, and these also may be discordant with the histopathologic findings.[4] While there is an excellent clinicopathologic correlation in the more advanced stages of reflux esophagitis, where friability and ulcers (Fig. 27-6) seen endoscopically correlate with necrosis and granulation tissue seen microscopically, it is in the more subtle cases that controversy still exists.[2,3,66–79] An excellent recent review of the controversy surrounding the histologic diagnosis of reflux esophagitis was reported by Mitros.[4] The pathologist should remember that these histopathologic changes are not specific for reflux per se but could result from any noxious stimulus that damages the esophageal mucosa (Table 27-1). As the histopathologic findings can be patchy, multiple biopsy frag-

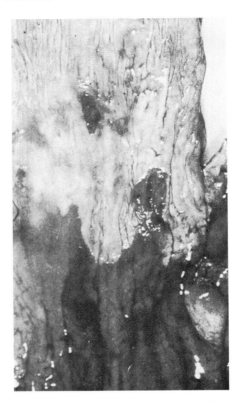

Fig. 27-6. Reflux esophagitis. The presence of two small ulcers and an irregular white patch of thickened, hyperemic mucosa can be appreciated in the distal esophagus.

TABLE 27-1. Histologic Features of Esophagitis: Relative Sensitivity and Specificity

Specificity	Sensitivity (%)
Definitive (100% specificity)	
Mucosal ulceration/necrosis	29–32
Neutrophils in epithelium or lamina propria	18–42
Barrett's epithelium	8–20
Highly suggestive (>80% specificity)	
Basal zone hyperplasia (>15%) and subepithelial papilla elongation (>67%)[a]	43–85
Intraepithelial eosinophils[b]	24–52
Possible (>50% specificity)	
Vascular dilation/congestion/intraepithelial hemorrhage	60–83
Undetermined (100% specificity, need more data)	
Balloon cells	100
Nondiagnostic	
Intraepithelial lymphocytes	
Lymphocytes, lymphoid aggregates, plasma cells, or eosinophils in lamina propria	

[a] In practice, biopsies obtained from greater than 2 to 3 cm above the esophagogastric junction fulfilling both of these criteria are considered consistent with esophagitis. If more than one biopsy fragment above this region demonstrates these changes, then the specificity approaches 100 percent.

[b] Similarly, if more than a rare intraepithelial eosinophil is found, the specificity of this finding probably approaches 100 percent.

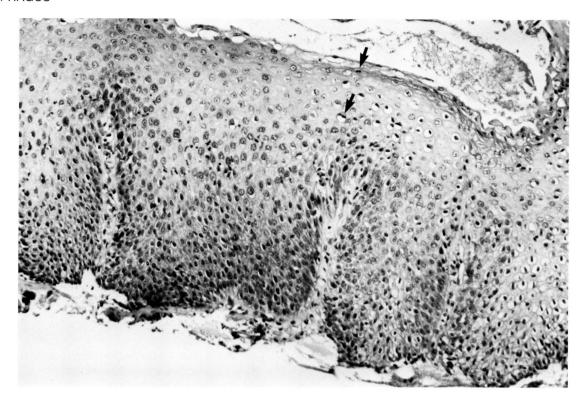

Fig. 27-7. Esophagitis. Note basal layer thickening (more than 15 percent) and elongation of the subepithelial papillae (more than 67 percent). Arrows indicate scattered eosinophils, which may be difficult to detect in Bouin's fixed specimens.

ments are encouraged.[67] Overall, the demonstration of reflux esophagitis by endoscopic biopsy is said to have a sensitivity of 77 percent and a specificity of 91 percent.[66] These figures are quite dependent on the type of biopsy (suction versus pinch), number of biopsy fragments, and the "gold standard."

The earliest microscopic changes in reflux esophagitis are recognized as an elongation of the subepithelial papillae and a widening of the basal zone (Fig. 27-7). Although the precise cutoff between controls and patients with reflux esophagitis in regard to these parameters has varied somewhat in different studies, the findings of papillary height and basal zone thickness greater than 67 percent and 15 percent of the total thickness of the epithelium, respectively, appear to be the most reproducible (approximately 80 percent intra- and interobserver variation).[2,3,66–79] As these mucosal findings have frequently been reported in the distal 2.5 cm of the esophagus in control subjects, they should not be used as the sole diagnostic criteria in this region.[68] Visual estimation of these parameters requires a well oriented histologic section, which is much more frequently encountered in suction rather than pinch (grasp) biopsies.[76] Multiple levels are often required to obtain optimal orientation. In one study, as few as 14 percent of all pinch biopsies were

suitable for assessment of these parameters.[74] A biopsy should have at least two well oriented papillae, the height of each being measured from the basal lamina at the base of the papilla to that at its apex.[71] A mean can then be determined.[4] A useful method for determining the thickness of the basal zone is measuring from the basal lamina to a point at which the epithelial nuclei are separated by a distance equal to their diameters.[71] The basal zone measurement is generally taken adjacent to the measured papillae.

While the presence of neutrophils within the lamina propria and/or epithelium is considered definitive evidence of esophagitis, the presence of other cell types is more controversial.[2,3,66–75] The presence of lymphocytes, lymphoid aggregates, plasma cells, and eosinophils in the lamina propria and of intraepithelial lymphocytes in normal biopsies has been well documented; thus, these findings have little diagnostic import.[2,3,69,70] The finding of even an occasional *intraepithelial eosinophil* has been reported as being a relatively sensitive and specific marker for esophagitis in children and adults, particularly in pinch biopsies, where criteria of papillary height and basal cell thickness often cannot be evaluated.[72–74] In one study, eosinophils were found to be more sensitive than neutrophils or necrosis, the frequencies being 52 percent,

42 percent, and 32 percent of biopsies, respectively. They were the only histologic finding of esophagitis in 23 percent of cases.[74] Since eosinophils are frequently sparse (70 percent less than or equal to five per biopsy fragment), the histologic slide must be carefully searched for these cells using the high-power objective.[74] This is particularly the case when Bouin's fixative is used, as this solution interferes with the staining of eosinophil granules. It should be noted, however, that a marked number of intraepithelial eosinophils may be found in reflux esophagitis. Recently, Tummala et al.[73] reported finding an exceedingly rare number of intra-epithelial eosinophils in roughly one third of biopsies from asymptomatic volunteers. The method of counting the number of eosinophils probably accounts for the low specificity in this particular study. Therefore, the finding of more than a rare intraepithelial eosinophil appears to be a useful marker for the histologic detection of reflux esophagitis, particularly in pinch biopsies. The diagnosis of idiopathic eosinophilic esophagitis, a quite rare disorder, can only be made in the absence of clinical reflux and the presence of peripheral eosinophilia and/or allergic phenomena.[78]

Dilation and congestion of capillaries and venules in the subepithelial papillae and intraepithelial extravasation of red blood cells (RBC) has also been reported with increased frequency in patients with reflux esophagitis.[75,77] This change is often found in control biopsies, particularly with the suction technique[75] and therefore suffers from lack of specificity.

Recently distended squamous cells with pale cytoplasm, termed balloon cells, have been described exclusively in patients with esophagitis, with a sensitivity of 60 to 70 percent.[79] These cells, which often possess pyknotic nuclei, are preferentially located in the prickle cell layer and are distinguished from the cells of glycogenic acanthosis by the relative paucity of cytoplasmic glycogen. They appear to correspond to what has previously been termed clear cell acanthosis[79] (see the section on squamous cell carcinoma, precursor lesions). Nonspecific cellular injury with uptake of surrounding plasma appears to account for the presence of intracytoplasmic plasma proteins as documented by the immunoperoxidase technique. In this study, the presence of balloon cells did not correlate with any of the other parameters of esophagitis. Further studies are required to confirm these data and to assess the role of the presence of balloon cells in the diagnosis of esophagitis.

The pathologist must be wary not to misinterpret reactive squamous atypia located adjacent to or at the base of an ulcer as squamous dysplasia or carcinoma. Typically, the reactive epithelium is quite thin, and although nucleoli may be prominent, the nuclei are quite vesicular and there is less hyperchromatism and nuclear pleomorphism. If there is any doubt, then deeper levels or perhaps a rebiopsy with concomitant cytologic studies should help resolve the dilemma. Use of the term dysplasia for reactive atypia or an uncertain diagnosis is to be avoided.

Complications

Reflux esophagitis may be associated with ulcers of various depths. Those located in the squamous mucosa are usually superficial. Deeper ulcers resembling peptic ulcers (Fig. 27-8A) are occasionally found in Barrett's mucosa and at the junction of squamous and columnar epithelium. Healing of deep ulcers is accompanied by fibrosis, which often results in stricture formation. Small inflammatory polyps have been described at the esophagogastric junction (see under Esophagogastric Polyp-Fold Complex). Barrett's esophagus (BE) is discussed below.

Barrett's Esophagus (Columnar-Lined Lower Esophagus)

In 1950, Barrett recognized a group of cases associated with hiatal hernia that he considered examples of congenital short esophagus with extension of the stomach into the mediastinum.[80] Three years later, Allison and Johnstone[81] concluded that the columnar mucosa actually was within the confines of the esophagus, and not in the stomach. In 1957 Barrett published a second paper agreeing with their findings.[82] Although Barrett was initially incorrect in his assumptions, the eponym Barrett's esophagus is well ensconced in the literature, generally indicating the presence of columnar mucosa in the distal esophagus in patients with gastroesophageal reflux (Table 27-2). The importance of the presence of BE is its known association with esophageal columnar dysplasia and adenocarcinoma, the latter reported with a prevalence of 0 to 47 percent (probably 5 to 10 percent).[11,65,83–87] The problems in defining the esophagogastric junction have been alluded to in the section on normal anatomy and histology.[10,11] The finding of columnar epithelium (without goblet cells) is considered within the range of normal in the distal 2 to 3 cm of the esophagus. Extension of columnar mucosa above this level, which coincides with the upper limits of the manometrically determined LES, or the presence of goblet cells (specialized columnar or intestinal metaplastic type of epithelium) anywhere in the distal esophagus is considered diagnostic of BE. If a biopsy obtained at 35 cm or less from the incisors in the absence of hiatal hernia or prior esophageal surgery contains columnar epithelium, it is generally considered to be diagnostic of BE.[4]

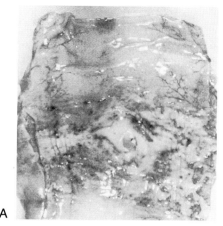

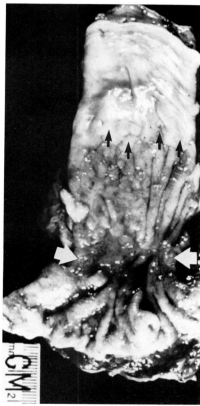

Fig. 27-8. **(A)** Peptic ulceration of the esophagus. A small, deeply penetrating peptic ulcer can be seen centrally in an area of severe inflammation. **(B)** BE. The velvety appearance of the 4 cm segment of metaplastic Barrett's mucosa in the distal esophagus contrasts with the pale gray squamous mucosa seen more proximally. White arrows indicate approximate level of the gastroesophageal junction. Black arrows indicate proximal boundary of the Barrett's mucosa. This esophagogastrectomy was performed for high-grade dysplasia (HGD). Extensive HGD, but not invasive adenocarcinoma, was found in the completely examined specimen.

TABLE 27-2. Barrett's Esophagus: Clinicopathologic Features and Diagnostic Criteria

Clinical features	
Prevalence	Esophagitis 8–20%
	Chronic peptic structure 44%
Age, sex (range)	Mean 55 yr (<1–88); M : F 2–3 : 1
Common symptoms	"Heartburn," dysphagia, odynophagia
Pathologic features	
Endoscopic/macroscopic	Pink, velvety mucosa in distal esophagus beginning at the EGJ and extending as a circumferential sheet, finger-like projections or detached islands
Histologic spectrum	
Atrophic fundic type	Atrophic glands with parietal/chief cells
Junctional (cardiac) type	Mucous glands identical to gastric cardia
Specialized columnar (intestinal metaplastic) type	Goblet cells, often villiform appearance, acidic mucin
Diagnostic criteria on biopsy	Columnar mucosa at least 2–3 cm above EGJ or intestinal metaplasia anywhere in distal esophagus; pathologist should indicate presence or absence of dysplasia
Prevalence of dysplasia	
In absence of adenocarcinoma	5–10%
In presence of adenocarcinoma	Approaches 100% with specimens that are totally examined.
Grading of dysplasia	
Negative	Usual columnar cell types, reactive/regenerative changes
Positive	
Low-grade	Enlarged hyperchromatic elongated (type 1) or round (type 2) nuclei confined to base of cell; increased nuclear-to-cytoplasmic ratio; nucleoli inconspicuous
High-grade	Type 1: Hyperchromatic nuclei, higher nuclear-to-cytoplasmic ratio, often conspicuous stratification; nucleoli more prominent
	Type 2: Large basal hyperchromatic nuclei, higher nuclear-to-cytoplasmic ratio; nucleoli more prominent
Indefinite	Atypical epithelium, but presence of acute inflammation or possibly regenerative changes precludes definitive diagnosis of dysplasia
Prevalence of adenocarcinoma	
Overall	0–47% (probably 5–10%)
In resection specimens for high-grade dysplasia	About 50%

Pathogenesis

Today it is accepted by virtually all investigators that BE, in contradistinction to embryonal rests of columnar epithelium, is an acquired condition.[11,88] Support for this assertion comes from several sources: (1) absence of typical cases in fetuses, (2) usual occurrence in adults,

(3) histologic demonstration of intestinal metaplasia, (4) strong association with gastroesophageal reflux (GER), and (5) decreased LES pressure. Virtually all patients (including children) with BE have GER. BE has been induced in animal models and in humans after surgery disrupting the gastroesophageal junction.[89]

The pathogenetic sequence is as follows.[88] Reflux esophagitis leads to repeated ulceration of the distal esophageal squamous mucosa. Columnar mucosa, being more resistant to acid-pepsin, proliferates and re-epithelializes the denuded mucosa, thus representing the process of metaplasia (i.e., replacement of one adult cell type by another). The source of the columnar epithelium can be from any one or more of the following sites: (1) upward growth of columnar cells from the gastric cardia, (2) foci of columnar lining epithelium and/or superficial glands of the distal esophagus, (3) multipotential undifferentiated cells of unknown origin, (4) basal (reserve) cells of the squamous epithelium, and (5) esophageal submucosal glands, with the first three sites being most likely.

Clinical Aspects

The prevalence of BE in the general population is unknown. It has been noted in 8 to 20 percent of patients with esophagitis and in 44 percent of patients with chronic peptic strictures.[11] Thus, an increased prevalence can be expected in populations with more severe GI reflux, such as those with scleroderma.[63]

Barrett's esophagus most commonly occurs in mid-adult life, but the age range varies from less than 1 year to the ninth decade. Males are more commonly affected (2 to 3 : 1), and 90 percent of patients are caucasian.[11,85,90] As one might expect, the presenting symptoms are those of GER or its complications. Duration of symptoms is quite variable, averaging 6 to 8 years. Patients presenting with adenocarcinoma and BE may not complain of reflux symptoms, thus leading to delay in diagnosis. Although an increased risk of colonic neoplasia has been reported in patients with BE, this association is controversial.[91,92] Current radiographic techniques cannot distinguish squamous from columnar mucosa, limiting their usefulness in diagnosis. However, double contrast esophagography may be a useful screening procedure.[93]

Macroscopic/Endoscopic Findings and Method of Biopsy

Barrett's epithelium has a velvety red appearance characteristic of gastric-type mucosa, in contrast to the pale pink, glossy appearance of squamous mucosa (Fig. 27-8B). The columnar mucosa merges imperceptibly with the stomach and extends proximally as a circumferential sheet, irregular finger-like projections, or possibly detached islands. Histologic documentation of columnar epithelium in the esophagus is the sine qua non of BE; hence, endoscopic biopsy is necessary for diagnosis. At the time of initial diagnosis, multiple biopsies should be obtained beginning at the gastroesophageal junction and extending approximately at 1 to 2 cm intervals to assess the extent of BE. The clinician must indicate the precise site of the biopsies for proper interpretation by the pathologist and to give an estimation of the length of the segment of BE. This is best recorded as centimeters above the EGJ.

Histologic Spectrum

One or more histologic types of columnar epithelium may be found in the esophagus of patients with BE, as originally described by Paull et al.[94] in 1976 (Fig. 27-9): (1) atrophic gastric fundic type, (2) junctional or cardiac type, and (3) specialized columnar (intestinal metaplastic) type. Many investigators using endoscopic biopsy data believe that distinct but interdigitating zones of these three types of epithelia exist, with the atrophic fundic type being most distal, specialized columnar type most proximal and the junctional type residing in between.[11] It appears, however, that a great deal of microscopic heterogeneity exists in what appear to be well defined but somewhat serpiginous zones, as mapped out by a limited number of biopsies. Thompson et al.,[95] in a study of resection specimens from patients with BE and associated adenocarcinoma, found a mosaic of epithelial types with a slight tendency of the atrophic fundic type to be distally located.

The atrophic gastric fundic type is defined by the presence of parietal and/or chief cells in addition to columnar, mucin-containing surface lining cells and mucous neck cells in the gastric-like pits. This is the most common type found in biopsies of BE in children (80 to 100 percent), while it is the least common type found in adults (16 to 45 percent).[11,83,90]

The junctional (cardiac) type is histologically identical to that of the gastric cardia and is found in 30 to 65 percent of adult and 50 to 100 percent of pediatric BE biopsies. The foveolae are lined by columnar mucus-containing (neutral, periodic acid-Schiff (PAS) positive) epithelium, and a rudimentary villous architecture may be noted. By definition, no parietal or chief cells or evidence of intestinal metaplasia (goblet cells, acidic mucin, Paneth cells) are noted, but neuroendocrine cells may be found.[96,97] Occasionally, the columnar cells appear quite distended with mucus, but definite goblet cells are not found. The use of stains such as Alcian blue-PAS or high iron diamine (HID)-Alcian blue can be helpful in detecting the acidic mucin characteristic of intestinal metaplasia.

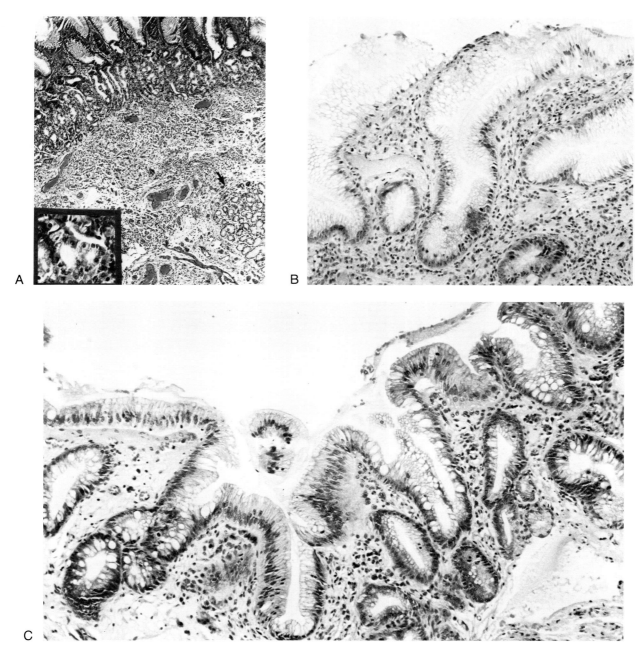

Fig. 27-9. Histologic spectrum of Barrett's esophagus. **(A)** Atrophic gastric fundic type. Note short gastric glands, which contain parietal cells, seen at higher magnification in the inset. The arrow points to a submucosal gland, indicating that the specimen is from the esophagus. **(B)** Junctional (cardiac) type. This mucosa is characterized by columnar cells containing mucus, without goblet, parietal, or chief cells. The mucous cells may appear distended, sometimes causing diagnostic confusion with goblet cells. High iron diamine-Alcian blue stain in this example did not demonstrate either sulfomucin or sialomucin, thus ruling out intestinal metaplasia. **(C)** Specialized columnar (intestinal metaplastic) type. Villiform architecture is characteristic, while the presence of goblet cells is diagnostic. True absorptive cells with well developed brush borders are only very rarely seen; therefore, it is an example of incomplete intestinal metaplasia. An esophageal biopsy containing this type of epithelium is considered diagnostic of BE.

The specialized columnar (intestinal metaplastic) type is probably the most common histologic type of BE found in adult biopsies (50 to 80 percent); however, it is the least common in children (12 to 45 percent).[11,83,90] It usually has a villiform surface lined by columnar and goblet cells containing sialo- and/or sulfomucin, thus resembling intestinal mucosa.[98–100] Goblet, Paneth, and neuroendocrine cells may also be found in mucosal glands, which resemble intestinal crypts.[95] An important difference exists, however, between the intestinal-type mucosa seen in the normal bowel and that seen in the specialized columnar epithelium of BE. In the first instance, the columnar absorptive cells possess a brush border and lack mucin, whereas in the latter, well defined brush borders are rarely seen and the apical cytoplasm contains mucin droplets (incomplete intestinal metaplasia). Scanning electron microscopy has found a heterogeneous population of cells described as gastric, intestinal, and variant, all of which contain mucin at the light microscopic level.[100]

The significance of finding specialized columnar epithelium in an esophageal biopsy is twofold. First, it is the only histologic type of columnar epithelium considered pathognomonic of BE when found in an esophageal biopsy. Although it may occasionally be obtained from the gastric cardia at the time of a presumed esophageal biopsy, its classification as BE is not unreasonable, as these patients may also be at risk of developing adenocarcinoma in the region of the EGJ.[101] Second, this epithelium is by far the most likely type to develop dysplastic changes.[86,102–104]

Dysplasia and Other Markers for Precancer in Barrett's Esophagus

Epithelial dysplasia in patients with BE may be defined in a manner similar to that in inflammatory bowel disease, that is, as an unequivocal neoplastic alteration of the columnar mucosa, which may be a marker for subsequent development of carcinoma or by itself may be associated with invasive disease.[86,102–106] In the absence of associated adenocarcinoma, dysplasia is detected in 5 to 10 percent of biopsies in patients with BE.[11] The dysplastic foci are usually noted in endoscopically unremarkable

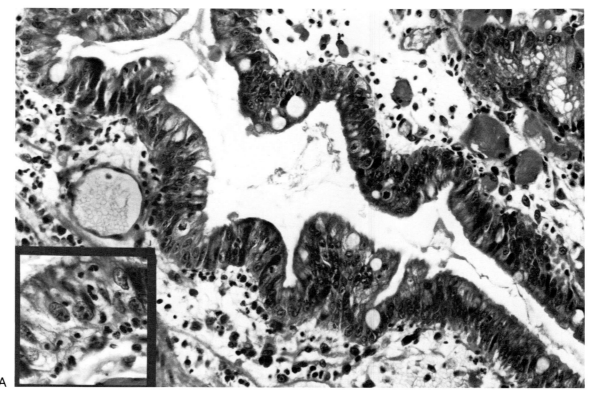

Fig. 27-10. Grading of dysplasia in Barrett's esophagus. **(A)** Indefinite for dysplasia. There is nuclear crowding and enlargement; however, the nuclei are quite vesicular and well oriented. The epithelium and lamina propria are both infiltrated with neutrophils. These features are demonstrated at higher magnification in the inset. The biopsy is not unequivocally dysplastic and the histologic features may represent a degenerative/regenerative phenomenon. Rebiopsy within a few months after treatment of esophagitis is indicated. (*Figure continues.*)

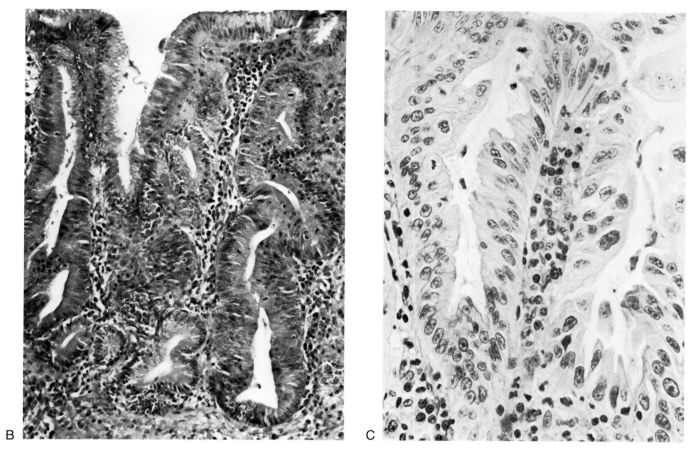

Fig. 27-10 (*Continued*). **(B)** Low-grade dysplasia. Enlarged hyperchromatic nuclei with minimal stratification are found, although tangential cutting of glands as seen here can occasionally cause diagnostic confusion. Rebiopsy in a few months is indicated. **(C)** High-grade dysplasia. The cells lining the villiform mucosa are markedly atypical, with loss of polarity, pleomorphism, nuclear hyperchromasia, and prominent and multiple nucleoli. These changes are consistent with carcinoma in situ, which is included in the category of high-grade dysplasia. If the diagnosis is confirmed, then esophagogastrectomy should strongly be considered in good surgical candidates.

flat mucosa, although rarely polypoid dysplastic lesions known as Barrett's adenomas may be found.[102–104] Dysplasia may be graded as positive (high- or low-grade), negative, or indefinite, although another system recognizes three grades of dysplasia[103] (Fig. 27-10). Recently, the features of dysplastic Barrett's epithelium have been described in cytologic specimens.[105]

Riddell[104] recognizes two different histologic types of dysplasia, one indistinguishable from that seen in adenomas found in other parts of the GI tract (type 1) and one characterized by large round hyperchromatic basal nuclei and a lack of cytoplasmic maturation (type 2). These histologic types may occur separately or together. Low-grade dysplasia is characterized by cells with enlarged hyperchromatic nuclei that are usually confined to the base. In high-grade dysplasia (which includes intraepithelial carcinoma in situ), there is a significant increase in the

nuclear/cytoplasmic ratio and in general an increased number of mitoses. Nuclear stratification may be prominent, particularly in type 1. Mucosa graded as indefinite has atypical nuclear and/or architectural features but cannot be unequivocally stated to be neoplastic. Neutrophils are often found in and around the epithelium of this type, suggesting the possibility that in some cases these changes are reactive. Usual Barrett's epithelium or actively regenerating columnar mucosa is termed negative for dysplasia.

The distinction of dysplastic from nondysplastic and indefinite Barrett's mucosa may at times be quite difficult, particularly in the face of significant acute inflammation and reactive epithelial atypia and especially for the pathologist who reviews only occasional biopsies of this nature. Although under optimal circumstances a panel of experts from several universities were able to reproducibly distinguish high grade dysplasia and intramucosal carcinoma from lesser lesions, there was considerable disagreement on separating indefinite from low-grade dysplasia.[107] Approximately 50 percent of patients undergoing esophagectomy for high-grade dysplasia alone will be found to harbor invasive foci of adenocarcinoma.[86,102,103,106] The relationship of low-grade dysplasia to adenocarcinoma is not clear. Prior to any surgical intervention, a diagnosis of high-grade dysplasia should be confirmed by a second pathologist, preferably one with expertise in GI pathology.

Other markers, such as the flow cytometric DNA analysis of aneuploidy and/or increased growth fraction,[108] lectin binding,[109] pepsinogen isoenzymes,[110] and the presence of sulfomucin,[98–100,104] have been described as having potential value in detecting neoplastic changes in BE. Currently, data generated from these parameters have not been found to be as useful as the histologic diagnosis of dysplasia in terms of patient management, although some of them may potentially play an adjunctive role.

Surveillance

The data regarding the incidence and prevalence of adenocarcinoma and the natural history of dysplasia in BE are rather limited. Prudent patient management suggests that endoscopic surveillance is indicated until further information is available.[11,83,103,104,111] Although several studies have suggested that BE may at least partially regress (replaced by squamous mucosa) after antireflux surgery, this remains a controversial issue.[11,104,112] All patients with nondysplastic BE should have endoscopy with biopsy performed at 1 to 2 year intervals. If high-grade dysplasia is detected and confirmed, then esophagogastrectomy should strongly be considered. The operative status of the patient, however, must be carefully reviewed and therapy individualized. If low-grade dysplasia is present and confirmed, repeat biopsy should be performed within 3 to 6 months after intense treatment of esophagitis.

Intramural Pseudodiverticulosis

Intramural pseudodiverticulosis, an uncommon condition, is better known to the radiologist than to the pathologist.[2,8,113–115] In a recent study, this condition was detected in 0.15 percent of patients undergoing radiographic examination of the esophagus.[114] One hundred or so cases have been reported, typically occurring in middle-aged and elderly patients who present with a long history of mild dysphagia. The classic finding on barium swallow is the presence of numerous small (1 to 4 mm) flask-shaped or collar-button outpouchings affecting the esophagus in a diffuse or segmental fashion (Fig. 27-11). Associated lesions include esophageal strictures, usually

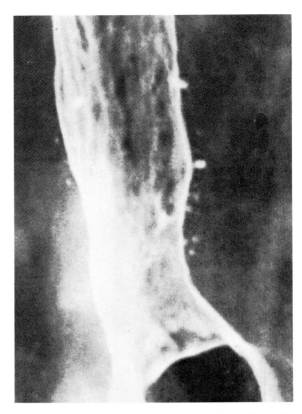

Fig. 27-11. Intramural pseudodiverticulosis. This radiograph demonstrates the presence of numerous flask-shaped outpouchings of the esophagus which represent dilated submucous glands. (From Laufer,[148] with permission.)

involving the upper esophagus, and esophagitis, each found in up to 90 percent of cases. The diverticula do not extend into the muscularis propria. Although the etiology remains obscure, esophageal intramural pseudodiverticulosis appears to arise from distention of the excretory ducts of the submucosal esophageal glands. This possibly results from plugging by viscous mucus, inflammatory material, or desquamated epithelium. Extrinsic ductal compression by periductal inflammation and fibrosis has also been postulated. Individual lesions are identical to the previously discussed esophageal retention cysts. *Candida albicans* has been cultured from 34 to 48 percent of affected esophagi; however, this organism is regarded as a secondary invader.[8] Candidiasis can itself produce an esophagitis that on barium esophagram may appear similar, but the apparent outpouchings in that condition are larger and more irregular.[113]

Infectious Esophagitis

The esophagus is quite resistant to primary infection under normal conditions. Infectious esophagitis, virtually always due to *Candida* species or to *herpes simplex* virus

(HSV), is nearly always a disorder of the debilitated and/or immunocompromised host. Currently this disorder is frequently seen in patients with the acquired immunodeficiency syndrome (AIDS).[116–118] Coexistent infection with multiple pathogens may occur.

Bacterial Esophagitis (Other Than Tuberculous)

This form of esophagitis is quite uncommon but has been reported due to *Klebsiella* species and *Lactobacillus acidophilis*.[2] In the latter instance, the disorder mimics esophageal candidiasis.[119] Diphtheria and streptococcal pharyngitis may also lead to esophagitis.[120] Recently, *Campylobacter pylori* has been reported in the esophagi of patients with Barrett's esophagus.[121] Whether it has a pathogenetic role in inducing or exacerbating esophagitis in this setting is unknown at this time.

Fungal Esophagitis

Fungal infections, usually candidal, have become a common cause of dysphagia and odynophagia (pain) in patients who are immunosuppressed, on chemotherapy, or chronically debilitated and occasionally in patients after a course of antibiotics. Other fungi such as *Torulopsis* and *Blastomyces* may rarely involve the esophagus.[118,122,123]

Candidal esophagitis may or may not be associated with oral candidiasis and characteristically involves the mid- and distal esophagus.[2,124] It produces shallow ulcers that typically are covered with a thick fibrinopurulent pseudomembrane (Fig. 27-12). The endoscopic/macroscopic appearance consists of rather discrete or confluent elevated white-green plaques on a background of otherwise friable and ulcerated mucosa. In advanced cases, the esophagus may be narrowed, shaggy, or cobblestoned and may be confused with pseudodiverticulosis, varices, or carcinoma.[125] Perforation during endoscopy is a risk. Grocott methenamine silver or other fungal stains should be performed on biopsy specimens that show a fibrinous exudate, even if there are only a minimal number of neutrophils. Mitros notes that the presence of elongated desquamated epithelial cells near the mucosal surface may be a clue to candidal infection on hematoxylin and eosin (H&E)-stained sections.[4] The finding of the pseudohyphal form is a reliable indication of an invasive lesion as opposed to simple contamination; however, actual tissue invasion is only occasionally demonstrated in biopsy material. Brush cytology specimens will increase the yield of diagnosis, as fungus-rich exudate may be lost in biopsy specimen preparation. With appropriate treatment, all lesions may disappear, although the development of strictures has been reported. Mixed infection with *Cryptosporidium* has been reported in the AIDS population.[117]

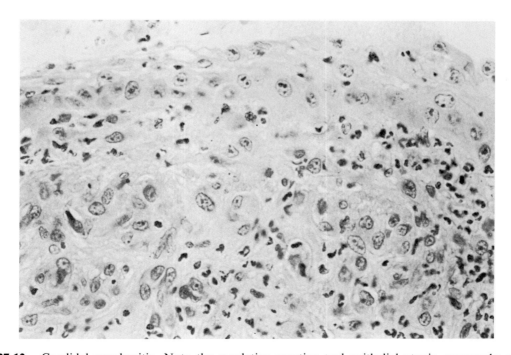

Fig. 27-12. Candidal esophagitis. Note the exudative reaction and epithelial atypia commonly seen in candidiasis. Organisms are not easily appreciated on hematoxylin and eosin-stained sections, such as this, but were readily demonstrable by Grocott stain.

Viral Esophagitis

As in fungal infection, viral esophagitis is being recognized more frequently antemortem with the increased use of endoscopy for obtaining histologic and cytologic material.[126–130] It occurs in the same clinical milieu as fungal esophagitis, produces similar symptomatology, and again is usually found in the mid- and distal esophagus. Herpes simplex type 1 (HSV-1) infection is the most common form seen.[128] Cytomegalovirus (CMV) is also reported and may coexist with HSV or with *Candida*.[116,128] Several reports have stated that 2 to 25 percent of all benign esophageal ulcers encountered histologically are herpetic.[128,130]

In the early stages, one sees multiple, small, punched-out ulcers, which later may become confluent. With HSV, two types of characteristic inclusions may be found within epithelial cells: (1) multinucleated epithelial cells with molded nuclei possessing a ground-glass appearance and a thickened nuclear membrane; and (2) large intranuclear eosinophilic bodies surrounded by a halo bordered by a thickened nuclear membrane—the classic Cowdry type A owl eye inclusion. Both types of inclusions are most frequently found in the epithelium at the margin of the ulcer, and biopsies should therefore be obtained from this region. In equivocal cases, immunohistochemical staining for herpes simplex antigen can be performed.

With CMV, on the other hand, nuclear and cytoplasmic inclusions are found in the ulcer base, usually in markedly enlarged endothelial or other mesenchymal cells. Nash and Ross found that 13 of 94 cases of herpetic esophagitis had or developed a herpetic pneumonia that simulated bacterial pneumonitis. This was the major cause of death in their series.[128]

Postirradiation Esophagitis

Esophagitis is a well known complication of radiation therapy to the chest. Although chronic lesions such as strictures do not typically occur below 6,000 rads, symptomatic esophagitis with mucosal ulceration may occur at lower radiation doses, particularly with simultaneous administration of chemotherapy.[2,131] The histopathologic features are nonspecific, although fibroblasts with marked nuclear atypia and hyalinized blood vessels are suggestive of radiation damage. Marked squamous atypia should not be misinterpreted as dysplasia or carcinoma.

Crohn's Disease and Granulomatous Esophagitis

Involvement of the esophagus by Crohn's disease (CD) has been reported in less than 20 cases and many of these are probably examples of something else.[132–134] Clinically, CD is usually considered to represent carcinoma, because of its appearance as an irregular stenotic segment of esophagus. Perhaps a half-dozen cases seem well doc-

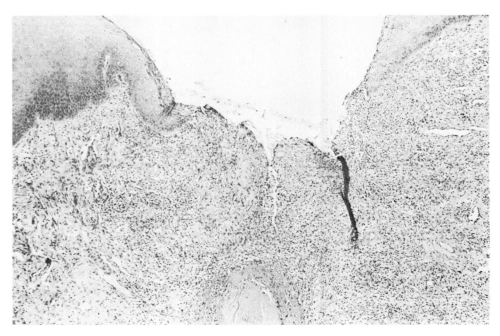

Fig. 27-13. Crohn's disease of the esophagus. Marked inflammation, ulceration, and sinus tract formation are noted in this case of Crohn's disease of the esophagus.

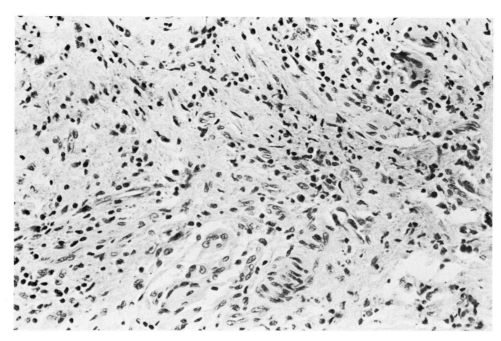

Fig. 27-14. Crohn's disease of the esophagus. (same case as Fig. 27-13). In a section deep to that pictured in Figure 27-13 a characteristic granuloma composed of epithelioid histiocytes and giant cells is seen.

umented with sinus tracts, granulomas, neuromatous hyperplasia, and muscular hypertrophy (Figs. 27-13 and 27-14). Most have evidence of disease elsewhere in the GI tract, but it may be isolated to the esophagus.[132] A confident diagnosis of isolated esophageal CD can only be made in the presence of epithelioid granulomas and the exclusion of other possible causes of granulomatous esophagitis such as tuberculosis[135] and sarcoidosis.[136] Barrett's esophagus is a reported complication.[134]

Other Causes of Esophagitis

Various drugs have been reported to cause esophagitis. This occasionally can result in stricture formation.[137,138] The ingestion of caustic substances, such as lye, strong acids, or other agents, typically results in acute (erosive) esophagitis.[139] Seventy-five percent of caustic esophageal "burns" result from accidental ingestions in children, while the remainder are related to suicide attempts in adults. The degree of injury varies from hyperemia to ulceration and transmural necrosis and can be graded endoscopically in a manner analogous to cutaneous burns. Strictures and squamous carcinoma are potential long-term complications (see the section squamous carcinoma). Rarely, BE has been reported.[140]

Chronic graft-versus-host (GVH) disease was associated with severe dysphagia and odynophagia in 13 percent of patients in one series.[141] The esophageal mucosa is described endoscopically as friable and peeling (desquamating), occasionally forming webs. The upper and middle thirds of the esophagus are characteristically involved. Microscopically, lymphocytes infiltrating the epithelium and individual necrotic (apoptotic) squamous cells in noninflamed regions, similar to the findings of GVH at other sites, are frequently present. Other nonspecific features of esophagitis are also found. Sclerotherapy is now frequently being employed for the treatment of esophageal varices.[142–144] The resultant thrombosis, perivenular fibrosis and denudation of the overlying esophageal mucosa probably contribute to the reduced frequency of bleeding. However, extensive areas of necrosis including deep ulcers and perforation may result and thus contribute to the 10 to 15 percent complication rate of this treatment modality. Esophagitis with histologic changes similar to those seen in the skin can be found in a number of mucocutaneous disorders such as pemphigus vulgaris and others.[2,4] Discrete nonspecific esophageal ulcers have occasionally been described in Behçet's disease.[2]

TUMORS, PSEUDOTUMORS, AND HYPERPLASIAS

Squamous cell carcinoma and adenocarcinoma are overwhelmingly the most frequent and most important tumors of the esophagus and will be discussed in detail.

All other tumors and pseudotumors are uncommon to exceedingly rare entities; nevertheless, they are of interest and of surprising diversity. Some of these are asymptomatic and are discovered incidentally in the course of clinical work-up or are found at autopsy. Others may produce dysphagia, pain, or rarely bleeding. It is unfortunate that many reports purporting to be a certain entity lack the appropriate photographs or information on the pathologic findings to permit the reader an independent judgment. Follow-up information is too often sketchy.

Most nonepithelial lesions are benign, whereas the majority of epithelial lesions are malignant. Benign nonepithelial tumors will be discussed with their malignant counterparts, if any, and with easily confused nonepithelial pseudotumors. Ulceration and bleeding may occur in benign tumors, although they are usually a minor feature. Totten and co-workers[28] found it convenient to separate benign lesions into intraluminal polypoid growths and intramural cysts or nodules. Forty of their 163 (25 percent) cases presented as polypoid growths, often on long pedicles. Any noninvasive tumor that protrudes into the lumen tends to develop a pedicle. Unfortunately, certain malignant tumors (polypoid carcinoma, leiomyosarcoma, malignant melanoma) also manifest in this fashion. The usual epithelial hyperplasias and tumors will be discussed together, followed by sections on unusual epithelial tumors, hematopoietic tumors and, finally, secondary involvement of the esophagus by carcinoma. An attempt is made to clarify certain areas of special confusion in the literature.

Nonepithelial Tumors and Pseudotumors

Leiomyoma

Leiomyomas are by far the most common benign tumor of the esophagus,[25] accounting for about 60 percent of all cases (Table 27-3). The reported frequency at autopsy varies from 0.01 to 8 percent,[145,146] depending on

TABLE 27-3. Relative Incidence of Various Benign Esophageal Lesions

Lesion	No. of Cases (%)
Leiomyoma	145 (61)
Cysts	55 (23)
Polyp	12 (5)
Lipoma	5 (2)
Papilloma	5 (2)
Hemangioma	3 (1)
Adenoma	3 (1)
Miscellaneous	11 (5)
Total	239 (100)

(Modified from Mahour and Harrison,[25] with permission.)

the methods of detection. In the study with the highest frequency, all leiomyomas were solely microscopic findings less than 7 mm in diameter found in completely embedded esophagi (seedling leiomyomas).[146] In general, esophageal leiomyomas account for about 5 to 15 percent of all GI stromal tumors.[145,147] In an excellent review of the total reported experience with esophageal leiomyomas through 1972, Seremitis and co-workers[145] analyzed 838 cases. They estimated 50 carcinomas for each reported clinically significant leiomyoma. Statistics, unless otherwise noted, are from their report.

The average age of patients is 44 years (range 12 to 80 years). Men are more commonly affected in a ratio of 1.9 : 1. At least one half of patients with routinely identified lesions are asymptomatic. In symptomatic patients, 60 percent complain of pain and dysphagia of at least 2 years duration. Interestingly, only 10 cases of bleeding secondary to leiomyoma have been reported, in sharp contrast to gastric leiomyoma. This most likely relates to the relatively small size of esophageal tumors with less frequent ulceration. The barium esophagram usually shows a smooth-surfaced crescent-shaped defect forming a characteristic obtuse angle with the esophageal wall[148] (Fig. 27-15). The lesion may pulsate due to the proximity

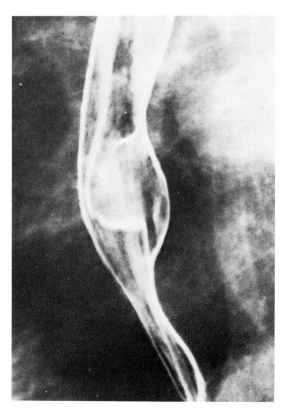

Fig. 27-15. Leiomyoma of the esophagus. This radiograph demonstrates the characteristic right angle tumor junction seen with leiomyomas on double contrast radiography. Also note the lesion's smooth surface. (From Laufer,[148] with permission.)

of the aorta, and an aortogram may be required for the differential diagnosis from an aneurysm. Coexisting hiatal hernia and diverticula may obscure the typical findings.

The vast majority of tumors (97 percent) are single intramural lesions having a predilection for the lower esophagus. The rare cases with multiple tumors should be distinguished from diffuse leiomyomatosis (which is discussed separately). Seremitis and co-workers[145] report a frequency of 11 percent in the upper third, 33 percent in the middle third, and 56 percent in the lower third of the esophagus. Only rarely do these tumors present as pedunculated polyps (1 percent) or as mediastinal masses attached to the serosa (2 percent).

Macroscopically, they are found to be ovoid or spherical, gray-white, bosselated, circumscribed masses that partially encircle the esophagus (Fig. 27-16). Size generally varies from 2 to 5 cm with occasional giant tumors weighing more than 1,000 g reported.[145] They resemble uterine leiomyomas histologically (plump spindle cells with a rather low cellularity), ultrastructurally (abundant microfilaments with focal densities, basal lamina, pinocytotic vesicles), and immunohistochemically (desmin and muscle actin immunoreactivity).[147,149,150] These features

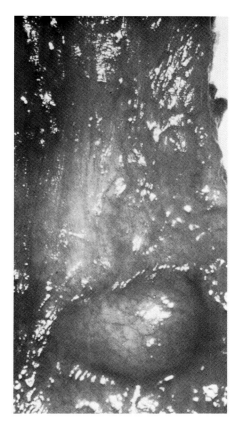

Fig. 27-16. Leiomyoma of the esophagus. A gross photograph of an esophageal leiomyoma shows a smooth surface.

are uncommon for stromal tumors at other GI sites, except perhaps for the gastric cardia and colorectum.[147,151] Calcification is distinctly uncommon (1.8 percent). The marked necrosis, cystic change, and hemorrhage of gastric leiomyomas (stromal tumors) are not a feature of those in the esophagus. Distinction from rare tumors of neural origin may potentially be a problem.[147,151] As in any smooth muscle tumor, one should carefully check for the presence of mitoses, anaplasia, and necrosis. Size of gastrointestinal stromal tumors in general is a good predictor of metastatic potential.[149] Distinction of leiomyoma from leiomyosarcoma may be impossible, particularly in biopsy specimens (see the following section on leiomyosarcoma).

Leiomyosarcoma

There were 43 reported cases of primary leiomyosarcoma of the esophagus as of 1981.[152] The histologic criteria, however, for diagnosis of this tumor have not been uniform, and it is uncertain how many of these cases represent polypoid carcinomas (see the section on unusual epithelial tumors) or, alternatively, leiomyomas. Reports of associated squamous cell carcinoma should be viewed with suspicion.[2,153] Patients reported with leiomyosarcoma have been in the fifth or sixth decade and have been predominantly men.[6] This tumor may arise anywhere in the esophagus, although it is perhaps more frequently found distally. It manifests as large polypoid tumors (sometimes pedunculated), infiltrative intramural growths, or rarely as a mediastinal mass[2,156] (Fig. 27-17).

Microscopically, the tumors are composed of pleomorphic spindle cells usually with easily identifiable mitotic figures (Fig. 27-18). Polypoid carcinoma must be excluded by searching carefully for foci of squamous differentiation. Immunoreactivity for desmin and/or antimuscle actin, but not cytokeratin, in spindle cells supports a

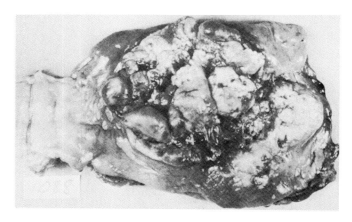

Fig. 27-17. Leiomyosarcoma. This leiomyosarcoma has a polypoid shape similar to that seen in some adenocarcinomas and squamous cell carcinomas.

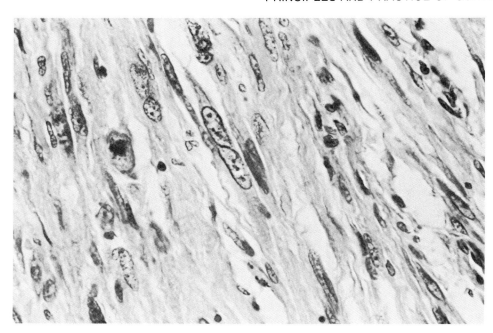

Fig. 27-18. Leiomyosarcoma. The tumor is composed of fascicles of spindle-shaped tumor cells with pleomorphic blunt-ended nuclei. Mitoses are relatively common.

smooth muscle rather than epithelial origin; however, problems in interpretation of these immunohistochemical stains may potentially arise.[147,150,154,155] Ultrastructural examination may also be helpful in the differential diagnosis. Distinction between these two entities may be impossible in biopsy material alone. Malignant melanoma can also be excluded by the absence of melanin pigment, immunoreactivity for desmin, the absence of S-100 immunoreactivity, and the absence of premelanosomes on EM examination. At the other end of the spectrum, as mentioned earlier in the section on leiomyoma, distinction of benign from malignant smooth muscle (stromal) tumors may occasionally be difficult. Although particular details for this distinction at this site are lacking, by analogy with stromal tumors at other GI sites it would appear that size greater than 6 cm and/or a mitotic rate of greater than 2 per 10 HPF supports the diagnosis of sarcoma.[149] The finding of any mitotic figures in a GI stromal tumor should at least make one suspicious of malignancy.

Survival has been poor overall, with 60 percent of patients dead within 1 year in one study.[156] In the review of Ranier and Brus, 8 of 12 patients surviving more than 1 year had polypoid tumors.[157] Metastases are said to be rare[6] or delayed[156]—at least for the polypoid forms. Again, the survival figures may reflect confusion among polypoid carcinoma, carcinosarcoma, and leiomyosarcoma.

Idiopathic Muscular Hypertrophy and Leiomyomatosis

These disorders, characterized by a diffuse prominence of esophageal smooth muscle, may be classified as three clinicopathologic types: (1) idiopathic muscular hypertrophy; (2) leiomyomatosis; and (3) esophagogastric-vulvar leiomyomatosis, a subset of the second type. These three conditions have been reported under various headings in the literature and are thus confusing. They can be sharply separated from the occasional patient who is shown to have more than one discrete leiomyoma (sometimes many) in an otherwise normal esophagus.

In summary, the literature suggests the presence of two distinct processes. One is best termed idiopathic (diffuse) muscular hypertrophy. It involves the distal esophagus, typically of elderly men and probably represents the pathologic correlate of diffuse esophageal spasm (see Fig. 27-3). This has been discussed previously under that heading. Leiomyomatosis is seen in young women and is characterized by confluent myomatous nodules that merge with a markedly hypertrophic muscularis propria (particularly the inner circular layer) in the lower two thirds of the esophagus and proximal stomach. In the literature, both conditions are occasionally referred to as diffuse leiomyomatosis, but they are dubiously neoplastic and more probably represent a peculiar myopathy or a response to an unknown primary neuropathic process.

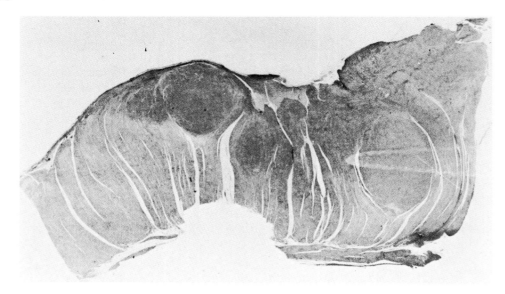

Fig. 27-19. Esophageal-vulvar leiomyomatosis. A low-power photomicrograph reveals several partly confluent nodules of smooth muscle within the hypertrophied circular muscle layer (cf. Fig. 27-3 for idiopathic, diffuse, muscular hypertrophy).

Esophageal-vulvar leiomyomatosis represents a subset of diffuse leiomyomatosis in which the vulvar region is similarly affected (Fig. 27-19). Further work is needed to clarify the pathogenesis and classification of these disorders.[2,41–44,158–163]

Neurogenic Tumors

Although there have been reports of benign nerve sheath tumors in the esophagus, their existence is controversial.[2,6,147,150,151] More likely, most of these represent leiomyomas with nuclear palisading. Trapped nerve twigs and smooth muscle demonstrating S-100 and desmin/antimuscle actin immunoreactivity, respectively, can cause diagnostic confusion.[147,150] Melanocytic schwannoma is discussed in the section on malignant melanoma.[164]

Granular Cell Tumor

Granular cell tumor, previously known as granular cell myoblastoma, is a rare esophageal tumor that virtually always has a neurogenic origin (Fig. 27-20). More than 60 cases have been reported in the esophagus, representing approximately one third of all GI tract granular cell tumors.[165,166] Although they are most frequently incidental findings, these nodular or stenotic lesions may cause dysphagia. The age range is reported as 19 to 65 years, and the tumors can be found anywhere in the esophagus. There is one case report quoted by Ming[6] of a granular

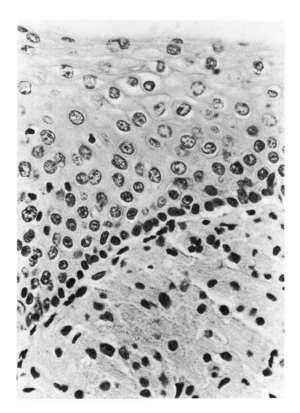

Fig. 27-20. Granular cell tumor. Just below the basal layer of epithelium, typical large, round, eosinophilic cells with a granular cytoplasm are noted. (Courtesy of Dr. Raymond Schiffman, Cooper Hospital, Camden, NJ.)

cell tumor invading the trachea and metastasizing to cervical lymph nodes (malignant granular cell tumor). As when this tumor is found at other sites, the pathologist should avoid misdiagnosing associated pseudoepitheliomatous hyperplasia as squamous cell carcinoma. Recently, a granular cell tumor and a contiguous well documented squamous cell carcinoma were reported in the region of the gastroesophageal junction.[167] The characteristic histopathologic features of granular cell tumor have been described in detail elsewhere in this book.

Fibroma

The existence of a true fibroma of the esophagus is dubious. Most sessile "fibromas" are probably collagenized leiomyomas or possibly neurilemmomas. Most of the polypoid "fibromas" are probably fibrovascular polyps.

Fibrosarcoma

Fibrosarcoma, as currently defined, is an exceedingly rare tumor of the esophagus, which has been reported following radiation.[168] Some other reports are dubious.

Fibrovascular Polyp

Although rare, fibrovascular polyps (fibroma, fibromyxoma, fibrolipoma, fibrous polyp) are second only to leiomyoma in clinical frequency. They classically manifest as pedunculated smooth-surfaced intramural masses.[2,28,169–171] Nearly 90 percent arise in the upper esophagus, particularly in the region of the cricoid,[28] although they also have been reported in the lower esophagus.[169] In about 75 percent of cases, the polyp is larger than 7 cm, and in some cases the pedicle may reach 20 cm in length.[2] The head of the polyp is surfaced by nonneoplastic squamous mucosa. Ulceration and inflammation are absent or minimal except for those polyps that extend into the gastroesophageal junction and cardia and are thus exposed to acid-pepsin. The stroma is composed of bland fibrous tissue with a quite variable myxoid and/or vascular (thin-walled blood vessels) component. Foci of adipose tissue may also be present, and when this is a predominant feature the term lipoma can be used.

These polyps may result in dysphagia, weight loss, and anginal pain, typically in middle-aged or elderly men. They may present dramatically when regurgitated into, or rarely, outside the mouth, or are aspirated into the larynx.[170,171] Despite their size, they may be easily overlooked on radiographic or endoscopic examination. Surgical and not endoscopic removal is generally considered to be the treatment of choice to avoid potential bleeding complications.[171]

One often quoted theory of origin is that they represent the end result of peristaltic action on the loose mucosa and submucosa of the subcricoid area.[28,171] Although they potentially could be hamartomatous, it is unlikely that they are neoplastic. There is one report in which a focus of squamous cell carcinoma was present.[172]

Various benign tumors, such as leiomyoma and lipoma, which may form pedunculated masses should be considered in the differential diagnosis. Inflammatory pseudotumor (inflammatory fibroid polyp) is distinguished from the fibrovascular polyp by (1) its rarity in the proximal esophagus; (2) its lack of a stalk; (3) the typical presence of ulceration; (4) proliferating fibrous tissue and reactive blood vessels; (5) the uniform presence of a polymorphous inflammatory infiltrate, which is often rich in eosinophils; and (6) the absence of fat.[173] Inflammatory pseudotumor is further discussed in Chapter 28. While grossly resembling some pedunculated malignant tumors, fibrovascular polyps lack the cellular pleomorphism of polypoid carcinoma, leiomyosarcoma and malignant melanoma, which may have this macroscopic appearance.

Esophagogastric Polyp-Fold Complex (Inflammatory Reflux Polyp)

Small (1 to 2 cm) sessile polyps have been found radiographically and endoscopically at the esophagogastric junction typically in association with a sentinal gastric fold (polyp-fold complex).[174,175] Associated findings of reflux esophagitis are typically present. The pathology of these polyps has not been well characterized. They are usually described as either nonspecific granulation tissue or inflamed gastric-type mucosa. Severe hematemesis has occasionally been reported.

Lipoma

Lipomas, which may be sessile or pedunculated, are extremely rare.[176,177] The overlap with fibrovascular polyp has been discussed above. Liposarcoma has not been reported.

Rhabdomyosarcoma and Related Lesions

As of 1980, there were five well documented cases of rhabdomyosarcoma of the esophagus in the literature.[178] A definitive diagnosis is made by demonstrating cross-striations on histologic examination, thick and thin filaments with Z-bands on electron microscopy, or most easily by the presence of myoglobin by immunohistochemistry. Desmin or antimuscle actin immunoreactivity in the cytoplasm of characteristic tumor cells suggests rhabdomyosarcoma, but leiomyosarcoma must be excluded. The presence of high-grade squamous dysplasia in some cases without a documented invasive epithelial component suggests the possibility, but does not prove, that the tumor is a carcinosarcoma.[178–180] The presence of other mesenchymal components classifies the tumor as a malignant mesenchymoma.[180] One example of a malignant Triton tumor (malignant peripheral nerve sheath tumor with rhabdomyoblastic differentiation) has been reported in the esophagus.[181] Rhabdomyoma of the esophagus has not been reported.

Synovial Sarcoma

Three cases of polypoid esophageal synovial sarcoma have been reported.[182] Two of the three cases were in patients 25 years of age or less.

Vascular Tumors

The esophagus is the least common site of GI hemangiomas.[25,183] They comprise 1 to 3 percent of all benign esophageal neoplasms. Most are small lesions found incidentally at autopsy.[183] Twenty-four symptomatic cases were reported through 1981.[183] Any portion of the esophagus may be involved. Symptomatic patients often complain of dysphagia or bleeding. Tumor size is typically 2 to 3 cm, although larger pedunculated lesions have been reported.[183] Although bleeding may be a potential problem with endoscopic biopsy, there were no serious sequelae in nine patients in the series of Hanel et al.[183] Histologically, the hemangiomas can be of the capillary or cavernous types.[183,184] Involvement of the esophagus has been reported in a patient with blue rubber bleb nevus syndrome.[185] Similarly, esophageal telangiectasias can be found in Rendu-Osler-Weber disease.[2] Rare reports of lymphangioma,[186] glomus tumor,[6] and possibly angiosarcoma[187] have appeared in the literature. Kaposi's sarcoma may also be found, particularly in AIDS patients.[188–190] With this disorder there is almost always evidence of associated cutaneous or lymph node disease. Endoscopic biopsies are frequently negative.[190]

Cartilaginous and Osseous Tumors

Benign cartilaginous or osteocartilaginous tumors have rarely been reported.[2,6,25,191] Mahour and Harrison[25] favored a tracheobronchial choristoma as the likely origin. The term chondroma is reasonable if the lesion is entirely cartilaginous.[2,192] Tracheobronchial remnant (tracheobronchial choristoma, chondroepithelial choristoma, cartilaginous esophageal ring), described earlier in this chapter, should also be considered.[31,33,34] Chondrosarcoma and osteosarcoma have rarely been reported.[193,194]

Epithelial Hyperplasias, Tumors, and Tumor-like Lesions

Glandular Lesions and Tumors

Cysts

Cysts are second to smooth muscle tumors in frequency of nonmalignant masses. They are discussed in the beginning of this chapter and in Chapter 24.

Ectopic Thyroid

Ectopic thyroid tissue has been described rarely within the wall of the esophagus.[169]

Adenoma

There are no well documented reports of adenomas arising from the submucosal glands which mimic those of the salivary glands, such as pleomorphic or monomorphic adenoma. The only well documented examples of adenoma (polypoid dysplasia) are those arising in BE (Barrett's adenoma).[102–104,195] These are discussed earlier in the section on precancer in BE.

Adenocarcinoma

Theoretically, esophageal adenocarcinoma could arise from several different origins, including the columnar mucosa of the distal 2 cm of the esophagus, the superficial (cardiac) glands, the submucosal glands, and their ducts or Barrett's epithelium. However, it is in the latter situation that the overwhelming majority of these tumors arise. An exception does exist in the upper esophagus, where esophageal adenocarcinoma may arise in association with ectopic gastric mucosa in the absence of reflex esophagitis and Barrett's mucosa.[21] This unusual situation has been discussed in the section on embryonic remnants and heterotopias.

Adenocarcinoma has been reported as comprising anywhere from 4 to 34 percent (19 percent in our institution) of all esophageal carcinomas and its frequency currently appears to be increasing.[84,196,197] The wide variation in reported frequencies may be related to one or more of the following factors: (1) many of the adenocarcinomas arising in the region of the EGJ in earlier series were considered to have originated in the gastric cardia; (2) geographic variability; (3) type of series, surgical versus autopsy; and (4) true recent increases in incidence. Tumor may be considered esophageal in origin when the majority of the neoplasm lies within the grossly recognizable esophagus. In about 10 percent of cases, the origin of the tumor from the esophagus or stomach cannot be determined with certainty, as it straddles the EGJ and may obliterate the adjacent mucosa[198] (Fig. 27-21A). As carcinomas arising in BE and those arising in the gastric cardia

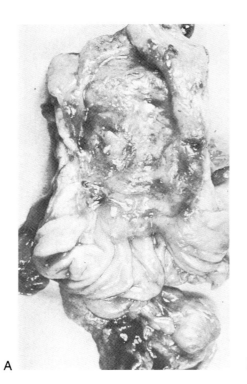

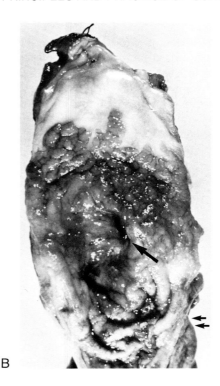

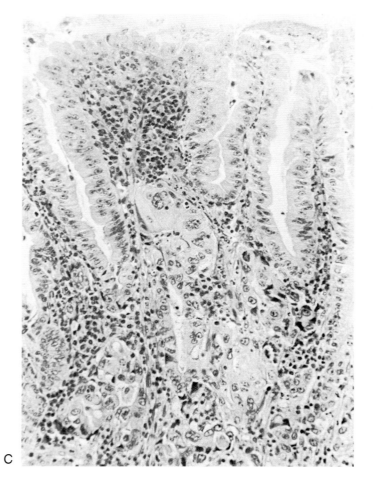

Fig. 27-21. (A) Adenocarcinoma of gastroesophageal junction. A large bulky, partly ulcerated tumor is seen at the gastroesophageal junction. Differentiation between gastric or esophageal origin is difficult. (B) Ulcerating adenocarcinoma arising in BE. Single arrow indicates central ulcer. Tumor extended into the adventitia and was associated with positive lymph nodes. Note nodular Barrett's mucosa proximally, where it interdigitates with the gray-white squamous mucosa. Double arrows demonstrate location of the gastroesophageal junction. (C) Microscopic appearance of invasive adenocarcinoma arising from a highly dysplastic villiform surface mucosa.

have virtually identical morphologic spectra and biologic behavior, as a practical matter their distinction is not important.[84,196,198] Both tumors appear to arise in a background of mucosal dysplasia, with carcinoma arising in BE perhaps having a stronger association with intestinal metaplasia.

Epidemiologic and Clinical Features. The prevalence of adenocarcinoma arising in the patients with BE reported in the literature is quite variable (0 to 47 percent) with an average of about 5 to 10 percent in the most nonselected series.[11,65,83–87] The fact that most patients reported in the literature present with BE at the time of discovery of their adenocarcinoma makes it difficult to assess the cancer risk of BE alone (incidence of adenocarcinoma arising in BE). Retrospectively obtained incidence data indicate that patients with BE have a 30- to 40-fold increased risk of developing esophageal adenocarcinoma.[87,199] As discussed in the section on BE, currently an endoscopic surveillance program is recommended for these patients.[11,83,103,104,111]

The mean age at presentation with adenocarcinoma is 58 years, roughly 6 years older than uncomplicated BE.[200] Eighty to 90 percent of patients are male, and nearly all cases have been reported in Caucasians. Smoking and drinking have been incriminated as potentiating factors.[11,199] About one third of patients lack a history of symptomatic reflux esophagitis.[200]

Pathologic Findings. Nearly 90 percent of adenocarcinomas arising in BE occur in the distal esophagus.[65,84,95,198,201] In general, surface ulceration is noted and the average tumor size is 4 cm in diameter (range less than 1 cm to 9 cm) (Fig. 27-21B). Although 35 percent of these tumors are polypoid or fungating, making them easily identifiable at the time of endoscopy, 65 percent are flat or nodular and may be difficult to distinguish from the surrounding Barrett's mucosa. Five to 10 percent of invasive cancers are multiple.

Biopsy and brush cytology, especially when used together in the upper GI tract, are highly sensitive (about 95 percent) diagnostic tools with only rare false positive results.[202] The new technique of endoscopic fine needle aspiration biopsy may possibly increase diagnostic accuracy.[203]

Microscopically, nearly all tumors are found to arise in dysplastic Barrett's mucosa when extensive sectioning of the adjacent mucosa is performed.[65,84,95,201] They have a glandular, or less commonly papillary, architecture (mixtures do exist) (Fig. 27-21C). The degree of differentiation is variable, even within a given tumor. Those that are predominantly moderately or poorly differentiated using architectural and cytologic criteria account for about 90 percent of all cases. Tumor cells may be found forming small tubules, infiltrating as individual cells or forming solid masses. By contrast, about 10 percent of tumors have a significant well differentiated tubular component. Occasionally, the neoplastic glands are composed of cells with clear cytoplasm and a single layer of nuclei resembling the pylorocardiac gland cell carcinoma described in the gastric cardia.[84] Rarely, focal squamous or neuroendocrine differentiation (adenosquamous carcinoma and adenocarcinoid, respectively) has been noted.[84,201] A case with synchronous independent tumors, adenocarcinoma and squamous cell carcinoma, the latter arising in a squamous remnant in BE, has also been described.[201] Flow cytometric DNA analysis demonstrated aneuploidy in all seven cases of Barrett's adenocarcinomas in one study.[108]

In unselected series, 80 percent of adenocarcinomas arising in BE have extended through the wall into the surrounding adventitia at surgical resection.[65,84,86,95,201] Lymph nodes are positive in two thirds of cases. Only 5 to 10 percent of tumors do not extend beyond the submucosa and thus could be classified as early esophageal cancers if lymph nodes were negative[204,205] (Fig. 27-22). Surgical margins are positive for tumor in one third of cases, probably related to insidious submucosal lymphatic permeation of the esophageal wall and problems with surgical technique.[201] When at all possible, esophageal margins should be free of tumor, dysplasia, and also all columnar epithelium.

Outcome. In one large surgical series, survival at 2 and 5 years was 34 percent and 14.5 percent, respectively.[206] Early squamous esophageal cancer (see below) has been associated with survival rates approaching 90 percent.[204,205] Several series have documented that surveillance programs, by performing esophageal resection for high-grade dysplasia or intramucosal carcinoma in appropriate surgical candidates, can detect adenocarcinomas that have not penetrated beyond the submucosa in at least 50 percent of patients.[86,102,103,106] Although 5 year survival data are currently not available on this select group of patients, it is hoped that their prognosis will be as good as that of early squamous esophageal carcinoma. More general features of prognosis and outcome for esophageal carcinoma are discussed under squamous cell carcinoma.

Squamous Hyperplasias and Tumors

Glycogenic Acanthosis

Multiple white plaque-like elevated mucosal lesions of the esophagus varying in size from a few millimeters up to 1.5 cm in diameter have been demonstrated in 5 to 15 percent of endoscopic examinations[207] and in up to 100 percent of autopsies.[208] Double-contrast barium studies have detected this mucosal abnormality in 28 percent of

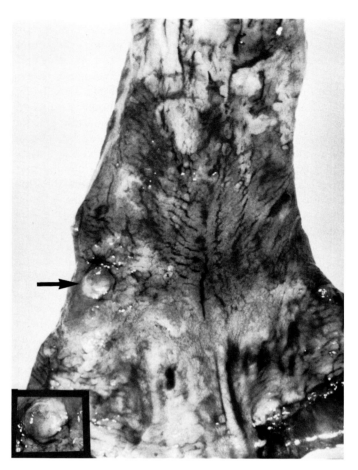

Fig. 27-22. Esophagogastrectomy specimen resected for a biopsy diagnosis of high-grade dysplasia. In addition to extensive areas of high-grade dysplasia, a single nodule, 0.5 cm in diameter, was found (arrow), which demonstrated adenocarcinoma extending only into the submucosa, with negative lymph nodes (early esophageal cancer). A closeup of this nodule is seen in the inset.

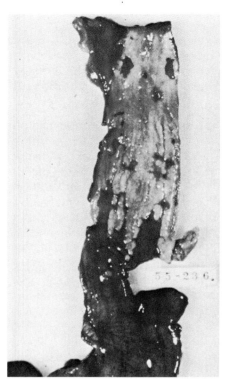

Fig. 27-23. Glycogenic acanthosis. Irregular islands of thickened squamous epithelium appear as white plaques and ridges.

examinations.[209] These lesions are distributed most commonly in the distal esophagus along the longitudinal mucosal ridges, and in about 10 percent of cases numerous plaques become confluent, appearing as large cobblestone areas[2,208] (Fig. 27-23). Critical histologic review of these plaques has shown them to be composed invariably of mucosa marked by thickening (acanthosis) due primarily to an increased number of enlarged cells of the prickle cell layer that contain large amounts of glycogen[207-210] (Fig. 27-24). The mucosa may be up to three times normal thickness. The increased glycogen content can easily be demonstrated with the PAS stain before and after diastase. Although referred to as leukoplakia in the past, the use of this clinical term is to be discouraged. Dysplastic changes, keratosis, and parakeratosis are not seen. There is no known relationship to carcinoma, and the pathogenesis is obscure.

On gross examination, these plaques may be confused with inflammatory pseudomembranes of candidiasis, but the lack of surrounding erythema and edema aids in the differential diagnosis. Obviously, histologic examination facilitates differentiation. Glycogenic acanthosis should also be distinguished from the balloon cells of clear cell acanthosis.[79] These lack or have minimal glycogen, and cytoplasmic serum proteins can be demonstrated immunohistochemically (see the sections on reflux esophagitis and precursor lesions of squamous carcinoma).

Dysplasia of Squamous Mucosa

A variety of dysplastic changes including squamous cell carcinoma in situ have been described. These lesions are discussed in the sections on precursor lesions of squamous cell carcinoma.

Squamous Papilloma and Papillomatosis

Squamous papillomas of the esophagus are rare benign tumors that have been detected endoscopically in recent years, leading to an increased number of case reports and small series.[211-220] About 50 well documented cases may be found in the literature. They have only rarely been reported before the age of 40 years and about 75 percent of cases have been in men. The overwhelming majority of

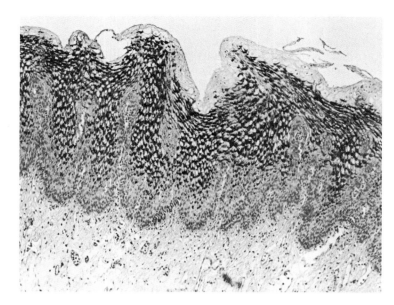

Fig. 27-24. Glycogenic acanthosis. A low-power photomicrograph shows the white plaques noted in Figure 27-23. The acanthotic surface matures normally and should not be confused with leukoplakia. (PAS stain.)

patients lack symptoms directly attributable to the papilloma, undergoing endoscopy typically for symptoms of reflux esophagitis.

These tumors are detected most commonly in the distal esophagus (66 percent). About two thirds are solitary, while some instances of multiple tumors warrant the designation of papillomatosis.[2,211,218,219] The mean size is 6 to 7 mm (range 2 to 100 mm)[212,214] and, although generally considered sessile, one third of lesions can be snared endoscopically and entirely removed.[214] Microscopically they are characterized by hyperplastic stratified squamous epithelium growing in a papillary pattern. The stromal element is relatively inconspicuous and is composed of vascular elements with scanty connective tissue. Papillomas should be separated from lesions such as the fibrovascular polyp, in which the primary element is stromal, surfaced by the usual esophageal squamous mucosa. This distinction has not always been made in prior reported cases. As at other sites, distinction from verrucous carcinoma may be impossible on small biopsies.

The etiology of these tumors is uncertain; however, viral, chemical, mechanical, and genetic factors have been considered. Although a viral etiology has been postulated, similar to squamous papillomas at other anatomic sites in humans,[2,216] to date immunoperoxidase studies performed in a limited number of esophageal cases have failed to detect human papillomavirus (HPV).[216,219] Winkler et al.[216] did, however, find HPV immunoreactivity in 4 of 11 cases (36 percent) of flat and spiked epithelial hyperplasias of the esophagus. The presence of reflux esophagitis in most patients and the common location of the tumor in the distal esophagus suggest that chemical irritation by acid/pepsin may be important. Papillomas were not reported until after bougienage in the case of Parnell et al.,[217] suggesting that mechanical irritation may also be a predisposing factor. The fact that these tumors have been reported in association with acanthosis nigricans[220] and focal dermal hypoplasia (Goltz-Gorlin syndrome)[219] raises the possibility of a genetic predisposition in some cases.

Squamous Cell Carcinoma

Incidence and Epidemiology. Most epidemiologic and incidence reports fail to identify the histologic type of cancer of the esophagus. For practical purposes, however, as most adenocarcinomas involving the distal esophagus were considered to have arisen from the gastric cardia and thus were excluded from statistical analysis, the various studies can be said to refer to squamous cell carcinoma.

There is an extraordinary range in frequency of cancer of the esophagus geographically and a large variation in the sex ratio. Overall, this cancer affects mainly those in the sixth to eighth decades,[221,222] and men more frequently than women, but great geographic variability exists. There were an estimated 8,800 deaths in the United States from esophageal carcinoma in 1985, accounting for about 1 percent of all cancer deaths, while in subsets of high-incidence regions, this disease may account for nearly 40 percent of cancer deaths.[2,221–223] Mortality is so high that mortality and incidence figures are nearly the same. In the United States, a region of low incidence, rates per 100,000 are 2.5 to 5 for men and 1.5 to 2.5 for women. The figures are slightly higher overall in Western Europe; however, in regions of France (particularly Normandy and Brittany), the incidence may exceed 50 per 100,000. Even within the United States there are great differences in regard to race. The average age-adjusted incidence rates per 100,000 as determined by the Surveillance Epidemiology and End Results (SEER) program for 1983 were 5.0 and 19.9 for white and black men and 1.5 and 4.0 for white and black women, respectively.[223] From the period between 1951 to 1953 and 1976 to 1978 the age-adjusted mortality rate in black men rose 92 percent,[221] while in the past decade it has risen more than 10 percent.[223]

The high incidence belt extends from northwestern China (130 per 100,000) through south central Asia to northwestern Iran and the shores of the Caspian sea (165 per 100,000 men; 195 per 100,000 women). In the southern and eastern areas of Africa (Transkei and Eastern Kenya) another high incidence area is found. Marked variation in incidence is noted in areas adjacent to both regions.[2,221–223]

Etiologic Factors. Although the evidence strongly suggests the importance of environmental factors in the pathogenesis of this tumor, none of the factors listed below is universally applicable—factors of seeming importance in one region do not seem to be significant in another. Therefore, various unique predisposing factors, mutagens and promoters probably determine the risk of squamous esophageal cancer in a given locale.[224]

Genetic Factors. Pour and Ghadirian[225] reported 14 patients with esophageal carcinoma from one small village in northeastern Iran, 13 of whom were members of one family. Precession was noted (the cancers in each generation occurred at earlier ages). These investigators suggested an unusual genetic susceptibility to environmental influences; however, common exposure to a carcinogen alone cannot be ruled out. Tylosis (keratosis palmaris et plantaris), a genodermatosis inherited in an autosomal-dominant fashion, has been reported associated with esophageal carcinoma in 17 family members.[221,226] This disorder, characterized by symmetric thickening (hyperkeratosis) of the palms and soles, has also been associated with squamous cell carcinoma of the larynx, lung, oral cavity, and skin.[227] Tylosis represents the single well documented example of a genetic association with esophageal carcinoma.

Alcohol. There is an association between alcohol consumption and esophageal carcinoma in the United States and Western Europe, particularly France (Brittany, Normandy), but not in Iran and parts of Asia.[221–223,225] For habitual consumers of alcohol in the United States, the risk is 10 to 25 times that of nondrinkers, depending on the ethanol content of the alcoholic beverage.[222,228] Alcohol and tobacco are implicated in 80 to 90 percent of cases in regions of low and moderate incidence. Although ethanol alone has not been shown to be carcinogenic, it may exert its effects by acting as a solvent for tobacco and other carcinogens or by increasing the permeability of the esophageal mucosa to these substances. The poor nutritional status of many alcoholics and the effects of various dietary factors used in the production of local beverages also appear to be important.[229,230]

Tobacco. Wynder and Mabuchi[228] found an association between smoking (cigarettes, cigars, and pipes) and esophageal carcinoma in the United States. The increased risk is two to six times that of nonsmokers. Auerbach and co-workers[231] reported finding acanthosis, basal layer changes, dysplasia, and carcinoma in situ in the esophageal mucosa of smokers as compared with nonsmokers. In India and central Asia, tobacco products are smoked and chewed in various concoctions and appear to be associated with high risk. In other areas, such as Iran, tobacco smoking does not seem to be a factor, but opium smoking may be important.[221]

Dietary Factors. Dietary factors appear to have an important role in the development of esophageal squamous carcinoma in regions of high incidence. In northern China, an interesting parallel in incidence of esophageal carcinoma in humans and chickens has been reported, with a correspondence of low- and high-incidence areas for both.[232] Dietary factors of potential importance have recently been summarized as follows[2]: (1) diets high in nitrosamines or compounds that can be converted into nitrosamines; (2) diets that include moldy foods, particularly those containing *Geotrichum candidum* and *Fusarium* species; (3) consumption of foods raised in soil deficient in trace elements, notably molybdenum, iron, and zinc; and (4) diets deficient in vitamins C and A and riboflavin, protein, and overall caloric content. The use of hot or spicy foods has been suspected in some parts of the world.

Overall, dietary factors are not considered to be as important in Western countries. However, the Plummer-Vinson (Paterson-Kelly) syndrome, also known as sideropenic dysphagia,[2,36,222,233–235] is an exception. This syndrome occurs in middle-aged northern European (particularly Swedish) women and is characterized by iron deficiency anemia, atrophic glossopathy, and dysphagia (with or without an upper esophageal web). Affected patients have an increased risk of hypopharyngeal and upper esophageal (10 percent) carcinoma. The precise relationship of different components of the syndrome is controversial, as the dysphagia has been reported in the absence of iron deficiency and/or an upper esophageal web. Various vitamin deficiencies have been reported in patients with this syndrome. Although this syndrome is rarely reported today, perhaps related to the marked reduction in iron deficiency anemia and changes in dietary pattern, relatively high rates of esophageal carcinoma in women persist in northern Norway and rural Wales.[222,235] This may relate to the high prevalence of the Plummer-Vinson syndrome seen in these regions 40 to 50 years ago.[235]

Human Papillomavirus Infection. Although human papillomavirus (HPV) has occasionally been detected in hyperplastic esophageal mucosa, a defined role in esophageal carcinogenesis has not to date been elucidated.[216]

Specific Known Associated Diseases—Conditions Causing Esophageal Stasis.

An increase in squamous cell carcinoma has been reported in most conditions in which there is a lesion leading to chronic esophageal stasis.

Achalasia. In 1975, Carter and Brewer[236] reviewed the literature and cited 221 cases of carcinoma associated with achalasia. The frequency in various reported series has varied widely, depending on whether they were clinical (0 to 7.7 percent) or autopsy (20 to 29 percent) studies.[236–239] The carcinomas are virtually always squamous and, similar to the usual carcinoma, about 85 percent arise in the middle or distal esophagus. The occasional adenocarcinoma that has been reported probably has arisen in the setting of prior therapy that has damaged the LES, resulting in reflux and Barrett's esophagus.[50] The esophageal carcinomas arising in achalasia patients usually present 20 to 28 years after the onset of disease and occur one decade earlier than those of nonachalasia patients.

Pharyngoesophageal (Zenker's) Diverticulum. An association between squamous cell carcinoma and Zenker's diverticulum has been reported (0.3 to 0.7 percent).[54,55] These tumors occur chiefly in patients over 60 years of age with longstanding diverticula in whom changes in symptoms develop, including dysphagia and hemoptysis.

Strictures Related to Ingestion of Caustic Substances (Lye Stricture). Carcinoma is known to occur at the site of lye stricture after a latent period averaging 41 years (12 to 71 years).[2,6,139,240] Since the ingestion typically occurs in childhood, the tumors may be found at rather an early age. They typically arise in the mid-esophagus in the region of the stricture. There is perhaps a 1,000-fold increase in expected frequency of esophageal carcinoma after caustic ingestion; however, currently these tumors account for only 0.2 to 0.5 percent of all esophageal cancers.[222]

Specific Known Associated Diseases—Other Conditions.

Squamous Cell Carcinoma of the Head and Neck. Ten percent of squamous cell carcinomas of the esophagus are associated with squamous cell carcinoma of the pharynx, larynx and, most commonly, the oral cavity.[241] Similarly, when a second primary occurs, in 60 percent of cases it will be in these areas.

Celiac Disease. Although small bowel lymphoma is the most common neoplastic complication of this disease, the frequency of esophageal cancer is also increased.[235,242] This association may be either a genetic or an environmental susceptibility.

Plummer-Vinson Syndrome and Tylosis. For discussions of Plummer-Vinson syndrome and tylosis, see the earlier sections on dietary and genetic factors, respectively.

Symptoms. The most common symptoms are dysphagia (83 percent), weight loss (60 percent), and pain (50 percent).[243] These symptoms are usually progressive and typically indicate advanced disease.[223,244] Other symptoms, such as cough, hoarseness, and bleeding, may represent manifestations of local invasion of the tracheo-bronchial tree, the recurrent laryngeal nerve, or mediastinal vasculature. Even in cases of early esophageal cancer (defined below), about 90 percent of patients have a history of mild retrosternal pain and a sense of friction on swallowing. These symptoms have often been present for 2 to 3 years, indicating the long natural history of this disease.[244]

In high-risk populations, in symptomatic patients, and in those patients with predisposing conditions, screening with radiologic, endoscopic, and cytologic techniques may help to diagnose early disease.[202,244–253]

Diagnosis. Diagnosis is usually made after esophagography (Fig. 27-25), followed by endoscopic examination with biopsy and brush cytologic studies.[202,244–253] The use of dyes such as toluidine blue and Lugol's iodine during endoscopy may aid in identifying neoplastic foci; however, false positive and false negative results can occur.[202,244,254] Overall, the combination of biopsy and brush cytology gives a diagnostic accuracy rate of about 95 percent.[202,249] Several diagnostic pitfalls do exist. Squamous cell carcinoma tends to invade longitudinally within the submucosa for long distances from the site of origin. The entire segment of involved esophagus may be narrowed and prevent passage of the endoscope, thus making it potentially impossible to obtain tissue biopsy specimens in some cases. Brush cytology specimens are quite useful in areas distal to a stricture, where mucosal involvement is present; thus, cytologic studies are more likely to be positive in these cases. Therefore, positive cytologic results in the face of a negative biopsy should not be ignored, but should be followed with repeat biopsies and cytologic studies. Macroscopically, narrowed areas in some cases may appear involved, but the presence of an intact nonneoplastic epithelium may lead to false negative results with either brushings or superficial biopsies (Fig. 27-26). The new technique of endoscopic

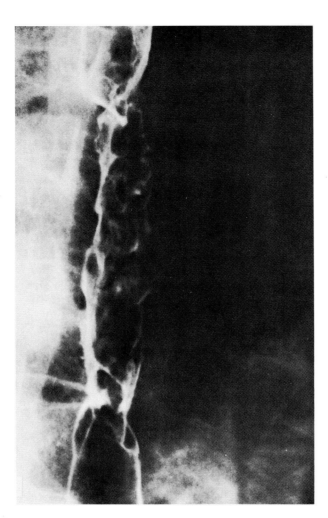

Fig. 27-25. Squamous cell carcinoma. This radiograph of an esophageal squamous cell carcinoma reveals the tremendous longitudinal submucosal spread typically seen with this lesion. (From Laufer,[148] with permission.)

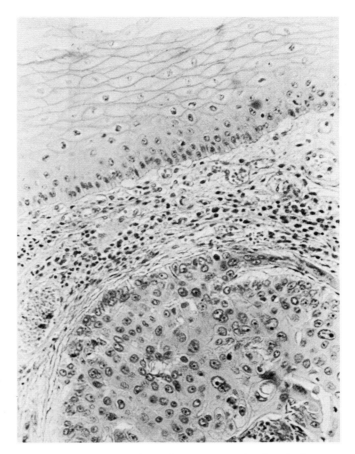

Fig. 27-26. Biopsy specimen from the proximal end of a narrowed esophagus reveals a normal surface mucosa but a large ball of tumor cells in a submucosal lymphatic. A superficial biopsy at this point would probably fail to reveal tumor.

fine needle aspiration biopsy may permit sampling of these more deep-seated tumor foci.[203] The balloon cytology technique has been found to be useful in screening programs in regions of high incidence. It has the advantage of sampling the entire esophagus and of being relatively inexpensive.[253]

Site. Evaluation of the site of occurrence of squamous cell carcinoma is complicated by three problems: (1) many series lump all carcinomas of the esophagus together because of a similarity in prognosis, (2) some series arbitrarily exclude lesions of the EGJ and the cervical esophagus, and (3) many tumors extend longitudinally for large distances and are difficult to assign to a specific site. Because of these differences, many studies are not comparable.

The American Joint Committee on Cancer has recommended dividing the esophagus into three portions as follows[255]: (1) the upper third (cervical portion) begins at the pharyngoesophageal junction and extends to the thoracic inlet, approximately 18 cm from the incisor teeth; (2) the middle third includes the upper and mid-thoracic esophagus, which extends from the thoracic inlet to a point 10 cm above the EGJ, a point approximated by the lower edge of the eighth thoracic vertebra, or roughly 31 cm from the incisor teeth; and (3) the lower third extends from a point 10 cm above the EGJ to the cardiac orifice of the stomach, approximately 40 cm from the incisor teeth.

Using these arbitrary divisions and extrapolating the data from several series,[6,243,245,256–262] one finds approximately 50 to 60 percent of cases in the middle third, 30 to 40 percent in the lower third, and 5 to 10 percent in the upper third. Incidence by site may vary in different geographic areas.[243] In some series, the cervical site is more frequent in women.[263] This may relate to an association with the Plummer-Vinson syndrome. Several unusual sites have also been described, including squamous cell carcinoma arising in an intramural squamous-lined cyst.[264]

Precursor Lesions. Precursor and associated lesions of esophageal squamous carcinoma have been described, particularly in regions of high incidence.[224,231,235,246,265] The earliest lesions are non-neoplastic (esophagitis, clear cell acanthosis, and epithelial atrophy), while these appear to be followed by histologic evidence of neoplasia (dysplasia and carcinoma in situ [CIS]).

Esophagitis. Histologic evidence of esophagitis has been found in 60 to 85 percent of patients in screening studies in China and Iran. The histologic findings are similar to those in low incidence regions; however, parakeratosis appears to be quite common.[266] The esophagitis typically involves the middle and lower thirds of the esophagus but spares the region of the EGJ.[246] The location of the esophagitis in areas of high incidence is therefore quite dissimilar from the ubiquitous presence of terminal esophageal involvement in reflux esophagitis, which is by far the most common form of esophagitis in regions of low incidence.

Clear Cell Acanthosis. Clear cell acanthosis is characterized macroscopically by white patches and microscopi-cally by thickened squamous mucosa containing swollen (ballooned) cells containing little glycogen (PAS-negative).[79,235,246] These foci are present in 65 to 81 percent of screened patients and should be distinguished from glycogenic acanthosis (PAS-positive).[2,207–210]

Epithelial Atrophy. Foci of atrophic squamous mucosa are found in about 10 percent of cases.

Intraepithelial Neoplasia (Dysplasia and Carcinoma in Situ. Intraepithelial neoplasia is considered the most important precursor lesion for the development of esophageal carcinoma[235,246,265–270] (Figs. 27-27 and 27-28). Dysplastic foci have been detected in 3 to 14 percent of randomly screened patients in high-incidence regions.[235,246,265] In one study, 1 percent of patients had severe dysplasia, while an equal number had squamous cell carcinoma. Carcinoma typically occurred one decade later than dysplasia, supporting a dysplasia-carcinoma sequence.[265] In this same study, nearly 30 percent of cases of severe dysplasia were found to progress to carcinoma over a period of several years. Of the cases of mild dysplasia, 15 percent progressed to severe dysplasia, 42 percent remained the same, and 45 percent returned to normal.[265] In autopsy studies from regions of low incidence, the frequency of CIS has been estimated at 0.3 percent and a direct correlation was found between the quantity of smoking and the chance of finding dysplasia

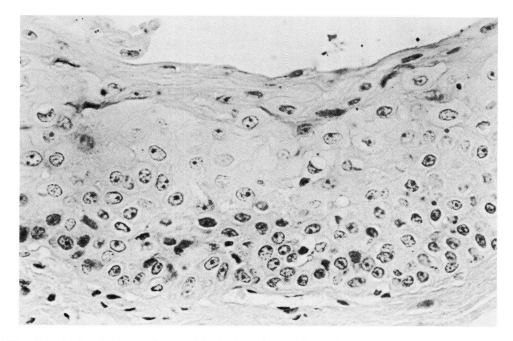

Fig. 27-27. Dysplasia of the esophagus. The lesion pictured here shows atypicality of nuclei within the bottom third of the mucosa. Such a lesion corresponds to mild dysplasia as defined in the uterine cervix. Comparison with Figure 27-12 should be made. The atypical cells in inflammatory processes seem to be more superficial in location and to show a relative sparing of the basal layer.

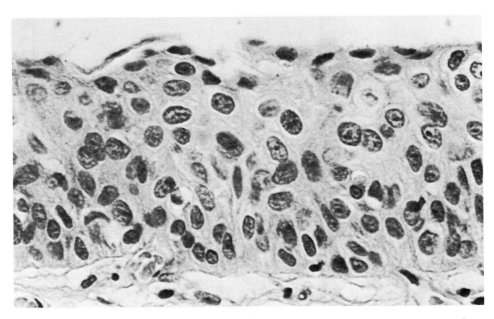

Fig. 27-28. Dysplasia of the esophagus. The dysplastic cells in this lesion demonstrate only one to two layers of cell maturation and correspond to severe dysplasia in the cervix. The lesion borders on carcinoma in situ.

or CIS.[231,267] The association of esophageal carcinoma and intraepithelial neoplasia is further supported by the study of Mandard et. al.[266] These investigators found at least one focus of intraepithelial neoplasia, usually adjacent to the invasive tumor, in 95% of esophagi resected for squamous cell carcinoma. Using cytofluorometry, Mukada et al.[269] found progressive changes from euploidy to tetraploidy in mild and moderate dysplasia and to octaploidy and progressive aneuploidy in severe dysplasia and CIS. Scanning electron microscopy (SEM) has also shown progressive changes from mild to severe dysplasia.[270] The cytologic and histologic features of esophageal intraepithelial neoplasia are in general similar to those of the cervix.[253,266,268] The neoplastic epithelium may contain small basaloid (undifferentiated) cells or larger nonkeratinized or keratinized cells. However, as in squamous intraepithelial neoplasia at other sites in the upper aerodigestive tract, the diagnosis of severe dysplasia/CIS can occasionally be made in the presence of marked cytologic abnormalities in the absence of full-thickness involvement.

In summary, it appears that esophagitis of varied etiology damages the epithelium, causing increased cell turnover, leading to foci of hyperplasia and atrophy. The rapid turnover facilitates the expression of mutagenic influences, which may result in the formation of neoplastic clones with more aggressive potential.[224] Multifactorial and multistage theories of esophageal carcinogenesis have been postulated.[224,235]

Pathologic Features

Advanced Esophageal Carcinoma

Gross Appearance. Most classic descriptions of esophageal carcinoma refer to the common morphologic findings of tumors that have infiltrated at least into the muscularis propria and usually into the adventitia and surrounding structures, *i.e.*, advanced esophageal carcinoma (AEC).[6] The specific criteria and morphologic features of early esophageal carcinoma, which are usually detected in patients in surveillance programs in regions of high incidence, are discussed subsequently.

Ming[6] described three basic macroscopic types of AEC: the fungating type (60 percent), the ulcerating type (25 percent), and the infiltrating type (15 percent).[6] A rare verrucous or papillary variant has also been described.[6,271,272] Although there is overlap among the three major types, these categories are useful in describing a given lesion. Tumor size is quite variable but is often 5 to 7 cm in its greatest diameter. Multiple foci of invasive carcinoma have been described in 13 percent of resection specimens.[266] Polypoid carcinoma with dominant spindle cell elements is reviewed toward the end of this chapter.

The fungating type of squamous carcinoma has a prominent intraluminal component composed of multiple polypoid masses, often with zones of ulceration (Fig. 27-29). In some foci, the lesion may appear plaque-like. Often the tumor appears to have a sharply defined border, but

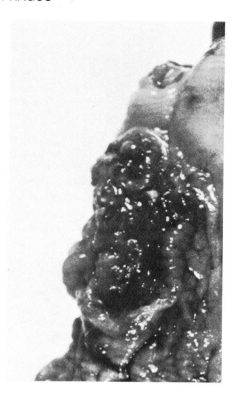

Fig. 27-29. Fungating squamous cell carcinoma. This form of squamous cell carcinoma manifests as an irregular polypoid mass admixed with foci of ulceration.

microscopic examination frequently indicates submucosal extension that was not grossly appreciated (see Fig. 27-26). The ulcerating type of lesion has an ulcer of variable depth with irregular edges and a shaggy, hemorrhagic central crater (Fig. 27-30). Penetration into surrounding viscera and the mediastinum is not uncommon. Intramural extension is also frequently present in this type. The infiltrating type of tumor primarily demonstrates intramural growth similar to the growth pattern seen in the "leather bottle stomach" (linitis plastica) (Fig. 27-31). A focus of ulceration is usually seen in addition, but is relatively insignificant in comparison to the degree of intramural growth. The lesion causes a narrowing of the esophagus and the strictured segment may cause obstruction with proximal dilatation.

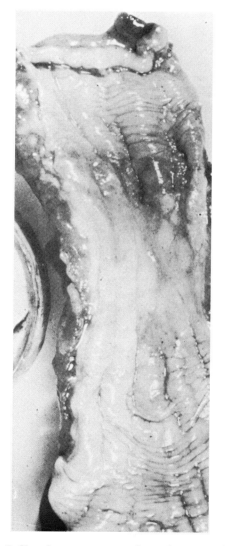

Fig. 27-31. Infiltrating squamous cell carcinoma. This form of squamous carcinoma is largely submucosal and narrows the esophageal lumen (see Figs. 27-25 and 27-26). The mucosa here is largely normal, and a site of mucosal origin is hard to identify.

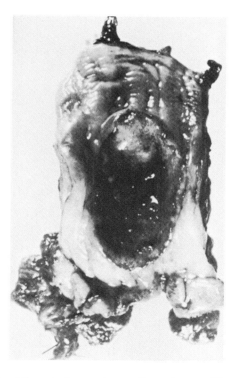

Fig. 27-30. Ulcerated squamous cell carcinoma. The ulcerated form of squamous cell carcinoma manifests as a deeply penetrating ulcer with shaggy margins.

Only eight examples of the rare verrucous type of squamous carcinoma had been reported as of 1984.[272] These lesions have a bulky papillary surface. Biopsy often reveals a deceptively bland well differentiated squamous carcinoma which may be misdiagnosed as benign epithelium. The pushing bulbous wedges of tumor, rather than the infiltrating nests of the usual squamous cell carcinoma, are much more easily recognized in resection than in biopsy specimens. Although the natural history of this tumor in the esophagus, similar to other sites, may be longer than the usual carcinoma, virtually all reported patients with esophageal lesions have died soon after their clinical presentation.[272] It appears that the term verrucous carcinoma has been used somewhat loosely at this site, as some of the published cases have had infiltrating tumor nests and lymph node metastases.[271]

On gross examination squamous cell carcinoma may mimic a benign stricture, the large folds sometimes seen in a hiatal hernia or the nodular lesions occasionally encountered in esophagitis.[245] An irregularity of the surface is usually seen at some point in squamous carcinoma and is a useful differential feature. Clandestine foci of intramural growth, not infrequently extending longitudinally for 5 to 6 cm or more, usually in a cephalad direction, can be seen in any of the macroscopic types.[273] This emphasizes the need for frozen section examination of the margins and explains the inadequacy of most segmental resections.

Microscopic Appearance. Squamous cell carcinoma of the esophagus is indistinguishable microscopically from squamous cell carcinoma at other sites (see Fig. 27-26). Depending on the ease with which keratinization can be demonstrated, the frequency of intercellular bridges, and the degree of cytologic pleomorphism, these tumors can be classified as well, moderately, or poorly differentiated. If keratinization or intercellular bridges are not identified (and mucin stains are negative), the lesion is classified as an undifferentiated carcinoma. Although statistically an esophageal biopsy demonstrating undifferentiated carcinoma is most likely to be primary, the possibility of a metastasis from another site should at least be considered. Most tumors are considered to be well differentiated[6]; however, frequently marked variability in differentiation exists in different regions of the tumor, often making tumor grading quite a subjective exercise. Although most authors believe that tumor differentiation does not affect prognosis, this is somewhat controversial.[273] Lymphatic and/or vascular invasion are detected in about 75 percent of esophagectomy specimens.

In well differentiated squamous carcinoma, intercellular bridges are easily found, and the degree of cellular pleomorphism is minimal. Keratinization is easily identified but may vary considerably in degree. On cytologic examination, well differentiated tumors are easy to identify. The cells exfoliate in great numbers and are seen on smears as pleomorphic cells with dark, irregular nuclei

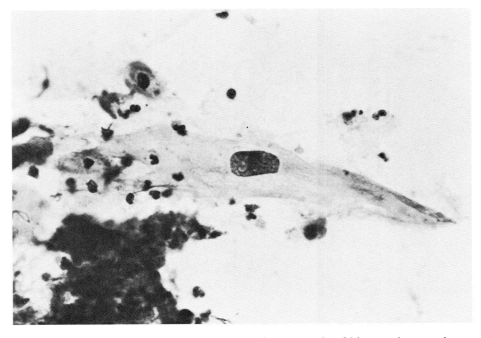

Fig. 27-32. Cytology of squamous cell carcinoma. This squame is of bizarre shape and contains a large nucleus with ill-defined areas of parachromatin clearing and a large nucleolus. These cells are commonly seen in well differentiated lesions and may assume unusual tadpole shapes.

demonstrating areas of ill defined clearing. The cytoplasm stains pink or orange and may be scant, or it may be ample and form long tadpole shapes (Fig. 27-32).[253,274,275]

Moderately and poorly differentiated tumors show progressive degrees of pleomorphism and demonstrate loss of keratinization and fewer intercellular bridges. They generally demonstrate areas of sheeting as they invade and may show prominent areas of necrosis within the sheets. Occasionally, this pattern of central necrosis in more poorly differentiated tumors resembles an acinar arrangement; however, mucin stains are negative. This change is best termed squamous cell carcinoma with pseudoglandular degeneration. On cytologic preparations the cells of moderately differentiated tumors are round to oval and resemble parabasal cells. The nuclear-to-cytoplasmic ratio is moderately increased, the amount of cytoplasm is relatively abundant, and nucleoli are often present. Cells exfoliated from poorly differentiated tumors can be large or small and are often irregular.[253,274,275] The nuclear-to-cytoplasmic ratio is usually quite high, nucleoli may be present or absent, and the cytoplasm is typically scant or even absent (naked nuclei).[253,273,275] Small sheets of these cells may mimic the balls of cells seen in adenocarcinoma (Fig. 27-33). The specific cytologic diagnosis of tumor type is not quite as accurate in these poorly differentiated lesions.

Early Esophageal Carcinoma. Because of the grim prognosis of advanced esophageal carcinoma, a major effort has been made, particularly in regions of high incidence, to recognize this tumor at a relatively early stage when it has invaded no further than the submucosa: early or superficial esophageal carcinoma (EEC).[273–282] In areas of China in which large-scale screening is performed, EEC may account for nearly 90 percent of all esophageal carcinomas. However, in other portions of China and in general throughout the rest of the world, EEC accounts for only 0.75 to 7 percent of all resected cases.[273,277–282] In one study, 32 percent of cases were intraepithelial (CIS), 39 percent intramucosal (in lamina propria), and 29 percent had penetrated the submucosa.[273] The first evidence of invasion into the submucosa may arise subsequent to the intraepithelial spread of neoplastic cells into the ducts and acini of the submucosal glands.[283] Although the literature varies somewhat as to whether patients with positive lymph nodes can be considered in this diagnostic category, as survival appears to be markedly affected by lymph nodal metastases (as discussed later in this chapter) the term EEC should probably be reserved for lymph-node-negative cases, in contrast to cases of early gastric carcinoma.[279,280–282]

Four macroscopic types, similar to those of AEC, have been recognized[273,276,278]:

1. *Plaque-like (superficially elevated):* The involved mucosa is slightly elevated and granular and may demonstrate small erosions. After fixation, it becomes pale. These lesions may be circumferential, measuring up to 4

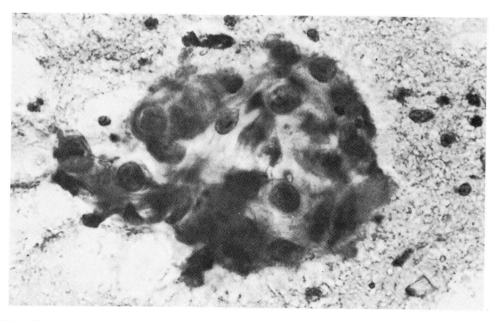

Fig. 27-33. Cytology of squamous cell carcinoma. More poorly differentiated squamous carcinomas may exfoliate as ball-like clusters of dark irregular cells with irregular nuclei showing parachromatin clearing and angular nucleoli. A differential diagnosis of adenocarcinoma must be entertained. Usually, a further search of the smear will reveal sheets and single cells more typical of squamous carcinoma.

cm in greatest dimension. This is the most common pattern (50 percent) in resection specimens of EEC.[273]

2. *Erosive (ulcerative) type:* The center of the lesion is slightly depressed. It accounts for one third of all cases.

3. *Papillary (protuberant):* There is a polypoid or papillary protrusion of tumor into the lumen with a well demarcated border; this type is usually 1 to 3 cm in diameter and represents about 8 percent of EEC.

4. *Flat (occult):* In this barely perceptible flat focus of pink congested mucosa, the tumor foci are nearly always less than 1 cm in greatest dimension. This pattern is the least common, representing about 7 percent of EEC. All 11 cases in one study demonstrated only intraepithelial carcinoma, while 56 percent, 82 percent, and 92 percent of plaque-like, erosive, and papillary tumors, respectively, showed foci of invasion.[273]

The histologic features of EEC are similar to those described under AEC. The entire lesion should be submitted for microscopic evaluation as invasive foci may be quite focal.

Spread and Complications. Because of the intimate relationship between the esophagus and the tracheobronchial tree, lungs, aorta, major vessels, and other mediastinal structures, local spread of disease is an important factor in determining prognosis. Squamous carcinoma in several large surgical series was found to have transgressed the esophageal wall and extended into the periesophageal soft tissues in 11 to 72 percent of cases.[6,260,266,279,280,283] Forty-one to 76 percent of unselected cases demonstrate lymph node metastases. Similar figures are found in autopsy studies.[262,282] There is a progressive relationship between depth of invasion and the frequency of lymph node metastases. Tumors invading the submucosa have been reported to metastasize to lymph nodes in 0 to 50 percent of cases,[266,276,278-280,283] while those extending into the periesophageal tissues demonstrate such metastases in 72 to 88 percent of cases. Fistulous involvement of the tracheobronchial tree and aorta/arterial system is seen in approximately 13 percent and 6 percent of cases, respectively.[6,262,284,285] The pattern of nodal metastases seen depends on the location of the primary tumor, although variation does exist.[6,262,280] Tumors of the cervical region tend to drain to the deep cervical, paraesophageal, and posterior mediastinal groups. Tumors of the upper and mid-thoracic esophagus commonly drain to the paraesophageal, posterior mediastinal, and tracheobronchial nodes. Tumors of the lower thoracic esophagus tend to drain toward the paraesophageal, celiac, and splenic groups. Overall, intrathoracic lymph node metastases are most common, followed by those to the subdiaphragmatic and supraclavicular regions.[286]

Visceral metastases are commonly seen only after nodal metastasis occurs.[6] The most common sites detected at autopsy are liver (30 percent), lungs (25 percent), kidneys (8 percent), and adrenal glands (4 percent).[6,262,286] Although uncommon in most prior studies, gastric metastases have more recently been reported in 15 to 20 percent of cases, typically in association with marked esophageal and gastric lymphatic invasion.[282,287] It appears that most visceral metastases are actually present at initial diagnosis.[286] Ectopic hormone production has occasionally been reported. Most commonly reported is hypercalcemia secondary to production of a parathyroid hormone-like substance(s).[288-291]

Survival and Prognostic Indicators. Without treatment esophageal cancer is uniformly fatal, with virtually no survivors at 2 years.[292] Attempts to evaluate survival with various modes of therapy in squamous carcinoma of the esophagus are complicated by several factors. First, many studies have excluded large numbers of patients from evaluation because of unsuitability (inoperability, evidence of nodal or mediastinal involvement, age, nutritional status). While the exclusion of various groups of patients may be clinically reasonable, large biases are introduced, which make comparison of various treatments impossible.[223] Second, to date, no prospective randomized study of various modalities has been performed. A review of 122 surgical series from 1960 to 1978 showed that only 61 percent of patients with esophageal carcinoma were resectable.[293] Perioperative mortality was quite variable, with a mean of 29 percent. More recent reports have found perioperative mortality to be as low as 2 to 5 percent.[260,261] Despite therapy, only 5 to 10 percent of all patients with esophageal carcinoma are alive at 5 years.[294] Five-year survivorship ranging from 5 to 35 percent can be found in selected surgical series (excluding those solely for early esophageal carcinoma),[243,256,259-261,279,280,281] with a similar percentage in patients treated with radiotherapy alone.[295] The role of surgery with adjuvant radiotherapy and/or chemotherapy is currently being explored.[295] Palliation with endoscopic ND:YAG laser therapy is another option.[296]

Several morphologic features appear to affect prognosis and should therefore be clearly stated in the pathology report. Of these, the most important are the presence of lymph node metastases and the depth of mural invasion.[260,273,279,280,281] The 5-year survival after resection of early esophageal carcinoma as defined above has been reported at 60 to 90 percent.[273,276-280,281] This is not surprising, as most patients with EEC will survive more than 5 years without treatment.[297] Overall, patients with and without lymph node metastases are reported as having 5-year survivals in the range of 4 to 22 percent and 40 to 49 percent, respectively.[273,279,280,281] Tumors located in the proximal esophagus are more difficult to resect and may therefore be associated with a poorer prognosis. A tumor length of 7 cm or more is also associated with a poor prognosis, related to the increased frequency of deep mural penetration and lymph node metastases in these tumors.[260,273,279,280] Positive margins of resection are also poor prognostic factors. The controversy regarding histologic grading has been mentioned above.[6,273,279] Recent studies have suggested that aneuploid EEC and AEC with high hyperploid DNA content have relatively poorer prognoses than do corresponding near-diploid tumors.[298,299] This parameter may be an independent predictor of prognosis.

Unusual Epithelial Tumors

Carcinoma with Adenoid Cystic Features

More than 40 cases have been reported in the literature as either adenoid cystic carcinoma or carcinoma with adenoid cystic differentiation,[6,300-304] accounting for less than 1 percent of all esophageal carcinomas.[300] Similar to esophageal squamous carcinoma, this tumor occurs most frequently in men in the sixth or seventh decades, typically arising as a fungating or ulcerative lesion of the mid- or distal esophagus.

Microscopically (similar to adenoid cystic carcinomas arising in salivary gland tissue), one sees a spectrum of histologic appearances including cystic, cribriform, trabecular, and solid patterns. Occasional well formed tubules (ducts) and focal deposition of hyaline-like material may also be seen. The cystic spaces and hyaline material contain acidic and neutral proteoglycans, respectively.[301] The tumor cells are basaloid, with only scant cytoplasm. The chromatin is dispersed and nucleoli are small. This tumor should be distinguished from squamous carcinomas with necrosis, which may simulate a cribriform pattern (pseudoglandular squamous cell carcinoma).[2] By contrast, small solid foci of basaloid tumor cells may strongly resemble small cell carcinoma. In fact, occasional neurosecretory granules have been described by electron microscopy in these tumors.[302]

In contrast to the usual adenoid cystic carcinoma, Epstein et al.[300] found in their series of cases and in a review of the literature that the esophageal tumors had (1) a predominance of solid (basaloid) foci with focal necrosis; (2) a greater degree of nuclear pleomorphism and crowding; (3) commonly two or more mitoses per HPF; (4) the occasional presence of direct continuity with the surface epithelium, which may demonstrate CIS (other investigators have favored an origin from submucosal glands or interculated ducts)[302-304]; and (5) a median survival of

only 9 months after diagnosis, with frequent lymph node and distant metastases.

Although potentially an adenoid cystic carcinoma with clinicopathologic features similar to those of salivary gland origin may arise in the esophagus, to date such a tumor has not been adequately described. It is suggested that the term esophageal carcinoma with adenoid cystic features be used to emphasize both the clinicopathologic similarities with other esophageal carcinomas and the differences with the usual rather low grade behavior of the adenoid cystic carcinoma of the salivary glands. Biopsy diagnosis is often difficult, as the characteristic architectural pattern of this tumor may be absent.

Mucoepidermoid Carcinoma: Adenoacanthoma, Adenosquamous Carcinoma, and Squamous Cell Carcinoma with Pseudoglandular Features

Rarely, malignant esophageal tumors contain areas with both squamous and glandular differentiation.[304-308] Diagnostic terms applied to these tumors vary considerably, causing confusion.

These neoplasms are preferentially found in the lower esophagus of men in the fifth to eighth decades of life. Some of the reported cases have arisen in the setting of BE.[201,309] Unlike mucoepidermoid carcinoma of the salivary glands and lung, the prognosis has been dismal. Nearly all patients have died within 2 years of diagnosis, usually with lymph node and distal metastases. One patient reported by Azzopardi and Menzies was alive and well 14 years after esophageal resection.[304]

It appears that if the term mucoepidermoid carcinoma is to have clinical significance, it should be confined to tumors identical to the descriptions of the better differentiated mucoepidermoid carcinomas of the salivary glands. The cases reported by Osamura et al.[308] and case 2 of Azzopardi and Menzies[304] and perhaps a few others would appear to fit in this category.

While theoretically any poorly differentiated squamous cell carcinoma with some glandular differentiation may indeed be considered mucoepidermoid, it would be preferable to term these simply adenosquamous carcinoma or squamous cell carcinoma with focal glandular differentiation. Adenoacanthoma is best used, as Kay[306] and Ming[6] have suggested, for primary glandular tumors with focal areas of bland squamous differentiation. This is also consistent with the use of this term in the gynecologic literature, in which such tumors are common. Certain squamous cell carcinomas of the esophagus may show areas suggesting gland formation, but fail to stain for proteoglycans. These are best termed squamous cell carcinoma with pseudoglandular features (degeneration) as described in the section on carcinoma with adenoid cystic features.

Rarely, an esophageal carcinoma may demonstrate two clearly different patterns—usually squamous in one area and glandular in another—often with an interdigitating border zone. An example would be a squamous cell carcinoma of the distal esophagus and adenocarcinoma of the cardia.[310,311] This particular variant of adenosquamous carcinoma potentially could represent either multicentric growth (collision tumor) or a change in the phenotype of one of the tumor nodules (composite tumor).[6]

Small Cell Carcinoma: Oat Cell Carcinoma, Small Cell Undifferentiated Carcinoma, and Anaplastic Carcinoma

As of 1984, 65 cases of primary esophageal small cell carcinoma (SCC) had been reported.[312–319] Usually these have been described as being of the oat cell type, although the intermediate cell type has also been reported.[315] SCC accounted for 2.4 percent of 955 primary esophageal carcinomas in one large study.[315] The mean age of onset was 65 years (range 29 to 88 years) and, contrary to pulmonary SCC, there appears to be a slight female predominance.[314] About 90 percent of tumors arise in the middle or lower third of the esophagus and they may be ulcerative, fungating, or polypoid. Rarely, multiple tumor nodules or coexistence with a separate invasive squamous cell carcinoma have been described.[316,317] ACTH and calcitonin have been detected in these tumors, but without an associated endocrine syndrome.[313,317] Of the 64 cases reviewed by Ibrahim et al.,[314] 52 percent demonstrated argyrophilia, and 50 percent demonstrated neurosecretory granules by electron microscopy. Eighty percent of cases were considered pure SCC, while the remaining cases had a squamous and/or glandular component. Some of the published photomicrographs of tumor foci demonstrating glandular differentiation[315] looked quite similar to foci described in so-called adenoid cystic carcinoma of the esophagus. Foci of carcinoid differentiation have also been reported in 13 percent of cases.[315]

Ho has postulated that esophageal SCC arises from totipotential cells which, under the usual scenario of carcinogenic stimulation, differentiate into squamous and, less commonly, adenocarcinoma.[316] Rarely, they may remain as small cells either with or without the presence of neurosecretory granules. A direct transformation of argyrophil cells, which are found scattered in the squamous mucosa of 28 percent of esophagi, is another possibility.[320]

Like pulmonary and other extrapulmonary SCC, these are aggressive tumors. Five-year survival has not been reported to date. Seventy percent of patients are dead within 6 months, frequently with widespread disease.[314] Perhaps early diagnosis and treatment with combination chemotherapy, possibly in conjunction with radiotherapy, will lead to increased survival.[318] Obviously, a primary lung SCC should always be excluded clinically prior to assuming an esophageal origin for this tumor.

Carcinoid

Several cases have been reported as primary carcinoids; however, the pathologic features of some of these, such as a relative paucity of cytoplasm and an increased mitotic rate, suggest that they are at least atypical carcinoids or neuroendocrine carcinomas.[2,321] Few follow-up data are supplied. Any diagnosis of primary esophageal carcinoid should be viewed with suspicion, as 13 percent of small cell carcinomas had foci of carcinoid in one study.[313] An adenocarcinoid has been reported in a series of patients with BE.[201]

Choriocarcinoma

There are three case reports of apparently primary choriocarcinoma of the esophagus to date, one of these being associated with an adenocarcinoma.[322–324] Primary choriocarcinoma as an entity is well established in the stomach, with about one half of cases being admixed with adenocarcinoma.[325]

Polypoid Carcinoma with Dominant Spindle Cell Elements: Polypoid Squamous Carcinoma, Spindle Cell Carcinoma, Carcinosarcoma, Pseudosarcoma, Pseudosarcomatous Carcinoma

More than 17 terms have been applied to the unusual polypoid esophageal neoplasm characterized histologically by a predominant spindle cell component, and typically, small foci of squamous carcinoma.[2,6,155,326–334] Identical tumors have been described in the oral cavity and larynx.[335] It accounts for 0.3 to 2.3 percent of all esophageal cancers, usually occurring in elderly men.[155,326]

Virtually all reported cases occur as bulky polypoid masses attached to the esophageal wall by a broad base or a short pedicle. Multiple tumors have occasionally been described.[334] They are nearly equally distributed between the mid- and lower esophagus, with only rare cases reported from the upper region. Tumor diameter is often 5 to 10 cm; however, larger masses are not uncommon.

The bulk of the tumor is composed of spindle cell elements, usually with admixed bizarre, often multinucleated giant cells (Fig. 27-34). The latter may possess abundant eosinophilic cytoplasm, thus mimicking rhabdomyoblasts, but they nearly always lack cross striations and immunoreactivity for desmin and myoglobin. The stromal element may be heavily collagenized. Rare reported cases have demonstrated osseous, chondroid, or rhabdomyoblastic differentiation.[179,333] The histologi-

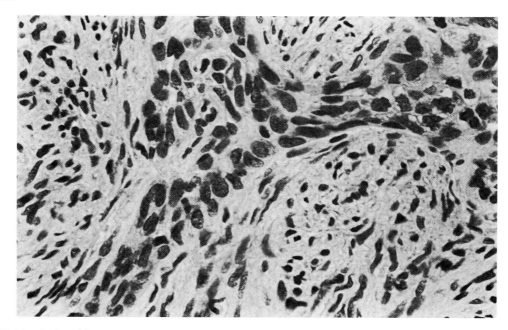

Fig. 27-34. Polypoid squamous carcinoma with dominant spindle cell elements. An admixture of neoplastic epithelial and spindle cells is seen. As the tumor was composed largely of spindle cells, a biopsy might be difficult to interpret. In specimens containing only a spindle cell element, immunoreactivity for cytokeratin and the absence of S-100 protein and markers indicative of muscle differentiation support a diagnosis of carcinoma over melanoma and leiomyosarcoma or rhabdomyosarcoma, respectively. Survival appears related to the degree of mural infiltration.

cally recognizable foci of carcinoma are usually inconspicuous and present at or near the base of the pedicle as in situ or invasive SCC. Rarely undifferentiated carcinoma or even adenocarcinoma may be found. When the two components appear distinctly separate the term carcinoma with pseudosarcoma has been used, whereas an intermingling of these elements has often been interpreted as carcinosarcoma. More likely we are dealing with one process demonstrating a spectrum of microscopic changes.[2,6,327,334] Extensive sectioning may be required to demonstrate the epithelial component, especially in tumors with prominent ulceration. Although bulky, these neoplasms are frequently reported to invade no further than the muscularis propria or even to be limited to the submucosa (early esophageal cancer).

The variety of diagnostic terms used for this entity reflects the varying views regarding the nature of the spindle cell component. Although earlier reports doubted the metastatic potential of the spindle cell element (pseudosarcoma), this has been shown not to be the case.[2,327,334] Therefore, this term should be abandoned. Several ultrastructural studies have demonstrated epithelial features such as tonofilaments and desmosomes, usually in a small proportion of the spindle cells.[327,330] More recently, immunohistochemical studies have also supported an epithelial origin of the spindle cell component.

Gal et al.[155] found that five of their eight cases (62 percent) had occasional spindle cells with immunoreactivity for cytokeratin, while an identical frequency was found by Ellis et al.[335] in their study of 21 similar lesions of the upper aerodigestive tract. The inability of Linder et al.[332] to detect cytokeratin immunoreactivity in the spindle cells may be related to the lack of prior trypsinization, other circumstances known to quench immunoreactivity, or sampling. It remains to be clarified whether the cases that demonstrate a differentiated neoplastic mesenchymal component (e.g., cartilage, bone) represent true carcinosarcomas or also originate via metaplasia of the epithelial component.[330,333]

Metastases have been reported in about 20 percent of cases.[327,334] It is difficult to predict prognosis based on much of the previously reported data, as the numbers of cases are relatively small, the follow-up information rather sketchy, and current improvements in operative technique would certainly decrease the perioperative mortality in prior series.[2,336] In the review of 51 cases by Hinderlieder et al.,[336] only three patients were found to have survived more than 5 years. It does appear, however, that the extent of mural invasion is an important prognostic factor, as analysis of two series shows that two thirds of patients with tumors extending no deeper than the submucosa were listed as survivors with only one tumor-related death, while about 90 percent of patients with deeper invasion were dead; half of the deaths were directly attributable to tumor.[2,327,334] Tumors with the smallest content of histologically recognizable carcinoma and the greatest amount of spindle cell elements (pseudosarcoma) tend to have less extensive mural invasion. This may account for their reported better survival as compared to cases called carcinosarcoma.[2,327,334,336]

Malignant Melanoma and Other Pigmented Lesions

Primary malignant melanoma accounts for less than 0.1 percent of all primary esophageal neoplasms.[326] Mills and Cooper[337–339] accepted 48 cases in their review of the literature as of 1983; since that time, several other cases have been reported. A melanoma may be definitively regarded as primary if an in situ component (radial growth phase, junctional component) is found in the overlying or adjacent mucosa.[337] A junctional component is found in perhaps 40 percent of reported cases.[340] Invasion of the epithelium by a secondary deposit may simulate a junctional component and should be ruled out. It is not unusual for primary melanomas to have extensive areas of ulceration; thus, an in situ component may not be detected. If the esophageal tumor is the dominant lesion, other sources (particularly the skin) are eliminated by careful evaluation, and metastases (if present) are local or regional, the tumor may be considered primary.[337] The progenitor cells of these tumors appear to be nonneoplastic melanocytes, which have been found in the basal layer of the esophageal mucosa in 4 to 8 percent of nonselected esophagi and in 25 percent of primary esophageal melanomas.[320,340,341]

With the exception of one case in a 7-year-old boy,[342] the tumors have occurred in middle-aged to elderly patients (mean 62 years). They present as large (mean 7 cm), distinctly polypoid tumors that are usually heavily pigmented.[337–340,342–344] Adjacent plaque-like zones of melanosis may be seen, occasionally involving the entire esophagus.[337,344] Eighty-five percent of cases occur in the mid- or lower esophagus.

Outcome is quite dismal as indicated in the review of Jawaleker and Tretter, in which 34 of 40 (85 percent) cases were dead within 1 year and only one patient survived 5 years in spite of various therapeutic interventions including surgical resection.[343] Nearly 45 percent of patients have metastases at the time of diagnosis, usually involving the periesophageal lymph nodes, but distant sites as well.[337]

Benign nevi have not as yet been reported. Benign melanin-containing tumors, however, do appear to exist.[164,345] The two reported cases to date were encapsulated intramural black tumors demonstrating spindle cells and occasional polygonal cells containing coarse melanin granules. Palisading was seen in one case,[164] and both contained fat and occasional psammoma bodies. No mitoses were seen in either case. Their precise nature is unclear, but they may represent melanotic schwannomas.

India ink injected into the esophagus in order to indicate a biopsy site may initially cause diagnostic confusion. In one case that we saw recently, an esophagectomy was performed for high-grade dysplasia in BE. At the site of a biopsy taken several weeks previously, there was a nodule containing spindle cells with cytoplasmic black granular pigment that was Fontana-Masson negative and lacked S-100 immunoreactivity. Consultation with the clinician revealed that India ink had been instilled at the site of previous biopsy.

Melanoma metastatic to the esophagus is uncommon. Antemortem metastases from cutaneous melanoma to the GI tract were found in 4.4 percent of cases in one study.[346] Only 1 percent of the metastases were found in the esophagus. An autopsy study also found the esophagus to be the least likely GI site of metastases, being present in only 4 percent of all cases versus 58 percent, 26 percent, and 22 percent for small intestine, stomach, and colon, respectively.[347]

Hematopoietic Tumors

Involvement of the esophagus by lymphoma (either non-Hodgkin's or Hodgkin's types) is nearly always a secondary phenomenon, frequently related to spread from adjacent mediastinal lymph nodes. It occurs with reported frequencies of less than 1 percent to 7.4 percent.[348,349] Rare cases of primary lymphoma have been reported.[350,351] Prominent lymphoid hyperplasia (pseudolymphoma) should be distinguished from lymphoma.[352] A solitary plasmacytoma has also been described.[353]

Secondary Malignant Epithelial Tumors

Secondary esophageal cancer is found in about 3 percent of patients dying with carcinoma.[2,354–356] Direct extension from the lung, upper aerodigestive tract, stomach, and involved mediastinal lymph nodes is relatively frequent, with breast and lung the most common primary sites of true metastatic disease. The esophagus typically appears strictured but, in contrast to primary carcinomas, rarely contains a large fungating or ulcerating mass. Superficial biopsies may not detect the submucosal tumor deposits.

REFERENCES

1. Johns BAE: Developmental changes in the oesophageal epithelium in man. J Anat 86:431, 1952
2. Enterline HT, Thompson JT: Pathology of the Esophagus. Springer-Verlag, New York, 1984

3. Ismail-Beigi F, Horton PF, Pope CE: Histological consequences of gastroesophageal reflux in man. Gastroenterology 58:163, 1970

4. Mitros FA: Inflammatory and neoplastic diseases of the esophagus. p. 1. In Appelman HD (ed): Pathology of the Esophagus, Stomach and Duodenum. Contemporary Issues in Surgical Pathology. Vol. 4. Churchill Livingstone, New York, 1984

5. Geboes K, De Wolf-Peeters C, Rutgeerts P, et al: Lymphocytes and Langerhans cells in the human oesophageal epithelium. Virchows Arch [A] 401:45, 1983

6. Ming SC: Tumors of the Esophagus and Stomach. Atlas of Tumor Pathology. Series 2. Fasc. 7. Armed Forces Institute of Pathology, Washington, DC, 1973, pp. 11–80

7. Ham AW: Esophagus. p. 652. In Histology. 7th Ed. JB Lippincott, Philadelphia, 1974

8. Umlas J, Sakhuja R: The pathology of esophageal intramural pseudodiverticulosis. Am J Clin Pathol 65:314, 1976

9. Vianna A, Hayes P, Moscoso G, et al: Normal venous circulation of the gastroesophageal junction. Gastroenterology 93:876, 1987

10. Goyal RK: Columnar cell-lined (Barrett's) esophagus. A historical perspective. p. 1. In Spechler SJ, Goyal RK (eds): Barrett's Esophagus. Pathophysiology, Diagnosis, and Management. Elsevier, New York, 1985

11. Spechler SJ, Goyal RK: Barrett's esophagus. N Engl J Med 315:362, 1986

12. Haagensen CD, Feind CR, Herter FP, et al: The Lymphatics in Cancer. WB Saunders, Philadelphia, 1972, p. 245

13. Hurwitz AL, Duranceau A: Upper-esophageal sphincter dysfunction. Pathogenesis and treatment. Am J Dig Dis 23:275, 1978

14. Cohen S: Motor disorders of the esophagus. N Engl J Med 301:184, 1979

15. Wesdorp ICE: Reflux oesophagitis: A review. Postgrad Med J 62:43, 1986

16. Aggestrup S, Uddman R, Jensen SL, et al: Regulatory peptides in lower esophageal sphincter of pig and man. Dig Dis Sci 31:1370, 1986

17. Pope CE II: Esophageal physiology. Med Clin North Am 58:1181, 1974

18. Rector LE, Connerley ML: Aberrant mucosa in the esophagus in infants and in children. Arch Pathol 31:285, 1941

19. Jabbari M, Goresky C, Lough J, et al: The inlet patch: Heterotropic gastric mucosa in the upper esophagus. Gastroenterology 89:352, 1985

20. Schridde H: Uber magenschleimhautinseln vom bau der cardialdrusenzone und fundusdrusenregion und den unteren, oesophagealen cardialdrusen gleichende drusen im obersten oesophagusabschnitt. Virchows Arch 175:1, 1904

21. Christensen W, Sternberg SS: Adenocarcinoma of the upper esophagus arising in ectopic gastric mucosa. Am J Surg Pathol 11:397, 1987

22. De La Pava S, Pickren JW: Ectopic sebaceous glands in the esophagus. Arch Pathol 73:397, 1962

23. Ramakrishnan T, Brinker JE: Ectopic sebaceous glands in the esophagus. Gastrointest Endosc 24:293, 1978

24. Merino M, Brand M, LiVolsi VA, McCallum R: Sebaceous glands in the esophagus diagnosed in a clinical setting. Arch Pathol Lab Med 106:47,1982

25. Mahour CH, Harrison EG Jr: Osteochondroma (tracheobronchial-choristoma) of the esophagus. Cancer 20:1489, 1967

26. Salyer DC, Salyer WR, Eggleston JC: Benign developmental cysts of the mediastinum. Arch Pathol Lab Med 101:136, 1977

27. Mindelzun R, Long P: Mediastinal bronchiogenic cysts with esophageal communication. Radiology 126:28, 1977

28. Totten RS, Stout AP, Humphreys GH II, et al: Benign tumors and cysts of the esophagus. J Thorac Surg 25:606, 1953

29. Biovin Y, Cholette J-P, Lefebvre R: Accessory esophagus complicated by an adenocarcinoma. Can Med Assoc J 90:1414, 1964

30. Cohen SR, Thompson JW, Geller KA, et al: Foregut cysts in infants and children. Diagnosis and Management. Ann Otol Rhinol Laryngol 91:622, 1982

31. Dehner LP: Pediatric Surgical Pathology. 2nd Ed. Williams & Wilkins, Baltimore, 1987, p. 335

32. Girdany BR: The esophagus in infancy: Congenital and acquired diseases. Radiol Clin North Am 1:557, 1963

33. Groote AD, Laurini RN, Polman HA: A case of congenital esophageal stenosis. Hum Pathol 16:1170, 1985

34. Benedict EB, Lever WF: Stenosis of the esophagus in benign mucous membrane pemphigus. Ann Otol Rhinol Laryngol 61:1120, 1952

35. Shamma'A MH, Benedict EB: Esophageal webs; report of 58 cases and an attempt at classification. N Engl J Med 259:378, 1978

36. Goyal RK, Glancy JJ, Spiro HM: Lower esophageal ring. N Engl J Med 282:1298, 1970

37. Goyal RK, Bauer JL, Spiro HM: The nature and location of lower esophageal ring. N Engl J Med 284:1175, 1971

38. Burns TW: Motor disorders of the esophagus: Diagnosis and treatment. South Med J 77:956, 1984

39. McCallum RW: The spectrum of esophageal motility disorders. Hosp Pract 22:71, 1987

40. Cohen S: Esophageal motility disorders and their response to calcium channel antagonists. The sphinx revisited. Gastroenterology 93:201, 1987

41. Ferguson TB, Woodbury JD, Roper CL: Giant muscular hypertrophy of the esophagus. Ann Thorac Surg 8:209, 1969

42. Demian SDE, Varges-Cortes F: Idiopathic muscular hypertrophy of the esophagus: Post mortem incidental finding in six cases. Chest 73:28, 1978

43. Iyer S, Chandrasekhara K, Sutton A: Diffusé muscular hypertrophy of esophagus. Am J Med 80:849, 1986

44. Friesen DL, Henderson RD, Hanna W: Ultrastructure of the esophageal muscle in achalasia and diffuse esophageal spasm. Am J Clin Pathol 79:319, 1983

45. Fernandes JP, Mascarenhas MJ, da Costa JC: Diffuse leiomyomatosis of the esophagus. Dig Dis 20:684, 1975

46. Cassella RR, Brown AL, Sayre GP, Ellis FH: Achalasia of the esophagus: Pathologic and etiologic considerations. Ann Surg 160:474, 1964

47. Csendes A, Smok G, Braghetto I, et al: Gastroesophageal

sphincter pressure and histological changes in distal esophagus in patients with achalasia of the esophagus. Dig Dis Sci 30:941, 1985

48. Qualman SJ, Haupt HM, Yang P, Hamilton SR: Esophageal lewy bodies associated with ganglion cell loss in achalasia. Gastroenterology 87:848, 1984

49. Spiro HM: Clinical Gastroenterology. 3rd Ed. Macmillan, London, 1983, p. 69

50. Gallez JF, Berger F, Moulinier B, Partensky C: Esophageal adenocarcinoma following Heller myotomy for achalasia. Endoscopy 19:76, 1987

51. Weaver DH, Maxwell JG, Castleton KB: Mallory-Weiss syndrome. Am J Surg 118:887, 1969

52. Sugawa C, Benishek D, Walt A: Mallory-Weiss syndrome. A study of 224 patients. Am J Surg 145:30, 1983

53. Bradley L, Pairolero PC, Payne WS, Gracey DR: Spontaneous rupture of the esophagus. Arch Surg 116:755, 1981

54. Belsey R: Functional disease of the esophagus. J Thorac Cardiovasc Surg 52:164, 1966

55. Wychulis AR, Gunnlaugsson GH, Clagett OT: Carcinoma occurring in pharyngeo-esophageal diverticulum: Report of three cases. Surgery 66:976, 1969

56. Payne WS, King RM: Pharyngoesophageal (Zenker's) diverticulum. Surg Clin North Am 63:815, 1983

57. Kaye MD: Oesophageal motor dysfunction in patients with diverticula of the mid-thoracic oesophagus. Thorax 29:666, 1974

58. Evander A, Little AG, Ferguson MK, Skinner DB: Diverticula of the mid- and lower esophagus: Pathogenesis and surgical management. World J Surg 10:820, 1986

59. Eckardt VF, Nix W, Kraus W, Bohl J: Esophageal motor function in patients with muscular dystrophy. Gastroenterology 90:628, 1986

60. Bevans M: Changes in the musculature of the gastrointestinal tract and in the myocardium in progressive muscular dystrophy. Arch Pathol 40:225, 1945

61. Rodnan GP, Schumacher R: Primer on Rheumatic Diseases. 8th Ed. Arthritis Foundation, Atlanta, 1983

62. Cohen S, Fisher R, Lipshutz W, et al: Pathogenesis of esophageal dysfunction in scleroderma and Raynaud's disease. J Clin Invest 51:2663, 1972

63. Katzka DA, Reynolds JC, Saul SH, et al: Barrett's metaplasia and adenocarcinoma of the esophagus in scleroderma. Am J Med 82:46, 1987

64. Nebel OT, Fornes MF, Castell DO: Symptomatic gastroesophageal reflux. Incidence and precipitating factors. Dig Dis Sci 21:953, 1976

65. Haggitt R, Tryzelaar J, Ellis FH, Colcher H: Adenocarcinoma complicating columnar epithelium-lined (Barrett's) esophagus. Am J Clin Pathol 70:1, 1978

66. Richter JE, Castell DO: Gastroesophageal reflux. Pathogenesis, diagnosis, and therapy. Ann Intern Med 97:93, 1982

67. Ismail-Beigi F, Pope CE: Distribution of the histological changes of gastroesophageal reflux in the distal esophagus of man. Gastroenterology 66:1109, 1974

68. Weinstein WM, Bogoch ER, Bowes KL: The human esophageal mucosa: A histological reappraisal. Gastroenterology 68:40, 1975

69. Behar J, Sheahan DC: Histologic abnormalities in reflux esophagitis. Arch Pathol 99:387, 1975

70. Seefeld U, Krejs GJ, Siebenmann RE, Blum AL: Esophageal histology in gastroesophageal reflux. Morphometric findings in suction biopsies. Dig Dis 22:956, 1977

71. Johnson LF, Demeester TR, Haggitt RC: Esophageal epithelial response to gastroesophageal reflux. A quantitative study. Dig Dis 23:498, 1978

72. Winter HS, Madara JL, Stafford RJ, et al: Intraepithelial eosinophils: A new diagnostic criterion for reflux esophagitis. Gastroenterology 83:818, 1982

73. Tummala V, Barwick KW, Sontag SJ, et al: The significance of intraepithelial eosinophils in the histologic diagnosis of gastroesophageal reflux. Am J Clin Pathol 87:43, 1987

74. Brown LF, Goldman H, Antonioli DA: Intraepithelial eosinophils in endoscopic biopsies of adults with reflux esophagitis. Am J Surg Pathol 8:899, 1984

75. Collins BJ, Elliott H, Sloan JM, et al: Oesophageal histology in reflux oesophagitis. J Clin Pathol 38:1265, 1985

76. Knuff TE, Benjamin SB, Worsham GF, et al: Histologic evaluation of chronic gastroesophageal reflux. An evaluation of biopsy methods and diagnostic criteria. Dig Dis Sci 29:194, 1984

77. Geboes K, Desmet V, Vantrappen G, Mebis J: Vascular changes in the esophageal mucosa. Early histologic sign of esophagitis. Gastrointest Endosc 26:29, 1980

78. Lee RG: Marked eosinophilia in esophageal mucosal biopsies. Am J Surg Pathol 9:475, 1985

79. Jessurun J, Yardley JH, Giardiello FM, Hamilton SR: Intracytoplasmic plasma proteins in distended esophageal squamous cells (Balloon cells). Mod Pathol 1:175, 1988

80. Barrett NR: Chronic peptic ulcer of the oesophagus and ''oesophagitis.'' Br J Surg 38:175, 1950

81. Allison PR, Johnstone AS: The oesophagus lined by gastric mucous membrane. Thorax 8:87, 1963

82. Barrett NR: The lower esophagus lined by columnar epithelium. Surgery 41:881, 1957

83. Reid BJ, Weinstein WM: Barrett's esophagus and adenocarcinoma. Annu Rev Med 38:477, 1987

84. Haggitt RC, Dean P: Adenocarcinoma in Barrett's epithelium. p. 153. In Spechler SJ, Goyal RK (eds): Barrett's Esophagus. Pathophysiology, Diagnosis, and Management. Elsevier, New York, 1985

85. Sjogren RW, Johnson LF: Barrett's esophagus: A review. Am J Med 74:313, 1983

86. Skinner DB, Walther BC, Riddell RH, et al: Barrett's esophagus. Comparison of benign and malignant cases. Ann Surg 198:554, 1983

87. Cameron AJ, Ott BJ, Payne WJ: The incidence of adenocarcinoma in columnar-lined (Barrett's) esophagus. N Engl J Med 318:857, 1985

88. Hamilton SR: Pathogenesis of columnar cell-lined (Barrett's) esophagus. p. 29. In Spechler SJ, Goyal RK (eds): Barrett's Esophagus. Pathophysiology, Diagnosis, and Management. Elsevier, New York, 1985

89. Bremner CG, Lynch VP, Ellis FH Jr: Barrett's esophagus: Congenital or acquired? An experimental study of

esophageal mucosal regeneration in the dog. Surgery 68:209, 1970

90. Hassall E, Weinstein WM, Ament ME: Barrett's esophagus in childhood. Gastroenterology 89:1331, 1985

91. Sontag SJ, Chljfec G, Stanley MM, et al: Barrett's esophagus and colonic tumors. Lancet 1:946, 1985

92. Ramage JK, Hall J, Williams JG: Barrett's esophagus. Lancet 2:851, 1987

93. Gilchrist AM, Levine MS, Carr RF, et al: Barrett's esophagus: Diagnosis by double contrast esophagography. AJR 150:97, 1988

94. Paull A, Trier JS, Dalton MD, et al: The histologic spectrum of Barrett's esophagus. N Engl J Med 295:476, 1976

95. Thompson JJ, Zinsser KR, Enterline H: Barrett's metaplasia and adenocarcinoma of the esophagus and gastroesophageal junction. Hum Pathol 14:42, 1983

96. Buchan AMJ, Grant S, Freeman HJ: Regulatory peptides in Barrett's oesophagus. J Pathol 146:227, 1985

97. Dayal Y, Wolfe HJ: Endocrine cells in Barrett's epithelium. p. 59. In Spechler SJ, Goyal RK (eds): Barrett's Esophagus. Pathophysiology, Diagnosis, and Management. Elsevier, New York, 1985

98. Peuchmaur M, Potet F, Goldfain D: Mucin histochemistry of the columnar epithelium of the esophagus (Barrett's esophagus): A prospective biopsy study. J Clin Pathol 37:607, 1984

99. Lee RG: Mucins in Barrett's esophagus. A histochemical study. Am J Clin Pathol 81:500, 1981

100. Zwas F, Shields HM, Doos WG, et al: Scanning electron microscopy of Barrett's epithelium and its correlation with light microscopy and mucin stains. Gastroenterology 90:1932, 1986

101. Kalish RJ, Clancy PE, Osringer MD, Appelman HD: Clinical, epidemiologic, and morphologic comparison between adenocarcinomas arising in Barrett's esophageal mucosa and in the gastric cardia. Gastroenterology 86:461, 1984

102. Lee RG: Dysplasia in Barrett's esophagus. A clinicopathologic study of six patients. Am J Surg Pathol 9:845, 1985

103. Hamilton SR, Smith RRL: The relationship between columnar epithelial dysplasia and invasive adenocarcinoma arising in Barrett's esophagus. Am J Clin Pathol 87:301, 1987

104. Riddell RH: Dysplasia and regression in Barrett's epithelium. p. 143. In Spechler SJ, Goyal RK (eds): Barrett's Esophagus. Pathophysiology, Diagnosis, and Management. Elsevier, New York, 1985

105. Robey SS, Hamilton SR, Gupta RK, Erozan YS: Diagnostic value of cytopathology in Barrett esophagus and associated carcinoma. Am J Clin Pathol 89:493, 1988

106. Reid BJ, Weinstein WM, Lewin KJ, et al: Endoscopic biopsy can detect high-grade dysplasia or early adenocarcinoma in Barrett's esophagus without grossly recognizable neoplastic lesions. Gastroenterology 94:81, 1988

107. Reid BJ, Haggitt RC, Rubin CE, et al: Criteria for dysplasia in Barrett's esophagus. A cooperative consensus study. Gastroenterology 90:A117, 1985

108. Reid BJ, Haggitt RC, Rubin CE, Rabinovitch PS: Flow cytometry complements histology in detecting patients at risk for Barrett's adenocarcinoma. Gastroenterology 93:1, 1987

109. Shimomoto C, Weinstein WW, Boland CR: Glycoconjugate (GC) in metaplastic and dysplastic epithelium in Barrett's esophagus (BE). Gastroenterology 90:A17, 1986

110. Westerveld BD, Pals G, Bosma A, et al: Gastric proteases in Barrett's esophagus. Gastroenterology 93:774, 1987

111. Spechler SJ: Endoscopic surveillance for patients with Barrett esophagus: Does the cancer risk justify the practice? Ann Intern Med 106:902, 1987

112. Pope CE: Regression of Barrett's epithelium. p. 223. In Spechler SJ, Goyal RK (eds): Barrett's Esophagus. Pathophysiology, Diagnosis, and Management. Elsevier, New York, 1985

113. Castillo S, Aburashed A, Kimmelman J, et al: Diffuse intramural esophageal pseudodiverticulosis. New cases and review. Gastroenterology 72:541, 1977

114. Levine MS, Moolten DN, Herlinger H, Laufer I: Esophageal intramural pseudodiverticulosis: A reevaluation. AJR 147:1165, 1986

115. Sabanathan S, Salama FD, Morgan WE: Oesophageal intramural pseudodiverticulosis. Thorax 40:849, 1985

116. Rotterdam H, Sommers SC: Alimentary tract biopsy lesions in the acquired immune deficiency syndrome. Pathology 17:181, 1985

117. Kazlow PG, Shah K, Benkov KJ, et al: Esophageal cryptosporidiosis in a child with acquired immune deficiency syndrome. Gastroenterology 91:1301, 1986

118. Tom W, Aaron JS: Esophageal ulcers caused by *Torulopsis glabrata* in a patient with acquired immune deficiency syndrome. Am J Gastroenterol 82:766, 1987

119. McManus JPA, Webb JN: A yeast-like infection of the esophagus caused by *Lactobacillus acidophilus*. Gastroenterology 68:583, 1975

120. Jass JR: The esophagus. p. 136. In Morson BC (ed): Alimentary Tract. Systemic Pathology. Vol. 3. 3rd Ed. Churchill Livingstone, London, 1987

121. Paull G, Yardley JH: Gastric and esophageal *Campylobacter pylori* in patient with Barrett's esophagus. Gastroenterology 95:216, 1988

122. Khandekar A, Moser D, Fidler WJ: Blastomycosis of the esophagus. *Ann Thorac Surg* 30:76, 1980

123. Jacobs DH, Macher AB, Handler R, et al: Esophageal cryptococcosis in a patient with the hyperimmunoglobulin E—Recurrent infection (Job's) syndrome. Gastroenterology 87:201, 1984

124. Kodsi BE, Wickremesinghe PC, Kozinn PJ, et al: Candida esophagitis. A prospective study of 27 cases. Gastroenterology 71:715, 1976

125. Lewicki AM, Moore JP: Esophageal moniliasis. A review of common and less frequent characteristics. AJR 125:218, 1975

126. Lightdale CJ, Wolf DJ, Marcucci RA, et al: Herpetic esophagitis in patients with cancer: Ante mortem diagnosis by brush cytology. Cancer 39:223, 1977

127. Lasser A: Herpes simplex virus esophagitis. Acta Cytol 31:301, 1977

128. Nash G, Ross JS: Herpetic esophagitis. A common cause of esophageal ulceration. Hum Pathol 5:339, 1974

129. Desigan N, Schneider R: Herpes simplex esophagitis in healthy adults. South Med J 78:1135, 1985

130. Matsumoto J, Sumiyoshi A: Herpes simplex esophagitis—A study in autopsy series. Am J Clin Pathol 84:96, 1985

131. Berthrong M, Fajardo LF: Radiation injury in surgical pathology. Am J Surg Pathol 5:153, 1981

132. LiVolsi VA, Jaretzki A III: Granulomatous esophagitis. A case of Crohn's disease limited to the esophagus. Gastroenterology 64:313, 1973

133. Haggitt RC, Meissner WA: Crohn's disease of the upper gastrointestinal tract. Am J Clin Pathol 59:613, 1973

134. Lee C-S, Mangla JC, Lee S-SC: Crohn's disease in Barrett's esophagus. Am J Gastroenterol 69:646, 1978

135. Damtew B, Frengley D, Wolinsky E, Spagnuolo PJ: Esophageal tuberculosis: Mimicry of gastrointestinal malignancy. Rev Infect Dis 9:140, 1987

136. Wiesner PJ, Kleinman MS, Condemi JJ, et al: Sarcoidosis of the esophagus. Am J Dig Dis 16:943, 1971

137. Bott S, Prakash C, McCallum RW: GI drug column. Medication induced esophageal injury: Survey of the literature. Am J Gastroenterol 82:758, 1987

138. Bonavina L, DeMeester TR, McChesney L, et al: Drug-induced esophageal strictures. Ann Surg 206:173, 1987

139. Rothstein FC: Caustic injuries to the esophagus in children. Pediatr Clin North Am 33:665, 1986

140. Spechler SJ, Schimmel EM, Dalton JW, et al: Barrett's epithelium complicating lye ingestion with sparing of the distal esophagus. Gastroenterology 81:580, 1981

141. McDonald GB, Sullivan KM, Schuffler MD, et al: Esophageal abnormalities in chronic graft-versus-host disease in humans. Gastroenterology 80:914, 1981

142. Fleischer D: Endoscopic therapy of upper gastrointestinal bleeding in humans. Gastroenterology 90:217, 1986

143. Pushpanathan C, Idikio H: Pathological findings in the esophagus after endoscopic sclerotherapy for variceal bleeding. Am J Gastroenterol 81:9, 1986

144. Kitano S, Koyanagi N, Iso Y, et al: Prevention of recurrence of esophageal varices after endoscopic injection sclerotherapy with ethanolamine oleate. Hepatology 7:810, 1987

145. Seremitis MG, Lyons WS, de Guzman VC, et al: Leiomyomata of the esophagus. An analysis of 838 cases. Cancer 38:2166, 1976

146. Takubo K, Nakagawa H, Tsuchiya S, et al: Seedling leiomyoma of the esophagus and esophagogastric junction zone. Hum Pathol 12:1006, 1981

147. Saul SH, Rast ML, Brooks JJ: The immunohistochemistry of gastrointestinal stromal tumors. Am J Surg Pathol 11:464, 1987

148. Laufer I (ed): Double Contrast Gastrointestinal Radiology with Endoscopic Correlation. WB Saunders, Philadelphia, 1979

149. Appelman HD: Stromal tumors of the esophagus, stomach and duodenum. p. 195. In Appelman HD (ed): Pathology of the Esophagus, Stomach and Duodenum. Contemporary Issues in Surgical Pathology. Vol. 4. Churchill Livingstone, New York, 1984

150. Miettinen M: Gastrointestinal stromal tumors: An immunohistochemical study of cellular differentiation. Am J Clin Pathol 89:601, 1988

151. Saitoh K, Nasu M, Kamiyama R, et al: Solitary neurofibroma of the esophagus. Acta Pathol Jpn 35:527, 1985

152. Partyka EK, Sanowski RA, Kozarek RA: Endoscopic diagnosis of a giant esophageal leiomyosarcoma. Am J Gastroenterol 75:132, 1981

153. Gaede JT, Postlethwait RW, Shelburne JT, et al: Leiomyosarcoma of the esophagus. Report of two cases, one with associated squamous cell carcinoma. J Thorac Cardiovasc Surg 75:740, 1978

154. Norton AJ, Thomas JA, Isaacson PG: Cytokeratin-specific monoclonal antibodies are reactive with tumours of smooth muscle derivation. An immunocytochemical and biochemical study using antibodies to intermediate filament cytoskeletal proteins. Histopathology 11:487, 1987

155. Gal AA, Martin SE, Kernen JA, Patterson MJ: Esophageal carcinoma with prominent spindle cells. Cancer 60:2244, 1987

156. Berk RN, Scher GS, Bode DF: Unusual tumors of the gastrointestinal tract. AJR 113:159, 1971

157. Rainer WG, Brus R: Leiomyosarcoma of the esophagus: Review of the literature and report of three cases. Surgery 58:343, 1965

158. Marston EL, Bradshaw HH: Idiopathic muscular hypertrophy of the esophagus. J Thorac Cardiovasc Surg 38:248, 1959

159. Fernandes JP, Mascarenhas MJ, Costa CD, et al: Diffuse leiomyomatosis of the esophagus: A case report and review of the literature. Am J Dig Dis 20:684, 1975

160. Kabuto T, Taniguchi K, Iwanaga T, et al: Diffuse leiomyomatosis of the esophagus. Dig Dis Sci 25:388, 1980

161. Heald J, Moussalli H, Hasleton PS: Diffuse leiomyomatosis of the oesophagus. Histopathology 10:755, 1986

162. Schapiro RL, Sandrock AR: Esophagogastric and vulvar leiomyomatosis: A new radiologic syndrome. J Can Assoc Radiol 24:184, 1973

163. Wahlen T, Astedt B: Familial occurrence of coexisting leiomyoma of vulva and oesophagus. Acta Obstet Gynecol Scand 44:197, 1965

164. Assor D: A melanocytic tumor of the esophagus. Cancer 35:1438, 1975

165. Johnston J, Helwig EB: Granular cell tumors of the gastrointestinal tract and perianal region. A study of 74 cases. Dig Dis Sci 26:807, 1981

166. Vuyk HD, Snow GB, Tiwari RM, et al: Granular cell tumor of the proximal esophagus. A rare disease. Cancer 55:445, 1985

167. Mannion P, Honan RP, Fitzgerald MD, Haselton PS: Contiguous granular cell myoblastoma and squamous cell carcinoma in the oesophagus. Thorax 40:551, 1985

168. Goolden AWG: Radiation cancer of pharynx. Br Med J 2:1110, 1951

169. Plachta A: Benign tumors of the esophagus. Review of literature and report of 99 cases. Am J Gastroenterol 38:639, 1962

170. Bernatz PE, Smith SL, Ellis FH Jr, et al: Benign, pedunculated, intraluminal tumors of the esophagus. J Thorac Surg 35:503, 1958

171. Patel J, Kieffer RW, Martin M, Avant GR: Giant fibrovascular polyp of the esophagus. Gastroenterology 87:953, 1984

172. Stout AP, Lattes R: p. 25. In Atlas of Tumor Pathology. Series 1. Fasc. 20. Armed Forces Institute of Pathology, Washington, DC, 1957

173. LiVolsi VA, Perzin KH: Inflammatory pseudotumors (inflammatory fibrous polyps) of the esophagus. Am J Dig Dis 20:475, 1975

174. Bleshman MH, Banner MP, Johnson RC: The inflammatory esophagogastric polyp and fold. Radiology 128:589, 1978

175. Branski D, Gardner RV, Fisher JE, et al: Gastroesophageal polyp as a cause of hematemesis in adolescence. Am J Gastroenterol 73:448, 1980

176. Nora PF: Lipoma of the esophagus. Am J Surg 108:353, 1964

177. Allen MS Jr, Talbot WH: Sudden death due to regurgitation of a pedunculated esophageal lipoma. J Thorac Cardiovasc Surg 54:756, 1967

178. Vartio T, Nickels J, Hockerstedt K, Scheinin TM: Rhabdomyosarcoma of the Oesophagus. Virchows Arch [A] 386:357, 1980

179. Ende M, Pizzolato P, Raider L, Ziskind J: An unusual carcinosarcoma. AJR 65:227, 1951

180. Haratake J, Jimi A, Horie A, et al: Malignant mesenchymoma of the esophagus. Acta Pathol Jpn 34:925, 1984

181. Brooks JSJ, Freeman M, Enterline HT: Malignant ''Triton'' tumors. Natural history and immunohistochemistry of nine new cases with literature review. Cancer 55:2543, 1985

182. Bloch MJ, Iozzo RV, Edmunds LH, Brooks JJ: Polypoid synovial sarcoma of the esophagus. Gastroenterology 92:229, 1987

183. Hanel K, Talley NA, Hunt DR: Hemangioma of the esophagus: An unusual cause of upper gastrointestinal bleeding. Dig Dis Sci 26:257, 1981

184. Okumura T, Tanoue S, Chiba K, Tanaka S: Lobular capillary hemangioma of the esophagus. A case report and review of the literature. Acta Pathol Jpn 33:1303, 1983

185. Rosenblum WI, Nakoneczna I, Konerding HS, et al: Multiple vascular malformation in the ''blue rubber bleb naevus'' syndrome: A case with aneurysm of the vein of Galen and vascular lesions suggesting a link to the Weber-Osler-Rendu syndrome. Histopathology 2:301, 1978

186. Armengol-Miro JR, Ramentol F, Salord J, et al: Lymphangioma of the oesophagus. Diagnosis and treatment by endoscopic polypectomy. Endoscopy 3:185, 1979

187. Palanker HK, Constantine AB, Paine JR: Successful resection of an angioendothelioma of the cervical esophagus. Arch Surg 62:627, 1951

188. Siegel JH, Janis R, Alper JC, et al: Disseminated visceral Kaposi's sarcoma appearance after human renal homograft operation. JAMA 207:1493, 1969

189. Umerah BD: Kaposi sarcoma of the oesophagus. Br J Radiol 53:807, 1980

190. Saltz RK, Kurtz RC, Lightdale CJ, et al: Kaposi's sarcoma: Gastrointestinal involvement correlation with skin findings and immunologic function. Dig Dis Sci 29:817, 1984

191. Stout AP, Lattes R: Tumors of the Esophagus. Atlas of Tumor Pathology. Series 1. Fasc. 20. Armed Forces Institute of Pathology, Washington, DC, 1957

192. Beckerman RC, Taussig LM, Froede RC, et al: Fibromuscular hamartoma of the esophagus in an infant. Am J Dis Child 134:153, 1980

193. Yaghami I, Ghahremani GG: Chondrosarcoma of the esophagus. AJR 126:1175, 1976

194. McIntyre M, Webb JN, Browning GCP: Osteosarcoma of the esophagus. Hum Pathol 13:680, 1982

195. McDonald GB, Brand DL, Thorning DR: Multiple adenomatous neoplasms arising in columnar-lined (Barrett's) esophagus. Gastroenterology 72:1317, 1977

196. Wang HH, Antonioli DA, Goldman H: Comparative features of esophageal and gastric adenocarcinomas: Recent changes in type and frequency. Hum Pathol 17:482, 1986

197. Levine MS, Caroline D, Thompson JJ, et al: Adenocarcinoma of the esophagus: Relationship to Barrett mucosa. Radiology 150:305, 1984

198. Appelman HD, Kalish RJ, Clancy PE, Orringer MB: Distinguishing features of adenocarcinoma in Barrett's esophagus and in the gastric cardia. p. 167. In Spechler SJ, Goyal RK (eds): Barrett's Esophagus. Pathophysiology, Diagnosis, and Management. Elsevier, New York, 1985

199. Spechler SJ, Robbins AH, Rubins HB, et al: Adenocarcinoma and Barrett's esophagus. An overrated risk? Gastroenterology 87:927, 1984

200. Sjogren RW, Johnson LF: Clinical features of Barrett's esophagus. p. 75. In Spechler SJ, Goyal RK (eds): Barrett's Esophagus. Pathophysiology, Diagnosis, and Management. Elsevier, New York, 1985

201. Smith RRL, Boitnott J, Hamilton SR, Rogers EL: The spectrum of carcinoma arising in Barrett's esophagus. A clinicopathologic study of 26 patients. Am J Surg Pathol 8:563, 1984

202. Chambers LA, Clark WE: The endoscopic diagnosis of gastroesophageal malignancy. A cytologic review. Acta Cytol 30:110, 1986

203. Kochhar R, Gupta SK, Malik AK, Mehta SK: Endoscopic fine needle aspiration biopsy. Acta Cytol 31:481, 1987

204. Levine MS, Dillon EC, Saul SH, Laufer I: Early esophageal cancer. AJR 146:507, 1986

205. Schmidt LW, Dean PJ, Wilson RT: Superficially invasive squamous cell carcinoma of the esophagus. A study of seven cases in Memphis, Tennessee. Gastroenterology 91:14561, 1986

206. Sanfey H, Hamilton SR, Smith RRL, Cameron JL: Carcinomas arising in Barrett's esophagus. Surg Gynecol Obstet 161:570, 1985

207. Stern Z, Sharon P, Ligumsky M, et al: Glycogenic acanthosis of the esophagus. Am J Gastroenterol 74:261, 1980

208. Rywlin AM, Ortega R: Glycogenic acanthosis of the esophagus. Arch Pathol 90:439, 1970

209. Glick SN, Teplick SK, Goldstein J, et al: Glycogenic acanthosis of the esophagus. AJR 139:683, 1982

210. Bender MD, Allison J, Cuartas F, et al: Glycogenic acanthosis of the esophagus: A form of benign epithelial hyperplasia. Gastroenterology 65:373, 1973

211. Colina F, Solis JA, Munoz MT: Squamous papilloma of the esophagus. Am J Gastroenterol 74:410, 1980

212. Walker JH: Giant papilloma of the thoracic esophagus. AJR 131:519, 1978

213. Franzin G, Musola R, Zamboni G, et al: Squamous papillomas of the esophagus. Gastrointest Endosc 29:104, 1983

214. Fernandez-Rodriguez CM, Badia-Figuerola N, Ruiz el Arbol L, et al: Squamous papilloma of the esophagus: Report of six cases with long-term follow-up in four patients. Am J Gastroenterol 81:1059, 1986

215. Javdan P, Pitman ER: Squamous papilloma of esophagus. Dig Dis Sci 29:317, 1984

216. Winkler B, Capo V, Reumann W, et al: Human papillomavirus infection of the esophagus. A clinicopathologic study with demonstration of papillomavirus antigen by the immunoperoxidase technique. Cancer 55:149, 1985

217. Parnell SAC, Peppercorn MA, Antonioli DA, et al: Squamous cell papilloma of esophagus. Report of a case after peptic esophagitis and repeated bougienage with a review of the literature. Gastroenterology 74:910, 1978

218. Waterfall WE, Somers S, Desa DJ: Benign oesophageal papillomatosis. A case report with review of the literature. J Clin Pathol 31:111, 1978

219. Brinson RR, Schuman BM, Mills LR, et al: Multiple squamous papillomas of the esophagus associated with Goltz syndrome. Am J Gastroenterol 82:1177, 1987

220. Itai Y, Kogure T, Okuyama Y: Radiologic manifestations of esophageal involvement in acanthosis nigricans. Br J Radiol 49:592, 1976

221. Schottenfeld D: Epidemiology of cancer of the esophagus. Semin Oncol 11:92, 1984

222. Sons HU: Etiologic and epidemiologic factors of carcinoma of the esophagus. Surg Gynecol Obstet 165:183, 1987

223. Spechler SJ: Overview of esophageal cancer. p. 243. In Levin B (ed): Gastrointestinal Cancer. Current Approaches to Diagnosis and Treatment. University of Texas Press, Austin, 1988

224. Correa P: Precursors of gastric and esophageal cancer. Cancer 50:2554, 1982

225. Pour P, Ghadirian P: Familial cancer of the esophagus in Iran. Cancer 33:1649, 1974

226. Tyldesley WR: Oral leukoplakia associated with tylosis and esophageal carcinoma. J Oral Pathol 3:62, 1974

227. Ritter SB, Peterson G: Esophageal cancer, hyperkeratosis and oral leukoplakia: Occurrence in a 25-year-old woman. JAMA 235:1723, 1976

228. Wynder EL, Mabuchi K: Etiologic and environmental factors (cancer of esophagus) JAMA 226:1546, 1973

229. Burrell RJW, Roach WA, Shadwell A: Esophageal cancer in the Bantu of the Transkei associated with mineral deficiency in garden plants. J Natl Cancer Inst 36:201, 1966

230. McGlashan ND: Oesophageal cancer and alcoholic spirits in central Africa. Gut 10:643, 1969

231. Auerbach O, Stout AP, Hammond EC, et al: Histologic changes in esophagus in relation to smoking habits. Arch Environ Health 11:4, 1965

232. Miller RW: High esophageal cancer rates in humans and chickens in north China. J Natl Cancer Inst 54:535, 1975

233. Wynder EL, Hultberg S, Jacobsson E, et al: Environmental factors in cancer of the upper alimentary tract. A Swedish study with special reference to Plummer-Vinson (Paterson-Kelly) syndrome. Cancer 10:470, 1957

234. Wynder EL, Fryer JN: Etiologic considerations of Plummer-Vinson (Paterson-Kelly) syndrome. Ann Intern Med 49:1106, 1958

235. Munoz N, Crespi M: High-risk conditions and precancerous lesions of the oesophagus. p. 53. In Sherlock P, Morson B, Barbara L, Veronesi U (eds): Precancerous Lesions of the Gastrointestinal Tract. Raven Press, New York, 1983

236. Carter R, Brewer LA III: Achalasia and esophageal carcinoma: Studies in early diagnosis for improved surgical management. Am J Surg 130:114, 1975

237. Lortat-Jacobs JL, Richard CA, Fekete F, et al: Cardiospasm and esophageal carcinoma. A report of 24 cases. Surgery 66:969, 1970

238. Wychulis AR, Woolam GL, Andersen HA, et al: Achalasia and carcinoma of the esophagus. JAMA 215:1638, 1971

239. Bolivar JC, Herendeen TL: Carcinoma of the esophagus and achalasia. Ann Thorac Surg 10, 81, 1970

240. Applequist JS, Brick HG: Lye corrosion carcinoma of the esophagus. Cancer 45:2655, 1980

241. DuPlessis LS, Nunn JR, Roach WA: Carcinogen in a Transkeian Bantu food additive. Nature (Lond) 222:1198, 1969

242. Holmes GKT, Stokes PL, Sorahan TM, et al: Coeliac disease, gluten free diet, and malignancy. Gut 17:612, 1976

243. Shani M, Modau B: Esophageal cancer in Israel: Selected clinical and epidemiologic aspects. Am J Dig Dis 20:951, 1975

244. Huang GJ, K'ai WY: Clinical diagnosis. p. 237. In Huang GJ, K'ai WY (eds): Carcinoma of the Esophagus and Gastric Cardia. Springer-Verlag, New York, 1984

245. Rubin P: Cancer of the gastrointestinal tract. I. Esophagus: Detection and diagnosis. JAMA 226:1544, 1973

246. Munoz N, Grassi A, Qiong S, et al: Precursor lesions of oesophageal cancer in high-risk populations in Iran and China. Lancet 1:876, 1982

247. Wiot JW, Felson B: Cancer of the gastrointestinal tract. Radiologic differential diagnosis. JAMA 226:1548, 1973

248. Morrissey JF: Cancer of the gastrointestinal tract. Endoscopic diagnosis. JAMA 226:1552, 1973

249. Prolla JC: Cancer of the gastrointestinal tract. Histopathology and cytology in detection. JAMA 226:1554, 1973

250. Rubin P: Cancer of the gastrointestinal tract. Comment: Cancer epidemiology. JAMA 226:1557, 1973

251. Proll JC, Reilly RW, Kirsner JB, et al: Direct vision endoscopic cytology and biopsy in the diagnosis of esophageal and gastric tumors: Current experience. Acta Cytol 21:399, 1977

252. Nabeya K: Markers of cancer risk in the esophagus and surveillance of high risk groups. p. 71. In Sherlock P, Morson B, Barbara L, Veronesi U (eds): Precancerous Lesions of the Gastrointestinal Tract. Raven Press, New York, 1983

253. Shen Q: Diagnostic cytology and early detection. p. 155. In Huang GJ, K'ai WY (eds): Carcinoma of the Esophagus and Gastric Cardia. Springer-Verlag, New York, 1984

254. Jessun K, Paolucci P, Classen M: Endoscopic vital staining of the oesophagus in high risk patients: Detection of dysplasia and early carcinoma. p. 65. In Sherlock P, Morson B, Barbara L, Veronesi U (eds): Precancerous Lesions of the Gastrointestinal Tract. Raven Press, New York, 1983

255. Beahrs OH, Myers MH: Manual for Staging of Cancer. 2nd Ed. JB Lippincott, Philadelphia, 1983

256. Parker EF, Gregorie HB: Carcinoma of the esophagus. JAMA 235:1018, 1976

257. Stone R, Rangel DM, Gordon HE, et al: Carcinoma of the gastroesophageal junction. Am J Surg 134:70, 1977

258. Pearson JG: The value of radiotherapy in the management of esophageal cancer. AJR 105:500, 1969

259. Parker EF, Gregorie HB Jr, Arrants JE, et al: Carcinoma of the esophagus. Ann Surg 171:746, 1970

260. Lu YK, Li YM, Gu YZ: Cancer of esophagus and esophagogastric junction: Analysis of results of 1,025 resections after 5 to 20 years. Ann Thorac Surg 43:176, 1987

261. Akiyama H, Tsurumaru M, Watanabe G, et al: Development of surgery for carcinoma of the esophagus. Am J Surg 147:9, 1984

262. Sons HU, Borchard F: Esophageal cancer. Arch Pathol Lab Med 108:983, 1984

263. Pearson JG: Cancer of the gastrointestinal tract. The value of radiation therapy. JAMA 227:181, 1974

264. McGregor DH, Mills G, Baudet RA: Intramural squamous cell carcinoma of the esophagus. Cancer 37:1556, 1976

265. The Coordinating Groups for the Research of Esophageal Carcinoma, Honan Province and Chinese Academy of Medical Sciences: Studies on relationship between epithelial dysplasia and carcinoma of the esophagus. Chin Med J 1:110, 1975

266. Mandard AM, Marnay J, Gignoux M, et al: Cancer of the esophagus and associated lesions: Detailed pathologic study of 100 esophagectomy specimens. Hum Pathol 15:6609, 1984

267. Postlethwait RW, Musser AW: Changes in the esophagus in 1000 autopsy specimens. J Thorac Cardiovasc Surg 68:953, 1974

268. Bishop D, Lushpihan, A: The cytology of carcinoma-in-situ and early invasive carcinoma of the esophagus. Acta Cytol 21:298, 1977

269. Mukada T, Sasano N, Sato E: Evaluation of esophageal dysplasia by cytofluorometric analysis. Cancer 41:1399, 1978

270. Goran DA, Shields HM, Bates ML, et al: Esophageal dysplasia. Assessment by light microscopy and scanning electron microscopy. Gastroenterology 86:39, 1984

271. Minielly JA, Harrison EG, Fontana RS, Payne WS: Verrucous squamous cell carcinoma of the esophagus. Cancer 20:2078, 1967

272. Agha FP, Weatherbee L, Sams JS: Verrucous carcinoma of the esophagus. Am J Gastroenterol 79:844, 1984

273. Liu FS, Zhou CN: Pathology of carcinoma of the esophagus. p. 77. In Huang GJ, K'ai WY (eds): Carcinoma of the Esophagus and Gastric Cardia. Springer-Verlag, New York, 1984

274. Schickendantz GA, Sabaugh RA, Ramos Mejia MM, Terzano G: Cytologic-histopathologic correlation in esophageal cancer. Acta Cytol 11:64, 1967

275. Shu YJ: Cytopathology of the esophagus. An overview of esophageal cytopathology in China. Acta Cytol 27:7, 1983

276. Tumor Prevention, Treatment and Research Groups: Pathology of early esophageal squamous cell carcinoma. Chin Med J 3:180, 1977

277. Guojun H, Lingfang S, Dawei Z, et al: Diagnosis and surgical treatment of early esophageal carcinoma. Chin Med J 94:229, 1981

278. Benasco C, Combalia N, Pou JM, Miquel JM: Superficial esophageal carcinoma: A report of 12 cases. Gastrointest Endosc 31:64, 1985

279. Watson A: Pathologic changes affecting survival in esophageal cancer. p. 90. In Delarue NC, Wilkins EW, Wong J (eds): Esophageal Cancer. International Trends in General Thoracic Surgery. Vol. 4. CV Mosby, St Louis, 1988

280. Mountain CF: Rationale in staging of cancer of the esophagus. p. 73. In Delarue NC, Wilkins, EW, Wong J (eds): Esophageal Cancer. International Trends in Thoracic Surgery. Vol. 4. CV Mosby, St Louis, 1988

281. Barge J, Molas G, Maillard JN, et al: Superficial oesophageal carcinoma: An oesophageal counterpart of early gastric cancer. Histopathology 5:499, 1981

282. Japanese Society for Esophageal Diseases: Guidelines for the clinical and pathologic studies on carcinoma of the esophagus. Jpn J Surg 6:69, 1976

283. Takubo K, Takai A, Takayama S, et al: Intraductal spread of esophageal squamous cell carcinoma carcinoma. Cancer 59:1751, 1987

284. Martini N, Goodner JT, D'Angio GJ, et al: Tracheoesophageal fistula due to cancer. J Thorac Cardiovasc Surg 59:319, 1970

285. Soreide O, Janssen CW, Koam G, et al: Aorto-oesophageal fistula complicating carcinoma of the oesophagus. Scand J Thorac Cardiovasc Surg 10:79, 1976

286. Anderson LL, Lad TE: Autopsy findings in squamous cell carcinoma of the esophagus. Cancer 50:1587, 1982

287. Saito T, Iizuka T, Kato H, Watanabe H: Esophageal carcinoma metastatic to the stomach. A clinicopathologic study of 35 cases. Cancer 56:2235, 1985

288. Grajower M, Barel VS: Ectopic hyperparathyroidism (pseudohyperparathyroidism) in esophageal malignancy. Am J Med 61:134, 1976

289. Mundy GR, Ibbotson KJ, D'Souza SM: Tumor products and the hypercalcemia of malignancy. J Clin Invest 76:381, 1985

290. Hamilton JW, Hartman CR, McGregor DH, et al: Synthesis of parathyroid hormone-like peptides by a human squamous cell carcinoma. J Clin Endocrinol Metab 45:1023, 1977

291. Kumar GK, Naidu VG, Razzaque MA: Esophageal carcinoma with pseudohyperparathyroidism and hypercorticism. Am J Gastroenterol 65:222, 1976

292. Roberts JG: Cancer of the esophagus—How should tumor biology affect treatment? Br J Surg 67:791, 1980

293. Earlam R, Cunha-Melo JR: Oesophageal squamous cell

carcinoma: I. A critical review of surgery. Br J Surg 67:381, 1980

294. Sondik EJ, Young JL, Horm JW: 1985 annual cancer statistics review. National Cancer Advisory Board, National Institutes of Health, Bethesda, MD, 1985

295. Rich TA, Ajani JA: Radiotherapy for esophageal cancer. p. 261. In Levin B (ed): Gastrointestinal cancer. Current approaches to diagnosis and treatment. University of Texas Press, Austin, 1988

296. Lightdale CJ, Zimbalist E, Winawer SJ: Outpatient management of esophageal cancer with endoscopic Nd: YAG Laser. Am J Gastroenterol 82:46, 1987

297. Yanjin M, Xianzhi G, Guangyi L, Wenheng C: Detection and natural progression of early oesophageal carcinoma: Preliminary communication. J R Soc Med 74:884, 1981

298. Matsuura H, Sugimachi K, Ueo H, et al: Malignant potentiality of squamous cell carcinoma of the esophagus predictable by DNA analysis. Cancer 57:1810, 1986

299. Sugimachi K, Koga Y, Mori M, et al: Comparative data on cytophotometric DNA in malignant lesions of the esophagus in the Chinese and Japanese. Cancer 59:1947, 1987

300. Epstein JI, Sears DL, Tucker RS, Eagan JW: Carcinoma of the esophagus with adenoid cystic differentiation. Cancer 53:1131, 1984

301. Akamatsu T, Honda T, Nakayama J, et al: Primary adenoid cystic carcinoma of the esophagus. Report of a case and its histochemical characterization. Acta Pathol Jpn 36:1707, 1986

302. Sweeney EC, Cooney T: Adenoid cystic carcinoma of the esophagus. A light and electron microscopic study. Cancer 45:1516, 1980

303. O'Sullivan JP, Cockburn JS, Drew CE: Adenoid cystic carcinoma of the oesophagus. Thorax 30:476, 1975

304. Azzopardi JG, Menzies T: Primary oesophageal adenocarcinoma. Confirmation of its existence by the finding of mucous gland tumours. Br J Surg 49:497, 1962

305. Woodard BH, Shelburne JD, Vollmer RT, et al: Mucoepidermoid carcinoma of the esophagus: A case report. Human Pathol 9:352, 1978

306. Kay S: Mucoepidermoid carcinoma of the esophagus. Report of two cases. Cancer 22:1053, 1968

307. Weitzner S: Mucoepidermoid carcinoma of esophagus. Arch Pathol 90:271, 1970

308. Osamura RY, Sato S, Miwa M, et al: Mucoepidermoid carcinoma of the esophagus. Report of an unoperated autopsy case and review of literature. Am J Gastroenterol 69:467, 1978

309. Pascal RR, Clearfield HR: Mucoepidermoid (adenosquamous) carcinoma arising in Barrett's esophagus. Dig Dis Sci 32:428, 1987

310. Dodge OG: Gastro-oesophageal carcinoma of mixed histological type. J Pathol Bacteriol 81:459, 1961

311. Spagnolo DV, Heenan PJ: Collision carcinoma at the esophagogastric junction: Report of two cases. Cancer 46:2702, 1980

312. Matsusaka T, Watanabe H, Enjoji M: Anaplastic carcinoma of the esophagus. Report of three cases and their histogenic consideration. Cancer 37:1352, 1976

313. Horai T, Kobayashi A, Tateishi R, et al: A cytologic study on small cell carcinoma of the esophagus. Cancer 41:1890, 1978

314. Ibrahim NBN, Briggs JC, Corbishley CM: Extrapulmonary oat cell carcinoma. Cancer 54:1645, 1984

315. Briggs JC, Ibrahim NBN: Oat cell carcinoma of the esophagus: a clinico-pathological study of 23 cases. Histopathology 7:261, 1983

316. Ho K-J, Herrera GA, Jones JM, Alexander CB: Small cell carcinoma of the esophagus: Evidence for a unified histogenesis. Hum Pathol 15:460, 1984

317. Johnson FE, Clawson MC, Bashiti HM, et al: Small cell undifferentiated carcinoma of the esophagus. Case report with hormonal studies. Cancer 53:1746, 1984

318. Rosenthal SN, Lemkin JA: Multiple small cell carcinomas of the esophagus. Cancer 51:1944, 1983

319. Sato T, Mukai M, Ando N, et al: Small cell carcinoma (non-oat cell type) of the esophagus concomitant with invasive squamous cell carcinoma and carcinoma in situ. A case report. Cancer 57:328, 1986

320. Tateishi R, Taniguchi H, Wade A, et al: Argyrophil cells and melanocytes in esophageal mucosa. Arch Pathol 98:87, 1974

321. Rankin R, Nirodi NS, Browne MK: Carcinoid tumour of the oesophagus: Report of a case. Scott Med J 25:245, 1980

322. Sasano N, Abe S, Satake O, et al: Choriocarcinoma mimicking of an esophageal carcinoma with urinary gonadotropic activities. Tohoku J Exp Med 100:153, 1970

323. McKechnie JC, Fechner RE: Choriocarcinoma and adenocarcinoma of the esophagus with gonadotropin secretion. Cancer 27:694, 1971

324. Trillo AA, Accettullo LM, Yeiter TL: Choriocarcinoma of the esophagus: Histologic and cytologic findings. A case report. Acta Cytol (Baltimore) 23:69, 1979

325. Jindrak K, Bochetto JF, Alpert LI: Primary gastric choriocarcinoma. Case report and review of world literature. Hum Pathol 7:595, 1976

326. Turnbull AD, Rosen P, Goodner JT, et al: Primary malignant tumors of the esophagus other than typical epidermoid carcinoma. Ann Thorac Surg 15:463, 1973

327. Osamura RY, Watanabe K, Shimamura K, et al: Polypoid carcinoma of the esophagus. A unifying term for "carcinosarcoma" and "pseudosarcoma." Am J Surg Pathol 2:201, 1978

328. Martin MR, Kahn LB: So-called pseudosarcoma of the esophagus. Nodal metastasis of the spindle cell element. Arch Pathol Lab Med 101:604, 1977

329. Stout AP, Humphreys GH III, Rottenberg LA: A case of carcinosarcoma of the esophagus. AJR 61:469, 1949

330. Battifora H: Spindle cell carcinoma. Ultrastructural evidence of squamous origin and collagen production by the tumor cells. Cancer 37:2275, 1976

331. Takubo K, Tsuchiya S, Nakagawa H, et al: Pseudosarcoma of the esophagus. Hum Pathol 13:503, 1982

332. Linder J, Stein RB, Roggli VL, et al: Polypoid tumor of the esophagus. Hum Pathol 18:692, 1987

333. Hanada M, Nakano K, Ii Y, Yamashita H: Carcinosarcoma of the esophagus with osseous and cartilagenous

production. A combined study of keratin immunohisto-chemistry and electron microscopy. Acta Pathol Jpn 34:669, 1984

334. Matsusaka T, Watanabe H, Enjoji M: Pseudosarcoma and carcinosarcoma of the esophagus. Cancer 37:1546, 1976

335. Ellis GL, Langlos JM, Heffner DK, Hyams VJ: Spindle-cell carcinoma of the aerodigestive tract. An immunohistochemical analysis of 21 cases. Am J Surg Pathol 11:335, 1987

336. Hinderleider CD, Aguam AS, Wilder JR: Carcinosarcoma of the esophagus. A case report and review of the literature. Int Surg 64:13, 1979

337. Mills SE, Cooper PH: Malignant melanoma of the digestive system. p. 1. In Sommers S, Rosen PP (eds): Pathology Annual. Vol. 18. Part 2. Appleton-Century-Crofts, East Norwalk, CT, 1983

338. DiCostanzo DP, Urmacher C: Primary malignant melanoma of the esophagus. Am J Surg Pathol 11:46, 1987

339. Takubo K, Kanda Y, Ishii M, et al: Primary malignant melanoma of the esophagus. Hum Pathol 14:727, 1983

340. Kreuser E-D: Primary malignant melanoma of the esophagus. Virchows Arch [A] 385:49, 1979

341. de la Pava S, Nigogosyan G, Pickren JW, Cabrera A: Melanosis of the esophagus. Cancer 16:48, 1963

342. Basque GJ, Boline JE, Holyoke JB: Malignant melanoma of the esophagus: First reported case in a child. Am J Clin Pathol 53:609, 1970

343. Jawalekar K, Tretter P: Primary malignant melanoma of the esophagus. Report of two cases. J Surg Oncol 12:19, 1979

344. Piccone VA, Klopstock R, LeVeen HH, Sika J: Primary malignant melanoma of the esophagus associated with melanosis of the entire esophagus. First case report. J Thorac Cardiovasc Surg 59:864, 1970

345. Kim SD: Lipomelanotic choristoma. A case report. J Natl Med Assoc 66:211, 1974

346. Reintgen DS, Thompson W, Garbutt J, Seigler HF: Radiologic, endoscopic, and surgical considerations of melanoma metastatic to the gastrointestinal tract. Surgery 95:635, 1984

347. Das Gupta TK, Brasfield RD: Metastatic melanoma of the gastrointestinal tract. Arch Surg 88:969, 1964

348. Rosenberg SA, Diamond HD, Jaslowitz B: Lymphosarcoma: Review of 1269 cases. Medicine (Baltimore) 40:31, 1961

349. Ehrlich AN, Stalder G, Geller W: Gastrointestinal manifestations of malignant lymphoma. Gastroenterology 54:1115, 1968

350. Matsuura H, Saito R, Nakajima S, et al: Non-Hodgkin's lymphoma of the esophagus. Am J Gastroenterol 80:941, 1985

351. Stein HA, Murray D, Warner HA: Primary Hodgkin's disease of the esophagus. Dig Dis Sci 26:457, 1981

352. Sheahan DG, West AB: Focal lymphoid hyperplasia (pseudolymphoma) of the esophagus. Am J Surg Pathol 9:141, 1985

353. Ahmed N, Ramos S, Sika J, et al: Primary extramedullary esophageal plasmacytoma. Cancer 38:943, 1976

354. Abrams HL, Spiro R, Goldstein N: Metastases in carcinoma. Analysis of 1000 autopsied cases. Cancer 3:74, 1950

355. Toreson WE: Secondary carcinoma of the esophagus as a cause of dysphagia. Arch Pathol 38:82, 1944

356. Nussbaum M, Grossman M: Metastases to the esophagus causing gastrointestinal bleeding. Am J Gasteroenterol 66:467, 1976

INDEX

Page numbers followed by f refer to figures; those followed by t refer to tables.

giant cell reaction from joint prostheses, 495, 495f
oily
    intestinal granulomas from, 1150
    and postlymphangiography granuloma, 394, 394f
    reactions to, in breast, 322
Formaldehyde-induced fluorescence of catecholamines in tumor diagnosis, 126t, 127
Formalin as fixative, 107
Fouchet stain in tumor diagnosis, 126t
Fractures
    healing of, 476, 477f
    stress, 476
Frozen sections, 106
    brain tissue, 2162
    for enzyme histochemical studies, 126
    intestinal, 1119
    liver biopsy specimens, 1244
    muscle, 547, 547f, 551f
    pancreatic, 1353
    preparation and processing of, 108–109
Fuchs' dystrophy of cornea, 2060, 2060f
Fucosidosis, 2156
Fuller's earth, pneumoconiosis from, 696t
Fungating carcinoma
    squamous cell, of esophagus, 1052, 1053f
    of stomach, 1104, 1104f
Fungus balls, pulmonary, 755
Fungus infections
    in AIDS, 65, 65f
    culture of tissue specimens in, 22t
    ear infections in, 2027
    endocarditis in, 812
    esophagitis in, 1035
    folliculitis in, 174f, 174–175
    gastritis in, 1084–1085
    granulomas in, 173
    keratitis in, 2060
    of lungs, 667–669, 753–755
    lymph nodes in, 390
    placenta in, 1838t
    tissue reactions in, 27t, 42–44, 43f–44f
    vaginal, 1701
Furriers' lung, 686
Furunculosis, 174
    of vulva, 1699

Galactocele, 320
Galactography, 317
Galactosylceramide lipidosis, 2158
Gallbladder, 1382–1388
    adenomas of, 1388, 1388f
    adenomyoma of, 1384, 1386
    carcinoma of, 1386–1387
    carcinosarcoma of, 1387
    cholecystitis of
        acute, 1382–1383, 1383f
        chronic, 1383–1385, 1384f
    cholelithiasis, 1385–1386, 1386f
    cholesterolosis of, 1385, 1385f
    congenital anomalies of, 1382
    melanoma of, 1387–1388
    polyps of, inflammatory, 1385
    porcelain, 1384
    sarcoma of, 1387
    tumors of, 1378t, 1386–1388
Gallstones, 1385–1386, 1386f
    in ampulla of Vater, 1378
    in cholecystitis, 1383–1384, 1384f

Galton's prolymphocytic leukemia, 449
Gamma heavy chain disease, 452
Gangliocytic paraganglioma in duodenum, 1203, 1203f, 1377
Gangliocytoma, dysplastic, of Lhermitte Duclos, 2140
Gangliogliomas, 2139–2140, 2140f
    immunostain of, 2165t
    ultrastructure of, 2149t
Ganglion, 497, 2001
    intraosseous, 535
Ganglion cell tumors, 2139–2140
Ganglioneuroblastoma
    adrenal, 1973, 1974f
    mediastinal, 965, 966f
    ultrastructure of, 2149t
Ganglioneuroma, 2140
    adrenal, 1974
    of bladder, 1503
    bone lesions in, 535
    mediastinal, 965–967, 966f
    retroperitoneal, 998
    ultrastructure of, 2149t
Gangliosidoses, 2157
Gangrene
    in cystitis, 1492
    of stomach, 1079, 1079f–1080f
Gardner syndrome
    desmoid tumors in, 265
    intestinal adenomas in, 1190
Gardnerella vaginalis infection, vaginitis in, 1697
Gartner's duct cysts, 1695, 1695f
Gastrectomy, 1073–1075, 1075f
    malabsorption after, 1160
Gastrin cells of stomach, 1073
    hyperplasia of, 1101–1102
Gastrin secretion
    by carcinoid tumors of small bowel, 1198
    by pancreatic tumors, 1373, 1375
Gastritis, 1080–1086
    acute noninfectious, 1081–1082, 1082f
    chronic nonspecific, 1085–1086
        antral, 1085
        atrophic, 1086, 1086f
        fundal, 1085
        superficial, 1085–1086
    classification of, 1081t
    cystica
        polyposa, 1096
        profunda, 1096
    erosive
        acute, 1081, 1082f
        chronic, 1085
    granulomatous, 1084, 1089
    hypersecretory, 1091–1092, 1092f
    hypertrophic, 1091f, 1091–1092
    infectious, 1083–1085
Gastroenteric cysts, 1021–1022
    thoracic, 938
Gastroenteritis
    eosinophilic, 1089f, 1089–1090, 1146
    infantile, 1134, 1139
    viral, 1139
Gastroenterostomy sites, polyps in, 1095–1096
Gastroesophageal reflux, esophagitis in, 1026f–1027f, 1026–1028
Gastrointestinal epithelium in lungs, 771
Gaucher's disease, 2158
    bone in, 485
    and foamy cells in marrow, 455f
    heart in, 798

hepatic reticuloendothelial storage in, 1289t
    and histiocytes in lymph nodes, 416, 416f
    liver in, 1301
    spleen in, 421
Gay bowel syndrome, 1171
Gelfoam, reactions to, 79, 79f
Gemistocytic astrocytoma, 2119, 2120f
Genitalia, external
    in females. 1691–1721
    in males, 1531–1575
Genotyping, 8, 383
Germ cell tumors
    of bladder, 1504
    of liver, malignant, 1331
    of mediastinum, 959–960
    metastatic, differential diagnosis of, 122
    of ovary, 1803–1808
    pineal, 2137–2138, 2138f
    retroperitoneal, 1001
    testicular, 1548–1563
Germinal cell hypoplasia, 1542–1543
Germinal centers
    of lymph nodes, 384
        transformation in Hodgkin's disease, 402
    of spleen, 417
Germinoma
    immunostain of, 2165t
    mediastinal, 959
    pineal, 2137–2138, 2138f
    ultrastructure of, 2149t
Ghost cells, in calcifying odontogenic cyst, 843, 844f
Giant cell(s)
    in arteritis, 169, 819–820, 820f
        in necrotizing sarcoid granulomatosis, 762
        uterine cervix in, 1644
    in foreign-body reaction, 495, 495f
    in granuloma of oral cavity, 879–882, 881f
    in hepatitis, postinfantile, 1274–1275, 1275f
    in interstitial pneumonia, 678
    macrophage, 381
    Touton-type
        in lipid granulomas, 455
        in malignant fibrous histiocytoma of bone, 532, 533f
Giant cell tumors, 124t
    astrocytoma, subependymal, 2119, 2120f, 2123
    of bone, 521–523, 522f
    carcinoma
        of lung, 738, 729f
        of pancreas, 1360–1361, 1361f–1362f
        of thyroid, 1912, 1912–1913f
    fibroblastoma, 267
    glioblastoma, 2119
        ultrastructure of, 2148
    histiocytoma, malignant fibrous, 270–271, 272f
    nasal, 618
    of tendon sheath, 271–273, 273f, 495
Giant lymph node hyperplasia, 939–941, 940f–941f
    retroperitoneal, 1001, 1002f
Giant pigmented nevi, 2145, 2146t
Giant pore, 222
Giardia lamblia, 1137
Giardiasis, 1137, 1137f
Giemsa stain, 23t, 25t
    in amyloidosis, 176
Gigantiform cementoma, 859
Gigantism, 1858
Gigantocellular glioma, 2123